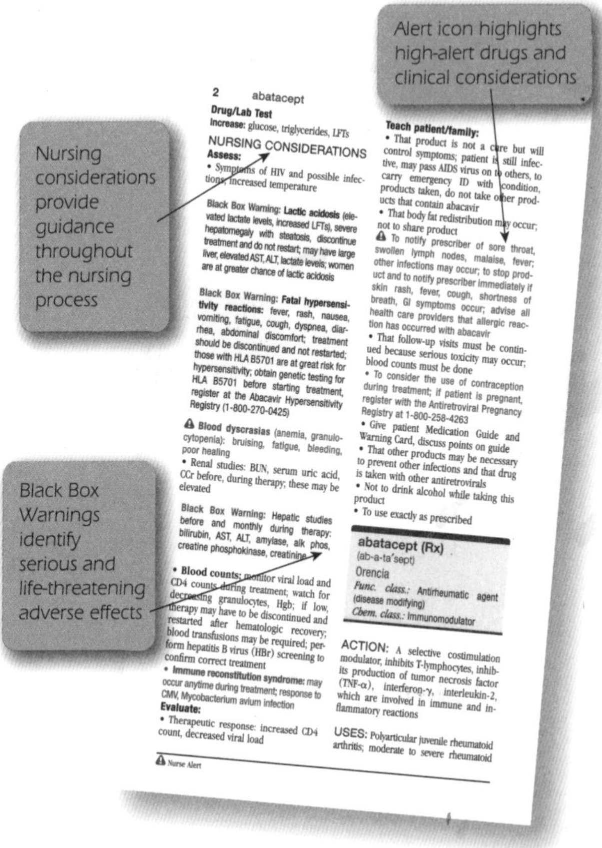
Alert icon highlights high-alert drugs and clinical considerations
Nursing considerations provide guidance throughout the nursing process
Black Box Warnings identify serious and life-threatening adverse effects

2 abatacept

Drug/Lab Test
Increase: glucose, triglycerides, LFTs

NURSING CONSIDERATIONS
Assess:
• Symptoms of HIV and possible infections, increased temperature

Black Box Warning: **Lactic acidosis** (elevated lactate levels, increased LFTs), severe hepatomegaly with steatosis, discontinue treatment and do not restart; may have large liver, elevated AST, ALT, lactate levels; women are at greater chance of lactic acidosis

Black Box Warning: **Fatal hypersensitivity reactions:** fever, rash, nausea, vomiting, fatigue, cough, dyspnea, diarrhea, abdominal discomfort; treatment should be discontinued and not restarted; those with HLA B5701 are at great risk for hypersensitivity; obtain genetic testing for HLA B5701 before starting treatment, register at the Abacavir Hypersensitivity Registry (1-800-270-0425)

⚠ **Blood dyscrasias** (anemia, granulocytopenia): bruising, fatigue, bleeding, poor healing
• Renal studies: BUN, serum uric acid, CCr before, during therapy; these may be elevated

Black Box Warning: Hepatic studies before and monthly during therapy: bilirubin, AST, ALT, amylase, alk phos, creatine phosphokinase, creatinine

• **Blood counts:** monitor viral load and CD4 counts during treatment; watch for decreasing granulocytes, Hgb; if low, therapy may have to be discontinued and restarted after hematologic recovery; blood transfusions may be required; perform hepatitis B virus (HBr) screening to confirm correct treatment
• **Immune reconstitution syndrome:** may occur anytime during treatment; response to CMV, Mycobacterium avium infection

Evaluate:
• Therapeutic response: increased CD4 count, decreased viral load

Teach patient/family:
• That product is not a cure but will control symptoms; patient is still infective, may pass AIDS virus on to others, to carry emergency ID with condition, products taken, do not take other products that contain abacavir
• That body fat redistribution may occur; not to share product
⚠ To notify prescriber of sore throat, swollen lymph nodes, malaise, fever; other infections may occur; to stop product and to notify prescriber immediately if skin rash, fever, cough, shortness of breath, GI symptoms occur; advise all health care providers that allergic reaction has occurred with abacavir
• That follow-up visits must be continued because serious toxicity may occur; blood counts must be done
• To consider the use of contraception during treatment; if patient is pregnant, register with the Antiretroviral Pregnancy Registry at 1-800-258-4263
• Give patient Medication Guide and Warning Card, discuss points on guide
• That other products may be necessary to prevent other infections and that drug is taken with other antiretrovirals
• Not to drink alcohol while taking this product
• To use exactly as prescribed

abatacept (Rx)
(ab-a-ta′sept)
Orencia
Func. class.: Antirheumatic agent (disease modifying)
Chem. class.: Immunomodulator

ACTION: A selective costimulation modulator, inhibits T-lymphocytes, inhibits production of tumor necrosis factor (TNF-α), interferon-γ, interleukin-2, which are involved in immune and inflammatory reactions

USES: Polyarticular juvenile rheumatoid arthritis; moderate to severe rheumatoid

⚠ Nurse Alert

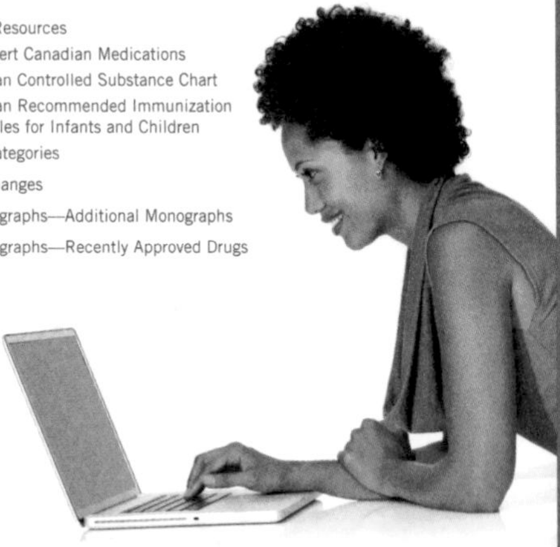

Mosby's

2017 NURSING DRUG REFERENCE

30TH EDITION

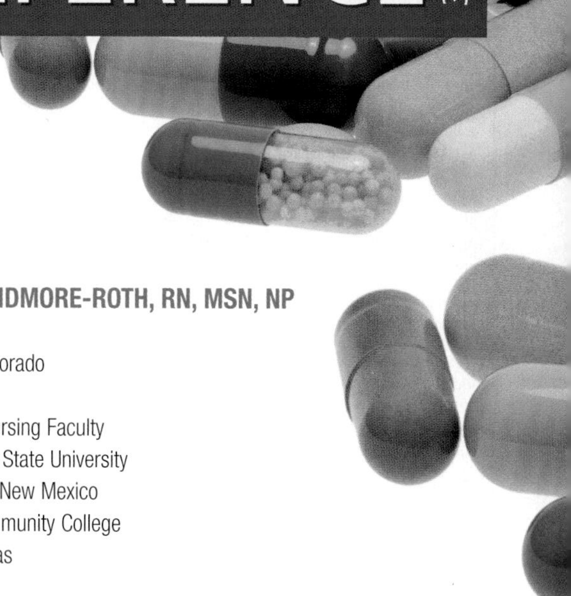

LINDA SKIDMORE-ROTH, RN, MSN, NP
Consultant
Littleton, Colorado

Formerly, Nursing Faculty
New Mexico State University
Las Cruces, New Mexico
El Paso Community College
El Paso, Texas

ELSEVIER

ELSEVIER

3251 Riverport Lane
St. Louis, Missouri 63043

MOSBY'S 2017 NURSING DRUG REFERENCE,
THIRTIETH EDITION

ISBN: 978-0-323-44826-0
ISSN: 1044-8470

Notices

Knowledge and best practice in this field are constantly changing. As new research and experience broaden our understanding, changes in research methods, professional practices, or medical treatment may become necessary.

Practitioners and researchers must always rely on their own experience and knowledge in evaluating and using any information, methods, compounds, or experiments described herein. In using such information or methods, they should be mindful of their own safety and the safety of others, including parties for whom they have a professional responsibility.

With respect to any drug or pharmaceutical products identified, readers are advised to check the most current information provided (i) on procedures featured or (ii) by the manufacturer of each product to be administered, to verify the recommended dose or formula, the method and duration of administration, and contraindications. It is the responsibility of practitioners, relying on their own experience and knowledge of their patients, to make diagnoses, to determine dosages and the best treatment for each individual patient, and to take all appropriate safety precautions.

To the fullest extent of the law, neither the Publisher nor the authors, contributors, or editors assume any liability for any injury and/or damage to persons or property as a matter of product liability, negligence or otherwise, or from any use or operation of any methods, products, instructions, or ideas contained in the material herein.

Previous editions copyrighted 2016, 2015, 2014.
International Standard Book Number: 978-0-323-44826-0

Executive Content Strategist: Sonya Seigafuse
Content Development Manager: Billie Sharp
Associate Content Development Specialist: Sarah Vora
Publishing Services Manager: Jeff Patterson
Senior Project Manager: Jodi M. Willard
Design Direction: Paula Catalano

Printed in the United States of America
Last digit is the print number: 9 8 7 6 5 4 3 2 1

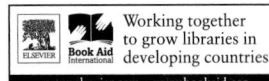

Consultants

Amanda Buckallew, PharmD, BCPS
Pharmacist
Inpatient Pharmacy
Missouri Baptist Medical Center
Saint Louis, Missouri

David Chun, PharmD, BCPS
Pharmacist in Charge
Omnicare of St. Louis
Florissant, Missouri

Joshua J. Neumiller, PharmD, CDE, CGP, FASCP
Associate Professor
Washington State University
Spokane, Washington

Travis Sonnett, PharmD, FASCP
Clinical Pharmacy Specialist/Inpatient Pharmacy Supervisor
Mann-Grandstaff VA Medical Center
Spokane, Washington
Adjunct Clinical Professor
Pharmacotherapy
Washington State University
Spokane, Washington

Patricia A. Talbert, AAS Nursing, AAS Horticulture, AA
Employee Health Nurse
Wellness
Baxter Regional Medical Center
Mountain Home, Arkansas
Aromatherapist
Gainesville, Missouri

Shamim Tejani, PharmD, CPHQ
Director of Quality Improvement
Adelante Healthcare
Phoenix, Arizona

Preface

Increasingly, patients are relying on nurses to know every detail of health care. More important, nurses are expected to have these answers, especially when it comes to medication. Let *Mosby's 2017 Nursing Drug Reference* be your answer. Our indispensable, yet compact, resource contains hundreds of monographs with several easy-to-use features.

NEW FEATURES

This edition features:

- Twenty recent FDA-approved drugs located in **Appendix A** (see Contents for a complete list). Included are monographs for:
  - albiglutide (Tanzeum)—for diabetes mellitus
  - ceritinib (Zykadia)—for metastatic lung cancer
  - daclatasvir (Daklinza)—for hepatitis C
  - sonidegib (Odomzo)—for locally advanced basal cell carcinoma
- **A new ebook** with easy-to-use navigation for quick access to drug categories and monographs of your choice

NEW FACTS

This edition features more than 2000 new drug facts, including:

- New drugs and dosage information
- Newly researched side effects and adverse reactions
- New and revised Black Box Warnings
- The latest precautions, interactions, and contraindications
- IV therapy updates
- Revised nursing considerations
- Updated patient/family teaching guidelines

ORGANIZATION

This reference is organized into two main sections:

- Individual drug monographs (in alphabetical order by generic name)
- Appendixes (identified by the wide thumb tabs on the edge)

The guiding principle behind this book is to provide fast, easy access to drug information and nursing considerations. Every detail—the paper, typeface, cover, binding, use of color, and appendixes—has been carefully chosen with the user in mind.

INDIVIDUAL DRUG MONOGRAPHS

This book contains monographs for more than 1300 generic and 4500 trade medications. Common trade names are given for all drugs regularly used in the United States and Canada, with drugs available only in Canada identified by a maple leaf ✱.

The following information is provided, whenever possible, for safe, effective administration of each drug:

High-alert status: Identifies high-alert drugs with a label and icon. Visit the Institute for Safe Medication Practices (ISMP) at http://www.ismp.org/tools/highalert-medications.pdf for a list of medications and drug classes with the greatest potential for patient harm if they are used in error.

Tall man lettering: Uses the capitalization of distinguishing letters to avoid medication errors and is required by the FDA for drug manufacturers.

Pronunciation: Helps the nurse master complex generic names.

Rx/OTC: Identifies prescription or over-the-counter drugs.

Functional and chemical classifications: Allow the nurse to see similarities and dissimilarities among drugs in the same functional but different chemical classes.

Do not confuse: Presents drug names that might easily be confused within each appropriate monograph.

Action: Describes pharmacologic properties concisely.

Uses: List the conditions the drug is used to treat.

Unlabeled uses: Describe drug uses that may be encountered in practice but are not yet FDA approved.

Dosages and routes: List all available and approved dosages and routes for adult, pediatric, and geriatric patients.

Available forms: Include tablets, capsules, extended-release, injectables (IV, IM, SUBCUT), solutions, creams, ointments, lotions, gels, shampoos, elixirs, suspensions, suppositories, sprays, aerosols, and lozenges.

Side effects: Groups these reactions by body system, with common side effects *italicized* and life-threatening reactions (those that are potentially fatal and/or permanently disabling) in **bold, red type** for emphasis.

Contraindications: List conditions under which the drug absolutely should not be given, including FDA pregnancy safety categories D or X.

Precautions: List conditions that require special consideration when the drug is prescribed, including FDA pregnancy safety categories A, B, or C.

Black Box Warnings: Identify FDA warnings that highlight serious and life-threatening adverse effects.

Pharmacokinetics: Outline metabolism, distribution, and elimination.

Interactions: Include confirmed drug interactions, followed by the drug or nutrient causing that interaction, when applicable.

Drug/herb: Highlights potential interactions between herbal products and prescription or OTC drugs.

Drug/food: Identifies many common drug interactions with foods.

Drug/lab test: Identifies how the drug may affect lab test results.

Nursing considerations: Identify key nursing considerations for each step of the nursing process: Assess, Administer, Evaluate, and Teach Patient/Family. Instructions for giving drugs by various routes (e.g., PO, IM, IV) are included, with route subheadings in bold.

Compatibilities: List syringe, Y-site, and additive compatibilities and incompatibilities. If no compatibilities are listed for a drug, the necessary compatibility testing has not been done and that compatibility information is unknown. To ensure safety, assume that the drug may not be mixed with other drugs unless specifically stated.

"Nursing Alert" icon ⚠: Highlights a critical consideration.

Treatment of overdose: Provides drugs and treatment for overdoses where appropriate.

APPENDIXES

Selected new drugs: Includes comprehensive information on 20 key drugs approved by the FDA during the past 12 months.

Ophthalmic, otic, nasal, and topical products: Provides essential information for more than 80 ophthalmic, otic, nasal, and topical products commonly used today, grouped by chemical drug class.

Vaccines and toxoids: Features an easy-to-use table with generic and trade names, uses, dosages and routes, and contraindications for over 40 key vaccines and toxoids.

I am indebted to the nursing and pharmacology consultants who reviewed the manuscript and thank them for their criticism and encouragement. I would also like to thank Billie Sharp and Sarah Vora, my editors, whose active encouragement and enthusiasm have made this book better than it might otherwise have been. I am likewise grateful to Jodi Willard and Graphic World Inc. for the coordination of the production process and assistance with the development of the new edition. A special "thank-you" to my son, Craig Roth, for completing the electronic files.

Linda Skidmore-Roth

FDA pregnancy categories

A	No risk demonstrated to the fetus in any trimester
B	No adverse effects in animals; no human studies available
C	Only given after risks to the fetus are considered; animal studies have shown adverse reactions; no human studies available
D	Definite fetal risks, may be given in spite of risks if needed in life-threatening conditions
X	Absolute fetal abnormalities; not to be used at any time during pregnancy

Note: **UK** = Unknown fetal risk (used in this text but not an official FDA pregnancy category)

Contents

⚠ HIGH ALERT

abacavir (Rx)

(ah-bak′ah-veer)

Ziagen

Func. class.: Antiretroviral

Chem. class.: Nucleoside reverse transcriptase inhibitor (NRTI)

Do not confuse:
abacavir/amprenavir

ACTION:
Inhibitory action against HIV-1; inhibits replication of the virus by incorporating into cellular DNA by viral reverse transcriptase, thereby terminating the cellular DNA chain

USES:
In combination with other antiretroviral agents for HIV-1 infection

Unlabeled uses: HIV prophylaxis following occupational exposure

CONTRAINDICATIONS

Black Box Warning: Hypersensitivity, moderate/severe hepatic disease, lactic acidosis

Precautions: Pregnancy (C), breastfeeding, children <3 mo, granulocyte count <1000/mm^3 or Hgb <9.5 g/dl, severe renal disease, impaired hepatic function, HLA B5701+ (black, Caucasian, Asian patients), abrupt discontinuation; Guillain-Barré syndrome, immune reconstitution syndrome, MI, obesity, polymyositis

DOSAGE AND ROUTES

• **Adult and adolescent ≥16 yr: PO** 300 mg bid or 600 mg/day with other antiretrovirals

• **Adolescent <16 yr and child ≥3 mo: PO** 8 mg/kg bid or 16 mg/kg daily, max 300 mg bid with other antiretrovirals

Hepatic dose

• **Adult: PO** (Child-Pugh 5-6) (oral sol) 200 mg bid; moderate to severe hepatic disease, do not use

HIV prophylaxis (unlabeled)

• **Adult: PO** 600 mg daily as an alternative

Available forms: Tabs 300 mg; oral sol 20 mg/ml

Administer:

• Give in combination with other antiretrovirals; do not use triple therapy as a beginning treatment, resistance may occur

• May give without regard to food

• Reduce dose in hepatic disease, use oral sol

• Storage in cool environment; protect from light; oral sol stored at room temperature; do not freeze

SIDE EFFECTS

CNS: *Fever, headache, malaise, insomnia,* paresthesia

GI: *Nausea, vomiting, diarrhea, anorexia,* cramps, abdominal pain, increased AST, ALT, **hepatotoxicity, hepatomegaly with steatosis**

HEMA: **Granulocytopenia, anemia, lymphopenia**

INTEG: *Rash,* urticaria, hypersensitivity reactions

META: **Lactic acidosis**

OTHER: **Fatal hypersensitivity reactions, MI, fat redistribution, immune reconstitution, decreased bone density**

RESP: Dyspnea

PHARMACOKINETICS

Rapid/extensive absorption, distributed to extravascular space, then erythrocytes; 50% protein binding; extensively metabolized to inactive metabolites; half-life 1½ hr; excreted in urine, feces (unchanged); onset, peak, duration unknown

INTERACTIONS

• Do not coadminister with abacavir-containing products, ribavirin, interferon

⚠ **Increase:** possible lactic acidosis—ribavirin

Increase: abacavir levels—alcohol

Decrease: abacavir levels—tipranavir

Decrease: levels of—methadone

Drug/Lab Test

Increase: glucose, triglycerides, LFTs

NURSING CONSIDERATIONS

Assess:

• Symptoms of HIV and possible infections; increased temperature

> **Black Box Warning: Lactic acidosis** (elevated lactate levels, increased LFTs), severe hepatomegaly with steatosis, discontinue treatment and do not restart; may have large liver, elevated AST, ALT, lactate levels; women are at greater chance of lactic acidosis

> **Black Box Warning: Fatal hypersensitivity reactions:** fever, rash, nausea, vomiting, fatigue, cough, dyspnea, diarrhea, abdominal discomfort; treatment should be discontinued and not restarted; those with HLA B5701 are at great risk for hypersensitivity; obtain genetic testing for HLA B5701 before starting treatment, register at the Abacavir Hypersensitivity Registry (1-800-270-0425)

⚠ **Blood dyscrasias** (anemia, granulocytopenia): bruising, fatigue, bleeding, poor healing

• Renal studies: BUN, serum uric acid, CCr before, during therapy; these may be elevated

> **Black Box Warning:** Hepatic studies before and monthly during therapy: bilirubin, AST, ALT, amylase, alk phos, creatine phosphokinase, creatinine

• **Blood counts;** monitor viral load and CD4 counts during treatment; watch for decreasing granulocytes, Hgb; if low, therapy may have to be discontinued and restarted after hematologic recovery; blood transfusions may be required; perform hepatitis B virus (HBr) screening to confirm correct treatment

• **Immune reconstitution syndrome:** may occur anytime during treatment; response to CMV, Mycobacterium avium infection

Evaluate:

• Therapeutic response: increased CD4 count, decreased viral load

Teach patient/family:

• That product is not a cure but will control symptoms; patient is still infective, may pass AIDS virus on to others, to carry emergency ID with condition, products taken, do not take other products that contain abacavir

• That body fat redistribution may occur; not to share product

⚠ To notify prescriber of sore throat, swollen lymph nodes, malaise, fever; other infections may occur; to stop product and to notify prescriber immediately if skin rash, fever, cough, shortness of breath, GI symptoms occur; advise all health care providers that allergic reaction has occurred with abacavir

• That follow-up visits must be continued because serious toxicity may occur; blood counts must be done

• To consider the use of contraception during treatment; if patient is pregnant, register with the Antiretroviral Pregnancy Registry at 1-800-258-4263

• Give patient Medication Guide and Warning Card, discuss points on guide

• That other products may be necessary to prevent other infections and that drug is taken with other antiretrovirals

• Not to drink alcohol while taking this product

• To use exactly as prescribed

abatacept (Rx)

(ab-a-ta′sept)

Orencia

Func. class.: Antirheumatic agent (disease modifying)

Chem. class.: Immunomodulator

ACTION: A selective costimulation modulator, inhibits T-lymphocytes, inhibits production of tumor necrosis factor (TNF-α), interferon-γ, interleukin-2, which are involved in immune and inflammatory reactions

USES: Polyarticular juvenile rheumatoid arthritis; moderate to severe rheumatoid arthritis; acute, chronic rheumatoid arthritis that has not responded to other disease-modifying agents; may use in combination with DMARDs; do not use with TNF antagonists (adalimumab, etanercept, infliximab), anakinra

CONTRAINDICATIONS: Hypersensitivity

Precautions: Pregnancy (C), breastfeeding, children, geriatric patients, recurrent infections, COPD, TB, viral hepatitis, immunosuppression, neoplastic disease, respiratory infection

DOSAGE AND ROUTES

Rheumatoid arthritis

- **Adult: SUBCUT** 125 mg within 1 day after single IV loading dose, then 125 mg weekly; weekly subcut dose may be initiated without an IV loading dose for those unable to receive an infusion
- **Adult >100 kg (220 lb): IV INFUSION** 1 g over 30 min, give at 2, 4 wk after first infusion, then q4wk
- **Adult 60-100 kg (132-220 lb): IV INFUSION** 750 mg over 30 min, give at 2, 4 wk after first infusion, then q4wk
- **Adult <60 kg (132 lb): IV INFUSION** 500 mg over 30 min, give at 2, 4 wk after first infusion, then q4wk

Juvenile rheumatoid arthritis (JRA)/ juvenile idiopathic arthritis (JIA)

- **Adolescent and child ≥6 yr and >100 kg: IV INFUSION** 1 g over 30 min q2wk × 3 doses, then 1 g over 30 min q4wk starting at wk 8
- **Adolescent and child ≥6 yr and 75-100 kg: IV INFUSION** 750 mg over 30 min q2wk × 2 doses, then 750 mg over 30 min q4wk starting at wk 8
- **Adolescent and child ≥6 yr and <75 kg: IV INFUSION** 10 mg/kg over 30 min q2wk × 3 doses, then 10 mg/kg q4wk starting at wk 8

Available forms: Lyophilized powder, single-use vials 250 mg; sol for subcut inj 125 mg/ml

Administer:

- Storage in refrigerator; do not use expired vials, protect from light, do not freeze

Intermittent IV INFUSION route

- **To reconstitute,** use 10 ml sterile water for injection; insert syringe needle into vial and direct stream of sterile water for inj on the wall of vial; rotate vial until mixed; vent with needle to rid foam after reconstitution (25 mg/ml); **further dilute** in 100 ml NS from a 100-ml infusion bag/bottle; withdraw the needed volume (2 vials remove 20 ml; 3 vials remove 30 ml, 4 vials remove 40 ml); slowly add the reconstituted sol from each vial into the infusion bag/bottle using the same disposable syringe supplied; mix gently; discard unused portions of vials; do not use if particulate is present or discolored; **give** over 30 min; use non–protein-binding filter (0.2-1.2 microns); protect from light
- Do not admix with other sol or medications

SUBCUT route

- Use prefilled syringe for subcut only (do not use for IV); allow syringe to warm to room temperature (30-60 min); do not speed up warming process; the amount of liquid should be between the 2 lines on the barrel; do not use the syringe if there is more or less liquid; inject into fronts of thighs, outer area of upper arm, or abdomen except for 2-inch area around the navel; do not inject into tender, bruised area
- Gently pinch skin and hold firmly; insert needle at 45-degree angle; inject full amount in 125-mg syringe
- Rotate injection sites

SIDE EFFECTS

CNS: Headache, asthenia, dizziness
CV: *Hypo/hypertension*
GI: Abdominal pain, dyspepsia, nausea
INTEG: Rash, *inj site reaction,* flushing, urticaria, pruritus
RESP: *Pharyngitis, cough, URI,* non-URI, *rhinitis,* wheezing
SYST: **Anaphylaxis, malignancies, serious infections, antibody development**

PHARMACOKINETICS
Terminal half-life IV 13 days, subcut 14.3 days, steady-state 60 days; clearance increases with increased body weight

INTERACTIONS
- Do not give concurrently with vaccines; immunizations should be brought up to date before treatment
- Do not use with TNF antagonists: adalimumab, etanercept, infliximab; anakinra
- Avoid use with corticosteroids, immunosuppressives, atropine, scopolamine, halothane, nitrous oxide

NURSING CONSIDERATIONS
Assess:
- **RA:** pain, stiffness, ROM, swelling of joints during treatment
- For latent/active TB, viral hepatitis before beginning treatment
- For inj site pain, swelling
- Patient's overall health at each visit; product should not be given with active infections; parenteral product contains maltose, glucose monitoring must be done with glucose-specific testing

⚠ **Infection:** sinusitis, urinary tract infection, influenza, bronchitis; serious infections have occurred

Evaluate:
- Therapeutic response: decreased inflammation, pain in joints

Teach patient/family:
- That product must be continued for prescribed time to be effective
- To use caution when driving; dizziness may occur
- Not to have vaccinations while taking this product or use alcohol, TNF antagonists, other immunosuppressants
- About patient information included in packaging
- How to inject and rotate inj sites
- To report signs of infection

⚠ HIGH ALERT

abiraterone
(a′bir-a′ter-one)
Zytiga
Func. class.: Antineoplastic
Chem. Class.: Androgen inhibitor

ACTION: Converted to abiraterone, which inhibits CYP17, the enzyme required for androgen biosynthesis; androgen-sensitive prostate cancer responds to treatment that decreases androgens

USES: Metastatic castration-resistant prostate cancer in combination with predniSONE

CONTRAINDICATIONS: Pregnancy (X), women, children

Precautions: Adrenal insufficiency, cardiac disease, MI, heart failure, hepatic disease, hypertension, hypokalemia, infection, surgery, ventricular dysrhythmia

DOSAGE AND ROUTES
- **Adult males: PO** 1000 mg/day with predniSONE 5 mg bid

Hepatic dose
- **Adult males (Child-Pugh B, 7-9): PO** 250 mg/day with predniSONE, permanently discontinue if AST/ALT >5 × the upper normal limit (ULN) or total bilirubin >3 × (ULN) (Child-Pugh C, >10) do not use

Available forms:
Tabs 250 mg

Administer:

PO route
- Give whole, on empty stomach 2 hr before or 1 hr after meals with full glass of water

⚠ Women who are pregnant or may become pregnant should not touch tabs without gloves
- Store tabs at room temperature

SIDE EFFECTS
CV: Angina, dysrhythmia exacerbation, atrial flutter/fibrillation/tachycardia, AV

block, chest pain, edema, heart failure, MI, hypertension, QT prolongation, sinus tachycardia, supraventricular tachycardia, ventricular tachycardia
ENDO: Hot flashes
GI: Diarrhea, dyspepsia, hepatotoxicity
GU: Increased urinary frequency, nocturia, urinary tract infection
META: Adrenocortical insufficiency, hyperbilirubinemia, hypertriglyceridemia, hypokalemia, hypophosphatemia
MS: Arthralgia, myalgia
RESP: Cough, upper respiratory infection
SYST: Infection

PHARMACOKINETICS

99% protein binding, converted to abiraterone (active metabolite), mean terminal half-life 12 hr; excreted 88% (feces), 5% (urine); high-fat food increases effect, give on empty stomach; increased effect in hepatic disease

INTERACTIONS

• Decrease: abiraterone effect—CYP3A4 inhibitors (clarithromycin, atazanavir, nefazodone, saquinavir, telithromycin, ritonavir, indinavir, nelfinavir, voriconazole, ketoconazole, itraconazole), loperamide, naprosen, pioglitazone, pitavastin, repaglinide, rosiglitazone
• Avoid use with: CYP3A4 inducers (carBAMazepine, phenytoin, rifampin, rifabutin, rifapentine, PHENobarbital)
• Increase: action of CYP2D6 substrates—dextromethorphan, thioridazine; dose of these products should be reduced

Drug/Food

Increase: abiraterone action—must be taken on an empty stomach

Drug/Lab

Increase: ALT, AST, bilirubin, triglycerides, cholesterol, alk phos

Decrease: potassium, phosphate, testosterone

NURSING CONSIDERATIONS

Assess:

• **Prostate cancer:** monitor prostate-specific antigen (PSA), serum potassium, serum bilirubin

⚠ **Hepatotoxicity:** monitor liver function tests (AST/ALT) at baseline, every 2 wk for 3 mo, monthly thereafter in patients with no known hepatic disease; interrupt treatment in patients without known hepatic disease at baseline who develop ALT/AST >5 × ULN or total bilirubin >3 × ULN; patients with moderate hepatic disease at baseline, measure ALT, AST, bilirubin before the start of treatment, every wk for 1 mo, every 2 wk for the following 2 mo, monthly thereafter; if elevations in ALT and/or AST >5 × ULN or total bilirubin >3 × ULN occur in patients with moderate hepatic impairment at baseline, discontinue and do NOT restart; measure serum total bilirubin, AST/ALT if hepatotoxicity is suspected; elevations of AST, ALT, bilirubin from baseline should prompt more frequent monitoring

• **Musculoskeletal pain, joint swelling, discomfort:** arthritis, arthralgia, joint swelling, and joint stiffness, some severe; muscle discomfort that includes muscle spasms, musculoskeletal pain, myalgia, musculoskeletal discomfort, and musculoskeletal stiffness may be relieved with analgesics

• Signs, symptoms of adrenocorticoid insufficiency; monthly for hypertension, hypokalemia, fluid retention

⚠ **QT prolongation:** Monitor ECG for QT prolongation, ejection fraction in patients with cardiac disease, small increases in the QTc interval such as <10 ms have occurred; monitor for arrhythmia exacerbation such as sinus tachycardia, atrial fibrillation, supraventricular tachycardia (SVT), atrial tachycardia, ventricular tachycardia, atrial flutter, bradycardia, AV block complete, conduction disorder, bradyarrhythmia

Teach patient/family:

⚠ That women must not come in contact with tabs; wear gloves if product needs to be handled, pregnancy (X)

• To report chest pain, swelling of joints, burning/pain when urinating

• Not to use with other meds, herbs without prescriber approval

acamprosate

(a-kam-pro′sate)

Func. class.: Alcohol deterrent

Chem. class.: Synthetic amino acid neurotransmitter analog

ACTION: Not completely understood; in vitro data suggest it has affinity for type A and type B GABA receptors, lowers neuronal excitability, centrally mediated

USES: Alcohol abstinence management

CONTRAINDICATIONS

Hypersensitivity to this product or sulfites, creatinine clearance ≤30 ml/min

Precautions: Pregnancy (C), breastfeeding, infants, children, ethanol intoxication, renal impairment, depression, suicidal ideation, driving or operating machinery, geriatric patients

DOSAGE AND ROUTES

- **Adult: PO** 666 mg tid

Renal dosage

- **Adult: PO** CCr 30-50 ml/min 333 mg tid; CCr <30 ml/min do not use

Available forms: Del-rel tabs 333 mg

Administer:

- Without regard to food; do not crush, chew, break del-rel tab
- Use only after alcohol is stopped
- Store at room temperature

SIDE EFFECTS

CNS: Anxiety, depression, dizziness, headache, insomnia, paresthesias, suicidal ideation, tremors, abnormal thoughts, chills, drowsiness

CV: Palpitations, hypertension, peripheral edema

EENT: Rhinitis, pharyngitis, abnormal vision

GI: Anorexia, constipation, diarrhea, dry mouth, abdominal pain, flatulence, nausea, vomiting, taste change, weight gain

GU: Impotence

INTEG: Rash, pruritus, increased sweating

MISC: Infection, flulike symptoms

MS: Back pain, myalgias, arthralgia

RESP: Dyspnea, bronchitis

PHARMACOKINETICS

Peak 3-8 hr, half-life 20-33 hr

INTERACTIONS

Drug/Lab

Increase: LFTs, blood glucose, bilirubin, uric acid

Decrease: Hgb/Hct, platelets

NURSING CONSIDERATIONS

Assess:

- Mental status: depression, abnormal thinking, suicidal thoughts/behaviors, length of alcohol use, date of discontinuing alcohol use
- B/P baseline and periodically

Evaluate:

- Therapeutic response: continued alcohol abstinence

Teach patient/family:

- To notify prescriber of depression, abnormal thoughts, suicidal thoughts/behaviors
- To take without regard to food; not to break, crush, chew del-rel tabs
- To notify prescriber if pregnancy is planned or suspected; to use effective contraception
- Not to engage in hazardous activities until effect is known, may impair thinking, monitor skills
- Not to use alcohol, continue treatment for alcohol addiction

acarbose (Rx)

(ay-car′bose)

Glucobay ✦, Prandase ✦, Precose

Func. class.: Oral antidiabetic

Chem. class.: α-Glucosidase inhibitor

Do not confuse:

Precose/preCare

ACTION: Delays digestion/absorption of ingested carbohydrates by inhibiting α-glucosidase, results in smaller rise in postprandial blood glucose after meals; does not increase insulin production

USES:
Type 2 diabetes mellitus, alone or in combination with a sulfonylurea, metformin, insulin

Unlabeled uses: Adjunct in type 1 diabetes mellitus

CONTRAINDICATIONS:
Breastfeeding, hypersensitivity, diabetic ketoacidosis, cirrhosis, inflammatory bowel disease, ileus, colonic ulceration, partial intestinal obstruction, chronic intestinal disease, serum creatinine >2 mg/dl, CCr <25 ml/min

Precautions: Pregnancy (B), children, renal/hepatic disease

DOSAGE AND ROUTES
- **Adult >60 kg (>132 lb): PO** 25 mg tid initially, with 1st bite of meal; maintenance dose may be increased to 50-100 mg tid; dosage adjustment at 4- to 8-wk intervals, individualized
- **Adult <60 kg (<132 lb): PO** max 50 mg tid

Type 1 diabetes mellitus (unlabeled)
- **Adult: PO** 50 mg tid with meals × 2 wk, then 100 mg tid with meals

Available forms: Tabs 25, 50, 100 mg

Administer:

PO route
- With 1st bite of each meal 3×/day
- Store in a tight container, cool environment

SIDE EFFECTS
GI: *Abdominal pain, diarrhea, flatulence*

PHARMACOKINETICS
Poor systemic absorption, peak 1 hr, duration 2-4 hr, metabolized in GI tract, excreted as intact product in urine, half-life 2 hr

INTERACTIONS
- Do not use with gatifloxacin

Increase: acetaminophen toxicity—acetaminophen combined with alcohol

Increase or decrease: glycemic control—androgens, lithium, bortezomib, quinolones

Decrease: effect of digoxin

Increase: hypoglycemia—sulfonylureas, insulin, MAOIs, salicylates, fibric acid derivatives, bile acid sequestrants, ACE inhibitors, angiotensin II receptor antagonists, β-blockers

Decrease: effect, increase hyperglycemia—digestive enzymes, intestinal absorbents, thiazide diuretics, loop diuretics, corticosteroids, estrogen, progestins, oral contraceptives, sympathomimetics, isoniazid, phenothiazines; protease inhibitors, atypical antipsychotics, carbonic anhydrase inhibitors, cycloSPORINE, tacrolimus, baclofen

Drug/Herb

Increase: hypoglycemia—chromium, garlic, horse chestnut

Drug/Lab Test

Increase: ALT, AST

Decrease: calcium, vit B_6, Hgb, Hct

Interference: urine glucose tests, 1,5-AG assay

NURSING CONSIDERATIONS
Assess:
- **Hypoglycemia** (weakness, hunger, dizziness, tremors, anxiety, tachycardia, sweating), hyperglycemia; even though product does not cause hypoglycemia, if patient is on sulfonylureas or insulin, hypoglycemia may be additive; if hypoglycemia occurs, treat with dextrose, or, if severe, with IV glucose or glucagon
- For stress, surgery, or other trauma that may require change in dose
- Monitor AST, ALT q3mo × 1 yr and periodically thereafter; if elevated, dose may need to be reduced or discontinued, usually increased with doses ≥300 mg/day; dose-related elevations may occur and patients are usually asymptomatic; if symptomatic, dosage reduction or withdrawal is needed; A1c q3mo, monitor serum glucose, 1 hr PP throughout treatment
- GI side effects for tolerability/compliance

Evaluate:
- Therapeutic response: improved signs/symptoms of diabetes mellitus

(decreased polyuria, polydipsia, polyphagia; clear sensorium, absence of dizziness, stable gait)

Teach patient/family:

- The symptoms of hypo/hyperglycemia; what to do about each
- That medication must be taken as prescribed; that must be taken with food; explain consequences of discontinuing medication abruptly; that insulin may need to be used for stress, including trauma, surgery, fever
- To avoid medications and herbal supplements unless approved by health care provider
- That diabetes is a lifelong illness; that the diet and exercise regimen must be followed; that this product is not a cure
- To carry emergency ID and a glucose source; to avoid sugar, because sugar is blocked by acarbose
- That blood glucose monitoring is required to assess product effect
- To avoid breastfeeding if using acarbose with other antidiabetics
- That GI side effects may occur

acetaminophen (OTC) (Paracetamol)

(a-seat-a-mee′noe-fen)

222AF 🍁, Abenol 🍁, Acephen, ACET 🍁, Acetab 🍁, Apacet, APAP, Apra, Atasol 🍁, Children's FeverAll, Equaline Children's Pain Relief, Equaline Infant's Pain Relief, Fortolin 🍁, Genapap, GoodSense Acetaminophen, GoodSense Children's Pain Relief, Infantaire, Leader Children's Pain Reliever, Mapap, NeoPAP, Novo-Gesic 🍁, Ofirmev, Pediaphen 🍁, Pediatrix 🍁, Q-Pap, Q-Pap Children's, Rapid Action Relief 🍁, Redutemp, Ridenol, Robigesic 🍁, Rounox 🍁, Silapap, Taminol 🍁, Tempra 🍁, T-Painol, Tylenol, Vick's Custom Care Body Aches 🍁, Walgreen's Non-Aspirin, XS pain reliever

Func. class.: Nonopioid analgesic, antipyretic

Chem. class.: Nonsalicylate, paraaminophenol derivative

ACTION: May block pain impulses peripherally that occur in response to inhibition of prostaglandin synthesis; does not possess antiinflammatory properties; antipyretic action results from inhibition of prostaglandins in the CNS (hypothalamic heat-regulating center)

USES: Mild to moderate pain or fever, arthralgia, dental pain, dysmenorrhea, headache, myalgia, osteoarthritis

Unlabeled uses: Migraine

CONTRAINDICATIONS: Hypersensitivity to this product or phenacetin

Precautions: Pregnancy (B), (C) IV; breastfeeding, geriatric patients, anemia, renal/hepatic disease, chronic alcoholism

DOSAGE AND ROUTES

• **Adult/child >12 yr: PO/RECT** 325-650 mg q4-6hr prn, max 4 g/day; weight ≥50 kg IV 1000 mg q6hr or 650 mg q4hr prn, max single dose 1000 mg, min dosing interval 4 hr; weight <50 kg IV 15 mg/kg/dose q6hr or 12.5 mg/kg/dose q4hr, max single dose 15 mg/kg, min dosing interval 4 hr, max 75 mg/kg/day from all sources, ext rel 650-1300 mg q8hr as needed, max 4 g/day

• **Child ≥2 yr and <50 kg: IV** 15 mg/kg/dose q6hr or 12.5 mg/kg/dose q4hr, max single dose 15 mg/kg, min dosing interval 4 hr, max 75 mg/kg/day from all sources

Migraine (unlabeled)

• **Adult and adolescent: PO/RECT** 500-1000 mg, max 1 g/dose or max 4 g/day

Available forms: Rect supp 120, 325, 650 mg; soft chew tabs 80 mg; caps 500 mg; elix 120, 160, 325 mg/5 ml; oral disintegrating tab 80, 160 ml; oral drops 80 mg/0.8 ml, liquid 500 mg/5 ml, 160/5 ml, 1000/30 ml; ext rel 650 mg, 80 mg/ml; tabs 325, 500, 650 mg; sol for inj 1000 mg/100 ml

Administer:

PO route

• Do not confuse 2 × 325 (650 mg), with 650 mg ER tab

• Crushed or whole, do not crush EXT REL product; chewable tabs may be chewed; give with full glass of water

• With food or milk to decrease gastric symptoms if needed

• Susp after shaken well; check elixir, liquid, suspension concentration carefully; susp and cups are bioequivalent

Rectal route

• Store suppositories <80° F (27° C)

Intermittent IV INFUSION route

• No further dilution needed; do not add other medications to vial or infusion device

• For doses equal to single vial, averted IV set may be used to deliver directly from vial; for doses less than a single vial, withdraw dose and place in an empty sterile syringe, plastic IV container, or glass bottle; infuse over 15 min

• Discard unused portion; if seal is broken, vial penetrated, or drug transferred to another container, give within 6 hr

Black Box Warning: Check IV dose carefully to prevent dosing errors

SIDE EFFECTS

GI: Nausea, vomiting, abdominal pain; **hepatotoxicity, hepatic seizure (overdose), GI bleeding**

GU: **Renal failure (high, prolonged doses)**

HEMA: **Leukopenia, neutropenia, hemolytic anemia (long-term use), thrombocytopenia, pancytopenia**

INTEG: Rash, urticaria, inj site pain

SYST: **Stevens-Johnson syndrome, toxic epidermal necrolysis**

TOXICITY: **Cyanosis, anemia, neutropenia, jaundice, pancytopenia, CNS stimulation, delirium followed by vascular collapse, seizures, coma, death**

PHARMACOKINETICS

85%-90% metabolized by liver, excreted by kidneys; metabolites may be toxic if overdose occurs; widely distributed; crosses placenta in low concentrations; excreted in breast milk; half-life 1-4 hr

PO: Onset 10-30 min, peak ½-2 hr, duration 4-6 hr, well absorbed

IV: Peak 30-120 min

RECT: Onset slow, peak 1-2 hr, duration 4-6 hr, absorption varies

INTERACTIONS

• Avoid use with salicylates

Increase: renal adverse reactions—NSAIDs, salicylates

Increase: hypoprothrombinemia—warfarin, long-term use, high doses of acetaminophen

Increase: hepatotoxicity—barbiturates, alcohol, carBAMazepine, hydantoins, rifampin, rifabutin, isoniazid, diflunisal, zidovudine, lamoTRIgine, imatinib, dasatinib, mipomersen

Decrease: absorption—colestipol, cholestyramine
Decrease: zidovudine effect
Drug/Herb
Increase: heptatotoxicity—St. John's wort, due to acetaminophen metabolism
Drug/Lab Test
Interference: urinary 5-HIAA
Increase: LFTs, potassium, bilirubin, LDH, pro-time
Decrease: Hgb/Hct, WBC, RBC, platelets; albumin, magnesium, phosphate (pediatrics)

NURSING CONSIDERATIONS

Assess:

- **Hepatic studies:** AST, ALT, bilirubin, creatinine before therapy if long-term therapy is anticipated; may cause hepatic toxicity at doses >4 g/day with chronic use
- **Renal studies:** BUN, urine creatinine, occult blood, albumin, if patient is on long-term therapy; presence of blood or albumin indicates nephritis
- **Blood studies:** CBC, PT if patient is on long-term therapy
- I&O ratio; decreasing output may indicate renal failure (long-term therapy)
- **For fever and pain:** type of pain, location, intensity, duration
- **Chronic poisoning:** rapid, weak pulse; dyspnea; cold, clammy extremities; report immediately to prescriber

Black Box Warning: Hepatotoxicity: dark urine; clay-colored stools; yellowing of skin, sclera; itching; abdominal pain; fever; diarrhea if patient is on long-term therapy; doses >4 g/day

- **Potentially fatal hypersensitivity: Allergic reactions:** rash, urticaria; if these occur, product may have to be discontinued
- Stevens-Johnson syndrome, toxic epidermal necrolysis may occur during beginning treatment or any other dose

Evaluate:

- Therapeutic response: absence of pain using pain scoring; fever

Teach patient/family:

Black Box Warning: Not to exceed recommended dosage; the elixir, liquid, suspension come in several concentrations, read label carefully; acute poisoning with liver damage may result; tell parents of children to check products carefully; that acute toxicity includes symptoms of nausea, vomiting, abdominal pain and that prescriber should be notified immediately; that toxicity may occur when used with other combination products

- Not to use with alcohol, herbals, OTC products without approval of prescriber
- May be used when breastfeeding, short-term
- To recognize signs of chronic overdose: bleeding, bruising, malaise, fever, sore throat
- That those with diabetes may notice blood glucose monitoring changes
- To notify prescriber of pain or fever lasting more than 3 days, not to be used in patients <2 yr unless approved by prescriber

TREATMENT OF OVERDOSE:

Product level, gastric lavage, activated charcoal; administer oral acetylcysteine to prevent hepatic damage *(see acetylcysteine monograph)*; monitor for bleeding

acetaZOLAMIDE (Rx)

(a-set-a-zole′a-mide)

Diamox ✦, Novo-Zolamide ✦

Func. class.: Diuretic, carbonic anhydrase inhibitor, antiglaucoma agent, antiepileptic

Chem. class.: Sulfonamide derivative

Do not confuse:
acetaZOLAMIDE/acetoHEXAMIDE
Diamox/Trimox/Dobutrex

ACTION: Inhibits carbonic anhydrase activity in proximal renal tubules to decrease reabsorption of water, sodium, potassium, bicarbonate resulting in increased urine volume and alkalinization of urine; decreases carbonic anhydrase in CNS, increasing seizure threshold; able to decrease secretion of aqueous humor in eye, which lowers intraocular pressure

USES:
Open-angle glaucoma, angle-closure glaucoma (preoperatively, if surgery delayed), mixed, tonic-clonic, myoclonic, refractory, epilepsy (petit mal, grand mal, absence), edema in CHF, product-induced edema, acute altitude sickness

Unlabeled uses: Urine alkalinization, metabolic alkalosis in mechanical ventilation, decrease CSF production in infants with hydrocephalus, familial periodic paralysis, nystagmus

CONTRAINDICATIONS:
Hypersensitivity to sulfonamides, severe renal/hepatic disease, electrolyte imbalances (hyponatremia, hypokalemia), hyperchloremic acidosis, Addison's disease, long-term use for closed-angle glaucoma, adrenocortical insufficiency, metabolic acidosis, acidemia, anuria

Precautions: Pregnancy (C), breastfeeding, hypercalciuria, respiratory acidosis, pulmonary obstruction/emphysema, COPD

DOSAGE AND ROUTES

Angle-closure glaucoma

• **Adult: PO/IV** 250 mg q4hr or 250 mg bid for short-term therapy

Chronic open-angle glaucoma

• **Adult: PO/IV** 250 mg 1-4 times per day or 500 mg **EXT REL** bid, max 1 g/day

• **Child (Unlabeled): PO** 8-30 mg/kg/day in divided doses tid or qid, or 300-900 mg/m^2/day, max 1 g/day; **IV** 5-10 mg q6hr, max 1 g/day

Edema in CHF

• **Adult: PO/IV** 250-375 mg/day or 5 mg/kg in AM, give for 2 days, then 1-2 days drug free

• **Child (Unlabeled): PO/IV** 5 mg/kg/day or 150 mg/m^2 in AM

Seizures

• **Adult: PO/IV** 8-30 mg/kg/day, in 1-4 divided doses, usual range 375-1000 mg/day; **ER** not recommended with seizures

Altitude sickness

• **Adult: PO** 125 mg bid, start therapy 24-48 hr before ascent and give for ≥48 hr after arrival at high altitude

• **Geriatric: PO** 250 mg bid, use lowest effective dose

Renal dose

• **Adult: PO/IV** CCr 50-80 ml/min give dose ≥q6hr regular release or IV; CCr 10-50 ml/min give dose q12hr; CCr <10 ml/min, avoid use

Urine alkalinization (unlabeled)

• **Adult: IV** 5 mg/kg/dose, repeat 2-3× over 24 hr

Familial periodic paralysis (unlabeled)

• **Adult: PO** 250-375 mg/day in divided doses

Metabolic alkalosis in mechanical ventilation (unlabeled)

• **Adult: IV** 500 mg as a single dose or 250 mg q6hr × 4 doses

Vestibular nystagmus (unlabeled)

• **Adult: PO** 250 mg, increase by 250 mg q3days; max 3 g/day in divided doses

Available forms: Tabs 125, 250 mg; ext rel caps 500 mg; inj 500 mg

Administer:

• In AM to avoid interference with sleep if using product as diuretic

• Potassium replacement if potassium level is <3 mg/dl

PO route

• Do not break, crush, or chew ext rel caps; this product should be used for altitude sickness, glaucoma; store at room temperature

• With food if nausea occurs; absorption may be decreased slightly

IV route

• Reconstitute with 500 mg in ≥5 ml sterile water for inj; **direct IV:** give at 100-500 mg/min

• Store in cool, dark area; use reconstituted solution within 24 hr

Additive compatibilities: cimetidine, ranitidine

SIDE EFFECTS

CNS: Anxiety, *confusion,* seizures, *depression,* dizziness, *drowsiness, fatigue,* headache, *paresthesia,* stimulation
EENT: Myopia, tinnitus
ENDO: *Hyper/hypoglycemia*
GI: *Nausea, vomiting, anorexia, diarrhea,* melena, *weight loss,* hepatic insufficiency, cholestatic jaundice, fulminant hepatic necrosis, *taste alterations,* bleeding
GU: *Frequency, polyuria,* uremia, glucosuria, hematuria, dysuria, crystalluria, renal calculi
HEMA: Aplastic anemia, hemolytic anemia, leukopenia, thrombocytopenia, purpura, pancytopenia
INTEG: *Rash,* pruritus, urticaria, fever, Stevens-Johnson syndrome, photosensitivity, flushing, toxic epidermal necrolysis
META: *Hypokalemia, hyperchloremic acidosis,* hyponatremia, sulfonamide-like reactions, metabolic acidosis, growth inhibition in children, hyperuricemia, hypercalcemia

PHARMACOKINETICS

65% absorbed if fasting (oral), 75% absorbed if given with food; half-life $2^1/_2$-$5^1/_2$ hr; excreted unchanged by kidneys (80% within 24 hr), crosses placenta
PO: Onset 1-$1^1/_2$ hr, peak 1-4 hr, duration 8-12 hr
PO-EXT REL: Onset 2 hr, peak 3-6 hr, duration 18-24 hr
IV: Onset 2 min, peak 15 min, duration 4-5 hr

INTERACTIONS

Increase: action of—amphetamines, flecainide, memantine, phenytoin, procainamide, quiNIDine, anticholinergics, methenamine, mecamylamine, ePHEDrine, memantine, mexiletine, folic acid antagonists
Increase: excretion of lithium, primidone
Increase: acidosis (respiratory disorders)—β-blockers
Increase: osteomalacia—carBAMazepine, ethotoin
Increase: toxicity—salicylates, cycloSPORINE
Increase: hypokalemia—corticosteroids, amphotericin B, corticotropin, ACTH
Increase: cardiac toxicity if hypokalemia develops—arsenic trioxide, cardiac glycosides, levomethadyl
Increase: renal stone formation, heat stroke—topiramate (avoid concurrent use)
Decrease: primidone levels
Drug/Lab Test
Increase: glucose, uric acid
Decrease: thyroid iodine uptake, sodium, Hct/Hgb, WBC, platelets
False positive: urinary protein, 17 hydroxysteroid

NURSING CONSIDERATIONS

Assess:

Black Box Warning: Severe reactions: Stevens-Johnson syndrome, toxic epidermal necrolysis, blood dyscrasias, discontinue if these occur

- Edema: weight daily, I&O daily to determine fluid loss; effect of product may be decreased if used daily; monitor geriatric patients for dehydration
- Ocular status: intraocular pressure, ophthalmologic examination
- B/P lying, standing; postural hypotension may occur
- Electrolytes: potassium, sodium, chloride; also BUN, blood glucose, CBC, serum creatinine, blood pH, ABGs, LFTs; I&O, platelet count, patient may need to be on a high-potassium diet; identify signs of hypokalemia (vomiting, fatigue, weakness)
- **Seizures:** neurologic status, provide seizure precaution

Evaluate:

- Therapeutic response: improvement in edema of feet, legs, sacral area daily if medication is being used for CHF; decrease in aqueous humor if medication is being used for glaucoma; decreased frequency of seizures, prevention of altitude sickness

Teach patient/family:

- To take exactly as prescribed; if dose is missed, take as soon as remembered; do not double dose

- Altitude sickness: to avoid rapid ascent
- Diabetic: that drug may alter blood glucose and to monitor blood glucose
- To use sunscreen to prevent photosensitivity
- To avoid prolonged sun exposure
- To avoid hazardous activities if drowsiness occurs
- To increase fluids to 2-3 L/day if not contraindicated

⚠ **To report nausea, vertigo, rapid weight gain, change in stools, weakness, numbness, rash, sore throat, bleeding/bruising; Stevens-Johnson syndrome, toxic epidermal necrolysis (blistering, red rash that spreads)**

TREATMENT OF OVERDOSE:
Lavage if taken orally; monitor electrolytes; administer dextrose in saline; monitor hydration, CV, renal status

acetylcholine ophthalmic
See Appendix B

acetylcysteine (Rx)
(a-se-teel-sis′tay-een)

Acetadote, Airbron ✦, Mucomyst ✦, Parvolex ✦

Func. class.: Mucolytic; antidote—acetaminophen

Chem. class.: Amino acid L-cysteine

Do not confuse:
acetylcysteine/acetylcholine
Mucomyst/Mucinex

ACTION: Decreases viscosity of secretions by breaking disulfide links of mucoproteins; serves as a substrate in place of glutathione, which is necessary to inactivate toxic metabolites with acetaminophen overdose

USES: Acetaminophen toxicity; bronchitis; cystic fibrosis; COPD; atelectasis

Unlabeled uses: Prevention of contrast medium nephrotoxicity, meconium ileus

CONTRAINDICATIONS: Hypersensitivity

Precautions: Pregnancy (B), breastfeeding, hypothyroidism, Addison's disease, CNS depression, brain tumor, asthma, renal/hepatic disease, COPD, psychosis, alcoholism, seizure disorders, bronchospasms, anaphylactoid reactions, fluid restriction, weight <40 kg, increased intracranial pressure, status asthmaticus

DOSAGE AND ROUTES
Acetaminophen toxicity

- **Adult and child >40 kg: PO** 140 mg/kg, then 70 mg/kg q4hr × 17 doses to total of 1330 mg/kg; **>40 kg: IV** loading dose 150 mg/kg over 60 min (dilution 150 mg/kg in 200 ml of D_5W); then 50 mg/kg over 4 hr (dilution 50 mg/kg in 500 ml D_5W); then 100 mg/kg over 16 hr (dilution 100 mg/kg in 1000 D_5W)
- **Child/Adolescent 21-40 kg: IV** 150 mg/kg in 100 ml diluent over 1 hr, then 50 mg/kg in 250 ml over 4 hr, then 100 mg/kg in 500 mg over 16 hr
- **Infant/Child 5-20 kg: IV** 150 mg/kg in 3 ml/kg diluent over 1 hr, then 50 mg/kg in 7 ml/kg diluent over 4 hr, then 100 mg/kg in 14 ml/kg diluent over 16 hr

Mucolytic

- **Adult and child: INSTILL** 1-2 ml (10%-20% sol) q6-8hr prn or 3-5 ml (20% sol) or 6-10 ml (10% sol) tid or qid; nebulization (face mask, mouthpiece, tracheostomy) 1-10 ml of a 20% sol, or 2-20 ml of a 10% sol, q2-8hr; nebulization (tent, croupette) may require large dose, up to 300 ml/treatment

Contrast-induced nephrotoxicity (unlabeled)

- **Adult: PO** 600-1200 mg bid × 2 days (beginning the day before the procedure)

Available forms: Oral sol 10%, 20%; inj 20% (200 mg/ml)

Administer:

PO route

- **Antidotal use:** give within 24 hr; dilute 10% or 20% sol to a 5% sol with diet soda, may use water if giving via gastric tube; dilution of 10% sol 1:1, 20% sol 1:3, store open undiluted solution refrigerated ≤96 hr

Direct intratracheal instill route

- By syringe: 1-2 ml of 10%-20% sol up to q1hr
- Decreased dose to geriatric patients; metabolism may be slowed
- Only if suction machine is available
- Only after patient clears airway by deep breathing, coughing
- Assistance with inhaled dose: bronchodilator if bronchospasm occurs; mechanical suction if cough insufficient to remove excess bronchial secretions

IV route

- **21-hr regimen:** loading dose: dilute 150 mg/kg in 200 ml D_5W; maintenance dose 1: dilute 50 mg/kg in 500 ml D_5W; maintenance dose 2: dilute 100 mg/kg in 1000 ml D_5W; give loading dose over 15 min; give maintenance dose 1 over 4 hr; give maintenance dose 2 over 16 hr, administer sequentially without time between doses
- Store in refrigerator; use within 96 hr of opening

SIDE EFFECTS

CNS: *Dizziness, drowsiness,* headache, fever, chills
CV: Hypotension, flushing tachycardia
EENT: *Rhinorrhea,* tooth damage
GI: *Nausea,* stomatitis, constipation, vomiting, anorexia, diarrhea
INTEG: Urticaria, rash, fever, clamminess, pruritus
RESP: Bronchospasm, burning, hemoptysis, chest tightness, cough, dyspnea
MISC: Anaphylaxis, angioedema, unpleasant odor

PHARMACOKINETICS

IV: Excreted in urine, half-life 5.6 hr (adult), 11 hr (newborn), protein binding 83%, peak ½-1 hr

INTERACTIONS

- Do not use with activated charcoal

NURSING CONSIDERATIONS

Assess:

- **Mucolytic use:** cough—type, frequency, character, including sputum; bronchospasm
- Rate, rhythm of respirations, increased dyspnea; sputum; discontinue if bronchospasm occurs
- VS, cardiac status including checking for dysrhythmias, increased rate, palpitations
- ABGs for increased CO_2 retention in asthma patients
- **Antidotal use:** LFTs, PT, BUN, creatinine, glucose, electrolytes, acetaminophen levels; inform prescriber if dose is vomited or vomiting is persistent; 150 mg/kg may be toxic, check acetaminophen level q4hr
- **Hypersensitivity:** Anaphylaxis may occur with IV dose; if present, stop infusion, treat, restart
- Nausea, vomiting, rash; notify prescriber if these occur

Evaluate:

- Therapeutic response: absence of purulent secretions when coughing, clear lung sounds (mucolytic use); absence of hepatic damage with acetaminophen toxicity

Teach patient/family:

- That foul odor and smell may be unpleasant
- To clear airway for inhalation
- To report vomiting because dose may need to be repeated

aclidinium

(a′kli-din′ee-um)

Tudorza Pressair

Func. class.: Anticholinergic, bronchodilator

Chem. class.: Synthetic quaternary ammonium compound

ACTION: Inhibits interaction of acetylcholine at receptor sites on the bronchial smooth muscle, thereby resulting in decreased cGMP and bronchodilation

USES:
Long-term maintenance treatment of bronchospasm in COPD, emphysema, chronic bronchitis, not indicated for initial treatment of acute episodes

CONTRAINDICATIONS:
Hypersensitivity

Precautions: Pregnancy (C), breastfeeding, milk sensitivity, contact lenses, narrow-angle glaucoma, neonates, ocular exposure, prostatic hypertrophy, bladder obstruction

DOSAGE AND ROUTES

- **Adults, including geriatric patients:** Oral inhalation 400 mcg (1 actuation) bid; doses should be 12 hours apart

Available forms: Powder for inhalation 400 mcg/actuation

Administer:

Oral inhalation route

- Before initial use, remove inhaler from pouch; remove the cap by squeezing the arrows marked on each side and pulling outward; instruct the patient to hold the inhaler with the mouthpiece facing patient but not inside the mouth; the green button should be facing straight up
- Before placing the inhaler into the mouth, the green button should be pushed all the way down and then released; patient should not continue to hold it down; once the green button is pressed, the control window changes from red to green, indicating that the medication is ready for inhalation; if the control window remains red, repeat the press-and-release actions until the control window is green
- Before inhaling the dose, have patient breathe out completely away from the inhaler; patient should never breathe out into the inhaler
- Instruct patient to put his/her lips tightly around the mouthpiece and to breathe in quickly and deeply through the mouth until a clicking sound is heard
- The patient should remove the inhaler from the mouth and hold breath for as long as is comfortable, then breathe out slowly through the nose
- The control window should turn red after the full dose has been inhaled. If it remains green after the dose is inhaled, the inhalation process should be repeated. If correct inhalation has not been achieved after several attempts, the doctor or health care professional should be contacted
- Once the window has turned red, the protective cap should be placed back onto the inhaler by pressing it back onto the mouthpiece
- The dose indicator displays how many doses are left. The first time the inhaler is used, the indicator displays the number 60. The indicator number counts down as the patient uses the inhaler
- Discard inhaler when the marking "0" with red background shows in the middle of the dose indicator, the device locks out after 45 days (whichever comes first); the inhaler does not need to be cleaned

SIDE EFFECTS

CNS: *Anxiety, dizziness, headache,* nervousness

CV: Palpitation

EENT: Dry mouth, blurred vision, nasopharyngitis congestion

GI: *Nausea, vomiting, diarrhea*

INTEG: Rash

RESP: *Cough, worsening of symptoms,* **bronchospasm**

PHARMACOKINETICS

Half-life 5-8 hr

INTERACTIONS

Increase: toxicity—other bronchodilators

NURSING CONSIDERATIONS

Assess:

- Tolerance over long-term therapy; dose might have to be increased or changed
- Respiratory status: rate, rhythm, auscultate breath sounds before and after administration; pulmonary function tests at baseline and periodically

Evaluate:

- Therapeutic response: ability to breathe adequately

Teach patient/family:

- That compliance is necessary with number of inhalations/24 hr or overdose can occur; that max therapeutic effects can take 2-3 mo
- About the correct method of inhalation
- To report any visual effects or urinary retention

acyclovir (Rx)

(ay-sye′kloe-veer)

Sitavig, Zovirax

Func. class.: Antiviral

Chem. class.: Purine nucleoside analog

Do not confuse:
Zovirax/Zyvox/Valtrex/Zostrix

ACTION: Interferes with DNA synthesis by conversion to acyclovir triphosphate, thereby causing decreased viral replication

USES: Mucocutaneous herpes simplex virus, herpes genitalis (HSV-1, HSV-2), varicella infections, herpes zoster, herpes simplex encephalitis

Unlabeled uses: Bell's palsy, prevention of CMV, Epstein-Barr virus, esophagitis, hairy leukoplakia, prevention of herpes labialis, herpes simplex, herpes simplex ocular prophylaxis, keratoconjunctivitis, pharyngitis, pneumonitis, prevention of postherpetic neuralgia, proctitis, stomatitis, tracheobronchitis, varicella prophylaxis

CONTRAINDICATIONS: Hypersensitivity to this product, valacyclovir

Precautions: Pregnancy (B), breastfeeding, renal/hepatic/neurologic disease, electrolyte imbalance, dehydration, hypersensitivity to famciclovir, ganciclovir, penciclovir, valganciclovir, obesity

DOSAGE AND ROUTES

Base dose in obese patients on ideal body weight, not actual body weight

Herpes simplex (recurrent)

- **Adult: PO** 400 mg 3×/day for 5 days or 200 mg 5×/day × 5 days
- **Adult and child >12 yr: IV INFUSION** 5 mg/kg over 1 hr q8hr × 7 days
- **Infant >3 mo/child <12 yr: IV INFUSION** 10 mg/kg q8hr × 7 day; if HIV infected 5-10 mg/kg q8hr (moderate to severe)
- **Neonate: IV INFUSION** 10 mg/kg q8hr × 10 days, may use higher dose

Genital herpes

- **Adult: PO** 200 mg q4hr (5×/day while awake) for 5 days to 12 mo depending on whether initial, recurrent, or chronic; **IV** 5 mg/kg q8hr × 5 days

Genital herpes, initial limited, mucocutaneous HSV in immunocompromised patients, non–life-threatening

- **Adult/child ≥12 yr: TOP** cover lesions q3hr 6 times/day

Herpes simplex encephalitis

- **Adult: IV** 10 mg/kg over 1 hr q8hr × 10 days
- **Child 3 mo-12 yr: IV** 20 mg/kg q8hr × 10 days
- **Child birth-3 mo: IV** 20 mg/kg q8hr × 21 days

Herpes labialis, recurrent

- **Adult/child ≥12 yr:** top apply cream 5×/day for 4 days, start as soon as symptoms appear

Herpes, labialis, recurrent in immunocompetent patients

- **Adult: Buccal** 50 mg as a single dose in upper gum region within 1 hr after prodromal symptoms and before cold sore formation

Herpes zoster

- **Adult: PO** 800 mg q4hr 5×/day while awake × 7-10 days; **IV** 10 mg/kg q8hr × 7 days

Herpes zoster (shingles) immunocompromised patients

- **Adult/adolescent: PO** 800 mg q4hr 5×/day for 7-10 days; **IV** 10 mg/kg q8hr × 7 days
- **Child ≥12 yr: IV** 10 mg/kg/dose q8hr × 7 days
- **Infant/child <12 yr: IV** 20 mg/kg/dose q8hr × 7-10 days

Herpes zoster (shingles) immunocompetent

- **Adult: PO** 800 mg q4hr 5×/day × 7-10 days; start within 48-72 hr of rash onset

Varicella (chickenpox) immunocompetent

- **Adult/adolescent/child: PO** 800 mg 4×/day × 5 days
- **Child ≥2 yr: PO** 20 mg/kg/dose (max 800 mg) 4×/day × 5 days

Mucosal/cutaneous herpes simplex infections in immunosuppressed patients

- **Adult and child >12 yr: IV** 5 mg/kg q8hr × 7 days
- **Infant >3 mo/child <12: IV** 10 mg/kg q8hr × 7 days

Renal dose

- **Adult and child: PO/IV** CCr >50 ml/min 100% dose q8hr, CCr 25-50 ml/min 100% dose q12hr, CCr 10-25 ml/min 100% dose q24hr, CCr 0-10 ml/min 50% dose q24hr

Recurrent ocular herpes, prevention (unlabeled)

- **Adult/child ≥12 yr: PO** 600-800 mg every day × 8-12 mo

CMV prophylaxis (unlabeled)

- **Adult: IV** 500 mg/m^2 q8hr

Herpes simplex in pneumonitis/esophagitis/tracheobronchitis/proctitis/stomatitis/pharyngitis (unlabeled)

- **Adult and adolescent: IV** 5-10 mg/kg q8hr × 2-7 days or **PO** 200 mg q4hr 5×/day × 7-10 days or 400 mg 3-5×/day × ≥10 days
- **Child 6 mo-12 yr: IV** 1000 mg/day in 3-5 divided doses × 7-14 days

Herpes simplex prophylaxis for chronic suppression therapy (unlabeled)

- **Adult and adolescent: PO** 400 mg bid up to 12 mo

Available forms: Caps 200 mg; tabs 400, 800 mg; powder for inj 500, 1000 mg; sol for inj 50 mg/ml; oral susp 200 mg/5 ml; ointment/cream 5%; buccal tab 50 mg

Administer:

PO route

- Do not break, crush, or chew caps
- May give without regard to meals, with 8 oz of water
- Shake susp before use

Topical route

- Use finger cot or glove to cover all lesions completely; do not get in eye; wash hands after use

Intermittent IV INFUSION route

- Increase fluids to 3 L/day to decrease crystalluria; most critical during first 2 hr after IV
- Reconstitute with 10 ml compatible sol/500 mg or 20 ml/1 g of product, concentrations of 50 mg/ml, shake, further dilute in 50-125 ml compatible sol; use within 12 hr; give over at least 1 hr (constant rate) by infusion pump to prevent nephrotoxicity; do not reconstitute with sol containing benzyl alcohol in neonates
- Store at room temperature for up to 12 hr after reconstitution; if refrigerated, sol may show a precipitate that clears at room temperature; yellow discoloration does not affect potency

Solution compatibilities: D_5W, LR, or NaCl (D_5 0.9% NaCl, 0.9% NaCl) sol

Y-site compatibilities: Alemtuzumab, alfentanil, allopurinol, amikacin, aminophylline, amphotericin B cholesteryl, amphotericin B liposome, ampicillin, anidulafungin, argatroban, atracurium, bivalirudin, buprenorphine, busulfan, butorphanol, calcium chloride/gluconate, CARBOplatin, cefazolin, cefonicid, cefotaxime, cefoxitin, ceftazidime, ceftizoxime, cefTRIAXone, cefuroxime, chloramphenicol, cholesteryl sulfate complex, cimetidine, clindamycin, dexamethasone sodium phosphate, dimenhyDRINATE, DOXOrubicin, doxycycline, erythromycin, famotidine, filgrastim, fluconazole, gallium, gentamicin, granisetron, heparin, hydrocortisone sodium succinate, hydromorphone, imipenem/cilastatin, LORazepam, magnesium sulfate, melphalan, methylPREDNISolone sodium succinate, metoclopramide, metroNIDAZOLE, multivitamin, nafcillin, oxacillin, paclitaxel, penicillin G potassium, PENTobarbital, perphenazine, piperacillin, potassium chloride, propofol, ranitidine, remifentanil, sodium bicarbonate, tacrolimus, teniposide, theophylline, thiotepa, ticarcillin, tobramycin, trimethoprim-sulfamethoxazole, vancomycin, vasopressin, voriconazole, zidovudine

SIDE EFFECTS

CNS: Tremors, confusion, lethargy, hallucinations, **seizures**, dizziness, headache, encephalopathic changes
EENT: Gingival hyperplasia
GI: Nausea, vomiting, diarrhea, increased ALT/AST, abdominal pain, glossitis, colitis
GU: **Oliguria, proteinuria, hematuria**, vaginitis, moniliasis, **glomerulonephritis, acute renal failure**, changes in menses, polydipsia
HEMA: **Thrombotic thrombocytopenia purpura, hemolytic uremic syndrome** (immunocompromised patients)
INTEG: Rash, urticaria, pruritus, pain or phlebitis at IV site, unusual sweating, alopecia, **Stevens-Johnson syndrome**
MS: Joint pain, leg pain, muscle cramps

PHARMACOKINETICS

Distributed widely; crosses placenta; CSF concentrations are 50% plasma; protein binding 9%-33%
PO: Absorbed minimally, onset unknown, peak 1.5-2 hr, terminal half-life 2.5-3.3 hr
IV: Onset immediate, peak immediate, duration unknown, half-life 20 min-3 hr (terminal); metabolized by liver, excreted by kidneys as unchanged product (95%)

INTERACTIONS

Increase: CNS side effects—zidovudine
Increase: levels, toxicity—probenecid
Increase: nephrotoxicity—aminoglycosides
Increase: concentrations of—entecavir, pemetrexed, tenofovir
Decrease: action of—hydantoins, valproic acid
Drug/Lab Test
Increase: BUN, creatinine

NURSING CONSIDERATIONS

Assess:

- Signs of infection, anemia
- **Toxicity:** any patient with compromised renal system because product is excreted slowly with poor renal system function; toxicity may occur rapidly
- Hepatic, renal studies: AST, ALT; urinalysis, protein, BUN, creatinine, CCr, watch for increasing BUN and serum creatinine or decreased CCr; I&O ratio; report hematuria, oliguria, fatigue, weakness; may indicate **nephrotoxicity;** check for protein in urine during treatment
- Bowel pattern before, during treatment; if severe abdominal pain with bleeding occurs, product should be discontinued
- Skin eruptions: rash, urticaria, itching
- Allergies before treatment, reaction of each medication; place allergies on chart in bright red letters
- Neurologic status with herpes encephalitis
- Provide adequate intake of fluids (2 L) to prevent deposits in kidneys, more likely to occur with rapid administration or in dehydration

Evaluate:

- Therapeutic response: absence of itching, painful lesions; crusting and healed lesions; decreased symptoms of chickenpox; healing, decreased pain with herpes zoster

Teach patient/family:

- To take as prescribed; if dose is missed, take as soon as remembered up to 1 hr before next dose; do not double dose
- That product may be taken orally before infection occurs; product should be taken when itching or pain occurs, usually before eruptions
- That sexual partners need to be told that patient has herpes because they can become infected; condoms must be worn to prevent reinfections
- Not to touch lesions to avoid spreading infection to new sites
- That product does not cure infection, just controls symptoms and does not prevent infecting others
- That product must be taken in equal intervals around the clock to maintain blood levels for duration of therapy

• To seek dental care during treatment to prevent gingival hyperplasia
• That women with genital herpes are more likely to develop cervical cancer; to keep all gynecologic appointments

TREATMENT OF OVERDOSE:

Discontinue product, hemodialysis, resuscitate if needed

adalimumab (Rx)

(add-a-lim′yu-mab)

Humira

Func. class.: Antirheumatic agent (disease modifying), immunomodulator, anti-TNF

Chem. class.: Recombinant human IgG1 monoclonal antibody, DMARD

Do not confuse:
Humira/Humulin/Humalog

ACTION: A form of human IgG1 monoclonal antibody specific for human tumor necrosis factor (TNF-α); elevated levels of TNF-α are found in patients with rheumatoid arthritis

USES: Reduction of signs and symptoms and inhibition of progression of structural damage in patients with moderate to severe active rheumatoid arthritis who are ≥18 years of age and who have not responded to other disease-modifying agents, juvenile rheumatoid arthritis (JRA), psoriatic arthritis, Crohn's disease, moderate to severe plaque psoriasis, ankylosing spondylitis, ulcerative colitis

CONTRAINDICATIONS: Hypersensitivity

Precautions: Pregnancy (B), breastfeeding, children, geriatric patients, CNS demyelinating disease, lymphoma, CHF, hepatitis B carriers, manitol hypersensitivity, latex allergy, neoplastic disease

Black Box Warning: Active infections, risk of lymphomas/leukemias, TB

DOSAGE AND ROUTES

Rheumatoid arthritis/ankylosing spondylitis/psoriatic arthritis
• **Adult: SUBCUT** 40 mg every other wk or every wk if not combined with methotrexate

Juvenile rheumatoid arthritis
• **Child ≥2 yr/adolescent ≥30 kg: SUBCUT** 40 mg every other wk
• **Child ≥2 yr/adolescent ≥15 kg to <30 kg: SUBCUT** 20 mg every other wk
• **Child ≥2 yr/adolescent 10-<15 kg: SUBCUT** 10 mg every other wk

Crohn's disease/ulcerative colitis
• **Adult: SUBCUT** 160 mg given as 4 inj, on day 1 or 2 inj each on days 1 and 2, then 80 mg at wk 2 and 40 mg every other wk starting at wk 4

Plaque psoriasis
• **Adult: SUBCUT** 80 mg baseline as 2 inj, then 40 mg every other wk starting 1 wk after initial dose × 16 wk

Available form: Inj 40 mg/0.8 ml; 20 mg/0.4 ml (pediatric)

Administer:

SUBCUT route
• Do not admix with other sol or medications; do not use filter; protect from light; give at 45-degree angle using abdomen, thighs; rotate inj sites; discard unused portions

SIDE EFFECTS

CNS: *Headache,* **Guillain-Barré syndrome**
CV: *Hypertension,* CHF
EENT: *Sinusitis*
GI: Abdominal pain, nausea, hepatic damage, **GI bleeding**
HEMA: **Leukopenia pancytopenia, aplastic anemia, agranulocytopenia, thrombocytopenia**
INTEG: *Rash, inj site reaction*
MISC: Flulike symptoms, UTI, back pain, lupus-like syndrome, **increased cancer risk,** *antibody development to this drug;* **risk of infection (TB, invasive fungal infections, other opportunistic**

infections), may be fatal, Stevens-Johnson syndrome, anaphylaxis, hypercholesterolemia, hyperlipidemia
RESP: *URI,* pulmonary fibrosis, bronchitis

PHARMACOKINETICS

Absorption 65%, terminal half-life 2 wk, lower clearance with advancing age (40-75 yr)

INTERACTIONS

Black Box Warning: Increase: serious infections—other TNF blockers, rilonacept

- Do not use with anakinra; serious infections may occur
- Do not give concurrently with live virus vaccines; immunizations should be brought up to date before treatment

Drug/Lab Test
Increase: ALT, cholesterol, lipids

NURSING CONSIDERATIONS

Assess:

- **RA:** pain, stiffness, ROM, swelling of joints before, during treatment
- For inj site pain, swelling, redness—usually occur after 2 inj (4-5 days)—use cold compress to relieve pain/swelling

Black Box Warning: For infections (fever, flulike symptoms, dyspnea, change in urination, redness/swelling around any wounds), stop treatment if present; some serious infections including sepsis may occur, may be fatal; patients with active infections should not be started on this product

- May reactivate hepatitis B in chronic carriers, may be fatal

Black Box Warning: Latent TB before therapy, treat before starting this product

- **Anaphylaxis, latex allergy:** stop therapy if lupus-like syndrome develops
- **Blood dyscrasias:** CBC, differential periodically

Black Box Warning: For neoplastic disease (lymphomas/leukemia) in children, adolescents, hepatosplenic T-cell lymphoma is more likely in adolescent males with Crohn's disease or ulcerative colitis

Evaluate:

- Therapeutic response: decreased inflammation, pain in joints, decreased joint destruction

Teach patient/family:

- About self-administration if appropriate: inj should be made in thigh, abdomen, upper arm; rotate sites at least 1 inch from old site; do not inject in areas that are bruised, red, hard
- That if medication is not taken when due, inject next dose as soon as remembered and inject next dose as scheduled
- Not to take any live virus vaccines during treatment
- To report signs of infection, allergic reaction, or lupus-like syndrome, immediately

adefovir (Rx)

(add-ee-foh′veer)

Hepsera

Func. class.: Antiviral
Chem. class.: Nucleoside

ACTION: Inhibits hepatitis B virus DNA polymerase by competing with natural substrates and by causing DNA termination after its incorporation into viral DNA; causes viral DNA death

USES: Chronic hepatitis B

CONTRAINDICATIONS: Hypersensitivity
Precautions: Pregnancy (C), labor, breastfeeding, children, geriatric patients, dialysis, females, obesity, organ transplant

Black Box Warning: Severe renal disease, impaired hepatic function, lactic acidosis, HIV

DOSAGE AND ROUTES

- **Adult/adolescent: PO** 10 mg/day, optimal duration unknown

Renal dose

- **Adult: PO** CCr ≥50 ml/min 10 mg q24hr; CCr 30-49 ml/min 10 mg q48hr; CCr 10-29 ml/min 10 mg q72hr; hemodialysis 10 mg q7days after dialysis

Available forms: Tabs 10 mg

Administer:

- By mouth without regard for food
- Take with full glass of water
- Store in cool environment; protect from light

SIDE EFFECTS

CNS: *Headache*

GI: *Dyspepsia,* abdominal pain, nausea, vomiting, diarrhea, hepatomegaly, flatulence, pancreatitis

GU: Hematuria, glycosuria, nephrotoxicity, Fanconi syndrome, renal failure

MISC: Fever, rash, weight loss, cough

PHARMACOKINETICS

PO: Rapidly absorbed from GI tract, peak 1¾ hr, excreted by kidneys 45%, terminal half-life 7.48 hr

INTERACTIONS

- Do not use in combination with emtricitabine/tenofovir, emtricitabine/rilpivirine, emtricitabine/efavirenz/tenofovir

Increase: serum concentrations and possible nephrotoxicity—aminoglycosides, memantine, emtricitabine, efavirenz, dofetilide, digoxin, cycloSPORINE, aMILoride, quiNINE, quiNIDine, procainamide, PEMEtrexed, midodrine, metFORMIN, NSAIDs, vancomycin, trospium, triamterene, tenofovir, tacrolimus, ranitidine, cimetidine, morphine

Black Box Warning: Increase: lactic acidosis, severe hepatomegaly, NNRTIs, NRTIs, antiretroviral protease inhibitors

Drug/Lab Test

Increase: ALT, AST, amylase, creatine kinase

NURSING CONSIDERATIONS

Assess:

Black Box Warning: Nephrotoxicity: increasing CCr, BUN

Black Box Warning: HIV antibody testing before beginning treatment, HIV resistance may occur in chronic hepatitis B patients

Black Box Warning: For lactic acidosis, severe hepatomegaly with stenosis; for use of NNRTIs, NRTIs, antiretroviral protease inhibitors (PIs), lactic acidosis with severe hepatomegaly is more common in females, obese patients, and with prolonged nucleoside use

- Geriatric patients more carefully; may develop renal, cardiac symptoms more rapidly

Black Box Warning: For exacerbations of hepatitis after discontinuing treatment, monitor LFTs, hepatitis B serology

- Pregnancy: If planned or suspected; if pregnant call the Pregnancy Registry: 800-258-4263

Evaluate:

- Therapeutic response: decreased symptoms of chronic hepatitis B, improving LFTs

Teach patient/family:

- That optimal duration of treatment is unknown; that product is not a cure; that transmission may still occur
- To avoid use with other medications unless approved by prescriber
- To notify prescriber of decreased urinary output
- Not to stop abruptly unless directed; worsening of hepatitis may occur
- To report immediately dyspnea, nausea, vomiting, abdominal pain, weakness, dizziness, cold extremities

• To notify prescriber if pregnancy is planned or suspected; avoid breastfeeding

⚠ HIGH ALERT

adenosine (Rx)

(a-den′oh-seen)

Adenocard

Func. class.: Antidysrhythmic

Chem. class.: Endogenous nucleoside

Do not confuse:
adenosine/adeosine phosphate

ACTION: Slows conduction through AV node, can interrupt reentry pathways through AV node, and can restore normal sinus rhythm in patients with paroxysmal supraventricular tachycardia; decreases cardiac oxygen demand, decreasing hypoxia

USES: PSVT, as a diagnostic aid to assess myocardial perfusion defects in CAD, Wolff-Parkinson-White syndrome
Unlabeled uses: Wide-complex tachycardia diagnosis

CONTRAINDICATIONS: Hypersensitivity, 2nd- or 3rd-degree AV block, sick sinus syndrome, bradycardia
Precautions: Pregnancy (C), breastfeeding, children, geriatric patients, asthma, atrial flutter, atrial fibrillation, ventricular tachycardia, bronchospastic lung disease, symptomatic bradycardia, bundle branch block, heart transplant, unstable angina, COPD, hypotension, hypovolemia, vascular heart disease, CV disease

DOSAGE AND ROUTES

Antidysrhythmic

• **Adult and child >50 kg: IV BOL** 6 mg; if conversion to normal sinus rhythm does not occur within 1-2 min, give 12 mg by rapid **IV BOL;** may repeat 12-mg dose again in 1-2 min

• **Infant and child <50 kg: IV BOL** 0.1 mg/kg; if not effective, increase dose by 0.05-0.1 mg/kg q2min to a max of 0.3 mg/kg/dose

• **Neonate: IV BOL** 0.05 mg/kg by rapid IV BOL, may increase by 0.05 mg/kg q2min, max 0.3 mg/kg/dose

Available forms: 3 mg/ml

Administer:

IV, direct route

• Warm to room temperature; crystals will dissolve
• Undiluted; give 6 mg or less by rapid inj over 1-2 sec; if using an IV line, use port near insertion site, flush with NS (20 ml), then elevate arm
• Store at room temperature; sol should be clear; discard unused product

Y-site compatibilities: abciximab
Solution compatibilities: D_5LR, D_5W, LR, 0.9% NaCl

SIDE EFFECTS

CNS: Lightheadedness, dizziness, arm tingling, numbness, headache
CV: Chest pain, pressure, atrial tachydysrhythmias, sweating, palpitations, hypotension, *facial flushing,* AV block, cardiac arrest, ventricular dysrhythmias, atrial fibrillation
GI: *Nausea,* metallic taste
RESP: *Dyspnea, chest pressure,* hyperventilation, bronchospasm (asthmatics)

PHARMACOKINETICS

Cleared from plasma in <30 sec, half-life 10 sec, converted to inosine/adenosine monophosphate

INTERACTIONS

Increase: risk for higher degree of heart block—carBAMazepine
Increase: risk for ventricular fibrillation—digoxin, verapamil
• Smoking: increase tachycardia
Increase: effects of adenosine—dipyridamole
Decrease: activity of adenosine—theophylline or other methylxanthines (caffeine)

Drug/Herb
Increase: adenosine effect—ginger
Decrease: adenosine effect—guarana, green tea

NURSING CONSIDERATIONS

Assess:

- **Cardiopulmonary status:** B/P, pulse, respiration, rhythm, ECG intervals (PR, QRS, QT); check for transient dysrhythmias (PVCs, PACs, sinus tachycardia, AV block)
- Respiratory status: rate, rhythm, lung fields for crackles; watch for respiratory depression; bilateral crackles may occur in **CHF** patient; increased respiration, increased pulse, product should be discontinued
- CNS effects: dizziness, confusion, psychosis, paresthesias, seizures; product should be discontinued

Evaluate:

- Therapeutic response: normal sinus rhythm or diagnosis of perfusion defect

Teach patient/family:

- To report facial flushing, dizziness, sweating, palpitations, chest pain; usually transient

TREATMENT OF OVERDOSE: Defibrillation, vasopressor for hypotension, theophylline

⚠ HIGH ALERT

ado-trastuzumab

(a′doe-tras-tooz′ue-mab)

Kadcyla

Func. class: Antineoplastic-biologic response modifier

Chem. class: Signal transduction inhibitors (STIs), humanized anti-HER2 antibody

Do not confuse:
ado-trastuzumab/trastuzumab

ACTION: Humanized anti-HER2 monoclonal antibody that is linked to DM1, a small molecule microtubular inhibitor; once the antibody is bound to the HER2 receptor, the complex is internalized and the DM1 is released to bind with tubulin to lead to apoptosis

USES: Breast cancer; metastatic with overexpression of HER2, who previously received trastuzumab and a taxane, separately or in combination

CONTRAINDICATIONS: Hypersensitivity to this product, Chinese hamster ovary cell protein, pregnancy (D)

Precautions: Breastfeeding, children, pulmonary disease, acute bronchospasm, anticoagulant, Asian patients, asthma, COPD, extravasation, fever, hepatitis, human anti-human antibody, hypotension, neuropathy, hepatotoxicity; cardiomyopathy/CHF; interstitial lung disease/pneumonitis; extravasation; thrombocytopenia

DOSAGE AND ROUTES

- **Adult:** IV 3.6 mg/kg over 30-90 min q3wk; give first infusion over 90 min; if tolerated, give over 30 min

Dosage adjustments for toxicities:
Hepatotoxicity:

- AST/ALT >5 to ≤20 × ULN: withhold, resume at a reduced dose when AST/ALT is ≤5 × ULN; first dose reduction: reduce the dose to 3 mg/kg; second dose reduction: reduce the dose to 2.4 mg/kg; requirement for further dose reduction: discontinue
- AST/ ALT >20× ULN: discontinue
- Total bilirubin >3 to ≤10× ULN: withhold, resume treatment at a reduced dose when total bilirubin recovers to ≤1.5; first dose reduction: reduce the dose to 3 mg/kg; second dose reduction: reduce the dose to 2.4 mg/kg; requirement for further dose reduction: discontinue treatment
- Total bilirubin >10× ULN: permanently discontinue; permanently discontinue treatment in patients with AST/ALT >3× ULN and total bilirubin >2× ULN; permanently discontinue treatment in patients diagnosed with nodular regenerative hyperplasia (NRH)
- Left ventricular ejection fraction *(LVEF); LVEF 40%-45% and decrease is <10%*

points from baseline: continue treatment; repeat LVEF assessment within 3 wk; *LVEF 40%-45% and decrease is ≥10% points from baseline:* withhold; repeat LVEF assessment within 3 wk; if LVEF remains ≥10% points from baseline, discontinue; *LVEF <40%:* withhold; repeat LVEF assessment within 3 wk; if LVEF remains <40%, discontinue; *symptomatic congestive heart failure (CHF):* discontinue

Thrombocytopenia:

- Platelet count 25,000/mm^3 to <50,000/mm^3: withhold; resume treatment at same dose when platelet count recovers to ≥75,000/mm^3
- Platelet count <25,000/mm^3: withhold; resume treatment at a reduced dose when platelet count recovers to ≥75,000/mm^3: first dose reduction: reduce the dose to 3 mg/kg; second dose reduction: reduce the dose to 2.4 mg/kg; requirement for further dose reduction: discontinue

Pulmonary toxicity:

- Permanently discontinue in patients diagnosed with interstitial lung disease or pneumonitis

Peripheral neuropathy:

- Withhold in patients experiencing grade 3 or 4 peripheral neuropathy; resume treatment upon resolution to ≤grade 2

Available forms: Lyophilized powder 100, 160 mg

Administer:

IV route

- Visually inspect for particulate matter and discoloration before use
- Give as (IV) infusion with a 0.2 or 0.22 micron in-line filter; do not administer as an IV push or bolus
- Use cytotoxic handling procedures; do not mix with, or administer as an infusion with, other IV products

Reconstitution:

- Slowly inject 5 ml of sterile water for injection into each 100-mg vial, or 8 ml of sterile water for injection into each 160-mg vial to yield a single-use solution of 20 mg/ml
- Direct the stream of sterile water toward the wall of the vial and not directly at the cake or powder
- Gently swirl the vial to aid in dissolution; do not shake
- After reconstitution, withdraw desired amount from the vial and dilute immediately in 250 ml of 0.9% sodium chloride; do not use dextrose 5% solution; gently invert the bag to mix the solution in order to avoid foaming
- The reconstituted single-use product does not contain a preservative; use the diluted solution immediately or store at 2-8° C (36-46° F) for up to 24 hr after reconstitution; discard any unused drug after 24 hr; do not freeze

IV infusion

- Closely monitor for possible subcutaneous infiltration during drug administration
- **First infusion**: give over 90 min; the infusion rate should be slowed or interrupted if the patient develops an infusion-related reaction; patients should be observed for at least 90 min following the initial dose for fever, chills, or other infusion-related reactions; permanently discontinue for life-threatening infusion-related reactions
- **Subsequent infusions**: administer over 30 min if prior infusions were well tolerated; the infusion rate should be slowed or interrupted if the patient develops an infusion-related reaction; patients should be observed for at least 30 min after the infusion; permanently discontinue for life-threatening infusion-related reactions

SIDE EFFECTS

CNS: Dizziness, insomnia, neuropathy, chills, fatigue, fever, flushing, headache, neuropathy

CV: Heart failure, tachycardia

EENT: Blurred vision, conjunctivitis, stomatitis

GI: Diarrhea, nausea, vomiting, abdominal pain, constipation, dyspepsia, hepatotoxicity

HEMA: Anemia, bleeding, thrombocytopenia

INTEG: Rash
MS: Arthralgia
RESP: Cough, dyspnea, **bronchospasm, pneumonitis, interstitial lung disease**
SYST: **Anaphylaxis**
Other: Elevated LFTs, **hand-foot syndrome**

PHARMACOKINETICS

93% protein binding, metabolized in the liver

INTERACTIONS

Increase: bleeding risk—warfarin; avoid use with CYP3A4 inhibitors with strong CYP3A4 inhibitors; platelet inhibitors; anticoagulants

• Do not give with other IV products; do not give with 5% dextrose

NURSING CONSIDERATIONS

Assess:

• Pregnancy test CBC, HER2 overexpression, differential

Black Box Warning: CHF, other cardiac symptoms: dyspnea, coughing; gallop; obtain full cardiac workup including ECG, echo, MUGA, ejection fraction

• Symptoms of infection; may be masked by product

• CNS reaction: LOC, mental status, dizziness, confusion

Black Box Warning: Hypersensitive reactions, anaphylaxis

• **Infusion reactions that may be fatal: fever, chills, nausea, vomiting, pain, headache, dizziness, hypotension; discontinue product**

• **Pulmonary toxicity: dyspnea, interstitial pneumonitis, pulmonary hypertension, ARDs; can occur after infusion reaction; those with lung disease may have more severe toxicity, discontinue**

• **Bleeding: Monitor for bleeding, grade 3 or 4 bleeding with fatalities have occurred, check platelets baseline and before each dose**

Evaluate:

• Therapeutic response: decrease in size of tumors

Black Box Warning: Hepatic disease: may be fatal, monitor LFTs, bilirubin baseline and before each dose

Teach patient/family:

• To take acetaminophen for fever

• To avoid hazardous tasks because confusion, dizziness may occur

• To report signs of infection: sore throat, fever, diarrhea, vomiting; bleeding; decreased heart function/SOB with exertion

• That emotional lability is common; to notify prescriber if severe or incapacitating

Black Box Warning: To use contraception while taking this product and for additional 7 mo after discontinuing this drug; pregnancy (D); not to breastfeed

• To report pain at infusion site

⚠ HIGH ALERT

afatinib

(a-fat′i-nib)

Gilotrif

Func. class.: Antineoplastic biologic response modifiers

Chem. class.: Signal transduction inhibitors (STIs), epidermal growth factor receptor, tyrosine kinase inhibitor

Do not confuse:

Afatinib/afinitor/axitinib

ACTION: Selective inhibitor of EGFR (ErbB1), HER2 (ErbB2), and HER4 (ErbB4); irreversible, covalent binding of intracellular tyrosine kinase inhibiting (and causing regression) tumor growth by decreasing EGFR signal transduction, cell cycle arrest, and inhibition of angiogenesis

USES: Treatment of non-small cell lung cancer whose tumors have epidermal growth factor receptor Exon 19 deletions or 21 substitution mutations

CONTRAINDICATIONS: Pregnancy (D), hypersensitivity

Precautions: Contact lens, dehydration, inflammation, keratitis, ocular disease, pneumonitis, pulmonary disease, renal disease, respiratory distress syndrome, serious rash, skin disease, diarrhea, hepatic disease, ocular disease

DOSAGE AND ROUTES

- **Adult: PO** 40 mg daily

Dose adjustments for toxicities:

- **Hepatotoxicity:** Hold therapy in patients who develop worsening liver function; when toxicity resolves to grade 1 or less, resume therapy at a reduced dose (10 mg/day less than the dose causing hepatotoxicity); permanently discontinue for severe drug-induced hepatic impairment or if hepatotoxicity persists at a dose of 20 mg/day
- **Grade 2 or higher renal toxicity (CCr >1.5 × ULN):** Hold until the toxicity resolves to grade 1 or less (CCr <1.5 × ULN), then resume at a reduced dose (10 mg/day less than the dose causing nephrotoxicity); permanently discontinue if nephrotoxicity persists at a dose of 20 mg/day
- **Grade 2 diarrhea, lasting 2 or more consecutive days while taking antidiarrheal medication, or any grade 3 diarrhea:** Hold until the toxicity resolves to grade 1 or less, then resume therapy at a reduced dose (10 mg/day less than the dose causing toxicity); antidiarrheal therapy should continue until no loose bowel movement for 12 hr; permanently discontinue if toxicity persists at a dose of 20 mg/day
- **Grade 2 cutaneous reactions that last more than 7 days or are intolerable:** Hold until the toxicity resolves to grade 1 or less, then resume at a reduced dose (10 mg/day less than the dose causing toxicity); permanently discontinue for life-threatening bullous, blistering, or exfoliative skin lesions, or if toxicity persists at a dose of 20 mg/day
- **Confirmed interstitial lung disease, persistent ulcerative keratitis, symptomatic left ventricular dysfunction, or any severe/intolerable adverse reaction occurring at a dose of 20 mg/day:** Permanently discontinue
- **Any grade 3 or higher adverse event:** Hold until the toxicity resolves to grade 1 or less, then resume therapy at a reduced dose (10 mg/day less than the dose causing toxicity); permanently discontinue if toxicity persists at a dose of 20 mg/day
- **Permanently discontinue for any severe or intolerable adverse event that occurs at a dose of 20 mg/day.**

Dosage Guidance in Patients on P-glycoprotein (P-gp) inhibitors/inducers:

- P-gp inhibitors: If use of a P-gp inhibitor is required, reduce the initial daily afatinib dosage to 30 mg/day if not tolerated; resume original dose after discontinuation of the P-gp inhibitor as tolerated
- P-gp inducers: If use of a P-gp inducer is required, increase the initial daily afatinib dosage to 50 mg/day as tolerated; resume original dose 2-3 days after discontinuation of the P-gp inducer

Available forms: Tabs 20, 30, 40 mg

Administer:

PO route

- Give on empty stomach 1 hr before, 2 hr after food; give at same time of day
- Do not take a missed dose if within 12 hr of the next dose

SIDE EFFECTS

CNS: Fatigue, fever

CV: Heart failure

EENT: Blurred vision, conjunctivitis

GI: Diarrhea, nausea, vomiting, stomatitis, decreased appetite

HEMA: Anemia, neutropenia, leukopenia, epistaxis

INTEG: Rash, pruritus, acne vulgaris, photosensitivity, nail bed infections

MS: Arthralgia

A

RESP: Cough, dyspnea, acute respiratory distress syndrome, interstitial lung disease, pneumonitis
Other: Elevated LFTs, infection, hand and foot syndrome, dehydration, renal failure, cystitis, hypokalemia

PHARMACOKINETICS
95% protein binding, half-life 37 hr, primarily excreted as unchanged drug in feces; peak 2-5 hr after dose; time to steady-state is approximately 8 days

INTERACTIONS
Increase: afatinib—P-gp inhibitors effect
Drug/Herb
Increase: afatinib concentration—St. John's wort
Drug/Food Test
Increase: afatinib effect—grapefruit juice; avoid use while taking product

NURSING CONSIDERATIONS
Assess:

Black Box Warning: Myelosuppression: anemia, neutropenia; obtain weekly × 1 mo, then monthly as needed; LFTs every mo × 3 mo, then as clinically indicated; hepatic failure may occur

Evaluate: Therapeutic response: decrease in progression of disease
Teach patient/family:
- To report adverse reactions immediately; bleeding
- About reason for treatment, expected results
- To use effective contraception during treatment and up to 30 days after discontinuing treatment
- To treat skin rash with topicals and oral antibiotics; use loperamide for diarrhea; if any side effect is severe or persistent, contact prescriber
- That complicated dosing changes may occur based on toxicity or drug-drug interaction
- To take on empty stomach 1 hr before or 2 hr after meal; not to take missed dose within 12 hr of next scheduled dose

aflibercept
(a-fli-ber′sept)
EYLEA
Func. class.: Biologic response modifier; signal transduction inhibitor (STIs) (Ophthalmic)

ACTION: A recombinant fusion protein consisting of portions of human VEGF receptors 1 and 2 extracellular domains fused to human IgG1; acts as a soluble decoy receptor that binds vascular endothelial growth factor-A (VEGF-A) and placental growth factor (PIGF); can act as mitogenic, chemotactic, vascular permeability factors for endothelial cells; VEGF-A interacts with VEGFR-1 and VEGFR-2 on the surface of endothelial cells; results in neovascularization and vascular permeability; binding of aflibercept to VEGF-A and PIGF prevents activation of these receptors

USES: For treatment of neovascular (wet) age-related macular degeneration (AMD), macular edema after central retinal vein, diabetic retinopathy with diabetic macular edema

CONTRAINDICATIONS: Hypersensitivity, ocular/periocular infection, active intraocular inflammation
Precautions: Neonates, infants, children, adolescents, pregnancy (C), breastfeeding; history of glaucoma, ocular surgery; driving or operating machinery, increased intraocular pressure

DOSAGE AND ROUTES
- **Adult: Intravitreal INJ** 2 mg (0.05 ml) into affected eye(s) q4wk × 12 wk, then 2 mg (0.05 ml) q8wk

Available forms: Solution for injection 2 mg/0.05 ml
Administer:
Intravitreal route
- Visually inspect for particulate matter, discoloration before use; do not use if particulates, cloudiness, discoloration

are visible; only for use by physicians trained in administration

- Use controlled aseptic conditions (sterile gloves, sterile drape, sterile eyelid speculum); adequate anesthesia, topical broad-spectrum antiinfective should be given before use
- Use each vial for treatment of single eye only; if other eye is being treated, use new vial and change the sterile field, syringe, gloves, drapes, eyelid speculum, filter, injection needles before administering to the other eye
- Use aseptic technique: withdraw all of vial contents through a 5-micron 19-G filter needle attached to 1-ml syringe supplied by manufacturer; after vial contents are withdrawn, discard filter needle and replace with sterile 30-G × ½ inch needle for intravitreal injection; expel any air bubbles and contents of syringe until plunger tip is aligned with line that marks 0.05 ml
- Immediately after the intravitreal injection, monitor patient for elevation in intraocular pressure (IOP); appropriate monitoring may consist of a check for perfusion of optic nerve head or tonometry; sterile paracentesis needle should be available if required
- Storage: do not freeze, protect from light, refrigerate, store in original package until time of use

SIDE EFFECTS

CV: Arterial thromboembolism, nonfatal stroke, nonfatal myocardial infarction, vascular death

EENT: *Ocular hemorrhage, ocular pain, cataracts, vitreous detachment, vitreous floaters,* conjunctival hyperemia, corneal erosion, detachment of retinal pigment epithelium, injection site pain, foreign body sensation, increased lacrimation, blurred vision, retinal pigment epithelium tear, injection site hemorrhage, blepharedema, corneal edema, increased intraocular pressure/ocular hypertension

SYST: Hypersensitivity

PHARMACOKINETICS

Absorbed into systemic circulation; present in its unbound form and stable inactive form bound with endogenous VEGF; elimination by binding to free endogenous VEGF; metabolism by proteolysis; terminal half-life in plasma 5-6 days

NURSING CONSIDERATIONS

Assess:

- **Infection:** monitor for infection during week after injection to permit early treatment of any ocular infection that may develop; proper aseptic injection technique should be used to minimize infection
- **Increased intraocular pressure:** monitor for acute increases in intraocular pressure within 60 min of injection; sustained increases in intraocular pressure have been reported after repeated intravitreal dosing; monitor intraocular pressure and optic nerve head perfusion, a sterile paracentesis needle should be available

Evaluate:

- Prevention of further vision loss

Teach patient/family:

⚠ To seek immediate care if symptoms of endophthalmitis or retinal detachment develop (ocular pain, hyperemia of the conjunctiva, photophobia, blurry vision)

albumin, human 5% (Rx)

(al-byoo′min)

Albumarc, Albuminar-5, Albutein 5%, Buminate 5%, Plasbumin-5

albumin, human 25%

Albuminar-25, Albutein 25%, Buminate 25%, Plasbumin-25

Func. class.: Plasma volume expander

ACTION: Exerts oncotic pressure, which expands volume of circulating blood and maintains cardiac output

USES: Restores plasma volume after burns, hyperbilirubinemia, shock, hypoproteinemia, prevention of cerebral edema, cardiopulmonary bypass procedures, ARDS, nephrotic syndrome

CONTRAINDICATIONS:
Hypersensitivity, CHF, severe anemia, renal insufficiency, pulmonary edema

Precautions: Pregnancy (C), decreased salt intake, decreased cardiac reserve, lack of albumin deficiency, renal/hepatic disease, chronic anemia

DOSAGE AND ROUTES

Burns

- **Adult: IV** dose to maintain plasma albumin at 3-4 mg/dl

Hypovolemic Shock

- **Adult: IV** rapidly give 5% sol, when close to normal infusion at ≤2-4 ml/min (25% sol ≤1 ml/min)
- **Child: IV** 0.5-1 g/kg/dose 5% sol, may repeat as needed, max 6 g/kg/day

Nephrotic Syndrome

- **Adult: IV** 100-200 ml of 25% and loop diuretic × 7-10 days

Hypoproteinemia

- **Adult: IV** 25 g, may repeat in 15-30 min, or 50-75 g of 25% albumin infused at ≤2 ml/min
- **Child and infant: IV** 0.5-1 g/kg/dose over 2-4 hr, may repeat q1-2days

Hyperbilirubinemia/erythroblastosis fetalis

- **Child: IV** 1 g/kg 1-2 hr before transfusion

Available forms: Inj (5%) 50 mg/ml, (25%) 250 mg/ml

Administer:

IV route

- Slowly, to prevent fluid overload; dilute with NS for injection or D_5W; 5% is given undiluted; 25% may be given diluted or undiluted; give over 30-60 min, use infusion pump, use large-gauge needle; infusion must be completed within 4 hr
- 5% solution may be used with hypovolemic/intravascular depletion
- 25% solution may be used with sodium/fluid restrictions

Solution compatibilities: LR, NaCl, Ringer's, D_5W, $D_{10}W$, $D_{2 1/2}W$, NaCl 0.9%, dextrose/Ringer's, dextrose/LR

Y-site compatibilities: Diltiazem, LORazepam

SIDE EFFECTS

CNS: Fever, chills, flushing, headache
CV: Fluid overload, hypotension, erratic pulse, tachycardia
GI: Nausea, vomiting, increased salivation
INTEG: Rash, urticaria
RESP: Altered respirations, **pulmonary edema**

PHARMACOKINETICS

In hyponutrition states, metabolized as protein/energy source; terminal half-life 16-24 hr

INTERACTIONS

Drug/Lab Test

Increase: serum albumin

NURSING CONSIDERATIONS

Assess:

- Blood studies Hct, Hgb; if serum protein declines, dyspnea, hypoxemia can result
- Decreased B/P, erratic pulse, respiration
- I&O ratio: urinary output may decrease
- Adequate hydration before, during administration
- Check type of albumin; some stored at room temperature; some need to be refrigerated; use within 4 hr of opening
- ⚠ **Circulatory/pulmonary overload:** CVP, pulmonary wedge pressure distended neck veins indicate circulatory overload; shortness of breath, anxiety, insomnia, expiratory crackles, frothy blood-tinged cough, cyanosis indicate pulmonary overload
- Allergy: fever, rash, itching, chills, flushing, urticaria, nausea, vomiting, hypotension, requires discontinuation of infusion, use of new lot if therapy reinstituted; premedicate with diphenhydrAMINE

Evaluate:

- Therapeutic response: increased B/P, decreased edema, increased serum albumin levels, increased plasma protein

Teach patient/family:

- Reason for product; to report hypersensitivity

albuterol (Rx)

(al-byoo′ter-ole)

Accuneb, Airomir ✱, ProAir HFA, ProAir RespiClick, Proventil, Proventil HFA, ReliOn, Salbutamol ✱, Ventolin HFA, VoSpire ER

Func. class.: Adrenergic β_2-agonist, sympathomimetic, bronchodilator

Do not confuse:
albuterol/atenolol/Albutein
Ventolin/Vantin
Proventil/Prinivil

ACTION: Causes bronchodilation by action on β_2 (pulmonary) receptors by increasing levels of cAMP, which relaxes smooth muscle; produces bronchodilation, CNS, cardiac stimulation as well as increased diuresis and gastric acid secretion; longer acting than isoproterenol

USES: Prevention of exercise-induced asthma, acute bronchospasm, bronchitis, emphysema, bronchiectasis, or other reversible airway obstruction

Unlabeled uses: Hyperkalemia in dialysis patients, COPD, emphysema

CONTRAINDICATIONS: Hypersensitivity to sympathomimetics

Precautions: Pregnancy (C), breastfeeding, cardiac/renal disease, hyperthyroidism, diabetes mellitus, hypertension, prostatic hypertrophy, angle-closure glaucoma, seizures, exercise-induced bronchospasm (aerosol) in children <12 yr, hypoglycemia, tachydysrhythmias, severe cardiac disease, heart block

DOSAGE AND ROUTES

Bronchospasm prophylaxis/treatment

- **Adult and child ≥4 yr: INH** (metered-dose inhaler) 2 puffs (180 mcg) q4-6hr as needed; **INH** (powdered inhaler) (ProAir RespiClick) **>12 yr:** 180 mcg (2 INH) q4-6hr as needed

Other respiratory conditions

- **Adult and child ≥12 yr: INH** (metered-dose inhaler) 1 puff q4-6hr; **PO** 2-4 mg tid-qid, max 32 mg; **NEB/IPPB** 2.5 mg tid-qid
- **Geriatric: PO** 2 mg tid-qid, may increase gradually to 8 mg tid-qid
- **Child 2-12 yr: INH** (metered-dose inhaler) 0.1 mg/kg tid (max 2.5 mg tid-qid); **NEB/IPPB** 0.1-0.15 mg/kg/dose tid-qid or 1.25 mg tid-qid for child 10-15 kg or 2.5 mg tid-qid for child >15 kg

Hyperkalemia (unlabeled)

- **Adult: ORAL INH** (albuterol nebulizer sol) 10-20 mg

Available forms: INH aerosol 108 mcg/actuation; oral syr 2 mg/5 ml; tabs 2, 4 mg; ext rel 4, 8 mg; INH sol 0.63 mg/3 ml, 1.25 mg/3 ml; 0.083%, 0.5%, 0.042%, 0.021%; powder inhaler 90 mcg/actuation

Administer:

- Store in light-resistant container; do not expose to temperatures of more than 86° F (30° C)

PO route

- Do not break, crush, or chew ext rel tabs; give with meals to decrease gastric irritation
- **Oral sol** to children (no alcohol, sugar)

Inhalation route

- For geriatric patients and children, a spacing device is advised
- After shaking metered-dose inhaler, exhale, place mouthpiece in mouth, inhale slowly while depressing inhaler, hold breath, remove, exhale slowly; give INH at least 1 min apart

ProAir Respistick: Instruct patient on inhalation use; before using for the first time, check the dose counter window that the number "200" is in the window. The dose counter will count down each time the mouthpiece cap is opened and closed. The dose counter only displays even numbers; hold the inhaler upright while opening the cap fully; when the cap is opened, a dose will be activated for delivery; make sure a "click" is heard; do not open the cap unless ready to give dose; the patient should breathe out through the mouth and push as much air from the lungs as he/she can; be careful that the patient does not breathe out into the inhaler mouthpiece; put the mouthpiece in the mouth and have patient close lips around it; the patient should breathe in deeply through the mouth, until his/her lungs feel completely full of air; ensure that the vent above the mouthpiece is not blocked by the patient's lips or fingers; hold breath for about 10 sec; remove the inhaler ; check dose counter on the back of the inhaler to make sure the dose was received; close the cap over the mouthpiece after each use of the inhaler; make sure the cap closes firmly into place; to inhale another dose, close the cap and then repeat inhaler steps; do not wash or put any part of the inhaler in water; if the mouthpiece needs cleaning, gently wipe with a dry cloth or tissue; when there are "20" doses left, the counter will change to red; refill

- **NEB/IPPB** diluting 5 mg/ml sol/2.5 ml 0.9% NaCl for INH; other sol do not require dilution; for neb O_2 flow or compressed air 6-10 L/min

SIDE EFFECTS

CNS: *Tremors, anxiety,* insomnia, headache, dizziness, stimulation, *restlessness,* hallucinations, flushing, irritability
CV: Palpitations, tachycardia, angina, hypo/hypertension, dysrhythmias
EENT: Dry nose, irritation of nose and throat
GI: Heartburn, nausea, vomiting
MISC: Flushing, sweating, anorexia, bad taste/smell changes, hypokalemia, metabolic acidosis
MS: Muscle cramps
RESP: Cough, wheezing, dyspnea, paradoxical bronchospasm, dry throat

PHARMACOKINETICS

Extensively metabolized in the liver and tissues, crosses placenta, breast milk, blood-brain barrier
PO: Onset ½ hr, peak 2-3 hr, duration 4-6 hr, half-life 2.7-6 hr, well absorbed
PO-ER: Onset ½ hr; peak 2-3 hr; duration 8-12 hr
INH: Onset 5-15 min, peak 1½-2 hr, duration 2-6 hr, half-life 4 hr

INTERACTIONS

Increase: QTc prolongation—other drugs that increase QT prolongation
Increase: digoxin level—digoxin
Increase: CNS stimulation—CNS stimulants
Increase: ECG changes/hypokalemia—potassium-losing diuretics
Increase: severe hypotension—oxytocics
Increase: toxicity—theophylline
Increase: action of aerosol bronchodilators
Increase: action of albuterol—tricyclics, MAOIs, other adrenergics; do not use together
Increase: CV effects—atomoxetine, selegiline
Decrease: albuterol—other β-blockers
Drug/Herb
Increase: stimulation—caffeine (cola nut, green/black tea, guarana, yerba maté, coffee, chocolate)
Drug/Lab Test
Decrease: potassium

NURSING CONSIDERATIONS

Assess:

- **Respiratory function:** vital capacity, forced expiratory volume, ABGs; lung sounds, heart rate and rhythm, B/P, sputum (baseline and peak); whether patient has not received theophylline therapy before giving dose
- Patient's ability to self-medicate
- For evidence of allergic reactions
- For paradoxical bronchospasm; hold medication, notify prescriber if bronchospasm occurs

Evaluate:

- Therapeutic response: absence of dyspnea, wheezing after 1 hr, improved airway exchange, improved ABGs

Teach patient/family:

- To use exactly as prescribed; to take missed dose when remembered, alter

dosing schedule; not to use OTC medications; that excess stimulation may occur
- About use of inhaler: review package insert with patient; use demonstration; return demonstration; shake, prime before 1st use and when not used for >2 wk; release 4 test sprays into air, away from the face; about when empty and when to renew
- To avoid getting aerosol in eyes (blurring of vision may result) or using near flames or sources of heat
- To wash inhaler in warm water daily and dry; to track number of inhalations used and to discard product when labeled inhalations have been used
- To avoid smoking, smoke-filled rooms, persons with respiratory infections

⚠ That **paradoxical bronchospasm** may occur; to stop product immediately, call prescriber
- To limit caffeine products such as chocolate, coffee, tea, colas

TREATMENT OF OVERDOSE:
Administer β_1-adrenergic blocker, IV fluids

RARELY USED

alemtuzumab
(al′em-tooz′ue-mab)

Lemtrada

Func. class.: Biologic response modifier

USES: Reserved for those with multiple sclerosis with inadequate response to ≥2 drugs because of severe adverse reactions

CONTRAINDICATIONS: HIV

DOSAGE AND ROUTES
- **Adults: IV** 12 mg daily 5 consecutive days (total 60 mg) for a first treatment course; follow 12 months later with 12 mg daily for 3 consecutive days (total 36 mg) for a second treatment course

alendronate (Rx)
(al-en-drone′ate)

Binosto, Fosamax, Fosamax plus D

Func. class.: Bone-resorption inhibitor
Chem. class.: Bisphosphonate

Do not confuse:
Fosamax/Flomax

ACTION: Decreases rate of bone resorption and may directly block dissolution of hydroxyapatite crystals of bone; inhibits osteoclast activity

USES: Treatment and prevention of osteoporosis in postmenopausal women, treatment of osteoporosis in men, Paget's disease, treatment of corticosteroid-induced osteoporosis in postmenopausal women not receiving estrogen and in men who are on continuing corticosteroid treatment with low bone mass

CONTRAINDICATIONS: Hypersensitivity to bisphosphonates, delayed esophageal emptying, inability to sit or stand for 30 min, hypocalcemia

Precautions: Pregnancy (C), breastfeeding, children, CCr <35 ml/min, esophageal disease, ulcers, gastritis, poor dental health, increased esophageal cancer risk

DOSAGE AND ROUTES
Osteoporosis in postmenopausal women
- **Adult and geriatic: PO** 10 mg/day or 70 mg/wk

Paget's disease
- **Adult and geriatric: PO** 40 mg/day × 6 mo, consider retreatment for relapse

Prevention of osteoporosis
- **Adult/postmenopausal female: PO** 5 mg/day or 35 mg/wk

Renal dose
- **Adult: PO** CCr ≤35 ml/min, not recommended

Available forms: Tabs 5, 10, 35, 40, 70 mg; tabs 70 mg with 2800 IU vit D_3, 70 mg with 5600 IU vit D_3; oral sol 70 mg/75 ml, effervescent tab 70 mg

Administer:

- For 6 mo to be effective for Paget's disease
- Store in cool environment, out of direct sunlight
- **Tablet:** take with 8 oz of water 30 min before 1st food, beverage, or medication of the day
- Do not lie down for ≥30 min after dose; do not take at bedtime or before rising
- **Liquid:** use oral syringe or calibrated device; give in AM with ≥2 oz of water ≥30 min before food, beverage, or medication

SIDE EFFECTS

CNS: Headache

GI: Abdominal pain, constipation, nausea, vomiting, esophageal ulceration, acid reflux, dyspepsia, **esophageal perforation**, diarrhea, **esophageal cancer**

META: Hypophosphatemia, hypocalcemia

MS: Bone pain, osteonecrosis of the jaw, bone fractures

SYST: **Angioedema, Stevens-Johnson syndrome, toxic epidermal necrolysis**

PHARMACOKINETICS

Protein binding 78%, rapidly cleared from circulation, taken up mainly by bones, eliminated primarily through kidneys, bound to bone, half-life >10 yr

INTERACTIONS

Increase: GI adverse reactions—NSAIDs, salicylates, H_2 blockers, proton pump inhibitors, gastric mucosal agents

Decrease: absorption—antacids, calcium supplements

Drug/Food

Decrease: absorption when used with caffeine, orange juice, food

Drug/Lab Test

Decrease: calcium, phosphate

NURSING CONSIDERATIONS

Assess:

⚠ **Serious reactions: angioedema, Stevens-Johnson syndrome, toxic epidermal necrolysis, atrial fibrillation**

- Hormonal status in women, before treatment
- **For osteoporosis:** bone density test before and during treatment
- **For Paget's disease:** increased skull size, bone pain, headache; decreased vision, hearing
- Electrolytes; BUN/creatinine; calcium, phosphorous, magnesium, potassium
- **For hypercalcemia:** paresthesia, twitching, laryngospasm; Chvostek's, Trousseau's signs
- Alk phos levels, baseline and periodically, 2× upper limit of normal is indicative of Paget's disease
- Dental status: regular dental exams should be performed; dental extractions (cover with antiinfectives before procedure)

Evaluate:

- Therapeutic response: increased bone mass, absence of fractures

Teach patient/family:

- To remain upright for 30 min after dose to prevent esophageal irritation; if dose is missed, skip dose, do not double doses or take later in day; to take in AM before food, other meds; to take with 6-8 oz of water only (no mineral water)
- To take calcium, vit D if instructed by health care provider
- To perform weight-bearing exercise to increase bone density
- To let health care provider know if pregnant or if pregnancy is planned or if breastfeeding; to inform dentist of the use of this product
- To maintain good oral hygiene

alfuzosin (Rx)

(al-fyoo′zoe-sin)

Uroxatral, Xatral ✤

Func. class.: Urinary tract, antispasmodic, α_1-agonist

Chem. class.: Quinazolone

ACTION: Binds to α_{1A}-adrenoceptor subtype located mainly in the prostate, relaxing smooth muscles

USES: Symptoms of benign prostatic hyperplasia

Unlabeled uses: Erectile dysfunction with sildenafil

CONTRAINDICATIONS: Hypersensitivity, moderate to severe hepatic impairment; not indicated for use in women or children, breastfeeding

Precautions: Pregnancy (B) but not used in females, geriatric patients; CAD, coronary insufficiency, mild hepatic disease, mild/moderate/severe renal disease, history of QT prolongation or coadministration with meds known to prolong QT interval, torsades de pointes, syncope, surgery, prostate cancer, orthostatic hypotension, ocular surgery, dysrhythmias, angina

DOSAGE AND ROUTES

• **Adult: PO EXT REL** 10 mg/day, taken after same meal each day

Available forms: Ext rel tabs 10 mg

Administer:

PO route

• Do not break, crush, chew tabs; give with food; take at same time each day

• Store in tight container in cool environment

SIDE EFFECTS

CNS: *Dizziness, headache,* fatigue, flushing

CV: Postural hypotension (dizziness, lightheadedness, fainting) within a few hours of administration, chest pain, tachycardia, angina

GI: Nausea, abdominal pain, dyspepsia, constipation, diarrhea, liver injury, jaundice

GU: Impotence, priapism

HEMA: Thrombocytopenia

INTEG: Rash, urticaria, angioedema, pruritus, toxic epidermal necrolysis

MISC: Body pain in general, xerostomia, rhinitis

RESP: Upper respiratory infection, pharyngitis, bronchitis, sinusitis

PHARMACOKINETICS

Peak 8 hr, elimination half-life 10 hr, extensively metabolized in liver by CYP3A4 enzyme, excreted via urine (11% unchanged), moderately protein binding (82%-90%)

INTERACTIONS

• Not to be taken with prazosin, terazosin, doxazosin

Increase: QT prolongation (slight)—class IA/III antidysrhythmics

Increase: effects of alfuzosin—alcohol

Increase: effects—CYP3A4 inhibitors (ketoconazole, itraconazole, cimetidine and ritonavir); do not use together

Increase: hypotension—β-blockers, phosphodiesterase type 5 inhibitors, nitrates, antihypertensives

NURSING CONSIDERATIONS

Assess:

• **Prostatic hyperplasia:** change in urinary patterns (hesitancy, dribbling, dysuria, urgency), baseline and throughout treatment

• **Serious skin reactions:** angioedema, **toxic epidermal necrolysis**

Evaluate:

• Therapeutic response: decreased symptoms of benign prostatic hyperplasia

Teach patient/family:

• To take at same time each day with food; to not double doses

• Not to drive or operate machinery for 4 hr after 1st dose or after dosage increase, dizziness may occur

- About orthostatic hypotension; to rise slowly from sitting or lying
- To avoid all OTC products, meds, herbs unless approved by prescriber
- To notify prescriber of fainting, dizziness
- That erectile dysfunction is a side effect and is temporary

aliskiren (Rx)

(a-lis′kir-en)

Rasilez ✱, Tekturna

Func. class.: Antihypertensive

Chem. class.: Direct renin inhibitor

ACTION: Renin inhibitor that acts on the renin-angiotensin system (RAS)

USES: Hypertension, alone or in combination with other antihypertensives

CONTRAINDICATIONS: Hypersensitivity

Black Box Warning: Pregnancy (D)

Precautions: Breastfeeding, children, geriatric patients, angioedema, aortic/renal artery stenosis, cirrhosis, CAD, dialysis, hyper/hypokalemia, hyponatremia, hypotension, hypovolemia, renal/hepatic disease, surgery, diabetes

DOSAGE AND ROUTES

- **Adult: PO** 150 mg/day, may increase to 300 mg/day if needed, max 300 mg/day

Available forms: Tabs 150, 300 mg

Administer:

- May use with other antihypertensives
- Do not use with a high-fat meal
- Daily with a full glass of water, titrate up to achieve correct dose
- Do not discontinue abruptly, correct electrolyte/volume depletion before treatment
- Store in tight container at room temperature

SIDE EFFECTS

CV: Orthostatic hypotension, hypotension

CNS: Headache, dizziness, **seizures**

GI: *Diarrhea*

GU: Renal stones, increased uric acid

INTEG: Rash

META: Hyperkalemia

MISC: Angioedema, cough

PHARMACOKINETICS

Poorly absorbed, bioavailability 2.5%, peak 1-3 hr, steady state 7-8 days, 91% excreted unchanged in the feces, half-life 24 hr

INTERACTIONS

- Do not use with ACE inhibitors, angiotensin II receptor antagonists in diabetes mellitus

Increase: potassium levels—ACE inhibitors, angiotensin II receptor antagonists, potassium supplements, potassium-sparing diuretics

Increase: hypotension—other antihypertensives, diuretics

Increase: aliskiren levels—atorvastatin, itraconazole, ketoconazole, cycloSPORINE; concurrent use is not recommended

Decrease: levels of warfarin

Drug/Food

Decrease: aliskiren effect—high-fat meal, grapefruit

Drug/Lab Test

Increase: uric acid, BUN, serum creatinine, potassium

NURSING CONSIDERATIONS

Assess:

- Renal studies: uric acid, serum creatinine, BUN may be increased; potassium, hyperkalemia may occur

⚠ **Allergic reactions: angioedema** may occur (swelling of face; trouble breathing, swallowing)

- Daily dependent edema in feet, legs; weight, B/P, orthostatic hypotension
- **Diabetes:** identify the use of ACE inhibitors, angiotensin II receptor antagonists if in use, do not use aliskiren

Evaluate:

- Therapeutic response: decrease in B/P

Teach patient/family:

- About the importance of complying with dosage schedule even if feeling better; that if dose is missed, take as soon as possible; that if it is almost time for the next dose, take only that dose; do not double dose

Black Box Warning: To notify if pregnancy is planned or suspected; if pregnant, product will need to be discontinued, pregnancy (D)

- How to take B/P and normal reading for age group
- Not to use OTC products including herbs, supplements unless approved by prescriber
- To report to prescriber immediately: dizziness, faintness, chest pain, palpitations, uneven or rapid heart beat, headache, severe diarrhea, swelling of tongue or lips, trouble breathing, difficulty swallowing, tightening of the throat
- Not to operate machinery or perform hazardous tasks if dizziness occurs
- To rise slowly; to avoid faintness

allopurinol (Rx)

(al-oh-pure′i-nole)

Alloprin ✤, Aloprim, Purinol 1, Zyloprim

Func. class.: Antigout drug, antihyperuricemic

Chem. class.: Xanthine oxidase inhibitor

Do not confuse:
Zyloprim/Zovirax/Zorprin/zolpidem

ACTION: Inhibits the enzyme xanthine oxidase, reducing uric acid synthesis

USES: Chronic gout, hyperuricemia associated with malignancies, recurrent calcium oxalate calculi, uric acid calculi

CONTRAINDICATIONS: Hypersensitivity

Precautions: Pregnancy (C), breastfeeding, children, renal/hepatic disease

DOSAGE AND ROUTES

Increased uric acid levels in malignancies

- **Adult: PO** 600-800 mg/day in divided doses for 2-3 days; start up to 1-2 days before chemotherapy; **IV INFUSION** 200-400 mg/m^2/day, max 600 mg/day 24-48 hr before chemotherapy, may be divided at 6-, 8-, 12-hr intervals
- **Child 6-10 yr: PO** 300 mg/day, adjust dose after 48 hr
- **Child <6 yr: PO** 150 mg/day, adjust dose after 48 hr
- **Child: IV INFUSION** 200 mg/m^2/day, initially as a single dose or divided q6-12hr

Recurrent calculi

- **Adult: PO** 200-300 mg/day in a single dose or divided bid-tid

Uric acid nephropathy prevention

- **Adult and child >10 yr: PO** 600-800 mg/day × 2-3 days

Gout (mild)

- **Adult: PO** 200-300 mg/day, increase weekly based on uric acid levels, max 800 mg/day

Gout (moderate-severe)

- **Adult: PO** 400-600 mg/day in a single dose or divided bid-tid, max 800 mg/day, doses >300 mg should be given in divided doses, may start during an acute attack as long as antiinflammatory drugs are being used

Renal dose

- **Adult: PO/IV** CCr 81-100 ml/min 300 mg/day; CCr 61-80 ml/min 250 mg/day; CCr 41-60 ml/min 200 mg/day; 21-40 ml/min 150 mg/day; CCr 10-20 ml/min 100-200 mg/day; CCr 3-9 ml/min 100 mg/day or 100 mg every other day; CCr <3 ml/min 100 mg q24hr or longer or 100 mg every 3rd day

Available forms: Tabs, scored 100, 300 mg; powder for inj 500 mg/vial

Administer:

PO route

- With meals to prevent GI symptoms; may crush, add to foods or fluids
- Begin 1-2 days before antineoplastic therapy

Intermittent IV INFUSION route

• Reconstitute 30-ml vial with 25 ml of sterile water for inj; dilute to desired concentrations (≤6 mg/ml) with 0.9% NaCl for inj or D_5 for inj; begin infusion within 10 hr

Y-site compatibilities: Acyclovir, aminophylline, amphotericin B lipid complex, anidulafungin, argatroban, atenolol, aztreonam, bivalirudin, bleomycin, bumetanide, buprenorphine, butorphanol, calcium gluconate, CARBOplatin, caspofungin, ceFAZolin, cefoTEtan, cefTAZidime, ceftizoxime, cefTRIAXone, cefuroxime, CISplatin, cyclophosphamide, DACTINomycin, DAUNOrubicin citrate liposome, dexamethasone, dexmedetomidine, DOCEtaxel, DOXOrubicin liposomal, enalaprilat, etoposide, famotidine, fenoldopam, filgrastim, fluconazole, fludarabine, fluorouracil, furosemide, gallium, ganciclovir, gatifloxacin, gemcitabine, gemtuzumab, granisetron hydrochloride, heparin, hydrocortisone phosphate, hydrocortisone succinate, HYDROmorphone, ifosfamide, linezolid injection, LORazepam, mannitol, mesna, methotrexate, metroNIDAZOLE, milrinone, mitoXANtrone, morphine, nesiritide, octreotide, oxytocin, PACLitaxel, pamidronate, pantoprazole, PEMEtrexed, piperacillin, piperacillin-tazobactam, plicamycin, potassium chloride, ranitidine, sodium acetate, sulfamethoxazole-trimethoprim, teniposide, thiotepa, ticarcillin, ticarcillin-clavulanate, tigecycline, tirofiban, vancomycin, vasopressin, vinBLAStine, vinCRIStine, voriconazole, zidovudine, zoledronic acid

SIDE EFFECTS

GI: *Nausea, vomiting, malaise,* cramps, diarrhea
INTEG: Rash
MS: Acute gouty attack

PHARMACOKINETICS

Protein binding <1%, half-life 1-2 hr
PO: Peak 1.5 hr; excreted in feces, urine
IV: Peak up to 30 min

INTERACTIONS

Increase: kidney stone formation—ammonium chloride, vit C, potassium/sodium phosphate
Increase: rash—ampicillin, amoxicillin, avoid concurrent use
Increase: action of oral anticoagulants, oral antidiabetics, theophylline
Increase: hypersensitivity, toxicity—ACE inhibitors, thiazides
Increase: bone marrow depression—antineoplastics (mercaptopurine, azaTHIOprine)
Increase: xanthine nephropathy, calculi—rasburicase

NURSING CONSIDERATIONS

Assess:

• **For gout:** joint pain, swelling; may use with NSAIDs for acute gouty attacks; uric acid levels q2wk; uric acid levels should be ≤6 mg/dl, effect may take several wk
• CBC, AST, BUN, creatinine before starting treatment, periodically
• I&O ratio; increase fluids to 2 L/day to prevent stone formation and toxicity
• For rash, hypersensitivity reactions, discontinue allopurinol

Evaluate:

• Therapeutic response: decreased pain in joints, decreased stone formation in kidneys, decreased uric acid levels

Teach patient/family:

• To take as prescribed; if dose is missed, take as soon as remembered; do not double dose; tabs may be crushed
• To increase fluid intake to 2 L/day
• To report skin rash, stomatitis, malaise, fever, aching; product should be discontinued
• To avoid hazardous activities if drowsiness or dizziness occurs
• To avoid alcohol, caffeine; will increase uric acid levels
• To avoid large doses of vit C; kidney stone formation may occur
• To reduce dairy products, refined sugars, sodium, meat if taking for calcium oxalate stones

almotriptan (Rx)

(al-moh-trip′tan)

Axert

Func. class.: Antimigraine agent, abortive

Chem. class.: $5\text{-}HT_1$-receptor agonist, triptan

Do not confuse:
Axert/Antivert

ACTION: Binds selectively to the vascular $5\text{-}HT_{1B/1D/1F}$-receptors, exerts antimigraine effect

USES: Acute treatment of migraine with or without aura (adult/adolescent/child ≥12 yr)

CONTRAINDICATIONS: Hypersensitivity, acute MI, angina, CV disease, CAD, stroke, vasospastic angina, ischemic heart disease or risk for, peripheral vascular syndrome, uncontrolled hypertension, basilar or hemiplegic migraine

Precautions: Pregnancy (C), postmenopausal women, men >40 yr, breastfeeding, children <18 yr, geriatric patients, risk factors for CAD, MI; hypercholesterolemia, obesity, diabetes, impaired renal/hepatic function, sulfonamide hypersensitivity, cardiac dysrhythmias, Raynaud's disease, tobacco smoking, Wolff-Parkinson-White syndrome

DOSAGE AND ROUTES

- **Adult, adolescent, and child ≥12 yr: PO** 6.25 or 12.5 mg; may repeat dose after 2 hr; max 2 doses/24 hr, 25 mg/day or 4 treatment cycles within any 30-day period

Hepatic/renal dose CCr 10-30 ml/min

- **Adult: PO** 6.25 mg initially, max 12.5 mg

Available forms: Tabs 6.25, 12.5 mg

Administer:

- Avoid using more than 2×/24 hr; rebound headache may occur
- Swallow tabs whole; do not break, crush, chew, without regard to food

SIDE EFFECTS

CNS: *Dizziness,* headache, seizures, paresthesias

CV: *Flushing,* palpitations, tachycardia, coronary artery vasospasm, MI, ventricular fibrillation, ventricular tachycardia

EENT: Throat, mouth, nasal discomfort; vision changes

GI: Nausea, xerostomia

INTEG: Sweating, rash

MS: *Weakness, neck stiffness,* myalgia

RESP: Chest tightness, pressure

PHARMACOKINETICS

Onset of pain relief 2 hr; peak 1-3 hr; duration 3-4 hr; bioavailability 70%; protein binding 35%; metabolized in the liver (metabolite), metabolized by MAO-A, CYP2D6, CYP3A4; excreted in urine (40%), feces (13%); half-life 3-4 hr

INTERACTIONS

Increase: serotonin syndrome—SSRIs, SNRIs, serotonin-receptor agonists, sibutramine

Increase: vasospastic effects—ergot, ergot derivatives, other $5\text{-}HT_1$ agonists; avoid concurrent use

⚠ **Increase:** almotriptan effect—MAOIs, do not use together

Increase: plasma concentration of almotriptan—(CYP3A4 inhibitors) itraconazole, ritonavir, erythromycin, ketoconazole, avoid concurrent use in renal/hepatic disease

Drug/Herb

- Avoid use with feverfew

Increase: serotonin syndrome—St. John's wort

NURSING CONSIDERATIONS

Assess:

- **Migraine:** pain location, aura, duration, intensity, nausea, vomiting
- **Serotonin syndrome:** occurs in those taking SSRIs, SNRIs; agitation, confusion, hallucinations, diaphoresis, hypertension, diarrhea, fever, tremors, usually occurs when dose is increased
- B/P; signs/symptoms of coronary vasospasms

- For stress level, activity, recreation, coping mechanisms
- Neurologic status: LOC, blurring vision, nausea, vomiting, tingling, hot sensation, burning, feeling of pressure, numbness, flushing preceding headache
- **Tyramine foods** (pickled products, beer, wine, aged cheese), food additives, preservatives, colorings, artificial sweeteners, chocolate, caffeine, which may precipitate these types of headaches
- Quiet, calm environment with decreased stimulation from noise, bright light, excessive talking

Evaluate:

- Therapeutic response: decrease in severity of migraine

Teach patient/family:

- To report chest pain, drowsiness, dizziness, tingling, flushing
- To use contraception while taking product, to notify prescriber if pregnancy is planned or suspected, to avoid breastfeeding
- That if one dose does not relieve migraine, to take another after 2 hr, max 4 doses/30 days, do not take MAOIs for ≥ 24 hrs
- That product does not prevent or reduce number of migraine attacks; use to relieve attack only

alogliptin

(al′oh-glip′tin)

Nesina

Func. class.: Antidiabetic

Chem. class.: Dipeptidyl peptidase-4 (DPP-4) inhibitor

ACTION: A dipeptidyl-peptidase-IV (DDP-IV) inhibitor for the treatment of type 2 diabetes mellitus (monotherapy or in combination with other antidiabetic agents), potentiates the effects of the incretin hormones by inhibiting their breakdown by DDP-IV

USES: Type 2 diabetes mellitus (T2DM)

CONTRAINDICATIONS: Hypersensitivity

Precautions: Pregnancy (B), breastfeeding, hepatic disease, burns, ketoacidosis, diarrhea, fever, GI obstruction, hyper/hypoglycemia, hyper/hypothyroidism, type 1 diabetes, hypercortisolism, children, ileus, malnutrition, pancreatitis, surgery, trauma, vomiting, kidney disease, adrenal insufficiency, angioedema

DOSAGE AND ROUTES

- **Adult: PO** 25 mg/day; when used in combination, a lower dose of the other antidiabetic may be needed

Renal dose

- **Adult: PO** CCr 30–59 ml/min: 12.5 mg every day; CCr <30 ml/min: 6.25 mg every day; intermittent hemodialysis: 6.25 mg every day; give without regard to the timing of hemodialysis

Available forms: Tabs 6.25, 12.5, 25 mg

Administer:

- Without regard to food

SIDE EFFECTS

CNS: Headache

GI: Pancreatitis

META: Hypoglycemia

RESP: Upper respiratory infection, nasopharyngitis

SYST: Rash, hypersensitivity, angioedema, Stevens–Johnson syndrome, anaphylaxis

PHARMACOKINETICS

20% protein binding, excreted unchanged (urine), peak 1-2 hr, effect decreased in liver disease and increased in kidney disease, half-life 21 hr

INTERACTIONS

Increase: hypoglycemia-insulin, sulfonylureas

Drug/Lab Test

Increase: LFTs

Decrease: glucose

NURSING CONSIDERATIONS

Assess:

- **Diabetes:** monitor blood glucose, glycosylated hemoglobin A1c (A1c), LFTs, serum creatinine/BUN

⚠ **Pancreatitis:** can occur during use

⚠ **Hypersensitivity reactions:** angioedema, Stevens–Johnson syndrome; product should be discontinued

Evaluate:

- Positive therapeutic response: decrease in polyuria, polydipsia, polyphagia, clear sensorium, absence of dizziness, improvement in A1c, daily blood glucose monitoring

Teach patient/family:

- That diabetes is a life-long condition, product does not cure disease
- That all food in diet plan must be eaten to prevent hypoglycemia; to continue with weight control, dietary medical nutrition therapy, physical activity, hygiene
- To carry emergency ID with prescriber, medications, and condition listed
- To test blood glucose using a blood glucose meter
- To report allergic reactions, nausea, vomiting, abdominal pain, dark urine

alosetron

(ah-loss′a-tron)

Lotronex

Func. class.: Antidiarrheal, anti-IBS agent

Chem. class.: Serotonin receptor antagonist

Do not confuse:

Lotronex/Lovenox

ACTION: A potent and selective antagonist at serotonin 5-HT_3 receptors, which are extensively distributed on enteric neurons in GI tract. Antagonism at these receptors in the GI tract modulates the regulation of visceral pain, colonic transit, and GI secretions

USES: Severe, chronic, diarrhea-predominant irritable bowel syndrome (IBS) in women who have failed conventional therapy

CONTRAINDICATIONS: Crohn's disease, severe hepatic disease, diverticulitis, toxic megacolon, GI adhesions/strictures/obstruction/perforation, thrombophlebitis, ulcerative colitis

Black Box Warning: Ischemic colitis, severe constipation

Precautions: Breastfeeding, pregnancy (B), child <18 yr, mild-moderate hepatic disease

DOSAGE AND ROUTES

- **Adult woman: PO** 0.5 mg bid, may increase to 1 mg bid after 4 wk if well tolerated; if symptoms are not controlled after 4 wk of treatment with 1 mg bid, discontinue

Available forms:

Tab 0.5 mg, 1 mg

Administer:

- Without regard to meals with full glass of water

Black Box Warning: Only after "Physician–Patient Agreement Form" is signed and patient receives official Medication Guide

- Store at room temperature, protect from light and moisture

SIDE EFFECTS

CNS: Fatigue, headache

GI: Constipation, abdominal pain, distention, reflux, nausea, obstruction, impaction, ischemic colitis, ileus perforation, small-bowel mesenteric ischemia

GU: Urinary tract infection

MS: Muscle spasm

RESP: Cough, nasopharyngitis, upper respiratory tract infection

PHARMACOKINETICS

Peak 1 hr, half-life 1½ hr, metabolized extensively in the liver, mainly excreted in urine

INTERACTIONS

- Do not use with fluvoxaMINE

Increase: Alosetron metabolism—CYP3A4, 1A2, 2C9 inducers

Increase: serious adverse reactions, drugs that decrease GI motility—drugs with anticholinergic effect such as TCAs, H1-blockers, orphenadrine, OLANZapine, maprotiline, disopyramide, cyclobenzaprine, cloZAPine, buPROPion, amoxapine, amantadine

Decrease: Alosetron metabolism—CYP3A4, 1A2, 2C9 inhibitors, hydrALAZINE, procainamide

Drug/Lab Test

Increase: ALT

NURSING CONSIDERATIONS

Assess:

Black Box Warning: Irritable bowel syndrome—constipation, diarrhea, abdominal pain, fecal incontinence; discontinue immediately if bloody diarrhea, severe constipation, rectal bleeding, or severe abdominal pain occur

Black Box Warning: Only clinicians enrolled in the Prometheus Prescribing Program for Lotronex should use this product

- Geriatric female patients can experience more severe side effects

Evaluate:

- Therapeutic response: decreasing symptoms of IBS

Teach patient/family:

Black Box Warning: Immediately report severe constipation, bloody diarrhea, rectal bleeding, or worsening abdominal pain

- Not to double doses; if a dose is missed skip it; do not take with other meds or herbs without prescriber approval
- That product may be taken without regard to food
- That product does not cure disorder, only controls symptoms
- Provide medication guide and clarify, if needed, that improvement in symptoms can take 1-4 wk
- That product is only used for women with IBS
- To report if pregnancy is planned or suspected; product should not be used during pregnancy, effects are unknown

ALPRAZolam (Rx)

(al-pray′zoe-lam)

Apo-Alpraz ✦, Niravam, Novo-Alprazol ✦, Nu-Alpraz ✦, Xanax, Xanax XR

Func. class.: Antianxiety

Chem. class.: Benzodiazepine (short/intermediate acting)

Controlled Substance Schedule IV

Do not confuse:

ALPRAZolam/LORazepam

Xanax/Lanoxin/Tylox/Zantac

ACTION: Depresses subcortical levels of CNS, including limbic system, reticular formation

USES: Anxiety, panic disorders with or without agoraphobia, anxiety with depressive symptoms

Unlabeled uses: Premenstrual dysphoric disorders, insomnia, PMS, alcohol withdrawal syndrome

CONTRAINDICATIONS: Pregnancy (D), breastfeeding, hypersensitivity to benzodiazepines, closed-angle glaucoma, psychosis, addiction

Precautions: Geriatric patients, debilitated patients, hepatic disease, obesity, severe pulmonary disease

DOSAGE AND ROUTES

Anxiety disorder

- **Adult: PO** 0.25-0.5 mg tid, may increase q3-4days if needed, max 4 mg/day in divided doses
- **Geriatric: PO** 0.25 mg bid; increase by 0.125 mg as needed

Panic disorder

• **Adult: PO** 0.5 mg tid, may increase up to 1 mg/day q3-4days, max 10 mg/day; **EXT REL** (Xanax XR) give daily in AM, 0.5-1 mg initially, maintenance 3-6 mg/day, max 10 mg/day

Hepatic dose

• Reduce dose by 50%-60%

Premenstrual dysphoric disorders/ PMS (unlabeled)

• **Adult: PO** 0.25 mg bid-tid starting on day 16-18 of menses, taper over 2-3 days when menses occurs, max 4 mg/day

Available forms: Tabs 0.25, 0.5, 1, 2 mg; ext rel tabs (Xanax XR) 0.5, 1, 2, 3 mg; orally disintegrating tabs 0.25, 0.5, 1, 2 mg; oral sol 1 mg/ml

Administer:

• Tabs may be crushed, mixed with food, fluids if patient is unable to swallow medication whole; do not break, crush, chew ext rel (XR), give ext rel tab in AM

• With food or milk for GI symptoms; high-fat meal will decrease absorption

• To discontinue, decrease by 0.5 mg q3days

• May divide total daily doses into more times/day if anxiety occurs between doses

• **Orally disintegrating tabs** on tongue to dissolve and swallow, protect from moisture

SIDE EFFECTS

CNS: *Dizziness, drowsiness,* confusion, headache, anxiety, tremors, stimulation, fatigue, depression, insomnia, hallucinations, memory impairment, poor coordination, suicide

CV: *Orthostatic hypotension,* ECG changes, tachycardia, hypotension

EENT: *Blurred vision,* tinnitus, mydriasis

GI: Constipation, dry mouth, nausea, vomiting, anorexia, diarrhea, weight gain/loss, increased appetite, ileus perforation, ischemic colitis

GU: Decreased libido

INTEG: Rash, dermatitis, itching, angioedema

PHARMACOKINETICS

PO: Well absorbed; widely distributed; onset 30 min; peak 1-2 hr; duration 4-6 hr; *oral disintegrating tab* peak 1.5-2 hr; therapeutic response 2-3 days; metabolized by liver (CYP3A4), excreted by kidneys; crosses placenta, breast milk; half-life 12-15 hr, protein binding 80%

INTERACTIONS

Increase: ALPRAZolam action—CYP3A4 inhibitors (cimetidine, disulfiram, erythromycin, FLUoxetine, isoniazid, itraconazole, ketoconazole, metoprolol, propranolol, valproic acid)

Increase: CNS depression—anticonvulsants, alcohol, antihistamines, sedative/hypnotics, opioids

Decrease: sedation—xanthines

Decrease: ALPRAZolam action—CYP3A4 inducers (barbiturates, rifampin)

Decrease: action of levodopa

Decrease: product level—cigarette smoking

Drug/Herb

Increase: CNS depression—kava, melatonin, St. John's wort, valerian

Drug/Food

Increase: product level—grapefruit juice, avoid concurrent use

Drug/Lab Test

Increase: AST/ALT, alk phos

NURSING CONSIDERATIONS

Assess:

• Mental status: anxiety, mood, sensorium, orientation, affect, sleeping pattern, drowsiness, dizziness, especially in geriatric patients both before and during treatment, suicidal thoughts, behaviors

• B/P lying, standing; pulse; if systolic B/P drops 20 mm Hg, hold product, notify prescriber

• Hepatic, blood studies: AST, ALT, bilirubin, creatinine, LDH, alk phos, CBC; may cause neutropenia, decreased Hct, increased LFTs

⚠ **Physical dependency, withdrawal symptoms:** anxiety, panic attacks, agitation, seizures, headache, nausea, vomiting, muscle pain, weakness; withdrawal seizures may occur after rapid decrease in dose or abrupt discontinuation; because duration of action is short, considered to be the product of choice for geriatric patients

• Pregnancy: if planned or suspected, pregnancy (D), to avoid breastfeeding

Evaluate:

• Therapeutic response: decreased anxiety, restlessness, sleeplessness

Teach patient/family:

• Not to double doses; take exactly as prescribed; if dose is missed, take within 1 hr as scheduled; that product may be taken with food

• Not to use for everyday stress or for more than 4 mo unless directed by prescriber; not to take more than prescribed amount; that product may be habit forming; that memory impairment is a result of long-term use

• To avoid OTC preparations unless approved by prescriber

• Not to use during pregnancy (D), to avoid breastfeeding

• Not to discontinue medication abruptly after long-term use

• To avoid driving, activities that require alertness because drowsiness may occur

• To avoid alcohol, other psychotropic medications unless directed by prescriber

• To rise slowly or fainting may occur, especially among geriatric patients

• That drowsiness may worsen at beginning of treatment

TREATMENT OF OVERDOSE:
Lavage, VS, supportive care, flumazenil

RARELY USED

alprostadil (Rx)

(al-pros′ta-dil)

Caverject, Caverject Impulse, Edex, Muse, Prostin VR Pediatric

Func. class.: Hormone

USES: To maintain patent ductus arteriosus (temporary treatment), erectile dysfunction

CONTRAINDICATIONS: Hypersensitivity, respiratory distress syndrome, those at risk for priapism

DOSAGE AND ROUTES

Patent ductus arteriosus

• **Infant: IV INFUSION** 0.05-0.1 mcg/kg/min until desired response, then reduce to lowest effective amount, max 0.4 mcg/kg/min

Erectile dysfunction of vasculogenic or mixed etiology, psychogenic

• **Men: INTRACAVERNOSAL** 2.5 mcg, may increase by 2.5 mcg, may then increase by 5-10 mcg until adequate response occurs (max 60 mcg/dose); **INTRAURETHRAL** 125-250 mcg, max 2 doses/24 hr, max dose 1000 mcg; administer as needed to achieve erection

⚠ HIGH ALERT

alteplase (Rx)

(al-ti-plaze′)

Activase, Cathflo

Func. class.: Thrombolytic enzyme

Chem. class.: Tissue plasminogen activator (TPA)

Do not confuse:

alteplase/Altace

Activase/Cathflo Activase

ACTION: Produces fibrin conversion of plasminogen to plasmin; able to bind to fibrin, convert plasminogen in thrombus to plasmin, which leads to local fibrinolysis, limited systemic proteolysis

USES: Lysis of obstructing thrombi associated with acute MI, ischemic conditions that require thrombolysis (i.e., PE, unclotting arteriovenous shunts, acute ischemic CVA), central venous catheter occlusion (Cathflo)

Unlabeled uses: Arterial thromboembolism, deep vein thrombosis (DVT), occlusion prophylaxis, percutaneous coronary intervention (PCI)

CONTRAINDICATIONS: Active internal bleeding, history of CVA, severe uncontrolled hypertension, intracranial/

intraspinal surgery/trauma (within 3 mo), aneurysm, brain tumor, platelets <100,000 mm^3, bleeding diathesis including INR >1.7 or PR >15 sec, arteriovenous malformation, subarachnoid hemorrhage, intracranial hemorrhage, uncontrolled hypertension, seizure at onset of stroke

Precautions: Pregnancy (C), breastfeeding, children, geriatric patients, neurologic deficits, mitral stenosis, recent GI/GU bleeding, diabetic retinopathy, subacute bacterial endocarditis, arrhythmias, diabetic hemorrhage retinopathy, CVA, recent major surgery, hypertension, acute pericarditis, hemostatic defects, significant hepatic disease, septic thrombophlebitis, occluded AV cannula at seriously infected site

DOSAGE AND ROUTES

MI (standard infusion) (Activase)

• **Adult >65 kg:** 100 mg total given over 3 hr as follows: 6- to 10-mg IV BOL over 1-2 min; remaining 50-54 mg given over the remainder of the hr; during 2nd, 3rd hr 20 mg given by **CONT IV INFUSION** (20 mg/hr)

• **Adult <65 kg:** 1.25 mg/kg over 3 hr: 60% during 1st hr (6%-10% as bolus); remaining 50% given over remainder of hr; during 2nd hr, 20% of dose given by CONT IV INFUSION; 20% given during 3rd hr by CONT IV INFUSION

MI (accelerated infusion) (Activase)

• **Adult >67 kg:** 100 mg total dose: give 15-mg IV bolus, then 50 mg over 30 min, then 35 mg over 60 min

• **Adult <67 kg:** 15-mg IV bolus, then 0.75 mg/kg (max 50 mg) over 30 min, then 0.5 mg/kg (max 35 mg) over next 60 min

Pulmonary embolism (Activase)

• **Adult: IV** 100 mg over 2 hr, then heparin

Acute ischemic stroke (Activase)

• **Adult: IV** 0.9 mg/kg, max 90 mg; give as **INFUSION** over 1 hr, give 10% of dose **IV BOL** over 1st min

Occluded venous access devices (Cathflo Activase)

• **Adult/child ≥30 kg: IV** 2 mg/2 ml instilled in occluded catheter, may repeat if needed after 2 hr

• **Child 10-29 kg: IV** 110% of lumen volume, max 2 mg/2 ml instilled in occluded catheter, may repeat if needed after 2 hr

Deep venous thrombosis (DVT) (Activase) (unlabeled)

• **Adult: IV** 4 mcg/kg/min as 2-hr infusion, then 1 mcg/kg/min × 33 hr

Percutaneous coronary intervention (PCI) (unlabeled)

• **Adult: INTRACARDIAC** 20 mg over 5 min, then 50 mg over the next 60 min

Occlusion prophylaxis (unlabeled) (Cathflo Activase)

• **Adult >30 kg:** Do not exceed 2 mg in 2 ml; may use up to 2 doses 120 min apart

Complicated pleural effusions (unlabeled)

• **Adult:** Intrapleural 10 mg in 30 ml NS bid in well time of 1 hr × 3 days, then after ≥2 hr intrapleural dornase alfa

Available forms: Powder for inj 50 mg (29 million international units/vial), 100 mg (58 million international units/vial); Cathflo Activase: lyophilized powder for inj 2 mg

Administer: (Activase)

Intermittent IV INFUSION route

• After reconstituting with provided diluent, add appropriate amount of sterile water for inj (no preservatives) 20-mg vial/20 ml or 50-mg vial/50 ml to make 1 mg/ml, mix by slow inversion or dilute with NaCl, D_5W to a concentration of 0.5 mg/ml; 1.5 to <0.5 mg/ml may result in precipitation of product; use 18G needle; flush line with NaCl after administration, give over 3 hr for MI, 2 hr for PE

• Heparin therapy after thrombolytic therapy is discontinued, TT, ACT, or APTT less than 2× control (about 3-4 hr); treatment can be initiated before coagulation study results obtained, infusion should be discontinued if pretreatment INR >1.7, PT >15 sec, or elevated APTT is identified

• Use reconstituted IV solution within 8 hr or discard

• Avoid invasive procedures, inj, rectal temperature

- Pressure for 30 sec to minor bleeding sites; 30 min to sites of atrial puncture followed by pressure dressing; inform prescriber if this does not attain hemostasis; apply pressure dressing
- Store powder at room temperature or refrigerate; protect from excessive light

Y-site compatibilities: Eptifibatide, lidocaine, metoprolol, propranolol

- **Cathflo Activase:** Use this product after other options used for declotting a line; reconstitute by using 2.2 ml of sterile water provided and injecting in vial, direct flow into powder (1 mg/ml), foam will disappear after standing; swirl, do not shake, sol will be pale yellow or clear, use within 8 hr, instill 2 ml of reconstituted sol into occluded catheter, try to aspirate after ½ hr; if unable to remove, allow 2 hr, a 2nd dose may be used; aspirate 5 ml of blood to remove clot and product, irrigate with normal saline

SIDE EFFECTS

CV: Sinus bradycardia, cholesterol microembolization, ventricular tachycardia, accelerated idioventricular rhythm, bradycardia, recurrent ischemic stroke, hypotension

EENT: Orolingual angioedema

INTEG: Urticaria, rash

SYST: GI, GU, intracranial, retroperitoneal bleeding, *surface bleeding,* anaphylaxis, fever

PHARMACOKINETICS

Cleared by liver, 80% cleared within 10 min of product termination, onset immediate, half-life 35 min

INTERACTIONS

Increase: bleeding—anticoagulants, salicylates, dipyridamole, other NSAIDs, abciximab, eptifibatide, tirofiban, clopidogrel, ticlopidine, some cephalosporins, plicamycin, valproic acid

Increase: orolingual angioedema—ACE inhibitors

Decrease: effect—nitroglycerin

Drug/Herb

Increase: risk for bleeding—feverfew, garlic, ginger, ginkgo, ginseng, green tea

Drug/Lab Test

Increase: PT, APTT, TT

NURSING CONSIDERATIONS

Assess:

- Treatment is not recommended for patients with acute ischemic stroke >3 hr after symptom onset or with minor neurologic deficits or rapidly improving symptoms
- VS, B/P, pulse, respirations, neurologic signs, temperature at least q4hr; temperature >104° F (40° C) indicates internal bleeding; monitor rhythm closely; ventricular dysrhythmias may occur with hyperfusion; monitor heart, breath sounds, neurologic status, peripheral pulses; assess neurologic status, neurologic change may indicate intracranial bleeding; those with severe neurologic deficit (NIH SS >22) at presentation have increased risk of hemorrhage

⚠ **For bleeding** during 1st hour of treatment and 24 hr after procedure: hematuria, hematemesis, bleeding from mucous membranes, epistaxis, ecchymosis; guaiac all body fluids, stools; do not use 150 mg or more total dose because intracranial bleeding may occur; do not use in severe uncontrolled hypertension, aneurysm, head trauma, for MI, pulmonary embolism

⚠ **Hypersensitivity:** fever, rash, itching, chills, facial swelling, dyspnea, notify prescriber immediately; stop product, keep resuscitative equipment nearby; mild reaction may be treated with antihistamines

- Previous allergic reactions or streptococcal infection; alteplase may be less effective
- Blood studies (Hct, platelets, PTT, PT, TT, APTT) before starting therapy; PT or APTT must be less than 2× control before starting therapy TT or PT q3-4hr during treatment
- **MI:** ECG continuously, cardiac enzymes, radionuclide myocardial scanning/coronary angiography; chest pain intensity, character; monitor those with major early infarct

signs on CT scan with substantial edema, mass effect, midline shift

• **PE:** pulse, B/P, ABGs, rate/rhythm of respirations

• **Occlusion:** have patient exhale then hold breath when connecting/disconnecting syringe to prevent air embolism

• **Cholesterol embolism:** purple toe syndrome, acute renal failure, gangrenous digits, hypertension, livedo reticularis, pancreatitis, MI, cerebral infarction, spinal cord infarction, retinal artery occlusion, bowel infarction, rhabdomyolysis

Evaluate:

• Therapeutic response: lysis of thrombi

Teach patient/family:

• The purpose and expected results of the treatment; to report adverse reactions, bleeding

aluminum hydroxide (OTC)

Func. class.: Antacid, hypophosphatemic
Chem. class.: Aluminum product, phosphate binder

ACTION: Neutralizes gastric acidity; binds phosphates in GI tract; these phosphates are then excreted

USES: Antacid, hyperphosphatemia in chronic renal failure; adjunct in gastric, peptic, duodenal ulcers; hyperacidity, reflux esophagitis, heartburn, stress ulcer prevention in critically ill, GERD

Unlabeled uses: GI bleeding

CONTRAINDICATIONS: Hypersensitivity to product or aluminum products

Precautions: Pregnancy (C), breastfeeding, geriatric patients, fluid restriction, decreased GI motility, GI obstruction, dehydration, renal disease, sodium-restricted diets, GI bleeding, hypokalemia

DOSAGE AND ROUTES

Antacid

• **Adult: PO** 500-1500 mg 3-6× daily, max 6 doses/day

Hyperphosphatemia

• **Adult: PO** 300-600 mg tid

• **Child: PO** 50-150 mg/kg/day in 4-6 divided doses

Available forms: Susp 320 mg/5 ml, 600 mg/5 ml

Administer:

• 2 tsp (10 ml) will neutralize 20 mEq of acid

PO route

• **Hyperphosphatemia:** give with 8 oz water, meals unless contraindicated

• Laxatives or stool softeners if constipation occurs, especially for geriatric patients

• After shaking susp

NG route: By nasogastric tube if patient unable to swallow

SIDE EFFECTS

GI: *Constipation,* anorexia, obstruction, fecal impaction

META: *Hypophosphatemia,* hypercalciuria, hypomagnesemia, aluminum toxicity

PHARMACOKINETICS

PO: Onset 20-40 min, duration 1-3 hr, excreted in feces

INTERACTIONS

Decrease: effectiveness of—allopurinol, amprenavir, cephalosporins, corticosteroids, delavirdine, digoxin, gabapentin, gatifloxacin, H_2-antagonists, iron salts, isoniazid, ketoconazole, penicillamine, phenothiazines, phenytoin, quiNIDine, quinolones, tetracyclines, thyroid hormones, ticlopidine, anticholinergics; separate by at least 4-6 hr

Drug/Food

Decrease: product effect—high-protein meal

Drug/Lab Test

Decrease: phosphate interference: Tc-99m

NURSING CONSIDERATIONS

Assess:

• **Pain:** location, intensity, duration, character, aggravating, alleviating factors

• Phosphate, calcium levels because product is bound in GI system

• **Hypophosphatemia:** anorexia, weakness, fatigue, bone pain, hyporeflexia

- Constipation; increase bulk in diet if needed, may use stool softeners or laxatives; record amount and consistency of stools
- **Aluminum toxicity:** severe renal disease, may also be used for hyperphosphatemia

Evaluate:

- Therapeutic response: absence of pain, decreased acidity, healed ulcers, decreased phosphate levels

Teach patient/family:

- Not to use for prolonged periods for patients with low serum phosphate or patients on low-sodium diets; to shake liquid well
- That stools may appear white or speckled
- To check with prescriber after 2 wk of self-prescribed antacid use
- To separate from other medications by 2 hr
- **Hyperphosphatemia:** to avoid phosphate foods (most dairy products, eggs, fruits, carbonated beverages) during product therapy
- To notify prescriber of black tarry stools, which may indicate bleeding

alvimopan

(al-vim′oh-pan)

Entereg

Func. class.: Functional GI disorder agent

Chem. class.: Peripheral mu-opioid receptor antagonist

ACTION: A peripherally selective mu-opioid receptor antagonist with activity restricted to the GI tract

USES: Prevention of postoperative ileus

Unlabeled uses: Opiate-agonist–induced constipation

CONTRAINDICATIONS: Those who have taken therapeutic doses of opioids for more than 7 consecutive days immediately before starting alvimopan, end-stage renal disease, Child-Pugh C

Precautions: Risk for MI, surgery for complete GI obstruction, hepatic disease, renal disease, pregnancy B, breastfeeding

DOSAGE AND ROUTES

- **Adult/geriatric patient: PO** 12 mg 30 min-5 hr before surgery, then 12 mg bid beginning the day after surgery; max 7 days or hospital discharge; max 15 doses

Opiate agonist–induced constipation (unlabeled)

- **Adult: PO** 0.5 mg or 1 mg every day

Renal/hepatic dosage

- **Adult: PO** Do not use in end-stage renal disease or Child-Pugh Class C

Available forms: Cap 12 mg

Administer:

- Without regard to food

Black Box Warning: Only in a hospital setting approved for the ENTEREG Access Support and Education (E.A.S.E.) program, MI

- Store at room temperature

SIDE EFFECTS

GI: *Constipation, dyspepsia,* flatulence, diarrhea, abdominal pain, cramping

HEMA: *Anemia*

META: Hypokalemia

MISC: Back pain, urinary retention, MI

PHARMACOKINETICS

Half-life 10-17 hr, extended in hepatic/renal disease, protein binding 80%-94%

INTERACTIONS

Increase: Alvimopan concentrations, toxicity—amiodarone, bepridil, cycloSPORINE, diltiazem, itraconazole, quiNIDine, quiNINE, spironolactone, verapamil

Black Box Warning: Do not use if opiate agonists have been used for 7 consecutive days before alvimopan

Black Box Warning: Do not use concurrently with other opiate antagonists

NURSING CONSIDERATIONS

Assess:

- Blood studies: Hgb/Hct, potassium; hyperkalemia occurs
- Recent opioid use, do not use within 7 consecutive days

Black Box Warning: Opioid use for chronic pain; MI is more common in this population

Evaluate:

- Therapeutic response: absence of postoperative ileus

Teach patient/family:

- To notify prescriber if pregnancy is planned or suspected, avoid breastfeeding
- That product is only used for a limited time in a hospital setting
- To report constipation, abdominal pain, cramping

amantadine (Rx)

(a-man′ta-deen)

Func. class.: Antiviral, antiparkinsonian agent

Chem. class.: Tricyclic amine

Do not confuse:

amantadine/ranitidine/rimantidine

ACTION: Prevents uncoating of nucleic acid in viral cell, thereby preventing penetration of virus to host; causes release of DOPamine from neurons

USES: Prophylaxis or treatment of influenza type A, EPS, parkinsonism, Parkinson's disease

Unlabeled uses: Neuroleptic malignant syndrome, MS-associated fatigue

CONTRAINDICATIONS: Hypersensitivity, breastfeeding, children <1, eczematic rash

Precautions: Pregnancy (C), geriatric patients, epilepsy, CHF, orthostatic hypotension, psychiatric disorders, renal/hepatic disease, peripheral edema, CV disease

DOSAGE AND ROUTES

Influenza type A

- **Adult and child >9 yr: PO** 200 mg/day in single dose or divided bid
- **Geriatric: PO** No more than 100 mg/day
- **Child 1-8 yr: PO** 4.4-8.8 mg/kg/day divided bid-tid, max 150 mg/day

Drug induced EPS

- **Adult: PO** 100 mg bid, up to 300 mg/day in divided doses
- **Adult: PO** 100 mg bid up to 400 mg/day in divided doses in EPS

Renal dose

- **Adult: PO** CCr 30-50 ml/min 200 mg 1st day then 100 mg/day; CCr 15-29 ml/min 100 mg 1st day, then 100 mg on alternate days; CCr 15 ml/min reduce dose and interval to 200 mg q7days

MS-associated fatigue (unlabeled)

- **Adult: PO** 200 mg/day or 100 mg bid

Neuroleptic malignant syndrome (unlabeled)

- **Adult: PO** 100 mg bid × 3 wk

Available forms: Caps 100 mg; oral sol 50 mg/5 ml; tab 100 mg

Administer:

- **Prophylaxis:** before exposure to influenza; continue for 10 days after contact; **treatment:** initiate within 24-48 hr of onset of symptoms, continue for 24-48 hr after symptoms disappear
- After meals for better absorption to decrease GI symptoms; at least 4 hr before bedtime to prevent insomnia
- In divided doses to prevent CNS disturbances: headache, dizziness, fatigue, drowsiness
- Store in tight, dry container

SIDE EFFECTS

CNS: *Headache, dizziness*, drowsiness, fatigue, *anxiety*, psychosis, *depression, hallucinations*, tremors, seizures, confusion, *insomnia*

CV: *Orthostatic hypotension*, CHF

EENT: Blurred vision

GI: *Nausea, vomiting,* constipation, dry mouth, anorexia

GU: *Frequency, retention*

HEMA: Leukopenia, agranulocytosis

INTEG: Photosensitivity, dermatitis, livedo reticularis

PHARMACOKINETICS

PO: Onset 48 hr, peak 1-4 hr, half-life 24 hr, not metabolized, excreted in urine (90%) unchanged, crosses placenta, excreted in breast milk

INTERACTIONS

Increase: anticholinergic response—atropine, other anticholinergics
Increase: CNS stimulation—CNS stimulants
Decrease: amantadine effect—metoclopramide, phenothiazines
Decrease: renal excretion of amantadine—triamterene, hydrochlorothiazide
Decrease: effect—S/B H1N1 influenza A virus vaccine; avoid use 2 wk before or 48 hr after amantadine

Drug/Lab Test
Increase: BUN, creatinine, alk phos, CK, LDH, bilirubin, AST, ALT, GGT

NURSING CONSIDERATIONS

Assess:
- Mental status: may cause increased psychiatric disorders especially in the elderly
- **CHF** (weight gain, jugular venous distention, dyspnea, crackles)
- Skin eruptions, photosensitivity after administration of product
- Serum creatinine, BUN in renal impairment
- Reaction to each medication
- Signs of infection
- **Livedo reticularis:** mottling of the skin, usually red; edema; itching in lower extremities, usually in Parkinson's disease
- **Parkinson's disease:** gait, tremors, akinesia, rigidity, may be effective if anticholinergics have not been effective

⚠ **Toxicity:** confusion, behavioral changes, hypotension, seizures

Evaluate:
- Therapeutic response: absence of fever, malaise, cough, dyspnea with infection; tremors, shuffling gait with Parkinson's disease

Teach patient/family:
- To change body position slowly to prevent orthostatic hypotension
- About aspects of product therapy: to report dyspnea, weight gain, dizziness, poor concentration, dysuria, complex sleep behaviors
- To avoid hazardous activities if dizziness, blurred vision occurs
- To take product exactly as prescribed; parkinsonian crisis may occur if product is discontinued abruptly; not to double dose; if a dose is missed, not to take within 4 hr of next dose; caps may be opened and mixed with food
- To avoid alcohol

TREATMENT OF OVERDOSE:

Withdraw product, maintain airway, administer EPINEPHrine, aminophylline, O_2, IV corticosteroids, physostigmine

ambrisentan (Rx)

(am-bri-sen′tan)

Letairis, Volibris ✤

Func. class.: Antihypertensive
Chem class.: Vasodilator/endothelin receptor antagonist

ACTION: Endothelin-A receptor antagonist; endothelin-A is a vasoconstrictor

USES: Pulmonary arterial hypertension, alone or in combination with other antihypertensives in WHO class II (significant exertion), III (mild exertion)

CONTRAINDICATIONS: Breastfeeding, hypersensitivity, idiopathic pulmonary fibrosis (IPF)

Black Box Warning: Pregnancy (X)

Precautions: Children, females, geriatric patients, hepatitis, anemia, heart failure, jaundice, peripheral edema, hepatic disease, pulmonary disease

DOSAGE AND ROUTES

- **Adult: PO** 5 mg/day; may increase to 10 mg/day if needed

Hepatic dose
- **Adult: PO** Discontinue if AST/ALT >5× ULN, or if elevations are accompanied by

bilirubin >2× ULN, or other signs of liver dysfunction

Available forms: Tabs 5, 10 mg

Administer:

- Do not break, crush, chew tabs
- Daily with a full glass of water without regard to food
- Do not discontinue abruptly
- Only those facilities enrolled in the LEAP program (866-664-5327) may administer this product
- Store in tight container at room temperature

SIDE EFFECTS

CNS: *Headache,* fever, flushing, fatigue
CV: Orthostatic hypotension, hypotension, *peripheral edema,* palpitations
EENT: Sinusitis, rhinitis
GI: Abdominal pain, constipation, anorexia, hepatotoxicity
GU: Decreased sperm counts
HEMA: *Anemia*
INTEG: Rash, angioedema
RESP: Pharyngitis, dyspnea, pulmonary edema, veno-occlusive disease (VOD)

PHARMACOKINETICS

Rapidly absorbed, peak 2 hr, protein binding 99%, metabolized by CYP3A4, CYP2C19, UGTa, terminal half-life 15 hr, effective half-life 9 hr

INTERACTIONS

- Possibly increase ambrisentan: cimetidine, clopidogrel, efavirenz, felbamate, FLUoxetine, modafinil, OXcarbazepine, ticlopidine

Increase: hypotension—other antihypertensives, diuretics, MAOIs

Increase: ambrisentan—CYP3A4 inhibitors (amprenavir, aprepitant, atazanavir, clarithromycin, conivaptan, cycloSPORINE, dalfopristin, danazol, darunavir, erythromycin, estradiol, imatinib, itraconazole, ketoconazole, nefazodone, nelfinavir, quinupristin, ritonavir, RU-486, saquinavir, tamoxifen, telithromycin, troleandomycin, zafirlukast); CYP2C19/CYP3A4 (chloramphenicol, delavirdine, fluconazole, fluvoxaMINE, isoniazid, voriconazole)

Decrease: ambrisentan—CYP3A4 inducers (carBAMazepine, PHENobarbital, phenytoin, rifampin)

Decrease: ambrisentan absorption—mefloquine, niCARdipine, propafenone, quiNIDine, ranolazine, tacrolimus, testosterone

Drug/Herb

- Need for ambrisentan dosage change: St. John's wort, ephedra (ma huang)

Drug/Food

- Avoid use with grapefruit products

Drug/Lab Test

Increase: LFTs, bilirubin
Decrease: Hct, Hgb

NURSING CONSIDERATIONS

Assess:

- **Pulmonary status:** improvement in breathing, ability to exercise; pulmonary edema that may indicate veno-occlusive disease
- Blood studies: CBC with differential; Hct, Hgb may be decreased
- Liver function tests: AST, ALT, bilirubin

Black Box Warning: Assess pregnancy status before giving this product and monthly; pregnancy (X)

- Hepatotoxicity: nausea, vomiting, abdominal pain/cramping, jaundice, anorexia, itching

Evaluate:

- Therapeutic response: decrease in B/P; decreased shortness of breath; importance of follow up with labs

Teach patient/family:

- The importance of complying with dosage schedule even if feeling better

Black Box Warning: To notify if pregnancy is planned or suspected (if pregnant, product will need to be discontinued, pregnancy test done monthly); to use 2 contraception methods while taking this product

- Not to use OTC products including herbs, supplements unless approved by prescriber

• To report to prescriber immediately: dizziness, faintness, chest pain, palpitations, uneven or rapid heart rate, headache, edema, weight gain
• To report hepatic dysfunction: nausea/vomiting, anorexia, fatigue, jaundice, right upper quadrant abdominal pain, itching, fever, malaise

amikacin (Rx)

(am-i-kay′sin)
Func. class.: Antiinfective
Chem. class.: Aminoglycoside

Do not confuse:
Amikacin/anakinra

ACTION: Interferes with protein synthesis in bacterial cells by binding to ribosomal subunits, which causes misreading of genetic code; inaccurate peptide sequence forms in protein chain, thereby causing bacterial death

USES: Severe systemic infections of CNS, respiratory tract, GI tract, urinary tract, bone, skin, soft tissues caused by *Staphylococcus aureus* (MSSA), *Pseudomonas aeruginosa, Escherichia coli, Enterobacter, Acinetobacter, Providencia, Citrobacter, Serratia, Proteus, Klebsiella pneumoniae*
Unlabeled uses: *Mycobacterium avium* complex (MAC) (intrathecal or intraventricular) in combination; actinomycotic mycetoma, febrile neutropenia, cystic fibrosis

CONTRAINDICATIONS: Pregnancy (D), hypersensitivity to aminoglycosides, sulfites
Precautions: Breastfeeding, neonates, geriatric patients, myasthenia gravis, Parkinson's disease, mild to moderate infections, dehydration

Black Box Warning: Hearing impairment, renal/neuromuscular disease

DOSAGE AND ROUTES

Severe systemic infections
• **Adult and child: IV INFUSION** 15 mg/kg/day in 2-3 divided doses q8-12hr in 100-200 ml D_5W over 30-60 min, max 1.5 g/day; **pulse dosing** (once-daily dosing) may be used with some infections; **IM** 10-15 mg/kg/day in divided doses q8-12hr; or extended-interval dosing as an alternative dosing regimen
• **Neonate: IV/IM** 10 mg/kg initially, then 7.5 mg/kg q8-12hr

Severe urinary tract infections
• **Adult: IM** 10-15 mg/kg/day divided q8-12hr

Hemodialysis
• **Adult: IM/IV** 7.5 mg/kg followed by 5 mg/kg 3×/wk after each dialysis session (for TIW dialysis)

Renal dose (extended interval dosing)
• **Adult: IV** CCr 40-59 ml/min 15 mg/kg q36hr; CCr 20-39 ml/min 15 mg/kg q48hr; <20 ml/min adjust based on serum concentrations and MIC (use traditional dosing)

Traditional dosing
• Decrease dose and maintain interval or maintain dose and decrease interval

***Mycobacterium avium* complex (MAC) (unlabeled)**
• **Adult and adolescent: IM/IV** 15-20 mg/kg/day or 5× per wk
• **Child: IV** 15-30 mg/kg/day divided q12-24hr as part of multiple-drug regimen, max 1.5 g/day

Actinomycotic mycetoma (unlabeled)
• **Adult: IM/IV** 15 mg/kg/day in 2 divided doses × 3 wk with co-trimoxazole for 5 wk; repeat cycle once, may be repeated 2×

Available forms: Inj 50, 250 mg/ml

Administer:
• Obtain C&S before administration; begin treatment before results

IM route
• Inj in large muscle mass; rotate inj sites
• Obtain peak 1 hr after IM, trough before next dose

Intermittent IV INFUSION route
• Dilute 500 mg of product/100-200 ml of D_5W, 0.9% NaCl and give over ½-1 hr; dilute in sufficient volume to allow for

infusion over 1-2 hr (infants); flush after administration with D_5W or 0.9% NaCl; sol clear or pale yellow; discard if precipitate or dark color develops
• In children, amount of fluid will depend on ordered dose; in infants, infuse over 1-2 hr
• In evenly spaced doses to maintain blood level, separate from penicillins by at least 1 hr

Y-site compatibilities: Acyclovir, alatrafloxacin, aldesleukin, alemtuzumab, alfentanil, amifostine, aminophylline, amiodarone, amsacrine, anidulafungin, argatroban, ascorbic acid, atracurium, atropine, aztreonam, benztropine, bivalirudin, bumetanide, buprenorphine, butorphanol, calcium chloride/gluconate, CARBOplatin, caspofungin, ceFAZolin, cefepime, cefonicid, cefotaxime, cefoTEtan, cefOXitin, cefTAZidime, ceftizoxime, cefTRIAXone, cefuroxime, chloramphenicol, chlorproMAZINE, cimetidine, cisatracurium, CISplatin, clindamycin, codeine, cyanocobalamin, cyclophosphamide, cycloSPORINE, cytarabine, DACTINomycin, DAPTOmycin, dexamethasone, dexmedetomidine, digoxin, diltiazem, diphenhydrAMINE, DOBUTamine, DOCEtaxel, DOPamine, doripenem, doxacurium, DOXOrubicin, doxycycline, eftifibatide, enalaprilat, ePHEDrine, EPINEPHrine, epirubicin, epoetin alfa, ertapenem, erythromycin, esmolol, etoposide, famotidine, fentaNYL, filgrastim, fluconazole, fludarabine, fluorouracil, foscarnet, furosemide, gemcitabine, gentamicin, glycopyrrolate, granisetron, hydrocortisone, HYDROmorphone, IDArubicin, ifosfamide, IL-2, imipenem/cilastin, isoproterenol, ketorolac, labetalol, levofloxacin, lidocaine, linezolid, LORazepam, magnesium sulfate, mannitol, mechlorethamine, melphalan, meperidine, metaraminol, methotrexate, methoxamine, methyldopate, methylPREDNISolone, metoclopramide, metoprolol, metroNIDAZOLE, midazolam, milrinone, mitoXANtrone, morphine, multivitamins, nafcillin, nalbuphine, naloxone, niCARdipine, nitroglycerin, nitroprusside, norepinephrine, octreotide, ondansetron, oxaliplatin, oxytocin, PACLitaxel, palonosetron, pantoprazole, papaverine, PEMEtrexed, penicillin G, pentazocine, perphenazine, PHENobarbital, phenylephrine, phytonadione, piperacillin/tazobactam, potassium chloride, procainamide, prochlorperazine, promethazine, propranolol, protamine, pyridoxime, quinupristin/dalfopristin, rantidine, remifentanil, riTUXimab, rocuromium, sargramostim, sodium acetate, sodium bicarbonate, succinylcholine, SUFentanil, tacrolimus, teniposide, theophylline, thiamine, thiotepa, ticarcillin/clavulanate, tigecycline, tirofiban, tobramycin, tolazoline, trimethaphan, urokinase, vancomycin, vasopressin, vecuronium, verapamil, vinCRIStine, vinorelbine, voriconazole, warfarin, zidovudine, zoledronic acid

SIDE EFFECTS

CNS: Confusion, depression, numbness, tremors, **seizures**, muscle twitching, **neurotoxicity**, dizziness, vertigo, tinnitus, **neuromuscular blockade with respiratory paralysis**
CV: Hypo/hypertension
EENT: *Ototoxicity,* deafness
GI: *Nausea, vomiting, anorexia;* bilirubin
GU: **Oliguria, hematuria, renal damage, azotemia, renal failure, nephrotoxicity**
HEMA: **Eosinophilia, anemia**
INTEG: *Rash,* burning, urticaria, dermatitis, alopecia

PHARMACOKINETICS

IM: Onset rapid, peak 1 hr, leads to unpredictable concentrations, IV preferred
IV: Onset immediate, peak 15-30 min, half-life 2 hr, prolonged up to 7 hr in infants; not metabolized; excreted unchanged in urine; crosses placenta; removed by hemodialysis

INTERACTIONS

Increase: masking ototoxicity: dimenhyDRINATE, ethacrynic acid
Increase: serum trough and peak—NSAIDs

Black Box Warning: Increase: nephrotoxicity—cephalosporins, acyclovir, vancomycin, amphotericin B, cycloSPORINE, loop diuretics, cidofovir

Black Box Warning: Increase: Ototoxicito-IV loop diuretics

Increase: neuromuscular blockade, respiratory depression—anesthetics, nondepolarizing neuromuscular blockers
Decrease: amikacin effect—parenteral penicillins, do not combine

Drug/Lab Test

Increase: BUN, creatinine, urea levels (urine)

NURSING CONSIDERATIONS

Assess:

- Weight before treatment; calculation of dosage is usually based on ideal body weight but may be calculated on actual body weight, in those underweight and not obese, use total body weight (TBW) instead of ideal body weight
- I&O ratio; urinalysis daily for proteinuria, cells, casts; report sudden change in urine output
- VS during infusion; watch for hypotension, change in pulse
- IV site for thrombophlebitis including pain, redness, swelling q30min; change site if needed; apply warm compresses to discontinued site

Black Box Warning: Renal impairment; obtain urine for CCr, BUN, serum creatinine; lower dosage should be given with renal impairment; nephrotoxicity may be reversible if product stopped at 1st sign

Black Box Warning: Deafness: audiometric testing, ringing, roaring in ears, vertigo; assess hearing before, during, after treatment

- Dehydration: high specific gravity, decrease in skin turgor, dry mucous membranes, dark urine
- Overgrowth of infection: increased temperature, malaise, redness, pain, swelling, perineal itching, diarrhea, stomatitis, change in cough, sputum
- Vestibular dysfunction: nausea, vomiting, dizziness, headache; product should be discontinued if severe

Black Box Warning: Neuromuscular blockade; respiratory paralysis may occur

- Provide adequate fluids of 2-3 L/day, unless contraindicated, to prevent irritation of tubules

Evaluate:

- Therapeutic response: absence of fever, draining wounds, negative C&S after treatment

Teach patient/family:

- To report headache, dizziness, symptoms of overgrowth of infection, renal impairment, symptoms of neurotoxicity, hepatotoxicity

⚠ To report loss of hearing; ringing, roaring in ears; feeling of fullness in head

- To report hypersensitivity: rash, itching, trouble breathing, facial edema; notify health care provider

TREATMENT OF HYPERSENSITIVITY: Hemodialysis, exchange transfusion in the newborn, monitor serum levels of product, may give ticarcillin or carbenicillin

aMILoride (Rx)

(a-mill′oh-ride)

Apo-Amilzide ♣, Midamor, Moduret ♣, Novamilor ♣, Nu-Amilzide ♣

Func. class.: Potassium-sparing diuretic
Chem. class.: Pyrazine

Do not confuse:
aMILoride/amLODIPine/amiodarone

ACTION: Inhibits sodium, potassium ion exchange in the distal tubule, cortical collecting duct resulting in inhibition of sodium reabsorption and decreasing potassium secretion

USES: Edema in CHF in combination with other diuretics, for hypertension, adjunct with other diuretics to maintain potassium

Unlabeled uses: Ascites

CONTRAINDICATIONS: Anuria, hypersensitivity, diabetic nephropathy, renal failure

Black Box Warning: Hyperkalemia

Precautions: Pregnancy (B), breastfeeding, children, geriatric patients, dehydration, diabetes, respiratory acidosis, hyponatremia, impaired renal function

DOSAGE AND ROUTES

- **Adult: PO** 5-10 mg/day in 1-2 divided doses; may be increased to 10-20 mg/day if needed
- **Infant/child (6-20 kg): PO** 0.625 mg/kg/day

Renal dose

- **Adult: PO** CCr 10-50 ml/min reduce dose by 50%; however, avoid if possible; CCr <10 ml/min contraindicated

Ascites (unlabeled)

- **Adult: PO** 10 mg/day, max 40 mg

Available forms: Tabs 5 mg

Administer:

- In AM to avoid interference with sleep if using as diuretic; if 2nd daily dose is needed, give in late afternoon
- With food; if nausea occurs, absorption may be decreased slightly

SIDE EFFECTS

CNS: *Headache,* dizziness, fatigue, weakness, paresthesias, tremors, depression, anxiety, encephalopathy

CV: *Orthostatic hypotension,* dysrhythmias, chest pain

EENT: Blurred vision, increased intraocular pressure

ELECT: Hyperkalemia, dehydration, hyponatremia, hypochloremia

GI: *Nausea, diarrhea,* dry mouth, *vomiting, anorexia,* cramps, constipation, abdominal pain, jaundice

GU: *Polyuria,* dysuria, urinary frequency, impotence

HEMA: Aplastic anemia, neutropenia

INTEG: *Rash, pruritus,* alopecia, urticaria

MS: Cramps

RESP: *Cough, dyspnea,* shortness of breath

PHARMACOKINETICS

50% absorbed from GI tract; widely distributed; onset 2 hr; peak 6-10 hr; duration 24 hr; excreted in urine, feces; half-life 6-9 hr

INTERACTIONS

Black Box Warning: Hyperkalemia: other potassium-sparing diuretics, potassium products, ACE inhibitors, salt substitutes, cycloSPORINE, tacrolimus; avoid concurrent use, if using together monitor potassium level

Increase: lithium toxicity: lithium, monitor lithium levels

Increase: action of antihypertensives

Decrease: effect of aMILoride—NSAIDs, avoid concurrent use

Drug/Herb

Increase: effect—hawthorn, horse chestnut

Drug/Food

- Possible hyperkalemia: foods high in potassium, potassium-based salt substitutes

Drug/Lab Test

Increase: LFTs, BUN, potassium, sodium

Interference: GTT

NURSING CONSIDERATIONS

Assess:

- Heart rate, B/P lying, standing; postural hypotension may occur
- Electrolytes: potassium, sodium, chloride; glucose (serum), BUN, CBC, serum creatinine, blood pH, ABGs, periodic ECG

A

Black Box Warning: Discontinue potassium-sparing diuretics 3 days before GTT, hyperkalemia may occur

• **Hypokalemia:** weakness, polyuria, polydipsia, fatigue, ECG U wave

Black Box Warning: Hyperkalemia: fatigue, weakness, paresthesia, confusion, dyspnea, dysrhythmias, ECG changes

Evaluate:
• Therapeutic response: improvement in edema of feet, legs, sacral area daily if medication is being used for CHF; decreased B/P; prevention of hypokalemia (diuretics)

Teach patient/family:
• To take as prescribed; if dose is missed, to take when remembered within 1 hr of next dose; to take with food or milk for GI symptoms; to take early in day to prevent nocturia; to avoid alcohol
• About adverse reactions: muscle cramps, weakness, nausea, dizziness, blurred vision
• To avoid potassium-rich foods: oranges, bananas, salt substitutes, dried fruits, potassium supplements
• To rise slowly from sitting to standing to avoid orthostatic hypotension
• To avoid hazardous activities if dizziness occurs

TREATMENT OF OVERDOSE:
Lavage if taken orally, monitor electrolytes, administer sodium bicarbonate for potassium >6.5 mEq/L, IV glucose, kayoxalate as needed; monitor hydration, CV, renal status

amino acids
(a-mee′noe)

amino acid infusions (crystalline)
Aminosyn, Aminosyn II, Aminosyn-PF, Clinisol, FreAmine III, Premasol, Travasol, TrophAmine

amino acid infusions/ dextrose
Aminosyn II with dextrose, Clinimix, Amino Acid Infusions/ electrolytes

aminosyn with electrolytes
Aminosyn II with electrolytes, FreAmine III with electrolytes, ProcalAmine with electrolytes, Travasol with electrolytes

amino acid infusions/ electrolytes/dextrose
Aminosyn II with electrolytes in dextrose

amino acid infusions (hepatic failure)
HepatAmine, Hepatasol

amino acid infusions (high metabolic stress)
Aminosyn-HBC, FreAmine HBC

amino acid infusions (renal failure)
Aminosyn-RF, NephrAmine

Func. class.: Nutritional supplement/ protein
Chem. class.: n/a

ACTION: Needed for anabolism to maintain structure, decrease catabolism, promote healing

Black Box Warning: Central infusions: Administration by central venous catheter should be used only by those familiar with this technique and its complications

USES:
Hepatic encephalopathy, cirrhosis, hepatitis, nutritional support in cancer; burn or solid organ transplant patients; to prevent nitrogen loss when adequate nutrition by mouth, gastric, or duodenal tube cannot be obtained

CONTRAINDICATIONS:
Hypersensitivity, severe electrolyte imbalances, anuria, severe liver damage, maple syrup urine disease, PKU, azotemia, genetic disease of amino acid metabolism

Precautions: Pregnancy (C), breastfeeding, children, renal disease, diabetes mellitus, CHF, sulfite sensitivity

DOSAGE AND ROUTES

Nutritional support (cirrhosis, hepatic encephalopathy, hepatitis)

- **Adult: IV** 80-120 g/day amino acids/12-18 g nitrogen of hepatic failure formula

TPN

- **Adult: IV** 1-1.5 g/kg/day

Metabolic stress (severe)

- **Adult: IV** 1.5 g/kg, use formula for high metabolic stress

Renal failure (nutritional support)

- **Adult: IV** Minosyn-RF 300-600 ml/70% dextrose/day; NephrAmine 250-500 ml/70% dextrose/day; the total daily dosage is calculated based on the daily protein requirements, as well as the patient's metabolic and clinical response. Check product instructions for specific directions
- **Child: IV** 2-3 g/kg/day
- The dosage and constant infusion rate of IV dextrose must be selected with caution in children, particularly neonates and low birth weight infants, because of the increased risk of hyper/hypoglycemia. Owing to their concentration, these solutions are not recommended for use in children younger than 1 year
- The total daily dosage is calculated based on the daily protein requirements, as well as the patient's metabolic and clinical response. Check each product's instructions for specific directions

Available forms:

Injection: 250, 500, 1000, 2000 ml, containing amino acids in various concentrations; amino acid infusions, crystalline: Aminosyn: 3.5%, 5%, 7%, 8.5%, 10%; Aminosyn II: 3.5%, 5%, 7%, 8.5%, 10%, 15%; Aminosyn-PF: 7%, 10%; Clinisol: 15%; FreAmine III: 8.5%, 10%; Premasol: 6%, 10%; Travasol: 10%; TrophAmine: 6%, 10%

Amino acid infusion/dextrose:
Aminosyn II: 3.5% in 5% dextrose, 4.25% in 20% dextrose, 4.25% in 10% dextrose, 4.25% in 25% dextrose; Clinimix: 2.75% in 5% dextrose, 4.25% in 5% dextrose, 4.25% in 10% dextrose, 4.25% in 20% dextrose, 4.25% in 25% dextrose, 5% in 10% dextrose, 5% in 15% dextrose, 5% in 20% dextrose, 5% in 25% dextrose, 5 amino acid infusions/electrolytes: Aminosyn: 3.5%, 7%, 8.5%; Aminosyn II: 3.5%, 7%, 8.5%; FreAmine III: 3%, 8.5%; ProcalAmine: 3%; Travasol: 3.5%, 5.5%, 8.5%

Amino acid infusions/electrolytes/dextrose:
Aminosyn II: 3.5% with electrolytes in 5% dextrose, 3.5% with electrolytes in 25% dextrose, 4.25% with electrolytes in 10% dextrose, 4.25% with electrolytes in 20% dextrose, 4.25% with electrolytes in 25% dextrose; Amino acid infusions (hepatic failure): HepatAmine: 8%; Hepatasol: 8%

Amino acid infusions (high metabolic stress):
Aminosyn-HBC 7%; Freamine HBC: 6.9%; Amino acid (renal failure): Aminosyn-RF:5.2%; NephrAmine: 5.4%

Administer:

Continuous IV INFUSION route

- Up to 40% protein and dextrose (up to 12.5%) via peripheral vein; stronger sol requires central IV administration
- TPN only mixed with dextrose to promote protein synthesis
- Immediately after mixing under strict aseptic technique, use infusion pump, in-line filter (0.22 μm) unless mixed with fat emulsion and dextrose (3 in 1); using careful monitoring technique; do

not speed up infusion; pulmonary edema, glucose overload will result

SIDE EFFECTS

CNS: Dizziness, headache, confusion, loss of concentration, fever

CV: Hypertension, **CHF/pulmonary edema**, flushing, **thrombosis**

ENDO: Hyperglycemia, rebound hypoglycemia, electrolyte imbalances, hyperosmolar hyperglycemic nonketotic syndrome, alkalosis, hypophosphatemia, hyperammonemia, dehydration, hypocalcemia

GI: Nausea, abdominal pain, cholestasis

GU: Glycosuria osmotic diuresis

INTEG: **Extravasation necrosis, phlebitis at inj site**

INTERACTIONS

Individual Drugs

Decrease: Protein-sparing effects—tetracycline

Drug/Lab Test

Increase: LFTs, ammonia glucose

Decrease: Potassium, phosphate, glucose

NURSING CONSIDERATIONS

Assess:

- Electrolytes (potassium, sodium, phosphate, chloride, magnesium, bicarbonate, blood glucose, ammonia, ketones)
- Renal/hepatic studies: BUN, creatinine, ALT, AST, bilirubin
- Weight changes, triglycerides before and after infusion; vit A level with renal disease
- **Inj site for extravasation: redness along vein, edema at site, necrosis, pain, hard tender area; site should be changed immediately**
- Discontinue infusion, culture tubing and sol
- **Sepsis: chills, fever, increased temperature, if sepsis is suspected**
- **For impending hepatic coma: asterixis, confusion, uremic fetor, lethargy**
- **Hyperammonemia: nausea, vomiting, malaise, tremors, anorexia, seizures**
- Change of dressing and IV tubing to prevent infection every 24-48 hr if chills, fever, other signs of infection occur

Evaluate:

- Therapeutic response: weight gain, decrease in jaundice with liver disorders, increased LOC

Teach patient/family:

- Reason for use of TPN
- **If chills, sweating are experienced to report at once, risk for infection is higher**
- About infusion pump, how to care for tubing/site; and blood glucose

⚠ *HIGH ALERT*

amiodarone (Rx)

(a-mee-oh′da-rone)

Cordarone, Nexterone, Pacerone

Func. class.: Antidysrhythmic (class III)

Chem. class.: Iodinated benzofuran derivative

Do not confuse:

amiodarone/Inamrinone

Cordarone/Inocor

ACTION: Prolongs duration of action potential and effective refractory period, noncompetitive α- and β-adrenergic inhibition; increases PR and QT intervals, decreases sinus rate, decreases peripheral vascular resistance

USES: Hemodynamically unstable ventricular tachycardia, supraventricular tachycardia, ventricular fibrillation not controlled by 1st-line agents

Unlabeled uses: Atrial fibrillation treatment/prophylaxis, atrial flutter, cardiac arrest, cardiac surgery, CPR, heart failure, PSVT, Wolff-Parkinson-White (WPW) syndrome, supraventricular tachycardia

CONTRAINDICATIONS: Pregnancy (D), breastfeeding, neonates, infants, severe sinus node dysfunction, hypersensitivity to this product/iodine/benzyl alcohol, cardiogenic shock

Black Box Warning: 2nd- to 3rd-degree AV block, bradycardia

Precautions: Children, goiter, Hashimoto's thyroiditis, electrolyte imbalances, CHF, respiratory disease, torsades de pointes

Black Box Warning: Severe hepatic disease, cardiac arrhythmias, pneumonitis, pulmonary fibrosis

DOSAGE AND ROUTES

Ventricular dysrhythmias

- **Adult: PO** Loading dose 800-1600 mg/day for 1-3 wk, then 600-800 mg/day for 1 mo, maintenance 400 mg/day; **IV** loading dose (1st rapid) 150 mg over the first 10 min, then slow 360 mg over the next 6 hr, maintenance 540 mg given over the remaining 18 hr, decrease rate of the slow infusion to 0.5 mg/min

Supraventricular dysrhythmias (atrial fibrillation, atrial flutter, PSVT, WPW syndrome) (unlabeled)

- **Adult: PO** 1.2-1.8 g/day divided until a total of 10 g has been given, then 200-400 mg/day (class IIa recommendation); **IV** 5-7 mg/kg over 30-60 min, then 1.2-1.8 g as **CONT IV INFUSION** or in divided PO dose's until 10 g, then 200-400 mg/day (class IIa recommendation)
- **Child and infant: PO** 10-20 mg/kg/day in divided doses for 7-10 days, then 5-10 mg/kg/day once daily

Available forms: Tabs 100, 200, 400 mg; inj 50 mg/ml

Administer:

PO route

- May be used with/without food but be consistent

IV, direct route

- **Peripheral:** max 2 mg/ml for more than 1 hr; preferred through central venous line with in-line filter; concentrations of more than 2 mg/ml should be given by central line
- **Cardiac arrest:** give 300 mg IV bol; diluted to a total volume of 20 ml D_5W; may repeat 150 mg after 3-5 min

Intermittent IV INFUSION route

- **Rapid loading:** add 3 ml (150 mg), 100 ml D_5W (1.5 mg/ml), give over 10 min
- **Slow loading:** add 18 ml (900 mg), 500 ml D_5W (1.8 mg/ml), give over next 6 hr

Continuous IV INFUSION route

- After 24 hr, dilute 50 ml to 1-6 mg/ml, give 1-6 mg/ml at 1 mg/min for the 1st 6 hr, then 0.5 mg/min

Y-site compatibilities: Amikacin, clindamycin, DOBUTamine, DOPamine, doxycycline, erythromycin, esmolol, gentamicin, insulin, isoproterenol, labetalol, lidocaine, metaraminol, metroNIDAZOLE, midazolam, morphine, nitroglycerin, norepinephrine, penicillin G potassium, phenylephrine, potassium chloride, procainamide, tobramycin, vancomycin

Solution compatibility: D_5W, 0.9% NaCl

SIDE EFFECTS

CNS: *Headache, dizziness,* involuntary movement, *tremors, peripheral neuropathy,* malaise, *fatigue,* ataxia, *paresthesias,* insomnia

CV: *Hypotension, bradycardia,* sinus arrest, CHF, dysrhythmias, SA node dysfunction, AV block, increased defibrillation energy requirement

EENT: Blurred vision, halos, photophobia, *corneal microdeposits,* dry eyes

ENDO: *Hypo*/hyperthyroidism

GI: *Nausea, vomiting,* diarrhea, abdominal pain, *anorexia, constipation,* hepatotoxicity

GU: Epididymitis, ED

INTEG: Rash, photosensitivity, blue-gray skin discoloration, alopecia, spontaneous ecchymosis, toxic epidermal necrolysis, urticaria, pancreatitis, phlebitis (IV)

MISC: Flushing, abnormal taste or smell, edema, abnormal salivation, coagulation abnormalities

MS: Weakness, pain in extremities

RESP: Pulmonary fibrosis/toxicity, pulmonary inflammation, ARDS; gasping syndrome if used with neonates

PHARMACOKINETICS

PO: Onset 1-3 wk, peak 3-7 hr, half-life 26-107 days, increased in geriatric patients, metabolized by liver (an inhibitor of CYP1A2, CYP3A4, CYP2C8, CYP2C9, CYP2C19, CYP2A6, CYP2B6, CYP2D6, P-glycoprotein), organic cation transporter, excreted by kidneys, 99% protein binding

A

INTERACTIONS

Increase: QT prolongation—azoles, fluoroquinolones, macrolides

Increase: amiodarone concentrations, possible serious dysrhythmias-protease inhibitors, reduce dose

Increase: myopathy—HMG-CoA reductase inhibitors

Increase: bradycardia—β-blockers, calcium channel blockers

Increase: levels of cycloSPORINE, dextromethorphan, digoxin, disopyramide, flecainide, methotrexate, phenytoin, procainamide, quiNIDine, theophylline, class I antidysrhythmics

Increase: anticoagulant effects—dabigatran, warfarin

Drug/Food

- Toxicity: grapefruit juice

Drug/Lab Test

Increase: T_4, ALT, AST, GGT alk phos, cholesterol, lipids, PT, INR

Decrease: T_3

NURSING CONSIDERATIONS

Assess:

Black Box Warning: Pulmonary toxicity: dyspnea, fatigue, cough, fever, chest pain; product should be discontinued; for ARDS, pulmonary fibrosis, crackles, tachypnea, increased at higher doses, toxicity is common

Black Box Warning: ECG continuously to determine product effectiveness; measure PR, QRS, QT intervals; check for PVCs, other dysrhythmias, B/P continuously for hypo/hypertension; report dysrhythmias, slowing heart rate; monitor amiodarone level: therapeutic 1-2.5 mcg/ml; toxic >2.5 mcg/ml

- Electrolytes (sodium, potassium, chloride); hepatic studies: AST, ALT, bilirubin, alk phos; for dehydration, hypovolemia, monitor PT, INR if using warfarin
- Chest x-ray, thyroid function tests
- CNS symptoms: confusion, psychosis, numbness, depression, involuntary movements; product should be discontinued
- **Hypothyroidism:** lethargy; dizziness; constipation; enlarged thyroid gland; edema of extremities; cool, pale skin
- **Hyperthyroidism:** restlessness; tachycardia; eyelid puffiness; weight loss; frequent urination; menstrual irregularities; dyspnea; warm, moist skin
- Ophthalmic exams at baseline and periodically (PO); to prevent corneal deposits, use methylcellulose
- Cardiac rate, respirations: rate, rhythm, character, chest pain; start with patient hospitalized and monitored up to 1 wk; for rebound hypertension after 1-2 hr

Evaluate:

- Therapeutic response: decrease in ventricular tachycardia, supraventricular tachycardia, fibrillation

Teach patient/family:

- To take this product as directed; to avoid missed doses; not to use with grapefruit juice; not to discontinue abruptly, not to use other drugs, herbs without prescriber approval, many interactions
- To use sunscreen or stay out of sun to prevent burns; that dark glasses may be needed for photophobia
- To report side effects immediately; more common at high dose
- That skin discoloration is usually reversible

TREATMENT OF OVERDOSE:

O_2, artificial ventilation, ECG, administer DOPamine for circulatory depression, administer diazepam, thiopental for seizures, isoproterenol

amitriptyline (Rx)

(a-mee-trip′ti-leen)

Elavil ✱, Levate ✱, Novo-Triptyn ✱

Func. class.: Antidepressant—tricyclic

Chem. class.: Tertiary amine

Do not confuse:

amitriptyline/nortriptyline/aminophylline

ACTION: Blocks reuptake of norepinephrine, serotonin into nerve endings, thereby increasing action of norepinephrine, serotonin in nerve cells

USES: Major depression

Unlabeled uses: Neuropathic pain, prevention of cluster/migraine headaches, fibromyalgia, ADHD, bulimia nervosa, diabetic neuropathy, enuresis, insomnia, panic disorder, postherpetic neuralgia, hiccups, social phobia

CONTRAINDICATIONS: Hypersensitivity to tricyclics; recovery phase of myocardial infarction

Precautions: Pregnancy (C), breastfeeding, geriatric patients, seizure disorders, prostatic hypertrophy, schizophrenia, psychosis, severe depression, increased intraocular pressure, closed-angle glaucoma, urinary retention, renal/hepatic/cardiac disease, hyperthyroidism, electroshock therapy, elective surgery

Black Box Warning: Children <12 yr, suicidal patients

DOSAGE AND ROUTES

Depression

- **Adult/adolescent: PO** 25-75 mg/day as single dose at bedtime or in divided doses, may increase to 200 mg/day; max 300 mg/day (if hospitalized)
- **Geriatric: PO** 10-25 mg at bedtime, may be increased to 150 mg/day

Cluster/migraine headache (unlabeled)

- **Adult: PO** 25-200 mg/day, initiate at lowest dose, titrate

Pain (unlabeled)

- **Adult: PO** 75-300 mg/day

Fibromyalgia/insomnia (unlabeled)

- **Adult: PO** 10-50 mg nightly

Enuresis (unlabeled)

- **Child 11-14 yr: PO** 50 mg at bedtime
- **Child 6-10 yr: PO** 25 mg at bedtime

ADHD/bulimia nervosa (unlabeled)

- **Adult: PO** 25 mg tid, titrate to 150 mg/day by 25-50 mg at weekly intervals
- **Child 6-12 yr: PO** 10-30 mg/day or 1-5 mg/kg/day in divided doses

Available forms: Tabs 10, 25, 50, 75, 100, 150 mg

Administer:

- Increase fluids, bulk in diet if constipation, urinary retention occur, especially in geriatric patients
- With food, milk for GI symptoms
- Crushed if patient unable to swallow medication whole
- Dosage at bedtime if oversedation occurs during day; may take entire dose at bedtime; geriatric patients may not tolerate once daily dosing
- Store at room temperature; do not freeze

SIDE EFFECTS

CNS: *Dizziness, drowsiness,* confusion, headache, anxiety, tremors, stimulation, weakness, *insomnia,* nightmares, EPS (geriatric patients), increased psychiatric symptoms, seizures, suicidal thoughts, anxiety

CV: *Orthostatic hypotension,* ECG changes, tachycardia, hypertension, palpitations, dysrhythmias

EENT: *Blurred vision,* tinnitus, mydriasis, ophthalmoplegia, amblyopia

GI: *Constipation, dry mouth,* weight gain, nausea, vomiting, paralytic ileus, increased appetite, cramps, epigastric distress, jaundice, hepatitis, stomatitis

GU: *Urinary retention,* sexual dysfunction

HEMA: Agranulocytosis, thrombocytopenia, eosinophilia, leukopenia, aplastic anemia

INTEG: Rash, urticaria, sweating, pruritus, photosensitivity

RESP: Asthma, exacerbation, rhinitis

SYST: Neuroleptic malignant syndrome, serotonin syndrome

PHARMACOKINETICS

Onset 45 min; peak 2-12 hr; therapeutic response 4-10 days; metabolized by liver to nortriptyline; excreted in urine, feces; crosses placenta; excreted in breast milk; half-life 10-46 hr

INTERACTIONS

⚠ Hyperpyretic crisis, seizures, hypertensive episode: MAOIs, do not use within 14 days of MAOIs

Increase: risk for agranulocytosis—antithyroid agents

Increase: QT prolongation—procainamide, quiNIDine, amiodarone, tricyclics, class IA, III antidysrhythmics

Increase: amitriptyline levels, toxicity—cimetidine, FLUoxetine, phenothiazines, oral contraceptives, antidepressants, carBAMazepine, class IC antidysrhythmics

Increase: effects of direct-acting sympathomimetics (EPINEPHrine), alcohol, barbiturates, benzodiazepines, CNS depressants, opioids, sedative/hypnotics

Increase: serotonin syndrome, linezolid, methyline blue, use cautiously

Decrease: effects of guanethidine, cloNIDine, indirect-acting sympathomimetics (ePHEDrine)

Drug/Herb

Increase: serotonin syndrome—SAM-e, St. John's wort, yohimbe

Increase: CNS depression—kava, hops, chamomile, lavender, valerian

Drug/Lab Test

Increase: serum bilirubin, blood glucose, alk phos, LFTs

Decrease: WBCs, platelets, granulocytes

NURSING CONSIDERATIONS

Assess:

- B/P lying, standing; pulse q4hr; if systolic B/P drops 20 mm Hg, hold product, notify prescriber; take vital signs q4hr with CV disease; ECG for flattening of T wave, prolongation of QTc interval, bundle branch block, AV block, dysrhythmias in cardiac patients, avoid use immediately after MI
- **Blood studies:** CBC, leukocytes, differential, cardiac enzymes if patient is receiving long-term therapy, thyroid function tests
- **Hepatic studies:** AST, ALT, bilirubin
- Weight weekly; appetite may increase with product
- EPS primarily in geriatric patients: rigidity, dystonia, akathisia
- Paralytic ileus, glaucoma exacerbation

Black Box Warning: Mental status: mood, sensorium, affect, suicidal tendencies; increase in psychiatric symptoms: depression, panic; suicidal tendencies are higher in those ≤24 yr, restrict amount of product available

- **Serotonin syndrome:** may occur with other serotonergic products (hyperthermia, hypertension, rigidity, delirium)
- Urinary retention, constipation; constipation is most likely to occur in children and geriatric patients
- **Withdrawal symptoms:** headache, nausea, vomiting, muscle pain, weakness; do not usually occur unless product was discontinued abruptly
- **Alcohol consumption:** if alcohol is consumed, hold dose until morning
- **Pain syndromes (unlabeled):** intensity, location, severity; use pain scale; product may be taken for 1-2 mo before effective
- **Sexual dysfunction:** erectile dysfunction, decreased libido

Evaluate:

- Therapeutic response: decrease in depression, absence of suicidal thoughts

Teach patient/family:

- To take medication as directed; not to double dose; that therapeutic effects may take 2-3 wk; not to discontinue medication quickly after long-term use: may cause nausea, headache, malaise
- To use caution when driving, performing other activities that require alertness because of drowsiness, dizziness, blurred vision; to avoid rising quickly from sitting to standing (especially geriatric patients); how to manage anticholinergic effects
- The symptoms of serotonin syndrome
- To avoid alcohol, other CNS depressants

- To wear sunscreen or large hat when outdoors, photosensitivity occurs
- That contraception is recommended during treatment; to avoid breastfeeding
- To watch for suicide

TREATMENT OF OVERDOSE:
ECG monitoring, lavage; administer anticonvulsant, sodium bicarbonate

amLODIPine (Rx)
(am-loe′di-peen)

Norvasc

Func. class.: Antianginal, antihypertensive, calcium channel blocker

Chem. class.: Dihydropyridine

Do not confuse:
amLODIPine/aMILoride

ACTION: Inhibits calcium ion influx across cell membrane during cardiac depolarization; produces relaxation of coronary vascular smooth muscle, peripheral vascular smooth muscle; dilates coronary vascular arteries; increases myocardial O_2 delivery in patients with vasospastic angina

USES: Chronic stable angina pectoris, hypertension, variant angina (Prinzmetal's angina); may coadminister with other antihypertensives, antianginals

Unlabeled uses: Hypertension (pediatric patients)

CONTRAINDICATIONS: Hypersensitivity to this product or dihydropyridine, severe aortic stenosis, severe obstructive CAD

Black Box Warning: Hypersensitivity to dihydropyridine

Precautions: Pregnancy (C), breastfeeding, children, geriatric patients, CHF, hypotension, hepatic injury, GERD

DOSAGE AND ROUTES
Coronary artery disease
- **Adult: PO** 5-10 mg/day
- **Geriatric: PO** 5 mg/day, max 10 mg/day

Hypertension
- **Adult: PO** 2.5-5 mg/day initially, max 10 mg/day
- **Geriatric: PO** 2.5 mg/day, may increase to 5 mg/day, max 10 mg/day
- **Child 6-16 yr (unlabeled): PO** 2.5-5 mg/day
- **Child <6 yr (unlabeled): PO** 0.05-0.2 mg/kg/day in 1-2 divided doses

Hepatic dose
- **Adult: PO** 2.5 mg/day; may increase to 10 mg/day (antihypertensive); 5 mg/day, may increase to 10 mg/day (antianginal)

Available forms: Tabs 2.5, 5, 10 mg

Administer:
- Once a day without regard to meals

SIDE EFFECTS
CNS: *Headache,* fatigue, dizziness, asthenia, anxiety, depression, insomnia, paresthesia, somnolence

CV: *Peripheral edema,* bradycardia, hypotension, palpitations, syncope, chest pain

GI: Nausea, vomiting, diarrhea, gastric upset, constipation, flatulence, anorexia, gingival hyperplasia, dyspepsia

GU: Nocturia, polyuria, sexual difficulties

INTEG: Rash, pruritus, urticaria, alopecia

OTHER: Flushing, muscle cramps, cough, weight gain, tinnitus, epistaxis, pulmonary edema, dyspnea

PHARMACOKINETICS
Peak 6-12 hr; half-life 30-50 hr; increased in geriatric patients, hepatic disease; metabolized by liver (CYP3A4); excreted in urine (90% as metabolites); protein binding >93%

INTERACTIONS
Increase: amLODIPine level—diltiazem, conivaptan; CYP3A4 inhibitors

Increase: level of cycloSPORINE

Increase: myopathy simvastatin

NURSING CONSIDERATIONS

Assess:

• Cardiac status: B/P, pulse, respirations, ECG; some patients have developed severe angina, acute MI after calcium channel blockers if obstructive CAD is severe

• Peripheral edema, dyspnea, jugular vein distention, crackles

• **Angina:** intensity, location, duration of pain

Evaluate:

• Therapeutic response: decreased anginal pain, decreased B/P, increased exercise tolerance

Teach patient/family:

• To take product as prescribed, not to double or skip dose

• To avoid hazardous activities until stabilized on product, dizziness is no longer a problem

• To avoid OTC products unless directed by prescriber

• To comply in all areas of medical regimen: diet, exercise, stress reduction, product therapy, smoking cessation

• To notify prescriber of irregular heartbeat; shortness of breath; swelling of feet, face, hands; severe dizziness; constipation; nausea; hypotension; if chest pain does not improve, use nitroglycerin when angina is severe

• To use correct technique when monitoring pulse; to contact prescriber if pulse <50 bpm

• To change positions slowly to prevent orthostatic hypotension

• To continue with good oral hygiene to prevent gingival disease

• To use sunscreen, protective clothing to prevent photosensitivity

• To notify all health care providers of use of this product

TREATMENT OF OVERDOSE:

Defibrillation, β-agonists, IV calcium inotropic agents, diuretics, atropine for AV block, vasopressor for hypotension

amoxicillin (Rx)

(a-mox-i-sill′in)

Amoxil ✱, Apo-Amoxi ✱, Larotid, Lin-Amox ✱, Moxatag, Novamoxin ✱, Nu-Amoxil ✱

Func. class.: Antiinfective, antiulcer

Chem. class.: Aminopenicillin

Do not confuse:

amoxicillin/amoxapine/Amoxil

Trimox/Diamox/Tylox

Wymox/Tylox

ACTION: Interferes with cell wall replication of susceptible organisms; bactericidal: lysis mediated by bacterial cell wall autolysins

USES: Treatment of skin, respiratory, GI, GU infections, otitis media, gonorrhea; for gram-positive cocci *(Staphylococcus aureus, Streptococcus pyogenes, Streptococcus faecalis, Streptococcus pneumoniae)*, gram-negative cocci *(Neisseria gonorrhoeae, Neisseria meningitidis)*, gram-positive bacilli *(Corynebacterium diphtheriae, Listeria monocytogenes)*, gram-negative bacilli *(Haemophilus influenzae, Escherichia coli, Proteus mirabilis, Salmonella)*; gastric ulcer, β-lactase–negative organisms

Unlabeled uses: Lyme disease, anthrax treatment and prophylaxis, cervicitis, *Chlamydia trachomatis,* dental abscess/infection, dyspepsia, non-gonococcal urethritis, periodontitis, typhoid fever; prophylaxis of bacterial endocarditis; in combination with other products for treatment of *Helicobacter pylori*

CONTRAINDICATIONS: Hypersensitivity to penicillins

Precautions: Pregnancy (B), breastfeeding, neonates, hypersensitivity to cephalosporins, carbapenems; severe renal disease, mononucleosis, phenylketonuria, diabetes, geriatric patients, asthma, child, colitis, dialysis, eczema, pseudomembranous colitis, syphilis

DOSAGE AND ROUTES

Upper respiratory infections

- **Adult/adolescent/child (≥40 kg): (mild-moderate infections) PO** 500 mg q12hr, or 250 mg q8hr; **(severe infections)** 875 mg q12hr or 500 mg q8hr
- **Child (<40 kg): (mild-moderate infections)** 25 mg/kg/day individual doses q12hr; **(severe infections)** 40 mg/kg/day divided q8hr or 45 mg/kg/day divided q12hr

***S. pyogenes* infection (pharyngitis/tonsillitis)**

- **Adult/child >12 yr: PO EXT REL** 775 mg every day with meal × 10 days

Otitis Media

- **Adult: PO** 500 mg q12hr or 250 mg q8hr
- **Infants >3 mo/children/adolescents: PO** 80-90 mg/kg/day in divided doses q8-12hr, max 500 mg/dose if given q8hr or 875 mg/dose if given q12hr

Gonorrhea (not CDC approved)

- **Adult: PO** 3 g given with 1 g probenecid as a single dose followed by tetracycline or erythromycin therapy

C. trachomatis

- **Adult: PO** 500 mg/tid × 1 wk

Duodenal/gastric ulcer/dyspepsia from *H. pylori* infection (unlabeled)

- **Adult: PO** 1000 mg bid with lansoprazole or clarithromycin/omeprazole

Bacterial endocarditis prophylaxis (unlabeled)

- **Adult: PO** 2 g 1 hr before procedure
- **Child: PO** 50 mg/kg 1 hr before procedure; max 2 g

Lyme disease (unlabeled)

- **Adult: PO** 500 mg tid × 14-21 days
- **Child: PO** 50 mg/kg/day in divided doses q8hr × 14-21 days

Anthrax treatment/prophylaxis (unlabeled)

- **Adult and child >20 kg: PO** 500 mg q8hr × 10-14 days (prophylaxis), 60 days (treatment)
- **Child <20 kg: PO** 80 mg/kg divided in 3 doses q8hr × 60 days (treatment)

Renal disease

- **Adult: PO** CCr 10-30 ml/min 250-500 mg q12hr; CCr <10 ml/min 250-500 mg q24hr; do not use 775, 875 mg strength if CCr <30 ml/min

Available forms: Caps 250, 500 mg; chew tabs 125, 200, 250, 400 mg; tabs, 500, 875 mg; ext rel tab (Moxatag) 775 mg; susp 125, 200, 250, 400 mg/5 ml

Administer:

PO route

- Identify allergies before use
- **Susp:** shake well before each dose; use calibrated spoon, oral syringe, or measuring cup; may be used alone, mixed in drinks; use immediately; discard unused portion after 14 days, store in refrigerator
- Give around the clock; caps may be emptied, mixed with liquids if needed without regard to food
- **Ext rel:** do not crush, chew, break; take with food

SIDE EFFECTS

CNS: Headache, seizures, agitation, confusion, dizziness, insomnia

GI: *Nausea, vomiting, diarrhea,* increased AST, ALT, abdominal pain, glossitis, colitis, pseudomembranous colitis, jaundice, cholestasis

HEMA: Anemia, increased bleeding time, bone marrow depression, granulocytopenia, hemolytic anemia, eosinophilia, thrombocytopenia, agranulocytosis

INTEG: *Urticaria, rash*

SYST: Anaphylaxis, respiratory distress, serum sickness, Stevens-Johnson syndrome, toxic epidermal necrolysis, exfoliative dermatitis

PHARMACOKINETICS

PO: Peak 1-2 hr, duration 6-8 hr, half-life 1-1$^{1}/_{3}$ hr extended in renal disease metabolized in liver, excreted in urine, crosses placenta, enters breast milk

INTERACTIONS

Increase: rash—allopurinol

Increase: amoxicillin level—probenecid

Increase: anticoagulant action—warfarin

Increase: methotrexate levels—methotrexate

Drug/Lab Test

Increase: AST/ALT, alk phos, LDH, eosinophils

Decrease: Hgb, WBC, platelets

Interference: urine glucose test (Clinitest, Benedict's reagent, cupric SO_4)

NURSING CONSIDERATIONS

Assess:

- Report hematuria, oliguria, penicillin products, in high doses are nephrotoxic
- Hepatic studies: AST, ALT
- Blood studies: WBC, RBC, Hgb, Hct, bleeding time
- Renal studies: urinalysis, protein, blood, BUN, creatinine
- C&S before product therapy; product may be given as soon as culture is taken

⚠ **Pseudomembranous colitis:** bowel pattern before, during treatment; diarrhea, cramping, blood in stools; report to prescriber

- Skin eruptions after administration of penicillin to 1 wk after discontinuing product; rash is more common if allopurinol is taken concurrently

⚠ **Anaphylaxis:** rash, itching, dyspnea, facial/laryngeal edema

Evaluate:

- Therapeutic response: absence of infection; prevention of endocarditis, resolution of ulcer symptoms

Teach patient/family:

- That caps may be opened, contents taken with fluids; that chewable form is available; to take as prescribed, not to double dose
- All aspects of product therapy: to complete entire course of medication to ensure organism death (10-14 days); that culture may be taken after completed course of medication

⚠ To report sore throat, fever, fatigue, diarrhea **(superinfection or agranulocytopenia),** blood in stool, abdominal pain **(pseudomembranous colitis),** decreased urinary output

- That product must be taken in equal intervals around the clock to maintain blood levels; to take without regard to food
- To wear or carry emergency ID if allergic to penicillins

TREATMENT OF ANAPHYLAXIS: Withdraw product, maintain airway; administer EPINEPHrine, aminophylline, O_2, IV corticosteroids

amoxicillin/clavulanate (Rx)

(a-mox-i-sill′in)

Apo-Amoxi Clav ✦, Augmentin, Augmentin XR, Clavulin ✦

Func. class.: Broad-spectrum antiinfective

Chem. class.: Aminopenicillin β-lactamase inhibitor

Do not confuse:

Augmentin/amoxicillin

ACTION: Bacteriocidal, interferes with cell wall replication of susceptible organisms; lysis mediated by bacterial cell wall autolytic enzymes, combination increases spectrum of activity against β-lactamase–resistant organisms

USES: Lower respiratory tract infections, sinus infections, pneumonia, otitis media, impetigo, skin infection, UTI; effective for *Actinomyces* sp., *Bacillus anthracis, Bacteroides* sp., *Bordetta pertassis, Borrelia burdofer; Brucella* sp., *Burkholderia pseudomallei, Clostridium perfringens/tetani, Corynebacterium diphtheriae, Eikenella corodens, Enterobacter* sp., *Enterococcus faecalis, Erysipelothrix rhusioputhae, Escherichiacoli, Eubacterium* sp., *Fusobacterium* sp., *Haemophilus ducrey/parainfluenzal (positive/negative beta-lactamase), Heliobacter pylori, Klebsiella* sp., *Lactobacillus* sp., *Listeria* *monocytogenes, Moraxella catarrholis, Neisseria gonorrheal/meningitis, Nocardia brasilensis, Peptococcus* sp., *Peptostreptococcus* sp., *Prevotella melaninogemica, Propionibacterium* sp., *shigella* sp., *Staphylococcus aureus (MSSA)/epidermidis/ Saprophyticus, streptococcus agalactial (group B Streptococci)/dysglactial/ pneumonia/pygenes (group A Streptococci) reponema pallidium, Vibrocholeral, viridans streptococci*

Unlabeled uses: Actinomycotic mycetoma, chancroid, dental infections, dentoalveolar infection, melioidosis, pericoronitis, SARS

CONTRAINDICATIONS:

Hypersensitivity to penicillins, severe renal disease, dialysis

Precautions: Pregnancy (B), breastfeeding, neonates, children, hypersensitivity to cephalosporins; renal/GI disease, asthma, colitis, diabetes, eczema, leukemia, mononucleosis, viral infections, phenylketonuria

DOSAGE AND ROUTES

- **Adult: PO** 250-500 mg q8hr or 500-875 mg q12hr, depending on severity of infection
- **Child ≤40 kg: PO** 20-90 mg/kg/day in divided doses q8-12hr

Community-acquired pneumonia or acute bacterial sinusitis

- **Adult: PO** 2000 mg/125 mg (Augmentin XR) q12 hr × 7-10 days (pneumonia), 10 days (sinusitis)

Renal disease

- **Adult: PO** CCr 10-30 ml/min dose q12hr; CCr <10 ml/min dose q24hr; do not use 875-mg strength or ext rel if CCr <30 ml/min; Augmentin XR is contraindicated with renal disease

Available forms: Tabs 250, 500, 875 mg/125 mg clavulanate; chew tabs 200/28.5, 400/57 mg; powder for oral susp 250/28.5, 200/28.5, 400/57, 600/42.9 mg/5 ml; ext rel tabs (XR) 1000 mg amoxicillin, 62.5 mg clavulanate; powder for oral susp (ES) 600 mg amoxicillin, 42.9 mg clavulanate

Administer:

PO route

- Do not break, crush, chew ext rel product

⚠ Only as directed; two 250-mg tabs not equivalent to one 500-mg tab due to strength of clavulanate

- Shake susp well before each dose; may be used alone, mixed in drinks; use immediately, discard unused portion of susp after 14 days, store in refrigerator
- Give around the clock
- Give with light meal for increased absorption, fewer GI effects, confusion, behavioral changes

SIDE EFFECTS

CNS: Headache, fever, seizures, agitation, insomnia

GI: *Nausea, diarrhea, vomiting,* increased AST/ALT, abdominal pain, glossitis, colitis, black tongue, pseudomembranous colitis, jaundice

GU: Oliguria, proteinuria, hematuria, *vaginitis, moniliasis,* glomerulonephritis

HEMA: Anemia, bone marrow depression, granulocytopenia, leukopenia, eosinophilia, thrombocytopenic purpura

INTEG: *Rash,* urticaria, dermatitis, toxic epidermal necrolysis

META: Hypo/hyperkalemia, alkalosis, hypernatremia

SYST: Anaphylaxis, respiratory distress, serum sickness, Stevens-Johnson syndrome, superinfection, candidiasis

PHARMACOKINETICS

PO: Peak 1-2.5 hr, duration 6-8 hr, half-life 1-1⅓ hr, metabolized in liver, excreted in urine, crosses placenta, excreted in breast milk, removed by hemodialysis

INTERACTIONS

Increase: amoxicillin levels—probenecid

Increase: anticoagulant effect—warfarin; monitor closely, dose adjustment may be needed

Increase: skin rash—allopurinol

Drug/Food
Decrease: absorption by a high-fat meal
Drug/Lab Test
Increase: AST/ALT, alk phos, LDH
Interference: urine glucose tests (Clinitest, Benedict's reagent, Cupric SO_4)

NURSING CONSIDERATIONS

Assess:

⚠ Nephrotoxicity at high doses: I&O ratio; report hematuria, oliguria

- Hepatic studies: AST, ALT
- Blood studies: WBC, RBC, Hgb, Hct, bleeding time
- Renal studies: urinalysis, protein, blood, BUN, creatinine; if urine output decreases, long-acting products should not be used
- C&S before product therapy; product may be given as soon as culture is taken

⚠ **Pseudomembranous colitis:** bowel pattern before, during treatment; diarrhea, cramping, blood in stools; report to prescriber

⚠ **Anaphylaxis:** rash, itching, dyspnea, facial/laryngeal edema; skin eruptions after administration of penicillin to 1 wk after discontinuing product

- Adrenaline, suction, tracheostomy set, endotracheal intubation equipment on unit
- Adequate intake of fluids (2 L) during diarrhea episodes

Evaluate:

- Therapeutic response: absence of infection

Teach patient/family:

- To take as prescribed, not to double dose
- All aspects of product therapy: to complete entire course of medication to ensure organism death (10-14 days); that culture may be taken after completed course of medication

⚠ To report sore throat, fever, fatigue **(superinfection or agranulocytosis);** diarrhea, cramping, blood in stools **(pseudomembranous colitis)**

- That product must be taken in equal intervals around the clock to maintain blood levels
- To wear or carry emergency ID if allergic to penicillins

TREATMENT OF HYPERSENSITIVITY: Withdraw product, maintain airway, administer EPINEPHrine, aminophylline, O_2, IV corticosteroids for anaphylaxis

⚠ HIGH ALERT

amphotericin B lipid complex (ABLC)

(am-foe-ter′i-sin)

Abelcet

Func. class.: Antifungal
Chem. class.: Amphoteric polyene

ACTION: Increases cell membrane permeability in susceptible fungi by binding sterols; alters cell membrane, thereby causing leakage of cell components, cell death

USES: Indicated for the treatment of invasive fungal infections in patients who cannot tolerate or have failed conventional amphotericin B therapy; broad-spectrum activity against many fungal, yeast and mold pathogen infections, including *Aspergillus, Zygomycetes, Fusarium, Cryptococcus,* and many hard-to-treat *Candida* species; *Aspergillus fumigatus, Aspergillus* sp., *Blastomyces dermatitidis, Candida albicans, Candida guilliermondii, Candida* sp., *Candida stellatoidea, Candida tropicalis, Coccidioides immitis, Cryptococcus* sp., *Histoplasma* sp., *sporotiaichosis*

CONTRAINDICATIONS: Hypersensitivity

Precautions: Anemia, breastfeeding, cardiac disease, children, electrolyte imbalance, geriatric, hematologic/hepatic/renal disease, hypotension, pregnancy (B)

DOSAGE AND ROUTES

- **Adult: IV** 3-5 mg/kg/day as a single infusion given at 2.5 mg/kg/hr

Renal dose

Adult: IV CCr <10 ml/min give 5 mg/kg q24-36hr

Available forms: Susp for inj 100 mg/20-ml vial

Administer:

⚠ Do not confuse four different types; these are not interchangeable: conventional amphotericin B, amphotericin B cholesteryl, amphotericin B lipid complex, amphotericin B liposome

- May premedicate with acetaminophin, diphenhydrAMINE
- Use only after C&S confirms organism

IV route

- Give product only after C&S confirms organism, product needed to treat condition; make sure product is used for life-threatening infections
- Handle with aseptic technique because amphotericin B lipid complex (ABLC) has no preservatives; visually inspect parenteral products for particulate matter and discoloration before use

Filtration and dilution:

- Before dilution, store at 36°-46° F (2°-8° C), protected from moisture and light; do not freeze; the diluted, ready-for-use admixture is stable for up to 48 hours at 36°-46° F (2°-8° C) and an additional 6 hr at room temperature; do not freeze
- Prepare the admixture for infusion by first shaking the vial until there is no evidence of yellow sediment on the bottom of the vial
- Transfer the appropriate amount of drug from the required number of vials into one or more sterile syringes using an 18-gauge needle
- Attach the provided 5-micron filter needle to the syringe; inject the syringe contents through the filter needle, into an IV bag containing the appropriate amount of D_5W injection; each filter needle may be used on the contents of no more than four 100-mg vials
- The suspension must be diluted with D_5W injection to a final concentration of 1 mg/ml; for pediatric patients and patients with cardiovascular disease, the final concentration may be 2 mg/ml; DO NOT USE SALINE SOLUTIONS OR MIX WITH OTHER DRUGS OR ELECTROLYTES
- The diluted ready-for-use admixture is stable for up to 48 hr at 2-8° C (36-46° F) and an additional 6 hr at room temperature; do not freeze

IV INFUSION

- Flush IV line with D_5W injection before use or use a separate IV line; DO NOT USE AN IN-LINE FILTER
- Before infusion, shake the bag until the contents are thoroughly mixed; max rate 2.5 mg/kg/hr; if the infusion time exceeds 2 hr, mix the contents by shaking the infusion bag every 2 hr

Y-site compatibilities: acyclovir, allopurinol, aminocaproic acid, aminophylline, amiodarone, anidulafungin, argatroban, arsenic trioxide, atracurium, azithromycin, aztreonam, bumetanide, buprenorphine, busulfan, butorphanol, CARBOplatin, carmustine, ceFAZolin, cefepime, cefotaxime, cefoTEtan, cefOXitin, cefTAZidime, ceftizoxime, cefTRIAXone, cefuroxime, chloramphenicol, chlorproMAZINE, cimetidine, cisatracurium, clindamycin, cyclophosphamide, cycloSPORINE, cytarabine, DACTINomycin, dexamethasone, digoxin, diphenhydrAMINE, DOCEtaxel, doxacurium, DOXOrubicin liposomal, enalaprilat, EPINEPHrine eptifibatide, ertapenem, etoposide, famotidine, fentaNYL, fludarabine, fluorouracil, fosphenytoin, furosemide, ganciclovir, granisetron, heparin, hydrocortisone, HYDROmorphone, ifosfamide, insulin, regular ketorolac, lepirudin, lidocaine, linezolid, LORazepam, mannitol, melphalan, meperidine, methotrexate, methylPREDNISolone, metoclopramide, mitoMYcin, mivacurium, nafcillin, nesiritide, nitroglycerin, nitroprusside, octreotide, oxaliplatin, PACLitaxel, pamidronate, pantoprazole, PEMEtrexed, pentazocine, PENTobarbital, PHENobarbital, phentolamine, piperacillin-tazobactam, procainamide, ranitidine, succinylcholine, SUFentanil, tacrolimus, telavancin, teniposide, theophylline, thiopental, thiotepa, ticarcillin, ticaracillin-clavulanate, trimethobenzamide, verapamil, vinBLAStine, vinCRIStine, zidovudine, zoledronic acid

SIDE EFFECTS

CNS: *Headache, fever, chills,* peripheral nerve pain, paresthesias, peripheral neuropathy, **seizures**, dizziness
CV: Bradycardia, hypotension, **cardiac arrest**, chest pain, hypertension
EENT: Tinnitus, deafness, diplopia, blurred vision
GI: *Nausea, vomiting, anorexia,* diarrhea, cramps, **hemorrhagic gastroenteritis, acute liver failure**, jaundice, bilirubinemia
GU: *Hypokalemia,* **azotemia, hyposthenuria, renal tubular acidosis, nephrocalcinosis, permanent renal impairment, anuria, oliguria**
HEMA: **Normochromic, normocytic anemia, thrombocytopenia, agranulocytosis, leukopenia, eosinophilia**
INTEG: *Burning, irritation,* pain, **necrosis at inj site with extravasation**, flushing, dermatitis
META: Hyponatremia, hypomagnesemia, hypokalemia
MS: Arthralgia, myalgia, generalized pain, weakness, weight loss
RESP: **Bronchospasm, dyspnea**
SYST: **Toxic epidermal neurolysis, exfoliative dermatitis, anaphylaxis, sepsis, infection, infusion reactions**

PHARMACOKINETICS

IV: terminal half-life lipid complex mean 7 days

INTERACTIONS

- **Do not use with cidofovir**

Increase: nephrotoxicity—other nephrotoxic antibiotics (aminoglycosides, CISplatin, vancomycin, cycloSPORINE, polymyxin B), antineoplastics, pentamidine, salicylates, tacrolimus, tenofovir
Increase: hypokalemia—corticosteroids, digoxin, skeletal muscle relaxants, thiazides, loop diuretics
Decrease: amphotericin B lipid complexazole antifungals may still be used concurrently in serious resistant infections

Drug/Lab Test
Increase: AST/ALT, alk phos, BUN, creatinine, LDH, bilirubin
Decrease: magnesium, potassium, Hgb, WBC, platelets

NURSING CONSIDERATIONS

Assess:

- VS every 15-30 min during first infusion; note changes in pulse, B/P
- I&O ratio; watch for decreasing urinary output, change in specific gravity; discontinue product to prevent permanent damage to renal tubules
- Blood studies: CBC, potassium, sodium, calcium, magnesium every 2 wk; BUN, creatinine 2-3 ×/wk
- Weight weekly; if weight increases by more than 2 lb/wk, edema is present; renal damage should be considered
- **For renal toxicity: increasing BUN, serum creatinine; if BUN is >40 mg/dl or if serum creatinine is >3 mg/dl, product may be discontinued, dosage reduced**
- **For hepatotoxicity: increasing AST, ALT, alk phos, bilirubin**
- **For allergic reaction: dermatitis, rash; product should be discontinued, antihistamines (mild reaction) or EPINEPHrine (severe reaction) should be administered**
- For hypokalemia: anorexia, drowsiness, weakness, decreased reflexes, dizziness, increased urinary output, increased thirst, paresthesias
- Infusion reactions: fever, chills, pain, swelling at site
- For ototoxicity: tinnitus (ringing, roaring in ears), vertigo, loss of hearing (rare)

Evaluate:

- Therapeutic response: decreased fever, malaise, rash, negative C&S for infecting organism

Teach patient/family:

- That long-term therapy may be needed to clear infection (2 wk-3 mo, depending on type of infection)
- **To notify prescriber of bleeding, bruising, or soft-tissue swelling, neurologic, renal symptoms**

⚠ HIGH ALERT

amphotericin B liposomal (LAmB)

(am-foe-ter′i-sin)

AmBisome

Func. class.: Antifungal

Chem. class.: Amphoteric polyene

ACTION: Increases cell membrane permeability in susceptible fungi by binding to membrane sterols; alters cell membrane, thereby causing leakage of cell components, cell death

THERAPEUTIC OUTCOME

Resolution of infection

USES: Empirical therapy for presumed fungal infection in febrile neutropenic patients; treatment of *Cryptococcal* meningitis in HIV-infected patients; treatment of *Aspergillus* species, *Candida* species, and/or *Cryptococcus* species infections refractory to amphotericin B deoxycholate, or in patients where renal impairment or unacceptable toxicity precludes the use of amphotericin B deoxycholate *(Aspergillus flavus, Aspergillus fumigatus, Blastomyces dermatitidis, Candida albicans, Candida krusei, Candida lusitaniae, Candida parapsilosis, Candida tropicalis, Cryptococcus neoformans)*; treatment of visceral leishmaniasis

Unlabeled uses: Coccidioidomycosis, histoplasmosis

CONTRAINDICATIONS

Hypersensitivity

Precautions: Anemia, breastfeeding, cardiac disease, children, electrolyte imbalance, geriatric, hematologic/hepatic/renal disease, hypotension pregnancy (B), severe bone marrow depression

DOSAGE AND ROUTES

Visceral leishmaniasis

- **Adult and child ≥1 mo: IV** 3 mg/kg every 24 hr days 1-5, and days 14, 21 (immunocompetent), 4 mg/kg every 24 hr days 1-5, and days 10, 17, 24, 31, 38 (immunocompromised)

Cryptococcal meningitis in HIV

- **Adult and child ≥1 mo: IV** 6 mg/kg/day

Fungal infection, empirical

- **Adult and child ≥1 mo: IV** 3 mg/kg/day

Fungal infection, systemic

- **Adult and child ≥1 mo: IV** 3-5 mg/kg/day

Renal dose

- **Adult: IV** CCr <10 ml/min use 3 mg/kg q24hr

Available forms: Powder for inj 50-mg vial

Administer:

⚠ Do not confuse four different types; these are not interchangeable: conventional amphotericin B, amphotericin B cholesteryl, amphotericin B lipid complex, amphotericin B liposome

- May premedicate with acetaminophen, diphenhydrAMINE

IV route

- Make sure product is used for life-threatening infections
- Administer by IV infusion only; handle with aseptic technique as LAmB does not contain any preservatives
- Visually inspect products for particulate matter and discoloration

Reconstitution

- LAmB *must* be reconstituted using sterile water for injection (without a bacteriostatic agent); DO NOT RECONSTITUTE WITH SALINE OR ADD SALINE TO THE RECONSTITUTED SUSPENSION, DO NOT MIX WITH OTHER DRUGS; doing so can cause a precipitate to form
- Reconstitute vials containing 50 mg of LAmB /12 ml of sterile water (4 mg/ml)
- Immediately after the addition of water, SHAKE THE VIAL VIGOROUSLY for 30 sec; the suspension should be yellow and translucent; visually inspect vial for particulate matter and continue shaking until product is completely dispersed
- Store suspension for up to 24 hours refrigerated if using sterile water for injection; do not freeze

Filtration and dilution
- Calculate the amount of reconstituted (4 mg/ml) suspension to be further diluted and withdraw this amount into a sterile syringe
- Attach the provided 5-micron filter to the syringe; inject the syringe contents through the filter, into the appropriate amount of D_5W injection; use only one filter per vial
- The suspension must be diluted with D_5W injection to a final concentration of 1-2 mg/ml before administration; for infants and small children, lower concentrations (0.2-0.5 mg/ml) may be appropriate to provide sufficient volume for infusion
- Use injection of LAmB within 6 hr of dilution with D_5W

IV INFUSION
- Flush intravenous line with D_5W injection before infusion; if this cannot be done, then a separate IV line must be used
- An inline membrane filter may be used provided the mean pore diameter of the filter is not less than 1 micron
- Administer by IV infusion using a controlled infusion device over a period of approximately 120 min; infusion time may be reduced to approximately 60 min in patients who tolerate the infusion; if discomfort occurs during infusion, the duration of infusion may be increased
- Store protected from moisture and light; diluted solution is stable for 24 hr at room temperature

Acetaminophen and diphenhydrAMINE
- 30 min before infusion to reduce fever, chills, headache

Y-site compatibilities:
Acyclovir, amifostine, aminophylline, anidulafungin, atropine, azithromycin, bivalirudin, bumetanide, buprenorphine, busulfan, butorphanol, CARBOplatin, carmustine, ceFAZolin, ceFOXitin, ceftizoxime, cefTRIAXone, cefuroxime, cimetidine, clindamycin, cyclophosphamide, cytarabine, DACTINomycin, DAPTOmycin, dexamethasone, dexmedetomidine, diphenhydrAMINE, doxacurium, enalaprilat, ePHEDrine, EPINEPHrine, eptifibatide, ertapenem, esmolol, etoposide, famotidine, fenoldopam, fentaNYL, fludarabine, fluorouracil, fosphenytoin, furosemide, granisetron, haloperidol, heparin, hydrocortisone, HYDROmorphone, ifosfamide, isoproterenol, ketorolac, levorphanol, lidocaine, linezolid, mesna, methotrexate, methylPREDNISolone, metoprolol, milrinone, mitoMYcin, nesiritide, nitroglycerin, nitroprusside, octreotide, oxaliplatin, oxytocin, palonosetron, pancuronium, pantoprazole, PEMEtrexed, PENTobarbital, PHENObarbital, phenylephrine, piperacillin/tazobactam, potassium chloride, procainamide, ranitidine, SUFentanil, tacrolimus, theophylline, thiopental, thiotepa, ticarcillin/clavulanate, tigecycline, trimethoprim-sulfamethoxazole, vasopressin, vinCRIStine, voriconazole, zidovudine

SIDE EFFECTS

CNS: *Headache, fever, chills,* peripheral nerve pain, paresthesias, peripheral neuropathy, **seizures**, dizziness, insomnia
CV: Bradycardia, hypotension, cardiac arrest
EENT: Tinnitus, deafness, diplopia, blurred vision
ENDO: Hyperglycemia
GI: *Nausea, vomiting, anorexia,* diarrhea, cramps, **hemorrhagic gastroenteritis, acute liver failure**
GU: *Hypokalemia,* **azotemia, hyposthenuria,** renal tubular acidosis, **nephrocalcinosis, permanent renal impairment, anuria,** oliguria
HEMA: **Normochromic normocytic anemia, thrombocytopenia, agranulocytosis, leukopenia, eosinophilia,** hyponatremia, hypomagnesemia
INTEG: *Burning, irritation,* pain, **necrosis at inj site with extravasation,** flushing, dermatitis, skin rash (topical route)
MS: Arthralgia, myalgia, generalized pain, weakness, weight loss
RESP: Dyspnea

SYST: Stevens–Johnson syndrome, toxic epidermal neurolysis, exfoliative dermatitis, anaphylaxis

PHARMACOKINETICS

IV: Initial half-life (LAmB) mean 4-6 days; metabolized in liver; excreted in urine (metabolites), breast milk; protein binding 90%; poorly penetrates CSF, bronchial secretions, aqueous humor, muscle, bone; terminal half-life mean 4-6 days

INTERACTIONS

Increase: nephrotoxicity—other nephrotoxic antibiotics (aminoglycosides, CISplatin, vancomycin, cycloSPORINE, polymyxin B)

Increase: hypokalemia—corticosteroids, digoxin, skeletal muscle relaxants, thiazides

NURSING CONSIDERATIONS

Assess:

- VS every 15-30 min during first infusion; note changes in pulse, B/P
- I&O ratio; watch for decreasing urinary output, change in specific gravity; discontinue product to prevent permanent damage to renal tubules
- Blood studies: CBC, potassium, sodium, calcium, magnesium every 2 wk, BUN, creatinine 2-3 ×/wk
- Weight weekly; if weight increases by more than 2 lb/wk, edema is present; renal damage should be considered
- **For renal toxicity:** increasing BUN, serum creatinine; if BUN is >40 mg/dl or if serum creatinine is >3 mg/dl, product may be discontinued, dosage reduced
- **For hepatotoxicity:** increasing AST, ALT, alk phos, bilirubin, monitor LFTs
- **For allergic reaction:** dermatitis, rash; product should be discontinued, antihistamines (mild reaction) or EPINEPHrine (severe reaction) administered
- **For hypokalemia:** anorexia, drowsiness, weakness, decreased reflexes, dizziness, increased urinary output, increased thirst, paresthesias
- **For ototoxicity:** tinnitus (ringing, roaring in ears), vertigo, loss of hearing (rare)
- **Infusion reaction:** chills, fever, pain, swelling at site

Evaluate:

- Therapeutic response: decreased fever, malaise, rash, negative C&S for infecting organism

Teach patient/family:

- That long-term therapy may be needed to clear infection (2 wk-3 mo, depending on type of infection)
- To notify prescriber of bleeding, bruising, or soft-tissue swelling, renal, neurologic side effects

ampicillin (Rx)

(am-pi-sill′in)

Ampicin ✱, Apo-Ampi ✱, Nu-Ampi ✱, Penbritin ✱

Func. class.: Antiinfective—broad-spectrum

Chem. class.: Aminopenicillin

Do not confuse:
Omnipen/imipenem

ACTION: Interferes with cell wall replication of susceptible organisms; the cell wall, rendered osmotically unstable, swells, bursts from osmotic pressure; lysis mediated by cell wall autolysins

USES: Effective for gram-positive cocci *(Staphylococcus aureus, Streptococcus pyogenes, Streptococcus faecalis, Streptococcus pneumoniae)*, gram-negative cocci *(Neisseria meningitidis)*, gram-negative bacilli *(Haemophilus influenzae, Proteus mirabilis, Salmonella, Shigella, Listeria monocytogenes)*, gram-positive bacilli; meningitis, GI/GU/respiratory infections, endocarditis, septicemia, otitis media, skin infection, bacterial endocarditis

Unlabeled uses: Biliary tract infection, shigellosis, typhoid fever, PID, OB/GYN infections, leptospirosis

CONTRAINDICATIONS: Hypersensitivity to penicillins, antimicrobial resistance

Precautions: Pregnancy (B), breastfeeding, neonates, hypersensitivity to cephalosporins, renal disease, mononucleosis

DOSAGE AND ROUTES

Systemic infections

- **Adult and child ≥40 kg: PO** 250-500 mg q6hr; **IV/IM** 2-8 g/day in divided doses q4-6hr
- **Child <40 kg: PO** 50-100 mg/kg/day in divided doses q6-8hr; **IV/IM** 50-500 mg/kg/day in divided doses q6-8hr

Bacterial meningitis

- **Adult and adolescent: IM/IV** 150-200 mg/kg/day in divided doses q3-4hr; IDSA dose IV 12 g in divided doses q4hr
- **Infant and child: IM/IV** 150-200 mg/kg/day in divided doses q3-4hr; IDSA dose IV 300 mg/kg/day in divided doses q6hr
- **Neonates >7 days and >2000 g: IM/IV** 200 mg/kg/day in divided doses q6hr; IDSA dose IV 200 mg/kg/day in divided doses q6-8hr

Prevention of bacterial endocarditis

- **Adult: IM/IV** 2 g 30 min before procedure
- **Child: IM/IV** 50 mg/kg 30 min before procedure, max 2 g

GI/GU infections other than *N. gonorrhoeae*

- **Adult and child >20 kg: PO** 500 mg q6hr, may use larger dose for more serious infections
- **Child <40 kg: PO** 50 mg/kg/day in divided doses q6-8hr

Renal disease

- **Adult and child:** CCr 10-50 ml/min extend to q6-12hr; CCr <10 ml/min extend to q12-16hr

Typhoid fever (unlabeled)

- **Adult/adolescent/child: IV** 100 mg/kg/day in divided doses q6hr × 14 days or more

Available forms: Powder for inj 125, 250, 500 mg, 1, 2, 10 g; IV inj 500 mg, 1, 2 g; caps 250, 500 mg; powder for oral susp 125, 250 mg/5 ml

Administer:

PO route

- On empty stomach with plenty of water for best absorption (1-2 hr before meals or 2-3 hr after meals)
- Shake susp well before each dose; store after reconstituting in refrigerator up to 2 wk, 1 wk room temperature

IM route (painful)

- **Reconstitute** by adding 0.9-1.2 ml/125-mg vial; 0.9-1.9 ml/250-mg vial; 1.2-1.8 ml/500-mg vial; 2.4-7.4 ml/1-g vial; 6.8 ml/2-g vial

IV route

IV direct

- After diluting with sterile water 0.9-1.2 ml/125 mg product, administer over 3-5 min (up to 500 mg), 10-15 min (>500 mg)

Intermittent IV INFUSION route

- May be diluted in 50 ml or more of D_5W, D_5 0.45% NaCl to a concentrations of 30 mg/ml or less; IV sol is stable for 1 hr; give at prescribed rate, do not give in same tubing as aminoglycosides, separate by ≥1 hr

Y-site compatibilities: Acyclovir, alemtuzumab, alprostadil, amifostine, aminocaproic acid, anidulafungin, argatroban, atenolol, azithromycin, bivalirudin, bleomycin, CARBOplatin, carmustine, CISplatin, clarithromycin, cyclophosphamide, cytarabine, DACTINomycin, DAPTOmycin, DAUNOrubicin liposome, dexmedetomidine, dexrazoxane, DOCEtaxel, doxacurium, doxapram, DOXOrubicin liposome, eptifibatide, etoposide, etoposide phosphate, filgrastim, fludarabine, fluorouracil, foscarnet, gallium, gatafloxacin, gemcitabine, gemtuzumab, granisetron, hetastarch, ifosfamide, irinotecan, lepirudin, leucovorin, levofloxacin, linezolid, mannitol, mechlorethamine, melphalan, methotrexate, metroNIDAZOLE, milrinone, octreotide, ofloxacin, oxaliplatin, PACLitaxel, palonosetron, pamidronate, pancuronium, pantoprazole, PEMEtrexed, penicillin G potassium, perphenazine, potassium acetate, propofol, remifentanil, riTUXimab, rocuronium, sodium acetate, teniposide, thiotepa, tigecycline, tirofiban,

TNA, trastuzumab, vecuronium, vinBLAStine, vinCRIStine, vit B/C, voriconazole, zoledronic acid

SIDE EFFECTS

GI: *Nausea, vomiting, diarrhea,* pseudomembranous colitis, stomatitis, black hairy tongue
GU: Oliguria, proteinuria, hematuria, *vaginitis, moniliasis,* glomerulonephritis
HEMA: Anemia, increased bleeding time, bone marrow depression, granulocytopenia, leukopenia, eosinophilia, hemolysis
INTEG: *Rash, urticaria,* erythema multiforme
MISC: Anaphylaxis, serum sickness, Stevens-Johnson syndrome, toxic epidermal necrolysis

PHARMACOKINETICS

Half-life 50-110 min; excreted in urine, bile, breast milk; crosses placenta; removed by dialysis
PO: Peak 2 hr, duration 6-8 hr
IM: Peak 1 hr
IV: Peak rapid

INTERACTIONS

Increase: bleeding, oral anticoagulants, monitor INR/PIJ
Increase: ampicillin concentrations—probenecid
Increase: ampicillin-induced skin rash—allopurinol, monitor for rash
Decrease: ampicillin level—H2 antagonists, proton pump inhibitors

Drug/Lab Test

Increase: eosinophil
Decrease: conjugated estrone during pregnancy, conjugated estriol, Hgb, WBC, platelets
False positive: urine glucose
Interference: urine glucose, (Clinitest, Benedict's reagent, cupric SO4)

NURSING CONSIDERATIONS

Assess:

• **Infection:** characteristics of wound, sputum, WBC; baseline, periodically; C&S before product therapy, product may be taken as soon as culture is taken
⚠ **Nephrotoxicity:** I&O ratio; report hematuria, oliguria; renal studies: urinalysis, protein, blood, BUN, creatinine
• Hepatic studies: AST, ALT
• Blood studies: WBC, RBC, Hgb, Hct, bleeding time
• Bowel pattern before, during treatment
• Skin eruptions after administration of penicillin to 1 wk after discontinuing product; identify allergies before using
• Respiratory status: rate, character, wheezing, tightness in chest
⚠ **Anaphylaxis:** rash, itching, dyspnea, facial swelling; stop product, notify prescriber, have emergency equipment available
• Adequate intake of fluids (2 L) during diarrhea episodes
• Scratch test to assess allergy after securing order from prescriber; usually done when penicillin is only product of choice
• Store in tight container; after reconstituting, oral suspension refrigerated for 2 wk or stored at room temperature for 1 wk

Evaluate:

• Therapeutic response: absence of fever, draining wounds, other symptoms of infection

Teach patient/family:

• To take oral ampicillin on empty stomach with full glass of water; to use alternate contraception
• All aspects of product therapy: to complete entire course of medication to ensure organism death (10-14 days); that culture may be taken after completed course of medication
⚠ To report sore throat, fever, fatigue, diarrhea (may indicate **superinfection**); to report rash, other signs of allergy
• That product must be taken in equal intervals around the clock to maintain blood levels
• To wear or carry emergency ID if allergic to penicillins
• **Pseudomembranous colitis:** diarrhea with blood or pus; notify prescriber

TREATMENT OF ANAPHYLAXIS: Withdraw product, maintain airway; administer EPINEPHrine, aminophylline, O_2, IV corticosteroids

ampicillin, sulbactam (Rx)

Unasyn

Func. class.: Antiinfective—broad-spectrum

Chem. class.: Aminopenicillin with β-lactamase inhibitor

ACTION: Interferes with cell wall replication of susceptible organisms; the cell wall, rendered osmotically unstable, swells, bursts from osmotic pressure; lysis due to cell wall autolytic enzymes; combination extends spectrum of activity by β-lactamase inhibition

USES: Skin infections, intraabdominal infections, cellulitis, diabetic foot ulcer, nosocomial pneumonicus, gynecologic infections; *acinetobacter* sp., *actinomyces* sp., *Bacillus anthracias, Bacteroides* sp., *Bifidobacterium* sp., *Bordetella pertussis, Borrelia burgdorferi, Brucella* sp., *Clostridium* sp., *Corynebacterium diptherial/xerosis, Eikenella corrodens, Entercoccus faecalis, Erysipelothrix rhusiopathial, Escherichia coli, Eubacterium* sp., *Fusobacterium* sp., *Gardnerella vaginalis, Haemophilas influenzal (beta-lactamase negative/ positive) Helicobacter pylori, Klebsiella* sp., *Lactobacillus* sp., *Leptospira* sp., *Listeria monocytogenes, Moraxella catarrhalis, Morganella morganii, Neisseria gonorrhoeae, Pasteurella multocida Peptococcus* sp., *Pepto streptococcus* sp., *Porphyromonas* sp., *Prevotella* sp., *Propionibacterium Sp. Proteus mirabilis, Proteus vulgaris, Provedencia rettgeri, Provedencia stuarti, Salmonella* sp., *Shigella* sp., *Staphylococcus aureus (MSSA)/epidermidis/saprophyticus, Streptococcus agalactinel, dysgalactial pneumonial/pyogenes, Treponema pallidum, Viridans Streptococci*

Unlabeled uses: Aspiration pneumonia, bone/joint infections, asthma, diabetes mellitus, dialysis, diarrhea, eczema, IBS, leukemia, pseudomembranous colitis, ulcerative colitis, hospital/community-acquired pneumonia, infective endocarditis, pelvic inflammatory disease

CONTRAINDICATIONS: Hypersensitivity to penicillins, sulbactam

Precautions: Pregnancy (B), breastfeeding, neonates, hypersensitivity to cephalosporins/carbapenems, renal disease, mononucleosis, viral infections, syphilis

DOSAGE AND ROUTES

- **Adult/adolescent/child ≥40 kg: IM/IV** 1.5-3 g q6hr, max 4 g/day sulbactam
- **Child ≤40 kg: IV** 150-300 mg/kg/day divided q6hr

Renal disease

- **Adult ≥40 kg: IM/IV** CCr 15-30 ml/min dose q12hr; CCr 5-15 ml/min dose q24hr

Community-acquired pneumonia (unlabeled)

- **Adult: IV** 3 g q12hr in combination × ≥5 days

Endocarditis (unlabeled)

- **Adult: IV** 12 g divided q8hr
- **Child: IV** 300 mg/kg/day divided q8hr

Pelvic inflammatory disease (unlabeled)

- **Adult/Adolescent: IV** 3 g q6hr in combination

Available forms: Powder for inj 1.5 g (1 g ampicillin, 0.5 g sulbactam), 3 g (2 g ampicillin, 1 g sulbactam), 15 g (10 g ampicillin, 5 g sulbactam)

Administer:

- Scratch test to assess allergy after securing order from prescriber; usually done when penicillin is only product choice
- Store at room temperature

IM route

- Reconstitute by adding 3.2 ml sterile water/1.5-g vial; 6.4 ml/3-g vial, give deep in large muscle, aspirate
- Do not use IM in child

Direct IV route

- After diluting 1.5 g/3.2 ml sterile water for inj or 3 g/6.4 ml (250 mg ampicillin/125 mg sulbactam), allow to stand until foaming stops; may give over 15 min, inject slowly

Intermittent IV INFUSION route

- Dilute further in 50 ml or more of D_5W, NaCl; administer within 1 hr after reconstitution; give over 15-30 min, separate doses from aminoglycosides by ≥1 hr

Y-site compatibilities: Alemtuzumab, amifostine, aminocaproic acid, anidulafungin, argatroban, atenolol, bivalirudin, bleomycin, CARBOplatin, carmustine, cefepime, CISplatin, codeine, cyclophosphamide, cytarabine, DAPTOmycin, DAUNOrubicin liposome, dexmedetomidine, DOCEtaxel, doxacurium, DOXOrubicin liposomal, eptifibatide, etoposide, fenoldopam, filgrastim, fludarabine, fluorouracil, foscarnet, gallium, gatifloxacin, gemcitabine, granisetron, hetastarch, irinotecan, levofloxacin, linezolid, methotrexate, metroNIDAZOLE, octreotide, oxaliplatin, PACLitaxel, palonosetron, pamidronate, pancuronium, pantoprazole, PEMEtrexed, remifentanil, riTUXimab, rocuronium, tacrolimus, teniposide, thiotepa, tigecycline, tirofiban, TNA, TPN, trastuzumab, vencuronium, vinCRIStine, voriconazole, zoledronic acid

SIDE EFFECTS

CNS: Lethargy, hallucinations, anxiety, depression, twitching, coma, seizures

GI: *Nausea, vomiting, diarrhea,* increased AST/ALT, abdominal pain, glossitis, colitis, pseudomembranous colitis, hepatic necrosis/failure, black hairy tongue

GU: Oliguria, proteinuria, hematuria, *vaginitis, moniliasis,* glomerulonephritis, dysuria

HEMA: Anemia, increased bleeding time, bone marrow depression, granulocytopenia, leukopenia, eosinophilia, hemolysis

INTEG: Injection site reactions, rash, edema, urticaria

MISC: Anaphylaxis, serum sickness, toxic epidermal necrolysis, Stevens-Johnson syndrome, hypoalbuminemia

PHARMACOKINETICS

IV: Peak 5 min, IM 1 hr; half-life 50-110 min, little metabolized in liver, 75%-85% of both products excreted in urine, diffuses to breast milk, crosses placenta

INTERACTIONS

Increase: bleeding risk—oral anticoagulants; check, INR, PT

Increase: ampicillin-induced skin rash—allopurinol, check for rash

Increase: ampicillin level—probenecid

Increase: methotrexate level—methotrexate

Drug/Lab Test

False positive: urine glucose, urine protein

NURSING CONSIDERATIONS

Assess:

- **Infection:** characteristics of wound, sputum; take temperature, WBC count; C&S before product therapy, product may be given as soon as culture is taken
- Bowel pattern before, during treatment
- I&O ratio; report hematuria, oliguria because penicillin in high doses is nephrotoxic

⚠ Any patient with compromised renal system, because product excreted slowly with poor renal system function; toxicity may occur rapidly

- Hepatic studies: AST, ALT if on long-term therapy
- Blood studies: WBC, RBC, Hct, Hgb, bleeding time
- Renal studies: urinalysis, protein, blood, BUN, creatinine

⚠ **Anaphylaxis:** skin eruptions after administration of ampicillin to 1 wk after discontinuing product

- Allergies before treatment; reaction to each medication; report allergies

Evaluate:

• Therapeutic response: absence of fever, draining wounds; negative C&S

Teach patient/family:

• To report superinfection: vaginal itching; loose, foul-smelling stools; black furry tongue

⚠ **Pseudomembranous colitis:** fever, diarrhea with pus, blood, mucus; may occur up to 4 wk after treatment; report immediately to health care provider

• To wear or carry emergency ID if allergic to penicillin products

TREATMENT OF ANAPHYLAXIS: Withdraw product, maintain airway; administer EPINEPHrine, aminophylline, O_2, IV corticosteroids

anakinra (Rx)

(an-ah-kin′rah)

Kineret

Func. class.: Antirheumatic (DMARD), immunomodulator

Chem. class.: Recombinant form of human interleukin-1 receptor antagonist (IL-1Ra)

Do not confuse:

Anakinra/amikacin

ACTION: A form of human interleukin-1 receptor antagonist (IL-1Ra) produced by DNA technology; blocks activity of IL-1, thereby resulting in decreased inflammation, cartilage degradation, bone resorption

USES: Reduction in signs and symptoms of moderate to severe active rheumatoid arthritis in patients ≥18 yr who have not responded to other disease-modifying agents, neonatal-onset multisystem inflammatory disease. **Unlabeled uses:** Cryopyrin-associated periodic syndromes

CONTRAINDICATIONS: Hypersensitivity to *Escherichia coli*–derived proteins, product, latex; sepsis

Precautions: Pregnancy (B), breastfeeding, children, geriatric patients, renal impairment, active infections, immunosuppression, neoplastic disease, asthma

DOSAGE AND ROUTES

Rheumatoid arthritis

• **Adult: SUBCUT** 100 mg/day

Renal dose

• **Adult:** CCr <30 ml/min **SUBCUT** 100 mg every other day

Neonatal-onset multisystem inflammatory disease

• **Adult/Child: SUBCUT** 1-2 mg/kg/day, may increase by 0.5-1 mg to max 8 mg/kg/day (adult) or 7.6 mg/kg/day (child)

Available form: Inj 100 mg/0.67 ml prefilled glass syringe

Administer:

SUBCUT route

• Do not use if cloudy, discolored, if particulate is present; protect from light

• Do not admix with other sol or medications; do not use filter; give at same time each day

• Apply cold compress before, after inj, allow sol to warm to room temperature before use

• Use middle thigh, abdomen (outside 2 inches from navel), upper outer buttocks, upper outer area of arm; rotate sites, give inj at least 1 inch from old site; do not give in skin that is bruised, red, tender, hard; remove needle cover immediately before use, pull gently back on plunger, if no blood appears, inject entire contents of prefilled syringe; discard any unused portion

SIDE EFFECTS

CNS: *Headache*

EENT: *Sinusitis*

GI: *Abdominal pain, nausea, diarrhea*

HEMA: Neutropenia

INTEG: Rash, *inj site reaction,* allergic reaction

MISC: Flulike symptoms, infection

MS: *Worsening of RA, arthralgia*

RESP: *URI*

PHARMACOKINETICS
Terminal half-life 4-6 hr; eliminated renally

INTERACTIONS
- Do not use rilonacept

Increase: risk for severe infection—TNF-blocking agents, do not use together
Decrease: antibody reactions—vaccines, avoid concurrent use

NURSING CONSIDERATIONS
Assess:
- **Rheumatoid arthritis:** pain, stiffness, ROM, swelling of joints, baseline, periodically during treatment
- For inj site pain, swelling; usually occurs after 2 inj (4-5 days)
- For infections (increased WBC, fever, flulike symptoms); stop treatment if present; do not start if patient has active infection
- CBC with differential, neutrophil counts before treatment, monthly × 3 mo, quarterly for up to 1 yr thereafter
- For allergic reactions (rash, dyspnea), discontinue if severe
- For urinary status: decreasing urinary output

Evaluate:
- Therapeutic response: decreased inflammation, pain in joints

Teach patient/family:
- Not to receive vaccines while taking this product; to update vaccines before treatment
- About self-administration, if appropriate: inj should be made in thigh, abdomen, upper arm; rotate sites at least 1 inch from old site; give at same time of day, store in refrigerator, do not freeze
- To notify prescriber if pregnancy is planned, suspected; to avoid breastfeeding; to notify prescriber of allergic reaction, decreasing urine output, signs/symptoms of infection

⚠ HIGH ALERT

anastrozole (Rx)
(an-a-stroh′zole)

Arimidex

Func. class.: Antineoplastic
Chem. class.: Aromatase inhibitor

ACTION: Highly selective nonsteroidal aromatase inhibitor that lowers serum estradiol concentrations; many breast cancers have strong estrogen receptors

USES: Advanced breast carcinoma in estrogen-receptor–positive patients (postmenopausal); patients with advanced disease taking tamoxifen, adjunct therapy
Unlabeled uses: Uterine leiomyomata, endometriosis

CONTRAINDICATIONS: Pregnancy (X), breastfeeding, hypersensitivity
Precautions: Children, geriatric patients, premenopausal women, osteoporosis, hepatic/cardiac disease

DOSAGE AND ROUTES
- **Adult: PO** 1 mg/day, max 5 yrs, may also combine with tamoxifen for up to 10 yrs

Available forms: Tabs 1 mg
Administer:
- Give without regard to meals at same time of day
- Store in light-resistant container at room temperature

SIDE EFFECTS
CNS: *Hot flashes, headache, lightheadedness,* depression, dizziness, confusion, insomnia, anxiety, fatigue, mood changes
CV: Chest pain, *hypertension,* thrombophlebitis, *edema,* angina, MI, cerebral infarct, CVA, *vasodilation*, PE, DVT
GI: *Nausea, vomiting,* altered taste leading to anorexia, diarrhea, constipation, abdominal pain, dry mouth, weight gain

GU: Vaginal bleeding, vaginal dryness, pelvic pain, pruritus vulvae, UTI
HEMA: Leukopenia, anemia
INTEG: *Rash,* Stevens-Johnson syndrome
MISC: Hypercholesterolemia
MS: Bone pain, myalgia, *asthenia,* bone loss/osteoporosis, arthralgia, fractures
RESP: Cough, sinusitis, dyspnea, pulmonary embolism

PHARMACOKINETICS

Peak 2 hr; half-life 50 hr; metabolized in liver, excreted in feces, urine, terminal half-life 50 hr

INTERACTIONS

• Do not use with oral contraceptives, estrogen, tamoxifen, androstenedione, DHEA

Drug/Lab Test

Increase: GGT, AST, ALT, alk phos, cholesterol, LDL

NURSING CONSIDERATIONS

Assess:

• Bone mineral density, cholesterol, lipid panel, periodically

⚠ **Serious skin reactions:** Stevens-Johnson syndrome

• Not effective in hormone-receptor–negative disease, use only in postmenopausal women

Evaluate:

• Therapeutic response: decreased tumor size, spread of malignancy

Teach patient/family:

• To report any complaints, side effects to prescriber

• That vaginal bleeding, pruritus, hot flashes reversible after discontinuing treatment

• To report continued vaginal bleeding immediately

• That **tumor flare**—increase in size of tumor, increased bone pain—may occur and will subside rapidly; may take analgesics for pain

• To take adequate calcium and vitamin D due to risk for bone loss/fractures

anidulafungin (Rx)

(a-nid-yoo-luh-fun′jin)

Eraxis

Func. class.: Antifungal, systemic
Chem. class.: Echinocandin

ACTION:

Inhibits fungal enzyme synthesis; causes direct damage to fungal cell wall

USES:

Esophageal candidiasis, *Candida albicans, C. glabrata, C. parapsilosis, C. tropicalis*

Unlabeled uses: Fungal prophylaxis, disseminated candidiasis, oropharyngeal candidiasis, *Aspergillosis* sp.

CONTRAINDICATIONS:

Hypersensitivity to product, other echinocandins

Precautions: Pregnancy (C), breastfeeding, children, severe hepatic disease

DOSAGE AND ROUTES

Candidemia and other *Candida* infections; serious systemic infections (unlabeled)

• **Adult: IV** 200 mg loading dose on day 1, then 100 mg/day × 14 days or more until last positive culture

Esophageal candidiasis

• **Adult: IV** 100 mg loading dose on day 1, then 50 mg/day × 14 days, for at least 7 days after symptoms resolved

Available forms: Powder for inj, lyophilized 50, 100 mg

Administer:

IV route

• Visually inspect prepared infusions for particulate matter and discoloration, do not use if present; give by IV infusion only, after dilution

• **Reconstitution:** Reconstitute each 50 mg or 100 mg vial/15 ml or 30 ml of sterile water for injection, respectively (3.33 mg/ml)

• **Storage:** Reconstituted solutions are stable for up to 24 hours at room temperature

• **Dilution:** Do not use any other diluents besides D_5W or sodium chloride 0.9% (NS)
• **Preparation of the 200 mg loading dose infusion:** Withdraw the contents of either four 50 mg reconstituted vials OR two 100 mg reconstituted vials and add to an IV infusion bag or bottle containing 200 ml of D_5W or NS to give a total infusion volume of 260 ml
• **Preparation of the 100 mg daily infusion:** Withdraw the contents of one 100 mg reconstituted vial OR two 50-mg reconstituted vials and add to an IV infusion bag or bottle containing 100 ml of D_5W or NS to give a total infusion volume of 130 ml
• **Preparation of a 50 mg daily infusion:** Withdraw the contents of one 50 mg reconstituted vial and add to an IV infusion bag or bottle containing 50 ml of D_5W or NS to give a total infusion volume of 65 ml
• **Storage:** Diluted solutions are stable for up to 48 hr at temperatures up to 77° F (25° C) or for 72 hours if stored frozen

Intermittent IV Infusion

• Do not mix or co-infuse with other medications
• Administer as a slow IV infusion at a rate of 1.4 ml/min or 84 ml/h; the minimum duration of infusion is 180 min for the 200 mg dose, 90 min for the 100 mg dose, and 45 min for the 50 mg dose
• Store reconstituted vials at 59° F-86° F for up to 24 hr, do not freeze (dehydrated alcohol); store reconstituted vials at 36° F-46° F (sterile water) for up to 24 hr, do not freeze

Y-site compatibilities: Acyclovir, alemtuzumab, alfentanil, allopurinol, amifostine, amikacin, aminocaproic acid, aminophylline, amiodarone, amphotericin B lipid complex, amphotericin B liposome, ampicillin, ampicillin sulbactam, argatroban, arsenic trioxide, atenolol, atracurium, azithromycin, aztreonam, bivalirudin, bleomycin, bumetanide, buprenorphine, busulfan, butorphanol, calcium chloride/gluconate, CARBOplatin, carmustine, caspofungin, ceFAZolin, cefepime, cefotaxime, cefoTEtan, cefOXitin, cefTAZidime, ceftizoxime, cefTRIAXone, cefuroxime, chloramphenicol, chlorproMAZINE, cimetidine, ciprofloxacin, cisatracurium, CISplatin, clindamycin, cyclophosphamide, cycloSPORINE, cytarabine, dacarbazine, DACTINomycin, DAUNOrubicin liposome, DAUNOrubicin hydrochloride, dexamethasone, dexmedetomidine, dexrazoxane, digoxin, diltiazem, diphenhydrAMINE, DOBUtamine, DOCEtaxel, dolasetron, DOPamine, doripenem, doxacurium, DOXOrubicin, DOXOrubicin liposomal, doxycycline, droperidol, enalaprilat, ePHEDrine, EPINEPHrine, epirubicin, eptifibatide, erythromycin, esmolol, etoposide, etoposide phosphate, famotidine, fenoldopam, fentaNYL, fluconazole, fludarabine, fluorouracil, foscarnet, fosphenytoin, furosemide, gallium nitrate, ganciclovir, gatifloxacin, gemcitabine, gentamicin, glycopyrrolate, granisetron, haloperidol, heparin, hydrALAZINE, hydrocortisone, HYDROmorphone, hydrOXYzine, IDArubicin, ifosfamide, imipenem-cilastatin, inamrinone, insulin (regular), irinotecan, isoproterenol, ketorolac, labetalol, leucovorin, levofloxacin, lidocaine, linezolid injection, LORazepam, mannitol, mechlorethamine, melphalan, meperidine, meropenem, mesna, metaraminol, methotrexate, methyldopate, methylPREDNISolone, metoclopramide, metoprolol, metroNIDAZOLE, midazolam, milrinone, mitoMYcin, mitoXANtrone, mivacurium, morphine, moxifloxacin, mycophenolate mofetil, nafcillin, naloxone, nesiritide, niCARdipine, nitroglycerin, nitroprusside, norepinephrine, octreotide, ondansetron, oxaliplatin, oxytocin, PACLitaxel, palonosetron, pamidronate, pancuronium, pantoprazole, PEMEtrexed, pentamidine, pentazocine, PENTobarbital, PHENobarbital, phentolamine, phenylephrine, piperacillin-tazobactam, polymyxin B, potassium acetate/chloride, procainamide, prochlorperazine, promethazine, propranolol, quiNIDine, quinupristin-dalfopristin, ranitidine, remifentanil, rocuronium, sodium acetate, streptozocin, succinylcholine, SUFentanil, sulfamethoxazole-trimethoprim, tacrolimus, teniposide, theophylline, thiopental, thiotepa, ticarcillin, ticarcillin-clavulanate, tirofiban, tobramycin, topotecan, trimethobenzamide, vancomycin, vasopressin, vecuronium, verapamil, vinBLAStine, vinCRIStine, vinorelbine, voriconazole, zidovudine, zoledronic acid

SIDE EFFECTS

Candidemia/other Candida infections

CNS: Seizures, dizziness, *headache*

CV: DVT, **atrial fibrillation, right bundle branch block,** hypotension, **sinus arrhythmia, thrombophlebitis superficial, ventricular extrasystoles, QT prolongation (rare)**

GI: *Nausea, anorexia, vomiting, diarrhea, increased AST, ALT*

META: Hypokalemia

Esophageal candidiasis

CNS: *Headache*

GI: *Nausea, anorexia, vomiting, diarrhea,* **hepatic necrosis**

HEMA: **Neutropenia, thrombocytopenia, leukopenia, coagulopathy**

INTEG: *Rash,* urticaria, itching, flushing

META: Hypocalcemia, hyperglycemia, hyperkalemia, hypernatremia, hypomagnesium (rare)

MS: *Back pain, rigors*

PHARMACOKINETICS

Steady state after loading dose, distribution half-life 0.5-1 hr, terminal half-life 40-50 hr, protein binding 99%

INTERACTIONS

Drug/Lab Test

Increase: amylase, bilirubin, CPK, creatinine, ECG, lipase, PT, alk phos

Decrease: platelets, magnesium, potassium, transferase, urea

NURSING CONSIDERATIONS

Assess:

• **Infection:** clearing of cultures during treatment; obtain culture at baseline and throughout treatment; product may be started as soon as culture is taken, those with HIV pharyngeal candidiasis may need antifungals

⚠ **Blood dyscrasias (rare): CBC (RBC, Hct, Hgb), differential, platelet count periodically; notify prescriber of results**

• Hepatic studies before, during treatment: bilirubin, AST, ALT, alk phos, as needed; also uric acid

⚠ **Bleeding: hematuria, heme-positive stools, bruising/petechiae of mucosa or orifices; blood dyscrasias can occur**

• GI symptoms: frequency of stools, cramping; if severe diarrhea occurs, electrolytes may need to be given

Evaluate:

• Therapeutic response: decreased symptoms of *Candida* infection, negative culture

Teach patient/family:

• To notify prescriber if pregnancy is suspected, planned; use nonhormonal form of contraception while taking this product

• To avoid breastfeeding while taking this product

• To inform prescriber of renal/hepatic disease

• To report bleeding

• To report signs of infection: increased temperature, sore throat, flulike symptoms

• To notify prescriber of nausea, vomiting, diarrhea, jaundice, anorexia, clay-colored stools, dark urine; hepatotoxicity may occur

RARELY USED

antihemophilic factor Fc fusion protein

(an-tee-hee-moe-fil′ik fak′tor)

Eloctate

Func. class.: Hemostatic

USES: Hemophilia A (congenital factor VIII deficiency), control/prevention of bleeding, perioperative management of surgical bleeding

DOSAGE AND ROUTES

Hemophilia A (congenital factor VIII deficiency)

• **Adults, adolescents, children, infants, and neonates: IV INFUSION** Infuse dose ≤10 ml/min; Dose (IU) = body weight (kg) × desired factor VIII increase (IU/dl or % of normal) × 0.5 (IU/kg per IU/dl) *OR* estimated increment of factor VIII (IU/dl or % of normal) = [total dose (IU)/body weight (kg)] × 2 (IU/dl per IU/kg)

Control/prevention of bleeding

• **Adults, adolescents, children, infants, and neonates:** Dose and duration of treatment depend on the severity of the factor VIII deficiency, the location and extent of bleeding, and the patient's clinical condition

Perioperative management of surgical bleeding

• **Adults, adolescents, children, infants, and neonates:** Dose and duration of treatment depend on the severity of the factor VIII deficiency, the location and extent of bleeding, and the patient's clinical condition

Routine bleeding prophylaxis to prevent/reduce the frequency of bleeding episodes: IV Initially, 50 IU/kg q4days; adjust dose based on response

antithymocyte

See lymphocyte immune globulin

⚠ HIGH ALERT

apixaban

a-pix'-a-ban

Eliquis

Func. class.: Anticoagulant

Chem. class: Factor Xa inhibitor

ACTION: Inhibits factor Xa and thereby decreases thrombin and clot formation

USES: Deep venous thrombosis (DVT) after hip or knee replacement, to prevent stroke and embolism in atrial fibrillation (nonvalvular)

CONTRAINDICATIONS: Hypersensitivity, active bleeding

Precautions: Breastfeeding, dialysis, hepatic/renal disease, labor, pregnancy, surgery, prosthetic heart valves

Black Box Warning: Abrupt discontinuation, epidural, spinal anesthesia, lumbar puncture

DOSAGE AND ROUTES

DVT or pulmonary embolism (PE)

• **Adults: PO** 10 mg bid × 7 days, then 5 mg bid ≥6 mo

Stroke prophylaxis and systemic embolism prophylaxis in patients with nonvalvular atrial fibrillation

• **Adults: PO** 5 mg bid; in those with any 2 of the following: age ≥ 80 years; body weight ≤ 60 kg; or serum creatinine ≥ 1.5 mg/dL, reduce the dose to 2.5 mg bid. Also decrease the dose to 2.5 mg bid (strong inhibitor of both CYP3A4 and P-glycoprotein)

Reduction in risk of recurrent DVT and/or PE after completion of treatment for acute DVT or PE

• **Adults:** 2.5 mg bid daily after at least 6 months of treatment for DVT or PE

DVT prophylaxis and PE prophylaxis in patients undergoing knee or hip replacement surgery

• **Adults:** 2.5 mg bid × 12 days after knee replacement surgery or for 35 days after hip replacement surgery. Give initial dose 12-24 hr after surgery

Renal dose: nonvalvular atrial fibrillation

• No dosage adjustment needed when used for treatment/prevention of venous thromboembolism. **Adult: PO** serum CCr ≥ 1.5 mg/dL: ≤60 kg and/or are ≥80 yr, then decrease dose to 2.5 mg bid

Hemodialysis end-stage renal disease maintained on hemodialysis
• 5 mg bid reduce, to 2.5 mg bid if patient is ≥80 yr or ≤60 kg
Available forms: Tabs 2.5, 5 mg
Administer:
• May be taken without regard to food
• If unable to swallow whole, may crush and suspend the tablet in 60 ml 5% dextrose solution; give immediately via NG
• If a dose is missed, it should be taken as soon as possible on the same day. Twice daily dosing should be resumed. Do not double the dose to make up for a missed dose.

SIDE EFFECTS

CNS: Syncope, intracranial bleeding
CV: Hypotension
HEMA: Severe bleeding
INTEG: Rash
MISC: Hypersensitivity

PHARMACOKINETICS

Peak 3-4 hr, half-life 12 hr

INTERACTIONS

Increase: bleeding risk—antiplatelets, other anticoagulants, salicylates, NSAIDs, SNRIs, SSRIs, thrombolytics, avoid concurrent use
Decrease: apixaban effect—strong inducers of CYP3A4 and also P-glycoprotein (carbamazepine, ketoconazole, itraconazole, phenytoin, rifampin), use lower dose
Drug/Herb
Decrease: apixaban effect—St. John's Wort, avoid concurrent use
Drug/Lab Test
Increase: PT, PTT, INR, coagulation studies

NURSING CONSIDERATIONS

Assess:

Black Box Warning: **Bleeding:** bleeding may occur from any body system, may be fatal if severe

Neurological status: monitor for impairment, including numbness, paresthesia, weakness, confusion, back pain, bowel/bladder impairment, notify prescriber immediately

Black Box Warning: **Abrupt discontinuation:** do not discontinue abruptly, if bleeding occurs, consider using another anticoagulant to prevent thromboembolic events

Black Box Warning: **Epidural, spinal anesthesia, lumbar puncture:** avoid use in these conditions, risk of hematoma and permanent paralysis, may be increased with use of other anticoagulants, thrombolytics, antiplatelets

Hypersensitivity: rash, itching, chills, fever, report to prescriber
Evaluate:
Therapeutic response: prevention/treatment of DVT, adequate anticoagulation
Teach Patient/Family:
• To avoid breastfeeding, it is not known if the product appears in breast milk, to notify prescriber if pregnancy is planned or suspected

Black Box Warning: Not to discontinue without prescriber approval

Black Box Warning: Bleeding: to report bleeding, bruising, confusion, weakness, numbness of limbs

• To avoid OTC products, supplements, herbs, unless approved by prescriber, serious product interactions may occur
• To carry emergency ID with product taken
• To report hypersensitivity reactions: rash, chills, fever, itching

RARELY USED

apomorphine

(ah-poe-more′feen)

Apokyn

Func. class.: Antiparkinson agent

Chem. class.: Dopamine agonist, non-ergot

USES: For use as rescue of "off" episodes associated with advanced Parkinson's disease

CONTRAINDICATIONS: Hypersensitivity to this product, sulfites, or benzyl alcohol, IV use, major psychotic disorder; concurrent treatment with drugs of the 5-HT_3 antagonist class (e.g., ondansetron, granisetron, alosetron)

DOSAGE AND ROUTES

- **Adult: Test dose: SUBCUT** 0.2 ml (2 mg) (test dose) where B/P can be closely monitored (before dose and 20, 40, 60 min after); if tolerated and patient response, then begin with 0.2 ml (2 mg); may increase by 1 mg every few days, max 0.6 ml (6 mg); if the test dose of 0.2 ml (2 mg) is tolerated but the patient does not respond, give a test dose of 0.4 ml (4 mg) no sooner than 2 hr after the 0.2 ml (2 mg) test dose, where BP can be closely monitored (before dose and 20, 40, and 60 min after the dose); if the 0.4 ml (4 mg) test dose is tolerated, the starting dose should be 0.3 ml (3 mg); may be increased by 1 mg every few days as required, max 0.6 ml (6 mg). If the 0.4 ml (4 mg) test dose is not tolerated, administer a test dose of 0.3 ml (3 mg) no sooner than 2 hr after the 0.4 ml (4 mg) test dose where BP can be closely monitored (before dose and 20, 40, and 60 min after the dose); if the 0.3 ml (3 mg) test dose is tolerated, begin with 0.2 ml (2 mg); may be increased by 0.1 ml (1 mg) every few days as required, max 0.4 ml (4 mg; outpatient)
- **Usual dosage:** 0.3-0.6 ml (3-6 mg), average frequency three times a day

apraclonidine ophthalmic

See Appendix B

apremilast

(a-pre′mi-last)

Otezla

Func. class.: Musculoskeletal agents: disease-modifying antirheumatic drugs (DMARDs)

ACTION: A phosphodiesterase-4 (PDE4) inhibitor specific for cyclic adenosine monophosphate (cAMP). Inhibition of PDE4 results in an increase in intracellular concentration of cAMP, with a partial inhibition of proinflammatory mediators and an increase in the production of some antiinflammatory mediators

USES: Treatment of active psoriatic arthritis; severe plaque psoriasis (in those not a candidate for phototherapy)

CONTRAINDICATIONS: Hypersensitivity

Precautions: Pregnancy (C), breastfeeding, depression/suicidal, renal disease (CrCl <30 ml/min)

SIDE EFFECTS

CNS: *Headache,* depression, suicidal ideation, fatigue, insomnia

GI: Diarrhea, nausea, vomiting, abdominal pain, frequent bowel movements, dyspepsia, weight loss

RESP: URI, pharyngitis, bronchitis

SYST: Hypersensitivity reactions

MS: Back pain

PHARMACOKINETICS

68% bound to plasma proteins; metabolized by CYP3A4, half-life is 6-9 hr; elimination in urine (58%), feces (39%); peak 2.5 hr

DOSAGES AND ROUTES

Treatment of active psoriatic arthritis/severe plaque psoriasis

• **Adults: PO** To reduce the risk for gastrointestinal symptoms, titrate to a final dose of 30 mg bid; day 1: 10 mg PO AM; day 2: 10 mg AM and PM; day 3: 10 mg AM and 20 mg PM; day 4: 20 mg AM and PM; day 5: 20 mg AM and 30 mg PM; day 6 and thereafter: 30 mg bid

Renal dose

• **Adult: PO** CrCl ≥ 30 ml/min: no change; CrCl < 30 ml/min: 30 mg every day. Initially, 10 mg AM days 1-3; 20 mg AM days 4 and 5; 30 mg every day for day 6 and thereafter

Available forms: Tab 30 mg; starter pack

INTERACTIONS

Decreased: apremilast—CYP3A4 inducers (rifampin, isoniazid, pyrazinamide, barbiturates, phenytoin, carbamazepine, enzalutamide), avoid concurrent use

Drug/Herb

Decreased: apremilast—CYP3A4 inducers (St. John's wort), avoid concurrent use

NURSING CONSIDERATIONS

Assess:

• **Psoriatic arthritis/severe plaque psoriasis:** assess for hypersensitivity reactions

• **Pregnancy and breastfeeding:** if used during pregnancy, call 1-877-311-8972; avoid use in breastfeeding

• For depression and suicidal ideation, mood changes; for renal failure or severe renal impairment (CrCl <30 ml/min), dosage reduction is required

Administer:

• Give whole, do not crush, break, or chew; give without regard to meals

Evaluate:

• Therapeutic response: resolution of symptoms of psoriatic arthritis or plaque psoriasis

Teach patient/family:

• To report rash, hypersensitivity reactions

• To avoid use in pregnancy and breastfeeding; if used during pregnancy, call 1-877-311-8972

• To be alert for depression and suicidal ideation, mood changes; if these occur, notify prescriber immediately

aprepitant (Rx)

(ap-re′pi-tant)

Emend

fosaprepitant

Emend

Func. class.: Antiemetic

Chem. class.: Miscellaneous

Do not confuse:

aprepitant/fosaprepitant

ACTION: Selective antagonist of human substance P/neurokinin 1 (NK_1) receptors that decreases emetic reflex

USES: Prevention of nausea/vomiting associated with cancer chemotherapy (highly emetogenic/moderately emetogenic), including high-dose CISplatin; used in combination with other antiemetics; postoperative nausea/vomiting

CONTRAINDICATIONS: Hypersensitivity to this product, polysorbate 80

Precautions: Pregnancy (B), breastfeeding, children, geriatric patients, hepatic disease

DOSAGE AND ROUTES

Prevention of nausea/vomiting after chemotherapy

• **Adult: PO** Day 1 (1 hr before chemotherapy) aprepitant 125 mg with 12 mg dexamethasone **PO,** with 32 mg ondansetron IV; day 2 aprepitant 80 mg with 8 mg dexamethasone **PO;** day 3 aprepitant 80 mg with 8 mg dexamethasone **PO;** day 4 only dexamethasone 8 mg **PO;** **IV INFUSION** 115 mg over 15 min,

30 min before chemotherapy as alternative to 1st dose of aprepitant on day 1 of regimen (fosaprepitant)

Prevention of postoperative nausea/vomiting

- **Adult: PO** 40 mg within 3 hr of induction of anesthesia

Available forms: Caps 40, 80, 125 mg; powder for inj 150 mg; combo pack cap 80-125 mg

Administer:

PO route

- Do not break, crush, or chew
- PO on 3-day schedule, give with full glass of water 1 hr before chemotherapy, with or without food, given with other antiemetics
- Store at room temperature; keep in original bottles, blisters

Intermittent IV INFUSION route

- Only approved as a substitute for the 1st dose of aprepitant in 3-day regimen
- **Reconstitution:** use aseptic technique; inject 5 ml 0.9% NaCl into the vial, directing stream to wall of vial to prevent foam; swirl (do not shake)
- Prepare infusion bag 145 ml/150 mg; do not dilute, reconstitute with any divalent cations such as calcium, magnesium, including LR, Hartmann's sol
- Withdraw entire volume from vial, transfer to infusion bag; total volume 115 ml (1 mg/1 ml)
- Gently invert bag 2-3 times; reconstituted sol stable for 24 hr at lower room temperature or <25° C
- Visually inspect for particulates, discoloration
- Infuse over 20-30 min, stable for 24 hr at room temperature

SIDE EFFECTS

CNS: *Headache, dizziness,* insomnia, anxiety, depression, confusion, peripheral neuropathy

CV: Bradycardia, tachycardia, DVT, hypo/hypertension

GI: *Diarrhea, constipation,* abdominal pain, anorexia, gastritis, increased AST, ALT, *nausea,* vomiting, heartburn

GU: Increased BUN, serum creatinine, proteinuria, dysuria

HEMA: Anemia, thrombocytopenia, neutropenia

INTEG: Pruritus, rash, urticaria, infection reaction

MISC: Asthenia, fatigue, dehydration, fever, hiccups, tinnitus, alopecia

SYST: Anaphylaxis

PHARMACOKINETICS

Absorption 60%-65%, peak 4 hr, metabolized in liver by CYP3A4 enzymes to active metabolite, half-life 9-12 hr, 95% protein bound, not excreted in kidneys, crosses blood-brain barrier

INTERACTIONS

Increase: aprepitant action—CYP3A4 inhibitors (ketoconazole, itraconazole, nefazodone, troleandomycin, clarithromycin, ritonavir, nelfinavir, diltiazem)

Increase: action of CYP3A4 substrates (pimozide, cisapride, dexamethasone, methylPREDNISolone, midazolam, ALPRAZolam, triazolam, DOCEtaxel, PACLitaxel, etoposide, irinotecan, imatinib, ifosfamide, vinorelbine, vinBLAStine, vinCRIStine)

Decrease: aprepitant action—CYP3A4 inducers (rifampin, carBAMazepine, phenytoin)

Decrease: action of CYP2C9 substrates (warfarin, TOLBUTamide, phenytoin), oral contraceptives

Decrease: action of both products—PARoxetine

Drug/Food

Decrease: effect—grapefruit juice

NURSING CONSIDERATIONS

Assess:

⚠ **For hypersensitive reactions:** pruritus, rash, urticaria, anaphylaxis

- CV status: hypo/hypertension, bradycardia, tachycardia, DVT
- For absence of nausea, vomiting during chemotherapy
- CBC, LFTs, creatinine baseline and periodically

Evaluate:
- Therapeutic response: absence of nausea, vomiting during cancer chemotherapy

Teach patient/family:
- To report diarrhea, constipation
- To take only as prescribed; to take 1st dose 1 hr before chemotherapy
- To report all medications and herbals to prescriber before taking this medication
- To use nonhormonal form of contraception while taking this agent and for 1 mo thereafter; oral contraceptive effect may be decreased
- That those patients also taking warfarin should have clotting monitored closely during 2-wk period after administration of aprepitant
- To avoid breastfeeding

arformoterol (Rx)
(ar-for-moe′ter-ole)
Brovana
Func. class.: Long-acting adrenergic β_2-agonist, sympathomimetic, bronchodilator

Do not confuse:
Brovana/Boniva

ACTION: Causes bronchodilation by action on β_2 (pulmonary) receptors by increasing levels of cAMP, which relaxes smooth muscle; produces bronchodilation and CNS, cardiac stimulation as well as increased diuresis and gastric acid secretion; longer acting than isoproterenol

USES: Maintenance bronchospasm prevention in COPD, including chronic bronchitis, emphysema

CONTRAINDICATIONS: Hypersensitivity to sympathomimetics, product, racemic formoterol; tachydysrhyhmias, severe cardiac disease, heart block, children, monotherapy in asthma

Precautions: Pregnancy (C), breastfeeding, cardiac disorders, hyperthyroidism, diabetes mellitus, hypertension, prostatic hypertrophy, angle-closure glaucoma, seizures, hypoglycemia

Black Box Warning: Asthma-related death

DOSAGE AND ROUTES
COPD
- **Adult: NEB** 15 mcg, bid, AM, PM

Available forms: Inh sol 15 mcg/2 ml

Administer:
- By nebulization only; no dilution needed; give over 5-10 min; sol should be colorless
- Store in refrigerator; if stored at room temperature, discard after 6 wk or if past expiration date, whichever is sooner

SIDE EFFECTS
CNS: *Tremors, anxiety,* insomnia, headache, dizziness, stimulation, *restlessness,* hallucinations, flushing, irritability

CV: Palpitations, tachycardia, hypertension, angina, hypotension, dysrhythmias, **AV block, heart failure, prolonged QT, supraventricular tachycardia**

EENT: Dry nose, irritation of nose, throat

GI: Heartburn, nausea, vomiting

MISC: Flushing, sweating, anorexia, bad taste/smell changes, hypokalemia, **anaphylaxis,** ***hypoglycemia***

MS: Muscle cramps, back pain

RESP: Cough, wheezing, dyspnea, **bronchospasm,** dry throat

PHARMACOKINETICS
Onset rapid; peak 1-1½ hr; duration 4-6 hr; terminal half-life (COPD) 26 hr; extensively metabolized by direct conjugation by CYP2D6, CYP2C19; crosses placenta; protein binding 52%-65%; excreted in urine 63%, feces 11%

INTERACTIONS
Increase: **QT prolongation—Class IA/III antidysrthymics, MAOIs, tricyclics**

Increase: severe hypotension—oxytocics

Increase: toxicity—theophylline

Increase: ECG changes/hypokalemia—potassium-losing diuretics

Increase: action of nebulized bronchodilators

Increase: action of arformoterol—tricyclics, MAOIs, other adrenergics; do not use together

Decrease: arformoterol action, asthma-related death—other β-blockers

Drug/Herb

Increase: stimulation—caffeine (cola nut, green/black tea, guarana, yerba maté, coffee, chocolate)

NURSING CONSIDERATIONS

Assess:

Black Box Warning: Respiratory function: vital capacity, forced expiratory volume, ABGs; lung sounds, heart rate, rhythm, B/P, sputum (baseline, peak); actively deteriorating COPD may occur; a rescue inhaler should be readily available

- Whether patient has received theophylline therapy, other bronchodilators before giving dose
- Patient's ability to self-medicate
- For evidence of allergic reactions
- For **paradoxical bronchospasm;** hold medication, notify prescriber if bronchospasm occurs

Evaluate:

- Therapeutic response: absence of dyspnea, wheezing after 1 hr, improved airway exchange, improved ABGs

Teach patient/family:

Black Box Warning: To use exactly as prescribed; that death has resulted from asthma with products similar to this one; to have a rescue inhaler always

- Not to use OTC medications because excess stimulation may occur
- That an opened unit-dose vial should be used right away
- To notify prescriber if there is more frequent use needed

⚠ HIGH ALERT

argatroban (Rx)

(are-ga-troe′ban)

Func. class.: Anticoagulant

Chem. class.: Thrombin inhibitor

Do not confuse:

argatroban/Aggrastat

ACTION: Direct inhibitor of thrombin, it reversibly binds to thrombin active site

USES: Anticoagulation prevention/treatment of thrombosis in heparin-induced thrombocytopenia; adjunct to percutaneous coronary intervention (PCI) in those with history of HIT, deep vein thrombosis, pulmonary embolism

Unlabeled uses: Acute MI, DIC, use in infants/children/adolescents

CONTRAINDICATIONS: Hypersensitivity, overt major bleeding

Precautions: Pregnancy (C), breastfeeding, children, intracranial bleeding, renal function impairment, hepatic disease, severe hypertension, after lumbar puncture, spinal anesthesia, major surgery/trauma, congenital/acquired bleeding, GI ulcers, abrupt discontinuation

DOSAGE AND ROUTES

DVT, Pulmonary Embolism

- **Adult: CONT IV INFUSION** 2 mcg/kg/min; adjust dose until steady-state aPTT is 1.5-3× initial baseline, max 100 sec, max dose 10 mcg/kg/min
- **Infant/child/adolescent (unlabeled): CONT IV INFUSION** 0.75 mcg/kg/min, monitor aPTT q2hr until stable, then at least daily

Hepatic dose

- **Adult: CONT INFUSION** 0.5 mcg/kg/min, adjust rate based on aPTT

Percutaneous coronary intervention (PCI) in HIT

- **Adult: IV INFUSION** 25 mcg/kg/min and bolus of 350 mcg/kg given over 3-5 min, check ACT 5-10 min after bolus completed, proceed if ACT >300 sec; if ACT <300 sec, give another 150 mcg/kg BOL, increase infusion rate to 30 mcg/kg/min, recheck ACT in 5-10 min; if ACT >450 sec, decrease infusion rate to 15 mcg/kg/min, recheck ACT in 5-10 min; when ACT is therapeutic, continue for duration of procedure

Acute MI (unlabeled)

- **Adult: IV** loading dose of 100 mcg/kg over 1 min, then 1-3 mcg/kg/min

DIC (unlabeled)

- **Adult: CONT IV** 0.7 mcg/kg/min

Available forms: Inj 100 mg/ml (2.5 ml; must dilute 100-fold), 50 mg/50 ml, 125 mg/125 ml

Administer:

- Avoid all IM inj that may cause bleeding

IV, direct route

- **For PCI:** 350 mg/kg bol and continuous infusion of 25 mcg/kg/min; check ACT 5-10 min after bolus

Intermittent IV INFUSION route

- **Dilute** in 0.9% NaCl, D_5W, LR to a final concentrations of 1 mg/ml; **dilute** each 2.5-ml vial 100-fold by mixing with 250 ml of diluent, mix by repeated inversion of the diluent bag for 1 min; may briefly be slightly hazy
- Dosage adjustment may be made after review of aPTT, max 10 mcg/kg/min

SIDE EFFECTS

CNS: *Fever,* intracranial bleeding, headache

CV: Atrial fibrillation, coronary thrombosis, MI, myocardial ischemia, coronary occlusion, ventricular tachycardia, bradycardia, *chest pain, hypotension*

GI: *Nausea, vomiting, abdominal pain, diarrhea,* GI bleeding

GU: Hematuria, abnormal kidney function, UTI

HEMA: Hemorrhage

MISC: *Back pain,* infection

RESP: Dyspnea, coughing, hemoptysis, pulmonary edema

SYST: Sepsis

PHARMACOKINETICS

Metabolized in liver, distributed to extracellular fluid, 54% plasma protein binding, half-life 39-51 min, excreted in feces, steady state 1-3 hr

INTERACTIONS

Increase: bleeding risk—antiplatelets, NSAIDs, salicylates, dipyridamole, clopidogrel, ticlopidine, heparin, warfarin, glycoprotein IIb/IIIa antagonists (abciximab, tirofiban, eptifibatide), thrombolytics (alteplase, reteplase, urokinase, tenecteplase), other anticoagulants

Drug/Herb

Increase: bleeding risk—ginger, garlic, ginkgo, horse chestnut

Drug/Lab

Decrease: Hgb/Hct

NURSING CONSIDERATIONS

Assess:

- Baseline aPTT before treatment; do not start treatment if aPTT ratio is ≥2.5; then check aPTT 2 hr after initiation of treatment and at least daily thereafter
- aPTT, which should be 1.5-3× control, draw blood for ACT every 20-30 min during long PCI

⚠ **Bleeding:** gums; petechiae; ecchymosis; black, tarry stools; hematuria/epistaxis; decreased B/P, Hct; vaginal bleeding, possible hemorrhage

⚠ **Anaphylaxis:** dyspnea, rash during treatment

- Fever, skin rash, urticaria

Evaluate:

- Therapeutic response: absence or decrease of thrombosis

Teach patient/family:

- To use a soft-bristle toothbrush to avoid bleeding gums; avoid contact sports; use electric razor; avoid IM inj
- To report any signs of bleeding: gums, under skin, urine, stools; trouble breathing wheezing, skin rash
- To notify prescriber if planning to become pregnant, breastfeeding
- Not to use OTC meds, herbal products unless approved by prescriber

ARIPiprazole (Rx)

(a-rip-ip-pra′zol)

Abilify, Abilify Discmelt, Abilify Maintena

Func. class.: Antipsychotic

Chem. class.: Quinolinone

ACTION: Exact mechanism unknown; may be mediated through both DOPamine type 2 (D_2, D_3) and serotonin type 2 ($5\text{-}HT_{1A}$, $5\text{-}HT_{2A}$) antagonism, DOPamine System Stabilizer

USES: Schizophrenia and bipolar disorder (adults and adolescents), mania, major depressive disorder, short-term mania or mixed episodes of bipolar disorder; irritability in patients with autism

CONTRAINDICATIONS: Breastfeeding, hypersensitivity, seizure disorders

Precautions: Pregnancy (C), geriatric patients, renal/hepatic/cardiac disease, neutropenia

Black Box Warning: Children with depression, dementia, suicidal ideation

DOSAGE AND ROUTES

Major depressive disorder

- **Adult: PO** 2-5 mg/day as an adjunct to other antidepressant treatment; adjust by 5 mg at ≥1 wk (range, 2-15 mg/day)

Schizophrenia

- **Adult: PO** 10-15 mg/day; if needed, dosage may be increased to 30 mg/day after 2 wk; maintenance 15 mg/day; periodically reassess; IM/ext rel monthly inj susp) 400 mg monthly
- **Adolescent 13-17 yr: PO** 2 mg/day, may increase to 5 mg after 2 days, then 10 mg after 2 more days, max 30 mg/day

Bipolar disorder

- **Adult: PO** 15 mg/day, may increase to 30 mg if needed (monotherapy); adjunctive to lithium or valproate PO 10-15 mg daily, may increase to 30 mg if needed
- **Child >10 yr, adolescents: PO** 2 mg, titrate to 5 mg/day after 2 days to target of 10 mg/day after another 2 days

Agitation with bipolar disorder/ schizophrenia

- **Adult: IM** 9.75 mg as a single dose, may start with a lower dose, max 30 mg/day

Irritability associated with autism

- **Child ≥6 yr, adolescents: PO** 2 mg/day, increase to 5 mg/day after 1 wk, may increase to 10-15 mg/day if needed; dose changes should not occur more frequently than q1wk

Potential CYP2D6 inhibitor, strong CYP3A4 inhibitors

- **Adult: PO** Reduce to 50% of usual dose; increase dose when CYP2D6, CYP3A4 inhibitor withdrawn

Combination of strong CYP3A4/ CYP2D6 inhibitors

- **Adult: PO** reduce to 25% of usual dose

Available forms: Tabs 2, 5, 10, 15, 20, 30 mg; inj 9.75 mg/1.3 ml; orally disintegrating tab 10, 15 mg; oral sol 1 mg/ml; susp for injection 441mg/1.6ml, 662mg/2.4ml, 882mg/3.2ml;

Administer:

PO route

- Store in tight, light-resistant container
- May be given without regard to meals
- **Orally disintegrating tabs;** do not open blister until ready to use, do not push tab through foil; place on tongue, allow to dissolve, swallow, do not divide
- **Oral liquid:** use calibrated measuring device
- **Oral solution:** can be substituted for tablet on a mg-per-mg, up to 25-mg dose. Patients receiving 30-mg tablets should receive 25 mg, immediate release of solution

IM route

- Give IM only; inject slowly, deeply into muscle mass; discard unused portion; do not give IV or subcut
- Available as ready to use
- Ext rel monthly (Abilify Maintena)

SIDE EFFECTS

CNS: *Drowsiness, insomnia, agitation, anxiety, headache,* seizures, neuroleptic malignant syndrome, *light-headedness, akathisia, asthenia, tremor,* stroke, suicidal ideation, dystonia, cogwheel rigidity

CV: Orthostatic hypotension, tachycardia, chest pain, hypertension, peripheral edema
EENT: *Blurred vision, rhinitis*
GI: *Constipation, nausea, vomiting,* jaundice, *weight gain*
INTEG: *Rash*
META: Hyperglycemia, dyslipidemia
MS: Musculoskeletal pain/stiffness, myalgia
RESP: *Cough*
SYST: Death among geriatric patients with dementia

PHARMACOKINETICS

PO: Absorption 87%; extensively metabolized by liver to a major active metabolite; plasma protein binding >99%; terminal half-life 75-146 hr; excretion via urine 25%, feces 55%; clearance decreased in geriatric patients

INTERACTIONS

Increase: effects of ARIPiprazole—CYP3A4 inhibitors (ketoconazole, erythromycin), CYP2D6 inhibitors (quiNIDine, FLUoxetine, PARoxetine); reduce dose of ARIPiprazole
Increase: sedation—other CNS depressants, alcohol
Increase: EPS—other antipsychotics, lithium
Decrease: ARIPiprazole level—famotidine, valproate
Decrease: effects of ARIPiprazole—CYP3A4 inducers (carBAMazepine)

Drug/Herb
Decrease: ARIPiprazole effect—St. John's wort

Drug/Lab
False positive: amphetephine drug screen

NURSING CONSIDERATIONS

Assess:

Black Box Warning: Mental status before initial administration, children/young adults may exhibit suicidal thoughts/behaviors, therefore smallest amount of product should be given; elderly patients with dementia-related psychosis are at increased risk of death

- Swallowing of PO medication; check for hoarding, giving of medication to other patients
- I&O ratio; palpate bladder if urinary output is low
- AIMS assessment, neurologic function, LFTs, weight, lipid profile, blood glucose monthly
- Affect, orientation, LOC, reflexes, gait, coordination, sleep pattern disturbances
- B/P standing and lying; also pulse, respirations; take q4hr during initial treatment; establish baseline before starting treatment; report drops of 30 mm Hg; watch for ECG changes
- Dizziness, faintness, palpitations, tachycardia on rising
- **EPS,** including akathisia (inability to sit still, no pattern to movements), tardive dyskinesia (bizarre movements of the jaw, mouth, tongue, extremities), pseudoparkinsonism (rigidity, tremors, pill rolling, shuffling gait)

⚠ **Neuroleptic malignant syndrome:** hyperthermia, increased CPK, altered mental status, muscle rigidity; notify prescriber immediately

- Constipation, urinary retention daily; if these occur, increase bulk, water in diet; stool softeners, laxatives may be needed
- Supervised ambulation until patient is stabilized on medication; do not involve patient in strenuous exercise program because fainting is possible; patient should not stand still for a long time

Evaluate:

- Therapeutic response: decrease in emotional excitement, hallucinations, delusions, paranoia; reorganization of patterns of thought, speech

Teach patient/family:

- That orthostatic hypotension may occur; to rise from sitting or lying position gradually
- To avoid hot tubs, hot showers, tub baths; hypotension may occur
- To avoid abrupt withdrawal of this product; EPS may result; product should be withdrawn slowly

- To avoid OTC preparations (cough, hay fever, cold) unless approved by prescriber because serious product interactions may occur; to avoid use with alcohol, CNS depressants because increased drowsiness may occur
- To avoid hazardous activities if drowsy, dizzy
- About compliance with product regimen
- To report impaired vision, tremors, muscle twitching, urinary retention
- That heat stroke may occur in hot weather; to take extra precautions to stay cool
- To notify prescriber if pregnant or intending to become pregnant; not to breastfeed

Black Box Warning: To report suicidal thoughts/behaviors, dementia immediately

TREATMENT OF OVERDOSE:
Lavage if orally ingested; provide airway; *do not induce vomiting*

RARELY USED

armodafinil (Rx)
(ar-moe-daf′in-il)

Nuvigil

Controlled Substance Schedule IV

USES: Narcolepsy, obstructive sleep apnea/hypoapnea syndrome, circadian rhythm disruption (shift-work sleep problems)

CONTRAINDICATIONS: Hypersensitivity to this product or modafinil

DOSAGE AND ROUTES
Narcolepsy, obstructive sleep apnea/hypoapnea syndrome
- **Adult and adolescent ≥17 yr: PO** 150-250 mg in AM

Circadian rhythm disruption (shift work sleep problems)
- **Adult and adolescent ≥17 yr: PO** 150 mg at start of shift

asenapine (Rx)
(a-sen′a-peen)

Saphris

Func. class.: Antipsychotic, atypical

Chem. class.: Dibenzapine

ACTION: Unknown; may be mediated through both DOPamine type 2 (D2) and serotonin type 2 (5-HT2A) antagonism

USES: Bipolar 1 disorder, schizophrenia

Unlabeled uses: Agitation

CONTRAINDICATIONS: Breastfeeding, hypersensitivity

Precautions: Pregnancy (C), children, geriatric patients, cardiac/renal/hepatic disease, breast cancer, Parkinson's disease, dementia, seizure disorder, CNS depression, agranulocytosis, QT prolongation, torsades de pointes, suicidal ideation, substance abuse, diabetes mellitus

Black Box Warning: Increased mortality in elderly patients with dementia-related psychosis

DOSAGE AND ROUTES
Schizophrenia
- **Adult: SL** 5 mg bid, max 20 mg/day

Bipolar 1 disorder
- **Adult: SL** 10 mg bid, may decrease to 5 mg bid as needed, max 20 mg/day

Available forms: SL tab 2.5, 5, 10 mg

Administer:
- Anticholinergic agent to be used for EPS
- Store in tight, light-resistant container
- **SL tab:** remove tab; place tab under tongue; after it dissolves, swallow; advise

patient not to chew, crush, swallow tabs, not to eat, drink for 10 min

SIDE EFFECTS

CNS: *EPS, pseudoparkinsonism, akathisia, dystonia, tardive dyskinesia; drowsiness, insomnia, agitation, anxiety, headache,* seizures, neuroleptic malignant syndrome, dizziness, suicidal ideation, drowsiness, depression
CV: Orthostatic hypotension, sinus tachycardia; heart failure, QT prolongation, stroke, bundle branch block
ENDO: Hyperglycemia, hyperlipidemia
GI: *Nausea,* vomiting, *constipation,* weight gain, increased appetite; oral hypoesthesia/parasthesia, mucosal ulcers, increased salivation (SL)
HEMA: Thrombocytopenia, agranulocytosis, anemia, leukopenia
INTEG: Serious allergic reactions (anaphylaxis, angioedema)

PHARMACOKINETICS

Extensively metabolized by liver, protein binding 95%, peak 0.5-1.5 hr, terminal half-life 24 hr

INTERACTIONS

Increase: sedation—other CNS depressants, alcohol
Increase: EPS—CYP2D6 inhibitors/substrates (SSRIs)
Increase: serotonin syndrome—SSRIs
Increase: Seizure risk—buPROPion
Increase: EPS—other antipsychotics
Increase: asenapine excretion—carBAMazepine
Increase: QT prolongation—class IA/III antidysrhythmics, some phenothiazines, β-agonists, local anesthetics, tricyclics, haloperidol, methadone, chloroquine, clarithromycin, droperidol, erythromycin, pentamidine
Decrease: asenapine action—CYP2D6 inducers (carBAMazepine, barbiturates, phenytoins, rifampin)

Drug/Herb
Increase: CNS depression—kava
Increase: EPS—betel palm, kava

Drug/Lab Test
Increase: prolactin levels, glucose LFTs, cholesterol, LFTs, lipids, triglycerides
Decrease: sodium

NURSING CONSIDERATIONS

Assess:

Black Box Warning: Mental status before initial administration; watch for suicidal thoughts and behaviors; dementia and death may occur among elderly patients

- Affect, orientation, LOC, reflexes, gait, coordination, sleep pattern disturbances
- B/P standing and lying; also pulse, respirations; take these q4hr during initial treatment; establish baseline before starting treatment; report drops of 30 mm Hg; watch for ECG changes; QT prolongation may occur
- Dizziness, faintness, palpitations, tachycardia on rising
- **EPS,** including akathisia, tardive dyskinesia (bizarre movements of the jaw, mouth, tongue, extremities), pseudoparkinsonism (rigidity, tremors, pill rolling, shuffling gait)
- **Neuroleptic malignant syndrome:** hyperthermia, increased CPK, altered mental status, muscle rigidity
- Constipation daily; increase bulk, water in diet if needed
- Weight, thyroid function studies, serum prolactin, lipid profile, serum electrolytes, creatinine, pregnancy test, neurologic function, LFTs, glycosylated hemoglobin A1c, CBC, blood glucose, AIMS assessment baseline and periodically
- Supervised ambulation until patient stabilized on medication; do not involve patient in strenuous exercise program because fainting is possible; patient should not stand still for a long time

Evaluate:

- Therapeutic response: decrease in emotional excitement, hallucinations, delusions, paranoia; reorganization of patterns of thought, speech

Teach patient/family:
- That orthostatic hypotension may occur; to rise from sitting or lying position gradually
- To avoid hot tubs, hot showers, tub baths; hypotension may occur
- To avoid abrupt withdrawal of this product; EPS may result; product should be withdrawn slowly
- To avoid OTC preparations (cough, hay fever, cold) unless approved by prescriber; serious product interactions may occur; to avoid use of alcohol; increased drowsiness may occur
- To avoid hazardous activities if drowsy, dizzy
- About compliance with product regimen
- That heat stroke may occur in hot weather; to take extra precautions to stay cool
- To use contraception; to inform prescriber if pregnancy is planned, suspected

Black Box Warning: To report suicidal thoughts/behaviors, dementia immediately

TREATMENT OF OVERDOSE:
Lavage if orally ingested; provide airway; *do not induce vomiting*

RARELY USED

asparaginase *Erwinia chrysanthemi*

Erwinaze

Func. class.: Antineoplastic, natural and semisynthetic

USES: Treatment of acute lymphocytic leukemia (ALL) in combination with other chemotherapeutic agents in patients who have developed hypersensitivity to *Escherichia coli*–derived asparaginase

CONTRAINDICATIONS: Hypersensitivity, breastfeeding, history of serious pancreatitis, bleeding, or serious thrombosis with prior L-asparaginase therapy

DOSAGE AND ROUTES
- **Adult, adolescent, child ≥2 yr (substitute for pegaspargase): IM** 25,000 IU/m² 3×/wk (Monday/Wednesday/Friday) × 6 doses for each planned dose of pegaspargase within a treatment
- **Adult (substitute for L-asparaginase *E. coli*): IM** 25,000 IU/m² for each scheduled dose of native *E. coli* asparaginase within a treatment

Available forms: Powder for inj 10,000 units

Administer:
- Slowly inject 1 or 2 ml of preservative-free sterile sodium chloride (0.9%) inj against inner vial wall; do not forcefully inject sol directly onto or into powder; if 1 ml of NS is used, concentrations is 10,000 IU/ml; if 2 ml of NS is used, concentrations is 5000 IU/ ml; dissolve contents by gentle mixing or swirling; do not shake or invert vial
- Reconstituted sol should be clear and colorless; discard if any visible particles or protein aggregates are present
- Calculate the volume needed to obtain dose; withdraw volume containing calculated dose from vial into polypropylene syringe within 15 min of reconstitution

IM route

Administer dose by IM inj within 4 hr of reconstitution; limit volume to 2 ml per inj site; multiple inj sites may be needed
- Do not freeze or refrigerate the reconstituted solution; discard any unused portions

A

aspirin (OTC)

(as′pir-in)

APC-ASA Coated Aspirin ✽, Apo-Asa ✽, Asaphen ✽, Asatab ✽, A.S.A., Ascriptin Enteric, Aspergum, Aspirin ✽, Aspir-Low, Aspir-trin ✽, Bayer Aspirin, Bayer Children's Aspirin, Bufferin, Ecotrin, Entrophen ✽, Equaline, Good Sense Aspirin, Halfprin, Lowprin ✽, Novasen ✽, PMS-ASA ✽, Rivasa ✽, St. Joseph Children's, St. Joseph's Adult, Walgreens Aspirin Adult

Func. class.: Nonopioid analgesic, nonsteroidal antiinflammatory, antipyretic, antiplatelet

Chem. class.: Salicylate

Do not confuse:
Aspirin/Ascendin/Afrin

ACTION: Blocks pain impulses by blocking COX-1 in CNS, reduces inflammation by inhibition of prostaglandin synthesis; antipyretic action results from vasodilation of peripheral vessels; decreases platelet aggregation

USES: Mild to moderate pain or fever including RA, osteoarthritis, thromboembolic disorders; TIAs, rheumatic fever, post-MI, prophylaxis of MI, ischemic stroke, angina, acute MI

Unlabeled uses: Prevention of cataracts (long-term use), prevention of pregnancy loss in women with clotting disorders, bone pain, claudication, colorectal cancer prophylaxis, Kawasaki disease, PCI, preeclampsia/thrombosis prophylaxis, vernal keratoconjunctivitis, pericarditis, polycythemia vera

CONTRAINDICATIONS: Pregnancy (D) 3rd trimester, breastfeeding, children <12 yr, children with flulike symptoms, hypersensitivity to salicylates, tartrazine (FDC yellow dye #5), GI bleeding, bleeding disorders, vit K deficiency, peptic ulcer, acute bronchospasm, agranulocytosis, increased intracranial pressure, intracranial bleeding, nasal polyps, urticaria

Precautions: Abrupt discontinuation, acetaminophen/NSAIDs hypersensitivity, acid/base imbalance, alcoholism, ascites, asthma, bone marrow suppression in elderly patients, dehydration, G6PD deficiency, gout, heart failure, anemia, renal/hepatic disease, pre/postoperatively, gastritis, pregnancy (C) 1st trimester

DOSAGE AND ROUTES

Arthritis

- **Adult: PO** 3 g/day in divided doses q4-6hr, target salicylate level 150-300 mcg/ml
- **Child: PO/RECT** 90-130 mg/kg/day in divided doses, target salicylate level 150-300 mcg/ml

Pain/fever

- **Adult: PO/RECT** 325-1000 mg q4hr prn, max 4 g/day
- **Child 2-11 yr: PO** 10-15 mg/kg/dose q4hr, max 4 g/day

Thromboembolic disorders

- **Adult: PO** 325-650 mg/day or bid

Transient ischemic attacks (risk)

- **Adult: PO** 50-325 mg/day (grade 1A)

Evolving MI with ST segment elevation (STEMI)

- **Adult: PO** 160-325 mg nonenteric, chewed and swallowed immediately, maintenance 75-162 mg daily

MI, stroke prophylaxis

- **Adult: PO** 50-325 mg/day

Prevention of recurrent MI

- **Adult: PO** 75-162 mg/day

CABG

- **Adult: PO** 325 mg/day starting 6 hr postprocedure, continue for 1 yr

PTCA

- **Adult: PO** 325 mg 2 hr before surgery, then 160-325 mg daily

Polycythemia vera (unlabeled)

- **Adult: PO** 75-100 mg/day during pregnancy and 6 wk after birth

Kawasaki disease (unlabeled)
- **Child: PO** 80-100 mg/kg/day in 4 divided doses, maintenance 3-5 mg/kg/day

Available forms: Tabs 81, 325, 500, 650, 800 mg; chewable tabs 81 mg; supp 300, 600 mg; gum 227 mg; enteric-coated tabs 81, 325, 500, 975 mg; ext rel tabs 800 mg; del rel tabs 325, 500 mg; suppository 300, 600 mg

Administer:

PO route
- Do not break, crush, or chew enteric product
- Crushed or whole, chewable tablets may be chewed
- 1/2 hr before planned exercise
- With food or milk to decrease gastric symptoms; separate by 2 hr from enteric products
- With 8 oz of water; sit upright for 1/2 hr after dose to facilitate product passing into stomach

Rectal route
- Place suppository in refrigerator for at least 30 minutes before removing wrapper

SIDE EFFECTS

CNS: Stimulation, drowsiness, dizziness, confusion, seizures, headache, flushing, hallucinations, coma, intracranial hemorrhage

CV: Rapid pulse, pulmonary edema, dysrhythmias

EENT: Tinnitus, hearing loss

ENDO: Hypoglycemia, hyponatremia, hypokalemia

GI: *Nausea, vomiting,* GI bleeding, diarrhea, heartburn, anorexia, hepatitis, GI ulcer

HEMA: Thrombocytopenia, agranulocytosis, leukopenia, neutropenia, hemolytic anemia, increased PT, aPTT, bleeding time

INTEG: *Rash,* urticaria, bruising

RESP: Wheezing, hyperpnea, bronchospasm

SYST: Reye's syndrome (children), anaphylaxis, laryngeal edema, angioedema

PHARMACOKINETICS

Enteric metabolized by liver; inactive metabolites excreted by kidneys; crosses placenta; excreted in breast milk; half-life 15-20 min, up to 9 hr in large dose; rectal products may be erratic, protein binding 90%

PO: Onset 15-30 min, peak 1-2 hr, duration 4-6 hr, well absorbed

PO: Enteric coated: onset 10-30 min, duration 2-4 hr; Solution: onset 10-30 min, peak 15-30 min, duration 2-4 hr

RECT: Onset slow, duration 4-6 hr

INTERACTIONS

Increase: gastric ulcer risk—corticosteroids, antiinflammatories, NSAIDs, alcohol

Increase: bleeding—alcohol, plicamycin, cefamandole, thrombolytics, ticlopidine, clopidogrel, tirofiban, eptifibatide, anticoagulants

Increase: effects of insulin, methotrexate, thrombolytic agents, penicillins, phenytoin, valproic acid, oral hypoglycemics, sulfonamides

Increase: salicylate levels—urinary acidifiers, ammonium chloride, nizatidine

Increase: hypotension—nitroglycerin

Decrease: effects of aspirin—antacids (high doses), urinary alkalizers, corticosteroids

Decrease: antihypertensive effect—ACE inhibitors

Decrease: effects of probenecid, spironolactone, sulfinpyrazone, sulfonylamides, NSAIDs, β-blockers, loop diuretics

Drug/Herb

Increase: risk of bleeding—feverfew, garlic, ginger, ginkgo, ginseng *(Panax)*, horse chestnut

Drug/Food

Increase: risk of bleeding—fish oil (omega-3 fatty acids)
- Foods that acidify urine may increase aspirin level

Drug/Lab Test

Increase: coagulation studies, LFTs, serum uric acid, amylase, CO_2, urinary protein

Decrease: serum potassium, cholesterol

Interference: VMA, 5-HIAA, xylose tolerance test, TSH, pregnancy test

A

NURSING CONSIDERATIONS

Assess:

- **Pain:** character, location, intensity; ROM before and 1 hr after administration
- **Fever:** temperature before and 1 hr after administration
- Hepatic studies: AST, ALT, bilirubin, creatinine if patient is receiving long-term therapy
- Renal studies: BUN, urine creatinine; I&O ratio; decreasing output may indicate renal failure (long-term therapy)
- Blood studies: CBC, Hct, Hgb, PT if patient is receiving long-term therapy

⚠ **Hepatotoxicity:** dark urine, clay-colored stools, yellowing of skin, sclera, itching, abdominal pain, fever, diarrhea if patient is receiving long-term therapy

- **Allergic reactions:** rash, urticaria; if these occur, product may have to be discontinued; patients with asthma, nasal polyps, allergies: severe allergic reaction may occur
- **Ototoxicity:** tinnitus, ringing, roaring in ears; audiometric testing needed before, after long-term therapy
- **Salicylate level:** therapeutic level 150-300 mcg/ml for chronic inflammation
- Edema in feet, ankles, legs
- Product history; many product interactions

Evaluate:

- Therapeutic response: decreased pain, inflammation, fever

Teach patient/family:

- To report any symptoms of hepatotoxicity, renal toxicity, visual changes, ototoxicity, allergic reactions, bleeding (long-term therapy)
- To avoid if allergic to tartrazine
- Not to exceed recommended dosage; acute poisoning may result
- To read labels on other OTC products because many contain aspirin, salicylates
- That the therapeutic response takes 2 wk (arthritis)
- To report tinnitus, confusion, diarrhea, sweating, hyperventilation
- To avoid alcohol ingestion; GI bleeding may occur
- That patients who have allergies, nasal polyps, asthma may develop allergic reactions
- To discard tabs if vinegar-like smell is detected
- That medication is not to be given to children or teens with flulike symptoms or chickenpox because Reye's syndrome may develop
- To take with a full glass of water
- Not to use during 3rd trimester of pregnancy (D)

TREATMENT OF OVERDOSE:

Lavage, activated charcoal, monitor electrolytes, VS

atazanavir (Rx)

(at-a-za-na′veer)

Reyataz

Func. class.: Antiretroviral

Chem. class.: Protease inhibitor

ACTION: Inhibits human immunodeficiency virus (HIV-1) protease, which prevents maturation of the infectious virus

USES: HIV-1 infection in combination with other antiretroviral agents

CONTRAINDICATIONS: Hypersensitivity, Child-Pugh Class C

Precautions: Pregnancy (B), breastfeeding, children, geriatric patients, hepatic disease, alcoholism, drug resistance, AV block, diabetes, dialysis, elderly, females, hemophilia, hypercholesterolemia, immune reconstitution syndrome, lactic acidosis, pancreatitis, cholelithiasis, serious rash

DOSAGE AND ROUTES

Antiretroviral-naive patients

- **Adult: PO** 400 mg/day (unable to take ritonavir); 300 mg with ritonavir 100 mg/day
- **Child ≥6 yr/adolescent ≥40 kg: PO** 300 mg with ritonavir 100 mg daily
- **Child ≥6 yr/adolescent 20 to <40 kg: PO** 200 mg with ritonavir 100 mg daily

- **Child ≥6 yr/adolescent 15 to <20 kg: PO** 150 mg with ritonavir 100 mg daily

Antiretroviral-experienced patients

- **Adult: PO** 300 mg with ritonavir 100 mg daily
- **Pregnant adults/adolescents (2nd/3rd trimester) with H2 blocker or tenofovir: PO** 400 mg with ritonavir 100 mg daily
- **Child ≥6 yr/adolescent ≥40 kg: PO** 300 mg with ritonavir 100 mg daily
- **Child ≥6 yr/adolescent 20 to <40 kg: PO** 200 mg with ritonavir 100 mg daily
- **Children and Adolescents ≥25 kg: PO** (oral powder) 300 mg q24hr with ritonavir 100 mg q24hr
- **Children 15 to 24 kg: PO** (oral powder) 250 mg q24hr with ritonavir 80 mg q24hr
- **Infants and Children ≥3 months and 5 to 14 kg: PO** (Oral Powder) 200 mg q24hr with ritonavir 80 mg q24hr

Hepatic dose

- **Adult: PO** Child-Pugh B: 300 mg/day; Child-Pugh C: do not use

Available forms: Caps 100, 150, 200, 300 mg; oral powder 50 mg

Administer:

- With food; 2 hr before or 1 hr after antacid or didanosine; swallow cap whole, do not open

SIDE EFFECTS

CNS: Headache, depression, dizziness, insomnia, peripheral neurologic symptoms

CV: Increased PR interval

EENT: Yellowing of sclera

GI: Vomiting, *diarrhea, abdominal pain, nausea,* hepatotoxicity, cholelithiasis

INTEG: *Rash,* Stevens-Johnson syndrome, *photosensitivity,* DRESS

MISC: Fatigue, fever, arthralgia, back pain, cough, lipodystrophy, pain, gynecomastia, nephrolithiasis; lactic acidosis, hyperbilirubinemia (pregnancy, females, obesity)

PHARMACOKINETICS

Rapidly absorbed, absorption increased with food, peak 2½ hr, 86% protein bound, extensively metabolized in liver by CYP3A4, 27% excreted unchanged in urine/feces (minimal), half-life 7 hr

INTERACTIONS

⚠ **Increase:** levels, toxicity of immunosuppressants (cycloSPORINE, sirolimus, tacrolimus, sildenafil), tricylic antidepressants, warfarin, calcium channel blockers, clarithromycin, chlorazepate, diazepam, irinotecan, HMG-CoA reductase inhibitors, antidysrhythmics, midazolam, triazolam, ergots, pimozide, other protease inhibitors

Increase: effects of estrogens, oral contraceptives (unboosted), decreased (boosted with ritonavir)

Increase: atazanavir levels—CYP3A4 substrates, CYP3A4 inhibitors

Increase: hyperbilirubinemia—indinavir

Decrease: teleprevir level when used with atazanavir and ritonavir

Decrease: atazanavir levels—CYP3A4 inducers, rifampin, antacids, didanosine, efavirenz, proton-pump inhibitors, H_2-receptor antagonists

Drug/Herb

Decrease: atazanavir levels—St. John's wort, avoid concurrent use

Increase: myopathy, rhabdomyolysis—red yeast rice

Drug/Lab Test

Increase: AST, ALT, total bilirubin, amylase, lipase, CK

Decrease: Hgb, neurophils, platelets

Drug/Food

- Increased drug bioavailability (to be taken with food)

NURSING CONSIDERATIONS

Assess:

⚠ For hepatic failure; hepatic studies: ALT, AST, bilirubin

- Immune reconstitution syndrome: when given with combination antiretroviral therapy
- For **lactic acidosis, hyperbilirubinemia** (females, pregnancy, obesity), if pregnant call Antiretroviral Pregnancy Registry 800-258-4263
- PR interval in those taking calcium channel blockers, digoxin
- For signs of infection, anemia, nephrolithiasis
- Bowel pattern before, during treatment; if severe abdominal pain with

bleeding occurs, product should be discontinued; monitor hydration
- Viral load, CD4 count throughout treatment
- **Serious rash (Stevens-Johnson syndrome, DRESS): most rashes last 1-4 wk; if serious, discontinue product**
- **Immune reconstitution syndrome: time of onset is variable**

Evaluate:
- Therapeutic response: increasing CD4 counts; decreased viral load, resolution of symptoms of HIV-1 infection

Teach patient/family:
- To take as prescribed with other antiretrovirals as prescribed; if dose is missed, to take as soon as remembered up to 1 hr before next dose; not to double dose, share with others
- That product must be taken daily to maintain blood levels for duration of therapy
- To report yellowing of skin, sclera
- To notify prescriber if diarrhea, nausea, vomiting, rash occurs; dizziness, lightheadedness may occur; ECG may be altered
- That product interacts with many products; St. John's wort; to advise prescriber of all products, herbal products used
- That redistribution of body fat may occur, the effect is not known
- That product does not cure HIV-1 infection, prevent transmission to others; only controls symptoms
- That, if taking phosphodiesterase type 5 inhibitor with atazanavir, there may be increased risk of phosphodiesterase type 5 inhibitor–associated adverse events (hypotension, prolonged penile erection); to notify physician promptly of these symptoms

atenolol (Rx)
(a-ten′oh-lole)

Tenormin

Func. class.: Antihypertensive, antianginal

Chem. class.: β-Blocker, $β_1$-, $β_2$-blocker (high doses)

Do not confuse:
atenolol/albuterol
Tenormin/thiamine/Imuran

ACTION:
Competitively blocks stimulation of β-adrenergic receptor within vascular smooth muscle; produces negative chronotropic activity (decreases rate of SA node discharge, increases recovery time), slows conduction of AV node, decreases heart rate, negative inotropic activity decreases O_2 consumption in myocardium; decreases action of renin-aldosterone-angiotensin system at high doses, inhibits $β_2$ receptors in bronchial system at higher doses

USES:
Mild to moderate hypertension, prophylaxis of angina pectoris; suspected or known MI (IV use); MI prophylaxis, atrial fibrillation/flutter

Unlabeled uses: Migraine prophylaxis, supraventricular tachycardia prophylaxis (PSVT), unstable angina, alcohol withdrawal, lithium-induced tremor

CONTRAINDICATIONS:
Pregnancy (D), hypersensitivity to β-blockers, cardiogenic shock, 2nd- or 3rd-degree heart block, sinus bradycardia, cardiac failure

Precautions: Breastfeeding, major surgery, diabetes mellitus, thyroid/renal disease, CHF, COPD, asthma, well-compensated heart failure, dialysis, myasthenia gravis, Raynaud's disease, pulmonary edema

Black Box Warning: Abrupt discontinuation

DOSAGE AND ROUTES
- **Adult: PO** 25-50 mg/day, increasing q1-2wk to 100 mg/day; may increase to 200 mg/day for angina, up to 100 mg/day for hypertension
- **Child: PO** 0.8-1 mg/kg/dose initially; range, 0.8-1.5 mg/kg/day; max 2 mg/kg/day
- **Geriatric: PO** 25 mg/day initially

Chronic stable angina

• **Adult: PO** 50 mg/day, then 100 mg/day as needed after 7 days, max 200 mg/day

Post MI, MI prophylaxis

• **Adult: PO** 100 mg/day in 1-2 divided doses; may need for 1-3 yr after MI

Renal disease

• **Adult: PO** CCr 15-35 ml/min, max 50 mg/day; CCr <15 ml/min, max 25 mg/day; hemodialysis 25-50 mg after dialysis

PSVT prophylaxis (unlabeled)

• **Child: PO** 0.3-1.3 mg/kg/day

Ethanol withdrawal prevention (unlabeled)

• **Adult: PO** 50-100 mg/day

Migraine prophylaxis (unlabeled)

• **Adult: PO** 50-150 mg/day, titrate to response

Lithium-induced tremor (unlabeled)

• **Adult: PO** 50 mg/day

Available forms: Tabs 25, 50, 100 mg

Administer:

PO route

• Before meals, at bedtime; tab may be crushed, swallowed whole, same time of day

• Reduced dosage with renal dysfunction

• Store protected from light, moisture; place in cool environment

SIDE EFFECTS

CNS: *Insomnia, fatigue, dizziness, mental changes,* memory loss, hallucinations, depression, lethargy, drowsiness, strange dreams, catatonia

CV: Profound hypotension, bradycardia, CHF, *cold extremities, postural hypotension, 2nd- or 3rd-degree heart block*

ENDO: Increased hypoglycemic response to insulin

GI: *Nausea, diarrhea,* vomiting, mesenteric arterial thrombosis, ischemic colitis

GU: Impotence, decreased libido

HEMA: Agranulocytosis, thrombocytopenia purpura

INTEG: Rash, fever, alopecia

RESP: Bronchospasm, dyspnea, wheezing, pulmonary edema

PHARMACOKINETICS

PO: Peak 2-4 hr; onset 1 hr; duration 24 hr; half-life 6-7 hr; excreted unchanged in urine, feces (50%); protein binding 5%-15%

INTERACTIONS

• Mutual inhibition: sympathomimetics (cough, cold preparations)

Increase: hypotension, bradycardia—reserpine, hydrALAZINE, methyldopa, prazosin, anticholinergics, digoxin, diltiazem, verapamil, cardiac glycosides, antihypertensives

Increase: hypoglycemia—insulins, oral antidiabetics

Increase: hypertension—amphetamines, ePHEDrine, pseudoephedrine

Decrease: effect—insulin, oral antidiabetic agents, theophylline, DOPamine, MAOIs

Drug/Herb

Increase: atenolol effect—hawthorn

Decrease: atenolol effect—ephedra (ma huang)

Drug/Lab Test

Increase: BUN, potassium, triglycerides, uric acid, ANA titer, platelets alkaline phosphatase, creatinine, LDH, AST/ALT

Decrease: glucose

NURSING CONSIDERATIONS

Assess:

• I&O, weight daily; watch for CHF (rales/crackles, jugular vein distention, weight gain, edema)

• **Hypertension:** B/P, pulse q4hr; note rate, rhythm, quality; apical/radial pulse before administration; notify prescriber of any significant changes (<50 bpm); ECG

• **Hypotension:** may be caused in hemodialysis

• **Hypoglycemia:** may be masked in diabetes mellitus

• Baselines in renal/hepatic studies before therapy begins

Black Box Warning: Taper gradually, do not discontinue abruptly, may precipitate angina, MI

Evaluate:

• Therapeutic response: decreased B/P after 1-2 wk, increased activity tolerance, decreased anginal pain

Teach patient/family:

Black Box Warning: Not to discontinue product abruptly, taper over 2 wk (angina); to take at same time each day as directed

- Not to use OTC products unless directed by prescriber
- To report bradycardia, dizziness, confusion, depression, fever
- To take pulse at home; advise when to notify prescriber
- To limit alcohol, smoking, sodium intake
- To comply with weight control, dietary adjustments, modified exercise program
- To carry emergency ID to identify product, allergies, conditions being treated
- To avoid hazardous activities if dizziness is present
- To change position slowly
- That product may mask symptoms of hypoglycemia in diabetic patients
- To use contraception while taking this product, pregnancy (D); to avoid breastfeeding

TREATMENT OF OVERDOSE: Lavage, IV atropine for bradycardia, IV theophylline for bronchospasm, dextrose for hypoglycemia, digoxin, O_2, diuretic for cardiac failure, hemodialysis

atomoxetine (Rx)

(at-o-mox′eh-teen)

Strattera

Func. class.: Psychotherapeutic—miscellaneous

Chem. class.: Selective norepinephrine reuptake inhibitor

ACTION: Selective norepinephrine reuptake inhibitor; may inhibit the presynaptic norepinephrine transporter

USES: Attention deficit hyperactivity disorder

CONTRAINDICATIONS: Hypersensitivity, closed-angle glaucoma, MAOI therapy, history of pleochromocytoma

Precautions: Pregnancy (C), breastfeeding, hepatic disease, angioedema, bipolar disorder, dysrhythmias, CAD, hypo/hypertension, arteriosclerosis, cardiac disease, cardiomyopathy, heart failure, jaundice

Black Box Warning: Children <6 yr, suicidal ideation

DOSAGE AND ROUTES

- **Child ≤70 kg >6 yrs: PO** 0.5 mg/kg/day, increase after 3 days to target daily dose of 1.2 mg/kg in AM or evenly divided doses AM, late afternoon; max 1.4 mg/kg/day or 100 mg/day, whichever is less
- **Adult and child >70 kg: PO** 40 mg/day, increase after 3 days to target daily dose of 80 mg in AM or evenly divided doses AM, late afternoon; max 100 mg/day

Maintenance

- **Adolescent ≤15 yr and child ≥6 yr: PO** 1.2-1.8 mg/kg/day

Initial dose titration with strong CYP2D6 inhibitors

- **Adult and child >6 yr weighing >70 kg: PO** 40 mg/day each AM or 2 evenly divided doses, titrate to target of 80 mg/day if symptoms do not improve after 4 wk and dose is well tolerated

Hepatic dose

- Child-Pugh B: reduce dose by 50%; Child-Pugh C: reduce dose by 75%

Available forms: Caps 10, 18, 25, 40, 60, 80, 100 mg

Administer:

- Whole; do not break, crush, chew
- Gum, hard candy, frequent sips of water for dry mouth
- Without regard to food

SIDE EFFECTS

CNS: *Insomnia,* dizziness, headache, irritability, crying, mood swings, fatigue, hypoesthesia, lethargy, paresthesia

CV: *Palpitations,* hot flushes, tachycardia, increased B/P, palpitations

ENDO: Growth retardation

GI: Dyspepsia, nausea, anorexia, dry mouth, weight loss, vomiting, diarrhea, constipation, hepatic injury

GU: Urinary hesitancy, retention, dysmenorrhea, erectile disturbance, ejaculation failure, impotence, prostatitis, abnormal orgasm, male pelvic pain

INTEG: Exfoliative dermatitis, sweating, rash

MISC: Cough, rhinorrhea, dermatitis, ear infection, rhabdomyolysis

PHARMACOKINETICS

Peak 1-2 hr, metabolized by liver, excreted by kidneys, 98% protein binding, half-life 5 hr

INTERACTIONS

Increase: hypertensive crisis—MAOIs or within 14 days of MAOIs, vasopressors

Increase: cardiovascular effects of albuterol, pressor agents

Increase: QT prolongation, torsade de pointes dofetilide, grepafloxacin, mesoridazine, pimozide, probucol, sparfloxacin, ziprasidone

Increase: effects of atomoxetine—CYP2D6 inhibitors (amiodarone, cimetidine [weak], clomipramine, delavirdine, gefitinib, imatinib, propafenone, quiNIDine [potent], ritonavir, citalopram, escitalopram, FLUoxetine, sertraline, PARoxetine, thioridazine, venlafaxine)

Increase: B/P pressor agents

NURSING CONSIDERATIONS

Assess:

- VS, B/P; check patients with cardiac disease more often for increased B/P
- **Hepatic injury:** may cause liver failure: monitor LFT; assess for jaundice, pruritus, flulike symptoms, upper right quadrant pain

⚠ Mental status: mood, sensorium, affect, stimulation, insomnia, aggressiveness, suicidal ideation in children/young adults

- Appetite, sleep, speech patterns
- For increased attention span, decreased hyperactivity with ADHD, growth rate, weight, therapy may need to be discontinued

Evaluate:

- Therapeutic response: decreased hyperactivity (ADHD)

Teach patient/family:

- To avoid OTC preparations, other medication, herbs, supplements unless approved by prescriber, no tapering needed when discontinuing product
- To avoid alcohol ingestion
- To avoid hazardous activities until stabilized on medication
- To get needed rest; patients will feel more tired at end of day; not to take dose late in day, insomnia may occur

Black Box Warning: To report suicidal ideation

- To notify prescriber immediately if erection >4 hr

atorvastatin (Rx)

(a-tore′va-stat-in)

Lipitor

Func. class.: Antilipidemic

Chem. class.: HMG-CoA reductase inhibitor (statin)

Do not confuse:

Lipitor/Levatol

ACTION: Inhibits HMG-CoA reductase enzyme, which reduces cholesterol synthesis; high doses lead to plaque regression

USES: As adjunct for primary hypercholesterolemia (types Ia, Ib), dysbetalipoproteinemia, elevated triglyceride levels, prevention of CV disease by reduction of heart risk in those with mildly elevated cholesterol

CONTRAINDICATIONS: Pregnancy (X), breastfeeding, hypersensitivity, active hepatic disease

Precautions: Previous hepatic disease, alcoholism, severe acute infections, trauma, severe metabolic disorders, electrolyte imbalance

DOSAGE AND ROUTES

• **Adult: PO** 10-20 mg/day, usual range 10-80 mg/day, dosage adjustments may be made in 2- to 4-wk intervals, max 80 mg/day; patients who require >45% reduction in LDL may be started at 40 mg/day

Heterozygous familial hypercholesterolemia

• **Child 10-17 yr: PO** 10 mg daily, adjust q4wk, max 20 mg/day

Available forms: Tabs 10, 20, 40, 80 mg

Administer:

• Total daily dose at any time of day without regard to meals

• Store in cool environment in tight container protected from light

SIDE EFFECTS

CNS: Headache, asthenia, insomnia

EENT: Lens opacities

GI: *Abdominal cramps, constipation, diarrhea, flatus, heartburn,* dyspepsia, liver dysfunction, pancreatitis, nausea, increased serum transaminase

GU: Impotence

INTEG: Rash, pruritus, alopecia; photosensitivity (rare)

MISC: Hypersensitivity; gynecomastia (child)

MS: Arthralgia, myalgia, rhabdomyolysis, myositis

RESP: Pharyngitis, sinusitis

PHARMACOKINETICS

Peak 1-2 hr, metabolized in liver, highly protein-bound, excreted primarily in urine, half-life 14 hr, protein binding 98%

INTERACTIONS

Increase: rhabdomyolysis—azole antifungals, cycloSPORINE, erythromycin, niacin, gemfibrozil, clofibrate

Increase: serum level of digoxin

Increase: levels of oral contraceptives

Increase: levels of atorvastatin, myopathy—CYP3A4 inhibitors

Increase: effects of warfarin

Decrease: atorvastatin levels—colestipol

Drug/Herb

Decrease: effect—St. John's wort

Drug/Food

• Possible toxicity when used with grapefruit juice; oat bran may reduce effectiveness

Drug/Lab Test

Increase: ALT, AST, CK

Interference: thyroid function tests

NURSING CONSIDERATIONS

Assess:

• **Hypercholesterolemia:** diet, obtain diet history including fat, cholesterol in diet; cholesterol triglyceride levels periodically during treatment; check lipid panel 6-12 wk after changing dose

• Hepatic studies q1-2mo, at initiation, 6, 12 wk after initiation or change in dose, periodically thereafter; AST, ALT, LFTs may be increased

• Renal studies in patients with compromised renal system: BUN, I&O ratio, creatinine

• Bowel status: constipation, stool softeners may be needed; if severe, add fiber, water to diet

⚠ **Rhabdomyolysis:** for muscle pain, tenderness, obtain CPK baseline; if markedly increased, product may need to be discontinued

Evaluate:

• Therapeutic response: decrease in LDL, total cholesterol, triglycerides, CAD; increase in HDL

Teach patient/family:

• That blood work and eye exam will be necessary during treatment

• To report blurred vision, severe GI symptoms, headache, muscle pain, weakness, avoid alcohol

• That previously prescribed regimen will continue: low-cholesterol diet, exercise program, smoking cessation

• Not to take product if pregnant (X), breastfeeding; to avoid alcohol

• To stay out of the sun; to use sunscreen, protective clothing to prevent photosensitivity (rare)

atovaquone (Rx)

(a-toe′va-kwon)

Mepron

Func. class.: Antiprotozoal

Chem. class.: Analog of ubiquinone

ACTION: Interferes with DNA/RNA synthesis in protozoa

USES: *Pneumocystis jiroveci* infections in patients intolerant of trimethoprim-sulfamethoxazole, prophylaxis, *Toxoplasma gondii,* toxoplasmosis

Unlabeled uses: Babesiosis, malaria treatment/prophylaxis, toxoplasmosis prophylaxis, *Plasmodium* sp.

CONTRAINDICATIONS: Hypersensitivity or history of developing life-threatening allergic reactions to any component of the formulation, benzyl alcohol sensitivity

Precautions: Pregnancy (C), breastfeeding, neonates, hepatic disease, GI disease, respiratory insufficiency

DOSAGE AND ROUTES

Acute, mild, moderate *Pneumocystis jiroveci* pneumonia

- **Adult and adolescent 13-16 yr: PO** 750 mg with food bid for 21 days

***Pneumocystis jiroveci* pneumonia, prophylaxis**

- **Adult and adolescent: PO** 1500 mg/day with meal

Babesiosis (unlabeled)

- **Adult: PO** 750 mg q12hr with azithromycin (1000 mg on day 1, then 250 mg/day × 7-14 days)

Toxoplasmosis prophylaxis in AIDS (unlabeled)

- **Adult: PO** 1500 mg alone or in combination

***Plasmodium falciparum* (unlabeled)**

- **Adult: PO** 250 mg with proguanil daily
- **Child: PO** 17 mg/kg with proguanil daily

Available forms: Susp 750 mg/5 ml

Administer:

- With high-fat food to increase absorption of product and higher plasma concentrations
- Oral susp; shake before using
- All contents of foil pouch

SIDE EFFECTS

CNS: *Dizziness, headache, anxiety, insomnia,* asthenia, fever

CV: Hypotension

GI: *Nausea, vomiting, diarrhea,* anorexia, increased AST/ALT, acute pancreatitis, constipation, abdominal pain

HEMA: Anemia, neutropenia

INTEG: Pruritus, urticaria, *rash*

META: Hypoglycemia, hyponatremia

OTHER: Cough, dyspnea

PHARMACOKINETICS

Excreted unchanged in feces (94%), highly protein bound (99%), half-life 2-3 days

INTERACTIONS

Increase: level of—zidovudine, monitor for toxicity

Decrease: effect of atovaquone—rifampin, rifabutin, tetracycline, avoid concurrent use

Drug/Lab Test

Increase: AST, ALT, alk phos

Decrease: glucose, neutrophils, Hgb, sodium

NURSING CONSIDERATIONS

Assess:

Infection: WBC, vital signs; sputum baseline, periodically; obtain specimens needed before giving 1st dose

- Bowel pattern before, during treatment
- Respiratory status: rate, character, wheezing, dyspnea; risk for respiratory infection
- Allergies before treatment, reaction to each medication

Evaluate:

- Therapeutic response: decreased temperature, ability to breathe

Teach patient/family:

• To take with food to increase plasma concentrations

atovaquone/proguanil

(a-toe′va-kwon)

Malarone, Malarone Pediatric

Func. class.: Antiprotozoal

Chem. class.: Aromatic diamide derivative

ACTION: The constituents of Malarone, atovaquone, and proguanil hydrochloride interfere with 2 different pathways involved in DNA/RNA synthesis in protozoa

USES: Malaria, malaria prophylaxis

CONTRAINDICATIONS: Hypersensitivity to this product, malaria prophylaxis in patients with severe renal impairment

Precautions: Pregnancy (C), breastfeeding, children, hepatic/GI/renal disease

DOSAGE AND ROUTES

Treatment of acute, uncomplicated *P. falciparum* malaria

Malarone adult strength tabs

• **Adult/adolescent/child >40 kg: PO** 4 adult strength tabs every day as a single dose × 3 consecutive days

• **Child 31-40 kg: PO** 3 adult strength tabs every day as a single dose × 3 consecutive days

• **Child 21-30 kg: PO** 2 adult strength tabs every day as a single dose × 3 consecutive days

• **Infant/child 11-20 kg: PO** 1 adult strength tab every day × 3 consecutive days

Malarone Pediatric Tabs

• **Infant/child 11-20 kg: PO** 4 pediatric tabs every day × 3 consecutive days

• **Infant/child 9-10 kg: PO** 3 pediatric tabs every day × 3 consecutive days

• **Infant/child 5-8 kg: PO** 2 pediatric tabs every day every 3 consecutive days

***P. falciparum* malaria prophylaxis, including chloroquine resistance areas**

Malarone adult strength tabs

• **Adult/adolescent/child >40 kg: PO** 1 adult strength tab every day; begin prophylaxis 1-2 days before entering the endemic area; continue daily during the stay and for 7 days after leaving the area

Malarone Pediatric Tab

• **Child 31-40 kg: PO** 3 pediatric tabs every day; begin prophylaxis 1-2 days before entering the endemic area; continue daily during the stay and for 7 days after leaving the area

• **Child 21-30 kg: PO** 2 pediatric tabs every day; begin prophylaxis 1-2 days before entering the endemic area; continue daily during the stay and for 7 days after leaving the area

• **Infant/child 11-20 kg: PO** 1 pediatric tab every day; begin prophylaxis 1-2 days before entering the endemic area; continue daily during the stay and for 7 days after leaving the area

Renal dose

• **Adult: PO** CCr <30 ml/min, do not use for prophylaxis

Available forms: Tabs (adult) 250 mg atovaquone/proguanil 100 mg; tabs (pediatric) 62.5 atovaquone/proguanil 25 mg

Administer:

• Give with food or with milk or milk-based drink (nutritional supplement shake) to enhance oral absorption of atovaquone; food with high fat content is desired

• Give dose at the same time each day; administer a repeat dose if vomiting occurs within 1 hr after dosing

• Tabs may be crushed and mixed with condensed milk for children unable to swallow whole tablets

SIDE EFFECTS

CNS: *Dizziness, headache, anxiety, insomnia,* asthenia, fever

CV: Hypotension

GI: *Nausea, vomiting, diarrhea,* anorexia, increased AST/ALT, **acute pancreatitis,** constipation, abdominal pain

HEMA: Anemia, neutropenia

INTEG: Pruritus, urticaria, *rash*, photosensitivity
META: Hypoglycemia, hyponatremia
OTHER: Cough, dyspnea

PHARMACOKINETICS

Atovaquone excreted unchanged in feces (94%), highly protein-bound (99%), proguanil 75% protein-bound, 40%-60% excreted in urine, hepatic metabolism; half-life 2-3 days

INTERACTIONS

Increase: level of indinavir
Decrease: effect of atovaquone-rifampin, rifabutin, tetracycline, metoclopramide
Drug/Lab
Increase: AST, ALT, alk phos
Decrease: glucose, neutrophils, Hgb

NURSING CONSIDERATIONS

Assess:

- **Malaria:** identify when the patient will be entering an area with malaria
- Bowel pattern before, during treatment
- Respiratory status: rate, character, wheezing, dyspnea; risk for respiratory infection
- Allergies before treatment, reaction to each medication
- CBC, LFTs, serum amylase, creatinine/BUN, sodium; increases in LFTs can persist for 4 wk after discontinuation of treatment

Evaluate:

Therapeutic response:

- Resolution/prevention of malaria

Teach patient/family:

- To take with food to increase plasma concentrations, at same time of day
- To take whole course of treatment

RARELY USED

atracurium (Rx)

(a-tra-kyoor′ee-um)
Func. class.: Neuromuscular blocker (nondepolarizing)

USES: Facilitation of endotracheal intubation, skeletal muscle relaxation during mechanical ventilation, surgery, or general anesthesia

CONTRAINDICATIONS: Hypersensitivity

Black Box Warning: Respiratory insufficiency

DOSAGE AND ROUTES

- **Adult and child >2 yr: IV BOL** 0.4-0.5 mg/kg, then 0.08-0.1 mg/kg 20-45 min after 1st dose if needed for prolonged procedures; give smaller doses with halothane
- **Child 1 mo-2 yr: IV BOL** 0.3-0.4 mg/kg

HIGH ALERT

atropine (Rx)

(a′troe-peen)
Func. class.: Antidysrhythmic, anticholinergic parasympatholytic, antimuscarinic
Chem. class.: Belladonna alkaloid

Do not confuse:
atropine/Akarpine

ACTION: Blocks acetylcholine at parasympathetic neuroeffector sites; increases cardiac output, heart rate by blocking vagal stimulation in heart; dries secretions by blocking vagus

USES: Bradycardia <40-50 bpm, bradydysrhythmia, reversal of anticholinesterase agents, insecticide poisoning, blocking cardiac vagal reflexes, decreasing secretions before surgery, antispasmodic with GU, biliary surgery, bronchodilator, AV heart block
Unlabeled uses: Cardiac arrest, CPR, pulseless electrical activity, ventricular asystole, asthma, irinotecan-induced diarrhea, rapid-sequence intubation

CONTRAINDICATIONS:
Hypersensitivity to belladonna alkaloids, closed-angle glaucoma, GI obstructions, myasthenia gravis, thyrotoxicosis, ulcerative colitis, prostatic hypertrophy, tachycardia/tachydysrhythmias, asthma, acute hemorrhage, severe hepatic disease, myocardial ischemia, paralytic ileus

Precautions: Pregnancy (C), breastfeeding, children <6 yr, geriatric patients, renal disease, CHF, hyperthyroidism, COPD, hypertension, intraabdominal infection, Down syndrome, spastic paralysis, gastric ulcer

DOSAGE AND ROUTES

Bradycardia/bradydysrhythmia

- **Adult: IV BOL** 0.5-1 mg given q3-5min, max 2 mg
- **Child: IV BOL** 0.02 mg/kg, may repeat ×1; min dose 0.1 mg to avoid paradoxical reaction, max single dose 0.5 mg, max total dose 1 mg

Organophosphate poisoning

- **Adult and child: IM/IV** 1-2 mg q20-30min muscarinic symptoms disappear; may need 6 mg every hr
- **Adult and child >90 lb, usually >10 yr: AtroPen** 2 mg
- **Child 40-90 lb, usually 4-10 yr: AtroPen** 1 mg
- **Child 15-40 lb: AtroPen** 0.5 mg
- **Infant <15 lb: IM/IV** 0.05 mg/kg q5-20min as needed

Presurgery

- **Adult and child >20 kg: SUBCUT/IM/IV** 0.4-0.6 mg 30-60 min before anesthesia
- **Child <20 kg: IM/SUBCUT** 0.01 mg/kg up to 0.4 mg ½-1 hr preop, max 0.6 mg/dose

Available forms: Inj 0.05, 0.1, 0.4, 0.5, 0.8, 1 mg/ml; AtroPen 0.5, 1, 2 mg inj prefilled autoinjectors

Administer:

- Without regard to meals

IM route

- Atropine flush may occur in children and is not harmful

AtroPen

- Use no more than 3 AtroPen inj unless under the supervision of trained medical provider
- Use as soon as symptoms appear (tearing, wheezing, muscle fasciculations, excessive oral secretions), may use through clothing

IV route

- Undiluted or diluted with 10 ml sterile water; give at 0.6 mg/min through Y-tube or 3-way stopcock; do not add to IV sol; may cause paradoxical bradycardia for 2 min

Y-site compatibilities: Amrinone, etomidate, famotidine, heparin, hydrocortisone, meropenem, nafcillin, potassium chloride, sufentanil, vit B/C

SIDE EFFECTS

CNS: Headache, dizziness, involuntary movement, confusion, psychosis, anxiety, **coma**, flushing, drowsiness, insomnia, weakness; delirium (geriatric patients)

CV: Hypo/hypertension, paradoxical bradycardia, angina, PVCs, **tachycardia**, ectopic ventricular beats, **bradycardia**, palpitations

EENT: Blurred vision, photophobia, glaucoma, eye pain, pupil dilation, nasal congestion, increased intraocular pressure

GI: Dry mouth, nausea, vomiting, abdominal pain, anorexia, constipation, **paralytic ileus**, abdominal distention, altered taste

GU: Retention, hesitancy, impotence, dysuria

INTEG: Rash, urticaria, contact dermatitis, dry skin, flushing

MISC: Suppression of lactation, decreased sweating, **anaphylaxis**

PHARMACOKINETICS
Half-life 2-3 hr, terminal 12.5 hr, excreted by kidneys unchanged (70%-90% in 24 hr), metabolized in liver, 40%-50% crosses placenta, excreted in breast milk

IM/SUBCUT: Onset 15-50 min, peak 30 min, duration 4-6 hr, well absorbed

IV: Peak 2-4 min, duration 4-6 hr

INTERACTIONS

Increase: mucosal lesions—potassium chloride tab

Increase: anticholinergic effects—tricyclics, amantadine, antiparkinson agents

Decrease: absorption—ketoconazole, levodopa
Decrease: effect of atropine—antacids

NURSING CONSIDERATIONS

Assess:

- I&O ratio; check for urinary retention, daily output
- **ECG** for ectopic ventricular beats, PVC, tachycardia in cardiac patients
- For bowel sounds, constipation
- Respiratory status: rate, rhythm, cyanosis, wheezing, dyspnea, engorged neck veins
- **Increased intraocular pressure:** eye pain, nausea, vomiting, blurred vision, increased tearing
- Cardiac rate: rhythm, character, B/P continuously
- Allergic reaction: rash, urticaria

Evaluate:

- Therapeutic response: decreased dysrhythmias, increased heart rate, secretions; GI, GU spasms; bronchodilation

Teach patient/family:

- To report blurred vision, chest pain, allergic reactions, constipation, urinary retention, to use sunglasses to protect the eyes
- Not to perform strenuous activity in high temperatures; heat stroke may result
- To take as prescribed; not to skip or double doses
- Not to operate machinery if drowsiness occurs
- Not to take OTC products without approval of prescriber
- Not to freeze or expose to light (AtroPen)

TREATMENT OF OVERDOSE:

O_2, artificial ventilation, ECG; administer DOPamine for circulatory depression; administer diazepam or thiopental for seizures; assess need for antidysrhythmics

atropine ophthalmic

See Appendix B

avanafil

(a-van′a-fil)

Stendra

Func. class.: Impotence agent
Chem. class.: Phosphodiesterase type 5 inhibitor

ACTION: Inhibits phosphodiesterase type 5 (PDE5); enhances erectile function by increasing the amount of cGMP causing smooth muscle relaxation and increasing blood flow to the corpus cavernosum

USES: Treatment of erectile dysfunction

CONTRAINDICATIONS: Hypersensitivity, severe renal/hepatic disease, current nitrates/nitrites, patients <18 yr

Precautions: Pregnancy (C) although not indicated for women, anatomic penile deformities, sickle cell anemia, leukemia, multiple myeloma, renal/hepatic/CV disease, bleeding disorders, active peptic ulcer, prolonged erection, aortic stenosis, HIV, stroke, geriatric patients, tinnitus, MI, visual disturbances, retinitis pigmentosa

DOSAGE AND ROUTES

Erectile dysfunction

- **Adult: PO** 100 mg 30 min before sexual activity, dose may be reduced to 50 mg or increased to 200 mg; usual max dose frequency is 1 time/day

Potent CYP3A4 inhibitors/nitrates

- Do not use

Moderate CYP3A4 inhibitors/α-blockers

- **Adult: PO** Max 50 mg/day

Hepatic dosage/severe renal disease

- **Adult: Child-Pugh C: PO** not recommended

Available forms: Tabs 50, 100, 200 mg

Administer:

PO route

- May be taken 30 min before sexual activity on an as-needed basis, but no more than once per day
- May be used without regard to meals
- Products should not be used with nitrates or strong CYP3A4 inhibitors

SIDE EFFECTS

CNS: *Headache, flushing*

EENT: Nasal congestion, nasopharyngitis, sudden hearing/vision loss

MISC: Back pain

PHARMACOKINETICS

99% protein binding, metabolized by CYP3A4, excreted as metabolites; urine 62%; 21% feces, half-life 5 hr, peak 30-45 min

INTERACTIONS

Do not use with nitrates/nitrites because of unsafe drop in B/P, which could result in MI, stroke

Do not use with strong CYP3A4 inhibitors (ketoconazole, ritonavir, atazanavir, clarithromycin, indivinavir, itraconazole, nefazodone, nelfinavir, saquinavir, telithromycin, isoniazid, boceprevir, delavirdine, telaprevir, tipranavir)

Avoid use with other phosphodiesterase type inhibitors (vardenafil, sildenafil, tadalafil)

Increase: Avanafil level—moderate CYP3A4 inhibitors (erythromycin, amprenavir, aprepitant, diltiazem, fluconazole, fosamprenavir, verapamil, amiodarone, crizotinib, darunavir, dasantinib, dronedarone, imatinib, lapatinib, ticagrelor, voriconazole)

Decrease: B/P—alcohol, α-blockers, amLODIPine

Increase: Avanafil effect—grapefruit juice

NURSING CONSIDERATIONS

Assess:

Erectile dysfunction: Assess for underlying cause before treatment; use of organic nitrates that should not be used with this product; any loss of vision/hearing while taking this product, hypersensitivity reactions

Evaluate:

Therapeutic response: Ability to engage in sexual intercourse

Teach patient/family:

- Sexual dysfunction: may be taken 30 min before sexual activity on an as-needed basis, but no more than once per day
- May be used without regard to meals
- ⚠ That products should not be used with nitrates/nitrates, or strong CYP3A4 inhibitors
- That product does not protect against sexually transmitted disease including HIV
- That product has no effect in the absence of sexual stimulation; to seek help if erection lasts >4 hr
- To tell prescriber about all medication, vitamins, herbs being taken, especially ritonavir, indinavir, ketoconazole, itraconazole, erythromycin, nitrates, α-blockers
- Not to drink large amounts of alcohol
- ⚠ To notify prescriber immediately and to stop taking product if vision or hearing loss occurs, if erection lasts >4 hr, or if chest pain occurs

⚠ HIGH ALERT

axitinib

Inlyta

Func. class.: Antineoplastics, biologic response modifiers, signal transduction inhibitors (STIs)

Chem. class.: Tyrosine kinase inhibitor

ACTION:
Inhibits receptor tyrosine kinases including vascular endothelial growth factor receptors (VEGFR)-1, VEGFR-2, and VEGFR-3; inhibits tumor growth and phosphorylation of VEGFR-2 and VEGF-mediated endothelial cell proliferation

USES:
Treatment of advanced renal cell cancer after failure of 1 prior systemic therapy

CONTRAINDICATIONS:
Pregnancy (D), breastfeeding

Precautions Risk for or history of thromboembolic disease, recent bleeding, untreated brain metastasis, recent GI bleeding, GI perforation, fistula, surgery, moderate hepatic disease, uncontrolled hypertension, hyper/hypothyroidism, proteinuria, infertility, end-stage renal disease (CrCl $<$15 ml/min); not intended for use in adolescents, children, infants, neonates

DOSAGE AND ROUTES

• **Adult:** PO 5 mg bid (at 12-hr intervals), may increase to 7 mg bid and then to 10 mg bid in those not receiving antihypertensives who tolerate the lower dosage for at least 2 consecutive wk with no more than grade 2 adverse reactions; reduce to 3 mg bid if a dose reduction is needed; if further reduction is necessary, reduce to 2 mg bid

• **Adult receiving a strong CYP3A4/5 inhibitor:** Reduce dose by 1/2, adjust as needed

Available forms: Tabs 1, 5 mg

Administer:

• Give with or without food; swallow tablet whole with a glass of water

• If patient vomits or misses a dose, an additional dose should not be taken; the next dose should be taken at the usual time

• Store at room temperature

SIDE EFFECTS

CNS: Dizziness, headache, reversible posterior leukoencephalopathy syndrome (RPLS), fatigue

CV: Hypertension, arterial thromboembolic events (ATE), venous thromboembolic events (VTE)

ENDO: Hypothyroidism, hyperthyroidism

GI: Lower GI bleeding/perforation/fistula, abdominal pain, constipation, diarrhea, dysgeusia, dyspepsia, dysphonia, hemorrhoids, nausea, mucosal inflammation, stomatitis, vomiting, increased ALT/AST

GU: Proteinuria

HEMA: Bleeding, intracranial bleeding, anemia, polycythemia, decreased/increased hemoglobin, lymphopenia thrombocytopenia, neutropenia

INTEG: Palmar-plantar erythrodysesthesia (hand and foot syndrome) rash, dry skin, pruritus, alopecia, erythema

MISC: Weight loss, dehydration, metabolic and electrolyte laboratory abnormalities

MS: Asthenia, arthralgia, musculoskeletal pain, myalgia

RESP: Cough, dyspnea

PHARMACODYNAMICS

Absorption: bioavailability 58%; distribution: protein binding $>$99%; metabolized in liver by CYP3A4/5, CYP1A2, CYP2C19, and UGT1A1; metabolites are carboxylic acid, sulfoxide, and *N*-glucuronide; excretion 41% in feces and 23% in urine, 12% unchanged; half-life: 2.5-6.1 hr; steady state 2-3 days; onset unknown, peak 2.5-4.1 hr, increased in moderate hepatic disease; duration unknown

INTERACTIONS

Increase: effect of axitinib—CYP3A4/5 inhibitor, strong, moderate (ketoconazole, boceprevir, chloramphenicol, conivaptan, delavirdine, fosamprenavir, imatinib, indinavir, isoniazid itraconazole, dalfopristin, quinupristin, posaconazole, ritonavir, telithromycin, tipranavir (boosted with ritonavir), darunavir (boosted with ritonavir), aldesleukin, IL-2, amiodarone, aprepitant, fosaprepitant atazanavir, bromocriptine, clarithromycin, crizotinib, danazol, diltiazem, dronedarone, erythromycin, fluvoxaMINE, lanreotide, lapatinib, miconazole, mifepristone, nefazodone, nelfinavir, niCARdipine, octreotide, pantoprazole, saquinavir, tamoxifen, verapamil, voriconazole, grapefruit juice)

Decrease: effect of axitinib—CYP3A4/5 inducers, strong/moderate (rifampin, carBAMazepine, dexamethasone, phenytoin, PHENobarbital, rifabutin, rifapentine, St. John's wort, ethanol, bexarotene, bosentan, efavirenz, etravirine, griseofulvin, metyrapone, modafinil, nafcillin, nevirapine, OXcarbazepine, vemurafenib, pioglitazone, topiramate)

Increase or decrease: effect of axitinib—CYP3A4/5 inhibitor and inducers (quiNINE)

Drug/Lab Test

Increase: creatinine, lipase, amylase, potassium

Decrease: bicarbonate, calcium, albumin, glucose, phosphate, sodium

Increase or decrease: sodium, glucose

Drug/Food

Increase: drug effect—grapefruit or grapefruit juice

Drug/Herb

Decrease: effect of axitinib—St. John's wort

NURSING CONSIDERATIONS

Assess:

- **Bleeding:** monitor for GI bleeding or perforation; temporarily discontinue therapy if a patient develops any bleeding that requires treatment
- **Surgery:** discontinue ≥24 hr before surgery; may be resumed after adequate wound healing
- **Hepatic/renal disease:** dosage should be reduced in patients with moderate (Child-Pugh Class B) hepatic disease; monitor liver function tests (ALT, AST, bilirubin) before and periodically during therapy; monitor CCr before and during treatment
- **Hypertension:** B/P should be well controlled before starting treatment; monitor patients for hypertension and administer antihypertensive therapy as needed before and during therapy; dose should be reduced for persistent hypertension; therapy should be discontinued if B/P remains elevated after a dosage reduction or if there is evidence of hypertensive crisis; after discontinuation monitor B/P for hypotension in those receiving antihypertensives
- **Hyper/hypothyroidism:** monitor thyroid function tests before and periodically during therapy; thyroid disease should be treated with thyroid medications
- Monitor for proteinuria before and periodically during therapy; product may need to be decreased or discontinued if moderate to severe proteinuria occurs

⚠ **Pregnancy/breastfeeding:** pregnancy (D); determine if the patient is pregnant or breastfeeding before using this product; may also cause infertility

Evaluate:

- Decreased spread of malignancy

Teach patient/family:

⚠ To use contraception during treatment (pregnancy [D]) or to avoid use of this product; to notify prescriber if pregnancy is planned or suspected, not to breastfeed

⚠ To notify prescriber of bleeding that is severe or that requires treatment

- That product will be discontinued ≥24 hr before surgery; may be resumed after adequate wound healing
- That laboratory testing will be required before and periodically during product use
- How to monitor B/P and that B/P products should be continued as directed by prescriber

⚠ HIGH ALERT

azaCITIDine (Rx)

(a-za-sie-ti′deen)

Vidaza

Func. class.: Antineoplastic

Chem. class.: Pyrimidine nucleoside analogue

Do not confuse:
azaCITIDine/azaTHIOprine

ACTION: Cytotoxic by producing damage to double-strand DNA during DNA synthesis

USES: Myelodysplastic syndrome (MDS)
Unlabeled uses: Acute myelogenous leukemia (AML), chronic myelogenous leukemia (CML)

CONTRAINDICATIONS: Pregnancy (D), hypersensitivity to product or mannitol, advanced malignant hepatic tumors

Precautions: Breastfeeding, children, geriatric patients, renal/hepatic disease, baseline albumin <30 g/L; a man should not father a child while taking product

DOSAGE AND ROUTES

• **Adult: SUBCUT/IV** 75 mg/m²/day × 7 days q4wk, dose may be increased to 100 mg/m² if no response seen after 2 treatment cycles; minimum treatment, 4 cycles

Available forms: Powder for inj 100 mg

Administer:

• Use cytotoxic handling procedures

SUBCUT route

• **Reconstitute** with 4 ml sterile water for inj (25 mg/ml), inject diluents slowly into vial, invert vial 2-3 times, gently rotate; sol will be cloudy, use immediately; divide doses >4 ml into 2 syringes; invert contents 2-3 times, gently roll syringe between the palms for 30 sec immediately before administration, rotate inj site

Intermittent IV INFUSION route

• **Reconstitute** each vial with 10 ml sterile water for inj, shake well until all solids are dissolved, withdraw sol (10 mg/ml), inject in 50-100 NS or LR infusion run over 10-40 min

SIDE EFFECTS

CNS: *Anxiety, depression, dizziness, fatigue, headache, fever, insomnia*

CV: Cardiac murmur, hypotension, tachycardia, peripheral edema, *chest pain*

GI: *Diarrhea, nausea, vomiting,* anorexia, *constipation,* abdominal pain, distention, tenderness, hemorrhoids, mouth hemorrhage, tongue ulceration, stomatitis, dyspepsia, hepatotoxicity, hepatic coma

GU: Renal failure, renal tubular acidosis, dysuria, UTI

HEMA: Leukopenia, anemia, thrombocytopenia, neutropenia, febrile neutropenia, ecchymosis, petechiae

INTEG: *Irritation at site, rash,* sweating, pyrexia, pruritus

META: Hypokalemia

MS: Weakness, arthralgia, muscle cramps, myalgia, back pain

RESP: Cough, *dyspnea, pharyngitis,* pleural effusion

PHARMACOKINETICS

Rapidly absorbed, peak ½ hr, metabolized in the liver, half-life 4 hr, excreted in urine

INTERACTIONS

Increase: bone marrow depression—other antineoplastics

Increase: bleeding—anticoagulants

Drug/Lab

Increase: BUN/Creatinine

Decrease: WBC, platelets, neutrophils, potassium

NURSING CONSIDERATIONS

Assess:

• For CNS symptoms: fever, headache, chills, dizziness

• **Bone marrow suppression/hematologic response:** CBC with differential, baseline WBC ≥3000/mm³, absolute neutrophil count (ANC) ≥1500/mm³, platelets >75,000/mm³, adjust dose based on nadir; ANC <500/mm³, platelets <25,000/mm³, give 50% dose next course; ANC 500-1500/mm³, platelets 25,000-50,000/mm³, give 67% next course; bruising, bleeding, blood in stools, urine, sputum, emesis; myelodysplastic syndrome (MDS), splenomegaly

• Buccal cavity q8hr for dryness, sores, or ulceration, white patches, oral pain, bleeding, dysphagia

• **Myelodysplastic syndrome:** severe anemia, cytopenias, splenomegaly

• Blood studies: BUN, bicarbonate, creatine, LFTs

• Increased fluid intake to 2-3 L/day to prevent dehydration unless contraindicated

• Rinsing of mouth tid-qid with water, club soda; brushing of teeth bid-tid with soft brush or cotton-tipped applicator for stomatitis; use unwaxed dental floss

Evaluate:

• Therapeutic response: improvement in blood counts with refractory anemia or refractory anemia with excess blasts

Teach patient/family:

• To avoid crowds, persons with known infections; not to receive immunizations

• To avoid foods with citric acid or hot or rough texture if stomatitis is present; to drink adequate fluids

• To report stomatitis; any bleeding, white spots, ulcerations in mouth; to examine mouth daily, report symptoms, infection site reactions, pruritus, fever

• To use contraception during and for several months after therapy (pregnancy [D]); not to breastfeed; not to father a child while receiving product

azaTHIOprine (Rx)

(ay-za-thye′oh-preen)

Azasan, Imuran

Func. class.: Immunosuppressant

Chem. class.: Purine antagonist

Do not confuse:

Imuran/Imferon/Elmiron/IMDUR/Enduron/Tenormin

azaTHIOprine/azaCITIDine

ACTION: Produces immunosuppression by inhibiting purine synthesis in cells

USES: Renal transplants to prevent graft rejection, refractory rheumatoid arthritis

Unlabeled uses: Myasthenia gravis, chronic ulcerative colitis, Crohn's disease, Behçet's disease, autoimmune hepatitis, dermatomyositis, thrombocytopenic purpura, lupus nephritis, polymyositis, pulmonary fibrosis, systemic lupus erythematosus (SLE), Wegener's granulomatosis, vasculitis, atopic dermatitis

CONTRAINDICATIONS: Pregnancy (D), hypersensitivity, breastfeeding

Precautions: Severe renal/hepatic disease, geriatric patients, thiopurine methyltransferase deficiency, infection

Black Box Warning: Bone marrow suppression, neoplastic disease, must be used by experienced clinician

DOSAGE AND ROUTES

Prevention of rejection

• **Adult and child: IV** 3-5 mg/kg/day, then maintenance (**PO**) of ≥1-3 mg/kg/day

Renal Dose

• **Adult: PO** Give lower dose in tubular necrosis in immediate post-cadaveric transplant period

Refractory rheumatoid arthritis

• **Adult: PO** 1 mg/kg/day, may increase dose after 2 mo by 0.5 mg/kg/day and then q4wk, max 2.5 mg/kg/day

Lupus nephritis/SLE/Wegener's granulomatosis/idiopathic pulmonary fibrosis/multiple sclerosis (unlabeled)

• **Adult: PO** 2-3 mg/kg/day

Atopic dermatitis (unlabeled)

• **Adult/adolescent ≥16 yr: PO** 2.5 mg/kg/day

Idiopathic thrombocytopenic purpura (unlabeled)

• **Adult: PO** 1-2 mg/kg/day × 3-6 mo, max 150 mg/day

Available forms: Tabs 50, 75, 100 mg; inj 100 mg

Administer:

• For several days before transplant surgery

• All medications PO if possible; avoid IM inj because bleeding may occur

PO route

• With meals to reduce GI upset

IV route

• Prepare in biologic cabinet with gown, gloves, mask

Direct IV

• **Dilute** to 10 mg/ml with 0.9% NaCl, 0.45% NaCl, D_5W, **give** over 5 min

Intermittent IV INFUSION route

• **Reconstitute** 100 mg/10 ml of sterile water for inj; rotate to dissolve; **further dilute** with 50 ml or more saline or glucose in saline, **give** over ½-1 hr

Y-site compatibilities: Alfentanil, atracurium, atropine, benztropine, calcium gluconate, cycloSPORINE, enalaprilat, epoetin alfa, erythromycin, fentaNYL, fluconazole, folic acid, furosemide, glycopyrrolate, heparin, insulin, mannitol,

mechlorethamine, metoprolol, naloxone, nitroglycerin, oxytocin, penicillin G, potassium chloride, propranolol, protamine, SUFentanil, trimetaphan, vasopressin
Solution compatibilities: D_5W, NaCl 0.9%, NaCl 0.45%

SIDE EFFECTS

GI: *Nausea, vomiting,* stomatitis, esophagitis, pancreatitis, hepatotoxicity, jaundice, hepatic veno-occlusive disease
HEMA: Leukopenia, thrombocytopenia, anemia, pancytopenia, bleeding
INTEG: Rash, alopecia
MISC: Serum sickness, Raynaud's symptoms, secondary malignancy, infection
MS: Arthralgia, muscle wasting

PHARMACOKINETICS

Metabolized in liver, excreted in urine (active metabolite), crosses placenta, half-life 3 hr

INTERACTIONS

Increase: leukopenia—ACE inhibitors, sulfamethoxazole-trimethoprim
Increase: myelosuppression—cycloSPORINE, mercaptopurine
Increase: action of azaTHIOprine—allopurinol
Decrease: immune response—vaccines, toxoids
Decrease: action of warfarin—warfarin
• Do not admix with other products

Drug/Lab Test
Increase: LFTs
Decrease: uric acid
Interference: CBC, differential count

NURSING CONSIDERATIONS

Assess:
• **For infection:** increased temperature, WBC; sputum, urine
• I&O, weight daily, report decreasing urine output; toxicity may occur

Black Box Warning: Bone marrow suppression: severe leukopenia, pancytopenia, thrombocytopenia; Hgb, WBC, platelets during treatment monthly; if leukocytes are <3000/mm³ or platelets <100,000/mm³, product should be discontinued, CBC

⚠ **Hepatotoxicity:** if dark urine, jaundice, itching, light-colored stools, increased LFTs, product should be discontinued; hepatic studies: alk phos, AST, ALT, bilirubin
• **Arthritis:** pain, ROM, swelling, mobility before, during treatment

Evaluate:
• Therapeutic response: absence of graft rejection, immunosuppression in autoimmune disorders

Teach patient/family:
• To take as prescribed; not to miss doses; if dose is missed on daily regimen, to skip dose; if taking multiple doses/day, to take as soon as remembered
• That therapeutic response may take 3-4 mo with RA; to continue with prescribed exercise, rest, other medications
• To report fever, rash, severe diarrhea, chills, sore throat, fatigue because **serious infections** may occur; report unusual bleeding, bruising; signs/symptoms of **renal/hepatic toxicity**
• To use contraceptive measures during treatment, for 16 wk after ending therapy (pregnancy [D]); to avoid vaccinations
• To avoid crowds to reduce risk for infection
• To take with food to decrease GI intolerance
• About multiple significant drug–drug interactions
• To use soft-bristled toothbrush to prevent bleeding
• That treatment is ongoing to prevent transplant rejection

RARELY USED

azelaic acid

(aze-eh-lay′ik)

Azelex, Finacea

Func. class.: Antiacne agent

Chem. class.: Dicarboxylic acid

USES: Mild to moderate inflammatory acne vulgaris, rosacea

CONTRAINDICATIONS: Hypersensitivity

DOSAGE AND ROUTES

Adult/child ≥12 yr:

- Apply a thin film and massage into affected areas bid AM and PM

Available forms:

Cream 20%, Gel 15%

azelastine (ophthalmic)

(ah-zell′ah-steen)

Optivar

Func. class.: Antihistamine (ophthalmic)

Chem. class.: H1 receptor antagonist

ACTION: Decreases the allergic response by inhibiting histamine release

USES: Pruritus from allergic conjunctivitis

CONTRAINDICATIONS: Hypersensitivity

Precautions: Pregnancy (C), breastfeeding, child <3 yr

DOSAGE AND ROUTES

- **Adult/child ≥3 yr: OPHTH** 1 drop into each affected eye bid

Available forms: Ophthalmic sol: 0.05%

Administer:

- Tip of dropper should not touch the eye
- Store upright and tightly closed at room temperature

SIDE EFFECTS

CNS: Headache

EENT: Eye burning/stinging/irritation, blurred vision, rhinitis, bitter taste

INTEG: Pruritus

RESP: Asthma, dyspnea, wheezing

PHARMACOKINETICS

Onset 3 min, duration 8 hr, half-life 22 hr, protein binding 88%

NURSING CONSIDERATIONS

Assess:

- Eyes: for itching, redness, use of soft or hard contact lenses

Evaluate:

- Therapeutic response: absence of redness, itching in the eyes

Teach patient/family:

- To use in the eyes only; not to touch dropper to eye/eyelid
- Not to wear contact lenses if eyes are red and itching
- To wait at least 10 min before inserting contact lenses; soft contact lenses can absorb preservative

azelastine nasal agent

See Appendix B

azilsartan

Edarbi

Func. class.: Antihypertensive

Chem. class.: Angiotensin II receptor antagonist

ACTION: Antagonizes angiotensin II at the AT_1 receptor in tissues like vascular smooth muscle and the adrenal gland; two angiotensin II receptors, AT_1 and AT_2, have been identified; azilsartan exhibits more than 10,000-fold greater affinity for the AT_1 receptor than the AT_2 receptor

USES: Hypertension, alone or in combination with other antihypertensives

CONTRAINDICATIONS

Black Box Warning: Pregnancy (D) 2nd/3rd trimesters

Precautions: Pregnancy (C) 1st trimester, breastfeeding, children, geriatric patients, angioedema, African descent, renal disease, renal artery stenosis, heart failure, hypovolemia

DOSAGE AND ROUTES

- **Adult: PO** 80 mg/day, may give an initial dose of 40 mg/day in patients receiving high-dose diuretic therapy

Available forms: Tabs 40, 80 mg

Administer:

- May administer without regard to food
- Use original package to protect from light and moisture, heat

SIDE EFFECTS

CNS: Dizziness, fatigue, asthenia, syncope
CV: Hypotension, orthostatic hypotension
GI: Nausea, diarrhea
HEMA: Anemia
INTEG: Angioedema, rash, pruritus
MS: Muscle cramps
RESP: Cough

PHARMACOKINETICS

Protein binding >99% to serum albumin; metabolized by CYP2C9; elimination half-life 11 hr, steady-state within 5 days and no accumulation in plasma occurs with once-daily dosing; elimination 55% in feces, 42% in urine; hydrolyzed to the active metabolite, azilsartan, in GI tract during absorption, rapidly absorbed, peak 1.5-3 hr; absolute bioavailability (60%) not affected by food

INTERACTIONS

Increase: hypotensive effect—other antihypertensives, other angiotensin receptor antagonists, MAOIs

Increase: hypoglycemia—antidiabetics

⚠ **Increase:** renal failure risk—cyclosporine, diuretics, NSAIDs in those with poor renal function; monitor closely

⚠ **Increase:** lithium toxicity—lithium

⚠ **Increase:** phosphate nephropathy—sodium phosphate monobasic monohydrate; sodium phosphate dibasic anhydrous

Drug/Herb:

Increase: antihypertensive effect—Hawthorn

Decrease: antihypertensive effect—ephedra

NURSING CONSIDERATIONS

Assess:

⚠ **Angioedema:** Assess for facial swelling, difficulty breathing

Black Box Warning: For pregnancy (D) 2nd/3rd trimester, can cause fetal death

- Response and adverse reactions especially in renal disease
- B/P, pulse when beginning therapy and periodically thereafter; note rhythm, rate, quality; obtain electrolytes before beginning therapy

Evaluate:

- Therapeutic response: decreased B/P

Teach patient/family:

- To comply with dosage schedule even if feeling better

⚠ To notify prescriber of facial swelling; if pregnancy is planned or suspected (category D 2nd/3rd trimester)

- That diarrhea, dehydration, excessive perspiration, vomiting, may lead to fall in B/P; to consult prescriber if these occur
- To rise slowly from lying or sitting to minimize orthostatic hypotension; that product may cause dizziness
- To avoid OTC medications unless approved by prescriber; to inform all health care providers of product use
- To use proper technique for obtaining B/P

azithromycin (Rx)

(ay-zi-thro-my′sin)

AzaSite, Zithromax, Zmax, Zithromax Tri Pak, Zithromax Z Pak

Func. class.: Antiinfective

Chem. class.: Macrolide (azalide)

Do not confuse:
azithromycin/erythromycin
Zithromax/Zinacef

ACTION: Binds to 50S ribosomal subunits of susceptible bacteria and suppresses protein synthesis; much greater spectrum of activity than erythromycin; more effective against gram-negative organisms

USES: Mild to moderate infections of the upper respiratory tract, lower respiratory tract; uncomplicated skin and skin structure infections caused by *Bacillus anthracias, Bacteroides bivius, Bordetella paertassis, Borrelia burgdorferi, Campylobacter jun juni, CDC coryneform group G, Chlamydia trachomatis, Chlamydophila pneumonial, Clostridium perffringes, Gardnerella vaginalis, Haemophilisducreyi, influenzal* (beta-lactamase negative/positive) *Helicobacter pylori, Klebsiella granulomatis, Legionella pnemohila moraxella catarrhalis, Mycobacterium arium/intracellulare, Mycoplasma genitalium/homonis/pneumonial, Neisseria gonorrhoel, Peptostreptococcus* sp., *Prevotella bivia, Rickettsia tsutsugamushi, Salmonella typhi, Staphylococcus aureus (MSSA)/epidermidis, Streptococcus* sp., *Toxoplasma gondi, Treponema pallidium, Ureaplasma urealytican, Vibriocholerae, Viridancs streptococci;* **PO;** acute pharyngitis/tonsillitis (group A streptococcal); acute skin/soft-tissue infections; community-acquired pneumonia; pharyngitis/tonsillitis; **Ophthalmic:** bacterial conjunctivitis

Unlabeled uses: Babesiosis, cholera, cystic fibrosis, dental abscess/infection, endocarditis prophylaxis, granuloma inguinale, Legionnaire's disease, Lyme disease, lymphogranuloma venereum, MAC, periodontitis, pertussis, prostatitis, shigellosis, syphilis, toxoplasmosis, typhoid fever

CONTRAINDICATIONS: Hypersensitivity to azithromycin, erythromycin, any macrolide, hepatitis, jaundice

Precautions: Pregnancy (B), breastfeeding; geriatric patients; renal/hepatic/cardiac disease; <6 mo for otitis media; <2 yr for pharyngitis, tonsillitis, QT prolongation, ulcerative colitis, torsades de pointes, sunlight exposure, sodium restriction, myasthenia gravis, *Pseudomembranous colitis,* contact lenses, hypokalemia, hypomagnesemia

DOSAGE AND ROUTES

Most infections

- **Adult: PO** 500 mg on day 1, then 250 mg/day on days 2-5 for a total dose of 1.5 g or 500 mg a day × 3 days
- **Child 2-15 yr: PO** 10 mg/kg on day 1, then 5 mg/kg × 4 days

Disseminated MAC infections

- **Adult: PO** 600 mg/day with ethambutol 15 mg/kg/day

Pelvic inflammatory disease

- **Adult: PO/IV** 500 mg **IV** q24hr × 2 doses, then 250 mg **PO** q24hr × 7-10 days

Cervicitis, chlamydia, chancroid, nongonococcal urethritis, syphilis

- **Adult: PO** 1 g single dose

Gonorrhea

- **Adult: PO** 2 g single dose

Lower respiratory tract infections

- **Adult: PO** 500 mg day 1, then 250 mg × 4 days
- **Child: PO** 5-12 mg/kg/day × 5 days

Acute otitis media

- **Child >6 mo: PO** 30 mg/kg as a single dose or 10 mg/kg/day × 3 days or 10 mg/kg as a single dose on day 1 (max 500 mg/day), then 5 mg/kg on days 2-5 (max 250 mg/day)

Prevention of acute otitis media

- **Child: PO** 10 mg/kg q wk × 6 mo

MAC in HIV

- **Adult/adolescent: PO** 1.2 g q1wk, alone or with rifabutin

Bacterial Conjunctivitis

- **Adult/Child ≥1 yr: Ophthalmic** Instill 1 drop in affected eye bid × 2 days, then 1 drop in eye daily × 5 days

Legionnaire's disease/early Lyme disease (unlabeled)

- **Adult: PO** 500 mg/day

Pertussis (unlabeled)

- **Adult: PO** 500 mg on day 1, then 250 mg/day for 2-5 days
- **Infant ≥6 mo and child: PO** 10 mg/kg/day (max 500 mg) on day 1, then 5 mg/kg/day (max 250 mg) on days 2-5
- **Infant <6 mo: PO** 10 mg/kg/day × 5 days

Available forms: Tabs 250, 500, 600 mg; powder for inj 500 mg; susp 100, 200 mg/5 ml 1 g single-dose powder for susp; ext rel powder for susp 2 g; ophthalmic drops 1% solution

Administer:

Ophthalmic route

- Store in refrigerator
- Do not touch dropper to eye

PO route

- **Susp** 1 hr before meal or 2 hr after meal; reconstitute 1 g packet for susp with 60 ml water, mix, rinse glass with more water and have patient drink to consume all medication; packets not for pediatric use
- Store at room temperature

Intermittent IV INFUSION route

- **Reconstitute** 500 mg of product with 4.8 ml sterile water for inj (100 mg/ml); shake, **dilute** with 250 or 500 ml 0.9% NaCl, 0.45% NaCl, or LR to 1-2 mg/ml; diluted sol stable for 24 hr or 7 days if refrigerated
- **Give** 1 mg/ml sol over 3 hr or 2 mg/ml sol over 1 hr; never give IM or as bolus
- Reconstituted product is stable for 24 hr at room temperature or 7 days refrigerated

Y-site compatibilities: Acyclovir, alatrofloxacin, alemtuzumab, alfentanol, aminocaproic acid, aminophyllum, amphotericin B liposome/complex, ampicillin, ampicillin-sulbactum, anidulafungin, atenolol, bivalirudin, bleomycin, bumetanide, buprenorphine, butorphanol, calcium chloride/gluconate, CARBOplatin, carmustine, ceFAZolin, cefepime, cefoTEtan, cefoxitin, ceftaroline, cefTAZidime, ceftizoxime, cimetidine, cisatracurium, CISplatin, cyclophosphamide, cycloSPORINE, cytarabine, DAPTOmycin, DAUNOrubicin liposome, dexamethasome, dexmedetomidine, dexrazoxane, digoxin, diltiazem, diphenhydrAMINE, DOBUTamine, DOCEtaxel, dolasetron, doripenem, doxacurium, DOXOrubicin liposomal, doxycycline, droperidol, enalaprilat, EPINEPHrine, epirubicin, eptifibatide, ertapenem, esmolol, etoposide, etoposide phosphate, fenoldopam, fluconozole, fluorouracil, foscarnet, fosphenytoin, gallium, ganciclovir, gatifloxacin, gemcitabine, granisetron, haloperidol, heparin, hydrocortisone phosphate/succinate, HYDROmorphone, hydrOXYzine, IDArubicin, ifosfamide, inamrinone, irinotecan, isoproterenol, labetalol, lepirudin, magnesium sulfate, mannitol, meperidine, meropenem, mesna, methochlorethamine, methohexital, methotrexate, methylPREDNISolone, metoclopramide, metroNIDAZOLE, milrinone, minocycline, miralacurium, nalbuphine, naloxone, nesiritide, nitroglycerin, nitroprusside, octreotide, ofloxacin, ondansetron, oxaliplatin, oxytocin, PACLitaxel, palonosetron, pamidronate, pantoprazole, PEMEtrexed, PENTobarbital, phenylephrine, piperacillin, potassium acetate/phosphates, proclinimide, proclorperazine, promethazine, propranolol, ranitidine, remifentanil, rocuronium, sodium acetate, succinylcholine, SUFentanil, sulfamethoxazole-trimethoprim, tacrolimus, telavancin, teniposide, thiotepa, ticarcillin, tigecycline, tirofiban, TPN, trimethobenzamide, vancomycin, vasopressin, vecuronium, verapamil, vinCRIStine, voriconazole, zidovudine, zoledronic acid

SIDE EFFECTS

CNS: Dizziness, headache, vertigo, somnolence, fatigue
CV: Palpitations, chest pain, QT prolongation, torsades de pointes (rare)
EENT: Hearing loss, tinnitus, loss of smell (anosmia)
GI: *Nausea, diarrhea,* hepatotoxicity, abdominal pain, stomatitis, heartburn, dyspepsia, flatulence, melena, cholestatic jaundice, pseudomembranous colitis, tongue discoloration
GU: Vaginitis, moniliasis, nephritis
HEMA: Anemia
INTEG: Rash, urticaria, pruritus, photosensitivity, pain at inj site
SYST: Angioedema, Stevens-Johnson syndrome, toxic epidermal necrolysis

PHARMACOKINETICS

PO: Peak 2-4 hr, duration 24 hr
IV: Peak end of infusion; duration 24 hr; half-life 11-57 hr; excreted in bile, feces, urine primarily as unchanged product; may be inhibitor of P-glycoprotein

INTERACTIONS

Increase: ergot toxicity—ergotamine
⚠ **Increase:** dysrhythmias—pimozide: fatal reaction, do not use concurrently
Increase: QT prolongation—amiodarone, quiNIDine, nilotinib, droperidol, methadone, propafenone, fluoroquinolones, lithium, paliperidone
Increase: effects of oral anticoagulants, digoxin, theophylline, methylPREDNISolone, cycloSPORINE, bromocriptine, disopyramide, triazolam, carBAMazepine, phenytoin, tacrolimus, nelfinavir
Decrease: clearance of triazolam
Decrease: absorption of azithromycin—aluminum, magnesium antacids, separate by ≥2 hr

Drug/Lab Test
Increase: CPK, ALT, AST, bilirubin, BUN, creatinine, alk phos, potassium, blood glucose

Drug/Food
Decrease: absorption—food (susp)
Decrease: blood glucose, potassium, sodium

NURSING CONSIDERATIONS

Assess:
- I&O ratio; report hematuria, oliguria with renal disease
- Hepatic studies: AST, ALT, CBC with differential
- Renal studies: urinalysis, protein, blood
- C&S before product therapy; product may be taken as soon as culture is taken; C&S may be repeated after treatment
- **QT prolongation, torsades de pointes:** assess for patients with serious bradycardia, ongoing proarrhythmic conditions, or elderly; more common in these patients
- **Serious skin reactions:** Stevens-Johnson syndrome, toxic epidermal necrolysis, angioedema; discontinue if rash develops, treat symptomatically
- **Superinfection:** sore throat, mouth, tongue; fever, fatigue, diarrhea, anogenital pruritus
- **Pseudomembranous colitis:** diarrhea, abdominal pain, fever, fatigue, anorexia; obtain CBC, serum albumin
- Bowel pattern before, during treatment
- Respiratory status: rate, character; wheezing, tightness in chest: discontinue product
- Cardiovascular death has occurred in those with serious bradycardia or ongoing hypokalemia, hypomagnesemia, avoid use

Evaluate:
- Therapeutic response: C&S negative for infection; decreased signs of infection

Teach patient/family:
⚠ To report sore throat, fever, fatigue, severe diarrhea, anal/genital itching (may indicate superinfection)
- Not to take aluminum-magnesium–containing antacids simultaneously with this product (PO)

⚠ To notify nurse of diarrhea, dark urine, pale stools; yellow discoloration of eyes, skin; severe abdominal pain
- To complete dosage regimen
- To take ZMAX 1 hr before or 2 hr after a meal; shake well before use
- To use protective clothing or stay out of the sun, photosensitivity may occur

TREATMENT OF HYPERSENSITIVITY: Withdraw product, maintain airway; administer EPINEPHrine, aminophylline, O_2, IV corticosteroids

azithromycin ophthalmic

See Appendix B

RARELY USED

aztreonam (Rx)

(az-tree′oh-nam)

Azactam, Cayston

Func. class.: Antibiotic—miscellaneous

USES: Urinary tract infection; septicemia; skin, muscle, bone infection; lower respiratory tract, intraabdominal infections; other infections caused by gram-negative organisms

CONTRAINDICATIONS: Hypersensitivity to product, severe renal disease

DOSAGE AND ROUTES

Urinary tract infections

- **Adult: IM/IV** 500 mg-1 g q8-12hr

Systemic infections

- **Adult: IM/IV** 1-2 g q8-12hr
- **Child: IM/IV** 90-120 mg/kg/day in divided doses q6-8hr; max 8 g/day **IV**

Severe systemic infections

- **Adult: IM/IV** 2 g q6-8hr; max 8 g/day; continue treatment for 48 hr after negative culture or until patient is asymptomatic

Cystic fibrosis with *Pseudomonas aeruginosa*

- **Adult, adolescent, child ≥7 yr: NEB** 75 mg tid × 28 days, then 28 days off; give q4hr or more; give bronchodilator before aztreonam

bacitracin topical

See Appendix B

baclofen (Rx)

(bak′loe-fen)

Gablofen, Lioresal Intrathecal

Func. class.: Skeletal muscle relaxant, central acting

Chem. class.: GABA chlorophenyl derivative

Do not confuse:
Lioresal/Lotensin
baclofen/Bactroban

ACTION: Inhibits synaptic responses in CNS by stimulating GABAb receptor subtype, which decreases neurotransmitter function; decreases frequency, severity of muscle spasms

USES: Spasticity with spinal cord injury, multiple sclerosis
Unlabeled uses: Neuropathic pain, hiccups, trigeminal neuralgia/nystagmus, recurrent priapism

CONTRAINDICATIONS: Hypersensitivity
Precautions: Pregnancy (C), breastfeeding, geriatric patients, peptic ulcer disease, renal/hepatic disease, stroke, seizure disorder, diabetes mellitus, psychosis

Black Box Warning: Abrupt discontinuation

DOSAGE AND ROUTES

- **Adult: PO** 5 mg tid × 3 days, then 10 mg tid × 3 days, then 15 mg tid × 3 days, then 20 mg tid × 3 days, then titrated to response, max 80 mg/day; **INTRATHECAL** use implantable intrathecal infusion pump, use screening trial of 3 separate bol doses if needed 24 hr apart (50 mcg, 75 mcg, 100 mcg); patients who do not respond to 100 mcg should not be considered for chronic IT therapy; maintenance: spinal origin spasticity 12-2003 mcg/day, cerebral origin spasticity 22-1400 mcg/day
- **Child >2-7 yr: PO** 10-15 mg/day divided q8hr; titrate q3days by 5-15 mg/day to max 40 mg/day
- **Child ≥8 yr:** As above; max 60 mg/day
- **Child: INTRATHECAL** initial test dose same as adult; for small children, initial dose of 25 mcg/dose may be used; 25-1200 mcg/day infusion titrated to response in screening phase

Neuropathic pain including trigeminal neuralgia (unlabeled)

- **Adult: PO** 10 mg tid, may increase by 10 mg every other day; max 80 mg/day

Hiccups (unlabeled)

- **Adult: PO** 10 mg qid

Stuttering/recurrent priapism (unlabeled)

- **Adult: PO** 40 mg at bedtime

Available forms: Tabs 10, 20 mg; IT inj 10,000 mcg/20 ml, 20,000 mcg/20 ml, 40,000 mcg/20 ml; 50 mcg/ml, 0.5 mg/ml, 10 mg/20 ml, 10 mg/5 ml, 40 mg/20 ml; pharmacy can prepare extemperaneous liquid preparations

Administer:

PO route

- With meals for GI symptoms
- Store in a tight container at room temperature

IT route

- **For screening,** dilute to a concentration of 50 mcg/ml with NaCl for inj (preservative free); give test dose over 1 min; watch for decreasing muscle tone, frequency of spasm; if inadequate, use 2 more test doses q24hr; **maintenance infusion** via implantable pump of 500-2000 mcg/ml because individual titration is required
- Do not give IT dose by inj, IV, IM, SUBCUT, epidural

Additive compatibilities: CloNIDine, morphine, ziconotide

SIDE EFFECTS

CNS: *Dizziness, weakness, fatigue, drowsiness,* headache, *disorientation,* insomnia, paresthesias, tremors; **seizures,**

life-threatening CNS depression, coma; CNS infection , impaired cognition memory loss, insomnia, somnolence (IT)
CV: Hypotension, bradycardia, flushing, orthostatic hypotension, chest pain, palpitations, edema; cardiovascular collapse (IT)
EENT: Nasal congestion, blurred vision, mydriasis, tinnitus
GI: *Nausea,* constipation, *vomiting,* abdominal pain, dry mouth, anorexia, weight gain
GU: Urinary frequency, hematuria
INTEG: Rash, pruritus
RESP: Dyspnea; respiratory failure (IT)

PHARMACOKINETICS

PO: Peak 2-3 hr, duration >8 hr, half-life $2^1/_2$-4 hr, partially metabolized in liver, excreted in urine (unchanged)
INTRATHECAL: CSF levels with plasma levels 100 × that of the oral route, peak 4 hr, duration 4-8 hr

INTERACTIONS

Increase: CNS depression—alcohol, tricyclics, opiates, barbiturates, sedatives, hypnotics, MAOIs
Increase: hypotension—antihypertensives
Drug/Herb
Increase: CNS depression—kava, valerian
Drug/Lab Test
Increase: AST, ALT, alk phos, blood glucose, CK

NURSING CONSIDERATIONS

Assess:

Black Box Warning: **Abrupt discontinuation;** serious adverse reactions may occur

- **Multiple sclerosis:** spasms, spasticity, ataxia; improvement should occur with product
- B/P, weight, blood glucose, hepatic function periodically

⚠ **Seizures:** for increased seizure activity with seizure disorders; product decreases seizure threshold; EEG in epileptic patients

- I&O ratio; check for urinary frequency
- Allergic reactions: rash, fever, respiratory distress
- Severe weakness, numbness in extremities
- Tolerance: increased need for medication, more frequent requests for medication, increased pain
- **Withdrawal symptoms:** CNS depression, dizziness, drowsiness, psychiatric symptoms
- **Intrathecal:** have emergency equipment nearby; assess test dose and titration; if no response, check pump, catheter for proper functioning
- Assistance with ambulation if dizziness, drowsiness occurs

Evaluate:

- Therapeutic response: decreased pain, spasticity

Teach patient/family:

- Not to discontinue medication quickly; hallucinations, spasticity, tachycardia will occur; product should be tapered off over 1-2 wk
- Not to take with alcohol, other CNS depressants
- To avoid hazardous activities if drowsiness, dizziness occurs; to rise slowly to prevent orthostatic hypotension
- To avoid using OTC medications; not to take cough preparations, antihistamines unless directed by prescriber
- To notify prescriber if nausea, headache, tinnitus, insomnia, confusion, constipation, inadequate or painful urination continues
- **MS:** may require 1-2 mo for full response

TREATMENT OF OVERDOSE:

Induce emesis in conscious patient, activated charcoal, dialysis, physostigmine to reduce life-threatening CNS side effects

⚠ HIGH ALERT

basiliximab (Rx)

(bas-ih-liks′ih-mab)

Simulect

Func. class.: Immunosuppressant

Chem. class.: Murine/human monoclonal antibody (interleukin-2) receptor antagonist

ACTION: Binds to and blocks the IL-2 receptor, which is selectively expressed on the surface of activated T lymphocytes; impairs the immune system to antigenic challenges

USES: Acute allograft rejection in renal transplant patients when used with cycloSPORINE and corticosteroids

Unlabeled uses: Liver transplant rejection prophylaxis

CONTRAINDICATIONS: Breastfeeding

Precautions: Pregnancy (B), children, geriatric patients, human anti-murine antibody, hypersensitivity to mannitol/murine, exposure to viral infections

Black Box Warning: Infections

DOSAGE AND ROUTES

- **Adult/child ≥35 kg: IV** 20 mg × 2 doses; 1st dose within 2 hr before transplant surgery; 2nd dose 4 days after transplantation
- **Child/adolescent <35 kg: IV** 10 mg × 2 doses; 1st dose within 2 hr before transplant surgery; 2nd dose 4 days after transplantation

Available forms: Powder for inj 10, 20 mg

Administer:

Intermittent IV INFUSION route

- **Reconstitute** 10-mg vial/2.5 ml or 20-mg vial in 5 ml sterile water for inj; shake gently to dissolve; **dilute** reconstituted sol in 25 ml (10-mg vial) or 50 ml (20-mg vial) with 0.9% NaCl or D_5W; gently invert bag, do not shake; **give** over ½ hr, do not admix
- Store reconstituted sol refrigerated for up to 24 hr or at room temperature for 4 hr

SIDE EFFECTS

CNS: *Pyrexia, chills, tremors, headache, insomnia, weakness, dizziness*

CV: *Chest pain,* angina, cardiac failure, hypotension, *hypertension, edema*

GI: *Vomiting, nausea, diarrhea, constipation, abdominal pain,* GI bleeding, *gingival hyperplasia, stomatitis*

GU: Urinary retention/frequency

INTEG: *Acne,* pruritus, impaired wound healing

META: *Acidosis, hypercholesterolemia, hyperuricemia, hypo/hyperkalemia, hypocalcemia, hypophosphatemia*

MISC: *Infection, moniliasis,* anaphylaxis, anemia, allergic reaction, dysuria, CMV infection, candidiasis, abnormal vision

MS: *Arthralgia, myalgia*

RESP: *Dyspnea, wheezing,* pulmonary edema, *cough*

PHARMACOKINETICS

Peak ½ hr (adults); terminal half-life 7 days (adult), 9½ days (children)

INTERACTIONS

Increase: immunosuppression—other immunosuppressants

Drug/Herb

Decrease: St. John's wort, turmeric

Drug/Lab Test

Increase: cholesterol, BUN, uric acid, creatinine, potassium, calcium blood glucose, Hgb, Hct

Decrease: Hgb, Hct, platelets, magnesium, phosphate

NURSING CONSIDERATIONS

Assess:

Black Box Warning: For infection: increased temperature, WBC, sputum, urine; may be fatal (bacterial, protozoal, fungal)

- Blood studies: Hgb, WBC, platelets during treatment monthly; if leukocytes

are <3000/mm^3, product should be discontinued; electrolytes, B/P, edema assessment
- Hepatic studies: alk phos, AST, ALT, bilirubin

⚠ **Anaphylaxis, hypersensitivity:** dyspnea, wheezing, rash, pruritus, hypotension, tachycardia; if severe hypersensitivity reactions occur, product should not be used again

Evaluate:
- Therapeutic response: absence of graft rejection

Teach patient/family:

> **Black Box Warning:** To report fever, chills, sore throat, fatigue; serious infection may occur

- To avoid crowds, persons with known upper respiratory tract infections
- To use contraception during treatment
- To report GI symptoms, bleeding, allergic reactions

beclomethasone (Rx)

(be-kloe-meth′a-sone)

QVAR

Func. class.: Corticosteroid, synthetic

Chem. class.: Glucocorticoid

Do not confuse:
beclomethasone/betamethasone

ACTION: Prevents inflammation by suppression of the migration of polymorphonuclear leukocytes, fibroblasts and the reversal of increased capillary permeability and lysosomal stabilization; does not suppress hypothalamus and pituitary function

USES: Chronic asthma, allergic/vasomotor rhinitis, nasal polyps

CONTRAINDICATIONS: Hypersensitivity, status asthmaticus (primary treatment)

Precautions: Pregnancy (C), breastfeeding, children <12 yr, nasal disease/surgery, nonasthmatic bronchial disease; bacterial, fungal, viral infections of mouth, throat, lungs; HPA suppression, osteoporosis, Cushing's syndrome, diabetes mellitus, measles, cataracts, corticosteroid hypersensitivity, glaucoma, herpes infection

DOSAGE AND ROUTES
- **Adult and child >12 yr: INH** 40-80 mcg bid (alone) or 40-160 mcg bid (previous inhaled corticosteroids); max 320 mcg bid
- **Child 5-11 yr: INH** 40 mcg bid; max 80 mcg bid

Available forms: Oral inh 40, 80, 250 🍁 mcg/metered spray

Administer:
- Bronchodilator inhaler; if used, should be used 1st, then wait a few minutes, then use beclomethasone
- Prime before 1st use or if not used for 7-10 days; prime by spraying 2 actuations into the air, away from the face; do not share inhaler
- **Oral inhalation** (metered-dose non-CFC aerosol); shake well, use spacer; after using, rinse mouth, gargle if possible; clean weekly with dry cloth/tissue; do not wash inhaler
- Titrated dose, use lowest effective dose

SIDE EFFECTS
CNS: *Headache,* psychiatric/behavioral changes (child)

EENT: *Hoarseness, candidal infection of oral cavity, sore throat,* loss of taste/smell, dysgeusia, pharyngitis, rhinitis, sinusitis, cataracts, fungal infections, epistaxis

ENDO: HPA suppression

GI: Dry mouth, dyspepsia

MISC: Angioedema, adrenal insufficiency, facial edema, Churg-Strauss syndrome (rare)

RESP: Bronchospasm, wheezing, cough

PHARMACOKINETICS
INH: Onset 1-4 wk; excreted in feces, urine (metabolites); half-life 2.8 hr; crosses placenta; metabolized in lungs, liver (by CYP3A)

NURSING CONSIDERATIONS

Assess:

- For fungal infection in mucous membranes
- Adrenal function periodically for HPA axis suppression during prolonged therapy, monitor growth/development
- Gum, rinsing of mouth for dry mouth

Evaluate:

- Therapeutic response: decreased dyspnea, wheezing, dry crackles

Teach patient/family:

- To gargle/rinse mouth after each use to prevent oral fungal infections
- That during times of stress, systemic corticosteroids may be needed to prevent adrenal insufficiency; not to discontinue oral product abruptly, to taper slowly
- To notify prescriber if therapeutic response decreases; dosage adjustment may be needed
- Proper administration technique and cleaning technique, need for spacer or face mask
- About all aspects of product usage, including cushingoid symptoms
- About **adrenal insufficiency symptoms:** nausea, anorexia, fatigue, dizziness, dyspnea, weakness, joint pain, depression

beclomethasone (nasal)

(be-kloe-meth′a-sone)

Beconase AQ, Qnasl, Rivanase ✦

Func. class.: Nasal corticosteroid

ACTION: Readily crosses cell membranes and binds with high affinity to specific cytoplasmic receptors; inhibition of leukocyte infiltration at the site of inflammation, interference in the function of mediators of inflammatory response, and suppression of humoral immune responses

USES: To relieve symptoms of seasonal/perennial rhinitis, postsurgical nasal polyps prophylaxis

CONTRAINDICATIONS: Hypersensitivity

Precautions: Child <6 yr, untreated fungal infections, glaucoma and/or cataracts, nasal septum ulcers/surgery/trauma

DOSAGE AND ROUTES

- **Adult/child ≥12 yr:** Nasal 1-2 sprays in each nostril bid (42 mcg/spray); 2 sprays in each nostril every day (80 mcg/actuation)
- **Child 6-12 yr:** Nasal 1 spray (42 mcg) in each nostril bid

Available forms: Nasal spray 42 mcg/metered spray; nasal aerosol 40, 80 mcg/actuation

Administer:

- Products are not always interchangeable owing to differences in route of administration and in the amount of active drug released per spray
- To avoid the spread of infection, do not use the container for more than one person
- Product's effectiveness depends on regular use

Nasal inhalation (metered-dose aerosol) (Qnasal):

- Instruct patient to shake the canister well before administering
- Before first use, instruct the patient to prime the pump by actuating 4 times; after the initial priming, the dose-counter should read 120
- If the canister is not used for 7 consecutive days, instruct the patient to prime by actuating 2 times
- Instruct patient on proper administration technique

Nasal inhalation (pump spray) (Beconase AQ):

- Instruct patient to shake the nasal sprayer well before use
- Before first use, instruct the patient to prime the pump by actuating 6 times
- If the pump is not used for 7 days, prime until a fine spray appears
- Instruct patient on proper administration technique
- After use, rinse the tip of the bottle with hot water, taking care not to suck water

into the bottle, and dry with a clean tissue; replace the cap

SIDE EFFECTS

INTEG: Rash, urticaria
SYST: Decreased growth, HPA suppression
CNS: Headache, dizziness
EENT: Nasal burning, epistaxis, nasal fungal infections, nasal congestion, sneezing, irritation, loss of smell/taste, cataracts
GI: Nausea

PHARMACOKINETICS

Onset 5-7 days, peak 21 days, half-life 15 hr

NURSING CONSIDERATIONS

Assess:

- Nasal symptoms: assess for sneezing, running of nose before and after use; avoid use longer than 3 wk; check for fungal infections, changes in vision

Evaluate:

- Decrease nasal running, sneezing, other symptoms of seasonal/perennial rhinitis

Teach patient/family:

- That products are not always interchangeable owing to differences in route of administration and in the amount of active drug released per spray
- Not to use the container for more than one person, to avoid the spread of infection
- That product effectiveness depends on regular use

Nasal inhalation (metered-dose aerosol) (Qnasal):

- Instruct patient to shake the canister well before administering
- Before first use, instruct the patient to prime the pump by actuating 4 times; after the initial priming, the dose-counter should read 120
- If the canister is not used for 7 consecutive days, instruct the patient to prime by actuating 2 times
- Instruct patient on proper administration technique

Nasal inhalation (pump spray) (Beconase AQ):

- Instruct patient to shake the nasal sprayer well before use
- Before first use, instruct the patient to prime the pump by actuating 6 times
- If the pump is not used for 7 days, prime until a fine spray appears
- Instruct patient on proper administration technique
- After use, rinse the tip of the bottle with hot water, taking care not to suck water into the bottle, and dry with a clean tissue; replace the cap

bedaquiline

bed-ak'-wi-leen

Sirturo

Func. class.: Antiinfective/antituberculotic

Chem. class.: Diarylquinoline

ACTION: Inhibits an enzyme that binds to adenosine 5'-triphosphate (ATP) synthase and prevents ATP synthase from using the energy from hydrogen and/or sodium

USES: For use as part of a combination regimen to treat pulmonary multidrug-resistant tuberculosis infection (MDR-TB) when other effective treatment regimens are not available

CONTRAINDICATIONS: Hypersensitivity

Precautions: Alcoholism, bradycardia, breastfeeding, arrhythmias, cardiac disease, children, coronary artery disease, diabetes mellitus, females, geriatric, heart failure, hepatic disease, hypertension, hypocalcemia, hypokalemia, hypomagnesemia, malnutrition, MI, pregnancy (B), syncope, thyroid disease

Black Box Warning: QT prolongation

DOSAGE AND ROUTES

- **Adults:** PO 400 mg daily × 2 wk, then reduce dose to 200 mg 3×/wk with food (≥48 hr between doses). Total duration is 24 wk

Available forms: Tabs 100 mg

Administer:

• If a dose is missed during the first 2 wk of treatment, instruct patient not to make up the missed dose but to continue with the usual dosing schedule. If a dose is missed during treatment wk 3-24, the missed dose should be taken as soon as possible and then resume 3×/wk regimen

• Give in combination with at least 3 other drugs proven to be or at least 4 other drugs suspected of being effective against the patient's *Mycobacterium tuberculosis* isolate

• **Give with food, give with water, use whole, do not break, crush, chew**

• **Store at room temperature in light-resistant container**

SIDE EFFECTS

CNS: *Headache*

CV: QT-C prolongation, chest pain

GI: Nausea, anorexia

MISC: Arthralgia, rash, hemoptysis

PHARMACOKINETICS

Half-life 5 mo, peak 5 hr

INTERACTIONS

Increase: QT prolongation—other drugs that prolong QT (class IA/III antidysrhythmics, some phenothiazines, beta agonists, local anesthetics, tricyclics, haloperidol, chloroquine, droperidol; CYP3A4 inhibitors (amiodarone, clarithromycin, erythromycin); CYP3A4 substrates (methadone, pimozide, quetiapine, quinidine, risperidone, ziprasidone)

Increase: adverse reactions—lopinavir/ritonavir

Increase: bedaquiline effect—strong CYP3A4 inhibitors, avoid use over 14 days

Decrease: bedaquiline effect—strong CYP3A4 inducers, avoid concurrent use

Drug/Lab Test:

Increase: hepatic enzymes

NURSING CONSIDERATIONS

Assess:

• **Acute TB:** chest x-ray, sputum culture, blood culture

• **Liver function:** monitor LFTs baseline and monthly if needed, repeat if >3 × ULN, test for viral hepatitis before use; monitor for dark urine, anorexia, jaundice, nausea, fatigue, hepatomegaly

Black Box Warning: QT Prolongation: monitor ECG baseline, at 2, 12 and 24 wk or more often if QT prolongation is suspected; close monitoring of the ECG is needed in those with QT prolonging risk factors; if prolongation of the QT interval is detected, electrolyte monitoring and frequent ECG (to ensure QTc interval return to baseline) are recommended; those developing a clinically significant ventricular arrhythmia or a QTcF interval >500 ms (confirmed by repeat ECG) discontinue this product and all other QT prolonging products

• Monitor Ca, magnesium, K baseline and periodically, correct imbalances

Evaluate:

• Positive therapeutic outcome: negative culture

Teach Patient/Family:

• The importance of compliance with the entire course of therapy, that tabs should be swallowed whole, take with water and food and used as part of a multidrug regimen

• Avoid breastfeeding, to notify prescriber if pregnancy is planned or suspected (B)

• Avoid use of alcohol, and all medications, herbs unless approved by prescriber

• That scheduled appointments must be kept because relapse may occur

belatacept

(bel-a-ta′sept)

Nulojix

Func. class.: Biologic response modifier

Chem. class.: Fusion protein

ACTION:

Activated T-lymphocytes are the mediators of immunologic rejection. This product is a selective T-cell costimulation blocker; blocks the CD28 mediated costimulation of T-lymphocytes by binding to CD80 and CD86 on antigen-presenting cells; inhibits T-lymphocyte proliferation and the production of the cytokines interleukin-2, interferon-gamma, interleukin-4, and TNF-alpha.

USES:
Kidney transplant rejection prophylaxis given with basiliximab induction, mycophenolate mofetil, corticosteroids

CONTRAINDICATIONS:
Hypersensitivity, EBV seronegative, EBV status unknown

Precautions: Breastfeeding, child/infant/neonate, pregnancy (C), diabetes mellitus, progressive multifocal leukoencephalopathy, immunosuppression, sunlight exposure, TB

Black Box Warning: Infection, organ transplant, requires an experienced clinician, secondary malignancy, posttransplant lymphoproliferation disorder

DOSAGE AND ROUTES

- **Adult: IV** 10 mg/kg rounded to the nearest 12.5-mg increment; give over 30 min the day of transplantation (day 1) but before transplantation, on day 5 approximately 96 hours after the day 1 dose 1, at the end of wk 2, at the end of wk 4, at the end of wk 8, and at the end of wk 12; maintenance dosage is 5 mg/kg rounded to the nearest 12.5-mg increment; give over 30 min at the end of wk 16 and every 4 wk ± 3 days thereafter; doses should be calculated on actual body weight on the transplantation day unless the patient's weight varies by >10%

Available forms: Powder for inj 250 mg

Administer:

Black Box Warning: Only providers skilled in the use of immunosuppressant and management of transplant should use these products

IV route

- Visually inspect for particulate matter, discoloration; discard if present
- Calculate the number of drug vials required to provide total infusion dose
- Reconstitute each vial/10.5 ml of sterile water for injection, 0.9% sodium chloride, D_5W, using the silicone-free disposable syringe provided with each vial and an 18-21G needle; if silicone-free disposable syringe is dropped or becomes contaminated, use a new silicone-free disposable syringe; if you need additional silicone-free disposable syringes, call 1-888-685-6549; if the powder is accidentally reconstituted using a different syringe than the one provided, the sol may develop a few translucent particles; discard any sol prepared using siliconized syringes
- Using aseptic technique, inject the diluent into the vial and direct the stream of diluent to the glass wall of the vial; to minimize foaming, rotate the vial and invert with gentle swirling until the contents are dissolved; do not shake when reconstituted (25 mg/ml), should be clear to slightly opalescent and colorless to pale yellow; do not use if opaque particles, discoloration, or other foreign particles are present
- Calculate the total volume of the reconstituted 25 mg/ml sol required to provide the total infusion dose; further dilute this volume with a volume of infusion fluid equal to the volume of the reconstituted drug sol required; use either NS or D_5W if drug was reconstituted with SWFI; use NS if drug was reconstituted with NS; use D_5W if drug was reconstituted with D_5W; with the same silicone-free disposable syringe used for reconstitution, withdraw the required amount of belatacept sol from the vial, inject it into the infusion container, gently rotate; final concentrations in infusion container should range 2-10 mg/ml; volume of 100 ml will be appropriate for most doses, but total infusion volumes ranging from 50-250 ml may be used;

discard any unused sol; after reconstitution, immediately transfer the reconstituted sol from the vial to the infusion bag or bottle; complete within 24 hr

IV INFUSION route

- Give over 30 min, use an infusion set and a sterile, nonpyrogenic, low-protein-binding filter (0.2-1.2 mm), use a separate line
- Store refrigerated, protected from light ≤24 hr; max 4 hr of the total 24 hr can be at room temperature and room light

SIDE EFFECTS

CV: Hypo/hypertension

CNS: Guillain-Barré syndrome, anxiety, dizziness, headache, fever, insomnia, tremors

EENT: Pharyngitis, stomatitis

GI: Abdominal pain, constipation, diarrhea, nausea, vomiting

GU: Renal tubular necrosis, renal failure, proteinuria, urinary incontinence, dysuria, UTI

HEMA: Anemia, neutropenia, leucopenia, leukoencephalopathy

INTEG: Acne, alopecia, infusion reaction

META: Hypercholesterolemia, hyperglycemia, hyper/hypokalemia, hypocalcemia, hypophosphatemia, hypomagnesemia

MS: Arthralgia

SYST: Secondary malignancy, posttransplant lymphoproliferation disorder, wound dehiscence, BK-virus-associated neuropathy

PHARMACOKINETICS

Half-life, 6.1-15.1 days during receipt of 10 mg/kg IV doses; during receipt of 5 mg/kg IV doses, terminal half-life 3.1-11.9; steady state by wk 8 after transplantation and by mo 6 during maintenance phase

INTERACTIONS

- Do not use 30 days before or with this product: live virus vaccines
- Do not use with cyclophosphamide IV

NURSING CONSIDERATIONS

Assess:

Black Box Warning: Transplant rejection: flulike symptoms, decreasing urinary output, malaise; some may experience pain in area (rare; monitor BUN/creatinine)

Black Box Warning: Infection: monitor for fever, chills, increased WBC, **wound dehiscences**

Black Box Warning: Posttransplant lymphoproliferation disorder: may lead to secondary malignancy (lymphoma) or infectious mononucleosis-like lesions; may be treated with antivirals or immunosuppressant; product may need to be discontinued

- Hyperlipidemia: monitor cholesterol, triglycerides; an antilipidemic may be needed

Evaluate:

- Therapeutic response: absence of renal transplant rejection

Teach patient/family:

- Reason for product and expected result, use REMS guidelines
- To avoid exposure to sunlight, tanning beds, risk of secondary malignancy
- To avoid crowds, persons with known infections
- That repeated lab test will be needed
- To avoid with vaccines
- That immunosuppressants will be needed for life to prevent rejection; symptoms of rejection/infection and to call provider immediately

belimumab

(be-lim′ue-mab)

Benlysta

Func. class.: Monoclonal antibody

Chem. class.: Disease-modifying antirheumatic drugs (DMARDs)

ACTION: Inhibits B-lymphocyte stimulator (BLyS), needed for B-cell survival; normally, soluble BLyS binds to its receptors on B cells and allows B-cell survival; binds BLyS and prevents binding to its receptors on B-cells

USES:
Active, autoantibody-positive, systemic lupus erythematosus (SLE) in combination with standard therapy

CONTRAINDICATIONS:
Hypersensitivity

Precautions: Pregnancy (C), breastfeeding, children/infants, geriatric patients, African descent patients, depression, immunosuppression, infection, suicidal ideation, vaccination, secondary malignancy, cardiac disease; requires experienced clinician

DOSAGE AND ROUTES
- **Adult: IV** 10 mg/kg over 1 hr q2wk for the first 3 doses, then q4wk

Available forms: Powder for injection 120, 400 mg

Administer:
- Only health care providers prepared to manage anaphylaxis should administer this product; may give premedication for prophylaxis against infusion and hypersensitivity reactions

Intermittent IV INFUSION route
- Visually inspect particulate matter and discoloration whenever sol and container permits
- Give as IV infusion only; do not give IV bolus or push; give over 1 hr and slow or stop if infusion reactions occur
- Do not give with any other agents in the same IV line
- Allow to stand at room temperature for 10-15 min before using
- Reconstitute with the appropriate amount of sterile water for injection (80 mg/ml); add 1.5 ml of sterile water (120 mg/vial) or 4.8 ml of sterile water (400 mg/vial)
- Direct the stream of sterile water toward the side of the vial to minimize foaming; gently swirl for 60 sec, allow to sit during reconstitution, gently swirl for 60 sec q5min until the powder is dissolved; do not shake; reconstitution is complete in 10-30 min
- If a mechanical reconstitution device (swirler) is used, max 500 rpm swirled for ≤30 min
- Sol should be opalescent and colorless to pale yellow and without particles; small air bubbles are expected; protect from sunlight
- Dilution: only dilute in normal saline for injection; dilute reconstituted sol with enough normal saline to 250 ml; from a 250-ml infusion bag or bottle of normal saline, withdraw and discard a volume equal to the volume of the reconstituted sol required for dose; add the required volume of the reconstituted sol to the infusion bag/bottle; gently invert to mix
- Discard any unused sol
- Store in refrigerator or at room temperature; total time from reconstitution to completion of infusion max 8 hr

SIDE EFFECTS
CNS: Headache, dizziness, anxiety, depression, fever, insomnia, migraine, suicidal ideation

GU: UTI

CV: Bradycardia, hypotension

GI: Nausea, diarrhea

MISC: Rash, dyspnea, cystitis, leukopenia, myalgia, rash, bronchitis, nasopharyngitis, pharyngitis

SYST: Anaphylaxis, angioedema, antibody formation, secondary malignancy, infection, influenza, infusion reactions

PHARMACOKINETICS
Terminal half-life 19.4 days; distribution half-life 1.75 days

NURSING CONSIDERATIONS
Assess:
- **SLE:** monitor for decreasing fever, malaise, fatigue, joint pain, myalgias
- **Suicidal ideation:** more common in those with preexisting depression
- **Infection:** determine if a chronic or acute infection is present, may be fatal when used with this product; do not begin therapy if any products are being

used for a chronic infection; leukopenia may occur with this product and susceptibility to infections increased

- **Anaphylaxis,** infusion site reactions: if these occur, stop infusion
- **African descent patients:** use cautiously in these patients, may not respond to this product
- Cardiac disease: monitor closely for cardiovascular side effects, bradycardia, hypotension
- Pregnancy: determine if pregnant or if pregnancy is planned or suspected; if pregnant, call 1-877-681-6269 to enroll in registry

Evaluate:

- Positive response: decreasing symptoms of SLE: decreasing fatigue, fever, malaise

Teach patient/family:

- To notify prescriber if pregnancy is planned or suspected; to use reliable contraception during and for 4 mo after final treatment; to avoid breastfeeding
- To seek treatment immediately for serious hypersensitive reactions
- Not to receive live vaccinations during treatment

⚠ HIGH ALERT

belinostat

(beh-lih′noh-stat′)

Beleodaq

Func. class.: Antineoplastic-biologic response modifier

Chem. class.: Histone deacetylase inhibitors

ACTION: A class I and II inhibitor of the histone deacetylase (HDAC) enzymes. Overexpression of HDACs is present in some cancer cells. HDAC inhibitors have been shown to activate differentiation, inhibit the cell cycle, and induce apoptosis

USES: For the treatment of relapsed or refractory peripheral T-cell lymphoma (PTCL)

CONTRAINDICATIONS: Hypersensitivity, pregnancy (D)

Precautions: Hematologic toxicity (thrombocytopenia, leukopenia, neutropenia, lymphopenia, anemia), serious infections (pneumonia, sepsis), fatal hepatic toxicity, tumor lysis syndrome (TLS), breastfeeding

DOSAGE AND ROUTES

- **Adult: IV** 1000 mg/m^2 over 30 min on days 1-5 q21days. Reduce the dose to 750 mg/m^2 in those who are homozygous for the UGT1A1*28 allele. Cycles should be repeated until disease progression or unacceptable toxicity

Available forms: Powder for injection 500 mg

Administer:

Intermittent IV route

- Reconstitution: Add 9 ml of sterile water for injection/500 mg, swirl until there are no visible particles in the solution (50 mg/ml); stable at room temperature for up to 12 hr
- Withdraw the appropriate amount from the reconstituted vial and further dilute in 250 ml 0.9% sodium chloride for injection, the final solution is stable at room temperature for up to 36 hr, including infusion time; use a 0.22-micron in-line filter; give over 30 min, if pain occurs at infusion site, run over 45 min

Dose adjustments due to treatment-related toxicity

Hematologic toxicities:

- Do not begin the next cycle of treatment until the absolute neutrophil count (ANC) is ≥1000/mm^3 and platelet count ≥50,000/mm^3
- ANC nadir ≥500/mm^3 ***and*** platelet count nadir ≥25,000/mm^3: no dose adjustment
- ANC nadir <500/mm^3 (any platelet count): begin next cycle of treatment at a reduced dose of 750 mg/m^2. For the second occurrence of an ANC nadir <500/mm^3, reduce the dose of the next cycle to 500 mg/m^2, if the ANC nadir is <500/mm^3 after 2 dose reductions, discontinue therapy

- Platelet nadir <25,000/mm³ (any ANC): begin next cycle of treatment at a reduced dose of 750 mg/m². For the second occurrence of a platelet nadir <25,000/mm³, reduce the dose of the next cycle to 500 mg/m². If the platelet nadir is <25,000/mm³ after 2 dose reductions, discontinue therapy

Nonhematologic toxicities:

- Grade 3 or 4 nausea, vomiting, or diarrhea for >7 days with supportive management, or other grade 3 or 4 toxicity of any duration: hold treatment. When toxicity resolves to grade ≤2, restart the next cycle at a reduced dose of 750 mg/m². For the second occurrence of grade 3 or 4 toxicity (for a duration >7 days with supportive management for GI toxicities), resume therapy at 500 mg/m² upon resolution to grade ≤2. If the grade 3 or 4 toxicity recurs after 2 dose reductions, discontinue therapy

SIDE EFFECTS

CNS: Fatigue, headache, dizziness, fever, chills

CV: Hypotension, QT prolongation

GI: *Constipation, anorexia, abdominal pain, nausea, vomiting, diarrhea,* **hepatotoxicity**

HEMA: Anemia, thrombocytopenia, neutropenia

RESP: Dyspnea, cough

INTEG: Injection-site reactions, rash, phlebitis,

MISC: Hypokalemia

SYST: Multi-organ failure, TLS, serious infections

PHARMACOKINETICS

Half-life of 1.1 hr; 92.9%-95.8% protein bound, 80%-90% metabolized by hepatic UGT1A1; metabolized in the liver, 40% excreted renally, primarily as metabolites

INTERACTIONS

Increase: belinostat—strong UGT1A1 inhibitors

NURSING CONSIDERATIONS

Assess:

- **Hematologic toxicity (thrombocytopenia, leukopenia, neutropenia, lymphopenia, anemia):** Monitor CBC before starting therapy and then every week. Dose modifications may be necessary in patients with bone marrow suppression and should be determined by the ANC and platelet count nadirs of the previous cycle of therapy. Platelet counts should be ≥50,000/mm³ and ANC >1000/mm³ before starting each cycle
- **Serious infections (pneumonia, sepsis):** May be fatal. Do not use in those with an active infection. Use caution in patients with a history of extensive or intensive chemotherapy, as they may be at higher risk of life-threatening infections
- **Fatal hepatic toxicity:** Monitor LFTs before the start of each cycle. Those with signs of hepatic disease may require dose modification or discontinuation
- **TLS:** Those with high tumor burden or advanced stage disease are at greater risk for development of TLS; consider tumor lysis prophylaxis with antihyperuricemic agents and hydration beginning 12-24 hr before treatment; for TLS treatment, administer aggressive IV hydration, antihyperuricemic agents, correct electrolyte abnormalities, and monitor renal function
- **Pregnancy (D) and breastfeeding:** Consider discontinuing breastfeeding, identify whether the patient is pregnant before using
- **Renal studies:** Monitor BUN/creatinine periodically

Evaluate:

- **Therapeutic response:** Prevention of spread of disease

Teach patient/family:

- To avoid use in breastfeeding, and not to use in pregnancy (D)
- To report infusion-site reactions, rash, severe constipation or diarrhea, abdominal pain

B

benazepril (Rx)

(ben-aze′uh-pril)

Lotensin

Func. class.: Antihypertensive

Chem. class.: Angiotensin-converting enzyme (ACE) inhibitor

Do not confuse:
benazepril/Benadryl

ACTION: Selectively suppresses renin-angiotensin-aldosterone system; inhibits ACE, thus preventing conversion of angiotensin I to angiotensin II

USES: Hypertension, alone or in combination with thiazide diuretics

Unlabeled uses: CHF, diabetic nephropathy, proteinuria, renal impairment

CONTRAINDICATIONS: Breastfeeding, children, hypersensitivity to ACE inhibitors, angioedema

Black Box Warning: Pregnancy (D)

Precautions: Geriatric patients, impaired renal/hepatic function, dialysis patients, hypovolemia, blood dyscrasias, CHF, asthma, bilateral renal artery stenosis

DOSAGE AND ROUTES

- **Adult: PO** 10 mg/day initially, then 20-40 mg/day divided bid or daily (without a diuretic); reduce initial dose to 5 mg **PO** daily (with a diuretic); max 80 mg/day
- **Geriatric: PO** used on the basis of the clinical response
- **Child ≥6 yrs: PO** 0.2 mg/kg/day max 5 mg/day

Renal dose

- **Adult: PO** CCr <30 ml/min 5 mg **PO** daily, max 40 mg/day

Renal impairment due to diabetic nephropathy (unlabeled)

- **Adult: PO** 5-10 mg/day

Heart failure (unlabeled)

- **Adult: PO** 2-20 mg/day

Available forms: Tabs 5, 10, 20, 40 mg

Administer:

- May give without regard to food
- Do not discontinue product abruptly
- Store in tight container at 86° F (30° C) or less

SIDE EFFECTS

CNS: Anxiety, hypertonia, insomnia, paresthesia, headache, dizziness, fatigue

CV: Hypotension, postural hypotension, syncope, palpitations, angina

GI: Nausea, constipation, vomiting, gastritis, melena, diarrhea, **hepatotoxicity, pancreatitis**

GU: Increased BUN, creatinine, decreased libido, impotence, UTI, renal insufficiency

HEMA: **Agranulocytosis, neutropenia**

INTEG: Rash, flushing, sweating, alopecia

META: Hyperkalemia, hyponatremia

MISC: **Angioedema, Stevens-Johnson syndrome**, hypersensitivity

MS: Arthralgia, arthritis, myalgia

RESP: Cough, asthma, bronchitis, dyspnea, sinusitis

PHARMACOKINETICS

Peak 1-2 hr fasting, 2-4 hr after food; protein binding 89%-95%; half-life 10-11 hr; metabolized by liver (metabolites); excreted in urine 33%

INTERACTIONS

Increase: hypotension—phenothiazines, nitrates, acute alcohol ingestion, diuretics, other antihypertensives

Increase: hyperkalemia—potassium-sparing diuretics, potassium supplements

Increase: myelosuppression—azaTHIOprine

Increase: serum levels of lithium, digoxin

Decrease: hypotensive effects—NSAIDs

Drug/Herb

Increase: antihypertensive effect—hawthorn

Decrease: antihypertensive effect—ephedra (Ma huang)

Drug/Lab Test

Increase: AST, ALT, alk phos, bilirubin, uric acid, blood glucose, potassium

Positive: ANA titer

False positive: ANA titer

NURSING CONSIDERATIONS

Assess:

- **Hypertension:** B/P, pulse at baseline, periodically; orthostatic hypotension, syncope when used with diuretic; notify prescriber of changes; monitor compliance
- **Blood dyscrasias:** neutrophils, decreased platelets; WBC with differential at baseline, q3mo; if neutrophils <1000/mm^3, discontinue treatment; recommended with **collagen-vascular disease**
- Renal studies: protein, BUN, creatinine; increased levels may indicate nephrotic syndrome; monitor urine for protein; LFTs, uric acid, glucose may be increased; diuretic should be discontinued 3 days before initiation of benazepril, if hypertension is not controlled, a diuretic can be added; measure B/P at peak 2-4 hr and trough (before next dose); this product is less effective in African descent patients
- Potassium levels, although hyperkalemia rarely occurs
- **Allergic reactions:** rash, fever, pruritus, urticaria; product should be discontinued if antihistamines fail to help; Stevens-Johnson syndrome; angioedema is more common in patients of African descent
- Renal symptoms: polyuria, oliguria, frequency, dysuria
- **CHF (unlabeled):** edema in feet, legs daily; weight daily

Evaluate:

- Therapeutic response: decrease in B/P

Teach patient/family:

- Not to use OTC products (cough, cold, allergy) unless directed by prescriber; not to use salt substitutes that contain potassium without consulting prescriber
- The importance of complying with dosage schedule, even if feeling better

Black Box Warning: To notify prescriber of pregnancy (D); product will need to be discontinued

- To rise slowly to sitting or standing position to minimize orthostatic hypotension
- To notify prescriber of mouth sores, sore throat, fever, swelling of hands or feet, irregular heartbeat, chest pain, bruising, bleeding, swelling of face, tongue, lips, difficulty breathing
- To report excessive perspiration, dehydration, vomiting, diarrhea; may lead to fall in B/P; to use caution in hot weather
- That product may cause dizziness, fainting, lightheadedness; that this may occur during first few days of therapy
- That product may cause skin rash or impaired perspiration
- How to take B/P, and normal readings for age group
- To avoid potassium-containing products (salt substitutes)

TREATMENT OF OVERDOSE:

0.9% NaCl IV INFUSION, hemodialysis

⚠ HIGH ALERT

bendamustine (Rx)

(ben-da-muss′teen)

Treanda

Func. class.: Antineoplastic alkylating agent

Chem. class.: Mechlorethamine derivative

ACTION: Cross-linking DNA that causes single-strand and double-strand breaks, inhibits several mitotic checkpoints, combines alkylating and antimetabolite properties

USES: Chronic lymphocytic leukemia, non-Hodgkin's lymphoma

CONTRAINDICATIONS: Pregnancy (D), fetal harm may occur; breastfeeding, children, hepatic disease, renal impairment, hypersensitivity to product or mannitol

Precautions: Hyperuricemia, infusion-related reactions, myelosuppression, infection, skin reactions

B

DOSAGE AND ROUTES

Chronic lymphocytic leukemia

• **Adult: IV INFUSION** 100 mg/m^2 over 30 min on days 1, 2 q28days up to 6 cycles

Non-Hodgkin's lymphoma

• **Adult: IV INFUSION** 120 mg/m^2 over 60 min on days 1, 2 q21days up to 8 cycles

Mantle cell lymphoma (unlabeled)

• **Adult: IV INFUSION** 90 mg/m^2 on days 1, 2 with rituximab on day 1 q28days for 6 cycles

Renal/hepatic dose

• **Adult: IV INFUSION** CCr <40 ml/min, do not use; AST or ALT 2.5-10 3 upper limit normal or bilirubin 1.5-3 3 ULN, do not use

Available forms: Powder for inj 25, 100 mg; solution for injection 180 mg/2 ml, 45 mg/0.5 ml

Administer:

• Allopurinol for 1-2 wk to those at high risk for tumor lysis syndrome; usually develops in first treatment cycle

• Blood transfusions; RBC colony-stimulating factors to counter anemia unless cure is the intent

• Antiemetic 30-60 min before giving product to prevent vomiting

• All medications PO; if possible, avoid IM inj if platelets are <100,000/mm^3

Intermittent IV INFUSION route

• Prepare in biologic cabinet wearing gown, gloves, mask; avoid contact with skin, can cause burning, stain the skin brown; use cytotoxic handling procedures

• After **reconstituting** 100 mg product/20 ml or 25 mg/5 ml sterile water for inj (5 mg/ml), sol should be clear, colorless to pale yellow, completely dissolve in 5 min; if particulate is present, do not use

• Within 30 min of reconstitution, withdraw volume needed and **further dilute** in 500 ml NS or $D_{2.5/0.45}$%NS to a final concentration of 0.2-0.6 mg/ml; doses of ≤100 mg/m^2, **give** over 30 min; doses of >100 mg/m^2, **give** over 60 min

• Monitor for infusion reactions; may use antihistamines or corticosteroids for grade 1, 2 reactions; if grade 3 or 4 occurs, discontinue if needed

• Store reconstituted sol in refrigerator for 24 hr or at room temperature for 3 hr; protect from light; store vials at room temperature

SIDE EFFECTS

CNS: Asthenia, *fatigue,* fever, *headache,* chills, hypertension

CV: Hypertension, hypertensive crisis

GI: *Nausea, vomiting, diarrhea,* hyperbilirubinemia, *constipation,* stomatitis, *anorexia*, weight loss

GU: Renal failure

HEMA: Thrombocytopenia, leukopenia, anemia, lymphocytopenia, neutropenia, secondary malignancy

INTEG: *Bulbous rash, pruritus,* extravasation

META: Hyperuricemia

SYST: Anaphylaxis, infection, dehydration, severe skin toxicities, tumor lysis syndrome, Stevens-Johnson syndrome, toxic epidermal necrolysis, tumor lysis syndrome

PHARMACOKINETICS

95% protein binding, metabolized by hydrolysis via CYP450 1A2, 2 metabolites are produced, half-life 40 min, 90% excreted unchanged (feces)

INTERACTIONS

Increase: agranulocytosis risk—cloZAPine (do not use concurrently)

Increase: bleeding risk—aspirin, anticoagulants, NSAIDs, platelet inhibitors, thrombolytics

Increase: myelosuppression—myelosuppressive agents

Increase: toxicity—other antineoplastics, radiation

Increase: adverse reactions, decreased antibody reaction—live vaccines

Increase: bendamustine—CYP1A2 inhibitors (atazanavir, cimetidine, ciprofloxacin, enoxacin, ethyl estradiol, fluvoxaMINE, mexiletine, norfloxacin, tacrine, thiabendazole, zileuton)

Decrease: bendamustine—CYP1A2 inducers (barbiturates, carBAMazepine, rifampin)

Drug/Lab Test
Increase: LFTs

NURSING CONSIDERATIONS
Assess:
- **Blood dyscrasias:** CBC, differential, platelet count weekly; withhold product if WBC is <1000 or if platelet count is <75,000; notify prescriber of results
- Hepatic studies: AST, ALT, bilirubin
- Renal studies: BUN, serum uric acid, urine CCr before, during therapy; I&O ratio; report fall in urine output of 30 or 40 ml/hr; electrolytes
- Monitor for cold, cough, fever (may indicate beginning infection)
- For malignancy regression
- Bleeding: hematuria, guaiac, bruising, petechiae, mucosa, orifices q8hr
- **Serious skin toxicities:** toxic epidermal necrolysis, Stevens-Johnson syndrome; product should be discontinued
- **Tumor lysis syndrome:** monitor uric acid, potassium; may occur during 1st treatment cycle; use allopurinol for patients at high risk for this condition, usually during the 1st 2 wk; provide adequate hydration

Evaluate:
- Therapeutic response: improvement in blood counts, morphology

Teach patient/family:
- To avoid hazardous activity that requires mental alertness
- To avoid crowds, persons with upper respiratory infections
- To report immediately fever, sore throat, flulike symptoms; indicates infection
- To report immediately allergic reaction, facial swelling, difficulty breathing, itchy rash
- Until reaction is known, not to breastfeed; males should also use contraception during and for 3 mo after
- To use contraception during therapy and for 3 mo after pregnancy (D)
- To avoid use of aspirin, ibuprofen, razors, commercial mouthwash
- To report signs of anemia (fatigue, irritability, SOB, faintness)
- To report signs of infection, myelosuppression, skin toxicities, diarrhea, nausea, vomiting

benzocaine topical
See Appendix B

RARELY USED

benzonatate (Rx)
(ben-zoe′na-tate)

Tessalon Perles, Zonatuss

Func. class.: Antitussive, nonopioid

USES: Nonproductive cough

CONTRAINDICATIONS: Hypersensitivity

DOSAGE AND ROUTES
- **Adult and child: PO** 100 mg up to tid; max 600 mg/day

benztropine (Rx)
(benz′troe-peen)

Cogentin

Func. class.: Cholinergic blocker, antiparkinson's agent

Chem. class.: Tertiary amine

ACTION: Blockade of central acetylcholine receptors, balances cholinergic activity

USES: Parkinson's symptoms, EPS associated with neuroleptic products, acute dystonic reactions

Unlabeled uses: Hypersalivation

CONTRAINDICATIONS: Children <3 yr, hypersensitivity, closed-angle glaucoma, dementia, tardive dyskinesia

Precautions: Pregnancy (C), breastfeeding, geriatric patients, tachycardia, renal/hepatic disease, substance abuse history, dysrhythmias, hypo/hypertension, myasthenia gravis, GI/GU obstruction, peptic ulcer, megacolon, prostate hypertrophy, psychosis

DOSAGE AND ROUTES

Drug-induced EPS

- **Adult: IM/IV/PO** 1-4 mg daily/bid; give **PO** dose as soon as possible
- **Child >3 yr: IM/IV/PO** 0.02-0.05 mg/kg/dose 1-2×/day

Parkinson's symptoms

- **Adult: PO/IM** 0.5-1 mg at bedtime; increase by 0.5 mg q5-6days titrated to patient response, max 6 mg/day

Acute dystonic reactions

- **Adult: IM/IV** 1-2 mg, may increase to 1-2 mg bid **(PO)**

Available forms: Tabs 0.5, 1, 2 mg; inj 1 mg/ml

Administer:

PO route

- With or after meals to prevent GI upset; may give with fluids other than water
- At bedtime to avoid daytime drowsiness with parkinsonism
- Store at room temperature

IM route

- Inject deeply in muscle; use filtered needle to remove solution from ampule

IV, direct route

- Use in emergencies

Syringe compatibilities: Metoclopramide, perphenazine

Y-site compatibilities: Alfentanil, amikacin, aminophylline, ascorbic acid injection, atracurium, atropine, azaTHIOprine, aztreonam, bumetanide, buprenorphine, butorphanol, calcium chloride, gluconate, ceFAZolin, cefotaxime, cefoTEtan, cefOXitin, cefTAZidime, ceftizoxime, cefTRIAXone, cefuroxime, chlorproMAZINE, cimetidine, clindamycin, cyanocobalamin, cycloSPORINE, dexamethasone, digoxin, diphenhydrAMINE, DOBUTamine, DOPamine, doxycycline, enalaprilat, ePHEDrine, epinephrine, epoetin alfa, erythromycin lactobionate, esmolol, famotidine, fentaNYL, fluconazole, folic acid (as sodium salt), gentamicin, glycopyrrolate, heparin, hydrocortisone sodium succinate, hydrOXYzine, imipenem-cilastatin, inamrinone, insulin (regular), isoproterenol, ketorolac, labetalol, lactated Ringer's, lidocaine, magnesium sulfate, mannitol, meperidine, metaraminol, methyldopate, methylPREDNISolone, metoclopramide, metoprolol, midazolam, minocycline, morphine, multiple vitamins injection, nafcillin, nalbuphine, naloxone, netilmicin, nitroglycerin, nitroprusside, norepinephrine, ondansetron, oxacillin, oxytocin, papaverine, penicillin G potassium/sodium, pentamidine, pentazocine, PHENobarbital, phentolamine, phenylephrine, phytonadione, piperacillin, polymyxin B, potassium chloride, procainamide, prochlorperazine, promethazine, propranolol, protamine, pyridoxine, quiNIDine, ranitidine, Ringer's injection, sodium bicarbonate, succinylcholine, SUFentanil, tacrolimus, theophylline, thiamine, ticarcillin, ticarcillin-clavulanate, tobramycin, tolazoline, urokinase, vancomycin, vasopressin, verapamil

SIDE EFFECTS

CNS: Anxiety, restlessness, irritability, delusions, hallucinations, headache, sedation, depression, incoherence, dizziness, memory loss; *confusion;* delirium (geriatric patients)

CV: Palpitations, tachycardia, hypotension, bradycardia

EENT: Blurred vision, photophobia, dilated pupils, difficulty swallowing

GI: *Dryness of mouth, constipation,* nausea, vomiting, abdominal distress, **paralytic ileus**

GU: Urinary hesitancy/retention, dysuria

INTEG: Rash, urticaria, dermatoses

MISC: Increased temperature, flushing, decreased sweating, **hyperthermia, heat stroke**, numbness of fingers

PHARMACOKINETICS

PO: Onset 1 hr, duration 6-10 hr

IM/IV: Onset 15 min, duration 6-10 hr

INTERACTIONS

Increase: anticholinergic effect—amantadine; antihistamines, phenothiazines,

tricyclics, disopyramide, quiNIDine; reduce dose
Decrease: absorption—antidiarrheals, antacids
Decrease: anticholinergic effect of—cholinergics

NURSING CONSIDERATIONS

Assess:

- **Parkinsonism:** EPS, shuffling gait, muscle rigidity, involuntary movements, loss of balance
- **Paralytic ileus:** abdominal pain, intermittent constipation/diarrhea
- I&O ratio; commonly causes decreased urinary output; urinary hesitancy, retention; palpate bladder if retention occurs
- Constipation: increase fluids, bulk, exercise if this occurs
- Mental status: affect, mood, CNS depression, worsening of mental symptoms during early therapy
- Use caution during hot weather; product may increase susceptibility to heat stroke by decreasing sweating
- With benztropine "buzz" or "high," patients may imitate EPS
- Hard candy, gum, frequent drinks to relieve dry mouth

Evaluate:

- Therapeutic response: absence of involuntary movements after 2 days of treatment

Teach patient/family:

- To report urinary hesitancy/retention, dysuria
- That tabs may be crushed, mixed with food; may take whole dose at bedtime if approved by prescriber
- Not to discontinue product abruptly; to taper off over 1 wk or withdrawal symptoms may occur (EPS, tremors, insomnia, tachycardia, restlessness); to take as directed; not to double dose
- To avoid driving, other hazardous activities; drowsiness/dizziness may occur
- To avoid OTC medications: cough, cold preparations with alcohol, antihistamines, antacids, antidiarrheals within 2 hr unless directed by prescriber
- To change positions slowly to prevent orthostatic hypotension
- To use good oral hygiene, frequent sips of water, sugarless gum for dry mouth

bepotastine

(beh-pot′uh-steen)

Bepreve

Func. class.: Antihistamine (ophthalmic)
Chem. class.: Histamine 1 receptor antagonist

ACTION: A topically active, direct H_1-receptor antagonist and mast cell stabilizer; by reducing these inflammatory mediators, relieves the ocular pruritus associated with allergic conjunctivitis

USES: Ocular pruritus associated with signs and symptoms of allergic conjunctivitis

CONTRAINDICATIONS: Hypersensitivity
Precautions: Pregnancy (C), breastfeeding, children, contact lenses

DOSAGE AND ROUTES

- **Adult/Child ≥2 yrs: OPHTH** Instill 1 drop in affected eye bid, max 2 drops/day in each eye

Available forms: Ophthalmic solution 1.5%

Administer:

Ophthalmic route

- For topical ophthalmic use only
- Wash hands before and after use; tilt the head back slightly and pull the lower eyelid down with the index finger; squeeze the prescribed number of drops into the conjunctival sac and gently close eyes for 1-2 min; do not blink
- Do not touch the tip of the dropper to the eye, fingertips, or other surface
- Wait ≥10 min after instilling the ophthalmic solution before inserting contact lenses; contact lenses should not be worn if eye is red; the preservative in this

product may be absorbed by soft contact lenses
• Do not share ophthalmic drops with others

SIDE EFFECTS

CNS: Headache
EENT: Taste change, ocular irritation, pharyngitis
SYST: Hypersensitivity

NURSING CONSIDERATIONS

Assess:
• Eyes: for itching, redness, use of soft or hard contact lenses
Evaluate:
• Therapeutic response: absence of redness, itching in the eyes
Teach patient/family:
Ophthalmic route
• Product is for topical ophthalmic use only
• Wash hands before and after use; tilt the head back slightly and pull the lower eyelid down with the index finger; squeeze the prescribed number of drops into the conjunctival sac and gently close eyes for 1-2 min; do not blink
• Do not touch the tip of the dropper to the eye, fingertips, or other surface
• Wait ≥10 min after instilling the ophthalmic solution before inserting contact lenses; contact lenses should not be worn if eye is red
• Do not share ophthalmic drops with others
• Remove **contact lenses** before use because the preservative, benzalkonium chloride, may be absorbed by soft contact lenses; product should not be used to treat contact lens–related irritation

RARELY USED

beractant (Rx)

(ber-ak′tant)
Survanta
Func. class.: Natural lung surfactant

USES: Prevention and treatment (rescue) of respiratory distress syndrome in premature infants

DOSAGE AND ROUTES

• **Newborn: INTRATRACHEAL INSTILL** 4 doses can be administered during the 1st 48 hr of life; give doses no more frequently than q6hr; each dose is 100 mg of phospholipids/kg birth weight

betamethasone (topical)

(bay-ta-meth′a-sone)
betamethasone dipropionate
Diprolene, Diprolene AF
betamethasone augmented dipropionate
betamethasone valerate
Beta-Val, Luxiq
Func. class.: Corticosteroid, topical

ACTION: Crosses cell membrane to attach to receptors to decrease inflammation, itching; inhibits multiple inflammatory cytokines

USES: Inflammation/itching corticosteroid-responsive dermatoses on the skin/scalp

CONTRAINDICATIONS: Hypersensitivity, use of some preparations on face, axilla, groin
Precautions: Pregnancy (C), skin infections

DOSAGE AND ROUTES

• **Adult: TOP** 1-2 times/day (dipropionate) or 1-3 times/day (valerate)

Available forms: dipropionate: gel, lotion, ointment, cream 0.05%; valerate: cream, lotion, ointment 0.1%, foam 0.12%

SIDE EFFECTS

INTEG: Burning, folliculitis, pruritus, dermatitis, maceration, erythema
MISC: Hyperglycemia; glycosuria, Cushing syndrome, HPA axis suppression

PHARMACOKINETICS

Unknown

NURSING CONSIDERATIONS

Assess:
- **Skin reactions:** burning pruritus, folliculitis, dermatitis

Evaluate:
- Decreased itching, inflammation on the skin, scalp

Teach patient/family:

Topical route:
- That betamethasone valerate may be used with occlusive dressings for psoriasis or recalcitrant conditions; not to use dipropionate with occlusive dressings

Cream/ointment/lotion:
- To apply sparingly in a thin film, using gloves, and rub gently into the cleansed, slightly moist affected area
- Not to use on broken, wet skin, area of infection, face, or groin, axilla

Gel:
- To apply sparingly in a thin film, using gloves, and rub gently into the cleansed, slightly moist affected area

Scalp foam:
- To invert can and dispense a small amount of foam onto a saucer or other cool surface; not to dispense directly onto hands; to pick up small amounts of foam with fingers and gently massage into affected area until foam disappears; repeat until entire affected scalp area is treated
- That treatment should be limited to 2 wk

betamethasone (augmented) topical

See Appendix B

betaxolol (ophthalmic)

(beh-tax′oh-lol)

Betoptic-S, Kerlone

Func. class.: Antiglaucoma
Chem. class.: β-Blocker

ACTION: Can decrease aqueous humor and increase outflows

USES: Treatment of chronic open-angle glaucoma and ocular hypertension; **PO** for hypertension

CONTRAINDICATIONS: Hypersensitivity, AV block, heart failure, bradycardia, sick sinus syndrome
Precautions: Abrupt discontinuation, children, pregnancy, breastfeeding, asthma, COPD, depression, diabetes mellitus, myasthenia gravis, hyperthyroidism, pulmonary disease, angle-closure glaucoma

DOSAGE AND ROUTES

Chronic open-angle glaucoma
- **Adult:** Instill 1-2 drops in the affected eye(s) bid

Available forms: Ophthalmic sol 0.5%; ophthalmic susp 0.25%, tabs 10, 20 mg

SIDE EFFECTS

CNS: Insomnia, headache, dizziness
CV: Palpitations
EENT: Eye stinging/burning, tearing, photophobia
MISC: Bronchospasm

PHARMACOKINETICS

Ophthalmic: Onset 30 min, peak 2 hr, duration ≥12 hr
PO: Peak 3 hr

NURSING CONSIDERATIONS

Assess:

⚠ **Systemic absorption:** When used in the eye, systemic absorption is common,

with the same adverse reactions and interactions
- Glaucoma: monitor intraocular pressure

Evaluate:
- Decreasing intraocular pressure

Teach patient/family:
- That strength is expressed in betaxolol base
- That drug for ophthalmic use only; shake the ophthalmic suspension well before use
- Not to touch the tip of the dropper to the eye, fingertips, or other surface to prevent contamination
- To wash hands before and after use; tilt the head back slightly and pull the lower eyelid down with the index finger to form a pouch; squeeze the prescribed number of drops into the pouch; close eyes to spread drops; to avoid excessive systemic absorption, apply finger pressure on the lacrimal sac for 1-2 min following use
- That if more than one topical ophthalmic drug product is being used, the drugs should be administered at least 5 min apart
- To avoid contamination or the spread of infection, do not use dropper for more than one person
- To report symptoms of heart failure (PO)

bethanechol (Rx)

(be-than′e-kole)

Urecholine

Func. class.: Urinary tract stimulant, cholinergic

Chem. class.: Synthetic choline ester

ACTION: Stimulates muscarinic ACH receptors directly; mimics effects of parasympathetic nervous system stimulation; stimulates gastric motility, micturition; increases lower esophageal sphincter pressure

USES: Urinary retention (postoperative, postpartum), neurogenic atony of bladder with retention

Unlabeled uses: Ileus, GERD, anticholinergic syndrome

CONTRAINDICATIONS: Hypersensitivity, severe bradycardia, asthma, severe hypotension, hyperthyroidism, peptic ulcer, parkinsonism, seizure disorders, CAD, COPD, coronary occlusion, mechanical obstruction, peritonitis, recent urinary/GI surgery, GI/GU obstruction

Precautions: Pregnancy (C), breastfeeding, children <8 yr, hypertension

DOSAGE AND ROUTES
- **Adult: PO** 10-50 mg bid-qid
- **Child (unlabeled): PO** 0.6 mg/kg/day in 3-4 divided doses

Ileus (unlabeled)
- **Adult: PO** 10-20 mg tid-qid before meals

Available forms: Tabs 5, 10, 25, 50 mg

Administer:
- To avoid nausea, vomiting, take on an empty stomach
- Only after all other cholinergics have been discontinued
- Store at room temperature

SIDE EFFECTS
CNS: Dizziness, headache, malaise

CV: Hypotension, bradycardia, reflex tachycardia, **cardiac arrest, circulatory collapse**

EENT: Miosis, increased salivation, lacrimation, blurred vision

GI: *Nausea, bloody diarrhea, belching, vomiting, cramps, fecal incontinence*

GU: Urgency

INTEG: Rash, urticaria, flushing, increased sweating

RESP: **Acute asthma, dyspnea, bronchoconstriction**

PHARMACOKINETICS
PO: Onset 30-90 min, duration 6 hr

INTERACTIONS
Increase: severe hypotension—ganglionic blockers

Increase: action or toxicity—cholinergic agonists, anticholinesterase agents
Decrease: action of anticholinergics, procainamide, quiNIDine
Drug/Lab Test
Increase: AST, lipase/amylase, bilirubin

NURSING CONSIDERATIONS

Assess:
- **Urinary patterns:** retention, urgency
- B/P, pulse: observe after parenteral dose for 1 hr; may need to use atropine subcut 0.6 mg or IV push slowly for bronchoconstriction
- I&O ratio: check for urinary retention, urge incontinence
- **Toxicity:** bradycardia, hypotension, bronchospasm, headache, dizziness, seizures, respiratory depression; product should be discontinued if toxicity occurs

Evaluate:
- Therapeutic response: absence of urinary retention, abdominal distention

Teach patient/family:
- To take product exactly as prescribed; 1 hr before meals or 2 hr after meals
- To make position changes slowly; orthostatic hypotension may occur
- To avoid driving, hazardous activities until effects are known

TREATMENT OF OVERDOSE:
Administer atropine 0.6-1.2 mg IV or IM (adult)

⚠ HIGH ALERT

bevacizumab (Rx)
(beh-va-kiz′you-mab)

Avastin

Func. class.: Antineoplastic—miscellaneous
Chem. class.: Monoclonal antibody

Do not confuse:
Avastin/Astelin

ACTION: Monoclonal antibody selectively binds to and inhibits activity of human vascular endothelial growth factor (VEGF) to reduce microvascular growth and metastatic disease progression

USES: Non–small-cell lung cancer (NSCLC), metastatic carcinoma of the colon or rectum, renal cell carcinoma, glioblastoma
Unlabeled uses: Adjunctive for ovarian cancer; (wet) macular degeneration

CONTRAINDICATIONS: Hypersensitivity, serious bleeding, hypertensive crisis, recent surgery
Precautions: Pregnancy (C), breastfeeding, children, geriatric patients, CHF, blood dyscrasias, CV disease, hypertension, surgery, thromboembolic disease, hamster protein/murine hypersensitivity

Black Box Warning: GI perforation, wound dehiscence, bleeding

DOSAGE AND ROUTES

Non–small-cell lung cancer
- **Adult:** **IV** 15 mg/kg over 60-90 min with CARBOplatin and paclitaxel q3wk

Metastatic colorectal cancer
- **Adult:** **IV INFUSION** in combination with 5-fluorouracil 5-10 mg/kg q14days given over 90 min; if well tolerated, next infusion may be given over 60 min; if 60-min infusion well tolerated, subsequent infusion may be given over 30 min; (second line) 5 mg/kg q2wk or 7.5 mg/kg q3wk with fluoropyrimidine and irinotecan or fluoropyramide and oxaliplatin-based agent

Metastatic cervical cancer
- **Adult:** **IV** 15 mg/kg q3wk with paclitaxel and Cisplatin or paclitaxel and topotecan

Metastatic renal cell carcinoma
- **Adult:** **IV** 10 mg/kg q2wk with interferon alfa 9 million units SUBCUT 3×/wk up to 52 wk

Glioblastoma single agent
- **Adult:** **IV** 10 mg/kg q2wk given over 60-90 min; 28-day cycle

Metastatic breast cancer (unlabeled)

• **Adult:** IV 15 mg/kg on day 1 with docetaxel 100 mg/m² q3wk, up to 9 cycles (those who have not received previous chemotherapy)

Metastatic renal cell cancer (unlabeled)

• **Adult (single agent):** IV 10 mg/kg over 60-90 min q2wk; may be given in combination with other products

Ovarian cancer (unlabeled)

• **Adult:** IV 15 mg/kg q21days until unacceptable toxicity, disease progression

Neovascular (wet) macular degeneration (unlabeled)

• **Adult:** INTRAVITREOUS INJ 1.25 mg monthly

Available forms: Inj 25 mg/ml

Administer:

Intermittent IV INFUSION route

• Do not give by IV bolus, IV push; do not shake vial

• Withdraw amount of product to be given, dilute in 100 ml 0.9% NaCl, discard any unused portion

Black Box Warning: **Wound dehiscence:** do not give for ≥28 days after surgery; make sure wound is healed before giving product

• Give as IV infusion over 90 min for 1st dose and 60 min thereafter if well tolerated; subsequent infusion may be given over 30 min; do not admix with dextrose

• **Rapid infusion rate (unlabeled):** give at rate of 0.5 mg/kg/min for all doses including initial infusion (5 mg/kg over 10 min; 10 mg/kg over 20 min; 15 mg/kg over 30 min)

SIDE EFFECTS

CNS: *Asthenia, dizziness,* intracranial hemorrhage (malignant glioma), headache, fatigue, confusion, weakness

CV: Deep vein thrombosis, arterial thrombosis, hypo/hypertension, hypertensive crisis, heart failure

GI: Nausea, vomiting, *anorexia, diarrhea,* constipation, *abdominal pain,* colitis, taste change, dyspepsia, stomatitis, GI hemorrhage/perforation

GU: Proteinuria, urinary frequency/urgency, nephrotic syndrome, ovarian failure

HEMA: Leukopenia, neutropenia, thrombocytopenia, microangiopathic hemolytic anemia, thromboembolism, bleeding

META: Bilirubinemia, hypokalemia, hyponatremia

MISC: Exfoliative dermatitis, hemorrhage, non-GI fistula formation, *alopecia, impaired wound healing,* osteonecrosis of the jaw, antibody formation, back pain myalgia

RESP: Dyspnea, upper respiratory tract infection

INTEG: Skin discoloration, infusion reactions

PHARMACOKINETICS

Half-life 20 days, steady state 100 days

INTERACTIONS

• Avoid concurrent use with SUNItinib; microangiopathic hemolytic anemia may occur

NURSING CONSIDERATIONS

Assess:

• B/P; take frequently if hypertension develops

• For symptoms of infection; may be masked by product

• **CNS reaction:** dizziness, confusion

• **CHF:** crackles, jugular venous distention, dyspnea during treatment

⚠ **GU status** (proteinuria): nephrotic syndrome may occur; monitor urinalysis for increasing protein level; product should be held if protein ≥2 g/24 hr; resume when <2 g/24 hr

Black Box Warning: **Wound dehiscence:** Hold for ≥28 days until incision is healed

Black Box Warning: **GI perforation, serious bleeding, nephrotic syndrome, hypertensive crisis;** product should be discontinued permanently, surgery should be postponed

Black Box Warning: **Bleeding:** if severe, discontinue product, occurs primarily in small-cell lung cancer

- **Pregnancy/Breastfeeding:** Drug may lead to fetal harm, avoid pregnancy, do not breastfeed
- Reversible posterior leukoencephalopathy syndrome (RPLS): discontinue if this disorder develops

Evaluate:
- Therapeutic response: decrease in size of tumors

Teach patient/family:
- To avoid hazardous tasks because confusion, dizziness may occur
- To report signs of infection: sore throat, fever, diarrhea, vomiting
- To report bleeding, changes in urinary patterns, edema, abdominal pain
- To avoid immunizations
- Need to discontinue a month before surgery and not restarted until wound is healed
- **Pregnancy/Breastfeeding:** Fetal harm may occur, do not breastfeed, not to become pregnant while taking this product or for several months after discontinuing treatment

bimatoprost (ophthalmic/topical)

(by-mat′oh-prost)

Latisse, Lumigan

Func. class.: Antiglaucoma agent

Chem. class.: Prostaglandin agonist

Do not confuse:
latanoprost/travoprost

ACTION:

Latisse

Promotion of eyelash growth, thickness, and darkness: unknown; possible increase in the percent of hairs and an increase in the duration of the hair growth (anagen) phase

Lumigan

Reduction of intraocular pressure (IOP) in patients with ocular hypertension or open-angle glaucoma; selectively mimics endogenous prostamides to produce ocular hypotension

USES:
Increased intraocular pressure in those with open-angle glaucoma/ocular hypertension (Lumigan); eyelash hypotrichosis (Latisse)

CONTRAINDICATIONS:
Hypersensitivity to this product, benzalkonium chloride

Precautions: Children, intraocular inflammation, closed-angle glaucoma, macular edema, contact lenses, ocular infection, surgery, trauma; corneal abrasion, iritis, urethritis

DOSAGE AND ROUTES

Increased intraocular pressure/ocular hypertension (Lumigan)
- **Adult: OPHTH Instill** 1 drop in each affected eye (conjunctival sac) every night

Eyelash hypotrichosis (Latisse)
- **Adult: Apply** 1 drop to skin of upper eyelid margin at base of eyelashes every night using a new supplied disposable sterile applicator

Available forms: Ophthalmic solution 0.01%; topical solution 0.03%

SIDE EFFECTS

EENT: *Conjunctival hyperemia, growth of eyelashes (hypertrichosis), ocular pigment changes ocular pruritus,* xerophthalmia, visual disturbance, ocular irritation/burning, foreign body sensation, ocular pain, blepharitis, cataracts, superficial punctate keratitis

INTEG: Hyperpigmentation of the periocular skin, eyelash darkening, lacrimation, photophobia, conjunctivitis, asthenopia, iritis, macular edema

MISC: Influenza, upper respiratory tract infections, asthenia, headache, hirsutism

PHARMACOKINETICS
Ophthalmic: Onset 4 hr, peak 8-12 hr; half-life 45 min

INTERACTIONS

Decrease: Intraocular pressure–lowering effect—latanoprost, travoprost (no longer available in the U.S.)

Drug/Lab Test

Increase: LFTs

NURSING CONSIDERATIONS

Assess:

- **Intraocular pressure:** in those with ongoing increased IOP or those using latanoprost, travoprost (no longer available in the U.S.)

Evaluate:

- Decreasing IOP or increased growth of eyelashes

Teach patient/family:

Ophthalmic route (Lumigan):

- To wash hands before and after use; remove contact lenses before use and reinsert 15 min after use; Lumigan contains benzalkonium chloride, which can be absorbed by soft contact lenses
- To tilt the head back slightly and pull the lower eyelid down with the index finger to form a pouch; squeeze the prescribed number of drops into the pouch and gently close the eyes for 1-2 min; do not blink; to avoid contamination, do not touch the tip of the dropper to the eye, fingertips, or other surface
- That the solution may be used concomitantly with other topical ophthalmic drug products to lower IOP; if more than one topical ophthalmic drug is being used, the drugs should be administered at least 5 min apart

Topical route (Latisse):

- To ensure the patient's face is clean and makeup is removed before using Latisse; the disposable sterile applicator is the only applicator that should be used; each applicator should be used for 1 eye only; dispose of the applicator after each use; after applying 1 drop of solution to the applicator, apply evenly along the skin of the upper eyelid margin at the base of the eyelashes; blot excess solution runoff outside the upper eyelid margin with a tissue or other absorbent cloth; do not apply to the lower eyelash line

bisacodyl (Rx, OTC)

(bis-a-koe′dill)

Carter's Little Pills ✱, Codulax ✱, Dacodyl, Doxidan, Dulcolax, Ex-Lax Ultra, Femilax, Soflax-Ex ✱

Func. class.: Laxative, stimulant
Chem. class.: Diphenylmethane

ACTION: Acts directly on intestine by increasing motor activity; thought to irritate colonic intramural plexus

USES: Short-term treatment of constipation; bowel or rectal preparation for surgery, examination

CONTRAINDICATIONS: Hypersensitivity, abdominal pain, nausea, vomiting, appendicitis, acute surgical abdomen, ulcerated hemorrhoids, acute hepatitis, fecal impaction, intestinal/biliary tract obstruction

Precautions: Pregnancy (C), breastfeeding, rectal fissures, severe CV disease

DOSAGE AND ROUTES

- **Adult and child ≥12 yr: PO** 5-15 mg in PM or AM; may use up to 30 mg for bowel or rectal preparation; **RECT** 10 mg as a single dose; 30-ml enema
- **Child 3-11 yr: PO** 5-10 mg as a single dose; **RECT** 5-10 mg as a single dose

Available forms: Tabs del rel 5, 10 mg; enteric-coated tabs 5 mg; supp 5, 10 mg; enema 10 mg/30 ml

Administer:

PO route

- Swallow tabs whole with full glass of water; do not break, crush, chew tabs
- Alone only with water for better absorption; do not take within 1 hr of other products or within 1 hr of antacids, milk, H_2 antagonists; do not take enteric product with proton-pump inhibitors
- In AM or PM

Rectal route

- Insert high in rectum

SIDE EFFECTS

CNS: Muscle weakness

GI: *Nausea, vomiting, anorexia, cramps,* diarrhea, rectal burning (suppositories)

META: Protein-losing enteropathy, alkalosis, hypokalemia, tetany; electrolyte, fluid imbalances

PHARMACOKINETICS

Small amounts absorbed/metabolized by liver; excreted in urine, bile, feces, breast milk

PO: Onset 6-10 hr

RECT: Onset 15-60 min

INTERACTIONS

Increase: gastric irritation—antacids, milk, H_2-blockers, gastric acid pump inhibitors

Drug/Food

- Increase irritation—dairy products separate by 2 hr

Drug/Lab

Increase: Sodium phosphate

Decrease: Calcium, magnesium

NURSING CONSIDERATIONS

Assess:

- Blood, urine electrolytes if product is used often by patient
- I&O ratio to identify fluid loss
- Cause of constipation; identify whether fluids, bulk, exercise missing from lifestyle; determine use of constipating products
- **GI symptoms:** cramping, rectal bleeding, nausea, vomiting; if these symptoms occur, product should be discontinued
- Multiple products/routes may be used for bowel prep

Evaluate:

- Therapeutic response: decrease in constipation

Teach patient/family:

- Not to use laxatives for long-term therapy because bowel tone will be lost; 1-wk use is usually sufficient
- That normal bowel movements do not always occur daily
- Not to use in presence of abdominal pain, nausea, vomiting
- To notify prescriber if constipation is unrelieved or if symptoms of electrolyte imbalance occur: muscle cramps, pain, weakness, dizziness
- To take with a full glass of water; not to take with dairy products, separate by 1 hr
- Identify bulk, water, constipating products, exercise in patient's life

bismuth subsalicylate (OTC)

(bis′muth sub-sal-iss′uh-late)

Bismatrol, Bismed ✤, Bismylate ✤, Kaopectate, Kao-Tin, Peptic Relief, Pepto-Bismol, Pink Bismuth, Stomak-care ✤

Func. class.: Antidiarrheal, weak antacid

Chem. class.: Salicylate

Do not confuse:

Kaopectate/Kayoxalate

ACTION: Inhibits the prostaglandin synthesis responsible for GI hypermotility, intestinal inflammation; stimulates absorption of fluid and electrolytes; binds toxins produced by *Escherichia coli*

USES: Diarrhea (cause undetermined), prevention of diarrhea when traveling; may be included to treat *Helicobacter pylori,* heartburn, indigestion, nausea

Unlabeled uses: Traveler's diarrhea, gastric/duodenal ulcer, *H. pylori* eradication

CONTRAINDICATIONS: Children <3 yr, children with chickenpox, history of GI bleeding, flulike symptoms, hypersensitivity to product or salicylates, PUD

Precautions: Pregnancy (C), breastfeeding, geriatric patients, gout, diabetes mellitus, bleeding disorders, previous hypersensitivity to NSAIDs, *Clostridium-difficile*–associated diarrhea when used with antiinfectives for *H. pylori*

DOSAGE AND ROUTES

Antidiarrheal/Gastric Distress

• **Adult: PO** 2 tabs or 30 ml (15 ml extra/max strength) q30min or 2 tabs q60min, max 4.2 g/24 hr

Antiulcer (unlabeled)

• **Adult/adolescent: PO** 525 mg qid, max 4.2 g/24 hr; given with metroNIDAZOLE or tetracycline and acid-suppressive therapy × 14 days

Traveler's diarrhea (unlabeled)

• **Adult: PO** 30 ml q30min (8×/day regular strength, 4×/day max strength)

Available forms: Tabs 262 mg; chewable tabs 262 mg, liquid 262mg /15ml, 525 mg/15 ml

Administer:

PO route

• Increased fluids to rehydrate patient
• **Susp:** shake liquid before using, use measuring cup/syringe
• Tabs can be chewed, dissolved in mouth; caplets to be swallowed whole with water

SIDE EFFECTS

CNS: Confusion, twitching, **neurotoxicity (high doses)**

EENT: Hearing loss, tinnitus, metallic taste, blue gums, black tongue

GI: Increased fecal impaction (high doses), dark stools, constipation, diarrhea, nausea

HEMA: Increased bleeding time

PHARMACOKINETICS

PO: Onset 1 hr, peak 2 hr, duration 4 hr

INTERACTIONS

Increase: toxicity—salicylates, methotrexate

Increase: effect of anticoagulants (PO), antidiabetics (PO)

Decrease: absorption of tetracycline, quinolones, phenytoin, separate for ≥2 hr

Drug/Lab Test

Interference: radiographic studies of GI system

NURSING CONSIDERATIONS

Assess:

• **Diarrhea:** bowel pattern before product therapy, after treatment
• Electrolytes K, Na, Cl if diarrhea is severe or continues long term; assess skin turgor, other signs of dehydration

Evaluate:

• Therapeutic response: decreased diarrhea, absence of diarrhea when traveling; resolution of ulcers

Teach patient/family:

• To chew, dissolve medication in mouth; not to swallow whole; to shake liquid before using, maintain hydration
• To avoid other salicylates unless directed by prescriber; not to give to children, possibility of Reye's syndrome
• That stools may turn black; that tongue may darken; that impaction may occur in debilitated patients
• To stop use if symptoms do not improve within 2 days or become worse, or if diarrhea is accompanied by high fever
• Separate quinolones, phenytoin, tetracycline by ≥2 hr

bisoprolol (Rx)

(bis-oh′pro-lole)

Zebeta

Func. class.: Antihypertensive

Chem. class.: β_1-Blocker

Do not confuse:

Zebeta/DiaBeta/Zetia

ACTION: Preferentially and competitively blocks stimulation of β_1-adrenergic receptors within cardiac muscle (decreases rate of SA node discharge, increases recovery time), slows conduction of AV node, decreases heart rate, which decreases O_2 consumption in myocardium; decreases renin-angiotensin-aldosterone system; inhibits β_2-receptors in bronchial and vascular smooth muscle at high doses

USES: Mild to moderate hypertension

Unlabeled uses: Stable angina, stable CHF

CONTRAINDICATIONS: Hypersensitivity to β-blockers, cardiogenic

shock, heart block (2nd, 3rd degree), sinus bradycardia, acute cardiac failure
Precautions: Pregnancy (C), breastfeeding, children, major surgery, diabetes mellitus, CHF, thyroid/renal/hepatic disease, COPD, asthma, well-compensated heart failure, aortic or mitral valve disease, peripheral vascular disease, myasthenia gravis

Black Box Warning: Abrupt discontinuation

DOSAGE AND ROUTES

Hypertension
- **Adult: PO** 5 mg/day; reduce to 2.5 mg in bronchospastic disease; may increase to 20 mg/day if necessary; max 20 mg/day

Renal/hepatic dose
- **Adult: PO** CCr <40 ml/min 2.5 mg, titrate upward

Angina (unlabeled)
- **Adult: PO** 5-20 mg/day

Heart failure (unlabeled)
- **Adult: PO** 1.25 mg/day × 48 hr, then 2.5 mg/day for 1st mo, then 5 mg/day; max 10 mg/day

Available forms: Tabs 5, 10 mg
Administer:
- Tab may be crushed, swallowed whole; may give without regard to meals
- Reduced dosage with renal/hepatic dysfunction
- Store protected from light, moisture; place in cool environment

SIDE EFFECTS

CNS: Vertigo, headache, insomnia, fatigue, dizziness, mental changes, memory loss, hallucinations, depression, lethargy, drowsiness, strange dreams, catatonia, peripheral neuropathy
CV: Ventricular dysrhythmias, profound hypotension, bradycardia, CHF, cold extremities, postural hypotension, 2nd-or 3rd-degree heart block, peripheral edema
EENT: Sore throat; dry, burning eyes
ENDO: Increased hypoglycemic response to insulin
GI: Nausea, diarrhea, vomiting, mesenteric arterial thrombosis, ischemic colitis, flatulence, gastritis, gastric pain
GU: Impotence, decreased libido
HEMA: Agranulocytosis, thrombocytopenia, purpura, eosinophilia
INTEG: Rash, flushing, alopecia, pruritus, sweating
MISC: Facial swelling, weight gain, decreased exercise tolerance
MS: Joint pain, arthralgia
RESP: Bronchospasm, dyspnea, wheezing, cough, nasal stuffiness, upper respiratory infection

PHARMACOKINETICS

Peak 2-4 hr, half-life 9-12 hr, 50% excreted unchanged in urine, protein binding 30%-36%, metabolized in liver to inactive metabolites

INTERACTIONS

Increase: hypotension—reserpine, guanethidine
Increase: myocardial depression—calcium channel blockers
Increase: antihypertensive effect—ACE inhibitors, α-blockers, calcium channel blockers, diuretics
Increase: bradycardia—digoxin, amiodarone
Increase: peripheral ischemia—ergots
Increase: antidiabetic effect—antidiabetics; may make hypoglycemic symptoms
Decrease: antihypertensive effect—NSAIDs, salicylates
Drug/Herb
Increase: β-blocking effect—hawthorn
Decrease: β-blocking effect—ephedra
Drug/Lab Test
Increase: AST, ALT, ANA titer, blood glucose, BUN, uric acid, potassium, lipoprotein
Interference: glucose/insulin tolerance tests

NURSING CONSIDERATIONS

Assess:
- **Hypertension:** B/P during beginning treatment, periodically thereafter; pulse q4hr: note rate, rhythm, quality; apical/radial pulse before administration; notify

prescriber of any significant changes (pulse <50 bpm)

- Baselines of renal, hepatic studies before therapy begins
- **CHF:** I&O, weight daily; increased weight, jugular venous distention, dyspnea, crackles, edema in feet, legs daily
- Skin turgor, dryness of mucous membranes for hydration status, especially for geriatric patients

Evaluate:

- Therapeutic response: decreased B/P after 1-2 wk

Teach patient/family:

Black Box Warning: Not to discontinue product abruptly; may cause precipitate angina, rebound hypertension; evaluate noncompliance

- Not to use OTC products that contain α-adrenergic stimulants (e.g., nasal decongestants, OTC cold preparations) unless directed by prescriber
- To report bradycardia, dizziness, confusion, depression, fever, cold extremities
- To take pulse at home; advise when to notify prescriber
- To avoid alcohol, smoking, sodium intake
- To comply with weight control, dietary adjustments, modified exercise program
- To carry emergency ID to identify product, allergies
- To avoid hazardous activities if dizziness is present

⚠ To report symptoms of CHF: difficulty breathing, especially on exertion or when lying down, night cough, swelling of extremities

- That if diabetic, product may mask signs of hypoglycemia or alter blood glucose levels

TREATMENT OF OVERDOSE:

Lavage, IV atropine for bradycardia; IV theophylline for bronchospasm; digoxin, O_2, diuretic for cardiac failure; hemodialysis, IV glucose for hypoglycemia; IV diazepam or phenytoin for seizures

⚠ HIGH ALERT

bivalirudin (Rx)

(bye-val-i-rue′din)

Angiomax

Func. class.: Anticoagulant

Chem. class.: Thrombin inhibitor

B

ACTION:
Direct inhibitor of thrombin that is highly specific; able to inhibit free and clot-bound thrombin

USES:
Unstable angina in patients undergoing percutaneous transluminal coronary angioplasty (PTCA), used with aspirin; heparin-induced thrombocytopenia, with/without thrombosis syndrome, PCI with iib/iiia

Unlabeled uses: Acute MI, DVT prophylaxis

CONTRAINDICATIONS:
Hypersensitivity, active bleeding, cerebral aneurysm, intracranial hemorrhage, recent surgery, CVA

Precautions: Pregnancy (B), breastfeeding, children, geriatric patients, renal function impairment, hepatic disease, asthma, blood dyscrasias, thrombocytopenia, GI ulcers, hypertension, inflammatory bowel disease, vitamin K deficiency, asthma

DOSAGE AND ROUTES

- **Adult: IV BOL** 0.75 mg/kg, then **IV INFUSION** 1.75 mg/kg/hr for 4 hr; another **IV INFUSION** may be used at 0.2 mg/kg/hr for ≤20 hr; this product is intended to be used with aspirin (325 mg/day) adjusted to body weight

Renal dose

- **Adult: IV** CCr ≥30 ml/min no adjustment; CrL 10-29 ml/min consider reducing to 1 mL/kg/hr

Acute MI (unlabeled)

- **Adult: IV BOL** 0.25 mg/kg, then **CONT IV INFUSION** 0.5 mg/kg/hr × 12 hr

DVT prophylaxis (unlabeled)

• **Adult: SUBCUT** 1 mg/kg q8hr for those undergoing orthopedic surgery

Available forms: Inj, lyophilized 250 mg/vial

Administer:

• Before PTCA; give with aspirin (325 mg)

• Store reconstituted vials in refrigerator for up to 24 hr; store diluted concentrations at room temperature for 24 hr

IV, direct route

• Dilute by adding 5 ml of sterile water for inj/250 mg bivalirudin, swirl until dissolved, further dilute in 50 ml of D_5W or 0.9% NaCl (5 mg/ml), give by bolus inj 0.75 mg/kg, then intermittent infusion

Continuous IV INFUSION route

• To each 250-mg vial add 5 ml of sterile water for inj, swirl until dissolved, further dilute in 500 ml D_5W or 0.9% NaCl (0.5 mg/ml); give infusion after bolus dose at a rate of 1.75 mg/kg/hr; may give an additional infusion at 0.2 mg/kg/hr

• Do not mix other IV medications with bivalirudin or provide via the same IV line as bivalirudin

Y-site compatibilities: Abciximab, acyclovir, alfentanil, allopurinol, amifostine, amikacin, aminocaproic acid, aminophylline, amphotericin B liposome, ampicillin, ampicillin-sulbactam, anidulafungin, argatroban, arsenic trioxide, atenolol, atracurium, atropine, azithromycin, aztreonam, bleomycin, bumetanide, buprenorphine, busulfan, butorphanol, calcium chloride/gluconate, capreomycin, CARBOplatin, carmustine, ceFAZolin, cefepime, cefotaxime, cefoTEtan, cefOXitin, cefTAZidime, ceftizoxime, cefTRIAXone, cefuroxime, chloramphenicol, cimetidine, ciprofloxacin, cisatracurium, CISplatin, clindamycin, cyclophosphamide, cycloSPORINE, cytarabine, dacarbazine, DACTINomycin, DAPTOmycin, DAUNOrubicin, DAUNOrubicin liposome, dexamethasone, dexmedetomidine, dexrazoxane, digoxin, diltiazem, diphenhydrAMINE, DOCEtaxel, dolasetron, DOPamine, DOXOrubicin, DOXOrubicin liposomal, doxycycline, droperidol, enalaprilat, ePHEDrine, EPINEPHrine, epirubicin, epoprostenol, eptifibatide, ertapenem, erythromycin, esmolol, etoposide, etoposide phosphate, famotidine, fenoldopam, fentaNYL, fluconazole, fludarabine, fluorouracil, foscarnet, fosphenytoin, furosemide, gallium, ganciclovir, gatifloxacin, gemcitabine, gentamicin, glycopyrrolate, granisetron, haloperidol, heparin, hydrALAZINE, hydrocortisone, HYDROmorphone, hydrOXYzine, IDArubicin, ifosfamide, imipenem-cilastatin, inamrinone, insulin (regular), irinotecan, isoproterenol, ketorolac, labetalol, leucovorin, levofloxacin, lidocaine, linezolid, LORazepam, magnesium, mannitol, mechlorethamine, melphalan, meperidine, meropenem, mesna, methohexital, methotrexate, methyldopate, methylPREDNISolone, metoclopramide, metoprolol, metroNIDAZOLE, midazolam, milrinone, mitoMYcin, mitoXANtrone, mivacurium, morphine, moxifloxacin, mycophenolate mofetil, nafcillin, nalbuphine, naloxone, nesiritide, niCARdipine, nitroglycerin, nitroprusside, norepinephrine, octreotide, ofloxacin, ondansetron, oxaliplatin, oxytocin, PACLitaxel, palonosetron, pamidronate, pancuronium, PEMEtrexed, PENTobarbital, PHENobarbital, phenylephrine, piperacillin, piperacillin-tazobactam, polymyxin B, potassium acetate/chloride/phosphates, procainamide, promethazine, propranolol, ranitidine, remifentanil, rocuronium, sodium acetate/bicarbonate/phosphates, streptozocin, succinylcholine, SUFentanil, sulfamethoxazole-trimethoprim, tacrolimus, teniposide, theophylline, thiopental, thiotepa, ticarcillin, ticarcillin-clavulanate, tigecycline, tirofiban, tobramycin, topotecan, vasopressin, vecuronium, verapamil, vinBLAStine, vinCRIStine, vinorelbine, voriconazole, warfarin, zidovudine, zoledronic acid

SUBCUT injection (unlabeled)

• May be used for DVT prophylaxis

SIDE EFFECTS

CNS: *Headache, insomnia, anxiety, nervousness*

CV: *Hypo/hypertension, bradycardia,* ventricular fibrillation

GI: *Nausea, vomiting, abdominal pain, dyspepsia*
HEMA: Hemorrhage, thrombocytopenia
MISC: Pain at inj site, pelvic pain, urinary retention, fever, **anaphylaxis**, infection
MS: *Back pain*
GU: Urinary retention, **renal failure, oliguria**

PHARMACOKINETICS
Excreted in urine, half-life 25 min, duration 1 hr, no protein binding

INTERACTIONS
Increase: bleeding risk—anticoagulants, aspirin, treprostinil, thrombolytics, NSAIDs, salicylates, cephalosporins, antineoplastics, sulfinpyrazone, GPIIb/IIIa inhibitors
Drug/Herb
Increase: bleeding risk—angelica, chamomile, devil's claw, dong quai, garlic, ginger, ginkgo, ginseng, horse chestnut, licorice, saw palmetto

NURSING CONSIDERATIONS
Assess:
- Baseline and periodic ACT, APTT, PT, INR, TT, platelets, Hgb, Hct
- ⚠ **Bleeding:** check arterial and venous sites, IM inj sites, catheters; all punctures should be minimized; fall in B/P or Hct may indicate hemorrhage, hematoma, hemorrhage at puncture site are more common in the elderly
- Fever, skin rash, urticaria
- CV status: B/P, watch for hypo/hypertension, bradycardia
- Neurologic status: any focal or generalized deficits should be reported immediately
- PCI use: possible thrombosis, stenosis, unplanned stent, prolonged ischemia, decreased reflow

Evaluate:
- Therapeutic response: anticoagulation with PTCA; resolution of heparin-induced thrombocytopenia, thrombosis syndrome

Teach patient/family:
- About the reason for the product and expected results
- To report black, tarry stools; blood in urine; difficulty breathing
- Not to use any OTC, herbal products unless approved by prescriber
- Not to use hard-bristle toothbrush or regular razor to avoid any injury; hemorrhage may result

⚠ **HIGH ALERT**

bleomycin (Rx)
(blee-oh-mye′sin)
Blenoxane ✦
Func. class.: Antineoplastic, antibiotic
Chem. class.: Glycopeptide

ACTION: Inhibits synthesis of DNA, RNA, protein; derived from *Streptomyces verticillus;* phase specific to the G_2 and M phases; a nonvesicant, sclerosing agent

USES: Cancer of head, neck, penis, cervix, vulva of squamous cell origin; Hodgkin's/non-Hodgkin's disease; testicular carcinoma; as a sclerosing agent for malignant pleural effusion
Unlabeled uses: Cutaneous T-cell lymphoma, hemangioma, Kaposi's sarcoma, malignant ascites, verruca plantaris/vulgaris, osteogenic sarcoma

CONTRAINDICATIONS: Pregnancy (D), breastfeeding, hypersensitivity, prior idiosyncratic reaction
Precautions: Patients >70 yr old, renal/hepatic disease, respiratory disease, max lifetime dose 400 units

Black Box Warning: Idiosyncratic reaction, pulmonary fibrosis, fever, requires specialized care setting, experienced clinician

DOSAGE AND ROUTES
Test dose
- **Adult and child (unlabeled): IM/IV/SUBCUT** ≤2 units for first 2 doses followed by 24 hr of observation
- **Adult and child: SUBCUT/IV/IM** 0.25-0.5 unit/kg 1-2×/wk or 10-20 units/m²,

then 1 unit/day or 5 units/wk; may also be given by **CONT INFUSION;** max total dose of 400 units during lifetime

Hodgkin's lymphoma

- **Adult/Child: IV/IM/SUBCUT** 5-20 units/m^2, may give in combination

Testicular cancer

- **Adult: IV** 10-20 units/m^2 1-2×/wk, may be given in combination

Renal dose

- **Adult/child:** CCr 40-50 ml/min reduce dose by 30%; CCr 30-39 ml/min reduce dose by 40%; CCr 20-29 ml/min reduce dose by 45%; CCr 10-19 ml/min reduce dose by 55%; CCr 5-10 ml/min reduce dose by 60%

Kaposi's sarcoma (unlabeled)

- **Adult: IV** 15 units q2wk with DOXOrubicin and vinCRIStine

Available forms: Powder for inj, 15, 30 units/vial

Administer:

- Antiemetic 30-60 min before giving product to prevent vomiting
- Topical or systemic analgesics for pain of stomatitis as ordered; antihistamines and antipyretics for fever, chills
- May be given IM, subcut, IV, intrapleurally, intralesionally, intraarterially

IM/SUBCUT route

- After reconstituting 15 units/1-5 ml or 30 mg/2-10 ml of 0.9% NaCl or bacteriostatic water for inj, max concentrations 5 units/ml, rotate inj sites; do not use products that contain benzyl alcohol when giving to neonates or that contain dextrose because of loss of potency

IV route

- Use cytotoxic handling procedures
- After reconstituting 15- or 30-unit vial with 5 or 10 ml of NS, respectively, inj slowly over 10 min or after further dilution with 50-100 ml 0.9% NaCl; give 15 units or less over 10 min through Y-tube or 3-way stopcock
- For patients with lymphoma, give 2 test doses of 2-5 units before initial dose; monitor for anaphylaxis
- Store for 2 wk after reconstituting if refrigerated or for 24 hr at room temperature; discard unused portions

Y-site compatibilities: Acyclovir, alfentanil, allopurinol, amifostine, amikacin, aminocaproic acid, aminophylline, amiodarone, ampicillin, ampicillin-sulbactam, anidulafungin, atenolol, atracurium, azithromycin, aztreonam, bivalirudin, bumetanide, buprenorphine, busulfan, butorphanol, calcium chloride/gluconate, CARBOplatin, carmustine, caspofungin, ceFAZolin, cefepime, cefotaxime, cefoTEtan, cefOXitin, cefTAZidime, ceftizoxime, cefTRIAXone, cefuroxime, chloramphenicol, chlorproMAZINE, cimetidine, ciprofloxacin, cisatracurium, CISplatin, clindamycin, codeine, cyclophosphamide, cycloSPORINE, cytarabine, dacarbazine, DACTINomycin, DAPTOmycin, DAUNOrubicin, dexamethasone, dexmedetomidine, dexrazoxane, digoxin, diltiazem, diphenhydrAMINE, DOBUTamine, DOCEtaxel, DOPamine, doxacurium, DOXOrubicin, DOXOrubicin liposomal, doxycycline, droperidol, enalaprilat, ePHEDrine, EPINEPHrine, epirubicin, ertapenem, erythromycin, esmolol, etoposide, famotidine, fenoldopam, fentaNYL, filgrastim, fluconazole, fludarabine, fluorouracil, foscarnet, fosphenytoin, furosemide, ganciclovir, gatifloxacin, gemcitabine, gentamicin, glycopyrrolate, granisetron, haloperidol, heparin, hydrALAZINE, hydrocortisone sodium succinate, HYDROmorphone, hydrOXYzine, IDArubicin, ifosfamide, imipenem-cilastatin, inamrinone, insulin (regular), irinotecan, isoproterenol, ketorolac, labetalol, leucovorin, levofloxacin, levorphanol, lidocaine, linezolid, LORazepam, magnesium sulfate, mannitol, mechlorethamine, melphalan, meperidine, meropenem, mesna, metaraminol, methohexital, methotrexate, methyldopate, methylPREDNISolone, metoclopramide, metoprolol, metroNIDAZOLE, midazolam, milrinone, minocycline, mitoMYcin, mitoXANtrone, mivacurium, morphine, nafcillin, nalbuphine, naloxone, nesiritide, niCARdipine, nitroglycerin, nitroprusside, norepinephrine, octreotide, ondansetron, oxaliplatin, palonosetron, pamidronate, pancuronium, pantoprazole, PEMEtrexed, pentamidine, pentazocine, PENTobarbital, PHENobarbital, phenylephrine, piperacillin, piperacillin-tazobactam, polymyxin B, potassium chloride, potassium phosphates, procainamide, prochlorperazine, promethazine, propranolol, quiNIDine, ranitidine, remifentanil, riTUXimab, rocuronium, sargramostim, sodium acetate, sodium bicarbonate, sodium phosphates, succinylcholine, SUFentanil, sulfamethoxazole-trimethoprim, tacrolimus, teniposide, theophylline, thiopental, thiotepa, ticarcillin, ticarcillin-clavulanate, tirofiban, tobramycin, tolazoline, trastuzumab, trimethobenzamide, vancomycin, vasopressin, vecuronium, verapamil, vinBLAStine, vinCRIStine, vinorelbine, voriconazole, zidovudine

SIDE EFFECTS

CNS: Pain at tumor site, headache, confusion, fever, chills, malaise
CV: **MI, stroke**
GI: *Nausea, vomiting, anorexia, stomatitis, weight loss,* ulceration of mouth, lips
GU: **Hemolytic-uremic syndrome**
IDIOSYNCRATIC REACTION: Hypotension, *confusion, fever,* chills, wheezing
INTEG: *Rash, hyperkeratosis, nail changes, alopecia,* pruritus, acne, striae, peeling, hyperpigmentation, phlebitis
RESP: **Fibrosis, pneumonitis,** wheezing, **pulmonary toxicity**
SYST: **Anaphylaxis,** radiation recall, Raynaud's phenomenon

PHARMACOKINETICS

Half-life 2-4 hr; when CCr is >35 ml/min, half-life is increased with lower clearance; metabolized in liver; 50% excreted in urine (unchanged)

INTERACTIONS

- Avoid live virus vaccines concurrently

Increase: toxicity—other antineoplastics, radiation therapy, general anesthesia, filgrastim, sargramostim
Decrease: serum phenytoin levels—phenytoin, fosphenytoin
Drug/Lab Test
Increase: uric acid
Decrease: pulmonary function tests

NURSING CONSIDERATIONS

Assess:

- IM test dose in patients with lymphoma of 1-2 units before 1st 2 doses

Black Box Warning: Pulmonary toxicity/fibrosis: pulmonary function tests; chest x-ray before, during therapy, should be obtained q2wk during treatment; pulmonary diffusion capacity for carbon monoxide (DLCO) monthly, if <40% of pretreatment value, stop treatment; treat pulmonary infection before treatment; dyspnea, crackles, unproductive cough, chest pain, tachypnea, fatigue, increased pulse, pallor, lethargy, more common in the elderly, radiation therapy, pulmonary disease; usually occurs with cumulative doses >400 units

- Temperature; fever may indicate beginning infection
- Renal status: serum creatinine/BUN; CBC
- Effects of alopecia, skin color alterations on body image; discuss feelings about body changes
- Buccal cavity q8hr for dryness, sores, ulceration, white patches, oral pain, bleeding, dysphagia
- Local irritation, pain, burning, discoloration at inj site

⚠ **Anaphylaxis:** rash, pruritus, urticaria, purpuric skin lesions, itching, flushing, wheezing, hypotension; have emergency equipment available

Black Box Warning: Idiosyncratic reaction: hypotension, mental confusion, fever, chills, wheezing in lymphoma

- Rinsing of mouth tid-qid with water, club soda; brushing of teeth with soft brush or cotton-tipped applicators for stomatitis; use unwaxed dental floss

Evaluate:

- Therapeutic response: decrease in size of tumor

Teach patient/family:

- To report any changes in breathing, coughing, fever
- That hair may be lost during treatment and that wig or hairpiece may make

patient feel better; that new hair may be different in color, texture
- To avoid foods with citric acid, hot or rough texture
- To report any bleeding, white spots, ulcerations in mouth; to examine mouth daily and report symptoms; decreased urination
- To use contraception during treatment (pregnancy [D]), to avoid breastfeeding
- Not to receive vaccines during treatment

boceprevir

(boe-se′pre-vir)

Victrelis

Func. class.: Antiviral, antihepatitis agents

ACTION: Prevents hepatitis C viral (HCV) replication by blocking the activity of HCV NS3/4A serine protease. Hepatitis C virus NS3/4A serine protease is an enzyme responsible for the conversion of HCV-encoded polyproteins to mature/functioning viral proteins

USES: Hepatitis C infection in combination with peginterferon alfa and ribavirin with compensated liver function

CONTRAINDICATIONS: Pregnancy (X), male partners of women who are pregnant

Precautions: Breastfeeding, neonates, infants, children, adolescents <18 years of age, anemia, neutropenia, thrombocytopenia, HIV, hepatitis B, decompensated hepatic disease, in liver or other organ transplants, hypersensitivity

DOSAGE AND ROUTES

Chronic hepatitis C infection (genotype 1) compensated liver disease (without cirrhosis, previously untreated with interferon and ribavirin therapy)/(partial responders/relapsers/null responders)

- **Adults: PO** Before starting therapy peginterferon alfa and ribavirin must be given 4 wk, then add boceprevir 800 mg (four 200 mg caps) PO TID (7-9 hr); treatment length is determined by HCV RNA concentrations at treatment wk 4, 8, 12, and 24; if patient has undetectable HCV RNA concentrations at wk 8 and 24, discontinue all 3 medications at wk 28 (previously untreated); 36 wk (partial responders/relapsers); if HCV RNA is detectable at wk 8 but undetectable at wk 24, the 3-drug regimen through wk 36, then give only peginterferon alfa and ribavirin through treatment wk 48; if the patient has a poor response to peginterferon alfa and ribavirin during the initial 4 wk, continue treatment with all 3 medications for a total of 48 wk; discontinue the 3-drug regimen if the HCV RNA concentrations >100 international units/ml at treatment wk 12 or a detectable HCA RNA concentration at treatment wk 24

Chronic hepatitis C infection (genotype 1) compensated liver disease with cirrhosis

- **Adults: PO** Before starting therapy with boceprevir, peginterferon alfa and ribavirin must be given 4 wk; then add boceprevir 800 mg (four 200 mg caps) PO TID (7-9 hr) to peginterferon alfa and ribavirin for an additional 44 wk (48 wk total)

Available forms: Caps 200 mg

Administer:
- Only use in combination with peginterferon alfa and ribavirin; never give as monotherapy
- Discontinue in hepatitis C virus (HCV)if RNA concentrations ≥100 international units/ml at wk 12 or a confirmed detectable HCV RNA concentrations at wk 24
- Any contraindication to peginterferon alfa or ribavirin also applies to boceprevir
- Give with food

SIDE EFFECTS

When used in combination with peginterferon/ribavarin

CNS: *Fatigue, chills, asthenia,* insomnia, irritability, dizziness

GI: Nausea, vomiting, diarrhea, dysgeusia, decreased appetite, xerostomia
HEMA: **Anemia (Hgb < 10 g/dL), neutropenia, thrombocytopenia**
INTEG: *Alopecia, rash*, xerosis
MISC: *Arthralgia, exertional dyspnea,* **drug rash with eosinophilia and systemic symptoms (DRESS) syndrome, exfoliative dermatitis, Stevens-Johnson syndrome, toxic epidermal necrolysis**

INTERACTIONS

⚠ Increase: life-threatening reactions of each product: alfuzosin, ergots (dihydroergotamine, ergotamine, ergonovine, methylergonovine), cisapride, pimozide, lovastatin, simvastatin, ezetimibe, niacin with simvastatin and boceprevir; triazolam, oral midazolam; sildenafil, tadalafil (pulmonary arterial hypertension); do not use concurrently

Increase: adverse reactions of each product—phosphodiesterase type 5 (PDE5) inhibitors (for erectile dysfunction), acetaminophen, alfentanil, aliskiren, almotriptan, alosetron, ALPRAZolam, aminophylline, amiodarone, amitriptyline, amLODIPine, ARIPiprazole, astemizole, atorvastatin, atorvastin, bepridil, boceprevir, bosentan, budesonide, bupivacaine, buprenorphine, busPIRone, carvedilol, cevimeline, chloroquine, cilostazol, cinacalcet, citalopram, clarithromycin, clomiPRAMINE, clonazePAM, clopidogrel, cloZAPine, colchicine, cyclobenzaprine, cycloSPORINE, dapsone, DAUNOrubicin, desipramine, desloratadine, dexamethasone, dexlansoprazole, dextromethorphan, diazepam, diclofenac, digoxin, diltiazem, disopyramide, disulfiram, DOCEtaxel, dolasetron, donepezil, DOXOrubicin, droperidol, dutasteride, ebastine, eletriptan, eplerenone, erlotinib, erythromycin, estazolam, eszopiclone, ethosuximide, etoposide, exemestane, felodipine, fentaNYL, fexofenadine, finasteride, flecainide, flunitrazepam, flurazepam, galantamine, gefitinib, glyburide, granisetron, halofantrine, haloperidol, HYDROcodone, ifosfamide, imipramine, indiplon, irinotecan, isradipine, itraconazole, ivermectin, ixabepilone, ketoconazole, lansoprazole, lidocaine, loperamide, loratadine, losartan, maraviroc, mefloquine, meloxicam, mirtazapine, mitoMYcin, montelukast, morphine, nateglinide, niCARdipine, NIFEdipine, nisoldipine, nortriptyline, omeprazole, ondansetron, oxybutynin, oxyCODONE, PACLitaxel, palonosetron, paricalcitol, plicamycin, posaconazole, prasugrel, praziquantel, propafenone, quazepam, QUEtiapine, quinacrine, quiNIDine, ramelteon, repaglinide, rifabutin, risperiDONE, ropivacaine, salmeterol, selegiline, sertraline, sibutramine, silodosin, sirolimus, sitaxsentan, solifenacin, SUFentanil, SUNItinib, systemic corticosteroids, tacrolimus, telithromycin, teniposide, terfenadine, testosterone, theophylline, tiaGABine, tinidazole, tolterodine, tolvaptan, traMADol, traZODone, vardenafil, venlafaxine, verapamil, vinBLAStine, vinCRIStine, voriconazole, warfarin, and others; use cautiously, may need to reduce dose

Increase: hyperkalemia—drospirenone
Decrease: estrogen levels—ethinyl estradiol
Decrease: boceprevir effect—CYP3A4 inhibitors (phenytoin, carBAMazepine, PHENobarbital, rifampin)
Decrease: effect of—methadone
Possible treatment failure: efavirenz, ritonavir, atazanavir, lopinavir with ritonavir

Drug/Herb

- Do not use with St. John's wort

Drug/Lab Test

Decrease: Hgb, platelets

NURSING CONSIDERATIONS

Assess:

⚠ Pregnancy: obtain a pregnancy test before, monthly during, and for 6 mo after treatment is completed; those who are not willing to practice strict contraception should not receive treatment; report any cases of prenatal ribavirin exposure to the Ribavirin Pregnancy Registry at (800) 593-2214

- **Anemia:** monitor Hgb, CBC with differential before, at treatment wk 2, 8, 12, and as needed. If Hgb is <10 g/dL, decrease ribavirin dosage; if Hgb is <8.5 g/dL, discontinuation of therapy is recommended; dosage should not be altered based on adverse reactions; anemia may be managed through ribavirin dose modifications; never alter the dose of boceprevir; if anemia persists despite a reduction in ribavirin dose, consider discontinuing boceprevir; if management of anemia requires permanent discontinuation of ribavirin, treatment with boceprevir MUST also be permanently discontinued; once boceprevir has been discontinued, it must not be restarted; monitor CBC with differential at treatment wk 4, 8, 12, and at other treatment points as needed

- **Serious skin disorders (DRESS, Stevens-Johnson syndrome, toxic epidermal necrolysis, exfoliative dermatitis):** These reactions may be due to combination use with peginterferon alfa, ribavarin; if serious skin reactions occur, discontinue all 3 products

Teach patient/family:

- To take with food to increase absorption; do not start new meds/herbs without prescriber's approval
- To use precautions to prevent transmission of hepatitis C
- To inform prescriber of all medications, herbs, supplements used
- To use 2 forms of effective contraception (intrauterine devices and barrier methods) during treatment and for 6 mo after treatment (pregnancy [X]); to avoid breastfeeding

⚠ HIGH ALERT

bortezomib (Rx)

(bor-tez′oh-mib)

Velcade

Func. class.: Antineoplastic—miscellaneous

Chem. class.: Proteasome inhibitor

ACTION: Reversible inhibitor of chymotrypsin-like activity in mammalian cells; causes delay in tumor growth by disrupting normal homeostatic mechanisms of 26S proteasome

USES: Multiple myeloma previously untreated or when at least 2 other treatments have failed; mantle cell lymphoma who have received ≥1 prior therapy

Unlabeled uses: Non-Hodgkin's lymphoma (NHL)

CONTRAINDICATIONS: Pregnancy (D), breastfeeding; hypersensitivity to product, boron, mannitol

Precautions: Children, geriatric patients, peripheral neuropathy, cardiac/hepatic disease, hypotension, tumor lysis syndrome, thrombocytopenia, infection, diabetes mellitus, bone marrow suppression, intracranial bleeding, injection site irritation

DOSAGE AND ROUTES

Multiple myeloma (previously untreated)

- **Adult: IV BOL/SUBCUT** Give for nine 6-wk cycles; cycles 1-4, 1.3 mg/m^2/dose given on days 1, 4, 8, 11, then a 10-day rest period (days 12-21), then give again on days 22, 25, 29, 32, then a 10-day rest period (days 33-42); given with melphalan (9 mg/m^2/day on days 1-4) and predniSONE (60 mg/m^2/day on days 1-4); during cycles 5-9, give bortezomib 1.3 mg/m^2/dose on days 1, 8, 22, 29 with melphalan (9 mg/m^2/day on days 1-4) and predniSONE (60 mg/m^2/day on days 1-4); this 6-wk cycle is considered 1 course; at least 72 hr should elapse between consecutive doses

Mantle cell lymphoma in combination

• **Adult: IV BOL/SUBCUT** 1.3 mg/m²/ dose on days 1, 4, 8, 11 followed by a 10-day rest period (days 12-21); ×6 (3-wk) cycles with rituximab 375 mg/m², cyclophosphamide 750 mg/m², doxorubicin 50 mg/m² all on day 1, and prednisone 100 mg/m² daily on days 1-5, give bortezomib before rituximab

Relapsed mantle cell lymphoma patients who have received ≥1 prior therapy

• **Adult: IV BOL/SUBCUT** 1.3 mg/m²/ dose on days 1, 4, 8, 11 followed by a 10-day rest period

Hepatic dose

• **Adult: IV** bilirubin >1.5 × ULN, reduce to 0.7 mg/m² during cycle 1; consider dose escalation to 1 mg/m² or further reduction to 0.5 mg/m² during next cycles based on tolerability

Non-Hodgkin's Lymphoma (unlabeled)

• **Adult: IV BOL** 1.3 mg/m² on days 1, 4, 8, 11 repeated every 21 days

Available forms: Lyophilized powder for inj 3.5 mg

Administer:

SUBCUT route

• Use 2.5 mg/ml, rotate inj sites; if inj site reaction occurs, use 1 mg/ml

IV bolus route

• **Reconstitute** each vial with 3.5 ml of 0.9% NaCl (1 mg/ml); sol should be clear/colorless; **inj** as bolus over 3-5 sec

• Store unopened product at room temperature, protect from light

• Wear protective clothing during handling, preparation; avoid contact with skin

• Check for extravasation at inj site

SIDE EFFECTS

CNS: Anxiety, insomnia, dizziness, headache, *peripheral neuropathy,* rigors, paresthesia, fever, headache

CV: *Hypotension,* edema

GI: Abdominal pain, *constipation, diarrhea,* dyspepsia, *nausea, vomiting,* anorexia

HEMA: *Anemia,* **neutropenia, thrombocytopenia**

MISC: Dehydration, weight loss, herpes zoster, *rash,* pruritus, blurred vision

MS: *Fatigue, malaise, weakness,* arthralgia, bone pain, muscle cramps, myalgia, back pain, **tumor lysis syndrome**

RESP: Cough, pneumonia, dyspnea, URI, **ARDs, pneumonitis, interstitial pneumonia, lung infiltration**

PHARMACOKINETICS

Half-life 9-15 hr, protein binding 83%, metabolized by CYP450 enzymes (3A4, 2D6, 2C19, 2C9, 1A2)

INTERACTIONS

• Do not use hematopoietic progenitor cells (sargramostim, filgrastim) within 24 hr of chemotherapy

• Oral hypoglycemics: may result in hypo/hyperglycemia

Increase: risk for bleeding—anticoagulants, NSAIDs, platelet inhibitors, salicylates, thrombolytics

Increase: hypotension—antihypertensives

Increase: peripheral neuropathy—amiodarone, antivirals (amprenavir; atazanavir; didanosine, lamiVUDine, 3TC; ritonavir; stavudine, zidovudine), chloramphenicol, CISplatin, colchicine, cycloSPORINE, dapsone, disulfiram, DOCEtaxel, gold salts, HMG-CoA reductase inhibitors, iodoquinol, INH, metroNIDAZOLE, nitrofurantoin, oxaliplatin, PACLitaxel, penicillamine, phenytoin, sulfaSALAzine, thalidomide, vinBLAStine, vinCRIStine, zalcitabine ddc, isoniazid, statins, others

Increase: toxicity or decrease efficacy when administered with products that induce or inhibit CYP3A4

Decrease: effect of norethindrone, estradiol, combination oral contraceptives, another nonhormonal contraceptive should be used

Drug/Herb

Increase: toxicity or decrease efficacy—St. John's wort

NURSING CONSIDERATIONS

Assess:

Fatal pulmonary toxicity: assess for risk factors or new worsening pulmonary symptoms

Tumor lysis syndrome: usually with those with a high tumor burden

- Hematologic status: platelets, CBC throughout treatment; platelets $\geq 70 \times 10^9$/L and ANC $\geq 1.0 \times 10^9$/L before any cycle; nonhematologic toxicities should be grade 1 or baseline before any cycle
- B/P, fluid status, peripheral neuropathy symptoms

Evaluate:

- Therapeutic response: improvement of multiple myeloma symptoms

Teach patient/family:

- To use contraception while taking this product (pregnancy [D]); to avoid breast-feeding
- To monitor blood glucose levels if diabetic
- To contact prescriber about new or worsening peripheral neuropathy, severe vomiting, diarrhea, easy bruising, bleeding, infection
- To avoid driving, operating machinery until effect is known
- To avoid using other medications unless approved by prescriber
- To report peripheral neuropathy (burning, discomfort)
- Bleeding risk (report bruising, bleeding)

bosentan (Rx)

(boh′sen-tan)

Tracleer

Func. class.: Vasodilator

Chem. class.: Endothelin receptor antagonist

ACTION: Peripheral vasodilation occurs via the antagonism of the effect of endothelin on endothelium and vascular smooth muscle

USES: Pulmonary arterial hypertension with WHO class III, IV symptoms

Unlabeled uses: Septic shock to improve microcirculatory blood flow, functional class II pulmonary arterial hypertension

CONTRAINDICATIONS: Hypersensitivity, CVA, CAD

Black Box Warning: Pregnancy X

Precautions: Breastfeeding, children, geriatric patients, mitral stenosis, anemia, edema, jaundice, hypovolemia, hypotension

Black Box Warning: Hepatic disease

DOSAGE AND ROUTES

- **Adult and adolescent ≥40 kg: PO** 62.5 mg bid × 4 wk, then 125 mg bid
- **Adult and adolescent <40 kg: PO** 62.5 mg bid, max 125 mg/day

Hepatic dose

- **Adult: PO** baseline AST/ALT<3×ULN no dosage change, monitor LFTs monthly reduce or interrupt if elevated; AST/ALT>3 and ≤5× ULN repeat test, if confirmed reduce to 62.5 mg bid or interrupt; monitor LFTs q2wk, if interrupted, restart when LFTs <3× ULN, check LFTs within 3 days; increase in AST/ALT>5 and ≤5× ULN; during treatment repeat test to confirm, discontinue, monitor LFTs q2wk until LFTs <3× ULN, restart at starting dose; AST/ALT >8× ULN **discontinue permanently**

Available forms: Tabs 62.5, 125 mg

Administer:

- Give without regard to meals
- Only available through the TAP program; 866-228-3546
- Do not stop product abruptly; taper
- Store at room temperature

SIDE EFFECTS

CNS: Headache, flushing, fatigue, fever

CV: Hypotension, chest pain, palpitations, edema of lower limbs, fluid retention

GI: Abnormal hepatic function, diarrhea, dyspepsia, **hepatotoxicity**
HEMA: Anemia, leukopenia, neutropenia, lymphopenia, thrombocytopenia
INTEG: Pruritus, anaphylaxis, rash, **Stevens-Johnson syndrome, toxic epidermal necrolysis**
MISC: Oligospermia, tumor lysis syndrome, respiratory infection, arthralgia
SYST: Secondary malignancy

PHARMACOKINETICS

Metabolized by inducer of CYP2C9, CYP3A4, possibly CYP2C19; metabolized by the liver; terminal half-life 5 hr; steady state 3-5 days

INTERACTIONS

- Do not coadminister cycloSPORINE with bosentan; bosentan is increased, cycloSPORINE is decreased
- Do not coadminister glyBURIDE with bosentan; glyBURIDE is decreased significantly, bosentan is also decreased, hepatic enzymes may be increased

Increase: bosentan effects—CYP2C9, CYP3A4 inhibitors
Increase: bosentan level—ketoconazole
Decrease: effects of warfarin, hormonal contraceptives, statins

Drug/Lab Test

Black Box Warning: Increase: ALT, AST

Decrease: Hgb, Hct

NURSING CONSIDERATIONS

Assess:

- **Serious skin toxicities:** Angioedema occurring 8-21 days after initiating therapy
- B/P, pulse during treatment until stable
- Blood studies: Hct, Hgb after 1 mo, 3 mo, then every 3 mo may be decreased
- **Pulmonary hypertension/CHF:** Fluid retention, weight gain, increased leg edema; may occur within weeks

Black Box Warning: Hepatic toxicity: vomiting, jaundice; product should be discontinued; hepatic studies: AST, ALT, bilirubin; hepatic enzymes may increase; if ALT/AST >3× and ≤5× ULN, decrease dose or interrupt treatment and monitor AST/ALT q2wk; if bilirubin >2× ULN or signs of hepatitis or hepatic disease are present, stop treatment

Evaluate:

- Therapeutic response: decrease in pulmonary hypertension

Teach patient/family:

- To report jaundice, dark urine, joint pain, fatigue, malaise, bruising, easy bleeding, fluid retention

Black Box Warning: Pregnancy (X), monitor pregnancy test monthly; patient must use nonhormonal contraception during and ≥1 month after conclusion of treatment

- That lab work will be required periodically
- To take without regard to food, do not take new meds/herbs without prescriber approval

bosutinib

(boe-sue′ti-nib)

Bosulif

Func. class.: Antineoplastic biologic response modifiers
Chem. class.: Signal transduction inhibitors (STIs), tyrosine kinase inhibitor

ACTION:
Inhibits bcr-abl tyrosine kinase created in patients with chronic myeloid leukemia (CML)

USES:
Treatment of CML (chronic accelerator phase); Philadelphia-chromosome–positive patients in blast-cell crisis

CONTRAINDICATIONS:
Pregnancy (D), hypersensitivity

Precautions: Breastfeeding, children, diarrhea, geriatric patients, hepatic disease, bone marrow suppression, infection, thrombocytopenia, neutropenia, immunosuppression, fluid retention

DOSAGE AND ROUTES

• **Adult: PO** 500 mg daily with food, may increase to 600 mg/day in those who have not developed grade 3 toxicity or in patients who do not reach complete hematological response by wk 8 or complete cytogenic response (CCyR) by wk 12

Hepatic dosage

• **Adult: PO** Any baseline hepatic impairment: Start at 200 mg/day; liver transaminase $>5 \times$ ULN, hold dose until levels are $\leq 2.5 \times$ ULN, then resume at 400 mg/day; liver transaminase level $\geq 3 \times$ ULN and bilirubin $>2 \times$ ULN and alk phos $<2 \times$ ULN, discontinue

Dosage adjustments for treatment-related toxicity

Hematologic toxicity:

⚠ ***ANC $<1000 \times 10^6$/L or platelet count $<50{,}000 \times 10^6$/L:*** hold dose until ANC is $\geq 1000 \times 10^6$/L and platelets are $\geq 50{,}000 \times 10^6$/L; if recovery within 2 wk, resume therapy at the same dosage; if blood counts remain low after 2 wk, upon recovery, resume at 100 mg/day less than the previous dosage

Diarrhea:

⚠ ***Grade 3 or 4 diarrhea ($\geq$7 stools/day compared with baseline):*** hold therapy until recovery to grade 1 toxicity or lower; resume therapy at 400 mg/day

Other nonhematologic toxicity:

⚠ ***Significant or moderate or severe toxicity:*** hold therapy until toxicity resolves; resume therapy at 400 mg/day

Available forms: Tabs 100, 500 mg

Administer:

PO route

• Give with food; swallow whole
• If dose is missed, take within 12 hr of missed dose; if >12 hr have passed, skip dose
• Follow cytotoxic handling procedures

SIDE EFFECTS

CNS: Headache, dizziness, fever, fatigue, weakness

GI: Nausea, vomiting, anorexia, abdominal pain, diarrhea

HEMA: Neutropenia, thrombocytopenia, bleeding

INTEG: Rash, pruritus

MS: Arthralgia, myalgia

RESP: Cough, dyspnea, pleural effusion, edema

OTHER: Elevated LFTs

PHARMACOKINETICS

Protein binding 96%; metabolized by CYP3A4; half-life 22.5 hr

INTERACTIONS

Increase: bosutinib concentrations—CYP3A4 inhibitors (ketoconazole, itraconazole, erythromycin, clarithromycin), P-gb inhibitors

Increase: plasma concentrations of simvastatin, calcium channel blockers, ergots

Decrease: bosutinib concentrations—CYP3A4 inducers (dexamethasone, phenytoin, carBAMazepine, rifampin, PHENObarbital), antacids, proton-pump inhibitors

Drug/Food

Increase: increase bosutinib effect—grapefruit juice; avoid use while taking product

Drug/Herb

Decrease: bosutinib concentration—St. John's wort

Drug/Lab

Increase: LFTs, magnesium

Decrease: bicarbonates, magnesium

NURSING CONSIDERATIONS

Assess:

⚠ **Myelosuppression: anemia, thrombocytopenia, neutropenia; obtain a CBC weekly × 1 mo, then monthly as needed**

• LFTs every mo × 3 mo, then as clinically indicated

Evaluate:

• Therapeutic response: decrease in leukemic cells or size of tumor

Teach patient/family:

• To report adverse reactions immediately, bleeding; report diarrhea, hepatic, hematologic symptoms/toxicity

• About reason for treatment, expected results
• To use effective contraception during treatment and up to 30 days after discontinuing treatment

⚠ HIGH ALERT

brentuximab

(bren-tuk′see-mab)

Adcetris

Func. class.: Antineoplastic
Chem. class.: Monoclonal antibody

ACTION: The anticancer activity is due to the binding of the ADC to CD30-expressing cells, followed by the internalization and transportation of the ADC-CD30 complex to lysosomes and the release of MMAE via selective proteolytic cleavage; MMAE binds to tubulin and disrupts the microtubule network within the cell, inducing cell cycle arrest and apoptotic death of the cells

USES: For the treatment of Hodgkin's disease after failure of autologous stem cell transplant (ASCT) or after failure of at least 2 prior multiagent chemotherapy regimens in patients who are not ASCT candidates; for the treatment of non-Hodgkin's lymphoma (NHL); for the treatment of systemic anaplastic large cell lymphoma (sALCL) after failure of at least 1 prior multiagent chemotherapy regimen

CONTRAINDICATIONS Hypersensitivity, pregnancy (category D)

Precautions: Breastfeeding, children, infants, neonates, neutropenia, peripheral neuropathy, tumor lysis syndrome (TLS)

Black Box Warning: Progressive multifocal leukoencephalopathy

DOSAGE AND ROUTES

• **Adult:** **IV** 1.8 mg/kg over 30 min every 3 wk until disease progression, or unacceptable toxicity; for patients >100 kg, max weight used for dosage calculation should be 100 kg, which translates to no more than 180 mg/dose

Dose adjustments for toxicity due to peripheral neuropathy:

• For grade <3: no dosage adjustments are recommended; for new or worsening grade 2-3: interrupt treatment until toxicity resolves to grade ≤1; when resuming treatment, reduce dosage to 1.2 mg/kg IV q3wk; for grade 4: discontinue treatment

Dose adjustments for toxicity due to neutropenia:

• For neutropenia grade <3: no dosage adjustments; for grade 3-4 neutropenia: interrupt treatment until toxicity resolves to baseline or grade ≤2; consider the use of growth factors (CSFs) for subsequent cycles of therapy; for grade 4 neutropenia despite the use of growth factors: discontinue treatment or reduce the dose to 1.2 mg/kg IV q3wk

Available forms: Powder for inj 50 mg

Administer:

Intermittent IV INFUSION route

• Visually inspect for particulate matter and discoloration whenever sol and container permit
• Only as an IV infusion, do not give as an IV push or bolus
• Use cytotoxic handling procedures
• Do not mix, or administer as an infusion, with other IV products
• Calculate the dose (mg) and the number of vials required. For patients weighing >100 kg, use 100 kg to calculate the dose; reconstitute each 50-mg vial per 10.5 ml of sterile water for inj (5 mg/ml)
• Direct the stream of sterile water toward the wall of the vial and not directly at the cake or powder; gently swirl the vial to aid in dissolution, do not shake
• Discard any unused portion left in the vial
• After reconstitution, dilute immediately with ≥100 ml of 0.9% sodium chloride, 5% dextrose, or lactated Ringer's solution to a final concentration (0.4 mg/ml-1.8 mg/ml)
• Infuse over 30 min

• Use the diluted sol immediately or store in refrigerator for ≤24 hr after reconstitution; do not freeze

SIDE EFFECTS

CNS: Headache, dizziness, *fever,* peripheral neuropathy, anxiety, chills, confusion, *fatigue,* paresthesias, insomnia, night sweats, progressive multifocal leukoencephalopathy
CV: Peripheral edema, supraventricular arrhythmia
GI: *Abdominal pain, nausea, vomiting,* constipation, *diarrhea,* weight loss
INTEG: *Rash,* pruritus, alopecia, xerosis
RESP: Pneumothorax, pneumonitis, pulmonary embolism, dyspnea, *cough*
SYST: Anaphylaxis, tumor lysis syndrome, antibody formation, Stevens-Johnson syndrome, infusion reactions
HEMA: Anemia, neutropenia, thrombocytopenia, lymphadenopathy

PHARMACOKINETICS

Protein binding is 68%-82%, only a small amount is metabolized; potent inhibitors or inducers of CYP3A4 may alter action; ADC peak at end of infusion; MME peak 1-3 days; terminal half-life is 4-6 days; 3 components are released: MMAE (monomethyl auristatin E), ADC, and the total antibody; the half-life of MMAE a component is 3.43-3.6 days

INTERACTIONS

Increase: brentuximab action: CYP3A4 inducers, P-gb inhibitors, ketoconazole, boceprevir, delavirdine, isoniazid, indinavir, itraconazole, dalfopristin; quinupristin, telithromycin, tipranavir, rifampin, ritonavir
Increase: noninfectious pulmonary toxicity bleomycin, do not use together
Decrease: brentuximab action-CYP3A4 inducers
Drug/Herb
• Increased brentuximab component action: St. John's wort
Drug/Lab:
Increase: LFTs
Decrease: WBC, platelets, RBCs

NURSING CONSIDERATIONS

Assess:
• **Tumor lysis syndrome (TLS):** assess for hyperkalemia, hypophosphatemia, hypocalcemia; may develop renal failure; may use allopurinol or rasburicase to prevent TLS; monitor serum BUN/creatinine
• **Pregnancy: determine if pregnancy is planned or suspected, pregnancy category D**
• **Peripheral neuropathy, progressive multifocal leukoencephalopathy:** assess for weakness or paralysis, vision loss, impaired speech, and cognitive deterioration; often fatal
• Monitor CBC, and differential, LFTs, serum bilirubin (direct and indirect), electrolytes, uric acid, neurologic function
Evaluate:
• Decreasing symptoms of Hodgkin's disease (increased lymph nodes, night sweats, weight loss, splenomegaly, hepatomegaly)
Teach patient/family:
• To report immediately weakness, change in vision, impaired speech; peripheral neuropathy, neutropenia if severe
• To use reliable contraception (pregnancy [D]); to avoid breastfeeding

brimonidine (ophthalmic)

(bri-moe′ni-deen)

Alphagan P

Func. class.: Antiglaucoma
Chem. class.: Selective α-2 agonist

Do not confuse:
brimonidine/bimatoprost

ACTION: Select α-agonist that decreases aqueous humor and increases outflows

USES: Treatment of chronic open-angle glaucoma and ocular hypertension

CONTRAINDICATIONS: Hypersensitivity, AV block, heart failure, bradycardia, sick sinus syndrome, within 14 days of MAOIs therapy

Precautions: Breastfeeding, depression, cerebrovascular disease, hepatic/renal impairment, Raynaud's phenomenon, orthostatic hypotension, thromboangiitis obliterans

DOSAGE AND ROUTES

- **Adult/child >2 yr:** Instill 1 drop in the affected eye(s) tid

Available forms: Ophthalmic solution 0.1%, 0.15%, 0.2%

SIDE EFFECTS

RESP: Cough, dyspnea, bronchitis, pharyngitis

CNS: Headache, dizziness, somnolence

CV: Hyper/hypotension, hypercholesterolemia

EENT: Eye stinging/burning, tearing, photophobia, change in vision, sinus infection, blurred vision, pruritus, photophobia, eyelid erythema, ocular pain, nasal dryness

PHARMACOKINETICS

Peak ½-2 hr, half-life 2 hr

INTERACTIONS

Increase: intraocular pressure reduction—apraclonidine, dorzolamide, pilocarpine, timolol

Increase: effects of—CNS depressants

Decrease: B/P—β-blockers, antihypertensives

Decrease: brimonidine effect—tricyclic antidepressants, may cause HTN crisis MAOIs, linezolid

NURSING CONSIDERATIONS

Assess:

- Glaucoma: monitor intraocular pressure

Evaluate:

- Decreasing intraocular pressure

Teach patient/family:

- That drug is for ophthalmic use only
- Not to touch the tip of the dropper to the eye, fingertips, or other surface to prevent contamination
- To wash hands before and after use; to tilt the head back slightly and pull the lower eyelid down with the index finger to form a pouch; squeeze the prescribed number of drops into the pouch; close eyes to spread drops; to avoid excessive systemic absorption, apply finger pressure on the lacrimal sac for 1-2 min following use
- That if more than one topical ophthalmic drug product is being used, the drugs should be administered at least 10 min apart
- To avoid contamination or the spread of infection, do not use dropper for more than one person

brinzolamide ophthalmic

See Appendix B

bromfenac (ophthalmic)

(brom′fen-ak)

Prolensa

Func. class.: Antiinflammatory (ophthalmic)

Chem. class.: Nonsteroidal antiflammatory drug

ACTION: The mechanism of action is thought to be ability to block prostaglandin synthesis by inhibiting cyclooxygenase 1 and 2. In studies performed in animal eyes, prostaglandins have been shown to produce disruption of the blood–aqueous humor barrier, vasodilation, increased vascular permeability, leukocytosis, and increased intraocular pressure

USES: To reduce pain and inflammation after cataract surgery

CONTRAINDICATIONS: Hypersensitivity to this product, sulfites, NSAIDs, salicylates

Precautions: Bleeding disorders, complicated ocular surgery, corneal denervation, diabetes mellitus, rheumatoid

arthritis, dry eye syndrome, pregnancy (C), breastfeeding
Do not administer while wearing contact lenses

DOSAGE AND ROUTES

• **Adult:** Instill 1 drop into affected eye twice daily beginning 24 hr before cataract surgery, continued on the day of surgery and through the first 14 days of the postoperative period

Available forms: Ophthalmic solution 0.07%, 0.09%

Administer:

• Apply topically to the eye
• Remove contact lenses before instilling solution; contact lenses should not be worn during use of this product
• Instruct patient on proper instillation of eye solution
• Do not touch the tip of the dropper to the eye, fingertips, or other surface
• Do not share bottle with other patients
• If more than one ophthalmic medication is being used, the medications should be administered at least 5 min apart

SIDE EFFECTS

CNS: Headache
EENT: Abnormal sensation in eye, conjunctival hyperemia, ocular irritation, ocular pain, ocular pruritus, conjunctival hyperemia, iritis, keratitis

PHARMACOKINETICS

Unknown

INTERACTIONS

Increase: corneal erosion, poor healing—topical corticosteroids
Increase: bleeding—anticoagulants
Increase: intraocular pressure—latanoprost
Drug/Lab
Increase: bleeding time

NURSING CONSIDERATIONS

Assess:

• Eyes for pain, inflammation, burning, redness after cataract surgery
• Identify if patient is using topical corticosteroids, anticoagulants; use cautiously in those using these products

Evaluate:

• Decreased pain and inflammation after cataract surgery

Teach patient/family:

• To apply topically to the eye
• To remove contact lenses before instilling solution; contact lenses should not be worn during use of this product
• Proper instillation of eye solution
• Not to touch the tip of the dropper to the eye, fingertips, or other surface
• Not to share bottle with other patients
• That if more than one ophthalmic medication is being used, the medications should be administered at least 5 min apart

bromocriptine (Rx)

(broe-moe-krip′teen)

Cycloset, Parlodel

Func. class.: Antiparkinson agent
Chem. class.: Dopamine receptor agonist

Do not confuse:
Parlodel/pindolol/Provera
bromocriptine/benztropine/brimonidine

ACTION: Inhibits prolactin release by activating postsynaptic dopamine receptors; activation of striatal dopamine receptors may be reason for improvement in Parkinson's disease

USES: Parkinson's disease, amenorrhea/galactorrhea caused by hyperprolactinemia, infertility, acromegaly, pituitary adenomas, adjunct for type 2 diabetes

Unlabeled uses: Neuroleptic malignant syndrome, alcoholism, premenstrual syndrome, mastalgia, cocaine withdrawal, premenstrual breast symptoms

CONTRAINDICATIONS: Severe ischemic disease, uncontrolled hypertension, severe peripheral vascular disease;

hypersensitivity to ergot, bromocriptine; migraine, preeclampsia

Precautions: Pregnancy (B), breastfeeding, children, renal/hepatic disease, pituitary tumors, peptic ulcer disease, sulfite hypersensitivity, pulmonary fibrosis, dementia, GI bleeding, bipolar disorder

DOSAGE AND ROUTES

Parkinson's disease

• **Adult: PO** 1.25 mg bid with meals; may increase q2-4wk by 2.5 mg/day, max 100 mg/day; levodopa should be continued while bromocriptine is being instituted

Hyperprolactinemia

• **Adult: PO** 1.25-2.5 mg with meals; may increase by 2.5 mg q3-7days, usual range 2.5-15 mg/day, max 30 mg/day

Acromegaly

• **Adult: PO** 1.25-2.5 mg × 3 days at bedtime; may increase by 1.25-2.5 mg q3-7days; usual range 20-30 mg/day, max 100 mg/day

Pituitary adenoma

• **Adult: PO** 1.25 mg bid-tid; may increase over several wk to 10-20 mg/day

Type 2 diabetes (Cycloset only)

• **Adult: PO** (initially) 0.8 mg daily in AM within 2 hr of waking; titrate by 0.8 mg/day no more than weekly to max 1.6-4.8 mg/day

Available forms: Caps 5 mg; tabs 2.5 mg (Parodel), 0.8 mg (Cycloset)

Administer:

• With meal to prevent GI symptoms

• At bedtime so that dizziness, orthostatic hypotension do not occur

• Store at room temperature in tight, light-resistant container

SIDE EFFECTS

CNS: *Headache,* depression, restlessness, anxiety, nervousness, confusion, **seizures**, *hallucinations,* dizziness, fatigue, drowsiness, abnormal involuntary movements, psychosis, weakness

CV: Orthostatic hypotension, decreased B/P, palpitations, extrasystole, **shock**, dysrhythmias, bradycardia, **MI**

EENT: Blurred vision, diplopia, burning eyes, nasal congestion

GI: *Nausea, vomiting, anorexia,* cramps, constipation, diarrhea, dry mouth, **GI hemorrhage**

GU: Frequency, retention, incontinence, diuresis

INTEG: *Rash on face, arms;* alopecia; coolness, pallor of fingers, toes; peripheral edema

META: Hypoglycemia

PHARMACOKINETICS

Peak 1-3 hr, duration 4-8 hr, 90%-96% protein bound, half-life 3 hr, metabolized by liver (inactive metabolites), 85%-98% of dose excreted in feces, >90% of absorbed dose undergoes 1st-pass metabolism

INTERACTIONS

• Disulfiram-like reaction: alcohol

Increase: action of antihypertensives, levodopa, chloramphenicol, probenecid, salicylates, sulfonamides

Decrease: action of bromocriptine—phenothiazines, oral contraceptives, progestins, estrogens, haloperidol, loxapine, methyldopa, metoclopramide, MAOIs, reserpine

Decrease/increase: effect of Cyclosert-CYP3A4 inhibitors/inducers

Decrease: effect of Cyclosert-butyrophenones, metoclopramide, phenothiazine, thioxanthenes

Drug/Lab Test

Increase: growth hormone, AST, ALT, CK, BUN, uric acid, alk phos

NURSING CONSIDERATIONS

Assess:

• B/P; establish baseline, compare with other readings; this product decreases B/P and causes orthostatic hypotension

• **Parkinson's symptoms:** pill rolling, shuffling gait, restlessness, tremors, postural instability before and during treatment

• **Neuroleptic malignant syndrome: decreased temperature, seizures, sweating, pulse indicates resolution of symptoms**

• Change in size of soft-tissue volume with acromegaly
• **Pregnancy:** may cause postpartum conception, use pregnancy testing q4wk or if menstruation does not occur

Evaluate:
• Therapeutic response (Parkinson's disease): decreased dyskinesia, slow movements, drooling

Teach patient/family:
• That tabs may be crushed, mixed with food; Cycloset to be taken within 2 hr of rising
• To change position slowly to prevent orthostatic hypotension
• To use contraceptives during treatment with this product; that pregnancy may occur; to use methods other than oral contraceptives/subdermal implants
• That therapeutic effect for Parkinson's disease may take 2 mo, titrate slowly
• To avoid hazardous activity if dizziness occurs
• To report symptoms of MI immediately
• To take with food, avoid alcohol

budesonide (Rx)

(byoo-des′oh-nide)

Uceris, Entocort EC, Pulmicort, Pulmicort Flexhaler, Rhinocort Allergy, Rhinocort Aqua, Uceris

Func. class.: Glucocorticoid
Chem. class.: Nonhalogenated

ACTION: Prevents inflammation by depressing migration of polymorphonuclear leukocytes and fibroblasts, reversal of increased capillary permeability, and lysosomal stabilization; does not suppress hypothalamus or pituitary function

USES: Rhinitis; prophylaxis for asthma; Crohn's disease, ulcerative colitis
Unlabeled uses: Microscopic colitis, laryngotracheobronchitis (croup)

CONTRAINDICATIONS: Hypersensitivity, status asthmaticus, acute bronchospasm

Precautions: Pregnancy (C), inhaled form (B); breastfeeding; children; TB; fungal, bacterial, systemic viral infections; ocular herpes simplex; nasal septal ulcers; hepatic disease, diabetes, GI disease, increased intraocular pressure

DOSAGE AND ROUTES

Rhinitis
• **Adult and child >12 yr: SPRAY/INH** 2 sprays in each nostril AM, PM or 4 sprays in each nostril AM

Asthma
• **Adult: INH** 360 mcg bid, max 720 mcg bid
• **Child 1-8 yr previously taking bronchodilator alone:** (Respules) 0.5 mg daily or 0.25 mg bid; susp via jet nebulizer, max 0.5 mg daily; previously using inhaled corticosteroid 0.5 mg daily or 0.25 mg bid susp via jet nebulizer, max 0.5 mg bid

Crohn's disease/ulcerative colitis (Uceris)
• **Adult: PO** 9 mg/day AM × 8 wk

Laryngotracheobronchitis (croup) (unlabeled)
• **Infant ≥3 mo-child ≤5 yr: NEB** (Pulmicort Respules INH susp) 2 mg inhaled as a single dose

Available forms: Dry powder for INH 90, 180; 32 mcg/actuation (Rhinocort Aqua) nasal spray; susp for INH 0.5 mg/2 ml, 0.25 mg/2 ml; cap 3 mg; ext rel tab (Uceris) 9 mg, rectal foam 2 mg/actuation

Administer:

PO route (Crohn's disease/ulcerative colitis)
• Swallow caps whole; do not break, crush, chew, take in AM
• May repeat 8-wk course if needed; may taper to 6 mg/day for 2 wk before cessation
• Store at 59° F-86° F (15° C-30° C); keep away from heat, open flame

Rectal foam route
• Product is flammable, may use before bedtime, applicators are single use only

B

SIDE EFFECTS

CNS: *Headache,* insomnia, hypertonia, syncope, dizziness, drowsiness
CV: Chest pain, hypertension, sinus tachycardia, palpitation
EENT: *Sinusitis, pharyngitis,* rhinitis, oral candidiasis
ENDO: Adrenal insufficiency, growth suppression in children
GI: Dry mouth, dyspepsia, nausea, vomiting, abdominal pain
MISC: Ecchymosis, fever, *hypersensitivity,* flulike symptoms, epistaxis, dysuria
MS: Back pain, myalgias, fractures
RESP: Nasal irritation, cough, nasal bleeding, *respiratory infections,* **bronchospasm**

PHARMACOKINETICS

Peak: Respules 4-6 wk, Rhinocort Aqua 2 wk, half-life 2-3.6 hr
Onset: Respules 2-8 days, Rhinocort Aqua 10 hr
Enters breast milk

INTERACTIONS

Increase: budesonide effect, CYP3A inhibitors, dose adjustment may be needed
• Avoid concurrent use of varicella live vaccine in pediatric patients

NURSING CONSIDERATIONS

Assess:
• Respiratory status: rate, rhythm, increase in bronchial secretions, wheezing, chest tightness; provide fluids to 2 L/day to decrease thickness of secretions; check for oral candidiasis
• **Bronchospasm: stop treatment, give bronchodilator**
• Viral infections: corticosteroid use can mask infections
• Increased intraocular pressure: discontinue use if this occurs

Evaluate:
• Therapeutic response: absence of asthma, rhinitis

Teach patient/family:
• To notify prescriber of pharyngitis, nasal bleeding, oral candidiasis
• Not to exceed recommended dose because adrenal suppression may occur
• To carry emergency ID that identifies steroid use
• To read and follow package directions
• To prevent exposure to infections (especially viral)
• To use good oral hygiene if using nebulizer or inhaler
• To avoid breastfeeding
• That burning or stinging may occur with first few doses of inhalation use
• That product is not a bronchodilator and not to be used for asthma; to use regularly
• Teach how to use as described in "administer"
• To notify prescriber if symptoms persist after wks, that results usually take 2 wk
• To notify prescriber if exposure to measles, chickenpox occurs

budesonide nasal agent

See Appendix B

bumetanide (Rx)

(byoo-met′a-nide)

Bumex, Burinex ♣

Func. class.: Loop diuretic, antihypertensive

Chem. class.: Sulfonamide derivative

ACTION: Acts on ascending loop of Henle by inhibiting reabsorption of chloride, sodium

USES: Edema in CHF, heart failure
Unlabeled uses: Hypercalcemia, hypertension, ascites

CONTRAINDICATIONS: Hypersensitivity to sulfonamides, anuria, hepatic coma

Black Box Warning: Electrolyte imbalance

Precautions: Pregnancy (C), breastfeeding, neonates, ascites, severe renal disease, hepatic cirrhosis, blood dyscrasias, ototoxicity, hyperuricemia, hypokalemia, hyperglycemia, oliguria, hypomagnesemia, hypovolemia

Black Box Warning: Dehydration

DOSAGE AND ROUTES

- **Adult and adolescent: PO** 0.5-2 mg/day; may give 2nd or 3rd dose at 4-5 hr intervals, max 10 mg/day; may be given on alternate days or intermittently; **IV/IM** 0.5-1 mg; may give 2nd or 3rd dose at 2-3 hr intervals, not to exceed 10 mg/day
- **Child and infant (unlabeled): PO/IM/IV** 0.015-0.1 mg/kg daily or every other day, max 10 mg/day

Hypercalcemia (unlabeled)

- **Adult: IV** 1-2 mg q1-4hr to maintain urine output of 200-250 ml/hr; give saline before 1st dose of this product

Hypertension (unlabeled)

- **Adult and adolescent: PO** 0.5-2 mg/day, max 10 mg/day in 2 divided doses

Available forms: Tabs 0.5, 1, 2, 5 ✱ mg; inj 0.25 mg/ml

Administer:

- In AM to avoid interference with sleep if using product as a diuretic; without regard to meals
- Potassium replacement if potassium is <3.0

PO route

- Use in AM to prevent nocturia
- Without regard to food

IV, direct route

- Direct IV undiluted slowly over 1-2 min through Y-tube, 3-way stopcock, or heplock

Intermittent IV INFUSION route

- Dilute in LR, D_5W, 0.9% NaCl (rarely given by this method), give over 12 hr with renal disease

Syringe compatibilities: Doxapram

Y-site compatibilities: Acyclovir, alfentanil, allopurinol, amifostine, amikacin, aminocaproic acid, aminophylline, amiodarone, amoxicillin, amphotericin B lipid complex (Abelcet), amphotericin B liposome (AmBisome), anidulafungin, ascorbic acid injection, atenolol, atracurium, atropine, aztreonam, benztropine, bivalirudin, bleomycin, buprenorphine, butorphanol, calcium chloride/gluconate, CARBOplatin, caspofungin, cefamandole, ceFAZolin, cefepime, cefmetazole, cefonicid, cefotaxime, cefoTEtan, cefOXitin, cefTAZidime, ceftizoxime, ceftobiprole, cefTRIAXone, cefuroxime, cephapirin, chloramphenicol, cimetidine, cisatracurium, CISplatin, cladribine, clarithromycin, clindamycin, codeine, cyanocobalamin, cyclophosphamide, cycloSPORINE, cytarabine, DACTINomycin, DAPTOmycin, dexamethasone, dexmedetomidine, digoxin, diltiazem, diphenhydrAMINE, DOBUTamine, DOCEtaxel, DOPamine, doripenem, doxacurium, DOXOrubicin, doxycycline, enalaprilat, ePHEDrine, EPINEPHrine, epirubicin, epoetin alfa, eptifibatide, ertapenem, erythromycin, esmolol, etoposide, famotidine, fentaNYL, filgrastim, fluconazole, fludarabine, fluorouracil, folic acid, furosemide, gatifloxacin, gemcitabine, gentamicin, glycopyrrolate, granisetron, heparin, hydrocortisone sodium succinate, HYDROmorphone, hydrOXYzine, IDArubicin, ifosfamide, imipenem-cilastatin, indomethacin, insulin (regular), irinotecan, isoproterenol, ketorolac, labetalol, levofloxacin, lidocaine, linezolid, LORazepam, magnesium sulfate, mannitol, mechlorethamine, melphalan, meperidine, metaraminol, methotrexate, methoxamine, methyldopate, methylPREDNISolone, metoclopramide, metoprolol, metroNIDAZOLE, mezlocillin, micafungin, miconazole, milrinone, mitoXANtrone, morphine, moxalactam, multiple vitamins injection, mycophenolate, nafcillin, nalbuphine, naloxone, netilmicin, nitroglycerin, nitroprusside, norepinephrine, octreotide, ondansetron, oxacillin, oxaliplatin, oxytocin, palonosetron, pamidronate, pancuronium, pantoprazole, PEMEtrexed, penicillin G potassium/sodium, pentazocine, PENTobarbital, PHENobarbital, phenylephrine, phytonadione, piperacillin, piperacillin-tazobactam, polymyxin B, potassium chloride, procainamide, promethazine, propofol, propranolol, protamine, pyridoxine, quiNIDine, ranitidine, remifentanil, rifampin, ritodrine, riTUXimab, rocuronium, sodium acetate, sodium bicarbonate, succinylcholine, SUFentanil, tacrolimus, teniposide, theophylline, thiamine, thiotepa, ticarcillin, ticarcillin-clavulanate, tigecycline, tirofiban, TNA, tobramycin, tolazoline, TPN, traMADol, trastuzumab, trimetaphan, urokinase, vancomycin, vasopressin, vecuronium, verapamil, vinCRIStine, vinorelbine, voriconazole

SIDE EFFECTS

CNS: *Headache,* fatigue, weakness, *dizziness,* **encephalopathy**

CV: **Chest pain,** *hypotension,* **circulatory collapse,** ECG changes, dehydration

EENT: *Loss of hearing*

ELECT: *Hypokalemia, hypochloremic alkalosis, hypomagnesemia, hyperuricemia, hypocalcemia, hyponatremia*

ENDO: *Hyperglycemia*

GI: *Nausea,* diarrhea, dry mouth, vomiting, anorexia, cramps, upset stomach, abdominal pain

GU: *Polyuria,* **renal failure,** glycosuria, premature ejaculation, hypercholesterolemia

HEMA: **Thrombocytopenia, leukopenia, granulocytopenia, hemoconcentration**

INTEG: *Rash, pruritus,* purpura, **Stevens-Johnson syndrome,** sweating

MS: Muscular cramps, arthritis, stiffness

PHARMACOKINETICS

Excreted by kidneys (50% unchanged), feces (20%); crosses placenta; excreted in breast milk; protein binding >96%; half-life 1-1½ hr

PO: Onset ½-1 hr, peak 1-2 hr, duration 3-6 hr

IM: Onset 40 min, peak 1-2 hr, duration 4-6 hr

IV: Onset 5 min, peak 15-30 min, duration 3-6 hr

INTERACTIONS

- **Increase:** ototoxicity: aminoglycosides, cisplatin
- **Increase:** hypokalemia: potassium-wasting products

Increase: toxicity—lithium, digoxin

Increase: diuresis, electrolyte loss—metolazone

Decrease: diuretic effect—indomethacin, NSAIDs, probenecid, other diuretics

Decrease: antidiabetic effects—antidiabetics

Drug/Herb

Increase: effect—hawthorn, horse chestnut

Decrease: effect of bumetanide—ginseng, ephedra

Drug/Lab

Increase: glucose

Decrease: chloride, potassium, sodium, calcium, phosphorus

NURSING CONSIDERATIONS

Assess:

- For tinnitus; obtain audiometric testing for long-term IV treatment
- Weight, I&O daily to determine fluid loss; if urinary output decreases or azotemia occurs, product should be discontinued; safest dosage schedule is alternate days
- B/P lying, standing; postural hypotension may occur

Black Box Warning: Electrolyte imbalances: Potassium, sodium, calcium; include BUN, blood glucose, CBC, serum creatinine, blood pH, ABGs, uric acid, calcium, magnesium; severe electrolyte imbalances should be corrected before starting treatment

- Blood glucose if patient is diabetic; blood uric acid levels in those with gout
- Improvement in edema of feet, legs, sacral area daily if medication is being used for CHF
- Signs of metabolic alkalosis: drowsiness, restlessness
- **Hypokalemia:** postural hypotension, malaise, fatigue, tachycardia, leg cramps, weakness
- Rashes, temperature elevation daily
- Confusion, especially in geriatric patients; take safety precautions if needed

- **Digoxin toxicity** in patients taking digoxin products: anorexia, nausea, vomiting, confusion, paresthesia, muscle cramps; **lithium toxicity** in those taking lithium

Evaluate:

- Therapeutic response: decreased edema, B/P

Teach patient/family:

- To increase fluid intake to 2-3 L/day unless contraindicated; to take potassium supplement; to rise slowly from lying or sitting position
- To recognize adverse reactions: muscle cramps, weakness, nausea, dizziness, edema, weight gain
- To take with food, milk for GI symptoms; to avoid alcohol
- To take early in day to prevent nocturia
- To use sunscreen to prevent photosensitivity

TREATMENT OF OVERDOSE: Lavage if taken orally; monitor electrolytes; administer dextrose in saline; monitor hydration, CV, renal status

HIGH ALERT

buprenorphine (Rx)

(byoo-pre-nor′feen)

Belbuca, Buprenex, Butrans ✦

Func. class.: Opioid analgesic, partial agonist

Chem. class.: Thebaine derivative

Controlled Substance Schedule V (Parenteral); Schedule III (Tablet, TD)

Do not confuse:
Buprenex/Bumex

ACTION: Depresses pain impulse transmission at the spinal cord level by interacting with opioid receptors, partial agonist at μ-opioid receptor

USES: Moderate to severe pain, opiate agonist withdrawal/dependence

Unlabeled uses: Cocaine withdrawal

CONTRAINDICATIONS: Hypersensitivity, ileus, status asthmaticus

Black Box Warning: Respiratory depression

Precautions: Pregnancy (C), breastfeeding, substance abuse/alcoholism, increased intracranial pressure, MI (acute), severe heart disease, respiratory depression, renal/hepatic/pulmonary disease, hypothyroidism, Addison's disease

Black Box Warning: QT prolongation, accidental exposure, potential for overdose/poisoning, substance abuse

DOSAGE AND ROUTES

- **Adult: IM/IV** 0.3 mg q6-8hr prn, reduce dosage in geriatric patients, may repeat after 30-60 min; **EPIDURAL** (unlabeled) 4 mcg/kg or 2 mcg/kg (epidural inj); **TD** each patch is worn for 7 days (moderate-severe pain); **opioid-naive patients** (those taking <30 mg of oral morphine or equivalent before beginning treatment with TD buprenorphine), 5 mcg/hr q7days, overestimating dose can be fatal; **conversion from other opiate agonist therapy,** titrate from other opioids for up to 7 days to no more than 30 mg oral morphine or equivalent before beginning TD therapy, begin with 5 mcg/hr q7days; for those with daily dose of 30-80 mg oral morphine or equivalent, start with 10 mcg/hr q7days; for those taking >80 mg oral morphine or equivalent, start with 20 mcg/hr q7days
- **Child 2-12 yr: IM/IV** 2-6 mcg/kg q4-8hr

Available forms: Inj 0.3 mg/ml (1-ml vials); SL tab 2, 8 mg as base; TD system 5, 7.5, 10, 15, 20 mcg/hr (weekly); dissolving film 75, 300, 450, 600, 750, 900 mcg

Administer:

SL route

- Do not chew, dissolve under tongue, use 2 or more at same time

Transdermal route

- Apply to clean, dry, intact skin; each patch should be worn for 7 days; do not

apply direct heat source to patch, will increase absorption of product, may use first aid tape if edge of patch is not adhering
- Apply to upper outer arm, upper chest/back, or side of chest

IM route
- In deep muscle mass

IV, direct route
- **Give** undiluted over ≥2 min, titrate to patient response; rapid injection will increase side effects
- With antiemetic if nausea, vomiting occur
- When pain is beginning to return; determine dosage interval by patient response

Y-site compatibilities: Acyclovir, alfentanil, allopurinol, amifostine, amikacin, aminocaproic acid, amphotericin B liposome (AmBisone), anidulafungin, ascorbic acid injection, atenolol, atracurium, atropine, aztreonam, benztropine, bivalirudin, bleomycin, bumetanide, butorphanol, calcium chloride/gluconate, CARBOplatin, cefamandole, ceFAZolin, cefepime, cefotaxime, cefoTEtan, cefOXitin, cefTAZidime, ceftizoxime, cefTRIAXone, cefuroxime, chloramphenicol, chlorproMAZINE, cimetidine, cisatracurium, CISplatin, cladribine, clindamycin, cyanocobalamin, cyclophosphamide, cycloSPORINE, cytarabine, D_5W-dextrose 5%, DACTINomycin, DAPTOmycin, dexamethasone, dexmedetomidine, digoxin, diltiazem, diphenhydrAMINE, DOBUTamine, DOCEtaxel, DOPamine, doxacurium, DOXOrubicin HCl, doxycycline, enalaprilat, ePHEDrine, EPINEPHrine, epirubicin, epoetin alfa, eptifibatide, ertapenem, erythromycin, esmolol, etoposide, famotidine, fenoldopam, fentaNYL, filgrastim, fluconazole, fludarabine, gatifloxacin, gemcitabine, gentamicin, glycopyrrolate, granisetron, heparin, hydrocortisone, hydrOXYzine, IDArubicin, ifosfamide, imipenem-cilastatin, inamrinone, insulin (regular), irinotecan, isoproterenol, ketorolac, labetalol, lactated Ringer's injection, levofloxacin, lidocaine, linezolid, LORazepam, magnesium sulfate, mannitol, mechlorethamine, melphalan, meperidine, metaraminol, methicillin, methotrexate, methoxamine, methyldopate, methylPREDNISolone, metoclopramide, metoprolol, metroNIDAZOLE, mezlocillin, miconazole, midazolam, milrinone, minocycline, mitoXANtrone, morphine, moxalactam, multiple vitamins injection, mycophenolate mofetil, nafcillin, nalbuphine, naloxone, nesiritide, netilmicin, nitroglycerin, nitroprusside, norepinephrine, octreotide, ondansetron, oxacillin, oxaliplatin, oxytocin, palonosetron, pamidronate, pancuronium, papaverine, PEMEtrexed, penicillin G potassium/sodium, pentamidine, pentazocine, phenylephrine, phytonadione, piperacillin, piperacillin-tazobactam, polymyxin B, potassium chloride, procainamide, prochlorperazine, promethazine, propofol, propranolol, protamine, pyridoxine, quiNIDine, ranitidine, remifentanil, Ringer's injection, riTUXimab, rocuronium, sodium acetate, succinylcholine, SUFentanil, tacrolimus, teniposide, theophylline, thiamine, thiotepa, ticarcillin, ticarcillin-clavulanate, tigecycline, tirofiban, TNA (3-in-1), tobramycin, tolazoline, TPN, trastuzumab, trimetaphan, urokinase, vancomycin, vasopressin, vecuronium, verapamil, vinCRIStine, vinorelbine, voriconazole

SIDE EFFECTS

CNS: *Drowsiness, dizziness, confusion, headache, sedation, euphoria,* **increased intracranial pressure,** amnesia, weakness, CNS depression
CV: Palpitations, bradycardia, change in B/P, tachycardia, **QT prolongation,** hypo/hypertension
EENT: Tinnitus, blurred vision, *miosis,* diplopia
GI: *Nausea,* vomiting, anorexia, constipation, cramps, dry mouth, abdominal pain, **hepatotoxicity**
GU: Dysuria, urinary retention
INTEG: *Rash,* urticaria, bruising, flushing, diaphoresis, pruritus
RESP: **Respiratory depression,** dyspnea, hypo/hyperventilation

PHARMACOKINETICS

Metabolized in liver by CYP3A4, excreted by kidneys and in feces, crosses placenta, excreted in breast milk, half-life 2½-3½ hr, 96% bound to plasma proteins

IM: Onset 15 min, peak 1 hr, duration 6-10 hr

SL: Onset, peak, duration unknown, half-life 37 hr

IV: Onset 1 min, peak 5 min, duration 6 hr, half-life 2.2 hr

TD: Half-life 26 hr

Epidural: Duration dose dependent

INTERACTIONS

Increase: effect with other CNS depressants—alcohol, opioids, sedative/hypnotics, antipsychotics, skeletal muscle relaxants, MAOIs

Increase: buprenorphine effect—CYP3A4 inhibitors (erythromycin, indinavir, ketoconazole, ritonavir, saquinavir)

Increase: QT prolongation—class IA, III antidysrhythmics

Decrease: buprenorphine effect—CYP3A4 inducers (carBAMazepine, PHENobarbital, phenytoin, rifampin)

Drug/Herb

Increase: CNS depression—St. John's wort

NURSING CONSIDERATIONS

Assess:

- **Pain:** intensity, location, type before treatment, after 5 min (IV); need for pain medication, tolerance
- I&O ratio; check for decreasing output; may indicate urinary retention
- Bowel pattern; severe constipation can occur
- CNS changes, dizziness, drowsiness, hallucinations, euphoria, LOC, pupil reaction; withdrawal in opioid-dependent persons; if dependence occurs, within 2 wk of discontinuing product **withdrawal symptoms** will occur
- Allergic reactions: rash, urticaria
- Respiratory dysfunction: respiratory depression, character, rate, rhythm; notify prescriber if respirations are <12/min

Black Box Warning: Potential for overdose may occur from chewing, swallowing, snorting, or injecting extracted product from TD formulation

Black Box Warning: QT prolongation: in those taking class Ia, III antidysrhythmics; patients with hypokalemia, cardiac instability (TD), max TD 20 mcg/hr q7day

Evaluate:

- Therapeutic response: decrease in pain, absence of grimacing

Teach patient/family:

- To report any symptoms of CNS changes, allergic reactions

Black Box Warning: That psychologic dependence leading to substance abuse may result when used for extended periods; that long-term use not recommended

- To avoid hazardous activities such as driving unless reaction known
- Do not start new meds/herbs without prescriber approval
- Start stool softener/laxatives to lessen constipation

TREATMENT OF OVERDOSE:

Naloxone 0.4 mg ampule diluted in 10 ml 0.9% NaCl given by direct IV push 0.02 mg q2min (adult)

buPROPion (Rx)

(byoo-proe′pee-on)

Aplenzin, Budeprion XL, Buproban, Forfivo XL, Wellbutrin, Wellbutrin SR, Wellbutrin XL, Zyban

Func. class.: Antidepressant—miscellaneous smoking deterrent

Chem. class.: Aminoketone

Do not confuse:

buPROPion/busPIRone

Zyban/Diovan/Zagam

ACTION: Inhibits reuptake of DOPamine, norepinephrine, serotonin

USES: Depression (Wellbutrin), smoking cessation (Zyban); seasonal affective disorder, substance abuse, glaucoma, smoking, cardiac disease, heart failure

Unlabeled uses: Neuropathic pain, enhancement of weight loss, ADHD (attention-deficit/hyperactivity disorder)

CONTRAINDICATIONS: Hypersensitivity, head trauma, stroke, intracranial mass, eating disorders, seizure disorders

Precautions: Pregnancy (C), breastfeeding, geriatric patients, renal/hepatic disease, recent MI, cranial trauma, seizure disorder, substance abuse, glaucoma, smoking, cardiac disease, heart failure

Black Box Warning: Children <18 yr, suicidal thinking/behavior (young adults)

DOSAGE AND ROUTES

Depression

- **Adult: PO** 100 mg bid initially, then increase after 3 days to 100 mg tid if needed, max 150 mg single dose; **ER/SR** initially 150 mg AM, increase to 300 mg/day if initial dose is tolerated, after no less than 4 days; after several wk, titrate to 200 mg bid; Aplenzin 174 mg q AM, may increase to 348 mg q AM on day 4, may increase to 522 mg after several weeks if needed; Forfivo XL (not for initial treatment) 450 mg daily after titration with another product (300 mg/day × ≥2 wk)
- **Geriatric: PO** 50-100 mg/day, may increase by 50-100 mg q3-4days

Smoking cessation (Zyban)

- **Adult: SR** 150 mg daily × 3 days, then 150 mg bid for remainder of treatment, initiate 1-2 wk before targeted "quit day," continue for 7-12 wk; in combination with nicotine TD, 150 mg daily × 3 days, then 150 mg bid for remainder of treatment, give ≥8 hr apart, max 300 mg/day, initiate 1-2 wk before targeted "quit day," continue for 7-12 wk, may be continued for 8-20 wk

Seasonal affective disorder

- **Adult: PO**(Wellbutrin XL) 150 mg as a single dose in the AM, after 1 wk may be increased to 300 mg/day; (Aplenzin) 174 mg daily in AM, after 7 days may increase to 348 mg daily

ADHD (unlabeled) (Wellbutrin)

- **Adult: PO** 100 mg bid, after ≥3 days titrate to 100 mg tid; **SR** 300 mg/day, 200 mg 8 AM, 100 mg 4 PM

Diabetic neuropathy/postherpetic neuralgia (unlabeled)(Wellbutrin SR)

- **Adult: PO** SR 150-300 mg/day

Available forms: Tabs 75, 100 mg; sus rel tabs (SR) 100, 150, 200 ext rel tab (XL) 100, 150, 300, 450 mg; (SR-12 hr, XL-24 hr); tab ext rel (Aplenzin) 174, 348, 522 mg

Administer:

PO route

⚠ When switching to Aplenzin from Wellbutrin, Wellbutrin SR or XL, use these equivalents: 174 mg buPROPion HBr = 150 mg buPROPion HCl; 348 mg buPROPion HBr = 300 mg buPROPion HCl; 522 mg buPROPion HBr = 450 mg buPROPion HCl

- **Wellbutrin immediate rel,** separate by ≥6 hr, give in 3 divided doses; **Wellbutrin SR,** if multiple doses are used, separate by ≥8 hr; **Wellbutrin XL,** give daily in AM; **Zyban SR,** give in 2 divided doses, ≥8 hr apart; **Aplenzin ER,** give daily in AM, a larger dose of Aplenzin is needed because these products are not equivalent
- Do not break, crush, chew sus rel, ext rel tab
- At evenly spaced times to prevent seizures; seizure risk increases with high doses
- Increase fluids, bulk in diet if constipation occurs
- With food, milk for GI symptoms
- Sugarless gum, hard candy, frequent sips of water for dry mouth
- Avoid giving at night to prevent insomnia

SIDE EFFECTS

CNS: *Headache, agitation, dizziness, akinesia, bradykinesia, confusion,*

seizures, delusions, *insomnia, sedation, tremors,* suicidal ideation, mania, hot flashes, myoclonia, chest pain, flushing
CV: *Dysrhythmias, hypertension,* palpitations, *tachycardia,* hypotension, complete AV block; QRS prolongation (overdose)
EENT: *Blurred vision, auditory disturbance,* tinnitus
GI: *Nausea, vomiting,* anorexia, diarrhea, *dry mouth,* increased appetite, *constipation,* altered taste
GU: Impotence, urinary frequency, retention, *menstrual irregularities,* nocturia, altered libido
INTEG: *Rash,* pruritus, *sweating,* Stevens-Johnson syndrome
MISC: *Weight loss or gain*

PHARMACOKINETICS

Onset 1-4 wk, half-life 14 hr (immediate release), extensively metabolized by liver, some conversion to active metabolites, steady state 5-8 days, protein binding 84%, excreted in urine and feces

INTERACTIONS

- Do not use within 14 days of MAOIs

⚠ **Increase:** adverse reactions, seizures—levodopa, MAOIs, phenothiazines, antidepressants, benzodiazepines, alcohol, theophylline, systemic steroids
Increase: buPROPion toxicity—ritonavir
Increase: buPROPion level—cimetidine
Increase: buPROPion effect—CYP2D6/CYP2B6 inhibitors
Decrease: effect of tamoxifen
Decrease: buPROPion effect—carBAMazepine, cimetidine, PHENobarbital, phenytoin or other products (CYP2D6); CYP2B6 inducers
Drug/Herb
Increase: CNS depression—kava, valerian
Drug/Lab Test
Positive: urine drug screen for amphetamine possible

NURSING CONSIDERATIONS

Assess:

- Hepatic/renal function in patients with hepatic, kidney impairment
- For increased risk of seizures; if patient has excessively used CNS depressants and OTC stimulants, dosage of buPROPion should not be exceeded
- Monitor weight regularly
- For smoking cessation after 7-12 wk; if progress has not been made, product should be discontinued

Black Box Warning: Mental status: mood, sensorium, affect, suicidal tendencies, increase in psychiatric symptoms

- Assistance with ambulation during beginning therapy because sedation occurs
- Safety measures, primarily for geriatric patients

Evaluate:

- Therapeutic response: decreased depression, ability to perform daily activities, ability to sleep throughout the night, smoking cessation

Teach patient/family:

- That therapeutic effects may take 2-4 wk; not to increase dose without prescriber's approval; that treatment for smoking cessation lasts 7-12 wk
- To use caution when driving, performing other activities that require alertness; sedation, blurred vision may occur
- Report hearing, visual, CNS changes
- May need to use stool softener/laxative
- To avoid alcohol, other CNS depressants; alcohol may increase risk of seizures
- Not to use with nicotine patches unless directed by prescriber; may increase B/P
- To notify prescriber immediately if urinary retention occurs
- That risk of seizures increased when dose exceeded, if patient has seizure disorder

Black Box Warning: That suicidal ideas, behaviors, hostility, depression may occur in children or young adults

- To notify prescriber if pregnancy is suspected, planned

TREATMENT OF OVERDOSE:

ECG monitoring; lavage, activated charcoal; administer anticonvulsant

busPIRone (Rx)

(byoo-spye′rone)

BuSpar, BuSpar Dividose, Buspirex ✦, Bustab ✦

Func. class.: Antianxiety, sedative

Chem. class.: Azaspirodecanedione

Do not confuse:
busPIRone/buPROPion

ACTION: Acts by inhibiting the action of serotonin (5-HT); has shown little potential for abuse; a good choice with substance abuse

USES: Management and short-term relief of generalized anxiety disorders
Unlabeled uses: Autism

CONTRAINDICATIONS: Children <18 yr, hypersensitivity
Precautions: Pregnancy (B), breastfeeding, geriatric patients, impaired hepatic/renal function

DOSAGE AND ROUTES

- **Adult: PO** 7.5 mg bid; may increase by 5 mg/day q2-3 days, max 60 mg/day

Autism with anxiety (unlabeled)

- **Adult: PO** 5-15 mg tid after titration, max 60 mg/day
- **Child ≥5 yr: PO** 0.2-0.6 mg/kg/day, max 60 mg/day; titrate to higher dose

Hepatic/renal dose

- **Adult: PO** reduce by 25%-50% for mild-moderate hepatic disease; do not use for severe hepatic disease; CCr 11-70 ml/min reduce by 25%-50%, CCr <10 ml/min do not use

Available forms: Tabs 5, 7.5, 10, 15, 30 mg

Administer:

- With food, milk for GI symptoms; avoid grapefruit juice; give drug at same time of day, with/without food consistently
- Crushed if patient unable to swallow medication whole
- Sugarless gum, hard candy, frequent sips of water for dry mouth

SIDE EFFECTS

CNS: *Dizziness, headache, depression, stimulation, insomnia, nervousness, light-headedness, numbness, paresthesia, incoordination,* nightmares, *tremors,* excitement, involuntary movements, confusion, akathisia, hostility
CV: *Tachycardia, palpitations,* hypo/hypertension, CVA, CHF, MI, chest pain
EENT: *Sore throat, tinnitus, blurred vision, nasal congestion;* red, itching eyes; change in taste, smell
GI: *Nausea, dry mouth, diarrhea, constipation,* flatulence, increased appetite, rectal bleeding
GU: Frequency, hesitancy, menstrual irregularity, change in libido
INTEG: *Rash,* edema, pruritus, alopecia, dry skin
MISC: *Sweating,* fatigue, weight gain, fever, serotonin syndrome
MS: *Pain, weakness,* muscle cramps, spasms, myalgia
RESP: Hyperventilation, chest congestion, shortness of breath

PHARMACOKINETICS

Peak 40-90 min, terminal half-life 2-4 hr, rapidly absorbed, metabolized by liver (CYP3A4), excreted in feces, protein binding 86%

INTERACTIONS

Increase: busPIRone—product metabolized by CYP3A4 (erythromycin, itraconazole, nefazodone, ketoconazole, ritonavir, verapamil, diltiazem, several other protease inhibitors)
Increase: B/P—procarbazine, MAOIs; do not use together
Increase: CNS depression—psychotropic products, alcohol (avoid use)
Increase: serotonin syndrome—SSRIs, SNRIs, serotonin receptor agonists
Decrease: busPIRone effects—rifampin
Decrease: busPIRone action—products induced by CYP3A4 (rifampin, phenytoin, PHENobarbital, carBAMazepine, dexamethasone)

Drug/Food

Increase: peak concentration of busPIRone—grapefruit juice

NURSING CONSIDERATIONS

Assess:

- B/P lying, standing; pulse; if systolic B/P drops 20 mm Hg, hold product, notify prescriber
- CNS reactions because some may be unpredictable
- Mental status: mood, sensorium, affect, sleeping pattern, drowsiness, dizziness; withdrawal symptoms when dose reduced, product discontinued
- Safety measures if drowsiness, dizziness occurs

Evaluate:

- Therapeutic response: decreased anxiety, restlessness, sleeplessness

Teach patient/family:

- That product may be taken consistently with/without food
- To avoid OTC preparations, alcohol ingestion, other psychotropic medications unless approved by prescriber; to avoid large amounts of grapefruit juice
- To avoid activities that require alertness because drowsiness may occur
- Not to discontinue medication abruptly after long-term use; if dose missed, do not double
- To rise slowly because fainting may occur, especially among geriatric patients
- That drowsiness may worsen at beginning of treatment; that 2 wk of therapy may be required before therapeutic effects occur, max effect 3-6 wk
- Serotonin syndrome: to report immediately (fever, tremor, sweating, diarrhea, delirium)

HIGH ALERT

busulfan (Rx)

(byoo-sul′fan)

Busulfex, Myleran

Func. class.: Antineoplastic alkylating agent

Chem. class.: Bifunctional alkylating agent

Do not confuse:

Myleran/Leukeran

ACTION:

Changes essential cellular ions to covalent bonding with resultant alkylation; this interferes with the normal biological function of DNA; activity is not phase-specific; action is due to myelosuppression

USES:

Chronic myelocytic leukemia, bone marrow ablation, stem cell transplant preparation with CML

CONTRAINDICATIONS:

Pregnancy (D) 3rd trimester, breastfeeding, blastic phase of chronic myelocytic leukemia, hypersensitivity

Precautions: Women of childbearing age, leukopenia, anemia, hepatotoxicity, renal toxicity, seizures, tumor lysis syndrome, hyperkalemia, hyperphosphatemia, hypocalcemia, hyperuricemia, radiation, chemotherapy

Black Box Warning: Thrombocytopenia, neutropenia, secondary malignancy

DOSAGE AND ROUTES

Chronic myelocytic leukemia

- **Adult: PO** 4-8 mg/day or 1.8-4 mg/m^2/day initially, reduce dose if WBC reaches 30,000-40,000/mm^3, discontinue if WBC $\leq$20,000/mm^3, maintenance 1-3 mg/day
- **Child: PO** 0.06-0.12 mg/kg/day or 1.8-4.6 mg/m^2/day; reduce if WBC reaches 30,000-40,000/mm^3, discontinue if WBC $\leq$20,000/mm^3

Allogenic hemopoietic stem cell transplantation with chronic myelogenous leukemia

- **Adult: IV** 0.8 mg/kg over 2 hr, q6hr × 4 days (total 16 doses); give cyclophosphamide **IV** 60 mg/kg over 1 hr daily for 2 days starting after 16th dose of busulfan; **PO** (unlabeled) 1 mg/kg q6hr × 16 doses
- **Adolescent and child (unlabeled) >12 kg: IV** 0.8 mg/kg over 2 hr q6hr × 16 doses (4 days), then high-dose cyclophosphamide 50 mg/kg/day × 4 days
- **Infant/child ≤12 kg (unlabeled): IV** 1.1 mg/kg over 2 hr q6hr × 16 doses

(4 days), then high-dose cyclophosphamide 50 mg/kg/day × 4 days

Available forms: Tabs 2 mg; inj 6 mg/ml

Administer:

- Store in tight container

PO route

- Give at same time daily on empty stomach

Intermittent IV INFUSION route

- Prepare in biologic cabinet while wearing gloves, gown, mask; **dilute** with 10 times volume of product with D_5W, 0.9% NaCl (0.5 mg/ml); when withdrawing product, use needle with 5-micron filter provided, remove amount needed, remove filter, and **inject** product into diluent; always add product to diluent (not vice versa); stable for 8 hr at room temperature (using D_5W) or 12 hr refrigerated; **give** by central venous catheter over 2 hr q6hr × 4 days, use infusion pump, do not admix
- Give antiemetics before IV route on schedule
- In those with history of seizures, give phenytoin before IV drug to prevent seizures (using 0.9% NaCl)

Y-site compatibilities: Acyclovir, amphotericin B lipid complex, amphotericin B liposome, anidulafungin, atenolol, bivalirudin, bleomycin, caspofungin, codeine, DAPTOmycin, dexmedetomidine, diltiazem, DOCEtaxel, ertapenem, fenoldopam, gatifloxacin, granisetron, HYDROmorphone, levofloxacin, linezolid, LORazepam, meperidine, metroNIDAZOLE, milrinone, nesiritide, octreotide acetate, ondansetron, palonosetron, pancuronium, piperacillin-tazobactam, riTUXimab, sodium acetate, tacrolimus, tigecycline, tirofiban, trastuzumab, vasopressin

SIDE EFFECTS

CV: *Hypotension,* **thrombosis,** *chest pain,* **tachycardia, atrial fibrillation, heart block, pericardial effusion, cardiac tamponade** (high dose with cyclophosphamide)

GI: *Anorexia, constipation, diarrhea, dry mouth, nausea, vomiting*

RESP: **Alveolar hemorrhage,** atelectasis, cough, hemoptysis, hypoxia, pleural effusion, pneumonia, sinusitis, **pulmonary fibrosis**

CNS: *depression, dizziness, insomnia, headache*

EENT: blurred vision

GU: Impotence, sterility, amenorrhea, gynecomastia, **renal toxicity,** hyperuremia, adrenal-insufficiency–like syndrome

HEMA: **Thrombocytopenia, leukopenia, pancytopenia, severe bone marrow depression**

INTEG: Dermatitis, hyperpigmentation, alopecia

OTHER: **Chromosomal aberrations**

RESP: **Irreversible pulmonary fibrosis,** pneumonitis

PHARMACOKINETICS

Well absorbed orally, excreted in urine, crosses placenta, excreted in breast milk, half-life 2.5 hr

INTERACTIONS

Increase: cardiac tamponade—cyclophosphamide

Increase: toxicity—other antineoplastics, radiation

Increase: risk for bleeding—anticoagulants, salicylates

Increase: antibody response—live virus vaccines

Decrease: busulfan level—phenytoin

Decrease: busulfan clearance—acetaminophen, itraconazole

Drug/Lab Test

False positive: breast, bladder, cervix, lung cytology tests

NURSING CONSIDERATIONS

Assess:

Black Box Warning: CBC, differential, platelet count weekly; withhold product if WBC is <15,000/mm³ or platelet count is <150,000/mm³; notify prescriber of results; institute thrombocytopenia precautions; levels for withholding product will be different for children

Black Box Warning: Bone marrow status before chemotherapy; seizure history; bone marrow suppression may be prolonged (up to 2 mo)

- **Pulmonary fibrosis:** pulmonary function tests, chest x-ray films before, during therapy; chest film should be obtained q2wk during treatment; pulmonary fibrosis may occur up to 10 yr after treatment with busulfan
- Renal studies: BUN, serum uric acid, urine CCr before, during therapy; monitor ALT, alk phos, bilirubin, uric acid before and during treatment; I&O ratio; report fall in urine output of <30 ml/hr; hyperuricemia

Black Box Warning: For secondary malignancy within 5-8 yr of chronic oral therapy, long-term follow-up may be required

- Monitor for cold, fever, sore throat (may indicate beginning infection)
- Bleeding: hematuria, guaiac, bruising, petechiae; mucosa, orifices q8hr; no rectal temperatures
- Dyspnea, crackles, nonproductive cough, chest pain, tachypnea
- Inflammation of mucosa, breaks in skin; use viscous xylocaine for oral pain
- Comprehensive oral hygiene
- Strict medical asepsis, protective isolation if WBC levels low
- Increased fluid intake to 2-3 L/day to prevent urate deposits, calculi formation

Evaluate:
- Therapeutic response: decreased exacerbations of chronic myelocytic leukemia

Teach patient/family:
- To avoid use of products that contain aspirin, ibuprofen; razors; commercial mouthwash
- To use effective contraception during and for at least 3 mo after treatment; to avoid breastfeeding; may cause infertility, discuss family planning before initiating therapy, pregnancy (D)
- To report signs of **anemia** (fatigue, headache, irritability, faintness, shortness of breath); symptoms of **infection;** jaundice; persistent cough, congestion, skin pigmentation, darkening of skin; sudden weakness, weight loss (may resemble adrenal insufficiency)
- To report symptoms of bleeding (hematuria, tarry stools)
- To avoid vaccinations, crowds, persons with known infections
- That impotence, amenorrhea can occur; that these are reversible after discontinuing treatment

butoconazole vaginal antifungal

See Appendix B

HIGH ALERT

butorphanol (Rx)

(byoo-tor′fa-nole)

Stadol ✱

Func. class.: Opioid analgesic

Chem. class.: Mixed opioid antagonist, partial agonist

Controlled Substance Schedule IV

ACTION: Depresses pain impulse transmission at the spinal cord level by interacting with opioid receptors

USES: Moderate to severe pain, general anesthesia induction/maintenance, headache, migraine, preanesthesia

Unlabeled uses: Pruritus

CONTRAINDICATIONS: Hypersensitivity to product, preservative; addiction (opioid)

Precautions: Pregnancy (C), breastfeeding, children <18 yr, addictive personality, increased intracranial pressure, respiratory depression, renal/hepatic disease, ileus, COPD

B

DOSAGE AND ROUTES

Moderate-severe pain

- **Adult: IM** 1-4 mg q3-4hr prn; **IV** 0.5-2 mg q3-4hr prn; **INTRANASAL** 1 spray in 1 nostril, may give another dose 1-1½ hr later; repeat if needed 3-4hr after last dose
- **Geriatric: IV** ½ adult dose at 2× the interval; **INTRANASAL** if no relief after 90-120 min, may repeat with 1 spray

Renal/hepatic dose

- **Adult: INTRANASAL** max 1 mg followed by 1 mg after 90-120 min; **IM/IV** give 50% of dose (0.5 mg **IV**, 1 mg **IM**), do not repeat within 6 hr

Opioid-induced pruritus (unlabeled)

- **Adult: INTRANASAL** 1 mg (1 spray) in each nostril q4-6hr

Intractable pruritus with inflammatory skin or systemic disease (unlabeled)

- **Adult: INTRANASAL** 1-4 mg/day

Available forms: Inj 1, 2 mg/ml; nasal spray 10 mg/ml

Administer:

- With antiemetic if nausea, vomiting occur
- When pain beginning to return; determine dosage interval according to patient response
- Store in light-resistant container at room temperature

Nasal route

- Prime before first use, point sprayer away from the face, pump activator 7 × until a fine, wide spray occurs, if not used for 48 hr, reprime by pumping 1-2 ×
- If more than 1 spray is needed, use other nostril
- Do not share with others
- Nasal congestion/irritation may occur

IM route

- Deeply in large muscle mass

IV direct route

- Undiluted at a rate of <2 mg/>3-5 min, titrate to patient response; inject directly in vein or tubing of free-flowing compatible IV infusion

Y-site compatibilities: Acyclovir, alfentanil, allopurinol, amifostine, amikacin, aminocaproic acid, aminophylline, amphotericin B liposome (AmBisome), anidulafungin, ascorbic acid injection, atenolol, atracurium, atropine, aztreonam, benztropine, bivalirudin, bleomycin, bumetanide, buprenorphine, calcium chloride/gluconate, CARBOplatin, caspofungin, cefamandole, ceFAZolin, cefepime, cefotaxime, cefoTEtan, cefOXitin, cefTAZidime, ceftizoxime, cefTRIAXone, cefuroxime, cephalothin, chlorproMAZINE, cimetidine, cisatracurium, CISplatin, cladribine, clindamycin, cyanocobalamin, cyclophosphamide, cycloSPORINE, cytarabine, DACTINomycin, DAPTOmycin, dexamethasone phosphate, dexmedetomidine, digoxin, diltiazem, diphenhydrAMINE, DOBUTamine, DOCEtaxel, DOPamine, doxacurium, DOXOrubicin, DOXOrubicin liposomal, doxycycline, enalaprilat, ePHEDrine, EPINEPHrine, epirubicin, epoetin alfa, eptifibatide, ertapenem, erythromycin, esmolol, etoposide, famotidine, fenoldopam, fentaNYL, filgrastim, fluconazole, fludarabine, fluorouracil, gatifloxacin, gemcitabine, gentamicin, glycopyrrolate, granisetron, heparin, hydrocortisone, hydrOXYzine, IDArubicin, ifosfamide, imipenem-cilastatin, irinotecan, isoproterenol, ketorolac, labetalol, lactated Ringer's injection, levofloxacin, lidocaine, linezolid injection, LORazepam, magnesium, mannitol, mechlorethamine, melphalan, meperidine, metaraminol, methicillin, methotrexate, methoxamine, methyldopate, methylPREDNISolone, metoclopramide, metoprolol, metroNIDAZOLE, mezlocillin, milrinone, minocycline, mitoXANtrone, morphine, multiple vitamins injection, mycophenolate mofetil, nafcillin, nalbuphine, naloxone, nesiritide, netilmicin, niCARdipine, nitroglycerin, nitroprusside, norepinephrine, octreotide, ondansetron, oxacillin, oxaliplatin, oxytocin, palonosetron, pamidronate, pancuronium, papaverine, PEMEtrexed, penicillin G potassium/sodium, pentazocine, PHENobarbital, phenylephrine, phytonadione, piperacillin, piperacillin-tazobactam, polymyxin B, potassium chloride, procainamide, prochlorperazine, promethazine, propofol, propranolol, protamine, pyridoxine, quiNIDine, ranitidine, remifentanil, Ringer's injection, riTUXimab, rocuronium, sargramostim, sodium acetate, succinylcholine, SUFentanil, tacrolimus, teniposide, theophylline, thiamine, thiotepa, ticarcillin, ticarcillin-clavulanate, tigecycline, tirofiban, TNA, tobramycin, tolazoline, TPN, trastuzumab, urokinase, vancomycin, vasopressin, vecuronium, verapamil, vinCRIStine, vinorelbine, voriconazole

SIDE EFFECTS

CNS: *Drowsiness, dizziness, confusion, headache, sedation, euphoria, weakness, hallucinations,* insomnia (nasal)

CV: Palpitations, **bradycardia**, hypotension

EENT: Tinnitus, blurred vision, miosis, diplopia, nasal congestion, unpleasant taste

GI: *Nausea, vomiting, anorexia, constipation, cramps*

GU: Urinary retention

INTEG: Rash, urticaria, bruising, flushing, diaphoresis, pruritus

RESP: **Respiratory depression**

PHARMACOKINETICS

Metabolized by liver, excreted by kidneys, crosses placenta, excreted in breast milk, half-life 2-9 hr, protein binding 80%

IM: Onset 5-15 min, peak 30-60 min, duration 3-4 hr

INTRANASAL: Onset within 15 min, peak 1-2 hr, duration 4-5 hr

IV: Onset 1 min, peak 4-5 min, duration 2-4 hr

INTERACTIONS

Increase: CNS effects—alcohol, opioids, sedative/hypnotics, antipsychotics, skeletal muscle relaxants, other CNS depressants, MAOIs

NURSING CONSIDERATIONS

Assess:

- For decreasing output; may indicate urinary retention
- ⚠ **For withdrawal symptoms in opioid-dependent patients; PE, vascular occlusion, abscesses, ulcerations**
- CNS changes: dizziness, drowsiness, hallucinations, euphoria, LOC, pupil reaction
- Allergic reactions: rash, urticaria
- Respiratory dysfunction: respiratory depression, character, rate, rhythm; notify prescriber if respirations are <10/min
- Need for pain medication, physical dependence
- Safety measures: night-light, call bell within easy reach, assistance with ambulation, especially for geriatric patients

Evaluate:

- Therapeutic response: decrease in pain

Teach patient/family:

- To report any symptoms of CNS changes, allergic reactions
- That physical dependency may result when used for extended periods
- That withdrawal symptoms may occur: nausea, vomiting, cramps, fever, faintness, anorexia
- How to use nasal product
- To avoid hazardous activities

TREATMENT OF OVERDOSE:

Naloxone 0.4-2 mg IV, O_2, IV fluids, vasopressors

calcitonin (salmon) (Rx)

Fortical, Miacalcin

Func. class.: Parathyroid agents (calcium regulator)

Chem. class.: Polypeptide hormone

Do not confuse:
Calcitonin/calcitriol/calcifediol/calcium

ACTION: Decreases bone resorption, blood calcium levels; increases deposits of calcium in bones; opposes parathyroid hormone

USES: Paget's disease, postmenopausal osteoporosis, hypercalcemia
Unlabeled uses: Bone/neuropathic pain, diabetic neuropathy, osteolytic metastases, osteoporosis prophylaxis, phantom limb pain

CONTRAINDICATIONS: Hypersensitivity to this product, fish
Precautions: Pregnancy (C), breastfeeding, children, hypotension

DOSAGE AND ROUTES

Postmenopausal osteoporosis

• **Adult: SUBCUT/IM** 100 international units every other day; **INTRANASAL** 200 international units (1 spray) daily, alternating nostrils daily, activate pump before 1st dose

Paget's disease

• **Adult: SUBCUT/IM** 100 international units/day, maintenance 50 international units daily, every other day, or 3 × per wk

Hypercalcemia

• **Adult: SUBCUT/IM** 4 international units/kg q12hr, increase to 8 international units/kg q12hr if response is unsatisfactory, no more than 4-7 days

Neuropathic pain/phantom limb pain/diabetic neuropathy (unlabeled)

• **Adult: IV/SUBCUT** 100-200 international units/day for phantom limb pain; **IV** 200 international units over 20 min and 2nd infusion given

Bone pain due to osteoporosis, osteolytic metastases (unlabeled)

• **Adult: SUBCUT** 50-100 international units/day or **INTRANASAL** 200 international units in 1 nostril/day

Available forms: Inj 200 units/ml; nasal spray 200 units/actuation

Administer:

• Store at <77° F (25° C); protect from light

SUBCUT route

• Rotate inj sites; use within 6 hr of reconstitution; **give** at bedtime to minimize nausea, vomiting

IM route

• After test dose of 10 international units/ml, 0.1 ml intradermally; watch for 15 min; **give** only with EPINEPHrine, emergency meds available

• IM inj slowly into deep muscle mass; rotate sites; preferred route if volume is >2 ml

SIDE EFFECTS

CNS: Headache, tetany, chills, weakness, dizziness, fever, tremors
CV: Chest pressure, hypertension
EENT: Nasal congestion, eye pain
GI: Nausea, diarrhea, vomiting, anorexia, abdominal pain, salty taste, epigastric pain
GU: Diuresis, nocturia, urine sediment, frequency, cystitis
INTEG: Rash, flushing, pruritus of earlobes, edema of feet, reaction at inj site
MS: Swelling, tingling of hands, backache, myalgia
RESP: Dyspnea, flulike symptoms, **bronchospasm**
SYST: **Anaphylaxis**, infection

PHARMACOKINETICS

IM/SUBCUT: Onset 15 min, peak 4 hr, duration 8-24 hr, metabolized by kidneys, excreted as inactive metabolites via kidneys

INTERACTIONS

Decrease: lithium effect
Decrease: effect of nasal spray—bisphosphonates (Paget's disease)

NURSING CONSIDERATIONS

Assess:

⚠ **Anaphylaxis, hypersensitivity reaction** (rash, fever, inability to breathe); emergency equipment should be nearby

- GI symptoms, polyuria, flushing, head swelling, tingling, headache; may indicate hypercalcemia
- Nutritional status; diet for sources of vit D (milk, some seafood), calcium (dairy products, dark green vegetables), phosphates
- Vit D 50-135 international units/dl), alk phos baseline, q3-6mo; monitor urine hydroproline with Paget's disease, biochemical markers of bone formation/absorption, radiologic evidence of fracture; bone density (osteoporosis)
- **Toxicity (can occur rapidly),** increased drug level; have parenteral calcium on hand if calcium level drops too low; check for tetany (irritability, paresthesia, nervousness, muscle twitching, seizures, tetanic spasms)

Evaluate:

- Therapeutic response: calcium levels 9-10 mg/dl, decreasing symptoms of Paget's disease

Teach patient/family:

- About the method of inj if patient will be responsible for self-medication
- To report difficulty swallowing, any changes in side effects to prescriber immediately

Nasal

- To use alternating nostrils for nasal spray; use after allowing to warm to room temperature; prime to get full spray

calcitriol vitamin D_3 (Rx)

(kal-sih-try′ole)

Calcijex, Rocaltrol, Vectical

Func. class.: Parathyroid agent (calcium regulator)

Chem. class.: Vit D hormone

Do not confuse:

calcitriol/Calciferol/calcitonin/calcium

ACTION: Increases intestinal absorption of calcium; provides calcium for bones; increases renal tubular reabsorption of phosphate

USES: Hypocalcemia with chronic renal disease, hyperparathyroidism pseudohypoparathyroidism, psoriasis, renal osteodystrophy

Unlabeled uses: Osteopetrosis, osteoporosis, osteoporosis prophylaxis, rickets, familial hypophosphatemia

CONTRAINDICATIONS: Hypersensitivity, hyperphosphatemia, hypercalcemia, vit D toxicity

Precautions: Pregnancy (C), breastfeeding, renal calculi, CV disease

DOSAGE AND ROUTES

Hypocalcemia (stage 5 chronic kidney disease, on dialysis)

- **Adult and child ≥6 yr: PO** 0.25 mcg/day
- **Adults: IV** 1 mcg (0.02 mcg/kg) to 2 mcg 3×/wk, initial doses of 0.5-4 mcg 3×/wk have been used, may increase by 0.5-1 mcg at 2-4 wk intervals if needed
- **Child 1-5 yr: PO** 0.25-2 mcg/day

Renal osteodystrophy

- **Adult and child ≥3 yr: PO** 0.25 mcg/day, may increase to 0.5 mcg/day
- **Child <3 yr: PO** 0.01-0.015 mcg/kg/day

Hypoparathyroidism

- **Adult and child ≥6 yr: PO** 0.25 mcg/day, may increase q2-4wk, maintenance 0.5-2 mcg/day
- **Child 1-5 yr: PO** 0.25-0.75 mcg daily
- **Child <1 yr: PO** 0.04-0.08 mcg/kg/day

Rickets (unlabeled)

- **Adult and child: PO** 1 mcg/day

Familial hypophosphatemia (unlabeled)

- **Adult: PO** 2 mcg/day
- **Child: PO** 0.015-0.02 mcg/kg/day, maintenance 0.03-0.06 mcg/kg/day; max 2 mcg/day

Postmenopausal osteoporosis (unlabeled)
• **Adult: PO** 0.25 mcg bid, adjust to serum calcium levels
Osteopetrosis (unlabeled)
• **Child: PO** high-dose calcitriol 1-2 mcg/kg/day given in 4-6 divided doses
Osteoporosis prophylaxis in corticosteroid therapy (unlabeled)
• **Adult: PO** 0.5-1 mcg/day
Available forms: Caps 0.25, 0.5 mcg; inj 1 mcg/ml; oral sol 1 mcg/ml; top 3 mcg/g
Administer:
PO route
• Do not break, crush, chew caps
• Give without regard to meals
• Store protected from light, heat, moisture
IV route
• Give by direct IV over 1 min through catheter at hemodialysis conclusion

SIDE EFFECTS

CNS: Drowsiness, headache, vertigo, fever, lethargy, hallucinations
CV: Palpitations, hypertension
EENT: Blurred vision, photophobia
ENDO: Hypercalcemia
GI: Nausea, diarrhea, vomiting, jaundice, anorexia, dry mouth, constipation, cramps, metallic taste
GU: Polyuria, hypercalciuria, hyperphosphatemia, hematuria, thirst
MS: Myalgia, arthralgia, decreased bone development, weakness
SYST: Anaphylaxis
INTEG: Pain at injection site, rash, pruritus

PHARMACOKINETICS

IV: Duration up to 2 hr
PO: Absorbed readily from GI tract, peak 10-12 hr, duration 3-5 days, half-life 3-6 hr, undergoes hepatic recycling, excreted in bile

INTERACTIONS

• **Hypercalcemia:** thiazide diuretics, calcium supplements
• Cardiac dysrhythmias: cardiac glycosides, verapamil
• **Hypermagnesemia:** magnesium antacids/supplements
• **Toxicity:** other vit D products
Increase: metabolism of vit D—phenytoin
Decrease: absorption of calcitriol—cholestyramine, mineral oil, fat-soluble vitamins
Drug/Food
• Large amounts of high-calcium foods may cause hypercalcemia
Drug/Lab Test
Increase: AST/ALT
False increase: Cholesterol
Interference: Alk phos, electrolytes

NURSING CONSIDERATIONS

Assess:
• BUN, urinary calcium, PTH, creatinine, chloride, magnesium, electrolytes, phosphate; may increase calcium; should be kept at 9-10 mg/dl, vit D 50-135 international units/dl, phosphate 70 mg/dl; toxic reactions may occur rapidly
• **Hypercalcemia:** dry mouth, metallic taste, polyuria, bone pain, muscle weakness, headache, fatigue, change in level of consciousness, dysrhythmias, increased respirations, anorexia, nausea, vomiting, cramps, diarrhea, constipation; paresthesia, twitching, dysrhythmias, Chvostek's sign, Trousseau's sign **(hypocalcemia)**
• Renal status: decreased urinary output (oliguria, anuria), edema in extremities, weight gain 5-7 lb, periorbital edema
• Nutritional status, diet for sources of vit D (milk, some seafood); calcium (dairy products, dark green vegetables), phosphates (dairy products) must be avoided
• Restrict sodium, potassium if required; restriction of fluids if required for chronic renal failure
Evaluate:
• Therapeutic response: calcium 9-10 mg/dl; decreasing symptoms of hypocalcemia, hypoparathyroidism

Teach patient/family:
- **About symptoms of hypercalcemia:** renal stones, nausea, vomiting, anorexia, lethargy, thirst, bone, or flank pain, confusion
- To avoid products with sodium: cured meats, dairy products, cold cuts, olives, beets, pickles, soups, meat tenderizers with chronic renal failure; products with potassium: oranges, bananas, dried fruit, peas, dark green leafy vegetables, milk, melons, beans
- To avoid OTC products that contain calcium, potassium, sodium with chronic renal failure
- To monitor weight weekly; to maintain fluid intake

calcium carbonate (PO-OTC)

Alka-Mints, Amitone, Apo-Cal ✦, BioCal, Calcarb, Calci-Chew, Calci-Mix, Calciday, Calcite ✦, Calsan ✦, Caltrate ✦, Chooz, Maalox Antacid, Os-Cal, Rolaids Extra Strength Softchew, Tums, Tums E-X

calcium acetate (OTC)

(kal′see-um ass′e-tate)

Eliphos, PhosLo, Phoslyra

Func. class.: Antacid, calcium supplement

Chem. class.: Calcium product

Do not confuse:
Os-Cal/Asacol
Calcium/Calcitriol/Calcitonin

ACTION: Neutralizes gastric acidity

USES: Antacid, calcium supplement; not suitable for chronic therapy, hyperphosphatemia, hypertension during pregnancy, osteoporosis, prevention, treatment of hypocalcemia, hypoparathyroidism

Unlabeled uses: Duodenal ulcer, PMS, stress gastritis

CONTRAINDICATIONS: Hypersensitivity, hypercalcemia

Precautions: Pregnancy (C), breastfeeding, geriatric patients, fluid restriction, decreased GI motility, GI obstruction, dehydration, renal disease, hyperparathyroidism, bone tumors

DOSAGE AND ROUTES

Nutritional supplement including osteoporosis prophylaxis
- **Adult ≥51 yr: PO** 1000-1500 mg/day elemental calcium (2500-3750 mg/day calcium carbonate)
- **Adult 19-50 yr: PO** 1000 mg/day elemental calcium (2500 mg/day calcium carbonate)

Chronic hypocalcemia
- **Adult: PO** 2-4 g/day elemental calcium (5-10 g/day calcium carbonate) in 3-4 divided doses
- **Child: PO** 45-65 mg/kg/day elemental calcium (112.5-162.5 mg/kg/day calcium carbonate) in 4 divided doses
- **Neonate: PO** 50-150 mg/kg/day elemental calcium (125-375 mg/kg/day in 4-6 divided doses, max 1 g/day)

Supplementation
- **Adolescent and child 9-18 yr: PO** 1300 mg elemental calcium (3250 mg calcium carbonate)
- **Child 4-8 yr: PO** 800 mg/day elemental calcium (2000 mg/day calcium carbonate)
- **Child 1-3 yr: PO** 500 mg/day elemental calcium (1250 mg/day calcium carbonate)
- **Infant 6-12 mo: PO** 270 mg/day elemental calcium based on total intake
- **Neonates and infants <6 mo: PO** 210 mg/day elemental calcium based on total intake

Hyperphosphatemia
- **Adult: PO** Individualized on response

Heartburn, dyspepsia, hyperacidity (OTC)
- **Adult: PO** 1-2 tabs q2hr, max 9 tabs/24 hr (Alka-mints); chew 2-4 tab q1hr prn, max 16 tabs (Tums regular strength);

chew 2-4 tab q1hr prn, max 10 tabs (Tums E-X); chew 2-3 tabs q1hr prn, max 10 tabs/24 hr (Tums Ultra); chew 2 tabs q2-3hr, max 19 tabs/24 hr (Titralac Extra Strength)

Duodenal ulcer/stress gastritis (unlabeled)

• **Adult: PO** 80-140 mEq q3-6hr

PMS (unlabeled)

• **Adult: PO** (Tums E-X, Tums Calcium for Life PMS) Chew 2 tabs bid

Available forms: Calcium carbonate: chewable tabs 350, 420, 450, 500, 750, 1000, 1250 mg; tabs 500, 600, 650, 667, 1000, 1250, 1500 mg; **gum** 300, 450, 500 mg; **susp** 1250 mg/5 ml; **caps** 1250 mg; **powder** 6.5 g/packet; **calcium acetate: tabs** 667 mg (169 mg elemental Ca), **gelcaps:** 667 mg (169 mg elemental calcium); caps 500 mg (125 mg elemental Ca)

Administer:

PO route

• 1 g calcium carbonate = 400 mg elemental calcium = 10 mmol calcium = 20 mEq calcium

• Do not give enteric-coated within 1 hr of calcium carbonate

• For ulcer treatment (adjunct): give 1 and 3 hr after meals and at bedtime

• For a phosphate binder: give 1 hr after each meal or snack and at bedtime

• For supplement: give 1-1½ hr after meals; avoid oxalic acid foods (spinach, rhubarb), phytic acid (brans, cereals) or phosphorus (milk, dairy), may decrease calcium absorption

• Suspension: shake well; use calibrated measuring device

• Laxatives or stool softeners if constipation occurs

SIDE EFFECTS

GI: *Constipation,* anorexia, nausea, vomiting, flatulence, diarrhea, rebound hyperacidity, eructation

GU: Calculi, hypercalciuria

PHARMACOKINETICS

⅓ of dose absorbed by small intestine, excreted in feces and urine, crosses placenta, must have adequate vit D for absorption

INTERACTIONS

Increase: digoxin toxicity—hypercalcemia

Increase: plasma levels of quiNIDine, amphetamines

Increase: hypercalcemia—thiazide diuretics, calcium supplements

Decrease: levels of salicylates, calcium channel blockers, ketoconazole, iron salts, tetracyclines, fluoroquinolones, phenytoin, etidronate, risedronate, atenolol PO

Drug/Lab Test

Decrease: phosphates

False increase: chloride

False positive: benzodiazepines

False decrease: magnesium, oxylate, lipase

NURSING CONSIDERATIONS

Assess:

• Calcium (serum, urine), calcium should be 8.5-10.5 mg/dl, urine calcium should be 150 mg/day, monitor weekly; serum phosphate

⚠ **Milk-alkali syndrome:** nausea, vomiting, disorientation, headache

• Constipation; increase bulk in the diet if needed

• **Hypercalcemia:** headache, nausea, vomiting, confusion; hypocalcemia: paresthesia, twitching colic, dysrhythmias, Chvostek's sign, Trousseau's sign

• Those taking digoxin for toxicity

• Antacid—for abdominal pain, heartburn, indigestion before, after administration

Evaluate:

• Therapeutic response: absence of pain, decreased acidity; decreased hyperphosphatemia with renal failure

Teach patient/family:

• To increase fluids to 2 L unless contraindicated; to add bulk to diet for constipation; to notify prescriber of constipation

• Not to switch antacids unless directed by prescriber; not to use as antacid for >2 wk without approval by prescriber

• That therapeutic dose recommendations are figured as elemental calcium
• To avoid excessive use of alcohol, caffeine, tobacco
• To avoid spinach, cereals, dairy products in large amounts

CALCIUM SALTS

calcium chloride (Rx)
calcium gluceptate (Rx)
calcium gluconate (Rx)
calcium lactate (Rx)

Func. class.: Electrolyte replacement—calcium product

ACTION: Calcium needed for maintenance of nervous, muscular, skeletal function; enzyme reactions; normal cardiac contractility; coagulation of blood; affects secretory activity of endocrine, exocrine glands

USES: Prevention and treatment of hypocalcemia, hypermagnesemia, hypoparathyroidism, neonatal tetany, cardiac toxicity caused by hyperkalemia, lead colic, hyperphosphatemia, vit D deficiency, osteoporosis prophylaxis, calcium antagonist toxicity (calcium channel blocker toxicity)
Unlabeled uses: Electrolyte abnormalities in cardiac arrest, CPR

CONTRAINDICATIONS: Hypercalcemia, digoxin toxicity, ventricular fibrillation, renal calculi
Precautions: Pregnancy (C), breastfeeding, children, respiratory/renal disease, cor pulmonale, digitalized patient, respiratory failure, diarrhea, dehydration

DOSAGE AND ROUTES

Acute hypocalcemia

Calcium Chloride 10%

• **Adult: IV** 0.5-1 g; **for tetany**, give over 5-10 min. Repeat q4-6hr, as needed by calcium concentrations *or* **IV INFUSION** 15 mg/kg elemental calcium (37.5 mg/kg calcium chloride) over 4-6hr
• **Child/Infant: IV** Range from 2.7-5 mg/kg/dose (0.027-0.05 ml/kg/dose of 10%. **For tetany** Slow IV 10 mg/kg/dose over 5-10 minutes, may repeat initial dosage in 4-6 hr. The initial dose can be followed by a **CONT INFUSION** max 200 mg/kg/day

Calcium Gluconate

• **Adult: IV** 2-3 g slowly, max 5 ml/min (47.5 mg/min calcium ion); **For tetany** Give over 5-10 min, repeat q6hr, as needed, as determined by serum calcium concentrations, max 15 g/day or **IV INFUSION** 15 mg/kg elemental calcium (167 mg/kg) over 4-6 hr may be administered if symptoms recur after initial IV calcium replacement
• **Child/Infant: IV** 200-500 mg/kg/day **CONT INFUSION** or given in 4 divided doses, at max rate 5 ml/min (47.5 mg/min calcium ion); **For tetany** IV 100-200 mg/kg over 5-10 min, may repeat after 6 hr or followed by 500 mg/kg/day IV as a **CONT INFUSION** or in 3-4 divided doses
• **Neonate: IV** 200-800 mg/kg/day as a **CONT INFUSION** or given in 3-4 divided doses; **For tetany** 100-200 mg/kg IV is recommended, followed by 500 mg/kg/day **CONT INFUSION** or given in 3-4 divided doses

Calcium Lactate

• **Adult: IM** 10 ml 1-2×/wk for 4-5 wk, may repeat if needed
• **PO (calcium citrate):**
• **Adult: PO** 9.5-19 g/day PO in divided doses 2-4 times a day after meals
• **PO (calcium gluconate):**
• **Adults: PO** 22.5-45 g/day in 3-4 divided doses
• **Child/Infant: PO** 500-725 mg/kg/day in 4 divided doses
• **Neonate: PO** 500-1500 mg/kg/day in 4-6 divided doses
• **PO (calcium lactate):**
• **Adults: PO** 15.4-30.8 g/day divided q8hr
• **Child: PO** 345-500 mg/kg/day in divided doses q6-8hr, max 9 g/day

- **Infant: PO** 400-500 mg/kg/day in divided doses q4-6hr
- **CPR/cardiac arrest associated with hyperkalemia, hypermagnesemia, or ionized hypocalcemia (unlabeled)**
- **IV (calcium chloride 10%):**
- **Adult: IV** 5-10 ml of a 10% solution (500-1000 mg) or 8-16 mg/kg given by slow IV inj; may repeat
- **IV (calcium gluconate):**
- **Adult: IV** 500-800 mg of 10% solution (5-8 ml), max 3 g
- **Infant/Child:** IV 60-100 mg/kg or intraosseous (0.6-1 ml/kg), max 3 g
- **For nutritional supplementation:**
- **PO (any oral calcium salt; dosage expressed as elemental calcium):**
- **Adults ≥51 yr: PO** 1200 mg/day (range 1000-1500 mg/day)
- **Adults 19-50 yr: PO** 1000 mg/day
- **Children and Adolescents 9-18 yr: PO** 1300 mg/day
- **Children 4-8 yr: PO** 800 mg/day
- **Children 1-3 yr: PO** 500 mg/day
- **Infants 6-12 mo: PO** 270 mg/day based on total intake (consumption from breast milk/infant formula and solid food)
- **Neonate/Infant <6 mo: PO** 210 mg/day based on total intake (content in human milk/infant formula). Source of calcium intake should come from food/breast milk only to prevent high levels of intake

Administer:

PO route (only acetate, carbonate, citrate, glubionate, lactate, phosphate)

- Give in 3-4 divided doses with or 1 hr after meals, follow with full glass of water; if using as phosphate binder in renal dialysis, do not follow with water, do not give oral medications within 1 hr of oral calcium; **chew tab:** chew thoroughly; **effervescent tab:** dissolve in full glass of water; **oral powder:** mix and give with food; **oral solution:** give before meals; **oral suspension:** shake well
- Store at room temperature

IM route

- **Glycerophosphate,** lactate may be given IM
- **Do not give chloride, gluconate IM;** use only if IV is not feasible. Inject into gluteal region (adult), lateral thigh (child)
- Aspirate before inj
- Do not give chloride subcut

IV route

- Undiluted or diluted with equal amounts of NS to a 5% sol for inj, give 0.5-1 ml/min
- Through small-bore needle into large vein; if extravasation occurs, necrosis will result (IV)
- Remain recumbent ½ hr after IV dose

Calcium chloride

Y-site compatibilities: Acyclovir, alemtuzumab, alfentanil, amikacin, aminocaproic acid, aminophylline, amiodarone, anidulafungin, argatroban, arsenic trioxide, ascorbic acid injection, asparaginase, atenolol, atracurium atropine, azithromycin, aztreonam, benztropine, bivalirudin, bleomycin, bumetanide, buprenorphine, butorphanol, calcium gluconate, CARBOplatin, carmustine, caspofungin acetate, cefotaxime, cefoTEtan, cefOXitin, ceftaroline, ceftizoxime, chloramphenicol, chlorothiazide, chlorpheniramine, chlorproMAZINE, cimetidine, CISplatin, clindamycin, cloxacillin, colistimethate, cyanocobalamin, cyclophosphamide, cycloSPORINE, cytarabine, DACTINomycin, DAPTOmycin, DAUNOrubicin, dexmedetomidine, dexrazoxane, digoxin, diltiazem, diphenhydrAMINE, DOBUTamine, DOCEtaxel, dolasetron, DOPamine, doxacurium, doxapram, DOXOrubicin, doxycycline, edetate calcium disodium, enalaprilat, ePHEDrine, EPINEPHrine, epirubicin, epoetin alfa, eptifibatide, ergonovine, ertapenem, erythromycin, esmolol, etoposide, etoposide phosphate, famotidine, fenoldopam, fentaNYL, fluconazole, fludarabine, furosemide, gallamine, gallium, ganciclovir, gatifloxacin, gemcitabine, gentamicin, glycopyrrolate, granisetron, heparin sodium, HYDROmorphone, hydrOXYzine, IDArubicin, ifosfamide, inamrinone, insulin, regular, irinotecan, isoproterenol, isoproterenol, kanamycin, labetalol, lactated ringer's, lepirudin, leucovorin, lidocaine, lincomycin, linezolid, LORazepam, mannitol, meperidine, mephentermine, mesna, methohexital, methotrexate, methyldopate, metoclopramide, metoprolol, metronidazole, micafungin, midazolam, milrinone, minocycline, mitoMYcin mitoXANtrone, mivacurium, morphine, moxifloxacin, multiple vitamins injection, mycophenolate mofetil, nafcillin, nalbuphine, nalorphine, naloxone, nesiritide, niCARdipine, nitroglycerin, nitroprusside, norepinephrine, octreotide, ondansetron, oxytocin, PAClitaxel (solvent/surfactant) pancuronium, papaverine, penicillin G potassium/sodium, pentazocine, PENTobarbital, PHENobarbital, phentolamine, phenylephrine, phytonadione, piperacillin, piperacillin-tazobactam, polymyxin B, potassium potassium chloride, procainamide, prochlorperazine, promazine, promethazine, propranolol, protamine, pyridoxine, quinupristin-dalfopristin, ranitidine, ringer's injection, rocuronium, streptomycin, succinylcholine, SUFentanil, tacrolimus, teniposide, theophylline, thiamine, thiotepa, ticarcillin -clavulanate, tigecycline, tirofiban, tna (3-in-1), tobramycin, tolazoline, topotecan, trimetaphan, tubocurarine, urokinase, vancomycin, vasopressin vecuronium, verapamil, vinBLAStine, vinCRIStine, vinorelbine, voriconazole

Calcium gluconate

Acyclovir, aldesleukin, alemtuzumab, alfentanil, allopurinol, amifostine, amikacin, aminocaproic acid, aminophylline, amiodarone, anidulafungin, argatroban, arsenic trioxide, ascorbic acid injection, asparaginase, atenolol, atracurium, atropine, azaTHIOprine, azithromycin, aztreonam, benztropine, bivalirudin, bleomycin, bumetanide, buprenorphine, butorphanol, calcium chloride, carboplatin, carmustine, caspofungin, ceFAZolin, cefepime, cefoperazone, cefotaxime, cefoTEtan, cefOXitin, ceftaroline, cefTAZidime, ceftizoxime, cefuroxime, chloramphenicol sodium succinate, chlorothiazide, chlorpheniramine, chlorproMAZINE, cimetidine, ciprofloxacin, cisatracurium, CISplatin, cladribine, clindamycin, cloxacillin, codeine, colistimethate, cyanocobalamin, cyclophosphamide, cycloSPORINE, cytarabine, DACTINomycin, DAPTOmycin, DAUNOrubicin liposome, daunorubicin, dexmedetomidine, dexrazoxane, digoxin, diltiazem, dimenhyDRINATE, diphenhydrAMINE, DOBUTamine, DOCEtaxel, dolasetron, DOPamine, doripenem, doxacurium, doxapram, doxorubicin, DOXOrubicin liposomal, doxycycline, edetate calcium disodium, enalaprilat, ePHEDrine, EPINEPHrine, epirubicin, epoetin alfa, eptifibatide, ergonovine, ertapenem, erythromycin, esmolol, etoposide, etoposide phosphate, famotidine, fenoldopam, fentaNYL, filgrastim, fludarabine, fluorouracil, folic acid (as sodium salt), furosemide, gallamine, gallium, ganciclovir, gatifloxacin, gemcitabine, gentamicin, glycopyrrolate, granisetron, heparin sodium, HYDROmorphone, hydrOXYzine, IDArubicin, ifosfamide, insulin (regular), irinotecan, isoproterenol, kanamycin, ketamine, labetalol, lactated ringer's injection, lepirudin, leucovorin, levofloxacin, lidocaine, lincomycin, linezolid, LORazepam, magnesium sulfate, mannitol, melphalan, meperidine, mephentermine, mesna, methohexital, methotrexate, methyldopate, metoclopramide, metoprolol, metroNIDAZOLE, micafungin, midazolam, milrinone, mitoMYcin, mitoXANtrone, mivacurium, morphine, moxifloxacin, multiple vitamins injection, nafcillin, nalbuphine, nalorphine, naloxone, nesiritide, netilmicin, niCARdipine, nitroglycerin, nitroprusside, norepinephrine, octreotide, ondansetron, oritavancin, oxaliplatin, oxytocin, PACLitaxel (solvent/surfactant), palonosetron, pancuronium, papaverine, penicillin G potassium/sodium, pentamidine, pentazocine, PENTobarbital, PHENobarbital, phentolamine, phenylephrine, phytonadione, piperacillin, piperacillin, polymyxin B, potassium acetate/, chloride, procainamide, prochlorperazine, promazine, promethazine, propofol, propranolol, protamine, pyridoxine, quiNIDine, ranitidine, remifentanil, ringer's, riTUXimab, rocuronium, sargramostim, sodium acetate, streptomycin, succinylcholine, SUFentanil, tacrolimus, telavancin, teniposide, theophylline, thiamine, thiotepa, ticarcillin, ticarcillin -clavulanate, tigecycline, tirofiban, tna (3-in-1), tobramycin, tolazoline, tpn (2-in-1), trastuzumab, trimetaphan, tubocurarine, urokinase, vancomycin, vasopressin, vecuronium, verapamil, vinBLAStine, vinCRIStine, vinorelbine, vitamin B complex with C, voriconazole

SIDE EFFECTS

CV: **Shortened QT, heart block,** hypotension, bradycardia, **dysrhythmias; cardiac arrest (IV)**

GI: *Vomiting, nausea, constipation*

HYPERCALCEMIA: Drowsiness, lethargy, muscle weakness, headache, constipation, **coma,** anorexia, nausea, vomiting, polyuria, thirst

INTEG: Pain, burning at IV site, **severe venous thrombosis, necrosis, extravasation**

PHARMACOKINETICS

Crosses placenta, enters breast milk, excreted via urine and feces, half-life unknown, protein binding 40%-50%

PO: Onset, peak, duration unknown, absorption from GI tract

IV: Onset immediate, duration ½-2 hr

INTERACTIONS

Increase: milk-alkali syndrome—antacids

Increase: dysrhythmias—digoxin glycosides

Increase: toxicity—verapamil, diltiazem

Increase: hypercalcemia—thiazide diuretics

Decrease: absorption of fluoroquinolones, tetracyclines, iron salts, phenytoin, thyroid hormones when calcium is taken PO

Decrease: effects of atenolol, verapamil

Drug/Herb

Increase: action/side effects—lily of the valley, pheasant's eye, shark cartilage, squill

Drug/Lab Test

Increase: calcium

NURSING CONSIDERATIONS

Assess:

- **ECG for decreased QT and T wave inversion:** **hypercalcemia, product should be reduced or discontinued, consider cardiac monitoring**
- Calcium levels during treatment (8.5-11.5 g/dl is normal level); urine calcium if hypercaluria occurs
- Cardiac status: rate, rhythm, CVP (PWP, PAWP if being monitored directly)
- **Hypocalcemia:** muscle twitching, paresthesia, dysrhythmias, laryngospasm
- Digitalized patients frequently; an increase in calcium increases digoxin toxicity risk
- **Seizure precautions: padded side rails, decreased stimuli (noise, light); place airway suction equipment, padded mouth gag if calcium levels are low**
- Store at room temperature

Evaluate:

- Therapeutic response: decreased twitching, paresthesias, muscle spasms; absence of tremors, seizures, dysrhythmias, dyspnea, laryngospasm; negative Chvostek's sign, negative Trousseau's sign

Teach patient/family:

- To add foods high in vit D
- To add calcium-rich foods to diet: dairy products, shellfish, dark green leafy vegetables; to decrease oxalate- and zinc-rich foods: nuts, legumes, chocolate, spinach, soy
- To prevent injuries; to avoid immobilization

HIGH ALERT

canagliflozin

(kan′a-gli-floe′zin)

Invokana

Func. class.: Oral antidiabetic

Chem. class.: SGLT 2 inhibitor

ACTION: Blocks glucose reabsorption by the kidney, increases glucose excretion, lowers blood glucose concentrations

USES: Type 2 diabetes mellitus, with diet and exercise

CONTRAINDICATIONS: Dialysis, renal failure, hypersensitivity, breastfeeding, diabetic ketoacidosis

Precautions: Pregnancy (C), children, renal/hepatic disease, hypothyroidism, hyperglycemia, hypotension, pituitary insufficiency, type 1 diabetes mellitus, malnutrition, fever, dehydration, adrenal insufficiency, geriatric patients

DOSAGE AND ROUTES

- **Adult: PO** 100 mg/day, may increase to 300 mg/day

Renal Dose

- **Adult PO** eGFR 45-59 ml/min/1.73 m^2, max 100 mg/day; <45 ml/min/1.73 m^2 do not use

Available forms: Tabs 100, 300 mg

Administer:

PO route

- Once daily with first meal of the day
- Correct volume depletion before use

SIDE EFFECTS

CNS: Dizziness, fatigue

GI: Abdominal pain, **pancreatitis**, constipation, nausea

GU: Cystisis, candidiasis, urinary frequency, polyclipsia, polyuria

INTEG: Photosensitivity, rash, pruritus

META: Hypercholesterolemia, lipidemia, hypoglycemia, **hyperkalemia**, hypermagnesemia, hyperphosphatemia

MISC: Bone fractures

PHARMACOKINETICS

99% protein binding, metabolized by UGT1A9, UGT2B4, excreted 33% in urine, peak 1-2 hr, half-life 10.6-13 hr depending on dose

INTERACTIONS

- Do not use gatifloxacin

Increase: hypoglycemia-sulfonylureas, insulin, MAOIs, salycilates, fibric acid derivatives, bile acid sequestrants, ACE inhibitors, angiotensin II receptor antagonists, beta blockers, SSRIs

Increase or decrease: glycemic control-androgens, lithium, bortezomib, quinolones

Decrease: effect hyperglycemia—digestive enzymes, intestinal absorbents, thiazide diuretics, loop diuretics, corticosteroids, estrogen, progestins, oral contraceptives, sympathomimetics, isoniazid, phenothiazines; protease inhibitors, atypical antipsychotics, carbonic anhydrase inhibitors, cycloSPORINE, tacrolimus, baclofen

Drug/Lab

Increase: urine, glucose, potassium, lipids, cholesterol

Decrease: serum glucose

NURSING CONSIDERATIONS

Assess:

- Hypoglycemia (weakness, hunger, dizziness, tremors, anxiety, tachycardia, sweating), hyperglycemia; even though product does not cause hypoglycemia, if patient is on sulfonylureas or insulin, hypoglycemia may be additive; if hypoglycemia occurs, treat with dextrose, or, if severe, with IV glucagon
- For stress, surgery, or other trauma that may require a change in dose
- A1c q3mo, monitor serum glucose; 1 hr PP throughout treatment; serum cholesterol, serum creatinine/BUN, serum electrolytes

Evaluate:

- Therapeutic response: improved signs/symptoms of diabetes mellitus (decreased polyuria, polydipsia, polyphagia); clear sensorium, absence of dizziness, stable gait

Teach patient/family:

- The symptoms of hypo/hyperglycemia, what to do about each
- That medication must be taken as prescribed; explain consequences of discontinuing medication abruptly; that insulin may need to be used for stress, including trauma, fever, surgery
- To avoid OTC medications and herbal supplements unless approved by health care provider
- That diabetes is a lifelong illness; that the diet and exercise regimen must be followed; that this product is not a cure
- To carry emergency ID and glucose source; to avoid sugar, because sugar is blocked by acarbose
- That blood glucose monitoring is required to assess product effect
- That GI side effects may occur

candesartan (Rx)

(can-deh-sar′tan)

Atacand

Func. class.: Antihypertensive

Chem. class.: Angiotensin II receptor (type AT_1) antagonist

ACTION: Blocks the vasoconstrictor and aldosterone-secreting effects of angiotensin II; selectively blocks the binding of angiotensin II to the AT_1 receptor found in tissues

USES: Hypertension, alone or in combination; CHF NYHA Class II-IV and ejection fraction ≤40%

CONTRAINDICATIONS: Hypersensitivity

Black Box Warning: Pregnancy (D) 2nd/3rd trimesters

Precautions: Pregnancy (C) 1st trimester, breastfeeding, children, geriatric patients, hypersensitivity to ACE inhibitors, volume depletion, renal/hepatic impairment, renal artery stenosis, hypotension, electrolyte abnormalities

DOSAGE AND ROUTES

Hypertension

- **Adult: PO** single agent 16 mg/day initially in patients who are not volume depleted, range 8-32 mg/day, with diuretic or volume depletion 8-32 mg/day as single dose or divided bid
- **Adolescent and child ≥6 yr and weight >50 kg: PO** 8-16 mg/day or divided bid, adjust to B/P; usual range 4-32 mg/day, max 32 mg/day
- **Child ≥6 yr, weight <50 kg: PO** 2-16 mg/day divided 1-2 doses, max 16mg/day
- **Child ≥1 yr and <6 yr: PO** 0.2 mg/kg/day in 1 dose or in 2 divided doses, adjust to B/P, max 0.4 mg/kg/day

Heart failure

- **Adult: PO** 4 mg/day, may be doubled ≥2 wk, target dose 32 mg/day

Renal/hepatic disease

- **Adult: PO** ≤8 mg/day for severe renal disease/moderate hepatic disease, adjust dose as needed

Available forms: Tabs 4, 8, 16, 32 mg

Administer:

- Without regard to meals
- Oral liquid (compounded): shake well, do not freeze

SIDE EFFECTS

CNS: *Dizziness,* fatigue, headache, syncope

CV: Chest pain, peripheral edema, hypotension, palpitations

EENT: Sinusitis, rhinitis, pharyngitis

GI: *Diarrhea,* nausea, abdominal pain, vomiting

GU: Renal failure

MS: Arthralgia, pain

RESP: *Cough, upper respiratory infection*

SYST: Angioedema

PHARMACOKINETICS

Peak 3-4 hr, protein binding 99%, half-life 9-12 hr, duration 24 hr, extensively metabolized, excreted in urine (33%) and feces (67%)

INTERACTIONS

Increase: lithium level—lithium
Increase: hyperkalemia—potassium, potassium-sparing diuretics
Increase: hypotension—ACE inhibitors, β-blockers, calcium channel blockers, α-blockers, MAOIs
Decrease: effect—salicylates, NSAIDs

Drug/Herb

Increase: antihypertensive effect—hawthorn
Decrease: antihypertensive effect—ephedra

Drug/Lab

Increase: albumin, ALT/AST, potassium

NURSING CONSIDERATIONS

Assess:

⚠ **Serious hypersensitivity reaction:** angioedema, anaphylaxis: facial swelling, difficulty breathing (rare)

Black Box Warning: For pregnancy; this product can cause fetal death when given during pregnancy (D), 2nd/3rd trimester

- Response and adverse reactions, especially with renal disease
- B/P, pulse q4hr; note rate, rhythm, quality; electrolytes: potassium, sodium, calcium; baselines of renal/hepatic studies before therapy begins
- **Heart failure:** jugular venous distention, weight, edema, dyspnea, crackles

Evaluate:

- Therapeutic response: decreased B/P

Teach patient/family:

- To comply with dosage schedule, even if feeling better
- To notify prescriber of mouth sores, fever, swelling of hands or feet, irregular heartbeat, chest pain
- That excessive perspiration, dehydration, vomiting, diarrhea may lead to fall in B/P; to consult prescriber if these occur

Black Box Warning: To notify prescriber immediately if pregnant (D) 2nd/3rd trimester, (C) 1st trimester; to use if breastfeeding

- To avoid all OTC medications unless approved by prescriber; to inform all health care providers of medication use, full effect 4 wk, onset 2 wk
- To use proper technique for obtaining B/P; to understand acceptable parameters; to rise slowly to sitting or standing position to minimize orthostatic hypotension; that product may cause dizziness, fainting, light-headedness

⚠ HIGH ALERT

capecitabine (Rx)

(cap-eh-sit′ah-bean)

Xeloda

Func. class.: Antineoplastic, antimetabolite

Chem. class.: Fluoropyrimidine carbamate

Do not confuse:
Xeloda/Xenical

ACTION: Competes with physiologic substrate of DNA synthesis, thereby interfering with cell replication in the S phase of cell cycle (before mitosis); also interferes with RNA and protein synthesis; product is converted to 5-FU

USES: PACLitaxel and anthracycline-resistant metastatic breast, colorectal cancer when 5-FU monotherapy is preferred; treatment of colorectal cancer patients who have undergone complete resection of their primary tumors

Unlabeled uses: Gastric/biliary tract, ovarian cancer

CONTRAINDICATIONS:
Pregnancy (D), hypersensitivity to 5-FU, infants, severe renal impairment (CCr <30 ml/min)

Precautions: Breastfeeding, children, infections, radiation therapy, anticoagulation, geriatric patients, renal/hepatic/cardiac disease, DPD deficiency

DOSAGE AND ROUTES

Metastatic breast cancer resistant to both PACLitaxel and anthracycline or resistant to PACLitaxel and when further anthracycline therapy is not indicated

• **Adult: PO** 2500 mg/m^2/day divided q12hr after a meal × 2 wk, repeat q3wk

Breast cancer (locally advanced/metastatic) with DOCEtaxel, previously treated with anthracycline

• **Adult: PO** 2500 mg/m^2/day divided q12hr after a meal on days 1-14, with DOCEtaxel 75 mg/m^2 IV on day 1

Advanced/metastatic breast cancer (HER2 positive) previously treated with anthracycline, taxane, and trastuzumab

• **Adult: PO** 2000 mg/m^2/day divided q12hr after a meal on days 1-14 with lapatinib 1250 mg/day on days 1-21, repeat q21days

Metastatic/locally advanced breast cancer resistant to anthracycline, previously treated with a taxane or taxane resistant, and when further anthracycline is contraindicated

• **Adult: PO** 2000 mg/m^2/day divided q12hr on days 1-14 with ixabepilone 40 mg/m^2 IV over 3 hr, repeat q3wk

As an adjuvant for Dukes C colorectal cancer with a complete resection when fluoropyrimidine alone is preferred

• **Adult: PO** 2500 mg/m^2/day divided q12hr within 30 min of a meal × 2 wk, repeat q3wk for 8 cycles

First-line treatment of metastatic colorectal cancer when fluoropyrimidine alone is preferred

• **Adult: PO** 2500 mg/m^2/day divided q12hr after a meal × 2 wk, repeat q3wk

First-line treatment of metastatic colorectal cancer with oxaliplatin with or without bevacizumab (unlabeled)

• **Adult: PO** 2000 mg/m^2/day divided q12hr after a meal on days 1-14 with oxaliplatin on day 1, repeat q3wk

First-/second-line treatment of advanced colorectal cancer with oxaliplatin (unlabeled)

• **Adult: PO** 2000 mg/m^2/day divided q12hr on days 1-14 and oxaliplatin 130 mg/m^2 IV on day 1, repeat q3wk

Unresectable advanced/metastatic biliary tract cancer (unlabeled)

• **Adult: PO** 2500 mg/m^2 divided q12hr on days 1-14, then 7-day rest period; given with CISplatin 60 mg/m^2 IV over 1 hr on day 1, repeat q21days

Renal dose

• **Adult: PO** CCr 30-50 ml/min, decrease initial dose to 75% of usual dose; CCr <30 ml/min, contraindicated

Available forms: Tabs 150, 500 mg

Administer:

• **Dosage adjustments of capecitabine monotherapy based on most severe toxicity OR when used in combination with ixabepilone based on nonhematologic toxicity: Grade 1 toxicity:** maintain current dosage; **Grade 2 toxicity (1st appearance):** interrupt therapy until toxicity is resolved to Grade 0-1; do not replace missed doses, begin the next cycle with 100% of the starting dose; **Grade 2 toxicity (2nd appearance):** interrupt therapy until toxicity is resolved to Grade 0-1; do not replace missed doses, begin the next cycle with 75% of the starting dose; **Grade 2 toxicity (3rd appearance):** interrupt therapy until toxicity is resolved to Grade 0-1; do not replace missed doses, begin the next cycle with 50% of the starting dose; **Grade 2 toxicity (4th appearance):** discontinue treatment permanently; **Grade 3 toxicity (1st appearance):** interrupt therapy until toxicity is resolved to Grade 0-1

SIDE EFFECTS

CNS: Dizziness, *headache, paresthesia, fatigue,* insomnia

CV: Venous thrombosis

GI: *Nausea, vomiting, anorexia, diarrhea, stomatitis, abdominal pain, constipation, dyspepsia,* intestinal obstruction, necrotizing enterocolitis, hyperbilirubinemia, hepatic failure, GI bleeding

HEMA: Neutropenia, lymphopenia, thrombocytopenia, anemia

INTEG: *Hand and foot syndrome, dermatitis,* nail disorders, alopecia, rash

OTHER: *Eye irritation, edema, myalgia,* limb pain, *pyrexia,* dehydration, renal impairment

RESP: *Cough, dyspnea,* pulmonary embolism

PHARMACOKINETICS

Readily absorbed, peak 1½ hr, food decreases absorption, extensively metabolized in the liver, elimination half-life 45 min

INTERACTIONS

Increase: toxicity—leucovorin

Increase: capecitabine levels—antacids (aluminum, magnesium)

Increase: phenytoin level—phenytoin

Black Box Warning: Increase: bleeding risk—anticoagulants, NSAIDs, salicylates, platelet inhibitors, thrombolytics

Drug/Food

Increase: absorption; give within 30 min of a meal

Drug/Lab Test

Increase: bilirubin

Decrease: Hgb/HcT/RBC, neutrophils, platelets, WBC

NURSING CONSIDERATIONS

Assess:

- **Bone marrow suppression,** CBC (RBC, Hct, Hgb), differential, platelet count weekly; withhold product if WBC is <1000/mm^3, platelet count is <50,000/mm^3, or RBC, Hct, Hgb low; notify prescriber of these results; frequently monitor INR in those receiving warfarin concurrently
- Renal studies: BUN, serum uric acid, urine CCr, electrolytes before, during therapy
- Monitor temperature q4hr; fever may indicate beginning infection; no rectal temperatures
- Hepatic studies before, during therapy: bilirubin, ALT, AST, alk phos as needed or monthly

Black Box Warning: Bleeding: hematuria, heme-positive stools, bruising or petechiae of mucosa or orifices q8hr, monitor INR and PT in those taking anticoagulants

- Dyspnea, crackles, unproductive cough, chest pain, tachypnea, fatigue, increased pulse, pallor, lethargy; personality changes with high doses
- **Hand and foot syndrome:** paresthesia, tingling, painful/painless swelling, blistering, erythema with severe pain of hands or feet
- **Toxicity:** severe diarrhea (multiple times/day or at night), nausea, vomiting, stomatitis, fever
- Buccal cavity q8hr for dryness, sores, ulceration, white patches, oral pain, bleeding, dysphagia
- **GI symptoms:** frequency of stools, cramping; if severe diarrhea occurs, fluid, electrolytes may need to be given
- Rinsing of mouth tid-qid with water, club soda; brushing of teeth bid-tid with soft brush or cotton-tipped applicators for stomatitis; use unwaxed dental floss

Evaluate:

- Therapeutic response: decreased tumor size, spread of malignancy

Teach patient/family:

- To avoid foods with citric acid, hot or rough texture if stomatitis is present; take with water within 30 min of end of meal

- To notify prescriber if pregnancy is planned or suspected, pregnancy (D); to avoid pregnancy while taking this product; not to breastfeed
- Not to double dose if dose is missed
- ⚠ To immediately report severe diarrhea, vomiting, stomatitis, fever of more than 100° F (37.8° C), hand and foot syndrome, anorexia
- To report signs of **infection:** increased temperature, sore throat, flulike symptoms; signs of **anemia:** fatigue, headache, faintness, shortness of breath, irritability; **bleeding;** to avoid use of razors, commercial mouthwash
- OTC antidiarrheals for mild diarrhea (4-6 stools/day or diarrhea at night)

captopril (Rx)

(kap′toe-pril)

Apo-Capto ♣

Func. class.: Antihypertensive
Chem. class.: Angiotensin-converting enzyme (ACE) inhibitor

Do not confuse:
captopril/Capitrol/carvedilol

ACTION: Selectively suppresses renin-angiotensin-aldosterone system; inhibits ACE; prevents conversion of angiotensin I to angiotensin II

USES: Hypertension, CHF, left ventricular dysfunction after MI, diabetic nephropathy, proteinuria
Unlabeled uses: Acute MI, hypertensive emergency/urgency, scleroderma renal crisis (SRC)

CONTRAINDICATIONS: Breastfeeding, children, hypersensitivity, heart block, potassium-sparing diuretics, bilateral renal artery stenosis, angioedema

Black Box Warning: Pregnancy (D) 2nd/3rd trimester

Precautions: Dialysis patients, hypovolemia, leukemia, scleroderma, SLE, blood dyscrasias, CHF, diabetes mellitus, thyroid/renal/hepatic disease, African descent, pregnancy (C) 1st trimester, collagen vascular disease, hyperkalemia, hyponatremia

DOSAGE AND ROUTES

Hypertension
- **Adult: PO** initial dose: 12.5-25 mg bid-tid; may increase to 50 mg bid-tid at 1-2 wk intervals; usual range: 25-150 mg bid-tid; max 450 mg/day
- **Child (unlabeled): PO** 0.3-0.5 mg/kg/dose, may titrate up to 6 mg/kg/day in 2-4 divided doses
- **Infant (unlabeled): PO** 0.15-0.3 mg/kg/dose initially, max 6 mg/kg/day
- **Neonate (unlabeled): PO** 0.01-0.1 mg/kg/dose, may increase as needed

CHF
- **Adult: PO** 25 mg bid; may increase to 50 mg tid; after 14 days, may increase to 150 mg tid if needed
- **Adolescent (unlabeled): PO** 6.25-12.5 mg q8-12hr titrated up to max 50-75 mg/dose
- **Child (unlabeled): PO** 0.1-2 mg/kg/dose q6-12hr, max 6 mg/kg/day
- **Infant (unlabeled): PO** 0.15-0.3 mg/kg/dose, max 6 mg/kg/day in 1-4 divided doses
- **Neonates (unlabeled): PO** 0.05-0.1 mg/kg q8-24hr titrate to 0.5 mg/kg q6-24hr, max 2 mg/kg/day

Diabetic nephropathy
- **Adult: PO** 25 mg tid

Renal dose
- **Adult: PO** CCr >50 ml/min, no change; CCr 10-50 ml/min, decrease dose by 25%; CCr <10 ml/min, decrease dose by 50%

Acute MI (unlabeled) or post-MI
- **Adult: PO** 6.25-12.5 mg tid, increase to 25 mg tid gradually

Hypertensive emergency/urgency (unlabeled)
- **Adult: PO** 25 mg, may repeat q30min

Available forms: Tabs 12.5, 25, 50, 100 mg

Administer:

- Store in tight container at 86° F (30° C) or less
- 1 hr before or 2 hr after meals
- **Oral sol:** may crush 25 mg tab, dissolve in 50-100 ml water; give within ½ hr; make sure tab completely dissolved

SIDE EFFECTS

CNS: Fever, chills

CV: *Hypotension,* postural hypotension, *tachycardia,* angina

GI: Loss of taste, increased LFTs

GU: Impotence, dysuria, nocturia, proteinuria, nephrotic syndrome, acute reversible renal failure, polyuria, oliguria, urinary frequency

HEMA: Neutropenia, agranulocytosis, pancytopenia, thrombocytopenia, anemia

INTEG: Rash, pruritus

MISC: Angioedema, hyperkalemia

RESP: Bronchospasm, *dyspnea, cough*

PHARMACOKINETICS

Peak 1 hr; duration 2-6 hr; half-life <2 hr, increased in renal disease; metabolized by liver (metabolites); excreted in urine; crosses placenta; excreted in breast milk, small amounts; protein binding 25%-30%

INTERACTIONS

- Do not use with potassium-sparing diuretics, sympathomimetics, potassium supplements

Increase: possible toxicity—lithium, digoxin

Increase: hypoglycemia—insulin, oral antidiabetics

Increase: hypotension—diuretics, other antihypertensives, phenothiazines, nitrates, acute alcohol ingestion, MAOIs

Decrease: captopril effect—antacids, NSAIDs, salicylates

Drug/Herb

Increase: antihypertensive effect—hawthorn

Decrease: antihypertensive effect—ephedra

Drug/Food

Decrease: absorption of captopril

Drug/Lab Test

Increase: AST, ALT, alk phos, bilirubin, uric acid, potassium

Decrease: platelets, WBC, RBC, Hgb/HcT

False positive: urine acetone, ANA titer

NURSING CONSIDERATIONS

Assess:

- **Blood dyscrasias:** blood studies: decreased platelets; WBC with differential at baseline and periodically q3mo; if neutrophils <1000/mm^3, discontinue treatment (recommended with collagen-vascular or renal disease)
- **Hypertension:** B/P, pulse rates at baseline, frequently
- Renal studies: protein, BUN, creatinine; watch for raised levels, may indicate nephrotic syndrome; increased LFTs, uric acid; glucose, potassium
- **Allergic reaction:** rash, fever, pruritus, urticaria; discontinue product if antihistamines fail to help
- **CHF:** edema, dyspnea, wet crackles, increased B/P, weight gain

Evaluate:

- Therapeutic response: decrease in B/P with hypertension; decreased edema, moist crackles (CHF)

Teach patient/family:

- To take 1 hr before or 2 hr after meals; not to discontinue product abruptly; if dose is missed, take as soon as remembered but not if almost time for next dose; not to double doses
- Not to use OTC products (cough, cold, or allergy) unless directed by prescriber; avoid salt substitutes, high-potassium or high-sodium foods
- To adhere to dosage schedule, even if feeling better
- To rise slowly to sitting or standing position to minimize orthostatic hypotension
- To notify prescriber of mouth sores, sore throat, fever, swelling of hands or feet, irregular heartbeat, chest pain, signs of angioedema, rash, hoarseness, difficulty breathing
- That excessive perspiration, dehydration, vomiting, diarrhea may lead to fall

in B/P; to consult prescriber if these occur

- That dizziness, fainting, light-headedness may occur during first few days of therapy; to avoid activities that require concentration
- How to take B/P and when to notify prescriber

Black Box Warning: To report if pregnancy is suspected or planned, pregnancy (D)

TREATMENT OF OVERDOSE: 0.9% NaCl IV/INFUSION; hemodialysis

carbachol ophthalmic

See Appendix B

carBAMazepine (Rx)

(kar-ba-maz′e-peen)

Carbatrol, Equetro, Mazepine ✤, Novo-Carbamaz ✤, TEGretol, TEGretol-XR

Func. class.: Anticonvulsant

Chem. class.: Iminostilbene derivative

Do not confuse:
TEGretol/Toradol

ACTION: Exact mechanism unknown; appears to decrease polysynaptic responses and block posttetanic potentiation

USES: Tonic-clonic, complex-partial, mixed seizures; trigeminal neuralgia; bipolar disorder

Unlabeled uses: Neurogenic pain, diabetic neuropathy, hiccups

CONTRAINDICATIONS: Pregnancy (D), hypersensitivity to carBAMazepine or tricyclics

Black Box Warning: Bone marrow suppression

Precautions: Breastfeeding, children <6 yr, glaucoma, AV or bundle branch block, cardiac/renal/hepatic disease, psychosis, alcoholism, hepatic porphyria

Black Box Warning: Hematologic disease, Asian patients, agranulocytosis, leukopenia, neutropenia, thrombocytopenia

DOSAGE AND ROUTES

Seizures

- **Adult and child >12 yr: PO** 200 mg bid, may be increased by 200 mg/day in weekly intervals, give in divided doses q6-8hr; maintenance 800-1200 mg/day, max 1600 mg/day (adult); max child 12-15 yr 1000 mg/day; max child >15 yr 1200 mg/day; adjust to minimum dose to control seizures; **EXT REL** give bid; rectal administration of **ORAL SUSP** 200 mg/10 ml or 6 mg/kg as a single dose
- **Child 6-12 yr: PO** tabs 100 mg bid or susp 50 mg qid; may increase by <100 mg weekly; max 1000 mg/day, usual dose 15-30 mg/kg/day; **EXT REL** tabs daily-bid
- **Child <6 yr: PO** 10-20 mg/kg/day in 2-3 divided doses or 4 divided dose (susp), may increase every wk, do not use ext rel

Trigeminal neuralgia

- **Adult: PO** 100 mg bid with meals; may increase 100 mg q12hr until pain subsides, max 1200 mg/day; maintenance 200-400 mg bid

Diabetic neuropathy (unlabeled)

- **Adult: PO** 100 mg bid or 50 mg qid, titrate to 600-800 mg/day

Bipolar disorder

- **Adult: PO** (Equetro only [regular release]) 200 mg bid, may adjust dose q3-4days to achieve carBAMazepine level to 8-12 mcg/ml micro response, max 1600 mg/day

Hiccups (unlabeled)
- **Adult: PO** 200 mg tid

Available forms: Chewable tabs 100 mg; tabs 200 mg; ext rel tabs (XR) 100, 200, 400 mg; oral susp 100 mg/5 ml; ext rel caps 100, 200, 300 mg

Administer:

PO route
- Do not crush, chew ext rel tab; ext rel cap may be opened and beads sprinkled over food; patient should chew chewable tab, not swallow it whole
- With food, milk to decrease GI symptoms; shake oral susp before use
- **(Susp):** Turn off NG/enteral feeding 15 min before and hold for 15 min after
- Mix an equal amount of water, D_5W, 0.9% NaCl when giving by NG tube; flush tube with 15-30 ml of above sol, do not give at same time as other liquid products or diluents
- Store at room temperature

SIDE EFFECTS

CNS: *Drowsiness,* dizziness, unsteadiness, confusion, fatigue, paralysis, headache, hallucinations, worsening of seizures, speech disturbance, suicidal thoughts/behaviors, neuroleptic malignant syndrome (when used with psychotropics), tremor

CV: Hypertension, CHF, dysrhythmias, AV block, hypotension, aggravation of cardiac artery disease

EENT: Tinnitus, dry mouth, blurred vision, diplopia, nystagmus, conjunctivitis

ENDO: SIADH (geriatric patients)

GI: *Nausea, constipation, diarrhea,* anorexia, vomiting, abdominal pain, stomatitis, glossitis, increased hepatic enzymes, hepatitis, hepatic porphyria, hypercholesterolemia, pancreatitis

GU: Frequency, retention, albuminuria, glycosuria, impotence, increased BUN, renal failure

HEMA: Thrombocytopenia, leukopenia, agranulocytosis, leukocytosis, aplastic anemia, eosinophilia, increased PT, lymphadenopathy

INTEG: *Rash,* Stevens-Johnson syndrome, urticaria, photosensitivity, toxic epidermal necrolysis, DRESS, alopecia, pruritus

MS: Osteoporosis

RESP: Pulmonary hypersensitivity (fever, dyspnea, pneumonitis)

PHARMACOKINETICS

Onset slow; peak 4-5 hr (PO), 1.5 hr (susp) metabolized by liver; excreted in urine, feces; crosses placenta, blood-brain barrier; excreted in breast milk; half-life 18-65 hr, then 8-29 hr after 1st month; protein binding 76%; metabolized by CYP3A4

INTERACTIONS

- CNS toxicity: lithium

⚠ Fatal reaction: MAOIs

- Do not use with: NNRTIs (non-nucleoside reverse transcriptase inhibitors nefazodone)

Increase: carBAMazepine levels—CYP3A inhibitors (cimetidine, clarithromycin, danazol, diltiazem, erythromycin, FLUoxetine, fluvoxamine, isoniazid, valproic acid, verapamil, voriconazole)

Increase: effects of desmopressin, lithium, lypressin, vasopressin

Decrease: carBAMazepine effect—CYP1A2, CYP2C9 substrates

Decrease: effect of CYP3A inducers

Decrease: effects of benzodiazepines, doxycycline, felbamate, haloperidol, oral contraceptives, PHENobarbital, phenytoin, primidone, theophylline, thyroid hormones, warfarin

Decrease: carBAMazepine levels—CYP3A4 inducers (CISplatin, darunavir, delavirdine, DOXOrubicin, felbamate, nefazodone, OXcarbazepine, PHENobarbital, phenytoin, primidone, rifampin, theophylline)

Drug/Herb

Decrease: carBAMazepine metabolism, increased levels—echinacea

Decrease: anticonvulsant effect—St. John's wort

Drug/Food

Increase: peak concentration of carBAMazepine—grapefruit juice

Drug/Lab Test
Decrease: serum calcium, sodium
Increase: cholesterol

NURSING CONSIDERATIONS

Assess:

Black Box Warning: Asian patients for serious skin reaction; genetic test for HLA-B1502 allele before administration

- **Seizures:** character, location, duration, intensity, frequency, presence of aura, in mixed seizure disorder, worsening of symptoms may occur
- **Trigeminal neuralgia:** facial pain including location, duration, intensity, character, activity that stimulates pain
- Renal studies: urinalysis, BUN, urine creatinine q3mo
- **Serious skin, multiorgan hypersensitivity (Stevens-Johnson syndrome, toxic epidermal necrolysis, DRESS):** may be increased in HLA-A 3101 gene and may be fatal

Black Box Warning: Bone marrow depression: blood studies: CBC reticulocyte counts every wk for 4 wk, then q3-6mo if on long-term therapy; if myelosuppression occurs, product should be discontinued; blood dyscrasias: fever, sore throat, bruising, rash, jaundice, agranulocytosis and aplastic anemia may occur

- Blood studies: ALT, AST, bilirubin; serum calcium, may be decreased and lead to osteoporosis; cholesterol periodically
- Product levels during initial treatment or when changing dose; should remain at 4-12 mcg/ml; anorexia may indicate increased blood levels
- ⚠ Mental status: mood, sensorium, affect, behavioral changes, **suicidal thoughts/behaviors;** if mental status changes, notify prescriber
- Eye problems: need for ophthalmic examinations before, during, after treatment (slit lamp, funduscopy, tonometry)
- Allergic reaction: purpura, red, raised rash; if these occur, product should be discontinued; increased risk if past hypersensitivity to hydantoins
- ⚠ Toxicity: bone marrow depression, nausea, vomiting, ataxia, diplopia, CV collapse
- Hard candy, gum, frequent rinsing for dry mouth

Evaluate:

- Therapeutic response: decreased seizure activity; document on patient's chart

Teach patient/family:

- To carry emergency ID stating patient's name, products taken, condition, prescriber's name, and phone number
- To avoid driving, other activities that require alertness usually for the first 3 days of treatment
- Not to discontinue medication quickly after long-term use, seizures may occur
- To immediately report chills, rash, light-colored stools, dark urine, yellowing of skin and eyes, abdominal pain, sore throat, mouth ulcers, bruising, blurred vision, dizziness, skin rash, fever
- That urine may turn pink to brown
- To notify if pregnancy is planned or suspected, pregnancy (D), avoid breastfeeding

TREATMENT OF OVERDOSE:

Lavage, VS

⚠ HIGH ALERT

CARBOplatin (Rx)

(kar-boe-pla′-tin)

Func. class.: Antineoplastic alkylating agent

Chem. class.: Platinum coordination compound

Do not confuse:
CARBOplatin/CISplatin

ACTION: Produces interstrand DNA cross-links and, to a lesser extent, DNA-protein cross-links; activity is not cell-cycle–phase specific

USES: Initial treatment of advanced ovarian cancer in combination with other agents; palliative treatment of ovarian carcinoma recurrent after treatment with other antineoplastic agents

Unlabeled uses: Acute lymphocytic leukemia (ALL), acute myelogenous leukemia (AML), bladder/breast/head/neck/lung/testicular cancer, bone marrow ablation, malignant glioma, neuroblastoma, non-Hodgkin's lymphoma, osteogenic sarcoma, soft-tissue sarcoma, stem-cell transplant preparation, Wilms' tumor, stage I seminoma

CONTRAINDICATIONS: Pregnancy (D), breastfeeding, hypersensitivity, significant bleeding, aluminum products used to prepare or administer CARBOplatin

Black Box Warning: Severe bone marrow depression, platinum compound hypersensitivity (anaphylaxis)

Precautions: Geriatric patients, radiation therapy within 1 mo, other cancer chemotherapy within 1 mo, renal/hepatic disease, hearing impairment

Black Box Warning: Anemia, infection

DOSAGE AND ROUTES

Dosing with the Calvert equation

GFR capped at max 12.5 ml/min

• **Adult:** The total CARBOplatin dose in mg for adults may be calculated using the Calvert equation:

Total dose (mg) = target AUC × (GFR + 25)

• **Children:** Calculate CARBOplatin dosage (mg/m²) in children:

Total dose (mg/m²) = target AUC × [(0.93 × GFR) + 15]

Advanced ovarian cancer

• **Adult (single agent): IV INFUSION** initially 300 mg/m² on day 1 with cyclophosphamide, 600 mg/m² **IV** on day 1, repeat q4wk × 6 cycles; refractory tumors 360 mg/m² single dose, may repeat q4wk as needed, do not repeat until neutrophils >2000/mm³ and platelets >100,000/mm³

Renal dose

• **Adult (single agent): IV INFUSION** CCr 41-59 ml/min, 250 mg/m², CCr 16-40 ml/min, 200 mg/m², do not use if CCr <15 ml/min

ALL (unlabeled)

• **Adult <21 yr/adolescent/child: IV** 635 mg/m² on day 3 with ifosfamide, mesna, etoposide

Relapsed Wilms' tumor (unlabeled)

• **Child: IV** 400 mg/m² × 2 days with etoposide, ifosfamide

Osteogenic sarcoma (unlabeled)

• **Adult/adolescent/child: IV** 560 mg/m² on day 1 with ifosfamide 2.65 g/m²/day **IV** on days 1-3

Neuroblastoma/soft-tissue sarcoma (unlabeled)

• **Child: IV** 300-600 mg/m² q4wk or 400 mg/m²/day for 2 days q4wk or 160 mg/m²/day × 5 days q4wk

Available forms: Lyophilized powder for inj 50-, 150-, 450-mg vials; aqueous sol for inj 50 mg/5-ml vial, 150 mg/15-ml vial, 450 mg/45-ml vial, 600 mg/60-ml vial

Administer:

• Antiemetic 30-60 min before product and prn for vomiting

IV route

• Do not use needles or IV administration sets that contain aluminum; may cause precipitate or loss of potency

• Use cytotoxic handling procedures

• Store protected from light at room temperature; reconstituted vials stable for 24 hr at room temperature, solutions further diluted in D_5W or NS are stable for 8 hr at room temperature. Paraplatin multidose (10 mg/ml) vials stable for up to 14 days after entry into vial

• **Reconstitute** CARBOplatin 50, 150, or 450 mg with 5, 15, or 45 ml, respectively, of sterile water for inj, D_5W, or NaCl (10 mg/ml); then further **dilute** with the same sol to 0.5-4 mg/ml; **give** over 15 min-1 hr (intermittent INFUSION)

• **Continuous IV INFUSION** give over 24 hr; max dose based on (GFR=125 mg/ml)

Solution compatibilities: D_5/0.2% NaCl, D_5/0.45% NaCl, D_5/0.9% NaCl, 0.9% NaCl, D_5W, sterile water for inj

Y-site compatibilities: Acyclovir, alfentanil, allopurinol, amifostine, amikacin, aminocaproic acid, aminophylline, amiodarone, amphotericin B lipid complex, amphotericin B liposome, ampicillin, ampicillin-sulbactam, anidulafungin, atenolol, atracurium, azithromycin, aztreonam, bivalirudin, bleomycin, bumetanide, buprenorphine, butorphanol, calcium chloride/gluconate, caspofungin, ceFAZolin, cefepime, cefotaxime, cefoTEtan, cefOXitin, cefTAZidime, ceftizoxime, cefTRIAXone, cefuroxime, cimetidine, ciprofloxacin, cisatracurium, CISplatin, cladribine, clindamycin, codeine, cyclophosphamide, cycloSPORINE, cytarabine, DAPTOmycin, DAUNOrubicin, dexamethasone, dexmedetomidine, dexrazoxane, digoxin, diltiazem, diphenhydrAMINE, DOBUTamine, DOCEtaxel, DOPamine, doripenem, doxacurium, DOXOrubicin, DOXOrubicin liposomal, doxycycline, droperidol, enalaprilat, ePHEDrine, EPINEPHrine, epirubicin, ertapenem, erythromycin, esmolol, etoposide, famotidine, fenoldopam, fentaNYL, filgrastim, fluconazole, fludarabine, fluorouracil, foscarnet, fosphenytoin, furosemide, ganciclovir, gatifloxacin, gemcitabine, gentamicin, granisetron, haloperidol, heparin, hydrocortisone, HYDROmorphone, hydrOXYzine, IDArubicin, ifosfamide, imipenem-cilastatin, inamrinone, insulin (regular), irinotecan, isoproterenol, ketorolac, labetalol, levofloxacin, levorphanol, lidocaine, linezolid injection, LORazepam, magnesium sulfate, mannitol, melphalan, meperidine, meropenem, mesna, methohexital, methotrexate, methylPREDNISolone, metoclopramide, metoprolol, metroNIDAZOLE, micafungin, midazolam, milrinone, minocycline, mitoXANtrone, mivacurium, morphine, nafcillin, nalbuphine, naloxone, nesiritide, niCARdipine, nitroglycerin, nitroprusside, norepinephrine, octreotide, ofloxacin, ondansetron, oxaliplatin, PACLitaxel, palonosetron, pamidronate, pancuronium, pantoprazole, PEMEtrexed, pentamidine, PENTobarbital, PHENobarbital, phenylephrine, piperacillin, piperacillin-tazobactam, potassium chloride, potassium phosphates, prochlorperazine, promethazine, propofol, propranolol, ranitidine, remifentanil, riTUXimab, rocuronium, sargramostim, sodium acetate, sodium bicarbonate, sodium phosphates, succinylcholine, SUFentanil, sulfamethoxazole-trimethoprim, tacrolimus, teniposide, theophylline, thiotepa, ticarcillin, ticarcillin-clavulanate, tigecycline, tirofiban, TNA, tobramycin, topotecan, TPN, trastuzumab, trimethobenzamide, vancomycin, vasopressin, vecuronium, verapamil, vinBLAStine, vinCRIStine, vinorelbine, voriconazole, zidovudine

SIDE EFFECTS

CNS: **Seizures, central neurotoxicity,** *peripheral neuropathy,* dizziness, confusion

CV: **Cardiac abnormalities (fatal CV events), stroke**

EENT: Tinnitus, hearing loss, *vestibular toxicity,* visual changes

GI: *Severe nausea, vomiting,* diarrhea, weight loss, mucositis, anorexia, constipation, taste change

HEMA: **Thrombocytopenia, leukopenia, pancytopenia, neutropenia, anemia,** bleeding

INTEG: *Alopecia,* dermatitis, rash, erythema, pruritus, urticaria

META: Hypomagnesemia, hypocalcemia, hypokalemia, hyponatremia, hyperuremia

SYST: **Anaphylaxis**

PHARMACOKINETICS

Initial half-life 1-2 hr, postdistribution half-life $2^1/_2$-6 hr, not bound to plasma proteins, excreted by the kidneys

INTERACTIONS

Increase: nephrotoxicity or ototoxicity—aminoglycosides, amphotericin B

Increase: bleeding risk—aspirin, NSAIDs, thrombolytics, anticoagulants, platelet inhibitors

Increase: toxicity—radiation, bone marrow suppressants
Increase: myelosuppression—myelosuppressives
Decrease: phenytoin levels, monitor levels

Drug/Lab Test

Increase: AST, BUN, alk phos, bilirubin, creatinine
Decrease: platelets, neutrophils, WBC, RBC, Hgb/HCT, calcium, potassium, magnesium, phosphate

NURSING CONSIDERATIONS

Assess:

Black Box Warning: To only be used by person experienced in the use of chemotherapeutic products, in a specialized care setting

Black Box Warning: Bone marrow depression: CBC, differential, platelet count weekly; withhold product if neutrophil count is <2000/mm^3 or platelet count is <100,000/mm^3; notify prescriber of results; calcium, magnesium, phosphate, potassium, sodium, uric acid, CCR, bilirubin; CCr <60 ml/min may be responsible for increased bone marrow suppression; assess frequently for infection and treat active infection before use

- Renal studies: BUN, creatinine, serum uric acid; urine CCr before, during therapy; I&O ratio; report fall in urine output to <30 ml/hr
- Monitor temperature q4hr (may indicate beginning infection)
- Hepatic studies before, during therapy (bilirubin, AST, ALT, LDH) as needed or monthly; jaundice of skin, sclera; dark urine, clay-colored stools, itchy skin, abdominal pain, fever, diarrhea

Black Box Warning: Anaphylaxis: hypotension, rash, pruritus, wheezing, tachycardia may occur within a few mins of use; notify prescriber after discontinuing product; resuscitation equipment, corticosteroids, epinephrine should be available

- Delay dental work until blood counts have returned to normal; regular toothbrushes, dental floss, and toothpicks should not be used; use soft bristle toothbrush
- **Peripheral neuropathy:** may be increased in geriatric patients
- **Bleeding;** hematuria, stool guaiac, bruising, petechiae, mucosa or orifices; avoid all IM injections if platelets <50,000/mm^3
- Effects of alopecia on body image; discuss feelings about body changes

Evaluate:

- Therapeutic response: decreasing size of tumor, spread of malignancy

Teach patient/family:

- To report ringing/roaring in the ears; numbness, tingling in face, extremities; weight gain
- That impotence or amenorrhea can occur; that this is reversible after treatment is discontinued; to notify prescriber if pregnancy is suspected or planned; pregnancy (D), that contraception should be used if patient is fertile
- Not to breastfeed during treatment
- To avoid OTC products with aspirin, NSAIDs, alcohol; not to receive vaccinations during treatment

⚠ To notify prescriber immediately of fever, fatigue, sore throat, bleeding, bruising, chills, back pain, blood in stools, dyspnea

- That hair may be lost during treatment; that a wig or hairpiece may make the patient feel better; that new hair may be different in color, texture
- To avoid crowds, persons with known infections; to avoid the use of razors, stiff-bristle toothbrushes

carboprost (Rx)

(kar′boe-prost)

Hemabate

Func. class.: Oxytocic, abortifacient
Chem. class.: Prostaglandin

ACTION: Stimulates uterine contractions, causes complete abortion in approximately 16 hr

USES: Abortion at 13-20 wk gestation, postpartum hemorrhage caused by uterine atony not controlled by other methods
Unlabeled uses: Hemorrhagic cystitis

CONTRAINDICATIONS: Hypersensitivity to this product or benzyl alcohol, severe CV/respiratory/renal/hepatic disease, PID
Precautions: Pregnancy (C), asthma, anemia, jaundice, diabetes mellitus, hypo/hypertension, seizure disorders, past uterine surgery

DOSAGE AND ROUTES

Pregnancy termination between 13-20 wk gestation
- **Adult: IM** 100 mcg (0.4 ml) test dose, then 250 mcg, then 250 mcg q1½-3½hr; may increase to 500 mcg if no response, max 12 mg total dose

Postpartum hemorrhage
- **Adult: IM** 250 mcg, repeat at 15- to 90-min intervals; max total dosage 2 mg

Hemorrhagic cystitis (unlabeled)
- **Adult: INTRAVESICULAR** 0.8 mg/dl in 50 ml of saline instilled into the bladder for 60 min, q6hr × 4 doses

Available forms: Inj 250 mcg/ml
Administer:
- Only by trained personnel in a hospital that can provide emergency services
- Incomplete abortion may occur in 20% of patients
- Give antiemetics to prevent nausea/vomiting
- Store in refrigerator
- In deep muscle mass; aspirate before inj, rotate inj sites if additional doses given

SIDE EFFECTS

CNS: *Fever, chills,* headache, anxiety, weakness
GI: *Nausea, vomiting, diarrhea*
CV: Hypertension
GU: **Uterine rupture,** vaginal pain, breast tenderness
MS: Back pain, leg cramps
RESP: Wheezing
INTEG: Sweating, rash

PHARMACOKINETICS

Peak 15-60 min, duration 24 hr, excreted in urine (major metabolites)

INTERACTIONS

Increase: action—other oxytocics

NURSING CONSIDERATIONS

Assess:
- B/P, pulse; watch for change that may indicate hemorrhage
- For length, duration of contractions; notify prescriber of contractions that last more than 1 min or absence of contractions; watch for signs of uterine rupture
- For incomplete abortion, pregnancy must be terminated by another method; product is teratogenic

Evaluate:
- Therapeutic response: expulsion of fetus, control of bleeding

Teach patient/family:
- To report increased blood loss, abdominal cramps, increased temperature, foul-smelling lochia

carfilzomib

(car-fil′zoe-mib)

Kyprolis

Func. class.: Antineoplastic biologic response modifiers

Chem. class.: Signal transduction inhibitors (STIs)

ACTION: Antiproliferative and pro-apoptotic activity

USES: Multiple myeloma in those who have received ≥2 therapies (including bortezomib and immunomodulatory agents)

CONTRAINDICATIONS: Pregnancy (D), hypersensitivity

Precautions: Breastfeeding, children, cardiac disease, cardiac arrest, dysrhythmias, MI, infusion-related reactions, pulmonary/hepatic disease, edema, thrombocytopenia, neutropenia, tumor lysis syndrome

DOSAGE AND ROUTES

- **Adult: IV** 20 mg/m^2 over 2-10 min on days 1, 2, 8, 9, 15, 16, then 12 day rest (days 17-28), then may increase to 27 mg/m^2 on days 1, 2, 8, 9, 15, 16 repeated every 28 days

⚠ **Refer to package insert for dosage adjustments for treatment-related toxicity**

Available forms: Powder for injection 60 mg

Administer:

- Premedicate with dexamethasone 4 mg PO/IV before all carfilzomib 20-mg/m^2 doses during cycle 1 and before all carfilzomib 27-mg/m^2 doses in cycle 2; dexamethasone may be given in subsequent cycles if infusion-related reactions occur
- Hydration with 250-500 ml of NS or other IV fluids before each dose in cycle 1; additional hydration with 250-500 ml may be given after the carfilzomib infusion in cycle 1, continue hydration as needed
- Do not mix with other products
- Flush IV line with NS or D_5W for injection, before and after use

Reconstitution:

- Add 29 ml of sterile water for injection to the inside wall of the vial to minimize foaming (2 mg/mL); to mix, gently swirl and/or invert the vial slowly for about 1 min or until the cake or powder completely dissolves; do not shake; if foaming occurs, allow the solution to rest for 2 to 5 min or until foaming subsides; visually inspect for particulate and discoloration before use

IV injection route

- Give over 2-10 min; do not give as an IV bolus; the reconstituted sol may be stored in the vial/syringe at room temperature × 4 hr or ≤24 hr refrigerated

IV infusion route

- May further dilute in D_5W; measure and inject the correct dose from the reconstituted vial into 50 ml D_5W
- Administer IV over 2-10 min
- The diluted solution may be stored at room temperature × 4 hr or ≤24 hr refrigerated

SIDE EFFECTS

CNS: Headache, dizziness, insomnia

CV: **Heart failure**, hypertension

GI: Nausea, vomiting, dyspepsia, anorexia, diarrhea, **hepatic failure**, constipation

HEMA: **Neutropenia, thrombocytopenia**

META: Hyperglycemia, hypercalcemia, hypomagnesemia, hyponatremia, hypophosphatemia

MISC: Fatigue, infusion-related reactions

MS: Arthralgia, myalgia

PHARMACOKINETICS

Protein binding 97%

NURSING CONSIDERATIONS

Assess:

⚠ **Tumor lysis syndrome (TLS):** hydrate well; assess for hyperuricemia, hyperkalemia, hyperphosphatemia, hypocalcemia, uremia

⚠ **Hematologic toxicity** grade 3 and 4 neutropenia and thrombocytopenia; platelet nadirs occur day 8 of each 28-day cycle; counts return to baseline before the start of the next cycle; monitor blood and platelet counts frequently; hold dose for grade 3 or 4 neutropenia or grade 4 thrombocytopenia, may require dosage reduction

⚠ **Serious liver toxicity:** AST/ALT and bilirubin elevations and rare cases of fatal hepatic failure have occurred; monitor hepatic enzymes frequently; withhold doses until resolution or return to baseline in grade 3 or 4-AST/ALT or bilirubin elevations

⚠ **Serious cardiac toxicity:** fatal cardiac arrest, CHF with decreased left ventricular function/ejection fraction, myocardial ischemia, and pulmonary edema; those with NYHA class III/IV CHF, MI within 6 mo, cardiac arrhythmias (conduction abnormalities) may be at increased risk; monitor for cardiac complications; withhold doses until resolution or return to baseline for grade 3 or 4 cardiac toxicity

⚠ **Infusion-related reactions:** may occur ≤24 hr after dose; premedication with dexamethasone is recommended; assess for fever, chills, arthralgia, myalgia, facial flushing, facial edema, vomiting, weakness, shortness of breath, hypotension, syncope, chest tightness, angina

Evaluate:

• Decreased spread of multiple myeloma

Teach patient/family:

• To promptly report infusion-related symptoms (fever, chills, arthralgia, myalgia, facial flushing, facial edema, vomiting, weakness, shortness of breath, hypotension, syncope, chest tightness, angina), report renal/liver symptoms, avoid infections

carglumic acid

(kar-gloo′mik)

Carbaglu

Func. class.: Antihyperammonemic agent

ACTION: The enzyme *N*-acetylglutamate synthase (NAGS) produces *N*-acetylglutamate (NAG), which is an essential activator of carbamoyl phosphate synthetase 1 (CPS 1); CPS 1 is the first enzyme of the urea cycle, and the enzyme converts ammonia to urea; patients with NAGS deficiency do not produce enough NAG, resulting in hyperammonemia; carglumic acid is a synthetic structural analog of NAG that works to activate CPS 1 and thus convert ammonia to urea

USES: Acute or chronic hyperammonemia in persons with *N*-acetylglutamate synthetase deficiency

Precautions: Breastfeeding, pregnancy (C), geriatric patients

DOSAGE AND ROUTES

• **Adult/child:** PO 100-250 mg/kg/day (rounded to the nearest 100 mg) initially, divided; bid-qid, given immediately before meals, titrate to ammonia level; usual maintenance dose <100 mg/kg/day

Available forms: Tabs 200 mg

Administer:

• Do not give whole or crushed tablets, disperse each tab in ≥2.5 ml of water immediately before use; the tabs do not dissolve completely in water, and undissolved tab particles can remain; rinse the mixing container with water and give to the patient, do not mix with foods or other fluids

Nasogastric tube

• Mix each tab in ≥2.5 ml of water (80 mg/ml), shake gently, give the correct volume immediately through the NG tube, flush with additional water, discard any unused portion

Oral syringe

• Mix each tab in ≥2.5 ml of water (80 mg/ml), shake gently, draw up the appropriate volume in an oral syringe and give immediately, refill syringe with ≥1-2 ml and give immediately, discard any unused portion

SIDE EFFECTS

CNS: Headache, fever, asthenia
EENT: Tonsillitis, ear infections
GI: Abdominal pain, vomiting, taste change, anorexia, diarrhea
OTHER: Infection, anemia, weight loss, rash

PHARMACOKINETICS

Peak 3 hr, half-life 5.6 hr

INTERACTIONS

Drug/Lab Test
Decrease: Hgb level

NURSING CONSIDERATIONS

Assess:

Neurologic symptoms and ammonia levels: Headache, fever, change in level of consciousness
Infection: Assess for upper respiratory infections, influenza, pneumonia

Evaluate:

• Decreasing ammonia levels

Teach patient/family:

• Not to swallow whole or crush, but disperse in water
• That blood for lab tests will be drawn regularly
• To advise prescriber if pregnancy is planned or suspected, not to breastfeed
• That a high-calorie, low-protein diet is necessary when ammonia levels are elevated
• To report adverse reactions of vomiting, infection, ear pain, headache
• To store unopened containers in refrigerator; opened bottle may be stored at room temperature for up to 1 mo; product stored at controlled room temperature should not be returned to a refrigerator; protect from moisture; discard opened bottle after 30 days

carisoprodol (Rx)

(kar-eye-soe-proe′dole)

Soma

Func. class.: Skeletal muscle relaxant, central acting
Chem. class.: Meprobamate congener

Controlled Substance Schedule IV

Do not confuse:
Soma/Soma Compound

ACTION: Depresses CNS by blocking interneuronal activity in descending reticular formation, spinal cord, thereby producing sedation

USES: Relieving pain, stiffness with musculoskeletal disorders

CONTRAINDICATIONS: Hypersensitivity to these products or carbamates, intermittent porphyria
Precautions: Pregnancy (C), breastfeeding, geriatric patients, Asian patients, renal/hepatic disease, substance abuse, seizure disorder, CNS depression, abrupt discontinuation

DOSAGE AND ROUTES

• **Adult/adolescent ≥16 yr: PO** 250-350 mg tid and at bedtime, max 3 wk of use

Available forms: Tabs 250, 350 mg

Administer:

• With meals for GI symptoms
• For short term (2-3 wk), potential for habituation
• Store in tight container at room temperature

SIDE EFFECTS

CNS: *Dizziness, weakness, drowsiness,* headache, tremor, depression, insomnia, ataxia, irritability, seizures, confusion, flushing
CV: Postural hypotension, tachycardia
EENT: Diplopia, temporary loss of vision

GI: *Nausea,* vomiting, hiccups, epigastric discomfort
HEMA: Eosinophilia, pancytopenia
INTEG: Rash, pruritus, fever, facial flushing, erythema multiforme
RESP: Asthmatic attacks
SYST: Angioedema, anaphylaxis

PHARMACOKINETICS

PO: Onset ½ hr; peak 4 hr; duration 4-6 hr; extensively metabolized by liver, substrate of CYP2C19; excreted in urine; crosses placenta; excreted in breast milk (large amounts); half-life 8 hr

INTERACTIONS

- Do not use together with meprobamate

Increase: CNS depression—alcohol, tricyclics, opioids, barbiturates, sedatives, hypnotics
Increase: carisoprodol effect—CYP2C19 inhibitors (FLUoxetine, fluvoxaMINE, isoniazid, modafinil)
Decrease: carisoprodol effect—CYP219 inducers (rifampin)
Drug/Herb
Increase: CNS depression—kava, valerian
Increase: metabolism of carisoprodol—St. John's wort
Drug/Lab Test
Increase: eosinophils
Increase: RBC, WBC, platelets

NURSING CONSIDERATIONS

Assess:
- **Pain,** stiffness, mobility, activities of daily living at baseline and throughout treatment
- **ECG in seizure patients:** poor seizure control has occurred among patients taking this product
- BUN, creatinine at baseline and periodically
- **Idiosyncratic reaction:** (weakness, dizziness, blurred vision, confusion, euphoria), anaphylaxis within a few minutes or hours of 1st to 4th dose, withhold and notify prescriber
- **Allergic reactions:** rash, fever, respiratory distress, anaphylaxis, angioedema
- **CNS depression:** dizziness, drowsiness, psychiatric symptoms, abuse potential
- **Abrupt discontinuation:** withdrawal reactions do occur but may be mild, dependence may occur
- Assistance with ambulation if dizziness, drowsiness occurs, especially for geriatric patients

Evaluate:
- Therapeutic response: decreased pain, spasticity; increased ROM

Teach patient/family:
- To avoid hazardous activities if drowsiness, dizziness occur; not to drive while taking product; to avoid rapid position changes, postural hypotension occurs, not to use for >2-3 wk
- To avoid using OTC medications (cough preparations, antihistamines) unless directed by prescriber; not to take with alcohol, other CNS depressants
- **Idiosyncratic reaction:** To report weakness, dizziness, blurred vision, confusion, euphoria, if these occur, to withhold product and call prescriber
- To report allergic reaction immediately: rash, swelling of tongue/lips, hives, dyspnea
- To take with food or milk for GI symptoms

TREATMENT OF OVERDOSE:

Activated charcoal, dialysis, lavage

⚠ HIGH ALERT

carmustine (Rx)

(kar-mus′teen)

BiCNU, Gliadel

Func. class.: Antineoplastic alkylating agent
Chem. class.: Nitrosourea

ACTION: Alkylates DNA, RNA; able to inhibit enzymes that allow for the synthesis of amino acids in proteins; activity is not cell-cycle–phase specific

USES:
Brain tumors such as glioblastoma, medulloblastoma, brain stem glioma, astrocytoma, ependymoma, metastatic brain tumors; multiple myeloma (with predniSONE), non-Hodgkin's disease, Hodgkin's disease, other lymphomas; GI, breast, bronchogenic, renal carcinomas; wafer, as adjunct to surgery/radiation for patients newly diagnosed with high-grade malignant glioma

Unlabeled uses: Ablation, mycosis fungoides, stem cell transplant preparation

CONTRAINDICATIONS:
Pregnancy (D), breastfeeding, hypersensitivity, leukopenia, thrombocytopenia

Precautions: Dental disease, extravasation, females, infection, secondary malignancy, thrombocytopenia, renal disease

Black Box Warning: Bone marrow suppression, pulmonary fibrosis, bleeding, infection

DOSAGE AND ROUTES
Brain tumors, Hodgkin's disease, malignant lymphoma, multiple myeloma

- **Adult: IV** 75-100 mg/m² over 1-2 hr × 2 days or 150-200 mg/m² × 1 dose q6-8wk or 30-75 mg/m²/day 40-75 mg/m²/day × 5 days q6wk **INTRACAVITARY** up to 8 wafers inserted into resection cavity
- **Child (unlabeled): IV** 200-250 mg/m² as a single dose q4-6wk

Stem cell transplant/bone marrow ablation (unlabeled)

- **Adult: IV** 450-600 mg/m² as a single dose or 2 divided doses q12hr at a rate of no more than 3 mg/m²/min

Available forms: Powder for inj 100 mg; wafer 7.7 mg (intracavitary)

Administer:

- Store reconstituted sol in refrigerator for 24 hr or at room temperature for 8 hr; protect from light
- Blood transfusions, RBC colony-stimulating factors to counter anemia
- Antiemetic, serotonin antagonists, dexamethasone
- All medications PO, if possible; avoid IM inj if platelets are <100,000/mm³

Black Box Warning: Carmustine should not be given until platelets >100,000/mm³ and WBC >4000/mm²

Wafer route

- Use cytotoxic handling procedures
- If wafers are broken into several pieces, they should not be used
- Foil pouches may be kept at room temperature for 6 hr if unopened

Intermittent IV INFUSION route

- Use cytotoxic handling procedures; do not use if an oil film appears on vial (decomposition)
- Do not use with PVC IV tubing, do not admix
- After **diluting** 100 mg product/3 ml ethyl alcohol (provided), **further dilute** with 100-500 ml 0.9% NaCl or D_5W, **give** over 1 hr or more, reduce rate if discomfort is felt; use only glass containers, protect from light
- **Flush** IV line after carmustine with 10 ml 0.9% NaCl to prevent irritation at site

Y-site compatibilities: Amifostine, amphotericin B lipid complex, amphotericin B liposome, anidulafungin, aztreonam, bivalirudin, bleomycin, caspofungin, cefepime, codeine, DAPTOmycin, dexmedetomidine, DOCEtaxel, ertapenem, etoposide, fenoldopam, filgrastim, fludarabine, gemcitabine, granisetron, levofloxacin, melphalan, meperidine, mitoXANtrone, nesiritide, octreotide, ondansetron, PACLitaxel, palonosetron, pamidronate, pantoprazole, PEMEtrexed, piperacillin-tazobactam, riTUXimab, sargramostim, sodium acetate, tacrolimus, teniposide, thiotepa, tigecycline, tirofiban, trastuzumab, vinCRIStine, vinorelbine, voriconazole

SIDE EFFECTS
GI: *Nausea, vomiting, anorexia, stomatitis,* hepatotoxicity

GU: *Azotemia,* renal failure
HEMA: Thrombocytopenia, leukopenia, myelosuppression, anemia
INTEG: Pain, burning, hyperpigmentation at inj site, alopecia
RESP: Fibrosis, pulmonary infiltrate
SYST: Secondary malignant neoplastic disease

PHARMACOKINETICS

Degraded within 15 min; crosses blood-brain barrier; 70% excreted in urine within 96 hr; 10% excreted as CO_2, fate of 20% is unknown

INTERACTIONS

Increase: bleeding risk—aspirin, anticoagulants, platelets inhibitors
Increase: myelosuppression—myelosuppressive agents, cimetidine
Increase: toxicity: other antineoplastics, radiation, cimetidine
Increase: adverse reactions, decreased antibody reaction—live vaccines
Decrease: effects of digoxin, phenytoins

Drug/Lab Test
Increase: bilirubin, prolactin, uric acid, LFTs
Decrease: platelets, WBC, neutrophils, HCT

NURSING CONSIDERATIONS

Assess:

Black Box Warning: Bone marrow suppression: CBC, differential, platelet count weekly; withhold product if WBC is <4000 or platelet count is <100,000; notify prescriber of results

- Hepatic studies: AST, ALT, bilirubin, monitor regularly, hepatotoxicity occurs rarely

Black Box Warning: Pulmonary fibrosis/infiltrate: pulmonary function tests, chest x-ray films before, during therapy; chest film should be obtained q2wk during treatment; monitor for dyspnea, cough, pulmonary fibrosis; infiltrate occurs after high doses or several low-dose courses (>1400 mg/m^2 cumulative dose), may occur months or years after treatment

Black Box Warning: Only to be used by an experienced clinician in cases of cancer, immune suppression

- Renal studies: BUN, serum uric acid, urine CCr before, during therapy; I&O ratio; report fall in urine output of 30 ml/hr, may use allopurinol for hyperuricemia with increased fluids
- Monitor for cold, cough, fever (may indicate beginning infection)
- **Bleeding:** hematuria, guaiac, bruising, petechiae, mucosa, orifices q8hr
- Rinsing of mouth tid-qid with water or club soda; use of sponge brush for stomatitis
- Warm compresses at inj site for inflammation; reduce flow rate if patient complains of burning at infusion site

Evaluate:
- Therapeutic response: decreasing size of tumor, spread of malignancy

Teach patient/family:

Black Box Warning: To report any changes in breathing or coughing; to avoid smoking

- To avoid foods with citric acid, hot or rough texture if stomatitis is present; to report any bleeding, white spots, ulceration in mouth to prescriber; to examine mouth daily
- To avoid aspirin, ibuprofen, razors, commercial mouthwash
- To report signs of anemia (fatigue, irritability, shortness of breath, faintness); to report signs of infection (sore throat, fever); pulmonary toxicity can occur up to 15 yr after treatment

- To use contraception during treatment; to avoid breastfeeding, pregnancy (D)
- Not to receive live vaccines during treatment
- Infusion can be painful to veins and product contains ethanol, report chest pain

carteolol (ophthalmic)

(kar′tee-oh-lol)

Func. class.: Antiglaucoma

Chem. class.: β-Blocker

ACTION: May decrease aqueous humor and increase outflows

USES: Treatment of chronic open-angle glaucoma and ocular hypertension

CONTRAINDICATIONS: Hypersensitivity, AV block, heart failure, bradycardia, sick sinus syndrome

Precautions: Abrupt discontinuation, children, pregnancy, breastfeeding, COPD, depression, diabetes mellitus, myasthenia gravis, hyperthyroidism, pulmonary disease, angle-closure glaucoma

DOSAGE AND ROUTES

- **Adult:** Instill 1 drop in the affected eye(s) bid

Available forms: Ophthalmic solution 1%

Administer:

- For ophthalmic use only
- Do not touch the tip of the dropper to the eye, fingertips, or other surface to prevent contamination
- Wash hands before and after use; tilt head back slightly and pull the lower eyelid down with the index finger; squeeze the prescribed number of drops into the pouch; close eyes to spread; to avoid excessive systemic absorption, apply finger pressure on the lacrimal sac for 1-2 min after use
- If more than one topical ophthalmic drug product is being used, the drugs should be administered at least 5 min apart
- Decreased intraocular pressure can take several weeks; monitor IOP after 1 mo

SIDE EFFECTS

CNS: Insomnia, headache, dizziness

CV: Palpitations

EENT: Eye stinging/burning, tearing, photophobia, sinusitis

INTERACTIONS

Increase: β-blocking effect—oral β-blockers

Increased: intraocular pressure reduction—topical miotics, dipivefrin, EPINEPHrine, carbonic anhydrase inhibitors, this may be beneficial

Increase: B/P, severe—when abruptly stopping cloNIDine

Increase: depression of AV nodal conduction, bradycardia, or hypotension—adenosine, cardiac glycosides, disopyramide, other antiarrhythmics, class 1C antiarrhythmic drugs (flecainide, propafenone, moricizine, encainide, quiNIDine or drugs that significantly depress AV nodal conduction)

Increase: AV block nodal conduction, induce AV block—high doses of procainamide

Increase: antihypertensive effect—other antihypertensives

NURSING CONSIDERATIONS

Assess:

- **Systemic absorption:** when used in the eye, systemic absorption is common with the same adverse reactions and interactions
- Glaucoma: monitor intraocular pressure

Evaluate:

- Decreasing intraocular pressure

Teach patient/family:

- For ophthalmic use only
- Not to touch the tip of the dropper to the eye, fingertips, or other surface to prevent contamination
- To wash hands before and after use; tilt the head back slightly and pull the lower eyelid down with the index finger to form

a pouch; squeeze the prescribed number of drops into the pouch; close eyes to spread drops; to avoid excessive systemic absorption, apply finger pressure on the lacrimal sac for 1-2 min following use
• If more than one topical ophthalmic drug product is being used, the drugs should be administered at least 5 min apart

carvedilol (Rx)

(kar-ved′i-lole)

Coreg, Coreg CR

Func. class.: Antihypertensive, α-/β-adrenergic blocker

Do not confuse:
carvedilol/captopril/carteolol

ACTION: A mixture of nonselective α-/β-adrenergic blocking activity; decreases cardiac output, exercise-induced tachycardia, reflex orthostatic tachycardia; causes vasodilation, reduction in peripheral vascular resistance

USES: Essential hypertension alone or in combination with other antihypertensives, CHF, LV dysfunction after MI, cardiomyopathy

Unlabeled uses: Angina, pediatric patients, atrial fibrillation/flutter

CONTRAINDICATIONS: Hypersensitivity, asthma, class IV decompensated cardiac failure, 2nd- or 3rd-degree heart block, cardiogenic shock, severe bradycardia, pulmonary edema, severe hepatic disease, sick sinus symptoms

Precautions: Pregnancy (C), breastfeeding, children, geriatric patients, cardiac failure, hepatic injury, peripheral vascular disease, anesthesia, major surgery, diabetes mellitus, thyrotoxicosis, emphysema, chronic bronchitis, renal disease

Black Box Warning: Abrupt discontinuation

DOSAGE AND ROUTES

Essential hypertension

• **Adult: PO** 6.25 mg bid × 7-14 days; if tolerated well, then increase to 12.5 mg bid × 7-14 days; if tolerated well, may be increased (if needed) to 25 mg bid; not to exceed 50 mg/day; **EXT REL** cap 20 mg/day, may increase after 7-14 days to 40 mg/day, max 80 mg/day

Congestive heart failure

• **Adult: PO** 3.125 mg bid × 2 wk; if tolerated well, give 6.25 mg bid × 2 wk, then double q2wk to max dose of 25 mg bid <85 kg or 50 mg bid >85 kg; **EXT REL** caps (Coreg CR) 10 mg/day × 2 wk, increase to 20, 40, 80 mg/day over successive intervals of 2 wk

Postmyocardial infarction

• **Adult: PO** 6.25 mg bid with food × 3-10 days, lower starting dose may be used if indicated; titrate upward as tolerated; may increase to 12.5 mg bid, then titrate to 25 mg bid; **PO EXT REL** 20 mg daily with food, lower starting dose of 10 mg/day may be used, titrate upward after 3-10 days, increase to 40 mg daily as required

Angina (unlabeled)

• **Adult: PO** 25-50 mg bid

Available forms: Tabs 3.125, 6.25, 12.5, 25 mg; ext rel cap 10, 20, 40, 80 mg

Administer:

• With food to minimize orthostatic hypotension; tabs may be crushed or swallowed whole; give ext rel every AM with food; do not break, crush, chew ext rel cap; separate alcohol (including OTC products that contain ethanol) by ≥2 hr; caps may be opened and sprinkled over applesauce

Black Box Warning: Do not discontinue before surgery

SIDE EFFECTS

CNS: *Dizziness, fatigue,* weakness, somnolence, insomnia, ataxia, hyperesthesia, paresthesia, vertigo, depression, headache

CV: Bradycardia, *postural hypotension,* dependent edema, *peripheral edema,* AV block, extrasystoles, hypo/hypertension, palpitations, peripheral ischemia, CHF, pulmonary edema
GI: *Diarrhea,* abdominal pain, increased alk phos, ALT, AST, nausea, vomiting
GU: Decreased libido, *impotence,* UTI
INTEG: Rash, Stevens-Johnson syndrome
MISC: Injury, back pain, viral infection, hypertriglyceridemia, thrombocytopenia, *hyperglycemia,* abnormal weight gain, aplastic anemia
RESP: Rhinitis, pharyngitis, dyspnea, bronchospasm, cough, lung edema

PHARMACOKINETICS

Peak 1-2 hr; duration 7-9 hr; ext rel onset 30 min, peak 5 hr, readily and extensively absorbed PO; >98% protein binding; extensively metabolized by liver; excreted through bile into feces; terminal half-life 7-10 hr with increases in geriatric patients, hepatic disease

INTERACTIONS

Increase: conduction disturbances—calcium channel blockers
Increase: bradycardia, hypotension—levodopa, MAOIs, reserpine
Increase: hypoglycemia—antidiabetic agents
Increase: concentrations of digoxin, cycloSPORINE, CYP2D6 inhibitors (FLUoxetine, quiNIDine)
Increase: toxicity of carvedilol—cimetidine, other antihypertensives, nitrates, acute alcohol ingestion
Decrease: heart rate, B/P—cloNIDine
Decrease: carvedilol levels—rifampin, NSAIDs, thyroid medications

Drug/Herb
Increase: antihypertensive effect—hawthorn
Decrease: antihypertensive effect—ephedra (ma huang)

Drug/Lab Test
Increase: blood glucose, BUN, potassium, triglycerides, uric acid, bilirubin, cholesterol, creatinine, LFTs
Decrease: sodium, HDL

NURSING CONSIDERATIONS

Assess:

- **Hypertension:** B/P when beginning treatment, periodically thereafter; pulse: note rate, rhythm, quality; apical/radial pulse before administration; notify prescriber of significant changes
- **CHF:** edema in feet, legs daily; fluid overload: dyspnea, weight gain, jugular venous distention, fatigue, crackles

Evaluate:

- Therapeutic response: decreased B/P with hypertension; decrease anginal pain

Teach patient/family:

- To comply with dosage schedule even if feeling better; that improvement may take several weeks
- To rise slowly to sitting or standing position to minimize orthostatic hypotension
- To report bradycardia, dizziness, confusion, depression, fever, weight gain, SOB, cold extremities, rash, sore throat, bleeding, bruising
- To weigh, take pulse, B/P at home; to advise if weight gain of >2 lb/day or 5 lb/wk and when to notify prescriber

Black Box Warning: Not to discontinue product abruptly; to taper over 1-2 wk; life-threatening dysrhythmias may occur

- To avoid hazardous activities until stabilized on medication; dizziness may occur
- To avoid all OTC medications unless approved by prescriber
- To carry emergency ID with product name, prescriber information at all times
- To inform all health care providers of products, supplements taken
- To report if pregnancy is planned or suspected, pregnancy (C), avoid breastfeeding
- That product may mask hypoglycemia

caspofungin (Rx)

(cas-po-fun′gin)

Cancidas

Func. class.: Antifungal, systemic

Chem. class.: Echinocandin

ACTION: Inhibits an essential component in fungal cell walls; causes direct damage to fungal cell wall

USES: Treatment of invasive aspergillosis and candidemia that has not responded to other treatment, including peritonitis, intraabdominal abscesses; susceptible species: *Aspergillus flavus, A. fumigatus, A. terreus, Candida albicans, C. glabrata, C. krusei, C. lusitaniae, C. parapsilosis, C. tropicalis,* esophageal candidiasis; empirical therapy for presumed fungal infection in febrile, neutropenic patients

Unlabeled uses: *Aspergillus niger,* fungal infections in premature neonates, neonates, infants, children <2 yr

CONTRAINDICATIONS: Hypersensitivity

Precautions: Pregnancy (C), breastfeeding, children, geriatric patients, severe hepatic disease

DOSAGE AND ROUTES

- **Adult: IV** loading dose 70 mg on day 1, then 50 mg/day maintenance dose, depending on condition; max 70 mg/day
- **Adolescent/child/infant ≥3 mo: IV INFUSION** 70 mg/m² loading dose, then 50 mg/m²/day; max 70 mg/day
- **Neonate and infant <3 mo (unlabeled): IV** 25 mg/m²/day

Esophageal candidiasis

- **Adult: IV** 50 mg × 7-14 days over 1 hr
- **Child:** 3 mo-17 yr: **IV** 70 mg/m² loading dose, then 50 mg/m² daily; max 70 mg/m²

Available forms: Powder for inj 50, 70 mg

Administer:

- Do not mix or confuse with other medications, do not use dextrose-containing products to dilute, do not give as bolus
- Store at room temperature for up to 24 hr or refrigerated for 48 hr; store reconstituted sol at room temperature for 1 hr before preparation of sol for administration

Intermittent IV INFUSION route

- Allow to warm to room temperature
- May administer loading dose on day 1
- **Reconstitute** 50-mg vial or 70-mg vial with 10.8 ml 0.9% NaCl, sterile water for inj or bacteriostatic water for inj (5 mg/ml or 7 mg/ml), respectively; **swirl** to dissolve, withdraw 10 ml reconstituted sol, and **further dilute** with 250 ml 0.9% NaCl, 0.45% NaCl, 0.225% NaCl, RL; **run** over 1 hr or more

SIDE EFFECTS

CNS: Dizziness, *headache,* fever, chills

CV: Sinus tachycardia, hypertension

GI: Abdominal pain, *nausea, anorexia, vomiting, diarrhea, increased AST/ALT, alk phos*

GU: Renal failure

HEMA: Thrombophlebitis, vasculitis, anemia

INTEG: *Rash, pruritus, inj site pain*

META: Hypokalemia

MS: Myalgia

RESP: Acute respiratory distress syndrome (ARDS), pleural effusions

SYST: Anaphylaxis, histamine-related reactions, Stevens-Johnson syndrome

PHARMACOKINETICS

Metabolized in liver to inactive metabolites; excretion in feces, urine; phase II terminal half-life 9-11 hr; phase III terminal half-life 40-50 hr; protein binding 97%

INTERACTIONS

Increase: caspofungin levels—cycloSPORINE; may need dosage reduction

Decrease: levels of tacrolimus, sirolimus

Decrease: caspofungin levels—carBAMazepine, dexamethasone, efavirenz, nelfinavir, nevirapine, phenytoin, rifampin

Drug/Lab Test

Increase: AST, ALT, RBC, eosinophils, glucose, bilirubin

Decrease: HCT/Hgb, WBC, potassium, magnesium

NURSING CONSIDERATIONS

Assess:

- **Infection;** clearing of cultures during treatment; obtain culture at baseline, throughout treatment; product may be started as soon as culture is taken (esophageal candidiasis); monitor cultures during HSCT for prevention of *Candida* infections
- Blood studies before, during treatment: bilirubin, AST, ALT, alk phos, as needed; obtain baseline renal studies; CBC with differential, serum potassium
- **Hypersensitivity:** rash, pruritus, facial swelling; also for phlebitis; anaphylaxis (rare)
- GI symptoms: frequency of stools, cramping; if severe diarrhea occurs, electrolytes may need to be given

Evaluate:

- Therapeutic response: decreased symptoms of *Candida, Aspergillus* infections

Teach patient/family:

- To notify prescriber if pregnancy is suspected or planned
- To inform prescriber of renal/hepatic disease
- To report bleeding, facial swelling, wheezing, difficulty breathing, itching, rash, hives, increasing warmth, flushing; anaphylaxis can occur

cefaclor

See cephalosporins—2nd generation

cefadroxil
ceFAZolin

See cephalosporins—1st generation

cefdinir
cefditoren pivoxil
cefepime
cefixime
cefotaxime

See cephalosporins—3rd generation

cefoTEtan
cefOXitin

See cephalosporins—2nd generation

cefpodoxime

See cephalosporins—3rd generation

cefprozil

See cephalosporins—2nd generation

cefTAZidime
ceftibuten
ceftizoxime
cefTRIAXone

See cephalosporins—3rd generation

cefuroxime

See cephalosporins—2nd generation

ceftaroline (Rx)

(sef-tar′oh-leen)

Teflaro

Func. class.: Cephalosporin action: Inhibits cell wall synthesis through binding to essential penicillin-binding protein (PBP)

USES: Acute bacterial skin/skin structure infections (ABSSI), bacterial community-acquired pneumonia

CONTRAINDICATIONS:
Cephalosporin hypersensitivity

Precautions: Child/infant/neonate, breastfeeding, elderly patients, antimicrobial resistance, carbapenem/penicillin hypersensitivity, coagulopathy, colitis, dialysis, diarrhea, GI disease, hypoprothrombinemia, IBS, pregnancy (B), pseudomembranous colitis, renal disease, ulcerative colitis, viral infection, vit K deficiency

DOSAGE AND ROUTES

- **Adult: IV** 600 mg q12hr × 5-14 days (skin/skin-structure infections) or × 5-7 days (bacterial community-acquired pneumonia)

Renal dose

- **Adult: IV** CCr >30-≤50 ml/min, 400 mg q12hr; CCr ≥15-≤30 ml/min, 300 mg q12hr, CCr <15 ml/min, 200 mg q12hr

Available forms: Powder for inj 400 mg, 600 mg

Administer:

- Obtain culture specimen before use
- Identify allergies before use

Intermittent IV INFUSION route

- Visually inspect for particulate matter, discoloration
- **Reconstitute:** add 20 mg of sterile water to 400- or 600-mg vial (20 mg/ml for 400 mg; 30 mg/ml for 600 mg), mix gently until dissolved; **dilute** in 250 ml of 0.9% NaCl, 0.45% NaCl, LR, D_5W, dextrose 2.5%, **give** over 1 hr, do not admix, use within 6 hr at room temperature or 24 hr refrigerated

SIDE EFFECTS

CNS: Dizziness, **seizures**

CV: **Phlebitis, palpitations, bradycardia**

ENDO: Hypo/hyperkalemia

GI: Diarrhea, nausea, vomiting, constipation, abdominal pain, **pseudomembranous colitis (rare)**

HEMA: **Thrombocytopenia, neutropenia,** anemia, eosinophilia

INTEG: Rash, **anaphylaxis**

GU: **Renal failure**

META: Hypokalemia, **hyperkalemia,** hyperglycemia

PHARMACOKINETICS

Protein binding 20%; excreted in urine 88%, feces 6%; half-life 1.6 hr; not hepatically metabolized

INTERACTIONS

Increase: prothrombin time risk—anticoagulants

Drug/Lab Test

Increase: LFTs, glucose, potassium

Decrease: potassium, eosinophils, platelets

NURSING CONSIDERATIONS

Assess:

- **Infection:** vital signs, sputum, WBC before, during therapy
- **Hypersensitivity: before use, obtain a history of hypersensitivity reactions to cephalosporins, carbapenems, penicillins; cross-sensitivity may occur**
- **Anaphylaxis (rare): rash, pruritus, laryngeal edema, dyspnea, wheezing; discontinue product, notify health care provider immediately, keep emergency equipment nearby**
- **Pseudomembranous colitis: diarrhea, abdominal pain, fever, bloody stools; report immediately if these occur; may occur several weeks after terminating therapy**
- Monitor BUN, creatinine baseline, periodically; elderly and those with renal disease are at greater risk of renal dysfunction

Evaluate:

- Therapeutic response: negative C&S, resolution of symptoms of infection

Teach patient/family:

- About the reason for treatment and expected result
- **To immediately report rash, itching, difficulty breathing, bloody diarrhea, fever, abdominal pain**

⚠ HIGH ALERT

celecoxib (Rx)

(sel-eh-cox′ib)

CeleBREX

Func. class.: Nonsteroidal antiinflammatory, antirheumatic

Chem. class.: COX-2 inhibitor

Do not confuse:
CeleBREX/CeleXA/Cerebra/Cerebyx

ACTION: Inhibits prostaglandin synthesis by selectively inhibiting cyclooxygenase-2 (COX-2), an enzyme needed for biosynthesis

USES: Acute, chronic rheumatoid arthritis, osteoarthritis, acute pain, primary dysmenorrhea, ankylosing spondylitis, juvenile rheumatoid arthritis (JRA)
Unlabeled uses: Colorectal adenoma prophylaxis

CONTRAINDICATIONS: Pregnancy (D) 3rd trimester; hypersensitivity to salicylates, iodides, other NSAIDs, sulfonamides, severe hepatic impairment

Black Box Warning: For perioperative pain in CABG

Precautions: Pregnancy (C) 1st/2nd trimesters, breastfeeding, children <18 yr, geriatric patients, bleeding, GI/renal/hepatic/cardiac disorders, PVD, hypertension, severe dehydration, asthma

Black Box Warning: GI bleeding/perforation, peptic ulcer disease, MI, stroke

DOSAGE AND ROUTES

Do not exceed recommended dose; deaths have occurred

Acute pain/primary dysmenorrhea
- **Adult: PO** 400 mg initially, then 200 mg if needed on 1st day, then 200 mg bid prn on subsequent days; start with ½ dose for poor CYP2C9 metabolizers

Osteoarthritis
- **Adult: PO** 200 mg/day as a single dose or 100 mg bid; start with ½ dose for poor CYP2C9 metabolizers
- **Geriatric: PO** use lowest possible dose

Rheumatoid arthritis
- **Adult: PO** 100-200 mg bid; start with ½ dose for poor CYP2C9 metabolizers

Ankylosing spondylitis
- **Adult: PO** 200 mg/day or in divided doses (bid); start with ½ dose for poor CYP2C9 metabolizers

Juvenile rheumatoid arthritis (JRA)
- **Adolescent and child ≥2 yr (>25 kg): PO** 100 mg bid; start with ½ dose for poor CYP2C9 metabolizers
- **Child ≥2 yr (10-25 kg): PO** 50 mg bid; start with ½ dose for poor CYP2C9 metabolizers

Hepatic disease
- **Adult: PO** (Child-Pugh B) reduce dose by 50%; (Child-Pugh C) do not use

Colorectal adenoma prophylaxis (unlabeled)
- **Adult: PO** 200-400 mg bid for up to 3 yr

Available forms: Caps 50, 100, 200, 400 mg

Administer:
- Do not break, crush, chew, or dissolve caps; give with a full glass of water to enhance absorption; caps may be opened into applesauce or soft food, ingest immediately with water
- With food, milk to decrease gastric symptoms (with higher doses [400 mg bid]); do not increase dose

SIDE EFFECTS

CNS: *Fatigue, anxiety, depression, nervousness, paresthesia,* dizziness, insomnia, headache

CV: Stroke, MI, tachycardia, CHF, angina, palpitations, dysrhythmias, hypertension, fluid retention

EENT: Tinnitus, hearing loss, blurred vision, glaucoma, cataract, conjunctivitis, eye pain

GI: Nausea, anorexia, vomiting, constipation, dry mouth, diverticulitis, gastritis, gastroenteritis, hemorrhoids, hiatal hernia, stomatitis, **GI bleeding/ulceration**
GU: **Nephrotoxicity:** *dysuria,* **hematuria, azotemia,** cystitis, UTI, **renal papillary necrosis**
HEMA: **Blood dyscrasias,** epistaxis, anemia
INTEG: **Serious (sometimes fatal) Stevens-Johnson syndrome, toxic epidermal necrolysis,** purpura, rash, pruritus, sweating, erythema, petechiae, photosensitivity, alopecia, bruising, hot flashes
RESP: Pharyngitis, SOB, pneumonia, coughing

PHARMACOKINETICS

Well absorbed, crosses placenta, bound to plasma proteins, metabolized by CYP2C9 in liver, very little excreted by kidneys/in feces, peak 3 hr, half-life 11 hr, protein binding ~97%

INTERACTIONS

Increase: bleeding risk—anticoagulants, SSRIs, antiplatelets, thrombolytics, salicylates, alcohol
Increase: adverse reactions—glucocorticoids, NSAIDs, aspirin
Increase: toxicity—lithium, antineoplastics, bisphosphonates, cidofovir
Increase: celecoxib blood level—fluconazole
Decrease: effect of aspirin, ACE inhibitors, thiazide diuretics, furosemide
Drug/Herb
Decrease: effect of feverfew
Increase: bleeding risk—garlic, ginger, ginkgo
Drug/Lab Test
Increase: ALT, AST, BUN, cholesterol, glucose, potassium, sodium
Decrease: glucose, sodium, WBC, platelets

NURSING CONSIDERATIONS

Assess:

- **Pain** of rheumatoid arthritis, osteoarthritis; check ROM, inflammation of joints, characteristics of pain

Black Box Warning: For cardiac disease that may be worse after taking product; MI, stroke; do not use with coronary artery bypass graft (CABG)

- CBC during therapy; watch for decreasing platelets; if low, therapy may need to be discontinued, restarted after hematologic recovery; LFTs, serum creatinine/BUN, stool guaiac

Black Box Warning: For blood dyscrasias (thrombocytopenia): bruising, fatigue, bleeding, poor healing

- **GI toxicity:** black, tarry stools; abdominal pain
- ⚠ **Serious skin disorders:** Stevens-Johnson syndrome, toxic epidermal necrolysis; may be fatal

Evaluate:

- Therapeutic response: decreased pain, inflammation in arthritic conditions; decreased number of polyps

Teach patient/family:

Black Box Warning: Not to exceed recommended dose; to notify prescriber immediately of chest pain, skin eruptions; to stop product if these occur

- To check with prescriber to determine when product should be discontinued before surgery
- That product must be continued for prescribed time to be effective; to avoid other NSAIDs, aspirin, sulfonamides

Black Box Warning: To notify prescriber of GI symptoms: black, tarry stools; cramping or rash; edema of extremities; weight gain

Black Box Warning: To report bleeding, bruising, fatigue, malaise because blood abnormalities do occur

- **To report possible respiratory infection: fever, SOB, coughing, painful swallowing**

• To report if pregnancy is planned or suspected, pregnancy (C) before 30 wk, (D) after 30 wk

cephalexin
See cephalosporins—1st generation

CEPHALOSPORINS—1ST GENERATION

cefadroxil (Rx)
(sef-a-drox′ill)
ceFAZolin (Rx)
(sef-a′zoe-lin)
cephalexin (Rx)
(sef-a-lex′in)
Keflex, Panixine
Func. class.: Antiinfective
Chem. class.: Cephalosporin (1st generation)

Do not confuse:
cephalexin/cefaclor

ACTION: Inhibits bacterial cell wall synthesis; renders cell wall osmotically unstable, leads to cell death; lysis mediated by cell wall autolytic enzymes

USES: **cefadroxil:** Gram-negative bacilli: *Escherichia coli, Proteus mirabilis, Klebsiella* (UTI only); gram-positive organisms: *Streptococcus pneumoniae, Streptococcus pyogenes, Staphylococcus aureus;* upper, lower respiratory tract, urinary tract, skin infections; otitis media; tonsillitis; UTIs
ceFAZolin: Gram-negative bacilli: *Haemophilus influenzae, Escherichia coli, Proteus mirabilis, Klebsiella, pneumonial;* gram-positive organisms: *Staphylococcus aureus/epidermidis;* upper, lower respiratory tract, urinary tract, skin infections; bone, joint, biliary, genital infections; endocarditis, surgical prophylaxis, septicemia; *Streptococcus Sp.*
cephalexin: Gram-negative bacilli: *Haemophilus influenzae, Escherichia coli, Proteus mirabilis, Klebsiella pneumoniae;* gram-positive organisms: *Streptococcus pneumoniae, Streptococcus pyogenes, Streptococcus agalactial, Staphylococcus aureus;* upper, lower respiratory tract, urinary tract, skin, bone infections; otitis media

CONTRAINDICATIONS: Hypersensitivity to cephalosporins, infants <1 mo
Precautions: Pregnancy (B), breastfeeding, hypersensitivity to penicillins, renal disease

DOSAGE AND ROUTES
cefadroxil
• **Adult: PO** 1-2 g/day or divided q12hr; loading dose of 1 g initially
• **Child: PO** 30 mg/kg/day in divided doses bid, max 2 g/day
Renal dose
• **Adult: PO** CCr 25-50 ml/min, 1 g, then 500 mg q12hr; CCr 10-24 ml/min, 1 g, then 500 mg q24hr; CCr <10 ml/min, 1 g, then 500 mg q36hr
Available forms: Caps 500 mg; tabs 1 g; oral susp 250, 500 mg/5 ml

ceFAZolin
Surgical prophylaxis
• **Adult: IM/IV** 1 g 30-60 min before surgery, then 0.5-1 g q6-8hr × 24 hr
Life-threatening infections
• **Adult: IM/IV** 1-2 g q6-8hr; max 12 g/day
• **Child >1 mo: IM/IV** 75-100 mg/kg/day in 3-4 divided doses; max 6 g/day
Mild/moderate infections
• **Adult: IM/IV** 250 mg-1 g q8hr, max 12 g/day
• **Child >1 mo: IM/IV** 50 mg/kg in 3-4 equal doses, max 6 g/day, or 2 g as a single dose
Renal dose
• **Adult: IM/IV** after loading dose, CCr 35-54 ml/min, dose q8hr; CCr 10-34 ml/min, 50% of dose q12hr; CCr <10 ml/min, 50% of dose q18-24hr

• **Child: IM/IV** CCr >70 ml/min, no dosage adjustment; CCr 40-70 ml/min after loading dose, reduce dose to 7.5-30 mg/kg q12hr; CCr 20-39 ml/min, give 3.125-12.5 mg/kg after loading dose q12hr; CCr 5-19 ml/min, 2.5-10 mg/kg after loading dose q24hr

Available forms: Inj 500 mg, 1, 10, 20 g; infusion 500 mg, 1 g/50-ml, 500 mg/50 ml vial

cephalexin

Moderate infections

• **Adult: PO** 250-500 mg q6hr, max 4 g/day

• **Child: PO** 25-100 mg/kg/day in 4 equal doses, max 4 g/day

Moderate skin infections

• **Adult: PO** 500 mg q12hr

Endocarditis prophylaxis

• 2 g 1 hr before procedure

Severe infections

• **Adult: PO** 500 mg-1 g q6hr, max 4 g

• **Child: PO** 50-100 mg/kg/day in 4 equal doses, max 4 g/day

Community-acquired pneumonia (unlabeled)

• **Child:** >3 mo **PO** 75-100 mg/kg/day divided in 3 or 4 doses × 10 days

Renal dose

• **Adult: PO** CCr 10-40 ml/min, 250-500 mg then 250-500 mg q8-12hr; CCr <10 ml/min, 250-500 mg, then 250 mg q12-24hr

Available forms: Caps 250, 500, 750 mg; tabs 250, 500 mg; oral susp 125 mg, 250 mg/5 ml

Administer:

cefadroxil

• For prescribed time to ensure organism death, prevent superinfection

• With food if needed for GI symptoms

• Shake susp, refrigerate, discard after 2 wk

• Identify allergies before use

• After C&S specimen is obtained

ceFAZolin

• Obtain C&S specimen before use

• Identify allergies before use

IV route

• Check for irritation, extravasation often; dilute in 2 ml/500 mg or 2.5 ml/1 g sterile water for inj, inject over 3-5 min; may be further diluted with 50-100 ml of NS, D_5W sol, run over 10 min-1 hr by Y-tube or 3-way stopcock

• After C&S completed

Y-site compatibilities: Acyclovir, alfentanil, allopurinol, alprostadil, amifostine, amikacin, aminocaproic acid, aminophylline, amphotericin B liposome, anidulafungin, ascorbic acid injection, atenolol, atracurium, atropine, aztreonam, benztropine, bivalirudin, bleomycin, bumetanide, buprenorphine, butorphanol, calcium gluconate, CARBOplatin, cefamandole, cefmetazole, cefonicid, cefoTEtan, cefOXitin, cefpirome, cefTAZidime, ceftizoxime, cefTRIAXone, cefuroxime, chloramphenicol, cimetidine, CISplatin, clindamycin, codeine, cyanocobalamin, cyclophosphamide, cycloSPORINE, cytarabine, DACTINomycin, DAPTOmycin, dexamethasone, dexmedetomidine, digoxin, diltiazem, DOCEtaxel, doxacurium, doxapram, DOXOrubicin liposomal, enalaprilat, ePHEDrine, EPINEPHrine, epirubicin, epoetin alfa, eptifibatide, esmolol, etoposide, fenoldopam, fentaNYL, filgrastim, fluconazole, fludarabine, fluorouracil, folic acid (as sodium salt), foscarnet, furosemide, gallium, gatifloxacin, gemcitabine, gentamicin, glycopyrrolate, granisetron, heparin, hydrocortisone, hydrOXYzine, IDArubicin, ifosfamide, imipenem-cilastatin, indomethacin, insulin (regular), irinotecan, isoproterenol, ketorolac, lidocaine, linezolid, LORazepam, LR's injection, mannitol, mechlorethamine, melphalan, meperidine, methotrexate, methyldopate, methylPREDNISolone, metoclopramide, metoprolol, metroNIDAZOLE, miconazole, midazolam, milrinone, morphine, moxalactam, multiple vitamins injection, nafcillin, nalbuphine, naloxone, nesiritide, niCARdipine, nitroglycerin, nitroprusside, norepinephrine, octreotide, ondansetron, oxacillin, oxaliplatin, oxytocin, PACLitaxel, palonosetron, pamidronate, pancuronium, pantoprazole, penicillin G potassium/sodium, peritoneal dialysis solution, perphenazine, PHENobarbital, phenylephrine, phytonadione, piperacillin, Plasma-Lyte M in dextrose 5%, polymyxin B, potassium chloride, procainamide, propofol, propranolol, ranitidine, remifentanil, Ringer's injection, ritodrine, riTUXimab, sargramostim, sodium acetate, sodium bicarbonate, succinylcholine, SUFentanil, tacrolimus, teniposide, tenoxicam, theophylline, thiamine, thiotepa, ticarcillin, ticarcillin-clavulanate, tigecycline, tirofiban, TNA, tolazoline, trastuzumab, trimetaphan, urokinase, vasopressin, vecuronium, verapamil, vinCRIStine, vitamin B complex with C, voriconazole, warfarin, zoledronic acid

cephalexin

- Shake susp, refrigerate, discard after 2 wk; use calibrated oral syringe, spoon, or measuring cup
- With food if needed for GI symptoms
- After C&S specimen is obtained
- Identify allergies before use

SIDE EFFECTS

CNS: Headache, dizziness, weakness, paresthesia, fever, chills, seizures (with high doses)

GI: Nausea, vomiting, *diarrhea, anorexia,* pain, glossitis, bleeding; increased AST, ALT, bilirubin, LDH, alk phos; abdominal pain, pseudomembranous colitis

GU: Proteinuria, vaginitis, pruritus, candidiasis, increased BUN, nephrotoxicity, renal failure

HEMA: Leukopenia, thrombocytopenia, agranulocytosis, anemia, neutropenia, lymphocytosis, eosinophilia, pancytopenia, hemolytic anemia

INTEG: Rash, urticaria, dermatitis

MS: Arthralgia, arthritis

RESP: Dyspnea

SYST: Anaphylaxis, serum sickness, superinfection, Stevens-Johnson syndrome

PHARMACOKINETICS

cefadroxil: Peak 1-1½ hr, duration 12-24 hr, half-life 1-2 hr, 20% bound by plasma proteins, crosses placenta, excreted in breast milk

ceFAZolin

IV: Peak 10 min, duration 6-12 hr, eliminated unchanged in urine, 75%-85% protein bound

IM: Peak 1-2 hr, duration 6-12 hr, half-life 1½-2 hr

cephalexin: Peak 1 hr, duration 6-12 hr, half-life 30-72 min, 5%-15% bound by plasma proteins, 80%-100% eliminated unchanged in urine, crosses placenta, excreted in breast milk

INTERACTIONS

Increase: prothrombin time—anticoagulants; use cautiously

Increase: toxicity—aminoglycosides, loop diuretics, probenecid

Decrease: oral contraceptives possible, use another form of contraception

Drug/Lab Test

Increase: AST, ALT, alk phos, LDH, BUN, creatinine, bilirubin

False positive: urinary protein, direct Coombs' test, urine glucose

Interference: cross-matching

NURSING CONSIDERATIONS

Assess:

- Sensitivity to penicillin and other cephalosporins

⚠ **Nephrotoxicity**: increased BUN, creatinine; urine output: if decreasing, notify prescriber

- I&O daily
- Blood studies: AST, ALT, CBC, Hct, bilirubin, LDH, alk phos, Coombs' test monthly if patient is on long-term therapy
- Electrolytes: potassium, sodium, chlorine monthly if patient is on long-term therapy
- **Pseudomembranous colitis:** bowel pattern daily; if severe diarrhea occurs, product should be discontinued

⚠ **Anaphylaxis:** rash, urticaria, pruritus, chills, fever, joint pain; angioedema; may occur a few days after therapy begins;

discontinue product, notify prescriber immediately, keep emergency equipment nearby

• Bleeding: ecchymosis, bleeding gums, hematuria, stool guaiac daily

⚠ **Overgrowth of infection:** perineal itching, fever, malaise, redness, pain, swelling, drainage, rash, diarrhea, change in cough, sputum

Evaluate:

• Therapeutic response: decreased symptoms of infection, negative C&S

Teach patient/family:

• To use yogurt or buttermilk to maintain intestinal flora, decrease diarrhea

• To take all medication prescribed for length of time ordered

⚠ To report sore throat, bruising, bleeding, joint pain (may indicate **blood dyscrasias** [rare]); diarrhea with mucus, blood (may indicate **pseudomembranous colitis**)

TREATMENT OF ANAPHYLAXIS: EPINEPHrine, antihistamines; resuscitate if needed

C

CEPHALOSPORINS—2ND GENERATION

cefaclor (Rx)

(sef′a-klor)

Ceclor ✱

cefoTEtan (Rx)

(sef′oh-tee-tan)

Cefotan

cefOXitin (Rx)

(se-fox′i-tin)

Mefoxin

cefprozil (Rx)

(sef-proe′zill)

Cefzil

cefuroxime (Rx)

(sef-yoor-ox′eem)

Ceftin, Zinacef

Func. class.: Antiinfective

Chem. class.: Cephalosporin (2nd generation)

Do not confuse:

cefaclor/cephalexin

Cefotan/Ceftin

cefprozil/ceFAZolin/cefuroxime

Cefzil/Ceftin

ACTION: Inhibits bacterial cell wall synthesis, renders cell wall osmotically unstable, leads to cell death by binding to cell wall membrane

USES:

cefaclor: Gram-negative bacilli: *Haemophilus influenzae, Escherichia coli, Proteus mirabilis, Klebsiella;* gram-positive organisms: *Streptococcus pneumoniae, Streptococcus pyogenes, Staphylococcus aureus;* respiratory tract, urinary tract, skin, infections; otitis media

cefoTEtan: Gram-negative organisms: *Haemophilus influenzae, Escherichia coli, Enterobacter aerogenes, Proteus mirabilis, Klebsiella, Citrobacter, Salmonella, Shigella, Acinetobacter, Bacteroides fragilis, Neisseria, Serratia;*

gram-positive organisms: *Streptococcus pneumoniae, Streptococcus pyogenes, Staphylococcus aureus;* lower, serious respiratory tract, urinary tract, skin, bone, joint, gynecologic, gonococcal, intraabdominal infections

cefOXitin: Gram-negative bacilli: *Haemophilus influenzae, Escherichia coli, Proteus, Klebsiella, Bacteroides fragilis, Neisseria gonorrhoeae;* gram-positive organisms: *Streptococcus pneumoniae, Streptococcus pyogenes, Staphylococcus aureus;* anaerobes including *Clostridium;* lower respiratory tract, urinary tract, skin, bone, gynecologic, gonococcal infections; septicemia, peritonitis

cefprozil: Pharyngitis/tonsillitis; otitis media; secondary bacterial infection of acute bronchitis; acute bacterial exacerbation of chronic bronchitis; uncomplicated skin and skin-structure infections; acute sinusitis

cefuroxime: Gram-negative bacilli: *Haemophilus influenzae, Escherichia coli, Neisseria, Proteus mirabilis, Klebsiella;* gram-positive organisms: *Streptococcus pneumoniae, Streptococcus pyogenes, Staphylococcus aureus;* serious lower respiratory tract, urinary tract, skin, bone, joint, gonococcal infections; septicemia, meningitis, surgery prophylaxis

CONTRAINDICATIONS:
Hypersensitivity to cephalosporins or related antibiotics; seizures

Precautions: Pregnancy (B), breastfeeding, children, GI/renal disease, diabetes mellitus, coagulopathy, pseudomembranous colitis

DOSAGE AND ROUTES

cefaclor

- **Adult: PO** 250-500 mg q8hr, ext rel 500 mg q12hr; max 1.5 g/day (cap, oral susp); 1 g/day (ext rel)
- **Child >1 mo: PO** 20-40 mg/kg/day in divided doses q8hr or total daily dose may be divided and given q12hr, max 1 g/day

Available forms: Caps 250, 500 mg; oral susp 125, 250, 375 mg/5 ml; ext rel tab 500 mg

cefoTEtan

- **Adult: IM/IV** 1-3 g q12hr × 5-10 days
- **Adult: CCr** 30-50 ml/min, 1-2 g, then 1-2 g q8-12hr; **IM/IV** CCr 10-29 ml/min 1-2 g, then 1-2 g q12-24hr; **CCr** 5-9 ml/min 1-2 g, then 0.5-1 g q12-24hr; **CCr** <5 ml/min 1-2 g, then 0.5-1 g q24-48hr

Perioperative prophylaxis

- **Adult: IV** 1-2 g ½-1 hr before surgery

Available forms: Inj 1, 2, 10 g

cefOXitin

- **Adult: IM/IV** 1-2 g q6-8hr

Renal dose

- **Adult: IM/IV** after loading dose, CCr 30-50 ml/min, 1-2 g q8-12hr; CCr 10-29 ml/min, 1-2 g q12-24hr; CCr <10 ml/min, 0.5-1 g q12-24hr

Uncomplicated gonorrhea (outpatient)

- **Adult/adolescent/child ≥45 kg: IM** 2 g as single dose with 1 g **PO** probenecid at same time

Severe infections

- **Adult: IM/IV** 2 g q4hr
- **Child ≥3 mo: IM/IV** 80-160 mg/kg/day divided q4-6hr; max 12 g/day

Available forms: Powder for inj 1, 2, 10 g

cefprozil

Upper respiratory infections

- **Adult: PO** 500 mg q24hr × 10 days

Otitis media

- **Child 6 mo-12 yr: PO** 15 mg/kg q12hr × 10 days

Lower respiratory infections

- **Adult: PO** 500 mg q12hr × 10 days

Skin/skin-structure infections

- **Adult: PO** 250-500 mg q12hr × 10 days

Renal dose

- CCr <30 ml/min, 50% of dose

Available forms: Tabs 250, 500 mg; susp 125, 250 mg/5 ml

cefuroxime

- **Adult and child: PO** 250 mg q12hr; may increase to 500 mg q12hr for serious infections
- **Adult: IM/IV** 750 mg-1.5 g q8hr for 5-10 days

Urinary tract infections
- **Adult: PO** 125 mg q12hr; may increase to 250 mg q12hr if needed

Otitis media
- **Child <2 yr: PO** 125 mg bid
- **Child >2 yr: PO** 250 mg bid

Surgical prophylaxis
- **Adult: IV** 1.5 g ½-1 hr before surgery

Severe infections
- **Adult: IM/IV** 1.5 g q6hr; may give up to 3 g q8hr for bacterial meningitis
- **Child >3 mo: IM/IV** 50-100 mg/kg/day or IM in divided doses q6-8hr

Uncomplicated gonorrhea
- **Adult: IM** 1.5 g as single dose in 2 separate sites with oral probenecid

Renal dose
- Dosage reduction indicated with severe renal impairment (CCr <20 ml/min)

Available forms: Tabs 250, 500 mg; solution for inj 1.5 g/50 ml, 750 mg/50 ml; susp 125, 250 mg/5 ml

Administer:
- Do not break, crush, or chew ext rel tabs or caps
- On an empty stomach 1 hr before or 2 hr after a meal

cefaclor
- Identify allergies before use
- Obtain C&S specimen before use
- Shake susp, refrigerate, discard after 2 wk
- For 10-14 days to ensure organism death, prevent superinfection
- With food if needed for GI symptoms
- After C&S completed
- Swallow ext rel whole

cefoTEtan
- Identify allergies before use
- Obtain C&S specimen before use
- IV direct after diluting 1 g/10 ml sterile water for inj, give over 3-5 min; may be diluted further with 50-100 ml NS or D_5W; shake; run over ½-1 hr by Y-tube or 3-way stopcock; discontinue primary infusion during administration
- May be stored 96 hr refrigerated or 24 hr at room temperature

Y-site compatibilities: Allopurinol, amifostine, aztreonam, diltiazem, famotidine, filgrastim, fluconazole, fludarabine, heparin, insulin (regular), melphalan, meperidine, morphine, PACLitaxel, remifentanil, sargramostim, tacrolimus, teniposide, theophylline, thiotepa

cefOXitin
IV route
- After diluting 1 g/10 ml or more D_5W, NS and give over 3-5 min; may be diluted further with 50-100 ml NS or D_5W; run over ½-1 hr by Y-tube or 3-way stopcock; discontinue primary infusion during administration; give by cont infusion at prescribed rate; may store 96 hr refrigerated or 24 hr at room temperature
- For 10-14 days to ensure organism death, prevent superinfection
- After C&S completed

Syringe compatibilities: Heparin, insulin

Y-site compatibilities: Acyclovir, amifostine, amphotericin B cholesteryl sulfate complex, aztreonam, cyclophosphamide, diltiazem, DOXOrubicin liposome, famotidine, fluconazole, foscarnet, HYDROmorphone, magnesium sulfate, meperidine, morphine, ondansetron, perphenazine, remifentanil, teniposide, thiotepa

cefprozil
- Identify allergies before use
- Obtain C&S specimen before use
- For 10-14 days to ensure organism death, prevent superinfection
- After C&S
- Refrigerate/shake susp before use, discard after 14 days

cefuroxime
- Identify allergies before use
- Obtain C&S specimen before use
- For 10-14 days to ensure organism death, prevent superinfection
- With food if needed for GI symptoms
- After C&S obtained

Y-site compatibilities: Acyclovir, allopurinol, amifostine, atracurium, aztreonam, cyclophosphamide, diltiazem, famotidine, fludarabine, foscarnet, HYDROmorphone, melphalan, meperidine, morphine, ondansetron, pancuronium, perphenazine, remifentanil, sargramostim, tacrolimus, teniposide, thiotepa, vecuronium

SIDE EFFECTS

CNS: Dizziness, headache, fatigue, paresthesia, fever, chills, confusion
GI: *Diarrhea,* nausea, vomiting, anorexia, dysgeusia, glossitis, bleeding; increased AST, ALT, bilirubin, LDH, alk phos; abdominal pain, loose stools, flatulence, heartburn, stomach cramps, colitis, jaundice, pseudomembranous colitis
GU: Vaginitis, pruritus, candidiasis, increased BUN, nephrotoxicity, renal failure, pyuria, dysuria, reversible interstitial nephritis
HEMA: Leukopenia, thrombocytopenia, agranulocytosis, anemia, neutropenia, lymphocytosis, eosinophilia, pancytopenia, hemolytic anemia, leukocytosis, granulocytopenia
INTEG: Rash, urticaria, dermatitis, Stevens-Johnson syndrome
RESP: Dyspnea
SYST: Anaphylaxis, serum sickness, superinfection

PHARMACOKINETICS

cefaclor
PO: Peak ½-1 hr, half-life 36-54 min, 25% bound by plasma proteins, 60%-85% eliminated unchanged in urine in 8 hr, crosses placenta, excreted in breast milk (low concentrations)
cefoTEtan
IM/IV: Peak 1½-3 hr, half-life 3-5 hr, 75%-90% bound by plasma proteins, 50%-80% eliminated unchanged in urine, crosses placenta, excreted in breast milk
cefOXitin
Half-life 0.75-1 hr; 65%-80% bound by plasma proteins; 90%-100% eliminated unchanged in urine; crosses placenta, blood-brain barrier; eliminated in breast milk; not metabolized
IM: Peak 15-30 min
IV: Peak 5 min
cefprozil
PO: Peak 1.5 hr, protein binding 36%, elimination half-life 1.3 hr (normal renal function), 2 hr (hepatic disease), 5½-6 hr (end-stage renal disease), extensively metabolized to an active metabolite, eliminated in urine 60%
cefuroxime
Peak PO 2 hr, IM 45 min, IV 2-3 min, 66% excreted unchanged in urine, half-life 1-2 hr in normal renal function

INTERACTIONS

Increase: effect/toxicity—aminoglycosides, furosemide, probenecid
Increase: bleeding risk (cefoTEtan)—anticoagulants, thrombolytics, NSAIDs, antiplatelets, plicamycin, valproic acid
Decrease: oral contraceptive, possible—use additional form of contraception
Decrease: absorption of cephalosporin—antacids
Decrease: effect of cephalosporin—H_2-blockers
Drug/Lab Test
False increase: creatinine (serum urine), urinary 17-KS
False positive: urinary protein, direct Coombs' test, urine glucose testing (Clinitest)
Interference: cross-matching

NURSING CONSIDERATIONS

Assess:
⚠ **Nephrotoxicity:** increased BUN, creatinine
- I&O ratio
- Blood studies: AST, ALT, CBC, Hct, bilirubin, LDH, alk phos, Coombs' test monthly if patient is on long-term therapy
- Electrolytes: potassium, sodium, chlorine monthly if patient is on long-term therapy
- Bowel pattern daily; if severe diarrhea occurs, product should be discontinued; may indicate pseudomembranous colitis
- Urine output; if decreasing, notify prescriber (may indicate nephrotoxicity)

⚠ **Anaphylaxis:** rash, flushing, urticaria, pruritus, dyspnea; discontinue product, notify prescriber, have emergency equipment available
- **Bleeding:** ecchymosis, bleeding gums, hematuria, stool guaiac daily

⚠ **Overgrowth of infection:** perineal itching, fever, malaise, redness, pain, swelling, drainage, rash, diarrhea, change in cough, sputum

Evaluate:

• Therapeutic response: negative C&S

Teach patient/family:

• If diabetic, to use blood glucose testing

• To complete full course of product therapy; to report persistent diarrhea

• To use yogurt, buttermilk to maintain intestinal flora, decrease diarrhea

• To notify prescriber if breastfeeding or of any side effects

⚠ To report sore throat, bruising, bleeding, joint pain (may indicate blood dyscrasias [rare]); diarrhea with mucus, blood (pseudomembranous colitis); symptoms of hypersensitivity

TREATMENT OF ANAPHYLAXIS: EPINEPHrine, antihistamines; resuscitate if needed

CEPHALOSPORINS—3RD/4TH GENERATION

cefdinir (Rx)
(sef′dih-ner)

cefditoren pivoxil (Rx)
(sef-dit′oh-ren pih-vox′il)
Spectracef

cefepime (Rx)
(sef′e-peem)
Maxipime (4th generation)

cefixime (Rx)
(sef-icks′ime)
Suprax

cefotaxime (Rx)
(sef-oh-taks′eem)
Claforan

cefpodoxime (Rx)
(sef-poe-docks′eem)

cefTAZidime (Rx)
(sef′tay-zi-deem)
Fortaz, Tazicef

ceftibuten (Rx)
(sef-ti-byoo′tin)
Cedax

cefTRIAXone (Rx)
(sef-try-ax′one)
Rocephin

Func. class.: Broad-spectrum antibiotic
Chem. class.: Cephalosporin (3rd generation)

Do not confuse:
cefTAZidime/ceftizoxime
Vantin/Ventolin

ACTION: Inhibits bacterial cell wall synthesis, renders cell wall osmotically unstable, leads to cell death

USES:
cefdinir: Community-acquired pneumonia, otitis media, sinusitis, pharyngitis, skin and skin-structure infections, acute

exacerbations of chronic bronchitis, pneumonia, tonsillitis, citrobacter diversus, escherichia coli, Klebsiella pneumonial, proteus mirabilis, Staphylococcus epidermidis, streptococcus agalactial (group B), viridans Streptococci alpha: *Haemophilus influenzae, Haemophilus parainfluenzae, Moraxella catarrhalis;* gram-positive organisms: *Streptococcus pneumoniae, Streptococcus pyogenes, Staphylococcus aureus* (MSSA)

cefditoren pivoxil: Acute bacterial exacerbations of chronic bronchitis caused by *Haemophilus influenzae, Haemophilus parainfluenzae, Streptococcus pneumoniae, Moraxella catarrhalis*; pharyngitis/tonsillitis caused by *Streptococcus pyogenes*; uncomplicated skin and skin-structure infections caused by *Staphylococcus aureus, Streptococcus pyogenes;* community-acquired pneumonia, viridans streptococci

cefepime: *Escherichia coli, Proteus, Klebsiella; Acinetobacter calcoaceticus, Acinetobacter lwoffii, Aeromonas hydrophilia, Citrobacter diversus, Citrobacter freundii, Enterobacter sp., Escherichia coli, Gardnerella vaginalis, Hafnia alvei, moraxella catarrhalis, Morganella morganii, Neisseria gonorrhoeal, Meningitidis, Providencia rettgeri, Stuartii, Pseudomonas aeruginosa, Salmonella sp., Serratia liquefaciens, Serratia marcescens, Shigella sp., Staphylococcus epidermidis, Staphylococcus saprophyticus, Streptococcus agalactial, Bovis, Viridans streptococci, Yersinia entercolitica: Streptococcus pneumoniae, Streptococcus pyogenes, Staphylococcus aureus;* lower respiratory tract, urinary tract, skin, bone infections; febrile neutropenia intraabdominal infection

cefixime: Uncomplicated UTI *(Escherichia coli, Proteus mirabilis)*, pharyngitis and tonsillitis *(Streptococcus pyogenes)*, otitis media *(Haemophilus influenzae), Moraxella catarrhalis,* acute bronchitis and acute exacerbations of chronic bronchitis *(Streptococcus pneumoniae, H. influenzae),* uncomplicated gonorrhea

cefotaxime: *Haemophilus influenzae, Haemophilus parainfluenzae, Escherichia coli, Enterococcus faecalis, Neisseria gonorrhoeae, Neisseria meningitidis, Proteus mirabilis, Klebsiella, Citrobacter, Serratia, Salmonella, Shigella Pseudomonas; Streptococcus pneumoniae, Streptococcus pyogenes, Staphylococcus aureus;* serious lower respiratory tract, urinary tract, skin, bone, gonococcal infections; bacteremia, septicemia, meningitis, skin, skin-structure infections; CNS infections; perioperative prophylaxis, intraabdominal infections, PID, UTI, ventriculitis

cefpodoxime: Bacteroides, *Neisseria gonorrhoeae, Haemophilus influenzae, Escherichia coli, Proteus mirabilis, Klebsiella;* gram-positive organisms: *Streptococcus pneumoniae, Streptococcus pyogenes, Staphylococcus aureus;* upper and lower respiratory tract, urinary tract, skin infections; otitis media; sexually transmitted diseases

cefTAZidime: *Haemophilus influenzae, Escherichia coli, Enterobacter aerogenes, Pseudomonas aeruginosa, Proteus mirabilis, Klebsiella, Citrobacter, Enterobacter, Salmonella, Shigella, Acinetobacter, Bacteroides fragilis, Neisseria, Serratia; Streptococcus pneumoniae, Streptococcus pyogenes, Staphylococcus aureus;* serious lower respiratory tract, urinary tract, skin, gynecologic, bone, joint, intraabdominal infections; septicemia, meningitis

ceftibuten: Pharyngitis/tonsillitis, otitis media, secondary bacterial infection of acute bronchitis

cefTRIAXone: Gram-negative bacilli: *Haemophilus influenzae, Escherichia coli, Enterobacter aerogenes, Proteus mirabilis, Klebsiella, Citrobacter, Enterobacter, Salmonella, Shigella, Acinetobacter, Bacteroides fragilis, Neisseria, Serratia;* gram-positive organisms: *Streptococcus pneumoniae, Streptococcus pyogenes, Staphylococcus aureus;* serious lower respiratory tract, urinary tract, skin, gonococcal, intraabdominal infections; septicemia, meningitis, bone, joint infections; otitis media; PID

CONTRAINDICATIONS: Hypersensitivity to cephalosporins, infants <1 mo

Precautions: Pregnancy (B), breastfeeding, children, hypersensitivity to penicillins, GI/renal disease, geriatric patients, pseudomembranous colitis, viral infection, vit K deficiencies, diabetes

DOSAGE AND ROUTES

cefdinir

Uncomplicated skin and skin-structure infections/community-acquired pneumonia

- **Adult and child ≥13 yr: PO** 300 mg q12hr × 10 days
- **Child 6 mo-12 yr: PO** 7 mg/kg q12hr or 14 mg/kg q24hr × 10 days

Acute exacerbations of chronic bronchitis/acute maxillary sinusitis

- **Adult and child ≥13 yr: PO** 300 mg q12hr or 600 mg q24hr × 10 days

Pharyngitis/tonsillitis

- **Adult and child ≥13 yr: PO** 300 mg q12hr or 600 mg q24hr × 10 days
- **Child 6 mo-12 yr: PO** 7 mg/kg q12hr × 5-10 days or 14 mg/kg q24hr × 10 days

Renal dose

- **Adult: PO** CCr <30 ml/min, 300 mg/day (adult); 7 mg/kg/day (child)

Available forms: Caps 300 mg; susp 125 mg, 250 mg/5 ml

cefditoren pivoxil

- **Adult: PO** 200-400 mg bid × 10-14 days

Renal dose

- **Adult: PO** CCr 30-49 ml/min, max 200 mg bid; CCr <30 ml/min, max 200 mg daily

Available forms: Tabs 200, 400 mg

cefepime

Febrile neutropenia

- **Adult/adolescent >16 yrs/child ≥ 40 kg: IV** 2 g q8hr × 7 days or until neutropenia resolves
- **Infant ≥2 mo/child/adolescent ≤16 yr and ≤40 kg: IV** 50 mg/kg/dose q8hr × 7 days or until neutropenia resolves

Urinary tract infections (mild to moderate)

- **Adult: IV/IM** 0.5-1 g q12hr × 7-10 days

Urinary tract infections (severe)

- **Adult/adolescent >16 yr/child ≥40 kg: IV** 2 g q12hr × 10 days

Pneumonia (moderate to severe)

- **Adult: IV** 1-2 g q12hr × 10 days

Available forms: Powder for inj 500 mg, 1, 2 g; 1 g/50 ml, 2 g/100 ml

cefixime

Mild to moderate pharyngitis, tonsillitis, bronchitis

- **Adult/adolescent/child >45 kg: PO** 400 mg/day divided q12-24hr
- **Children ≤45 kg infants ≥6 months: PO** 8 mg/kg/day divided q12-24hr

Uncomplicated urinary tract infection (UTI)

- **Adult/adolescent/child >45 kg: PO** 400 mg/day divided q12-24hr
- **Children ≤45 kg and infants ≥6 mo: PO** 8 mg/kg/day divided q12-24hr max: 400 mg/day × 7-14 days is recommended by the American Academy of Pediatrics (AAP) for the treatment of initial UTI in febrile infants and young children 2-24 mo
- **Infants 2-5 mo (unlabeled): PO** 8 mg/kg/day × 7-14 days is recommended by the American Academy of Pediatrics (AAP) for the treatment of initial UTI in febrile infants and young children

Mild to moderate otitis media

- **Adult/adolescent/child >45 kg: PO** 400 mg/day divided q12-24hr
- **Children ≤45 kg: PO** 8 mg/kg/day divided q12-24hr, max 400 mg/day
- **Infants ≥6 months: PO** 8 mg/kg/day divided q12-24hr

Gonorrhea of uncomplicated cervicitis, or urethritis due to *N. gonorrhoeae*

- **Adult/adolescent: PO** as alternative therapy, 400 mg as a single dose with a regimen effective against uncomplicated genital *C. trachomatis* infection (e.g., azithromycin as a single dose or doxycycline for 7 days) if chlamydial infection is not ruled out; the CDC states that cefixime is only acceptable if IM cefTRIAXone is not an option because of rising cefixime MICs for gonorrhea; if cefixime is used, test-of-cure should be done at the infected site 1 wk after treatment; cefixime is not recommended for infections of the pharynx

• **Children ≥45 kg: PO** 400 mg as a single dose with a regimen effective against uncomplicated genital *C. trachomatis* infection (e.g., azithromycin as a single dose or doxycycline for 7 days) if chlamydial infection is not ruled out; cefixime is not recommended for infections of the pharynx; cefixime is an alternative to cefTRIAXone per AAP

Gonorrhea prophylaxis (victims of sexual assault) (unlabeled)

• **Adult/adolescent:** The CDC recommends 400 mg as a single dose with metroNIDAZOLE (for trichomoniasis and bacterial vaginosis prophylaxis) plus either azithromycin or doxycycline (for chlamydia prophylaxis); the CDC states that cefixime is only acceptable if IM cefTRIAXone is not an option because of rising cefixime MICs for gonorrhea

Typhoid fever caused by multidrug-resistant *Salmonella typhi* (unlabeled)

• **Adult/adolescent/child:** 100-200 mg **PO BID** or 15-20 mg/kg/day **PO** in 2 divided doses for 7-14 days; for quinolone-resistant organisms, 20 mg/kg/day **PO** in 2 divided doses for 7-14 days should be used

• **Children <50 kg:** should receive weight-based dosing, max adult dosages

Acute bacterial sinusitis (unlabeled)

• **Infants ≥6 mo/child/adolescent: PO** 8 mg/kg/day **PO** divided q12hr, max 400 mg/day, with clindamycin for 10-14 days

Renal dose

• **Adult: PO** CCr 21-59 ml/min, give 65% of dose; CCr <20 ml/min, give 50% of dose

Available forms: Tabs 400 mg; powder for oral susp 100 mg/5 ml, chew tabs 100, 200 mg, 200 mg/5 ml, cap 400 mg

cefotaxime

• **Adult/adolescent/child ≥50 kg: IV/IM** (uncomplicated infections) 1 g q12hr, (moderate-severe infection) 1-2 g q8hr, (severe infections) 2 g q6-8hr, (life-threatening infections) 2 g q4hr, max 12 g/day

• **Adolescent/child <50 kg and infants: IV/IM** 50-180 mg/kg/day divided q6-8hr, max 2 g/dose; (severe infections) 200-225 mg/kg/day divided q4-6hr max 12 g

• **Neonates >7 days: IV/IM** 50 mg/kg/dose q8-12hr

Uncomplicated gonorrhea

• **Adult: IM** 500 mg as a single dose

Renal Dose

• **Adult: IM** CCr <20 ml/min 50% dose reduction

Available forms: Powder for inj 500 mg, 1, 2, 10 g; inj 1, 2 g premixed frozen

cefpodoxime

Pneumonia

• **Adult >12 yr: PO** 200 mg q12hr × 14 days

Skin and skin structure

• **Adult >13 yr: PO** 400 mg q12hr × 7-14 days

Pharyngitis and tonsillitis

• **Adult >13 yr: PO** 100 mg q12hr × 5-10 days

• **Child 5 mo-12 yr: PO** 5 mg/kg q12hr (max 100 mg/dose or 200 mg/day) × 5-10 days

Uncomplicated UTI

• **Adult >13 yr: PO** 100 mg q12hr × 7 days; dosing interval increased with severe renal impairment

Acute otitis media

• **Child 5 mo-12 yr: PO** 5 mg/kg q12hr × 5 days

Available forms: Tabs 100, 200 mg; granules for susp 50 mg, 100 mg/5 ml

cefTAZidime

- **Adult: IV/IM** 1-2 g q8
- **Child: IV** 30-50 mg/kg q8hr, max 6 g/day
- **Neonate: IV** 30-50 mg/kg q8-12hr

Renal dose

- **Adult: IM/IV** CCr 31-50 ml/min 1 g q12hr; CCr 16-30 ml/min 1 g q24hr; CCR 6-15 ml/min 1 g loading dose, then 0.5 g q24hr; CCr <5 ml/min 1 g loading dose, then 0.5 g q48hr

Available forms: Inj 250, 500 mg, 1, 2, 6 g

ceftibuten

- **Adult: PO** 400 mg/day × 10 days
- **Child 6 mo-12 yr: PO** 9 mg/kg/day × 10 days

Renal dose

- **Adult: PO** CCr 30-49 ml/min, give 200 mg q24hr; CCr 5-29 ml/min, give 100 mg q24hr

Available forms: Caps 400 mg; susp 90 mg, 180 mg/5 ml

cefTRIAXone

- **Adult: IM/IV** 1-2 g/day, max 4 g/24 hr
- **Child: IM/IV** 50-75 mg/kg/day in equal doses q12-24hr

Uncomplicated gonorrhea

- **Adult:** 250 mg **IM** as single dose
- Reduce dosage in severe renal impairment (CCr <10 ml/min)

Available forms: Inj 250, 500 mg, 1, 2, 10 g

Administer:

- Change IV site q72hr

cefdinir

- Oral susp after adding 39 ml water to the 60-ml bottle or 65 ml water to the 120-ml bottle; discard unused portion after 10 days; give without regard to food, do not give within 2 hr of antacids, iron supplements
- After C&S completed

cefditoren pivoxil

- For 10-14 days to ensure organism death, prevent superinfection
- With food; do not give with antacids
- After C&S completed

cefepime

Intermittent IV INFUSION route

- IV after diluting in 50-100 ml or more D_5, NS; give over 30 min
- For 7-10 days to ensure organism death, prevent superinfection

Solution compatibilities: 0.9% NaCl, D_5, D_5W, 0.5%, 10% lidocaine, bacteriostatic water for inj with parabens/benzyl alcohol

Y-site compatibilities: DOXOrubicin liposome

cefixime

- For 10-14 days to ensure organism death, prevent superinfection
- Without regard to food
- Chew tabs before swallowing

cefotaxime

IV route

- IV after **diluting** 1 g/10 ml D_5W, NS, sterile water for inj, **give** over 3-5 min by Y-tube or 3-way stopcock; may be **diluted further** with 50-100 ml NS or D_5W; **run** over ½-1 hr; discontinue primary infusion during administration; may be **diluted** in larger vol of sol, given as a cont infusion
- For 10-14 days to ensure organism death, prevent superinfection
- Thaw frozen container at room temperature or refrigeration; do not force thaw by immersion or microwave; visually inspect container for leaks

Syringe compatibilities: Caffeine, diphenhyDRINATE, heparin, ofloxacin

Y-site compatibilities: Acyclovir, alfentanil, alprostadil, amifostine, amikacin, aminocaproic acid, aminophylline, anidulafungin, ascorbic acid injection, atenolol, atracurium, atropine, aztreonam, benztropine, bivalirudin, bleomycin, bumetanide, buprenorphine, butorphanol, caffeine, calcium chloride/gluconate, CARBOplatin, cefamandole, cefmetazole, cefonicid, cefoperazone, cefoTEtan, cefOXitin, cefTAZidime (L-arginine), cefTRIAXone sodium, cefuroxime, cimetidine, CISplatin, clindamycin, codeine, cyanocobalamin, cyclophosphamide, cycloSPORINE, cytarabine, DACTINomycin, DAPTOmycin, dexamethasone, dexmedetomidine, digoxin, diltiazem, DOCEtaxel, DOPamine, doxacurium, doxycycline, enalaprilat, ePHEDrine, EPINEPHrine, epirubicin, epoetin alfa, eptifibatide, erythromycin, esmolol, etoposide, famotidine, fenoldopam, fentaNYL, fludarabine, fluorouracil, folic acid, furosemide, gatifloxacin, gentamicin, glycopyrrolate, granisetron, heparin, hydrocortisone, HYDROmorphone, ifosfamide, imipenem-cilastatin, insulin (regular), isoproterenol, ketorolac, lidocaine, linezolid, LORazepam, LR, magnesium sulfate, mannitol, mechlorethamine, melphalan, meperidine, metaraminol, methicillin, methotrexate, methoxamine, methyldopate, metoclopramide, metoprolol, metroNIDAZOLE, mezlocillin, miconazole, midazolam, milrinone, minocycline, mitoXANtrone, morphine, moxalactam, multiple vitamins, mycophenolate, nafcillin, nalbuphine, naloxone, nesiritide, netilmicin, nitroglycerin, nitroprusside, norepinephrine, normal saline, octreotide, ofloxacin, ondansetron, ornidazole, oxacillin, oxaliplatin, oxytocin, PACLitaxel, palonosetron, pamidronate, pancuronium, pantoprazole, papaverine, pefloxacin, PEMEtrexed, penicillin G potassium/sodium, pentamidine, pentazocine, PENTobarbital, peritoneal dialysis solution, perphenazine, PHENobarbital, phenylephrine, phenytoin, phytonadione, piperacillin, polymyxin B, potassium chloride, procainamide, prochlorperazine, promethazine, propofol, propranolol, protamine, pyridoxine, quiNIDine, quinupristin, ranitidine, remifentanil, Ringer's injection, ritodrine, riTUXimab, rocuronium, sargramostim, sodium acetate/bicarbonate, sodium fusidate, sodium lactate, succinylcholine, SUFentanil, sulfamethoxazole-trimethoprim, tacrolimus, teniposide, theophylline, thiamine, thiotepa, ticarcillin, ticarcillin-clavulanate, tigecycline, tirofiban, TNA, tobramycin, tolazoline, TPN, trastuzumab, trimetaphan, urokinase, vancomycin, vasopressin, vecuronium, verapamil, vinorelbine, voriconazole

cefpodoxime

- Do not break, crush, or chew tabs due to taste
- For 10-14 days to ensure organism death, prevent superinfection
- With food for better absorption; do not give within 2 hr of antacids, H_2-receptor antagonists
- Shake susp well, refrigerate, discard after 2 wk

cefTAZidime

IM route

- **Fortaz, Tazidime vials:** reconstitute 500 mg or 1 g with 1.5 or 3 ml, respectively, of sterile or bacteriostatic water for inj or 0.5%-1% lidocaine (approx 280 mg/ml)
- **Tazicef vials:** reconstitute 1 g/3 ml sterile water for inj (approx 280 mg/ml)
- **Ceptaz vials:** reconstitute 1 g/3 ml sterile or bacteriostatic water for inj or 0.5%-1% lidocaine (approx 250 mg/ml)
- **Withdraw** dose while making sure needle remains in vial; **ensure** no CO_2 bubbles present; **inject** deeply in large muscle mass, **aspirate** before injection

IV route

- Visually inspect for particulate matter, discoloration, if possible
- **Fortaz, Tazicef, Tazidime packs: reconstitute** 1 or 2 g/100 ml sterile water for inj or other compatible IV sol (10 or 20 mg/ml, respectively); reconstitution is done in two stages: first, **inject** 10 ml of the diluent into the pack and **shake** well to dissolve and become clear; CO_2 pressure inside container will occur, **insert** vent needle to release pressure; **add** remaining diluents, **remove** vent needle
- **Fortaz, Tazicef, Tazidime vials: reconstitute** 500 mg, 1 g, 2 g with 5, 10, 10 ml, respectively, of sterile water for inj or other compatible IV solution (100, 95-100, or 170-180 mg/ml, respectively); **shake** well to dissolve
- **Fortaz, Tazidime ADD-Vantage vials (for IV only): reconstitute** 1 or 2 g with NS, ½ NS, D_5W in either 50- or 100-ml flexible diluent container; to release

CO_2 pressure, **insert** vent needle after dissolving, **remove** vent before using

- **Ceptaz packs: reconstitute** 1 or 2 g/100 ml sterile water for inj or compatible IV sol (10 or 20 mg/ml, respectively); reconstitution is done in two stages: first, **inject** 10 ml of the diluent into the pack and **shake** well to dissolve, **add** the remaining diluent, **insert** vent needle before giving
- **Ceptaz vials: reconstitute** 1 or 2 g/10 ml of sterile water for inj or compatible IV sol (90-95, or 170-180 mg/ml, respectively)
- **Ceptaz ADD-Vantage vials (for IV only): reconstitute** 1 or 2 g with NS, ½ NS, or D_5W in either 50- or 100-ml diluent container

Direct Intermittent IV INFUSION route

- **Vials: withdraw** dose while making sure needle remains in sol; make sure there are no CO_2 bubbles in syringe before inj; **inject** directly over 3-5 min or slowly into tubing of a free-flowing compatible IV solution

Intermittent IV INFUSION route

- **Vials: withdraw** dose while making sure needle opening remains in sol; make sure there are no CO_2 bubbles in syringe before inj; infusion packs and ADD-Vantage systems ready for infusion after reconstitution, **infuse** over 15-30 min

Syringe compatibilities: Cimetidine, dimenhyDRINATE, HYDROmorphone

Y-site compatibilities: Acyclovir, alfentanil, allopurinol, amifostine, amikacin, aminocaproic acid, aminophylline, amphotericin B lipid complex, anakinra, anidulafungin, atenolol, atropine sulfate, aztreonam, benzotropine, bivalirudin, bleomycin, bumetanide, buprenorphine, butorphanol, calcium gluconate, CARBOplatin, cefamandole, ceFAZolin, cefonicid, cefoperazone, cefoTEtan, cefOXitin, cefTAZidime, ceftizoxime, cefTRIAXone, cefuroxime, cephalothin, cephapirin, cimetidine, ciprofloxacin, CISplatin, clindamycin, codeine, cyanocobalamin, cyclophosphamide, cycloSPORINE, cytarabine, DACTINomycin, DAPTOmycin, dexamethasone, dexmedetomidine, digoxin, diltiazem, DOCEtaxel, DOPamine, doxacurium, doxapram, enalaprilat, ePHEDrine, EPINEPHrine, epoetin alfa, eptifibatide, esmolol, etoposide, famotidine, fenoldopam, fentaNYL, filgrastim, fludarabine, fluorouracil, folic acid, foscarnet, furosemide, gallium, gatifloxacin, gemcitabine, gentamicin, glycopyrrolate, granisetron, heparin, HYDROmorphone, ifosfamide, imipenem-cilastatin, indomethacin, insulin (regular), irinotecan, isepamicin, isoproterenol, isosorbide, ketamine, ketorolac, labetalol, levofloxacin, lidocaine, linezolid, LORazepam, LR, magnesium sulfate, mannitol, mechlorethamine, melphalan, meperidine, metaraminol, methicillin, methotrexate, methoxamine, methyldopate, methylPREDNISolone, metoclopramide, metoprolol, metroNIDAZOLE, miconazole, milrinone, morphine, moxalactam, multiple vitamin inj, nafcillin, nalbuphine, PACLitaxel, ranitidine, remifentanil, tacrolimus, teniposide, theophylline, thiotepa, vinorelbine, zidovudine

ceftibuten

- For 10 days to ensure organism death, prevent superinfection
- On empty stomach

cefTRIAXone

- For 10-14 days to ensure organism death, prevent superinfection
- **IM** inj deeply in large muscle mass

IV route

- **IV** after **diluting** 250 mg/2.4 ml, 500 mg/4.8 ml, 1 g/9.6 ml, 2 g/19.2 ml D_5W, water for inj, 0.9% NaCl; may be **further diluted** with 50-100 ml NS, D_5W, $D_{10}W$; shake; **run** over ½ hr
- Do not mix with calcium salts

Y-site compatibilities: Acetaminophen, acyclovir, alfentanil, allopurinol, amifostine, amikacin, aminocaproic acid, aminophylline, amiodarone, amphotericin B liposome, anidulafungin, argatroban, atenolol, atracurium, atropine, aztreonam, benztropine, bivalirudin, bleomycin, bumetanide, buprenorphine, butorphanol, CARBOplatin, cefamandole, ceFAZolin, cefmetazole, cefonicid, cefoperazone, cefoTAXime, cefoTEtan, cefOXitin, cefTAZidime, ceftizoxime, cefuroxime, cephalothin, cephapirin, cimetidine, cisatracurium, CISplatin, codeine, cyanocobalamin, cyclophosphamide, cycloSPORINE, cytarabine, DACTINomycin, DAPTOmycin, dexamethasone, dexmedetomidine, digoxin, diltiazem, DOCEtaxel, DOPamine, doxacurium, DOXOrubicin liposomal, doxycycline, drotrecogin alfa, enalaprilat, ePHEDrine, EPINEPHrine, epoetin alfa, eptifibatide, erythromycin, esmolol, etoposide, fenoldopam, fludarabine, fluorouracil, folic acid, foscarnet, furosemide, gallium, gatifloxacin, gemcitabine, gentamicin, glycopyrrolate, granisetron, heparin, hydrocortisone, HYDROmorphone, ifosfamide, indomethacin, insulin (regular), isoproterenol, ketorolac, lansoprazole, levofloxacin, lidocaine, linezolid, LORazepam, mannitol, mechlorethamine, melphalan, meperidine, metaraminol, methicillin, methotrexate, methoxamine, methyldopate, methylPREDNISolone, metoclopramide, metoprolol, metroNIDAZOLE, mezlocillin, miconazole, midazolam, milrinone, morphine, moxalactam, multiple vitamins injection, nafcillin, nalbuphine, naloxone, nesiritide, netilimicin, nitroglycerin, nitroprusside, norepinephrine, octreotide, oxacillin, oxaliplatin, oxytocin, PACLitaxel, palonosetron, pamidronate, pancuronium, pantoprazole, PEMEtrexed, penicillin G potassium/sodium, PHENobarbital, phenylephrine, phytonadione, piperacillin, polymyxin B, potassium chloride, procainamide, propofol, propranolol, pyridoxine, ranitidine, remifentanil, ritodrine, riTUXimab, rocuronium, sargramostim, sodium acetate/bicarbonate, succinylcholine, SUFentanil, tacrolimus, teniposide, theophylline, thiamine, thiotepa, ticarcillin, ticarcillin-clavulanate, tigecycline, tirofiban, tolazoline, trastuzumab, trimetaphan, urokinase, vasopressin, vecuronium, verapamil, vinCRIStine, voriconazole, warfarin, zidovudine

SIDE EFFECTS

CNS: Headache, dizziness, weakness, paresthesia, fever, chills, **seizures,** dyskinesia (cefdinir); **neurotoxicity (renal disease) cefepime**

CV: **Heart failure,** syncope (cefdinir)

EENT: *Oral candidiasis*

GI: *Nausea, vomiting, diarrhea, anorexia,* pain, glossitis, **bleeding;** increased AST, ALT, bilirubin, LDH, alk phos; abdominal pain, **pseudomembranous colitis;** cholestasis (cefotaxime)

GU: **Proteinuria,** vaginitis, pruritus, *candidiasis,* increased BUN, **nephrotoxicity, renal failure**

HEMA: **Leukopenia, thrombocytopenia, agranulocytosis,** anemia, **neutropenia, lymphocytosis, eosinophilia, pancytopenia, hemolytic anemia**

INTEG: Rash, urticaria, dermatitis

MS: Arthralgia (cefditoren)

RESP: Dyspnea

SYST: **Anaphylaxis, serum sickness, Stevens-Johnson syndrome, toxic epidermal necrolysis**

PHARMACOKINETICS

cefdinir

Unchanged in urine; crosses placenta, blood-brain barrier; eliminated in breast milk, not metabolized; 60%-70% protein binding, half-life 1.7 hr

cefditoren pivoxil

Well absorbed when broken down (prodrug), wide distribution, half-life 100 min, onset rapid, peak 1.5-3 hr, duration 12 hr, 88% protein binding

cefepime

Peak 79 min; half-life 2 hr; 20% bound by plasma proteins; 90% excreted unchanged in urine; crosses placenta, blood-brain barrier; excreted in breast milk, not metabolized

cefixime

PO: Peak 2-8 hr, half-life 3-4 hr, 65%-70% protein binding, 50% eliminated unchanged in urine, crosses placenta, excreted in breast milk

cefotaxime

Half-life 1 hr, 35%-65% is bound by plasma proteins, 40%-65% is eliminated

unchanged in urine in 24 hr, 25% metabolized in the liver to active metabolites, excreted in breast milk (small amounts)
IM: Onset 30 min
IV: Onset 5 min
cefpodoxime
Half-life 1-1.5 hr, 13%-38% bound by plasma proteins, 30% eliminated unchanged in urine in 8 hr, crosses placenta, excreted in breast milk
cefTAZidime
IM/IV:
Half-life 1½-2 hr, 10% bound by plasma proteins, 80% eliminated unchanged in urine, crosses placenta, excreted in breast milk
ceftibuten
PO: Peak 2-3 hr; plasma protein binding 65%, elimination half-life 2 hr, extensively metabolized to an active metabolite
IM: Peak 1 hr
IV: Onset 5 min
cefTRIAXone
Half-life 6-9 hr, 58%-96%, eliminated unchanged in urine, crosses placenta, excreted in breast milk
IM: Peak 1½-4 hr
IV: Peak 30 min

INTERACTIONS

Many products should not be used with calcium salts (mixed or administered) or H2 blockers antacids (PO)
Increase: cycloSPORINE levels—cycloSPORINE
Increase: bleeding—anticoagulants, thrombolytics, plicamycin, valproic acid, NSAIDs
Increase: toxicity—aminoglycosides, furosemide, probenecid
Decrease: absorption of cefdinir—iron
Drug/Food
Decrease: absorption—iron-rich cereal, infant formula
Drug/Lab Test
Increase: ALT, AST, alk phos, LDH, bilirubin, BUN, creatinine
False increase: creatinine (serum urine), urinary 17-KS
False positive: urinary protein, direct Coombs' test, urine glucose
Interference: cross-matching

NURSING CONSIDERATIONS

Assess:
- Sensitivity to penicillin, other cephalosporins

⚠ **Nephrotoxicity:** increased BUN, creatinine; urine output: if decreasing, notify prescriber
- Blood studies: AST, ALT, CBC, Hct, bilirubin, LDH, alk phos, Coombs' test monthly if patient is on long-term therapy
- Electrolytes: potassium, sodium, chloride monthly if patient is on long-term therapy
- **Pseudomembranous colitis:** bowel pattern daily; if severe diarrhea occurs, product should be discontinued
- IV site for extravasation, phlebitis

⚠ **Anaphylaxis:** rash, urticaria, pruritus, chills, fever, joint pain, angioedema; may occur a few days after therapy begins
- Bleeding: ecchymosis, bleeding gums, hematuria, stool guaiac

⚠ **Overgrowth of infection:** perineal itching, fever, malaise, redness, pain, swelling, drainage, rash, diarrhea, change in cough, sputum
- Monitor heart rate during direct IV infusion (cefotaxime)

Evaluate:
- Therapeutic response: decreased symptoms of infection; negative C&S

Teach patient/family:
- If diabetic, to check blood glucose

⚠ To report sore throat, bruising, bleeding, joint pain, may indicate **blood dyscrasias (rare);** diarrhea with mucus, blood, may indicate **pseudomembranous colitis**
- That cefditoren can be taken with oral contraceptives

TREATMENT OF ANAPHYLAXIS:
EPINEPHrine, antihistamines; resuscitate if needed

cephradine

See cephalosporins—1st generation

certolizumab pegol (Rx)

(ser′tue-liz′oo-mab pegh′ol)

Cimzia

Func. class.: Biologic response modifier

Chem. class.: Antitissue necrosis factor (anti-TNF) agent

ACTION:

Monoclonal antibody that neutralizes the activity of tumor necrosis factor α (TNF-α) found in Crohn's disease; decreases infiltration of inflammatory cells

USES:

Crohn's disease (moderate to severe) that has not responded to conventional therapy, rheumatoid arthritis (moderate to severe), psoriatic arthritis, ankylosing spondylitis

Unlabeled uses: Moderate to severe chronic plaque psoriasis, fistulizing Crohn's disease

CONTRAINDICATIONS:

Influenza, IV administration, sepsis, hypersensitivity

Precautions: Pregnancy (B), breastfeeding, children, geriatric patients, AIDS, coagulopathy, diabetes, fungal infection, heart failure, hepatitis, human antichimeric antibody, immunosuppression, leukopenia, MS, cancer, neurologic/renal disease, surgery, thrombocytopenia, TB, vaccinations

Black Box Warning: Infection, neoplastic disease

DOSAGE AND ROUTES

Crohn's disease (moderate to severe)

- **Adult: SUBCUT** 400 mg given as 2 inj at wk 0, 2, 4; if clinical response occurs, give 400 mg q4wk

Rheumatoid arthritis (moderate to severe)

- **Adult: SUBCUT** 400 mg q2wk × 3 doses, then 200 mg q2wk; given with methotrexate

Crohn's disease (fistulizing)/intolerant to infliximab (unlabeled)

- **Adult: SUBCUT** 400 mg wk 0, 2, 4, then 400 mg q4wk

Available forms: Powder for inj 200-, 400-mg kit

Administer:

SUBCUT route

- Give by subcut inj only
- Reconstitution: allow to warm to room temperature; add 1 ml sterile water for inj to each vial; 2 vials will be needed for patients with Crohn's disease
- Gently swirl; do not shake; full reconstitution may take up to 30 min; reconstituted product may remain at room temperature for up to 2 hr or refrigerated up to 24 hr
- If reconstituted product has been refrigerated, allow to warm to room temperature
- Use 2 syringes and two 20G needles
- Withdraw reconstituted sol from each vial into separate syringes; each will contain 200 mg; switch 20G to 23G needle; inject into 2 separate sites in abdomen or thigh
- Store in refrigerator; do not freeze

SIDE EFFECTS

CNS: *Dizziness,* syncope, peripheral neuropathy, fever, **seizures, demyelinating disease of CNS**

CV: **Heart failure, MI, cardiac dysrhythmia**

EENT: Optic neuritis, retinal hemorrhage, uveitis

GI: Increased LFTs, **hepatitis, bowel obstruction**

GU: UTI, renal disease

HEMA: **Anemia, aplastic anemia, pancytopenia, thrombocytopenia**

INTEG: *Rash, urticaria,* angioedema

MISC: **Anaphylaxis,** antibody formation, arthralgia, bleeding, infection, lupuslike symptoms, lymphadenopathy, **malignancies, serum sickness, suicidal ideation**

RESP: Dyspnea, upper respiratory tract infection

PHARMACOKINETICS
Peak 54-171 hr, terminal half-life 14 days

INTERACTIONS
- Do not administer live vaccines, toxoids concurrently

Increase: possible infections—abatacept, adalimumab, anakinra, etanercept, immunosuppressive agents, infliximab, rilonacept; do not use concurrently
Increase: possible malignancies—adalimumab, etanercept, infliximab

NURSING CONSIDERATIONS
Assess:
- Antinuclear antibody test (ANA), hepatitis B serology, CBC
- For rheumatoid arthritis, ROM, pain
- GI symptoms: nausea, vomiting, abdominal pain, hepatitis, increased LFTs
- Periodic blood counts (CBC)
- CV status: B/P, pulse, chest pain

⚠ **Allergic reaction, anaphylaxis:** rash, dermatitis, urticaria, dyspnea, hypotension, fever, chills; discontinue if severe; administer EPINEPHrine, corticosteroids, antihistamines; assess for allergies to murine proteins before starting therapy

Black Box Warning: Infection: discontinue if infection occurs; do not administer to patients with active infection

Black Box Warning: Identify TB, risk for HBV before beginning treatment; TB test should be obtained; if present, TB should be treated before certolizumab treatment

Evaluate:
- Therapeutic response: absence of fever, mucus in stools

Teach patient/family:
- Not to breastfeed while taking this product

Black Box Warning: To notify prescriber of GI symptoms, hypersensitivity reactions, infections, fluid retention; redness, pain, swelling at inj site

Black Box Warning: Not to operate machinery, drive if dizziness, vertigo occur

C

cetirizine (Rx, OTC)
(se-teer′i-zeen)

All Day Allergy, All Day Allergy Children's, Reactine ✦, ZyrTEC, ZyrTEC Children's

Func. class.: Antihistamine (2nd generation, peripherally selective)
Chem. class.: Piperazine, H_1-histamine antagonist

Do not confuse:
ZyrTEC/Xanax/Zantac

ACTION:
Acts on blood vessels, GI, respiratory system by competing with histamine for H_1-receptor site; decreases allergic response by blocking pharmacologic effects of histamine; minimal anticholinergic, sedative action

USES:
Rhinitis, allergy symptoms, chronic idiopathic urticaria
Unlabeled uses: Asthma, atopic dermatitis

CONTRAINDICATIONS:
Breastfeeding, newborn or premature infants, hypersensitivity to this product or hydrOXYzine, severe hepatic disease
Precautions: Pregnancy (B), children, geriatric patients, respiratory disease, angle-closure glaucoma, prostatic hypertrophy, bladder neck obstruction, asthma

DOSAGE AND ROUTES
Perennial/seasonal allergic rhinitis or idiopathic urticaria
- **Adult and child ≥6 yr: PO** 5-10 mg/day

- **Child 2-5 yr: PO** 2.5 mg/day, may increase to 5 mg/day or 2.5 mg bid
- **Child 1-2 yr: PO** 2.5 mg/day, may increase to 2.5 mg q12hr
- **Geriatric: PO** 5 mg/day, may increase to 10 mg/day

Self-treatment of hay fever/other respiratory allergies

- **Adult/adolescent/child ≥6 yr: PO** 10 mg/day; **ORAL SOL** 5-10 mg/day

Renal dose/hemodialysis/hepatic dose

- **Adult: PO** CCr 11-31 ml/min, 5 mg/day

Atopic dermatitis (unlabeled)

- **Child 6-12 yr: PO** 5-10 mg/day
- **Child 1-2 yr: PO** 0.25 mg/kg bid

Available forms: Tabs 5, 10 mg; syr 5 mg/5 ml, prefilled spoons 1 mg/ml; oral sol 5 mg/ml; liquid-filled caps 10 mg; chew tabs 5, 10 mg; oral disintegrating tab 10 mg

Administer:

- Without regard to meals
- Store in tight, light-resistant container
- **Caps:** swallow whole; do not break, cut, chew, crush
- **Chew tabs:** chew before swallowing; may use with or without water
- **Oral liquid:** use calibrated measuring device

SIDE EFFECTS

CNS: *Headache,* stimulation, *drowsiness,* sedation, *fatigue,* confusion, blurred vision, tinnitus, restlessness, tremors; paradoxical excitation in children, geriatric patients

GI: *Dry mouth,* increased LFTs, constipation

INTEG: Rash, eczema, photosensitivity, urticaria

RESP: *Thickening of bronchial secretions,* dry nose, throat

PHARMACOKINETICS

Absorption rapid; onset ½ hr; peak 1-2 hr; duration 24 hr; protein binding 93%; half-life decreased in children, increased in renal/hepatic disease

INTERACTIONS

Increase: CNS depression—alcohol, opiates, sedative/hypnotics, other CNS depressants

Increase: anticholinergic/sedative effect—MAOIs

Increase: cetirizine effect—ritonavir

Drug/Food

- Food prolongs absorption by 1.7 hr

Drug/Lab Test

False negative: skin allergy tests

NURSING CONSIDERATIONS

Assess:

- **Allergy symptoms:** pruritus, urticaria, watering eyes at baseline and during treatment
- Respiratory status: rate, rhythm, increase in bronchial secretions, wheezing, chest tightness
- Blood studies: LFTs, BUN, creatinine at baseline, periodically
- Hard candy, gum, frequent rinsing of mouth for dryness

Evaluate:

- Therapeutic response: absence of running or congested nose, rashes

Teach patient/family:

- About all aspects of product use; to notify prescriber if confusion, sedation, hypotension occur
- To avoid driving, other hazardous activity if drowsiness occurs
- To avoid alcohol, other CNS depressants, OTC antihistamines
- To avoid exposure to sunlight; burns may occur
- To use sugarless gum, candy, frequent sips of water to minimize dry mouth
- Not to breastfeed

TREATMENT OF OVERDOSE:

Administer diazepam, vasopressors, phenytoin IV

⚠ HIGH ALERT

cetrorelix (Rx)

(set-roe-ree′lix)

Cetrotide

Func. class.: Gonadotropin-releasing hormone antagonist

Chem. class.: Synthetic decapeptide

ACTION: Inhibitor of pituitary gonadotropin secretion; initially increases LH and FSH; induces a rapid suppression of gonadotropin secretion

USES: For inhibition of premature LH surges in women undergoing controlled ovarian hyperstimulation

Unlabeled uses: Benign prostatic hyperplasia (BPH), endometriosis

CONTRAINDICATIONS: Pregnancy (X), breastfeeding, hypersensitivity, latex allergy, renal disease, KRA5 mutation

Precautions: Geriatric patients, bronchospasm

DOSAGE AND ROUTES

Single-dose regimen

- **Adult: SUBCUT** 3 mg when serum estradiol level at appropriate stimulation response, usually on stimulation day 7; if hCG not given within 4 days after inj of 3 mg cetrorelix, give 0.25 mg daily until day of hCG administration

Multiple-dose regimen

- **Adult: SUBCUT** 0.25 mg given on stimulation day 5 (either morning or evening) or 6 (morning) and continued daily until day hCG is given

BPH (unlabeled)

- **Adult (male): SUBCUT** 5 mg bid × 2 days, then 1 mg/day

Endometriosis (unlabeled)

- **Adult (female): SUBCUT** 3 mg weekly

Available forms: Inj 0.25 mg

Administer:

SUBCUT route

- Attach yellow-marked needle to diluent syringe; dilute powder by injecting liquid from syringe into vial, leaving syringe on vial; gently swirl until clear, avoid bubbles; withdraw contents of vial back into syringe, replace yellow-marked needle with gray-marked needle
- SUBCUT using abdomen, 1 inch away from navel or upper thigh; swab inj area with disinfectant; clean a 2-inch circle and allow to dry; pinch up area between thumb and finger; insert needle 45-90 degrees to surface; if positioned correctly, no blood will be drawn back into syringe; reposition needle without removing it; rotate inj sites
- Protect from light

SIDE EFFECTS

CNS: Headache, hot flashes

CV: Edema

ENDO: Ovarian hyperstimulation syndrome, abdominal pain (gyn)

GI: Nausea, vomiting, diarrhea

INTEG: Pain on inj; local site reactions, bruising, pruritus

Other: Rapid weight gain

RESP: Shortness of breath

SYST: **Fetal death, anaphylaxis**

PHARMACOKINETICS

Excreted in feces/urine, half-life depends on dosage, metabolized to metabolites, protein binding 86%

NURSING CONSIDERATIONS

Assess:

- Serum progesterone, LH; ovarian ultrasound day 7-14; pelvic exam, serum estradiol/gonadotropin; weight
- **For suspected pregnancy, product should not be used, pregnancy (X)**
- **For latex allergy, product should not be used**

⚠ **For anaphylaxis during first infusion**

Evaluate:

- Therapeutic response: pregnancy

Teach patient/family:

- To report abdominal pain, vaginal bleeding, nausea, vomiting, diarrhea, SOB, peripheral edema
- How to perform self-administration technique if needed

⚠ HIGH ALERT

cetuximab (Rx)

(se-tux′i-mab)

Erbitux

Func. class.: Antineoplastic—miscellaneous, monoclonal antibody

Chem. class.: Epidermal growth factor receptor inhibitor

ACTION: Not fully understood; binds to epidermal growth factor receptors (EGFRs); inhibits phosphorylation and activation of receptor-associated kinase, thereby resulting in inhibition of cell growth

USES: Alone or in combination with irinotecan for EGFRs expressing metastatic colorectal carcinoma, head/neck cancer

Unlabeled uses: Front-line use for non–small-cell lung cancer in combination with CISplatin and vinorelbine

CONTRAINDICATIONS: Hypersensitivity to this product, murine proteins

Precautions: Pregnancy (C), breastfeeding, children, geriatric patients; CV/renal/hepatic disease; ocular, pulmonary disorders

Black Box Warning: Arrhythmias, CAD, infusion-related reactions, radiation/platinum-based therapy, cardiac, respiratory arrest

DOSAGE AND ROUTES

- **Adult: IV INFUSION** 400 mg/m^2 loading dose given over 120 min, max infusion rate 5 ml/min; weekly maintenance dose (all other infusion) is 250 mg/m^2 given over 60 min, max infusion rate 5 ml/min (10 mg/min); premedicate with an H_1-antagonist (diphenhydrAMINE 50 mg IV); dosage adjustments made for infusion reactions or dermatologic toxicity; other protocols used

Non–small-cell lung cancer (NSCLC) (unlabeled)

- **Adult: IV** 400 mg/m^2 over 120 min (max 5 ml/min) week 1 with weekly infusion of 250 mg/m^2 over 60 min (max 5 ml/min) with CISplatin 80 mg/m^2 on day 1 and vinorelbine 25 mg/m^2 on days 1, 8

Available forms: Sol for inj 100 mg/50 ml, 200 mg/100 ml

Administer:

Intermittent IV INFUSION route

- Use cytoxic handling procedures
- By IV infusion only; do not give by IV push or bolus; do not shake or dilute
- Do not dilute with other products
- Store refrigerated at 36° F-46° F, discard unused portions
- **Infusion pump:** draw up volume of vial using appropriate syringe/needle (vented spike or other appropriate transfer device); fill Erbitux into sterile evacuated container/bag, repeat until calculated volume put into the container; use new needle for each vial; give through in-line filter (low protein binding 0.22 micrometer); affix infusion line and prime before starting infusion, max rate 5 ml/min; flush line at end of infusion with 0.9% NaCl, use a low protein binding 0.22-micrometer in-line filter
- **Syringe pump:** draw up volume of vial using appropriate syringe/needle (vented spike); place syringe into syringe driver of syringe pump and set rate; use in-line filter (low protein binding 0.22-micrometer); connect infusion line, start infusion after priming; repeat until calculated volume given
- Use new needle and filter for each vial, max 5 ml/min rate; use 0.9% NaCl to flush line after infusion
- Do not piggyback to patient infusion line
- Observe patient for adverse reactions for 1 hr after infusion

Black Box Warning: Infusion reactions: if mild (grade 1 or 2), reduce all doses by 50%; if severe (grade 3 or 4), permanently discontinue

SIDE EFFECTS

CNS: *Headache, insomnia, depression,* aseptic meningitis
CV: Cardiac arrest
GI: *Nausea, diarrhea, vomiting, anorexia, mouth ulceration, dehydration, constipation, abdominal pain*
HEMA: Leukopenia, anemia, neutropenia
INTEG: Rash, pruritus, acne, dry skin, toxic epidermal necrolysis, angioedema, *blepharitis, cheilitis, cellulitis, cysts, alopecia, skin/nail disorder,* acute infusion reactions, other skin toxicities
MISC: *Conjunctivitis, asthma, malaise, fever,* renal failure, hypomagnesemia
MS: *Back pain*
RESP: Interstitial lung disease, *cough, dyspnea,* pulmonary embolus, *peripheral edema,* respiratory arrest
SYST: Anaphylaxis, sepsis, infection, mucosal inflammation, Stevens-Johnson syndrome, toxic epidermal necrolysis

PHARMACOKINETICS

Half-life 114 hr, steady state by 3rd wkly infusion, peak 168-235 g/ml

INTERACTIONS

Drug/Lab:
Increase: LFTs

NURSING CONSIDERATIONS

Assess:

Black Box Warning: Pulmonary changes: lung sounds, cough, dyspnea; interstitial lung disease may occur, may be fatal; discontinue therapy if confirmed

- Cardiac arrest: monitor electrolytes, in those undergoing radiation therapy, electrolytes may be decreased; monitor cardiac patients that receive this product and radiation therapy or platinum based therapy with 5-FU (head, neck, cancer)

⚠ **Serious hypersensitivity reactions:** toxic epidermal necrosis, angioedema, anaphylaxis, Stevens-Johnson syndrome

- GI symptoms: frequency of stools, dehydration, abdominal pain, stomatitis
- **K-RAS mutations** with metastatic colorectal carcinoma; if K-RAS mutation on codon 12 or 13 detected, patient should not receive anti-EGFR antibody therapy

Evaluate:

- Therapeutic response: decreased growth, spread of EGFR-expressing metastatic colorectal, head/neck carcinoma

Teach patient/family:

Black Box Warning: To report adverse reactions immediately: shortness of breath, severe abdominal pain, skin eruptions

- About the reason for treatment, expected results

Black Box Warning: To use contraception during treatment (pregnancy [C]), not to breastfeed

- To wear sunscreen and hats to limit sun exposure; sun exposure can exacerbate any skin reactions
- To avoid crowds, persons with known infections

chlordiazePOXIDE (Rx)

(klor-dye-az-e-pox′ide)

Librium, Solium ✤

Func. class.: Antianxiety

Chem. class.: Benzodiazepine, long-acting

Controlled Substance Schedule IV

Do not confuse:
Librium/Librax

ACTION: Potentiates the actions of GABA, especially in the limbic system, reticular formation

USES: Short-term management of anxiety, acute alcohol withdrawal, preoperatively for relaxation

CONTRAINDICATIONS:
Pregnancy (D), breastfeeding, children <6 yr, hypersensitivity to benzodiazepines, closed-angle glaucoma, psychosis

Precautions: Geriatric patients, debilitated, renal/hepatic disease, suicidal ideation, abrupt discontinuation, respiratory depression, Parkinson's disease, myasthenia gravis

DOSAGE AND ROUTES
Mild anxiety
- **Adult: PO** 5-10 mg tid-qid
- **Geriatric: PO** 5 mg bid initially, increase as needed
- **Child >6 yr: PO** 5 mg bid-qid, max 10 mg bid-tid

Severe anxiety
- **Adult: PO** 25-50 mg tid-qid

Preoperatively
- **Adult: PO** 5-10 mg tid-qid on day before surgery

Alcohol withdrawal
- **Adult: PO** 50-100 mg q4-6hr prn, max 300 mg/day

Renal disease
- **Adult: PO** CCr <10 ml/min, give 50% dose

Available forms: Caps 5, 10, 25 mg

Administer:

PO route
- With food or milk for GI symptoms

SIDE EFFECTS
CNS: *Dizziness, drowsiness,* confusion, headache, anxiety, tremors, stimulation, fatigue, depression, insomnia, hallucinations

CV: *Orthostatic hypotension,* edema, ECG changes, tachycardia, hypotension

EENT: *Blurred vision,* tinnitus, mydriasis

GI: Constipation, dry mouth, nausea, vomiting, anorexia, diarrhea

GU: Irregular periods, decreased libido

HEMA: Agranulocytosis

INTEG: Rash, dermatitis, itching

PHARMACOKINETICS
PO: Onset 30 min, peak within 2 hr, duration 4-6 hr, metabolized by liver, excreted by kidneys, crosses placenta, excreted in breast milk, half-life 5-30 hr (increased in geriatric patients)

INTERACTIONS
Increase: CNS depression—CNS depressants, alcohol

Increase: chlordiazePOXIDE—cimetidine, disulfiram, FLUoxetine, isoniazid, ketoconazole, metoprolol, oral contraceptives, propranolol, valproic acid

Decrease: action of levodopa

Decrease: action of chlordiazePOXIDE—CYP3A4 inhibitors (protease inhibitors, barbiturates, rifamycins)

Drug/Lab Test

Increase: LFTs

False increase: 17-OHCS

False positive: pregnancy test (some methods)

NURSING CONSIDERATIONS
Assess:
- B/P (lying, standing), pulse; if systolic B/P drops 20 mm Hg, hold product, notify prescriber
- Blood studies: CBC during long-term therapy; **blood dyscrasias** have occurred rarely
- Hepatic studies: AST, ALT, bilirubin, creatinine, LDH, alk phos during long-term therapy
- For ataxia, oversedation of geriatric patients, debilitated patients
- Physical dependency, withdrawal symptoms: headache, nausea, vomiting, muscle pain, weakness after long-term use
- Mental status: mood, sensorium, affect, sleeping pattern, drowsiness, dizziness; suicidal tendencies; paradoxic reactions such as excitement, stimulation, acute rage
- For pregnancy; product should not be used during pregnancy (D)
- Assistance with ambulation during beginning therapy because drowsiness, dizziness occur
- Check to confirm that PO medication has been swallowed if patient is depressed, suicidal

• Sugarless gum, hard candy, frequent sips of water for dry mouth

Evaluate:

• Therapeutic response: decreased anxiety, restlessness, sleeplessness

Teach patient/family:

• That product may be taken with food
• Not to use product for everyday stress or use for more than 4 mo unless directed by prescriber, tolerance occurs
• Not to take more than prescribed amount; may be habit forming
• To avoid OTC preparations unless approved by prescriber
• To avoid driving, activities that require alertness because drowsiness may occur
• To avoid alcohol ingestion, other psychotropic medications unless directed by prescriber
• Not to discontinue medication abruptly after long-term use because this may precipitate seizures
• To rise slowly because fainting may occur, especially among geriatric patients
• That drowsiness may be worse at beginning of treatment
• To notify prescriber if pregnancy is suspected or planned
• To immediately report suicidal thoughts/behaviors

TREATMENT OF OVERDOSE:

Lavage, VS, supportive care, give flumazenil

chloroquine (Rx)

(klor′oh-kwin)

Aralen

Func. class.: Antimalarial

Chem. class.: Synthetic 4-aminoquinoline derivative

ACTION: Inhibits parasite replication, transcription of DNA to RNA by forming complexes with DNA of parasite

USES: Malaria of *Plasmodium vivax, P. malariae, P. ovale, P. falciparum* (some strains); amebiasis

Unlabeled uses: Discoid lupus erythematosus, polymorphous light eruption, rheumatoid arthritis, ulcerative colitis

CONTRAINDICATIONS: Hypersensitivity, retinal field changes

Precautions: Pregnancy (C), breastfeeding, children, blood dyscrasias, severe GI/neurologic/cardiac disease, alcoholism, hepatic disease, G6PD deficiency, psoriasis, eczema, seizures, preexisting auditory damage, torsades de pointes

Black Box Warning: Infection

DOSAGE AND ROUTES

Acute malaria attacks

• **Adult: PO** 1000 mg (600-mg base), then 500 mg (300-mg base) in 6-8 hr, then 500 mg (300-mg base) daily × 2 days for a total of 2.5 g (1.5-g base) in 3 days
• **Adult/adolescent of low body weight, child/infant: PO** 16.5 mg (10-mg base)/kg, max 600-mg base, then 8.3 mg (5-mg base)/kg, max 300-mg base 6 hr after 1st dose, then 8.3 mg (5-mg base)/kg, max 300-mg base 24 hr after 1st dose, then 8.3 mg (5-mg base)/kg, max 300-mg base 36 hr after 1st dose

Malaria prophylaxis (in areas with chloroquine-sensitive *P. falciparum*)

• **Adult: PO** 500 mg (300-mg base) weekly on same day of each wk starting 2 wk before travel and for 8 wk after leaving

Extraintestinal amebiasis

• **Adult: PO** 1 g (600-mg base) daily × 2 days, then 500 mg (300-mg base) for ≥2-3 wk
• **Child (unlabeled): PO** 16.6 mg (10-mg base)/kg (max 300-mg base) daily × 2-3 wk

Rheumatoid arthritis/discoid lupus erythematosus (unlabeled)

• **Adult: PO** 250 mg (150-mg base) daily

Available forms: Tabs 250 mg (150-mg base), 500 mg (300-mg base) phosphate

Administer:

- Product in mg or base; they are different

PO route

- Before or after meals at same time each day to maintain product level
- Store in tight, light-resistant container at room temperature; keep inj in cool environment

SIDE EFFECTS

CNS: Headache, stimulation, fatigue, **seizures**, psychosis, hallucinations, insomnia

CV: Hypotension, **heart block, asystole with syncope**, ECG changes, cardiomyopathy

EENT: *Blurred vision, corneal changes, retinal changes, difficulty focusing,* tinnitus, vertigo, deafness, photophobia, corneal edema

GI: *Nausea, vomiting, anorexia,* diarrhea, cramps

HEMA: **Thrombocytopenia, agranulocytosis, hemolytic anemia, leukopenia**

INTEG: Pruritus, pigmentary changes, skin eruptions, lichen-planus–like eruptions, eczema, **exfoliative dermatitis**

PHARMACOKINETICS

Metabolized in liver; excreted in urine, feces, breast milk; crosses placenta

PO: Peak 1-3 hr, half-life 3-5 days

INTERACTIONS

- Reduced oral clearance and metabolism of chloroquine: cimetidine

Increase: **QT prolongation, torsades de pointes—class IA, III antidysrhythmics**

Increase: effects—2D6 inhibitors (amiodarone, chlorpheniramine, FLUoxetine, haloperidol, ritonavir, PARoxetine, terbinafine, ticlopidine); CYP3A4 inhibitors (diltiazem, verapamil, itraconazole, ketoconazole, erythromycin, doxycycline, clarithromycin)

Decrease: action of chloroquine—magnesium, aluminum compounds, kaolin; do not use concurrently

Decrease: effects of ampicillin, rabies vaccine (ID)

Drug/Lab Test

Decrease: Hgb, platelets, WBC

NURSING CONSIDERATIONS

Assess:

Black Box Warning: Infection: resistance is common, not to be used for *P. falciparum* acquired in areas of resistance or where prophylaxis has failed

- Ophthalmic test if long-term treatment or dosage of >150 mg/day, baseline and periodically
- Blood studies: CBC, as blood dyscrasias occur
- **ECG during therapy; watch for depression of T waves, widening of QRS complex**
- **Allergic reactions:** pruritus, rash, urticaria
- **Blood dyscrasias:** malaise, fever, bruising, bleeding (rare)
- **For ototoxicity (tinnitus, vertigo, change in hearing); audiometric testing should be done before, after treatment**

⚠ **For toxicity: blurring vision; difficulty focusing; headache; dizziness; decreased knee, ankle reflexes; seizures, CV collapse; product should be discontinued immediately and IV fluids given**

Evaluate:

- Therapeutic response: decreased symptoms of infection

Teach patient/family:

- To take with meals or immediately after meals
- To use sunglasses in bright sunlight to decrease photophobia
- That urine may turn rust or brown color
- **To report hearing, visual problems; fever, fatigue, bruising, bleeding; may indicate blood dyscrasias**

TREATMENT OF OVERDOSE:

Administer barbiturate (ultrashort-acting), vasopressor; tracheostomy may be necessary

- **Keep away from pets, children; overdose is fatal**

chlorpheniramine (OTC, Rx)

(klor-fen-ir′a-meen)

AHIST, Aller-Chlor, Allergy, Chlor-Pheniton, Chlor-Trimeton, Diabetic Tussin Allergy Relief, ED-Chlor-Tann, Equaline Allergy, Equate Chlortabs Allergy, Novo-Pheniram ✱, P-Tann, Tana Hist-PD, Teldrin, Tripolon ✱

Func. class.: Antihistamine (1st generation, nonselective)

Chem. class.: Alkylamine, H_1-receptor antagonist

Do not confuse:
Teldrin/Tedral

ACTION: Acts on blood vessels, GI system, respiratory system by competing with histamine for H_1-receptor site; decreases allergic response by blocking histamine

USES: Allergy symptoms, rhinitis, conjunctivitis (allergic)

Unlabeled uses: Nausea, vomiting due to motion sickness, pruritus, urticaria

CONTRAINDICATIONS: Newborns/neonates

Precautions: Pregnancy (B), breastfeeding, children, geriatric patients, increased intraocular pressure, cardiac/renal disease, hypertension, asthma, seizure disorder, hyperthyroidism, prostatic hypertrophy, GI obstruction, peptic ulcer disease, emphysema, hypersensitivity to H_1-receptor antagonists, lower respiratory tract disease, stenosed peptic ulcers, bladder neck obstruction, closed-angle glaucoma

DOSAGE AND ROUTES

- **Adult and child ≥12 yr: PO** 4 mg tid-qid, max 24 mg/day; **EXT REL** 8-12 mg bid-tid, max 24 mg/day
- **Child 6-12 yr: PO** 2 mg q4-6hr, max 12 mg/day; **EXT REL** 8 mg bedtime or daily; **EXT REL** not recommended for child <6 yr

Available forms: Chewable tabs 2 mg; tabs 4, 8, 12 mg; ext rel tabs 8, 12 mg; ext rel caps 8, 12 mg; syr 1 mg/5 ml, 2 mg/5 ml, 2.5 mg/5 ml; 2 mg/ml drops

Administer:

- Avoid concurrent use with other CNS depressants
- Do not break, crush, or chew ext rel forms
- Without regard to meal
- Avoid use in children <6 yr
- Store in tight container at room temperature
- **Syrup:** Use dosing utensil to measure correct dose

SIDE EFFECTS

CNS: *Dizziness, drowsiness,* poor coordination, fatigue, anxiety, euphoria, confusion, paresthesia, neuritis

EENT: Blurred vision; dilated pupils; tinnitus; nasal stuffiness; dry nose, throat, mouth

GI: Nausea, anorexia, diarrhea

GU: *Retention,* dysuria, urinary frequency

HEMA: **Thrombocytopenia, agranulocytosis, hemolytic anemia**

INTEG: Photosensitivity

RESP: Increased thick secretions, wheezing, chest tightness

PHARMACOKINETICS

Detoxified in liver, excreted by kidneys (metabolites/free drug), half-life 12-15 hr

PO: Onset ½ hr, duration 4-12 hr

PO-ER: Duration 8-24 hr

INTERACTIONS

Increase: CNS depression—barbiturates, opiates, hypnotics, tricyclics, alcohol

Increase: effect of chlorpheniramine—MAOIs

Increase: anticholinergic action—atropine, phenothiazines, quiNIDine, haloperidol

Drug/Lab Test
False negative: skin allergy tests

NURSING CONSIDERATIONS
Assess:
- Be alert for urinary retention, frequency, dysuria; product should be discontinued
- Respiratory status: rate, rhythm, increase in bronchial secretions, wheezing, chest tightness
- Hard candy, gum, frequent rinsing of mouth for dryness

Evaluate:
- Therapeutic response: absence of running, congested nose, rashes, conjunctivitis

Teach patient/family:
- About all aspects of product use; to notify prescriber of confusion, sedation, hypotension, difficulty voiding
- To avoid driving, other hazardous activity if drowsiness occurs, especially geriatric patients
- To avoid concurrent use of alcohol

TREATMENT OF OVERDOSE:
Administer diazepam, vasopressors, phenytoin IV

chlorproMAZINE (Rx)
(klor-proe′ma-zeen)
Func. class.: Antipsychotic/antiemetic
Chem. class.: Phenothiazine-aliphatic

Do not confuse:
chlorproMAZINE/chlorproPAMIDE/prochlorperazine

ACTION: Depresses cerebral cortex, hypothalamus, limbic system, which control activity aggression; blocks neurotransmission produced by DOPamine at synapse; exhibits a strong α-adrenergic, anticholinergic blocking action; mechanism for antipsychotic effects is unclear

USES: Psychotic disorders, mania, schizophrenia, anxiety, intractable hiccups in adults, nausea, vomiting; preoperatively for relaxation; acute intermittent porphyria, behavioral problems in children, nonpsychotic, demented patients, Tourette's syndrome
Unlabeled uses: Vascular headache, agitation, dementia, neonatal abstinence syndrome

CONTRAINDICATIONS: Children <6 mo, hypersensitivity, circulatory collapse, liver damage, cerebral arteriosclerosis, coronary disease, coma
Precautions: Pregnancy (C), breastfeeding, geriatric patients, seizure disorders, hypertension, hepatic/cardiac disease, prostatic enlargement, Parkinson's disease, pulmonary disease, severe hypo/hypertension, blood dyscrasias, brain damage, bone marrow depression, alcohol/barbiturate withdrawal, closed-angle glaucoma

Black Box Warning: Dementia; increased mortality in geriatric patients with dementia-related psychosis

DOSAGE AND ROUTES
Psychosis
- **Adult: PO** 10-50 mg q1-4hr initially then increase up to 2 g/day if necessary; **IM** 10-50 mg q1-4hr, usual dose 300-800 mg/day
- **Geriatric:** 10-25 mg daily-bid, increase by 10-25 mg/day q4-7days, max 800 mg/day
- **Child >6 mo: PO** 0.55 mg/kg q4-6hr; **IM** 0.5 mg/kg q6-8hr

Nausea and vomiting
- **Adult: PO** 10-25 mg q4-6hr prn; **IM** 12.5-25 mg, then 25-50 mg if no hypotension q3hr prn; q6-8hr prn, max 400 mg/day; **IV** 25-50 mg daily-qid
- **Child ≥6 mo: PO** 0.55 mg/kg q4-6hr; **IM** q6-8hr; **IM** ≤5 yr or ≤22.7 kg, 40 mg; max **IM** 5-10 yr or 22.7-45.5 kg, 75 mg

Intractable hiccups/acute intermittent porphyria
- **Adult: PO** 25-50 mg tid-qid; **IM** 25-50 mg (only if PO dose does not work); **IV**

25-50 mg in 500-1000 ml **NS** (only for severe hiccups)

Available forms: Tabs 10, 25, 50, 100, 200 mg; inj 25 mg/ml

Administer:

- Anticholinergic agent for EPS if ordered

PO route

- With full glass of water, milk or with food to decrease GI upset
- Periodically attempt dosage reduction in those with behavioral problems
- Store in tight, light-resistant container
- **Syrup:** Use calibrated measuring device, do not spill on skin or clothes

IM route

- Use gloves to prepare product; if product touches skin, wash with soap and water to prevent contact dermatitis
- IM, inject in deep muscle mass with patient recumbent, do not give SUBCUT, no dilution needed; if irritation occurs, may dilute in NS or procaine 2%
- Avoid skin contact with injection solution—may cause contact dermatitis

IV route

Direct IV: After **diluting** 1 mg/1 ml with NS, **give** 1 mg or less/2 min or more with patient recumbent, never give undiluted

Intermittent IV INFUSION: Dilute 25-50 mg/500-1000 NS or other compatible large IV sol, **give** over ½ hour, protect from light

Syringe compatibilities: Atropine, benztropine, butorphanol, diphenhydrAMINE, doxapram, droperidol, fentaNYL, glycopyrrolate, HYDROmorphone, hydrOXYzine, meperidine, metoclopramide, midazolam, morphine, pentazocine, perphenazine, prochlorperazine, promazine, promethazine, scopolamine

Y-site compatibilities: Alfentanil, amikacin, amphotericin B lipid complex, amsacrine, anidulafungin, ascorbic acid injection, atenolol, atracurium, atropine, benztropine, bleomycin sulfate, buprenorphine, butorphanol, calcium chloride/gluconate, caspofungin, cimetidine, cisatracurium, CISplatin, cladribine, codeine, cyanocobalamin, cyclophosphamide, cycloSPORINE, cytarabine, DACTINomycin, DAPTOmycin, dexmedetomidine, digoxin, diltiazem, diphenhydrAMINE, DOBUTamine, DOCEtaxel, DOPamine, doxacurium, DOXOrubicin, DOXOrubicin liposomal, doxycycline, enalaprilat, ePHEDrine, EPINEPHrine, epirubicin, erythromycin, esmolol, etoposide, famotidine, fenoldopam, fentaNYL, filgrastim, fluconazole, gatifloxacin, gemcitabine, gentamicin, glycopyrrolate, granisetron, hydrocortisone, HYDROmorphone, hydrOXYzine, IDArubicin, ifosfamide, isoproterenol, labetalol, levofloxacin, lidocaine, LORazepam, LR, magnesium sulfate, mannitol, mechlorethamine, meperidine, methicillin, methoxamine, methyldopate, methylPREDNISolone, metoclopramide, metoprolol, metroNIDAZOLE, miconazole, midazolam, milrinone, minocycline, mitoXANtrone, morphine, multiple vitamins injection, mycophenolate mofetil, nafcillin, nalbuphine, naloxone, netilmicin, nitroglycerin, norepinephrine, octreotide, ondansetron, oxacillin, oxaliplatin, palonosetron, pamidronate, pancuronium, papaverine, penicillin G potassium, pentamidine, pentazocine, phytonadione, polymyxin B, potassium chloride, procainamide, prochlorperazine, promethazine, propofol, propranolol, protamine sulfate, pyridoxine, quiNIDine, quinupristin-dalfopristin, ranitidine, Ringer's injection, ritodrine, riTUXimab, rocuronium, sodium acetate, succinylcholine, SUFentanil, tacrolimus, teniposide, theophylline, thiamine, thiotepa, tirofiban, TNA, tolazoline, TPN, trimetaphan, vancomycin, vasopressin, vecuronium, verapamil, vinCRIStine, vinorelbine, vitamin B complex with C, voriconazole, zoledronic acid

SIDE EFFECTS

CNS: *EPS: pseudoparkinsonism, akathisia, dystonia, tardive dyskinesia,* seizures, *headache,* neuroleptic malignant syndrome, dizziness

CV: *Orthostatic hypotension,* hypertension, cardiac arrest, ECG changes, tachycardia

EENT: Blurred vision, glaucoma, dry eyes
ENDO: SIADH
GI: *Dry mouth, nausea, vomiting, anorexia, constipation,* diarrhea, cholestatic jaundice, weight gain
GU: Urinary retention, enuresis, impotence, amenorrhea, gynecomastia, breast engorgement
HEMA: Anemia, leukopenia, leukocytosis, agranulocytosis
INTEG: *Rash,* photosensitivity, dermatitis
RESP: Laryngospasm, dyspnea, respiratory depression
SYST: Death in geriatric patients with dementia

PHARMACOKINETICS

Metabolized by liver, excreted in urine (metabolites), crosses placenta, enters breast milk, 95% bound to plasma proteins, elimination half-life 23-37 hr
PO: Absorption variable, widely distributed, onset erratic 30-60 min, duration 4-6 hr
PO-ER: Onset 30-60 min, peak unknown, duration 10-12 hr
IM: Well absorbed, peak 15-20 min, duration 4-8 hr
IV: Onset 5 min, peak 10 min, duration unknown

INTERACTIONS

Increase: CNS depression—other CNS depressants, alcohol, barbiturate anesthetics, antihistamines, sedatives/hypnotics, antidepressants
Increase: toxicity—EPINEPHrine
Increase: agranulocystosis—antithyroid agents
Increase: effects of both products—β-adrenergic blockers, alcohol
Increase: anticholinergic effects—anticholinergics, antidepressants, antiparkinsonian agents, MAOIs
Increase: valproic acid level
Decrease: seizure threshold—anticonvulsants
Decrease: absorption—aluminum hydroxide, magnesium hydroxide antacids, cimetidine
Decrease: antiparkinson activity—levodopa, bromocriptine
Decrease: serum chlorproMAZINE—lithium, barbiturates
Decrease: anticoagulant effect—warfarin

Drug/Lab Test
Increase: hepatic studies
Decrease: WBC, platelets, Hgb/HcT
False positive: pregnancy tests, PKU
False negative: urinary steroids, 17-OHCS

NURSING CONSIDERATIONS

Assess:

- Mental status: orientation, mood, behavior, presence and type of hallucinations before initial administration and monthly
- Any potentially reversible causes of behavior problems in geriatric patients before and during therapy
- Swallowing of PO medication; check for hoarding or giving of medication to other patients
- I&O ratio; palpate bladder if low urinary output occurs, especially in geriatric patients
- Bilirubin, CBC, LFTs, ocular exam; agranulocytosis, glaucoma, cholestatic jaundice may occur
- Respirations q4hr during initial treatment; establish baseline before starting treatment; report drops of 30 mm Hg; obtain baseline ECG; Q-wave and T-wave changes
- Dizziness, faintness, palpitations, tachycardia on rising

⚠ **Neuroleptic malignant syndrome:** hyperpyrexia, muscle rigidity, increased CPK, altered mental status, for acute dystonia (check chewing, swallowing, eyes, pill rolling)

- **EPS:** akathisia (inability to sit still, no pattern to movements), tardive dyskinesia (bizarre movements of the jaw, mouth, tongue, extremities), pseudoparkinsonism (rigidity, tremors, pill rolling, shuffling gait)
- Constipation, urinary retention daily; increase bulk, water in diet

⚠ Nurse Alert

• Supervised ambulation until stabilized on medication; do not involve in strenuous exercise program because fainting is possible; patient should not stand still for long periods
• Increased fluids, roughage to prevent constipation
• Candy, gum, sips of water for dry mouth

Evaluate:
• Therapeutic response: decrease in emotional excitement, hallucinations, delusions, paranoia; reorganization of patterns of thought, speech; increase in target behaviors

Teach patient/family:
• To use good oral hygiene; to use frequent rinsing of mouth, sugarless gum, candy, ice chips for dry mouth
• To avoid hazardous activities until product response is determined
• That orthostatic hypotension occurs often; to rise gradually from sitting or lying position
• To remain lying down for at least 30 min after IM inj
• To avoid hot tubs, hot showers, tub baths because hypotension may occur; that, during hot weather, heat stroke may occur; to take extra precautions to stay cool
• To avoid abrupt withdrawal of product or EPS may result; product should be withdrawn slowly
• To avoid OTC preparations (cough, hay fever, cold) unless approved by prescriber since serious product interactions may occur; avoid use with alcohol, increased drowsiness may occur
• To use a sunscreen and sunglasses to prevent burns
• To take antacids 2 hr before or after this product
• **To report sore throat, malaise, fever, bleeding, mouth sores; CBC should be drawn and product discontinued**
• To employ contraceptive measures
• That urine may turn pink or reddish brown

TREATMENT OF OVERDOSE: Lavage if orally ingested; provide airway; *do not induce vomiting or use EPINEPHrine*

C

cholestyramine (Rx)
(koe-less-tir′a-meen)
Prevalite, Questran, Questran Light
Func. class.: Antilipemic
Chem. class.: Bile acid sequestrant

Do not confuse:
Questran/Quarzan

ACTION: Adsorbs, combines with bile acids to form insoluble complex that is excreted through feces; loss of bile acids lowers LDL, cholesterol levels

USES: Primary hypercholesterolemia (esp. type IIa/IIb hyperlipoproteinemia), pruritus associated with biliary obstruction
Unlabeled uses: Diarrhea caused by excess bile acid

CONTRAINDICATIONS: Hypersensitivity; complete biliary obstruction; hyperlipidemia III, IV, V
Precautions: Pregnancy (C), breastfeeding, children, PKU, renal disease, coagulopathy

DOSAGE AND ROUTES
• **Adult: PO** 4 g/day or bid, max 24 g/day
• **Child: PO** 240 mg/kg/day in 3 divided doses with food or drink, max 8 g/day titrated up over several weeks to decrease GI effects

Available forms: Powder for susp 4 g cholestyramine/packet or scoop; tab 1 g

Administer:
• Product daily or bid; give all other medications 1 hr before or 4-6 hr after cholestyramine to avoid poor absorption
• Product mixed with applesauce or stirred into beverage (2-6 oz), let stand for 2 min; do not take dry, avoid inhaling powder, avoid GI tube administration, take with food

• Supplemental doses of vit A, D, K if levels are low
• Doses are expressed in anhydrous cholestyramine resin; amount of resin varies with each product

SIDE EFFECTS

CNS: Headache, dizziness, drowsiness, vertigo, tinnitus, anxiety
GI: *Constipation, abdominal pain, nausea,* fecal impaction, hemorrhoids, flatulence, vomiting, steatorrhea, peptic ulcer
HEMA: Bleeding, increased PT
INTEG: Rash, irritation of perianal area, tongue, skin
META: Decreased vit A, D, K, red cell folate content; hyperchloremic acidosis
MS: Muscle, joint pain

PHARMACOKINETICS

PO: Excreted in feces, LDL lowered within 4-7 days, serum cholesterol lowered within 1 mo, duration 2-4 wk

INTERACTIONS

Decrease: absorption of warfarin; thiazides; cardiac glycosides; propranolol; corticosteroids; iron; thyroid hormones; acetaminophen; amiodarone; penicillin G; tetracyclines; clofibrate; gemfibrozil; oral vancomycin, glipiZIDE; vit A, D, E, K
Drug/Lab Test
Increase: AST, ALT, alk phos
Decrease: sodium, potassium

NURSING CONSIDERATIONS

Assess:
• Cardiac glycoside level if both products administered, may need to adjust dose of cardiac glycoside, if this product is increased or decreased
• For signs of vit A, D, K deficiency
• **Hypercholesterolemia:** fasting LDL, HDL, total cholesterol, triglyceride levels, electrolytes if receiving extended therapy; diet history
• **Pruritus:** for signs of itching
• Bowel pattern daily; increase bulk, water in diet for constipation; diarrhea may also occur

Evaluate:
• Therapeutic response: decreased LDL, cholesterol level (hyperlipidemia); diarrhea, pruritus (excess bile acids)

Teach patient/family:
⚠ About the symptoms of hypoprothrombinemia: bleeding mucous membranes, dark tarry stools, hematuria, petechiae; report immediately
• To take with food, never use dry
• That PKU patients should avoid Questran Light (contains aspartame and phenylalanine)
• About the importance of compliance
• That risk factors should be decreased: high-fat diet, smoking, alcohol consumption, absence of exercise
• That GI side effects will resolve with continued use

cidofovir (Rx)

(si-doh-foh′veer)
Vistide
Func. class.: Antiviral
Chem. class.: Nucleotide analog

ACTION: Suppresses cytomegalovirus (CMV) replication by selective inhibition of viral DNA synthesis

USES: CMV retinitis in patients with HIV; used with probenecid
Unlabeled uses: Adenovirus, condylomata acuminata, eczema vaccination, Epstein-Barr virus, generalized vaccinia, herpes genitalis/simplex, HPV, molluscum contagiosum, vaccinia necrosum, vaccinia, varicella-zoster, variola

CONTRAINDICATIONS: Hypersensitivity to this product, probenecid, sulfa products; direct intraocular injection

Black Box Warning: Proteinuria, renal disease/failure

Precautions: Pregnancy (C), breastfeeding, children <6 mo, geriatric patients, preexisting cytopenias, renal function impairment, platelet count $<25,000/mm^3$, dehydration

Black Box Warning: Neutropenia, infertility, secondary malignancy

DOSAGE AND ROUTES

• **Adult: IV** 5 mg/kg weekly × 2 wk then 3 mg/kg q2wk, give with probenecid

Renal dose

• **Adult: IV** CCr ≤55 ml/min, do not use; SCr increase of 0.3-0.4 mg/dl above baseline, decrease dose to 3 mg/kg; SCr increase of ≥0.5 mg/dl above baseline or ≥221 proteinuria, discontinue

Available forms: Inj 75 mg/ml

Administer:

Black Box Warning: Use cytotoxic handling procedures

• Allow to warm to room temperature
• If product comes in contact with skin, wash with soap and water immediately
• If zidovudine is used, reduce dose to 50% on cidofovir treatment days

Intermittent IV INFUSION route

• **Dilute** in 100 ml 0.9% saline sol before administration; probenecid must be given PO 2 g 3 hr before the cidofovir infusion and 1 g at 2 and 8 hr after ending the cidofovir infusion; **give** 1 L of 0.9% saline sol IV with each INFUSION of cidofovir, give saline INFUSION over 1-2 hr period immediately before cidofovir; patient should be given a 2nd L if the patient can tolerate the fluid load (2nd L given at time of cidofovir or immediately afterward, should be given over 1-3 hr)
• **Give** slowly; do not give by bolus IV, SUBCUT inj
• Use diluted sol within 24 hr, do not freeze; do not use sol with particulate matter or discoloration
• Do not admix

SIDE EFFECTS

CNS: *Fever, chills,* coma, confusion, abnormal thoughts, *dizziness*, bizarre dreams, *headache*, psychosis, tremors, somnolence, paresthesia, *amnesia, anxiety, insomnia*, seizures

CV: Dysrhythmias, hypo/hypertension

EENT: Retinal detachment with CMV retinitis

GI: Abnormal LFTs, *nausea, vomiting, anorexia, diarrhea*, abdominal pain, hemorrhage

GU: Hematuria, increased creatinine, BUN, nephrotoxicity

HEMA: Granulocytopenia, thrombocytopenia, irreversible neutropenia, anemia, eosinophilia

INTEG: *Rash, alopecia, pruritus, acne*, urticaria, pain at inj site, phlebitis

RESP: Dyspnea

PHARMACOKINETICS

Terminal half-life 2.6 hr

INTERACTIONS

Black Box Warning: Nephrotoxicity: amphotericin B, foscarnet, aminoglycosides, pentamidine IV, NSAIDs, salicylates; wait 7 days after use to begin cidofovir

NURSING CONSIDERATIONS

Assess:

• Culture before treatment is initiated; cultures of blood, urine, and throat may all be taken; CMV not confirmed by this method; diagnosis made by ophthalmic exam

Black Box Warning: Renal, hepatic, increased hemopoietic studies, BUN; serum creatinine, AST, ALT, creatinine, CCr, A-G ratio, baseline and drip treatment, blood counts should be done q2wk; watch for decreasing granulocytes, Hgb; if low, therapy may have to be discontinued and restarted after hematologic recovery; blood transfusions may be required, renal failure can occur also, Fanconi syndrome

• For GI symptoms: severe nausea, vomiting, diarrhea; severe symptoms may necessitate discontinuing product

• Electrolytes and minerals: calcium, phosphorus, magnesium, sodium, potassium; watch closely for tetany during 1st administration

Black Box Warning: Blood dyscrasias (anemia, granulocytopenia); bruising, fatigue, bleeding, poor healing; leukopenia, neutropenia, thrombocytopenia: WBCs, platelets q2days during 2×/day dosing and every wk thereafter; check for leukopenias with daily WBC count in patients with prior leukopenia, with other nucleoside analogs, or for whom leukopenia counts are <1000 cells/mm^3 at start of treatment

• Allergic reactions: flushing, rash, urticaria, pruritus
• Monitor serum creatinine or CCr at least q2wk; give only to those with creatinine levels ≤1.5 mg/dl, CCr >55 ml/min, urine protein <100 mg/dl

Evaluate:
• Therapeutic response: decreased symptoms of CMV

Teach patient/family:
• To notify prescriber if sore throat, swollen lymph nodes, malaise, fever occur; may indicate other infections
• To report perioral tingling, numbness in extremities, paresthesias; report rash immediately, mental/vision changes, urinary problems, abnormal bleeding
• That serious product interactions may occur if OTC products are ingested; check with prescriber
• That product is not a cure but will control symptoms
• That regular ophthalmic exams, renal studies must be continued
• That major toxicities may necessitate discontinuing product
• To use contraception during treatment, that infertility may occur, and that men should use barrier contraception for 90 days after treatment

TREATMENT OF OVERDOSE:
Discontinue product; use hemodialysis; increase hydration

cilostazol (Rx)
(sih-los′tah-zol)
Pletal
Func. class.: Platelet aggregation inhibitor
Chem. class.: Quinolinone derivative

Do not confuse:
Pletal/Plendil

ACTION:
Multifactorial effects (antithrombotic, antiplatelet vasodilation)

USES:
Intermittent claudication associated with PVD
Unlabeled uses: Buerger's disease, percutaneous coronary intervention (PCI)

CONTRAINDICATIONS:
Hypersensitivity, acute MI, active bleeding conditions, hemostatic conditions

Black Box Warning: CHF

Precautions: Pregnancy (C), breastfeeding, children, geriatric patients, previous hepatic disease, cardiac/renal disease, increased bleeding risk, low platelet count, platelet dysfunction, smoking

DOSAGE AND ROUTES
• **Adult: PO** 100 mg bid taken ≥30 min before or 2 hr after breakfast and dinner or 50 mg bid if using products that inhibit CYP3A4 and CYP2C19; 12 wk of treatment may be needed for beneficial effect

PCI to prevent acute coronary thrombosis/Buerger's disease (unlabeled)
• **Adult: PO** 100 mg bid

Available forms: Tabs 50, 100 mg

Administer:
• Give bid 30 min before or 2 hr after meals with a full glass of water; do not give with grapefruit juice

SIDE EFFECTS

CNS: *Dizziness, headache*
CV: *Palpitations, tachycardia,* nodal dysrhythmia, postural hypotension, chest pain
EENT: Blindness, diplopia, ear pain, tinnitus, retinal hemorrhage
GI: *Nausea,* vomiting, *diarrhea,* GI discomfort, colitis, cholelithiasis, ulcer, esophagitis, gastritis, anorexia, *flatulence, dyspepsia*
GU: Cystitis, frequency, vaginitis, **vaginal hemorrhage,** hematuria
HEMA: Bleeding (epistaxis, hematuria, retinal hemorrhage, GI bleeding), thrombocytopenia, anemia, **polycythemia, aplastic anemia**
INTEG: *Rash,* urticaria, dry skin, **Stevens-Johnson syndrome**
MISC: *Back pain, headache, infection, myalgia, peripheral edema,* chills, fever, malaise, diabetes mellitus
RESP: *Cough, pharyngitis, rhinitis,* asthma, pneumonia

PHARMACOKINETICS

95%-98% protein binding; metabolism: hepatic extensively by CYP3A4, 2C19 enzymes (active metabolite); excreted in urine (74%), feces (20%); half-life 11-13 hr

INTERACTIONS

Increase: bleeding tendencies—anticoagulants, NSAIDs, thrombolytics, abciximab, eptifibatide, tirofiban, ticlopidine
Increase: cilostazol levels—CYP3A4, CYP2C19 inhibitors; diltiazem, erythromycin, clarithromycin, verapamil, protease inhibitors, omeprazole; exercise caution when coadministering with fluvoxaMINE, FLUoxetine, ketoconazole, isoniazid, gemfibrozil, omeprazole, itraconazole, voriconazole, fluconazole; reduce dose to 50 mg bid
Decrease: cilostazol levels—CYP3A4 inducers

Drug/Herb

Decrease: action—chamomile, coenzyme Q10, feverfew, garlic, ginger, ginko biloba, flax, goldenseal, St. John's wort

Drug/Food

• Do not use with grapefruit juice, toxicity may occur
Increase: cilostazol action—fatty meal, avoid giving with food

NURSING CONSIDERATIONS

Assess:

Black Box Warning: For underlying CV disease because CV risk is great; for CV lesions with repeated oral administration; do not administer to patients with CHF of any severity; for severe headache, signs of toxicity

• Blood studies: CBC q2wk, Hct, Hgb, PT

Evaluate:

• Therapeutic response: improved walking distance, duration; decreased pain

Teach patient/family:

• To avoid hazardous activities until effect is known
• To report any unusual bleeding
• To report side effects such as diarrhea, skin rashes, subcutaneous bleeding
• That effects may take 2-4 wk; treatment of up to 12 wk may be required for necessary effect
• That reading the patient package insert is necessary
• That it is best to discontinue tobacco use, not to use grapefruit juice
• **That there are many drug and herb interactions; obtain approval from prescriber before use**

cimetidine (OTC, Rx)

(sye-met′i-deen)

Acid Reducer, Equaline Acid Reducer, Nu-Cimet ✦, Tagamet, Tagamet HB

Func. class.: H_2-histamine receptor antagonist
Chem. class.: Imidazole derivative

ACTION: Inhibits histamine at H_2-receptor site in the gastric parietal cells, which inhibits gastric acid secretion

USES: Short-term treatment of duodenal and gastric ulcers and maintenance; management of GERD (PO) and Zollinger-Ellison syndrome; prevention of upper GI bleeding; prevent, relieve heartburn, acid indigestion, upper GI bleeding

Unlabeled uses: Prevention of aspiration pneumonitis, stress ulcers, angioedema, molluscum contagiosum, NSAID-induced ulcer prophylaxis, verruca vulgaris

CONTRAINDICATIONS: Hypersensitivity to this product, H2 blockers, benzyl alcohol

Precautions: Pregnancy (B), breastfeeding, children <16 yr, geriatric patients, organic brain syndrome, renal/hepatic disease

DOSAGE AND ROUTES

Short-term treatment of active ulcers

- **Adult/adolescents ≥16 yr: PO** 300 mg qid with meals, at bedtime × 8-12 wk or 400 mg bid, 800 mg at bedtime; after 8 wk, give bedtime dose only; **IV BOL** 300 mg/20 ml 0.9% NaCl over 1-2 min q6hr; **IV INFUSION** 300 mg/50 ml D_5W over 15-20 min; **IM** 300 mg q6hr, max 2400 mg/day
- **Child: PO** 20-40 mg/kg/day, divided q6hr; **IM/IV** 5-10 mg/kg q6-8hr

Prophylaxis of duodenal ulcer

- **Adult and child >16 yr:** 400 mg at bedtime or 300 mg bid

GERD

- **Adult: PO** 800-1600 mg/day in divided doses × up to 12 wk

Hypersecretory conditions (Zollinger-Ellison syndrome)

- **Adult: PO/IM/IV** 300-600 mg q6hr; may increase to 12 g/day if needed; OTC use ≤200 mg daily or bid, max 2×/wk

Upper GI bleeding prophylaxis

- **Adult: IV** 50 mg/hr; lowered in renal disease

Heartburn

- **Adult/child ≥12 yrs: PO** 200 mg Tagamet Hb up to bid, may use before eating, max 400 mg/day, max daily use up to 2 wk

Renal disease

- **Adult: PO/IV** CCr <30 ml/min, 300 mg q12hr

Verruca vulgaris (unlabeled)

- **Child: PO** 30-40 mg/kg/day divided tid × 2 mo

Available forms: Tabs 100, 200, 300, 400, 800 mg; liq 200, 300 mg/5 ml; inj 300 mg/2 ml, 300 mg/50 ml 0.9% NaCl

Administer:

PO route

- With meals for prolonged product effect; antacids 1 hr before or 1 hr after cimetidine

IM route

- May give undiluted
- Give at end of dialysis
- Inject deeply in large muscle mass, aspirate

IV route

- After **diluting** 300 mg/20 ml of 0.9% NaCl for inj; give by **direct IV over** ≥5 min; **Intermittent IV INFUSION** may be **diluted** 300 mg/50 ml of D_5W; **run** ≥30 min; or total daily dose (900 mg) diluted in 100-1000 ml D_5W given over 24 hr **Continuous IV INFUSION**
- Storage of diluted sol at room temperature up to 48 hr

Y-site compatibilities: Acetaminophen acyclovir, alfentanil, amifostine, amikacin, aminocaproic acid, aminophylline, amphotericin B lipid complex/liposome, anakinra, anidulafungin, ascorbic acid injection, atenolol, atracurium, atropine, aztreonam, benztropine, bivalirudin, bleomycin, bumetanide, buprenorphine, butorphanol, calcium chloride/gluconate, CARBOplatin, caspofungin, cefamandole, ceFAZolin, cefmetazole, cefonicid, cefotaxime, cefoTEtan, cefOXitin, cefTAZidime, ceftizoxime, cefTRIAXone, cefuroxime, cephalothin, cephapirin, chlorproMAZINE, cisatracurium, CISplatin, cladribine, clarithromycin, clindamycin, codeine, cyanocobalamin, cyclophosphamide, cycloSPORINE, cytarabine, DACTINomycin, DAPTOmycin, dexamethasone, dexmedetomidine, digoxin, diltiazem, diphenhydrAMINE, DOBUTamine, DOCEtaxel, DOPamine, doripenem, doxacurium, doxapram, DOXOrubicin, DOXOrubicin liposome, enalaprilat, ePHEDrine, EPINEPHrine, epirubicin, epoetin alfa, eptifibatide, ertapenem, erythromycin, esmolol, etoposide, famotidine, fenoldopam, fentaNYL, filgrastim, fluconazole, fludarabine, fluorouracil, folic acid, foscarnet, gallium, gatifloxacin, gemcitabine, gentamicin, gycopyrrolate, granisetron, heparin, hydrocortisone, HYDROmorphone, hydrOXYzine, IDArubicin, ifosfamide, imipenem-cilastatin, irinotecan, isoproterenol, ketorolac, labetalol, levofloxacin, lidocaine, linezolid, LORazepam, LR, magnesium sulfate, mannitol, mechlorethamine, melphalan, meperidine, metaraminol, meropenem, methicillin, methotrexate, methoxamine, methyldopate, methylPREDNISolone, metoclopramide, metoprolol, metroNIDAZOLE, mezlocillin, miconazole, midazolam, milrinone, minocycline, mitoXANtrone, morphine, moxalactum, multiple vitamin injection, mycophenolate, nafcillin, nalbuphine, naloxone, nesiritide, netilmicin, niCARdipine, nitroglycerin, nitroprusside, norepinephrine, octreotide, ondansetron, oxacillin, oxaliplatin, oxytocin, PACLitaxel, palonosetron, pamidronate, pancuronium, pantoprazole, papaverine, PEMEtrexed, penicillin G sodium/potassium, pentamidine, pentazocine, phenylephrine, phytonadione, pipercillin, piperacillin/tazobactam, polymyxin B, potassium chloride, procainamide, prochlorperazine, promethazine, propofol, propranolol, protamine, pyridoxine, quiNIDine, quinupristin-dalfopristin, ranitidine, remifentanil, Ringers' ritodrine, riTUXimab, rocuronium, sargramostim, sodium acetate/bicarbonate, succinylcholine, SUFentanil, tacrolimus, teniposide, theophylline, thiamine, thiotepa, ticarcillin, ticarcillin-clavulanate, tigecycline, tirofiban, TNA, tobramycin, tolazoline, topotecan, TPN, trastuzumab, trimetaphan, urokinase, vancomycin, vasopressin, vecuronium, verapamil, vinCRIStine, vinorelbine, voriconazole, zidovudine, zoledronic acid

SIDE EFFECTS

CNS: *Confusion, headache,* depression, dizziness, anxiety, weakness, psychosis, tremors, **seizures**

CV: Bradycardia, tachycardia, **dysrhythmias**

GI: *Diarrhea,* abdominal cramps, **paralytic ileus, jaundice**

GU: Gynecomastia, galactorrhea, impotence, increase in BUN, creatinine

HEMA: **Agranulocytosis, thrombocytopenia, neutropenia, aplastic anemia, increase in PT**

INTEG: Urticaria, rash, alopecia, sweating, flushing, **exfoliative dermatitis**

RESP: **Pneumonia**

PHARMACOKINETICS

Half-life $1^1/_2$-2 hr; 30%-40% metabolized by liver, excreted in urine (unchanged), crosses placenta, enters breast milk

PO: Onset 30 min, peak 45-90 min; duration 4-5 hr, well absorbed

IM/IV: Onset 10 min, peak ½ hr, duration 4-5 hr, well absorbed (IM)

INTERACTIONS

Increase: toxicity due to CYP450 pathway—benzodiazepines, β-blockers, calcium channel blockers, carBAMazepine, chloroquine, lidocaine, metroNIDAZOLE, moricizine, phenytoin, quiNIDine, quiNINE, sulfonylureas, theophylline, tricyclics, valproic acid, warfarin

Increase: bone marrow suppression—carmustine

Decrease: absorption of cimetidine—antacids, sucralfate

Decrease: absorption—ketoconazole, itraconazole

Drug/Lab Test

Increase: alk phos, AST, creatinine, prolactin

False positive: gastroccult, hemoccult tests

False negative: TB skin tests

NURSING CONSIDERATIONS

Assess:

- **Ulcer symptoms:** epigastric pain, duration, intensity; aggravating, ameliorating factors

Evaluate:

- Therapeutic response: decreased pain in abdomen; healing of ulcers; absence of gastroesophageal reflux, gastric pH of 5

Teach patient/family:

- That gynecomastia, impotence may occur, are reversible
- To avoid driving, other hazardous activities until stabilized on this medication; drowsiness or dizziness may occur
- To avoid OTC preparations: aspirin; cough, cold preparations; condition may worsen, OTC therapy is used for short term (2 wk)
- That smoking decreases effectiveness of product
- That product must be taken exactly as prescribed and continued for prescribed time to be effective; not to double dose
- To report bruising, fatigue, malaise; blood dyscrasias may occur
- To report diarrhea, black tarry stools, sore throat, rash to prescriber

cinacalcet (Rx)

(sin-a-kal′set)

Sensipar

Func. class.: Calcium receptor agonist

Chem. class.: Polypeptide hormone

ACTION: Directly lowers PTH levels by increasing sensitivity of calcium-sensing receptors to extracellular calcium

USES: Hypercalcemia with parathyroid carcinoma, secondary hyperparathyroidism with chronic kidney disease for patient on dialysis, primary hyperparathyroidism

CONTRAINDICATIONS: Hypersensitivity, hypocalcemia

Precautions: Pregnancy (C), breastfeeding, children, seizure disorders, hepatic disease

DOSAGE AND ROUTES

Parathyroid carcinoma

- **Adult: PO** 30 mg bid, titrate q2-4wk, with sequential doses of 30 mg bid, 60 mg bid, 90 mg bid, 90 mg tid-qid to normalize calcium levels

Secondary hyperparathyroidism

- **Adult: PO** 30 mg/day, titrate no more frequently than q2-4wk with sequential doses of 30, 60, 90, 120, 180 mg/day

Available forms: Tabs 30, 60, 90 mg

Administer:

- Swallow tabs whole; do not break, crush, or chew; use with food or right after a meal
- Can be used alone or in combination with vit D sterols, phosphate binders
- Storage at <77° F (25° C)

Secondary hyperthyroidism

- Titrate q2-4wk to target iPTH consistent with National Kidney Foundation–Kidney Disease Outcomes Quality Initiative (NKF-K/DOQI) for chronic kidney disease patient on dialysis of 150-300 pg/ml; if iPTH <150-300 pg/ml, reduce dose of cinacalcet and/or vit D sterols or discontinue treatment

SIDE EFFECTS

CNS: Dizziness, asthenia, **seizures**, tetany, hallucinations, depression, headache

CV: Hypertension, dysrhythmia exacerbation

GI: Nausea, diarrhea, vomiting, anorexia

MISC: Access infection, noncardiac chest pain, hypocalcemia

MS: Myalgia, bone fractures

PHARMACOKINETICS

93%-97% bound to plasma; proteins metabolized by CYP3A4, 2D6, 1A2; half-life 30-40 hr; renal excretion of metabolites (80% renal, 15% in feces)

INTERACTIONS

Increase: cinacalcet levels: CYP3A4 inhibitors (ketoconazole, erythromycin, itraconazole)

Increase: levels of CYP2D6 inhibitors (flecainide, vinBLAStine, thioridazine, tricyclics)

Drug/Food
Increase: action by high-fat meal

NURSING CONSIDERATIONS

Assess:

- **Hypocalcemia:** cramping, seizures, tetany, myalgia, paresthesia; calcium, phosphorous within 1 wk and iPTH 1-4 wk after initiation or dosage adjustment when maintenance established; measure calcium, phosphorus monthly; iPTH q1-3mo, target range 150-300 pg/ml for iPTH level; biochemical markers of bone formation/resorption; radiologic evidence of fracture; serum testosterone
- **Renal disease (without dialysis): these patients should not receive treatment with this product, high risk of hypocalcemia**
- If calcium <8.4 mg/dl, do not start therapy

Evaluate:

- Therapeutic response: calcium levels 9-10 mg/dl, decreasing symptoms of hypercalcemia

Teach patient/family:

- To take with food or shortly after a meal; to take tabs whole, not to take any other meds, supplements without prescriber approval
- To report cramping, seizures, muscle pain, tingling, tetany immediately

ciprofloxacin (Rx)

(sip-ro-floks′a-sin)

Cipro, Cipro XR

Func. class.: Antiinfective—broad spectrum

Chem. class.: Fluoroquinolone

Do not confuse:
ciprofloxacin/cephalexin

ACTION: Interferes with conversion of intermediate DNA fragments into high-molecular-weight DNA in bacteria; DNA gyrase inhibitor

USES: Infection caused by susceptible *Escherichia coli, Enterobacter cloacae, Proteus mirabilis, Klebsiella pneumoniae, Proteus vulgaris, Citrobacter freundii, Serratia marcescens, Pseudomonas aeruginosa, Staphylococcus aureus, Staphylococcus epidermidis, Enterobacter, Campylobacter jejuni, Salmonella;* chronic bacterial prostatitis, acute sinusitis, postexposure inhalation anthrax, infectious diarrhea, typhoid fever, complicated intraabdominal infections, nosocomial pneumonia, urinary tract infections

Unlabeled uses: *Acinetobacter/woffii, Aeromonas hydrophila,* brucellosis, *Burkholderia, pseudomallei,* chancroid, cholera, dental infection, *Edwardsiella tarda,* endocarditis, *Enterobacter aerogenes,* granuloma inguinale, *Klebsiella oxytoca,* Legionnaire's disease, melioidosis, meningococcal infection prophylaxis, *Pasteurella multocida,* PID, periodontitis, pharyngitis, *Salmonella sp., Stenotrophomonas maltophilia,* tularemia, *Vibrio cholerae/parahaemolyticus/vulnificus, Yersinia enterocolitica*

CONTRAINDICATIONS: Hypersensitivity to quinolones

Precautions: Pregnancy (C), breastfeeding, children, geriatric patients, renal disease, seizure disorder, stroke, CV disease, hepatic disease, QT prolongation, hypokalemia, colitis

Black Box Warning: Tendon pain/rupture, tendinitis, myasthenia gravis

DOSAGE AND ROUTES

Uncomplicated urinary tract infections

- **Adult: PO** 250 mg q12hr × 3 days or XL 500 mg q24hr × 3 days

Complicated/severe urinary tract infections

- **Adult: PO** 500 mg q12hr or XL 1000 mg q24hr × 7-14 days; **IV** 400 mg q12hr

Respiratory, bone, skin, joint infections (mild-moderate)

• **Adult: PO** 500-750 mg q12hr × 7-14 days; **IV** 400 mg q12hr

Nosocomial pneumonia

• **Adult: IV** 400 mg q8hr × 10-14 days

Intraabdominal infections, complicated

• **Adult: PO** 500 mg q12hr × 7-14 days; **IV** 400 mg q12hr × 7-14 days, usually given with metroNIDAZOLE

Acute sinusitis, mild/moderate

• **Adult: PO** 500 mg q12hr × 10 days; **IV** 400 mg q12hr × 10 days

Inhalational anthrax (postexposure)

• **Adult: PO** 500 mg q12hr × 60 days; **IV** 400 mg q12hr × 60 days

• **Child: PO** 15 mg/kg/dose q12hr × 60 days, max 500 mg/dose; **IV** 10 mg/kg q12hr, max 400 mg/dose

Infectious diarrhea

• **Adult: PO** 500-750 mg q12hr × 5-7 days

Chronic bacterial prostatis

• **Adult: PO** 500 mg q12hr × 28 days; **IV** 400 mg q12hr × 28 days

Renal disease

• **Adult:** CCr 30-50 ml/min, **PO** 250-500 mg q12hr; CCr 5-29 ml/min, **PO** 250-500 mg q18hr; **IV** 200-400 mg q18-24hr

Available forms: Tabs 100, 250, 500, 750 mg; ext rel tabs (XR) 500, 1000 mg; inj 200 mg/100 ml D_5, 400 mg/200 ml D_5; inj 200, 400 mg; oral susp 250 mg, 500 mg/5 ml

Administer:

• Obtain C&S before use

• Use caution when giving with antidysrhythmics IA, III

PO route

• Do not break, crush, chew XR (ext rel) product, use adequate fluids to prevent crystalluria

• 2 hr before or 6 hr after antacids, zinc, iron, calcium

• Do not give oral susp by GI tube

IV route

• Over 1 hr as an infusion, comes in premixed plastic infusion container or diluted 20- or 40-ml vial to a final concentration of 0.5-2 mg/ml of NS or D_5W; give through Y-tube or 3-way stopcock, diluted vials can be stored for 14 days at room temperature or refrigerator; do not freeze

Y-site compatibilities: Amifostine, anakinra, anidulafungin, argatroban, arsenic, atenolol, aztreonam, bivalirudin, bleomycin, calcium gluconate, CARBOplatin, caspofungin, cefTAZidime, cisatracurium, CISplatin, clarithromycin, codeine, cytarabine, DACTINomycin, DAPTOmycin, dexmedetomidine, digoxin, diltiazem, diphenhydrAMINE, DOBUTamine, DOCEtaxel, doripenem, DOPamine, doxacurium, DOXOrubicin, epirubicin, eptifibatide, ertapenem, etoposide, fenoldopam, fludarabine, gallium, gemcitabine, gentamicin, granisetron, HYDROmorphone, hydrOXYzine, IDArubicin, ifosfamide, irinotecan, lidocaine, linezolid, LORazepam, LR, mechlorethamine, meperidine, methotrexate, metoclopramide, metroNIDAZOLE, midazolam, midodrine, milrinone, mitoXANtrone, mycophenolate, nesiritide, octreotide, ondansetron, oxaliplatin, oxytocin, PACLitaxel, palonosetron, pamidronate, pancuronium, piperacillin, potassium acetate/chloride, promethazine, ranitidine, remifentanil, rocuronium, sodium chloride, tacrolimus, teniposide, thiotepa, tigecycline, tirofiban, TNA, tobramycin, trastuzumab, vasopressin, vecuronium, verapamil, vinCRIStine, vinorelbine, voriconazole

SIDE EFFECTS

CNS: *Headache*, dizziness, fatigue, insomnia, depression, *restlessness,* seizures, confusion, hallucinations

GI: *Nausea, diarrhea*, increased ALT/AST, dry mouth, flatulence, heartburn, *vomiting*, oral candidiasis, dysphagia, **pseudomembranous colitis, abdominal pain, pancreatitis**

GU: Crystalluria, interstitial neuritis

HEMA: **Bone marrow depression**, agranulocytosis, eosinophils

INTEG: *Rash*, pruritus, urticaria, photosensitivity, flushing, fever, chills, **toxic epidermal necrolysis**, injection site reactions

MISC: **Anaphylaxis, Stevens-Johnson syndrome**, visual impairment, **QT prolongation, pseudotumor cerebri**

MS: Tremor, arthralgia, tendinitis, tendon rupture

PHARMACOKINETICS

PO: Peak 1-2 hr; half-life 4 hr; excreted in urine as active product, metabolites 35%-40%, 20%-40% protein binding

INTERACTIONS

Black Box Warning: Increase: tendonitis, tendon rupture—corticosteroids

Increase: nephrotoxicity—cycloSPORINE
Increase: ciprofloxacin levels—probenecid; monitor for toxicity
Increase: levels of theophylline, warfarin, monitor blood levels, reduce dose
Increase: levels of CYP1A2 inhibitors
Increase: QT prolongation—astemizole, droperidol, class IA/III antidysrhythmics, tricyclics, tetracyclines, local anesthetics, phenothiazines, haloperidol, risperiDONE, sertindole, ziprasidone, alfuzosin, arsenic trioxide, β-agonists, chloroquine, cloZAPine, cyclobenzapine, dasatinib, dolasetron, droperidol, flecainide, halogenated anesthetics, lapatinib, levomethadyl, macrolides, methadone, octreotide, ondansetron, paliperidone, palonosetron, pentamidine, propafenone, ranolazine, SUNItinib, tacrolimus, terfenadine, vardenafil, vorinostat; less likely than other quinolones
Decrease: ciprofloxacin absorption—antacids that contain magnesium, aluminum; zinc, iron, sucralfate, enteral feedings, calcium, sevelamer

Drug/Food
Increase: effect of caffeine
Decrease: absorption—dairy products, food

Drug/Lab Test
Increase: AST, ALT, BUN, creatinine, LDH, bilirubin, alk phos, glucose, proteinuria, albuminuria
Decrease: WBC, glucose

NURSING CONSIDERATIONS

Assess:

- **Infection:** WBC, temperature before treatment, periodically
- **QT Prolongation:** Monitor for changes in QTc if taking other products that increase QT

Black Box Warning: Myasthenia gravis: Avoid use in these patients, increases muscle weakness

- **CNS symptoms:** headache, dizziness, fatigue, insomnia, depression, seizures
- Renal, hepatic studies: BUN, creatinine, AST, ALT
- I&O ratio, urine pH <5.5 is ideal

Black Box Warning: Tendonitis, tendon rupture: discontinue at first sign of tendon pain, inflammation; increased in those >60 yr, those taking corticosteroids, organ transplants

- ⚠ **Anaphylaxis:** fever, flushing, rash, urticaria, pruritus, dyspnea
- **Pseudomotor Cerebri:** may occur at excessive doses
- Limited intake of alkaline foods, products: milk, dairy products, alkaline antacids, sodium bicarbonate; caffeine intake if excessive cardiac or CNS stimulation
- Increase fluids to 3 L/day to avoid crystallization in kidneys

Evaluate:

- Therapeutic response: decreased pain, frequency, urgency, C&S; absence of infection

Teach patient/family:

- Not to take any products that contain magnesium, calcium (such as antacids), iron, aluminum with this product or 2 hr before, 6 hr after product; to drink fluids to prevent crystals in urine

Black Box Warning: To report tendon pain, chest pain, palpitations

- To ambulate, perform activities with assistance if dizziness occurs
- To complete full course of product therapy; not to double or miss doses
- To notify prescriber if rash occurs, discontinue product

- To notify prescriber if pregnancy is planned or suspected pregnancy (C); not to breastfeed
- To frequently rinse mouth; use sugarless candy, gum for dry mouth
- To contact prescriber if taking theophylline, warfarin
- Extended release and regular release are not interchangeable
- Not to add or stop products without prescriber's approval
- To use calibrated measuring device for suspension

ciprofloxacin (ophthalmic)

(sip-roe-flox′a-sin)

Ciloxan

Func. class.: ophthalmic antiinfective

Chem. class.: fluoroquinolone

Do not confuse:
ciprofloxacin/gatifloxacin/levofloxacin/moxifloxacin/ofloxacin

ACTION: Inhibits DNA gyrase, thereby decreasing bacterial replication

USES: Corneal ulcers, bacterial conjunctivitis

CONTRAINDICATIONS: Hypersensitivity to this product or fluoroquinolones

Precautions: Pregnancy (C), breastfeeding

DOSAGE AND ROUTES

Bacterial conjunctivitis

- **Adult/adolescent/child ≥1 yr:** Ophthalmic (sol): 1-2 drops in affected eye(s) every 2 hr while awake × 2 days, then every 4 hr while awake for the next 5 days
- **Adult/adolescent/child ≥2 yr:** Ophthalmic (ointment): 1/2-inch ribbon to conjunctival sac tid × 2 days, then 1/2 inch bid for next 5 days

Ophthalmic infection associated with corneal ulcer

- **Adult/adolescent/child ≥1 yr:** Ophthalmic (solution): 2 drops in affected eye(s) every 15 min × 6 hr, then every 30 min for the remainder of the first day; for the second day, 2 drops every hr; for days 3-14, 2 drops every 4 hr

Available forms: Ophthalmic ointment, solution 0.3%

Administer:

- Commercially available ophthalmic solutions are not for injection subconjunctivally or into the anterior chamber of the eye

Ophthalmic route

- Apply topically to the eye, taking care to avoid contamination
- Do not touch the tip of the dropper to the eye, fingertips, or other surface
- Apply pressure to lacrimal sac for 1 min after instillation
- Avoid wearing contact lens(es) while treating eye infection
- Protect from light, store at room temperature

SIDE EFFECTS

EENT: Burning, hypersensitivity, pruritus, precipitate in those with corneal ulcers, lid margin crusting

NURSING CONSIDERATIONS

Assess:

Allergic reaction:

- Assess for hypersensitivity, discontinue product

Evaluate:

- Decreased ophthalmic infection

Teach patient/family:

Ophthalmic route:

- To apply topically to the eye, taking care to avoid contamination; for ophthalmic use only
- Not to touch the tip of the dropper to the eye, fingertips, or other surface
- To apply pressure to lacrimal sac for 1 min after instillation
- To avoid wearing contact lens(es) while treating eye infection

⚠ HIGH ALERT

cisatracurium

(sis-ah-trah-kyoo′ree-um)

Nimbex

Func. class.: Skeletal muscle relaxant

Chem. class.: Nondepolarizing neuromuscular blocker

ACTION:

Antagonizes acetylcholine by binding to cholinergic receptors on the motor end plate, resulting in neuromuscular blockade

USES:

To maintain neuromuscular blockade during mechanical ventilation and as an adjunct to general anesthesia

CONTRAINDICATIONS:

Hypersensitivity

Precautions: Pregnancy (B), breastfeeding, children, benzyl alcohol hypersensitivity, electrolyte imbalances, long-term use in ICU, trauma, or burns, dehydration, metabolic alkalosis, respiratory acidosis, myopathy, myasthenia gravis

DOSAGE AND ROUTES

For neuromuscular blockade, as an adjunct to general anesthesia, to facilitate endotracheal intubation, and to provide skeletal muscle relaxation during surgery or mechanical ventilation in the ICU

Endotracheal intubation

- **Adult/adolescent (healthy): IV** 0.15-0.2 mg/kg, one time
- **Adult with myasthenia gravis: IV** use peripheral nerve stimulator monitoring and an initial dose ≤0.02 mg/kg
- **Child 2-12 yr: IV** 0.1-0.15 mg/kg over 5-10 sec during either halothane or opioid anesthesia
- **Infant/child ≤23 mo: IV** 0.15 mg/kg over 5-10 sec during either halothane or opioid anesthesia

To maintain neuromuscular blockade during prolonged surgical procedures:

- **Adult/adolescent/child ≥2 yr (healthy): IV** Maintenance dose 0.03 mg/kg; maintenance dosing is generally required 40-50 min after an initial dose of 0.15 mg/kg IV or 50-60 min after an initial dose of 0.2 mg/kg; the need for maintenance doses should be determined by clinical criteria

Available forms: Injection solution 2, 10 mg/ml

Administer:

IV route

- Visually inspect for particulate matter and discoloration before use
- Only experienced clinicians, familiar with the use of neuromuscular blocking drugs, should administer or supervise the use of this product
- Use by rapid IV injection or by continuous IV infusion

IV INFUSION route

- Inject IV over 5-10 sec

Continuous IV INFUSION route

- Dilute with NS, D_5W, or D_5NS (0.1-0.4 mg/ml); adjust the rate of infusion according to peripheral nerve stimulation
- The amount of infusion sol required per minute depends on the concentration of cisatracurium in the infusion sol, the desired dose of cisatracurium, and the patient's weight
- Store Nimbex injection diluted to 0.1 mg/ml either under refrigeration or at room temperature for 24 hr; dilutions to 0.1 mg/ml or 0.2 mg/ml in D_5W/LR injection may be stored under refrigeration for 24 hr
- Not an analgesic, treat pain with other agents

SIDE EFFECTS

CV: Bradycardia, flushing, hypotension

RESP: **Apnea, bronchospasm, prolonged neuromuscular block**

PHARMACOKINETICS

Onset 2 min, peak 3-5 min, duration 25-44 min, half-life 22-30 min

INTERACTIONS

Increase: neuromuscular blockade—aminoglycosides, clindamycin, lithium, local anesthetics, magnesium salts, colistin, colistimethate, procainamide, quiNIDine, tetracyclines, bacitracin, capreomycin, polymyxin B, vancomycin; amphotericin B, CISplatin, corticosteroids, loop/thiazide diuretics (if hypokalemia is present)

Decrease: neuromuscular blockade—carBAMazepine, phenytoin

NURSING CONSIDERATIONS

Assess:

Neuromuscular function:

- Use nerve stimulator to monitor neuromuscular function; if no response, stop until response; not to be used for rapid-sequence endotracheal intubation

Electrolyte:

- Electrolytes and acid-base balance may be altered

Malignant hyperthermia: Assess for malignant hyperthermia; those with a family history of this condition should not receive this product or it should be used cautiously

Evaluate:

- Maintenance of neuromuscular blockade

Teach patient/family:

- Reason for product and expected results

HIGH ALERT

CISplatin (Rx)

(sis′pla-tin)

Func. class.: Antineoplastic alkylating agent

Chem. class.: Platinum complex

Do not confuse:

CISplatin/CARBOplatin

ACTION: Alkylates DNA, RNA; inhibits enzymes that allow for the synthesis of amino acids in proteins; activity not cell-cycle–phase specific

USES: Advanced bladder cancer; adjunct in metastatic testicular cancer; adjunct in metastatic ovarian cancer

Unlabeled uses: Astrocytoma; breast, gastric, head, neck, hepatocellular, lung, penile cancer; carcinoid, desmoid tumor; Hodgkin's disease, malignant glioma, malignant melanoma, neuroblastoma, non-Hodgkin's lymphoma (NHL), osteogenic sarcoma, osteosarcoma; soft-tissue sarcomas; head, neck cancer; esophagus, prostate, lung, cervical cancer; lymphoma

CONTRAINDICATIONS: Pregnancy (D), breastfeeding

Black Box Warning: Preexisting hearing impairment, bone marrow suppression, platinum compound hypersensitivity, renal disease/failure

Precautions: Geriatric patients, vaccination, infections, extravasation, peripheral neuropathy, radiation therapy

DOSAGE AND ROUTES

Dosage protocols may vary

Metastatic testicular cancer

- **Adult: IV** 20 mg/m²/day × 5 days, repeat q3wk for 2 cycles or more, depending on response

Advanced bladder cancer

- **Adult: IV** 50-70 mg/m² q3-4wk

Metastatic ovarian cancer

- **Adult: IV** 100 mg/m² q4wk or 75-100 mg/m² q3wk with cyclophosphamide

Hodgkin's/non-Hodgkin's lymphoma (unlabeled)

- **Adult and child: IV INFUSION** 100 mg/m² 24 hr continuous infusion day 1 of 4-day regimen with cytarabine/dexamethasone q3-4wk

Gastric cancer (unlabeled)

- **Adult: IV** 75 mg/m² on day 1 with DOCEtaxel 75 mg/m² and fluorouracil 750 mg/m² on days 1-5, q21days

Available forms: Inj 0.5 ♣, 1 mg/ml

Administer:

IV route

- Do not use aluminum equipment during any preparation or administration, will form precipitate; do not refrigerate unopened powder or solution; protect from sunlight
- Prepare in biologic cabinet using gown, gloves, mask; do not allow product to come in contact with skin; use soap and water if contact occurs; use cytotoxic handling procedures
- Hydrate patient with 0.9% NaCl over 8-12 hr before treatment
- EPINEPHrine, antihistamines, corticosteroids for hypersensitivity reaction
- Antiemetic 30-60 min before product and prn; allopurinol to maintain uric acid levels, alkalinization of urine; diuretic (furosemide 40 mg IV) or mannitol after INFUSION

Intermittent IV INFUSION route

- **Dilute** 10 mg/10 ml or 50 mg/50 ml sterile water for inj, withdraw prescribed dose; **dilute** ½ dose with 1000 ml D_5 0.2 NaCl, D_5 0.45 NaCl with 37.5 g mannitol; IV INFUSION is **given** over 3-4 hr; use a 0.45-μm filter; total dose 2 L over 6-8 hr; check site for irritation, phlebitis

Continuous IV INFUSION route

- **Give** over 24 hr × 5 days

Solution compatibilities: D_5/0.225% NaCl, D_5/0.45% NaCl, D_5/0.9% NaCl, D_5/0.45% NaCl with mannitol 1.875%, D_5/0.33% NaCl with KCl 20 mEq and mannitol 1.875%, 0.9% NaCl, 0.45% NaCl, 0.3% NaCl, 0.225% NaCl

Y-site compatibilities: Acyclovir, alfentanil, allopurinol, amikacin, aminophylline, amiodarone, ampicillin, ampicillin-sulbactam, anidulafungin, atenolol, atracurium, azithromycin, aztreonam, bivalirudin, bleomycin, bumetanide, buprenorphine, butorphanol, calcium chloride/gluconate, carmustine, caspofungin, ceFAZolin, cefoperazone, cefotaxime, cefoTEtan, cefOXitin, cefTAZidime, ceftizoxime, cefTRIAXone, cefuroxime, chlorproMAZINE, cimetidine, ciprofloxacin, cisatracurium, cladribine, clindamycin, codeine, cyclophosphamide, cycloSPORINE, cytarabine, DACTINomycin, DAPTOmycin, DAUNOrubicin, dexamethasone, dexmedetomidine, dexrazoxane, digoxin, diltiazem, diphenhydrAMINE, DOBUTamine, DOCEtaxel, DOPamine, doripenem, doxacurium, DOXOrubicin, DOXOrubicin liposomal, doxycycline, droperidol, enalaprilat, ePHEDrine, EPINEPHrine, epirubicin, ertapenem, erythromycin, esmolol, etoposide, famotidine, fenoldopam, fentaNYL, filgrastim, fluconazole, fludarabine, fluorouracil, foscarnet, fosphenytoin, furosemide, ganciclovir, gatifloxacin, gemcitabine, gentamicin, glycopyrrolate, granisetron, haloperidol, heparin, hydrocortisone, HYDROmorphone, IDArubicin, ifosfamide, imipenem-cilastatin, inamrinone, indomethacin, irinotecan, isoproterenol, ketorolac, labetalol, leucovorin, levofloxacin, levorphanol, lidocaine, linezolid, LORazepam, magnesium sulfate, mannitol, melphalan, meperidine, meropenem, methohexital, methotrexate, methylPREDNISolone, metoclopramide, metoprolol, metroNIDAZOLE, midazolam, milrinone, minocycline, mitoMYcin, mitoXANtrone, mivacurium, nafcillin, naloxone, nesiritide, niCARdipine, nitroglycerin, nitroprusside, norepinephrine, octreotide, ofloxacin, ondansetron, oxaliplatin, PACLitaxel, palonosetron, pamidronate, pancuronium, PEMEtrexed, pentamidine, pentazocine, PENTobarbital, PHENobarbital, phenylephrine, phenytoin, piperacillin, polymyxin B, potassium chloride/phosphates, procainamide, prochlorperazine, promethazine, propofol, propranolol, quiNIDine, quinupristin-dalfopristin, ranitidine, remifentanil, riTUXimab, sargramostim, sodium acetate/bicarbonate/phosphates, succinylcholine, SUFentanil, sulfamethoxazole-trimethoprim, tacrolimus, teniposide, theophylline, thiopental, ticarcillin, ticarcillin-clavulanate, tigecycline, tirofiban, TNA, tobramycin, topotecan, trastuzumab, vancomycin, vasopressin, vecuronium, verapamil, vinBLAStine, vinCRIStine, vinorelbine, voriconazole, zidovudine, zoledronic acid

SIDE EFFECTS

CNS: Seizures, *peripheral neuropathy*
CV: Cardiac abnormalities
EENT: *Tinnitus, hearing loss, vestibular toxicity,* blurred vision, altered color perception
GI: *Severe nausea, vomiting, diarrhea, weight loss*
GU: Renal tubular damage, *renal insufficiency,* impotence, sterility, amenorrhea, gynecomastia, hyperuremia
HEMA: Thrombocytopenia, leukopenia, pancytopenia
INTEG: *Alopecia,* dermatitis
META: *Hypomagnesemia,* hypocalcemia, hypokalemia, hypophosphatemia
RESP: Fibrosis
SYST: Anaphylaxis

PHARMACOKINETICS

Absorption complete, metabolized in liver, excreted in urine, half-life 20 min first phase, 48-70 min second phase, 24 hr terminal phase, accumulates in body tissues for several months, enters breast milk

INTERACTIONS

Increase: bleeding risk—aspirin, NSAIDs, alcohol
Increase: ototoxicity—bumetanide, ethacrynic acid, furosemide
Increase: myelosuppression—myelosuppressive agents, radiation
Increase: nephrotoxicity—aminoglycosides, loop diuretics, salicylates
Decrease: effects of phenytoin
Decrease: antibody response—live virus vaccines

Drug/Lab Test
Increase: uric acid, BUN, creatinine
Decrease: CCr, calcium, phosphate, potassium, magnesium
Positive: Coombs' test

NURSING CONSIDERATIONS

Assess:

Black Box Warning: Bone marrow depression: CBC, differential, platelet count weekly; withhold product if WBC is <4000 or platelet count is <100,000; notify prescriber of results

Black Box Warning: Renal toxicity: BUN, creatinine, serum uric acid, urine CCr before, electrolytes during therapy; dose should not be given if BUN <25 mg/dl; creatinine <1.5 mg/dl; I&O ratio; report fall in urine output of <30 ml/hr

⚠ **Anaphylaxis:** wheezing, tachycardia, facial swelling, fainting; discontinue product, report to prescriber; resuscitation equipment should be nearby, may occur within minutes; often EPINEPHrine, corticosteroids, antihistamines may alleviate symptoms
• Monitor temperature q4hr; may indicate beginning infection
• Hepatic studies before, during therapy (bilirubin, AST, ALT, LDH) as needed
⚠ **Bleeding:** hematuria, guaiac, bruising, petechiae, mucosa, or orifices q8hr; obtain prescription for viscous lidocaine (Xylocaine)

Black Box Warning: Ototoxicity: more common in genetic variants TPMT 3B and 3C in children; use audiometric testing baseline and before each dose

• Effects of alopecia on body image; discuss feelings about body changes
• Comprehensive oral hygiene
• All medications PO, if possible; avoid IM inj when platelets <100,000/mm^3
• **Hyperuricemia in lymphoma:** Increase fluid intake to 2-3 L/day to prevent urate deposits, calculi formation; promote elimination of product, usually occurs between 3-5 days after a dose, may use allopurinol

Evaluate:
• Therapeutic response: decreased tumor size, spread of malignancy

Teach patient/family:

- To report signs of infection: increased temperature, sore throat, flulike symptoms
- To report signs of anemia: fatigue, headache, faintness, SOB, irritability
- To report bleeding, bruising, petechiae; to avoid use of razors, commercial mouthwash; to avoid aspirin, ibuprofen, NSAIDs, alcohol; may cause GI bleeding
- That impotence or amenorrhea can occur but is reversible after discontinuing treatment

Black Box Warning: Ototoxicity: to report loss of hearing, ringing or roaring in the ears

- To maintain adequate fluids; to report decreased urine output, flank pain
- That hair may be lost during treatment; a wig or hairpiece may make patient feel better; new hair may be different in color, texture
- To report numbness, tingling in face or extremities; poor hearing; joint pain, swelling
- Not to receive vaccinations during treatment
- To use contraception during treatment and for 4 mo after (pregnancy [D]); product may cause infertility; to avoid breastfeeding

citalopram (Rx)

(sigh-tal′oh-pram)

CeleXA

Func. class.: Antidepressant

Chem. class.: Selective serotonin reuptake inhibitor (SSRI)

Do not confuse:
CeleXA/CeleBREX/Cerebyx/Cerebra/Zyprexa

ACTION: Inhibits CNS neuron uptake of serotonin but not of norepinephrine; weak inhibitor of CYP450 enzyme system, thus making it more appealing than other products

USES: Major depressive disorder

Unlabeled uses: Premenstrual disorders, panic disorder, social phobia, obsessive-compulsive disorder in adolescents; anxiety, hot flashes, menopause; adjunct in schizophrenia, PTSD

CONTRAINDICATIONS: Hypersensitivity

Precautions: Pregnancy (C), breastfeeding, geriatric patients, renal/hepatic disease, seizure disorder, hypersensitivity to escitalopram, bradycardia, recent MI, abrupt discontinuation, QT prolongation

Black Box Warning: Children, suicidal ideation

DOSAGE AND ROUTES

Depression

- **Adult: PO** 20 mg/day AM or PM, may increase if needed to 40 mg/day after 1 wk; maintenance: after 6-8 wk of initial treatment, continue for 24 wk (32 wk total), reevaluate long-term usefulness (max 40 mg/day)

Hepatic dose/geriatric

- **Adult: PO** 20 mg/day

Panic disorder (unlabeled)

- **Adult: PO** 20-40 mg/day

Premenstrual dysphoria/social phobia (unlabeled)

- **Adult: PO** 10-30 mg/day, used intermittently in premenstrual dysphoria

Available forms: Tabs 10, 20, 40 mg; oral sol 10 mg/5 ml

Administer:

- With food or milk for GI symptoms
- Crushed if patient is unable to swallow medication whole
- Dosages at bedtime if oversedation occurs during the day; may take entire dose at bedtime
- Do not give within 14 days of MAOIs
- Store at room temperature; do not freeze

SIDE EFFECTS

CNS: *Headache, nervousness, insomnia, drowsiness, anxiety, tremor, dizziness, fatigue, sedation, poor concentration, abnormal dreams, agitation,* **seizures**, apathy, euphoria, hallucinations, delusions, psychosis, **suicidal attempts, neuroleptic malignant-like syndrome reactions**

CV: *Hot flashes, palpitations,* angina pectoris, **hemorrhage**, hypertension, tachycardia, 1st-degree AV block, bradycardia, **MI, thrombophlebitis, QT prolongation**, orthostatic hypotension, **torsades de pointes**

EENT: Visual changes, ear/eye pain, photophobia, tinnitus

GI: *Nausea, diarrhea, dry mouth, anorexia, dyspepsia, constipation, cramps, vomiting, taste changes, flatulence, decreased appetite*

GU: *Dysmenorrhea, decreased libido, urinary frequency, UTI,* amenorrhea, cystitis, impotence, urine retention

INTEG: *Sweating, rash, pruritus,* acne, alopecia, urticaria, photosensitivity

MS: *Pain,* arthritis, twitching

RESP: *Infection, pharyngitis, nasal congestion, sinus headache, sinusitis, cough, dyspnea, bronchitis,* asthma, hyperventilation, pneumonia

SYST: *Asthenia, viral infection, fever, allergy, chills;* hyponatremia (geriatric patients), **serotonin syndrome, neonatal abstinence syndrome**

PHARMACOKINETICS

Metabolized in liver by CYP3A4, CYP2C19; excreted in urine; steady state 1 wk; peak 4 hr; half-life 35 hr

INTERACTIONS

⚠ **Fatal reactions: do not use with MAOIs**

⚠ **Increase: QTc interval—dofetilide, halofantrine, probucol, pimoside, quinolones, ziprasidone; do not use together**

Increase: effect of tricyclics; use cautiously

Increase: serotonin syndrome—serotonin receptor agonists, SSRIs, traMADol, lithium, MAOIs, traZODone, SNRIs (venlafaxine, DULoxetine)

Increase: bleeding risk—NSAIDs, salicylates, thrombolytics, anticoagulants, antiplatelets

Increase: CNS effects—barbiturates, sedative/hypnotics, other CNS depressants

Increase: citalopram levels—macrolides, azole antifungals

Increase: plasma levels of β-blockers

Decrease: citalopram levels—carBAMazepine, cloNIDine

Drug/Herb

⚠ **Increase: serotonin syndrome—St. John's wort, SAM-e; fatal reaction may occur; do not use concurrently**

Increase: CNS stimulation—yohimbe

Drug/Lab Test

Increase: serum bilirubin, blood glucose, alk phos

Decrease: VMA, 5-HIAA

False increase: urinary catecholamines

NURSING CONSIDERATIONS

Assess:

Black Box Warning: Mental status: mood, sensorium, affect, suicidal tendencies, increase in psychiatric symptoms, depression, panic

⚠ **Serotonin syndrome: increased heart rate, sweating, dilated pupils, tremors, twitching, hyperthermia, agitation**

- B/P lying, standing, pulse q4hr; if systolic B/P drops 20 mm Hg, hold product, notify prescriber; take vital signs q4hr in patients with CV disease
- Weight weekly; appetite may decrease or increase with product
- **Torsades de pointes, QT prolongation: is dose-dependent, ECG for flattening of T wave, bundle branch, AV block, dysrhythmias in cardiac patients**
- Alcohol consumption; if alcohol is consumed, hold dose until AM
- Sexual dysfunction: erectile dysfunction, decreased libido
- Assistance with ambulation during therapy, as drowsiness, dizziness occur
- Safety measures, primarily for geriatric patients

• Sugarless gum, hard candy, frequent sips of water for dry mouth

Evaluate:

• Therapeutic response: decreased depression

Teach patient/family:

• That therapeutic effect may take 4-6 wk; that patient may have increased anxiety 1st 5-7 days of therapy; not to discontinue abruptly

• To use caution when driving, performing other activities that require alertness because of drowsiness, dizziness, blurred vision; to report signs, symptoms of bleeding

• To avoid alcohol, other CNS depressants

Black Box Warning: That suicidal ideas, behavior may occur in children or young adults

• To notify prescriber if pregnant, planning to become pregnant, or breastfeeding

⚠ About the effects of serotonin syndrome: nausea/vomiting, tremors; if symptoms occur, to discontinue immediately, notify prescriber

clarithromycin (Rx)

(klare-ith′row-my-sin)

Biaxin, Biaxin XL

Func. class.: Antiinfective

Chem. class.: Macrolide

ACTION: Binds to 50S ribosomal subunits of susceptible bacteria and suppresses protein synthesis

USES: Mild to moderate infections of the upper and lower respiratory tract, uncomplicated skin and skin-structure infections caused by *Streptococcus pneumoniae, Mycoplasma pneumoniae, Legionella pneumophila, Moraxella catarrhalis, Neisseria gonorrhoeae, Corynebacterium diphtheriae, Listeria monocytogenes, Haemophilus influenzae, Streptococcus pyogenes, Staphylococcus aureus, Mycobacterium avium* complex (MAC); complex infection in AIDS patients; *Mycobacterium avium intracellulare, Helicobacter pylori* in combination with omeprazole, *H. parainfluenzae*

Unlabeled uses: Endocarditis prophylaxis, dyspepsia, gastric ulcer, Legionnaire's disease, pertussis, SARS

CONTRAINDICATIONS: Hypersensitivity to this product or macrolide antibiotics, torsades de pointes, QT prolongation

Precautions: Pregnancy (C), breastfeeding, geriatric patients, renal/hepatic disease

DOSAGE AND ROUTES

Acute exacerbation of chronic bronchitis

• **Adult: PO** 250-500 mg q12hr × 7-14 days or 1000 mg/day × 7 days (XL)

Pharyngitis/tonsillitis

• **Adult: PO** 250 mg q12hr × 10 days

Community-acquired pneumonia

• **Adult: PO** 250 mg q12hr × 7-14 days or 1000 mg/day × 7 days (XL)

MAC prophylaxis/treatment

• **Adult: PO** 500 mg bid; will require an additional antiinfective for active infection

***H. pylori* infection**

• **Adult: PO** 500 mg with 30 mg lansoprazole and 1 g amoxicillin together q12hr × 10-14 days or 500 mg with omeprazole 20 mg and 1 g amoxicillin together q12hr × 10 days or 500 mg q8hr and omeprazole 40 mg daily × 14 days, continue omeprazole for 14 more days

Acute maxillary sinusitis

• **Adult: PO** 500 mg q12hr × 14 days

Most infections

• **Child: PO** 7.5 mg/kg q12hr × 10 days, max 500 mg/dose for MAC

Renal dose

• **Adult and child: PO** CCr 30-60 ml/min decrease dose by 50% if using with ritonavir; <30 ml/min, reduce dose by 50%, if used with ritonavir reduce by 75%

Legionnaire's disease/SARS/ whooping cough/gastric ulcer/ dyspepsia *(H. pylori)* (unlabeled)
• **Adult: PO** 500 mg q12hr; may be used in combination for some of these conditions

Endocarditis prophylaxis (unlabeled)
• **Adult: PO** 500 mg 1 hr before procedure

Available forms: Tabs 250, 500 mg; oral susp 125 mg/5 ml, 250 mg/5 ml; ext rel tab (XL) 500 mg

Administer:
• Do not break, crush, or chew ext rel
• Adequate intake of fluids (2 L) during diarrhea episodes
• q12hr to maintain serum levels
• Store at room temperature

Susp: Shake well, store at room temperature, discard after 2 wk
Ext Rel: Give with food

SIDE EFFECTS

CV: Ventricular dysrhythmias, QT prolongation
GI: *Nausea, vomiting, diarrhea,* hepatotoxicity, *abdominal pain,* stomatitis, heartburn, anorexia, *abnormal taste,* pseudomembranous colitis, tooth/tongue discoloration, pancreatitis
GU: Vaginitis, moniliasis, interstitial nephritis, azotemia
HEMA: Leukopenia, thrombocytopenia, increased INR
INTEG: Rash, urticaria, pruritus, Stevens-Johnson syndrome, toxic epidermal necrolysis
MISC: *Headache,* hearing loss

PHARMACOKINETICS

Regular release: peak 2-2.5 hr; duration 12 hr; Ext release: peak 5-7 hr; half-life 5-7 hr; metabolized by liver; excreted in bile, feces; possible inhibition of P-glycoprotein

INTERACTIONS

Increase: dysrhythmias—cisapride, pimozide
Increase: levels, increase toxicity—ALPRAZolam, busPIRone, carBAMazepine, cycloSPORINE, digoxin, disopyramide, ergots, felodipine, fluconazole, omeprazole, tacrolimus, theophylline, antidiabetics, digoxin, theophylline, carBAMazepine
Increase: levels of HMG-CoA reductase inhibitors
Increase: action, risk for toxicity—all products metabolized by CYP3A enzyme system
Increase: effect of calcium channel blockers, midazolam, benzodiazepines, tacrolimus
Increase: QT prolongation—class IA, III antidysrhythmics or other products that prolong QT
Increase or decrease action: zidovudine
Decrease: clarithromycin action—CYP3A4 substrates
Decrease: levels—rifampin, rifabutin, nevirapine, etravirine, benzodiazepine

Drug/Food
• Do not use with grapefruit juice

Drug/Lab Test
Increase: 17-OHCS/17-KS, AST, ALT, BUN, creatinine, LDH, total bilirubin
Decrease: folate assay, WBC

NURSING CONSIDERATIONS

Assess:
• **Infection:** wound characteristics, urine, stool, sputum, WBC, temperature; C&S before product therapy; product may be given as soon as culture is taken; C&S may be repeated after treatment
• For ulcers: abdominal pain, bleeding in stools, emesis
• Renal, hepatic studies; report hematuria, oliguria
• Bowel pattern before, during treatment
• Respiratory status: rate, character, wheezing, tightness in chest; discontinue product
• Bleeding: check INR if anticoagulants are taken
• Allergies before treatment, reaction to each medication
• **QT prolongation, ventricular dysrhythmias:** monitor ECG, cardiac status

in those with underlying cardiac abnormalities

- **Serious skin reaction:** Stevens-Johnson syndrome, toxic epidermal necrolysis; product should be discontinued immediately

Evaluate:

- Therapeutic response: C&S negative for infection

Teach patient/family:

- To take with full glass of water; may give with food to decrease GI symptoms, ext rel with food
- ⚠ To report sore throat, fever, fatigue; may indicate superinfection
- ⚠ To notify prescriber of diarrhea, dark urine, pale stools, yellow discoloration of eyes or skin, severe abdominal pain
- To take at evenly spaced intervals; to complete dosage regimen; to notify prescribers of all products used
- To notify prescriber if pregnancy is suspected or planned

TREATMENT OF HYPERSENSITIVITY: Withdraw product, maintain airway, administer EPINEPHrine, aminophylline, O_2, IV corticosteroids

clevidipine (Rx)

(klev-id'i-peen)

Cleviprex

Func. class.: Calcium channel blocker (L-type)

Chem. class.: Dihydropyridine

ACTION: L-type calcium channels mediate the influx of calcium during depolarization in arterial smooth muscle; reduces mean arterial B/P by decreasing systemic vascular resistance

USES: Reduction of B/P when oral therapy not feasible

CONTRAINDICATIONS: Hypersensitivity to this product, eggs, soya lecithin; defective lipid metabolism; severe aortic stenosis, pancreatitis

Precautions: Pregnancy (C), labor, breastfeeding, children <18 yr, heart failure, hyperlipidemia, chronic hypertension, pheochromocytoma

DOSAGE AND ROUTES

- **Adult: CONT IV** 1-2 mg/hr; dose may be doubled q90sec initially; as B/P reaches goal, adjust dose less frequently (q5-10min) with smaller increases in dose; most patients require 4-6 mg/hr, max 32 mg/hr; no more than 1000 ml should be infused per 24-hr period due to lipid load restrictions

Available forms: Single-dose vial 50, 100 ml (0.5 mg/ml)

Administer:

Intermittent IV INFUSION route

- Do not give through same line as other medications; do not dilute, do not filter
- Gently invert several times before use; do not use if discolored or if particulate matter is present
- Give through central or peripheral line at 1-2 mg/hr; use infusion device
- Store vials in refrigerator; do not freeze; leave vials in carton until use; product is photosensitive, but protection from light during administration is not required

SIDE EFFECTS

CNS: Headache

CV: **MI, sinus tachycardia,** syncope, **reflex tachycardia, atrial fibrillation**

GI: Nausea, vomiting

PHARMACOKINETICS

Onset 2-4 min; half-life initially 1 min, terminal 15 min; metabolized via esterases in blood, extravascular tissues; excreted in urine 63%-74%, feces 7%-22%; protein binding >99%

NURSING CONSIDERATIONS

Assess:

- Cardiac status: B/P, pulse, respiration, ECG; some patients have developed severe angina, acute MI after calcium channel blockers if obstructive CAD is severe; if not transitioned to other antihypertensive therapies after clevidipine infusion, patients should be monitored ≥8 hr for rebound hypertension; monitor for rebound hypertension after product stoppage

Evaluate:

- Therapeutic response: decreased B/P

Teach patient/family:

- **To notify prescriber immediately if neurological symptoms, visual changes, or symptoms of CHF occur**
- To continue follow-up for hypertension
- To notify prescriber if pregnancy is planned, suspected, or if breastfeeding

clindamycin HCl (Rx)

(klin-da-my′sin)

Cleocin HCl, Dalacin C ♣

clindamycin palmitate (Rx)

Cleocin Pediatric, Dalacin C Flavored Granules ♣

clindamycin phosphate (Rx)

Cleocin Phosphate, Dalacin C Phosphate Sterile Solution ♣

Func. class.: Antiinfective—miscellaneous

Chem. class.: Lincomycin derivative

ACTION: Binds to 50S subunit of bacterial ribosomes, suppresses protein synthesis

USES: Infections caused by staphylococci, streptococci, *Rickettsia, Fusobacterium, Actinomyces, Peptococcus, Bacteroides, Pneumocystis jiroveci*

Unlabeled uses: Acne rosacea, *Bacillus anthracis,* dental infections, folliculitis, malaria, pemphigus, periodontitis, *Pneumocystis jiroveci* pneumonia (PCP), toxoplasmosis

CONTRAINDICATIONS: Hypersensitivity to this product or lincomycin, tartrazine dye; ulcerative colitis/enteritis

Black Box Warning: Pseudomembranous colitis

Precautions: Pregnancy (B), breastfeeding, GI/hepatic disease, asthma, allergy

Black Box Warning: Diarrhea

DOSAGE AND ROUTES

- **Adult: PO** 150-450 mg q6hr, max 2700 mg/day; **IM/IV** 1.2-2.7 g/day in 2-4 divided doses, max 4800mg/day severe infections
- **Child >1 mo: PO** 8-25 mg/kg/day in divided doses q6-8hr; **IM/IV** 20-40 mg/kg/day in 3-4 equal divided doses q6-8hr
- **Neonate: IM/IV** 15-20 mg/kg/day divided doses q6-8hr

PID

- **Adult: IV** 900 mg q8hr plus gentamicin

Bacterial endocarditis prophylaxis (unlabeled)

- **Adult:** 600 mg 1 hr before procedure

***P. jiroveci pneumonia* (unlabeled)**

- **Adult: PO** 1200-1800 mg/day in divided doses with 15-30 mg primaquine/day × 21 days

Available forms: HCl: caps 75, 150, 300 mg; **palmitate:** oral sol 75 mg/5 ml; **phosphate:** inj 150, 300, 600 mg base/16 ml; 900 mg base/ml; inj infusion in D_5 300 mg, 600 mg, 900 mg/16 ml

Administer:

- In equal intervals around the clock to maintain blood levels
- Obtain C&S before use

PO route

- Do not break, crush, chew caps
- Orally with at least 8 oz of water

Oral solution

- Do not refrigerate reconstituted product; store at room temperature ≤2 wk
- Reconstitute granules with most of 75 ml of water, shake well, add remaining water, shake well (75 mg/5 ml)

IM route

- IM deep inj; rotate sites; do not give >600 mg in single IM inj

IV route

- Visually inspect parenteral products for particulate matter and discoloration before use
- **Vials:** dilute 300 and 600 mg doses with 50 ml of a compatible diluent; dilute 900 mg doses with 50-100 ml of a compatible diluent; dilute 1200 mg doses with 100 ml of a compatible diluent, final concentration max 18 mg/ml
- **ADD-vantage vials:** dilute 600 and 900 mg ADD-vantage containers with 50 or 100 mg, respectively, of NS or D_5W
- **Storage:** when diluted in D_5W, NS, or LR, solutions with concentrations of 6, 9, or 12 mg/ml are stable for 16 days at room temperature or 32 days under refrigeration when stored in glass bottles or minibags; when diluted in D_5W, solutions with a concentration of 18 mg/ml are stable for 16 days at room temperature

Intermittent IV infusion route

- Infuse over at least 10-60 min, infusion rates max 30 mg/min and ≤1.2 g should be infused in a 1 hr period
- Infuse 300 mg doses over 10 min; 600 mg doses over 20 min, 900 mg doses over 30 min, and 1200 mg doses over 40 min

Continuous IV infusion route

- Give first dose rapidly, then follow with continuous infusion
- Rate is based on desired serum clindamycin levels:
- To maintain serum concentrations above 4 mcg/ml, use a rapid infusion rate of 10 mg/min for 30 min and a maintenance rate of 0.75 mg/min; to maintain serum concentrations above 5 mcg/ml, use a rapid infusion rate of 15 mg/min for 30 min and a maintenance rate of 1 mg/min; to maintain serum concentrations above 5 mcg/ml, use a rapid infusion rate of 20 mg/min for 30 min and a maintenance rate of 1.25 mg/min

Y-site compatibilities: Acyclovir, alfentanil, amifostine, amikacin, aminocaproic acid, aminophylline, amiodarone, amphotericin B cholesteryl, amphotericin B lipid complex, amsacrine, anakinra, anidulafungin, ascorbic acid injection, atenolol, atracurium, atropine, aztreonam, benztropine, bivalirudin, bleomycin, bumetanide, buprenorphine, butorphanol, calcium chloride/gluconate, CARBOplatin, cefamandole, ceFAZolin, cefmetazole, cefonicid, cefoperazone, cefotaxime, cefoTEtan, cefOXitin, cefpirome, cefTAZidime, ceftizoxime, ceftobiprole, cefuroxime, cephalothin, cephapirin, chloramphenicol, cimetidine, cisatracurium, CISplatin, codeine, cyanocobalamin, cyclophosphamide, cycloSPORINE, cytarabine, DACTINomycin, DAPTOmycin, dexamethasone, dexmedetomidine, digoxin, diltiazem, diphenhydrAMINE, DOCEtaxel, DOPamine, doxacurium, DOXOrubicin, DOXOrubicin liposomal, doxycycline, enalaprilat, ePHEDrine, EPINEPHrine, epirubicin, epoetin alfa, eptifibatide, esmolol, etoposide, famotidine, fenoldopam, fentaNYL, fludarabine, fluorouracil, folic acid, foscarnet, furosemide, gatifloxacin, gemcitabine, gemtuzumab, gentamicin, glycopyrrolate, granisetron, heparin, hydrocortisone, HYDROmorphone, ifosfamide, imipenem-cilastatin, indomethacin, insulin (regular), irinotecan, isoproterenol, ketorolac, levofloxacin, lidocaine, linezolid, LORazepam, LR, magnesium sulfate, mannitol, mechlorethamine, melphalan, meperidine, metaraminol, methicillin, methotrexate, methoxamine, methyldopate, methylPREDNISolone, metoclopramide, metoprolol, metroNIDAZOLE, mezlocillin, miconazole, milrinone, morphine, moxalactam, multiple vitamins injection, nafcillin, nalbuphine, naloxone, nesiritide, netilmicin, niCARdipine, nitroglycerin, nitroprusside, norepinephrine, octreotide, ondansetron, oxacillin, oxaliplatin, oxytocin, PACLitaxel, palonosetron, pamidronate, pancuronium, pantoprazole, PEMEtrexed, penicillin G potassium/sodium, pentazocine, perphenazine, PHENobarbital, phenylephrine, phytonadione, piperacillin, piperacillin-tazobactam, potassium chloride, procainamide, propofol, propranolol, protamine, pyridoxine, ranitidine, remifentanil, Ringer's, ritodrine, riTUXimab, rocuronium, sargramostim, sodium acetate/bicarbonate, succinylcholine, SUFentanil, tacrolimus, teniposide, theophylline, thiamine, thiotepa, ticarcillin, ticarcillin-clavulanate, tigecycline, tirofiban, TNA, tobramycin, tolazoline, TPN, trimetaphan, urokinase, vancomycin, vasopressin, vecuronium, verapamil, vinCRIStine, vinorelbine, vitamin B complex/C, voriconazole, zidovudine, zoledronic acid

SIDE EFFECTS

GI: *Nausea, vomiting, abdominal pain, diarrhea,* pseudomembranous colitis, anorexia, weight loss, increased AST/ALT, bilirubin, alk phos; jaundice

GU: *Vaginitis,* urinary frequency

INTEG: Rash, urticaria, pruritus, erythema, pain, abscess at inj site

SYST: Stevens-Johnson syndrome, exfoliative dermatitis

PHARMACOKINETICS

PO: Peak 45 min, duration 6-8 hr

IM: Peak 3 hr (adult), 1 hr (child); duration 8-12 hr; half-life 2½ hr; metabolized in liver; excreted in urine, bile, feces as inactive metabolites; crosses placenta; excreted in breast milk

INTERACTIONS

- May block clindamycin effect: erythromycin, chloramphenicol

Increase: neuromuscular blockade—neuromuscular blockers

Decrease: absorption—kaolin

Drug/Lab Test

Increase: alk phos, bilirubin, CPK, AST, ALT

NURSING CONSIDERATIONS

Assess:

- **Infection:** C&S before product therapy; product may be given as soon as culture is taken
- VS, urine, stools, sputum
- Hepatic studies: AST, ALT if on long-term therapy
- B/P, pulse in patient receiving product parenterally

Black Box Warning: Pseudomembranous colitis: bowel pattern before, during treatment; if severe diarrhea occurs, product should be discontinued, may occur several wk after therapy is terminated

- Respiratory status: rate, character, wheezing, tightness in chest
- **Serious skin reactions:** Stevens-Johnson syndrome, exfoliative dermatitis

Evaluate:

- Therapeutic response: decreased temperature, negative C&S

Teach patient/family:

- To take oral product with full glass of water; that antiperistaltic products may worsen diarrhea
- About all aspects of product therapy; to complete entire course of medication to ensure organism death (10-14 days); culture may be taken after medication course completed
- ⚠ To report sore throat, fever, fatigue; may indicate **superinfection**
- To take with food to reduce GI symptoms
- To notify nurse or prescriber of diarrhea with pus, mucous

TREATMENT OF HYPERSENSITIVITY:

- Withdraw product; maintain airway; administer EPINEPHrine, aminophylline, O_2, IV corticosteroids

clindamycin (topical, vaginal)

(klin-da-mye′sin)

Cleocin, Cleocin-T, Clindacin-P, Clindagel, ClindaMax, Clindasol ✤, Clinda-T ✤, Clindesse, Clindets, Dalacin ✤, Evoclin

Func. class.: Topical antiinfective

Chem. class.: Lincosamide derivative

ACTION: Antibacterial activity results from inhibition of protein synthesis; bacteriostatic

USES: For the treatment of acne vulgaris; treatment of bacterial vaginosis and anaerobic bacteria

CONTRAINDICATIONS: Hypersensitivity to this product or lincomycin, history of antibiotic-associated colitis or ulcerative colitis

Precautions: Breastfeeding, children <12 yr

DOSAGE AND ROUTES

Acne vulgaris

- **Adult/adolescent: TOP** (gel, lotion, solution) Apply a thin film of 1% to affected areas bid
- **Adult/adolescent/child ≥12 yr: TOP (foam)** Apply 1% topical foam to affected areas once daily; if there is no improvement after 6-8 weeks or if the condition worsens, discontinue treatment
- **TOP** (medicated pledgets) Use a pledget to apply a thin film to the affected area bid; more than one pledget may be used, but each pledget should be used only once and then discarded

Bacterial vaginosis and anaerobic bacteria

Nonpregnant adult/adolescent/postmenarchal females:

- **Intravaginal cream:** one applicatorful (100 mg clindamycin/5 g cream) intravaginally, preferably at bedtime, for 3 or 7 consecutive days in nonpregnant women and for 7 consecutive days in pregnant women; clindesse is administered as a single dose at any time of the day
- **Intravaginal ovules/suppositories:** as an alternative to first-line therapies, the CDC recommends one ovule (100 mg clindamycin) inserted intravaginally at bedtime for 3 days

Available forms: Topical gel, foam, lotion, pledget, solution 1%; vaginal cream 2%, vaginal suppositories 100 mg

Administer:

Topical route:

- Improvement occurs after 6 wk but can require 8-12 wk
- Topical skin products are not for intravaginal therapy and are for external use only; do not use skin products near the eyes, nose, or mouth
- Wash hands before and after use; wash affected area and gently pat dry

Cream/ointment/lotion:

- Shake well before use (lotion); apply a thin film to the cleansed affected area; massage gently into affected areas

Foam formulations:

- Do not dispense foam directly onto hands or face; the warmth of the skin will cause the foam to melt; instead, dispense desired amount directly into the cap or onto a cool surface; make sure enough foam is dispensed to cover the affected area(s); if the can feels warm or the foam seems runny, run the can under cold water; to apply, pick up small amounts of the foam with the fingertips and gently massage into the affected areas until the foam disappears

Solution formulations:

- Shake well before use; apply a thin film to the cleansed affected area; massage gently into affected areas; if using a solution-soaked pledget, patient may use more than 1 pledget per application as needed to treat affected areas, but each pledget should be used only once and then discarded

Intravaginal route:

- Only use dosage formulations specified for intravaginal use; intravaginal dosage forms are not for topical therapy; do not ingest

Suppository:
- Unwrap vaginal ovule (suppository) before insertion; use applicator(s) supplied by the manufacturer

Cream:
- Use applicator(s) supplied by the manufacturer

SIDE EFFECTS

GU: Colitis, diarrhea, overgrowth, vaginitis, vaginal moniliasis, UTI
INTEG: Redness, burning, dermatitis, rash, pruritus

NURSING CONSIDERATIONS

Assess:
Allergic reaction: Assess for hypersensitivity; product may need to be discontinued
- Contact prescriber immediately if severe diarrhea, stomach cramps/pain, or bloody stools occur

Infection: Assess for number of lesions, severity in acne, itching in vaginosis
Evaluate:
- Decreased lesions in acne, infection in vaginosis

Teach patient/family:
Topical route:
- That improvement occurs after 6 wk but can require 8-12 wk
- That topical skin products are not for intravaginal therapy and are for external use only; not to use skin products near the eyes, nose, or mouth
- To wash hands before and after use; wash affected area and gently pat dry

Cream/ointment/lotion:
- Shake well before use; **lotion:** apply a thin film to the cleansed affected area; massage gently into affected areas

Foam formulations:
- Do not dispense foam directly onto hands or face; the warmth of the skin will cause the foam to melt; instead, dispense desired amount directly into the cap or onto a cool surface; make sure enough foam is dispensed to cover the affected area(s); if the can feels warm or the foam seems runny, run the can under cold water; to apply, pick up small amounts of the foam with the fingertips and gently into the affected areas until the foam disappears

Solution formulations:
- Shake well before use; apply a thin film to the cleansed affected area; massage gently into affected areas; if using a solution-soaked pledget, patient may use more than one pledget per application as needed to treat affected areas, but each pledget should be used only once and then discarded

Intravaginal route:
- Only use dosage formulations specified for intravaginal use; intravaginal dosage forms are not for topical therapy; do not ingest

Suppository:
- Unwrap vaginal ovule (suppository) before insertion; use applicator(s) supplied by the manufacturer

Cream:
- Use applicator(s) supplied by the manufacturer

clobetasol

(kloe-bay′ta-sol)

Clobex, Cormax, Olux, Olux-E, Temovate, Temovate-E

Func. class.: Corticosteroid, topical

ACTION: Crosses cell membrane to attach to receptors to decrease inflammation, itching

USES: Inflammation/itching in corticosteroid-responsive dermatoses on the skin/scalp

CONTRAINDICATIONS: Hypersensitivity, use of some preparations on face, axilla, groin; monotherapy for primary bacterial infections
Precautions: Pregnancy (C), breastfeeding, children <12 yr

DOSAGE AND ROUTES

- **Adult: TOP** Apply to infected areas bid (shampoo: daily up to 4×/wk)

Available forms: Gel, lotion, ointment, cream, shampoo, solution, spray, foam 0.05%

Administer

Topical route

⚠ Do not use with occlusive dressings

⚠ Treatment should be limited to 2 wk

- **Cream/Ointment/Lotion:** using gloves, apply sparingly in a thin film and rub gently into the cleansed, slightly moist affected area
- **Gel:** using gloves, apply sparingly in a thin film and rub gently into the cleansed, slightly moist affected area
- **Scalp foam:** invert can and dispense a small amount of foam onto a saucer or other cool surface; do not dispense directly onto hands; pick up small amounts of foam with fingers and gently massage into affected area until foam disappears; repeat until entire affected scalp area is treated
- **Shampoo:** apply onto dry scalp in thin film, leave lather on scalp for 15 min, rinse off

SIDE EFFECTS

GU: Glycosuria

INTEG: Burning, folliculitis, pruritus, dermatitis, irritation, erythema, hypertrichosis, acne

MISC: Hyperglycemia, HPA axis suppression

NURSING CONSIDERATIONS

Assess:

- Skin reactions: burning, pruritus, folliculitis, dermatitis

Evaluate:

- Decreasing itching, inflammation on the skin, scalp

Teach patient/family:

Topical route

⚠ Do not use with occlusive dressings

⚠ Treatment should be limited to 2 wk

- **Cream/Ointment/Lotion:** to apply sparingly in a thin film and rub gently into the cleansed, affected area
- **Gel:** to apply sparingly in a thin film and rub gently into the cleansed, slightly moist affected area
- **Scalp foam:** to invert can and dispense a small amount of foam onto a saucer or other cool surface; not to dispense directly onto hands; to pick up small amounts of foam with fingers and gently massage into affected area until foam disappears; repeat until entire affected scalp area is treated

clomiPHENE (Rx)

(kloe′mi-feen)

Clomid, Serophene

Func. class.: Ovulation stimulant

Chem. class.: Selective estrogen receptor modulator (SERM)

Do not confuse:

clomiPHENE/clomiPRAMINE

Serophen/Sarafem

ACTION: Increases LH, FSH release from the pituitary, which increases the maturation of the ovarian follicle, ovulation, and the development of the corpus luteum

USES: Female infertility (ovulatory failure)

Unlabeled uses: Oligospermia

CONTRAINDICATIONS: Pregnancy (X), hypersensitivity, hepatic disease, undiagnosed uterine bleeding, uncontrolled thyroid or adrenal dysfunction, intracranial lesion, ovarian cysts, endometrial carcinoma

Precautions: Hypertension, depression, seizures, diabetes mellitus, abnormal ovarian enlargement, ovarian hyperstimulation

DOSAGE AND ROUTES

- **Adult: PO** 50 mg/day × 5 days or 50 mg/day beginning on day 5 of menstrual cycle, may increase to 100 mg daily × 5 days with next cycle; may be repeated until conception occurs or max 6 cycles of therapy

Oligospermia (unlabeled)
- **Adult (men): PO** 25 mg/day × 25 days, then 5 days off cycle each mo

Available forms: Tabs 50 mg

Administer:
- After discontinuing estrogen therapy
- At same time daily to maintain product level, without regard to food
- Avoid heat, moisture, light; store at room temperature

SIDE EFFECTS

CNS: *Headache, depression,* restlessness, anxiety, nervousness, fatigue, insomnia, dizziness, flushing
CV: Vasomotor flushing, phlebitis, deep venous thrombosis
EENT: Blurred vision, diplopia, photophobia
GI: *Nausea, vomiting, constipation,* abdominal pain, bloating, hepatitis
GU: Polyuria, urinary frequency, birth defects, spontaneous abortions, multiple ovulation, breast pain, oliguria, abnormal uterine bleeding, ovarian cyst, hypertrophy of ovary, hot flashes
INTEG: *Rash, dermatitis,* urticaria, alopecia

PHARMACOKINETICS

Metabolized in liver, excreted in feces

INTERACTIONS

Drug/Herb
Decrease: clomiPHENE effect—DHEA, black cohosh, chaste tree fruit
Drug/Food
Decrease: clomiPHENE effect—soy
Drug/Lab Test
Increase: LFTs

NURSING CONSIDERATIONS

Assess:
- Verify infertility workup, pelvic exam
- LFTs before therapy: AST, ALT, alk phos
- Serum progesterone, urinary excretion of pregnanediol to identify occurrence of ovulation
- Ovarian size, cervical condition by pelvic examination
- Rule out endometrial carcinoma in women >35 yr by endometrial biopsy

Evaluate:
- Therapeutic response: fertility

Teach patient/family:
- That multiple births are common
- To notify prescriber immediately if low abdominal pain occurs; may indicate ovarian cyst, cyst rupture
- To notify prescriber of photophobia, blurred vision, diplopia, abnormal bleeding
- That, if dose is missed, to double it next time; if more than one dose is missed, to call prescriber
- That response usually occurs 4-10 days after last day of treatment
- About the method for taking, recording basal body temperature to determine whether ovulation has occurred
- If ovulation can be determined (there is a slight decrease in temperature then a sharp increase with ovulation), to attempt coitus 3 days before and every other day until after ovulation
- If pregnancy is suspected, to notify prescriber immediately (X)

clomiPRAMINE (Rx)

(kloe-mip′ra-meen)

Anafranil

Func. class.: Antidepressant, tricyclic
Chem. class.: Tertiary amine

Do not confuse:
clomiPRAMINE/clomiPHENE/chlorproMAZINE/desipramine/Norpramin

ACTION: Potentiates serotonin and norepinephrine; moderate anticholinergic effect

USES: Obsessive-compulsive disorder
Unlabeled uses: Autism, depression, premature ejaculation

CONTRAINDICATIONS: Hypersensitivity to this product, carBAMazepine, tricyclics, immediate post-MI, MAOI therapy
Precautions: Pregnancy (C), breastfeeding, geriatric patients, seizures,

cardiac disease, glaucoma, prostatic hypertrophy, urinary retention

Black Box Warning: Children, suicidal ideation

DOSAGE AND ROUTES

Obsessive-compulsive disorder

- **Adult: PO** 25 mg at bedtime, increase gradually over 4 wk to 75-250 mg/day in divided doses
- **Child 10-18 yr: PO** 25 mg/day gradually increase over 2 wk; max 3 mg/kg/day or 200 mg/day, whichever is smaller

Autism (unlabeled)

- **Adult: PO** 25 mg/day, may increase to 75-100 mg/day, max 250 mg/day
- **Child: PO** 25 mg/day, may increase if needed

Premature ejaculation (unlabeled)

- **Adult: PO** 25-50 mg/day

Depression (unlabeled)

- **Adult: PO** 25 mg at bedtime and increase gradually over 4 wk to 75-250 mg/day in divided doses
- **Child 10-18 yr: PO** 25-50 mg/day gradually increased; max 3 mg/kg/day or 200 mg/day, whichever is smaller

Available forms: Caps 25, 50, 75 mg

Administer:

- Do not break, crush, or chew caps
- Increased fluids, bulk in diet for constipation, especially for geriatric patients
- Without regard to food, during initial dosing and titration give with meals
- After titration, may be given as a single dose at bedtime to reduce daytime sedation
- Store in tight container, at room temperature; do not freeze

SIDE EFFECTS

CNS: *Dizziness, tremors, mania,* **seizures**, aggressiveness, EPS, drowsiness, headache, **neuroleptic malignant syndrome,** insomnia, agitation, anxiety, impaired memory

CV: Hypotension, tachycardia, **cardiac arrest,** hypertension, palpitations

EENT: Blurred vision, altered taste, tinnitus, increased intraocular pressure

ENDO: Galactorrhea, hyperprolactinemia

GI: *Constipation, dry mouth, nausea, dyspepsia,* weight gain, **hepatic toxicity**

GU: *Delayed ejaculation, anorgasmia,* urinary retention, decreased libido

HEMA: **Agranulocytosis, neutropenia, pancytopenia**

INTEG: Diaphoresis, photosensitivity, abnormal skin order, flushing, rash, pruritus

META: Hyponatremia

RESP: **Pharyngitis, rhinitis, bronchospasm**

SYST: **Suicide in children, adolescents**

PHARMACOKINETICS

Onset ≥2 wk (depression), 4-10 wk (OCD); peak 2-6 hr; extensively bound to tissue and plasma proteins; demethylated in liver; active metabolites excreted in urine (50%-60%), feces (24%-32%); half-life 32 hr; steady state 1-2 wk

INTERACTIONS

Increase: **hypertensive crisis, seizures, hypertensive episode—MAOIs**

Increase: **serotonin syndrome—SSRIs, SNRIs serotonin syndrome, linezolid, methylene blue IV**

Increase: clomiPRAMINE levels—cimetidine, FLUoxetine, fluvoxaMINE, sertraline; do not use together

Increase: hypertensive effect—cloNIDine, EPINEPHrine, norepinephrine

Increase: clomiPRAMINE level—CYP1A2, CYP2D6

Increase: CNS depression—alcohol, CNS depressants, general anesthetics

Increase: **QT prolongation—other tricyclics, phenothiazines, quinolones, antidysrhythmics, droperidol, mefloquine, mesoridazine, moxifloxacin, pentamidine, pimozide, tacrolimus, ziprasidone**

Decrease: effect of cloNIDine, levodopa, skeletal muscle relaxants, haloperidol, opiates

Decrease: clomiPRAMINE levels—barbiturates, carBAMazepine, phenytoin

Drug/Herb

Increase: serotonin syndrome—St. John's wort; do not use concurrently

Increase: CNS depression—hops, kava, valerian

Drug/Lab Test

Increase: prolactin, TBG, AST, ALT, blood glucose

Decrease: serum thyroid hormone (T_3, T_4)

NURSING CONSIDERATIONS

Assess:

- B/P lying, standing; pulse q4hr; if systolic B/P drops 20 mm Hg, withhold product, notify prescriber; take VS q4hr in patients with CV disease
- **Serotonin syndrome:** hyperpyrexia, rigidity, irregular pulse, diaphoresis
- **ECG** for flattening of T wave, QTc prolongation, bundle branch block, AV block, dysrhythmias in cardiac patients, may lead to cardiac collapse
- Blood studies: CBC, leukocytes, differential, cardiac enzymes if patient is receiving long-term therapy and signs of blood dyscrasias
- Hepatic studies: AST, ALT, bilirubin

Black Box Warning: Mental status: mood, sensorium, affect, suicidal tendencies; increase in psychiatric symptoms: depression, panic, frequency of obsessive-compulsive behaviors; watch closely for evidence of suicidal thoughts in children, adolescents; seizure disorders

- Urinary retention, constipation; constipation more likely in children
- **Withdrawal symptoms:** headache, nausea, vomiting, muscle pain, weakness; not usual unless product discontinued abruptly
- Alcohol consumption; if alcohol consumed, withhold dose until AM
- Assistance with ambulation during beginning therapy, since drowsiness, dizziness occurs
- Gum, hard candy, or frequent sips of water for dry mouth

Evaluate:

- Therapeutic response: decreased anxiety, depression

Teach patient/family:

- That the effects may take 4-6 wk to appear
- About risk for seizures
- To use caution when driving, performing other activities that require alertness because drowsiness, dizziness, blurred vision may occur
- To avoid alcohol, other CNS depressants
- Not to discontinue medication quickly after long-term use because this may cause nausea, headache, malaise

Black Box Warning: That suicidal thoughts/behaviors may occur in children, young adults; report immediately

- To wear sunscreen, protective clothing to prevent photosensitivity
- To notify prescriber if pregnancy is planned, suspected
- That men may experience a high incidence of sexual dysfunction
- **Serotonin syndrome:** report immediately sweating, diarrhea, twitching
- **Abrupt discontinuation:** do not stop abruptly

TREATMENT OF OVERDOSE:

ECG monitoring; induce emesis; lavage, activated charcoal; anticonvulsant; diazepam IV

HIGH ALERT

clonazePAM (Rx)

(kloe-na′zi-pam)

KlonoPIN, Rivotril ✦

Func. class.: Anticonvulsant

Chem. class.: Benzodiazepine derivative

Controlled Substance Schedule IV

Do not confuse:

clonazePAM/LORazepam/clorazepate/cloNIDine

KlonoPIN/cloNIDine

ACTION:
Inhibits spike, wave formation during absence seizures (petit mal); decreases amplitude, frequency, duration, spread of discharge during minor motor seizures

USES:
Absence, atypical absence, akinetic, myoclonic seizures; Lennox-Gastaut syndrome, panic disorder
Unlabeled uses: Anxiety, insomnia, nystagmus, restless leg syndrome

CONTRAINDICATIONS:
Pregnancy (D), hypersensitivity to benzodiazepines, acute closed-angle glaucoma, psychosis, severe hepatic disease
Precautions: Breastfeeding, geriatric patients, open-angle glaucoma, chronic respiratory disease, renal/hepatic disease

DOSAGE AND ROUTES
Lennox-Gastaut syndrome/atypicals absence seizures/akinetic and myclonic seizures
- **Adult: PO** up to 1.5 mg/day in 3 divided doses; may be increased 0.5-1 mg q3days until desired response, max 20 mg/day
- **Geriatric: PO** 0.25 daily-bid initially, increase by 0.25/day q7-14days as needed
- **Child <10 yr or <30 kg: PO** initial 0.01-0.03 mg/kg/day in divided doses q8hr, max 0.05 mg/kg/day; may be increased 0.25-0.5 mg q3days until desired response, max 0.1-0.2 mg/kg/day

Panic disorder
- **Adult: PO** 0.25 mg bid increase to 1 mg daily after 3 days, max 4 mg/day

Restless leg syndrome (RLS) (unlabeled)
- **Adult: PO** 0.5 mg tid or 0.5 mg in the evening and 30 min before bedtime

Insomnia/anxiety (unlabeled)
- **Adult: PO** 0.125-0.25 mg at bedtime, titrate up q3-4days as needed

Available forms: Tabs 0.5, 1, 2 mg; orally disintegrating tabs 0.125, 0.25, 0.5, 1, 2 mg
Administer:
PO route
- With food, milk for GI symptoms
- **Orally disintegrating tablets:** open pouch by peeling back foil on blister pack (do not push tab through foil), place on tongue, allow to dissolve; may be swallowed with/without water
- Store at room temperature

SIDE EFFECTS
CNS: *Drowsiness,* dizziness, confusion, behavioral changes, tremors, insomnia, headache, **suicidal tendencies,** slurred speech, anterograde amnesia, fatigue, poor coordination
CV: Palpitations, bradycardia, tachycardia
EENT: *Increased salivation, nystagmus, diplopia,* abnormal eye movements
GI: *Nausea, constipation,* polyphagia, anorexia, xerostomia, diarrhea, gastritis, sore gums, blurred vision
GU: Dysuria, enuresis, nocturia, retention, libido changes
HEMA: **Thrombocytopenia, leukocytosis, eosinophilia**
INTEG: Rash, alopecia, hirsutism
RESP: **Respiratory depression,** dyspnea, congestion
MS: myalgia, muscle weakness

PHARMACOKINETICS
PO: Peak 1-2 hr, metabolized by liver, excreted in urine, half-life 18-50 hr, duration 6-12 hr, protein binding 85%

INTERACTIONS
Increase: clonazePAM effects—CYP3A4 inhibitors (azoles, cimetidine, clarithromycin, diltiazem, erythromycin, FLUoxetine), oral contraceptives
Increase: CNS depression—alcohol, barbiturates, opiates, antidepressants, other anticonvulsants, general anesthetics, hypnotics, sedatives
Decrease: clonazePAM effect—CYP3A4 inducers (carBAMazepine, PHENobarbital, phenytoin)
Drug/Herb
Increase: CNS depression—kava, chamomile, valerian
Increase: clonazePAM effect—ginkgo, melatonin

Decrease: clonazePAM effect—ginseng, St. John's wort

Drug/Lab Test

Increase: AST, alk phos, bilirubin

Decrease: platelets, WBC

NURSING CONSIDERATIONS

Assess:

- **Seizures:** duration, type, intensity, with/without aura
- Blood studies: RBC, Hct, Hgb, reticulocyte counts every wk for 4 wk, then monthly
- Hepatic studies: ALT, AST, bilirubin, creatinine
- **Abrupt discontinuation:** do not discontinue abruptly; seizures may increase
- Signs of physical withdrawal if medication suddenly discontinued

⚠ **Mental status:** mood, sensorium, affect, oversedation, behavioral changes, **suicidal thoughts/behaviors;** if mental status changes, notify prescriber

- Eye problems: need for ophthalmic exam before, during, after treatment (slit lamp, funduscopy, tonometry)
- Allergic reaction: red, raised rash; product should be discontinued

⚠ **Blood dyscrasias:** fever, sore throat, bruising, rash, jaundice

- **Toxicity:** bone marrow depression, nausea, vomiting, ataxia, diplopia, CV collapse; drug levels during initial treatment (therapeutic 20-80 ng/ml)
- Assistance with ambulation during early part of treatment; dizziness occurs, especially among geriatric patients

Evaluate:

- Therapeutic response: decreased seizure activity

Teach patient/family:

- To carry emergency ID bracelet stating name, products taken, condition; prescriber's name, phone number, discuss tolerance, withdrawal
- To avoid driving, other activities that require alertness
- To avoid alcohol, other CNS depressants; increased sedation may occur
- Not to discontinue medication quickly after long-term use; to taper off over several wk
- To notify prescriber of yellowing of skin/eyes, clay-colored stools, bleeding, fever, extreme fatigue, sore throat, suicidal thoughts/behaviors

TREATMENT OF OVERDOSE:
Lavage, activated charcoal, flumazenil, monitor electrolytes, VS, administer vasopressors

cloNIDine (Rx)
(klon′i-deen)

Catapres, Catapres-TTS, Duraclon, Kapvay

Func. class.: Antihypertensive

Chem. class.: Central α-adrenergic agonist

Do not confuse:

cloNIDine/KlonoPIN/clonazePAM

Catapres/Cataflam/Catarase

ACTION: Inhibits sympathetic vasomotor center in CNS, which reduces impulses in sympathetic nervous system; blood pressure, pulse rate, cardiac output decrease, prevents pain signal transmission in CNS by α-adrenergic receptor stimulation of the spinal cord

USES: Mild to moderate hypertension, used alone or in combination; severe pain in cancer patients (epidural), attention-deficit/hyperactivity disorder (ADHD)

Unlabeled uses: Opioid withdrawal, prevention of vascular headaches, treatment of menopausal symptoms, dysmenorrhea, autism, cycloSPORINE nephrotoxicity prophylaxis, diabetic neuropathy, ethanol/nicotine/opiate agonist withdrawal, Tourette's syndrome, hypertensive emergency, neonatal abstinence syndrome, scleroderma renal crisis

CONTRAINDICATIONS: Hypersensitivity; (epidural) bleeding disorders, anticoagulants

Precautions: Pregnancy (C), breastfeeding, children <12 yr (transdermal), geriatric patients, noncompliant patients, MI (recent), diabetes mellitus, chronic renal failure, Raynaud's disease, thyroid disease, depression, COPD, asthma, pheochromocytoma

Black Box Warning: Labor (epidermal clonidine)

DOSAGE AND ROUTES

Hypertension

- **Adult: PO** 0.1 mg bid then increase by 0.1-0.2 mg/day at weekly intervals until desired response; max 2.4 mg; range 0.2-0.6 mg/day in divided doses or **TRANSDERMAL** q7days, start 0.1 mg and adjust q1-2wk
- **Geriatric: PO** 0.1 mg at bedtime; may increase gradually
- **Child: PO** 5-10 mcg/kg/day in divided doses q8-12hr, max 0.9 mg/day

Severe pain

- **Adult: CONT EPIDURAL INFUSION** 30 mcg/hr
- **Child: CONT EPIDURAL INFUSION** 0.5 mcg/kg/hr, then titrate to response

Opioid withdrawal (unlabeled)

- **Adult: PO** 0.3-1.2 mg/day; may decrease by 50% × 3 days, then decrease by 0.1-0.2 mg/day or discontinue

ADHD

- **Adolescent/child ≥6 yr: PO** 0.05 mg/kg/day in 3-4 divided doses may increase in 0.1 mg/day weekly up to 0.4 mg/day; ext rel 0.1 mg at bedtime, increase dose by 0.1 mg/day up to 0.4 mg/day

Menopausal symptoms (unlabeled)

- **Adult: TRANSDERMAL** 0.1-mg patch q1wk; **PO** 0.05-0.4 mg/day

Tourette's syndrome (unlabeled)

- **Adult: PO** 0.15-0.2 mg/day

Hypertensive emergency (unlabeled)

- **Adult: PO** 0.1-0.2 mg q1hr to a total of 0.6 mg

Available forms: Tabs 0.025 ✦, 0.1, 0.2, 0.3 mg; transdermal 2.5, 5, 7.5 mg delivering 0.1, 0.2, 0.3 mg/24 hr, respectively; inj 100, 500 mcg/ml; ext rel tab 0.1 mg (Kapvay)

Administer:

- Store patches in cool environment, tablets in tight container

PO route

- Give last dose at bedtime
- Do not crush, cut, chew, or break ext rel tabs; Kapvay is not interchangeable with other products

Transdermal route

- Once weekly; apply to site without hair; best absorption over chest or upper arm; rotate sites with each application; clean site before application; apply firmly, especially around edges; may secure with adhesive tape if loosen, fold sticky sides together and discard
- Should be removed before MRI

Epidural route

- Used for severe cancer pain
- May be used with opiates
- Use only if familiar with epidural infusion devices

Black Box Warning: Do not use for labor

SIDE EFFECTS

CNS: *Drowsiness, sedation, headache, fatigue,* nightmares, insomnia, mental changes, anxiety, depression, hallucinations, delirium, syncope, dizziness

CV: *Orthostatic hypotension, palpitations,* CHF, ECG abnormalities, sinus tachycardia

EENT: Taste change, parotid pain

ENDO: Hyperglycemia

GI: *Nausea, vomiting, malaise,* constipation, *dry mouth*

GU: Impotence, dysuria, nocturia, gynecomastia

INTEG: *Rash,* alopecia, facial pallor, pruritus, hives, edema, burning papules, excoriation (transdermal patches)

MISC: Withdrawal symptoms

MS: Muscle, joint pain; leg cramps

PHARMACOKINETICS

Absorbed well

PO: Onset ½ to 1 hr, peak 2-4 hr, duration 8-12 hr, half-life 6-12 hr

TRANSDERMAL: Onset 3 days; duration 1 wk; metabolized by liver (metabolites); excreted in urine (45% unchanged, inactive metabolites), feces; crosses blood-brain barrier; excreted in breast milk

INTERACTIONS

- AV block: verapamil, diltiazem

⚠ Life-threatening elevations of B/P: tricyclics, β-blockers

Increase: CNS depression—opiates, sedatives, hypnotics, anesthetics, alcohol

Increase: hypotensive effects—diuretics, other antihypertensive nitrates

Decrease: hypotensive effects—tricyclics, MAOIs, appetite suppressants, amphetamines, prazosin, antipsychotics

Decrease: effect of levodopa

Drug/Herb

Increase: antihypertensive effect—hawthorn

Decrease: antihypertensive effect—ephedra, ginseng

Drug/Lab Test

Increase: blood glucose

Decrease: VMA, urinary catecholamines, aldosterone

NURSING CONSIDERATIONS

Assess:

- **Hypertension:** B/P, pulse; report significant changes
- **Opiate withdrawal (unlabeled):** fever, diarrhea, nausea, vomiting, cramps, insomnia, shivering, dilated pupils
- **Cancer pain:** location, intensity, character; alleviating, aggravating factors at baseline and frequently
- Edema in feet, legs daily; monitor I&O; check for falling output
- **Allergic reaction:** rash, fever, pruritus, urticaria; product should be discontinued if antihistamines fail to help
- **CHF:** edema, dyspnea, wet crackles, B/P, more common in geriatric patients
- **ADHD:** B/P, pulse, palpitations, syncope
- Renal symptoms: polyuria, oliguria, frequency

Evaluate:

- Therapeutic response: decrease in B/P with hypertension, decrease in withdrawal symptoms (opioid), decrease in pain

Teach patient/family:

- To avoid hazardous activities, since product may cause drowsiness
- To notify all health care providers of medication use
- Not to discontinue product abruptly or **withdrawal symptoms** may occur: anxiety, increased B/P, headache, insomnia, increased pulse, tremors, nausea, sweating; to comply with dosage schedule even if feeling better
- Not to use OTC (cough, cold, or allergy), alcohol or CNS depressant products unless directed by prescriber
- To rise slowly to sitting or standing position to minimize orthostatic hypotension, especially among geriatric patients
- To notify prescriber of mouth sores, sore throat, fever, swelling of hands or feet, irregular heartbeat, chest pain, signs of **angioedema**
- About excessive perspiration, dehydration, vomiting; diarrhea may lead to fall in B/P; consult prescriber if these occur; that product may cause dizziness, fainting; that light-headedness may occur during first few days of therapy
- That product may cause dry mouth; to use hard candy, saliva product, sugarless gum, or frequent rinsing of mouth
- That compliance is necessary; not to skip or stop product unless directed by prescriber; tolerance may develop with long-term use
- **Transdermal:** how to use patch; that patch comes in two parts: product patch and overlay to keep patch in place; not to trim or cut patch; that response may take 2-3 days if product is given transdermally; on administration of patch, if switching from tabs to patch, to taper tabs to avoid withdrawal, remove for MRI, can use during bathing, swimming

TREATMENT OF OVERDOSE:

Supportive treatment; administer tolazoline, atropine, DOPamine prn

clopidogrel (Rx)

(klo-pid′oh-grel)

Plavix

Func. class.: Platelet aggregation inhibitor

Chem. class.: Thienopyridine derivative

Do not confuse:
Plavix/Paxil/Elavil

ACTION: Inhibits ADP-induced platelet aggregation

USES: Reducing the risk of stroke, MI, vascular death, peripheral arterial disease in high-risk patients, acute coronary syndrome, transient ischemic attack (TIA), unstable angina

Unlabeled uses: Cardiac surgery (infant and child), Kawasaki disease

CONTRAINDICATIONS: Hypersensitivity, active bleeding

Precautions: Pregnancy (B), breastfeeding, children, previous hepatic disease, increased bleeding risk, neutropenia, agranulocytosis, renal disease, Asian/Black/Caucasian patients

Black Box Warning: CYP2C19 allele (poor metabolizers)

DOSAGE AND ROUTES

Recent MI, stroke, peripheral arterial disease, TIA

- **Adult: PO** 75 mg/day with/without aspirin

Acute coronary syndrome

- **Adult: PO** loading dose 300 mg, then 75 mg/day with aspirin

Cardiac surgery/other cardiac conditions (unlabeled)

- **Child ≤2 yr, infant, neonate: PO** 0.2 mg/kg/day for platelet inhibition

Available forms: Tabs 75, 300 mg

Administer:

- Without regard to food
- Should be discontinued 5 days before elective surgery if an antiplatelet action is not desired

SIDE EFFECTS

CNS: Headache, dizziness, depression, syncope, hypesthesia, neuralgia, confusion, hallucinations

CV: Edema, hypertension, chest pain

GI: Nausea, vomiting, diarrhea, constipation, GI discomfort, **GI bleeding, pancreatitis, hepatic failure**

GU: **Glomerulonephritis**

HEMA: Epistaxis, purpura, **bleeding (major/minor from any site), neutropenia, aplastic anemia, agranulocytosis, thrombotic thrombocytopenic purpura**

INTEG: Rash, pruritus, **anaphylaxis**

MISC: UTI, hypercholesterolemia, chest pain, fatigue, **intracranial hemorrhage, toxic epidermal necrolysis, Stevens-Johnson syndrome,** flulike syndrome

MS: Arthralgia, back pain

RESP: Upper respiratory tract infection, dyspnea, rhinitis, bronchitis, cough, **bronchospasm**

PHARMACOKINETICS

Rapidly absorbed; metabolized by liver (CYP3A4, CYP2B6, CYP1A2, CYP2C8); excreted in urine, feces; half-life 6 hr; plasma protein binding 95%; effect on platelets after 3-7 days

INTERACTIONS

Black Box Warning: Avoid use with CYP2C19 inhibitors (omeprazole, esomeprazole)

Increase: bleeding risk—anticoagulants, aspirin, NSAIDs, abciximab, eptifibatide, tirofiban, thrombolytics, ticlopidine, SSRIs, treprostinil, rifampin

Increase: action of some NSAIDs, phenytoin, TOLBUTamide, tamoxifen, torsemide, fluvastatin, warfarin

Decrease: clopidogrel effect—proton pump inhibitor (PPIs)

Decrease: CYP3A4 inhibitors/substrates—atorvastatin, simvastatin, cerivastatin

Drug/Herb

Increase: clopidogrel effect—feverfew, fish oil, omega-3 fatty acid, garlic, ginger, ginkgo biloba, green tea, horse chestnut

Decrease: clopidogrel effect—bilberry, saw palmetto

Drug/Lab Test

Increase: AST, ALT, bilirubin, uric acid, total cholesterol, nonprotein nitrogen (NPN)

NURSING CONSIDERATIONS

Assess:

⚠ **Thrombotic/thrombocytic purpura,** fever, thrombocytopenia, neurolytic anemia

Black Box Warning: CYP2C19 Allele (poor metabolizers): Consider using another antiplatelet product, higher CV reaction occurs after acute coronary syndrome or PCI, tests are available to determine CYP2C19 allele

- Symptoms of stroke, MI during treatment
- Hepatic studies: AST, ALT, bilirubin, creatinine (long-term therapy)
- Blood studies: CBC, differential, Hct, Hgb, PT, cholesterol (long-term therapy)

Evaluate:

- Therapeutic response: absence of stroke, MI

Teach patient/family:

- That blood work will be necessary during treatment
- To report any unusual bruising, bleeding to prescriber; that it may take longer to stop bleeding
- To take without regard to food
- To report diarrhea, skin rashes, subcutaneous bleeding, chills, fever, sore throat
- To tell all health care providers that clopidogrel is being used; may be held for 5 days before surgery

clotrimazole (topical, vaginal, oral)

(kloe-trim′a-zole)

Cruex, Gyne-Lotrimin, Lotrimin, Lotrimin AF, MyCelex, MyCelex-7, Trivagizole 3, Desenex

Func. class.: Topical antifungal

Chem. class.: Imidazole derivative

Do not confuse: clotrimazole/miconazole/clobetasol

ACTION: Antifungal activity results from altering cell wall permeability

USES: Vulvovaginal, oropharyngeal candidiasis; topical fungal infections

CONTRAINDICATIONS: Hypersensitivity, ophthalmic use

Precautions: Hepatic impairment (oral)

DOSAGE AND ROUTES

Tinea corporis, cruris, pedis, versicolor; candidiasis

- **Adult/child ≥2 yr:** Apply to affected area and rub into area AM/PM × 2-4 wk

Vulvovaginal candidiasis

- **Adult/child ≥12 yr: Vag cream** 1 applicator at bedtime × 3 days (2%) or 7 days (1%)

Oropharyngeal candidiasis

- **Adult/child ≥3 yr: Lozenge** 1 PO dissolved 5×/day × 2 wk or adults 1 lozenge dissolved tid (prevention)

Available forms: Topical cream, solution, 1%; vaginal cream 1%, 2%; lozenges, troches 10 mg

Administer:

Topical route

- Topical skin products are not for intravaginal therapy and are for external use only; do not use skin products near the eyes, nose, or mouth
- Wash hands before and after use; wash affected area and gently pat dry

- **Cream/solution:** apply to the cleansed affected area; massage gently into affected areas
- **Troches:** allow to dissolve; do not chew or swallow whole

Intravaginal route

- Only use dosage formulations specified for intravaginal use; intravaginal dosage forms are not for topical therapy; do not ingest
- **Cream:** use applicator(s) supplied by the manufacturer

SIDE EFFECTS

GI: Nausea, vomiting
GU: Vaginal burning, irritation
INTEG: Burning, peeling, rash, pruritus

PHARMACOKINETICS

PO duration 3 hr

INTERACTIONS

Drug/Lab Test
Increase: LFTs

NURSING CONSIDERATIONS

Assess:

- **Allergic reaction:** assess for hypersensitivity; product might need to be discontinued
- **Infection:** assess for severity of infection, itching
- Hepatic function studies periodically if using oral troches

Evaluate:

- Decreased infection, itching

Teach patient/family:

Topical route:

- That topical skin products are not for intravaginal therapy and are for external use only; do not use skin products near the eyes, nose, or mouth; do not use occlusive dressings
- To wash hands before and after use; wash affected area and gently pat dry
- **Cream:** to shake well before use; apply a thin film to the cleansed affected area; massage gently into affected areas

PO route:

- **Troches**: allow to dissolve; do not chew or swallow whole

Intravaginal route: To use only dosage formulations specified for intravaginal use; intravaginal dosage forms are not for topical therapy; do not ingest; abstain from sexual contact; may damage condoms, diaphragms

- **Cream:** to use applicator(s) supplied by the manufacturer

C

cloZAPine (Rx)

(kloz′a-peen)

Clozaril, FazaClo, Versacloz

Func. class.: Antipsychotic

Chem. class.: Tricyclic dibenzodiazepine derivative

Do not confuse:
Clozaril/Colazal
cloZAPine/cloNIDine/clofazimine/clonazePAM/Klonopin

ACTION:
Interferes with DOPamine receptor binding with lack of EPS; also acts as an adrenergic, cholinergic, histaminergic, serotonergic antagonist

USES:
Management of psychotic symptoms for schizophrenic patients for whom other antipsychotics have failed; recurrent suicidal behavior

Unlabeled uses: Agitation, bipolar disorder, psychosis in dementia, psychosis in Parkinson's disease

CONTRAINDICATIONS:
Hypersensitivity, severe granulocytopenia (WBC <3500 before therapy), coma

Black Box Warning: Myeloproliferative disorders, severe CNS depression, agranulocytosis, leukopenia, neutropenia, seizure disorder

Precautions: Pregnancy (B), breastfeeding, children <16 yr, geriatric patients; CV, pulmonary, cardiac, renal, hepatic disease; seizures, prostatic enlargement, closed-angle glaucoma, stroke

Black Box Warning: Bone marrow suppression, hypotension, myocarditis, orthostatic hypotension, geriatric patients with dementia-related psychosis

DOSAGE AND ROUTES

Schizophrenia

- **Adult: PO** 12.5 mg daily or bid; may increase by 25-50 mg/day; normal range 300-450 mg/day after 2 wk; dose >500 mg require 3 divided doses; do not increase dose more than 2×/wk; max 900 mg/day; use lowest dose to control symptoms; if dose is to be discontinued, taper over 1-2 wk
- **Child ≥9 yr, adolescents (unlabeled): PO** 6.25-12.5 mg initially slowly titrate

Dementia with multiple behavioral disturbances (unlabeled)

- **Geriatric: PO** 12.5 mg daily at bedtime, may increase by 12.5 mg every other day, max 50 mg/day

Available forms: Tabs 12.5, 25, 50, 100, 200 mg; orally disintegrating tabs 12.5, 25, 100, 150, 200 mg; oral suspension 50 mg/ml

Administer:

- May be taken with or without food
- Patient-specific registration required before administration; if WBC <3500 cells/mm^3 or ANC <2000 cells/mm^3, therapy should not be started; may only dispense the 7, 14, 28 day supply upon receipt of lab report that is appropriate
- Check to confirm PO medication swallowed; monitor for hoarding or giving of medication to other patients, if hospitalized; avoid giving patient >7 days' worth of medication if outpatient
- Store in tight, light-resistant container
- **Orally disintegrating tab:** do not push through foil; leave in foil blister until ready to take, peel back foil, place tab in mouth; allow to dissolve, swallow; water is not needed
- **Oral suspension:** Shake before using, use oral syringe and syringe adapter

SIDE EFFECTS

CNS: Neuroleptic malignant syndrome, *sedation, salivation, dizziness, headache, tremors, sleep problems, akinesia, fever,* seizures, *sweating, akathisia, confusion, fatigue, insomnia,* depression, slurred speech, anxiety, *agitation,* dystonia, obsessive-compulsive symptoms

CV: *Tachycardia, hypo/hypertension,* chest pain, ECG changes, orthostatic hypotension

EENT: *Blurred vision*

GI: *Drooling or excessive salivation, constipation, nausea, abdominal discomfort, vomiting, diarrhea,* anorexia, *weight gain, dry mouth,* heartburn, *dyspepsia, gastroesophageal reflux*

GU: *Urinary abnormalities,* incontinence, ejaculation dysfunction; frequency, urgency, retention, dysuria

HEMA: Leukopenia, agranulocytosis, eosinophilia

MS: Weakness; pain in back, neck, legs; spasm, *rigidity*

OTHER: *Diaphoresis*

RESP: Dyspnea, nasal congestion, lower respiratory tract infection

SYST: Death among geriatric patients with dementia, aggravation of diabetes mellitus

PHARMACOKINETICS

Bioavailability 27%-47%; 97% protein bound; completely metabolized by liver enzymes involved in metabolism CYP1A2, 2D6, 3A4; excreted in urine (50%), feces (30%) (metabolites); half-life 8-12 hr

INTERACTIONS

Increase: CNS depression—CNS depressants, psychoactives, alcohol

Increase: cloZAPine level—caffeine, citalopram, FLUoxetine, sertraline, ritonavir, risperiDONE, CYP1A2 inhibitors (fluvoxaMINE), CYP3A4 inhibitors (ketoconazole, erythromycin)

Increase: plasma concentration—warfarin, digoxin, other highly protein-bound products

Increase: QT prolongation—β blockers, class IA/III antidysrhythmias, and other drugs that increase QT
Increase: hypotension, respiratory, cardiac arrest, collapse—benzodiazepines
Decrease: cloZAPine level—CYP1A2 inducers (carBAMazepine, omeprazole, rifampin); PHENobarbital

Drug/Lab Test
Increase: LFTs, cardiac enzymes, cholesterol, blood glucose, bilirubin, PBI, cholinesterase, ^{131}I, Hct/Hgb, erythrocyte sedimentation rate
Decrease: WBC
False positive: pregnancy tests, PKU
False negative: urinary steroids, 17-OHCS

NURSING CONSIDERATIONS

Assess:

Black Box Warning: Myocarditis; if suspected, discontinue use; myocarditis usually occurs during 1st month of treatment

Black Box Warning: Seizures; usually occur with higher doses >600 mg/day or dosage change >100 mg/day; do not use in uncontrolled seizure disorder, use cautiously in those with a predisposition to seizures

- AIMS assessment, blood glucose, CBC differential, glycosylated hemoglobin A1c, LFTs, neurologic function, pregnancy test, serum creatinine, electrolytes, lipid profile, prolactin, thyroid function tests, weight

Black Box Warning: Bone marrow depression: bilirubin, CBC, LFTs monthly; discontinue treatment if WBC <3000-3500/mm^3 or ANC <1500/mm^3; test weekly; may resume when normal; if WBC <2000/mm^3 or ANC <1000/mm^3, discontinue; if agranulocytosis develops, never restart product

- Affect, orientation, LOC, reflexes, gait, coordination, sleep pattern disturbances

Black Box Warning: Hypotension: B/P standing and lying; take pulse, respirations q4hr during initial treatment; establish baseline before starting treatment; report drops of 30 mm Hg

- Dizziness, faintness, palpitations, tachycardia on rising
- **EPS** including akathisia (inability to sit still, no pattern to movements), tardive dyskinesia (bizarre movements of the jaw, mouth, tongue, extremities), pseudoparkinsonism (rigidity, tremors, pill rolling, shuffling gait)

⚠ **Neuroleptic malignant syndrome:** tachycardia, seizures, fever, dyspnea, diaphoresis, increased/decreased B/P; notify prescriber immediately

- Constipation, urinary retention daily; if these occur, increase bulk, water in diet, especially for geriatric patients; stool softeners, laxatives may be needed
- Do not involve patient in strenuous exercise program fainting is possible; patient should not stand still for long periods

Evaluate:

- Therapeutic response: decrease in emotional excitement, hallucinations, delusions, paranoia, reorganization of patterns of thought, speech

Teach patient/family:

- About symptoms of agranulocytosis and need for blood tests weekly for 6 mo, then q2wk; to report flulike symptoms
- That orthostatic hypotension often occurs; to rise gradually from sitting or lying position; to avoid hot tubs, hot showers, tub baths; hypotension may occur
- To avoid abrupt withdrawal of this product because EPS may result; that product should be withdrawn over 1-2 wk
- To avoid OTC preparations (cough, hay fever, cold) unless approved by prescriber, since serious product interactions may occur; to avoid use with alcohol or CNS depressants, increased drowsiness may occur
- About compliance with product regimen
- About EPS and necessity for meticulous oral hygiene, since oral candidiasis may occur

Black Box Warning: To report sore throat, malaise, fever, bleeding, mouth sores; if these occur, CBC should be drawn and product discontinued

- That heat stroke may occur in hot weather; to take extra precautions to stay cool
- To avoid driving, other hazardous activities; seizures may occur
- To notify prescriber if pregnant or if pregnancy is intended; not to breastfeed

TREATMENT OF OVERDOSE:
Lavage, activated charcoal; provide an airway; do not induce vomiting

codeine (Rx)

(koe′deen)

Func. class.: Opiate analgesic, antitussive

Chem. class.: Opiate, phenathrene derivative

Controlled Substance Schedule II, III, IV, V (depends on content)

Do not confuse:
codeine/Lodine/iodine/Cardene

ACTION:
Depresses pain impulse transmission at the spinal cord level by interacting with opioid receptors; decreases cough reflex, GI motility

USES:
Mild to moderate pain

Unlabeled uses: Diarrhea, arthralgia, bone/dental pain, headache, migraine, myalgia, nonproductive cough

CONTRAINDICATIONS:
Breastfeeding, hypersensitivity to opiates, respiratory depression, increased intracranial pressure, seizure disorders, severe respiratory disorders

Black Box Warning: Children (tonsillectomy/adenoidectomy)

Precautions: Pregnancy (C), geriatric patients, cardiac dysrhythmias, prostatic hypertrophy, bowel impaction

DOSAGE AND ROUTES

Pain
- **Adult: PO/IM/IV** 15-60 mg q4hr prn, use phosphate product for IM/IV
- **Child 6-17 yr: PO** 3 mg/kg/day in divided doses q4hr prn

Renal disease
- **Adult: PO** CCr 10-50 ml/min, 75% of dose; CCr <10 ml/min, 50% of dose

Cough (unlabeled)
- **Adult: PO** 10-20 mg q4-6hr, max 120 mg/day

Diarrhea (unlabeled)
- **Adult: PO** 30 mg; may repeat qid prn

Arthralgia/bone pain/back pain/dental pain/headache/migraine/myalgia (unlabeled)
- **Adult: PO** 15-60 mg q4-6hr
- **Child ≥3 yr: PO** 0.5-1 mg/kg or 15 mg/m^2 (max 60 mg/dose) q4-6hr

Available forms: Tabs 15, 30 mg; inj 15, 30, 60 mg/ml; oral sol 30 mg/5 ml; syrup 5 mg/ml ✱

Administer:
- Discontinue gradually after long-term use, use stool softener, laxative for constipation
- Store in light-resistant container at room temperature

SIDE EFFECTS

CNS: *Drowsiness, sedation,* dizziness, agitation, dependency, lethargy, restlessness, euphoria, seizures, hallucinations, headache, confusion

CV: Bradycardia, palpitations, orthostatic hypotension, tachycardia, circulatory collapse

GI: *Nausea, vomiting, anorexia, constipation,* dry mouth

GU: Urinary retention

INTEG: Flushing, rash, urticaria, pruritus

RESP: Respiratory depression, respiratory paralysis, dyspnea

SYST: Anaphylaxis

PHARMACOKINETICS
Bioavailability 60%-90%; peak ½-1 hr; duration 4-6 hr; metabolized by liver (CYP3A4 to morphine); excreted by kidneys, in

breast milk; crosses placenta; half-life 3 hr; protein binding 7%; altered codeine metabolism occurs in different ethnic groups
PO: Onset 30-60 min

INTERACTIONS

Increase: CNS depression—CYP2D6, alcohol, opiates, sedative/hypnotics, antipsychotics, skeletal muscle relaxants
⚠ **Increase:** toxicity—MAOIs; use cautiously
Drug/Lab Test
Increase: lipase, amylase

NURSING CONSIDERATIONS

Assess:
- **Pain:** intensity, type, location, aggravating, alleviating factors; need for pain medication, tolerance; use pain scoring
- I&O ratio; check for decreasing output; may indicate urinary retention, especially among geriatric patients
- GI function: nausea, vomiting, constipation
- **Cough:** type, duration, ability to raise secretion for productive cough; do not use to suppress productive cough
- CNS changes, dizziness, drowsiness, hallucinations, euphoria, LOC, pupil reaction
- Allergic reactions: rash, urticaria

Black Box Warning: Children (tonsillectomy/adenoidectomy): Deaths have occurred; use is contraindicated

⚠ **Respiratory dysfunction:** respiratory depression, character, rate, rhythm; notify prescriber if respirations are <10/min, shallow; obstructive sleep apnea (children) (tonsillectomy/adenoidectomy)
Evaluate:
- Therapeutic response: decrease in pain, absence of grimacing, decreased cough, decreased diarrhea

Teach patient/family:
- Not to breastfeed
- To report any symptoms of CNS changes, allergic reactions
- That physical dependency may result after extended periods
- To decrease dry mouth use sugarless gum, rinse mouth often
- To change position slowly; orthostatic hypotension may occur
- To avoid hazardous activities if drowsiness, dizziness occurs
- To avoid alcohol, other CNS depressants unless directed by prescriber

TREATMENT OF OVERDOSE:

Naloxone 0.4-mg ampule diluted in 10 ml 0.9% NaCl and given by direct IV push, 0.02 mg q2min (adult)

colchicine (Rx)

(kol′chih-seen)
Colcrys
Func. class.: Antigout agent
Chem. class.: ***Colchicum autumnale*** alkaloid

ACTION: Inhibits microtubule formation of lactic acid in leukocytes, which decreases phagocytosis and inflammation in joints

USES: Gout, gouty arthritis (prevention, treatment); to arrest the progression of neurologic disability in those with MS, Mediterranean fever
Unlabeled uses: Hepatic cirrhosis, pericarditis, amyloidosis, Behçet's syndrome, biliary cirrhosis, dermatitis herpetiformis, idiopathic thrombocytopenic purpura, Paget's disease, pseudogout, pulmonary fibrosis

CONTRAINDICATIONS: Pregnancy (D) (injectable), serious GI, severe cardiac/renal/hepatic disorders, hypersensitivity
Precautions: Pregnancy (C) (PO), breastfeeding, children, geriatric patients, blood dyscrasias, hepatic disease

DOSAGE AND ROUTES

Gout prevention
- **Adult: PO** 0.6-1.2 mg/day in 1-2 divided doses, depending on severity

Gout treatment

• **Adult: PO** 1.2 mg initially, then 0.6 mg 1 hr later (1.8 mg); for those on strong CYP3A4 inhibitor (during past 14 days), 0.6 mg initially, then 0.3 mg 1 hr later

Renal dose

• **Adult: PO** CCr <30 ml/min, for acute gout, do not repeat course for 2 wk; for familial Mediterranean fever, 0.3 mg daily, increase cautiously

Pericarditis (unlabeled)

• **Adult: PO** 0.5 mg bid

Mediterranean fever (unlabeled)

• **Adult on no interacting products: PO** 1.2-2.4 mg/day in 1-2 divided doses; strong CYP3A4 inhibitor; P-glycoprotein inhibitors within 14 day: max 0.6 mg/day in 1-2 divided doses; moderate CYP3A4 inhibitors with 14 day: max 1.2 mg/day in 1-2 divided doses

• **Adolescent: PO** 1.2-2.4 mg/day in 1-2 divided doses, titrate by 0.3 mg/day

• **Child > 6-12 yr: PO** 0.9-1.8 mg/day in 1-2 divided doses

• **Child 4-6 yr: PO** 0.3-1.8 mg/day in 1-2 divided doses

Amyloidosis/biliary cirrhosis/ dermatitis herpetiformis/Paget's disease/Behçet's syndrome/chronic idiopathic thrombocytopenic purpura/pulmonary fibrosis (unlabeled)

• **Adult: PO** 0.5-0.6 mg bid-tid

Available forms: Tabs 0.6 mg; cap 0.6 mg

Administer:

PO route

• Without regard to food

• Cumulative doses ≤4 mg, renal patients ≤2 mg; when reached, administer only for 3 wk

SIDE EFFECTS

GI: *Nausea, vomiting, anorexia, malaise,* metallic taste, cramps, peptic ulcer, diarrhea

GU: Hematuria, oliguria, renal damage

HEMA: Agranulocytosis, thrombocytopenia, aplastic anemia, pancytopenia

INTEG: Chills, dermatitis, pruritus, purpura, erythema

MISC: Myopathy, alopecia, reversible azoospermia, peripheral neuritis

PHARMACOKINETICS

PO: Peak ½-2 hr, half-life 4.4 hr, deacetylates in liver, excreted in feces (metabolites/active product)

INTERACTIONS

Increase: colchicine level/toxicity—moderate/strong CYP3A4 inhibitors, reduce dose

Increase: GI effects—NSAIDs, ethanol

Increase: bone marrow depression—radiation, bone marrow depressants, cycloSPORINE

Decrease: action of vit B_{12}; may cause reversible malabsorption

Drug/Food

Increase: colchicine level—grapefruit juice

Drug/Lab Test

Increase: alk phos, AST

Decrease: platelets, WBC, granulocytes

False positive: urine Hgb

Interference: urinary 17-hydroxycorticosteroids

NURSING CONSIDERATIONS

Assess:

• Relief of pain, uric acid levels returning to normal

• I&O ratio; observe for decrease in urinary output

⚠ CBC, platelets, reticulocytes before, during therapy (q3mo); may cause aplastic anemia, agranulocytosis, decreased platelets

• **Toxicity:** weakness, abdominal pain, nausea, vomiting, diarrhea; product should be discontinued, report symptoms immediately

Evaluate:

• Therapeutic response: decreased stone formation, decreased pain in kidney region, absence of hematuria, decreased pain in joints

Teach patient/family:

• To avoid alcohol, OTC preparations that contain alcohol

• To report any pain, redness, hard areas, usually in legs; rash, sore throat, fever, bleeding, bruising, weakness, numbness, tingling, nausea, vomiting, abdominal pain
• About the importance of complying with medical regimen (diet, weight loss, product therapy); about the possibility of bone marrow depression occurring
• Advise all providers of product use; surgery may increase possibility of acute gout symptoms

TREATMENT OF OVERDOSE:
D/C medication; may need opioids to treat diarrhea

colesevelam (Rx)
(koe-leh-seve′eh-lam)
WelChol
Func. class.: Antilipemic
Chem. class.: Bile acid sequestrant

ACTION: Adsorbs, combines with bile acids to form insoluble complex excreted through feces; loss of bile acids lowers cholesterol levels

USES: Elevated LDL cholesterol, alone or in combination with HMG-COA reductase inhibitor; type 2 diabetes (adjunct)

CONTRAINDICATIONS: Hypersensitivity, bowel disease, primary biliary cirrhosis, triglycerides >500 mg/dl, bowel obstruction, pancreatitis, biliary obstruction, dysphagia, fat-soluble vitamin deficiency
Precautions: Pregnancy (B), breastfeeding, children

DOSAGE AND ROUTES
Monotherapy
• **Adult: PO** three 625-mg tabs bid with meals or 6 tabs daily with meal; may increase to 7 tabs if needed
Combination therapy
• **Adult: PO** 3 tabs bid with meals or 6 tabs daily with meal given with an HMG-CoA reductase inhibitor
Type 2 diabetes, adjunct (to improve glycemic control)
• **Adult and geriatric: PO** Approx 3.8 g (6 tabs)/day or approx 1.9 g (3 tabs) bid
Heterozygous familial hypercholesterolemia
• **Females (postmenarchal and >10 yr) and males ≥10 yr: PO** 1.875-g packet bid or 3.75-g packet daily dissolved in 4-8 oz of water with meal
Available forms: Tabs 625 mg; powder for oral susp 3.75 g/packet
Administer:
• Swallow tabs whole; do not break, crush, or chew
• Give product daily or bid with meals; give all other medications 4 hr before colesevelam; with liquid to avoid poor absorption
• **Powder for oral susp:** empty contents of packet into a cup/glass, add ½-1 cup (4-8 oz) of water, fruit juice, diet soda; stir well before drinking

SIDE EFFECTS
GI: *Constipation, abdominal pain, nausea,* fecal impaction, hemorrhoids, flatulence, vomiting, GI obstruction
MISC: Hypertriglycerides, hypoglycemia
MS: Muscle, joint pain

PHARMACOKINETICS
Excreted in feces, peak response 2 wk

INTERACTIONS
Decrease: absorption of diltiazem, gemfibrozil, mycophenolate, phenytoin, propranolol, warfarin, thiazides, digoxin, penicillin G, tetracyclines, corticosteroids, iron, thyroid, fat-soluble vitamins, glyBURIDE, fluoroquinolones
Decrease: action of—oral contraceptives
Drug/Lab Test
Increase: LFTs

NURSING CONSIDERATIONS
Assess:
• Cardiac glycoside level, if both products administered
• Fasting LDL, HDL, total cholesterol, triglyceride levels, electrolytes if on extended therapy

• Bowel pattern daily; increase bulk, water in diet for constipation

Evaluate:

• Therapeutic response: decreased total cholesterol level, LDL cholesterol, apolipoproteins

Teach patient/family:

• About the importance of compliance; toxicity may result if doses missed; timing of dose 4 hr after other meds

• That risk factors should be decreased: high-fat diet, smoking, alcohol consumption, absence of exercise

conivaptan (Rx)

(kon-ih-vap′tan)

Vaprisol

Func. class.: Vasopressin receptor antagonist

ACTION:

Dual arginine vasopressin (AVP) antagonist with affinity for V_{1A}, V_2 receptors; level of AVP in circulating blood is critical for regulation of water, electrolyte balance and is usually elevated in euvolemic/hypervolemic hyponatremia

USES:

Euvolemia hyponatremia in hospitalized patients; not indicated for CHF, hypervolemic hyponatremia

CONTRAINDICATIONS:

Hypersensitivity, hypovolemia

Precautions: Pregnancy (C), breastfeeding, orthostatic disease, renal disease, heart failure, rapid correction of serum sodium

DOSAGE AND ROUTES

• **Adult: IV INFUSION** loading dose 20 mg given over 30 min then **CONT IV** over 24 hr; after 1 day, give for an additional 1-3 days as a **CONT INFUSION** of 20 mg/day total; can be titrated up to 40 mg/day if serum sodium is not rising at desired rate; max time 4 days

Hepatic/renal dose

• **Adult: IV Child-Pugh A-C or CCr 30-60 ml/min:** give IV loading dose over 10 min then **CONT IV INFUSION** 10 mg over 24 hr × 2-4 days

Available forms: Injection (premixed) 0.2 mg/ml in 100 ml D_5W

Administer:

IV route

• Withdraw 4 ml (20 mg), add to 100 ml D_5W, gently invert several times to mix, give over 30 min; in large vein, change site every 24 hr to minimize vascular irritation

Continuous IV INFUSION route

• Withdraw 4 ml (20 mg), add to 250 ml D_5W, gently invert several times to mix, give over 24 hr; or give 40 mg in 250 ml D_5W, gently invert several times to mix, give over 24 hr

SIDE EFFECTS

CNS: Headache, confusion, insomnia

CV: Atrial fibrillation, hypo/hypertension, *orthostatic hypotension,* phlebitis

GI: Nausea, vomiting, constipation, dry mouth

GU: Hematuria, polyuria, UTI, pollakiuria

HEMA: Anemia

INTEG: Erythemia, inj site reaction

META: Dehydration, hypo/hyperglycemia, hypokalemia, hypomagnesia, hyponatremia

MISC: Oral candidiasis, pain, peripheral edema, pneumonia

PHARMACOKINETICS

Protein binding 99%, metabolized by CYP3A4, terminal half-life 5 hr

INTERACTIONS

Increase: effect of—CYP3A4 substrates (alfuzosin, ARIPiprazole, bexarolene, bortezomib, bosentan, bupivacaine, buprenorphine, carBAMazepine, cevimeline, cilostazol, cinacalcet, clopidogrel, colchicine, cyclobenzaprine, dapsone, darifenacin, disopyramide, DOCEtaxel, donepezil, DOXOrubicin, dutasteride, eletriptan, eplerenone, ergots, erlotinib, eszopiclone, ethinyl estradiol, ethosuximide, etoposide, fentaNYL, galantamine, gefitinib, ifosfamide, irinotecan, lidocaine, loperimide, loratadine, mefloquine, methadone, modafinil, PACLitaxel, paricalcitrol, pimozide, praziquantel, quiNIDine, quiNINE, ramelteon, repaglinide, rifabutin, sibutramine, sildenafil, sirolimus, SUFentanil, SUNItinib, tacrolimus, tamoxifen, teniposide, testosterone, tiaGABine, tinidazole, trimetrexate, vardenafil, vinca alkaloids, ziprasidone, zolpidem, zonisamide); do not use concurrently

NURSING CONSIDERATIONS

Assess:

- Renal, hepatic function
- Frequent sodium volume status; overly rapid correction of sodium concentration (>12 mEq/L per 24 hr) may result in osmotic demyelination syndrome
- Neurologic status: confusion, headache
- CV status: atrial fibrillation, hypo/hypertension, orthostatic hypotension; monitor B/P, pulse
- Monitor other electrolytes (magnesium and potassium)

Evaluate:

- Therapeutic response: correction of serum sodium levels

Teach patient/family:

- To report neurologic changes: headache, insomnia, confusion
- About administration procedure and expected results
- To report inj site pain, redness, swelling

C

CONTRACEPTIVES, HORMONAL

Monophasic, Oral

ethinyl estradiol/ desogestrel (Rx)

Apri, Cesia, Desogen, Kariva, Mircette, Ortho-Cept, Reclipsen, Solia, Velivet

ethinyl estradiol/ drospirenone (Rx)

Yasmin, Yaz 28, Ocella

ethinyl estradiol/ ethynodiol (Rx)

Kelnor 1/35, Zovia 1/35, Zovia 1/50

ethinyl estradiol/ levonorgestrel (Rx)

Alesse, Aviane-28, Enpresse, Jolessa, Lessina, Levlen, Levlite, Levora, Lutera, Nordette, Portia, Quasense, Seasonique, Sronyx

ethinyl estradiol/ norethindrone (Rx)

Brevicon, Genora 1/35, Junel 21 1/20, Junel 21 1.5/20, Loestrin 21 1.5/30, Loestrin 21 1/20, Microgestin, Modicon, N.E.E 1/35, Necon 0.5/35, Norcept-E 1/35, Norinyl 1+35, Nortrel 1/35, Nortrel 7/7/7

ethinyl estradiol/ norgestimate (Rx)

MonoNessa, Ortho-Cyclen, Previfem, Sprintec, Tri-Sprintec

ethinyl estradiol/ norgestrel (Rx)

Cryselle, Lo/Ovral, Low-Ogestrel, Ogestrel, Ovral

mestranol/ norethindrone (Rx)
Norinyl 1+50

Biphasic, Oral

ethinyl estradiol/ norethindrone (Rx)
Ortho-Novum 10/11

Triphasic, Oral

ethinyl estradiol/ desogestrel (Rx)
Cyclessa

ethinyl estradiol/ norethindrone (Rx)
Nortrel 7/7/7, Ortho-Novum 7/7/7, Tri-Norinyl

ethinyl estradiol/ norgestimate (Rx)
Ortho Tri-Cyclen, Ortho Tri-Cyclen Lo

ethinyl estradiol/ levonorgestrel (Rx)
Enpresse, Tri-Levlen, Triphasil

Extended Cycle, Oral

ethinyl estradiol/ levonorgestrel (Rx)
Seasonale

Progestin, Oral

norethindrone (Rx)
Errin, Ortho Micronor, Camila, Jolivette, Nor-Q D

Progressive Estrogen, Oral

ethinyl estradiol/ norethindrone acetate (Rx)
Estrostep, Estrostep Fe

Emergency

levonorgestrel/ethinyl estradiol (Rx)
Preven

levonorgestrel (Rx)
Plan B

medroxyPROGESTERone (Rx)
Depo-Provera

Intrauterine

levonorgestrel (Rx)
Mirena

Implant

etonogestrel (Rx)
Implanon

Vaginal Ring

ethinyl estradiol/ etonogestrel (Rx)
NuvaRing

Transdermal

ethinyl estradiol/ norelgestromin (Rx)
Ortho Evra

ACTION: Prevents ovulation by suppressing FSH and LH; *monophasic:* estrogen/progestin (fixed dose) used during a 21-day cycle; ovulation is inhibited by suppression of FSH and LH; thickness of cervical mucus and endometrial lining prevents pregnancy; *biphasic:* ovulation is inhibited by suppression of FSH and LH; alteration of cervical mucus, endometrial lining prevents pregnancy; *triphasic:* ovulation is inhibited by suppression of FSH and LH; change of cervical mucus, endometrial lining prevents pregnancy; variable doses of estrogen/progestin combinations may be similar to natural hormonal fluctuations; *extended cycle:* estrogen/progestin continuous for 84 days, off for 7 days, results in 4 menstrual periods/yr; *progressive estrogen:* constant progestin with 3 progressive doses of estrogen; *progestin-only pill, implant, intrauterine:* change of cervical mucus and endometrial lining prevents pregnancy; ovulation may be suppressed

USES: To prevent pregnancy, regulation of menstrual cycle, treatment of acne in women >14 yr for whom other treatment has failed, emergency contraception; *injection:* inhibits gonadotropin secretion, ovulation, follicular maturation; *emergency:* inhibits ovulation and fertilization, decreases transport of sperm and egg from fallopian tube to uterus; *vaginal ring, transdermal:* inhibits ovulation, prevents sperm entry into uterus; *antiacne:* may decrease sex hormone binding globulin, results in decreased testosterone

CONTRAINDICATIONS: Pregnancy (X), breastfeeding, women ≥40 yr, reproductive cancer, thrombophlebitis, MI, hepatic tumors, hepatic disease, CAD, CVA, breast cancer, jaundice, stroke, vaginal bleeding

Precautions: Depression, hypertension, renal disease, seizure disorders, lupus erythematosus, rheumatic disease, migraine headache, amenorrhea, irregular menses, gallbladder disease, diabetes mellitus, heavy smoking, acute mononucleosis, sickle cell disease

Black Box Warning: Tobacco smoking

DOSAGE AND ROUTES

Monophasic

- **Adult: PO** Take first tab on Sunday after start of menses × 21 days; skip 7 days, then repeat cycle; start on 1st day of menses × 21 days; skip 7 days, then repeat cycle; may contain 7 placebo tabs when 1 tab is taken daily

Biphasic

- **Adult: PO** Take 10 days of small progestin, then large progestin; estrogen is the same during cycle; skip 7 days, then repeat cycle; may contain 7 placebo tabs when 1 tab is taken daily

Triphasic

- **Adult: PO** Estrogen dose remains constant; progestin changes throughout 21-day cycle; some products contain 28 tabs per month

Extended cycle

- **Adult: PO** Start taking on 1st day of menses; continue for 84 days of active tab, then 7 days of placebo; repeat cycle

Progestin

- **Adult: PO** Start on 1st day of menses, then daily and continuously

Progressive estrogen

- **Adult: PO** Progestin dose remains constant; estrogen increases q7days throughout 21-day cycle; may include 7 placebo tabs for 28-day cycle

Emergency

- **Adult/adolescent:** Give within 72 hr of intercourse, repeat 12 hr later; **Plan B** 1 tab, then 1 tab 12 hr later; **Preven** 2 tab, then 2 tab 12 hr later; **Ovral (unlabeled)** 2 white tabs; **Lo/Ovral (unlabeled)** 4 white tabs; **Levlen (unlabeled), Nordette (unlabeled)** 4 orange tabs; **Triphasil (unlabeled), Tri-Levlen (unlabeled)** 4 yellow tabs

Injectable

- **Adult: IM (Depo-Provera)** 150 mg within 5 days of start of menses or within 5 days postpartum (must not be breastfeeding); if breastfeeding, give 6 wk postpartum, repeat q3mo

Intrauterine

- **Adult:** To be inserted using the levonorgestrel-releasing intrauterine system (LRIS) by those trained in procedure; inserted into uterine cavity within 7 days of the onset of menstruation; use should not exceed 5 yr per implant

Vaginal ring

- **Adult: VAG** Insert 1 ring on or before day 5 of cycle; leave in place 3 wk; remove for 1 wk, then repeat

Transdermal

• **Adult: TD** Apply patch within 7 days of menses; change weekly × 3 wk; no patch wk 4; repeat cycle

Implant

• **Adult: SUBDERMAL** In inner side of upper arm on days 1-5 of menses, replace q3yr

Acne

• **Adult: PO (Ortho Tri-Cyclen)** Take daily × 21 days, off 7 days

Administer:

• PO with food for GI symptoms; give at same time each day

• Subdermal implant of 6 caps effective for 5 yr, then should be removed

• IM inj deep in large muscle mass after shaking suspension; ensure patient not pregnant if inj are 2 wk or more apart

SIDE EFFECTS

CNS: Depression, fatigue, dizziness, nervousness, anxiety, headache

CV: Increased B/P, cerebral hemorrhage, thrombosis, pulmonary embolism, fluid retention, edema, MI

EENT: Optic neuritis, retinal thrombosis, cataracts

ENDO: Decreased glucose tolerance, increased TBG, PBI, T_4, T_3, temporary infertility

GI: *Nausea,* vomiting, cramps, diarrhea, bloating, constipation, change in appetite, cholestatic jaundice, weight change

GU: Breakthrough bleeding, amenorrhea, spotting, dysmenorrhea, galactorrhea, endocervical hyperplasia, vaginitis, cystitis-like syndrome, breast changes

HEMA: Increased fibrinogen, clotting factor

INTEG: *Chloasma, melasma,* acne, rash, urticaria, erythema, pruritus, hirsutism, alopecia, photosensitivity

PHARMACOKINETICS

Excreted in breast milk

INTERACTIONS

Decrease: oral contraceptives effectiveness—anticonvulsants, rifampin, analgesics, antibiotics, antihistamines, griseofulvin

Decrease: oral anticoagulants action

Drug/Herb

• Altered action: black cohosh

Decrease: oral contraceptives effect—saw palmetto, St. John's wort

Drug/Food

Increase: peak level—grapefruit juice

Drug/Lab Test

Increase: PT; clotting factors VII, VIII, IX, X; TBG, PBI, T_4, platelet aggregability, BSP, triglycerides, bilirubin, AST, ALT

Decrease: T_3, antithrombin III, folate, metyrapone test, GTT, 17-OHCS

NURSING CONSIDERATIONS

Assess:

• Glucose, thyroid function, LFTs, BP

• Reproductive changes: changes in breasts, tumors; positive Pap smear; product should be discontinued

Evaluate:

• Therapeutic response: absence of pregnancy, endometriosis, hypermenorrhea

Teach patient/family:

• About detection of clots using Homan's sign

• To use sunscreen or avoid sunlight; photosensitivity can occur

• To take at same time each day to ensure equal product level

• To report GI symptoms that occur after 4 mo

• To use another birth control method during 1st week of oral contraceptive use

• To take another tablet as soon as possible if one is missed

• That, after product is discontinued, pregnancy may not occur for several months

• To report abdominal pain, change in vision, shortness of breath, change in menstrual flow, spotting, breakthrough bleeding, breast lumps, swelling, headache, severe leg pain

• That continuing medical care is needed: Pap smear and gynecologic examinations q6mo

• To notify health care providers and dentists of oral contraceptive use

Black Box Warning: Do not smoke; increased risk of CV side effects

⚠ HIGH ALERT

crizotinib

(kriz-oh′ti-nib)

XALKORI

Func. class.: Antineoplastic; biologic response modifiers

Chem. class.: Signal transduction inhibitors (STIs)

ACTION: Inhibits receptor tyrosine kinases (anaplastic lymphoma kinase (ALK), Hepatocyte Growth Factor Receptor (HGFR, c-Met), Recepteur d'Origine Nantais (RON)

USES: Locally advanced or metastatic non–small-cell lung cancer (NSCLC) that is anaplastic lymphoma kinase (ALK)-positive as detected by an FDA-approved test

CONTRAINDICATIONS: Pregnancy (D), breastfeeding, hypersensitivity

Precautions: Neonates, infants, children, adolescents, pneumonitis, severe hepatic disease, congenital long QT syndrome, severe renal impairment, end-stage renal disease, vision disorders

DOSAGE AND ROUTES

• **Adult: PO** 250 mg bid, continue as long as beneficial

Dose adjustments for hematologic toxicities

• **For Grade 1-2:** no dosage adjustment needed; **Grade 3:** interrupt treatment until toxicity resolves to grade ≤2, then continue with the same dosage schedule; in case of recurrence after a grade 4 event with dose reduction, interrupt treatment until toxicity resolves to grade ≤2; when resuming treatment, reduce dosage to 250 mg PO daily; **Grade 4:** interrupt treatment until toxicity resolves to grade ≤2; when resuming treatment, reduce dosage to 200 mg PO bid; in case of grade 4 recurrence, permanently discontinue treatment

Dose adjustments for hepatic laboratory abnormalities

• **For Grade 1:** No dosage adjustment necessary; **Grade 2 ALT/AST elevations with grade ≤1 total bilirubin elevations:** no dosage adjustment necessary; **Grade 3-4 ALT/AST elevations with grade ≤1 total bilirubin elevations:** interrupt treatment until toxicity resolves to grade ≤1 or baseline; when resuming treatment, reduce dosage to 200 mg PO bid; in case of recurrence, interrupt treatment until toxicity resolves to grade ≤1, and when resuming treatment, reduce dosage to 250 mg PO daily; permanently discontinue treatment in case of further recurrence; **Grade 2-4 ALT/AST elevations with concurrent Grade 2-4 total bilirubin elevations (in the absence of cholestasis or hemolysis):** permanently discontinue treatment

Dose adjustments for pneumonitis not attributable to NSCLC progression, other pulmonary disease, infection, or radiation effect

• **For any grade pneumonitis:** permanently discontinue

Dose adjustment for QTc prolongation:

• **For Grade 1-2 QTc prolongation:** no dosage adjustment necessary; **For Grade 3 QTc prolongation:** interrupt treatment until toxicity resolves to grade ≤1; when resuming treatment, reduce dosage to 200 mg PO bid; in case of recurrence, interrupt treatment until toxicity resolves to grade ≤1 and when resuming treatment, reduce dosage to 250 mg PO daily; permanently discontinue in case of further recurrence; **For Grade 4 QTc prolongation:** permanently discontinue

Available forms: Cap 200, 250 mg

Administer:

• May be taken orally with or without food

• Have the patient swallow capsule whole; do not crush or chew

• If a dose is missed, it can be taken up to 6 hr before the next dose is due to

maintain the twice daily regimen; do not take both doses at the same time
- Store at room temperature

SIDE EFFECTS

CNS: Dizziness, balance disorder, presyncope, neuropathy (motor and sensory), burning sensation, dysesthesia, hyperesthesia, hypoesthesia, neuralgia, paresthesias, peripheral neuropathy (motor and sensory), headache, insomnia
CV: QT prolongation, disseminated intravascular coagulation (DIC), septic shock, bradycardia
EENT: *Diplopia, photopsia,* photophobia, *blurred vision,* visual field defect, *vitreous floaters,* visual brightness, reduced *visual acuity;* esophageal disorders
GI: *Nausea, diarrhea, vomiting, constipation,* decreased appetite, dysgeusia, abdominal pain, abdominal discomfort/pain, stomatitis, oral ulceration, glossodynia, glossitis, cheilitis, mucosal inflammation, oropharyngeal pain/discomfort, oral pain, esophageal disorder, elevated hepatic enzymes and hyperbilirubinemia, hepatotoxicity, dyspepsia, dysphagia, epigastric discomfort/pain, burning, esophagitis, esophageal obstruction/pain/spasm, esophageal ulceration, gastroesophageal reflux, odynophagia, and reflux esophagitis
HEMA: Grade 3/4 neutropenia, thrombocytopenia, lymphopenia
MISC: Fatigue, fever, *edema,* localized/peripheral edema, chest pain (unspecified), chest discomfort, musculoskeletal chest pain, arthralgia, back pain, *rash*
RESP: Severe, life-threatening pneumonitis, pneumonia, hypoxia, acute respiratory distress syndrome (ARDS), dyspnea, empyema, pulmonary hemorrhage, pulmonary embolism, upper respiratory tract infection (nasopharyngitis, pharyngitis, rhinitis), cough

PHARMACOKINETICS

Protein binding 91%; distribution into the tissues and plasma; metabolized by the CYP3A4/5; primary metabolic pathways are oxidation to metabolites; terminal half-life 42 hr; excreted 63% feces, 22% urine; unchanged drug 53% feces, 2.3% urine; absolute bioavailability is 43%; peak is 4-6 hr; steady state is reached within 15 days; dosage adjustments may need to be made in hepatic/renal disease and Asian patients

INTERACTIONS

Increase: CYP2B6 substrates (prasugrel, selegiline, cyclophosphamide)
Increase: CYP3A4 inhibitors (ketoconazole, atazanavir, indinavir, itraconazole, nefazodone, nelfinavir, ritonavir, voriconazole, boceprevir, delavirdine, isoniazid, dalfopristin-quinupristin, tipranavir)
Decrease: CYP3A4 inducers (rifampin, carBAMazepine, PHENobarbital, phenytoin, rifabutin); antacids, H2-blockers, proton pump inhibitors (PPIs)
Increase: action of—midazolam
Avoid use with CYP3A4 substrates(alfentanil, cycloSPORINE, ergotamine, dihydroergotamine fentaNYL, sirolimus, colchicine)
Increase: QT prolongation, torsades de pointes—arsenic trioxide, certain phenothiazines (chlorproMAZINE, mesoridazine, thioridazine), grepafloxacin, pentamidine, probucol, sparfloxacin, troleandomycin, class IA antiarrhythmics (disopyramide, procainamide, quiNIDine), class III antiarrhythmics (amiodarone, dofetilide, ibutilide, sotalol), clarithromycin, ziprasidone, pimozide, haloperidol, halofantrine, quiNIDine, chloroquine, dronedarone, droperidol, erythromycin, methadone, posaconazole, propafenone, saquinavir, abarelix, amoxapine, apomorphine, asenapine, β-agonists, ofloxacin, eribulin, ezogabine, flecainide, gatifloxacin, gemifloxacin, halogenated anesthetics, iloperidone, levofloxacin, local anesthetics, magnesium sulfate, potassium sulfate, sodium, maprotiline, moxifloxacin, nilotinib, norfloxacin, ciprofloxacin, OLANZapine, paliperidone, some phenothiazines (fluPHENAZine, perphenazine, prochlorperazine, trifluoperazine), telavancin, tetrabenazine, tricyclic antidepressants, venlafaxine, vorinostat, citalopram, alfuzosin, cloZAPine,

cyclobenzaprine, dolasetron, palonosetron, QUEtiapine, rilpivirine, SUNItinib, tacrolimus, tacrolimus, vardenafil, indacaterol, dasatinib, fluconazole, lapatinib, lopinavir/ritonavir, mefloquine, octreotide, ondansetron, ranolazine, risperiDONE, telithromycin, vemurafenib

Drug/Herb

Do not use with St. John's wort

Drug/Food

Do not use with grapefruit juice

NURSING CONSIDERATIONS

Assess:

- **Severe, life-threatening, or fatal treatment-related** pneumonitis: all cases occurred within 2 mo of treatment initiation; monitor for pulmonary symptoms that may indicate pneumonitis, other causes of pneumonitis should be excluded; permanently discontinue in patients with treatment-related pneumonitis I
- **Hepatic disease:** liver function test (LFT) abnormalities, altered bilirubin levels may occur during treatment; monitor LFTs and bilirubin levels before treatment, then monthly; more frequent testing is needed in those presenting with grade 2 or greater toxicities; laboratory alterations should be managed with dose reduction, treatment interruption, or discontinuation
- **QT prolongation** has been reported with use of product; therefore, avoid crizotinib use in those patients; monitor ECG and electrolytes in patients with congestive heart failure, bradycardia, electrolyte imbalance (hypokalemia, hypomagnesemia), or in patients taking concomitant medications known to prolong the QT interval; treatment interruption, dosage adjustment, treatment discontinuation may be needed in patients who develop QT prolongation
- **Vision disorders,** generally start within 2 wk of the start of therapy; ophthalmological evaluation should be considered, particularly if patients experience photopsia or new or increased vitreous floaters; caution should be used when driving or operating machinery by patients who experience vision disorders
- **Pregnancy/breastfeeding:** identify if pregnancy is planned or suspected (pregnancy category D), do not breastfeed
- CBC with differential; BUN/creatinine

Evaluate:

- Decreasing spread of malignancy

Teach patient/family:

- That missed doses can be taken up to 6 hr before the next dose is due to maintain the twice daily regimen
- To use reliable contraception; both women and men of childbearing age should use adequate contraceptive methods during therapy and for at least 90 days after completing treatment, pregnancy category D
- To report immediately shortness of breath, cough, fatigue, visual changes
- Not to take with grapefruit juice
- To avoid activities requiring mental alertness until effects are known
- To report signs of QT prolongation (abnormal heartbeats, dizziness, syncope)
- To swallow caps whole and avoid contact with broken cap

crofelemer

(kroe-fel′e-mer)

Fulyzaq

Func. class.: Antidiarrheal

Chem. class.: Red sap of Croton lechleri plant

ACTION: Blocks chloride channel and high volume water loss in diarrhea

USES: Non-infectious diarrhea in those with HIV/AIDS using antiretrovirals

CONTRAINDICATIONS: Hypersensitivity

Precautions: Pregnancy (C), breastfeeding, black patients, children/adolescents, GI disease, infection, malabsorption syndrome, pancreatitis

DOSAGE AND ROUTES

- **Adult: PO** 125 mg bid

Available forms: Delayed rel tabs 125 mg

Administer:

- Do not break, crush, or chew
- Without regard to meals

SIDE EFFECTS

CNS: Dizziness, depression

GI: Nausea, constipation, abdominal pain, anorexia, flatulence

INTEG: Acne vulgaris, contact dermatitis

MISC: Arthralgia, cough, increased urinary frequency

INTERACTIONS

Increase: serious constipation, bowel obstruction—alosetron (IBS)

Increase: constipation—may occur with antimuscarinics, opiate agonists

NURSING CONSIDERATIONS

Assess:

- Stools: volume, color, characteristic, frequency; bowel pattern before protein rebound constipation
- Electrolytes (K, Na, Cl), hydration status
- Monitor effect in black patients; may be less effective

Evaluate: Therapeutic response: decreased diarrhea

Teach patient/family:

- To avoid OTC products unless directed by prescriber
- If drowsiness occurs, not to operate machinery

RARELY USED

crotamiton

(kroe-tam′-ih-tuhn)

Eurax

Func. class.: Scabicide/pediculicide

CONTRAINDICATIONS: Hypersensitivity; raw, inflamed skin

DOSAGE AND ROUTES

- **Adult: TOP** After routine bath, apply over the entire body from the chin to the soles; do not apply to the face or head; repeat in 24 hr; patient may take a cleansing bath 48 hr after the second dose

Treatment of pruritus

- **Adult: TOP** Apply topically by massaging gently into affected area until medication is completely absorbed; repeat if needed

Available forms: Lotion, cream 10%

cyanocobalamin (vit B_{12}) (OTC, Rx)

(sye-an-oh-koe-bal′a-min)

Nascobal, Rubramin PC

hydroxocobalamin (OTC, Rx)

CytoKit ✦

Func. class.: Vit B_{12}, water-soluble vitamin

ACTION: Needed for adequate nerve functioning, protein and carbohydrate metabolism, normal growth, RBC development, cell reproduction

USES: Vit B_{12} deficiency, pernicious anemia, vit B_{12} malabsorption syndrome, Schilling test, increased requirements with pregnancy, thyrotoxicosis, hemolytic anemia, hemorrhage, renal/hepatic disease, nutritional supplementation

CONTRAINDICATIONS: Hypersensitivity to this product, cobalt, benzyl alcohol, optic nerve atrophy

Precautions: Pregnancy (A), breastfeeding, children, renal/hepatic disease, folic acid/iron deficiency anemia, infection

DOSAGE AND ROUTES

Cyanocobalamin

- **Adult: PO** Up to 1000 mcg/day **SUBCUT/IM** 30-100 mcg/day × 1 wk, then 100-200 mcg/mo

Schilling test
- **Adult and child: IM** 1000 mcg in 1 dose
- **Child: PO** Up to 1000 mcg/day **SUBCUT/IM** 30-50 mcg/day × 2 wk, then 100 mcg/mo; **NASAL** 500 mcg weekly

Hydroxocobalamin
- **Adult: SUBCUT/IM** 30-50 mcg/day × 5-10 days, then 100-200 mcg/mo
- **Child: SUBCUT/IM** 30-50 mcg/day × 5-10 days, then 30-50 mcg/mo

Available forms: *Cyanocobalamin:* tabs 50, 100, 250, 500, 1000, 5000 mcg; ext rel tabs 1000 mcg; lozenges 100, 250, 500 mcg; nasal 500 mcg/spray; inj 100, 1000 mcg/ml; *hydroxocobalamin:* inj 1000 mcg/ml, powder for inj 5 g/vial

Administer:

PO route
- With fruit juice to disguise taste; immediately after mixing
- With meals if possible for better absorption; large doses should not be used because most is excreted
- Protect from light, heat

IM route
- By IM inj for pernicious anemia for life unless contraindicated

Intranasal route
- Avoid use within 1 hr of hot fluids, food, no primary needed

IV route
- IV route not recommended but may be admixed in TPN solution

Additive compatibilities: Ascorbic acid, chloramphenicol, hydrocortisone, vit B/C

Solution compatibilities: Dextrose/Ringer's or LR combinations, dextrose/saline combinations, D_5W, $D_{10}W$, 0.45% NaCl, Ringer's or LR sol

Y-site compatibilities: Alfentanil, amikacin, aminophylline, ascorbic acid, atracurium, atropine, azaTHIOprine, aztreonam, benztropine, bretylium, bumetanide, buprenorphine, butorphanol, calcium chloride/gluconate, ceFAZolin, cefmetazole, cefonicid, cefotaxime, cefoTEtan, cefOXitin, cefTAZidime, ceftizoxime, cefTRIAXone, cefuroxime, chloramphenicol, chlorproMAZINE, cimetidine, clindamycin, dexamethasone, digoxin, diphenhydrAMINE, DOBUTamine, DOPamine, doxycycline, enalaprilat, ePHEDrine, EPINEPHrine, epoetin alfa, erythromycin, esmolol, famotidine, fentaNYL, fluconazole, folic acid, furosemide, ganciclovir, gentamicin, glycopyrrolate, heparin, hydrocortisone, hydrOXYzine, imipenem-cilastatin, indomethacin, insulin (regular), isoproterenol hydrochloride, ketorolac, labetalol, lidocaine, magnesium, mannitol, meperidine, methoxamine, methyldopate, methylPREDNISolone, metoclopramide, metoprolol, miconazole, midazolam, minocycline, morphine, moxalactam, multiple vitamins injection, nafcillin, nalbuphine, naloxone, netilmicin, nitroglycerin, nitroprusside, norepinephrine, ondansetron, oxacillin, oxytocin, papaverine, penicillin G potassium/sodium, pentamidine, pentazocine, PENTobarbital, PHENobarbital, phentolamine, phenylephrine, phytonadione, piperacillin, polymyxin B, potassium chloride, procainamide, prochlorperazine, promethazine, propranolol, protamine, pyridoxine, quiNIDine, ranitidine, ritodrine, sodium bicarbonate, succinylcholine, SUFentanil, theophylline, thiamine, ticarcillin, ticarcillin-clavulanate, tobramycin, tolazoline, trimetaphan, urokinase, vancomycin, vasopressin, verapamil, vitamin B complex with C

SIDE EFFECTS

CNS: Flushing, optic nerve atrophy
CV: **CHF**, peripheral vascular thrombosis, **pulmonary edema**
GI: *Diarrhea*
INTEG: Itching, rash, pain at inj site
META: Hypokalemia
SYST: **Anaphylactic shock**

PHARMACOKINETICS

Gastric intrinsic factor must be present for absorption to occur; stored in liver, kidneys, stomach; 50%-90% excreted in urine; crosses placenta; excreted in breast milk

INTERACTIONS

Increase: absorption—predniSONE
Decrease: absorption—aminoglycosides, anticonvulsants, colchicine, chloramphenicol, aminosalicylic acid, potassium preparations, cimetidine

Drug/Herb
Decrease: vit B_{12} absorption—goldenseal
Drug/Lab Test
False positive: intrinsic factor

NURSING CONSIDERATIONS

Assess:

- For vit B_{12} deficiency: red, beefy tongue; psychosis; pallor; neuropathy
- GI function: diarrhea, constipation
- Potassium levels during beginning treatment in megaloblastic anemia; q6mo in pernicious anemia; folic acid, plasma vit B_{12} (after 1 wk), reticulocyte counts
- Nutritional status: egg yolks, fish, organ meats, dairy products, clams, oysters: good sources of vit B_{12}
- For pulmonary edema, worsening of CHF in cardiac patients

Evaluate:

- Therapeutic response: decreased anorexia, dyspnea on exertion, palpitations, paresthesias, psychosis, visual disturbances

Teach patient/family:

- That treatment must continue for life for pernicious anemia
- To eat a well-balanced diet
- To avoid contact with persons with infection; that infections are common

TREATMENT OF OVERDOSE:

Discontinue product

cyclobenzaprine (Rx)

(sye-kloe-ben′za-preen)

Amrix, Fexmid, Flexeril

Func. class.: Skeletal muscle relaxant, central acting

Chem. class.: Tricyclic amine salt

Do not confuse:
cyclobenzaprine/cyproheptadine

ACTION: Reduces tonic muscle activity at the brain stem; may be related to antidepressant effects

USES: Adjunct for relief of muscle spasm and pain in musculoskeletal conditions

Unlabeled uses: Fibromyalgia

CONTRAINDICATIONS: Children <12 yr, acute recovery phase of MI, dysrhythmias, heart block, CHF, hypersensitivity, intermittent porphyria, thyroid disease, QT prolongation

Precautions: Pregnancy (B), breastfeeding, geriatric patients, renal/hepatic disease, addictive personality

DOSAGE AND ROUTES

Muscloskeletal disorders

- **Adult/adolescent ≥15 yr: PO** 5 mg tid × 1 wk, max 30 mg/day × 3 wk
- **Adult: EXT REL** 15 mg/day, max 30 mg/day × 3 wk
- **Geriatric: PO** 5 mg tid

Hepatic dose

- **Adult (mild hepatic disease): PO** 5 mg, titrate slowly

Fibromyalgia (unlabeled)

- **Adult: PO** 10 mg at bedtime, titrated up

Available forms: Tabs 5, 7.5, 10 mg; ext rel tab 15, 30 mg

Administer:

- Without regard to meals, give with food for GI symptoms
- Do not crush, break, chew ext rel cap
- Store in tight container at room temperature

SIDE EFFECTS

CNS: *Dizziness, weakness, drowsiness,* headache, tremor, depression, insomnia, confusion, paresthesia, nervousness
CV: Postural hypotension, tachycardia, dysrhythmias
EENT: Diplopia, temporary loss of vision, blurred vision
GI: *Nausea,* vomiting, hiccups, dry mouth, constipation, hepatitis
GU: Urinary retention, frequency, change in libido
INTEG: Rash, pruritus, fever, facial flushing, sweating

PHARMACOKINETICS

PO: Onset 1 hr, peak 3-8 hr, duration 12-24 hr, half-life 1-3 days, 32 hr ext rel, metabolized by liver, excreted in urine, crosses placenta, excreted in breast milk

INTERACTIONS

• Do not use within 14 days of MAOIs, traMADol

Increase: QT interval—Class IA/III antidysrhythmics, and other products that increase QT interval

Increase: serotonin syndrome—SSRIs, SNRIs

Increase: CNS depression—alcohol, tricyclics, opiates, barbiturates, sedatives, hypnotics

Drug/Herb

Increase: CNS depression—kava

NURSING CONSIDERATIONS

Assess:

• **Serotonin syndrome:** If using with SSRIs, SNRIs, monitor closely, if syndrome occurs, discontinue both products immediately

• **Pain:** location, duration, mobility, stiffness at baseline, periodically

• **Allergic reactions:** rash, fever, respiratory distress

• Severe weakness, numbness in extremities

• Assistance with ambulation if dizziness, drowsiness occur, especially for geriatric patients

Evaluate:

• Therapeutic response: decreased pain, spasticity; muscle spasms of acute, painful musculoskeletal conditions generally short term; long-term therapy seldom warranted

Teach patient/family:

• Not to discontinue medication abruptly; that insomnia, nausea, headache, spasticity, tachycardia will occur; that product should be tapered off over 1-2 wk

• Not to take with alcohol, other CNS depressants

• To avoid hazardous activities if drowsiness, dizziness occur

• To avoid using OTC medication (cough preparations, antihistamines) unless directed by prescriber

• To use gum, frequent sips of water for dry mouth

TREATMENT OF OVERDOSE:

Administer activated charcoal; use anticonvulsants if indicated; monitor cardiac function

cyclopentolate ophthalmic

See Appendix B

⚠ **HIGH ALERT**

cyclophosphamide (Rx)

(sye-kloe-foss′fa-mide)

Cytoxan, Procytox ✦

Func. class.: Antineoplastic alkylating agent

Chem. class.: Nitrogen mustard

Do not confuse:

cyclophosphamide/cycloSPORINE

Cytoxan/Cytosar/Cytotec/cytarabine

ACTION: Alkylates DNA is responsible for cross-linking DNA strands; activity is not cell-cycle–phase specific

USES: Hodgkin's disease, lymphomas, leukemia; cancer of female reproductive tract, breast, multiple myeloma; neuroblastoma; retinoblastoma; Ewing's sarcoma; nephrotic syndrome

Unlabeled uses: Aplastic anemia, chronic idiopathic thrombocytopenic purpura, dermatomyositis, pneumonitis, polymyositis, SLE, scleroderma, RA, Behçet's syndrome, Churg-Strauss syndrome, polyarteritis nodosa, Wegener's granulomatosis, idiopathic pulmonary fibrosis, localized neuroblastoma, CLL

CONTRAINDICATIONS: Pregnancy (D), hypersensitivity, prostatic hypertrophy, bladder neck obstruction

Precautions: Radiation therapy, cardiac disease, anemia, dysrhythmias, child, dental disease/work, dialysis, geriatric patients, heart failure, hematuria, infections, leukopenia QT prolongation, secondary malignancy surgery, tumor lysis syndrome, vaccinations, breastfeeding, severely depressed bone marrow function

DOSAGE AND ROUTES

Acute lymphocytic leukemia (ALL) (induction therapy)

- **Adult/adolescent/child: IV** Total doses of IV 300-1500mg/m^2 have been incorporated into induction, intensification, consolidation regimens, possibly using vinCRIStine, predniSONE, or others; **PO** 1-5mg/kg/day depending on response

Neuroblastoma

- **Adult/Child: IV** For induction, 40-50 mg/kg in divided doses over 2-5 days or 10-15 mg/kg q7-10days, 3-5 mg/kg 2×/wk or 1-5 mg/kg daily
- **Child and infant: PO** 150 mg/m^2/day, days 1-7 with DOXOrubicin (**IV** 35 mg/m^2 on day 8) q21days × 5 cycles
- **Child: IV** 70 mg/kg/day with hydration on days 1, 2 with DOXOrubicin and vinCRIStine q21days for courses 1, 2, 4, 6 alternating with CISplatin and etoposide q21days for courses 3, 5, 7

Breast cancer

- **Adult: PO** 100-200 mg/m^2/day or 2 mg/kg/day × 4-14 days; **IV** 500-1000 mg/m^2 on day 1 in combination with fluorouracil and methotrexate or DOXOrubicin or DOXOrubicin alone, also cyclophosphamide 600 mg/m^2; may be given dose-dense on day 1 of q14days with DOXOrubicin (60 mg/m^2) with growth-factor support

Operable node-positive breast cancer IV (TAC regimen)

- **Adult: IV** 500 mg/m^2 with DOXOrubicin (50 mg/m^2 **IV**), then DOCEtaxel (75 mg/m^2) **IV** given 1 hr later q3wk × 6 cycles

Nephrotic syndrome

- **Child: PO** 2.5-3 mg/kg daily × 60-90 days

Aplastic anemia (unlabeled)

- **Adult: IV** 45-50 mg/kg divided over 4 days

Behçet's syndrome/Churg-Strauss syndrome/polyarteritis nodosa/uveitis/Wegener's granulomatosis (unlabeled)

- **Adult: PO** 1-2 mg/kg/day, **IV** 0.5-1 g/m^2

Rheumatoid arthritis (unlabeled)

- **Adult and child: PO** 1.5-2.5 mg/kg/day

CLL (unlabeled)

- **Adult: IV** 250 mg/m^2/day on days 1-3 with fludarabine 30 mg/m^2/day on days 1-3

Available forms: Inj ✱ 200, 500 mg, 1, 2 g vials; tabs 25, 50 mg

Administer:

- Use cytotoxic handling procedures
- In AM so product can be eliminated before bedtime
- Fluids IV or PO before chemotherapy to hydrate patient
- Antacid before oral agent; give after evening meal, before bedtime
- Antiemetic 30-60 min before product and prn
- Allopurinol or sodium bicarbonate to maintain uric acid levels, alkalinization of urine

PO route

- Take on empty stomach; do not crush, break, chew tabs; wash hands immediately if in contact with tab
- May be taken as a single dose or divided doses
- Take in AM or afternoon, avoid evening
- Store in tight container at room temperature

Direct IV route

- Reconstitute with NS only

Intermittent IV INFUSION route

- Use cytotoxic handling procedures
- IV after diluting 100 mg/5 ml of sterile water or bacteriostatic water; shake; let stand until clear; may be further diluted in ≤250 ml D_5 NS D_5/NS; 0.45% NaCl give 100 mg or less/min through 3-way stopcock of glucose or saline infusion
- Use 21, 23, 25G needle; check site for irritation, phlebitis

Solution compatibilities: Amino acids 4.25%/D_{25}, D_5/0.9% NaCl, D_5W, 0.9% NaCl

Syringe compatibilities: Bleomycin, CISplatin, doxapram, DOXOrubicin, droperidol, fluorouracil, furosemide, heparin, leucovorin, methotrexate, metoclopramide, mitoMYcin, vinBLAStine, vinCRIStine

Y-site compatibilities: Acyclovir, alfentanil, allopurinol, amifostine, amikacin, aminocaproic acid, aminophylline, amiodarone, amphotericin B lipid complex, amphotericin B liposome, ampicillin, ampicillin-sulbactam, anidulafungin, atenolol, atracurium, azlocillin, aztreonam, bivalirudin, bleomycin, bumetanide, buprenorphine, butorphanol, calcium chloride/gluconate, CARBOplatin, caspofungin, cefamandole, ceFAZolin, cefepime, cefoperazone, cefotaxime, cefoTEtan, cefOXitin, cefTAZidime, ceftizoxime, cefTRIAXone, cefuroxime, chloramphenicol, chlorproMAZINE, cimetidine, ciprofloxacin, cisatracurium, CISplatin, cladribine, clindamycin, codeine, cycloSPORINE, cytarabine, DACTINomycin, DAPTOmycin, DAUNOrubicin, dexamethasone, dexmedetomidine, dexrazoxane, digoxin, diltiazem, diphenhydrAMINE, DOBUTamine, DOCEtaxel, dolasetron, DOPamine, doripenem, doxacurium, DOXOrubicin, DOXOrubicin liposomal, doxycycline, droperidol, enalaprilat, ePHEDrine, EPINEPHrine, epirubicin, ertapenem, erythromycin, esmolol, etoposide, famotidine, fenoldopam, fentaNYL, filgrastim, fluconazole, fludarabine, fluorouracil, foscarnet, fosphenytoin, furosemide, gallium, ganciclovir, gatifloxacin, gemcitabine, gentamicin, granisetron, haloperidol, heparin, hydrocortisone, HYDROmorphone, hydrOXYzine, IDArubicin, imipenem-cilastatin, inamrinone, insulin (regular), irinotecan, isoproterenol, kanamycin, ketorolac, labetalol, leucovorin, levofloxacin, levorphanol, lidocaine, linezolid, LORazepam, magnesium sulfate, mannitol, melphalan, meperidine, meropenem, mesna, methohexital, methotrexate, methylPREDNISolone, metoclopramide, metoprolol, metroNIDAZOLE, midazolam, milrinone, minocycline, mitoMYcin, mitoXANtrone, mivacurium, morphine, nafcillin, nalbuphine, naloxone, nesiritide, nitroglycerin, nitroprusside, norepinephrine, octreotide, ondansetron, oxacillin, oxaliplatin, PACLitaxel, palonosetron, pamidronate, pancuronium, pantoprazole, PEMEtrexed, penicillin G potassium, pentamidine, PENTobarbital, PHENobarbital, phenylephrine, piperacillin, piperacillin-tazobactam, potassium chloride/phosphates, procainamide, prochlorperazine, promethazine, propofol, propranolol, quinupristin-dalfopristin, ranitidine, rapacuronium, remifentanil, riTUXimab, rocuronium, sargramostim, sodium acetate/bicarbonate/phosphates, succinylcholine, SUFentanil, sulfamethoxazole-trimethoprim, tacrolimus, teniposide, theophylline, thiopental, thiotepa, ticarcillin, ticarcillin-clavulanate, tigecycline, tirofiban, TNA, tobramycin, topotecan, TPN, trastuzumab, vancomycin, vasopressin, vecuronium, verapamil, vinBLAStine, vinCRIStine, vinorelbine, voriconazole, zidovudine, zoledronic acid

C

SIDE EFFECTS

CNS: Headache, dizziness

CV: **Cardiotoxicity (high doses), myocardial fibrosis, congestive heart failure, pericarditis**

ENDO: SIADH, gonadal suppression

GI: *Nausea, vomiting, diarrhea, weight loss,* colitis, **hepatotoxicity**

GU: **Hemorrhagic cystitis,** *hematuria, neoplasms, amenorrhea, azoospermia, sterility, ovarian fibrosis,* **renal tubular fibrosis**

HEMA: **Thrombocytopenia, leukopenia, pancytopenia; myelosuppression**

INTEG: *Alopecia,* dermatitis

META: Hyperuricemia

MISC: Secondary neoplasms, **anaphylaxis**

RESP: **Pulmonary fibrosis, interstitial pneumonia**

PHARMACOKINETICS

Metabolized by liver, excreted in urine, half-life 4-6½ hr, 50% bound to plasma proteins

INTERACTIONS

Increase: neuromuscular blockade—succinylcholine

Increase: cyclophosphamide toxicity—barbiturates

Increase: action of warfarin

Increase: bone marrow depression—allopurinol, thiazides
Increase: hypoglycemia—insulin
Decrease: digoxin levels—digoxin
Decrease: cyclophosphamide effect—chloramphenicol, corticosteroids
Decrease: antibody response—live virus vaccines

Drug/Herb
- Toxicity: St. John's wort

Drug/Lab Test
Increase: uric acid
False positive: Pap smear
False negative: PPD, mumps, trichophytin, *Candida, Trichophyton,* Pap smear

NURSING CONSIDERATIONS

Assess:
- **Hemorrhagic cystitis;** renal studies: BUN, serum uric acid, urine CCr before, during therapy; I&O ratio; report fall in urine output <30 ml/hr
- **Bone marrow depression:** CBC, differential, platelet count baseline, weekly; withhold product if WBC is <2500 or platelet count is <75,000; notify prescriber of results
- Pulmonary function tests, chest x-ray films before, during therapy; chest film should be obtained q2wk during treatment
- Monitor temperature q4hr; elevated temperature may indicate beginning infection
- **Hepatotoxicity:** hepatic studies before, during therapy (bilirubin, AST, ALT, LDH), as needed; jaundice of skin, sclera; dark urine, clay-colored stools; itchy skin; abdominal pain; fever; diarrhea
- **Bleeding:** hematuria, guaiac, bruising or petechiae, mucosa or orifices q8hr
- Dyspnea, crackles, unproductive cough, chest pain, tachypnea
- Effects of alopecia on body image, discuss feelings about body changes
- Buccal cavity q8hr for dryness, sores or ulceration, white patches, oral pain, bleeding, dysphagia; obtain prescription for viscous lidocaine (Xylocaine)

⚠ Symptoms that indicate severe allergic reaction: rash, pruritus, urticaria, purpuric skin lesions, itching, flushing

- Increase fluid intake to 2-3 L/day to prevent urate deposits, calculi formation, reduce incidence of hemorrhagic cystitis
- Rinsing of mouth tid-qid with water, club soda; brushing of teeth bid-tid with soft brush or cotton-tipped applicators for stomatitis; use unwaxed dental floss
- Warm compresses at inj site for inflammation

Evaluate:
- To take adequate fluids to eliminate product
- Therapeutic response: decreased tumor size, spread of malignancy

Teach patient/family:
- That amenorrhea can occur and may last up to 1 yr after therapy but is reversible after stopping treatment
- To report any changes in breathing or coughing
- That hair may be lost during treatment; a wig or hairpiece may make patient feel better; new hair may be different in color, texture
- To avoid foods with citric acid, hot, or rough texture
- To report signs of infection: increased temperature, sore throat, flulike symptoms
- To report signs of anemia: fatigue, headache, faintness, SOB, irritability
- To report bleeding (bruising, hematuria, petechiae); to avoid use of razors, commercial mouthwash
- To use reliable contraception during and for 4 mo after treatment; not to breastfeed
- To avoid use of aspirin products, ibuprofen
- To avoid vaccinations during therapy
- Advise patient on proper handling and disposal of chemotherapy drugs

C

cycloSPORINE (Rx)

(sye′kloe-spor-een)

Cyclosporine (modified), Gengraf, Neoral, Sandimmune

Func. class.: Immunosuppressant

Chem. class.: Fungus-derived peptide

Do not confuse:
cycloSPORINE/cycloSERINE/cyclophosphamide

ACTION: Produces immunosuppression by inhibiting lymphocytes (T)

USES: Organ transplants (liver, kidney, heart) (GVHD) to prevent rejection, rheumatoid arthritis, psoriasis

Unlabeled uses: Recalcitrant ulcerative colitis, aplastic anemia, Crohn's disease, thrombocytopenia purpura, lupus, nephritis, myasthenia gravis, psoriatic arthritis, atopic dermatitis

CONTRAINDICATIONS: Breastfeeding, hypersensitivity to polyxyethylated castor oil (inj only); psoriasis or RA in renal disease (Neoral/Gengraf); Gengraf/Neoral used with PUVA/UVB, methotrexate, coal tar; ocular infections

Black Box Warning: Uncontrolled, malignant hypertension; radiation in psoriasis, neoplastic disease, sunlight (UV) exposure, renal disease/failure

Precautions: Pregnancy (C), geriatric patients, severe hepatic disease

DOSAGE AND ROUTES

Prevention of transplant rejection (nonmodified)

- **Adult and child: PO** 15 mg/kg several hr before surgery, daily for 2 wk, reduce dosage by 2.5 mg/kg/wk to 5-10 mg/kg/day; **IV** 5-6 mg/kg several hr before surgery, daily, switch to PO form as soon as possible

Prevention of transplant rejection (modified)

- **Adult and child: PO** 4-12 mg/kg/day divided q12hr, depends on organ transplanted

Rheumatoid arthritis (Neoral/Gengraf)

- **Adult: PO** 2.5 mg/kg/day divided bid, may increase 0.5-0.75 mg/kg/day after 8-12 wk, max 4 mg/kg/day

Psoriasis (Neoral/Gengraf)

- **Adult: PO** 2.5 mg/kg/day divided bid, × 4 wk, then increase by 0.5 mg/kg/day q2wk, max 4 mg/kg/day

Idiopathic thrombocytopenia purpura (unlabeled)

- **Adult: PO** 1.25-2.5 mg/kg bid

Severe aplastic anemia (unlabeled)

- **Adult and child: PO** 12 mg/kg/day or 15 mg/kg/day (child) with antithymocyte globulin (ATG)

Atopic dermatitis (unlabeled)

- **Adult/adolescent/child ≥2 yr: PO** 5 mg/kg/day

Crohn's disease that is resistant to/intolerant of corticosteroids (unlabeled)

- **Adult: PO** 2.5-15 mg/kg/day (nonmodified)

Available forms: Oral sol 100 mg/ml; soft gel cap 25, 50, 100 mg; inj 50 mg/ml

Administer:

PO route

- Some brands are not interchangeable
- Do not break, crush, or chew caps
- Use pipette provided to draw up oral sol; may mix with milk or juice; wipe pipette, do not wash (Neoral)
- For several days before transplant surgery; give at same time of day
- With corticosteroids
- With meals for GI upset or in chocolate milk, milk, or orange juice (SandIMMUNE)

Rheumatoid arthritis

- Give Neoral or Gengraf 2.5 mg/kg/day divided bid; may use with salicylates, NSAIDs, PO corticosteroids
- Always give the daily dose of Neoral/Gengraf in 2 divided doses on consistent schedule

• Give initial SandIMMUNE PO dose 4-12 hr before transplantation as a single dose of 15 mg/kg, continue the single daily dose for 1-2 wk, then taper 5%/wk to a maintenance dose of 5-10 mg/kg/day

Intermittent IV INFUSION route

• After diluting each 50 mg/20-100 ml of 0.9% NaCl or D_5W; run over 2-6 hr, use an infusion pump, glass infusion bottles only

Continuous IV INFUSION route

• May run over 24 hr

• **For SandIMMUNE parenteral,** give 1/3 of PO dose, initial dose 4-12 hr before transplantation as a single IV dose 5-6 mg/kg/day, continue the single daily dose until PO can be used

Solution compatibilities: D_5W, NaCl 0.9%

Y-site compatibilities: Abciximab, alatrofloxacin, alfentanil, amikacin, aminocaproic acid, aminophylline, amphotericin B lipid complex, anidulafungin, argatroban, ascorbic acid injection, atenolol, atracurium, atropine, azaTHIOprine, aztreonam, benztropine, bivalirudin, bleomycin, bretylium, bumetanide, buprenorphine, butorphanol, calcium chloride/gluconate, CARBOplatin, carmustine, caspofungin, ceFAZolin, cefmetazole, cefonicid, cefotaxime, cefoTEtan, cefOXitin, cefTAZidime, ceftizoxime, cefTRIAXone, cefuroxime, chloramphenicol, chlorproMAZINE, cimetidine, ciprofloxacin, CISplatin, clindamycin, codeine, cyanocobalamin, cyclophosphamide, cytarabine, DACTINomycin, DAPTOmycin, DAUNOrubicin, dexamethasone, dexmedetomidine, digoxin, diltiazem, diphenhydrAMINE, DOBUTamine, DOCEtaxel, DOPamine, doripenem, doxacurium, DOXOrubicin, doxycycline, enalaprilat, ePHEDrine, EPINEPHrine, epirubicin, epoetin alfa, eptifibatide, ertapenem, erythromycin, esmolol, etoposide, famotidine, fenoldopam, fentaNYL, fluconazole, fludarabine, fluorouracil, folic acid, furosemide, gallium, ganciclovir, gatifloxacin, gemcitabine, gentamicin, glycopyrrolate, granisetron, heparin, hydrocortisone, HYDROmorphone, hydrOXYzine, ifosfamide, imipenem-cilastatin, indomethacin, irinotecan, isoproterenol, ketorolac, labetalol, lansoprazole, levofloxacin, lidocaine, linezolid, LORazepam, mannitol, mechlorethamine, meperidine, meropenem, methotrexate, methyldopate, methylPREDNISolone, metoclopramide, metoprolol, metroNIDAZOLE, micafungin, miconazole, midazolam, milrinone, minocycline, mitoXANtrone, morphine, multiple vitamins injection, nafcillin, naloxone, nesiritide, netilmicin, nitroglycerin, nitroprusside, norepinephrine, octreotide, ondansetron, oxacillin, oxaliplatin, oxytocin, PACLitaxel, palonosetron, pamidronate, pancuronium, pantoprazole, papaverine, PEMEtrexed, penicillin G potassium/sodium, pentamidine, pentazocine, phentolamine, phenylephrine, phytonadione, piperacillin, piperacillin-tazobactam, polymyxin B, potassium acetate/chloride, procainamide, prochlorperazine, promethazine, propofol, propranolol, protamine, pyridoxine, quiNIDine, quinupristin-dalfopristin, ranitidine, ritodrine, sargramostim, sodium acetate/bicarbonate, succinylcholine, SUFentanil, tacrolimus, teniposide, theophylline, thiamine, thiotepa, ticarcillin, ticarcillin-clavulanate, tigecycline, tirofiban, tobramycin, trimetaphan, urokinase, vancomycin, vasopressin, vecuronium, verapamil, vinCRIStine, vinorelbine, zoledronic acid

SIDE EFFECTS

CNS: *Tremors, headache,* seizures, confusion, encephalopathy, migraine

GI: Nausea, vomiting, diarrhea, *oral candida, gum hyperplasia,* hepatotoxicity, pancreatitis

GU: Albuminuria, hematuria, proteinuria, renal failure, hemolytic uremic syndrome, nephrotoxicity

INTEG: Rash, acne, *hirsutism,* pruritus

META: Hyperkalemia, hypomagnesemia, hyperlipidemia, hyperuricemia

MISC: *Infection, hypertension*

PHARMACOKINETICS

Peak 4 hr; highly protein bound; half-life (biphasic) 1.2 hr, 25 hr; metabolized in liver; excreted in feces, 6% in urine; crosses placenta; excreted in breast milk

INTERACTIONS

Increase: action, toxicity of cycloSPORINE—allopurinol, amiodarone, amphotericin B, androgens, azole antifungals, β-blockers, bromocriptine, calcium channel blockers, carvedilol, cimetidine, colchicine, corticosteroids, fluoroquinolones, foscarnet, imipenem-cilastatin, macrolides, metoclopramide, oral contraceptives, NSAIDs, melphalan, SSRIs

Increase: effects of aliskiren, digoxin, etoposide, HMG-CoA reductase inhibitors, methotrexate, potassium-sparing diuretics, sirolimus, tacrolimus

Increase: action toxicity of—digoxin, colchicine

Decrease: cycloSPORINE action—anticonvulsants, nafcillin, orlistat, PHENobarbital, phenytoin, rifamycins, sulfamethoxazole-trimethoprim, terbinafine, ticlopidine

Decrease: antibody reaction—live virus vaccines

Drug/Food

- Slowed metabolism of product: grapefruit juice, food

NURSING CONSIDERATIONS

Assess:

- Renal studies: BUN, creatinine at least monthly during treatment, 3 mo after treatment
- Product blood level during treatment 12 hr after dose, toxic >400 ng/ml
- Hepatic studies: alk phos, AST, ALT, bilirubin; hepatotoxicity: dark urine, jaundice, itching, light-colored stools; product should be discontinued
- Serum lipids, magnesium, potassium, cycloSPORINE blood concentrations, therapeutic range: 100-400 mg/ml

⚠ **Encephalopathy:** impaired cognition, seizures, visual changes including blindness, loss of motor function, movement disorders and psychiatric changes; dosage reduction or discontinuation may be needed in severe cases

⚠ **Nephrotoxicity:** 6 wk after surgery, acute tubular necrosis, CyA trough level >200 ng/ml, gradual rise in creatinine (0.15 mg/dl/day), creatinine plateau <25% above baseline, intracapsular pressure <40 mm Hg

⚠ Signs/symptoms of encephalopathy, lymphoma

Evaluate:

- Therapeutic response: absence of rejection

Teach patient/family:

- To report fever, chills, sore throat, fatigue, since serious infections may occur; tremors, bleeding gums, increased B/P
- To use contraceptive measures during treatment, for 12 wk after ending therapy; to notify prescriber if pregnancy is planned or suspected
- To take at same time of day, every day; not to skip doses or double dose; not to use with grapefruit juice or receive vaccines; that there are many drug interactions; not to add new products without approval of prescriber

Black Box Warning: To limit UV exposure

- That treatment is lifelong to prevent rejection; to identify signs of rejection
- To report severe diarrhea because drug loss may result
- About the signs of nephrotoxicity: increased B/P, tremors of the hands, changes in gums, increased hair on body, face
- To continue with all lab work and follow-up appointments
- That types of products are not interchangeable
- Not to wash syringe/container with water; variation in dose may result

⚠ HIGH ALERT

cytarabine (Rx)

(sye-tare′a-been)

Cytosar ✦

cytarabine liposomal (Rx)

DepoCyt

Func. class.: Antineoplastic, antimetabolite

Chem. class.: Pyrimidine nucleoside analog

Do not confuse:
Cytosar/Cytoxan/Cytovene

ACTION: Competes with physiologic substrate of DNA synthesis, thus interfering with cell replication in the S phase of the cell cycle (before mitosis)

USES: Acute myelocytic leukemia, acute nonlymphocytic leukemia, chronic myelocytic leukemia; lymphomatous meningitis (intrathecal/intraventricular)
Unlabeled uses: Hodgkin's/non-Hodgkin's lymphoma, malignant meningitis, mantle cell lymphoma

CONTRAINDICATIONS: Pregnancy (D), hypersensitivity
Precautions: Breastfeeding, children, renal/hepatic disease, tumor lysis syndrome, infection, hyperkalemia, hyperphosphatemia, hyperuricemia, hypocalcemia

Black Box Warning: Bone marrow suppression

DOSAGE AND ROUTES

Acute myelogenous leukemia (AML)
- **Adult: CONT IV INFUSION** 100 mg/m^2/day × 7 days q2wk as single agent or 2-6 mg/kg/day (100-200 mg/m^2/day) as a single dose or 2-3 divided doses for 5-10 days until remission, used in combination; maintenance 70-200 mg/m^2/day for 2-5 days monthly; **SUBCUT/IM** maintenance 100 mg/m^2/day × 5 days q28days

Meningeal leukemia
- **Adult/Child: IV** For induction, 40-50 mg/kg in divided doses over 2-5 days or 10-15 mg/kg q7-10days, 3-5 mg/kg 2×/wk or 1-5 mg/kg daily
- **Adult/child: INTRATHECAL** For induction 50 mg (liposomal) q14days × 2 doses (wk 1, 3); consolidation 50 mg (liposomal) q14days × 3 doses (wk 5, 7, 9), then another dose at wk 13; maintenance 50 mg (liposomal) q28days (wk 17, 21, 25, 29)

Refractory acute Hodgkin's/refractory non-Hodgkin's lymphoma (unlabeled)
- **Adult/child: IV** 2 g/m^2/day; on day 5 q21days, with etoposide, methylPREDNISolone, and CISplatin

Carcinomatous meningitis (liposoma)
- **Adult: IT** 50 mg over 1-5 min q14days, during induction and consolidation wk 1, 3, 5, 7, 9, give another 50 mg **IT** wk 13; maintenance 50 mg q28days on wk 17, 21, 25, 29 use with dexamethasone 4 mg **PO/IV** × 5 days on each day of cytarabine

Renal dose
- **Adult CCr ≤60 ml/min, serum creatinine 1.5-1.9 mg/dl or increase of 0.5-1.2 mg/dl from baseline during treatment:** reduce to 1 g/m^2/dose; **serum creatinine ≥2 mg/dl or change from baseline serum creatinine was 1.2 mg/dl:** reduce to 100 mg/m^2/day

Available forms: Solution for injection 20 mg/ml (DepoCyt) liposomal for intrathecal use 10 mg/ml

Administer:
- Antiemetic 30-60 min before product and prn
- Allopurinol to maintain uric acid levels and alkalinization of the urine

IT route
- Use preservative-free NS, add 5 ml/100-mg vial or 10 ml/500-mg vial; use immediately, discard unused product

IV route

- Use cytotoxic handling precautions

Direct IV route

- After diluting 100 mg/5 ml of sterile water for inj; given by direct IV over 1-3 min through free-flowing tubing (IV)

Intermittent IV INFUSION route

- May be further diluted in 50-100 ml NS or D_5W, given over 30 min to 24 hr, depending on dose

Continuous IV INFUSION route

- May also be given by continuous infusion

Solution compatibilities: Amino acids, D_5/LR, D_5/0.2% NaCl, D_5/0.9% NaCl, D_{10}/0.9% NaCl, D_5W, invert sugar 10% in electrolyte #1, Ringer's, LR, 0.9% NaCl, sodium lactate 1/6 mol/L, TPN #57

Y-site compatibilities: Acyclovir, alfentanil, amifostine, amikacin, aminocaproic acid, aminophylline, amphotericin B lipid complex, amphotericin B liposome, ampicillin, ampicillin-sulbactam, amsacrine, anidulafungin, atenolol, atracurium, azithromycin, aztreonam, bivalirudin, bleomycin, bumetanide, buprenorphine, butorphanol, calcium chloride/gluconate, CARBOplatin, ceFAZolin, cefepime, cefotaxime, cefoTEtan, cefOXitin, cefTAZidime, ceftizoxime, cefTRIAXone, cefuroxime, chlorproMAZINE, cimetidine, ciprofloxacin, cisatracurium, CISplatin, cladribine, clindamycin, codeine, cyclophosphamide, cycloSPORINE, DAUNOrubicin, dexamethasone, dexmedetomidine, dexrazoxane, digoxin, diltiazem, diphenhydrAMINE, DOBUTamine, DOCEtaxel, dolasetron, DOPamine, doxacurium, DOXOrubicin, DOXOrubicin liposomal, doxycycline, droperidol, enalaprilat, ePHEDrine, EPINEPHrine, ertapenem, erythromycin, esmolol, etoposide, famotidine, fenoldopam, fentaNYL, filgrastim, fluconazole, fludarabine, foscarnet, fosphenytoin, furosemide, gatifloxacin, gemcitabine, gemtuzumab, gentamicin, granisetron, haloperidol, heparin, hydrocortisone, HYDROmorphone, hydrOXYzine, IDArubicin, ifosfamide, imipenem-cilastatin, inamrinone, insulin (regular), irinotecan, isoproterenol, ketorolac, labetalol, leucovorin, levofloxacin, levorphanol, lidocaine, linezolid, LORazepam, magnesium sulfate, mannitol, melphalan, meperidine, meropenem, mesna, methohexital, methotrexate, methylPREDNISolone, metoclopramide, metoprolol, metroNIDAZOLE, midazolam, milrinone, minocycline, mitoXANtrone, mivacurium, morphine, nalbuphine, naloxone, nesiritide, niCARdipine, nitroglycerin, nitroprusside, norepinephrine, octreotide, ofloxacin, ondansetron, oxaliplatin, PACLitaxel, palonosetron, pamidronate, pancuronium, pantoprazole, PEMEtrexed, pentamidine, PENTobarbital, PHENobarbital, phenylephrine, piperacillin, piperacillin-tazobactam, potassium chloride/phosphates, procainamide, prochlorperazine, promethazine, propofol, propranolol, quinupristin-dalfopristin, ranitidine, rapacuronium, remifentanil, riTUXimab, rocuronium, sargramostim, sodium acetate/bicarbonate/phosphates, succinylcholine, SUFentanil, sulfamethoxazole-trimethoprim, tacrolimus, teniposide, theophylline, thiopental, thiotepa, ticarcillin, ticarcillin-clavulanate, tigecycline, tirofiban, TNA, tobramycin, trastuzumab, trimethobenzamide, vancomycin, vasopressin, vecuronium, verapamil, vinCRIStine, vinorelbine, voriconazole, zidovudine, zoledronic acid

SIDE EFFECTS

CNS: Neuritis, dizziness, headache, **cerebellar syndrome,** personality changes, ataxia, mechanical dysphasia, **coma; chemical arachnoiditis (IT)**

CV: Chest pain, **cardiopathy**

CYTARABINE SYNDROME: ***Fever,* myalgia, bone pain, chest pain, *rash,* conjunctivitis, malaise (6-12 hr after administration)**

EENT: Sore throat, conjunctivitis

GI: *Nausea, vomiting, anorexia, diarrhea, stomatitis,* **hepatotoxicity,** abdominal pain, hematemesis, **GI hemorrhage**

GU: Urinary retention, **renal failure, hyperuricemia**

HEMA: Thrombophlebitis, bleeding, thrombocytopenia, leukopenia, myelosuppression, anemia

INTEG: *Rash, fever,* freckling, cellulitis
META: Hyperuricemia
RESP: Pneumonia, dyspnea, pulmonary edema (high doses)
SYST: Anaphylaxis, tumor lysis syndrome

PHARMACOKINETICS

INTRATHECAL: Half-life 100-236 hr; metabolized in liver; excreted in urine (primarily inactive metabolite); crosses blood-brain barrier, placenta
IV/SUBCUT: Distribution half-life 10 min, elimination half-life 1-3 hr

INTERACTIONS

- Do not use with live virus vaccines
- Do not use within 24 hr of chemotherapy—sargramostim, GM-CSF, filgrastim, G-CSF

Increase: toxicity—immunosuppressants, methotrexate, flucytosine, radiation, or other antineoplastics
Increase: bleeding risk—anticoagulants, platelet inhibitors, salicylates, thrombolytics, NSAIDs
Decrease: effects of oral digoxin, gentamicin

NURSING CONSIDERATIONS

Assess:

Black Box Warning: **Bone marrow suppression:** CBC (RBC, Hct, Hgb), differential, platelet count weekly; withhold product if WBC is <1000/mm³, platelet count is <50,000/mm³, or RBC, Hct, Hgb low; notify prescriber of these results

- Renal studies: BUN, serum uric acid, urine CCr, electrolytes before and during therapy
- I&O ratio; report fall in urine output to <30 ml/hr
- Monitor temperature; fever may indicate beginning infection; no rectal temperatures
- **Hepatotoxicity:** hepatic studies before and during therapy: bilirubin, ALT, AST, alk phos, as needed or monthly; check for jaundice of skin, sclera; dark urine; clay-colored stools; pruritus; abdominal pain; fever; diarrhea
- Blood uric acid during therapy

⚠ **For anaphylaxis:** rash, pruritus, facial swelling, dyspnea; resuscitation equipment should be nearby

⚠ **Chemical arachnoiditis (IT):** headache, nausea, vomiting, fever; neck rigidity pain, meningism, CSF pleocytosis; may be decreased by dexamethasone

- Cytarabine syndrome 6-12 hr after infusion: fever, myalgia, bone pain, chest pain, rash, conjunctivitis, malaise; corticosteroids may be ordered
- Bleeding: hematuria, heme-positive stools, bruising or petechiae, mucosa or orifices q8hr

⚠ Dyspnea, crackles, unproductive cough, chest pain, tachypnea, fatigue, increased pulse, pallor, lethargy; personality changes, with high doses; pulmonary edema may be fatal (rare)

- Buccal cavity q8hr for dryness, sores or ulceration, white patches, oral pain, bleeding, dysphagia
- Local irritation, pain, burning, discoloration at inj site
- GI symptoms: frequency of stools, cramping; antispasmodic may be used
- Acidosis, signs of dehydration: rapid respirations, poor skin turgor, decreased urine output, dry skin, restlessness, weakness
- Increased fluid intake to 2-3 L/day to prevent urate deposits and calculi formation unless contraindicated
- Rinsing of mouth tid-qid with water, club soda; brushing of teeth bid-tid with soft brush or cotton-tipped applicators for stomatitis; use unwaxed dental floss

Evaluate:

- Therapeutic response: improvement of hematologic parameters

Teach patient/family:

- To report any coughing, chest pain, changes in breathing; may indicate beginning **pneumonia, pulmonary edema**
- To avoid foods with citric acid, spicy, or rough texture if stomatitis is present; use sponge brush and rinse with water after each meal; to report stomatitis: any

bleeding, white spots, ulcerations in mouth; to examine mouth daily, report any symptoms
- To report signs of **infection:** increased temperature, sore throat, flulike symptoms; to avoid crowds, persons with infections
- To report signs of **anemia:** fatigue, headache, faintness, SOB, irritability
- To report bleeding; to avoid use of razors, commercial mouthwash, salicylates, NSAIDs, anticoagulants
- To use thrombocytopenia precautions
- To take fluids to 3 L/day to prevent renal damage
- To use reliable contraception during treatment and for 4 mo thereafter; not to breastfeed
- To avoid receiving vaccines during treatment
- That fever, headache, nausea, vomiting likely to occur

dabigatran

(da-bye-gat′ran)

Pradaxa

Func. class.: Anticoagulant

Chem. class.: Thrombin inhibitor

ACTION: Direct thrombin inhibitor that inhibits both free and clot-bound thrombin, prevents thrombin-induced platelet aggregation and thrombus formation by preventing conversion of fibrinogen to fibrin

USES: Stroke/systemic embolism prophylaxis with nonvalvular atrial fibrillation, DVT, pulmonary embolism in hip replacement

CONTRAINDICATIONS: Hypersensitivity, bleeding, prosthetic heart valves

Precautions: Pregnancy (C), labor, obstetric delivery, breastfeeding, children, geriatric patients, abrupt discontinuation, anticoagulant therapy, renal disease, surgery

Black Box Warning: Abrupt discontinuation

DOSAGE AND ROUTES

Stroke prophylaxis

- **Adult: PO** 150 mg bid

For conversion from an alternative anticoagulant to dabigatran

- When converting from warfarin to dabigatran, discontinue warfarin and initiate dabigatran therapy when the INR is <2.0; when converting from a parenteral anticoagulant to dabigatran, initiate dabigatran 0-2 hr before the time of the next scheduled anticoagulant dose or at the time of discontinuation of a continuously administered anticoagulant (e.g., intravenous unfractionated heparin)

For conversion from dabigatran to warfarin

- **Adult:** CCr >50 ml/min, start warfarin 3 days before discontinuing dabigatran; CCr 31-50 ml/min, start warfarin 2 days before discontinuing dabigatran; CCr 15-30 ml/min, start warfarin 1 day before discontinuing dabigatran

For conversion from dabigatran to parenteral anticoagulants

- **Adult: PO** discontinue dabigatran; start parenteral anticoagulant 12 hr (CCr ≥30 ml/min) or 24 hr (CCr <30 ml/min) after the last dabigatran dose

Deep venous thrombus (DVT)/ pulmonary embolism (PE) prophylaxis

- **Adult: PO** 220 mg or 150 mg/day × 28-35 days, starting with ½ dose 1-4 hr after surgery (knee replacement); 110 on first day 1-4 hr after surgery, hemostasis achieved, then 220 mg qd × 28-35 days; those previously treated 150 mg bid (hip replacement)

Renal dose

- **Adult: PO** CCr 15-30 ml/min, 75 mg bid

DVT/PE/treated with a parenteral anticoagulant × 5-10 days

- **Adult: PO** 150 mg bid

Available forms: Caps 75, 150 mg

Administer:

- Do not crush, break, chew, or empty contents of capsule
- Without regard to food
- Store in original package at room temperature until time of use; discard after 30 days; protect from moisture

SIDE EFFECTS

CNS: Intracranial bleeding

CV: Myocardial infarction

GI: Abdominal pain, dyspepsia, peptic ulcer, esophagitis, GERD, gastritis, GI bleeding

HEMA: Bleeding (any site), hemorrhagic erosive gastritis

INTEG: Rash, pruritus

SYST: Anaphylaxis (rare)

PHARMACOKINETICS

Protein binding 35%, half-life 12-17 hr (extended in renal disease), peak 1 hr, high-fat meal delays peak

INTERACTIONS

Increase: bleeding risk—amiodarone, other anticoagulants, clopidogrel, ketoconazole, quiNIDine, thrombolytics, verapamil

Decrease: dabigatran effect—rifampin

Decrease: dabigatran effect—P-glycoprotein inducers (carBAMazepine, rifampin, tipranovir

Drug/Herb

Decrease: dabigatran—St. John's wort

Drug/Lab Test

Increase: thrombin time, aPTT

NURSING CONSIDERATIONS

Assess:

- **Bleeding:** blood in urine or emesis, dark tarry stools, lower back pain; caution with arterial/venous punctures, catheters, NG tubes; monitor vital signs frequently; elderly patients more prone to serious bleeding, monitor aPTT, ecarin clotting time baseline and during treatment
- **Thrombosis/MI/emboli:** swelling, pain, redness, difficulty breathing, chest pain, tachypnea, cough, coughing up blood, cyanosis
- **Postthrombotic syndrome:** pain, heaviness, itching/tingling, swelling, varicose veins, brownish/reddish skin discoloration, ulcers; use of ambulation, compression stockings, adequate anti-coagulation can prevent this syndrome
- **Surgery:** discontinue 24-48 hr before surgery in those with CCr ≥50 ml/min, 72-96 hr in those with CCr <50 ml/min; longer times may be needed in major surgery

Evaluate:

- Therapeutic response: decreased thrombus formation/extension, absence of emboli, postthrombotic effects

Teach patient/family:

- About the purpose and expected results of this product; to take at same time of day; not to skip or double doses; if dose is missed, take as soon as remembered if on the same day; do not administer if <6 hr before next dose; store in original container
- To take without regard to food, swallow cap whole, not to open
- To notify all providers that this product is being used, check with prescriber about when to discontinue
- To report any bleeding or bruising including blood in stool, emesis, urine; nosebleeds
- Not to use any other OTC products, herbs without prescriber approval
- That lab tests will be required during treatment
- To keep dry, do not use other containers

D

dabrafenib

(da-braf′e-nib)

Tafinlar

Func. class.: Antineoplastic

Chem. class.: Signal transduction inhibitor, kinase inhibitor

ACTION: Inhibits kinase, inhibitor against mutated forms of BRAF kinases in melanoma cells

USES: Unresectable or metastatic BRAD V600E-mutated malignant melanoma

CONTRAINDICATIONS: Pregnancy (D), hypersensitivity

Precautions: Breastfeeding, children, infection, dehydration, diabetes mellitus, fever, G6PD deficiency, hemolytic anemia, hyperglycemia, hypotension, infertility, iritis, renal failure, secondary malignancy

DOSAGE AND ROUTES

- **Adult: PO** 150 mg q12hr until disease progression; avoid strong CYP3A4/CYP2C8 inhibitors or inducers

Available forms: Caps 50, 75 mg

Administer:

PO route

- Swallow whole
- If dose is missed, take within 6 hr of missed dose; if >6 hr have passed, skip dose
- Space doses q12hr
- Take at least 1 hr before or 2 hr after a meal

SIDE EFFECTS

CNS: Headache, fever
GI: Pancreatitis
INTEG: Rash, alopecia
MISC: Arthralgia, myalgia, back pain
OTHER: Hyperglycemia, hypophosphatemia, hyponatremia, secondary malignancy, hand/foot syndrome

PHARMACOKINETICS

Protein binding 99.7%, half-life 8 hr (dabrafenib), 10 hr, 21-22 hr metabolites, excreted 71% (feces), 23% (urine)

INTERACTIONS

Altered: dabrafenib concentrations—CYP3A4 inhibitors (ketoconazole, itraconazole, erythromycin, clarithromycin)
Decrease: dabrafenib concentrations—CYP3A4 inducers (dexamethasome, phenytoin, carBAMazepine, rifampin, PHENobarbital), antacids, proton-pump inhibitors
Drug/Herb
Decrease: dabrafenib concentrations St. John's Wort
Drug/Food Test
Increase: dabrafenib effect—grapefruit juice; avoid use while taking product

NURSING CONSIDERATIONS

Assess:
- Toxicity: fever, grade 2, 3

Evaluate:
- Therapeutic response: decrease in melanoma progression

Teach patient/family:
- To report adverse reactions immediately
- About reason for treatment, expected results
- To use effective contraception during treatment and up to 30 days after discontinuing treatment, pregnancy (D)

HIGH ALERT

dacarbazine (Rx)

(da-kar′ba-zeen)

DTIC ✱, DTIC-Dome

Func. class.: Antineoplastic alkylating agent

Chem. class.: Cytotoxic triazine

ACTION:
Alkylates DNA, RNA; inhibits DNA, RNA synthesis; also responsible for breakage, cross-linking of DNA strands; activity is not cell-cycle–phase specific

USES:
Hodgkin's disease, malignant melanoma
Unlabeled uses: Malignant pheochromocytoma in combination with cyclophosphamide and vinCRIStine, metastatic soft-tissue sarcoma in combination with other agents, carcinoma meningitis, neuroblastoma

CONTRAINDICATIONS:
Breastfeeding, hypersensitivity
Precautions: Renal disease, infection

Black Box Warning: Pregnancy (C) 1st trimester, radiation therapy, hepatic disease, bone marrow suppression, secondary malignancy

DOSAGE AND ROUTES

Metastatic malignant melanoma
- **Adult:** **IV** 2-4.5 mg/kg/day × 10 days or 100-250 mg/m^2/day × 5 days; repeat q3-4wk depending on response

Hodgkin's disease
- **Adult:** **IV** 150 mg/m^2/day × 5 days with other agents, repeat q4wk; or 375 mg/m^2 on days 1 and 15 when given in combination, repeat q28days

Osteogenic sarcoma (unlabeled)
- **Adult and child:** **IV** 250 mg/m^2/day as continuous infusion × 4 days in combination with other agents q28days

Soft-tissue sarcoma (unlabeled)
- **Adult and child:** **IV** 250-300 mg/m^2/day as continuous infusion × 3 days q21-28days

Available forms: Powder for inj 100, 200 mg

Administer:

- Antiemetic 30-60 min before giving product to prevent vomiting, nausea; vomiting may subside after several doses, nausea/vomiting may be severe and last several hours
- Antibiotics for prophylaxis of infection

IV route

- Use cytotoxic handling precautions

Direct IV route

- After diluting 100 mg/9.9 or 200 mg/19.7 ml of sterile water for inj (10 mg/ml), give by direct IV over 2-3 min through **Y**-tube or 3-way stopcock

Intermittent IV INFUSION route

- May be further diluted in 50-250 ml D_5W or NS for inj, given as an infusion over 1/2 hr
- Watch for extravasation; stop infusion, apply ice to area
- Store in light-resistant container in a dry area

Y-site compatibilities: Amifostine, anidulafungin, atenolol, aztreonam, bivalirudin, bleomycin, caspofungin, DAPTOmycin, dexmedetomidine, DOCEtaxel, DOXOrubicin, ertapenem, etoposide, fenoldopam, filgrastim, fludarabine, gemtuzumab, granisetron, levofloxacin, mechlorethamine, melphalan, nesiritide, octreotide, ondansetron, oxaliplatin, PACLitaxel, palonosetron, pamidronate, quinupristin-dalfopristin, sargramostim, teniposide, thiotepa, tigecycline, tirofiban, vinorelbine, voriconazole, zoledronic acid

SIDE EFFECTS

CNS: Facial paresthesia, flushing, fever, malaise; confusion, headache, **seizures, cerebral hemorrhage,** blurred vision (high doses)

GI: *Nausea, anorexia, vomiting,* **hepatotoxicity** (rare)

HEMA: Thrombocytopenia, leukopenia, anemia

INTEG: *Alopecia,* dermatitis, pain at inj site, photosensitivity; severe sun reactions (high doses)

MISC: Flulike symptoms, malaise, fever, myalgia, hypotension

SYST: Anaphylaxis

PHARMACOKINETICS

Metabolized by liver; excreted in urine; terminal half-life 19 min; 5% protein bound

INTERACTIONS

Black Box Warning: Toxicity, bone marrow suppression: bone marrow suppressants, radiation, other antineoplastics

- Bleeding: salicylates, anticoagulants, NSAIDs

Increase: adverse reaction; decrease antibody reaction—live virus vaccines

Increase: nephrotoxicity—aminoglycosides

Increase: ototoxicity—loop diuretics

Decrease: dacarbazine effect—phenytoin, PHENobarbital

NURSING CONSIDERATIONS

Assess:

Black Box Warning: Bone marrow suppression: CBC, differential, platelet count weekly; notify prescriber of results

- Monitor temperature; may indicate beginning infection, I&O, for nausea, appetite

Black Box Warning: Secondary malignancy: assess for secondary malignancy that may occur with this product

- Bleeding: hematuria, guaiac, bruising, petechiae of mucosa or orifices q8hr
- Effects of alopecia on body image, discuss feelings about body changes

Black Box Warning: Hepatic disease: jaundice of skin, sclera; dark urine; clay-colored stools; itchy skin; abdominal pain; fever; diarrhea; hepatic studies before, during therapy (bilirubin, AST, ALT, LDH) as needed or monthly

- Inflammation of mucosa, breaks in skin
- IV site for irritation, redness, pain; if infiltration occurs, use hot packs at site

⚠ **Hypersensitivity reactions, anaphylaxis,** discontinue product, administer meds for anaphylaxis

- Increased fluid intake to 2-3 L/day to prevent urate deposits, calculi formation

Evaluate:

- Therapeutic response: decreased tumor size, spread of malignancy

Teach patient/family:

- That patient should avoid prolonged exposure to sun, wear sunscreen
- That hair may be lost during treatment; that a wig or hairpiece may make the patient feel better; that new hair may be different in color, texture
- To report signs of **infection:** fever, sore throat, flulike symptoms
- To report signs of **anemia:** fatigue, headache, faintness, SOB, irritability
- To report bleeding; to avoid use of razors, commercial mouthwash
- **Pregnancy:** to notify prescriber if pregnancy is planned or suspected pregnancy (D)
- To avoid aspirin products or ibuprofen

Black Box Warning: To use reliable contraceptives during and for several mo after therapy; not to breastfeed

dalbavancin

(dal-ba-van′sin)

Dalvance

Func. class.: Antiinfective-glycopeptide

ACTION: Binds to the bacterial cell walls, inhibiting their synthesis

USES: Treatment of acute bacterial skin and skin structure infections due to gram-positive organisms (cellulitis, major abscess, wound infections)

CONTRAINDICATIONS: Hypersensitivity

Precautions: Antimicrobial resistance, breastfeeding, colitis, diarrhea, GI disease, inflammatory bowel disease, infusion-related reactions, pregnancy, pseudomembranous colitis, ulcerative colitis, vancomycin hypersensitivity, viral infection

DOSAGE AND ROUTES

- **Adults: IV** 1000 mg once, then 500 mg IV 1 wk later

Available forms: Powder for injection 500 mg

Administer:

IV INFUSION route

- Visually inspect parenteral products for particulate matter and discoloration
- **Reconstitution:** Reconstitute each 500 mg/25 ml sterile water for injection, to avoid foaming, alternate between gentle swirling and inversion until completely dissolved, do not shake; further dilution is required
- **Storage:** Refrigerate or store at room temperature. Do not freeze. The total time from reconstitution to dilution to use should not exceed 48 hr
- **Dilution:** Transfer the dose of reconstituted solution from the vial(s) to an IV bag or bottle containing D_5W (1-5 mg/ml)

Intermittent IV INFUSION

- Give over 30 min, do not infuse with other medications or electrolytes, saline-based infusion solutions may cause precipitation and should not be used; if a common IV line is being used to administer other drugs, the line should be flushed before and after each dose

SIDE EFFECTS

CNS: Dizziness, headache, flushing

GI: Nausea, vomiting, pseudomembranous colitis, GI bleeding, abdominal pain, diarrhea

HEMA: Thrombocytopenia, neutropenia, leukopenia, anemia

SYST: Red man syndrome, hypersensitivity reactions

INTEG: Rash, urticaria, infusion-related reactions, pruritus

PHARMACOKINETICS
Protein binding 93%, primarily to albumin, with a protein binding of approximately 93%, excreted in feces and urine, metabolism decreased in renal disease

INTERACTIONS
Decrease: oral contraceptives may occur with prolonged use
Drug/lab test
Increase: LFTs

NURSING CONSIDERATIONS
Assess: BUN/creatinine, lower dose may be required in severe renal disease
Pseudomembranous colitis: bowel pattern daily, if severe diarrhea occurs, product should be discontinued
IV site for INFUSION-site reactions
Anaphylaxis: rash, urticaria, pruritus, wheezing, may occur a few days after administration
Red man syndrome: flushing, rash over upper torso and neck, may occur after a few minutes of infusion, may be treated with antihistamines and a slower infusion
Evaluate:
- Therapeutic response: decreased symptoms of infection, negative C&S

Teach patient/family:
- To report sore throat, bruising, bleeding, joint pain (**blood dyscrasias**); diarrhea with mucus, blood (**pseudomembranous colitis**)
- To use nonhormonal contraceptive if on long-term therapy (controversial)

dalfampridine (Rx)
(dal-fam′pri-deen)
Ampyra, Fampyra ♣
Func. class.: Neurological agent—multiple sclerosis
Chem. class.: Broad-spectrum potassium channel blocker

ACTION: Mechanism of action is not fully understood; a broad-spectrum potassium channel blocker that inhibits potassium channels and increased action potential conduction in demyelinated axions

USES: For improved walking in patients with multiple sclerosis

CONTRAINDICATIONS: Renal failure (CCr <50 ml/min), seizures
Precautions: Pregnancy (C), breastfeeding, geriatric patients, renal disease

DOSAGE AND ROUTES
- **Adult: PO** 10 mg q12hr

Renal dose
- **Adult: PO** CCr 51-80 ml/min, no dosage adjustment needed but seizure risk unknown; CCr ≤50 ml/min, do not use

Available forms: Ext rel tab 10 mg
Administer:
- Do not break, crush, or chew; give without regard to meals
- Do not give closer together than q12hr; seizures may occur
- Do not double doses; if a dose is missed, skip it

SIDE EFFECTS
CNS: **Seizures**, paresthesias, headache, dizziness, asthenia, insomnia
GI: Nausea, constipation, dyspepsia
GU: Urinary tract infection
MS: Back pain

PHARMACOKINETICS
Bioavailability 96%; peak 3-4 hr (fasting), longer if taken with food; largely unbound to plasma proteins; 96% recovered in urine

INTERACTIONS
- Do not use with fampridine, other 4-aminopyridine (4-AP)–containing products

NURSING CONSIDERATIONS
Assess:
- **Multiple sclerosis:** improved walking, including speed
- **Seizures:** more common in those with previous seizure disorder

Evaluate:
- Therapeutic response: ability to walk at improved speed in multiple sclerosis

Teach patient/family:
- To notify prescriber if pregnancy is planned or suspected; not to breastfeed
- Expected results; side effects, including seizures

HIGH ALERT

dalteparin (Rx)

(dahl′ta-pear-in)

Fragmin

Func. class.: Anticoagulant

Chem. class.: Low–molecular-weight heparin

ACTION: Inhibits factor Xa/IIa (thrombin), resulting in anticoagulation

USES: Unstable angina/non–Q-wave MI; prevention/treatment of deep venous thrombosis in abdominal surgery, hip replacement, or in those with restricted mobility during acute illness, pulmonary embolism

Unlabeled uses: Antiphospholipid antibody, arterial thromboembolism (after heart valve surgery), cerebral thromboembolism, acute MI

CONTRAINDICATIONS: Hypersensitivity to this product, heparin, or pork products; active major bleeding, hemophilia, leukemia with bleeding, thrombocytopenic purpura, cerebrovascular hemorrhage, cerebral aneurysm; those undergoing regional anesthesia for unstable angina, non–Q-wave MI, dalteparin-induced thrombocytopenia

Precautions: Hypersensitivity to benzyl alcohol, pregnancy (B), breastfeeding, children, recent childbirth, geriatric patients; hepatic disease; severe renal disease; blood dyscrasias; bacterial endocarditis; acute nephritis; uncontrolled hypertension; recent brain, spine, eye surgery; congenital or acquired disorders; severe cardiac disease; peptic ulcer disease; hemorrhagic stroke; history of HIT; pericarditis; pericardial effusion; recent lumbar puncture; vasculitis; other diseases in which bleeding is possible

Black Box Warning: Epidural anesthesia, lumbar puncture

DOSAGE AND ROUTES

DVT/pulmonary embolism
- **Adult:** **SUBCUT** 200 international units/kg daily during 1st mo (max single dose 18,000 international units), then 150 international units/kg daily for mo 2-6 (max single dose 18,000 international units), use prefilled syringe that is closest to calculated dose; if platelets are 50,000-100,000/mm^3, reduce dose by 2500 international units until platelets ≥100,000 mm^3; if platelets <50,000/mm^3, discontinue until >50,000/mm^3

Hip replacement surgery/DVT prophylaxis
- **Adult:** **SUBCUT** 2500 international units 2 hr before surgery and 2nd dose in the evening on the day of surgery (4-8 hr postop), then 5000 international units **SUBCUT** 1st postop day and daily × 5-10 days

Unstable angina/non–Q-wave MI
- **Adult:** **SUBCUT** 120 international units/kg q12hr × 5-8 days, max 10,000 international units q12hr × 5-8 days with concurrent aspirin; continue until stable

DVT, prophylaxis for abdominal surgery
- **Adult:** **SUBCUT** 2500 international units 1-2 hr before surgery; repeat daily × 5-10 days; for high-risk patients, >3400 international units should be used

Renal dose
- **Adult:** **SUBCUT** cancer patient with CCr <30 ml/min, monitor and adjust based on anti-factor Xa during extended treatment

APLA (unlabeled)
- **Adult (female):** **SUBCUT** Antepartum 5000 international units/day with aspirin; maintain anti-factor Xa of 0.2-0.6 international units/ml

Arterial thromboembolism prophylaxis (unlabeled)
• **Adult: SUBCUT** LMWH in combination with oral anticoagulants until INR is in therapeutic range × 2 consecutive days

Available forms: Prefilled syringes, 2500, 5000 international units/0.2 ml; 7500 international units/0.3 ml; 10,000, 12,500, 15,000, 18,000, 25,000 international units/ml

Administer:
• Cannot be used interchangeably (unit for unit) with unfractionated heparin or other LMWHs
• Do not give IM or IV product route; approved is SUBCUT only; do not mix with other inj or sol
• Have patient sit or lie down; SUBCUT inj may be 2 inches from umbilicus in a U-shape, upper outer side of thigh, around navel, or upper outer quadrangle of the buttocks; rotate inj sites
• Change inj site daily; use at same time of day

SIDE EFFECTS

CNS: **Intracranial bleeding**
HEMA: **Thrombocytopenia**
INTEG: Pruritus, superficial wound infection, skin necrosis, inj site reaction, alopecia
SYST: Hypersensitivity, **hemorrhage, anaphylaxis** possible, **hematoma**

PHARMACOKINETICS

87% absorbed, excreted by kidneys, elimination half-life 3-5 hr, peak 2-4 hr, onset 1-2 hr, duration >12 hr

INTERACTIONS

Increase: bleeding risk—aspirin, oral anticoagulants, platelet inhibitors, NSAIDs, salicylates, thrombolytics, some cephalosporins

Drug/Herb
Increase: bleeding risk—feverfew, garlic, ginger, ginkgo, horse chestnut

Drug/Lab Test
Increase: AST, ALT

NURSING CONSIDERATIONS

Assess:
• **Blood studies (Hct/Hgb, CBC, platelets, anti-Xa, stool guaiac) during treatment because bleeding can occur**
⚠ **Bleeding: Bleeding gums, petechiae, ecchymosis, black tarry stools, hematuria, epistaxis, decrease in Hct, B/P; may indicate bleeding, possible hemorrhage; notify prescriber immediately, product should be discontinued**

Black Box Warning: Epidural anesthesia: Neurologic impairment frequently in those when neuraxial anesthesia has been used, spinal/epidural hematomas can occur, with paralysis

• **Hypersensitivity: fever, skin rash, urticaria; notify prescriber immediately**
• Needed dosage change q1-2wk; dose may need to be decreased if bleeding occurs

Evaluate:
• Therapeutic response: absence of DVT

Teach patient/family:
• To avoid OTC preparations that contain aspirin; other anticoagulants, serious product interaction may occur unless approved by prescriber
• To use soft-bristle toothbrush to avoid bleeding gums; to avoid contact sports; to use electric razor; to avoid IM inj
• **To report any signs of bleeding (gums, under skin, urine, stools), unusual bruising**

TREATMENT OF OVERDOSE:

Protamine sulfate 1% given IV; 1 mg protamine/100 anti-Xa international units of dalteparin given

dantrolene (Rx)

(dan′troe-leen)

Dantrium, Revonto

Func. class.: Skeletal muscle relaxant, direct acting
Chem. class.: Hydantoin

Do not confuse:
Dantrium/danazol

ACTION: Interferes with intracellular release of calcium from the sarcoplasmic reticulum necessary to initiate contraction; slows catabolism in malignant hyperthermia

USES: Spasticity in multiple sclerosis, stroke, spinal cord injury, cerebral palsy, malignant hyperthermia
Unlabeled uses: Neuroleptic malignant syndrome

CONTRAINDICATIONS: Hypersensitivity, compromised pulmonary function, impaired myocardial function

Black Box Warning: Active hepatic disease

Precautions: Pregnancy (C), breastfeeding, geriatric patients, peptic ulcer disease, cardiac/renal/hepatic disease, stroke, seizure disorder, diabetes mellitus, ALS, COPD, MS, mannitol/gelatin hypersensitivity, labor, lactase deficiency, extravasation

Black Box Warning: Females >35 yr, with MS, or taking estrogens

DOSAGE AND ROUTES

Spasticity
- **Adult: PO** 25 mg/day; may increase to 25-100 mg bid-qid, max 400 mg/day, may be increased q 7 days as needed
- **Child: PO** 0.5 mg/kg/day given in divided doses bid, may be increased q 7 days as needed, max 400 mg/day

Prevention of malignant hyperthermia
- **Adult and child: PO** 4-8 mg/kg/day in 3-4 divided doses × 1-3 days before procedure, give last dose 4 hr preop; **IV** 2.5 mg/kg before anesthesia

Malignant hyperthermia
- **Adult and child: IV** 1-2.5 mg/kg, may repeat to total dose of 10 mg/kg; **PO** 4-8 mg/kg/day in 4 divided doses × 1-3 days

Neuroleptic malignant syndrome (unlabeled)
- **Adult: PO** 100-300 mg/day in divided doses; **IV** 1.25-1.5 mg/kg

Available forms: Caps 25, 50, 100 mg; powder for inj 20 mg/vial

Administer:
- Avoid use with other CNS depressants

PO route
- Do not crush or chew caps
- Caps may be opened, mixed with juice and swallowed
- With meals for GI symptoms

IV route
- IV after diluting 20 mg/60 ml sterile water for inj without bacteriostatic agent (333 mcg/ml); shake until clear; give by rapid IV push through Y-tube or 3-way stopcock; follow with prescribed doses immediately; may also give by intermittent infusion over 1 hr before anesthesia
- Considered incompatible in sol or syringe; compatibility unknown
- Store in tight container at room temperature; protect diluted sol from light, use reconstituted sol within 6 hr

SIDE EFFECTS

CNS: *Dizziness, weakness, fatigue, drowsiness,* headache, disorientation, insomnia, paresthesias, tremors, seizures
CV: Hypotension, chest pain, palpitations, tachycardia
EENT: Nasal congestion, blurred vision, mydriasis, excessive lacrimation
GI: Hepatic injury, *nausea,* constipation, vomiting, increased AST, alk phos, abdominal pain, dry mouth, anorexia, hepatitis, dyspepsia
GU: Urinary frequency, nocturia, impotence, crystalluria, hepatitis
HEMA: Eosinophilia, aplastic anemia, leukopenia, thrombocytopenia/lymphoma
INTEG: Rash, pruritus, photosensitivity, extravasation (tissue necrosis), phlebitis
RESP: Pleural effusion, pulmonary edema

PHARMACOKINETICS

PO: Peak 5 hr, highly protein bound, half-life 8 hr, metabolized in liver, excreted in urine (metabolites), absorption poor (35%)

INTERACTIONS

Increase: dysrhythmias—verapamil

Increase: hepatotoxicity—estrogens, other hepatotoxics
Increase: CNS depression—alcohol, tricyclics, opiates, barbiturates, sedatives, hypnotics, antihistamines, tramadol

NURSING CONSIDERATIONS

Assess:

- **Seizures:** increased seizure activity, ECG in epilepsy patient; poor seizure control has occurred
- I&O ratio; check for urinary retention, frequency, hesitancy, especially geriatric patients

Black Box Warning: Active hepatic disease: hepatic function by frequent determination of AST, ALT, bilirubin, alk phos, GGTP; renal function studies, BUN, creatinine, CBC, use lowest dose possible; check for jaundice, dark urine, diarrhea, weakness; product should be discontinued

- **Allergic reactions:** rash, fever, respiratory distress
- Severe weakness, numbness in extremities; prescriber should be notified and product discontinued
- Tolerance: increased need/more frequent requests for medication, increased pain
- CNS depression: dizziness, drowsiness, insomnia, psychiatric symptoms
- ⚠ **Signs of hepatotoxicity:** jaundice, yellow sclera, pain in abdomen, nausea, fever; prescriber should be notified, product discontinued

Evaluate:

- Therapeutic response: decreased pain, spasticity

Teach patient/family:

- Not to discontinue medication quickly because hallucinations, spasticity, tachycardia will occur; product should be tapered off over 1-2 wk; to notify prescriber of abdominal pain, jaundiced sclera, clay-colored stools, change in color of urine
- That if improvement does not occur within 6 wk, prescriber may discontinue product
- To avoid hazardous activities if drowsiness, dizziness occurs
- To report severe weakness, seizures, signs of liver insufficiency
- To avoid using OTC medications: cough preparations, antihistamines, other CNS depressants, alcohol unless directed by prescriber, to take with meals
- To use sunscreen or stay out of the sun to prevent burns

Malignant hyperthermia: To use a medical ID stating condition, products used

TREATMENT OF OVERDOSE:

Activated charcoal, supportive care

dapagliflozin

(dap′a-gli-floe′zin)

Farxiga

Func. class.: Oral antidiabetic
Chem. class.: SGLT 2 inhibitor

ACTION: Blocks reabsorption of glucose by the kidney, increases glucose excretion, lower blood glucose concentrations

USES: Type 2 diabetes mellitus, with diet and exercise

CONTRAINDICATIONS: Dialysis, renal failure, hypersensitivity, breastfeeding, diabetic ketoacidosis
Precautions: Pregnancy (C), children, renal/hepatic disease, hypothyroidism, hyperglycemia, hypotension, bladder cancer, hypercholesterolemia, pituitary insufficiency, type 1 diabetes mellitus, malnutrition, fever, dehydration, adrenal insufficiency, geriatrics, genital fungal infections, hypoglycemia

DOSAGE AND ROUTES

- **Adult: PO** 5 mg in AM; may increase to 10 mg daily if needed

Renal Dose

- **Adult: PO** eGFR ≥60 ml/min/1.73 m^2 no change, eGFR <60 ml/min, do not use

Available forms: Tabs 5, 10 mg

Administer:

PO route

- Once daily in AM without regard to food

SIDE EFFECTS

CNS: Dizziness, fatigue

GI: Abdominal pain, pancreatitis, constipation, nausea

GU: Cystitis, candidiasis, urinary frequency, polydipsia, polyuria, increased serum creatinine; renal impairment/failure; infections

INTEG: Photosensitivity, rash, pruritus

META: Hypercholesterolemia, lipidemia, hypoglycemia, hyperkalemia, hypomagnesemia, hypo/hyperphosphatemia

MISC: Bone fractures, hypotension; dehydration; orthostatic hypotension; hypersensitivity; new bladder cancer; increased hematocrit

PHARMACOKINETICS

91% protein binding, primary excretion in urine, half-life 12.9 hr; primarily metabolized by O-glucuronidation by UGT1A9; minor CYP3A4; Cmax is less than 2 hr

INTERACTIONS

- Do not use gatifloxacin

Increase: hypoglycemia—sulfonylureas, insulin, MAOIs, salicylates, fibric acid derivatives, bile acid sequestrates, ACE inhibitors, angiotensin II receptor antagonists, beta blockers

Increase or decrease: glycemic control—androgens, lithium, bortezomib, quinolones

Decrease: effect hyperglycemia—digestive enzymes, intestinal absorbents, thiazide diuretics, loop diuretics, corticosteroids, estrogen, progestins, oral contraceptives, sympathomimetics, isoniazid, phenothiazines, protease inhibitors, atypical antipsychotics, carbonic anhydrase inhibitors, cycloSPORINE, tacrolimus, baclofen

Drug/Lab Test

Increase: HCT, LDL

NURSING CONSIDERATIONS

Assess:

- **Hypoglycemia** (weakness, hunger, dizziness, tremors, anxiety, tachycardia, sweating), **hyperglycemia;** even though product does not cause hyperglycemia, if patient is on sulfonylureas or insulin, hypoglycemia may be additive; if hypoglycemia occurs, treat with dextrose, or, if severe, with IV glucagon; HbA1c; lipid panel; renal function tests; volume status; blood pressure
- Renal function: baseline and periodically, discontinue if renal function is reduced
- Hypersensitivity: discontinue immediately
- Hypotension: more frequent in those with poor renal function

Evaluate:

- Therapeutic response: improved signs/symptoms of diabetes mellitus (decreased polyuria, polydipsia, polyphagia); clear sensorium, absence of dizziness, stable gait; HbA1c WNL

Teach patient/family:

- The symptoms of hypo/hyperglycemia, what to do about each
- That medication must be taken as prescribed; explain consequences of discontinuing medication abruptly; that insulin may need to be used for stress, including trauma, fever, surgery
- To avoid OTC medications and herbal supplements unless approved by health care provider
- That diabetes is a lifelong illness; that the diet and exercise regimen must be followed; that this product is not a cure
- To carry emergency ID and glucose source
- That blood glucose monitoring is required to assess product effect
- That GI side effects may occur
- That there is a risk of renal impairment, dehydration, and bladder cancer
- To report fever, itching, change in urine output, light-headedness or feeling faint
- To use adequate fluids

DAPTOmycin (Rx)

(dap′toe-mye-sin)

Cubicin

Func. class.: Antiinfective—miscellaneous

Chem. class.: Lipopeptides

ACTION: A new class of antiinfective; it binds to the bacterial membrane and results in a rapid depolarization of the membrane potential, thereby leading to inhibition of DNA, RNA, and protein synthesis

USES: Bacteremia, endocarditis, UTI, complicated skin, skin-structure infections caused by *Staphylococcus aureus* (MRSA, MSSA) including methicillin-resistant strains, *Streptococcus pyogenes, Streptococcus agalactiae, Streptococcus dysgalactiae, Enterococcus faecalis* (vancomycin-susceptible strains), *Streptococcus pyogenes* (group A beta hemolytic), *Staphylococcus aureus, Staphylococcus epidermidis, Corynebacterium jeikeium, Staphylococcus haemolyticus*

Unlabeled uses: Vancomycin-resistant enterococci (VRE), bone, joint infection, infectious arthritis, orthopedic device-related infection, osteomyelitis

CONTRAINDICATIONS: Hypersensitivity

Precautions: Pregnancy (B), breastfeeding, children, geriatric patients, GI/renal disease, myopathy, ulcerative/pseudomembranous colitis, rhabdomyolysis, eosinophilic pneumonia

DOSAGE AND ROUTES

- **Adult: IV INFUSION** 4 mg/kg over ½ hr diluted in 0.9% NaCl, give q24hr × 7-14 days; some indications may use up to 6 mg/kg
- **Adolescent/child/infant ≥5 mo (unlabeled): IV** 4-6 mg/kg/day

***Staphylococcus aureus* bacteremia, including right-sided infective endocarditis**

- **Adult: IV INFUSION** 6 mg/kg daily × 2-6 wk, up to 8-10 mg/kg daily; treatment failures should use another agent

Renal dose

- **Adult: IV INFUSION** CCr <30 ml/min, hemodialysis, CAPD 4 mg/kg q48hr, 6 mg/kg q48hr (bacteremia)

Bacteremia, endocarditis, UTI (unlabeled)

- **Adult: IV** 6 mg/kg/day

VRE (unlabeled)

- **Adult: IV** 4 mg/kg/day

Available forms: Lyophilized powder for inj 500 mg

Administer:

IV route

- After reconstitution with 10 ml 0.9% NaCl (500 mg/10 ml); further dilution is needed with 0.9 NaCl; infuse over ½ hr or give reconstituted sol (50 mg/ml) by IV inj over 2 min; do not use dextrose-containing solutions
- Refrigerate vials, for single use only, discard unused portion; prepared solutions are stable for 12 hr at room temperature or 48 hr refrigerated

Y-site compatibilities: Alfentanil, amifostine, amikacin, aminocaproic acid, aminophylline, amiodarone, amphotericin B liposome, ampicillin, ampicillin-sulbactam, argatroban, arsenic trioxide, atenolol, atracurium, azithromycin, aztreonam, bivalirudin, bleomycin, bumetanide, buprenorphine, busulfan, butorphanol, calcium chloride/gluconate, CARBOplatin, carmustine, caspofungin, ceFAZolin, cefepime, cefotaxime, cefoTEtan, cefOXitin, cefTAZidime, ceftizoxime, cefTRIAXone, cefuroxime, chloramphenicol, chlorproMAZINE, cimetidine, ciprofloxacin, cisatracurium, CISplatin, clindamycin, cyclophosphamide, cycloSPORINE, dacarbazine, DACTINomycin, DAUNOrubicin, dexamethasone, dexmedetomidine, dexrazoxane, diazepam, digoxin, diltiazem, diphenhydrAMINE, DOBUTamine, DOCEtaxel,

DOPamine, doripenem, doxacurium, DOXOrubicin, DOXOrubicin liposomal, doxycycline, droperidol, enalaprilat, ePHEDrine, EPINEPHrine, epirubicin, eptifibatide, ertapenem, erythromycin, esmolol, etoposide, famotidine, fenoldopam, fentaNYL, fluconazole, fludarabine, fluorouracil, foscarnet, fosphenytoin, furosemide, ganciclovir, gentamicin, glycopyrrolate, granisetron, haloperidol, heparin, hydrALAZINE, hydrocortisone, HYDROmorphone, hydrOXYzine, IDArubicin, ifosfamide, inamrinone, insulin (regular), irinotecan, isoproterenol, ketorolac, labetalol, lepirudin, leucovorin, levofloxacin, lidocaine, linezolid, LORazepam, magnesium sulfate, mannitol, mechlorethamine, melphalan, meperidine, meropenem, mesna, metaraminol, methyldopate, methylPREDNISolone, metoclopramide, metoprolol, midazolam, milrinone, mitoXANtrone, mivacurium, morphine, moxifloxacin, mycophenolate mofetil, nafcillin, nalbuphine, naloxone, niCARdipine, nitroprusside, norepinephrine, octreotide, ondansetron, oxaliplatin, oxytocin, PACLitaxel, palonosetron, pamidronate, pancuronium, PEMEtrexed, pentamidine, PHENobarbital, phenylephrine, piperacillin-tazobactam, polymyxin B, potassium acetate/chloride/phosphates, procainamide, prochlorperazine, promethazine, propranolol, quinupristin-dalfopristin, ranitidine, rocuronium, sodium acetate/bicarbonate/citrate/phosphates, succinylcholine, sulfamethoxazole-trimethoprim, tacrolimus, teniposide, theophylline, thiotepa, ticarcillin, ticarcillin-clavulanate, tigecycline, tirofiban, tobramycin, topotecan, trimethobenzamide, vasopressin, vecuronium, verapamil, vinBLAStine, vinCRIStine, vinorelbine, voriconazole, zidovudine, zoledronic acid

Solution compatibilities: 0.9% NaCl, LR

SIDE EFFECTS

CNS: Headache, insomnia, dizziness, confusion, anxiety, fatigue, fever

CV: Hypo/hypertension, heart failure, chest pain

GI: Nausea, constipation, diarrhea, vomiting, dyspepsia, pseudomembranous colitis, abdominal pain, stomatitis, xerostomia, anorexia

GU: Nephrotoxicity

HEMA: Leukocytosis, anemia, thrombocytopenia

INTEG: Rash, pruritus

META: Electrolyte imbalances

MISC: Fungal infections, UTI, anemia, hypoglycemia

MS: Muscle pain or weakness, arthralgia, pain, myopathy, rhabdomyolysis

RESP: Cough, eosinophilic pneumonia, dyspnea

SYST: Anaphylaxis, DRESS, Stevens-Johnson syndrome

PHARMACOKINETICS

Site of metabolism unknown, protein binding 92%, terminal half-life 8-9 hr, 78% excreted unchanged (urine), breast milk

INTERACTIONS

Increase: tobramycin levels

Increase: daptomycin action-tobramycin

Increase: myopathy—HMG-CoA reductase inhibitors

Drug/Lab Test

Increase: CPK, AST, ALT, BUN, creatinine, albumin, LDH

Increase/Decrease: glucose

Decrease: alkaline phosphatase, magnesium, phosphate, bicarbonate

NURSING CONSIDERATIONS

Assess:

- **Eosinophilic pneumonia:** dyspnea, fever, cough, shortness of breath; if left untreated, can lead to respiratory failure and death
- ⚠ **Nephrotoxicity:** any patient with compromised renal system, toxicity may occur; BUN, creatinine
- **Rhabdomyolysis:** Check for myopathy CPK $>$ 1000 U/L (5 $\times$ ULN), discontinue product, muscle pain, weakness
- **Bowel function:** diarrhea, fever, abdominal pain report to prescriber; pseudomembranous colitis may occur

- I&O ratio: report hematuria, oliguria, nephrotoxicity may occur
- Blood studies: CBC, CPK
- C&S; product may be given as soon as culture taken
- B/P during administration; hypo/hypertension may occur
- Signs of infection
- Allergies before treatment, reaction of each medication

Evaluate:

- Therapeutic response: negative culture

Teach patient/family:

- About allergies before treatment, reaction to each medication
- To report sore throat, fever, fatigue; could indicate superinfection; diarrhea; muscle weakness, pain, shortness of breath
- Avoid breastfeeding

⚠ HIGH ALERT

darbepoetin (Rx)

(dar′bee-poh′eh-tin)

Aranesp

Func. class.: Hematopoietic agent

Chem. class.: Recombinant human erythropoietin

ACTION: Stimulates erythropoiesis by the same mechanism as endogenous erythropoietin; in response to hypoxia, erythropoietin is produced in the kidney and released into the bloodstream, where it interacts with progenitor stem cells to increase red-cell production

USES: Anemia associated with chronic renal failure, in patients on and not on dialysis, and anemia in nonmyeloid malignancies for patients receiving coadministered chemotherapy

CONTRAINDICATIONS: Hypersensitivity to hamster protein products, human albumin, polysorbate 80; uncontrolled hypertension; red-cell aplasia

Precautions: Pregnancy (C), breastfeeding, children, seizure disorder, porphyria, hypertension, sickle cell disease; vit B_{12}, folate deficiency; chronic renal failure, dialysis; latex hypersensitivity, CABG, angina, anemia

Black Box Warning: Hgb >11 g/dl, neoplastic disease

DOSAGE AND ROUTES

Correction of anemia in chronic renal failure

- **Adult: SUBCUT/IV** 0.45 mcg/kg as a single inj; every wk, titrate max target Hgb of 11 g/dl

Chemotherapy treatment

- **Adult: SUBCUT** 2.25 mcg/kg/wk or 500 mcg q3wk

Epoetin alfa to darbepoetin conversion

- **Adult: SUBCUT/IV** (epoetin alfa <2500 units/wk) 6.25 mcg/wk; (epoetin alfa 2500-4999 units/wk) 12.5 mcg/wk; (epoetin alfa 5000-10,999 units/wk) 25 mcg/wk; (epoetin alfa 11,000-17,999 units/wk) 40 mcg/wk; (epoetin alfa 18,000-33,999 units/wk) 60 mcg/wk; (epoetin alfa 34,000-89,999 units/wk) 100 mcg/wk; (epoetin alfa >90,000 units/wk) 200 mcg/wk

Available forms: Sol for inj 25, 40, 60, 100, 150, 200, 300, 500 mcg/ml

Administer:

- Transfusions may still be required for anemia, use iron supplements with this product

SUBCUT/IV route

- Without shaking; check for discoloration, particulate matter, do not use if present; do not dilute, do not mix with other products or sol, discard unused portion, do not pool unused portions
- Subcut typically used for those not requiring dialysis
- IV given direct undiluted or bolus into IV tubing or venous line after completion of dialysis; watch for clotting of line
- Adjust dosage every mo or more
- Store refrigerated, do not freeze; protect from light

SIDE EFFECTS

CNS: Seizures, sweating, headache, dizziness, stroke

CV: *Hypo/hypertension,* cardiac arrest, *angina pectoris,* thrombosis, CHF, acute MI, dysrhythmias, chest pain, transient ischemic attacks, edema

GI: *Diarrhea, vomiting, nausea, abdominal pain, constipation*

HEMA: Red-cell aplasia

MISC: *Infection, fatigue, fever,* death, *fluid overload,* vascular access hemorrhage, dehydration, sepsis

MS: *Bone pain, myalgia, limb pain, back pain*

RESP: *URI, dyspnea, cough, bronchitis,* PE

SYST: Allergic reactions, anaphylaxis

PHARMACOKINETICS

IV: Onset of increased reticulocyte count 2-6 wk; distributed to vascular space; absorption slow and rate limiting; terminal half-life 49 hr (SUBCUT), 21 hr (IV); peak concentrations at 34 hr; increased Hgb levels not generally observed until 2-6 wk after treatment initiated

INTERACTIONS

⚠ Do not use epoetin alfa with product

Increase: darbepoetin-alfa effect—androgens

Drug/Lab Test

Increase: WBC, platelets, Hgb

Decrease: bleeding time

NURSING CONSIDERATIONS

Assess:

- Symptoms of anemia: fatigue, dyspnea, pallor

⚠ **Serious allergic reactions:** rash, urticaria; if anaphylaxis occurs, stop product, administer emergency treatment (rare)

Black Box Warning: Renal studies: urinalysis, protein, blood, BUN, creatinine; monitor dialysis shunts; during dialysis, heparin may need to be increased, those with renal dysfunction may be at greater risk of death

Black Box Warning: Blood studies: ferritin, transferrin monthly; transferrin saturation ≥20%, ferritin ≥100 ng/ml; Hgb 2×/wk until stabilized in target range (30%-33%), then at regular intervals; those with endogenous erythropoietin levels of <500 units/L respond to this agent; iron stores should be corrected before beginning therapy; if there is lack of response, obtain folic acid, iron, B_{12} levels

Black Box Warning: Neoplastic disease: breast, non–small-cell lung, head and neck, lymphoid, or cervical cancers, increased tumor progression; use lowest dose to avoid RBC transfusion

- B/P: check for rising B/P as Hgb rises; antihypertensives may be needed

Black Box Warning: CV status: hypertension may occur rapidly, leading to **hypertensive encephalopathy**; Hgb >11 g/dl may lead to death, do not administer

- I&O; report drop in output to <50 ml/hr

Black Box Warning: Seizures: if Hgb is increased by 4 pts within 2 wk, institute seizure precautions

- CNS symptoms: sweating, pain in long bones
- **Dialysis patients:** thrill, bruit of shunts, monitor for circulation impairment

Black Box Warning: Facility must be enrolled in the ESA APPRISE oncology program 1-866-284-8089 to use this product in cancer

Evaluate:

- Therapeutic response: increase in reticulocyte count, Hgb/Hct; increased appetite, enhanced sense of well-being

Teach patient/family:

- To avoid driving or hazardous activity during beginning of treatment

- To monitor B/P, Hgb, max Hgb 11 g/dl
- To take iron supplements, vit B_{12}, folic acid as directed

Black Box Warning: To report chest pain, SOB, swelling/pain in legs, confusion in ability to speak to prescriber; to comply with treatment regimen

- That menses and fertility may return; to use contraception
- About home administration procedures, if appropriate

Black Box Warning: Seizures: discuss injury prevention in those who are prone to seizures

darifenacin

(da-ree-fen′ah-sin)

Enablex

Func. class.: Antispasmodic/ Guanticholinergic

ACTION: Bladder smooth muscle relaxation by decreasing the action of muscarinic receptors, thereby relieving overactive bladder

USES: Urge incontinence, frequency, urgency in overactive bladder

CONTRAINDICATIONS: Hypersensitivity, urinary retention, narrow-angle glaucoma (uncontrolled)

Precautions: Severe hepatic disease (Child-Pugh C), GI/GU obstruction, controlled narrow-angle glaucoma, ulcerative colitis, myasthenia gravis, moderate hepatic disease (Child-Pugh B), elderly

DOSAGE AND ROUTES

- **Adult: PO** 7.5 mg/day, initially; may increase to 15 mg/day after 14 days if needed

With CYP3A4 inhibitor

- **Adult: PO** max 7.5 mg/day

Hepatic dosage

- **Adult: PO** (Child-Pugh B) max 7.5 mg/day

Available forms: Tabs, ext rel 7.5, 15 mg

Administer:

- Without regard to meals, do not crush, break, chew extended-release tabs
- Store at room temperature

SIDE EFFECTS

CNS: Dizziness, headache

EENT: Blurred vision, drying eyes, sinusitis, rhinitis

GI: Constipation, dry mouth, abdominal pain, nausea, vomiting, dyspepsia

GU: UTI, urine retention, vaginosis

INTEG: Rash, pruritus, skin drying

MISC: Bronchitis, flulike symptoms

PHARMACOKINETICS

Peak 7 hr, half-life 12-19 hr

INTERACTIONS

Increase: level of—digoxin

Increase: anticholinergic effect—anticholinergics

Increase: darifenacin level—CYP3A4 and CYP2D6 inhibitors

Increase: levels of—drugs metabolized by CYP2D6

NURSING CONSIDERATIONS

Assess:

- Urinary function: urgency, frequency, retention in bladder-outflow obstruction

Evaluate:

- Decreasing urgency, frequency of urination

Teach patient/family:

- To take without regard to meals; do not crush, break, chew extended-release tabs, not to use other products unless approved by prescriber
- To store at room temperature
- To avoid breastfeeding; to notify prescriber if pregnancy (C) is planned or suspected
- About anticholinergic symptoms (dry mouth, constipation, dry eyes, heat prostration); not to become overheated
- To avoid hazardous activities until reaction is known; dizziness, blurred vision can occur

darunavir (Rx)

(dar-ue′na-vir)

Prezista

Func. class.: Antiretroviral

Chem. class.: Protease inhibitor

ACTION: Inhibits human immunodeficiency virus (HIV-1) protease; this prevents maturation of the virus

USES: HIV-1 in combination with ritonavir and other antiretrovirals

CONTRAINDICATIONS: Hypersensitivity

Precautions: Pregnancy (B), breastfeeding, children, geriatric patients, renal/hepatic disease, history of renal stones, diabetes, hypercholesterolemia, sulfonamide hypersensitivity, antimicrobial resistance, bleeding, immune reconstitution syndrome, pancreatitis

DOSAGE AND ROUTES

Treatment-naive patients

- **Adult: PO** 800 mg with ritonavir 100 mg daily
- **Child/Adolescent ≥ 40 kg and ≥12 yr: PO** 800 mg with ritonavir 100 mg q day, avoid once daily darunavir dosing in those <12 yr
- **Child/Adolescent 30 to 39 kg and ≥12 yr: PO** 675 mg with ritonavir 100 mg q day, avoid once daily darunavir dosing in those <12 yr
- **Children ≥3 yr, 15 to 29 kg: PO** 600 mg with ritonavir 100 mg q day, avoid once daily darunavir dosing in those <12 yr
- **Children ≥3 yr, <14 kg: PO** 490 mg with ritonavir 96 mg qd; **13 kg:** 455 mg with ritonavir 80 mg q day; **12 kg:** 420 mg with ritonavir 80 mg q day; **11 kg:** 385 mg with ritonavir 64 mg q day; **10 kg:** 350 mg with ritonavir 64 mg q day, avoid once daily dosing in those <12 yrs

Treatment-experienced patients with at least one darunavir resistance-associated substitution

- **Adult/adolescent/child ≥40 kg: PO** 600 mg bid; with ritonavir 100 mg bid with food
- **Adolescent ≥30 kg, <40 kg: PO** 450 mg bid with ritonavir 60 mg bid
- **Adolescent ≥15 kg, <30 kg: PO** 375 mg bid with ritonavir 50 mg bid
- **Child 3 to <6 yr (14 kg): PO** 280 mg (with ritonavir 48 mg) bid with food
- **Child 3 to <6 yr (13 kg): PO** 260 mg (with ritonavir 40 mg) bid with food
- **Child 3 to <6 yr (12 kg): PO** 240 mg (with ritonavir 40 mg) bid with food
- **Child 3 to <6 yr (11 kg): PO** 220 mg (with ritonavir 32 mg) bid with food
- **Child 3 to <6 yr (10 kg): PO** 200 mg (with ritonavir 32 mg) bid with food

Available forms: Tabs 75, 150, 400, 600, 800 mg; oral susp 100 mg/ml

Administer:

- With food and ritonavir
- Tab should be swallowed whole

SIDE EFFECTS

CNS: *Headache, insomnia,* dizziness, somnolence

GI: *Diarrhea, abdominal pain, nausea, vomiting,* anorexia, dry mouth, hepatitis, hepatotoxicity, pancreatitis

GU: Nephrolithiasis

INTEG: Rash, angioedema, Stevens-Johnson syndrome, toxic epidermal necrolysis, exanthematous pustulosis

MS: Pain

OTHER: Asthenia, insulin-resistant hyperglycemia, hyperlipidemia, ketoacidosis, lipodystrophy

PHARMACOKINETICS

95% protein binding; metabolized by CYP3A; peak 2.5-4 hr; terminal half-life 15 hr; excreted in feces 79.5%, urine 13.9%

INTERACTIONS

⚠ Life-threatening dysrhythmias: ergots, midazolam, rifampin, pimozide, triazolam; do not use concurrently

Increase: myopathy, rhabdomyolysis—HMG-CoA reductase inhibitors (atorvastatin, lovastatin, simvastatin)
Increase: darunavir levels—CYP3A4 inhibitors (ketoconazole, itraconazole)
Increase: levels of both products—clarithromycin, zidovudine
Increase: levels of telapravir, rilpivarine, monitor for adverse reactions
Increase: side effects—(CYP3A4 substrate) artemether/lumefantrine
Decrease: darunavir levels—CYP3A4 inducers (carBAMazepine, phenytoin, fosphenytoin, PHENobarbital), rifamycins, fluconazole, nevirapine, efavirenz
Decrease: levels of oral contraceptives
Decrease: levels of both products—tenofovir, avoid concurrent use

Drug/Herb

Decrease: darunavir levels—St. John's wort; avoid concurrent use
Increase: myopathy, rhabdomyolysis risk—red yeast rice

Drug/Food

Increase: darunavir absorption

Drug/Lab Test

Increase: LFTs, bilirubin, uric acid, amylase, lipase
Decrease: WBC, neutrophils, platelets

NURSING CONSIDERATIONS

Assess:

- Complaints of lower back, flank pain; indicates kidney stones
- Signs of infection, anemia, the presence of other sexually transmitted diseases
- **Serious skin reactions:** angioedema, Stevens-Johnson syndrome, toxic epidermal necrolysis; discontinue immediately, notify prescriber
- **Hepatotoxicity:** hepatic studies (ALT, AST, bilirubin, amylase); all may be elevated in those with underlying liver disease; product should be discontinued in those with increased LFTs
- Viral load, CD4, HIV RNA during treatment
- Bowel pattern before, during treatment; if severe abdominal pain with bleeding occurs, product should be discontinued; monitor hydration
- **Hyperlipidemia:** cholesterol, triglycerides, LDL may be elevated; monitor serum cholesterol, lipid panel throughout treatment

Evaluate:

- Therapeutic response: decreased viral load, increased CD4 count

Teach patient/family:

- To use nonhormonal birth control; not to breastfeed
- To take as prescribed; if dose is missed, to take as soon as remembered up to 1 hr before next dose; not to double dose
- That product must be taken at same time of day to maintain blood levels for duration of therapy
- ⚠ That **hyperglycemia** may occur; to watch for increased thirst, weight loss, hunger, dry, itchy skin; to notify prescriber if these occur
- To increase fluids to prevent kidney stones; that if stone formation occurs, treatment may need to be interrupted
- That product does not cure AIDS, only controls symptoms; not to donate blood; not to share medication; to notify all health care providers of use; not to use with any other products without prescriber's approval

dasatinib (Rx)

(da-si′ti-nib)

Sprycel

Func. class.: Antineoplastic—miscellaneous
Chem. class.: Protein-tyrosine kinase inhibitor

ACTION: Inhibits a tyrosine kinase enzyme, thereby reducing cell growth in leukemia, inhibitor of BCR-ABL and imatinib-resistant mutations of BCR-ABL

USES: Treatment of accelerated, chronic blast phase CML or acute lymphoblastic leukemia (ALL); chronic phase CML with resistance or intolerance to prior therapy; Philadelphia chromosome–positive CML in chronic phase

CONTRAINDICATIONS:
Pregnancy (D), hypersensitivity

Precautions: Breastfeeding, children, geriatric patients, QT prolongation, infection, thrombocytopenia, accidental exposure, edema, infertility, lactase deficiency, neutropenia, anemia, autoimmune disease with immune reconstitution syndrome

DOSAGE AND ROUTES

Accelerated or myeloid/lymphoid blast phase CML with resistance/intolerance to prior therapy

- **Adult: PO** 140 mg daily titrated up to 180 mg daily in those resistant to therapy

Chronic phase CML with resistance/intolerance to prior therapy

- **Adult: PO** 100 mg daily either AM or PM

Dosage reduction for those taking a strong CYP3A4 inhibitor

- **Adult: PO** 20-40 mg daily

Available forms: Tabs 20, 50, 70, 80, 100, 140 mg

Administer:

- Do not break, crush, or chew tab
- After meal and with large glass of water
- Separate from antacids by 2 hr before and 2 hr after; do not use with H2 blockers and PPIs

SIDE EFFECTS

CNS: CNS hemorrhage, headache, dizziness, insomnia, neuropathy, asthenia

CV: Dysrhythmias, chest pain, CHF, pericardial effusion, congestive cardiomyopathy, decreased injection fraction, QT prolongation

GI: *Nausea,* vomiting, *anorexia, abdominal pain,* constipation, diarrhea, GI bleeding, muscositis, stomatitis, hepatotoxicity

HEMA: Neutropenia, thrombocytopenia, bleeding

INTEG: *Rash, pruritus,* alopecia

META: Fluid retention, edema, hypocalcemia, hypophosphatemia

MISC: Increased/decreased weight, infection, fatigue

MS: Pain, arthralgia, myalgia

RESP: Cough, dyspnea, pulmonary edema/hypertension, pneumonia, upper respiratory tract infection, pleural effusion

PHARMACOKINETICS

Metabolized by CYP3A4; 96% protein bound; peak 0.5-6 hr; excreted in feces (85%), small amount in urine (4%); terminal half-life 3-5 hr

INTERACTIONS

- Altered action of CYP3A4 substrates: alfentanil, cycloSPORINE, ergots, fentaNYL, pimozide, quiNIDine, sirolimus, tacrolimus

Increase: dasatinib concentrations—CYP3A4 inhibitors: ketoconazole, itraconazole, erythromycin, clarithromycin, nefazodone, protease inhibitors, telithromycin

Increase: myopathy, rhabdomyolysis-HMG-CoA reductase inhibitors (rare)

Increase: plasma concentrations of simvastatin

Increase: QT prolongation—class IA/III antidysrhythmics and other products that increase QT prolongation

Decrease: dasatinib concentrations—CYP3A4 inducers (dexamethasone, phenytoin, carBAMazepine, rifampin, PHENobarbital), H_2 blockers (famotidine), proton pump inhibitors (omeprazole)

Drug/Food

- Grapefruit: do not use

Drug/Herb

Decrease: dasatinib concentrations—St. John's wort

NURSING CONSIDERATIONS

Assess:

- **Myelosuppression:** ANC, platelets; in chronic phase, if ANC $<1 \times 10^9$/L and/or platelets $<50 \times 10^9$/L, stop until ANC $>1.5 \times 10^9$/L and platelets $>75 \times 10^9$/L; in accelerated phase/blast crisis, if ANC $<0.5 \times 10^9$/L and/or platelets $<10 \times 10^9$/L, determine whether cytopenia is related to biopsy/aspirate, if not, reduce dose by 200 mg, if cytopenia continues, reduce dose by another 100 mg; if cytopenia continues for 4 wk, stop product until ANC $\geq 1 \times 10^9$/L, monitor CBC weekly $\times$ 8 wk, then monthly

- **Hepatotoxicity:** monitor LFTs before treatment and monthly; if liver transaminases >5 × IULN, withhold until transaminase levels return to <2.5 × IULN
- **Signs of fluid retention, edema:** weigh, monitor lung sounds, assess for edema; some fluid retention is dose dependent, may result in CHF, congestive cardiomyopathy, decreased injection failure
- **QT Prolongation:** more common in those with hypokalemia, hypomagnesemia, congenital long QT syndrome, those taking products that prolong QT; correct electrolyte imbalances before use

Evaluate:

- Therapeutic response: decrease in leukemic cells or size of tumor

Teach patient/family:

- To report adverse reactions immediately: SOB, swelling of extremities, bleeding, bruising
- About reason for treatment, expected results
- To use contraception (pregnancy [D]); to avoid breastfeeding; men should use condoms
- To take at same time of day; not to crush or chew; not to use grapefruit juice

HIGH ALERT

DAUNOrubicin (Rx)

(daw-noe-roo′bi-sin)

Cerubidine

DAUNOrubicin citrate liposomal (Rx)

DaunoXome

Func. class.: Antineoplastic, antibiotic
Chem. class.: Anthracycline glycoside

Do not confuse:
DAUNOrubicin/DOXOrubicin

ACTION: Inhibits DNA synthesis, primarily; derived from *Streptomyces coerulorubidus;* replication is decreased by binding to DNA, binds DNA causing confirmational changes; a vesicant

USES: Acute lymphocytic leukemia (ALL), acute myelogenous leukemia (AML); *liposomal:* Kaposi's sarcoma
Unlabeled uses: *Liposomal:* AML, non-Hodgkin's lymphoma

CONTRAINDICATIONS: Pregnancy (D), breastfeeding, hypersensitivity, systemic infections, cardiac disease, bone marrow depression

Black Box Warning: IM/SUBCUT use

Precautions: Tumor lysis syndrome, MI, infection, thrombocytopenia, renal/hepatic disease; gout

Black Box Warning: Bone marrow suppression, cardiac disease, extravasation, renal failure, hepatic disease; requires a specialized care setting and an experienced clinician

DOSAGE AND ROUTES

Use decreased dose for those >60 yr

DAUNOrubicin

- **Adult:** IV 45-60 mg/m²/day × 3 days, then 2 days of subsequent courses in combination, max 400-600 mg/m² total cumulative dose
- **Child:** IV 30-40 mg/m²/day depending on cycle (AML); ≤2 yr or <0.5 m²: 1 mg/kg on day 1 weekly in combination with vinCRIStine and predniSONE, base dose on body weight not surface area (ALL); >2 yr or 0.5 m²: 25 mg/m² day 1 weekly in combination with vinCRIStine and predniSONE (ALL)

DAUNOrubicin citrate liposomal

- **Adult:** IV 40 mg/m² q2wk (Kaposi's sarcoma); IV 100-140 mg/m² q3wk (non-Hodgkin's lymphoma, unlabeled); IV escalating doses of 75, 100, 125, 135, 150 mg/m²/day × 3 days (AML, unlabeled)

Renal dose

- **Adult:** IV serum CCr >3 mg/dl, reduce dose by 50%

Hepatic dose

- **Adult:** IV serum bilirubin 1.2-3 mg/dl, reduce dose by 50%; bilirubin >3 mg/dl, reduce dose by 75%; bilirubin >5 mg/dl, omit dose

Available forms: Inj 20 mg powder/vial, *liposomal:* solution for inj 2 mg/ml

Administer:

- Antiemetic 30-60 min before giving product to prevent vomiting

Black Box Warning: To be used in a care setting with emergency equipment available

Black Box Warning: To be used by a clinician knowledgeable in cytotoxic therapy

Black Box Warning: Do not give by IM/subcut injection

IV route (Cerubidine)

Do not confuse with liposome

- Use cytotoxic handling precautions
- After diluting 20 mg/4 ml sterile water for inj (5 mg/ml), rotate, further dilute in 10-15 ml 0.9% NaCl; give over 3-5 min by direct IV through Y-tube or 3-way stopcock of infusion of D_5W or 0.9% NaCl; or dilute in 50 ml 0.9% NaCl and give over 10-15 min; or dilute in 100 ml and give over 30 min, may use premix vial 5 mg/ml
- Apply ice compress after stopping infusion for extravasation

Solution compatibilities: $D_{3.3}\%$/0.3% NaCl, D_5W, Normosol R, LR, 0.9% NaCl

Y-site compatibilities: Amifostine, anidulafungin, atenolol, bivalirudin, bleomycin, CARBOplatin, caspofungin, CISplatin, codeine, cyclophosphamide, cytarabine, DACTINomycin, DAPTOmycin, dexmedetomidine, etoposide, fenoldopam, filgrastim, gemcitabine, gemtuzumab, granisetron, melphalan, meperidine, methotrexate, nesiritide, octreotide, ondansetron, oxaliplatin, PACLitaxel, palonosetron, quinupristin-dalfopristin, riTUXimab, sodium acetate/bicarbonate, teniposide, thiotepa, tigecycline, trastuzumab, vinCRIStine, vinorelbine, voriconazole, zoledronic acid

IV route (DaunoXome)

- Dilute with D_5W to (1 mg/ml), give over 1-2 hr, do not use in-line filter, reconstituted sol may be stored ≤6 hr refrigerated; do not admix

IV compatibilities: Anidulafungin, bivalirudin, meperidine, octreotide, sodium acetate, tirofiban, trastuzumab

SIDE EFFECTS

DAUNOrubicin

CNS: Fever, chills

CV: CHF, pericarditis, myocarditis, peripheral edema, fatal myocarditis, left ventricular failure, QT prolongation, ST-T wave changes, QRS voltage changes, tachycardia, SVT, PVCs

GI: *Nausea, vomiting, anorexia, mucositis,* hepatotoxicity

GU: Impotence, sterility, amenorrhea, gynecomastia

HEMA: Thrombocytopenia, leukopenia, anemia

INTEG: *Rash,* extravasation, dermatitis, reversible alopecia, cellulitis, thrombophlebitis at inj site

SYST: Anaphylaxis, tumor lysis syndrome, secondary malignancies

DAUNOrubicin citrate liposomal

CNS: *Fatigue, headache,* depression, insomnia, dizziness, *malaise, neuropathy*

CV: Chest pain, edema

GI: Abdominal pain, stomatitis, *nausea, vomiting, diarrhea,* constipation

INTEG: *Alopecia, pruritus,* sweating

MISC: *Allergic reactions, chest pain, fever,* edema, flulike symptoms

MS: *Rigors,* arthralgia, back pain

RESP: *Cough, dyspnea, rhinitis, sinusitis*

PHARMACOKINETICS

Half-life 18½ hr, liposome 55½ hr; metabolized by liver; crosses placenta; excreted in breast milk, urine, bile

INTERACTIONS

Increase: QT prolongation, torsades de pointes—arsenic trioxide, chloroquine, clarithromycin, class IA, class III antidysrhythmics, dasatinib, dolasetron, droperidol, erythromycin, flecainide, haloperidol, methadone, ondansetron, palonosetron, pentamidine, some phenothiazines, propafenone, risperiDONE, sparfloxacin; tricyclic antidepressants (high doses); vorinostat, ziprasidone

Increase: bleeding risk—NSAIDs, salicylates, anticoagulants, platelet inhibitors, thrombolytics
Increase: toxicity—other antineoplastics, radiation, cyclophosphamide
Decrease: DAUNOrubicin effects—hematopoietic progenitor cells given within 24 hr
Decrease: antibody reaction—live virus vaccines

Drug/Lab Test
Increase: uric acid

NURSING CONSIDERATIONS

Assess:

Black Box Warning: Bone marrow suppression: CBC, differential, platelet count weekly, leukocyte nadir within 2 wk after administration, recovery within 3 wk; do not administer if absolute granulocyte count is <750/mm³ (liposome)

- **Acute renal failure, uric acid nephropathy:** renal studies: BUN, urine CCr, electrolytes, uric acid baseline before each dose; I&O ratio; report fall in urine output to <30 ml/hr; provide aggressive alkalinization of urine and use of allopurinol; can prevent urate nephropathy
- Monitor temperature q4hr; fever may indicate beginning infection
- **Hepatotoxicity:** monitor hepatic studies baseline before each dose: bilirubin, AST, ALT, alk phos; check for jaundice of skin, sclera; dark urine, clay-colored stools; itchy skin, abdominal pain, fever; diarrhea

Black Box Warning: Cardiac toxicity: chest x-ray, echocardiography, radionuclide angiography, MUGA, ECG; watch for ST-T wave changes, low QRS and QT prolongation, possible dysrhythmias (sinus tachycardia, heart block, PVCs); watch for CHF (jugular vein distention, weight gain, edema, crackles), may occur after 2-6 mo of treatment, cumulative dose (400-550 mg/m²), 450 mg/m² if used in combination with radiation, cyclophosphamide

- Bleeding: hematuria, guaiac stools, bruising, petechiae, mucosa, or orifices q8hr
- Effects of alopecia on body image; discuss feelings about body changes
- Buccal cavity q8hr for dryness, sores, ulceration, white patches, oral pain, bleeding, dysphagia, rinse mouth tid-qid with water, club soda; brush teeth bid-qid with soft brush or cotton-tipped applicators for stomatitis; use unwaxed dental floss
- **Tumor lysis syndrome:** hyperkalemia, hyperphosphatemia, hyperuricemia, hypocalcemia

Black Box Warning: Extravasation: swelling, pain, decreased blood return; if extravasation occurs, stop infusion, remove tubing, attempt to aspirate the drug before removing the needle, elevate area, treat with ice pack

- GI symptoms: frequency of stools, cramping
- Increase fluid intake to 2-3 L/day to prevent urate and calculi formation

Evaluate:

- Therapeutic response: decreased tumor size, spread of malignancy

Teach patient/family:

- To report signs of infection, bleeding, bruising, SOB, swelling, change in heart rate
- That hair may be lost during treatment; that wig or hairpiece may make patient feel better; that new hair may be different in color, texture
- To avoid pregnancy (D) while taking product and for 4 mo thereafter; not to breastfeed
- To avoid foods with citric acid, hot, or rough texture if stomatitis is present
- To report any bleeding, white spots, ulcerations in mouth; to examine mouth daily
- That urine and other body fluids may be red-orange for 48 hr
- To avoid vaccines, alcohol, aspirin, NSAIDs while taking this product
- To avoid crowds, those with known infections

RARELY USED

deferasirox (Rx)

(def-a′sir-ox)

Exjade

Func. class.: Heavy-metal chelating agent

USES: Chronic iron overload, transfusion hemosiderosis

CONTRAINDICATIONS: Breastfeeding, children, hypersensitivity, severe renal/hepatic disease, GI hemorrhage

DOSAGE AND ROUTES

• **Adult and child >2 yr: PO** 20-30 mg/kg/day; oral dispersion tablet is dissolved in water <1 g in 3.5 oz; >1 g in 7 oz or more; give on empty stomach at least 30 min before meals

degarelix

(day-gah-rel′iks)

Firmagon

Func. class.: Antineoplastic

Chem. class.: GnRH-receptor antagonist

ACTION: Reduces gonadotropins release and testicular steroidogenesis by reversibly binding to GnRH receptors

USES: Advanced prostate cancer

CONTRAINDICATIONS: Hypersensitivity, QT prolongation, osteoporosis, severe hepatic/renal disease, pregnancy (X), breastfeeding

• Precautions: CV disease, electrolyte abnormalities, geriatric patients

DOSAGE AND ROUTES

• **Adult (male): SUBCUT** 240 mg given as two 120-mg injections; (40 mg/ml concentrations) maintenance 80 mg (20 mg/ml concentrations) every 28 days, starting 28 days after first dose

Available forms: Injection 80, 120 mg vial

Administer:

• Do not give IV, subcut only

General reconstitution information:

• Use gloves, aseptic technique during preparation and administration

• Keep vials vertical at all times; do *not* shake the vials; give reconstituted drug within 1 hr after addition of sterile water for injection

Reconstitution of 120-mg vial (240-mg dose *only*):

• For a 240-mg dose, use two 120-mg vials; repeat for each 120-mg vial: draw up 3 ml of sterile water for injection with a 2-inch, 21-G needle; do not use bacteriostatic water for injection; inject the sterile water slowly into vial containing 120 mg; to maintain sterility, do not remove the syringe or the needle from the vial; keep the vial in an upright position and swirl gently; avoid shaking; reconstitution can take up to 15 min; tilt the vial slightly and withdraw 3 ml (40 mg/ml); avoid turning the vial upside down; repeat with a new vial, needle, and syringe for the second 120-mg dose (total dose = 240 mg)

Reconstitution of 80-mg vial:

• Draw up 4.2 ml of sterile water for injection with a 2-inch, 21-G needle; do not use bacteriostatic water for injection; inject the sterile water slowly into vial containing 80 mg; do not remove the syringe or the needle from the vial; keep the vial upright, swirl gently; avoid shaking; reconstitution can take up to 15 min; tilt vial slightly and withdraw 4 ml (20 mg/ml); avoid turning upside down during withdrawal

Subcut injection:

• Exchange the reconstitution needle with a 1.25-inch, 27-G needle; remove air bubbles; give in the abdominal region; rotate injection site periodically; use area not exposed to pressure; grasp the skin of abdomen, elevate the subcutaneous tissue, and insert the needle deeply at an angle ≥45 degrees; aspirate before injection; inject the dose subcut; when giving the loading dose of two 120-mg doses, the second dose should be injected at a different site

SIDE EFFECTS

CNS: Chills, dizziness, fatigue, fever, headache, insomnia

CV: Increased QT prolongation, hypotension, hot flashes, hypertension

GI: Diarrhea, constipation, nausea

GU: ED, UTI, gynecomastia, testicular atrophy

INTEG: Injection site reactions, pain at site, redness, swelling

MS: Back pain, decreased bone density

SYST: Hypersensitivity, anaphylaxis, angioedema

PHARMACOKINETICS

Peak 2 days, duration 50 days, half-life 53 days

INTERACTIONS

Increase: QT prolongation—Class IA/III antidysrhythmics, methyldopa, metoclopramide, reserpine

Drug/Lab Test

Increase: PSA, LFTs

Decrease: bone density test

NURSING CONSIDERATIONS

Assess:

QT prolongation: More common in those taking Class IA/III antidysrhythmics, heart failure, congenital long QT syndrome; monitor cardiac status at baseline and often thereafter

Anaphylaxis angioedema (rash, trouble breathing): Discontinue treatment and do not restart in serious reactions

• Liver function studies, PSA, GGT that may be elevated; bone density that may be decreased; electrolytes

Evaluate:

• Decreasing spread, size of tumor

Teach patient/family:

• To notify all prescribers of cardiac disease or use of all cardiac products

• Injection technique if patient/family will be giving product (provide patient information)

• **Pregnancy:** Notify prescriber if pregnancy is planned or suspected, pregnancy (X), do not breastfeed

delavirdine (Rx)

(de-la-veer′deen)

Rescriptor

Func. class.: Antiretroviral

Chem. class.: Nonnucleoside reverse transcriptase inhibitor (NNRTI)

ACTION:
Binds directly to reverse transcriptase; blocks RNA-, DNA-dependent polymerase activities, causing a disruption of the enzyme's site

USES:
HIV-1 in combination with at least 2 other antiretrovirals

CONTRAINDICATIONS:
Hypersensitivity

Precautions: Pregnancy (C), breastfeeding, children, hepatic disease, achlorhydria, antimicrobial resistance, exfoliative dermatitis, hepatitis, immune reconstitution syndrome

DOSAGE AND ROUTES

• **Adult and adolescent ≥16 yr: PO** 400 mg tid, max 1200 mg/day

Available forms: Tabs 100, 200 mg

Administer:

• 100-mg tab: dispersion by adding 4 tab/3-4 oz water, let stand, stir, swallow, rinse glass, swallow; use only 100-mg tabs for dispersion; 200-mg tab take as intact tab

• Do not give within 1 hr of antacids or didanosine

• Always use as combination therapy; this product is not recommended for initial treatment; due to inferior, virologic effect, it is no longer listed as part of any preferred regimens

SIDE EFFECTS

CNS: Headache, fatigue, anxiety, insomnia, fever
GI: Diarrhea, abdominal pain, nausea, anorexia, vomiting, dyspepsia, **hepatotoxicity**
GU: **Nephrotoxicity**
HEMA: **Neutropenia, leukopenia, thrombocytopenia, anemia, granulocytopenia**
INTEG: Rash, pruritus
MISC: Cough
MS: Pain, myalgia, **rhabdomyolysis**
SYST: **Stevens-Johnson syndrome; immune reconstitution syndrome (combination therapy)**

PHARMOCOKINETICS

98% protein bound, half-life 5.8 hr, peak 1 hr, duration 8 hr, extensively metabolized by CYP3A4, excreted in urine, feces

INTERACTIONS

Do not coadminister with nevirapine, efavirenz, rilpivirine, combined use not beneficial

⚠ **Serious life-threatening adverse reaction: amphetamines, ergots, benzodiazepines, calcium channel blockers, sedative/hypnotics, antidysrhythmics, sildenafil, pimozide, ALPRAZolam, astemizole, midazolam, opiates, triazolam**

Increase: levels of ALPRAZolam, clarithromycin, dapsone, ergots, felodipine, midazolam, NIFEdipine, indinavir, saquinavir, lovastatin, simvastatin, atorvastatin, other CYP3A4, 2D6 inhibitors

Increase: delavirdine levels—FLUoxetine, ketoconazole

Increase: levels of both products—quiNIDine, warfarin, clarithromycin

Decrease: delavirdine levels—antacids, anticonvulsants, rifamycins, protease inhibitors, didanosine, H2 blockers, PPIs

Decrease: action of oral contraceptives, didanosine

Drug/Herb

Decrease: delavirdine level—St. John's wort

NURSING CONSIDERATIONS

Assess:

- **HIV:** obtain hepatitis B virus (HBV) screening to ensure proper treatment, if coinfected, a fully suppressive antiretroviral regimen with products against both; CBC, blood chemistry, plasma HIV RNA, absolute CD41/CD81/cell counts/%, serum β_2 microglobulin, serum ICD124 antigen levels
- **Immune reconstitution syndrome: when treated with combination therapy; development of opportunistic infections (*Mycobacterium avium complex* [MAC], cytomegalovirus [CMV], *Pneumocystis carinii* pneumonia [PCP], TB)**
- Signs of infection, anemia
- Hepatic studies: ALT, AST; renal studies
- Bowel pattern before, during treatment; if severe abdominal pain with bleeding occurs, product should be discontinued; monitor hydration
- Allergies before treatment, reaction to each medication; place allergies on chart
- Plasma delavirdine concentrations (trough 10 micromolar)
- **Toxicity: severe nausea/vomiting, maculopapular rash**
- **Serious skin reactions: Stevens-Johnson syndrome; rash may occur within 1-3 wk of beginning treatment; if rash is not severe, manage with diphenhydrAMINE, hydrOXYzine, topical corticosteroids**

Evaluate:

- Therapeutic response: increased CD4 cell count, decreased viral load, improvement in symptoms of HIV

Teach patient/family:

- To take as prescribed; if dose is missed, to take as soon as remembered up to 1 hr before next dose; not to double dose, do not take antacids concurrently, separate by 1 hr
- That tabs may be dissolved in ½ cup of water (100 mg only); to stir; when dissolved, drink right away; to rinse cup with water and drink to get all medication
- To make sure health care provider knows about all medications being taken

• That if severe rash, mouth sores, swelling, aching muscles/joints, or eye redness occur, to notify health care provider
• Not to breastfeed if taking this product
• That this product is not a cure, only controls symptoms

denosumab (Rx)

(den-oh′sue-mab)

Prolia, Xgeva

Func. class.: Bone resorption inhibitor
Chem. class.: Monoclonal antibody, bone resorption

ACTION: Neutralizes activity of receptor activator nuclear factor kappa-B ligand (RANKL) by binding to it and blocking its interaction with cell-surface receptors; use of a RANKL inhibitor may reduce bone turnover and decrease tumor burden

USES: Osteoporosis in postmenopausal women or men at high risk for fractures; increase bone mass in men who are receiving androgen deprivation therapy for prostate cancer and women receiving aromastase inhibitor therapy for breast cancer at high risk for fractures; prevention of skeletal-related events in bone metastases from solid tumors (Xgeva), giant cell tumor of bone

CONTRAINDICATIONS: Hypersensitivity, hypocalcemia, pregnancy (Xgeva) D; (Prolina) X

Precautions: Breastfeeding, child/infant/neonate, anemia, coagulopathy, diabetes mellitus, dialysis, eczema, hypoparathyroidism, immunosuppression, latex hypersensitivity, malabsorption syndrome, neoplastic disease, pancreatitis, parathyroid disease, dental/renal/thyroid disease, TB, vit D deficiency

DOSAGE AND ROUTES

Postmenopausal osteoporosis (Prolia)
• **Adult female: SUBCUT** 60 mg q6mo with 1000 mg calcium and 400 international units vit D, max 60 mg q6mo

Bone metastases from solid tumors (Xgeva)
• **Adult: SUBCUT** 120 mg q4wk, max 120 mg q4wk; administer with calcium and vit D as necessary to prevent hypocalcemia

Giant cell tumor (bone) (Xgeva)
• **Adult: SUBCUT** 120 mg, then 120 mg q 4 wk on day 1, 8, 15, use calcium, vit D as needed

Available forms: Sol for inj 60 mg/ml (Prolia); 120 mg/1.7 ml (Xgeva)

Administer:

SUBCUT route
• Give acetaminophen before and for 72 hr after to decrease pain
• Do not use if particulate matter or discoloration is present; sol is clear and colorless to slightly yellow with small white/opalescent particles; remove from refrigerator and allow to warm to room temperature (15-30 min)
• **Use of prefilled syringe with needle safety guard:** leave green guard in original position until after administration; remove and discard needle cap immediately before inj; give by subcut inj in upper arm/thigh or abdomen; after inj, point needle away from people and slide green guard over needle
• **Use of single-use vials:** use 27-G needle; give in upper arm/thigh or abdomen; do not reinsert needle in vial; discard supplies as appropriate
• Store and use out of direct sunlight/heat; do not freeze; use within 14 days after removal from refrigerator; store unopened containers in refrigerator

SIDE EFFECTS

CNS: Chills, fever, flushing, headache, vertigo, neuropathic pain
CV: Angina, **atrial fibrillation**
GI: Abdominal pain, constipation, *diarrhea,* flatulence, GERD, *vomiting, nausea*

GU: Cystitis, lactation suppression
HEMA: Anemia, neutropenia
INTEG: Atopic dermatitis, pruritus
META: Hypercholesterolemia, hypocalcemia, hypophosphatemia
MS: Back, bone pain; MS pain, myalgia, osteonecrosis of the jaw, atypical low trauma femoral fractures
RESP: Cough, *dyspnea*
SYST: Infection, secondary malignancy

PHARMACOKINETICS

Terminal half-life 25.4 days, bioavailability 62%, max serum concentrations 3-21 days, steady state 6 mo

INTERACTIONS

Increase: infection, possible—immunosupressives, corticosteroids
Increase: osteonecrosis of the jaw, possible—antineoplastics, corticosteroids

NURSING CONSIDERATIONS

Assess:

- **Acute phase reaction:** fever, myalgia, headache, flulike symptoms for 72 hr after inj; usually resolves after 72 hr
- **Blood tests:** serum calcium, creatitine, BUN, magnesium, phosphate
- **Hypocalcemia (may be fatal):** paresthesia, twitching, laryngospasm, Chvostek's and Trouseau's signs; preexisting hypocalcemia should be corrected before treatment; patient with vit D deficiency may require higher doses of vit D
- **Hypercalcemia:** nausea, vomiting, anorexia, weakness, thirst, constipation, dysrhythmias
- **Dental status:** correct dental complications before product use; good oral hygiene should be maintained; if dental work is to be performed, antiinfectives should be given to prevent osteonecrosis of the jaw
- **Infection:** do not start treatment in patients with active infections; infections should be resolved first

Evaluate:

- Therapeutic response: increased/maintained bone density, decreased calcium levels

Teach patient/family:

- To report hypercalcemic relapse: nausea, vomiting, bone pain, thirst
- To continue with dietary recommendations, including additional Ca 1000 mg/day and vit D ≥400 units (Prolia product labeling)
- To avoid use during pregnancy and breastfeeding; to notify prescriber if pregnancy is planned, suspected
- To use acetaminophen before and for 72 hr after inj to lessen bone pain
- About the purpose of this product and its expected results
- To avoid OTC, Rx medications and herbs and supplements unless approved by prescriber
- To exercise regularly, stop smoking, and avoid alcohol to maintain bone health
- To inform all health care providers of product use; to avoid dental procedures/surgery if possible; to practice good oral hygiene
- That lab tests and follow-up exams will be required

desipramine (Rx)

(dess-ip′ra-meen)

Norpramin

Func. class.: Antidepressant, tricyclic
Chem. class.: Dibenzazepine, secondary amine

ACTION: Blocks reuptake of norepinephrine, serotonin into nerve endings, thereby increasing action of norepinephrine, serotonin in nerve cells

USES: Depression

Unlabeled uses: Chronic pain, postherpetic neuralgia, ADHD, bulimia, diabetic neuropathy, panic disorder, social phobia

CONTRAINDICATIONS: Hypersensitivity to tricyclics, carBAMazepine, closed-angle glaucoma, acute MI, MAOIs

Precautions: Pregnancy (C), breastfeeding, geriatric patients, severe depression, increased intraocular pressure, seizure disorder, CV disease, urinary retention, cardiac dysrhythmias, cardiac conduction disturbances, family history of sudden death, prostatic hypertrophy, thyroid disease

Black Box Warning: Children <18 yr, suicidal patients

DOSAGE AND ROUTES

Major depression

- **Adult: PO** 50-75 mg/day in 1-4 divided doses; titrate by 25-50 mg weekly up to 300 mg/day in single or divided doses (inpatient), 200 mg/day (outpatient)
- **Geriatric: PO** 25 mg/day at bedtime, titrate weekly; may increase to 150 mg/day
- **Adolescent: PO** 25-50 mg/day in divided doses; max 150 mg/day
- **Child 6-12 yr: PO** 1-3 mg/kg/day in divided doses; give >3 mg/kg/day with close medical monitoring; max 5 mg/kg/day

Bulimia nervosa (unlabeled)

- **Adult: PO** 25 mg tid; may titrate to 200 mg/day by 25-50 mg/day at weekly intervals

ADHD (unlabeled)

- **Child ≥5 yr: PO** up to 3.5 mg/kg/day divided bid

Neuropathic pain/postherpetic neuralgia (unlabeled)

- **Adult: PO** 10-25 mg at bedtime, titrate to relief

Diabetic neuropathy (unlabeled)

- **Adult: PO** 75-150 mg

Available forms: Tabs 10, 25, 50, 75, 100, 150 mg

Administer:

- Increased fluids, bulk in diet for constipation, especially in geriatric patients; with food or milk for GI symptoms; crushed if patient is unable to swallow medication whole
- Dosage at bedtime if oversedation occurs during day; may take entire dose at bedtime; geriatric patients may not tolerate once-daily dosing

SIDE EFFECTS

CNS: *Dizziness, drowsiness,* confusion, headache, anxiety, tremors, stimulation, weakness, insomnia, nightmares, EPS (geriatric patients), increased psychiatric symptoms, paresthenia, **suicidal ideation,** impaired memory, **seizures, serotonin syndrome**

CV: *Orthostatic hypotension,* **ECG changes,** *tachycardia, hypertension,* palpitations

EENT: *Blurred vision,* tinnitus, mydriasis, ophthalmoplegia

ENDO: SIADH

GI: *Diarrhea, dry mouth,* nausea, vomiting, **paralytic ileus,** increased appetite, cramps, epigastric distress, jaundice, **hepatitis,** stomatitis, constipation, weight gain

GU: *Retention,* **acute renal failure**

HEMA: **Agranulocytosis, thrombocytopenia, eosinophilia, leukopenia**

INTEG: Rash, urticaria, sweating, pruritus, photosensitivity

PHARMACOKINETICS

Well absorbed, widely distributed, protein binding 92%, extensively metabolized in the liver to active metabolite of imipramine, half-life 7-60 hr

INTERACTIONS

Increase: **serotonin syndrome, neuroleptic malignant syndrome—SSRIs, SNRIs, serotonin-receptor agonists, other tricyclic antidepressants**

Increase: CNS depression—alcohol, barbiturates, opioids, CNS depressants, skeletal muscle relaxants

Increase: desipramine level—cimetidine, diltiazem, fluvoxaMINE, FLUoxetine, PARoxetine, sertraline, verapamil

Increase: life-threatening B/P elevations; do not use concurrently—cloNIDine

Increase: **hypertension—EPINEPHrine, norepinephrine**

Increase: **hyperpyrexia, seizures, excitation; do not use within 14 days of MAOIs**

Increase: **QT interval—tricyclics, SUNItinib, vorinostat, ziprasidone, gatifloxacin,**

levofloxacin, moxifloxacin, sparfloxacin, class IA/III antidysrhythmics

Drug/Herb

Increase: serotonin syndrome, avoid concurrent use—St. John's wort

Increase: CNS depression—kava, valerian

Drug/Lab Test

Increase: serum bilirubin, blood glucose, alk phos

Decrease: sodium

NURSING CONSIDERATIONS

Assess:

- B/P (lying, standing), pulse q4hr; if systolic B/P drops 20 mm Hg, hold product, notify prescriber; take VS q4hr in patients with cardiovascular disease
- Hepatic studies: AST, ALT, bilirubin; thyroid function studies
- Weight weekly; appetite may increase with product
- **ECG** for flattening T wave, bundle branch block, AV block, dysrhythmias in cardiac patients
- **EPS** primarily in geriatric patients: rigidity, dystonia, akathisia
- **Seizure activity** in those with a history of seizures

Black Box Warning: Mental status: mood, sensorium, affect, **suicidal tendencies,** increase in psychiatric symptoms (depression, panic); this product is not indicated for children, monitor mental status baseline and during first few months of treatment

- Urinary retention, constipation; constipation most likely in children
- **Withdrawal symptoms:** headache, nausea, vomiting, muscle pain, weakness; not usual unless product discontinued abruptly
- Alcohol consumption; if consumed, hold dose until morning
- Check to confirm that PO medication is swallowed

Evaluate:

- Therapeutic response: decreased depression

Teach patient/family:

- That therapeutic effects may take 2-3 wk

Black Box Warning: That suicidal thoughts/behaviors may occur; to notify prescriber immediately

- To use caution when driving, performing other activities requiring alertness because of drowsiness, dizziness, blurred vision
- To avoid alcohol, other CNS depressants
- Not to discontinue medication abruptly after long-term use because this may cause nausea, headache, malaise
- To wear sunscreen or large hat because photosensitivity occurs

TREATMENT OF OVERDOSE:

ECG monitoring; lavage, activated charcoal; administer anticonvulsant

desirudin

(deh-sihr′uh-din)

Iprivask

Func. class.: Anticoagulant

Chem. class.: Thrombin inhibitor

ACTION: Selectively inhibits free and clot-bound thrombin, prevents activation of clotting factors

USES: Prevents DVT in hip-replacement surgery

Unlabeled uses: Acute MI, PTCA, unstable angina

CONTRAINDICATIONS: Hypersensitivity to this product, mannitol (diluent), hirudin, active bleeding, coagulation disorders

Precautions: Renal disease (CCr <60 ml/min), hepatic disease, GI/respiratory bleeding ≤ 3 mo, severe uncontrolled hypertension, spinal/epidural anesthesia, bacterial endocarditis, children, geriatric patients, inflammatory bowel disease, labor, organ biopsy, trauma, pregnancy (C)

Black Box Warning: Epidural anesthesia, lumbar puncture

DOSAGE AND ROUTES

• **Adult: SUBCUT** 15 mg every 12 hr × 9-12 days; give first dose 5-15 min before surgery and after induction if a regional block is used

Renal dose

• **Adult: SUBCUT** CCr 31-60 ml/min 5 mg q12hr; CCr < 31 ml/min 1.7 mg q12hr

Available forms: Inj 15 mg and mannitol 3% in water

Administer:

• Visually inspect particulate matter and discoloration before use; do not use sols that are cloudy or contain particles

• Do not use IM

Subcut route

• Do not mix with other injections, solvents, or parenteral fluids

• **Reconstitute** each vial with 0.5 ml of provided diluent; shake gently until the drug is fully reconstituted; the injection should be clear, colorless; once reconstituted, each 0.5 ml contains 15.75 mg desirudin; use immediately; however, it remains stable ≤24 hr at room temperature and protected from light; discard any unused solution

• **Subcut injection:** have patient sit or lie down; using a syringe with a 26- or 27-G needle, which is approximately 0.5 inch long, withdraw the entire reconstituted sol into the syringe; inject total volume subcut (unless renal dose); alternate between the left and right anterolateral and left and right posterolateral thigh or abdominal wall; insert whole length of the needle in a skin fold held between the thumb and forefinger; the skin fold should be held throughout the injection; to minimize bruising, do not rub the site, rotate sites

SIDE EFFECTS

CNS: Dizziness, fever

CV: **Thrombosis**, **thrombophlebitis**, hypotension

EENT: Nosebleeds, ocular bleeding

GI: **Hematemesis**, nausea, vomiting

GU: Hematuria

HEMA: **Hemorrhage**, anemia

MISC: **Anaphylaxis**, impaired healing, edema, inj site reaction

PHARMACOKINETICS

Onset ½ hr, 1-1½ hr, half-life 2 hr (12 hr in severe renal disease)

INTERACTIONS

Increase: bleeding risk—other anticoagulants, salicylates, NSAIDs, thrombolytics, glycoprotein IIb/IIIa antagonists, corticosteroids, dextran 40

Drug/Herb

Increase: bleeding risk—feverfew, garlic, ginger, ginkgo, horse chestnut

Drug/Lab Test

Decrease: Hct/Hgb

NURSING CONSIDERATIONS

Assess:

Bleeding:

• Gums, black tarry stools, hematuria, epistaxis, decreased Hct/Hgb, guiac-positive stools, bleeding from hip-replacement site, notify prescriber if these occur; observe for thrombosis, ecchymosis

• Monitor aPTT daily in those with bleeding risk, CCr <60 ml/min, aPTT should not be >2× control

Black Box Warning: Epidural/spinal anesthesia sites for hematomas; can result in irreversible paralysis

• CCr baseline and daily if CCr >60 ml/min

Evaluate:

• Decreased occurrence of DVT in hip-replacement surgery

Teach patient/family:

• To report any signs of bleeding

• To use a soft-bristle toothbrush to avoid bleeding gums, to use an electric razor

desloratadine (Rx)

(des′lor-at′ah-deen)

Clarinex, Clarinex RediTabs

Func. class.: Antihistamine, 2nd generation

Chem. class.: Selective histamine (H_1)-receptor antagonist

ACTION: Binds to peripheral histamine receptors, thus providing antihistamine action without sedation

USES: Seasonal/perennial allergic rhinitis, chronic idiopathic urticaria, pruritus

CONTRAINDICATIONS: Hypersensitivity, infants/neonates

Precautions: Pregnancy (C), breastfeeding, child, asthma, renal/hepatic impairment, phenylketonuria

DOSAGE AND ROUTES

- **Adult and child ≥12 yr: PO** 5 mg/day
- **Child 6-11 yr: PO** 2.5 mg/day
- **Child 2-5 yr: PO** 1.25 mg/day
- **Child 6-11 mo: PO** 1 mg/day (urticaria, only)

Hepatic/renal dose

- **Adult: PO** 5 mg every other day

Available form: Tabs 5 mg; orally disintegrating tabs 2.5, 5 mg (RediTabs); syr 0.5 mg/ml

Administer:

- Without regard to meals
- Do not remove RediTabs from blister until ready to use
- RediTabs directly on tongue; may take with or without water
- Use calibrated device for syrup

SIDE EFFECTS

CNS: Sedation (more common with increased doses), headache, psychomotor hyperactivity, seizures, fatigue, dizziness

GI: Hepatitis, nausea, dry mouth

MISC: Flulike symptoms, pharyngitis, myalgias

PHARMACOKINETICS

Onset antihistamine effect 1 hr, peak 1½ hr, elimination half-life 8½-28 hr, metabolized in liver to active metabolites, excreted in urine

INTERACTIONS

Increase: CNS depression (rare)—alcohol, opiates, sedative/hypnotics, H_1 blockers, antipsychotics, tricyclic antidepressants, anxiolytics

Increase: desloratadine—nilotinib, etravirine

NURSING CONSIDERATIONS

Assess:

- **Allergy:** hives, rash, rhinitis; monitor respiratory status; stop product 4 days before antigen skin test

Evaluate:

- Therapeutic response: absence of running or congested nose, other allergy symptoms

Teach patient/family:

- To avoid driving, other hazardous activities if drowsiness occurs; to use caution until product's effects are known
- That product may cause photosensitivity; to use sunscreen or stay out of the sun to prevent burns
- Not to exceed max dose, take without regard to meals
- To use RediTab by removing from pack and allow to dissolve on tongue, without regard to water

desmopressin (Rx)

(des-moe-press′in)

DDAVP, Minirin, Octostim ✱, Stimate

Func. class.: Pituitary hormone

Chem. class.: Synthetic antidiuretic hormone

ACTION: Promotes reabsorption of water by action on renal tubular epithelium; causes smooth muscle constriction, increase in plasma factor VIII levels, which increases platelet aggregation, thereby resulting in vasopressor effect; similar to vasopressin

USES: Hemophilia A, von Willebrand's disease type 1, nonnephrogenic diabetes insipidus, symptoms of polyuria/polydipsia caused by pituitary dysfunction, nocturnal enuresis

Unlabeled uses: Cardiopulmonary bypass, sickle cell disease, uremic bleeding, primary nocturnal enuresis (intranasal)

CONTRAINDICATIONS: Hypersensitivity, nephrogenic diabetes insipidus, severe renal disease, hyponatremia

Precautions: Pregnancy (B), breastfeeding, coronary artery disease, hypertension, cystic fibrosis, thrombus, electrolyte imbalances, male infertility

DOSAGE AND ROUTES

Primary nocturnal enuresis

- **Adult and child ≥6 yr: PO** 20 mcg at bedtime, max 0.6 mg at bedtime; **intranasal** 0.2 ml at bedtime, half in each nostril (unlabeled)

Diabetes insipidus

- **Adult: INTRANASAL** 10-40 mcg in divided doses (1-4 sprays with pump); **PO** Initially 0.05 mg bid, adjust based on diurnal pattern of response; usual range (0.1-1.2 mg)/day in 2-3 divided doses IV/SUBCUT 2-4 mcg/day or SUBCUT in 2 divided doses
- **Child 3 mo to 12 yr: INTRANASAL** 5-30 mcg in divided doses

Hemophilia/von Willebrand's disease

- **Adult and child >3 mo: IV** 0.3 mcg/kg in 0.9% NaCl over 15-30 min; may repeat if needed

Antihemorrhagic

- **Adult and child >3 mo: IV/SUBCUT** 0.2-0.4 mcg/kg/dose
- **Adult and child <50 kg: INTRANASAL** 1 spray in 1 nostril
- **Adult and child >50 kg:** 1 spray in each nostril

Cardiopulmonary bypass (unlabeled)

- **Adult: IV** 0.3 mcg/kg with aminocaproic acid given as a single postop dose

Sickle cell disease (unlabeled)

- **Adult: SUBCUT/IV** 0.3 mcg/kg with a high fluid intake

Uremic bleeding (unlabeled)

- **Adult: SUBCUT/IV** 0.3-0.4 mcg/kg as a single inj

Available forms: Inj 4 mcg/ml, rhinal tube delivery 2.5 mg/vial (0.1 mg/ml); tabs 0.1, 0.2 mg; nasal spray pump (DDAVP) 10 mcg/spray (0.1 mg/ml); nasal spray (Stimate) 1.5 mg/ml (150 mcg/dose)

Administer:

PO route

- Store at room temperature

Nasal route

- DDAVP and Stimate are not interchangeable
- Prime before 1st dose (press down 4 times), pump stays primed for 1 wk, to reprime, press down 1 time

Direct IV route

- Undiluted over 1 min for diabetes insipidus

Intermittent IV INFUSION route

- Diluted single dose/50 ml of 0.9% NaCl (adult and child >10 kg), single dose/10 ml as IV infusion over 15-30 min for von Willebrand's disease or hemophilia A
- Store in refrigerator

SIDE EFFECTS

CNS: Drowsiness, headache, lethargy, flushing, seizures

CV: Increased B/P, palpitations, tachycardia
EENT: Nasal irritation, congestion, rhinitis
GI: Nausea, heartburn, cramps
GU: Vulval pain
META: Hyponatremia, hyponatremia-induced seizures
SYST: Anaphylaxis (IV)

PHARMACOKINETICS

PO: Onset 1 hr, peak 4-7 hr
INTRANASAL: Onset 1 hr; peak 1-4 hr; duration 8-20 hr
IV: Onset 1 min, peak 1/2 hr, duration >3 hr

INTERACTIONS

Increase: antidiuretic action—carBAMazepine, chlorproPAMIDE, clofibrate, SSRIs, lamotrigine
Increase: pressor effect—pressor products
Decrease: antidiuretic action—lithium, alcohol, demeclocycline, heparin, large doses of EPINEPHrine

NURSING CONSIDERATIONS

Assess:

- Pulse, B/P when giving IV or SUBCUT
- I&O ratio, weight daily; check for edema in extremities; if water retention severe, diuretic may be prescribed
- **Water intoxication:** lethargy, behavioral changes, disorientation, neuromuscular excitability
- **Intranasal use:** nausea, congestion, cramps, headache; usually decreased with decreased dose; for nasal mucosa changes: congestion, edema, discharge, scarring (nasal route)

⚠ For severe allergic reaction, including **anaphylaxis (IV route)**, notify prescriber, discontinue use

- **Nocturnal enuresis:** identify how often enuresis is occurring, avoid use in those prone to water intoxication or sodium depletion
- Urine volume/osmolality and plasma osmolality (diabetes insipidus)
- Factor VIII coagulant activity, bleeding time before using for hemostasis
- **Nocturnal enuresis:** frequency of enuresis before and during treatment

Evaluate:

- Therapeutic response: absence of severe thirst, decreased urine output, decreased osmolality

Teach patient/family:

- About the proper technique for nasal instillation: to insert tube into nostril to instill product, clear nasal passage before use
- To avoid OTC products (cough, hay fever) because these preparations may contain EPINEPHrine, decrease product response; not to use with alcohol because adverse reactions may occur
- To wear emergency ID specifying therapy
- That, if dose is missed, to take when remembered up to 1 hr before next dose; not to double dose; to avoid fluids from 1 hr to up to 8 hr after PO dose
- To report upper respiratory infection, nasal congestion to prescriber
- How to use subcut, rotate sites

desonide topical

See Appendix B

desoximetasone

(dess-ox′ee-met′ah-sone)

Topicort, Topicort Spray

Func. class.: Corticosteroid, topical

ACTION: Crosses cell membrane to attach to receptors to decrease inflammation, itching; inhibits multiple inflammatory cytokines

USES: Inflammation/itching of corticosteroid-responsive dermatoses on the skin; spray-plaque psoriasis

CONTRAINDICATIONS: Hypersensitivity, use of some preparations on face, axilla, groin, intertriginous areas; monotherapy in primary bacterial infection, TB

Precautions: Pregnancy (C), breastfeeding, children, skin infections, Cushing syndrome

DOSAGE AND ROUTES

Adult/child >10 yr:

- Apply to affected areas 2 times/day

Available forms: Cream 0.05%, 0.25%; ointment 0.05%, 0.25%; gel 0.05%; spray 0.25%

Administer:

Topical route

⚠ Do not use with occlusive dressings

- **Cream/ointment/lotion:** apply sparingly in a thin film and rub gently into the cleansed, affected area
- **Gel:** apply sparingly in a thin film and rub gently into the cleansed, affected area
- **Spray:** discard after 30 days; keep away from heat/flame; store at room temperature

SIDE EFFECTS

INTEG: Burning, folliculitis, pruritus, dermatitis, maceration

MISC: Hyperglycemia, glycosuria, systemic absorption, hypothalamic-pituitary-adrenal (HPA) axis suppression, Cushing syndrome

NURSING CONSIDERATIONS

Assess:

- Skin reactions: burning pruritus, folliculitis, dermatitis
- **Systemic absorption:** HPA suppression and possible adrenocortical insufficiency after stopping treatment

Evaluate:

- Decreasing itching, inflammation on the skin

Teach patient/family:

Topical route

⚠ Not to use with occlusive dressings

- **Cream/ointment/lotion:** apply sparingly in a thin film and rub gently into the cleansed, affected area
- **Gel:** apply sparingly in a thin film and rub gently into the cleansed, affected area
- **Spray:** discard after 30 days; keep away from heat/flame; store at room temperature

desvenlafaxine

Khedezla, Pristiq

Func. class.: Antidepressant, serotonin-receptor norepinephrine reuptake inhibitor (SNRI)

ACTION: May work by blocking the central presynaptic reuptake of 5-HT and NE, resulting in an increased sustained level of these neurotransmitters

USES: Major depressive disorder

Unlabeled uses: Vasomotor symptoms (hot flashes) associated with menopause

CONTRAINDICATIONS: Hypersensitivity to this product or venlafaxine, MAOI therapy

Precautions: CNS depression, abrupt discontinuation, hypertension, hepatic/renal disease, hyponatremia, geriatric patients, pregnancy (C), labor and delivery, breastfeeding, angina, bleeding, cardiac dysrhythmias, MI, stroke, mania, hypovolemia, dehydration, increased intraocular pressure

Black Box Warning: Children, suicidal ideation

DOSAGE AND ROUTES

- **Adult: PO** Initially, 50 mg/day; max 400 mg/day with adjustments as needed

Renal dose

- **Adult: PO** CCr 30-50 ml/min 50 mg daily; CCr < 30 ml/min or end stage renal disease 50 mg q other day

Available forms:

Extended release tabs 50, 100 mg

Administer:
- Without regard to food; food may minimize GI symptoms
- Extended release tab: do not crush, break, or chew
- Store at room temperature

SIDE EFFECTS

CNS: *Dizziness,* drowsiness, *headache,* tremor, paresthesias, asthenia, suicidal thoughts/behaviors, seizures, fatigue, chills, yawning, hot flashes, flushing, *irritability, insomnia, anxiety, abnormal dreams, fatigue*
CV: Palpitations, sinus tachycardia, increased blood pressure, orthostatic hypotension
EENT: Blurred vision, mydriasis, tinnitus, bruxism
GI: *Nausea,* xerostomia, *diarrhea,* constipation, vomiting, anorexia, weight loss, dysgeusia, hypercholesterolemia, hypertriglyceridemia
GU: Urinary retention/hesitancy, orgasm dysfunction, decreased libido, impotence, proteinuria
HEMA: Impaired platelet aggregation
INTEG: Photosensitivity, hyperhidrosis, diaphoresis, rash
SYST: Serotonin syndrome, neuroleptic malignant syndrome–like symptoms, toxic epidermal necrolysis, Stevens-Johnson syndrome, erythema multiforme, angioedema; neonatal abstinence syndrome (fetal exposure)

PHARMACOKINETICS

Protein binding 30%, elimination half-life 11 hr; elimination half-life is increased (hepatic/renal disease)

INTERACTIONS

Increase: serotonin syndrome, neuroleptic malignant syndrome–like reactions—SSRIs, other SNRIs, serotonin receptor agonists (almotriptan, eletriptan, frovatriptan, naratriptan, rizatriptan, SUMAtriptan, ZOLMitriptan), tricyclics, traZODone, sibutramine, SUMAtriptan, ergots, lithium, nefazodone, meperidine, phentermine, MAOIs, dextromethorphan, linezolid, promethazine, methylphenidate, dexmethylphenidate, mirtazapine, pentazocine, tryptophan, methylene blue IV; do not administer concurrently
Increase: bleeding risk—salicylates, thrombolytics, NSAIDs, platelet inhibitors, anticoagulants
Increase: CNS depression—alcohol, opioids, antihistamines, sedatives/hypnotics
Increase: hallucinations, delusions, disorientation—zolpidem

Drug/Herb
Increase: desvenlafaxine action—kava, valerian

Drug/Lab Test
Increase: sodium, cholesterol, triglycerides
False positive: amphetamine, phencyclidine

NURSING CONSIDERATIONS

Assess:

Black Box Warning: Suicidal thoughts/behaviors: mental status and mood; identify suicidal ideation

- **Serotonin syndrome, neuroleptic malignant syndrome–like symptoms:** assess for nausea/vomiting, sedation, dizziness, diaphoresis (sweating), facial flush, hallucinations, mental status changes, myoclonia, restlessness, shivering, elevated blood pressure, hyperthermia, muscle rigidity, autonomic instability, mental status changes; if serotonin syndrome occurs, discontinue desvenlafaxine and any other serotonergic agents
- Monitor B/P baseline and periodically during treatment, lipid levels, signs of glaucoma
- Appetite and nutritional intake, weight loss is common, change diet as need to support weight

Evaluate:
- Decreased depression, increased sense of well-being, renewed interest in activities

Teach patient/family:
- To take as directed, not to double or skip doses; if a dose is missed, take as soon as remembered unless close to next dose; do not discontinue abruptly, decrease gradually

Black Box Warning: To report immediately suicidal thoughts/behaviors; have family members look for symptoms of suicidal ideation

- Not to operate machinery or engage in hazardous activities until reaction is known, may cause dizziness, drowsiness
- To avoid all other products unless approval by prescriber
- To report if pregnancy is planned or suspected (pregnancy [C]) or if breastfeeding
- To report immediately allergic reactions, including rash, hives, difficulty breathing, or swelling of face, lips
- That continuing follow-up exams will be needed

dexamethasone (Rx)
(dex-ah-meth′a-sone)

Dexasone ✤

dexamethasone sodium phosphate (Rx)

Func. class.: Corticosteroid, synthetic
Chem. class.: Glucocorticoid, long acting

Do not confuse:
Decadron/Percodan

ACTION: Decreases inflammation by suppression of migration of polymorphonuclear leukocytes, fibroblasts, reversal of increased capillary permeability and lysosomal stabilization, suppresses normal immune response, no mineralocorticoid effects

USES: Inflammation, allergies, neoplasms, cerebral edema, septic shock, collagen disorders, dexamethasone suppression test for Cushing syndrome, adrenocortical insufficiency, TB, meningitis, acute exacerbations of MS

CONTRAINDICATIONS: Hypersensitivity to corticosteroids, sulfites, or benzyl alcohol; fungal infections, abrupt discontinuation, coagulopathy, ulcerative colitis, seizure disorders

Precautions: Pregnancy (C), breastfeeding, diabetes mellitus, osteoporosis, seizure disorders, ulcerative colitis, CHF, myasthenia gravis, renal disease, peptic ulcer, esophagitis, recent MI, hypertension, TB, active hepatitis, psychosis, sulfite hypersensitivity, thromboembolic disorders

DOSAGE AND ROUTES

Inflammation
- **Adult: PO** 0.75-9 mg/day in divided doses q6-12hr or phosphate **IM** 0.5-9 mg/day divided q6-12hr
- **Child: PO** 0.024-0.34 mg/kg/day in divided doses q6-12hr

Anaphylactic shock
- **Adult: IV** (phosphate) single dose 1-6 mg/kg or **IV** 40 mg q2-6hr as needed up to 72 hr

Cerebral edema
- **Adult: IV** (phosphate) 10 mg, then 4-6 mg **IM** q6hr × 2-4 days, then taper over 1 wk
- **Child:** loading dose 1-2 mg/kg **(PO/IM/IV)**, then 1-1.5 mg/kg/day, max 16 mg/day divided q4-6hr for 2-4 days, then taper down weekly

Adrenocortical insufficiency
- **Adult: PO** 0.75-9 mg/day in divided doses
- **Child: PO** 0.03-0.3 mg/kg/day in 2-4 divided doses

Suppression test
- **Adult: PO** 1 mg at 11 PM or 0.5 mg q6hr × 48 hr

ARDS (unlabeled)
- **Adult: IM/IV** (phosphate) 0.5-9 mg/day in 2-4 divided doses
- **Child: IM/IV** 0.06-0.3 mg/kg/day or 1.2-10 mg/m^2 in divided doses q6-12hr

Bone pain (unlabeled)
- **Adult: PO/IV** 12-20 mg/day in divided doses

Pediatric bacterial meningitis (unlabeled)
- **Child and infant >2 mo: IV** 0.15 mg/kg qid × first 2 days of antibiotics

Available forms: Dexamethasone: tabs 0.5, 0.75, 1, 1.5, 2, 4, 6 mg; elix 0.5 mg/5 ml; oral sol 0.5 mg/5 ml, 1 mg/1 ml; **sodium phosphate:** 4, 10 mg/ml; ophth implant 0.7 mg; ophth susp drops/solution 0.1%

Administer:

PO route
- Titrated dose; use lowest effective dose
- With food or milk to decrease GI symptoms, give once daily in AM for less toxicity, fewer adverse reactions

IM route
- IM inj deeply in large muscle mass; rotate sites; avoid deltoid; use 21-G needle
- In 1 dose in AM to prevent adrenal suppression; avoid SUBCUT administration, may damage tissue

Direct IV route (sodium phosphate)
- Undiluted direct over ≤1 min

Intermittent IV INFUSION route
- Diluted with 0.9% NaCl or D_5W, give as IV infusion at prescribed rate

Dexamethasone sodium phosphate

Syringe compatibilities: Acetaminophen, caffeine, dimenhydrAMINE, furosemide, granisetron, hyaluronidase, ketamine, metoclopramide, octreotide, oxyCODONE, palonosetron, ranitidine, salbutamol, SUFentanil, traMADol

Y-site compatibilities: Acetaminophen, acyclovir, alfentanil, allopurinol, amifostine, amikacin, aminocaproic acid, aminophylline, amphotericin B cholesteryl, amphotericin B lipid complex, amphotericin B liposome, amsacrine, anidulafungin, argatroban, ascorbic acid injection, atenolol, atracurium, atropine, aztreonam, benztropine, bivalirudin, bleomycin, bumetanide, buprenorphine, butorphanol, caffeine, CARBOplatin, carmustine, ceFAZolin, cefepime, cefmetazole, cefonicid, cefotaxime, cefoTEtan, cefOXitin, cefpirome, ceftaroline, cefTAZidime, ceftizoxime, cefTRIAXone, chloramphenicol, cimetidine, cisatracurium, CISplatin, cladribine, clindamycin, codeine, cyanocobalamin, cyclophosphamide, cycloSPORINE, cytarabine, DACTINomycin, DAPTOmycin, DAUNOrubicin, dexmedetomidine, digoxin, diltiazem, DOCEtaxel, DOPamine, doripenem, doxacurium, DOXOrubicin, DOXOrubicin liposomal, enalaprilat, ePHEDrine, EPINEPHrine, epoetin alfa, eptifibatide, ertapenem, etoposide, etoposide phosphate, famotidine, fentaNYL, filgrastim, fluconazole, fludarabine, fluorouracil, folic acid, fosaprepitant, foscarnet, furosemide, ganciclovir, gatifloxacin, gemcitabine, glycopyrrolate, granisetron, heparin, hydrocortisone, HYDROmorphone, ifosfamide, imipenem-cilastatin, indomethacin, insulin (regular), irinotecan, isoproterenol, ketorolac, lansoprazole, leucovorin, levofloxacin, lidocaine, linezolid, liposome, LORazepam, LR, mannitol, mechlorethamine, melphalan, meropenem, metaraminol, methadone, methicillin, methoxamine, methyldopate, methylPREDNISolone, metoclopramide, metoprolol, metroNIDAZOLE, mezlocillin, miconazole, milrinone, morphine, multiple vitamins injection, nafcillin, nalbuphine, naloxone, nitroglycerin, nitroprusside, norepinephrine, octreotide, ondansetron, oxacillin, oxaliplatin, oxyCODONE, oxytocin, PACLitaxel, palonosetron, pamidronate, pancuronium, PEMEtrexed, penicillin G potassium/sodium, PENTobarbital, PHENobarbital, phenylephrine, phytonadione, piperacillin, piperacillin-tazobactam, potassium chloride, procainamide, propofol, propranolol, pyridoxine, ranitidine, remifentanil, Ringer's, ritodrine, riTUXimab, sargramostim, sodium acetate/bicarbonate, succinylcholine, SUFentanil, tacrolimus, telavancin, teniposide, theophylline, thiamine, thiotepa, ticarcillin, ticarcillin-clavulanate, tigecycline, tirofiban, TNA, tolazoline, topotecan, trastuzumab, urokinase, vancomycin, vasopressin, vecuronium, verapamil, vinCRIStine, vinorelbine, vitamin B complex/C, voriconazole, zidovudine, zoledronic acid

SIDE EFFECTS

CNS: *Depression, flushing, sweating,* headache, mood changes, euphoria, psychosis, **seizures**, insomnia, **pseudotumor cerebri**

CV: *Hypertension,* **circulatory collapse**, tachycardia, edema, cardiomyopathy, **thromboembolism, heart failure, dysrhythmias**

EENT: Fungal infections, increased intraocular pressure, blurred vision, cataracts, glaucoma

ENDO: HPA suppression, hyperglycemia, sodium, fluid retention

GI: *Diarrhea, nausea, abdominal distention,* **GI hemorrhage,** *increased appetite,* **pancreatitis**

HEMA: **Thrombocytopenia,** transient leukocytosis, **thromboembolism**

INTEG: Acne, poor wound healing, ecchymosis, petechiae, hirsutism, **angioedema**

META: Hypokalemia

MS: Fractures, osteoporosis, weakness, arthralgia, myopathy

PHARMACOKINETICS

Half-life 1-2 days

PO: Onset 1 hr, peak 1-2 hr, duration $2^1/_2$ days

IM: Duration 2 days-3 wk

INTERACTIONS

Increase: toxicity—cycloSPORINE

Increase: side effects—alcohol, salicylates, amphotericin B, digoxin, cycloSPORINE, diuretics, NSAIDs

Increase: dexamethasone action—salicylates, estrogens, indomethacin, hormonal contraceptives, ketoconazole, macrolide antiinfectives, NSAIDs

Increase: tendinitis, tendon rupture risk—quinolones

Increase: effect of—antidiabetics

Decrease: dexamethasone action—cholestyramine, colestipol, barbiturates, rifampin, ePHEDrine, phenytoin, theophylline, antacids, bosentan, carBAMazepine, ethotoin

Decrease: anticoagulant effect—anticonvulsants, antidiabetics, ambenonium, neostigmine, isoniazid, toxoids, vaccines, anticholinesterases, salicylates, somatrem

Decrease: potassium levels—thiazide/loop diuretics, amphotericin B

Drug/Lab Test

Increase: cholesterol, sodium, blood glucose, uric acid

Decrease: calcium, potassium, T_4, T_3, thyroid ^{131}I uptake test, urine 17-OHCS, 17-KS, PBI

False negative: skin allergy tests

NURSING CONSIDERATIONS

Assess:

- Potassium, blood, urine glucose while receiving long-term therapy; hypo/hyperglycemia
- Weight daily; notify prescriber of weekly gain >5 lb
- B/P, pulse; notify prescriber of chest pain
- I&O ratio; be alert for decreasing urinary output, increasing edema
- **Epidural injections (unlabeled): may cause rare events (vision loss, paralysis, stroke, death)**
- **Cushingoid symptoms: assess for buffalo hump, moon face, increased B/P; monitor; plasma cortisol levels during long-term therapy (normal: 138-635 nmol/L SI units when drawn at 8 AM); prolonged use can cause cushingoid symptoms**
- **Infection:** fever, WBC even after withdrawal of medication; product masks infection
- **Potassium depletion:** paresthesias, fatigue, nausea, vomiting, depression, polyuria, dysrhythmias, weakness
- Edema, hypertension, cardiac symptoms
- **Mental status:** affect, mood, behavioral changes, aggression
- **Abrupt withdrawal: acute adrenal insufficiency and death may occur following**

abrupt discontinuation of systemic therapy; withdraw gradually

Evaluate:

- Therapeutic response: decreased inflammation

Teach patient/family:

- That ID as corticosteroid user should be carried
- To contact prescriber if surgery, trauma, stress occurs because dose may need to be adjusted
- To notify prescriber if therapeutic response decreases because dosage adjustment may be needed
- To take with food or milk
- That bruising may occur easily
- That if on long-term therapy, a high-protein diet may be needed

⚠ Not to discontinue abruptly because **adrenal crisis** can result

- About symptoms of adrenal insufficiency: nausea, anorexia, fatigue, dizziness, dyspnea, weakness, joint pain
- To avoid OTC products: salicylates, alcohol in cough products, cold preparations unless directed by prescriber
- About all aspects of product usage, including cushingoid symptoms; to notify health care provider of infection
- To avoid exposure to chickenpox or measles, persons with infection

dexamethasone (ophthalmic)

(dex-a-meth′a-sone)

Maxidex

Func. class.: Ophthalmic antiinflammatory

Chem. class.: Corticosteroid

Do not confuse:
dexamethasone/desoximetasone

ACTION: Exact mechanism of antiinflammatory action unknown; inhibits multiple inflammatory cytokines; decreases inflammation, collagen deposits, capillary dilation, edema

USES: Treatment of corticosteroid-responsive ophthalmic disorders

CONTRAINDICATIONS: Hypersensitivity to this product or sulfites, ocular TB, acute herpes simplex (superficial), fungal/viral infections of the eye, posterior lens capsule rupture

Precautions: Corneal infected abrasions, glaucoma, pregnancy (C), breastfeeding, migration of intravitreal implant risk, children

DOSAGE AND ROUTES

Corticosteroid-responsive ophthalmic disorders including allergic conjunctivitis (not controlled topically), allergic marginal corneal ulcer, anterior segment inflammation, chorioretinitis, cyclitis, Graves' ophthalmopathy, giant papillary conjunctivitis (GPC), ophthalmic herpes zoster (herpes zoster ophthalmicus, herpes zoster keratitis), iritis, keratitis, superficial punctate keratitis, postoperative ocular inflammation, optic neuritis, diffuse choroiditis, sympathetic ophthalmia, vernal keratoconjunctivitis, corneal injury (corneal abrasion):

- **Adult:** Instill 1 or 2 drops of 0.1% ophthalmic sol or susp every hr during the day and every 2 hr at night; reduce application to every 4 hr after response occurs

Available forms: Ophthalmic solution, suspension 0.1%

Administer:

- For ophthalmic use only
- Instruct patient on proper instillation of eye ointment or solution; do not touch the tip of the dropper to the eye, fingertips, or other surface; wait ≥15 min before inserting soft contact lens

SIDE EFFECTS

EENT: Burning, stinging, poor vision, corneal ulcerations, increased IOP, optic nerve damage

NURSING CONSIDERATIONS

Assess:

- **Corneal effects:** ulcerations, infections can worsen with this product

Evaluate:

- Decreased corneal inflammation

Teach patient/family:

- How to use products
- Not to share with others or use for other conditions
- To notify prescriber immediately if vision changes or if condition worsens
- To take as prescribed

dexlansoprazole (Rx)

(dex-lan-so-prey′zole)

Dexilant

Func. class.: Antiulcer, proton-pump inhibitor

Chem. class.: Benzimidazole

ACTION: Suppresses gastric secretion by inhibiting hydrogen/potassium ATPase enzyme system in gastric parietal cell; characterized as gastric acid pump inhibitor because it blocks final step of acid production

USES: Gastroesophageal reflux disease (GERD), severe erosive esophagitis, heartburn

CONTRAINDICATIONS: Hypersensitivity

Precautions: Pregnancy (B), breastfeeding, children, proton-pump hypersensitivity, gastric cancer, hepatic disease, vit B_{12} deficiency, colitis

DOSAGE AND ROUTES

Erosive esophagitis

- **Adult: PO** 60 mg daily for up to 8 wk; maintenance: **PO** 30 mg daily for up to 6 mo

GERD

- **Adult: PO** 30 mg daily × 4 wk

Hepatic disease

- **Adult: PO** (Child-Pugh B): max 30 mg/day

Available forms: Del rel caps 30, 60 mg

Administer:

- Swallow caps whole; do not crush, chew caps; caps may be opened, contents sprinkled on food, use immediately; do not chew contents of capsule; give without regard to food

D

SIDE EFFECTS

CNS: Headache, dizziness, confusion, agitation, amnesia, depression, anxiety, seizures, insomnia, migraine

CV: Chest pain, angina, bradycardia, palpitations, CVA, hypertension, MI

EENT: Tinnitus

GI: Diarrhea, abdominal pain, vomiting, nausea, constipation, flatulence, colitis, dysgeusia, **pseudomembranous colitis**

HEMA: Anemia, **neutropenia, thrombocytopenia, pernicious anemia, thrombosis**

INTEG: Rash, urticaria, pruritus

META: Gout

MS: Arthralgia, mylagia

RESP: Upper respiratory infections, cough, epistaxis, dyspnea, **pneumonia**

SYST: Anaphylaxis, Stevens-Johnson syndrome, toxic epidermal necrolysis, exfoliative dermatitis

PHARMACOKINETICS

Absorption 57%-64%; plasma half-life 1-2 hr; protein binding 96.1%-98.8%; extensively metabolized in liver; excreted in urine, feces; clearance decreased in geriatric patients, renal/hepatic impairment; peak dual 1-2 hr, 4-5 hr

INTERACTIONS

Increase: dexlansoprazole effect—CYP2C19, 3A4 inhibitors (fluvoxaMINE, voriconazole)

- Dexlansoprazole absorption: sucralfate

Decrease: absorption of ketoconazole, itraconazole, iron, delavirdine, ampicillin, calcium carbonate

Drug/Lab Test
Increase: LFTs, bilirubin, creatinine, glucose, lipids
Decrease: platelets, magnesium

NURSING CONSIDERATIONS

Assess:

- **Pseudomembranous colitis:** diarrhea, abdominal cramps, fever, report to prescriber promptly
- **Hepatotoxicity (rare):** hepatitis, jaundice, monitor hepatic studies (AST, ALT, alk phos) if hepatic adverse reactions occur
- **Hypomagnesemia:** usually 3 mo to 1 yr after beginning therapy; monitor magnesium level, assess for irregular heartbeats, muscle spasms; in children, fatigue, upset stomach, dizziness; magnesium supplement may be used
- **Anaphylaxis (rare), serious skin disorders:** require emergency intervention

Evaluate:

- Therapeutic response: absence of epigastric pain, swelling, fullness; healing of erosive esophagitis

Teach patient/family:

- **Pseudomembranous colitis:** report to prescriber at once abdominal cramps, bloody diarrhea, fever
- That diabetic patient should know that hypoglycemia may occur
- To avoid hazardous activities; dizziness may occur
- To avoid alcohol, salicylates, ibuprofen; may cause GI irritation
- To report allergic reactions, symptoms of low magnesium levels
- To notify prescriber if pregnancy is planned or suspected; not to breastfeed
- To swallow cap whole, not to chew, crush, to report all products being used to prescriber

dexmethylphenidate (Rx)

(dex′meth-ul-fen′ih-dayt)

Focalin, Focalin XR

Func. class.: Central nervous system (CNS) stimulant, psychostimulant

Controlled Substance Schedule II

Do not confuse:
dexmethylphenidate/methylphenidate

ACTION: Increases release of norepinephrine and DOPamine into the extraneuronal space; also blocks the reuptake of norepinephrine and DOPamine into the presynaptic neuron; mode of action for treating attention-deficit/hyperactivity disorder (ADHD) is unknown

USES: ADHD

CONTRAINDICATIONS: Hypersensitivity to methylphenidate, anxiety, history of Gilles de la Tourette's syndrome, tics, glaucoma, concurrent treatment with MAOIs or within 14 days of discontinuing treatment with MAOIs
Precautions: Pregnancy (C), hypertension, depression, seizures, CV disorders, breastfeeding, child <6 yr, geriatric patients, psychosis, thyrotoxicosis

Black Box Warning: Substance abuse, alcoholism

DOSAGE AND ROUTES

- **Adult/adolescent/child >6 yr: PO** 2.5 mg bid with doses at least 4 hr apart, gradually increase to a maximum of 20 mg/day (10 mg bid); for those taking methylphenidate, use 1/2 of methylphenidate dose initially, then increase as needed to a max of 20 mg/day
- **Adolescent and child ≥6 yr: EXT REL** 5 mg/day, may adjust to 20 mg/day in 5-mg increments, max 30 mg/day

• **Adult: PO EXT REL** 10 mg/day, may adjust to 20 mg/day in 10-mg increments, max 40 mg/day

Available forms: Tabs 2.5, 5, 10 mg; ext rel caps 5, 10, 15, 20, 25, 30, 35, 40 mg

Administer:

• Twice daily at least 4 hr apart; ext rel once a day; in the morning, ext rel cap may be opened and contents sprinkled onto applesauce and consumed without chewing

• Without regard to meals

• Do not break, crush, or chew ext rel product

• Med guide should be provided by dispenser

SIDE EFFECTS

CNS: Dizziness, headache, drowsiness, nervousness, insomnia, **toxic psychosis, neuroleptic malignant syndrome (rare),** Tourette's syndrome

CV: Palpitations, B/P changes, angina, **dysrhythmias, tachycardia, MI, stroke**

GI: *Nausea, anorexia,* abnormal hepatic function, **hepatic coma,** *abdominal pain*

HEMA: **Leukopenia, anemia, thrombocytopenic purpura**

INTEG: **Exfoliative dermatitis,** urticaria, rash, erythema multiforme

MISC: *Fever*, arthralgia, scalp hair loss, **rhabdomyolysis**

PHARMACOKINETICS

Readily absorbed, elimination half-life 2.2 hr, metabolized by liver, excreted by kidneys

PO: Peak 1½ hr, onset ½-1 hr

PO-ER: Onset unknown, peak 4 hr

INTERACTIONS

⚠ **Increase: hypertensive crisis—MAOIs or within 14 days of MAOIs, vasopressors**

Increase: sympathomimetic effect—decongestants, vasoconstrictors

Increase: effects of anticonvulsants, tricyclics, SSRIs, coumarin

Decrease: effects of antihypertensives

Drug/Herb

• Synergistic effect: melatonin

NURSING CONSIDERATIONS

Assess:

Black Box Warning: Substance abuse, past or current; psychotic episodes may occur, especially with parental abuse

• **Toxicity: rhabdomyolysis, headache, flushing, vomiting, agitation, tachycardia, tremor, euphoria, hallucinations, hyperreflexia**

• VS, B/P; may reverse antihypertensives; check patients with cardiac disease more often for increased B/P

• CBC, differential platelet counts during long-term therapy, urinalysis; with diabetes: blood glucose, urine glucose; insulin changes may have to be made because eating will decrease; platelets

• Height, growth rate q3mo in children; growth rate may be decreased

• Mental status: mood, sensorium, affect, stimulation, insomnia, aggressiveness, hostility

⚠ **Withdrawal symptoms: headache, nausea, vomiting, muscle pain, weakness**

• Appetite, sleep, speech patterns

• For attention span, decreased hyperactivity in persons with ADHD

Evaluate:

• Therapeutic response: decreased hyperactivity or ability to stay awake

Teach patient/family:

• To decrease caffeine consumption (coffee, tea, cola, chocolate); may increase irritability, stimulation

• To take early in day to prevent insomnia

• To avoid OTC preparations unless approved by prescriber; to avoid alcohol ingestion

• To taper off product over several wk to avoid depression, increased sleeping, lethargy

• To avoid hazardous activities until stabilized on medication

• To get needed rest; patients will feel more tired at end of day

• To notify all health care workers, including school nurse, of medication and schedule
• About information, instructions provided in patient information section
• To notify prescriber if pregnancy is planned or suspected; to avoid breastfeeding
• To report toxicity immediately: vomiting, agitation, tremor, hyperreflexia, euphoria, confusion, hallucinations, flushing, headache, tachycardia, rhabdomyolysis

TREATMENT OF OVERDOSE:
Administer fluids; hemodialysis or peritoneal dialysis; antihypertensive for increased B/P; administer short-acting barbiturate before lavage

dextroamphetamine (Rx)

(dex-troe-am-fet′a-meen)

Dexedrine, ProCentra

Func. class.: Cerebral stimulant

Chem. class.: Amphetamine

Controlled Substance Schedule II

ACTION: Increases release of norepinephrine, DOPamine in cerebral cortex to reticular activating system

USES: Narcolepsy, attention-deficit/hyperactivity disorder (ADHD)
Unlabeled uses: Obesity

CONTRAINDICATIONS: Hypersensitivity to sympathomimetic amines, hyperthyroidism, glaucoma, severe arteriosclerosis

Black Box Warning: Symptomatic CV disease, substance abuse

Precautions: Pregnancy (C), breastfeeding, children <3 yr, depression, Gilles de la Tourette's disorder, cardiomyopathy, bipolar disorder, abrupt discontinuation, acute MI; benzyl alcohol, salicylate hypersensitivity; hypercortisolism, obesity, psychosis, seizure disorder, hypertension, anxiety, anorexia nervosa, tartrazine dye hypersensitivity

DOSAGE AND ROUTES
Narcolepsy
• **Adult: PO** 5 mg bid, titrate daily dose by no more than 10 mg/wk, max 60 mg/day
• **Child 6-12 yr: PO** 5 mg/day, titrate daily dose by no more than 5 mg/day at weekly intervals, max 60 mg/day
ADHD
• **Adult: PO** 5-60 mg/day daily or divided bid, max 40 mg/day
• **Child 3-5 yr: PO** 2.5 mg/day increasing by 2.5 mg/day at weekly intervals, max 40 mg/day
• **Child >6-12 yr: PO** 5 mg daily-bid increasing by 5 mg/day at weekly intervals
Obesity, exogenous (unlabeled)
• **Adult and adolescent: PO** 5-30 mg/dose given 30-60 min before meals, use for 3-6 wk only
Available forms: Tabs 5, 10 mg; oral sol 5 mg/5 ml; caps: ext rel 5, 10, 15 mg
Administer:
• At least 6 hr before bedtime to avoid sleeplessness
• Use calibrated measuring device for oral sol
• Store all forms at room temperature

SIDE EFFECTS
CNS: *Hyperactivity, insomnia, restlessness, talkativeness,* dizziness, headache, chills, stimulation, dysphoria, irritability, aggressiveness, tremor, dependence, addiction
CV: *Palpitations, tachycardia,* hypertension, decrease in heart rate, dysrhythmias
GI: *Anorexia,* dry mouth, diarrhea, constipation, weight loss, metallic taste
GU: Impotence, change in libido
INTEG: Urticaria
MISC: Rhabdomyolysis

PHARMACOKINETICS

Onset 1 hr; peak 2 hr; ext rel onset 1 hr, peak 2 hr, duration 8 hr; metabolized by liver; urine excretion pH dependent; crosses placenta, breast milk; half-life 6-8 hr (child), 10-12 hr (adult)

INTERACTIONS

⚠ Hypertensive crisis: MAOIs or within 14 days of MAOIs

Increase: serotonin syndrome, neuroleptic malignant syndrome: SSRIs, SNRIs, serotonin-receptor agonists; do not use concurrently

Increase: dextroamphetamine effect—acetaZOLAMIDE, antacids, sodium bicarbonate

Increase: CNS effect—haloperidol, tricyclics, phenothiazines

Decrease: absorption of barbiturates, phenytoin

Decrease: dextroamphetamine effect—ascorbic acid, ammonium chloride

Decrease: effect of adrenergic blockers, antidiabetics, antihypertensives, antihistamines

Drug/Herb

- Serotonin syndrome: St. John's wort

Decrease: stimulant effect—eucalyptus

Drug/Food

Increase: amine effect—caffeine (cola, coffee, tea [green/black])

Drug/Lab Test

Increase: plasma corticosteroids, urinary steroids

NURSING CONSIDERATIONS

Assess:

Black Box Warning: Cardiac disease: VS, B/P; product may reverse antihypertensives; check patients with cardiac disease often

Black Box Warning: Substance abuse: use for prolonged periods may lead to dependence; sudden death or serious CV events can occur from misuse; chronic intoxication (insomnia, irritability, personality changes)

- CBC, urinalysis; with diabetes: blood glucose, urine glucose; insulin changes may be required because eating will decrease
- Height, growth rate in children; growth rate may be decreased, weight
- **Toxicity:** Symptoms may vary in children; anxiety, headache, flushing, vomiting, rhabdomyolysis, tremor, hyperreflexia, confusion, euphoria, tachycardia
- Mental status: mood, sensorium, affect, stimulation, insomnia, irritability
- Tolerance or dependency: increased amount may be used to get same effect; will develop after long-term use

Evaluate:

- Therapeutic response: increased CNS stimulation, decreased drowsiness

Teach patient/family:

- To take before meals (obesity)
- To decrease caffeine consumption (coffee, tea, cola, chocolate); may increase irritability, stimulation
- To avoid OTC preparations unless approved by prescriber, to avoid alcohol ingestion
- To taper product over several wk; depression, increased sleeping, lethargy may occur
- To avoid hazardous activities until stabilized on medication
- To get needed rest; patient will feel more tired at end of day

TREATMENT OF OVERDOSE:

Administer fluids, hemodialysis, or peritoneal dialysis; antihypertensive for increased B/P, ammonium chloride for increased excretion

dextromethorphan (OTC)

(dex-troe-meth-or′fan)

Balminil ✱, Buckley's Mixture, Delsym 12-Hour, ElixSure Cough, Koffex ✱, Robitussin, Robitussin Cough with honey, Robitussin Long Acting Strength, Scot-Tussin Diabetes CF, Triaminic Long Acting Cough, Vicks Formula 44, Wal-Tussin

Func. class.: Antitussive, nonopioid
Chem. class.: Levorphanol derivative

ACTION: Depresses cough center in medulla by direct effect

USES: Nonproductive cough caused by colds or inhaled irritants

CONTRAINDICATIONS: Hypersensitivity

Precautions: Pregnancy (C), fever, hepatic disease, asthma/emphysema, chronic cough

DOSAGE AND ROUTES

- **Adult and child ≥12 yr: PO** 10-20 mg q4hr or 30 mg q6-8hr, max 120 mg/day; **SUS-REL LIQ** 60 mg q12hr, max 120 mg/day
- **Child 6-11 yr: PO** 5-10 mg q4hr; **SUS REL LIQ** 30 mg bid, **LOZ** 5-10 mg q1-4hr; max 60 mg/day
- **Child 4-5 yr: PO** 2.5-7.5 mg q4-8hr, max 30 mg/day; **SUS REL LIQ** 15 mg bid

Available forms: Liq 7.5, 15 mg/5 ml; syr 10 mg/5 ml, 15 mg/5 ml, 30 mg/15 ml; gel caps 15 mg; caps 15 mg; ext rel susp: 30 mg/5 ml

Administer:

- **Chew tabs:** chew well; **syrup:** use calibrated measuring device; **ext rel susp:** shake well, use calibrated measuring device
- Decreased dose for geriatric patients; metabolism may be slowed

SIDE EFFECTS

CNS: *Dizziness,* sedation, confusion, ataxia, fatigue
GI: *Nausea*

PHARMACOKINETICS

PO: Onset 15-30 min, duration 3-6 hr
SUS: Duration 12 hr, terminal half-life 11 hr, metabolized by the liver, excreted via kidneys

INTERACTIONS

- **Do not give with MAOIs or within 2 wk of MAOIs; avoid furazolidone, linezolid, procarbazine (MAOI activity)**

Increase: CNS depression—alcohol, antidepressants, antihistamines, opioids, sedative/hypnotics
Increase: adverse reactions—amiodarone, quiNIDine, serotonin receptor agonist, sibutramine, SSRI

NURSING CONSIDERATIONS

Assess:

- **Cough:** type, frequency, character, including sputum
- Increase fluids to liquify secretions

Evaluate:

- Therapeutic response: absence of cough

Teach patient/family:

- To avoid driving, other hazardous activities until stabilized on medication
- To avoid smoking, smoke-filled rooms, perfumes, dust, environmental pollutants, cleaners that increase cough
- To avoid alcohol, CNS depressants
- To notify prescriber if cough persists over a few days

RARELY USED

dextrose (D-glucose) (Rx)

Func. class.: Caloric, parenteral solution

USES: Increases intake of calories; increases fluids in patients unable to take adequate fluids, calories orally; acute hypoglycemia

CONTRAINDICATIONS: Hyperglycemia, delirium tremens, hemorrhage (cranial/spinal), CHF, anuria, allergy to corn products (concentrated products)

DOSAGE AND ROUTES

Hypoglycemia

• **Adult: PO/IV** 10-25 mg g/dose (20-50 ml of a 50% sol), may need subsequent continuous IV infusion of 10% dextrose

Acute symptomatic hypoglycemia (infants/neonates)

• **Neonate/infant: IV** 250-500 mg/kg/dose (25% sol)

diazepam (Rx)

(dye-az′-e-pam)

Diazemuls ✤, Diastat, Valium

Func. class.: Antianxiety, anticonvulsant, skeletal muscle relaxant, central acting

Chem. class.: Benzodiazepine, long-acting

Controlled Substance Schedule IV

Do not confuse:
diazepam/Ditropan/LORazepam

ACTION: Potentiates the actions of GABA, especially in the limbic system, reticular formation; enhances presympathetic inhibition, inhibits spinal polysynaptic afferent paths

USES: Anxiety, acute alcohol withdrawal, adjunct for seizure disorders; preoperatively as a relaxant for skeletal muscle relaxation; rectally for acute repetitive seizures

Unlabeled uses: Agitation, benzodiazepine withdrawal, chloroquine overdose, insomnia, seizure prophylaxis

CONTRAINDICATIONS: Pregnancy (D), hypersensitivity to benzodiazepines, closed-angle glaucoma, coma, myasthenia gravis, ethanol intoxication, hepatic disease, sleep apnea

Precautions: Breastfeeding, children <6 mo, geriatric patients, debilitation, renal disease, asthma, bipolar disorder, COPD, CNS depression, labor, Parkinson's disease, neutropenia, psychosis, seizures, substance abuse, smoking

D

DOSAGE AND ROUTES

Anxiety/seizure disorders

• **Adult: PO** 2-10 mg bid-qid; **IM/IV** 2-5 mg q3-4hr

• **Geriatric: PO** 2-2.5 mg daily-bid, increase slowly as needed

• **Child >6 mo: PO** 1-2.5 mg tid/qid; **IM/IV** 0.04-0.3 mg/kg/dose q2-4hr, max 0.6 mg/kg in an 8-hr period

Precardioversion

• **Adult: IV** 5-15 mg 5-10 min precardioversion

Preendoscopy

• **Adult: IV** 2.5-20 mg; **IM** 5-10 mg ½ hr preendoscopy

Muscle relaxation

• **Adult: PO** 2-10 mg tid-qid or **EXT REL** 15-30 mg/day; **IV/IM** 5-10 mg, repeat in 2-4 hr

Tetanic muscle spasms

• **Child >5 yr: IM/IV** 5-10 mg q3-4hr prn

• **Infant >30 days: IM/IV** 1-2 mg q3-4hr prn

Status epilepticus

• **Adult: IV/IM** 5-10 mg, 2 mg/min, may repeat q10-15min, max 30 mg; may repeat in 2-4 hr if seizures reappear

• **Child >5 yr: IM** 1 mg q2-5min; **IV** 1 mg slowly

• **Child 1 mo-5 yr: IV** 0.2-0.5 mg slowly; **IM** 0.2-0.5 mg slowly q2-5min up to 5 mg, may repeat in 2-4 hr prn

Seizures other than status epilepticus

• **Adult: RECT** 0.2 mg/kg, may repeat in 4-12 hr

• **Child 6-11 yr: RECT** 0.3 mg/kg, may repeat in 4-12 hr

• **Child 2-5 yr: RECT** 0.5 mg/kg, may repeat in 4-12 hr

Alcohol withdrawal

- **Adult: IV** 10 mg initially, then 5-10 mg q3-4hr prn

Benzodiazepine withdrawal (unlabeled)

- **Adult: PO** Taper 0.5-2 mg over 4-16 wk

Febrile seizure prophylaxis (unlabeled)

- **Child 6 mo-5 yr: PO** 0.33 mg/kg q8hr until afebrile for ≥24 hr

Available forms: Tabs 2, 5, 10 mg; inj 5 mg/ml; oral sol 5 mg/5 ml, rectal 2.5 (pediatric), 10, 20 mg, twin packs; ext rel cap 15 mg, rectal gel

Administer:

- With food or milk for GI symptoms; crushed if patient is unable to swallow medication whole
- Reduced opioid dose by 1/3 if given concomitantly with diazepam
- **Concentrate:** use calibrated dropper only; mix with water, juice, pudding, applesauce; to be consumed immediately

Rectal route

- Do not use more than 5×/mo or for an episode q5days (Diastat)

Direct IV route

- Into large vein; give IV 5 mg or less/1 min or total dose over 3 min or more (children, infants); continuous infusion is not recommended; inject as close to vein insertion as possible; do not dilute or mix with other products

SIDE EFFECTS

CNS: *Dizziness, drowsiness,* confusion, headache, anxiety, tremors, stimulation, fatigue, depression, insomnia, hallucinations, ataxia, fatigue

CV: *Orthostatic hypotension,* ECG changes, tachycardia, hypotension

EENT: *Blurred vision,* tinnitus, mydriasis, nystagmus

GI: Constipation, dry mouth, nausea, vomiting, anorexia, diarrhea

HEMA: Neutropenia

INTEG: Rash, dermatitis, itching

RESP: Respiratory depression

PHARMACOKINETICS

Metabolized by liver via CYP2C19, CYP3A4; excreted by kidneys; crosses placenta; excreted in breast milk; crosses the blood-brain barrier; half-life 1-12 days; more reliable by mouth; 99% protein binding

PO: Rapidly absorbed, onset 1/2 hr, peak 2 hr, duration up to 24 hr

IM: Onset 15-30 min, duration 1-1 1/2 hr, absorption slow and erratic

RECT: Peak 1.5 hr

IV: Onset immediate, duration 15 min-1 hr

INTERACTIONS

Increase: diazepam effect—amiodarone, protease inhibitors, diltiazem, cimetidine, clarithromycin, dalfopristin-quinupristin, delavirdine, disulfiram, efavirenz, erythromycin, fluconazole, fluvoxaMINE, imatinib, itraconazole, ketoconazole, IV miconazole, nefazodone, niCARdipine, ranolazine, troleandomycin, valproic acid, verapamil, voriconazole, zafirlukast, zileuton

Increase: toxicity—barbiturates, SSRIs, cimetidine, CNS depressants, valproic acid, CYP3A4 inhibitors

Increase: CNS depression—CNS depressants, alcohol

Decrease: diazepam metabolism—oral contraceptives, valproic acid, disulfiram, isoniazid, propranolol

Decrease: diazepam effect—CYP3A4 inducers (rifampin, barbiturates, carBAMazepine, ethotoin, phenytoin, fosphenytoin), smoking

Drug/Lab Test

Increase: AST/ALT, serum bilirubin, alk phos

NURSING CONSIDERATIONS

Assess:

- B/P (lying, standing), pulse; respiratory rate; if systolic B/P drops 20 mm Hg, hold product, notify prescriber; respirations q5-15min if given IV
- Blood studies: CBC during long-term therapy; blood dyscrasias (rare); hepatic studies: AST, ALT, bilirubin, creatinine, LDH, alk phos

• **Degree of anxiety;** what precipitates anxiety and whether product controls symptoms
• **Alcohol withdrawal symptoms,** including hallucinations (visual, auditory), delirium, irritability, agitation, fine to coarse tremors
• Seizure control and type, duration, intensity of seizures
• For muscle spasms; pain relief
• IV site for thrombosis or phlebitis, which may occur rapidly
• Mental status: mood, sensorium, affect, sleeping pattern, drowsiness, dizziness, suicidal tendencies
• **Physical dependency, withdrawal symptoms:** headache, nausea, vomiting, muscle pain, weakness after long-term use

Evaluate:
• Therapeutic response: decreased anxiety, restlessness, insomnia

Teach patient/family:
• That product may be taken with food
• That product not to be used for everyday stress or for >4 mo unless directed by prescriber; to take no more than prescribed amount; that product may be habit forming
• To avoid OTC preparations unless approved by prescriber
• To avoid driving, activities that require alertness; drowsiness may occur
• To avoid alcohol, other psychotropic medications unless directed by prescriber; that smoking may decrease diazepam effect by increasing diazepam metabolism
• Not to discontinue medication abruptly after long-term use; to gradually taper
• To rise slowly or fainting may occur, especially in geriatric patients
• That drowsiness may worsen at beginning of treatment
• To notify prescriber if pregnancy is planned or suspected (D), avoid breastfeeding

TREATMENT OF OVERDOSE:
Lavage, VS, supportive care, flumazenil

dibucaine topical
See Appendix B

D

diclofenac epolamine (Rx)
(dye-kloe′fen-ak)
Flector

diclofenac potassium (Rx)
Cambia, Cataflam, Rapide ✤, Zipsor

diclofenac sodium (Rx)
Apo-Diclo ✤, Novo-Difenac ✤, Nu-Diclo ✤, PENNSAID, Sandoz Diclofenac ✤, Solaraze Topical Gel, Voltaren, Voltaren Topical Gel, Voltaren XR

Func. class.: Nonsteroidal antiinflammatory products (NSAIDs), nonopioid analgesic
Chem. class.: Phenylacetic acid

Do not confuse:
Cataflam/Catapres

ACTION: Inhibits COX-1, COX-2 by blocking arachidonate resulting in analgesic, antiinflammatory, antipyretic effects

USES: Acute, chronic RA; osteoarthritis; ankylosing spondylitis; analgesia; primary dysmenorrhea; patch: mild to moderate pain
Unlabeled uses: Arthralgia, headache, migraine, bone pain, myalgia

CONTRAINDICATIONS: Hypersensitivity to aspirin, iodides, other NSAIDs, bovine protein, asthma, serious CV disease; eczema, exfoliative dermatitis, skin abrasions (gel, patch)

Black Box Warning: Treatment of perioperative pain (CABG), surgery

Precautions: Pregnancy (C) (tabs, del rel tab, ext rel tab, top gel), (ophthalmic sol); pregnancy (B) (top gel) (solaraze); top patch, top sol, cap, powder for oral sol (C <30 wk, D >30 wk); breastfeeding, children, bleeding disorders, GI disorders, cardiac disorders, hypersensitivity to other antiinflammatory agents, CCr <30 ml/min, accidental exposure, acute bronchospasm, hypersensitivity to benzyl alcohol

Black Box Warning: GI bleeding, MI, stroke

DOSAGE AND ROUTES

Osteoarthritis

• **Adult: PO** (Cataflam) 50 mg bid-tid, max 150 mg/day; **DEL REL** (Voltaren) 50 mg bid-tid or 75 mg bid, max 150 mg/day; **EXT REL** (Voltaren-XR) 100 mg daily, max 150 mg/day; **TOP GEL** 1% (Voltaren gel) 4 g for each of lower extremities qid, max 16 g/day; 2 g for each of upper extremities qid, max 8 g/day; **TOP SOL** (Pennsaid) apply 40 drops to each affected knee qid; apply 10 drops at a time, spread over entire knee

Rheumatoid arthritis

• **Adult: PO** (Cataflam) 50 mg tid-qid, max 200 mg/day; **DEL REL** (Voltaren) 50 mg tid-qid or 75 mg bid, max 200 mg/day; **EXT REL** (Voltaren-XR) 100 mg daily, may increase to 200 mg/day, max 200 mg/day

Ankylosing spondylitis

• **Adult: PO DEL REL** (Voltaren) 25 mg qid and 25 mg at bedtime, max 125 mg/day

Acute migraine with/without aura

• **Adult: PO** (powder for oral sol) (Cambia) 50 mg as a single dose, mix contents of packet in 1-2 oz water

Mild to moderate pain

• **Adult: PO** (Zipsor) 25 mg qid

Dysmenorrhea or nonrheumatic inflammatory conditions

• **Adult: PO** (Cataflam) 50 mg tid or 100 mg initially, then 50 mg tid, max 200 mg 1st day, then 150 mg/day, immediate release only

Pain of strains/sprains

• **Adult: TOP PATCH** (Flector) apply patch to area bid

Actinic keratosis

• **Adult: TOP GEL** (Solaraze) apply to area bid

Prevention of heterotropic ossification (unlabeled)

• **Adult: PO** 50 mg tid × 3 wk

Renal dose

• **Avoid:** Use of topical gel, patch, sol, potassium oral tab for advanced renal disease

Available forms: Epolamine: topical patch 1.3%; **potassium:** tabs 50 mg; tabs liquid filled 25 mg; oral powder for sol 50 mg; **sodium:** delayed rel tabs (enteric-coated) 25, 50, 75 mg; Pennsaid: ext rel tabs, 100 mg

Administer:

PO route

• Do not break, crush, or chew enteric products

• Take with a full glass of water to enhance absorption, remain upright for ½ hr; if dose missed, take as soon as remembered within 2 hr if taking 1-2×/day; do not double doses

• Store at room temperature

Topical patch route (Flector)

• Wash hands before handling patch

• Remove and release liner before administration

• Use only on normal, intact skin

• Remove before bath, shower, swimming, do not use heat or occlusive dressings

• Discard removed patch in trash away from children, pets

• Store at room temperature

Topical gel route

• Apply to intact skin, do not use heat or occlusive dressings

• Use only for osteoarthritis, mild to moderate pain

• Store at room temperature, avoid heat, do not freeze

Topical solution route

• Apply to clean, dry skin

• Wait until dry before applying clothing, other creams/lotions

- Wait ≥30 min after use before bathing, swimming
- Store at room temperature

SIDE EFFECTS

CNS: *Dizziness, headache,* drowsiness, fatigue, tremors, confusion, insomnia, anxiety, depression, nervousness, paresthesia, muscle weakness
CV: **CHF**, tachycardia, peripheral edema, palpitations, **dysrhythmias**, hypo/hypertension, fluid retention, **MI**, **stroke**
EENT: Tinnitus, hearing loss, blurred vision, **laryngeal edema**
GI: Nausea, anorexia, vomiting, diarrhea, **jaundice, cholestatic hepatitis**, constipation, flatulence, cramps, dry mouth, peptic ulcer, **GI bleeding, hepatotoxicity,** hematemesis
GU: **Nephrotoxicity: dysuria, hematuria, oliguria, azotemia, cystitis**
HEMA: **Blood dyscrasias,** epistaxis, anemia
INTEG: Purpura, rash, pruritus, sweating, erythema, petechiae, photosensitivity, alopecia
META: **Hyperglycemia, hypoglycemia**
RESP: Dyspnea, **bronchospasm**
SYST: **Anaphylaxis, Stevens-Johnson syndrome**

PHARMACOKINETICS

PO: Peak 2-3 hr; **TOP Patch:** peak 12 hr; elimination half-life 1-2 hr, patch 12 hr, 99% bound to plasma proteins, metabolized in liver to metabolite, excreted in urine

INTERACTIONS

- Need for dosage adjustment: antidiabetics

Increase: hyperkalemia—potassium-sparing diuretics
Increase: anticoagulant effect—anticoagulants, NSAIDs, platelet inhibitors, salicylates, thrombolytics, SSRIs
Increase: **toxicity—phenytoin, lithium, cycloSPORINE, methotrexate, digoxin, lithium, cidofovir**
Increase: GI side effects—aspirin, other NSAIDs, bisphosphonates, corticosteroids
Decrease: antihypertensive effect—β-blockers, diuretics, ACE inhibitors
Decrease: effect of diuretics
Drug/Herb
Increase: bleeding risk—garlic, ginger, ginkgo; monitor for bleeding

NURSING CONSIDERATIONS

Assess:

Black Box Warning: CABG: do not use oral, top, gel, patch, in perioperative pain in coronary artery bypass graft surgery for 10-14 days

Black Box Warning: Stroke/MI: may increase CHF and hypertension, increased CV thrombotic events that may be fatal; those with CV disease may be at greater risk

- **Pain:** location, character, aggravating/alleviating factors, ROM before and 1 hr after dose
- Patients with asthma, aspirin hypersensitivity, nasal polyps; may develop hypersensitivity
- LFTs (may be elevated), uric acid (may be decreased—serum; increased—urine) periodically; also BUN, creatinine, electrolytes (may be elevated)

⚠ **Blood dyscrasias (thrombocytopenia): bruising, fatigue, bleeding, poor healing; blood counts during therapy; watch for decreasing platelets; if low, therapy may need to be discontinued, restarted after hematologic recovery; stool guaiac**

Evaluate:

- Therapeutic response: decreased inflammation in joints, after cataract surgery

Teach patient/family:

- That product must be continued for prescribed time to be effective; to contact prescriber before surgery regarding when to discontinue this product
- **To report bleeding, bruising, fatigue, malaise; blood dyscrasias do occur**
- To avoid aspirin, alcoholic beverages, NSAIDs, or other OTC medications unless approved by prescriber

- To take with food, milk, or antacids to avoid GI upset; to swallow whole
- To use caution when driving; drowsiness, dizziness may occur
- To report **hepatotoxicity:** flulike symptoms, nausea, vomiting, jaundice, pruritus, lethargy
- To use sunscreen to prevent photosensitivity
- To notify all providers of product use
- To notify prescriber if pregnancy is planned or suspected (C, tabs) (C, <30 wk, D, >30 wk caps, topical patch/solution, powder for oral solution)

diclofenac ophthalmic

See Appendix B

RARELY USED

dicyclomine (Rx)

(dye-sye′kloe-meen)

Bentyl, Bentylol ✤, Formulex ✤, Lomine ✤

Func. class.: Gastrointestinal anticholinergic

USES: IBS

CONTRAINDICATIONS: Hypersensitivity to anticholinergics, closed-angle glaucoma, GI obstruction, myasthenia gravis, paralytic ileus, GI atony, toxic megacolon, dementia

DOSAGE AND ROUTES

- **Adult: PO** 10-20 mg tid-qid; **IM** 20 mg q4-6hr; max 160 mg/day
- **Child >2 yr: PO** 10 mg tid-qid
- **Child 6 mo-2 yr: PO** 5 mg tid-qid

didanosine (Rx)

(dye-dan′oh-seen)

ddI, Videx Pediatric Powder, Videx EC

Func. class.: Antiretroviral

Chem. class.: Nucleoside reverse transcriptase inhibitor (NRTI)

ACTION: Nucleoside analog incorporating into cellular DNA by viral reverse transcriptase, thereby terminating the cellular DNA chain

USES: HIV-1 infection in combination with at least 2 other antiretrovirals

Unlabeled uses: HIV prophylaxis

CONTRAINDICATIONS: Hypersensitivity, lactic acidosis, pancreatitis, phenylketonuria

Precautions: Pregnancy (B), breastfeeding, children, renal disease, sodium-restricted diets, elevated amylase, preexisting peripheral neuropathy, hyperuricemia, gout, CHF, noncirrhotic portal hypertension

Black Box Warning: Hepatic disease, lactic acidosis, pancreatitis

DOSAGE AND ROUTES

- **Adult/adolescent/child ≥6 yr and ≥60 kg: PO EXT REL CAP** 400 mg/day; if used with tenofovir, reduce to 250 mg/day
- **Adult/adolescent/child ≥6 yr and 25 kg to <60 kg: PO EXT REL CAP** 250 mg/day; if used with tenofovir, reduce to 200 mg/day
- **Adolescent 20 kg to <25 kg: PO EXT REL CAP** 200 mg/day
- **Adult ≥60 kg: PO ORAL SOL** 200 mg bid or 400 mg/day; if used with tenofovir, reduce to 250 mg/day
- **Adult <60 kg: PO ORAL SOL** 125 mg bid or 250 mg/day; if used with tenofovir, reduce to 200 mg/day

- **Adolescent/child/infant >8 mo: PO ORAL SOL** 120 mg/m^2 every 12 hr, max adult dosing
- **Infant <8 mo/neonate ≥2 wk: PO ORAL SOL** 100 mg/m^2 every 12 hr for up to 3 months

Renal dose

- **Adult: PO** CrCl ≥60 ml/min: No change
- **Adult/adolescent ≥60 kg: PO** CCr 30-59 ml/min: reduce oral sol to 100 mg every 12 hr or 200 mg every 24 hr; reduce EXT-REL caps to 200 mg/day; CCr 10-29 ml/min: reduce oral sol to 150 mg every 24 hr; reduce EXT-REL caps to 125 mg/day; CCr <10 ml/min: reduce oral sol to 100 mg every 24 hr; reduce EXT-REL caps to 125 mg/day
- **Adult/adolescent <60 kg: PO** CCr 30-59 ml/min: reduce oral sol to 75 mg every 12 hr or to 150 mg every 24 hr; reduce EXT-REL caps to 125 mg/day; CCr 10-29 ml/min: reduce oral sol to 100 mg every 24 hr; reduce EXT-REL caps to 125 mg/day; CCr <10 ml/min: reduce oral sol to 75 mg every 24 hr; EXT-REL caps are not recommended

Intermittent hemodialysis/ continuous ambulatory peritoneal dialysis

- **Adult/adolescent >60 kg:** Give 100 mg oral sol or 125 mg EXT-REL CAPS every 24 hr
- **Adult/adolescent <60 kg:** Give 75 mg oral sol every 24 hr, EXT-REL CAPS are not recommended

Available forms: Powder for oral sol 10 mg/ml; del rel caps 125, 200, 250, 400 mg

Administer:

- Pediatric powder for oral sol after preparation by pharmacist; dilution required using purified USP water, then antacid (10 mg/ml), refrigerate, shake before use
- On an empty stomach ≥30 min before or 2 hr after meals
- Adjust dose with renal impairment
- Store tabs, caps in tightly closed bottle at room temperature; store oral sol after dissolving at room temperature ≤4 hr

SIDE EFFECTS

CNS: **Peripheral neuropathy, seizures,** confusion, *anxiety,* hypertonia, abnormal thinking, asthenia, *insomnia,* **CNS depression,** pain, dizziness, chills, fever

CV: Hypertension, vasodilation, dysrhythmia, syncope, **CHF,** palpitation

EENT: Ear pain, otitis, photophobia, visual impairment, retinal depigmentation, optic neuritis

GI: **Pancreatitis,** *diarrhea, nausea,* vomiting, *abdominal pain,* constipation, stomatitis, dyspepsia, liver abnormalities, flatulence, taste perversion, dry mouth, oral thrush, melena, increased ALT/AST, alk phos, amylase, **hepatic failure,** noncirrhotic portal hypertension

GU: Increased bilirubin, uric acid

HEMA: **Leukopenia, granulocytopenia, thrombocytopenia, anemia**

INTEG: *Rash, pruritus,* alopecia, ecchymosis, hemorrhage, petechiae, sweating

MS: Myalgia, arthritis, myopathy, muscular atrophy

RESP: Cough, pneumonia, dyspnea, asthma, epistaxis, hypoventilation, sinusitis

SYST: **Lactic acidosis, anaphylaxis**

PHARMACOKINETICS

PO: Peak 0.67 hr, del rel 2 hr; elimination half-life 48 min; extensive metabolism; administration within 5 min of food will decrease absorption (50%); excreted urine, feces

INTERACTIONS

Increase: didanosine level—allopurinol, tenofovir

Increase: side effects from magnesium, aluminum antacids

Increase: pancreatitis risk—stavudine

Decrease: absorption—ketoconazole, dapsone

Decrease: concentrations of fluoroquinolones, other antiretrovirals, itraconazole, tetracyclines

Black Box Warning: Increase: **fatal lactic acidosis—stavudine, tenofovir, other antiretrovirals**

• Do not use with these products PO: gatifloxacin, gemifloxacin, levofloxacin, moxifloxacin, norfloxacin

Drug/Food

• Any food decreases rate of absorption 50%, do not use with food
• Do not use with acidic juices

NURSING CONSIDERATIONS

Assess:

Black Box Warning: Pancreatitis: do not use in those with symptoms of pancreatitis; may be dose related in advanced HIV, alcoholism, history of pancreatitis

• **Peripheral neuropathy:** tingling or pain in hands and feet, distal numbness; onset usually occurs 2-6 mo after beginning treatment, may persist if product not discontinued

Black Box Warning: Lactic acidosis, severe hepatomegaly, pancreatitis: abdominal pain, nausea, vomiting, elevated hepatic enzymes; product should be discontinued because condition can be fatal

• Children by dilated retinal exam q6mo to rule out retinal depigmentation
• CBC, differential, platelet count monthly; notify prescriber of results; alk phos, monitor amylase; viral load, CD4 count
• Renal studies: BUN, serum uric acid, urine CCr before, during therapy
• Temperature may indicate beginning infection
• Hepatic studies before, during therapy (bilirubin, AST, ALT) as needed, monthly
• Clean up of powdered products; use wet mop or damp sponge

Evaluate:

• Therapeutic response: absence of infection; symptoms of HIV

Teach patient/family:

• To avoid use with alcohol; not to take with food
• To report numbness/tingling in extremities
• To take on an empty stomach; not to take dapsone at same time as ddI; not to mix powder with fruit juice; chew tab or crush and dissolve in water; to drink powder immediately after mixing
• To report signs of **infection:** increased temperature, sore throat, flulike symptoms
• To report signs of **anemia:** fatigue, headache, faintness, SOB, irritability
• To report **bleeding;** to avoid use of razors, commercial mouthwash
• That hair may be lost during therapy (rare); that a wig or hairpiece may make patient feel better
• That product does not cure, only controls symptoms

difluprednate (ophthalmic)

(die-flu′pred-nate)

Durezol

Func. class.: Ophthalmic antiinflammatory

Chem. class.: Corticosteroid

ACTION: Exact mechanism of antiinflammatory action unknown; inhibits multiple inflammatory cytokines; decreases release of arachidonic acid, which increases in inflammation

USES: For the treatment of postoperative ocular pain and postoperative ocular inflammation; for the treatment of endogenous anterior uveitis

CONTRAINDICATIONS: Hypersensitivity to this product, glycerin, polysorbate, ocular TB, acute herpes simplex (superficial), fungal/viral infections of the eye

Precautions: Pregnancy (C), breastfeeding, children, corneal infected abrasions, glaucoma

DOSAGE AND ROUTES

Postoperative ocular pain, postoperative ocular inflammation

• **Adult/geriatric/adolescents/children/infants: OPHTH** Instill 1 drop into the conjunctival sac of the affected eye(s) qid beginning 24 hr after surgery; continue giving 4 ×/day for the first 2 wk of the postoperative period, then administer bid × 1 wk; at the end of the third wk, taper dosage based on response

Endogenous anterior uveitis

• **Adult: OPHTH** Instill 1 drop into the conjunctival sac of the affected eye(s) qid × 14 days, followed by tapering based on response

Available forms: Ophthalmic emulsion 0.05%

Administer:

• Apply topically to the eye, shake well before use

• Do not touch the tip of the dropper to the eye, fingertips, or other surface

• Instruct patient on proper instillation of eye sol

• When using this product, the patient should not wear contact lenses

SIDE EFFECTS

EENT: Burning, stinging, poor vision, corneal ulcerations, increased IOP, optic nerve damage

NURSING CONSIDERATIONS

Assess:

• **Corneal effects:** ulcerations, infections can worsen with this product, monitor IOP used IO over 10 days

Evaluate:

• **Therapeutic response:** Decreased corneal inflammation

Teach patient/family:

• How to use product

• Not to share with others or use for other conditions

• To notify prescriber immediately if vision changes or if condition worsens

• To take as prescribed

⚠ HIGH ALERT

digoxin (Rx)

(di-jox′in)

APO-Digoxin ♣, Lanoxin

Func. class.: Cardiac glycoside, inotropic, antidysrhythmic

Chem. class.: Digoxin preparation

Do not confuse:

Lanoxin/Lasix/Lonox/Lomotil/Xanax/Levoxine

ACTION: Inhibits the sodium-potassium ATPase pump, which makes more calcium available for contractile proteins, thereby resulting in increased cardiac output (positive inotropic effect); increases force of contractions; decreases heart rate (negative chronotropic effect); decreases AV conduction speed

USES: Heart failure, atrial fibrillation

Unlabeled uses: Atrial flutter, paroxysmal supraventricular tachycardia (PSVT) treatment/prophylaxis

CONTRAINDICATIONS: Hypersensitivity to digoxin, ventricular fibrillation, ventricular tachycardia

Precautions: Pregnancy (C), breastfeeding, geriatric patients, renal disease, acute MI, AV block, severe respiratory disease, hypothyroidism, sinus nodal disease, hypokalemia, carotid sinus syndrome, 2nd- or 3rd-degree heart block, electrolyte disturbances, hypertension, cor pulmonale, Wolff-Parkinson-White syndrome

DOSAGE AND ROUTES

Loading dose, IV route

• **Adult/adolescent/child >10 yr: IV** 8-12 mcg/kg, divided into ≥3 doses, with the first dose equaling one-half the total, give subsequent doses every 6-8 hr

- **Child 5-10 yr: IV** 15-30 mcg/kg divided into ≥3 doses, with the first dose equaling one-half the total, give subsequent doses every 6-8 hr
- **Child 2-4 yr: IV** 25-35 mcg/kg, divided into ≥3 doses, with the first dose equaling one-half the total, give subsequent doses every 6-8 hr
- **Infant/child <2 yr: IV** 30-50 mcg/kg, divided into ≥3 doses, with the first dose equaling one-half the total, give subsequent doses every 6-8 hr
- **Full-term neonate: IV** 20-30 mcg/kg, divided into ≥3 doses, with the first dose equaling one-half the total, give subsequent doses every 6-8 hr
- **Premature neonate: IV** 15-25 mcg/kg, divided into ≥3 doses, with the first dose equaling one-half the total, give subsequent doses every 6-8 hr

Loading dose, PO (tablets): Tablets are 60%-80% bioavailable; oral elixir should be used to obtain the appropriate dose in infants, young pediatric patients, or patients with very low body weight

- **Adult/adolescent/child >10 yr: PO** Total dosage of 10-15 mcg/kg in 3 divided doses, give one-half the total loading dose initially, then one-fourth the loading dose every 4-8 hr × 2 doses
- **Child 5-10 yr: PO** Total dosage of 20-45 mcg/kg in 3 divided doses, give one-half the total loading dose initially, then one-fourth the loading dose every 4-8 hr × 2 doses

Loading dose, PO (elixir): Elixir is approximately 70%-85% bioavailable

- **Adult/adolescent/child >10 yr: PO** Total dosage of 10-15 mcg/kg, give one-half the total loading dose initially, then additional fractions of the planned total dose at 4-8 hr
- **Child 5-10 yr: PO** Total dosage of 20-35 mcg/kg, give one-half the total loading dose initially, then additional fractions of the planned total dose at 4-8 hr
- **Child 2-4 yr: PO** Total dosage of 30-45 mcg/kg, give one-half the total loading dose initially, then additional fractions of the planned total dose at 4-8 hr
- **Infant/child <2 yr: PO** Total dosage of 35-60 mcg/kg, give one-half the total loading dose initially, then additional fractions of the planned total dose at 4-8 hr
- **Full-term neonate: PO** Total dosage of 25-35 mcg/kg, give one-half the total loading dose initially, then additional fractions of the planned total dose at 4-8 hr
- **Premature neonate: PO** Total dosage of 20-30 mcg/kg, give one-half the total loading dose initially, then additional fractions of the planned total dose at 4-8 hr

Maintenance dose, IV

- **Adult: IV** 125-350 mcg/day, depending on CrCl, usual daily maintenance dosage for CHF based on corrected CrCl (ml/min/70 kg) and lean body weight (LBW) are listed below
- LBW 50-59 kg: CrCl ≥100 ml/min: 175 mcg/day; CrCl 70-99 ml/min: 150 mcg/day; CrCl 60-69 ml/min: 125 mcg/day
- LBW 60-69 kg: CrCl ≥90 ml/min: 200 mcg/day; CrCl 70-89 ml/min: 175 mcg/day; CrCl 60-69 ml/min: 150 mcg/day
- LBW 70-79 kg: CrCl ≥100 ml/min: 250 mcg/day; CrCl 90-99 ml/min: 225 mcg/day; CrCl 70-89 ml/min: 200 mcg/day; CrCl 60-69 ml/min: 175 mcg/day
- LBW 80-89 kg: CrCl ≥100 ml/min: 275 mcg/day; CrCl 80-99 ml/min: 250 mcg/day; CrCl 70-79 ml/min: 225 mcg/day; CrCl 60-69 ml/min: 200 mcg/day
- LBW 90-99 kg: CrCl ≥90 ml/min: 300 mcg/day; CrCl 80-89 ml/min: 275 mcg/day; CrCl 70-79 ml/min: 250 mcg/day; CrCl 60-69 ml/min: 225 mcg/day
- LBW ≥100 kg: CrCl ≥100 ml/min: 350 mcg/day; CrCl 90-99 ml/min: 325 mcg IV/day; CrCl 80-89 ml/min: 300 mcg/day; CrCl 70-79 ml/min: 275 mcg IV/day; CrCl 60-69 ml/min: 250 mcg/day
- **Full-term neonate to child >10 yr:** 25%-35% of the IV digitalizing dose bid

Maintenance dose, PO (tablets)

- **Adult/adolescent/child >10 yr: PO** 3.4-5.1 mcg/kg/day
- LBW 40-49 kg: CrCl ≥70 ml/min: 187.5 mcg/day; CrCl ≥60-69 ml/min: 125 mcg/day

• LBW 50-59 kg: CrCl ≥90 ml/min: 250 mcg/day; CrCl 60-89 ml/min: 187.5 mcg/day
• LBW 60-69 kg: CrCl ≥100 ml/min: 312.5 mcg/day; CrCl 60-99 ml/min: 250 mcg/day
• LBW 70-79 kg: CrCl ≥80 ml/min: 312.5 mcg/day; CrCl 60-79 ml/min: 250 mcg/day
• LBW 80-89 kg: CrCl ≥90 ml/min: 375 mcg/day; CrCl 60-89 ml/min: 312.5 mcg/day
• LBW 90-99 kg: CrCl ≥90 ml/min: 437.5 mcg/day; CrCl 70-89 ml/min: 375 mcg/day; CrCl 60-69 ml/min: 312.5 mcg/day
• LBW ≥100 kg: CrCl ≥100 ml/min: 500 mcg/day; CrCl 80-99 ml/min: 437.5 mcg/day; CrCl 60-79 ml/min: 375 mcg/day
• **Child 5-10 yr: PO** 6.4-12.9 mcg/kg/day in 2 divided doses is recommended starting maintenance dose

Maintenance dose, PO (elixir)

• **Adult/adolescent/child >10 yr: PO** 3-4.5 mcg/kg/day
• LBW 40-49 kg: CrCl ≥100 ml/min: 170 mcg/day; CrCl 90-99 ml/min: 160 mcg/day; CrCl 80-89 ml/min: 150 mcg/day; CrCl 70-79 ml/min: 140 mcg/day; CrCl 60-69 ml/min: 130 mcg/day
• LBW 50-59 kg: CrCl ≥100 ml/min: 213 mcg/day; CrCl 90-99 ml/min: 200 mcg/day; CrCl 80-89 ml/min: 188 mcg/day; CrCl 70-79 ml/min: 175 mcg/day; CrCl 60-69 ml/min: 163 mcg/day
• LBW 60-69 kg: CrCl ≥100 ml/min: 255 mcg/day; CrCl 90-99 ml/min: 240 mcg/day; CrCl 80-89 ml/min: 225 mcg/day; CrCl 70-79 ml/min: 210 mcg/day; CrCl 60-69 ml/min: 195 mcg/day
• LBW 70-79 kg: CrCl ≥100 ml/min: 298 mcg/day; CrCl 90-99 ml/min: 280 mcg/day; CrCl 80-89 ml/min: 263 mcg/day; CrCl 70-79 ml/min: 245 mcg/day; CrCl 60-69 ml/min: 228 mcg/day
• LBW 80-89 kg: CrCl ≥100 ml/min: 340 mcg/day; CrCl 90-99 ml/min: 320 mcg/day; CrCl 80-89 ml/min: 300 mcg/day; CrCl 70-79 ml/min: 280 mcg/day; CrCl 60-69 ml/min: 260 mcg/day
• LBW 90-99 kg: CrCl ≥100 ml/min: 383 mcg/day; CrCl 90-99 ml/min: 360 mcg/day; CrCl 80-89 ml/min: 338 mcg/day; CrCl 70-79 ml/min: 315 mcg/day; CrCl 60-69 ml/min: 293 mcg/day
• LBW ≥100 kg: CrCl ≥100 ml/min: 425 mcg/day; CrCl 90-99 ml/min: 400 mcg/day; CrCl 80-89 ml/min: 375 mcg/day; CrCl 70-79 ml/min: 350 mcg/day; CrCl 60-69 ml/min: 325 mcg/day
• **Child 5-10 yr: PO** 5.6-11.3 mcg/kg/day in 2 divided doses
• **Child 2-4 yr: PO** 9.4-13.1 mcg/kg/day in 2 divided doses
• **Infant/child <2 yr: PO** 11.3-18.8 mcg/kg/day in 2 divided doses
• **Full-term neonate: PO** 7.5-11.3 mcg/kg/day in 2 divided doses
• **Preterm neonate: PO** 4.7-7.8 mcg/kg/day in 2 divided doses

Renal dose, IV route

• **CrCl 50-59 ml/min:** LBW 50-59 kg: 125 mcg 1× daily; LBW 60-69 kg: 150 mcg 1× daily; LBW 70-79 kg: 175 mcg 1× daily; LBW 80-89 kg: 200 mcg 1× daily; LBW 90-99 kg: 225 mcg 1× daily; LBW ≥100 kg: 250 mcg 1× daily
• **CrCl 40-49 ml/min:** LBW 50-59 kg: 100 mcg 1× daily; LBW 60-69 kg: 125 mcg 1× daily; LBW 70-79 kg: 150 mcg 1× daily; LBW 80-89 kg: 175 mcg 1× daily; LBW 90-99 kg: 200 mcg 1× daily; LBW ≥100 kg: 225 mcg 1× daily
• **CrCl 30-39 ml/min:** LBW 50-59 kg: 100 mcg 1× daily; LBW 60-69 kg: 125 mcg 1× daily; LBW 70-89 kg: 150 mcg 1× daily; LBW 90-99 kg: 175 mcg 1× daily; LBW ≥100 kg: 200 mcg 1× daily
• **CrCl 20-29 ml/min:** LBW 50-69 kg: 100 mcg 1× daily; LBW 70-79 kg: 125 mcg 1× daily; LBW 80-99 kg: 150 mcg 1× daily; LBW ≥100 kg: 175 mcg 1× daily
• **CrCl 10-19 ml/min:** LBW 50-59 kg: 75 mcg 1× daily; LBW 60-79 kg: 100 mcg 1× daily; LBW 80-89 kg: 125 mcg 1× daily; LBW ≥90 kg: 150 mcg 1× daily
• **CrCl <10 ml/min** LBW 50-69 kg: 75 mcg 1× daily; LBW 70-89 kg: 100 mcg 1× daily; LBW 90-99 kg: 125 mcg 1× daily; LBW ≥100 kg: 150 mcg 1× daily

Renal dose, PO (tablets)

- **CrCl 40-59 ml/min:** LBW 50-69 kg: 187.5 mcg 1× daily
- **CrCl 30-39 ml/min:** LBW 50-59 kg: 125 mcg 1× daily; LBW 60-79 kg: 187.5 mcg 1× daily; LBW 80-99 kg: 250 mcg 1× daily; LBW ≥100 kg: 312.5 mcg 1× daily
- **CrCl 20-29 ml/min:** LBW 50-69 kg: 125 mcg 1× daily; LBW 70-89 kg: 187.5 mcg 1× daily; LBW ≥90 kg: 250 mcg 1× daily
- **CrCl <20 ml/min:** LBW 50-69 kg: 125 mcg 1× daily; LBW 70-99 kg: 187.5 mcg 1× daily; LBW ≥100 kg: 250 mcg 1× daily

Renal dose, PO (elixir)

- **CrCl 50-59 ml/min:** LBW 50-59 kg: 150 mcg 1× daily; LBW 60-69 kg: 180 mcg 1× daily; LBW 70-79 kg: 210 mcg 1× daily; LBW 80-89 kg: 240 mcg 1× daily; LBW 90-99 kg: 270 mcg 1× daily; LBW ≥100 kg: 300 mcg 1× daily
- **CrCl 40-49 ml/min:** LBW 50-59 kg: 138 mcg 1× daily; LBW 60-69 kg: 165 mcg 1× daily; LBW 70-79 kg: 193 mcg 1× daily; LBW 80-89 kg: 220 mcg 1× daily; LBW 90-99 kg: 248 mcg 1× daily; LBW ≥100 kg: 275 mcg 1× daily
- **CrCl 30-39 ml/min:** LBW 50-59 kg: 125 mcg 1× daily; LBW 60-69 kg: 150 mcg 1× daily; LBW 70-79 kg: 175 mcg PO 1× daily; LBW 80-89 kg: 200 mcg PO 1× daily; LBW 90-99 kg: 225 mcg 1× daily; LBW ≥100 kg: 250 mcg PO 1× daily
- **CrCl 20-29 ml/min:** LBW 50-59 kg: 113 mcg 1× daily; LBW 60-69 kg: 135 mcg 1× daily; LBW 70-79 kg: 158 mcg 1× daily; LBW 80-89 kg: 180 mcg PO 1× daily; LBW 90-99 kg: 203 mcg 1× daily; LBW ≥100 kg: 225 mcg PO 1× daily
- **CrCl <20 ml/min:** LBW 50-59 kg: 100 mcg 1× daily; LBW 60-69 kg: 120 mcg 1× daily; LBW 70-79 kg: 140 mcg 1× daily; LBW 80-89 kg: 160 mcg 1× daily; LBW 90-99 kg: 180 mcg 1× daily; LBW ≥100 kg: 200 mcg 1× daily

The daily maintenance dose can also be estimated using patient CrCl and loading dose (LD) according to the method of Jelliffe and Brooker: Daily % loss = 14 + CrCl/5

Available forms: Elix 0.05 mg/ml; tabs 0.0625, 0.125, 0.1875, 0.25, 0.5 mg; inj 0.5 ✱, 0.25 mg/ml; pediatric inj 0.1 mg/ml

Administer:

PO route

⚠ Bioavailability varies among different oral dosage forms of digoxin and among different brands of the same dosage form; changing from one preparation to another might require dosage adjustments

- **All dosage forms:** may be administered without regard to meals
- **Tab:** may be crushed and administered with food or fluids
- **Pediatric elixir:** administer using a calibrated measuring device

Injectable

- When changing from PO to IM/IV use 20%-25% less
- IV is preferred over IM because it is less painful and more rapid action
- PO should replace parenteral therapy as soon as possible
- Visually inspect parenteral products for particulate matter and discoloration before use

IM route

- Do not administer >2 ml at any one IM injection site
- Inject deeply into gluteal muscle, then massage area

IV route

- May be given undiluted or each 1 ml may be diluted in 4 ml of sterile water for injection, NS, D_5W, or LR; diluent volumes <4 ml will cause precipitation; use diluted solutions immediately
- Inject over ≥5 min via Y-site or 3-way stopcock; in patients with pulmonary edema, administer over 10-15 min; to avoid inadvertent overdosage, do not flush the syringe following administration

Additive compatibilities: Cimetidine, furosemide, lidocaine, potassium chloride, ranitidine, verapamil

Syringe compatibilities: Heparin, milrinone

Y-site compatibilities: Acyclovir, alfentanil, amikacin, aminocaproic acid, aminophylline, amphotericin B lipid complex, anidulafungin, ascorbic acid injection, atenolol, atracurium, atropine, aztreonam, benztropine, bivalirudin, bleomycin, bumetanide, buprenorphine, butorphanol, calcium chloride/gluconate, CARBOplatin, ceFAZolin, cefonicid, cefotaxime, cefoTEtan, cefOXitin, cefTAZidime, ceftizoxime, cefTRIAXone, cefuroxime, chloramphenicol, chlorproMAZINE, cimetidine, ciprofloxacin, cisatracurium, CISplatin, clindamycin, codeine, cyanocobalamin, cyclophosphamide, cycloSPORINE, cytarabine, DACTINomycin, DAPTOmycin, dexamethasone, dexmedetomidine, diltiazem, diphenhydrAMINE, DOBUTamine, DOCEtaxel, DOPamine, doripenem, doxacurium, doxycycline, enalaprilat, ePHEDrine, EPINEPHrine, epirubicin, epoetin alfa, eptifibatide, ertapenem, erythromycin, esmolol, etoposide, famotidine, fenoldopam, fentaNYL, fludarabine, fluorouracil, folic acid, furosemide, ganciclovir, gatifloxacin, gemcitabine, gentamicin, glycopyrrolate, granisetron, heparin, hydrocortisone, HYDROmorphone, hydrOXYzine, ifosfamide, imipenem-cilastatin, indomethacin, irinotecan, isoproterenol, ketorolac, labetalol, levofloxacin, lidocaine, linezolid, LORazepam, LR, magnesium sulfate, mannitol, mechlorethamine, meperidine, meropenem, methicillin, methotrexate, methyldopate, methylPREDNISolone, metoclopramide, metoprolol, metroNIDAZOLE, mezlocillin, miconazole, midazolam, milrinone, morphine, multiple vitamins injection, mycophenolate mofetil, nafcillin, nalbuphine, naloxone, nesiritide, metilmicin, nitroglycerin, nitroprusside, norepinephrine, octreotide, ondansetron, oxacillin, oxaliplatin, oxytocin, palonosetron, pamidronate, pancuronium, pantoprazole, papaverine, PEMEtrexed, penicillin G potassium/sodium, pentazocine, PENTobarbital, PHENobarbital, phenylephrine, phytonadione, piperacillin, piperacillin-tazobactam, polymyxin B, potassium chloride, procainamide, prochlorperazine, promethazine, propranolol, protamine, pyridoxine, quiNIDine, ranitidine, remifentanil, Ringer's, ritodrine, riTUXimab, rocuronium, sodium acetate/bicarbonate, succinylcholine, SUFentanil, tacrolimus, teniposide, theophylline, thiamine, thiotepa, ticarcillin, ticarcillin-clavulanate, tigecycline, tirofiban, TNA, tobramycin, tolazoline, TPN, trastuzumab, trimetaphan, urokinase, vancomycin, vasopressin, vecuronium, verapamil, vinCRIStine, vinorelbine, vitamin B complex, voriconazole, zoledronic acid

D

SIDE EFFECTS

CNS: *Headache,* drowsiness, apathy, confusion, disorientation, fatigue, depression, hallucinations

CV: **Dysrhythmias,** ***hypotension,*** bradycardia, **AV block**

EENT: Blurred vision, yellow-green halos, photophobia, diplopia

GI: Nausea, vomiting, anorexia, abdominal pain, diarrhea

PHARMACOKINETICS

Half-life 30-40 hr, excreted in urine, protein binding 20%-30%

PO: Onset ½-2 hr, peak 2-6 hr, duration 3-4 days

IV: Onset 5-30 min, peak 1-4 hr, duration variable

INTERACTIONS

Increase: toxicity—azole antifungals, macrolides, tetracyclines, ritonavir

Increase: hypercalcemia, hypomagnesemia, digoxin toxicity—thiazides, parenteral calcium

Increase: hypokalemia, digoxin toxicity—diuretics, amphotericin B, carbenicillin, ticarcillin, corticosteroids

Increase: digoxin levels—propantheline, quiNIDine, verapamil, amiodarone, anticholinergics, diltiazem, NIFEdipine, indomethacin

Increase: bradycardia—β-adrenergic blockers, antidysrythmics

Increase: cardiac dysrhythmia risk—sympathomimetics

Decrease: digoxin absorption—antacids, kaolin/pectin, cholestyramine, metoclopramide
Decrease: digoxin level—thyroid agents, cholestyramine, colestipol, metoclopramide, aMILoride

Drug/Food
Decrease: digoxin
Decrease: GI absorption—flaxseed, psyllium

Drug/Herb
Decrease: product effect—St. John's wort

Drug/Lab Test
Increase: CPK

NURSING CONSIDERATIONS

Assess:

- Apical pulse for 1 min before giving product; if pulse <60 in adult or <90 in infant, take again in 1 hr; if <60 in adult, call prescriber; note rate, rhythm, character; monitor ECG continuously during parenteral loading dose
- Electrolytes: potassium, sodium, chloride, magnesium, calcium; renal function studies: BUN, creatinine; blood studies: ALT, AST, bilirubin, Hct, Hgb before initiating treatment and periodically thereafter
- Monitor product levels; therapeutic level 0.5-2 ng/ml, draw ≥6-8 hr after last dose, optimally 12-24 hr after a dose

Evaluate:

- Therapeutic response: decreased weight, edema, pulse, respiration, crackles; increased urine output; serum digoxin level (0.5-2 ng/ml)

Teach patient/family:

- Not to stop product abruptly; about all aspects of product; to take exactly as ordered; how to monitor heart rate
- To avoid OTC medications, herbal remedies because many adverse product interactions may occur; not to take antacid at same time
- To notify prescriber of loss of appetite, lower stomach pain, diarrhea, weakness, drowsiness, headache, blurred or yellow vision, rash, depression, toxicity
- About the toxic symptoms of this product; when to notify prescriber
- To maintain a sodium-restricted diet as ordered
- To use one brand consistently

TREATMENT OF OVERDOSE:

Discontinue product; give potassium; monitor ECG; give adrenergic-blocking agent, digoxin immune FAB

RARELY USED

digoxin immune FAB (ovine) (Rx)

(di-jox′in im-myoon′ FAB)

DigiFab

Func. class.: Antidote—digoxin specific

USES:
Life-threatening digoxin toxicity

CONTRAINDICATIONS:
Mild digoxin toxicity, hypersensitivity to this product, papain or ovine protein

DOSAGE AND ROUTES

1 (40 mg) DigiFab binds 0.5 mg digoxin

Digoxin toxicity (known amount) (tabs, oral sol, IM)

- **Adult and child: IV** dose (mg) = dose ingested (mg) × 0.8/1000 × 38- or 40-mg vial

Toxicity (known amount) (cap, IV)

- **Adult and child: IV** dose = dose ingested (mg)/0.5 × 38- or 40-mg vial

Toxicity (known amount) by serum digoxin concentrations (SDCs)

- **Adult and child: IV** SDC (ng/ml) × kg of weight/100 × 38- or 40-mg vial

Digoxin toxicity (unknown amount)

- **Adult and child >20 kg: IV** 228 mg (6 vials)
- **Infant and child <20 kg: IV** 38 mg (1 vial)

Acute ingestion

- **Adult: IV** 380 mg (10 vials)

Life-threatening ingestion

- **Adult: IV** 760 mg (20 vials)

Skin test
- **Adult: ID** 0.1 ml of 1:100 dilution check after 20 min

⚠ HIGH ALERT

diltiazem (Rx)

(dil-tye′a-zem)

Apo-Diltiaz ♣, Cardizem, Cardizem CD, Cardizem LA, Cartia XT, Dilacor-XR, Dilt-CD, Diltia XR, Diltia XT, Diltzac, Taztia XT, Tiazac

Func. class.: Calcium channel blocker, antiarrhythmic class IV, antihypertensive

Chem. class.: Benzothiazepine

Do not confuse:
Cardizem/Cardene

ACTION: Inhibits calcium ion influx across cell membrane during cardiac depolarization; produces relaxation of coronary vascular smooth muscle, dilates coronary arteries, slows SA/AV node conduction times, dilates peripheral arteries

USES: **PO** angina pectoris due to coronary artery spasm, hypertension, **IV** atrial fibrillation, flutter, paroxysmal supraventricular tachycardia

Unlabeled uses: Unstable angina, proteinuria, cardiomyopathy, diabetic neuropathy

CONTRAINDICATIONS: Sick sinus syndrome, AV heart block, hypotension <90 mm Hg systolic, acute MI, pulmonary congestion, cardiogenic shock

Precautions: Pregnancy (C), breastfeeding, children, geriatric patients, CHF, aortic stenosis, bradycardia, GERD, hepatic disease, hiatal hernia, ventricular dysfunction

DOSAGE AND ROUTES

Prinzmetal's or variant angina, chronic stable angina
- **Adult: PO** 30 mg qid, increasing dose gradually to 180-360 mg/day in divided doses or **EXT REL** (LA, CD, XT, XR products) 180-360 mg, max 480-540 mg/day, depending on brand

Atrial fibrillation/flutter, paroxysmal supraventricular tachycardia
- **Adult: IV BOL** 0.25 mg/kg over 2 min initially, then 0.35 mg/kg may be given after 15 min; if no response, may give **CONT INFUSION** 5-15 mg/hr for up to 24 hr

Hypertension
- **Adult: PO** 30 mg TID, increase to max 480 mg/day; **EXT REL** 120-240 mg q day, max 540 mg/day; **SUS REL** 60 mg bid, max 360 mg/day

Rapid ventricular rate secondary to dysrhythmias (unlabeled)
- **Adolescent/child/infant >7 mo: IV BOL** 0.25 mg/kg over 5 min, then **CONT IV INFUSION** 0.11 mg/kg/hr

Available forms: Tabs 30, 60, 90, 120 mg; ext rel tabs 120, 180, 240, 300, 360, 420 mg; ext rel caps 60, 90, 120, 180, 240, 300, 360, 420 mg; inj 5 mg/ml (5, 10 ml); powder for inj 100 mg

Administer:

PO route
- Not all products are interchangeable
- Store at room temperature
- **Cardiazem LA** ext rel tab 24 hr: give daily, either AM or PM, without regard to meals
- **Dilacor XR/Diltia XT** ext rel cap 24 hr: give daily; take on empty stomach; swallow whole; do not cut, crush, chew, open
- **Tiazac, Tiztia XT:** give daily without regard to meals
- **Conventional regular-rel tab:** give before meals, at bedtime
- **Cardizem CD or equivalent (Cartia XT):** generic ext rel cap 24 hr: give daily, without regard to meals
- May crush, sprinkle regular tab on applesauce for administration

Direct IV route
- IV undiluted over 2 min

Continuous IV INFUSION route
- Diluted 125 mg/100 ml, 250 mg/250 ml of D_5W, 0.9% NaCl, $D_5/0.45\%$ NaCl, give 10 mg/hr, may increase by 5 mg/hr to 15 mg/hr, continue infusion up to 24 hr

Y-site compatibilities: Albumin, amikacin, amphotericin B, aztreonam, bumetanide, ceFAZolin, cefotaxime, cefoTEtan, cefOXitin, cefTAZidime, cefTRIAXone, cefuroxime, cimetidine, ciprofloxacin, clindamycin, digoxin, DOBUTamine, DOPamine, doxycycline, EPINEPHrine, erythromycin, esmolol, fentaNYL, fluconazole, gentamicin, hetastarch, HYDROmorphone, imipenem-cilastatin, labetalol, lidocaine, LORazepam, meperidine, metoclopramide, metroNIDAZOLE, midazolam, milrinone, morphine, multivitamins, niCARdipine, nitroglycerin, norepinephrine, oxacillin, penicillin G potassium, pentamidine, piperacillin, potassium chloride, potassium phosphates, ranitidine, sodium nitroprusside, theophylline, ticarcillin, ticarcillin/clavulanate, tobramycin, trimethoprim-sulfamethoxazole, vancomycin, vecuronium

SIDE EFFECTS

CNS: *Headache, fatigue, drowsiness,* dizziness, depression, weakness, insomnia, tremor, paresthesia
CV: Dysrhythmia, *edema,* CHF, bradycardia, hypotension, palpitations, heart block
GI: *Nausea,* vomiting, diarrhea, gastric upset, *constipation*, increased LFTs
GU: Nocturia, polyuria, acute renal failure
INTEG: *Rash,* flushing, photosensitivity, burning, pruritus at inj site
RESP: Rhinitis, dyspnea, pharyngitis

PHARMACOKINETICS

Onset 30-60 min; peak 2-3 hr immediate rel, 10-14 hr ext rel, 11-18 hr sus rel; half-life $3^1/_2$-9 hr; metabolized by liver; excreted in urine (96% as metabolites)

INTERACTIONS

Increase: effect, toxicity—theophylline
Increase: effects of β-blockers, digoxin, lithium, carBAMazepine, cycloSPORINE, anesthetics, HMG-CoA reductase inhibitors, benzodiazepines, lovastatin, methylPREDNISolone
Increase: effects of diltiazem—cimetidine

NURSING CONSIDERATIONS

Assess:
- **CHF:** dyspnea, weight gain, edema, jugular venous distention, rales; monitor I&O ratios daily, weight
- **Angina:** location, duration, alleviating factors, activity when pain starts
- **Dysrhythmias:** cardiac status: B/P, pulse, respiration, ECG and intervals PR, QRS, QT; if systolic B/P <90 mm Hg or HR <50 bpm, hold dose, notify prescriber

Evaluate:
- Therapeutic response: decreased anginal pain, decreased B/P

Teach patient/family:
- How to take pulse, B/P before taking product; that a record or graph should be kept
- To avoid hazardous activities until stabilized on product, dizziness is no longer a problem
- To limit caffeine consumption; to avoid grapefruit juice
- To avoid OTC products unless directed by prescriber
- About the importance of complying with all areas of medical regimen: diet, exercise, stress reduction, product therapy
- To change position slowly
- ⚠ To report dizziness, SOB, palpitations
- Not to discontinue abruptly

TREATMENT OF OVERDOSE:

Atropine for AV block, vasopressor for hypotension

dimenhyDRINATE (OTC, Rx)

(dye-men-hye′dri-nate)

Apo-DimenhyDRINATE ✦, Dramamine, Driminate, Gravol ✦

Motion Sickness

TripTone, Wal-Dram

Func. class.: Antiemetic, antihistamine, anticholinergic

Chem. class.: H_1-receptor antagonist, ethanolamine derivative

Do not confuse:
dimenhyDRINATE/diphenhydrAMINE

ACTION: Competes with histamine for H_1 receptors in GI tract, blood vessels, respiratory tract; central anticholinergic activity, which results in decreased vestibular stimulation and blockade of chemoreceptor trigger zone

USES: Motion sickness, nausea, vomiting, vertigo

Unlabeled uses: Hyperemesis gravidarum, Ménière's syndrome

CONTRAINDICATIONS: Hypersensitivity, infants, neonates, tartrazine dye hypersensitivity

Precautions: Pregnancy (B), breastfeeding, children, geriatric patients, cardiac dysrhythmias, asthma, prostatic hypertrophy, bladder-neck obstruction, closed-angle glaucoma, stenosing peptic ulcer, pyloroduodenal obstruction

DOSAGE AND ROUTES

- **Adult: PO** 50-100 mg q4hr; **IM/IV** 50 mg q4hr as needed (Canada only)
- **Child 6-12 yr: PO** 25-50 mg q6-8hr prn, max 150 mg/day
- **Child 2-5 yr: PO** 12.5-25 mg q6-8hr, max 75 mg/day

Available forms: Tabs 50 mg; inj 50 mg/ml ✦; elixir 15 mg/5 ml ✦; chew tabs 50 mg

Administer:

- IM inj in large muscle mass; aspirate to avoid IV administration (Canada only)
- Tablets may be swallowed whole, chewed, or allowed to dissolve

IV route (Canada only)

- After diluting 50 mg/10 ml of NaCl inj, give ≤50 mg over 2 min

SIDE EFFECTS

CNS: *Drowsiness,* restlessness, headache, dizziness, insomnia, confusion, nervousness, tingling, vertigo

CV: Hypertension, *hypotension*, palpitation

EENT: *Dry mouth,* blurred vision, diplopia, nasal congestion, photosensitivity, xerostomia

GI: Nausea, anorexia, vomiting, *constipation*

INTEG: Rash, urticaria, fever, chills, flushing

MISC: **Anaphylaxis**

PHARMACOKINETICS

PO/IM: Onset 15-30 min, duration 4-6 hr

INTERACTIONS

Increase: effect—alcohol, anticholinergic, tricyclics, MAOIs, opiates, sedative/hypnotics, other CNS depressants

Drug/Lab Test

False negative: Allergy skin testing

NURSING CONSIDERATIONS

Assess:

- VS, B/P; check patients with cardiac disease more often
- **Signs of toxicity** of other products or masking of symptoms of disease: brain tumor, intestinal obstruction
- Observe for drowsiness, dizziness

Evaluate:

- Therapeutic response: absence of nausea, vomiting, or vertigo

Teach patient/family:

- To avoid hazardous activities, activities requiring alertness because dizziness may occur; to request assistance with ambulation
- To avoid alcohol, other CNS depressants

dimethyl fumarate (Rx)

(dahy-meth'ul fyoo' muh-reyt)

Tecfidera

Func. class.: Immunomodulator

ACTION: Has beneficial effects on inflammation and oxidative stress. Induces an antioxidant effect–related neuronal death, and damage to myelin in the CNS may also improve mitochondrial function.

USES: Relapsing multiple sclerosis

CONTRAINDICATIONS: Hypersensitivity

Precautions: Pregnancy (C), breastfeeding, immunosuppression, infertility, male-mediated teratogenicity

DOSAGE AND ROUTES

- **Adult: PO** 120 mg bid × 7 days, may increase to 240 mg bid for maintenance

Available forms: Caps, del rel 120, 240 mg

Administer:

- Do not break, crush, or chew, do not open cap; give without regard to meals, use with food may decrease flushing

SIDE EFFECTS

CNS: *Flushing*

GI: Nausea, dyspepsia, abdominal pain, diarrhea, vomiting

GU: Albuminuria

INTEG: Rash, pruritus

HEMA: Lymphopenia, leukopenia

SYST: Anaphylaxis

PHARMACOKINETICS

Half-life 1 hr, peak 2½ hr

INTERACTIONS

None known

NURSING CONSIDERATIONS

Assess:

- **Multiple sclerosis:** monitor for improved number and severity of spasms, chronic pain, fatigue and weakness, balance and dizziness
- CBC with differential baseline and every 6 months thereafter; leukopenia and lymphopenia may occur
- **Anaphylaxis:** usually during first dose, but may occur any time during treatment; monitor for difficulty breathing, urticaria, and swelling of the throat and tongue
- **Pregnancy:** Identify if pregnancy is planned or suspected, pregnancy (C), or if breastfeeding

Evaluate:

- Therapeutic response: improved symptoms of multiple sclerosis

Teach patient/family:

- To notify prescriber if pregnancy is planned or suspected; not to breastfeed
- Expected results; side effects
- **Anaphylaxis:** discontinue the drug and seek immediate medical treatment if patient experiences difficulty breathing, urticaria, and swelling of the throat/tongue

dinoprostone (Rx)

(dye-noe-prost′one)

Cervidil, Prepidil, Prostin E-2

Func. class.: Oxytocic, abortifacient

Chem. class.: Prostaglandin E_2

Do not confuse:

Prepidil/bepridil

ACTION: Stimulates uterine contractions, causing abortion; acts within 30 hr for complete abortion

USES: Abortion during 2nd trimester, benign hydatidiform mole, expulsion of uterine contents in fetal deaths to 28 wk, missed abortion, to efface and dilate the cervix in pregnancy at term

CONTRAINDICATIONS:
Hypersensitivity, C-section, surgery, fetal distress, multiparity, vaginal bleeding, cephalopelvic disproportion

Precautions: Pregnancy (C), cardiac disease, asthma, anemia, jaundice, diabetes mellitus, seizure disorders, hypertension, glaucoma, uterine fibrosis, cervical stenosis, pelvic surgery, pelvic inflammatory disease, respiratory disease

Black Box Warning: Requires a specialized setting and an experienced clinician

DOSAGE AND ROUTES

Abortifacient/2nd trimester/missed abortion/benign hydatidiform mole/intrauterine fetal death

- **Adult:** VAG SUPP 20 mg, repeat q3-5hr until abortion occurs, max dose is 240 mg

Cervical ripening

- **Adult:** GEL 0.5 mg vag gel placed in cervical canal, may repeat after 6 hr, max 1.5 mg/24 hr; vag insert 10 mg high in vagina, remove at onset of active labor or within 12 hr

Available forms: VAG SUPP 20 mg; gel 0.5 mg/3 g (prefilled syringe); vag insert 10 mg

Administer:

- **By gel:** after warming to room temperature, remove seal from end of syringe, remove protective end cap and insert into plunger stopper assembly; make sure patient is in dorsal position; **insert:** must be kept frozen until use, warm to room temperature before use
- Antiemetic/antidiarrheal before administration of this product

SIDE EFFECTS

CNS: *Headache,* dizziness, chills, fever, flushing

CV: Hypotension, dysrhythmias, DIC

EENT: Blurred vision

SYST: Anaphylactoid syndrome of pregnancy

FETAL: Bradycardia (i.e., deceleration)

GI: *Nausea, vomiting, diarrhea*

GU: Vaginitis, vaginal pain, vulvitis, vaginismus

INTEG: Rash, skin color changes

MS: *Leg cramps, joint swelling,* weakness

GEL: Uterine contractile abnormality, GI side effects, back pain, fever

INSERT: Uterine hyperstimulation, fever, nausea, vomiting, diarrhea, abdominal pain

SUPPOSITORY: Uterine rupture, anaphylaxis

INTERACTIONS

Increase: effect—other oxytocics

Decrease: oxytocic effect—alcohol

PHARMACOKINETICS

Metabolized in spleen, kidney, lungs; excreted in urine

GEL: Onset 10 min, peak 30-45 min

SUPP: Onset 10 min, duration 2-3 hr

NURSING CONSIDERATIONS

Assess:

Black Box Warning: Specialized setting, specialized clinician: use only with emergency equipment nearby, by a clinician experienced when used in pregnancy termination; complete abortion should result within 17 hr

- **Cervical ripening:** dilation, effacement of cervix and uterine contraction, fetal heart tones, check for contractions over 1 min
- For fever that occurs $1/2$ hr after suppository insertion (abortion)
- Respiratory rate, rhythm, depth; notify prescriber of abnormalities, pulse, B/P, temperature
- **Vaginal discharge:** check for itching, irritation; indicates vaginal infection

Evaluate:

- Therapeutic response: expulsion of fetus

Teach patient/family:

- To remain supine for 10-15 min after insertion of supp, 2 hr after insert, 15-30 min after gel

- To report excessive cramping, bleeding, chills, fever
- About some methods of pain, comfort control
- To avoid intercourse, tub baths, douches, tampon use for at least 2 wk

diphenhydrAMINE (OTC, Rx)

(dye-fen-hye′dra-meen)

Allerdryl ✱, AllerMax ✱, Altaryl, Banophen, Benadryl, Benadryl Allergy, Benadryl Allergy Dye Free, Benadryl Children's Allergy, Buckley's Bedtime, Diphedryl, Diphenhist, Dytan, ElixSure Allergy, Equaline Allergy, Equaline Children's Allergy, Equate Allergy, Equate Children's Allergy, Genahist, Good Sense Children's Allergy Relief, Good Sense Diphedryl, Leader Complete Allergy, Nytol, PediaCare Children's Allergy, PediaCare Nighttime Cough, Q-Dryl Allergy, Select Brand Allergy, Siladryl, Silphen, Simply Sleep, Sleepinal, Sleep Tabs, Sominex, Unisom ✱, Valu-Dryl, Wal-dryl Allergy, Wal-dryl Allergy Dye Free, Wal-dryl Children's Allergy, ZzzQuil

Func. class.: Antihistamine (1st generation, nonselective)

Chem. class.: Ethanolamine derivative, H_1-receptor antagonist

Do not confuse:
diphenhydrAMINE/dicyclomine
diphenhydrAMINE/dimenhyDRINATE

ACTION: Acts on blood vessels, GI, respiratory system by competing with histamine for H_1-receptor site; decreases allergic response by blocking histamine

USES: Allergy symptoms, rhinitis, motion sickness, antiparkinsonism, nighttime sedation, infant colic, nonproductive cough, insomnia in children

Unlabeled uses: Nystagmus

CONTRAINDICATIONS: Hypersensitivity to H_1-receptor antagonist, neonates

Precautions: Pregnancy (B), breastfeeding, children <2 yr, increased intraocular pressure, cardiac/renal disease, hypertension, bronchial asthma, seizure disorder, stenosed peptic ulcers, hyperthyroidism, prostatic hypertrophy, bladder neck obstruction

DOSAGE AND ROUTES

- **Adult and child >12 yr: PO** 25-50 mg q4-6hr, max 300 mg/day; **IM/IV** 10-50 mg, max 300 mg/day
- **Child 6-12 yr: PO/IM/IV** 5 mg/kg/day in 4 divided doses, max 300 mg/day

Nighttime sleep aid

- **Adult and child ≥12 yr: PO** 25-50 mg at bedtime

Antitussive (syrup only)

- **Adult and child ≥12 yr: PO** 25 mg q4hr, max 150 mg/24 hr
- **Child 6-12 yr: PO** 12.5 mg q4hr, max 75 mg/24 hr

Peripheral vestibular nystagmus (unlabeled)

- **Adult: PO** 25-50 mg q4-6hr up to 48 hr

Available forms: Caps 25, 50 mg; tabs 25, 50 mg; chew tabs 12.5, 25 mg; elix 12.5 mg/5 ml; syr 12.5 mg/5 ml; inj 50 mg/ml; orally disintegrating tabs 12.5, mg; orally disintegrating strips 12.5, 25 mg

Administer:

⚠ Avoid use in children <2 yr; death has occurred; overdose has occurred with topical gel taken orally (adult/child)

- With meals for GI symptoms; absorption rate may slightly decrease
- At bedtime only if using for sleep aid

IM route

- Deep IM in large muscle; rotate site

Direct IV route

- Undiluted; give 25 mg/min or less

Intermittent IV INFUSION route

- Dilute with 0.9% NaCl, 0.45% NaCl, D_5W, 0.9% NaCl, $D_{10}W$, LR, Ringer's

Y-site compatibilities: Acetaminophen, aldesleukin, alfentanil hydrochloride, amifostine, amikacin sulfate, aminocaproic acid, amphotericin B lipid complex (Abelcet), amphotericin B liposome (AmBisome), amsacrine, anidulafungin, argatroban, ascorbic acid injection, atenolol, atracurium besylate, atropine sulfate, azithromycin, benztropine mesylate, bivalirudin, bleomycin, bumetanide, buprenorphine, butorphanol, calcium chloride/gluconate, CARBOplatin, caspofungin, cefTAZidime, ceftizoxime, chlorproMAZINE, cimetidine, ciprofloxacin, cisatracurium, CISplatin, cladribine, clindamycin, codeine, cyanocobalamin, cyclophosphamide, cycloSPORINE, cytarabine, DACTINomycin, DAPTOmycin, digoxin, diltiazem, DOBUTamine, DOCEtaxel, DOPamine, doripenem, doxacurium, DOXOrubicin, DOXOrubicin liposomal, doxycycline, enalaprilat, ePHEDrine, EPINEPHrine, epirubicin, epoetin alfa, eptifibatide, ertapenem, erythromycin, esmolol, etoposide, famotidine, fenoldopam, fentaNYL, filgrastim, fluconazole, fludarabine, folic acid, gallium, gatifloxacin, gemcitabine, gemtuzumab, gentamicin, glycopyrrolate, granisetron, HYDROmorphone, hydrOXYzine, IDArubicin, ifosfamide, imipenem-cilastatin, irinotecan, isoproterenol, labetalol, levofloxacin, lidocaine, linezolid, LORazepam, LR, magnesium sulfate, mannitol, mechlorethamine, melphalan, meperidine, meropenem, metaraminol, methadone, methicillin, methotrexate, methoxamine, methyldopate, metoclopramide, metoprolol, metroNIDAZOLE, miconazole, midazolam, minocycline, mitoXANtrone, morphine, multiple vitamins injection, mycophenolate, nalbuphine, naloxone, nesiritide, netilmicin, nitroglycerin, norepinephrine, octreotide, ondansetron, oxaliplatin, oxytocin, PACLitaxel, palonosetron, pamidronate, pancuronium, papaverine, PEMEtrexed, penicillin G potassium/sodium, pentamidine, pentazocine, phenylephrine, phytonadione, piperacillin, piperacillin-tazobactam, polymyxin B, potassium chloride, procainamide, prochlorperazine, promethazine, propofol, propranolol, protamine, pyridoxine, quiNIDine, quinupristin-dalfopristin, ranitidine, remifentanil, Ringer's, ritodrine, riTUXimab, rocuronium, sargramostim, sodium acetate, succinylcholine, SUFentanil, tacrolimus, teniposide, theophylline, thiamine, thiotepa, ticarcillin, ticarcillin-clavulanate, tigecycline, tirofiban, TNA, tobramycin, tolazoline, TPN, trastuzumab, trimetaphan, urokinase, vancomycin, vasopressin, vecuronium, verapamil, vinCRIStine, vinorelbine, vitamin B complex/C, voriconazole, zoledronic acid

SIDE EFFECTS

CNS: *Dizziness, drowsiness,* poor coordination, fatigue, anxiety, euphoria, confusion, paresthesia, neuritis, **seizures**
CV: Hypotension, palpitations
EENT: Blurred vision, dilated pupils, tinnitus, nasal stuffiness, dry nose, throat, mouth
GI: Nausea, anorexia, diarrhea
GU: *Retention,* dysuria, frequency
HEMA: **Thrombocytopenia, agranulocytosis, hemolytic anemia**
INTEG: Photosensitivity
MISC: **Anaphylaxis**
RESP: Increased thick secretions, wheezing, chest tightness

PHARMACOKINETICS

Metabolized in liver, excreted by kidneys, crosses placenta, excreted in breast milk, half-life 2-4 hr
PO: Peak 2-4 hr, duration 4-8 hr
IM: Onset ½ hr, peak 2-4 hr, duration 4-8 hr
IV: Onset immediate, duration 4-8 hr

INTERACTIONS

Increase: CNS depression—barbiturates, opiates, hypnotics, tricyclics, alcohol
Increase: diphenhydrAMINE effect—MAOIs

Drug/Lab Test
False negative: skin allergy tests

NURSING CONSIDERATIONS

Assess:

- Urinary retention, frequency, dysuria; product should be discontinued
- CBC during long-term therapy; blood dyscrasias may occur
- Respiratory status: rate, rhythm, increase in bronchial secretions, wheezing, chest tightness
- Product should be discontinued 4 days before skin allergy tests
- Store in tight container at room temperature

Evaluate:

- Therapeutic response: absence of running or congested nose or rashes, improved sleep

Teach patient/family:

- About all aspects of product use; to notify prescriber of confusion, sedation, hypotension
- To avoid driving, other hazardous activity if drowsiness occurs
- That photosensitivity may occur
- To avoid concurrent use of alcohol, other CNS depressants
- To avoid breastfeeding; not to breastfeed (injectable)
- To use hard candy, gum, frequent rinsing of mouth for dryness

TREATMENT OF OVERDOSE:

Administer diazepam, vasopressors, phenytoin IV

diphenoxylate/atropine (Rx)

(dye-fen-ox′ee-late/a′troe-peen)

Lomotil, Lonox

difenoxin/atropine (Rx)

(dye-fen-ox′in/a′troe-peen)

Motofen

Func. class.: Antidiarrheal

Chem. class.: Phenylpiperidine derivative opiate agonist

Controlled Substance Schedule V

diphenoxylate/atropine

Controlled Substance Schedule IV

difenoxin/atropine (US)

Do not confuse:

Lomotil/LaMICtal/LamISIL/Lanoxin/Lasix/Ludomil

ACTION: Inhibits gastric motility by acting on mucosal receptors responsible for peristalsis

USES: Acute nonspecific and acute exacerbations of chronic functional diarrhea

CONTRAINDICATIONS: Children <2 yr, hypersensitivity, pseudomembranous colitis, severe electrolyte imbalances, diarrhea associated with organisms that penetrate intestinal mucosa

Precautions: Pregnancy (C), breastfeeding, hepatic disease, ulcerative colitis, severe hepatic disease, substance abuse, dehydration

DOSAGE AND ROUTES

Diphenoxylate/atropine

- **Adult: PO** 5 mg qid titrated to patient response needed, max 8 tabs/day
- **Child 2-12 yr: PO** (liquid only) 0.3-0.4 mg/kg/day in 4 divided doses

Difenoxin/atropine

- **Adult: PO** 2 tabs, then 1 tab after each loose stool or q3-4hr prn, max 8 tabs/day

Available forms: Diphenoxylate/atropine: tabs 2.5 mg with atropine 0.025 mg; liquid 2.5 mg with atropine 0.025 mg/5 ml; **difenoxin/atropine:** tabs 1 mg difenoxin/0.025 atropine

Administer:

- For 48 hr only; if no response, product should be discontinued

SIDE EFFECTS

CNS: *Dizziness, drowsiness, lightheadedness, headache,* fatigue, nervousness, insomnia, confusion

EENT: Burning eyes, blurred vision

GI: *Nausea, vomiting, dry mouth, epigastric distress,* constipation, **paralytic ileus, toxic megacolon**

MISC: **Anaphylaxis, angioedema**

RESP: **Respiratory depression**

PHARMACOKINETICS

PO: Onset 40-60 min, peak 3 hr, duration 3-4 hr, terminal half-life 12-14 hr, metabolized in liver to active metabolite; excreted in urine and feces

INTERACTIONS

- **Do not use with MAOIs; hypertensive crisis may occur**

Increase: action of alcohol, opioids, barbiturates, other CNS depressants, anticholinergics

Decrease: GI motility, possible toxic megacolon—amantadine, antimuscarinics, amoxapine, diphenhydrAMINE, cloZAPine, clemastine, cyclobenzaprine, loperamide, maprotiline, phenothiazines, tricyclics, disopyramide, OLANZapine

NURSING CONSIDERATIONS

Assess:

- Electrolytes (potassium, sodium, chlorine) if receiving long-term therapy
- Bowel pattern before; for rebound constipation after termination of medication; bowel sounds
- Response after 48 hr; if none, product should be discontinued
- **Abdominal distention, toxic megacolon;** may occur in ulcerative colitis
- Hepatic studies if receiving long-term therapy

Evaluate:

- Therapeutic response: decreased diarrhea

Teach patient/family:

- To avoid OTC products unless directed by prescriber (may contain alcohol); not to use alcohol or CNS depressants
- Not to exceed recommended dose
- **That product may be habit forming**
- Not to engage in hazardous activities; that drowsiness may occur; not to use for longer than 48 hr for acute diarrhea

dipyridamole (Rx)

(dye-peer-id′a-mole)

Persantine

Func. class.: Coronary vasodilator, antiplatelet agent

Chem. class.: Nonnitrate

ACTION: Inhibits adenosine uptake, which produces coronary vasodilation; increases oxygen saturation in coronary tissues, coronary blood flow; acts on small resistance vessels with little effect on vascular resistance; may increase development of collateral circulation; decreases platelet aggregation by the inhibition of phosphodiesterase (an enzyme)

USES: Prevention of transient ischemic attacks, inhibition of platelet adhesion to prevent myocardial reinfarction, thromboembolism, with warfarin in prosthetic heart valves, prevention of coronary bypass graft occlusion with aspirin; IV form used to evaluate CAD; used as alternative to exercise with thallium myocardial perfusion imaging to evaluate CAD

Unlabeled uses: Cardiomyopathy, MI prophylaxis, proteinuria, TIA, valvular heart disease

CONTRAINDICATIONS: Hypersensitivity

Precautions: Pregnancy (B), breastfeeding, hypotension, unstable angina, asthma, hepatic disease, labor

DOSAGE AND ROUTES

Inhibition of platelet adhesion

• **Adult: PO** 75-100 mg qid in combination with warfarin, 75 mg qid with aspirin

Thallium myocardial perfusion imaging

• **Adult: IV** 570 mcg/kg, max 60 mg/day

TIA with aspirin (unlabeled)

• **Adult: PO** 225-400 mg/day max 400 mg/day

Available forms: Tabs 25, 50, 75 mg; inj 10 mg/2 ml

Administer:

PO route

• On empty stomach: 1 hr before meals or 2 hr after; give with 8 oz water for better absorption

• Store at room temperature

IV route

• IV after diluting to at least 1:2 ratio using D_5W, 0.45% NaCl, or 0.9% NaCl to a total vol of 20-50 ml; give over 4 min; do not give undiluted

• Inject thallium 201 within 5 min after product infusion

• Do not admix

SIDE EFFECTS

CNS: *Headache, dizziness, weakness, fainting, syncope;* IV: transient cerebral ischemia, weakness

CV: *Postural hypotension;* IV: MI

GI: *Nausea, vomiting,* anorexia, diarrhea

INTEG: *Rash,* flushing

PHARMACOKINETICS

PO: Peak 75 min; **IV** peak 2 min, therapeutic response may take several mo, metabolized in liver, excreted in bile, undergoes enterohepatic recirculation, protein binding 91%-99%, terminal half-life 12 hr

INTERACTIONS

• Prevention of coronary vasodilation: theophylline

Increase: digoxin effect—digoxin

Increase: bleeding risk—NSAIDs, cefoTEtan, valproic acid, salicylates, sulfinpyrazole, anticoagulants, thrombolytics

NURSING CONSIDERATIONS

Assess:

• B/P, pulse during treatment until stable; take B/P lying, standing; orthostatic hypotension is common

• Cardiac status: chest pain; what aggravates, ameliorates condition

Evaluate:

• Therapeutic response: decreased platelet adhesion

Teach patient/family:

• That medication is not a cure; may have to be taken continuously in evenly spaced doses only as directed

• To avoid hazardous activities until stabilized on medication; dizziness may occur

• To rise slowly from sitting or lying to prevent orthostatic hypotension

• Not to use alcohol or OTC medications unless approved by prescriber

HIGH ALERT

DOBUTamine (Rx)

(doe-byoo′ta-meen)

Func. class.: Adrenergic direct-acting β_1-agonist, cardiac stimulant

Chem. class.: Catecholamine

Do not confuse:

DOBUTamine/DOPamine

ACTION: Causes increased contractility, increased cardiac output without marked increase in heart rate by acting on β_1-receptors in heart; minor α and β_2 effects

USES: Cardiac decompensation due to organic heart disease or cardiac surgery

Unlabeled uses: Cardiogenic shock in children; congenital heart disease in children undergoing cardiac catheterization

CONTRAINDICATIONS:

Hypersensitivity, idiopathic hypertrophic subaortic stenosis

Precautions: Pregnancy (B), breastfeeding, children, hypertension, CAD, MI, hypovolemia, dysrhythmias, sulfite hypersensitivity, renal failure, geriatric patients

DOSAGE AND ROUTES

• **Adult and child: IV INFUSION** 0.5-1 mcg/kg/min; titrate to 2-20 mcg/kg/min may increase to 40 mcg/kg/min if needed

Available forms: Inj 12.5 mg/ml, 250 mg/20 ml

Administer:

Injectable

• Visually inspect parenteral products for particulate matter and discoloration before administration whenever solution and container permit

• Store reconstituted sol for 24 hr if refrigerated

IV route

Note: Infusions ≤72 hr have been given without development of tolerance; however, beta-receptor desensitization can occur with prolonged infusion of any beta-adrenergic agonist, including DOBUTamine, or as a consequence of sympathetic compensatory mechanisms associated with advanced congestive heart failure, resulting in alterations in DOBUTamine pharmacodynamics; experience with intravenous DOBUTamine in controlled trials does not extend beyond 48 hr of repeated boluses and/or continuous infusion

• Must be diluted before administration

• Infuse into a large vein

Dilution

• Concentrate for injection must be diluted with ≥50 ml of a compatible IV solution (strongly alkaline [e.g., sodium bicarbonate] solutions are incompatible); a common dilution is 500 mg (40 ml) in 210 ml D_5W or NS (withdraw 40 ml from a 250-ml bag) to produce a final concentration of 2000 mcg/ml; or 1000 mg (80 ml) in 170 ml D_5W or NS (withdraw 80 ml from a 250 ml bag) to produce a final concentration of 4000 mcg/ml; maximum concentrations should not exceed 5000 mcg/ml and should be adjusted according to the patient's fluid requirements

Infusion

• Administer diluted solution by IV infusion using a controlled-infusion device

• Premixed bags of DOBUTamine in D_5W solutions can exhibit a pink color that increases with time; this color change is due to slight oxidation of the drug, but there is no significant loss of potency

• Do not administer DOBUTamine simultaneously with solutions containing sodium bicarbonate or strong alkaline solutions (incompatible)

• Infusion of DOBUTamine should be started at a low rate and titrated frequently to reach the optimal dosage (see Dosage and Routes); dosage titration is guided by the patient's response, including systemic blood pressure, urine flow, frequency of ectopic activity, heart rate, and (whenever possible) measurements of cardiac output, central venous pressure, and/or pulmonary capillary wedge pressure

Y-site compatibilities: Alfentanil, alprostadil, amifostine, amikacin, aminocaproic acid, amiodarone, anidulafungin, argatroban, ascorbic acid injection, atenolol, atracurium, atropine, aztreonam, benztropine, bleomycin, bumetanide, buprenorphine, butorphanol, calcium chloride/gluconate, CARBOplatin, caspofungin, chlorproMAZINE, cimetidine, ciprofloxacin, cisatracurium, CISplatin, cladribine, clarithromycin, cloNIDine, codeine, cyanocobalamin, cyclophosphamide, cycloSPORINE, cytarabine, DACTINomycin, DAPTOmycin, dexmedetomidine, digoxin, diltiazem, diphenhydrAMINE, DOCEtaxel, DOPamine, doripenem, doxacurium, DOXOrubicin, DOXOrubicin liposomal, doxycycline, enalaprilat, ePHEDrine, EPINEPHrine, epirubicin, epoetin alfa, eptifibatide, erythromycin, esmolol, etoposide, famotidine, fenoldopam, fentaNYL, fluconazole, fludarabine, gatifloxacin, gemcitabine, gentamicin, glycopyrrolate, granisetron, HYDROmorphone, hydrOXYzine, IDArubicin, ifosfamide, irinotecan, isoproterenol, labetalol, levofloxacin, lidocaine, linezolid, LORazepam, LR, magnesium sulfate, mannitol, mechlorethamine, meperidine, meropenem, metaraminol, methoxamine, methyldopate, methylPREDNISolone, metoclopramide, metoprolol, metroNIDAZOLE, miconazole, milrinone, minocycline, mitoXANtrone, morphine, multiple vitamins injection, mycophenolate mofetil, nafcillin, nalbuphine, naloxone, netilmicin, niCARdipine, nitroglycerin, norepinephrine, octreotide, ondansetron, oxaliplatin, oxytocin, PACLitaxel, palonosetron, pamidronate, pancuronium, papaverine, pentamidine, pentazocine, phenylephrine, polymyxin B, potassium chloride, procainamide, prochlorperazine, promethazine, propofol, propranolol, protamine, pyridoxine, quiNIDine, ranitidine, remifentanil, Ringer's, ritodrine, riTUXimab, rocuronium, sodium acetate, succinylcholine, SUFentanil, tacrolimus, temocillin, teniposide, theophylline, thiamine, thiotepa, tigecycline, tirofiban, TNA, tobramycin, tolazoline, TPN, trastuzumab, trimetaphan, urokinase, vancomycin, vasopressin, vecuronium, verapamil, vinCRIStine, vinorelbine, voriconazole, zidovudine, zoledronic acid

SIDE EFFECTS

CNS: *Anxiety,* headache, dizziness, fatigue
CV: Palpitations, tachycardia, hypo/hypertension, PVCs, angina
ENDO: Hypokalemia
GI: Heartburn, nausea, vomiting
MS: Muscle cramps (leg)
RESP: Dyspnea

PHARMACOKINETICS

IV: Onset 1-2 min, peak 10 min, half-life 2 min, metabolized in liver (inactive metabolites), excreted in urine

INTERACTIONS

Increase: severe hypertension—guanethidine
Increase: dysrhythmias—general anesthetics
Increase: pressor effect, dysrhythmias—atomoxetine, COMT inhibitors, tricyclics, MAOIs, oxytocics
Decrease: DOBUTamine action—other β-blockers

NURSING CONSIDERATIONS

Assess:

• **Hypovolemia;** if present, correct first; administer cardiac glycoside before DOBUTamine
• **Oxygenation/perfusion deficit:** check B/P, chest pain, dizziness, loss of consciousness
• **Heart failure:** S_3 gallop, dyspnea, neck venous distention, bibasilar crackles in patients with CHF, cardiomyopathy, palpate peripheral pulses; report if extremities become cold or mottled or if peripheral pulses decrease
• **ECG** during administration continuously; if B/P increases, product is decreased; CVP or PCWP, cardiac output during infusion; report changes
• Serum electrolytes, urine output
⚠ **Sulfite sensitivity,** which may be life threatening

Evaluate:

• Therapeutic response: increased B/P with stabilization, increased urine output

Teach patient/family:

• About the reason for product administration; to report dyspnea, chest pain, numbness of extremities, headache, IV site discomfort

TREATMENT OF OVERDOSE:

Administer a β_1-adrenergic blocker; reduce IV or discontinue, ensure oxygenation/ventilation; for severe tachydysrhythmias (ventricular), give lidocaine or propranolol

⚠ HIGH ALERT

DOCEtaxel (Rx)

(doe-se-tax′el)

Docefrez, Taxotere

Func. class.: Antineoplastic—miscellaneous

Chem. class.: Taxane

Do not confuse:
Taxotere/Taxol

ACTION: Inhibits reorganization of microtubule network needed for interphase and mitotic cellular functions; also causes abnormal bundles of microtubules during cell cycle and multiple esters of microtubules during mitosis

USES: Locally advanced or metastatic breast cancer, non–small-cell lung cancer, androgen-independent metastatic prostate cancer, postsurgery operable node-positive breast cancer, induction treatment of locally advanced squamous cell of the head and neck, gastric adenocarcinoma

Unlabeled uses: Malignant melanoma, ovarian cancer, front-line use with bevacizumab for metastatic breast cancer, adjuvant treatment of breast cancer with CARBOplatin and trastuzumab

CONTRAINDICATIONS: Pregnancy (D), breastfeeding, hypersensitivity to this product, bilirubin exceeding upper normal limit

Black Box Warning: Other products with polysorbate 80, neutropenia of $<1500/mm^3$

Precautions: Children, cardiovascular disease, pulmonary disorders, bone marrow depression, herpes zoster, pleural effusion

Black Box Warning: Edema, hepatic disease, lung cancer, taxane hypersensitivity

DOSAGE AND ROUTES:
- Other regimens are used

Locally advanced or metastatic breast cancer after failure of other chemotherapy
- **Adult: IV** 60-100 mg/m^2 given over 1 hr q3wk; if neutrophil count is <500 cells/mm^3 for >1 wk, reduce dose by 25%

Operable node-positive breast cancer, adjuvant postsurgery treatment of operable node-positive breast cancer
- **Adult: IV** (TAC regimen) 75 mg/m^2 1 hr after DOXOrubicin 50 mg/m^2 and cyclophosphamide 500 mg/m^2 q3wk × 6 cycles

Adjuvant treatment of operable stage I-III invasive breast cancer in combination with cyclophosphamide
- **Adult: IV** (TC regimen) DOCEtaxel 75 mg/m^2 with cyclophosphamide 600 mg/m^2 q21days × 4 cycles

Locally advanced or metastatic non–small-cell lung cancer after failure of CISplatin chemotherapy
- **Adult: IV** 75 mg/m^2 over 1 hr q3wk; if neutrophil count is <500 cells/mm^3 for >1 wk, reduce dose to 55 mg/m^2; if patient develops grade 3 peripheral neuropathy, stop product

Unreactable, locally advanced, or metastatic non–small-cell lung cancer previously treated with chemotherapy
- **Adult: IV** 75 mg/m^2 over 1 hr, then CISplatin 75 mg/m^2 **IV** given over 30-60 min q3wk; reduce dose to 65 mg/m^2 in those with hematologic or non-hematologic toxicities

Androgen-independent metastatic prostate cancer
- **Adult: IV** 75 mg/m^2 given over 1 hr q3wk with 5 mg predniSONE **PO** bid continuously; give dexamethasone 8 mg **PO** at 12 hr, 3 hr, and 1 hr prior to DOCEtaxel; if neutrophil count is <500 cells/mm^3 for more than 1 wk or other toxicities occur, reduce dose to 60 mg/m^2

Squamous cell of head and neck
- **Adult: IV** 75 mg/m^2 over 1 hr, then CISplatin 100 mg/m^2 over 1 hr on day 1, then 5FU 1000 mg/m^2/day **CONT INFUSION** × 5 days, repeat cycle q3wk

Gastric adenocarcinoma
- **Adult: IV** 75 mg/m^2 q3wk, given with CISplatin, fluorouracil

Advanced ovarian cancer/ metastatic melanoma (unlabeled)
- **Adult: IV** 100 mg/m^2 over 1 hr q3wk

Available forms: Inj 10 mg/ml, 20 mg/0.5 ml, 20 mg/ml, 80 mg/2 ml, 80 mg/4 ml; 20, 80 mg powder for injection

Administer:
- Premedicate with dexamethasone 8 mg **PO** bid × 3 days starting 1 day before treatment
- Antiemetic 30-60 min before product and prn
- Confirmation that dexamethasone was given 12 hr and 6 hr before infusion begins
- Store prepared sol up to 27 hr in refrigerator

Intermittent IV INFUSION route
- Use cytotoxic handling procedures
- Use non-PVC bag and use non-DEHP tubing
- Allow vials to warm to room temperature; withdraw all diluent, inject in vial of DOCEtaxel; rotate gently to mix; allow to stand to decrease foaming, then withdraw the required amount (10 mg/ml), inject in 250 ml of 0.9% NaCl, D_5W; mix gently; give over 1 hr

Y-site compatibilities: Acyclovir, alfentanil, allopurinol, amifostine, amikacin, aminocaproic acid, aminophylline, amiodarone, amphotericin B lipid complex, ampicillin, ampicillin-sulbactam, anidulafungin, atenolol, atracurium, azithromycin, aztreonam, bivalirudin, bleomycin, bumetanide, buprenorphine, busulfan, butorphanol, calcium chloride/gluconate, CARBOplatin, carmustine, caspofungin, ceFAZolin, cefepime, cefonicid, cefotaxime, cefoTEtan, cefOXitin, cefTAZidime, ceftizoxime, cefTRIAXone, cefuroxime, chloramphenicol, chlorproMAZINE, cimetidine, ciprofloxacin, cisatracurium, CISplatin, clindamycin, codeine, cyclophosphamide, cycloSPORINE, cytarabine, dacarbazine, DACTINomycin, DAPTOmycin, dexamethasone, dexmedetomidine, dexrazoxane, diazepam, digoxin, diltiazem, diphenhydrAMINE, DOBUTamine, DOPamine, doripenem, doxacurium, DOXOrubicin HCL, doxycycline, droperidol, enalaprilat, ePHEDrine, EPINEPHrine, epirubicin, ertapenem, erythromycin, esmolol, etoposide, famotidine, fenoldopam, fentaNYL, fluconazole, fludarabine, fluorouracil, foscarnet, fosphenytoin, furosemide, ganciclovir, gatifloxacin, gemcitabine, gentamicin, glycopyrrolate, granisetron, haloperidol, heparin, hydrALAZINE, hydrocortisone, HYDROmorphone, hydrOXYzine, ifosfamide, imipenem-cilastatin, inamrinone, insulin (regular), irinotecan, isoproterenol, ketorolac, labetalol, leucovorin, levofloxacin, levorphanol, lidocaine, linezolid, LORazepam, LR, magnesium sulfate, mannitol, meperidine, meropenem, mesna, methotrexate, methyldopate, metoclopramide, metoprolol, metroNIDAZOLE, midazolam, milrinone, minocycline, mitoXANtrone, mivacurium, morphine, nafcillin, naloxone, nesiritide, netilmicin, niCARdipine, nitroglycerin, nitroprusside, norepinephrine, octreoide, ofloxacin, ondansetron, oxaliplatin, palonosetron, pamidronate, pancuronium, pantoprazole, PEMEtrexed, pentamidine, pentazocine, PENTobarbital, PHENobarbital, phenylephrine, piperacillin, piperacillin-tazobactam, polymyxin B, potassium chloride/phosphates, procainamide, prochlorperazine, promethazine, propranolol, quiNIDine, quinupristin-dalfopristin, ranitidine, remifentanil, riTUXimab, rocuronium, sodium acetate/bicarbonate/ phosphates, succinylcholine, SUFentanil, sulfamethoxazole-trimethoprim, tacrolimus, teniposide, theophylline, thiopental, thiotepa, ticarcillin, ticarcillin-clavulanate, tigecycline, tirofiban, tobramycin, tolazoline, trastuzumab, trimethobenzamide, vancomycin, vasopressin, vecuronium, verapamil, vinCRIStine, vinorelbine, voriconazole, zidovudine, zoledronic acid

SIDE EFFECTS

CNS: Seizures
CV: *Hypotension, fluid retention, peripheral edema,* flushing, MI, sinus tachycardia
GI: *Nausea, vomiting, diarrhea,* hepatotoxicity, stomatitis, colitis
HEMA: Neutropenia, leukopenia, thrombocytopenia, anemia, bleeding, infections, myelosuppression
INTEG: *Alopecia,* nail pain, rash, skin eruptions
MISC: Amenorrhea, fever of unknown origin, secondary malignancy, Stevens-Johnson syndrome, epiphora
MS: *Arthralgia, myalgia,* back pain, weakness
NEURO: *Peripheral neuropathy*
RESP: Dyspnea, pulmonary edema, fibrosis, embolism
SYST: *Hypersensitivity reactions*

PHARMACOKINETICS

Metabolized in liver, excreted in feces, terminal half-life 11.1 hr

INTERACTIONS

Increase: CYP3A inhibition: anastrozole (high doses), aprepitant, fosaprepitant, clarithromycin, conivaptan, delavirdine, efavirenz (induces or inhibits), erythromycin, fluconazole, FLUoxetine, fluvoxaMINE, imatinib, itraconazole, ketoconazole, nefazodone, voriconazole, and others
Increase: CYP3A induction: barbiturates, bosentan, carBAMazepine, nevirapine, phenytoin, fosphenytoin, rifabutin, rifampin, rifapentine
Increase: myelosuppression—other antineoplastics, radiation
Decrease: immune response—live virus vaccines

NURSING CONSIDERATIONS

Assess:

Black Box Warning: CBC, differential, platelet count before treatment and weekly; withhold product if WBC is <1500/mm^3 or platelet count is <100,000/mm^3; notify prescriber

Black Box Warning: DOCEtaxel, polysorbate 80 hypersensitivity: contraindicated

Black Box Warning: Edema: oral corticosteroids should be given as premedication, assess for fluid retention

Black Box Warning: Lung cancer: increased mortality in those with increased LFTs and a history of platinum-based products

- Monitor temperature; fever may indicate beginning of infection

Black Box Warning: **Hepatic disease:** hepatic studies before, during therapy (bilirubin, AST, ALT, LDH) prn or monthly; check for jaundiced skin and sclera, dark urine, clay-colored stools, itchy skin, abdominal pain, fever, diarrhea

- **CNS changes:** confusion, paresthesias, peripheral neuropathy, dysesthesia, pain, weakness; if severe, product should be discontinued
- VS during 1st hr of infusion, check IV site for signs of infiltration

Black Box Warning: **Hypersensitive reactions, anaphylaxis,** including hypotension, dyspnea, angioedema, generalized urticaria; discontinue infusion immediately

- **Bone marrow depression/bleeding:** hematuria, guaiac, bruising or petechiae, mucosa or orifices q8hr; obtain prescription for viscous lidocaine (Xylocaine); avoid invasive procedures
- Effects of alopecia on body image; discuss feelings about body changes

Evaluate:

- Therapeutic response: decreased tumor size, spread of malignancy

Teach patient/family:

- To report signs of **infection:** fever, sore throat, flulike symptoms
- To report signs of **anemia:** fatigue, headache, faintness, SOB, irritability

- To report **bleeding;** to avoid use of razors, commercial mouthwash
- To avoid use of aspirin, ibuprofen
- That hair may be lost during treatment; that a wig or hairpiece may make patient feel better; that new hair may be different in color and texture
- That pain in muscles and joints 2-5 days after infusion is common
- To use barrier contraception during and for several mo after treatment, pregnancy (D); to avoid breastfeeding
- To avoid receiving vaccinations while taking product

docosanol topical

See Appendix B

docusate calcium (OTC)

(dok′yoo-sate cal′see-um)

Kaopectate Stool Softener, Kao-Tin

docusate sodium (OTC)

Colace, Correctol, Diocto, Docu DOK, Doculace, Enemeez, Fleet Pedialax, Fleet Sof-Lax, Phillips Liquid-Gels, Selex ✦, Silace, Soflax ✦

Func. class.: Laxative, emollient; stool softener

Chem. class.: Anionic surfactant

ACTION: Increases water, fat penetration in intestine; allows for easier passage of stool

USES: Prevention of dry, hard stools

CONTRAINDICATIONS: Hypersensitivity, obstruction, fecal impaction, nausea/vomiting

Precautions: Pregnancy (C), breastfeeding

DOSAGE AND ROUTES

- **Adult: PO** 50-300 mg/day (sodium) or 240 mg (calcium); **ENEMA** 4 ml
- **Child >12 yr: ENEMA** 2 ml
- **Child 6-12 yr: PO** 40-150 mg/day (sodium) in divided doses
- **Child 3-6 yr: PO** 20-60 mg/day (sodium) in divided doses
- **Child <3 yr: PO** 10-40 mg/day (sodium) in divided doses

Available forms: *Calcium:* 240 mg; *sodium:* caps 50, 100, 250 mg; tabs 100 mg; syr 20 mg/5 ml; liquid 50 mg/5 ml, enema 283 mg

Administer:

- Swallow tabs whole; do not break, crush, or chew
- Oral sol: diluted in milk, fruit juice to decrease bitter taste
- In morning or evening (oral dose)
- Store in cool environment; do not freeze

SIDE EFFECTS

EENT: Bitter taste, throat irritation
GI: Nausea, anorexia, cramps, diarrhea
INTEG: Rash

PHARMACOKINETICS

Onset 12-72 hr

INTERACTIONS

- **Toxicity:** mineral oil

Drug/Herb

Increase: laxative action—flax, senna

NURSING CONSIDERATIONS

Assess:

- **Cause of constipation;** identify whether fluids, bulk, or exercise missing from lifestyle; constipating products
- Cramping, rectal bleeding, nausea, vomiting; if these occur, product should be discontinued

Evaluate:

- Therapeutic response: decrease in constipation

Teach patient/family:

- That normal bowel movements do not always occur daily

- Not to use in presence of abdominal pain, nausea, vomiting
- To notify prescriber if constipation unrelieved or if symptoms of electrolyte imbalance occur: muscle cramps, pain, weakness, dizziness, excessive thirst
- That product may take up to 3 days to soften stools
- To take oral preparations with a full glass of water (unless on fluid restrictions) and to increase fluid intake

⚠ HIGH ALERT

dofetilide (Rx)

Tikosyn

Func. class.: Antidysrhythmic (Class III)

ACTION: Blocks cardiac ion channel carrying the rapid component of delayed potassium current; no effect on sodium channels

USES: Atrial fibrillation, flutter, maintenance of normal sinus rhythm

CONTRAINDICATIONS: Children, hypersensitivity, digoxin toxicity, aortic stenosis, pulmonary hypertension, severe renal disease

Black Box Warning: QT prolongation, torsades de pointes, renal failure

Precautions: Pregnancy (C), breastfeeding, AV block, bradycardia, electrolyte imbalance

Black Box Warning: Renal disease, arrhythmias, ventricular arrhythmias/tachycardia

DOSAGE AND ROUTES

Conversion of atrial fibrillation/atrial flutter to normal sinus rhythm; maintenance therapy with highly symptomatic atrial fibrillation/atrial flutter of ≥1 wk duration

- **Adult: PO** Individualize dosage based on renal function and QTc in a monitored facility; refer to the step-by-step procedure for determining the initial dosage of dofetilide

Maintenance therapy of atrial fibrillation/atrial flutter after hospital discharge

- **Adult: PO** Continue dosage at discharge as from initial dosage titration; individualize dosage based on renal function and QTc, which should be re-evaluated every 3 mo or as medically warranted; if the QTc >500 msec (550 msec in patients with ventricular conduction abnormalities) at any time, discontinue; carefully monitor until QTc returns to baseline; if renal function deteriorates, adjust the dosage as described in the dosage guidelines for patients with renal impairment

Discontinuation of dofetilide before use of interacting drugs

- **Adult: PO** Discontinue dofetilide for ≥2 days before starting a potentially interacting drug

Renal dose

- **Adult: PO** CCr >60 ml/min, 500 mcg bid; CCr 40-60 ml/min, 250 mcg bid; CCr 20-39 ml/min, 125 mcg bid; CCr <20 ml/min, do not use

Available forms: Caps 125, 250, 500 mcg

Administer:

- Physician and pharmacy must be registered to use product

Black Box Warning: Step 1: Assess cardiac conduction: Before first dose, the QTc interval must be determined using an average of 5-10 beats; if the QTc interval is >440 msec (or >500 msec in ventricular conduction abnormalities), do not use; if baseline heart rate is <60 bpm, then the QT interval should be used

Black Box Warning: Step 2: Assess renal function: Before first dose, determine renal function using the Cockroft-Gault equation, use actual body weight to calculate creatinine clearance

Black Box Warning: Step 3: Adjust starting dose according to renal function: Refer to the renal dose section above to determine the appropriate initial dosage

Black Box Warning: Step 4: ECG monitoring: Begin continuous ECG monitoring starting with the first dose

Black Box Warning: Step 5: Dosage adjustments: Approximately 2-3 hr after the first dose, determine the QTc interval; if the QTc interval has increased by >15% (compared to baseline), or if the QTc interval is >500 msec (>550 msec in patients with ventricular conduction abnormalities), the initial dosage should be reduced by half as follows:

- Decrease an initial dose of 500 mcg bid to 250 mcg bid
- Decrease an initial dose of 250 mcg bid to 125 mcg bid
- Decrease an initial dose of 125 mcg bid to 125 mcg/day

Black Box Warning: Step 6: Reassess QTc interval: Reassess the QTc interval 2-3 hr after each subsequent dose; if the QTc interval lengthens to >500 msec (or >550 msec in patients with ventricular conduction abnormalities), *discontinue*

Black Box Warning: Step 7: ECG monitoring: Monitor continuous ECG for a minimum of 3 days or for 12 hr after conversion to normal sinus rhythm, whichever is greater

SIDE EFFECTS

CNS: *Syncope, dizziness,* headache, stroke
CV: *Hypotension, postural hypotension, bradycardia,* angina, PVCs, substernal pressure, transient hypertension, precipitation of angina, QT prolongation, torsades de pointes, ventricular dysrhythmias, chest pain
GI: *Nausea, vomiting,* severe diarrhea, anorexia
MISC: Angioedema
RESP: Dyspnea, respiratory infections

PHARMACOKINETICS

Well absorbed, max plasma concentrations 2-3 hr, steady state 2-3 days, half-life 10 hr, metabolized by liver, excreted by kidneys

INTERACTIONS

- Do not use with cimetidine, ketoconazole, verapamil, prochlorperazine, trimethoprim-sulfamethoxazole, megestrol, hydrochlorothiazide

Increase: QT prolongation, torsades de pointes—class IA/III antidysrhythmics, arsenic trioxide, chloroquine, clarithromycin, droperidol, erythromycin, halofantrine, haloperidol, methadone, pentamidine, some phenothiazines, ziprasidone, ciprofloxacin
Increase: hypokalemia—potassium-depleting diuretics
Increase: toxicity—aMILoride metFORMIN, entecavir, lamiVUDine, memantine, triamterene, procainamide, trospium
Increase: dofetilide levels—antiretroviral protease inhibitors

Drug/Food

- Do not use with grapefruit juice

NURSING CONSIDERATIONS

Assess:

- AF patients should receive anticoagulation prior to cardioversion
- Cardiac status: rate, rhythm, character, continuously; B/P

Black Box Warning: Severe renal impairment CCr <20 ml/min: do not use for mild to moderate renal disease; monitor BUN/creatinine; adjust dose based on creatinine clearance

Evaluate:

- Therapeutic response: control of atrial fibrillation

Teach patient/family:

- To make position changes slowly; orthostatic hypotension may occur
- To notify prescriber if fast heartbeats with fainting or dizziness occur
- To notify all prescribers of all medications, supplements taken
- That if dose is missed, not to double; to take next dose at usual time
- To avoid breastfeeding

dolasetron (Rx)

(do-la′se-tron)

Anzemet

Func. class.: Antiemetic

Chem. class.: 5-HT3 receptor antagonist

ACTION: Prevents nausea, vomiting by blocking serotonin peripherally, centrally, and in the small intestine

USES: Prevention of postoperative nausea, vomiting

Unlabeled uses: Radiotherapy-induced nausea/vomiting

CONTRAINDICATIONS: Hypersensitivity

Precautions: Pregnancy (B), breastfeeding, children, geriatric patients, hypokalemia, electrolyte imbalances; granisetron/ondansetron/palonosetron hypersensitivity, QT prolongation

DOSAGE AND ROUTES

Prevention of postoperative nausea and vomiting

- **Adult: IV** 12.5 mg as single dose 15 min before cessation of anesthesia; **PO** 100 mg 2 hr before surgery (prevention only)
- **Child 2-16 yr: IV** 0.35 mg/kg as single dose 15 min before cessation of anesthesia; **PO** 1.2 mg/kg 2 hr before surgery (prevention only)

Available forms: Tabs 50, 100 mg; inj 20 mg/ml, 12.5 mg/0.625 ml

Administer:

PO route

- Do not mix product for oral administration in apple or apple-grape juice until immediately before administration; diluted product can be kept for 2 hr at room temperature
- Store at room temperature 48 hr after dilution

Intermittent IV INFUSION route

- By inj 100 mg/30 sec or more or diluted in 50 ml compatible sol; give over 15 min
- Do not admix

SIDE EFFECTS

CNS: *Headache,* dizziness, fatigue, drowsiness

CV: Dysrhythmias, ECG changes, hypo/hypertension, tachycardia, bradycardia; **ventricular tachycardia/fibrillation, QT prolongation, torsades de pointes, cardiac arrest (IV)**

GI: *Diarrhea,* constipation, increased AST/ALT, abdominal pain, anorexia

GU: Urinary retention, oliguria

MISC: Rash, **bronchospasm**

PHARMACOKINETICS

Well absorbed, metabolized to active metabolite, half-life of active metabolite 8 hr, max concentrations after 1 hr

INTERACTIONS

- **QT Prolongation:** QRS, PR prolongation; do not use in those with congenital long QT syndrome, hypokalemia, hypomagnesemia, complete heart block

(unless a pacemaker is in place), correct electrolytes before use, monitor ECG in elderly patients, renal cardiac disease
Increase: dysrhythmias—antidysrhythmics
Increase: dolasetron levels—cimetidine
Increase: QT prolongation—thiazide/loop diuretics, antidysrhythmics—class IA, III, arsenic trioxide, chloroquine, clarithromycin, droperidol, erythromycin, halofantrine, haloperidol, methadone, pentamidine, some phenothiazines, ziprasidone; occurs at higher dose of dolasetron
Decrease: dolasetron levels—rifampin

NURSING CONSIDERATIONS

Assess:

- **Hypersensitivity reaction:** rash, bronchospasm
- Cardiac conduction conditions, electrolyte imbalances, dysrhythmias, heart rate

Evaluate:

- Therapeutic response: absence of nausea, vomiting during cancer chemotherapy

Teach patient/family:

- To report diarrhea, constipation, nausea, vomiting, rash, or changes in respirations
- May cause headache; use analgesic

dolutegravir

(dole-oo-teg′ra-vir)

Tivicay

Func. class: Antiretroviral
Chem class: HIV integrase strand transfer inhibitor (ISTIs)

ACTION: Inhibits catalytic activity of HIV integrase, which is an HIV-encoded enzyme needed for replication

USES: HIV in combination with other retrovirals

CONTRAINDICATIONS: Breastfeeding, hypersensitivity

Precautions: Pregnancy (C), children, geriatric patients, hepatic disease, immune reconstitution syndrome, hepatitis, antimicrobial resistance, lactase deficiency

DOSAGE AND ROUTES

- **Adult and child ≥12 yr and ≥40 kg (treatment naïve or treatment experienced but integrase strand transfer inhibitor naïve): PO** 50 mg daily; if given with efavirenz, fosamprenavir/ritonavir, tipranavir/ritonavir, or rifampin, give 50 mg bid

Available forms: Tabs 50 mg

Administer:

- May give without regard to meals, with 8 oz of water
- Store at room temperature
- Give 2 hr before or 6 hr after cation-containing antacids or laxatives, sucralfate, oral iron, oral calcium, or buffered products

SIDE EFFECTS

CNS: Fatigue, fever, dizziness, headache, asthenia, suicidal ideation
CV: MI
GI: Nausea, vomiting, diarrhea, abdominal pain, asthenia, gastritis, hepatitis
INTEG: Rash, pruritus, urticaria
META: Hyperglycemia
SYST: Immune reconstitution syndrome

PHARMACOKINETICS

Peak 2-3 hr, steady state 5 days, terminal half-life 14 hr, 98% protein binding, metabolized in the liver, excreted in feces 53%, urine 31%

INTERACTIONS

Decreased: effect of dolutegravir—antacids, laxatives/ sucralfate, oral iron, oral calcium, buffered products
Decreased: levels—rifampin efavirenz, tenofovir, tipranavir/ritonavir

Drug/Herb

- Avoid concurrent use with St. John's wort

NURSING CONSIDERATIONS

Assess:

- HIV infection: CD4, T-cell count, plasma HIV RNA, viral load; resistance testing before treatment, at treatment failure
- Drug resistance testing before use in treatment naïve patients
- **Immune reconstitution syndrome, usually during initial phase of treatment; may need antiinfective before starting**
- Monitor total HDL/LDL cholesterol baseline and periodically; all may be elevated

Evaluate:

- Therapeutic response: improvement in cell counts, T-cell counts

Teach patient/family:

- To take as prescribed; if dose missed to take as soon as remembered up to 1 hr before next dose; not to double dose; not to share with others
- That sexual partners need to be told that patient has HIV; that product does not cure infection, just controls symptoms, does not prevent infecting others
- To report sore throat, fever, fatigue (may indicate superinfection)
- To notify prescriber if pregnancy is planned or suspected; to avoid breastfeeding and to continue follow-up exams and work

donepezil (Rx)

(don-ep-ee′zill)

Aricept, Aricept ODT

Func. class.: Anti-Alzheimer's agent

Chem. class.: Reversible cholinesterase inhibitor

ACTION: Elevates acetylcholine concentrations (cerebral cortex) by slowing degradation of acetylcholine released in cholinergic neurons; does not alter underlying dementia

USES: Mild to severe dementia with Alzheimer's disease

Unlabeled uses: Subcortical, vascular dementia; dementia with Lewy bodies

CONTRAINDICATIONS: Hypersensitivity to this product or piperidine derivatives

Precautions: Pregnancy (C), breastfeeding, children, sick sinus syndrome, history of ulcers, GI bleeding, hepatic disease, bladder obstruction, asthma, seizures, COPD, abrupt discontinuation, AV block, GI obstruction, Parkinson's disease, surgery

DOSAGE AND ROUTES

- **Adult: PO** 5 mg/day at bedtime; may increase to 10 mg/day after 4-6 wk, may increase to 23 mg/day after 3 mo of 10 mg/day (moderate to severe)

Available forms: Tabs 5, 10, 23 mg; orally disintegrating tabs (Aricept ODT) 5, 10 mg

Administer:

- Daily in the evening before bedtime; swallow whole; do not cut, break, chew, or crush tab
- Dosage adjusted to response no more than q4-6wk; oral dosage forms are interchangeable
- **Orally disintegrating tabs:** allow to dissolve on tongue before swallowing; may be given with/without water

SIDE EFFECTS

CNS: Dizziness, *insomnia,* somnolence, *headache,* fatigue, abnormal dreams, syncope, **seizures**, drowsiness, agitation, depression, confusion, fever, hallucinations

CV: **Atrial fibrillation**, hypo/hypertension, **sinus bradycardia, AV block**

GI: *Nausea, vomiting,* anorexia, *diarrhea,* abdominal pain, **GI bleeding**, weight loss

GU: Urinary frequency, UTI, incontinence

INTEG: Rash, flushing, diaphoresis, bruising

META: Hyperlipidemia

MS: Cramps, arthritis, arthralgia, back pain

RESP: Rhinitis, URI, cough, pharyngitis, dyspnea

PHARMACOKINETICS

Well absorbed PO; metabolized by CYP2D6, CYP3A4; elimination half-life 10 hr single dose, 70 hr multiple doses; protein binding 96%

INTERACTIONS

Increase: donepezil effects—CYP2D6, CYP3A4 inhibitors
Increase: synergistic effect—succinylcholine, cholinesterase inhibitors, cholinergic agonists
Increase: GI intolerance—NSAIDs
Decrease: donepezil effects—CYP2D6, CYP3A4 inducers
Decrease: action of anticholinergics
Increase: QT prolongation—dofetilide, dronedarone, grepafloxacin, mesoridazine, pimozide, probucol, sparfloxacin, ziprasidone, do not use concurrently
Decrease: donepezil effect—carBAMazepine, dexamethasone, phenytoin, PHENObarbital, rifampin
Drug/Herb
Decrease: donepezil—St. John's wort

NURSING CONSIDERATIONS

Assess:
- B/P: hypo/hypertension, heart rate
- Mental status: affect, mood, behavioral changes, depression, complete suicide assessment; neurologic status
- GI status: nausea, vomiting, anorexia, diarrhea; monitor weight
- GU status: urinary frequency, incontinence, I&O
- Assistance with ambulation during beginning therapy; dizziness, ataxia may occur

Evaluate:
- Therapeutic response: decrease in confusion, improved mood

Teach patient/family:
- To report side effects: twitching, nausea, vomiting, sweating, dizziness; indicates cholinergic crisis or overdose
- To use product exactly as prescribed, not to use with other products, unless approved by prescriber
- To notify prescriber of nausea, vomiting, diarrhea (dose increase or beginning treatment), or rash
- Not to increase or abruptly decrease dose; serious consequences may result
- That product is not a cure, relieves symptoms

⚠ HIGH ALERT

DOPamine (Rx)

(doe′pa-meen)
Func. class.: Adrenergic
Chem. class.: Catecholamine

Do not confuse:
DOPamine/DOBUTamine

ACTION:
Causes increased cardiac output; acts on β_1- and α-receptors, causing vasoconstriction in blood vessels; low dose causes renal and mesenteric vasodilation; β_1 stimulation produces inotropic effects with increased cardiac output

USES:
Shock, increased perfusion, hypotension, cardiogenic/septic shock
Unlabeled uses: Bradycardia, cardiac arrest, CPR, acute renal failure, cirrhosis, barbiturate intoxication

CONTRAINDICATIONS:
Hypersensitivity, ventricular fibrillation, tachydysrhythmias, pheochromocytoma, hypovolemia
Precautions: Pregnancy (C), breastfeeding, geriatric patients, arterial embolism, peripheral vascular disease, sulfite hypersensitivity, acute MI

Black Box Warning: Extravasation

DOSAGE AND ROUTES

- **Adult: IV INFUSION** 2-5 mcg/kg/min, titrate upward in 5-10 mcg/kg/min increments, max 50 mcg/kg/min; titrate to patient's response
- **Child: IV** 1-5 mcg/kg/min initially; usual dosage range, 2-20 mcg/kg/min

CHF

- **Adult: IV** 3-10 mcg/kg/min

Bradycardia (unlabeled)

- **Adult: IV** 2-10 mcg/kg/min, titrate as needed

Available forms: Inj 40 mg, 80 mg, 160 mg/ml; concentrations for IV infusion 0.8, 1.6, 3.2 mg/ml in 250, 500 ml D_5W

Administer:

- Store reconstituted sol for up to 24 hr if refrigerated
- Do not use discolored sol; protect from light

IV route

- IV after diluting 200-400 mg/250-500 ml of D_5W, D_5 0.45% NaCl, D_5 0.9% NaCl, D_5LR, LR; use large vein
- After reconstituting, use infusion pump; give at rate of 0.5-5 mcg/kg/min, increase by 1-4 mcg/kg/min at 10-30 min intervals until desired response

Black Box Warning: Extravasation: if extravasation occurs, stop infusion, may inject area with phentolamine 10 mg/15 ml of NS

Y-site compatibilities: Alfentanil, alprostadil, amifostine, amikacin, aminocaproic acid, aminophylline, amiodarone, anidulafungin, argatroban, ascorbic acid injection, atenolol, atracurium, atropine, aztreonam, benztropine, bivalirudin, bleomycin, bumetanide, buprenorphine, butorphanol, calcium chloride/gluconate, CARBOplatin, caspofungin, cefmetazole, cefonicid, cefotaxime, cefoTEtan, cefOXitin, cefTAZidime, ceftizoxime, cefTRIAXone, cefuroxime, chlorproMAZINE, cimetidine, ciprofloxacin, cisatracurium, CISplatin, cladribine, clarithromycin, clindamycin, cloNIDine, codeine, cyanocobalamin, cyclophosphamide, cycloSPORINE, cytarabine, DACTINomycin, DAPTOmycin, dexamethasone, dexmedetomidine, digoxin, diltiazem, diphenhydrAMINE, DOBUTamine, DOCEtaxel, doripenem, doxacurium, DOXOrubicin, DOXOrubicin liposomal, doxycycline, droperidol, enalaprilat, ePHEDrine, EPINEPHrine, epirubicin, epoetin alfa, eptifibatide, ertapenem, erythromycin, esmolol, etoposide, famotidine, fenoldopam, fentaNYL, fluconazole, fludarabine, fluorouracil, folic acid, foscarnet, gatifloxacin, gemcitabine, gemtuzumab, gentamicin, glycopyrrolate, granisetron, heparin, hydrocortisone, HYDROmorphone, hydrOXYzine, IDArubicin, ifosfamide, imipenem-cilastatin, irinotecan, isoproterenol, ketorolac, labetalol, levofloxacin, lidocaine, linezolid, LORazepam, LR, magnesium sulfate, mannitol, mechlorethamine, meperidine, methicillin, methyldopate, methylPREDNISolone, metoclopramide, metoprolol, metroNIDAZOLE, micanfungin, miconazole, midazolam, milrinone, minocycline, mitoXANtrone, morphine, multiple vitamins injection, mycophenolate, nafcillin, nalbuphine, naloxone, netilmicin, niCARdipine, nitroglycerin, nitroprusside, norepinephrine, octreotide, ondansetron, oxacillin, oxaliplatin, oxytocin, PACLitaxel, palonosetron, pamidronate, pancuronium, pantoprazole, papaverine, PEMEtrexed, penicillin G potassium/sodium, pentamidine, pentazocine, PENTobarbital, PHENobarbital, phenylephrine, phytonadione, piperacillin, piperacillin-tazobactam, polymyxin B, potassium chloride, procainamide, prochlorperazine, promethazine, propofol, propranolol, protamine, pyridoxine, quiNIDine, ranitidine, remifentanil, Ringer's, ritodrine, riTUXimab, rocuronium, sargramostim, sodium acetate, succinylcholine, SUFentanil, tacrolimus, temocillin, teniposide, theophylline, thiamine, thiotepa, ticarcillin, ticarcillin-clavulanate, tigecycline, tirofiban, TNA, tobramycin, tolazoline, TPN, trastuzumab, trimetaphan, urokinase, vancomycin, vasopressin, vecuronium, verapamil, vinCRIStine, vinorelbine, vitamin B complex/C, voriconazole, warfarin, zidovudine, zoledronic acid

SIDE EFFECTS

CNS: *Headache,* anxiety
CV: *Palpitations,* tachycardia, *hypertension, ectopic beats, angina,* wide QRS complex, peripheral vasoconstriction, hypotension
GI: *Nausea, vomiting, diarrhea*
INTEG: Necrosis, tissue sloughing with extravasation, gangrene
RESP: Dyspnea

PHARMACOKINETICS

IV: Onset 5 min; duration <10 min; metabolized in liver, kidney, plasma; excreted in urine (metabolites); half-life 2 min

INTERACTIONS

- Do not use within 2 wk of MAOIs; hypertensive crisis may result

Increase: bradycardia, hypotension—phenytoin
Increase: dysrhythmias—general anesthetics
Increase: severe hypertension—ergots
Increase: B/P—oxytocics
Increase: pressor effect—tricyclics, MAOIs
Decrease: DOPamine action—β-/α-blockers

Drug/Lab Test
Increase: urinary catecholamine, serum glucose

NURSING CONSIDERATIONS

Assess:
- Hypovolemia; if present, correct first
- **Oxygenation/perfusion deficit:** check B/P, chest pain, dizziness, loss of consciousness
- **Heart failure:** S_3 gallop, dyspnea, neck venous distention, bibasilar crackles in patients with CHF, cardiomyopathy, palpate peripheral pulses
- I&O ratio: if urine output decreases without decrease in B/P, product may need to be reduced
- **ECG** during administration continuously; if B/P increases, product should be decreased; PCWP, CVP during infusion
- B/P, pulse q5min
- Paresthesias and coldness of extremities; peripheral blood flow may decrease
- Inj site: tissue sloughing; if this occurs, administer phentolamine mixed with NS

Evaluate:
- Therapeutic response: increased B/P with stabilization; increased urine output

Teach patient/family:
- About the reason for product administration

TREATMENT OF OVERDOSE:

Discontinue IV, may give a short-acting α-adrenergic blocker

doripenem (Rx)

(dore-i-pen′em)

Doribax

Func. class.: Antiinfective—miscellaneous
Chem. class.: Carbapenem

ACTION: Bactericidal; interferes with cell-wall replication of susceptible organisms; osmotically unstable cell-wall swells, bursts from osmotic pressure

USES: Serious infections caused by *Acinetobacter baumannii, Bacteroides caccae, Bacteroides fragilis, Bacteroides thetaiotaomicron, Bacteroides uniformis, Bacteroides vulgatus, Citrobacter freundii, Escherichia coli, Klebsiella pneumoniae, Peptostreptococcus micros, Proteus mirabilis, Pseudomonas aeruginosa, Serratia marcescens, Staphylococcus aureus, Streptococcus constellatus, Streptococcus intermedius*; complicated urinary tract infections, pyelonephritis, complicated intraabdominal infections

CONTRAINDICATIONS: Hypersensitivity to carbapenems (meropenem, doripenem, imipenem), penicillin, β-lactam; viral infection

Precautions: Pregnancy (B), breastfeeding, geriatric patients, renal disease, seizure disorder, pseudomembranous colitis, nebulizer or inhalation use, hypersensitivity to cephalosporins, children/adolescents

DOSAGE AND ROUTES

• **Adult: IV** 500 mg q8hr × 5-14 days; if improvement occurs after 3 days, switch to appropriate oral product

Renal dose

• **Adult: IV** CCr 30-50 ml/min, 250 mg over 1 hr, q8hr; CCr >10 to <30 ml/min, 250 mg over 1 hr q12hr; CCr ≤10 ml/min, no data

Available forms: Powder for inj 250, 500 mg

Administer:

IV route

• Visually inspect parenteral products for particulate matter and discoloration before use, diluted range in color from clear, colorless solutions to solutions that are clear and slightly yellow

• **Reconstitution:** no bacteriostatic preservative is present; observe aseptic technique while preparing the infusion

• **500-mg dose using the 500-mg vial**: reconstitute the vial with 10 ml of sterile water for injection or sodium chloride 0.9% (normal saline); gently shake (50 mg/ml); *the reconstituted suspension is not for direct injection; further dilution is required;* using a syringe with a 21-G needle, withdraw the suspension and add it to an infusion bag containing 100 ml of NS or D_5W; gently shake until clear: final concentrations: 4.5 mg/ml

• **250-mg dose using the 500-mg vial**: reconstitute the vial with 10 ml of sterile water for injection or sodium chloride 0.9% (normal saline); gently shake (50 mg/ml); *the reconstituted suspension is not for direct injection; further dilution is required;* using a syringe with a 21-G needle, withdraw 5 ml (250 mg) and add it to an infusion bag containing 100 ml of normal saline or D_5W; gently shake until clear; remove 55 ml of this solution and discard; the remaining infusion sol contains 250 mg (4.5 mg/ml)

• **250-mg dose using the 250-mg vial**: reconstitute the vial with 10 ml of sterile water for injection or sodium chloride 0.9% (normal saline); gently shake (25 mg/ml); *the reconstituted suspension is not for direct injection; further dilution is required;* using a syringe with a 21-G needle, withdraw the contents of the vial and add it to an infusion bag containing 50 or 100 ml of normal saline or D_5W; gently shake until clear; final concentrations 4.2 mg/ml (50 ml infusion bag) or 2.3 mg/ml (100 ml infusion bag)

• **Storage:** reconstituted suspensions may be held in vial for up to 1 hr before transfer and dilution in the infusion bag; including storage and infusion time, diluted infusion sols are stable for up to 12 hr (NS) or 4 hr (D_5W) at controlled room temperature; diluted infusion sols are stable for up to 72 hr (NS) or 24 hr (D_5W) refrigerated; do not freeze reconstituted solutions

• If Baxter Minibag Plus infusion bags are to be used, consult the instructions provided by the infusion bag manufacturer

Intermittent IV INFUSION route

• After C&S is taken

• Do not mix with or physically add to solutions containing other drugs; infuse over 1 hr

Y-site compatibilities: Acyclovir, amikacin, aminophylline, amiodarone, anidulafungin, atropine, azithromycin, bumetanide, calcium gluconate, CARBOplatin, caspofungin, ceftaroline, ceftobiprole, cimetidine, ciprofloxacin, CISplatin, cyclophosphamide, cycloSPORINE, DAPTOmycin, dexamethasone, digoxin, diltiazem, diphenhydrAMINE, DOBUTamine, DOCEtaxel, DOPamine, DOXOrubicin, enalaprilat, esmolol, esomeprazole, etoposide, famotidine, fentaNYL, fluconazole, fluorouracil, foscarnet, furosemide, gemcitabine, gentamicin, granisetron, heparin, hydrocortisone, HYDROmorphone, ifosfamide, insulin (regular), labetalol, levofloxacin, linezolid, LORazepam, magnesium sulfate, mannitol, meperidine, methotrexate, methylPREDNISolone, metoclopramide, metroNIDAZOLE, micafungin, midazolam, milrinone, morphine, moxifloxacin, norepinephrine,

ondansetron, PACLitaxel, pantoprazole, PHENobarbital, phenylephrine, potassium chloride, ranitidine, sodium bicarbonate/phosphates, tacrolimus, telavancin, tigecycline, tobramycin, vancomycin, voriconazole, zidovudine
Solution compatibilities: D_5W, 0.9% NaCl, sterile water for inj

SIDE EFFECTS

CNS: Seizures, headache
GI: *Diarrhea, nausea,* vomiting, pseudomembranous colitis, hepatitis
GU: Renal impairments/failure
HEMA: Neutropenia, leukopenia, anemia
INTEG: *Rash,* urticaria, phlebitis, erythema at inj site, Stevens-Johnson syndrome, toxic epidermal necrolysis, pruritus
RESP: Pneumonitis (inhalation)
SYST: Anaphylaxis, Stevens-Johnson syndrome, toxic epidermal necrolysis

PHARMACOKINETICS

IV: Distributed to most body fluids/tissue, excreted mainly unchanged in urine, 70% recovered in 48 hr, half-life 1 hr, half-life extended in renal disease

INTERACTIONS

Increase: doripenem plasma levels—probenecid
Decrease: effect of valproic acid, divalproex sodium
Drug/Lab Test
Increase: AST, ALT, LDH, BUN, alk phos, bilirubin, creatinine
False positive: direct Coombs' test

NURSING CONSIDERATIONS

Assess:
- Sensitivity to carbapenem antibiotics, penicillins, cephalosporins, other beta lactams
- Renal disease: lower dose may be required
- Bowel pattern daily; if severe diarrhea occurs, product should be discontinued; may indicate pseudomembranous colitis
- For infection: temperature; sputum; characteristics of wound before, during, and after treatment

⚠ **Allergic reactions, anaphylaxis:** rash, urticaria, pruritus; may occur few days after therapy begins
- **Overgrowth of infection:** perineal itching, fever, malaise, redness, pain, swelling, drainage, rash, diarrhea, change in cough, sputum

Evaluate:
- Therapeutic response: negative C&S; absence of symptoms and signs of infection

Teach patient/family:
- To report severe diarrhea; may indicate pseudomembranous colitis
- To report sore throat, bruising, bleeding, joint pain; may indicate blood dyscrasias (rare)
- To report overgrowth of infection: black, furry tongue; vaginal itching; foul-smelling stools
- To avoid breastfeeding; product is excreted in breast milk

TREATMENT OF HYPERSENSITIVITY: EPINEPHrine, antihistamines; resuscitate if needed (anaphylaxis)

dorzolamide (ophthalmic)

(dor-zole′ah-mide)

Trusopt

Func. class.: Antiglaucoma
Chem. class.: Carbonic anhydrase inhibitor

ACTION: Decreases aqueous humor secretion by decreasing bicarbonate, thus decreasing IOP

USES: For the treatment of elevated intraocular pressure in patients with ocular hypertension or open-angle glaucoma

CONTRAINDICATIONS: Hypersensitivity

Precautions: Hypersensitivity to sulfonamides, hepatic/renal disease, angle-closure glaucoma, electrolyte disturbances

DOSAGE AND ROUTES

Elevated intraocular pressure in patients with ocular hypertension or open-angle glaucoma

- **Adult/adolescent/child/infant/neonate ≥1 wk: Ophthalmic** Instill 1 drop of a 2% solution into the affected eye(s) tid

Available forms: Ophthalmic solution 2%

Administer:

- Wash hands before and after use, tilt the head back slightly and pull the lower eyelid down with the index finger to form a pouch, squeeze the prescribed number of drops into the pouch and gently close eyes for 1-2 min; do not blink
- Care should be taken to avoid contamination; do not touch the tip of the dropper to the eye, fingertips, or other surface
- The sol may be used concomitantly with other topical ophthalmic drug products to lower IOP; if more than one topical ophthalmic drug is being used, administer ≥10 min apart

SIDE EFFECTS

CNS: Headache

EENT: Blurred vision, tearing, allergy, burning/stinging, photophobia

GI: Bitter taste

PHARMACOKINETICS

Onset 1-2 hr, peak 3 hr, duration 8 hr, half-life 4 mo

INTERACTIONS

Increase: effects—carbonic anhydrase inhibitors (PO)

NURSING CONSIDERATIONS

Assess:

- Hypersensitivity
- Monitor IOP during treatment

Evaluate:

- Decreasing IOP

Teach patient/family:

- How to use product
- Not to share with others or use for other conditions
- **To notify prescriber immediately if vision changes or if condition worsens**
- To take as prescribed

doxazosin (Rx)

(dox-ay′zoe-sin)

Cardura, Cardura XL

Func. class.: Peripheral α_1-adrenergic receptor blocker

Chem. class.: Quinazoline

Do not confuse:
Cardura/Coumadin/Cardene/Ridaura

ACTION:
Dilates peripheral blood vessels, lowers peripheral resistance; reduction in B/P results from peripheral α_1-adrenergic receptors being blocked

USES:
Hypertension, urinary outflow obstruction, symptoms of benign prostatic hyperplasia

CONTRAINDICATIONS:
Hypersensitivity to quinazolines

Precautions: Pregnancy (C), breastfeeding, children, hepatic disease, geriatric patients

DOSAGE AND ROUTES

BPH

- **Adult: PO** 1 mg/day at bedtime; increase in stepwise manner to 2, 4, 8 mg/day as needed at 1-2 wk intervals, max 8 mg; ext rel tab (Cardura XL) 4 mg daily with breakfast, adjust dose q3-4wk, up to 8 mg daily

Hypertension

- **Adult: PO** 1 mg/day at bedtime; increasing up to 16 mg/day if required; usual range 4-16 mg/day
- **Geriatric: PO** 0.5 mg nightly, gradually increase

Available forms: Tabs 1, 2, 4, 8 mg; ext rel tabs 4, 8 mg

Administer:

- Store in tight container at room temperature
- **Tabs** broken, crushed, or chewed; if chewed, will be bitter; do not break, crush, chew XL tabs
- **Immediate release tab:** without regard to meals; **ext rel tabs:** give with breakfast; when switching from immediate release to ext rel, the final evening dose of immediate release should not be taken

SIDE EFFECTS

CNS: *Dizziness, headache,* drowsiness, anxiety, depression, *vertigo,* weakness, fatigue, asthenia, syncope

CV: Palpitations, *orthostatic hypotension*, tachycardia, *edema,* dysrhythmias, chest pain

EENT: Epistaxis, tinnitus, dry mouth, red sclera, pharyngitis, rhinitis

GI: *Nausea,* vomiting, diarrhea, constipation, abdominal pain, hepatitis

GU: Incontinence, polyuria, priapism, impotence

PHARMACOKINETICS

PO: Onset 2 hr, peak 2-3 hr, duration up to 24 hr, half-life 22 hr, metabolized in liver, excreted via bile/feces (<63%) and in urine (9%), extensively protein bound (98%)

INTERACTIONS

Increase: hypotensive effects—alcohol, other antihypertensives, nitrates, PDE-5 inhibitors

Decrease: antihypertensive effects of cloNIDine

NURSING CONSIDERATIONS

Assess:

- **Hypertension:** B/P (lying, standing), pulse 2-6 hr after each dose, with each increase; postural effects may occur, crackles, dyspnea, orthopnea with B/P; pulse; jugular venous distention during beginning treatment
- **BPH:** urinary pattern changes (hesitancy, dribbling, incomplete bladder emptying, dysuria, urgency, nocturia, urgency incontinence, intermittency) before and during treatment
- I&O, weight daily; edema in feet, legs daily

Evaluate:

- Therapeutic response: decreased B/P; decreased symptoms of BPH

Teach patient/family:

- That fainting occasionally occurs after 1st dose; not to drive, operate machinery for 4 hr after 1st dose, after dosage increase; to take 1st dose at bedtime; may take 1-2 wk to respond with BPH
- Rise slowly from sitting position

TREATMENT OF OVERDOSE:

Administer volume expanders or vasopressors; discontinue product; place patient in supine position

doxepin (Rx)

(dox′e-pin)

Prudoxin Cream, Silenor, Zonalon Topical Cream

Func. class.: Antidepressant, tricyclic, antihistamine (topical)

Chem. class.: Dibenzoxepin, tertiary amine

ACTION: Blocks reuptake of norepinephrine, serotonin into nerve endings, increasing action of norepinephrine, serotonin in nerve cells

USES: Major depression, anxiety; *topical:* lichen simplex, atopic dermatitis, eczema, insomnia, migraine prophylaxis

Unlabeled uses: Topical pruritus

CONTRAINDICATIONS: Hypersensitivity to tricyclics, urinary retention, closed-angle glaucoma, prostatic hypertrophy, acute recovery from MI

Precautions: Pregnancy (C) (PO) (B) (topical), breastfeeding, geriatric patients, seizures

Black Box Warning: Children, suicidal patients

DOSAGE AND ROUTES

Depression/anxiety

- **Adult: PO** 50-75 mg/day, may increase to 300 mg/day for severely ill; give in divided doses if >150 mg/day
- **Geriatric: PO** 25-50 mg at bedtime, increase weekly by 25-50 mg to desired dose, max 150 mg/day

Pruritus

- **Adult: PO** 10 mg at bedtime, may increase to 25 mg at bedtime; **TOP** apply thin film qid at least 3 hr apart

Insomnia (Silenor)

- **Adult: PO** 6 mg 30 min before bedtime, 3 mg may be sufficient, max 6 mg/night

Available forms: Caps 10, 25, 50, 75, 100, 150 mg; oral concentrations 10 mg/ml; cream 5%; tabs (Silenor) 3, 6 mg

Administer:

- **Oral concentrations:** should be diluted with 120 ml water, milk or orange, grapefruit, tomato, prune, or pineapple juice; do not mix with grape juice
- Increased fluids, bulk in diet for constipation
- With food, milk for GI symptoms; do not give with carbonated beverages
- Dosage at bedtime to avoid oversedation during day; may take entire dose at bedtime; geriatric patients may not tolerate daily dosing
- Gum, hard candy, or frequent sips of water for dry mouth
- Store in tight container protected from direct sunlight
- **Topical:** by applying to affected area, rub slightly; do not use occlusive dressings

SIDE EFFECTS

CNS: *Dizziness, drowsiness,* confusion, headache, anxiety, tremors, stimulation, weakness, insomnia, nightmares, EPS (geriatric patients), increased psychiatric symptoms, paresthesia, **suicidal ideation**

CV: *Orthostatic hypotension, ECG changes, tachycardia,* **hypertension,** palpitations, **dysrhythmias**

EENT: *Blurred vision,* tinnitus, mydriasis, ophthalmoplegia, glossitis

GI: *Diarrhea, dry mouth,* nausea, vomiting, **paralytic ileus,** increased appetite, cramps, epigastric distress, jaundice, **hepatitis,** stomatitis, constipation

GU: *Urinary retention,* **acute renal failure**

HEMA: **Agranulocytosis, thrombocytopenia, eosinophilia, leukopenia,** pancytopenia, purpuric disorder

INTEG: Rash, urticaria, sweating, pruritus, photosensitivity

PHARMACOKINETICS

PO: Peak 2 hr, metabolized by liver, excreted by kidneys, crosses placenta, excreted in breast milk, half-life 8-24 hr

INTERACTIONS

Increase: **hyperpyretic crisis, seizures, hypertensive episode—MAOIs**

Increase: hypertensive action—EPINEPHrine, norepinephrine

Increase: **hypertensive crisis—cloNIDine; do not use together**

Increase: doxepin effect—cimetidine, FLUoxetine, fluvoxaMINE, PARoxetine, sertraline

Increase: CNS depression—barbiturates, benzodiazepines, sedative/hypnotics, alcohol, other CNS depressants

Increase: **QT interval: class IC/III antiarrhythmics (propafenone, flecainide), quinolones**

Increase: serotonin syndrome, toxicity—SSRIs, SNRIs, serotonin-receptor agonists

Increase: anticholinergic effects—anticholinergics

Drug/Herb

- Serotonin syndrome: St. John's wort

Drug/Lab Test

Increase: serum bilirubin, blood glucose, alk phos, LFTs

NURSING CONSIDERATIONS

Assess:

- B/P (lying, standing), pulse q4hr; if systolic B/P drops 20 mm Hg, hold

product, notify prescriber; VS q4hr in patients with CV disease
- Blood studies: CBC, leukocytes, differential, cardiac enzymes if patient is receiving long-term therapy
- Hepatic studies: AST, ALT, bilirubin
- Weight weekly; appetite may increase with product
- **ECG** for flattening of T wave, bundle branch block, AV block, dysrhythmias in cardiac patients; product should be discontinued gradually several days before surgery
- **EPS** primarily in geriatric patients: rigidity, dystonia, akathisia
- **Depression:** mood, sensorium, affect, suicidal tendencies, increase in psychiatric symptoms
- **Chronic pain:** location, severity, type before and during treatment, alleviating/aggravating factors
- Urinary retention, constipation; constipation most likely in children, geriatric patients
- **Withdrawal symptoms:** headache, nausea, vomiting, muscle pain, weakness; not usual unless product is discontinued abruptly
- Alcohol consumption; if alcohol is consumed, hold dose until morning
- Assistance with ambulation during beginning therapy because drowsiness/dizziness occurs; safety measures primarily for geriatric patients

Evaluate:
- Therapeutic response: decreased anxiety, depression

Teach patient/family:
- That therapeutic effect (depression) may take 2-3 wk, antianxiety effects sooner
- To use caution when driving, during other activities requiring alertness because of drowsiness, dizziness, blurred vision
- To avoid alcohol, other CNS depressants; may potentiate effects
- Not to discontinue medication abruptly after long-term use; may cause nausea, headache, malaise
- To wear sunscreen or large hat; photosensitivity occurs
- That clinical worsening and suicide may occur
- To immediately report urinary retention

TREATMENT OF OVERDOSE:
ECG monitoring; lavage, activated charcoal; administer anticonvulsant, sodium bicarbonate

⚠ HIGH ALERT

DOXOrubicin
(dox-oh-roo′bi-sin)

Adriamycin

Func. class.: Antineoplastic, antibiotic
Chem. class.: Anthracycline glycoside

Do not confuse:
DOXOrubicin/DOXOrubicin liposomal/DAUNOrubicin

ACTION: Inhibits DNA synthesis primarily; replication is decreased by binding to DNA, which causes strand splitting; active throughout entire cell cycle; a vesicant

USES: Wilms' tumor; bladder, breast, lung, ovarian, stomach, thyroid cancer; Hodgkin's/non-Hodgkin's disease; acute lymphoblastic leukemia; myeloblastic leukemia; neuroblastomas; soft tissue/bone sarcomas

CONTRAINDICATIONS: Pregnancy (D) 1st trimester, breastfeeding, hypersensitivity, systemic infections, cardiac disorders, severe myelosuppression, lifetime dose of 550 mg/m^2

Black Box Warning: Hepatic disease

Precautions: Accidental exposure, cardiac disease, dental work, electrolyte imbalance, infection, hyperuricemia

Black Box Warning: Bone marrow suppression, extravasation, heart failure, secondary malignancy; requires an experienced clinician

DOSAGE AND ROUTES

- **Adult: IV** 60-75 mg/m² every 3 wk, or may be used in combination with other antineoplastics with 40-75 mg/m² every 21-28 days, max cumulative dose 550 mg/m² or 450 mg/m² if prior DAUNOrubicin, cyclophosphamide, mediastinal XRT

Hepatic dose

⚠ **Adult: IV** Bilirubin 1.2-3 mg/dl, give 50% of dose; bilirubin 3.1-5 mg/dl, give 25% of dose

Renal dose

⚠ **Adult: IV** CCr < 10 ml/min give 75% of dose

Available forms: Powder for inj 10, 20, 50 mg; inj 2 mg/ml

Administer:

IV route

- Give antiemetic 30-60 min before product to prevent vomiting
- Give allopurinol or sodium bicarbonate to maintain uric acid levels, alkalization of urine
- Use cytotoxic handling procedures: inspect for particulate and discoloration before use

Black Box Warning: Do not give IM, subcut

Black Box Warning: If extravasation occurs, stop infusion and complete via another vein, preferably in another limb, use dexrazoxane topically

- Aluminum needles may be used during administration; avoid aluminum during storage
- Rapid injection can cause facial flushing or erythema along the vein

Reconstitution:

- To avoid risks with reconstitution, the commercially available injection may be used; there are still risks involved in handling the injection
- Do not use diluents containing preservatives to reconstitute powder for injection
- Reconstitute 10, 20, 50, 100 mg of DOXOrubicin with 5, 10, 25, 50 ml, respectively, of nonbacteriostatic NS injection (2 mg/ ml), shake until completely dissolved; use reconstituted solution within 24 hr; do not expose to sunlight
- **IV injection** Inject reconstituted solution over >3-5 min via Y-site or 3-way stopcock into a free-flowing IV infusion of NS or D_5W; a butterfly needle inserted into a large vein is preferred

Black Box Warning: Care should be taken to avoid extravasation because the drug is extremely irritating to extravascular tissue

- Increased fluid intake to 2-3 L/day to prevent urate, calculi formation
- Store at room temperature for 24 hr after reconstituting

Y-site compatibilities: Alemtuzumab, alfentanil, amifostine, amikacin, anidulafungin, argatroban, aztreonam, bivalirudin, bleomycin, bumetanide, buprenorphine, butorphanol, calcium chloride/gluconate, CARBOplatin, carmustine, caspofungin, ceftizoxime, chlorproMAZINE, cimetidine, ciprofloxacin, CISplatin, cladribine, clindamycin, cyclophosphamide, cycloSPORINE, cytarabine, DACTINomycin, DAPTOmycin, dexamethasone, diltiazem, diphenhydrAMINE, DOBUTamine, DOCEtaxel, dolasetron, DOPamine, doripenem, doxycycline, droperidol, enalaprilat, ePHEDrine, EPINEPHrine, erythromycin, esmolol, etoposide, etoposide phosphate, famotidine, fenoldopam, fentaNYL, filgrastim, fluconazole, fludarabine, gemcitabine, gentamicin, granisetron, haloperidol, hydrocortisone, HYDROmorphone, ifosfamide, imipenem cilastatin, inamrinone, isoproterenol, ketorolac, labetalol, leucovorin, levorphanol, lidocaine, linezolid, LORazepam, mannitol, mechlorethamine, melphalan, meperidine, mesna, methotrexate, metoclopramide, metoprolol, metroNIDAZOLE, midazolam, milrinone, mitoMYcin, morphine, nalbuphine, naloxone, nesiritide, niCARdipine, nitroglycerin, nitroprusside, octreotide, ofloxacin, ondansetron, oxaliplatin, PACLitaxel, palonosetron, pancuronium, phenylephrine, potassium chloride, procainamide, prochlorperazine, promethazine, propranolol, quinupristin-dalfopristin, ranitidine, sargramostim, sodium acetate, tacrolimus, teniposide, theophylline, thiotepa, ticarcillin/clavulanate, tigecycline, tirofiban, tobramycin, topotecan, trastuzumab, trimethobenzamide, vancomycin, vasopressin, vecuronium, verapamil, vinBLAStine, vinCRIStine, vinorelbine, zidovudine, zoledronic acid

SIDE EFFECTS

CV: Increased B/P, sinus tachycardia, PVCs, chest pain, bradycardia, extrasystoles, irreversible cardiomyopathy, acute left ventricular failure

GI: *Nausea, vomiting,* anorexia, *mucositis,* hepatotoxicity

GU: Impotence, sterility, amenorrhea, gynecomastia, hyperuricemia, urine discoloration

HEMA: Thrombocytopenia, leukopenia, anemia

INTEG: *Rash,* necrosis at inj site, dermatitis, reversible *alopecia,* cellulitis, thrombophlebitis at inj site, radiation recall

SYST: Anaphylaxis, secondary malignancy

PHARMACOKINETICS

Half-life 30 min, terminal 16.5 hr; metabolized by liver; crosses placenta; excreted in urine, bile, breast milk

INTERACTIONS

Increase: life-threatening dysrhythmias—posaconazole, fluconazole, do not use together

Increase: QT prolongation—other drugs that increase QT prolongation

Increase: neutropenia, thrombocytopenia—progesterone

Increase: cardiomyopathy—calcium-channel blockers

Increase: toxicity—other antineoplastics, cycloSPORINE, radiation, mercaptopurine

Increase: hemorrhagic cystitis risk, cardiac toxicity—cyclophosphamide

Increase: effect of phenytoin, fosphenytoin

Increase: DOXOrubicin effect—streptozocin

Decrease: DOXOrubicin effect—PHENObarbital

Decrease: antibody response—live virus vaccine

Decrease: antineoplastic effect—hematopoietic progenitor cell; do not use 24 hr before or after treatment

Decrease: clearance of DOXOrubicin—PACLitaxel

Drug/Lab Test

Increase: uric acid

NURSING CONSIDERATIONS

Assess:

Black Box Warning: **Bone marrow depression:** CBC, differential, platelet count weekly; withhold or reduce dose of product if WBC is <1500/mm^3 or platelet count is <50,000/mm^3; notify prescriber of these results

Renal studies: BUN, serum uric acid, urine CCr, electrolytes before, during therapy

I&O ratio: Report fall in urine output to <30 ml/hr

Monitor temperature: Fever might indicate beginning infection

Black Box Warning: **Hepatotoxicity:** hepatic studies before, during therapy: bilirubin, AST, ALT, alk phos as needed or monthly; check for jaundice of skin and sclera, dark urine, clay-colored stools, itchy skin, abdominal pain, fever, diarrhea

Black Box Warning: Dysrhythmias: ECG; watch for ST-T wave changes, low QRS and T, possible dysrhythmias (sinus tachycardia, heart block, PVCs), ejection fraction before treatment, signs of irreversible cardiomyopathy, can occur up to 6 mo after treatment begins

- Bleeding: hematuria, guaiac, bruising, petechiae of mucosa or orifices every 8 hr
- Effects of alopecia on body image; discuss feelings about body changes; almost total alopecia is expected
- Buccal cavity every 8 hr for dryness, sores, ulceration, white patches, oral pain, bleeding, dysphagia
- Alkalosis if severe vomiting is present

Black Box Warning: Extravasation: local irritation, pain, burning at inj site; a vesicant; if extravasation occurs, stop drug, restart at another site, apply ice, elevate extremity to reduce swelling; if resolution does not occur, surgical debridement may be required

- GI symptoms: frequency of stools, cramping
- Rinsing of mouth tid-qid with water, club soda; brushing of teeth bid-tid with soft brush or cotton-tipped applicators for stomatitis; use unwaxed dental floss

Evaluate:
- Therapeutic response: decreased tumor size, spread of malignancy

Teach patient/family:
- To add 2-3 L of fluids unless contraindicated before and for 24-48 hr after to decrease possible hemorrhagic cystitis
- To report any complaints, side effects to nurse or prescriber
- That hair may be lost during treatment; that wig or hairpiece might make patient feel better; that new hair might be different in color, texture
- To avoid foods with citric acid, hot or rough texture
- To report any bleeding, white spots, ulcerations in mouth to prescriber; to examine mouth daily
- That urine, other body fluids may be red-orange for 48 hr
- To avoid crowds and persons with infections when granulocyte count is low
- That barrier contraceptive measures are recommended during therapy and for 4 mo after (pregnancy [D]); to avoid breastfeeding
- To avoid vaccinations

⚠ HIGH ALERT

DOXOrubicin liposomal

(dox-oh-roo′bi-sin)

Doxil, Lipodex

Func. class.: Antineoplastic, antibiotic

Chem. class.: Anthracycline glycoside

Do not confuse: DOXOrubicin/DOXOrubicin liposomal/DAUNOrubicin

ACTION: Inhibits DNA synthesis primarily; replication is decreased by binding to DNA, which causes strand splitting; active throughout entire cell cycle; a vesicant

USES: AIDS-related Kaposi's sarcoma, multiple myeloma, metastatic ovarian carcinoma

CONTRAINDICATIONS: Pregnancy (D), breastfeeding, hypersensitivity, systemic infections, cardiac disorders

Black Box Warning: Cardiotoxicity, infusion reactions, myelosuppression, hepatic disease

Precautions: Children, infection, leukopenia, stomatitis, thrombocytopenia

DOSAGE AND ROUTES

Max lifetime cumulative dose 550 mg/m^2; 400 mg/m^2 for those who have received other cardiotoxics or mediastinal radiation

Kaposi's sarcoma
- **Adult: IV** 20 mg/m^2 every 3 wk

Multiple myeloma

- **Adult: IV** 30 mg/m² IV infusion on day 4 every 3 wk plus bortezomib 1.3 mg/m²/dose IV bolus on days 1, 4, 8, 11 of each cycle; give DOXOrubicin liposomal after bortezomib receipt on day 4; administer up to 8 treatment cycles or until disease progression or unacceptable toxicity occurs

Breast cancer, metastatic (unlabeled)

- **Adult: IV** 50 mg/m² day 1, q4wk

Available forms: Liposomal dispersion for inj: 2 mg/ml

Administer:

- Prepared liposomal DOXOrubicin is a translucent, red liposomal dispersion; visually inspect for particulate matter and discoloration before use
- Pegylated liposomal DOXOrubicin (Doxil) is for IV INFUSION use only and should not be given IM/subcut, give under the supervision of a physician who is experienced in cancer chemotherapy

Black Box Warning: Care should be taken to avoid extravasation because the drug is irritating to extravascular tissue

- Premedication with antiemetics is recommended

IV route

- **Reconstitution (Doxil):** dilute the appropriate dose, not to exceed 90 mg/250 ml D_5W; do not mix with any other diluent, drugs, or bacteriostatic agent, use aseptic technique; product contains no preservative or bacteriostatic agent; diluted solution must be refrigerated and used within 24 hr
- **IV INFUSION (Doxil):** do not administer as a bolus injection or an undiluted solution; rapid injection can increase the risk of an infusion-related reaction

Black Box Warning: Care should be taken to avoid extravasation because the drug is irritating to extravascular tissue

- An acute infusion reaction can occur during the first infusion and is usually resolved by slowing the rate of infusion; most patients can tolerate subsequent infusion
- **Rate:** infuse at an initial rate of 1 mg/min; if no infusion-related action, the rate can be increased to complete the infusion over 1 hr; do not filter
- **For hematologic toxicity in patients with ovarian cancer or HIV-related Kaposi's sarcoma: Grade 1 (ANC of 1500-1900/mm³, platelets ≥75,000/mm³):** No dose reduction; **Grade 2 (ANC of 1000-1499/mm³, platelets ≥50,000/mm³ and <75,000/mm³:** Wait until ANC ≥1500 cells/mm³ and platelets ≥75,000 cells/mm³; redose with no dose reduction; **Grade 3 (ANC of 500-999/mm³, platelets ≥25,000/mm³ and <50,000/mm³):** Wait until ANC ≥1500 cells/mm³ and platelets ≥75,000 cells/mm³; redose with no dose reduction; **Grade 4 (ANC <500/mm³, platelets <25,000/mm³):** Wait until ANC ≥1500 cells/mm³ and platelets ≥75,000 cells/mm³; reduce dose by 25% or continue with full dose with colony-stimulating factor
- Give antiemetic 30-60 min before product to prevent vomiting
- Use allopurinol or sodium bicarbonate to maintain uric acid levels, alkalinization of urine
- Avoid mixing with other products
- Increase fluid intake to 2-3 L/day to prevent urate, calculi formation
- Store refrigerated for 24 hr after reconstituting

SIDE EFFECTS

CNS: Paresthesias, headache, depression, insomnia, fatigue, fever

CV: Chest pain, decreased B/P, cardiomyopathy, heart failure, dysrhythmias, tachycardia

EENT: Optic neuritis, rhinitis, pharyngitis, stomatitis

GI: *Nausea, vomiting,* anorexia, *mucositis,* hepatotoxicity, constipation, oral candidiasis, abdominal pain

HEMA: Thrombocytopenia, leukopenia, anemia, neutropenia

INTEG: *Rash*, necrosis at inj site, dermatitis, reversible *alopecia*, **exfoliative dermatitis, palmar-plantar erythrodysesthesia**, thrombophlebitis at inj site
RESP: Dyspnea, cough, respiratory infections

PHARMACOKINETICS

Half-life 55 hr; metabolized by liver; crosses placenta; excreted in urine, bile, breast milk

INTERACTIONS

Increase: life-threatening dysrhythmias—posaconazole, fluconazole, do not use together
Increase: QT prolongation—other drugs that increase QT prolongation
Increase: neutropenia, thrombocytopenia—progesterone
Increase: cardiomyopathy—calcium-channel blockers
Increase: toxicity—other antineoplastics, cycloSPORINE, radiation, mercaptopurine
Increase: hemorrhagic cystitis risk, cardiac toxicity—cyclophosphamide
Increase: effect of—phenytoin, fosphenytoin
Increase: DOXOrubicin effect—streptozocin
Decrease: DOXOrubicin effect—PHENobarbital
Decrease: antibody response—live virus vaccine
Decrease: antineoplastic effect—hematopoietic progenitor cell; do not use 24 hr before or after treatment
Decrease: clearance of DOXOrubicin—PACLitaxel

Drug/Lab Test
Increase: uric acid

NURSING CONSIDERATIONS

Assess:

Black Box Warning: **Bone marrow depression:** CBC, differential, platelet count weekly; withhold product if WBC is <4000/mm³ or platelet count is <75,000/mm³; notify prescriber of these results

- Renal studies: BUN, serum uric acid, urine CCr, electrolytes before, during therapy
- I&O ratio: report fall in urine output to <30 ml/hr
- Monitor temperature; fever can indicate beginning infection

Black Box Warning: **Hepatotoxicity:** Hepatic studies before, during therapy: bilirubin, AST, ALT, alk phos as needed or monthly; check for jaundice of skin and sclera, dark urine, clay-colored stools, itchy skin, abdominal pain, fever, diarrhea

Black Box Warning: **Dysrhythmias:** ECG: watch for ST-T wave changes, low QRS and T, possible dysrhythmias (sinus tachycardia, heart block, PVCs), ejection fraction before treatment, signs of irreversible cardiomyopathy, can occur up to 6 mo after treatment begins

- Bleeding: hematuria, guaiac, bruising, petechiae of mucosa or orifices every 8 hr
- Effects of alopecia on body image; discuss feelings about body changes; almost total alopecia is expected
- Inflammation of mucosa, breaks in skin
- Buccal cavity every 8 hr for dryness, sores, ulceration, white patches, oral pain, bleeding, dysphagia
- Alkalosis if severe vomiting is present

Black Box Warning: **Extravasation:** Local irritation, pain, burning at inj site; a vesicant; if extravasation occurs, stop drug, restart at another site, apply ice, elevate extremity to reduce swelling; if resolution does not occur, surgical debridement may be required

- GI symptoms: frequency of stools, cramping
- Rinsing of mouth tid-qid with water, club soda; brushing of teeth bid-tid with soft brush or cotton-tipped applicators for stomatitis; use unwaxed dental floss

Evaluate:
- Therapeutic response: decreased tumor size, spread of malignancy

Teach patient/family:
- To add 2-3 L of fluids unless contraindicated before and for 24-48 hr after to decrease possible **hemorrhagic cystitis**
- To report any complaints, side effects to nurse or prescriber
- That hair may be lost during treatment; that wig or hairpiece might make patient feel better; that new hair may be different in color, texture
- To avoid foods with citric acid, hot or rough texture
- To report any bleeding, white spots, ulcerations in mouth to prescriber; to examine mouth daily
- That urine, other body fluids may be red-orange for 48 hr
- To avoid crowds and persons with infections when granulocyte count is low
- That barrier contraceptive measures are recommended during therapy and for 4 mo after (pregnancy [D]); to avoid breastfeeding
- To avoid vaccinations because reactions can occur; to avoid alcohol

doxycycline (Rx)
(dox-i-sye′kleen)

Oracea

doxycycline calcium
Vibramycin

doxycycline hyclate
Adoxa, Apo-Doxy ♣, Doryx, Doxy, Doxycaps, Doxycin ♣, Periostat, Vibramycin, Vibra-Tabs

doxycycline monohydrate
Adoxa, Monodox, Vibramycin

Func. class.: Antiinfective
Chem. class.: Tetracycline

Do not confuse:
doxycycline/doxepin/dicyclomine

ACTION: Inhibits protein synthesis, phosphorylation in microorganisms by binding to 30S ribosomal subunits, reversibly binding to 30S ribosomal subunits; bacteriostatic

USES: *Acinetobacter* sp., *Actinomyces israelii, Bacillus anthracis, Bacteroides* sp., *Balantidium coli, Bartonella bacilliformis, Borrelia recurrentis, Brucella* sp., *Campylobacter fetus, Chlamydia psittaci, Chlamydia trachomatis, Clostridium* sp., *Entamoeba histolytica, Enterobacter aerogenes, Enterococcus* sp., *Escherichia coli, Francisella tularensis, Fusobacterium fusiforme, Haemophilus ducreyi, Haemophilus influenzae* (beta-lactamase negative), *Haemophilus influenzae* (beta-lactamase positive), *Klebsiella granulomatis, Klebsiella* sp., *Leptospira* sp., *Listeria monocytogenes, Mycoplasma pneumoniae, Neisseria gonorrhoeae, Neisseria meningitidis, Orientia tsutsugamushi, Plasmodium falciparum, Propionibacterium acnes, Rickettsia akari, Rickettsia prowazekii, Rickettsia rickettsii, Shigella* sp., *Staphylococcus aureus* (MSSA), *Streptococcus pneumoniae, Streptococcus pyogenes* (group A beta-hemolytic streptococci), *Streptococcus* sp., *Treponema pallidum, Treponema pertenue, Ureaplasma urealyticum, Vibrio cholerae, Viridans streptococci, Yersinia pestis;* syphilis, gonorrhea, lymphogranuloma venereum, uncommon gram-negative/gram-positive organisms, malaria prophylaxis

Unlabeled uses: Enterocolitis, biliary tract, intraabdominal infections; epididymitis *(Chlamydia trachomatis);* chronic prostatitis *(Ureaplasma urealyticum);* traveler's diarrhea (enterotoxigenic *Escherichia coli*); Legionnaire's disease *(Legionella pneumophila);* Lyme disease *(Borrelia burgdorferi),* Lyme disease (erythema migrans); Lyme arthritis; Lyme carditis; pleural effusion; malaria (chloroquine-resistant *Plasmodium falciparum*); pelvic inflammatory disease (PID), tubo-ovarian abscess in combination; acute dental infection, dentoalveolar infection, endodontic infection; aggressive juvenile periodontitis, plaque prophylaxis *(Yersinia pestis);* tularemia prophylaxis *(Francisella tularensis);* Bancroft's filariasis (elephantiasis) *(Wuchereria bancrofti):* melioidosis due to *Burkholderia pseudomallei; Burkholderia pseudomallei* bacteremia melioidosis; leptospirosis (*Leptospira* sp); infection prophylaxis for gynecologic procedures/surgical infection prophylaxis hysterosalpingogram or chromotubation/induced abortion/dilation and evacuation; methicillin-resistant *Staphylococcus aureus* (MRSA)-associated bone and joint infections

CONTRAINDICATIONS:

Pregnancy (D), children <8 yr, hypersensitivity to tetracyclines, esophageal ulceration

Precautions: Breastfeeding, hepatic disease, pseudomembranous colitis, ulcerative colitis, sulfite hypersensitivity, excessive sunlight

DOSAGE AND ROUTES

Most infections

- **Adult: PO/IV** 100 mg q12hr on day 1, then 100 mg/day; **IV** 200 mg in 1-2 infusion on day 1, then 100-200 mg/day
- **Child >8 yr, ≥45 kg: PO** 100 mg q12hr on day 1, then 100 mg daily; severe infections 100 mg q12hr; **IV** 200 mg on day 1, then 100-200 mg daily, give 200 mg dose as 1 or 2 infusion
- **Child ≥8 yr, <45 kg: PO** 2.2 mg/kg q12hr on day 1, then 2.2 mg/kg daily, severe infections 2.2 mg/kg q12hr; **IV** 4.4 mg/kg divided on day 1, then 2.2-4.4 mg/kg daily in 1 to 2 divided doses

Gonorrhea (uncomplicated) in patients allergic to penicillin

- **Adult: PO** 100 mg q12hr × 7 days or 300 mg followed 1 hr later by another 300 mg

Malaria prophylaxis

- **Adult: PO** 100 mg/day 1-2 days before travel, daily during travel, and for 4 wk after return
- **Adolescent/child ≥8 yr, <45 kg: PO** 2 mg/kg/day (up to 100 mg/day) begin 1-2 days before travel, continue for 4 wk after return

C. trachomatis

- **Adult: PO** 100 mg bid × 7 days

Syphilis

- **Adult: PO** 100 mg bid × 14 days

Anthrax

- **Adult and child >8 yr and ≥45 kg: IV** 100 mg q12hr; change to **PO** when able × 60 days
- **Adolescent/child ≥8 yr and <45 kg: PO** 2.2 mg/kg q12hr × 60 days; **IV** 100 mg q12hr, change to **PO** when able × 60 days

Lyme disease

- **Adult/adolescent/child ≥8 yr: PO** 100 mg bid × 10-21 days

Periodontitis

- **Adult:** 20 mg bid after scaling and root planing for ≤9 mo; give close to meal time AM or PM

Pleural effusion (unlabeled)

- **Adult: INTRACAVITARY** 500 mg diluted with 250 ml 0.9% NaCl given by chest tube lavage and drainage

Available forms: Doxycycline: cap 40 mg; doxycycline calcium: susp 50 mg/5 ml; doxycycline hyclate: cap 20, 50, 100 mg; del rel tabs 75, 100, 150 mg; del rel cap 75, 100 mg; inj 42.5, 100, 200 mg; tabs 20, 100 mg; doxycycline monohydrate: caps 50, 100, 150 mg; tabs 50, 75, 100 mg; oral susp 25 mg/5 ml

Administer:

PO route

- Do not break, crush, or chew caps; may crush tabs and mix with food
- On empty stomach or with full glass of water 2 hr before or after meals; avoid dairy products, antacids, laxatives, iron-containing products; if these must be taken, give 2 hr before or after product; avoid giving oral products within 1 hr of bedtime, esophageal uleration may occur
- **Delayed release cap:** Swallow whole or open and sprinkle on applesauce
- **Susp:** Shake well, use calibrated device, may give with food/milk for GI irritation, store at room temperature, discard after 14 days

Intermittent IV INFUSION route

- After diluting 100 mg or less/10 ml or 200 mg/20 ml of sterile water or NS for inj, each 100 mg must be further diluted with 100-1000 ml of NaCl, D_5W, Ringer's, LR D_5LR, Normosol-M, Normosol-R in D_5W; run 100 mg or less over 1-4 hr; infusion must be completed in 6 hr when diluted in LR sol or 12 hr with other sol; protect from light, heat
- Avoid rapid use, extravasation
- Store in tight, light-resistant container at room temperature; IV stable for 12 hr at room temperature, 72 hr refrigerated; discard if precipitate forms

Y-site compatibilities: Acyclovir, alemtuzumab, alfentanil, amifostine, amikacin, aminophylline, amiodarone, anidulafungin, ascorbic acid, atracurium, atropine, aztreonam, bivalirudin, bumetanide, buprenorphine, butorphanol, calcium chloride/gluconate, CARBOplatin, caspofungin, cefonicid, cefotaxime, cefTRIAXone, chlorproMAZINE, cimetidine, cisatracurium, CISplatin, clindamycin, codeine, cyanocobalamin, cyclophosphamide, cycloSPORINE, cytarabine, DACTINomycin, DAPTOmycin, dexmedetomidine, digoxin, diltiazem, diphenhydrAMINE, DOBUTamine, DOCEtaxel, DOPamine, doxacurium, DOXOrubicin, enalaprilat, ePHEDrine, EPINEPHrine, epirubicin, epoetin alfa, eptifibatide, ertapenem, esmolol, etoposide, etoposide phosphate, famotidine, fenoldopam, fentaNYL, filgrastim, fluconazole, fludarabine, gemcitabine, gemtuzumab, gentamicin, glycopyrrolate, granisetron, HYDROmorphone, IDArubicin, ifosfamide, imipenem/cilastatin, insulin, isoproterenol, labetalol, levofloxacin, lidocaine, linezolid, LORazepam, magnesium sulfate, mannitol, mechlorethamine, melphalan, meperidine, methyldopate, metoclopramide, metoprolol, metroNIDAZOLE, miconazole, midazolam, milrinone, mitoXANtrone, morphine, multivitamins, nalbuphine, naloxone, nesiritide, netilmicin, nitroglycerin, nitroprusside, norepinephrine, octreotide, ondansetron, oxaliplatin, oxytocin, PACLitaxel, pancuronium, pantoprazole, papaverine, pentamidine, pentazocine, perphenazine, phentolamine, phenylephrine, phytonadione, potassium chloride, procainamide, prochlorperazine, promethazine, propofol, propranolol, protamine, pyridoxime, quinupristin/dalfopristin, ranitidine, remifentanil, ritodrine, riTUXimab, rocuronium, sargramostim, sodium acetate, succinylcholine, SUFentanil, tacrolimus, telavancin, teniposide, theophylline, thiamine, thiotepa, tirofiban, tobramycin, tolazoline, TPN (2 in 1), trastuzumab, trimetaphan, urokinase, vancomycin, vasopressin, vecuronium, verapamil, vinCRIStine, vinorelbine, voriconazole, zoledronic acid

SIDE EFFECTS

CNS: Fever, headache
CV: **Pericarditis**
EENT: Dysphagia, glossitis, decreased calcification of deciduous teeth, oral candidiasis, tooth discoloration
GI: *Nausea, abdominal pain, vomiting, diarrhea,* anorexia, enterocolitis, **hepatotoxicity,** flatulence, abdominal cramps, gastric burning, stomatitis
GU: *Increased BUN*
HEMA: **Eosinophilia, neutropenia, thrombocytopenia, hemolytic anemia**
INTEG: *Rash, urticaria, photosensitivity, increased pigmentation,* **exfoliative dermatitis,** pruritus, phlebitis, injection site reaction
MS: Bone growth retardation (<8 yr old), muscle, joint pain
RESP: Cough
SYST: **Stevens-Johnson syndrome, angioedema, anaphylaxis, toxic epidermal necrolysis**

PHARMACOKINETICS

PO: Well absorbed widely distributed; peak $1^1/_2$-4 hr; half-life 1 day; excreted in urine, feces, bile; 90% protein bound; crosses placenta; enters breast milk

INTERACTIONS

Increase: effect of—anticoagulants, digoxin, methotrexate

Decrease: doxycycline effect—antacids, $NaHCO_3$, dairy products, alkali products, iron, kaolin/pectin, barbiturates, carBAMazepine, phenytoin, cimetidine sucralfate, cholestyramine, colestipol, rifampin, bismuth; iron, magnesium, zinc, calcium, aluminum salts, Sevelamer
Decrease: effects—penicillins, oral contraceptives, digoxin
Drug/Lab Test
Increase: BUN, alk phos, bilirubin, amylase, ALT, AST, eosinophils, WBC
Decrease: Hgb
False increase: urinary catecholamines

NURSING CONSIDERATIONS

Assess:

- I&O ratio
- Blood studies: PT, CBC, AST, ALT, BUN, creatinine
- Signs of infection
- **Allergic reactions:** rash, itching, pruritus, angioedema
- Nausea, vomiting, diarrhea; administer antiemetic, antacids as ordered
- **Overgrowth of infection:** fever, malaise, redness, pain, swelling, drainage, perineal itching, diarrhea, changes in cough or sputum
- IV site for phlebitis/thrombosis; product is highly irritating
- After C&S is obtained, do not wait for results

Evaluate:

- Therapeutic response: decreased temperature, absence of lesions, negative C&S

Teach patient/family:

- To avoid sun because burns may occur; that sunscreen does not seem to decrease photosensitivity
- That all prescribed medication must be taken to prevent superinfection; not to use outdated products because Fanconi syndrome may occur (reversible nephrotoxicity)
- That if children ≤8 yr old are undergoing tooth development, teeth will be permanently discolored
- Not to use with antacids, iron products, H2 blockers, Sevelamer
- To take with full glass of water; if nausea occurs take with food

RARELY USED

doxylamine/pyridoxine

(docks-ill'ah-meen/peer-reh-dock'seen)

Diclegis ✱

Func. class.: Antiemetic

USES: Nausea and vomiting of pregnancy in women who do not respond to other treatment

CONTRAINDICATIONS: Hypersensitivity

DOSAGE AND ROUTES

Adult pregnant females: PO 2 tabs (on an empty stomach) at bedtime, on day 1; if dose controls symptoms the next day, continue regimen. If symptoms persist on the afternoon of day 2, continue 2 tabs at bedtime, then take 3 tabs starting on day 3 (1 tab in AM and 2 tabs at bedtime); if symptoms are controlled, continue regimen. If symptoms persist, on day 4, take 4 tabs (1 tab in AM, 1 tab midafternoon, and 2 tabs at bedtime); max 4 tabs/day. Use only as needed
Available forms: tab 10 mg/10 mg

⚠ HIGH ALERT

dronedarone (Rx)

(drone′da′rone)

Multaq

Func. class.: Antidysrhythmic (class III)
Chem. class.: Iodinated benzofuran derivative

ACTION: Prolongs duration of action potential and effective refractory period, noncompetitive α- and β-adrenergic inhibition; increases RR and QT intervals, decreases sinus rate, decreases peripheral vascular resistance

USES:
Atrial fibrillation, atrial flutter

CONTRAINDICATIONS:
Pregnancy (X), breastfeeding; 2nd-, 3rd-degree AV block; bradycardia, severe sinus node dysfunction, hypersensitivity, heart failure, hepatic disease, QT prolongation, aminodarone-induced lung/liver toxicity

Black Box Warning: NYHA Class IV heart failure or Class II-III with recent decompensation requiring hospitalization, permanent atrial fibrillation (cannot restore sinus rhythm)

Precautions: Children, geriatric patients, Asian patients, females, electrolyte imbalances, atrial fibrillation/flutter

DOSAGE AND ROUTES
• **Adult: PO** 400 mg bid; discontinue class I, III antidysrhythmics or strong CYP3A4 inhibitors before beginning treatment; max 800 mg/day

Available forms: Tabs 400 mg

Administer:

PO route
• Give bid with morning, evening meals
• Give MedGuide; should be dispensed with each prescription, refill

SIDE EFFECTS
CNS: Weakness
CV: *Bradycardia,* heart failure, QT prolongation, torsades de pointes, atrial flutter
ENDO: Hypo/hyperthyroidism
GI: Nausea, vomiting, diarrhea, abdominal pain, severe hepatic injury, hepatic failure
INTEG: Rash, photosensitivity, anaphylaxis, angioedema
RESP: Interstitial pneumonitis, pulmonary fibrosis

PHARMACOKINETICS
Peak 3-6 hr, half-life 13-19 hr, metabolized by liver, excreted in feces (84%), via kidneys (6%), protein binding >98%

INTERACTIONS
Increase: dronedarone levels: CYP3A inhibitors/2D6 inhibitors
Decrease: dronedarone levels: 3A/2D6 inducers
Increase: bradycardia—β-blockers, calcium channel blockers
Increase: levels of cycloSPORINE, dextromethorphan, digoxin, disopyramide, flecainide, methotrexate, phenytoin, procainamide, quiNIDine, theophylline
Increase: anticoagulant effects—dabigatran, warfarin

Drug/Herb
Increase: anticoagulant effect—yohimbine
Decrease: dronedarone effect—St. John's wort

Drug/Food:
Increase: dronedarone effect, grapefruit; avoid use

Drug/Lab Test
Increase: T_4, creatinine, LFTs, bilirubin
Decrease: potassium, magnesium

NURSING CONSIDERATIONS
Assess:

Black Box Warning: NYHA Class IV heart failure or symptomatic heart failure with recent decomposition requiring hospitalization doubles risk of death

• **ECG** to determine product effectiveness; measure PR, QRS, QT intervals; check for PVCs, other dysrhythmias, B/P continuously for hypo/hypertension; report dysrhythmias, slowing heart rate
• Serum creatinine, potassium, magnesium
• I&O ratio; electrolytes (potassium, creatinine, magnesium)
• Dehydration or hypovolemia
• Rebound hypertension after 1-2 hr
• **Hypothyroidism:** lethargy, dizziness, constipation, enlarged thyroid gland, edema of extremities; cool, pale skin
• **Hyperthyroidism:** restlessness, tachycardia, eyelid puffiness, weight loss,

frequent urination, menstrual irregularities, dyspnea; warm, moist skin
• Cardiac rate, respiration: rate, rhythm, character, chest pain; start with patient hospitalized and monitored up to 1 wk

Evaluate:
• Therapeutic response: atrial fibrillation, flutter

Teach patient/family:
• To take this product as directed; to avoid missed doses; not to use with grapefruit juice, to avoid all other products without approval of provider
• To immediately report weight gain, edema, difficulty breathing
• To use effective contraception during treatment (pregnancy [X]) not to breastfeed

TREATMENT OF OVERDOSE:
O_2, artificial ventilation, ECG, administer DOPamine for circulatory depression; administer diazepam or thiopental for seizures, isoproterenol

droxidopa
(drox′-i-doe′-pa)
Northera
Func. class.: Cardiovascular agent-vasopressor

ACTION: A synthetic amino acid precursor of norepinephrine. It is used to increase blood pressure with symptomatic neurogenic orthostatic hypotension (NOH) caused by primary autonomic failure (e.g., Parkinson's disease, multiple system atrophy, and pure autonomic failure), dopamine β-hydroxylase deficiency, or nondiabetic autonomic neuropathy

USES: To increase blood pressure

CONTRAINDICATIONS: Hypersensitivity
Precautions: Angina, breastfeeding, cardiac arrhythmias, cardiac disease, children, coronary artery disease, heart disease, hyperthermia, infants, mental status changes, myocardial infarction, neonates, pregnancy, salicylate/tartrazine dye hypersensitivity

Black Box Warning: Hypertension

DOSAGE AND ROUTES
• **Adults: PO** 100 mg tid: upon arising in the morning, at midday, and in the late afternoon at least 3 hr before bedtime; titrate to response, by 100 mg tid q24-48hr up to a dose of 600 mg PO tid, max 1800 mg/day

Available forms: Caps 100, 200, 300 mg

Administer:
• Give tid at the following times: upon arising in the morning, at midday, and in the late afternoon at least 3 hr before bedtime (to reduce the potential for supine hypertension during sleep)
• Use without regard to food, but should be taken consistently in regard to food to ensure consistent absorption
• Swallow capsules whole

SIDE EFFECTS
CNS: Headache, dizziness, fatigue
CV: Supine hypertension, arrhythmia exacerbation, chest pain
MISC: Urinary tract infection, **neuroleptic malignant syndrome**

PHARMACOKINETICS
Peak 3-4 hr

INTERACTIONS
Increase: droxidopa effects—carbidopa, serotonin receptor agonists, sympathomimetics
Increase: hypertensive crisis—MAOIs

NURSING CONSIDERATIONS
Assess:
• Monitor supine B/P before and at every dosage increase, assess response periodically. Advise to elevate the head of the bed when resting or sleeping to lessen the risk for supine hypertension. B/P

should be monitored, in supine position and the recommended head-elevated sleeping position. Reduce or discontinue if supine hypertension persists

- **Neuroleptic malignant syndrome:** Hyperthermia, severe extrapyramidal dysfunction, alterations in consciousness, mental status changes, and autonomic instability (tachycardia, blood pressure fluctuations, diaphoresis). In those with Parkinson's disease, this condition may occur with abrupt reduction of products with dopaminergic properties
- **Arrhythmia exacerbation:** exacerbation of existing ischemic cardiac disease (coronary artery disease, angina, myocardial infarction, CHF); consider the potential risk before initiating therapy; if chest pain occurs during use, assess cardiac status

Evaluate:

- **Therapeutic response:** Increased B/P

Teach patient/family:

- Instruct patients to rest and sleep in an upper-body elevated position and to monitor blood pressure (to reduce the potential for supine hypertension)

DULoxetine (Rx)

(du-lox′uh-teen)

Cymbalta

Func. class.: Antidepressant

Chem. class.: Serotonin-norepinephrine reuptake inhibitor (SNRI)

ACTION: May potentiate serotonergic, noradrenergic activity in the CNS; in studies, DULoxetine is a potent inhibitor of neuronal serotonin and norepinephrine reuptake

USES: Major depressive disorder (MDD), neuropathic pain associated with diabetic neuropathy, generalized anxiety disorder, fibromyalgia, chronic low back pain, osteoarthritis pain

Unlabeled uses: Stress, urinary incontinence

CONTRAINDICATIONS: Alcohol intoxication, alcoholism, closed-angle glaucoma, hepatic disease, hepatitis, jaundice, hypersensitivity

Precautions: Pregnancy (C), breastfeeding, geriatric patients, mania, hypertension, renal/cardiac disease, seizures, increased intraocular pressure, anorexia nervosa, bleeding, dehydration, diabetes, hyponatremia, hypotension, hypovolemia, orthostatic hypotension, abrupt product withdrawal

Black Box Warning: Children, suicidal ideation

DOSAGE AND ROUTES

Depression

- **Adult: PO** 40-60 mg/day as single dose or 2 divided doses

Diabetic neuropathy

- **Adult: PO** 60 mg/day

Generalized anxiety disorder

- **Adult: PO** 60 mg/day, may start with 30 mg/day × 1 wk, then increase to 60 mg/day; maintenance 60-120 mg/day

Fibromyalgia

- **Adult: PO** 30 mg/day × 1 wk, then 60 mg/day

Musculoskeletal pain

- **Adult: PO** 60 mg/day or 30 mg/day × 1 wk, then 60 mg/day

Renal dose

- **Adult: PO** Start with 20 mg, gradually increase; avoid use in severe renal disease

Available forms: Caps 20, 30, 60 mg

Administer:

- Swallow cap whole; do not break, crush, or chew; do not sprinkle on food or mix with liquid
- Without regard to food
- Store in tight container at room temperature; do not freeze

SIDE EFFECTS

CNS: Insomnia, anxiety, dizziness, tremor, somnolence, fatigue, decreased

appetite, decreased weight, agitation, diaphoresis, hallucinations, **neuroleptic malignant–like syndrome reaction**, aggression, **seizures**, *headache,* abnormal dreams, flushing, hot flashes, chills
CV: **Thrombophlebitis**, peripheral edema, hypertension, palpitations, **supraventricular dysrhythmia**, orthostatic hypotension
EENT: *Abnormal vision*
ENDO: Hypo/hyperglycemia, SIADH
GI: Constipation, diarrhea, dysphagia, *nausea,* vomiting, anorexia, dry mouth, colitis, gastritis, abdominal pain, **hepatic failure**
GU: Abnormal ejaculation, urinary hesitation/retention/frequency, ejaculation delayed, erectile dysfunction, gynecologic bleeding
INTEG: Photosensitivity, bruising, sweating, **Stevens-Johnson syndrome**
MS: Gait disturbance, muscle spasm, restless leg syndrome, myalgia
SYST: **Anaphylaxis, angioedema, serotonin syndrome, Stevens-Johnson syndrome**

PHARMACOKINETICS

Well absorbed; extensively metabolized (CYP2D6, CYP1A2) in the liver to an active metabolite; 70% of product recovered in urine, 20% in feces; 90% protein binding; elimination half-life 9.2-19.1 hr

INTERACTIONS

• **Do not use with linezolid or methylene blue IV**
• **Narrow therapeutic index: CYP2D6 extensively metabolized products (flecainide, phenothiazines, propafenone, tricyclics, thioridazine)**
⚠ **Hyperthermia, rigidity, rapid fluctuations of vital signs, mental status changes, neuroleptic malignant syndrome—MAOIs, coadministration contraindicated within 14 days of MAOI use**
Increase: CNS depression—opioids, antihistamines, sedative/hypnotics
Increase: serotonin syndrome, neuroleptic malignant syndrome—SSRIs, serotonin-receptor agonists
Increase: bleeding risk—anticoagulants, antiplatelets, salicylates, NSAIDs
Increase: action of DULoxetine—CYP1A2 inhibitors (fluvoxamine, quinolone anti-infectives); CYP2D6 inhibitors (FLUoxetine, quiNIDine, PARoxetine)
Increase: ALT, bilirubin—alcohol
Drug/Herb
• Serotonin syndrome: St. John's wort
Increase: CNS depression—kava, valerian
Drug/Lab Test
Increase: blood glucose

NURSING CONSIDERATIONS

Assess:

Black Box Warning: Depression: mood, sensorium, affect, **suicidal tendencies,** increase in psychiatric symptoms; depression, panic, monitor children weekly face to face during first 4 wk, or dosage change, then every other wk for next 4 wk, then at 12 wk

• B/P lying, standing; pulse q4hr; if systolic B/P drops 20 mm Hg, hold product, notify prescriber; take VS q4hr in patients with CV disease
• Hepatic studies: AST, ALT, bilirubin
• Weight weekly; weight loss or gain; appetite may increase; peripheral edema may occur
• Sugarless gum, hard candy, frequent sips of water for dry mouth
• **Withdrawal symptoms:** headache, nausea, vomiting, muscle pain, weakness; not common unless product is discontinued abruptly
⚠ **Malignant neuroleptic-like syndrome reaction**
⚠ **Serotonin syndrome:** nausea/vomiting, dizziness, facial flush, shivering, sweating
• **Sexual dysfunction:** ejaculation dysfunction, erectile dysfunction, decreased libido, orgasm dysfunction
• Assistance with ambulation during beginning therapy; drowsiness, dizziness occur

Evaluate:

- Therapeutic response: decreased depression

Teach patient/family:

- To report urinary retention; about signs and symptoms of bleeding (GI bleeding, nosebleed, ecchymoses, bruising)
- To use with caution when driving, performing other activities requiring alertness because of drowsiness, dizziness, blurred vision
- To avoid alcohol ingestion, MAOIs, other CNS depressants
- Not to discontinue medication quickly after long-term use; may cause nausea, headache, malaise; taper

Black Box Warning: That clinical worsening and suicide risk may occur

- To wear sunscreen or large hat; photosensitivity may occur
- To notify prescriber if pregnancy planned or suspected, or if breastfeeding
- Improvement may occur in 4-8 wk or in up to 12 wk (geriatric patients)

dutasteride (Rx)

(doo-tass′ter-ide)

Avodart

Func. class.: Androgen inhibitor

Chem. class.: Synthetic 5α-reductase inhibitor, 4-azasteroid compound

ACTION: Inhibits both type 1 and type 2 forms of a steroid enzyme that converts testosterone to 5α-dihydrotestosterone (DHT), which is responsible for the initial growth of prostatic tissue

USES: Treatment of benign prostatic hyperplasia (BPH) in men with an enlarged prostate gland; may be used in combination with tamsulosin

Unlabeled uses: Alopecia

CONTRAINDICATIONS: Pregnancy (X), breastfeeding, women, children, hypersensitivity

Precautions: Hepatic disease

DOSAGE AND ROUTES

Benign prostatic hyperplasia (BPH)

- **Adult: PO** 0.5 mg/day

Alopecia (unlabeled)

- **Adult: PO** 0.5-2.5 mg/day

Available form: Caps 0.5 mg

Administer:

- Swallow caps whole; do not break, crush, chew
- Without regard to meals

SIDE EFFECTS

GU: Decreased libido, impotence, gynecomastia, ejaculation disorders (rare), mastalgia, teratogenesis

INTEG: Serious skin infections

PHARMACOKINETICS

Peak 2-3 hr, protein binding 99%, metabolized in liver by CYP3A4, excreted in feces, half-life 5 wk at steady state

INTERACTIONS

Increase: dutasteride concentrations—ritonavir, ketoconazole, verapamil, diltiazem, cimetidine, ciprofloxacin, antiretroviral protease inhibitors, or other products metabolized by CYP3A4

Drug/Lab Test

Decrease: PSA

NURSING CONSIDERATIONS

Assess:

- **For decreasing symptoms of BPH:** decreasing urinary retention, frequency, urgency, nocturia
- PSA levels; digital rectal, urinary obstruction; determine the absence of urinary cancer before starting treatment
- Blood studies: ALT, AST, bilirubin, CBC with differential, serum creatinine, serum electrolytes

Evaluate:

- Therapeutic response: decreasing symptoms of BPH; decreased urinary retention, frequency, urgency, nocturia

Teach patient/family:

- To read patient information leaflet before starting therapy; to reread it upon prescription renewal
- To notify prescriber if therapeutic response decreases, if edema occurs
- Not to discontinue product abruptly
- About changes in sex characteristics
- That men taking dutasteride should not donate blood for at least 6 mo after last dose to prevent blood administration to pregnant female
- That caps should not be handled by a woman who is pregnant or who may become pregnant because product can be absorbed through skin
- That ejaculate volume may decrease during treatment; that product rarely interferes with sexual function
- Should not be used or handled by breastfeeding women
- Swallow whole; do not crush, chew, or open
- May increase risk for developing high-grade prostate cancer

ecallantide

(ee-kal′an-tide)

Kalbitor

Func. class.: Hematological agents

Chem. class.: Kallikrein inhibitor

ACTION: Selectively, reversibly inhibits kallikrein within the inflammatory pathways, preventing excess production of bradykinin

USES: Acute attacks of hereditary angioedema (≥16 yr)

CONTRAINDICATIONS: Hypersensitivity to the drug or its components

Black Box Warning: Anaphylaxis has occurred after administrations (usually within first hour after dosing); drug should be administered only by health care provider with medical support available to treat anaphylaxis and hereditary angioedema; monitor patient closely

Precautions: Pregnancy (C), breastfeeding, geriatric patients, child <16 yr

DOSAGE AND ROUTES

- **Adult/adolescent ≥16 yr: SUBCUT** 30 mg given as three 10-mg injections; give additional 30-mg dose within 24 hours if attack persists

Available forms: Solution 10 mg/ml

Administer:

- Using aseptic technique, withdraw 1 ml (10 mg) using a large-bore needle; change the needle on the syringe to a needle suitable for subcut inj (27 gauge recommended)
- Inject into the skin of the abdomen, thigh, or upper arm
- Repeat the procedure for each of the three vials (30 mg total dose); the injection site for each of the three injections may be in the same or different anatomic location (abdomen, thigh, or upper arm); there is no need for site rotation; individual injections should be separated by at least 2 inches and away from the anatomical site of attack
- The same directions for administration apply if an additional dose is required within 24 hr; different injection sites or the same anatomical location as used for the first dose may be used
- Visually inspect parenteral products for particulate matter and discoloration before administration

SIDE EFFECTS

CNS: Fatigue, fever, headache, flushing

EENT: Nasopharyngitis

GI: Abdominal pain, diarrhea, nausea, vomiting

CV: Hypotension, chest pain

INTEG: Injection-site reactions, pruritus, rash, urticaria

RESP: Upper respiratory tract infection

Black Box Warning: Assess: anaphylaxis; usually within first hr after dosing

NURSING CONSIDERATIONS

Teach patient/family:

- To immediately report wheezing, cough, chest tightness, trouble breathing, dizziness, fainting, throat tightness, itchiness, hives, and swelling of tongue or throat
- Inform patient that drug must be given by health care provider in a health care setting in case serious allergic reaction occurs

econazole

(ee-koe′na-zole)

Func. class.: Topical antifungal

Chem. class.: Imidazole derivative

ACTION: Antifungal activity results from inhibiting cell-wall permeability

USES: Tinea corporis, cruris, pedis, versicolor; cutaneous candidiasis

CONTRAINDICATIONS:
Hypersensitivity

Precautions: Pregnancy (C)

DOSAGE AND ROUTES

Tinea corporis, cruris, pedis, versicolor

- **Adult/child: TOP** rub into affected areas daily × 2 wk, or × 4 wk (pedis)

Cutaneous candidiasis

- **Adult/child:** rub into affected areas bid × 2 wk

Available forms: Topical cream/foam 1%

Administer:

Topical route

- Do not use products near the eyes, nose, or mouth
- Wash hands before and after use; wash affected area and gently pat dry
- **Cream:** apply to the cleansed affected area; massage gently into affected areas

SIDE EFFECTS

INTEG: Burning, rash, pruritus, erythema

PHARMACOKINETICS

Unknown

NURSING CONSIDERATIONS

Assess:

- **Allergic reaction**: assess for hypersensitivity, product might need to be discontinued
- **Infection**: assess for itching, peeling

Evaluate:

- Decreased itching, peeling

Teach patient/family:

Topical route

- That product is for external use only; do not use skin products near the eyes, nose, or mouth
- To wash hands before and after use; to wash affected area and gently pat dry
- **Cream:** to apply a thin film to the cleansed affected area; massage gently into affected areas

econazole topical

See Appendix B

RARELY USED

edetate calcium disodium (Rx)

(ee′de-tate)

Calcium Disodium Versenate

Func. class.: Heavy-metal antagonist (antidote)

Do not confuse:

edetate calcium disodium/edetate disodium

USES:
Lead poisoning, acute lead encephalopathy

CONTRAINDICATIONS:
Hypersensitivity, anuria, poisoning of other metals, severe renal disease, hepatitis

Black Box Warning: Child <3 yr

DOSAGE AND ROUTES

Lead mobilization test (lead toxicity 25-45 mcg/dl)

- **Adult/adolescent: IV INFUSION** 500 mg/m^2 over 1 hr or **IM**
- **Child: IV INFUSION** 500 mg/m^2 over 1 hr or **IM** as single dose or 2 divided doses

Acute lead encephalopathy (blood levels >70 mcg/dl)

- **Adult/adolescent/child/infant: IM/IV** 1500 mg/m^2 as **IV INFUSION** over 12-24 hr in combination with dimercaprol **IM,** give 1st dose ≥4 hr after initial dimercaprol, when urine flow established

efavirenz (Rx)

(ef-ah-veer′enz)

Sustiva

Func. class.: Antiretroviral

Chem. class.: Nonnucleoside reverse transcriptase inhibitor (NNRTI)

ACTION:
Binds directly to reverse transcriptase and blocks RNA, DNA polymerase, thus causing a disruption of the enzyme's site

USES:
HIV-1 in combination with at least 2 other antivirals

Unlabeled uses: HIV prophylaxis

CONTRAINDICATIONS:
Pregnancy (D), hypersensitivity, moderate/severe hepatic disease

Precautions: Breastfeeding, children <3 yr, renal/hepatic disease, myelosuppression, depression, seizures

DOSAGE AND ROUTES

Given in combination with protease inhibitor or nucleoside analog reverse transcriptase inhibitors (NARTIs)

- **Adult and child >40 kg: PO** 600 mg/day at bedtime
- **Child ≥3 mo, 32.5-39.9 kg: PO** 400 mg/day at bedtime
- **Child ≥3 mo, 25-32.4 kg: PO** 350 mg/day at bedtime
- **Child ≥3 mo, 20-24.9 kg: PO** 300 mg/day at bedtime
- **Child ≥3 mo, 15-19.9 kg: PO** 250 mg/day at bedtime
- **Child ≥3 mo, 7.5-14.9 kg: PO** 200 mg/day at bedtime
- **Child ≥3 mo, 5-<7.5 kg: PO** 150 mg/day at bedtime
- **Child 3.5-≤5 kg:** 100 mg/day at bedtime

Available forms: Caps 50, 200 mg; 600-mg tabs

Administer:

- Give on empty stomach; give at bedtime to decrease CNS side effects
- Caps may be opened, added to grape jelly to disguise peppery taste, or sprinkled on food, do not cut/break tabs

SIDE EFFECTS

CNS: Fatigue, impaired cognition, insomnia, abnormal dreams, depression, headache, dizziness, anxiety, drowsiness, odd feeling, depersonalization

GI: *Diarrhea,* abdominal pain, *nausea,* hyperlipidemia, constipation, increased LFTs, vomiting, hepatotoxicity

GU: Hematuria, kidney stones

INTEG: Rash, erythema multiforme, Stevens-Johnson syndrome, toxic epidermal necrolysis, exfoliative dermatitis

PHARMACOKINETICS

Peak 3-5 hr, well absorbed, metabolized by liver; terminal half-life 40-76 hr; >99% protein binding, excreted in urine, feces; concentrations higher in females and those of African, Asian, and Hispanic descent

INTERACTIONS

- Avoid use with boceprevir, delavirdine, rilpivirine; dosage change may be needed if given with telaprevir
- Do not give together with benzodiazepines, ergots, midazolam, triazolam, pimozide

Increase: CNS depression—alcohol, antidepressants, antihistamines, opioids

Increase: levels of both products—ritonavir, estrogens, anticonvulsants

Increase: levels of warfarin, statins (except pravastatin, fluvastatin)

Decrease: levels of indinavir, amprenavir, lopinavir, oral contraceptives, ketoconazole, itraconazole, posaconazole, voriconazole, saquinavir, cyclosporine, tacrolimus, sirolimus, bupropion, sertraline

Decrease: efavirenz metabolism—CYP3A4 inhibitors (conivaptan, ambrisentan, SORAfenib)

Decrease: efavirenz effect—CYP3A4 inducers (carBAMazepine, rifamycins)

Drug/Herb

Decrease: efavirenz level—St. John's wort; do not use together

Drug/Food
Increase: absorption—high-fat foods
Drug/Lab Test
Increase: ALT
False positive: cannibinoids

NURSING CONSIDERATIONS
Assess:
- **Pregnancy:** Rule out pregnancy (D) before starting treatment; a type of contraception is needed, oral/non-oral contraceptives are decreased, use barrier methods also
- Bowel pattern before, during treatment; if severe abdominal pain with bleeding occurs, product should be discontinued; monitor hydration
- **Serious skin reactions:** Stevens-Johnson syndrome, toxic epidermal necrolysis, usually occurs during first 2 wk, mild rash may resolve within 30 days; severe skin reactions including blistering, fever, product should be discontinued immediately and corticosteroids started
- **HIV:** Monitor CBC, blood chemistry, plasma HIV RNA, absolute CD4+/CD8+ cell counts/%, serum β_2 microglobulin, serum ICD+24 antigen levels, cholesterol, hepatic enzymes
- **Signs of toxicity:** severe nausea/vomiting, maculopapular rash
- **Hepatotoxicity:** LFTs in those with liver disease, hold if LFTs are moderately elevated; if severe or if LFTs increase after product is restarted, discontinue permanently

Evaluate:
- Therapeutic response: increased CD4 cell counts; decreased viral load; slowing progression of HIV

Teach patient/family:
- To take as prescribed; if dose is missed, to take as soon as remembered; not to double dose; to take with water, juice; to take on empty stomach at bedtime
- To make sure health care provider knows all medications, supplements, OTC products taken
- That, if severe rash occurs, to notify health care provider; that adverse reactions (rash, dizziness, abnormal dreams, insomnia) lessen after 1 mo
- Not to breastfeed or become pregnant if taking this product; to use nonhormonal contraception because serious birth defects have occurred (pregnancy [D]), use barrier method for ≥12 wk after last dose
- To avoid hazardous activities if dizziness, drowsiness occur
- That product does not cure disease but controls symptoms; that HIV can be transmitted to others even while taking this product; to continue with safe-sex practices

E

efinaconazole topical
See Appendix B

eletriptan (Rx)
(el-ee-trip′tan)

Relpax

Func. class.: Antimigraine agent, abortive

Chem. class.: 5-HT_1-1B/1D receptor agonist, triptan

ACTION: Binds selectively to the vascular 5-HT_1-receptor subtype; causes vasoconstriction in cranial arteries

USES: Acute treatment of migraine with/without aura

CONTRAINDICATIONS: Hypersensitivity, coronary artery vasospasm, peripheral vascular disease, hemiplegic/basilar migraine, uncontrolled hypertension; ischemic bowel, heart disease; severe renal/hepatic disease, acute MI, stroke, angina, postmenopausal women, men >40 yr; risk factors of CAD, MI, or other cardiac disease; hypercholesterolemia, obesity, diabetes

Precautions: Pregnancy (C), breastfeeding, children, geriatric patients, impaired renal/hepatic function

DOSAGE AND ROUTES
- **Adult: PO** 20 or 40 mg, may increase if needed, max 40 mg (single dose); may

repeat in 2 hr if headache improves but returns, max 80 mg/24 hr

Available forms: Tabs 20, 40 mg

Administer:

• Swallow tabs whole; do not break, crush, or chew; use with 8 oz of water

• At beginning of headache; if headache returns, repeat dose after 2 hr of 1st dose if 1st dose is ineffective; treat no more than 3 headaches per 30 days

SIDE EFFECTS

CNS: *Dizziness,* headache, anxiety, paresthesia, asthenia, somnolence, flushing, fatigue, hot/cold sensation, chills, vertigo, hypertonia, seizures, serotonin syndrome

CV: Chest pain, palpitations, hypertension, MI, sinus tachycardia, stroke, ventricular fibrillation/tachycardia, atrial fibrillation, AV block, bradycardia, chest pressure syndrome, coronary vasospasm

GI: Nausea, dry mouth, vomiting

MS: *Weakness,* back pain

RESP: Chest tightness, pressure

PHARMACOKINETICS

Onset of pain relief ½ hr, peak 1½-2 hr, half-life 4 hr, metabolized in the liver, 70% excreted in urine and feces

INTERACTIONS

Increase: plasma concentrations of eletriptan—CYP3A4 inhibitors (clarithromycin, erythromycin, itraconazole, ketoconazole, nelfinavir, ritonavir), propranolol, ergots, avoid use within 72 hr of these products

Increase: serotonin syndrome—SSRIs, SNRIs, serotonin-receptor agonists

Increase: vasospastic reactions—ergots, ergot similar products, avoid use within 24 hr of these products

NURSING CONSIDERATIONS

Assess:

• **Migraine:** pain location, character, intensity, nausea, vomiting, aura; quiet, calm environment with decreased stimulation from noise, bright light, excessive talking

• B/P; signs, symptoms of coronary vasospasms, geriatric patients may be at higher risk

• Tingling, hot sensation, burning, feeling of pressure, numbness, flushing

• Stress level, activity, recreation, coping mechanisms

• Neurologic status: LOC, blurring vision, nausea, vomiting, tingling in extremities preceding headache

• Ingestion of tyramine foods (pickled products, beer, wine, aged cheese), food additives, preservatives, colorings, artificial sweeteners, chocolate, caffeine, which may precipitate these types of headaches

• Patients with CAD risk factors; 1st dose should be administered in prescriber's office or medical facility

• Determine whether CYP3A4 inhibitors or other ergot-type products have been given

Evaluate:

• Therapeutic response: decrease in frequency, severity of migraine

Teach patient/family:

• To report any side effects to prescriber

• To use contraception while taking product; to inform prescriber if pregnant or intending to become pregnant

• To provide dark, quiet environment

• That product does not prevent or reduce number of migraine attacks

RARELY USED

elvitegravir/cobicistat/emtricitabine/tenofovir

(el-vye-teg′gra-veer/koe-bik′-i-stat/em-tra-sye′tah-ben/te-noe′to-veer)

Stribild ⚠ 🍁

Func. class.: Antiretrovirals

USES: HIV in treatment-naïve patients

CONTRAINDICATIONS: Hypersensitivity, CCr <70 ml/min, severe hepatic disease

DOSAGE AND ROUTES

• **Adult: PO** 1 Tab daily

Renal Dose

• **Adult: PO** do not use in CCr <50 ml/min

RARELY USED

eltrombopag

(ell-trom-bow′pag)

Promacta

Func. class.: Hematopoietic

USES: Thrombocytopenia in chronic immune thrombocytopenic purpura when unresponsive to other treatment, chronic hepatitis C–associated thrombocytopenia

CONTRAINDICATIONS: Hypersensitivity

Black Box Warning: Hepatotoxicity

DOSAGE AND ROUTES

• **Adult: PO** 50 mg/day, adjust dosage to maintain platelets at $\geq 50 \times 10^9$, max 75 mg/day; 25 mg/day chronic hepatitis C; East Asian descent reduce dose to 25 mg daily

emedastine ophthalmic

See Appendix B

empagliflozin

(em-pa-gli-floe′zin)

Jardiance

Func. class.: Antidiabetic

Chem. class.: Sodium-glucose cotransporter 2 (SGLT2) inhibitors

ACTION: An inhibitor of sodium-glucose cotransporter 2 (SGLT2), the transporter responsible for reabsorbing the majority of glucose filtered by the tubular lumen in the kidney

USES: Type 2 diabetes mellitus with diet and exercise

CONTRAINDICATIONS: Hypersensitivity, dialysis, renal failure

Precautions: Adrenal insufficiency, breastfeeding, children, dehydration, diabetic ketoacidosis, fever, geriatric patients, hypercholesterolemia, hypercortisolism, hyperglycemia, hyperthyroidism, hypoglycemia, hypotension, hypothyroidism, hypovolemia, malnutrition, pituitary insufficiency, pregnancy, renal impairment, type 1 diabetes mellitus, vaginitis

DOSAGE AND ROUTES

• **Adults: PO** 10 mg daily, may increase to 25 mg daily

Available forms: Tabs 10, 25 mg

Administer:

• Give every day without regard to food in the AM

SIDE EFFECTS

MS: Arthralgia

ENDO: Hypercholesterolemia, hyperlipidemia, hypoglycemia

CV: Hypotension, orthostatic hypotension

GU: Increased urinary frequency, nocturia, polyuria, cystitis, dehydration, diuresis

GI: Nausea

CNS: Syncope

MISC: Infection

PHARMACOKINETICS

Protein binding 82.6%, terminal elimination half-life 12.4 hr, peak 1.5 hr

INTERACTIONS

Increase: hypoglycemic effect—Angiotensin II receptor antagonists, angiotensin-converting enzyme (ACE) inhibitors, loop diuretics, thiazide diuretics, fluoxetine, olanzapine, β-blockers, octreotide, fibric acid derivatives, MAOIs type A

Increase/Decrease: hypoglycemic effect—clonidine, androgens, bortezomib, lithium, alcohol, sulfonamides

Decrease: hypoglycemic effect—phenothiazines, atypical antipsychotics, baclofen, carbonic anhydrase inhibitors,

estrogens, progestins, oral contraceptives, dextrothyroxine, glucagon, corticosteroids, fenfluramine, dexfenfluramine, phenytoin, fosphenytoin, ethotoin, salicylates, cyclosporine, tacrolimus, tobacco
Do not use with gatifloxacin, thyroid hormones

Drug/Herb/Supplements
Increase: hypoglycemia—chromium, horse chestnut
Increase/Decrease: hypoglycemia—niacin
Decrease: hypoglycemia—green tea

NURSING CONSIDERATIONS

Assess:
- **Diabetes:** Monitor blood glucose, glycosylated hemoglobin A1c (HbA1c), serum cholesterol profile, serum creatinine/BUN, assess for polydipsia, other products taken by patient

Evaluate:
- Therapeutic response: decreasing blood glucose, A1c

Teach patient/family:
- How to check blood glucose, to continue with diet and exercise changes, to avoid smoking, alcohol
- To avoid other products unless approved by prescriber

emtricitabine (Rx)

(em-tri-sit′uh-bean)

Emtriva

Func. class.: Antiretroviral
Chem. class.: Nucleoside reverse transcriptase inhibitor (NRTI)

ACTION:
A synthetic nucleoside analog of cytosine; inhibits replication of HIV virus by competing with the natural substrate and then becoming incorporated into cellular DNA by viral reverse transcriptase, thereby terminating cellular DNA chain

USES:
HIV-1 infection with other antiretroviral

Unlabeled uses: HBV (hepatitis B virus) infection with HIV, HIV prophylaxis

CONTRAINDICATIONS:
Hypersensitivity

Black Box Warning: Lactic acidosis

Precautions: Pregnancy (B), breastfeeding, children, geriatric patients, renal disease

Black Box Warning: Hepatic insufficiency, chronic hepatitis B virus (HPV)

DOSAGE AND ROUTES

Oral cap and solution are not interchangeable
- **Adult: PO** Caps 200 mg/day; oral sol 240 mg (24 ml)/day
- **Adolescent/child >33 kg: PO** Caps 200 mg/day; **child 3 mo-17 yr:** oral sol 6 mg/kg/day, max 240 mg (24 ml)
- **Infants <3 mo: PO oral sol** 3 mg/kg daily, do not use caps

Renal dose
- **Adult: PO** Caps CCr 30-49 ml/min, 200 mg q48hr; oral sol 120 mg q24hr; caps CCr 15-29 ml/min, 200 mg q72hr; oral sol 80 mg q24hr; caps CCr <15 ml/min, 200 mg q96hr; oral sol 60 mg q24hr

Available forms: Cap 200 mg; oral sol 10 mg/ml

Administer:
- Give without regard to meals
- Oral cap and solution not interchangeable
- Store (caps) at 25° C (77° F); (oral sol) refrigerated, use within 3 mo

SIDE EFFECTS

CNS: *Headache,* abnormal dreams, *depression,* dizziness, *insomnia,* neuropathy, paresthesia, *asthenia*
GI: *Nausea, vomiting, diarrhea, anorexia, abdominal pain, dyspepsia,* hepatomegaly with steatosis (may be fatal)
INTEG: *Rash,* skin discolorization
MS: Arthralgia, myalgia
RESP: *Cough*

SYST: Change in body fat distribution, lactic acidosis

PHARMACOKINETICS

Rapidly, extensively absorbed; peak 1-2 hr; protein binding <4%; excreted unchanged in urine (86%), feces (14%); half-life 10 hr

INTERACTIONS

- Do not use with efavirenz, tenofovir, lamiVUDine, treatment duplication

Decrease: emtricitabine level—interferons

- Complex interactions—ribavirin, cautious use

Drug/Lab Test

Increase: AST/ALT, glucose, amylase, bilirubin, CK, lipase

Decrease: neutrophils

NURSING CONSIDERATIONS

Assess:

- Renal/hepatic function tests: AST, ALT, bilirubin, amylase, lipase, triglycerides periodically during treatment

Black Box Warning: **Lactic acidosis, severe hepatomegaly with steatosis;** if lab reports confirm these conditions, discontinue treatment; may be fatal, more common in females or those who are overweight, monitor lactic acid levels, LFTs

Black Box Warning: **Hepatotoxicity:** do not use in those with risk factors such as alcoholism, discontinue if hepatotoxicity occurs

Black Box Warning: Hepatitis B and HIV coinfection (unlabeled); perform HBV screening in any patient who has HIV to ensure appropriate treatment; avoid single-drug treatments in HBV

Evaluate:

- Therapeutic response: decreased signs, symptoms of HIV; decreased viral load, increased CP4 counts

Teach patient/family:

- That GI complaints resolve after 3-4 wk of treatment
- To report planned or suspected pregnancy; not to breastfeed while taking product
- That product must be taken at same time of day to maintain blood level; solution and cap are not interchangeable
- That product will control symptoms but is not a cure for HIV; patient still infectious, may pass HIV virus on to others; that other products may be necessary to prevent other infections
- That changes in body fat distribution may occur

Black Box Warning: Lactic acidosis: to notify prescriber immediately if fatigue, muscle aches/pains, abdominal pain, difficulty breathing, nausea, vomiting, change in heart rhythm occur

Black Box Warning: Hepatotoxicity: to notify prescriber of dark urine, yellowing of skin/eyes, clay-colored stools, anorexia, nausea, vomiting

enalapril/enalaprilat (Rx)

(e-nal′a-pril)/(e-nal′a-pril-at)

Vasotec

Func. class.: Antihypertensive

Chem. class.: Angiotensin-converting enzyme (ACE) inhibitor

Do not confuse:

enalapril/ramipril/Anafranil/Eldepryl

ACTION:
Selectively suppresses renin-angiotensin-aldosterone system; inhibits ACE; prevents conversion of angiotensin I to angiotensin II, dilation of arterial, venous vessels

USES:
Hypertension, CHF, left ventricular dysfunction

Unlabeled uses: Diabetic nephropathy, hypertensive emergency/urgency, post-MI, proteinuria, renal crisis in scleroderma

CONTRAINDICATIONS:
Hypersensitivity, history of angioedema

Black Box Warning: Pregnancy (D)

Precautions: Breastfeeding, renal disease, hyperkalemia, hepatic failure, dehydration, bilateral renal artery/aortic stenosis

DOSAGE AND ROUTES
Hypertension
- **Adult: PO** 2.5-5 mg/day, may increase or decrease to desired response, range 10-40 mg/day in 1-2 divided doses; **IV** 0.625-1.25 mg q6hr over 5 min
- **Child: PO** 0.08 mg/kg/day in 1-2 divided doses, max 0.58 mg/kg/day
- **Child: IV** 5-10 mcg/kg/dose q8-24hr

CHF
- **Adult: PO** 2.5-20 mg/day in 2 divided doses, max 40 mg/day in divided doses

Renal disease
- **Adult: PO** 2.5 mg/day (CCr <30 ml/min), increase gradually; **IV** CCr >30 ml/min, 1.25 mg q6hr; CCr <30 ml/min, 0.625 mg as one-time dose, increase as per B/P

Hypertensive emergency/urgency (unlabeled)
- **Adult: IV** 1.25-5 mg q6hr

Available forms: *Enalapril:* tabs 2.5, 5, 10, 20 mg; *enalaprilat:* inj 1.25 mg/ml

Administer:

PO route
- Tab may be crushed, given without regard to meals

IV route
- Prepare in sterile environment using aseptic technique
- Dilute each dose with ≤50 ml compatible sol
- For 25 mcg/ml dilution often used for neonatal or pediatric patients, combine 1 ml enalaprilat 1.25 mg/ml and 49 ml compatible sol for IV

IV, Direct/Intermittent IV INFUSION route
- Undiluted over ≥5 min, use diluent provided or 50 ml D_5W, 0.9% NaCl, 0.9% NaCl in D_5W or LR, Isolyte E; give through Y-tube of free-flowing infusion of 0.9% NaCl, D_5W, LR, Isolyte E

Y-site compatibilities: Acyclovir, alemtuzumab, alfentanil, allopurinol, amifostine, amikacin, aminophylline, amphotericin B liposome, anidulafungin, ascorbic acid, atracurium, atropine, azaTHIOprine, aztreonam, benztropine, bivalirudin, bretylium, bumetanide, buprenorphine, butorphanol, calcium chloride/gluconate, CARBOplatin, ceFAZolin, cefonicid, cefotaxime, cefoTEtan, cefOXitin, cefTAZidime, ceftizoxime, cefTRIAXone, cefuroxime, chloramphenicol, cimetidine, cisatracurium, cladribine, clindamycin, cyanocobalamin, cyclophosphamide, cycloSPORINE, cytarabine, DACTINomycin, DAPTOmycin, dexamethasone, dexmedetomidine, dextran 40, digoxin, diltiazem, diphenhydrAMINE, DOBUTamine, DOCEtaxel, DOPamine, doripenem, doxacurium, DOXOrubicin, DOXOrubicin liposome, doxycycline, ePHEDrine, EPINEPHrine, epirubicin, epoetin, ertapenem, erythromycin, esmolol, etoposide, etoposide phosphate, famotidine, fenoldopam, fentaNYL, filgrastim, fluconazole, fludarabine, fluorouracil, folic acid, furosemide, ganciclovir, gemcitabine, gentamicin, granisetron, heparin, hydrocortisone, HYDROmorphone, ifosfamide, imipenem-cilastatin, indomethacin, insulin, isoproterenol, ketorolac, labetalol, levofloxacin, lidocaine, linezolid, LORazepam, magnesium sulfate, mannitol, mechlorethamine, melphalan, meperidine, meropenem, metaraminol, methicillin, methotrexate, methoxamine, methyldopate, methylPREDNISolone, metoclopramide, metoprolol, metroNIDAZOLE, mezlocillin, miconazole, midazolam, milrinone, minocycline, mitoXANtrone, morphine, moxalactam, multiple vitamin injection, nafcillin, nalbuphine, naloxone, netilmicin, niCARdipine, nitroglycerin, nitroprusside, norepinephrine, octreotide, ondansetron, oxacillin, oxaliplatin, oxytocin, PACLitaxel, palonosetron, papaverine, PEMEtrexed, penicillin G potassium, pentamidine, pentazocine, PENTobarbital, PHENobarbital, phentolamine, phenylephrine, phytonadione, piperacillin-tazobactam, potassium chloride/phosphate, procainamide, prochlorperazine, promethazine, propofol, propranolol, protamine, pyridoxime, quinupristin-dalfopristin, ranitidine, remifentanil, ritodrine, riTUXimab, rocuronium, sodium acetate, sodium bicarbonate, succinylcholine, SUFentanil, tacrolimus, teniposide, tetracycline, theophylline, thiamine, thiotepa, ticarcillin/clavulanate, tigecycline, tirofiban, tobramycin, tolazoline, trastuzumab, trimetaphan, urokinase, vancomycin, vasopressin, vecuronium, verapamil, vinCRIStine, vinorelbine, voriconazole, zoledronic acid

SIDE EFFECTS

CNS: *Insomnia, dizziness,* paresthesias, headache, fatigue, anxiety
CV: *Hypotension,* chest pain, tachycardia, **dysrhythmias,** syncope, angina, **MI,** orthostatic hypotension
EENT: *Tinnitus;* visual changes; sore throat; double vision; dry, burning eyes
GI: Nausea, vomiting, colitis, cramps, diarrhea, constipation, flatulence, dry mouth, loss of taste, **hepatotoxicity**
GU: **Proteinuria, renal failure,** increased frequency of polyuria or oliguria
HEMA: **Agranulocytosis, neutropenia**
INTEG: Rash, purpura, alopecia, hyperhidrosis, photosensitivity
META: Hyperkalemia
RESP: Dyspnea, dry cough, crackles
SYST: **Toxic epidermal necrolysis, Stevens-Johnson syndrome, angioedema**

PHARMACOKINETICS

Enalapril: **PO:** Onset 1 hr, peak 4-6 hr, duration ≥24 hr
Enalaprilat: **IV:** Onset 5-15 min, peak up to 4 hr, duration 4-6 hr, half-life 35 hr, metabolized by liver to active metabolite, excreted in urine

INTERACTIONS

Increase: hypersensitivity—allopurinol
Increase: hypotension—diuretics, other antihypertensives, phenothiazines, nitrates, acute alcohol ingestion, general anesthesia
Increase: potassium levels—salt substitutes, potassium-sparing diuretics, potassium supplements, cycloSPORINE, NSAIDs
Increase: levels of lithium, digoxin
Decrease: effects of enalapril—antacids, rifampin

Drug/Lab Test
Increase: ALT, AST, bilirubin, alk phos, glucose, uric acid, BUN, creatine
False positive: ANA titer

NURSING CONSIDERATIONS

Assess:

- **Bone marrow depression (rare):** neutrophils, decreased platelets; WBC with differential baseline, q3mo; if neutrophils <1000/mm³, discontinue treatment (recommended with collagen-vascular disease)
- **Hypertension:** B/P, peak/trough level, orthostatic hypotension, syncope when used with diuretic, pulse q4hr; note rate, rhythm, quality
- Baselines of renal, hepatic studies before therapy begins and 1 wk into therapy; electrolytes: potassium, sodium, chloride during 1st 2 wk of therapy
- Skin turgor, dryness of mucous membranes for hydration status; edema in feet, legs daily
- **Symptoms of CHF: edema, dyspnea, wet crackles, weight gain, jugular venous distension, difficulty breathing**

Evaluate:

- Therapeutic response: decreased B/P

Teach patient/family:

- Not to use OTC (cough, cold, or allergy) products unless directed by prescriber; to avoid potassium, salt substitutes
- To avoid sunlight or wear sunscreen for photosensitivity
- To comply with dosage schedule even if feeling better
- **To notify prescriber of mouth sores, sore throat, fever, swelling of hands or feet, irregular heartbeat, chest pain, signs of angioedema**
- That excessive perspiration, dehydration, vomiting, diarrhea may lead to fall in

blood pressure; to consult prescriber if these occur, maintain adequate hydration
- That product may cause dizziness, fainting; that light-headedness may occur during 1st few days of therapy, avoid activities requiring coordination
- That product may cause skin rash, impaired perspiration or angioedema; to discontinue if angioedema occurs
- Not to discontinue product abruptly
- That CV adverse reactions may reoccur
- To rise slowly to sitting or standing position to minimize orthostatic hypotension

Black Box Warning: To notify prescriber if pregnancy is planned or suspected; to use contraception during treatment; pregnancy (D)

TREATMENT OF OVERDOSE:
Lavage, IV atropine for bradycardia, IV theophylline for bronchospasm, digoxin, O_2, diuretic for cardiac failure

enfuvirtide (Rx)
(en-fyoo′vir-tide)

Fuzeon

Func. class.: Antiretroviral

Chem. class.: Fusion Inhibitor

ACTION: Inhibitor of the fusion of HIV-1 with CD4+ cells

USES: Treatment of HIV-1 infection in combination with other antiretrovirals

Unlabeled uses: HIV prophylaxis after occupational exposure

CONTRAINDICATIONS: Breastfeeding, hypersensitivity

Precautions: Pregnancy (B) (must be enrolled in the Antiretroviral Pregnancy Registry: 1-800-258-4263), children <6 yr, liver disease, myelosuppression, infections

DOSAGE AND ROUTES
- **Adult: SUBCUT** 90 mg (1 ml) bid
- **Child 6-16 yr and <42.6 kg: SUBCUT** 2 mg/kg bid, max 90 mg bid; 11-15.5 kg 27 mg/0.3 ml bid; 15.6-20 kg 36 mg/0.4 ml bid; 20.1-24.5 kg 45 mg/0.5 ml bid; 24.6-29 kg 54 mg/0.6 ml bid; 29.1-33.5 kg 63 mg/0.7 ml bid; 33.6-38 kg 72 mg/0.8 ml bid; 38.1-42.5 kg 81 mg/0.9 ml bid

HIV prophylaxis (unlabeled)
- **Adult: SUBCUT** 90 mg bid added to PEP regimen

Available forms: Powder for inj, lyophilized 108 mg (90 mg/ml when reconstituted)

Administer:

SUBCUT route
- **Reconstitute** vial with 1.1 ml sterile water for inj; tap and roll to mix; allow to stand until completely dissolved, may take up to 45 min; after dissolved, immediately **inject** or refrigerate up to 24 hr
- Do not mix with other medications
- SUBCUT: give bid, rotate sites; preferred sites: upper arm, anterior thigh, abdomen

SIDE EFFECTS
CNS: Anxiety, peripheral neuropathy, taste disturbance, Guillain-Barré syndrome, insomnia, depression

GI: Nausea, abdominal pain, anorexia, constipation, pancreatitis

GU: Glomerulonephritis, renal failure

HEMA: Thrombocytopenia, neutropenia

INTEG: *Inj site reactions*

MISC: Influenza, cough, conjunctivitis, lymphadenopathy, myalgia, hyperglycemia, pneumonia, rhinitis, fatigue, hypersensitivity

PHARMACOKINETICS
Peak 8 hr, terminal half-life 3.8 hr, well absorbed, undergoes catabolism, 92% protein binding

INTERACTIONS
Drug/Lab

Increase: LFTs, lipase

Decrease: Hgb

NURSING CONSIDERATIONS
Assess:
- **Signs of infection, inj site reactions, use analgesics; bacterial pneumonia**

may occur if blood counts are low, or viral load is high

- **Glomerulonephritis/renal failure:** BUN, creatinine, renal failure may occur
- Bowel pattern before, during treatment; if severe abdominal pain or constipation occurs, notify prescriber; monitor hydration
- Skin eruptions, rash, urticaria, itching
- Allergies before treatment, reaction to each medication
- **Immune reconstitution syndrome:** with combination theory
- **HIV:** CBC, blood chemistry, plasma HIV RNA, absolute CD4+/CD8+ cell counts/%, serum β_2 microglobulin, serum ICD+24 antigen levels, cholesterol

Evaluate:

- Therapeutic response: increased CD4 cell counts; decreased viral load; slowing progression of HIV-1 infection

Teach patient/family:

- To notify prescriber if pregnancy is suspected or if breastfeeding
- That pneumonia may occur; to contact prescriber if cough, fever occur
- That hypersensitive reactions may occur; rash, pruritus; to stop product, contact prescriber
- That product is not a cure for HIV-1 infection but controls symptoms; HIV-1 can still be transmitted to others; that product is to be used in combination only with other antiretrovirals
- How to prepare and give using subcut inj, watch for site reactions, rotate sites

⚠ HIGH ALERT

enoxaparin (Rx)

(ee-nox′a-par-in)

Lovenox

Func. class.: Anticoagulant, antithrombotic

Chem. class.: Low-molecular-weight heparin (LMWH)

Do not confuse:

enoxaparin/enoxacin

Lovenox/Lotronex

ACTION: Binds to antithrombin III inactivating factors Xa/IIa, thereby resulting in a higher ratio of anti-factor Xa to IIa

USES: Prevention of DVT (inpatient or outpatient), PE (inpatient) in hip and knee replacement, abdominal surgery at risk for thrombosis; unstable angina, acute MI, coronary artery thrombosis

Unlabeled uses: Antiphospholipid antibody syndrome, arterial thromboembolism prophylaxis, cerebral thromboembolism, percutaneous coronary intervention

CONTRAINDICATIONS: Hypersensitivity to this product, heparin, pork; active major bleeding, hemophilia, leukemia with bleeding, thrombocytopenic purpura, heparin-induced thrombocytopenia

Precautions: Pregnancy (B), breastfeeding, children, geriatric patients, low weight men (<57 kg), women (<45 kg), severe renal/hepatic disease, severe hypertension, subacute bacterial endocarditis, acute nephritis, recent burn, spinal surgery, indwelling catheters, hypersensitivity to benzyl alcohol

Black Box Warning: Lumbar puncture, aneurysm, coagulopathy, epidural anesthesia, spinal anesthesia

DOSAGE AND ROUTES

DVT/PE prophylaxis

- **Adult:** (moderate risk—general surgery, nonsurgery 40-60 yr major surgery <40 yr with no risk factors)
- **Adult:** **SUBCUT** 20 mg daily; higher risk adults—abdominal surgery, geriatric—general surgery, major surgery <40 yr no risk factors; **SUBCUT** 30 mg q12hr or 40 mg daily

DVT prevention before hip or knee surgery

- **Adult: SUBCUT** 30 mg bid given 12-24 hr postop for 7-10 days until DVT risk is diminished

DVT prevention before hip replacement

• **Adult: SUBCUT** 40 mg/day started 9-15 hr preop or 30 mg q12hr started 12-24 hr postop, continued until DVT risk diminished or patient adequately on anticoagulant

DVT prophylaxis before abdominal surgery

• **Adult: SUBCUT** 40 mg/day starting 24 hr before surgery × 7-10 days to prevent thromboembolic complications

Treatment of DVT or PE

• **Adult: SUBCUT** 1 mg/kg q12hr (without PE, outpatient); 1 mg/kg q12hr or 1.5 mg/kg/day (with or without PE, inpatient); warfarin should be started within 72 hr, continued ≥5 days until INR is 2-3 (at least 3 days)

Prevention of ischemic complications in unstable angina or non–Q-wave MI/non-ST

• **Adult: SUBCUT/IV** 1 mg/kg q12hr until stable with aspirin 100-325 mg/day × ≥2 days

Renal dose

• **Adult: SUBCUT** CCr < 30 ml/min: 30 mg daily **(thrombosis prophylaxis in abdominal surgery, hip or knee replacement surgery, during acute illness)**; 1 mg/kg daily **(concurrently with aspirin to treat unstable angina or non-Q-wave myocardial infarction)**; 1 mg/kg daily **(STEMI in those ≥75 yr)**, 30 mg IV bolus plus 1 mg/kg SC, then 1 mg/kg daily **(STEMI in those <75 yr)**, or 1 mg/kg daily **(concurrently with warfarin for inpatient or outpatient treatment of acute deep vein thrombosis with or without pulmonary embolism)**

Available forms: Prefilled syringes/inj 30 mg/0.3 ml, 40 mg/0.4 ml, 60 mg/0.6 ml, 80 mg/0.8 ml, 100 mg/1 ml, 120 mg/0.8 ml, 150 mg/ml; multidose vials 100 mg/ml (3 ml)

Administer:

• Only after screening patient for bleeding disorders
• Do not mix with other products or infusion fluids

⚠ Only this product when ordered; not interchangeable with heparin or other LMWHs

• At same time each day to maintain steady blood levels
• Avoid all IM inj that may cause bleeding
• Prepare in a sterile environment using aseptic technique

SUBCUT route

• Do not give IM; begin 1 hr before surgery; do not aspirate; rotate sites; do not expel bubble from syringe before administration
• To recumbent patient, give SUBCUT; rotate inj sites (left/right anterolateral, left/right posterolateral abdominal wall)
• Insert whole length of needle into skin fold held with thumb and forefinger
• If withdrawing from multidose vial, use TB syringe for proper measurement
• Prefilled syringes (30, 40 mg) not graduated; do not use for partial doses
• Do not administer if particulate is present, do not use products with benzyl alcohol in pregnant women

Direct IV route

• Use multidose vial for IV administration; use TB syringe, other graduated syringe to measure dose; give IV BOL through IV line, flush after
• Dilution may be stored for up to 4 wk in glass vial at room temperature, up to 2 wk in TB syringes with rubber stoppers at room temperature or refrigerated

SIDE EFFECTS

CNS: Fever, confusion
GI: Nausea
HEMA: Hemorrhage from any site, hypochromic anemia, thrombocytopenia, bleeding
INTEG: Ecchymosis, inj site hematoma
META: Hyperkalemia in renal failure
MS: Osteoporosis
SYST: Edema, peripheral edema

PHARMACOKINETICS

SUBCUT: 90% absorbed, maximum antithrombin activity (3-5 hr), elimination half-life $4^1/_2$ hr, excreted in urine

INTERACTIONS

Increase: enoxaparin action—anticoagulants, salicylates, NSAIDs, antiplatelets, thrombolytics, RU-486

Drug/Lab Test
Increase: bleeding risk—feverfew, garlic, ginger, ginkgo, horse chestnut
Increase: AST, ALT
Decrease: platelet count

NURSING CONSIDERATIONS

Assess:
- Monitor anti-factor Xa activity in chronic therapy (renal disease)
- Blood studies (Hct/Hgb, CBC, coagulation studies, platelets, occult blood in stools), anti-factor Xa (should be checked 4 hr after inj); thrombocytopenia may occur
- Renal studies: BUN/creatinine baseline and periodically
- **Bleeding:** gums, petechiae, ecchymosis, black tarry stools, hematuria; notify prescriber
- **Hypersensitivity:** rash, fever, chills, report to prescriber
- **Neurologic status:** those with epidural catheters are at greater chance for impairments
- Injection-site reactions: inflammation, redness, hematomas

Black Box Warning: Neurologic symptoms in patients who have received spinal anesthesia, may develop spinal hematoma, those who have had trauma, spinal surgery are at greater risk

Evaluate:
- Therapeutic response: prevention of DVT/PE

Teach patient/family:
- To use soft-bristle toothbrush to avoid bleeding gums; to use electric razor
- To report any signs of bleeding: gums, under skin, urine, stools; do not rub injection site, easy bruising, dizziness, rash, breathing changes
- To avoid OTC products containing aspirin, NSAIDs unless approved by prescriber

TREATMENT OF OVERDOSE:

Protamine 1 mg for each mg of this product

entacapone (Rx)

(en′ta-kah-pone)

Comtan

Func. class.: Antiparkinson agent
Chem. class.: COMT inhibitor

E

ACTION: Inhibits COMT (catechol *O*-methyltransferase) and alters the plasma pharmacokinetics of levodopa; given with levodopa/carbidopa

USES: Parkinson's disease for those experiencing end of dose; decreased effect as adjunct to levodopa/carbidopa

CONTRAINDICATIONS: Hypersensitivity

Precautions: Pregnancy (C), breastfeeding, children, renal/hepatic disease, affective disorders, psychosis

DOSAGE AND ROUTES

- **Adult: PO** 200 mg given with carbidopa/levodopa, max 1600 mg/day; may allow for 25% dosage reduction in levodopa therapy

Available forms: Tabs, film coated 200 mg

Administer:
- Only after MAOIs have been discontinued for 2 wk
- Give with dose of levodopa/carbidopa; product has no effect on its own

SIDE EFFECTS

CNS: *Involuntary choreiform movements, hand tremors, fatigue, headache, anxiety, twitching, numbness, dyskinesia, hypokinesia, hyperkinesia, weakness, confusion, agitation, nightmares,* psychosis, hallucination, hypomania, severe depression, dizziness, **neuroleptic malignant syndrome**
CV: *Orthostatic hypotension*
GI: *Nausea, vomiting, anorexia, abdominal distress, dry mouth, flatulence, bitter taste, diarrhea, constipation, dyspepsia,* gastritis, GI disorder

INTEG: Rash, sweating, alopecia
MISC: Dark urine and other body fluids, back pain, dyspnea, purpura, fatigue, asthenia, bacterial infection, rhabdomyolysis

PHARMACOKINETICS

Duration up to 8 hr; excreted in urine, feces; well absorbed; protein binding 98%; metabolized in liver extensively; enters breast milk; half-life of levodopa extended, half-life 0.5 hr initial, 2.5 hr second

INTERACTIONS

- Prevents catecholamine metabolism—nonselective MAOIs; do not use together

Increase: B/P, tachycardia, dysrhythmias, avoid use—bitolterol, DOPamine, DOBUTamine, EPINEPHrine, methyldopa, isoetharine, norepinephrine
Decrease: excretion of entacapone—ampicillin, chloramphenicol, probenecid, erythromycin, rifampin
Drug/Herb
Increase: B/P—ma huang
Decrease: effect—kava

NURSING CONSIDERATIONS

Assess:

⚠ **Neuroleptic malignant syndrome:** high temperature, increased CPK, rigidity, change in LOC usually during rapid withdrawal

- **Involuntary movements of Parkinson's disease:** akinesia, tremors, staggering gait, muscle rigidity, drooling when given with levodopa/carbidopa
- B/P, respirations during initial treatment
- Mental status: affect, mood, behavioral changes, depression; complete suicide assessment
- **Rhabdomyolysis:** muscle pain, tenderness, weakness; swelling of affected muscles; may lead to decreased B/P, shock
- Assistance with ambulation during beginning therapy

Evaluate:

- Therapeutic response: decrease in akathisia, increased mood when given with levodopa/carbidopa

Teach patient/family:

- That hallucinations, mental changes, nausea, dyskinesia can occur; may mean patient is overmedicated
- To change positions slowly to prevent orthostatic hypotension; not to drive, operate machinery until stabilized on medication and mental performance not affected
- To use product exactly as prescribed; if dose is missed, to take as soon as remembered up to 2 hr before next dose; not to discontinue abruptly; to withdraw gradually
- That urine, sweat may darken
- To notify prescriber if pregnancy is suspected; if lactating, that product excreted in breast milk

entecavir (Rx)

(en-te′ka-veer)

Baraclude

Func. class.: Antiretroviral nucleoside reverse transcriptase inhibitor (NRTIs)
Chem. class.: Guanosine nucleoside analog

ACTION: Inhibits hepatitis B virus DNA polymerase by competing with natural substrates and by causing DNA termination after its incorporation into viral DNA; causes viral DNA death

USES: Chronic hepatitis B (HBV)

CONTRAINDICATIONS: Hypersensitivity
Precautions: Pregnancy (C), breastfeeding, children, geriatric patients, severe renal disease, liver transplant

Black Box Warning: Hepatic disease, hepatitis, HIV, lactic acidosis

DOSAGE AND ROUTES

Chronic hepatitis B (nucleoside treatment naive)

- **Adult and adolescent ≥16 yr: PO** Tab 0.5 mg/day

• **Adults: PO** (solution) 0.5 mg q day; **Child/Adolescents ≥2 yr >30 kg:** 0.5 mg (10 ml) q day; **Child ≥2 yr, 27 to 30 kg:** 0.45 mg (9 ml) q day; **Child ≥2 yr, 24 to 26 kg:** 0.4 mg (8 ml) q day; **Child ≥2 yr, 21 to 23 kg:** 0.35 mg (7 ml) q day; **Child ≥2 yr, 18 to 20 kg:** 0.3 mg (6 ml) q day; **Children ≥2 yr, 15 to 17 kg:** 0.25 mg (5 ml) q day; **Children 2 ≥yrs, 12 to 14 kg:** 0.2 mg (4 ml) q day.; **Child ≥2 yr,** 0.15 mg (3 ml) q day

Chronic hepatitis B with compensated liver disease and history of hepatitis B viremia while receiving lamiVUDine or known lamiVUDine/telbivudine-resistant mutations

• **Adult and adolescent ≥16 yr: PO** Tab 1 mg/day

• **Adults: PO** (solution) 1 mg q day; **Child/ Adolescent ≥2 yr, >30 kg:** 1 mg (20 ml) q day; **Children ≥2 yr, 27 to 30 kg:** 0.9 mg (18 ml) q day; **Children ≥2 yr, 24 to 26 kg:** 0.8 mg (16 ml) q day; **Children 2 years and older weighing 21 to 23 kg:** 0.7 mg (14 ml); **Child ≥2yr, 18 to 20 kg:** 0.6 mg (12 ml) q day; **Child ≥2 yr, 15 to 17 kg:** 0.5 mg (10 ml) q day; **Child ≥2 yr, 12 to 14 kg:** 0.4 mg (8 ml) q day; **Child ≥2 yr,** 10 to 11 kg: 0.3 mg (6 ml) q day

Renal dose

• **Adult: PO** CCr ≥50 ml/min, 0.5 mg/day; CCr 30-49 ml/min, 0.25 mg/day, 0.5 mg/day or 1 mg q48hr for lamiVUDine-refractory patient; CCr 10-29 ml/min, 0.15/day or 1 mg q72hr for lamiVUDine-refractory patient; CCr <10 ml/min, 0.05 mg/day, 0.1 mg/day or 1 mg q7day for lamiVUDine-refractory patient

Available forms: Tabs, film coated 0.5, 1 mg; oral sol 0.05 mg/ml

Administer:

• After hemodialysis
• By mouth on empty stomach 2 hr before or after food
• Store at room temperature
• **Oral liquid:** use calibrated oral dosing spoon provided; may be used interchangeably with tabs, do not dilute

SIDE EFFECTS

CNS: *Headache,* fatigue, dizziness, insomnia
ENDO: Hyperglycemia
GI: *Dyspepsia,* nausea, vomiting, diarrhea, elevated liver function enzymes
INTEG: Alopecia, rash
SYST: **Lactic acidosis, severe hepatomegaly with steatosis**

PHARMACOKINETICS

Peak 0.5-1.5 hr, steady state 6-10 days, 100% bioavailability, extensively distributed to tissues, protein binding 13%, terminal half-life 128-149 hr, excreted unchanged (62%-73%) via kidneys

INTERACTIONS

Drug/Food

Decrease: absorption—high-fat meal

Drug/Lab Test

Increase: ALT, AST, total bilirubin, amylase, lipase, creatinine, blood glucose, urine glucose
Decrease: platelets, albumin

NURSING CONSIDERATIONS

Assess:

• For nephrotoxicity: increasing CCr, BUN

Black Box Warning: For HIV before beginning treatment because HIV resistance may occur in chronic hepatitis B patients; monitor HIV RNA

Black Box Warning: For lactic acidosis and severe hepatomegaly with stenosis; increased serum lactate, increased hepatic enzymes, palpate line; discontinue if present, discontinue if signs occur

• Geriatric patients more carefully; may develop renal, cardiac symptoms more rapidly

Black Box Warning: For exacerbations of hepatitis (jaundice, pruritus, fatigue), anorexia after discontinuing treatment, and for several months monitor LFTs

Evaluate:

- Therapeutic response: decreased symptoms of chronic hepatitis B, improving LFTs

Teach patient/family:

- Not to take with food
- To take exactly as prescribed, read the "Patient Information," take missed dose when remembered unless close to time of next dose; compliance with dosage schedule is required; do not share product
- Not to stop medication without approval of prescriber
- That optimal duration of treatment is unknown
- To avoid use with other medications, supplements unless approved by prescriber
- To notify prescriber of decreased urinary output, blood in urine

Black Box Warning: Symptoms of lactic acidosis: muscle pain, severe tiredness, weakness, trouble breathing, stomach pain with nausea/vomiting, coldness in arms/legs, fast/irregular heartbeat, dizziness

Black Box Warning: Symptoms of hepatotoxicity: eyes/skin turning yellow, dark urine, light bowel movements, no appetite for days, nausea, stomach pain

- That product does not cure but lowers amount of HBV in body
- That product does not stop spread of HBV to others by sex, sharing needles, or being exposed to blood
- Not to breastfeed, to notify prescriber if pregnancy is planned or suspected
- Not to operate machinery until effect is known, dizziness may occur
- That regular follow-up and lab tests will be needed

RARELY USED

enzalutamide

(en-zal-u′ta-mide)

Xtandi

Func. class.: Antineoplastic hormone

Chem. class.: Nonsteroidal antiandrogen

USES: Metastatic castration-resistant prostate cancer in those who have received DOCEtaxel

CONTRAINDICATIONS: Pregnancy (X), women, hypersensitivity

DOSAGE AND ROUTES

- **Adult: PO** 160 mg (4 × 40-mg caps) daily
- If a patient experiences a grade 3 or higher toxicity or an intolerable adverse effect, withhold dosing for 1 wk or until symptoms improve to grade 2 or less, then resume at the same or a reduced dosage (120 or 80 mg), if warranted
- The concomitant use of strong cytochrome P450 (CYP-450) 2C8 inhibitors should be avoided if possible; if a strong CYP2C8 inhibitor must be coadministered, reduce the enzalutamide dosage to 80 mg once daily

Available forms: Tabs 40 mg

epinastine (ophthalmic)

(ep-ih-nas′teen)

Elestat

Func. class.: Antihistamine (ophthalmic)

Chem. class.: Histamine 1 receptor antagonist/mast cell stabilizer

ACTION: A topically active, direct H_1-receptor antagonist and mast cell stabilizer; by reducing these inflammatory mediators, it relieves the ocular pruritus associated with allergic conjunctivitis

USES:
Prevention of ocular pruritus associated with signs and symptoms of allergic conjunctivitis

CONTRAINDICATIONS:
Hypersensitivity

Precautions: Pregnancy (C), breastfeeding, children, contact lenses

DOSAGE AND ROUTES

- **Adult/child ≥3 yr: OPHTH** Instill 1 drop in each eye bid

Available forms: Ophthalmic sol 0.5%

Ophthalmic route

- For topical ophthalmic use only
- The preservative benzalkonium chloride may be absorbed by soft contact lenses; wait ≥10 min after instilling the ophthalmic solution before inserting contact lenses; contact lenses should not be worn if eye is red
- Do not share ophthalmic drops with others
- Keep bottle tightly closed when not in use
- Treatment should be continued throughout the period of exposure (i.e., until the pollen season is over or until exposure to the offending allergen is terminated), even when symptoms are absent

SIDE EFFECTS

EENT: Ocular irritation, folliculosis, hyperemia, ocular pruritus

MISC: Infection (including cold symptoms and upper respiratory infections), headache, rhinitis, sinusitis, increased cough, pharyngitis

PHARMACOKINETICS

Onset 3-5 min, peak 2 hr, duration 8 hr

NURSING CONSIDERATIONS

Assess:

- Eyes: for itching, redness, use of soft or hard contact lenses

Evaluate:

- Therapeutic response: absence of redness, itching in the eyes

Teach patient/family:

Ophthalmic route

- Product is for topical ophthalmic use only
- Wash hands before and after use; tilt the head back slightly and pull the lower eyelid down with the index finger; squeeze the prescribed number of drops into the conjunctival sac and gently close eyes for 1-2 min; do not blink
- Do not touch the tip of the dropper to the eye, fingertips, or other surface
- Wait ≥10 min after instilling the ophthalmic solution before inserting contact lenses; contact lenses should not be worn if eye is red
- Keep bottle tightly closed when not in use
- Do not share ophthalmic drops with others
- Remove contact lenses before use because the preservative benzalkonium chloride may be absorbed by soft contact lenses; product should not be used to treat contact lens–related irritation

⚠ HIGH ALERT

EPINEPHrine (Rx)

(ep-i-nef′rin)

Adrenaclick, Primatene Mist, Twinject, Walgreens Bronchial Mist

EPINEPHrine HCL

Adrenalin, EpiPen, EpiPen Jr.

Func. class.: Bronchodilator nonselective adrenergic agonist, vasopressor

Chem. class.: Catecholamine

Do not confuse:

EPINEPHrine/ePHEDrine

ACTION:
β_1- and β_2-agonist causing increased levels of cAMP, thereby producing bronchodilation, cardiac, and CNS stimulation; high doses cause vasoconstriction via α-receptors; low doses can cause vasodilation via β_2-vascular receptors

USES:
Acute asthmatic attacks, hemostasis, bronchospasm, anaphylaxis, allergic reactions, cardiac arrest, adjunct in anesthesia, shock

Unlabeled uses: Bradycardia, chloroquine overdose

CONTRAINDICATIONS:
Hypersensitivity to sympathomimetics, sulfites, closed-angle glaucoma, nonanaphylactic shock during general anesthesia

Precautions: Pregnancy (C), breastfeeding, cardiac disorders, hyperthyroidism, diabetes mellitus, prostatic hypertrophy, hypertension, organic brain syndrome, local anesthesia of certain areas, labor, cardiac dilation, coronary insufficiency, cerebral arteriosclerosis, organic heart disease

DOSAGE AND ROUTES

Anaphylaxis/severe asthma exacerbation

- **Adult: IM/SUBCUT** 0.3-0.5 mg, may repeat q10-15min (anaphylaxis) or q20min-4 hr (asthma)

Severe allergic reactions type I

- **Adult/child ≥30 kg: IM** 0.3 mg (EpiPen/EpiPen 2-Pak, 1:1000)
- **Child <30 kg: IM** 0.15 mg (EpiPen Jr/EpiPen Jr 2-Pak 1:2000)
- **Adult/child ≥66 lb: IM/SUBCUT** 0.3 mg (0.3 ml) initially (Twinject 1.1 ml 1:1000, 1 mg/ml, containing 2 doses of 0.3 mg)
- **Adult/child 33-66 lb: IM/SUBCUT** 0.15 mg (0.15 ml) initially, may give another 0.15 mg after 10 min (Twinject 1.1 ml 1:1000 [1 mg/ml] containing 2 doses of 0.15 mg)

Status asthmaticus

- **Adult/adolescent: SUBCUT** 0.3-0.5 mg (0.3-0.5 ml of the 1:1000 injection) q20min × 3 doses
- **Infant/child: SUBCUT** 0.01 mg/kg-0.5 mg q20min × 3 doses

Available forms: Nasal spray (sol) 1 mg/ml; sol for inj 1 mg/ml, 1:10,000, 1:1000; inh vapor (sol) 0.22 mg/actuation; pressurized inh (sol) 0.22 mg/actuation; sol for inj 0.15 mg/0.15 ml autoinjector, 0.3 mg/0.3 ml autoinjector, 0.15 mg/0.3 ml

Administer:

- Increased dose of insulin for diabetic patients if glucose is elevated
- Check for correct concentrations, route, dosage before administering
- Give subcut, IM, intraosseously, IV; suspensions are for subcut use only; do not give IV
- Visually inspect parenteral products for particulate matter and discoloration before use; do not use sols that are pinkish to brownish or that contain a precipitate
- Avoid extravasation during parenteral administration; if extravasation occurs, infiltrate the affected area with phentolamine diluted in NS
- Death has occurred from drug errors, make sure the right concentration is used
- Store reconstituted sol refrigerated ≤24 hr

Inhalation route

- Place in nebulizer (10 drops of a 1% base sol)
- Dilute racepinephrine 2.25% sol

IM route

- EPINEPHrine injection should preferably be into the deltoid or anterior thigh (vastus lateralis); do not administer into the gluteal muscle
- Twinject is light sensitive and should be stored in the carrying case provided; do not refrigerate; protect from freezing; replace if solution is discolored or contains a precipitate

SUBCUT route

- Inject, taking care not to inject intradermally; massage injection site well after use to enhance absorption and to decrease local vasoconstriction; injection can cause tissue irritation

Intraosseous INFUSION route (unlabeled)

- During CPR, the same EPINEPHrine dosage may be given via the intraosseous route when IV access is not available

Intracardiac route

- Intracardiac route should be reserved for extreme emergencies; intracardiac injection should only be performed by properly trained medical personnel

Endotracheal route

- Per the ACLS or PALS guidelines, the EPINEPHrine parenteral product is administered via endotracheal (ET) route;

ET administration should only be used if access to IV or intraosseous routes is not possible

- **Adult:** Dilute dose in 5-10 ml of NS or sterile distilled water; administer via ET tube; endotracheal absorption of EPINEPHrine may be improved by diluting with water instead of NS
- **Child:** after dose administration, flush the ET tube with a minimum of 5 ml NS

Direct IV INJ route

- Inject EPINEPHrine directly into a vein over 5-10 min for adults or 1-3 min for children; may be given IV push in cardiac arrest
- In neonates, may administer via the umbilical vein
- **During adult cardiopulmonary resuscitation (CPR):** Resuscitation drugs may be given IV by bolus injection into a peripheral vein, followed by an injection of 20 ml IV fluid; elevate the extremity for 10-20 sec to facilitate drug delivery to the central circulation

Continuous IV INFUSION route

- Dilute 1 mg EPINEPHrine in 250 or 500 ml of a compatible IV infusion sol to provide a concentration of 4 or 2 mcg/ml, respectively; give into a large vein, if possible; more-concentrated sols (16-32 mcg/ml) may be used in fluid-restricted patients when administered through a central line

Y-site compatibilities: Alfentanil, amikacin, amiodarone, amphotericin B liposome, anidulafungin, ascorbic acid, atracurium, atropine, aztreonam, benztropine, bivalirudin, bleomycin, bumetanide, buprenorphine, butorphanol, calcium chloride/gluconate, CARBOplatin, caspofungin, ceFAZolin, cefotaxime, cefoTEtan, cefOXitin, cefTAZidime, ceftizoxime, cefTRIAXone, cefuroxime, chloramphenicol, chlorproMAZINE, cimetidine, cisatracurium, CISplatin, clindamycin, cyanocobalamin, cyclophosphamide, cycloSPORINE, cytarabine, DACTINomycin, DAPTOmycin, dexamethasone, dexmedetomidine, digoxin, diltiazem, diphenhydrAMINE, DOBUTamine, DOCEtaxel, DOPamine, DOXOrubicin, doxycycline, enalaprilat, epirubicin, epoetin alfa, ertapenem, erythromycin, esmolol, etoposide, etoposide phosphate, famotidine, fenoldopam, fentaNYL, fluconazole, fludarabine, folic acid, furosemide, gemcitabine, gentamicin, glycopyrrolate, granisetron, heparin, hydrocortisone, HYDROmorphone, ifosfamide, imipenem-cilastatin, isoproterenol, ketorolac, labetalol, levofloxacin, lidocaine, linezolid, LORazepam, magnesium sulfate, mannitol, mechlorethamine, meperidine, metaraminol, methicillin, methotrexate, methoxamine, methyldopa, methylPREDNISolone, metoclopramide, metoprolol, metroNIDAZOLE, midazolam, milrinone, minocycline, mitoXANtrone, morphine, multiple vitamins, nafcillin, nalbuphine, naloxone, niCARdipine, nitroglycerin, nitroprusside, norepinephrine, octreotide, ondansetron, oxacillin, oxaliplatin, oxytocin, PACLitaxel, palonosetron, pancuronium, pantoprazole, PEMEtrexed, penicillin G potassium, pentamidine, pentazocine, phentolamine, phenylephrine, phytonadione, piperacillin/tazobactam, potassium chloride, procainamide, prochlorperazine, promethazine, propofol, propranolol, protamine, pyridoxime, quinupristin/dalfopristin, ranitidine, remifentanil, ritodrine, rocuronium, sodium acetate, streptomycin, succinylcholine, SUFentanil, tacrolimus, teniposide, theophylline, thiamine, thiotepa, ticarcillin/clavulanate, tigecycline, tirofiban, tobramycin, tolazoline, trimethaphan, urokinase, vancomycin, vasopressin, vecuronium, verapamil, vinCRIStine, vinorelbine, vitamin B complex with C, voriconazole, warfarin, zoledronic acid

SIDE EFFECTS

CNS: *Tremors, anxiety,* insomnia, headache, *dizziness,* confusion, hallucinations, **cerebral hemorrhage**, weakness, drowsiness

CV: *Palpitations, tachycardia,* hypertension, **dysrhythmias, increased T wave**

GI: *Anorexia, nausea, vomiting*

MISC: Sweating, dry eyes

RESP: *Dyspnea,* **paradoxical bronchospasm (inhalation)**

META: Hypoglycemia

PHARMACOKINETICS

Crosses placenta, metabolized in liver
IM: Onset variable, duration 1-4 hr
SUBCUT: Onset 5-15 min, duration 20 min-4 hr
INH: Onset 1-5 min, duration 1-3 hr

INTERACTIONS

- Do not use with MAOIs or tricyclics; hypertensive crisis may occur
- Toxicity: other sympathomimetics

Decrease: hypertensive effects—β-adrenergic blockers, stop β-blocker 3 days before starting product
Increase: hypotension—α-blockers
Increase: cardiac effects—antihistamines, thyroid replacement hormones
Increase: dysrhythmias—cardiac glycosides
Drug/Herb
- Increased stimulation: coffee, tea, guarana, yerba maté

NURSING CONSIDERATIONS

Assess:
- **Asthma:** auscultate lungs, pulse, B/P, respirations, sputum (color, character); monitor pulmonary function studies before and during treatment
- **Vasopressor: ECG** during administration continuously; if B/P increases, decrease dose; B/P, pulse q5min after parenteral route; CVP, ISVR, PCWP during infusion if possible; inadvertent high arterial B/P can result in angina, aortic rupture, cerebral hemorrhage
- Inj site: tissue sloughing; administer phentolamine with NS
- **Sulfite sensitivity;** may be life-threatening
- Cardiac status, I&O; blood glucose in diabetes
- **Allergic reactions, bronchospasms (swelling of face/lips/eyelids, rash, difficulty breathing):** withhold dose, notify prescriber

Evaluate:
- Therapeutic response: increased B/P with stabilization or ease of breathing

Teach patient/family:
- About the reason for product administration; how to administer
- To rinse mouth after use to prevent dryness after inhalation
- Not to take OTC preparations

TREATMENT OF OVERDOSE:

Administer α-blocker and β-blocker

EPINEPHrine nasal agent

See Appendix B

HIGH ALERT

epirubicin (Rx)

(ep-ih-roo′bi-sin)
Ellence, Pharmorubicin ♣
Func. class.: Antineoplastic, antibiotic
Chem. class.: Anthracycline

Do not confuse:
DOXOrubicin DAUNOrubicin, eribulin, IDArubicin
epirubicin/eribulin

ACTION: Inhibits DNA synthesis primarily; replication is decreased by binding to DNA, which causes strand splitting; maximum cytotoxic effects at S and for G_2 phases; a vesicant

USES: Adjuvant therapy for breast cancer with axillary node involvement after resection
Unlabeled uses: Used in combination for treatment of advanced forms of cancer: bladder, gastric, head and neck, hepatocellular, lung, ovarian, multiple myeloma, soft-tissue sarcoma

CONTRAINDICATIONS: Pregnancy (D), breastfeeding; hypersensitivity to product, anthracyclines, anthracenediones; baseline neutrophil count <1500 cell/mm³, severe myocardial insufficiency, recent MI, heart failure, cardiomyopathy

Black Box Warning: Severe hepatic disease, IM/SUBCUT use

Precautions: Children, geriatric patients, cardiac/renal/hepatic disease, accidental exposure, angina, dental disease, herpes, hyperkalemia, hyperphosphatemia, hypertension, hyperuricemia, hypocalcemia, infection, infertility, tumor lysis syndrome, ventricular dysfunction, previous anthracycline use

Black Box Warning: Bone marrow depression (severe), heart failure, extravasation, secondary malignancy, requires an experienced clinician

DOSAGE AND ROUTES

Breast cancer with axillary node involvement following resection of the primary tumor in combination with cyclophosphamide and fluorouracil

• **Adult: IV** 100 mg/m² on day 1 with fluorouracil and cyclophosphamide (FEC regimen) every 21 days × 6 cycles or 60 mg/m² on days 1 and 8 with oral cyclophosphamide and fluorouracil every 28 days × 6 cycles

Breast cancer in combination with cyclophosphamide

• **Adult: IV** 60 mg/m² day 1 with cyclophosphamide (500 mg/m² IV day 1), repeated every 21 days × 8 cycles or a higher-dose regimen of epirubicin 100 mg/m² IV day 1 with cyclophosphamide (830 mg/m² IV day 1), every 21 days × 8 cycles

Dosage adjustments based upon hematologic and non-hematologic toxicities

• **Nadir platelet counts <50,000/mm³, absolute neutrophil counts (ANC) <250/mm³, neutropenic fever, or grades 3/4 non-hematologic toxicities:** day 1 dose in subsequent cycles should be reduced by 25% of the previous dose

• **For patients receiving divided-dose epirubicin (i.e., days 1 and 8):** Day 8 dose should be reduced by 25% of the day 1 dose if the platelet counts are 75,000-100,000/mm³ and the ANC is 1000-1499/mm³; if day 8 platelet counts are <75,000/mm³, ANC <1000/mm³, or Grade 3/4 non-hematologic toxicity has occurred, omit the day 8 dose

Hepatic dose

• **Adult: IV** Bilirubin 1.2-3 mg/dl or AST 2-4× normal upper limit, 50% of starting dose; bilirubin >3-5 mg/dl or AST >4 × normal upper limit, 25% of starting dose

Available forms: Inj (2 mg/ml) 10 mg/5 ml, 50 mg/25 ml, 150 mg/75 ml, 200 mg/100 ml

Administer:

• Antiemetic 30-60 min before product to prevent vomiting

Black Box Warning: To be used by a clinician experienced in giving cytotoxic products

Black Box Warning: Do not use IM/SUBCUT because of severe tissue necrosis, give IV, only, subcut; a vesicant; if extravasation occurs stop and complete via another vein, preferably in another limb; avoid infusion into veins over joints or in extremities with compromised venous or lymphatic drainage

• Rapid injection can cause facial flushing or erythema along the vein; avoid administration time of <3 min

• Product should be given to those with neutrophils ≥1500/mm³, platelet count ≥100,000/mm³, and nonhematologic toxicities recovered to ≤grade 1

• When refrigerated, the preservative-free, ready-to-use solution can form a gelled product and will return to solution after 2-4 hr at room temperature

• Visually inspect for particulate matter and discoloration before use

IV route

• Use cytotoxic handling procedures; pregnant women must not handle product

• Reconstitute 50 mg and 200 mg powder for injection vials with 25 ml and 100 ml, respectively, of sterile water for injection (2 mg/ml), shake vigorously for up to 4 min; reconstituted sols are stable for 24 hr when stored refrigerated and protected from light or at room temperature in normal light

- Solution can be further diluted with sterile water for injection

IV INJ route

- Give doses of 100-120 mg/m^2 into tubing of a freely flowing 0.9% sodium chloride (NS) or D_5W IV infusion over 15-20 min; the infusion time may be decreased, proportionally, in those who require lower doses; infusion times <3 min are not recommended
- Direct injection into the vein is not recommended because of the risk of extravasation; avoid use with any solution of alkaline pH because hydrolysis will occur

IV INFUSION route

- Dilute dose in 0.9% sodium chloride (NS) or D_5W, infuse over 30-60 min, avoid use with any solution of alkaline pH because hydrolysis will occur

Y-site compatibilities: Alemtuzumab, alfentanil, amifostine, amikacin, aminocaproic acid, anidulafungin, argatroban, atracurium, aztreonam, bivalirudin, bleomycin, bumetanide, buprenorphine, butorphanol, calcium chloride/gluconate, CARBOplatin, caspofungin, ceFAZolin, cefotaxime, ceftizoxime, chlorproMAZINE, cimetidine, ciprofloxacin, cisatracurium, CISplatin, clindamycin, cyclophosphamide, cycloSPORINE, DAPTOmycin, dexrazoxane, digoxin, diltiazem, diphenhydrAMINE, DOBUTamine, DOCEtaxel, dolasetron, DOPamine, doxacurium, doxycycline, droperidol, enalaprilat, ePHEDrine, EPINEPHrine, ertapenem, erythromycin, etoposide, famotidine, fenoldopam, fentaNYL, fluconazole, gatifloxacin, gemcitabine, gentamicin, granisetron, haloperidol, hydrocortisone, HYDROmorphone, hydrOXYzine, ifosfamide, imipenem-cilastatin, inamrinone, insulin (regular), isoproterenol, labetalol, levofloxacin, levorphanol, lidocaine, linezolid, LORazepam, mannitol, meperidine, mesna, methotrexate, metoclopramide, metoprolol, metroNIDAZOLE, midazolam, milrinone, minocycline, mitoMYcin, mivacurium, morphine, moxifloxacin, nalbuphine, naloxone, nesiritide, niCARdipine, nitroglycerin, nitroprusside, norepinephrine, octreotide, ofloxacin, ondansetron, oxaliplatin, PACLitaxel, palonosetron, pamidronate, pancuronium, pentamidine, pentazocine, phenylephrine, potassium chloride, procainamide, prochlorperazine, promethazine, propranolol, quinupristin-dalfopristin, ranitidine, remifentanil, rocuronium, sodium acetate, succinylcholine, SUFentanil, tacrolimus, teniposide, theophylline, thiotepa, tigecycline, tirofiban, tobramycin, trimethobenzamide, vancomycin, vasopressin, vecuronium, verapamil, vinBLAStine, vinCRIStine, vinorelbine, voriconazole, zidovudine, zoledronic acid

SIDE EFFECTS

CV: Increased B/P, sinus tachycardia, PVCs, chest pain, bradycardia, extrasystoles, cardiomyopathy

GI: *Nausea, vomiting, anorexia, mucositis, diarrhea*

GU: *Amenorrhea, hot flashes, hyperuricemia, red urine*

HEMA: Thrombocytopenia, leukopenia, anemia, neutropenia, secondary AML

INTEG: *Rash,* necrosis, *pain at inj site, reversible alopecia*

MISC: *Infection, febrile neutropenia, lethargy, fever, conjunctivitis,* tumor lysis syndrome

PHARMACOKINETICS

Triphasic pattern of elimination; half-life 3 min, 1 hr, 30 hr; metabolized by liver; crosses placenta; excreted in urine, bile, breast milk

INTERACTIONS

- Give epirubicin before PACLitaxel if both are given

Increase: toxicity—other antineoplastics or radiation, cimetidine

Increase: ventricular dysfunction, CHF—trastuzumab

Increased: heart failure—calcium channel blockers

Decrease: antibody response—live virus vaccine

NURSING CONSIDERATIONS

Assess:

Black Box Warning: Bone marrow depression (severe): CBC, differential, platelet count weekly; withhold product if baseline neutrophil ≤1500/mm³; leukocyte nadir occurs 10-14 days after administration, recovery by day 21; notify prescriber of results

- **Infection:** treat before receiving this product if regimens >120 mg/m², prophylactic antibiotics should be given (trimethaprin-sulfamethoxazole or a quinolone)
- Blood, urine uric acid levels; swelling, joint pain primarily in extremities; patient should be well hydrated to prevent urate deposits
- Renal disease: BUN, serum uric acid, urine CCr, electrolytes before, during therapy; I&O ratio; report fall in urine output to <30 ml/hr; dosage adjustment needed if serum creatinine >5 mg/dl
- Increased fluid intake to 2-3 L/day to prevent urate, calculi formation

Black Box Warning: Hepatic studies before, during therapy: bilirubin, AST, ALT, alk phos as needed or monthly

Black Box Warning: Heart failure: B/P, pulse, character, rhythm, rate, ABGs, ECG, LVEF, MUGA scan, or ECHO; watch for ST-T wave changes, low QRS and T, possible dysrhythmias (sinus tachycardia, heart block, PVCs); identify cumulative amount of anthracycline received (lifetime)

- Bleeding: hematuria, guaiac, bruising, or petechiae, mucosa or orifices q8hr
- Effects of alopecia on body image; discuss feelings about body changes

Black Box Warning: Extravasation (vesicant): local irritation, pain, burning, necrosis at inj site, discontinue and start at another site

- GI symptoms: frequency of stools, cramping

Evaluate:

- Therapeutic response: decreased tumor size, spread of malignancy

Teach patient/family:

- That hair may be lost during treatment; that wig or hairpiece may make patient feel better; that new hair may be different in color, texture; new hair growth occurs in ≤3 mo after treatment
- To avoid crowds, persons with infections when granulocyte count is low
- That contraceptive measures recommended during therapy and for 4 mo thereafter for men and women; pregnancy (D)
- To avoid vaccinations because reactions may occur; to avoid cimetidine during therapy
- That urine may appear red for 2 days
- To avoid OTC medications, supplements unless approved by prescriber

Black Box Warning: That irreversible myocardial damage, leukopenia, menopause may occur

- To report rapid heartbeat, trouble breathing, fever, nausea, vomiting, oral sores
- To report pain at site immediately

eplerenone (Rx)

(ep-ler-ee′known)

Inspra

Func. class.: Antihypertensive

Chem. class.: Selective aldosterone receptor antagonist

Do not confuse:
Inspra, Spiriva

ACTION: Binds to mineralocorticoid receptor and blocks the binding of aldosterone, a component of the renin-angiotensin-aldosterone system (RAAS)

USES: Hypertension, alone or in combination with thiazide diuretics, CHF, post-MI

CONTRAINDICATIONS:
Hypersensitivity; increased serum creatinine >2 mg/dl (male), >1.8 mg/dl (female); potassium >5.5 mEq/L, type 2 diabetes with microalbuminuria, hepatic disease, CCr <30 ml/min; CCr <50 ml/min in hypertension

Precautions: Pregnancy (B), breastfeeding, children, geriatric patients, impaired renal/hepatic function, hyperkalemia

DOSAGE AND ROUTES

Hypertension

- **Adult: PO** 50 mg/day initially, may increase to 50 mg bid after 4 wk; start dose at 25 mg/day if patient is taking CYP3A4 inhibitors

CHF or post-MI

- **Adult: PO** 25 mg/day initially, may increase to 50 mg/day max after 4 wk

Available forms: Tabs 25, 50 mg

Administer:

- Without regard to food
- Do not use salt substitutes containing potassium
- Store in tight container at ≤86° F (30° C)

SIDE EFFECTS

CNS: Headache, *dizziness, fatigue*

CV: Angina, MI

GI: Increased GGT *diarrhea,* abdominal pain, increased ALT

GU: Gynecomastia, mastodynia (males), abnormal vaginal bleeding

META: *Hyperkalemia,* hyponatremia, hypercholesteremia, hypertriglyceridemia, increased uric acid

RESP: *Cough*

PHARMACOKINETICS

Peak 1½ hr; serum protein binding 50%; half-life 4-6 hr; metabolized in liver by CYP3A4; excreted in urine, feces

INTERACTIONS

Increase: hyperkalemia—ACE inhibitors, angiotensin II antagonists, NSAIDs, potassium supplements, potassium-sparing diuretics

Increase: serum levels of lithium

Increase: eplerenone levels—erythromycin, fluconazole, verapamil; reduce dose of eplerenone

Increase: levels of eplerenone—CYP3A4 inhibitors (ketoconazole, itraconazole, saquinavir, clarithromycin, imatinib, nelfinavir, nefazodone, ritonavir, troleandomycin; do not use concurrently); reduce dose of eplerenone

Decrease: antihypertensive effect—NSAIDs

Drug/Herb

Decrease: antihypertensive effect—ephedra

Drug/Food

- Grapefruit, grapefruit juice increase product level by 25%
- Do not use salt substitutes containing potassium

Drug/Lab Test

Increase: BUN, creatinine, potassium, cholesterol, lipids, uric acid

Decrease: sodium

NURSING CONSIDERATIONS

Assess:

- **Hypertension:** B/P at peak/trough level of product, orthostatic hypotension, syncope when used with diuretic; monitor lithium level in those also taking lithium
- **Renal studies:** protein, BUN, creatinine; increased LFTs, uric acid may be increased
- Potassium levels, hyperkalemia may occur

Evaluate:

- Therapeutic response: decreased B/P

Teach patient/family:

- Not to discontinue product abruptly
- Not to use OTC products (cough, cold, allergy) unless directed by prescriber; not to use salt substitutes containing potassium without consulting prescriber
- To comply with dosage schedule, even if feeling better

• That product may cause dizziness, fainting, light-headedness; may occur during first few days of therapy
• How to take B/P; and about normal readings for age group
• Avoid activities that require coordination

⚠ HIGH ALERT

epoetin alfa (Rx)

(ee-poe′e-tin)

Epogen, Eprex ✦, Procrit

Func. class.: Antianemic, biologic modifier, hormone

Chem. class.: Amino acid polypeptide

ACTION: Erythropoietin is a factor controlling the rate of red cell production; product is developed by recombinant DNA technology

USES: Anemia caused by reduced endogenous erythropoietin production, primarily end-stage renal disease; to correct hemostatic defect in uremia; anemia due to AZT treatment in patients with HIV or those receiving chemotherapy; reduction of allogenic blood transfusion in surgery patients

Unlabeled uses: Anemia in premature preterm infants, anemia due to ribavirin and interferon-alfa therapy in hepatitic C

CONTRAINDICATIONS: Hypersensitivity to mammalian-cell–derived products, human albumin; uncontrolled hypertension

Precautions: Pregnancy (C), breastfeeding, children <1 mo, seizure disorder; multidose preserved formulation contains benzyl alcohol and should not be used in premature infants; porphyria, CV disease, hemodialysis, latex allergy, hypertension, history of CABG

Black Box Warning: Hgb >11 g/dl, surgery, neoplastic disease

DOSAGE AND ROUTES

Anemia (chronic kidney disease including dialysis-dependent and dialysis-independent patients to decrease the need for red blood cell transfusion)

• **Adult/adolescent ≥17 yr: SUBCUT/IV** Initially, 50–100 units/kg 3×/wk; for patients on dialysis, administer IV; for patients on dialysis, initiate treatment when hemoglobin (Hgb) is <10 g/dl; if Hgb approaches or exceeds 11 g/dl, reduce or interrupt the dose; for patients not on dialysis, consider initiating treatment only when Hgb is <10 g/dl and the rate of Hgb decline indicates the likelihood of requiring RBC transfusion and reducing the risk of alloimmunization and/or other RBC transfusion–related risks is a goal; if Hgb is >10 g/dl, reduce or interrupt the dose, and use the lowest dose sufficient to reduce the need for RBC transfusions; if the Hgb rises >1 g/dl in any 2-wk period, reduce dose by 25% or more as needed to reduce rapid responses; in contrast, if Hgb has not increased >1 g/dl after 4 wk of therapy, increase the dose by 25%; for patients who do not respond adequately over a 12-wk escalation period, increasing the dose further is unlikely to improve response and can increase risks; use the lowest dose that will maintain a Hgb concentration sufficient to reduce the need for RBC transfusions; evaluate other causes of anemia, and discontinue if responsiveness does not improve

• **Infant/child/adolescent ≤16 yr: SUBCUT/IV** 50 units/kg 3×/wk initially; for dosage adjustments, see adult dosage

Zidovudine-induced anemia in HIV-infected patients with circulating endogenous erythropoietin concentrations ≤500 mUnits/ml who are receiving a dose of zidovudine ≤4200 mg/wk

• **Adult: SUBCUT/IV** Initially, 100 units/kg 3×/wk; if Hgb does not increase after 8 wk, increase by 50-100 units/kg at 4-8-wk intervals until Hgb is at a concentration to avoid RBC transfusions or a dose of 300 units/kg is reached; if the Hgb is >12 g/dl, withhold, once Hgb is <11 g/dl resume at a dose 25% below the previous dose

Anemia (non-myeloid malignancies when anemia is due to the effect of concomitantly administered chemotherapy and at least 2 additional mo of chemotherapy is planned)

• **Adult: SUBCUT** 150 units/kg 3×/wk or 40,000 units 1×/wk only when the hemoglobin is <10 g/dl and only until the chemotherapy course is completed; adjust the dosage to maintain the lowest Hgb concentration rise of <1-2 g/dl sufficient to avoid RBC transfusions; if no rise in Hgb ≥1 g/dl after 4 wk of therapy and Hgb is <10 g/dl, the dosage may be increased to 300 units/kg subcut 3×/wk or 60,000 units 1×/wk; discontinue if after 8 wk of therapy there is no response as measured by Hgb concentrations or if transfusions are still required; reduce the dosage by approximately 25% if Hgb increases by >1 g/dl in any 2-wk period or if Hgb reaches a concentration needed to avoid RBC infusion; if Hgb is increasing and exceeds a concentration necessary to avoid blood transfusions, hold therapy and reinstitute at a dose that is 25% lower when the Hgb reaches a concentration where transfusions may be needed

• **Adolescent/child ≥5 yr: IV** 600 units/kg/wk only when the hemoglobin is <10 g/dl and only until the chemotherapy course is completed; adjust the dosage to maintain the lowest Hgb concentrations sufficient to avoid RBC transfusions; if no rise in Hgb ≥1 g/dl after 4 wk of therapy and Hgb is <10 g/dl, the dosage may be increased to 900 units/kg (up to 60,000 units)/wk IV; discontinue if after 8 wk there is no response as measured by Hgb concentrations or if transfusions are still required; reduce the dosage by approximately 25% if Hgb increases by more than 1 g/dl in any 2-wk period or if Hgb reaches a concentration needed to avoid RBC infusion; if the Hgb is increasing and exceeds a concentration necessary to avoid blood transfusions, hold therapy and reinstitute at a dose that is 25% lower when the Hgb reaches a concentration where transfusions may be needed

To reduce the need for allogenic blood transfusions in anemic patients (hemoglobin >10 and ≤13 g/dl) scheduled to undergo elective, noncardiac, nonvascular surgery

• **Adult: SUBCUT** 300 units/kg/day × 10 days before surgery, on the day of surgery, and for 4 days after surgery (15 days total) or 600 units/kg 1×/wk, 21, 14, and 7 days before surgery plus 1 dose on the day of surgery

Available forms: Inj 2000, 3000, 4000, 10,000, 20,000, 40,000 units/ml

Administer:

• Do not shake vial

• Use 1 single-use vial/dose, once syringe has entered single-dose vial, sterility cannot be guaranteed, do not administer with other product, multidose vials can be stored in refrigerator up to 21 days once opened, do not use if discolored or particulates are present

SUBCUT route

• Before injecting preservative-free, single-dose formulation may be admixed using 0.9% NaCl with benzyl alcohol 0.9% at a 1:1 ratio to reduce inj-site discomfort, store solution in refrigerator, protect from light

Direct IV route

• Additional heparin to lower chance of clots

• By direct inj or bolus into IV tubing or venous line at end of dialysis

• Decrease dose by 25% if Hgb increases by 1 g/dl in 2 wk; increase dose if Hgb does not increase by 5-6 pts after 8 wk of therapy; suggested target Hgb range 30%-36%

Solution compatibilities: Do not dilute or administer with other sol

SIDE EFFECTS

CNS: Seizures, coldness, sweating, headache, fatigue, dizziness

CV: *Hypertension,* hypertensive encephalopathy, CHF, edema, DVT

INTEG: Pruritus, rash, inj site reaction
MISC: Iron deficiency
MS: Bone pain, arthralgia, myalgia
RESP: Cough

PHARMACOKINETICS

IV: Metabolized in body, extent of metabolism unknown, onset of increased reticulocyte count 2-6 wk, peak immediate; **Subcut:** Peak 5-24 hr

INTERACTIONS

- Need for increased heparin during hemodialysis

NURSING CONSIDERATIONS

Assess:

- Renal studies: urinalysis, protein, blood, BUN, creatinine; I&O, report drop in output <50 ml/hr

Black Box Warning: Blood studies: ferritin, transferrin, serum iron monthly; transferrin sat ≥20%, ferritin ≥100 ng/ml; Hct 2×/wk until stabilized in target range (30%-36%) then at regular intervals; those with endogenous erythropoietin levels of <500 units/L respond to product; monitor Hct 2×/wk with chronic renal failure; patients treated with zidovudine or patients with cancer should be monitored weekly, then periodically after stabilization; death may occur with Hgb >12 g/dl

- B/P; check for rising B/P as Hct rises, antihypertensives may be needed; hypertension may occur rapidly, leading to hypertensive encephalopathy
- CNS symptoms: coldness, sweating, pain in long bones; for seizures if Hct is increased within 2 wk by 4 pts
- Hypersensitivity reactions: skin rashes, urticaria (rare), antibody development does not occur

⚠ **Pure cell aplasia (PRCA)** in absence of other causes; evaluate by testing sera for recombinant erythropoetin antibodies; any loss of response to epoetin should be evaluated

- Dialysis patients: thrill, bruit of shunts; monitor for circulation impairment
- **Seizures:** place patient on seizure precautions if increase of ≥4 points HCT in 2 wk, increased B/P; more common in chronic renal failure during the first 90 days of treatment

Evaluate:

- Therapeutic response: increase in reticulocyte count in 2-6 wk, Hgb/Hct; increased appetite, enhanced sense of well-being

Teach patient/family:

- To avoid driving or hazardous activities during beginning of treatment
- To monitor B/P
- To take iron supplements, vit B_{12}, folic acid as directed

eprosartan (Rx)

(ep-roh-sar′tan)

Teveten

Func. class.: Antihypertensive
Chem. class.: Angiotensin II–receptor antagonist (Subtype AT_1)

ACTION:
Blocks the vasoconstrictive and aldosterone-secreting effects of angiotensin II; selectively blocks the binding of angiotensin II to the AT_1 receptor found in tissues

USES:
Hypertension, alone or with other antihypertensives

CONTRAINDICATIONS:
Hypersensitivity

Black Box Warning: Pregnancy (D)

Precautions: Breastfeeding, children, geriatric patients, hypersensitivity to ACE inhibitors; renal/hepatic disease, angioedema, hyperkalemia

DOSAGE AND ROUTES

- **Adult: PO** 600 mg/day; dose may be divided, given bid, with total daily doses from 400-800 mg, max 900 mg/day

Renal dose
- **Adult: PO** CCr ≤30 ml/min, max 600 mg/day

Available forms: Tabs 600 mg
Administer:
- Without regard to meals

SIDE EFFECTS

CNS: *Dizziness,* depression, *fatigue,* headache
CV: Chest pain, hypotension, palpitations
EENT: Sinusitis
GI: *Diarrhea, dyspepsia, abdominal pain*
GU: UTI
HEMA: Neutropenia
INTEG: Pruritus, angioedema
META: Hypertriglyceridemia
MS: *Myalgia,* arthralgia, rhabdomyolysis
RESP: *Cough, upper respiratory infection,* rhinitis, pharyngitis, viral infection
SYST: Anaphylaxis

PHARMACOKINETICS

Peak 1-2 hr, food delays absorption; protein binding 98%; moderate renal impairment increases product levels by 30%, hepatic impairment increases levels by 40%; excreted in urine and feces; half-life 5-9 hr

INTERACTIONS

Increase: hyperglycemia—antidiabetics
Increase: antihypertensive effect—other antihypertensives
Increase: hyperkalemia—ACE inhibitors, angiotensin II receptor antagonists, potassium-sparing diuretics, potassium supplements
Increase: lithium toxicity—lithium
Decrease: antihypertensive effect—NSAIDs, salicylates

Drug/Herb
Decrease: antihypertensive effect—ephedra
Increase: antihypertensive effect—hawthorn

Drug/Lab Test
Increase: ALT, AST, alk phos, potassium
Decrease: Hgb

NURSING CONSIDERATIONS

Assess:
- B/P with position changes, pulse q4hr; note rate, rhythm, quality
- ⚠ Hypersensitivity reactions, including anaphylaxis
- ⚠ Myalgia, arthralgia; may cause rhabdomyolysis
- Baselines of renal, hepatic studies before therapy begins
- Edema in feet, legs daily, weight
- Skin turgor, dryness of mucous membranes for hydration status

Evaluate:
- Therapeutic response: decreased B/P

Teach patient/family:
- To comply with dosage schedule, even if feeling better
- To notify prescriber of fever; chest pain; swelling of hands, feet, face, lip, or tongue
- That excessive perspiration, dehydration, diarrhea may lead to fall in B/P; consult prescriber if these occur, maintain adequate hydration
- That product may cause dizziness; to avoid hazardous activities until effect is known; to rise slowly from sitting

Black Box Warning: Not to take this product if pregnant or breastfeeding, or if have had an allergic reaction to product

- To take missed dose as soon as possible unless within 1 hr before next dose
- That therapeutic effect may take 2-3 wk

⚠ HIGH ALERT

eptifibatide (Rx)

(ep-tih-fib′ah-tide)

Integrilin

Func. class.: Antiplatelet agent
Chem. class.: Glycoprotein IIb/IIIa inhibitor

ACTION: Platelet glycoprotein antagonist; this agent reversibly prevents fibrinogen, von Willebrand's factor from binding to the glycoprotein IIb/IIIa receptor, thus inhibiting platelet aggregation

USES: Acute coronary syndrome including those undergoing percutaneous coronary intervention (PCI)

CONTRAINDICATIONS: Hypersensitivity, active internal bleeding; recent history of bleeding, stroke within 30 days or any hemorrhagic stroke; major surgery with severe trauma, severe hypertension, current or planned use of another parenteral GP IIb/IIIa inhibitor, dependence on renal dialysis, coagulopathy, AV malformation, aneurysm

Precautions: Pregnancy (B), breastfeeding, children, geriatric patients, bleeding, impaired renal function

DOSAGE AND ROUTES

Acute coronary syndrome

• **Adult: IV BOL** 180 mcg/kg as soon as diagnosed, max 22.6 mg, then **IV CONT** 2 mcg/kg/min or CABG discontinue ≥2-4 hr before procedure

PCI in patients without acute coronary syndrome

• **Adult: IV BOL** 180 mcg/kg given immediately before PCI, then 2 mcg/kg/min × 18 hr CONT IV INFUSION and a second 180-mcg/kg bolus by 10 min after 1st bolus; continue infusion for up to 18-24 hr

Renal dose

• **Adult: IV** maintenance CCr <50 ml/min, 1 mcg/kg/min, max rate 7.5 mg/hr; CCr <10 ml/min, contraindicated

Available forms: Sol for inj 2 mg/ml (10 ml), 0.75 mg/ml (100 ml)

Administer:

• Aspirin may be given with this product; check for bleeding

• D/C heparin before removing femoral artery sheath, after PCI

• Do not give discolored solutions, those with particulates; discard unused amount, protect from light

• Discontinue product before CABG

Direct IV route

• After withdrawing bolus dose from 10-ml vial, give IV push over 1-2 min

Continuous IV INFUSION route

• Follow bolus dose with continuous infusion using pump; give product undiluted directly from 100-ml vial, spike 100-ml vial with vented infusion set, use caution when centering spike on circle of stopper top, refrigerate vials, or may store vials ≤2 mo at room temperature

Y-site compatibilities: Alfentanil, alteplase, amikacin, aminophylline, amphotericin B lipid complex, amphotericin B liposome, ampicillin, ampicillin-sulbactam, anidulafungin, argatroban, atenolol, atracurium, atropine, azithromycin, aztreonam, bivalirudin, bumetanide, buprenorphine, butorphanol, calcium chloride/gluconate, ceFAZolin, cefepime, cefotaxime, cefoTEtan, cefOXitin, cefTAZidime, ceftizoxime, cefTRIAXone, cefuroxime, cimetidine, ciprofloxacin, cisatracurium, clindamycin, cycloSPORINE, DAPTOmycin, dexamethasone, D_5/NaCl 0.9%, diazepam, diltiazem, diphenhydrAMINE, DOBUTamine, dolasetron, DOPamine, doxycycline, droperidol, enalaprilat, ePHEDrine, EPINEPHrine, ertapenem, erythromycin, esmolol, famotidine, fentaNYL, fluconazole, fosphenytoin, ganciclovir, gatifloxacin, gentamicin, granisetron, haloperidol, heparin, hydrocortisone, HYDROmorphone, hydrOXYzine, imipenem-cilastatin, inamrinone, isoproterenol, ketorolac, labetalol, leucovorin, levofloxacin, levorphanol, lidocaine, linezolid, LORazepam, magnesium sulfate, mannitol, meperidine, meropenem, methylPREDNISolone, metoclopramide, metoprolol, metroNIDAZOLE, micafungin, midazolam, milrinone, minocycline, mivacurium, morphine, nalbuphine, naloxone, niCARdipine, nitroglycerin, nitroprusside, NS, octreotide, ofloxacin, ondansetron, oxytocin, palonosetron, pancuronium, PEMEtrexed, PENTobarbital, PHENobarbital, phenylephrine, piperacillin, piperacillin-tazobactam, potassium chloride/phosphates, procainamide, prochlorperazine, promethazine,

propranolol, ranitidine, remifentanil, rocuronium, sodium bicarbonate/phosphates, succinylcholine, SUFentanil, sulfamethoxazole-trimethoprim, teniposide, theophylline, ticarcillin, ticarcillin-clavulanate, tigecycline, tirofiban, tobramycin, trimethobenzamide, vancomycin, vecuronium, verapamil, zidovudine, zoledronic acid
Solution compatibilities: 0.9% NaCl, D_5/0.9% NaCl

SIDE EFFECTS

CV: Stroke, hypotension
GU: Hematuria
HEMA: Thrombocytopenia, platelet dysfunction
SYST: Major/minor bleeding from any site, anaphylaxis

PHARMACOKINETICS

Onset within 1 hr, protein binding 25%, half-life 1.5-2 hr, steady state 4-6 hr, metabolism limited, excretion via kidneys

INTERACTIONS

- Do not give with glycoprotein inhibitors IIb, IIIa

Increase: bleeding—aspirin, heparin, NSAIDs, anticoagulants, ticlopidine, clopidogrel, dipyridamole, thrombolytics, valproate, abciximab, SSRIs, SNRIs
Drug/Herb
Increase: Bleeding risk—feverfew, garlic, ginger, ginkgo, ginseng

NURSING CONSIDERATIONS

Assess:
⚠ **Thrombocytopenia:** platelets, Hgb, Hct, creatinine, APTT baseline within 6 hr of loading dose, daily therafter, patients undergoing PCI should have ACT monitored; maintain APTT 50-70 sec unless PCI to be performed; during PCI, ACT should be 200-300 sec; if platelets drop <100,000/mm³, obtain additional platelet counts; if thrombocytopenia is confirmed, discontinue product; draw Hct, Hgb, serum creatinine
⚠ **Bleeding:** gums, bruising, ecchymosis, petechiae; from GI, GU tract, cardiac cath sites, IM inj sites
Teach patient/family:
- About reason for medication and expected results
- To report bruising, bleeding, chest pain immediately

⚠ HIGH ALERT

eribulin
(er′i-bu′lin)
Halaven
Func. class.: Antineoplastics—non-taxane

Do not confuse:
eribulin/epirubicin/erlotinib

ACTION: Potent antimitotic agent, different from taxanes, vinca alkaloids, epothilones; blocks cell progression during G2-M phase; inhibits the growth phase of microtubules and sequesters tubules, leading to the disruption of mitotic spindles and apoptotic cell death

USES: Metastatic breast cancer in patients who have received at least 2 chemotherapy regimens

CONTRAINDICATIONS: Hypersensitivity, pregnancy (D)
Precautions: Breastfeeding, neonates, infants, children, bradycardia, electrolyte imbalances, heart failure, hypokalemia, hypomagnesemia, infertility, neutropenia, peripheral neuropathy, QT prolongation, hepatic/renal disease

DOSAGE AND ROUTES

- **Adult: IV** 1.4 mg/m² over 2-5 min on days 1 and 8, repeat q21days
- **Recommendations for dose delay:** for ANC <1000/mm³, platelets <75,000/mm³, or grade 3 or 4 nonhematologic toxicities: do not administer; the day 8 dose may be delayed a maximum of 1 wk; for the day 8 dose, if toxicities do not

resolve to ≤ Grade 2 by day 15: omit the dose; for the day 8 dose, if toxicities resolve or improve to ≤ Grade 2 by day 15: administer eribulin at reduced dose (see below), initiate the next cycle no sooner than 2 wk later

• **Dose adjustments for hematologic toxicity:** ANC <500/mm^3 for >7 days or ANC <1000/mm^3 with fever or infection: permanently reduce dose to 1.1 mg/m^2; platelets <25,000/mm^3 or <50,000/mm^3 requiring transfusion: permanently reduce dose to 1.1 mg/m^2; if day 8 of previous cycle omitted or delayed: permanently reduce dose to 1.1 mg/m^2; while receiving 1.1 mg/m^2, if recurrence of hematologic event occurs, or if day 8 of previous cycle omitted or delayed: permanently reduce dose to 0.7 mg/m^2; while receiving 0.7 mg/m^2, if recurrence of hematologic event occurs, or if day 8 of previous cycle omitted or delayed: discontinue

• **Dose adjustments of eribulin for nonhematologic toxicity during treatment:** any Grade 3 or 4 nonhematologic toxicity: permanently reduce dose to 1.1 mg/m^2; if day 8 of previous cycle omitted or delayed: permanently reduce dose to 1.1 mg/m^2; while receiving 1.1 mg/m^2, if recurrence of Grade 3 or 4 nonhematologic toxicity occurs, or if day 8 of previous cycle omitted or delayed: permanently reduce dose to 0.7 mg/m^2; while receiving 0.7 mg/m^2, if recurrence of Grade 3 or 4 nonhematologic toxicity occurs, or if day 8 of previous cycle omitted or delayed: discontinue

Available forms: Sol for inj 1 mg/2 ml

Administer:

IV direct, intermittent route

• Visually inspect for particulate matter, discoloration as solution and container permit; withdraw required amount (0.5 mg/ml) from single-use vial, give undiluted over 2-5 min or diluted in 100 ml 0.9% NaCl and give as intermittent infusion; do not give through line with dextrose or any other product

• Store at room temperature for 4 hr or 24 hr refrigerated

SIDE EFFECTS

CNS: Depression, dizziness, *fatigue*, fever, headache, insomnia, *peripheral neuropathy*

CV: QT prolongation, peripheral edema

GI: Abdominal pain, anorexia, constipation, diarrhea, dyspepsia, nausea, vomiting, weight loss

HEMA: Anemia, neutropenia, thrombocytopenia

INTEG: *Alopecia*, rash, stomatitis, infusion-related reactions

META: Hypokalemia

MS: Arthralgia, myalgia, bone/back pain

RESP: Cough, dyspnea

SYST: Infection

PHARMACOKINETICS

Protein binding 49%-65%; inhibits CYP3A4; excreted in feces 82%; urine 9%; elimination half-life 40 hr; increased levels in hepatic/renal disease

INTERACTIONS

Increase: QT prolongation—arsenic trioxide, bepridil, chloroquine, certain phenothiazines (chlorproMAZINE, mesoridazine, thioridazine), clarithromycin, class IA antiarrhythmics (disopyramide, procainamide, quiNIDine), class III antiarrhythmics (amiodarone, bretylium, dofetilide, ibutilide, sotalol), dextromethorphan; quiNIDine, dronedarone, droperidol, erythromycin, halofantrine, haloperidol, levomethadyl, methadone, pentamidine, pimozide, posaconazole, probucol, propafenone, saquinavir, sparfloxacin, troleandomycin, and ziprasidone; also to a lesser degree abarelix, alfuzosin, amoxapine, apomorphine, artemether; lumefantrine, asenapine, β-agonists, ofloxacin, cloZAPine, cyclobenzaprine, dasatinib, dolasetron, flecainide, gatifloxacin, gemifloxacin, halogenated anesthetics, iloperidone, lapatinib, levofloxacin, local anesthetics, lopinavir; ritonavir, magnesium sulfate; potassium sulfate; sodium sulfate, maprotiline, mefloquine, moxifloxacin, nilotinib, norfloxacin, octreotide, ciprofloxacin, OLANZapine, ondansetron, paliperidone, palonosetron, some phenothiazines (fluPHENAZine, perphenazine, prochlorperazine, trifluoperazine), QUEtiapine, ranolazine, risperiDONE, sertindole, SUNItinib, tacrolimus, telavancin, telithromycin, tetrabenazine, tricyclic antidepressants, venlafaxine, vardenafil, vorinostat

NURSING CONSIDERATIONS

Assess:

- Peripheral neuropathy: pain, numbness in extremities
- Infection: increased temperature, sore throat, flulike symptoms
- **QT prolongation:** assess for drug interactions that may occur; monitor ECG, heart rate
- **Bone marrow depression:** CBC, differential, serum creatinine, BUN, electrolytes, LFTs at baseline, periodically; increased AST/ALT >3 × ULN or total bilirubin >1.5 × ULN involve greater chance of Grade 4 or febrile neutropenia

Teach patient/family:

- **Infection:** to notify prescriber of increased temperature, sore throat, fatigue, flulike symptoms
- **QT prolongation:** to report extra heartbeats
- **Peripheral neuropathy:** to report tingling, pain in extremities
- About reason for product and expected results
- To avoid other medications, supplements unless approved by provider; serious drug interactions may occur
- About hair loss, use of wig or hairpiece
- To notify prescriber if pregnancy is planned or suspected (pregnancy [D]), to avoid breastfeeding

⚠ HIGH ALERT

erlotinib (Rx)

(er-loe′tye-nib)

Tarceva

Func. class.: Antineoplastic—miscellaneous

Chem. class.: Epidermal growth factor receptor inhibitor

ACTION: Not fully understood; inhibits intracellular phosphorylation of cell-surface receptors associated with epidermal growth factor receptors

USES: Non–small-cell lung cancer (NSCLC) including EGFR ex on 19 deletions or ex on 21 substitution mutations, pancreatic cancer

CONTRAINDICATIONS: Pregnancy (D), breastfeeding

Precautions: Children, geriatric patients, ocular/pulmonary/renal/hepatic disorders, diverticulitis

DOSAGE AND ROUTES

Non–small-cell lung cancer (NSCLC)

- **Adult: PO** 150 mg/day

Pancreatic cancer

- **Adult: PO** 100 mg/day in combination with gemcitabine 1000 mg/m^2 cycle 1, days 1, 8, 15, 22, 29, 36, 43 of 8-wk cycle; cycle 2 and subsequent cycle, days 1, 8, 15 of 4-wk cycle

CYP3A4 inducers concurrently (rifampin, phenytoin)

- Dosage increase is advised

CYP3A4 inhibitors (atazanavir, clarithromycin, indinavir, itraconazole, ketoconazole, telithromycin, ritonavir, saquinavir, troleandomycin, nelfinavir)

- Dosage reduction may be needed

Hepatic dose

- **Adult: PO** interrupt if total bilirubin >3 times ULN and/or transaminases >5 times ULN

Head or neck cancer (unlabeled)
- **Adult: PO** 150 mg daily

Available forms: Tabs 25, 100, 150 mg

Administer:
- 1 hr before or 2 hr after food; at same time of day

SIDE EFFECTS

CNS: CVA, anxiety, depression, headache, rigors, insomnia
CV: MI/ischemia
EENT: Ocular changes, *conjunctivitis, eye pain,* hypertrichosis
GI: *Nausea, diarrhea, vomiting, anorexia, mouth ulceration,* hepatic failure, GI perforation
GU: Renal impairment/failure
HEMA: Deep vein thrombosis, bleeding
INTEG: *Rash,* Stevens-Johnson–like skin reaction, toxic epidermal necrolysis
MISC: *Fatigue, infection*
RESP: Interstitial lung disease, *cough, dyspnea,* ARDS, pulmonary fibrosis
SYST: Hepatorenal syndrome

PHARMACOKINETICS

Slowly absorbed (60%); peak 3-7 hr; excreted in feces (86%), urine (<4%); metabolized by CYP3A4; elimination half-life 36 hr; protein binding 93%

INTERACTIONS

Increase: GI bleeding, may be fatal—warfarin, NSAIDs
Increase: erlotinib concentrations—CYP3A4 inhibitors (ketoconazole, itraconazole, erythromycin, clarithromycin, telithromycin)
Increase: plasma concentrations of warfarin, metoprolol
Increase: myopathy—HMG-CoA reductase inhibitors
Decrease: erlotinib levels—CYP3A4 inducers (phenytoin, rifampin, carBAMazepine, PHENobarbital), proton-pump inhibitors

Drug/Herb
Decrease: erlotinib levels—St. John's wort

Drug/Smoking
Decrease: erlotinib level; dose may need to be increased

Drug/Food
Increase: effect of erlotinib—grapefruit juice

Drug/Lab Test
Increase: INR, PT, AST, ALT, bilirubin

NURSING CONSIDERATIONS

Assess:
- Serious skin toxicities: toxic epidermal necrolysis, Stevens-Johnson syndrome, check for rash, blistering, discontinue treatment, may need corticosteroids
- ⚠ **MI/ischemia, CVA** in patients with pancreatic cancer
- ⚠ **Pulmonary changes:** lung sounds, cough, dyspnea; interstitial lung disease may occur, may be fatal; discontinue therapy if confirmed
- **Ocular changes:** eye irritation, corneal erosion/ulcer, aberrant eyelash growth
- GI symptoms: frequency of stools; if diarrhea is poorly tolerated, therapy may be discontinued for ≤14 days, monitor for dehydration, fluid status during period of vomiting and diarrhea
- Blood studies: INR, LFTs, PT
- **Hepatic failure:** interrupt dosing if severe changes to liver function occur (total bilirubin >3× ULN and/or transaminases >5× ULN when normal pretreatment LFTs)
- **GI perforation/bleeding:** some cases have been fatal, usually occurs in those using NSAIDs, taxanes; or those with diverticulitis or peptic ulcer disease, discontinue if these occur

Evaluate:
- Therapeutic response: decrease in NSCLC cells, pancreatic cancer cells

Teach patient/family:
- ⚠ To report adverse reactions immediately: SOB, severe abdominal pain, persistent diarrhea or vomiting, ocular changes, skin eruptions (face, upper chest/back pain)
- About reason for treatment, expected results
- To use reliable contraception during treatment (pregnancy D); to avoid breastfeeding

• To avoid use with other products, herbs, supplements unless approved by provider
• To avoid smoking, decreases effect of this product

ertapenem (Rx)

(er-tah-pen′em)

INVanz

Func. class.: Antiinfective—miscellaneous

Chem. class.: Carbapenem

Do not confuse:
INVanz/AVINza

ACTION: Interferes with cell-wall replication of susceptible organisms; bactericidal

USES: *Bacteroides distasonis, Bacteroides fragilis, Bacteroides ovatus, Bacteroides thetaiotaomicron, Bacteroides uniformis, Bacteroides vulgatus, Citrobacter freundii, Citrobacter koseri, Clostridium clostridioforme, Clostridium perfringens, Enterobacter aerogenes, Enterobacter cloacae, Escherichia coli, Eubacterium lentum, Fusobacterium* sp., *Haemophilus influenzae* (beta-lactamase negative), *Haemophilus influenzae* (beta-lactamase positive), *Haemophilus parainfluenzae, Klebsiella oxytoca, Klebsiella pneumoniae, Moraxella catarrhalis, Morganella morganii, Peptostreptococcus* sp., *Porphyromonas asaccharolytica, Prevotella bivia, Proteus mirabilis, Proteus vulgaris, Providencia rettgeri, Providencia stuartii, Serratia marcescens, Staphylococcus aureus* (MSSA), *Staphylococcus epidermidis, Streptococcus agalactiae* (group B streptococci), *Streptococcus pneumoniae, Streptococcus pyogenes* (group A beta-hemolytic streptococci); bacteremia, community-acquired pneumonia, diabetic foot ulcer, endometritis, gyn/intraabdominal skin/skin structure/urinary tract infections, surgical infection prophylaxis

CONTRAINDICATIONS: Hypersensitivity to this product, its components, amide-type local anesthetics (IM only); anaphylactic reactions to β-lactams, other carbapenems

Precautions: Pregnancy (B), breastfeeding, children, geriatric patients, GI/renal/hepatic disease, seizures

DOSAGE AND ROUTES

Complicated intraabdominal infections
• **Adult/adolescent: IM/IV** 1 g/day × 5-14 days
• **Infant ≥3 mo/child: IM/IV** 15 mg/kg bid (max 1 g/day) × 5-14 days

Complicated skin/skin-structure infections
• **Adult/adolescent: IM/IV** 1 g/day × 7-14 days
• **Child 3 mo-12 yr: IM/IV** 15 mg/kg bid × 7-14 days

Community-acquired pneumonia
• **Adult/adolescent: IM/IV** 1 g/day × 10-14 days
• **Child 3 mo-12 yr: IM/IV** 15 mg/kg bid × 10-14 days, max 1 g/day

Complicated UTI
• **Adult/adolescent: IM/IV** 1 g/day × 10-14 days
• **Child 3 mo-12 yr: IM/IV** 15 mg/kg bid × 10-14 days

Acute pelvic infections
• **Adult/adolescent: IM/IV** 1 g/day × 3-10 days
• **Child 3 mo-12 yr: IM/IV** 15 mg/kg bid 3-10 days

Surgical infection prophylaxis (unlabeled)
• **Adult: IV** 1 g as a single dose 1 hr before surgical incision

Renal dose
• **Adult: IM/IV** CCr ≤30 ml/min 500 mg daily

Available form: Powder, lyophilized, 1 g

Administer:

IM route
• Reconstitute the 1-g vial of ertapenem with 3.2 ml of 1% lidocaine HCl injection (without EPINEPHrine) (280 mg/ml), agitate well to form a solution; the

IM reconstituted formulation is not for IV use

• IM administration may be used as an alternative to IV administration in the treatment of infections where IM therapy is appropriate; only give via IM injection × 7 days

• **For a 1-g dose:** immediately withdraw the contents of the vial and inject deeply into a large muscle, aspirate before injection to avoid injection into a blood vessel

• **For a dose** <1 g (i.e., for pediatric patients 3 mo-12 yr): immediately withdraw a volume equal to 15 mg/kg (max 1 g/day) and inject deeply into a large muscle, aspirate before injection to avoid injecting into a blood vessel; use the reconstituted IM sol within 1 hr after preparation

IV route

• Visually inspect for particulate matter and discoloration before use, may be colorless to pale yellow; do not mix with other products; dextrose sols are not compatible

• **1-g vial:** For each gram reconstitute with 10 ml of either NS injection, sterile water for injection, or bacteriostatic water for injection to 100 mg/ml, shake

• **1 g dose**: immediately transfer contents of the reconstituted vial to 50 ml of NS injection; for a dose <1 g (pediatric patients 3 mo-12 yr): from the reconstituted vial, immediately withdraw a volume equal to 15 mg/kg of body weight (max 1 g/day) and dilute in NS injection to a concentrations of 20 mg/ml or less

IV INFUSION route

• Complete the infusion within 6 hr of reconstitution, infuse over 30 min; do not co-infuse with other medications

• The reconstituted IV sol may be stored at room temperature if used within 6 hr, or store under refrigeration for 24 hr and use within 4 hours after removal from refrigeration; do not freeze

Y-site compatibilities: Acyclovir, alfentanil, amifostine, amikacin, aminocaproic acid, aminophylline, amphotericin B lipid complex, amphotericin B liposome, argatroban, arsenic trioxide, atenolol, atracurium, azithromycin, aztreonam, bivalirudin, bleomycin, bumetanide, buprenorphine, busulfan, butorphanol, calcium chloride/gluconate, CARBOplatin, carmustine, chloramphenicol, cimetidine, ciprofloxacin, cisatracurium, CISplatin, cyclophosphamide, cycloSPORINE, cytarabine, dacarbazine, DACTINomycin, DAPTOmycin, dexamethasone, dexmedetomidine, dexrazoxane, digoxin, diltiazem, diphenhydrAMINE, DOCEtaxel, dolasetron, DOPamine, doxacurium, doxycycline, enalaprilat, ePHEDrine, EPINEPHrine, eptifibatide, erythromycin, esmolol, etoposide, etoposide phosphate, famotidine, fenoldopam, fluconazole, fludarabine, fluorouracil, foscarnet, fosphenytoin, furosemide, ganciclovir, gatifloxacin, gemcitabine, gemtuzumab, gentamicin, glycopyrrolate, granisetron, haloperidol, heparin, hydrocortisone, HYDROmorphone, ifosfamide, inamrinone, insulin (regular), irinotecan, isoproterenol, ketorolac, labetalol, lepirudin, leucovorin, levofloxacin, lidocaine, linezolid, LORazepam, magnesium sulfate, mannitol, mechlorethamine, melphalan, meperidine, mesna, metaraminol, methotrexate, methyldopate, methylPREDNISolone, metoclopramide, metroNIDAZOLE, milrinone, mitoMYcin, mivacurium, morphine, moxifloxacin, nalbuphine, naloxone, nesiritide, nitroglycerin, nitroprusside, norepinephrine, octreotide, oxaliplatin, oxytocin, PACLitaxel, pamidronate, pancuronium, pantoprazole, PEMEtrexed, PENTobarbital, PHENobarbital, phentolamine, phenylephrine, polymyxin B, potassium acetate/chloride/phosphates, procainamide, propranolol, ranitidine, remifentanil, rocuronium, sodium acetate/bicarbonate/phosphates, streptozocin, succinylcholine, SUFentanil, sulfamethoxazole-trimethoprim, tacrolimus, telavancin, teniposide, theophylline, thiotepa, tigecycline, tirofiban, tobramycin, trimethobenzamide, vancomycin, vasopressin, vecuronium, vinBLAStine, vinCRIStine, vinorelbine, voriconazole, zidovudine, zoledronic acid

SIDE EFFECTS

CNS: Insomnia, seizures, dizziness, *headache,* agitation, confusion, somnolence, disorientation, edema, hypotension
CV: Tachycardia, seizures
GI: *Diarrhea, nausea, vomiting,* pseudomembranous colitis, cholelithiasis, jaundice, abdominal pain
GU: *Vaginitis,* dysuria
INTEG: *Rash,* urticaria, *pruritus,* pain at inj site, *infused vein complication, phlebitis/thrombophlebitis,* erythema at inj site, dermatitis
RESP: Dyspnea, cough, pharyngitis, crackles, respiratory distress
SYST: Anaphylaxis, angioedema

PHARMACOKINETICS

IV: Onset immediate; peak dose dependent; half-life 4 hr; metabolized by liver; excreted in urine, feces, breast milk

INTERACTIONS

Increase: INR—warfarin
Increase: ertapenem levels—probenecid; do not coadminister
Decrease: effect of valproic acid
Drug/Lab Test
Increase: hepatic enzymes

NURSING CONSIDERATIONS

Assess:
- Renal disease: lower dose may be required
- **Pseudomembranous colitis:** bowel pattern daily: if severe diarrhea occurs, product should be discontinued
- For infection: temperature, sputum, characteristics of wound before, during, after treatment
- ⚠ **Allergic reactions, anaphylaxis;** rash, urticaria, pruritus; may occur a few days after therapy begins; sensitivity to carbapenem antibiotics, other β-lactam antibiotics, penicillins
- **Overgrowth of infection:** perineal itching, fever, malaise, redness, pain, swelling, drainage, rash, diarrhea, change in cough or sputum

Evaluate:
- Therapeutic response: negative C&S; absence of signs, symptoms of infection

Teach patient/family:
- To report severe diarrhea (may indicate **pseudomembranous colitis**), CNS side effects
- To report overgrowth of infection: black, furry tongue; vaginal itching; foul-smelling stools
- To avoid breastfeeding; product is excreted in breast milk

TREATMENT OF OVERDOSE:

EPINEPHrine, antihistamines; resuscitate if needed (anaphylaxis)

erythromycin (ophthalmic)

(e-rith′roe-mye′sin)

Ilotycin, Romycin

Func. class.: Ophthalmic antiinfective
Chem. class.: Macrolide

ACTION: Inhibits protein synthesis, thereby decreasing bacterial replication

USES: Conjunctivitis, eye infections, prevention of ophthalmic neonatorum

CONTRAINDICATIONS: Hypersensitivity to this product or macrolides
Precautions: Pregnancy (B), breastfeeding

DOSAGE AND ROUTES

Bacterial conjunctivitis
- **Adult/adolescent/child:** apply 1 cm of ointment directly to the eye up to 6 times a day ×7-10 days depending on severity of infection

Prevention of ophthalmic neonatorum
Neonate: Ointment apply 1-cm ribbon to lower conjunctival sac of each eye once after birth

Administer:
Ophthalmic route
- Apply ribbon of ointment directly to the eye; for ophthalmic use only

Available forms: ointment/ophthalmic 0.5%

SIDE EFFECTS
EENT: Hypersensitivity, irritation, redness

PHARMACOKINETICS
Unknown

NURSING CONSIDERATIONS
Assess:
- **Allergic reaction:** assess for hypersensitivity, discontinue product

Evaluate:
- Decreased ophthalmic infection

Teach patient/family:

Ophthalmic route:
- Apply ribbon of ointment directly to the eye; for ophthalmic use only

erythromycin base (Rx)
(eh-rith-roh-my′sin)

Apo-Erythro ✤, Ery-Tab, Novo-Rythro Encap ✤, PCE

erythromycin ethylsuccinate (Rx)
Apo-Erythro-Es ✤, E.E.S., Erythro-Es ✤, Ery Ped, Novo-Rythro ✤

erythromycin lactobionate (Rx)
Erythrocin

erythromycin stearate (Rx)
Apo-Erythro-S ✤, Erythrocin, My-E, Novo-Rythro ✤

Func. class.: Antiinfective
Chem. class.: Macrolide

Do not confuse:
erythromycin/azithromycin

ACTION: Binds to 50S ribosomal subunits of susceptible bacteria and suppresses protein synthesis

USES: Mild to moderate respiratory tract, skin, soft-tissue infections caused by *Bordetella pertussis, Borrelia burgdorferi, Chlamydia trachomatis; Corynebacterium diphtheriae, Haemophilus influenzae* (when used with sulfonamides); *Legionella pneumophila,* Legionnaire's disease, *Listeria monocytogenes; Mycoplasma pneumoniae, Streptococcus pneumoniae,* syphilis: *Treponema pallidum; Staphylococcus* sp.

Unlabeled uses: Bartonellosis, burn wound infection, chancroid, cholera, diabetic gastroparesis, endocarditis prophylaxis, gastroenteritis, granuloma inguinale, Lyme disease, tetanus

CONTRAINDICATIONS: Hypersensitivity, preexisting hepatic disease (estolate)

Precautions: Pregnancy (B), breastfeeding, geriatric patients, hepatic disease, GI disease, QT prolongation, seizure disorder, myasthenia gravis

DOSAGE AND ROUTES
Acne vulgaris
- **Adult: PO** 250 mg qid

Mild to moderately severe upper respiratory tract infections (otitis media, sinusitis) or lower respiratory tract infections (pneumonia, bronchitis) caused by susceptible organisms
- **Adult: PO** 250-500 mg (of base, estolate, or stearate) every 6 hr or 400-800 mg (ethylsuccinate) every 6 hr; **IV** 15-20 mg/kg/day in divided doses every 4-6 hr, max 4 g/day
- **Adolescent/child/infant: PO** 20-50 mg/kg/day divided every 6 hr, max adult doses; **IV** 15-20 mg/kg/day in divided doses every 4-6 hr, or as a continuous infusion, max dose 4 g/day
- **Neonate >7 days, ≥1200 g: PO** 30 mg/kg/day in divided doses every 8 hr
- **Neonates >7 days, <1200 g: PO** 20 mg/kg/day in divided doses every 12 hr
- **Neonates ≤7 days: PO** 20 mg/kg/day in divided doses every 12 hr

Pneumonia caused by *Chlamydia trachomatis*
- **Infant/neonate: PO** CDC recommends 50 mg/kg/day in 4 divided doses ×

14 days (erythromycin base or ethylsuccinate)

Mycoplasma infection such as *Mycoplasma pneumoniae* pneumonia

- **Adult: PO** 250-500 mg tid
- **Adult/adolescent/child/infant: IV** 15-20 mg/kg/day, given in divided doses every 4-6 hr, or as a continuous infusion, max dose 4 g/day; replace by oral dosage as soon as possible

Legionnaire's disease (caused by *Legionella pneumophila*)

- **Adult: PO/IV** 0.5-1 g every 6 hr × 21 days

Treatment of group A β-hemolytic streptococcal (GAS) pharyngitis (primary rheumatic fever prophylaxis)

- **Adult: PO** 250-500 mg (base, estolate, or stearate) every 6 hr or 400-800 mg (ethylsuccinate) every 6 hr × 10 days
- **Adolescent/child/infant: PO** 20-50 mg/kg/day, divided every 6 hr × 10 days, max adult dose

Secondary prevention of rheumatic fever (prevention of recurrent attacks of rheumatic fever)

- **Adult/adolescent/child: PO** 250 mg bid in patients allergic to penicillin and sulfADIAZINE for 10 yr or age 40, whichever is longer, secondary prophylaxis (American Heart Association)

Listeriosis

- **Adult: PO** 250-500 mg (base, estolate or stearate) every 6 hr or 400-800 mg (ethylsuccinate) every 6 hr
- **Adolescent/child/infant: PO** 20-50 mg/kg/day, divided every 6 hr, max adult doses

Cervicitis caused by *Chlamydia trachomatis*

- **Adult/adolescent: PO** CDC recommends erythromycin base 500 mg qid or erythromycin ethylsuccinate 800 mg qid × 7 days as alternatives to first-line agents doxycycline or azithromycin
- **Pregnant females: PO** As alternatives to first-line agents azithromycin or amoxicillin, CDC recommends base 500 mg q12hr, 333 mg q8hr, or 250 mg qid × 14 days
- **Child $\leq$45 kg: PO** CDC recommends base or ethylsuccinate 50 mg/kg/day in 4 doses × 14 days

Chlamydial conjunctivitis caused by *Chlamydia trachomatis* including trachoma and inclusion conjunctivitis

- **Pregnant/lactating woman/child $<$8 yr: PO** 250-500 mg qid × 10-14 days

Infant pneumonia caused by *Chlamydia trachomatis*

- **Infant/neonate: PO** (base or ethylsuccinate) CDC recommends 50 mg/kg/day 4 divided doses × 14 days
- **Pregnant female: PO** CDC recommends base 400 mg qid × 14 days

Non-gonococcal urethritis (NGU) caused by *Chlamydia trachomatis* or *Ureaplasma urealyticum*

- **Adult/adolescent: PO** CDC recommends 500 mg (base) qid or 800 mg (ethylsuccinate) qid × 7 days as alternatives to first-line agents doxycycline or azithromycin
- **Child $<$45 kg: PO** CDC recommends base 50 mg/kg/day in 4 divided doses × 14 days, second course of therapy may be required

Ophthalmia neonatorum caused by *Chlamydia trachomatis*

- **Neonate: PO** (erythromycin base or ethylsuccinate) CDC recommends 50 mg/kg/day qid × 14 days, may repeat if condition returns

Lymphogranuloma venereum caused by *Chlamydia trachomatis*

- **Adult: PO** (base) CDC recommends 500 mg qid × 21 days as an alternative to doxycycline

Adjunctive treatment of diphtheria to prevent establishment of carrier state and to eradicate *Corynebacterium diphtheriae* in carriers

- **Adult: PO** 500 mg every 6 hr × 10 days

Intestinal amebiasis (unable to take metroNIDAZOLE)

- **Adult: PO** 250 mg every 6 hr × 10-14 days
- **Adolescent/child: PO** 30-50 mg/kg/day, divided every 6 hr × 10-14 days, max adult dose

Pertussis (whooping cough) caused by *Bordetella pertussis* or for postexposure pertussis prophylaxis

- **Adult: PO** 500 mg qid (2 g total) × 14 days
- **Adolescent/child/infant: PO** 40-50 mg/kg/day (max 2 g/day) in 4 divided doses × 14 days

Primary or secondary syphilis (caused by *Treponema pallidum*) in penicillin-allergic nonpregnant patients

- **Adult: PO** 48-64 g (ethylsuccinate) or 30-40 g (base or stearate) in divided doses × 10-15 days

Surgical infection prophylaxis as a bowel preparation in combination with neomycin

- **Adult:** It is generally recommended that if surgery is scheduled for 8 AM, 1 g of erythromycin PO with neomycin sulfate PO should be given at 1 PM, 2 PM, and 11 PM on the day before surgery

Impetigo, burn wound infection (unlabeled)

- **Adult: PO** 250-500 mg q6hr (base, estolate, stearate) or 400-800 mg (ethylsuccinate) q6hr
- **Infant/child/adolescent:** 20-50 mg/kg/day divided q6hr

Available forms: *Base:* enteric-coated tabs 250, 333, 500 mg; film-coated tabs 250, 500 mg; enteric-coated caps 250, 333 mg; *stearate:* film-coated tabs 250 mg; *ethylsuccinate:* granules for oral susp 200, 400 mg/5 ml; powder for inj 500 mg, 1 g (lactobionate), 1 g (as gluceptate)

Administer:

- Do not break, crush, or chew time rel cap or tab; chew only chewable tabs; enteric-coated tablets may be given with food
- Do not give by IM or IV push
- Oral product with full glass of water; do not give with fruit juice
- Give 1 hr before or 2 hr after meals
- Store at room temperature; store susp in refrigerator
- Adequate intake of fluids (2 L) during diarrhea episodes

IV route

- After **reconstituting** 500 mg or less/10 ml sterile water without preservatives; dilute further in 100-250 ml of 0.9% NaCl, LR, Normosol-R; may be **further diluted** to 1 mg/ml and **given** as cont infusion; run 1 g or less/100 ml over ½-1 hr; cont infusion over 6 hr, may require buffers to neutralize pH if dilution is <250 ml, use infusion pump

Lactobionate

Y-site compatibilities: Acyclovir, alfentanil, amikacin, aminocaproic acid, aminophylline, amiodarone, anidulafungin, argatroban, atenolol, atosiban, atracurium, atropine, azaTHIOprine, benztropine, bivalirudin, bleomycin, bumetanide, buprenorphine, butorphanol, calcium chloride/gluconate, CARBOplatin, caspofungin, cefotaxime, cefTRIAXone, cefuroxime, chlorproMAZINE, cimetidine, CISplatin, cyanocobalamin, cyclophosphamide, cycloSPORINE, cytarabine, DACTINomycin, DAPTOmycin, dexmedetomidine, digoxin, diltiazem, diphenhydrAMINE, DOBUTamine, DOCEtaxel, DOPamine, doxacurium, doxapram, DOXOrubicin, enalaprilat, ePHEDrine, EPINEPHrine, epirubicin, epoetin alfa, eptifibatide, ertapenem, esmolol, etoposide, famotidine, fenoldopam, fentaNYL, fluconazole, fludarabine, fluorouracil, folic acid, foscarnet, gatifloxacin, gemcitabine, gentamicin, glycopyrrolate, granisetron, hydrocortisone, HYDROmorphone, hydrOXYzine, IDArubicin, ifosfamide, imipenem-cilastatin, insulin (regular), irinotecan, isoproterenol, labetalol, levofloxacin, lidocaine, LORazepam, LR, mannitol, mechlorethamine, meperidine, methicillin, methotrexate, methoxamine, methyldopate, methylPREDNISolone, metoclopramide, metroNIDAZOLE, miconazole, midazolam, milrinone, mitoXANtrone, morphine, multiple vitamins injection, mycophenolate, nafcillin, nalbuphine, naloxone, nesiritide, netilmicin, niCARdipine, nitroglycerin, norepinephrine, octreotide, ondansetron, oxacillin, oxaliplatin, oxytocin, PACLitaxel, palonosetron, pamidronate, pancuronium, papaverine, pentamidine, pentazocine, perphenazine, phenylephrine, phytonadione, piperacillin, piperacillin-tazobactam, polymyxin B, procainamide, prochlorperazine, promethazine, propranolol, protamine, pyridoxine, quiNIDine, ranitidine, Ringer's, ritodrine, sodium acetate/bicarbonate, succinylcholine, SUFentanil, tacrolimus, temocillin, teniposide, theophylline, thiamine, thiotepa, tigecycline, tirofiban, TNA, tobramycin, tolazoline, TPN, trimetaphan, urokinase, vancomycin, vasopressin, vecuronium, verapamil, vinCRIStine, vinorelbine, vitamin B complex/C, voriconazole, zidovudine, zoledronic acid

SIDE EFFECTS

CNS: Seizures
CV: Dysrhythmias, QT prolongation
EENT: Hearing loss, tinnitus
GI: *Nausea, vomiting, diarrhea,* hepatotoxicity, abdominal pain, stomatitis, heartburn, anorexia, pseudomembranous colitis, esophagitis, hepatotoxicity
GU: *Vaginitis, moniliasis*
INTEG: Rash, urticaria, pruritus, thrombophlebitis, inj-site reactions (IV site)
SYST: Anaphylaxis

PHARMACOKINETICS

Peak 1-4 hr (base); ½-2½ hr (ethylsuccinate); half-life 1-2 hr; metabolized in liver; excreted in bile, feces; protein binding 75%-90%; inhibitor of CYP3A4 and P-glycoprotein

INTERACTIONS

⚠ Serious dysrhythmias—diltiazem, itraconazole, ketoconazole, nefazodone, pimozide, protease inhibitors, verapamil
Increase: QT prolongation—products that increase QT prolongation
Increase: action, toxicity of alfentanil, ALPRAZolam, bromocriptine, busPIRone, carBAMazepine, cilostazol, clindamycin, cloZAPine, cycloSPORINE, diazepam, digoxin, disopyramide, ergots, felodipine, HMG-CoA reductase inhibitors, ibrutinib methylPREDNISolone, midazolam, quiNIDine, rifabutin, sildenafil, tacrolimus, tadalafil, theophylline, triazolam, vardenafil, vinBLAStine, warfarin

Drug/Lab Test
Increase: AST/ALT
Decrease: folate assay
False increase: 17-OHCS/17-KS

NURSING CONSIDERATIONS

Assess:
- **Infection:** temperature, characteristics of wounds, urine, stools, sputum, WBCs at baseline and periodically
- I&O ratio; report hematuria, oliguria in renal disease
- Hepatic studies: AST, ALT if patient is receiving long-term therapy
- Hearing at baseline and after treatment
- Renal studies: urinalysis, protein, blood
- C&S before product therapy; product may be given as soon as culture is taken; C&S may be repeated after treatment
- **Pseudomembranous colitis:** diarrhea with blood, mucus; abdominal pain, fever; product should be discontinued immediately, notify prescriber
- **Anaphylaxis:** generalized hives, itching, flushing, swelling of lips, tongue, throat, wheezing; have emergency equipment nearby
- **QT prolongation:** may occur (IV >15 mg/min); those with electrolyte imbalances, congenital QT prolongation, elderly at greater risk; correct electrolyte imbalances before treatment, ECG

Evaluate:
- Therapeutic response: decreased symptoms of infection

Teach patient/family:
- To report sore throat, fever, fatigue (could indicate superinfection), rhythm changes in the heart, hearing loss
- To notify nurse of diarrhea stools, dark urine, pale stools, jaundice of eyes or skin, severe abdominal pain
- To take at evenly spaced intervals; to complete dosage regimen; to take without food
- To avoid use with other products unless approved by prescriber

TREATMENT OF HYPERSENSITIVITY: Withdraw product; maintain airway; administer EPINEPHrine, aminophylline, O_2, IV corticosteroids

erythromycin (topical)

(e-rith-roe-mye′sin)

Akne-mycin, Ery-sol ✦

Func. class.: Topical antiinfective, anti-acne

Chem. class.: Macrolide

ACTION: Antibacterial activity results from inhibition of protein synthesis; bacteriostatic

USES: Treatment of acne vulgaris

CONTRAINDICATIONS: Hypersensitivity, children

DOSAGE AND ROUTES

Acne vulgaris

• **Adult/adolescent: TOP** Apply to affected areas bid, AM, PM

Available forms: Topical gel, ointment, pledget, solution 2%

Administer:

Topical route

• For external use only; do not use skin products near the eyes, nose, or mouth

• Wash hands before and after use. Wash affected area and gently pat dry before using

• **Gel/ointment/pledget/solution:** Apply to the cleansed affected area. Massage gently into affected areas

• Each pledget should be used once and discarded

SIDE EFFECTS

INTEG: Burning, rash, pruritus, peeling, irritation

NURSING CONSIDERATIONS

Assess:

• **Allergic reaction:** assess for hypersensitivity, product might need to be discontinued

• **Infection:** assess for number of lesions, severity in acne

Evaluate:

• Decreased lesions in acne

Teach patient/family:

Topical Route:

• That product is for external use only; do not use skin products near the eyes, nose, or mouth

• To wash hands before and after use, wash affected area and gently pat dry before using

• **Gel/pledget/solution/ointment/lotion:** To apply to the cleansed affected area; massage gently into affected areas

• That each pledget should be used once and discarded

escitalopram (Rx)

(es-sit-tal′oh-pram)

Cipralex ✦, Lexapro

Func. class.: Antidepressant, SSRI (selective serotonin reuptake inhibitor)

ACTION: Inhibits CNS neuron uptake of serotonin but not of norepinephrine

USES: General anxiety disorder; major depressive disorder in adults/adolescents

Unlabeled uses: Panic disorder, social phobia, autism

CONTRAINDICATIONS: Hypersensitivity to this product, citalopram, MAOIs

Precautions: Pregnancy (C), breastfeeding, geriatric patients, renal/hepatic disease, history of seizures, abrupt discontinuation, bleeding, anticoagulants

Black Box Warning: Children/adolescents ≤12 yr, suicidal ideation

DOSAGE AND ROUTES

• **Adult: PO** 10 mg/day in AM or PM; after 1 wk, if no clinical improvement is noted, dose may be increased to 20 mg/day PM;

maintenance 10-20 mg/day; reassess to determine need for treatment

Hepatic dose/geriatric

- **Adult: PO** 10 mg/day

Available forms: Tabs 5, 10, 20 mg; oral sol 5 mg (as base)/5 ml (contains sorbitol)

Administer:

- With food or milk for GI symptoms, give with full glass of water
- Crushed if patient is unable to swallow medication whole, scored tabs can be cut
- Dosage at bedtime if oversedation occurs during the day
- Gum, hard candy, frequent sips of water for dry mouth
- **Oral sol:** measure with calibrated device
- Store at room temperature; do not freeze

SIDE EFFECTS

CNS: *Headache, nervousness, insomnia,* suicidal ideation, *drowsiness, anxiety, tremor, dizziness, fatigue, sedation, poor concentrations, abnormal dreams, agitation,* seizures, apathy, euphoria, hallucinations, delusions, psychosis, neuroleptic malignant-like syndrome, ataxia, worsening depression

CV: *Hot flashes, palpitations,* angina pectoris, hemorrhage, hypertension, tachycardia, 1st-degree AV block, bradycardia, MI, thrombophlebitis, postural hypotension

EENT: Visual changes, ear/eye pain, photophobia, tinnitus, pupil dilation, dental pain

GI: *Nausea, diarrhea, dry mouth, anorexia, dyspepsia, constipation, cramps, vomiting, taste changes, flatulence, decreased appetite,* hepatitis

GU: *Dysmenorrhea, decreased libido, urinary frequency, UTI,* amenorrhea, cystitis, impotence, urine retention, ejaculation disorder

HEMA: Impaired platelet aggregation

INTEG: *Sweating, rash, pruritus,* acne, alopecia, urticaria, photosensitivity, bruising

MS: *Pain,* arthritis, twitching, osteopenia

RESP: *Infection, pharyngitis, nasal congestion, sinus headache, sinusitis, cough, dyspnea, bronchitis,* asthma, hyperventilation, pneumonia

SYST: *Asthenia, viral infection, fever, allergy, chills,* serotonin syndrome, neonatal abstinence syndrome, Stevens-Johnson syndrome

PHARMACOKINETICS

PO: Metabolized in liver; excreted in urine; 56% protein binding; metabolized by CYP2C19, 3A4, half-life 27-32 hr; half-life increased by 50% in geriatric patients

INTERACTIONS

- Paradoxical worsening of OCD: busPIRone

Increase: serotonin syndrome—tryptophan, amphetamines, busPIRone, lithium, amantadine, bromocriptine, SSRI, SNRIs, serotonin-receptor agonists, traMADol

⚠ Do not use pimozide, MAOIs, with or 14 days before escitalopram

Increase: CNS depression—alcohol, antidepressants, opioids, sedatives

Increase: side effects of escitalopram—highly protein-bound products

Increase: levels or toxicity of carBAMazepine, lithium, warfarin, phenytoin, antipsychotics, antidysrhythmics

Increase: levels of tricyclics, phenothiazines, haloperidol, diazepam

Increase: bleeding risk—NSAIDs, salicylates, anticoagulants, SSRIs, platelet inhibitors

Decrease: escitalopram effect—cyproheptadine

Drug/Herb

- St. John's wort: do not use together, serotonin syndrome may occur

Increase: CNS effect—kava, valerian

Drug/Food

- Grapefruit juice—increased escitalopram effect

Drug/Lab Test

Increase: serum bilirubin, blood glucose, alk phos

Decrease: VMA, 5-HIAA

False increase: urinary catecholamines

NURSING CONSIDERATIONS

Assess:

Black Box Warning: Mental status: mood, sensorium, affect, **suicidal tendencies,** increase in psychiatric symptoms, depression, panic, not approved for use in children

- Appetite with bulimia nervosa, weight daily; increase nutritious foods in diet, watch for binging and vomiting
- **Allergic reactions:** itching, rash, urticaria; product should be discontinued, may need to give antihistamine
- B/P (lying/standing), pulse q4hr; if systolic B/P drops 20 mm Hg, hold product, notify prescriber
- Blood studies: CBC, leukocytes, differential, cardiac enzymes if patient receiving long-term therapy; check platelets; bleeding can occur
- **Serotonin syndrome:** nausea, vomiting, sedation, dizziness, sweating, facial flushing, mental changes, shivering, increased B/P; discontinue product, notify prescriber
- Hepatic studies: AST, ALT, bilirubin, creatinine; thyroid function studies
- Weight weekly; appetite may decrease with product
- **ECG** for flattening of T wave, bundle branch, AV block, dysrhythmias in cardiac patients
- Alcohol consumption; if alcohol is consumed, hold dose until AM
- **Sexual dysfunction:** ejaculation dysfunction, erectile dysfunction, decreased libido, orgasm dysfunction, priapism
- Assistance with ambulation during therapy, since drowsiness, dizziness occur; safety measures primarily for geriatric patients

Evaluate:

- Therapeutic response: decreased depression

Teach patient/family:

- That therapeutic effect may take 1-4 wk, may have increased anxiety for first 5-7 days, do not abruptly discontinue
- **Serotonin syndrome:** To report immediately nausea, vomiting, sedation, dizziness, sweating, facial flushing, mental changes, shivering
- To use caution when driving, performing other activities requiring alertness because drowsiness, dizziness, blurred vision may occur
- To avoid alcohol, other CNS depressants; to avoid all OTC products unless approved by prescriber, to take without regard to meals
- To notify prescriber if pregnant or planning to become pregnant or breastfeeding, discuss sexual dysfunction
- To change positions slowly, orthostatic hypotension may occur
- To report signs of urinary retention immediately

Black Box Warning: That clinical worsening and suicide risk may occur especially in adolescents and young adults

- To use MedGuide provided

TREATMENT OF OVERDOSE:

Activated charcoal, supportive care, serotonin antagonist

⚠ HIGH ALERT

eslicarbazepine

(es′lye-kar-bay′ze-peen)

Aptiom

Func. class: Anticonvulsant, misc

Chem. class: Voltage-gated sodium channel (VGSC) blocker

ACTION: Exact mechanism unknown; a voltage-gated sodium-channel blocker inhibits repetitive neuronal firing

USES: Partial seizures, adjunctive treatment

CONTRAINDICATIONS: Hypersensitivity to this product or OXcarbazepine

Precautions: Breastfeeding, abrupt discontinuation, depression, driving/operating machinery, ethanol intoxication, hepatic disease, renal disease, hyponatremia, suicidal ideation, pregnancy (C)

DOSAGE AND ROUTES

• **Adult: PO** 400 mg daily; after 1 wk, increase to 800 mg daily, max 1600 mg daily

Renal dose

• **Adult: PO** CCr <50 ml/min 200 mg daily; after 2 wk, increase to 400 mg daily, max 600 mg daily

Available forms: Tab 200, 400, 600, 800 mg

Administer:

• May be taken without regard to food
• May be crushed or whole

SIDE EFFECTS

CNS: Drowsiness, dizziness, amnesia, depression, insomnia, lethargy, memory impairment, confusion, fatigue, headache, speech disturbance, suicidal thoughts/behaviors, tremors

CV: Hypertension, peripheral edema

EENT: Blurred vision, nystagmus, diplopia

GI: Nausea, constipation, diarrhea, hypercholesterolemia/hypertriglyceridemia, vomiting, hepatotoxicity

GU: Cystitis

INTEG: Rash, Stevens-Johnson syndrome, toxic epidermal necrolysis, anaphylaxis, angioedema

META: Hyponatremia

RESP: Cough

PHARMACOKINETICS

Peak 1-4 hr; metabolized by liver; moderate CYP2C19 inhibitor; weak/moderate CYP3A4 inducer; steady state 4-5 days; excreted in urine, feces; half-life 13-20 hr; protein binding <40%

INTERACTIONS

Decrease: effects of bedaquiline, boceprevir, bosutinib, cabozantinib, cobicistat, elvitegravir, emtricitabine, crizotinib, cycloSPORINE, dronedarone, erlotinib, fosamprenavir, galantamine, gefitinib, HYDROcodone, maraviroc, oxyCODONE, paliperidone, perm panel, pimozide, praziquantel, QUEtiapine, ranolazine, rilpivirine

Decrease: eslicarbazepine effect CYP1A2, CYP2C19 substrates

Decrease: effect of CYP3A inducers

NURSING CONSIDERATIONS

Assess:

• **Hyponatremia:** assess for nausea, vomiting, increased seizures, headache, weakness, confusion, irritability
• Seizures: character, location, duration, intensity, frequency, presence of aura
• Hepatic studies: ALT, AST, bilirubin; sodium

Black Box Warning: Mental status: mood, sensorium, affect, behavioral changes, suicidal thoughts/behaviors; if mental status changes, notify prescriber

• Eye problems: need for ophthalmic examinations before, during, after treatment (slit lamp, fundoscopy, tonometry)
• Allergic reaction: purpura, red, raised rash; if these occur, product should be discontinued
• **Pregnancy (C):** patient should enroll in North American Antiepileptic Drug Pregnancy Registry (1-888-233-2334)

Evaluate:

• Therapeutic response: decreased seizure activity; document on patient's chart

Teach patient/family:

• To carry emergency ID stating patient's name, products taken, condition, prescriber's name, and phone number
• To avoid driving, other activities that require alertness usually for the first 3 days of treatment
• Not to discontinue medication quickly after long-term use
• To notify if pregnancy is planned or suspected, pregnancy (C), to use additional contraceptives, if using hormonal contraceptives; to avoid breastfeeding
• Not to abruptly discontinue drug
• To report signs of decreased renal function, dizziness, increased cholesterol, ocular toxicity, suicide risk, skin rashes

- To take with or without food; that tablet can be crushed
- To report increased seizures, headache, nausea, vomiting, weakness, confusion, irritability (hyponatremia)

⚠ HIGH ALERT

esmolol (Rx)

(ez′moe-lole)

Brevibloc

Func. class.: β-Adrenergic blocker (antidysrhythmic II)

Do not confuse:
esmolol/Osmitrol
Brevibloc/Brevital

ACTION: Competitively blocks stimulation of β_1-adrenergic receptors in the myocardium; produces negative chronotropic, inotropic activity (decreases rate of SA node discharge, increases recovery time), slows conduction of AV node, decreases heart rate, decreases O_2 consumption in myocardium; also decreases renin-aldosterone-angiotensin system at high doses; inhibits β_2-receptors in bronchial system at higher doses

USES: Supraventricular tachycardia, noncompensatory sinus tachycardia, intraoperative and postoperative tachycardia and hypertension, atrial fibrillation/flutter

Unlabeled uses: Acute MI, ECT, thyroid storm, pheochromocytoma, hypertensive crisis/urgency, unstable angina, hypertensive crisis

CONTRAINDICATIONS: 2nd- or 3rd-degree heart block; cardiogenic shock, CHF, cardiac failure, hypersensitivity, severe bradycardia

Precautions: Pregnancy (C), breastfeeding, geriatric patients, hypotension, peripheral vascular disease, diabetes, hypoglycemia, thyrotoxicosis, renal disease, atrial fibrillation, bronchospasms, hyperthyroidism, myasthenia gravis, asthma, COPD, CV disease, pheochromocytoma, abrupt discontinuation

DOSAGE AND ROUTES

Atrial fibrillation/flutter

- **Adult:** **IV** loading dose 500 mcg/kg/min over 1 min; maintenance 50 mcg/kg/min for 4 min; if no response after 5 min, give 2nd loading dose, then increase infusion to 100 mcg/kg/min for 4 min; if no response, repeat loading dose, then increase maintenance infusion by 50 mcg/kg/min (max of 200 mcg/kg/min); titrate to patient response
- **Child:** **IV** total loading dose of 600 mcg/kg over 2 min, maintenance **IV INFUSION** 200 mcg/kg/min, titrate upward by 50-100 mcg/kg/min q5-10min until B/P, heart rate reduced by >10%

Perioperative hypertension/tachycardia

- **Adult:** **IV** Immediate control 80 mg (bolus) over 30 seconds, then 150 mcg/kg/min, adjust to response, max 300 mcg/kg/min

Hypertensive emergency (unlabeled)

- **Adult:** **IV** 250-500 mcg/kg over 1 min, then **IV INFUSION** 50-100 mcg/kg/min × 4 min

Available forms: Inj 10 mg, 20 mg/ml

Administer:

- Do not discontinue product suddenly
- Store protected from light, moisture; in cool environment

IV route

- Check that correct concentrations being given
- 10 mg/ml inj sol needs no dilution, may be used as an IV loading dose using a handheld syringe

Continuous IV INFUSION route

- Ready-to-use bags of premixed isotonic sol of 10 mg/ml and 20 mg/ml available in 100-, 250-ml bags; use controlled infusion device, central line preferred; rate is based on patient's weight

Y-site compatibilities: Amikacin, aminophylline, amiodarone, atracurium, butorphanol, calcium chloride, ceFAZolin, cefTAZidime, ceftizoxime, chloramphenicol, cimetidine, cisatracurium, clindamycin, diltiazem, DOPamine, enalaprilat, erythromycin, famotidine, fentaNYL, gentamicin, insulin (regular), labetalol, magnesium sulfate, methyldopate, metroNIDAZOLE, midazolam, morphine, nitroglycerin, nitroprusside, norepinephrine, pancuronium, penicillin G potassium, piperacillin, polymyxin B, potassium chloride, potassium phosphate, propofol, ranitidine, remifentanil, streptomycin, tacrolimus, tobramycin, trimethoprim-sulfamethoxazole, vancomycin, vecuronium, voriconazole, zoledronic acid

SIDE EFFECTS

CNS: Confusion, light-headedness, paresthesia, somnolence, fever, dizziness, fatigue, headache, depression, anxiety, seizures

CV: Hypotension, bradycardia, chest pain, peripheral ischemia, SOB, CHF, conduction disturbances; 1st-, 2nd-, 3rd-degree heart block

GI: *Nausea,* vomiting, anorexia, gastric pain, flatulence, constipation, heartburn, bloating

GU: Urinary retention, impotence, dysuria

INTEG: *Induration, inflammation at site,* discoloration, edema, erythema, burning pallor, flushing, rash, pruritus, dry skin, alopecia

RESP: Bronchospasm, dyspnea, cough, wheeziness, nasal stuffiness, pulmonary edema

PHARMACOKINETICS

Onset very rapid, duration short, half-life 9 min, metabolized by hydrolysis of ester linkage, excreted via kidneys

INTERACTIONS

• Avoid use with MAOIs, Sotalol

Increase: effect of antidiabetics

Increase: possible fatal B/P increase—clonidine

Increase: potentiate suppressive effects of diltiazem, verapamil

Increase: antihypertensive effect—general anesthetics

Increase: digoxin levels—digoxin

Increase: α-adrenergic stimulation—ePHEDrine, EPINEPHrine, amphetamine, norepinephrine, phenylephrine, pseudoePHEDrine

Decrease: action of thyroid hormones

Decrease: action of esmolol—thyroid hormone, salicylates

Drug/Herb

Increase: β-blocking effect—hawthorn

Decrease: antihypertensive effect—ephedra

Drug/Lab Test

Interference: glucose/insulin tolerance test

NURSING CONSIDERATIONS

Assess:

• **CHF:** I&O ratio, weight daily, jugular venous distention, weight gain, crackles, edema

• **Dysrhythmias:** B/P, pulse q4hr; note rate, rhythm, quality; rapid changes can cause shock; if systolic <100 or diastolic <60, notify prescriber before giving product; ECG continuously during infusion, hypotension common, if severe, slow or stop infusion

• Baselines in renal/hepatic studies, blood glucose before therapy begins

• **Bronchospasm:** breath sounds, respiratory pattern

Evaluate:

• Therapeutic response: lower B/P immediately, lower heart rate

Teach patient/family:

• About reason for use, expected results

• To notify prescriber if chest pain, SOB, wheezing, hypotension, bradycardia, pain, swelling at IV site occurs

TREATMENT OF OVERDOSE:

Discontinue product

esomeprazole (Rx)

(es′oh-mep′rah-zohl)

NexIUM

Func. class.: Antiulcer

Chem. class.: Proton-pump inhibitor, benzimidazole

Do not confuse:

NexIUM/NexAVAR

Nurse Alert

ACTION:
Suppresses gastric secretions by inhibiting hydrogen/potassium ATPase enzyme system in gastric parietal cell; characterized as gastric acid pump inhibitor because it blocks the final step of acid production

USES:
Gastroesophageal reflux disease (GERD), adult/child/infant; severe erosive esophagitis, adult/child; treatment of active duodenal ulcers in combination with antiinfectives for *Helicobacter pylori* infection; long-term use for hypersecretory conditions

CONTRAINDICATIONS:
Hypersensitivity to proton-pump inhibitors (PPIs)

Precautions: Pregnancy (B), breastfeeding, children, geriatric patients, hypomagnesemia, osteoporosis

DOSAGE AND ROUTES

Active duodenal ulcers associated with *H. pylori*

- **Adult: PO** 40 mg/day × 10-14 days in combination with clarithromycin 500 mg bid × 10 days and amoxicillin 1000 mg bid × 10 days

Hepatic dose

- **Adult: PO/IV** max 20 mg/day (severe hepatic disease)

GERD/erosive esophagitis

- **Adult: PO** 20 or 40 mg/day × 4-8 wk; no adjustment needed in renal/liver failure, geriatric patients; **IV** 20 or 40 mg/day up to 10 days
- **Adolescent and child 12-17 yr: PO** 20 or 40 mg/day 1 hr before meals for ≤8 wk
- **Child 1-11 yr and ≥20 kg: PO** 10 mg/day 1 hr before meals for ≤8 wk
- **Infant ≥1 mo: IV** 0.5 mg/kg over 10-30 min
- **Infant 1-11 mo (>7.5-12 kg): PO** 10 mg daily × up to 6 wk
- **Infant 1-11 mo (>5-7.5 kg): PO** 5 mg daily × up to 6 wk
- **Infant 1-11 mo (3-5 kg): PO** 2.5 mg daily × up to 6 wk

Available forms: Del rel caps 20, 40 mg; powder for IV inj 20, 40 mg/vial; del rel powder for oral susp 2.5, 5, 10, 20, 40 mg

Administer:

PO route

- Swallow caps whole; do not crush or chew; cap may be opened and sprinkled over Tbsp of applesauce
- Same time daily, 1 hr before meal
- **Oral susp (del rel):** empty contents of packet into container with 1 Tbsp of water, let stand 2-3 min to thicken, restir, give within 30 min of mixing; any residual product should be flushed with more water, taken immediately
- **NG tube (del rel oral susp):** add 15 ml water to contents of packet in syringe, shake, leave 2-3 min to thicken, shake, inject through NG tube within 30 min

IV, direct route

- Reconstitute each vial with 5 ml 0.9% NaCl, D_5W, LR; give over 3 min

Intermittent IV INFUSION route

- Dilute reconstituted sol to 50 ml, give over 30 min, do not admix, flush line with D_5W, 0.9% NaCl, LR after infusion

Solution compatibilities: D_5W, LR, 0.9% NaCl

SIDE EFFECTS

CNS: *Headache, dizziness*

GI: *Diarrhea, flatulence,* abdominal pain, constipation, dry mouth, **hepatic failure, hepatitis,** microscopic colitis

INTEG: *Rash,* dry skin

MISC: **Heart failure**

RESP: *Cough,* **pneumonia**

SYST: **Stevens-Johnson syndrome, toxic epidermal necrolysis, exfoliative dermatitis**

PHARMACOKINETICS
Well absorbed 90%; protein binding 97%; extensively metabolized in liver (CYP2C19); terminal half-life 1-1.5 hr; eliminated in urine as metabolites and in feces; in geriatric patients, elimination rate decreased, bioavailability increased

INTERACTIONS

Increase: effect, toxicity of diazepam, digoxin, penicillins, saquinavir, cilostazol, clozapine, those drugs metabolized by CYP2C19

Increase: effect of methotrexate, tacrolimus, warfarin

Decrease: effect—atazanavir, nelfinavir, dapsone, iron, itraconazole, ketoconazole, indinavir, calcium carbonate, vit B_{12}, clopidogrel, iron salts, mycophenolate

Drug/Lab Test

Interference: sodium, Hgb, WBC, platelets, magnesium

NURSING CONSIDERATIONS

Assess:

- **GI system:** bowel sounds, abdomen for pain, swelling, anorexia, bloody stools; pseudomembranous colitis may occur
- **Hepatic failure, hepatitis:** AST, ALT, alk phos at baseline and periodically during treatment
- **Serious skin disorders:** Stevens-Johnson syndrome, toxic epidermal necrolysis, exfoliative dermatitis

Evaluate:

- Therapeutic response: absence of epigastric pain, swelling, fullness

Teach patient/family:

- To report severe diarrhea; abdominal pain; black, tarry stools, rash; product may have to be discontinued
- That hypoglycemia may occur if diabetic
- To avoid hazardous activities; dizziness may occur
- To avoid alcohol, salicylates, NSAIDs; may cause GI irritation
- To take ≥1 hr before meal; not to crush, chew del rel product, if missed, take as soon as remembered if not almost time for next dose
- If cap is unable to be swallowed, whole contents may be mixed with a Tbsp of applesauce

estradiol (Rx)

(es-tra-dye′ole)

Estrace

estradiol cypionate (Rx)

Depo-Estradiol

estradiol gel (Rx)

Divigel, Elestrin, Estrogel

estradiol spray (Rx)

Evamist

estradiol topical emulsion (Rx)

Estrasorb

estradiol valerate (Rx)

Delestrogen

estradiol transdermal system (Rx)

Alora, Climara, Minivelle, Vivelle-Dot

estradiol vaginal tablet (Rx)

Vagifem

estradiol vaginal ring (Rx)

Estring, Femring

Func. class.: Estrogen, progestins

ACTION: Needed for adequate functioning of female reproductive system; affects release of pituitary gonadotropins; inhibits ovulation, adequate calcium use in bone

USES: Vasomotor symptoms (menopause), inoperable breast cancer (selected cases), prostatic cancer, atrophic vaginitis, kraurosis vulvae, hypogonadism, primary ovarian failure, prevention of osteoporosis, castration

CONTRAINDICATIONS: Pregnancy (X), breastfeeding, reproductive cancer, genital bleeding (abnormal, undiagnosed), protein S or C deficiency, antithrombin deficiency, angioedema, MI, stroke

Black Box Warning: Breast/endometrial cancer, thromboembolic disorders, MI, stroke

Precautions: Hypertension, asthma, blood dyscrasias, gallbladder/bone/renal/hepatic disease, CHF, diabetes mellitus, depression, migraine headache, seizure disorders, family history of cancer of breast or reproductive tract, smoking, uterine fibroids, vaginal irritation/infection, history of angioedema

Black Box Warning: Cardiac disease, dementia, accidental exposure pets/children (topical)

DOSAGE AND ROUTES

Hormone replacement/menopause symptoms

• **Adult: TRANSDERMAL** 1 patch delivering 0.025, 0.0375, 0.05, 0.075, or 0.1 mg/day 2×/wk (Alora, Estraderm, Vivelle-Dot); 1 patch delivering 0.025, 0.0375, 0.05, 0.06, 0.075, or 0.1 mg/day replace q7days (Climara); 1 patch delivering 0.025 mg/day, replace q7days, may increase to 2 patches after 4-6 wk; **GEL** apply entire unit-dose packet to 5 × 7-inch area of upper thigh/day, alternate thighs; **SPRAY** (Evamist) 1 spray to inner surface of forearm/day in AM

Menopause/hypogonadism/castration/ovarian failure

• **Adult: PO** 0.5-2 mg/day, 3 wk on, 1 wk off or continuously; **IM** (cypionate) 1-5 mg q3-4wk; (valerate) 10-20 mg q4wk

• **Adult: TOP** (Estraderm) 0.05 mg/24 hr applied 2×/wk; (Climara) 0.05 mg/hr applied 1×/wk in cyclic regimen; women with hysterectomy may use continuously

Prostatic cancer (inoperable)

• **Adult: IM** (valerate) 30 mg q1-2wk; **PO** (oral estradiol) 1-2 mg bid-tid

Breast cancer (palliative treatment)

• **Adult: PO** 10 mg tid × 3 mo or longer

Atropic vaginitis/kraurosis vulvae

• **Adult: VAG CREAM** 2-4 g/day × 1-2 wk, then 1 g 1-3×/wk cycled; vag tab 1/day × 2 wk, maintenance 1 tab 2×/wk; **VAG RING** inserted, left in place continuously for 3 mo

Vasomotor symptoms

• **Adult: TOP** after cleaning and drying skin on left thigh, calf, rub in contents of pouch using both hands until completely absorbed; wash hands

Available forms: ***Estradiol:*** tabs 0.5, 1, 2 mg; ***valerate:*** inj 10, 20, 40 mg/ml; ***transdermal:*** 0.014, 0.025, 0.0375, 0.05, 0.075, 0.1 mg/24 hr release rate; ***vag cream:*** 100 mcg/g; ***vag tab:*** 10 mcg; ***vag ring:*** 2 mg/90 days; ***topical emulsion:*** 2.5 mg; ***gel*** (Divigel) 0.06%, 0.1%; ***spray*** (Evamist) 1.53 mg/acuation

Administer:

• Titrated dose; use lowest effective dose

• IM inj deeply in large muscle mass

PO route

• With food or milk to decrease GI symptoms

Transdermal route

• May contain aluminum or other metals in backing of patch, can overheat in MRI scan and burn patients

• Apply to trunk of body 2×/wk; press firmly, hold in place for 10 sec to ensure good contact; do not apply to breasts

• On intermittent cycle schedule: 3 wk on, then 1 wk off; if patch falls off, reapply

Topical route

• Use Evamist daily; spray to inner upper arm; may increase to 2-3×/day based on response; allow to dry for 2 min, avoid secondary exposure to children, pets, caregivers

Vaginal route

• Use a new applicator daily, provided

SIDE EFFECTS

CNS: Dizziness, headache, migraines, depression, **seizures**

CV: Hypertension, thrombophlebitis, edema, **thromboembolism, stroke, pulmonary embolism, MI**, chest pain

EENT: Contact lens intolerance, increased myopia, astigmatism, throat swelling, eyelid edema

GI: *Nausea,* vomiting, diarrhea, anorexia, pancreatitis, cramps, constipation, increased appetite, increased weight, cholestatic jaundice, hepatic adenoma

GU: Amenorrhea, cervical erosion, breakthrough bleeding, dysmenorrhea, vaginal candidiasis, breast changes, *gynecomastia, testicular atrophy, impotence,* increased risk of breast cancer, endometrial cancer, changes in libido; toxic shock, vaginal wall ulceration/erosion (vag ring)

INTEG: Rash, urticaria, acne, hirsutism, alopecia, oily skin, seborrhea, purpura, erythema, pruritus, melasma; site irritation (transdermal)

META: Folic acid deficiency, hypercalcemia, hyperglycemia

PHARMACOKINETICS

PO/INJ/TRANSDERMAL: Degraded in liver, excreted in urine, crosses placenta, excreted in breast milk

INTERACTIONS

Increase: action of corticosteroids, tricyclics

Increase: toxicity—cycloSPORINE, dantrolene

Decrease: action of anticoagulants, oral hypoglycemics, tamoxifen

Decrease: estradiol action—anticonvulsants, barbiturates, phenylbutazone, rifampin, calcium

Drug/Herb

- Altered estrogen effect: black cohosh, DHEA

Decrease: estrogen effect—saw palmetto, St. John's wort

Drug/Food

Increase: estrogen level—grapefruit juice

Drug/Lab Test

Increase: BSP retention test, PBI, T_4, serum sodium, platelet aggregation, thyroxine-binding globulin (TBG), prothrombin; factors VII, VIII, IX, X; triglycerides

Decrease: serum folate, serum triglyceride, T_3 resin uptake test, glucose tolerance test, antithrombin III, pregnanediol, metyrapone test

False positive: LE prep, ANA

NURSING CONSIDERATIONS

Assess:

Black Box Warning: For previous breast/endometrial cancer, thrombo-embolic disorders, MI, stroke, dementia, use adequate screening for these conditions, estrogen increases the risk

- Blood glucose of diabetic patient; hyperglycemia may occur
- Weight daily; notify prescriber of weekly weight gain >5 lb; if increase, diuretic may be ordered
- B/P q4hr; watch for increase caused by water and sodium retention
- I&O ratio; decreasing urinary output, increasing edema, report changes
- Hepatic studies, including AST, ALT, bilirubin, alk phos at baseline, periodically; periodic folic acid level
- Hypertension, cardiac symptoms, jaundice, hypercalcemia
- Mental status: affect, mood, behavioral changes, aggression
- Female patient for intact uterus; if so, progesterone should be added to estrogen therapy to decrease risk of endometrial cancer

Evaluate:

- Therapeutic response: reversal of menopause symptoms; decrease in tumor size in prostatic, breast cancer

Teach patient/family:

- To weigh weekly; to report gain >5 lb
- ⚠ To report breast lumps, vaginal bleeding, edema, jaundice, dark urine, clay-colored stools, dyspnea, headache, blurred vision, abdominal pain, numbness or stiffness in legs, chest pain; tenderness, redness, and swelling in extremities; males to report impotence, gynecomastia; to report dermal rash with transdermal patch
- To avoid grapefruit or grapefruit juice (PO)
- That smoking increases CV conditions, encourage to stop

• To notify prescriber if pregnancy is planned or suspected, and not to become pregnant when using estrogen
• To report changes in blood glucose, if diabetic

estrogens, conjugated (Rx)

Cenestin, Premarin

estrogens, conjugated synthetic B (Rx)

Enjuvia

Func. class.: Estrogen, hormone

Do not confuse:
Premarin/Provera

ACTION: Needed for adequate functioning of female reproductive system; affects release of pituitary gonadotropins, inhibits ovulation, adequate calcium use in bone

USES: Vasomotor symptoms (menopause), inoperable breast cancer, prostatic cancer, abnormal uterine bleeding, hypogonadism, primary ovarian failure, prevention of osteoporosis, castration, atrophic vaginitis

Unlabeled uses: Hyperparathyroidism, infertility

CONTRAINDICATIONS: Pregnancy (X), breastfeeding, thromboembolic disorders, reproductive cancer, genital bleeding (abnormal, undiagnosed), hypersensitivity, MI, stroke, thrombophlebitis

Black Box Warning: Endometrial, breast cancer, thromboembolic diseases

Precautions: Hypertension, asthma, blood dyscrasias, CHF, diabetes mellitus, depression, migraine headache, seizure disorders, gallbladder/bone/hepatic/renal disease, family history of cancer of breast or reproductive tract, smoking, dementia, hypothyroidism, obesity, SLE

DOSAGE AND ROUTES

Estrogens conjugated

Vasomotor symptoms (menopause)
• **Adult: PO** 0.3-1.25 mg/day 3 wk on, 1 wk off

Prevention of osteoporosis
• **Adult: PO** 0.3 mg/day or in cycle

Atrophic vaginitis
• **Adult: VAG CREAM** 0.5 g/day × 21 days, off 7 days, repeat

Prostatic cancer
• **Adult: PO** 1.25-2.5 mg tid

Advanced inoperable breast cancer
• **Adult: PO** 10 mg tid × ≥3 mo

Abnormal uterine bleeding
• **Adult: IV/IM** 25 mg q6-12hr

Castration/primary ovarian failure
• **Adult: PO** 1.25 mg/day 3 wk on, 1 wk off

Hypogonadism
• **Adult: PO** 0.3 or 0.625 mg daily (3 wk on, 1 wk off), adjust to response

Estrogens conjugated synthetic B

Vasomotor symptoms (menopause)
• **Adult: PO** 0.625 mg/day initially; may increase based on response

Available forms: Tabs 0.3, 0.45, 0.625, 0.9, 1.25, 2.5 mg; inj 25 mg/vial; vag cream 0.625 mg/g; *synthetic B:* tabs 0.625, 1.25 mg

Administer:
• Titrated dose; use lowest effective dose

PO route
• Give with or immediately after food to reduce nausea

IM route
• IM reconstitute after withdrawing 5 ml of air from container, inject sterile diluent on vial side, rotate to dissolve; give inj deep in large muscle mass, aspirate before inj

Vaginal route
• Use applicator provided, wash after use

Direct IV route
• IV, after reconstituting as for IM, inject into distal port of running IV line of D_5W, 0.9% NaCl at ≤5 mg/min

Y-site compatibilities: Heparin, hydrocortisone, potassium chloride, vit B/C

SIDE EFFECTS

CNS: Dizziness, headache, migraine, depression, **seizures**, mood disturbances
CV: Hypertension, thrombophlebitis, edema, **thromboembolism, stroke, pulmonary embolism, MI**, chest pain
EENT: Contact lens intolerance, increased myopia, astigmatism
GI: *Nausea,* vomiting, diarrhea, anorexia, pancreatitis, cramps, constipation, increased appetite, **cholestatic jaundice, hepatic adenoma**, weight gain/loss
GU: Amenorrhea, cervical erosion, breakthrough bleeding, dysmenorrhea, vaginal candidiasis, breast changes, *gynecomastia, testicular atrophy, impotence,* **increased risk of breast cancer, endometrial cancer**, libido changes
INTEG: Rash, urticaria, acne, hirsutism, alopecia, oily skin, seborrhea, purpura, melasma
META: Folic acid deficiency, hypercalcemia, hyperglycemia

PHARMACOKINETICS

PO/IM/IV: Degraded in liver, excreted in urine, crosses placenta, excreted in breast milk

INTERACTIONS

Increase: toxicity—cycloSPORINE, dantrolene
Increase: action of corticosteroids
Decrease: action of estrogens—anticonvulsants, barbiturates, phenylbutazone, rifampin, bosentan
Decrease: action of anticoagulants, oral hypoglycemics, tamoxifen, thyroid, tricyclics

Drug/Food

Increase: estrogen level—grapefruit juice

Drug/Lab Test

Increase: BSP retention test, PBI, T_4, serum sodium, platelet aggregation, thyroxine-binding globulin (TBG), prothrombin; factors VII, VIII, IX, X; triglycerides
Decrease: serum folate, serum triglyceride, T_3 resin uptake test, glucose tolerance test, antithrombin III, pregnanediol, metyrapone test
False positive: LE prep, antinuclear antibodies

NURSING CONSIDERATIONS

Assess:

Black Box Warning: Breast, endometrial cancer: estrogens should not be used in known, suspected, or history of these disorders

Black Box Warning: Stroke, thromboembolic disease of MI: Should not be used in these conditions or known protein C deficiency, protein S deficiency, or antithrombin deficiency

- Blood glucose if diabetic patient; hyperglycemia may occur
- Weight daily; notify prescriber of weekly weight gain >5 lb; if increase, diuretic may be ordered; check for edema; B/P baseline and periodically
- Hepatic studies: AST, ALT, bilirubin, alk phos
- Hypertension, cardiac symptoms, jaundice, hypercalcemia
- Mental status: affect, mood, behavioral changes, aggression
- Female patient for intact uterus; if so, progesterone should be added to estrogen therapy to decrease risk of endometrial cancer; abnormal uterine bleeding, breast exam; Pap smear

Evaluate:

- Therapeutic response: absence of breast engorgement, reversal of menopause symptoms, decrease in tumor size with prostatic cancer

Teach patient/family:

- To avoid breastfeeding, since product excreted in breast milk
- To weigh weekly; to report gain >5 lb

Black Box Warning: To report breast lumps, vaginal bleeding, edema, jaundice, dark urine, clay-colored stools, dyspnea, headache, blurred vision, abdominal pain; leg pain and redness, numbness or stiffness; chest pain; males to report impotence or gynecomastia

- To avoid sunlight or wear sunscreen; burns may occur
- To notify prescriber if pregnancy is suspected
- That vasomotor symptoms improve in 2 wk, max relief in 8 wk

⚠ HIGH ALERT

eszopiclone (Rx)

(es-zop′i-klone)

Lunesta

Func. class.: Sedative/hypnotic, nonbenzodiazepine

Chem. class.: Cyclopyrrolone

Controlled Substance Schedule IV

ACTION: Interacts with GABA receptors

USES: Insomnia

CONTRAINDICATIONS: Hypersensitivity

Precautions: Pregnancy (C), breastfeeding, children, geriatric patients, severe hepatic disease, abrupt discontinuation, COPD, depression, labor, sleep apnea, substance abuse, suicidal ideation, ethanol intoxication

DOSAGE AND ROUTES

- **Adult: PO** 1 mg immediately before bed, may increase to 3 mg if needed

Hepatic dose/CYP3A4 inhibitors

- **Adult: PO** 1 mg immediately before bed with severe hepatic disease, max 2 mg/day

Available forms: Tabs 1, 2, 3 mg

Administer:

- Do not break, crush, or chew tab
- Immediately before bedtime; avoid use with food; for short-term use only

SIDE EFFECTS

CNS: Worsening depression, hallucinations, headache, daytime drowsiness, suicidal thoughts/actions, migraine, restlessness, anxiety, sleep driving, sleepwalking

CV: Peripheral edema, chest pain

GI: Dry mouth, bitter taste (dysgeusia)

GU: Gynecomastia, dysmenorrhea

INTEG: Rash, angioedema

PHARMACOKINETICS

Onset rapid; peak 1 hr; duration 6 hr; extensively metabolized in the liver by CYP3A4, CYP2E1; excreted via kidneys; half-life 6 hr, geriatric patients 9 hr, protein binding 52%-59%

INTERACTIONS

Increase: CNS depression—CNS depressants

Increase: toxicity due to decreased eszopiclone elimination—CYP3A4 inhibitors (clarithromycin, itraconazole, ketoconazole, nefazodone, nelfinavir, ritonavir, troleandomycin, SSRIs)

Decrease: eszopiclone effect—CYP3A4 inducers (dexamethasone, barbiturates, carbamazepine, oxcarbazepine, phenytoin, fosphenytoin, ethotoin)

Drug/Food

Decrease: product action—food

Drug/Herb

Decrease: eszopiclone effect—St. John's Wort

NURSING CONSIDERATIONS

Assess:

- **Sleep pattern:** ability to go to sleep, stay asleep, early morning awakenings, conservative methods used
- For abuse of this product, other products
- **Anaphylaxis, angioedema:** monitor during first dose
- Alternative methods to improve sleep: reading, quiet environment, warm bath, milk
- Assistance with ambulation, night light, call bell within reach

Evaluate:

- Therapeutic response: ability to fall asleep and stay asleep throughout the night

Teach patient/family:

- That daytime drowsiness may occur; not to engage in hazardous activities until effect is known; that memory problems may occur

- That all other medications and supplements should be avoided unless approved by prescriber; to avoid alcohol
- To notify prescriber if pregnancy is suspected or planned
- To avoid use after a high-fat meal
- To swallow tab whole
- Not to stop drug abruptly, tolerance may occur

etanercept (Rx)

(eh-tan′er-sept)

Enbrel

Func. class.: Antirheumatic agent (disease modifying) (DMARDs)

Chem. class.: Anti-TNF agent

ACTION: Binds tumor necrosis factor (TNF), which is involved in immune and inflammatory reactions

USES: Acute, chronic rheumatoid arthritis that has not responded to other disease-modifying agents, polyarticular course of juvenile rheumatoid arthritis (JRA), ankylosing spondylitis, plaque psoriasis, psoriatic arthritis

Unlabeled uses: Crohn's disease; plaque psoriasis (child ≥4 yr)

CONTRAINDICATIONS: Sepsis

Precautions: Pregnancy (B), breastfeeding, children <4 yr, geriatric patients, malignancies, CHF, seizures, multiple sclerosis, latex hypersensitivity

Black Box Warning: Infection, lymphoma, neoplastic disease, TB

DOSAGE AND ROUTES

Rheumatoid/psoriatic arthritis, ankylosing spondylitis

- **Adult: SUBCUT** 50 mg/wk or 25 mg 2×/wk, 3-4 days apart; may be used with methotrexate for psoriatic arthritis
- **Child 2-17 yr: SUBCUT** 0.8 mg/kg/wk, max 50 mg/wk

Plaque psoriasis

- **Adult: SUBCUT** 50 mg 2×/wk × 3 mo, then 50 mg q wk maintenance
- **Adolescent/child 4-17 yr (unlabeled): SUBCUT** 0.8 mg/kg/wk, max 50 mg/wk

Juvenile rheumatoid arthritis (JRA)

- **Adolescent/child 2-17 yr: SUBCUT** 0.8 mg/kg/wk, max 50 mg/wk

Available forms: Powder for inj 25 mg; inj 50 mg/ml; autoinjector, single use

Administer:

- May be administered by the patient or a caregiver. Assess the patient's or caregiver's ability to inject subcut and observe the first injection
- Administration of one 50-mg/ml prefilled syringe or autoinjector provides a dose equivalent to two 25-mg prefilled syringes or two 25-mg vials of lyophilized
- The needle cap on the prefilled syringe and on the SureClick autoinjector contain dry natural rubber (latex) and should not be handled by persons sensitive to this product

Route-Specific Use

Injectable Use

- Inspect for particulate matter and discoloration before use, solution should be clear and colorless, although small white particles may be noted in the autoinjector or prefilled syringe

Subcut Use

- Injection sites include front of the thigh, abdomen except the 2 in around the navel, or outer area of the upper arm; rotate injection sites; do not administer where skin is tender, bruised, red, or hard; do not inject directly into any raised, thick, red, or scaly skin patches or lesions related to psoriasis

Reconstitution and administration of the vial:

- Do not mix or transfer the contents of one vial into another vial; do not filter reconstituted product during preparation or administration; do not add other medications to solutions containing etanercept; ONLY use the supplied diluent

• A vial adaptor is supplied for use when reconstituting the powder; however, the adaptor should not be used if multiple doses are going to be withdrawn from the vial; to reconstitute using the vial adaptor, slide the plunger into the flange end of the syringe; attach the plunger to the gray rubber stopper in the syringe by turning the plunger clockwise until a slight resistance is felt; remove the twist-off cap from the prefilled diluent syringe by turning counterclockwise; once the twist-off cap is removed, twist the vial adapter onto the syringe clockwise until a slight resistance is felt; place the vial adapter over the top of the vial, being careful not to bump or touch the plunger, the plastic spike inside the vial adapter should puncture the gray stopper; push the plunger down until all the liquid from the syringe is in the vial and gently swirl to dissolve the powder; after the diluent is added, some foaming may occur; do not shake; generally, dissolution takes less than 10 min; the solution should be clear and colorless. Each reconstituted vial contains 25 mg/ml of etanercept; turn the vial upside down and slowly pull the plunger down to the unit markings on the side of the syringe that correspond with the needed dose; gently tap the syringe to make any air bubbles rise to the top of the syringe, and slowly push the plunger up to remove them; remove the syringe from the vial adapter by turning the syringe counterclockwise and attach the 27-gauge needle

• If the vial will be used for multiple doses, use a 25-gauge needle for reconstituting and withdrawing the solution; insert the 25-gauge needle or the vial adapter straight into the center of the gray stopper; a "pop" will be felt; inject the diluent very slowly; after the diluent is added, some foaming may occur; do not shake; swirl contents gently during dissolution; generally, dissolution takes less than 10 minutes; the solution should be clear and colorless; write the mixing date on the supplied sticker and attach to the vial; each reconstituted vial contains 25 mg/ml of etanercept; withdraw the correct dose of the solution into the syringe; remove any air bubbles; remove the 25-gauge needle from the syringe; attach a 27-gauge needle

• Hold the barrel of the syringe with one hand and pull the needle cover straight off; hold the syringe in one hand like a pencil and use the other hand to gently pinch a fold of skin at the cleaned injection site; insert the needle at a 45-degree angle to the skin; let go of the skin and hold the syringe near its base to stabilize it; push the plunger to inject all of the solution at a slow, steady rate; withdraw the needle at the same angle as insertion; do NOT rub the site

• Use as soon as possible after reconstitution; place reconstituted vials for multiple doses in the refrigerator at 36°-46° F (2°-8° C) within 4 hr of reconstitution and may be stored up to 14 days; DO NOT FREEZE

• **Use of the SureClick autoinjector:** allow to reach room temperature, do not shake; immediately before use, remove the needle shield by pulling it straight off

• Stretch the skin under and around the prefilled autoinjector, place the open end against the injection site at a 90-degree angle; without pushing the purple button on top, push the autoinjector firmly against the skin to unlock; press the purple button on top once and release the button; listen for the first click; wait for the second click or wait 15 seconds, and remove the autoinjector from injection site; do NOT rub the site

• Look at the inspection window; if it is not purple, call 1-888-436-2735; do not try to reuse the autoinjector

Use of the prefilled syringe:

• **Single-use:** allow to reach room temperature, do not shake; remove the needle shield; check to see if the amount of liquid in the prefilled syringe falls between the two purple fill level indicator lines on the syringe; if bubbles are seen, gently tap the syringe; turn the syringe so that the purple horizontal lines on the barrel are directly facing you; do not use if the syringe does not have the right amount of liquid

• Hold the barrel of the prefilled syringe with one hand and pull the needle cover straight off; holding the syringe with the needle pointing up, check the syringe for air bubbles; if there are bubbles, gently tap until the air bubbles rise to the top of the syringe; slowly push the plunger up to force the air bubbles out of the syringe

• Insert the needle at a 45-degree angle to the pinched skin; push the plunger to inject all of the solution at a slow, steady rate; withdraw the needle at the same angle as insertion; do NOT rub the site

SIDE EFFECTS

CNS: *Headache,* asthenia, dizziness, seizures

CV: Heart failure

GI: Abdominal pain, dyspepsia, vomiting, hepatitis, diarrhea

HEMA: Pancytopenia, anemia, thrombocytopenia, leukopenia, neutropenia

INTEG: Rash, *inj-site reaction,* keratoderma blenorrhagicum

RESP: *Pharyngitis, cough, URI, non-URI,* sinusitis, *rhinitis*

SYST: Serious infections, sepsis, death, malignancies, Stevens-Johnson syndrome, reactivation of hepatitis B virus, lupus-like syndrome

PHARMACOKINETICS

Elimination half-life 102 hr, 60% absorbed (SUBCUT)

INTERACTIONS

• **Increase:** neutropenia—sulfaSALAzine

• Do not give concurrently with live virus vaccines; immunizations should be brought up to date before treatment

• Avoid use with anakinra, cyclophosphamide, rilonacept

Drug/Lab Test

Increase: LFTs

NURSING CONSIDERATIONS

Assess:

• **RA:** pain, stiffness, ROM, swelling of joints before, during, after treatment

• For inj-site pain, swelling; usually occurs after 2 inj (4-5 days)

Black Box Warning: Infection: patients using immunosuppressives, corticosteroids, methotrexate at greater risk; assess for fever, discontinue in those who develop a serious infection, do not use in active infection

• **Hypersensitivity:** to this product, latex needle cap, benzyl alcohol; usual reactions to product last 3-5 days

Evaluate:

• Therapeutic response: decreased inflammation, pain in joints

Teach patient/family:

• That product must be continued for prescribed time to be effective

• To use caution when driving; dizziness may occur

• Not to receive live vaccinations during treatment

• About self-administration if appropriate: inj should be made in thigh, abdomen, upper arm; rotate sites at least 1 in from previous site, check for inj reactions that last 3-5 days

• To notify prescriber of possible infection (upper respiratory, other)

ethambutol (Rx)

(e-tham′byoo-tole)

Etibi ♣, Myambutol

Func. class.: Antitubercular

Chem. class.: Diisopropylethylene diamide derivative

Do not confuse:

ethambutol/Ethmozine

ACTION: Inhibits RNA synthesis, decreases tubercle bacilli replication

USES: Pulmonary TB as an adjunct, other mycobacterial infections

CONTRAINDICATIONS: Children <13 yr, hypersensitivity, optic neuritis

Precautions: Pregnancy (B), breastfeeding, renal disease, diabetic retinopathy, cataracts, ocular defects, hepatic and hematopoietic disorders

DOSAGE AND ROUTES

• **Adult/child >13 yr: PO** 15-25 mg/kg/day as single dose (treatment naive) or 25 mg/kg daily (treatment experienced)

Renal disease

• CCr 10-50 ml/min, dose q24-36hr; CCr <10 ml/min, dose q48hr

Retreatment

• **Adult: PO** 25 mg/kg/day as single dose × 2 mo with at least 1 other product, then decrease to 15 mg/kg/day as single dose, max 2.5 g/day

• **Child: PO** 15 mg/kg/day

Available forms: Tabs 100, 400 mg

Administer:

• With meals to decrease GI symptoms
• Antiemetic if vomiting occurs
• After C&S completed; monthly to detect resistance
• 4 hr between this product and antacids

SIDE EFFECTS

CNS: *Headache, confusion,* fever, malaise, dizziness, *disorientation,* hallucinations, peripheral neuropathy

EENT: Blurred vision, optic neuritis, photophobia, decreased visual acuity

GI: *Abdominal distress, anorexia, nausea, vomiting*

INTEG: Dermatitis, pruritus, **toxic epidermal necrolysis**, erythema multiforme

META: *Elevated uric acid, acute gout,* impaired hepatic function

MISC: **Thrombocytopenia**, joint pain, **anaphylaxis**

PHARMACOKINETICS

Peak 2-4 hr, half-life 3 hr, metabolized in liver, excreted in urine (unchanged product/inactive metabolites, unchanged product in feces)

INTERACTIONS

• Delayed absorption of ethambutol: aluminum salts, separate by 4 hr
• **Neurotoxicity: other neurotoxics**

NURSING CONSIDERATIONS

Assess:

• Hepatic studies weekly × 2 wk, then q2mo: ALT, AST, bilirubin; decreased appetite, jaundice, dark urine, fatigue
• Signs of anemia: Hct, Hgb, fatigue
• Mental status often: affect, mood, behavioral changes; psychosis may occur
• C&S, including sputum, before treatment
• Visual status: decreased activity, altered color perception
• **Serious skin reactions: toxic epidermal necrolysis**

Evaluate:

• Therapeutic response: decreased symptoms of TB, decrease in acid-fast bacteria

Teach patient/family:

• To avoid alcohol products
• That compliance with dosage schedule, duration is necessary
• That scheduled appointments must be kept or relapse may occur
• **To report to prescriber any visual changes; rash; hot, swollen, painful joints; numbness, tingling of extremities**

etodolac

(ee-toe′doe-lak)

Ultradol ♣

Func. class.: Nonsteroidal antiinflammatory/nonopioid analgesic

ACTION: Inhibits COX1,2; analgesic, antiinflammatory

USES: Mild to moderate pain, osteoarthritis, rheumatoid arthritis, arthralgia, myalgia, juvenile rheumatoid arthritis

CONTRAINDICATIONS: Hypersensitivity; patients in whom aspirin, iodides, or NSAIDs have produced asthma; urticaria

Black Box Warning: **Coronary artery bypass graft surgery (CABG)**

Precautions: Edema, renal/hepatic disease, children, GI ulcers, geriatric patients, bronchospasm, nasal polyps, alcoholism, bone marrow suppression, MI, hemophilia, neutropenia, ulcerative colitis

Black Box Warning: GI bleeding, perforation, MI, stroke

DOSAGE AND ROUTES

Osteoarthritis

- **Adult: PO** 300 mg bid-tid, or 400-500 mg bid initially, then adjust dosage to 600-1200 mg/day in divided doses; max 1200 mg/day; ext rel 400-1000 mg daily

Analgesia

- **Adult: PO** 200-400 mg every 6-8 hr up to 1000 mg daily; max 1200 mg/day; patients <60 kg, max 20 mg/kg; ext rel 400-1000 mg daily

Available forms: Caps 200, 300 mg; tabs 400, 500 mg; ext rel 400, 500, 600 mg

Administer:

- Without regard to food
- Store at room temperature

SIDE EFFECTS

CNS: Dizziness, headache, drowsiness, fatigue, tremors, confusion, insomnia, anxiety, depression, light-headedness, vertigo

CV: Tachycardia, peripheral edema, fluid retention, palpitations, dysrhythmias, CHF

EENT: Tinnitus, hearing loss, blurred vision, photophobia

GI: Nausea, anorexia, vomiting, diarrhea, jaundice, cholestatic hepatitis, constipation, flatulence, cramps, dry mouth, peptic ulcer, dyspepsia, GI bleeding

GU: Nephrotoxicity: dysuria, hematuria, oliguria, azotemia, cystitis, urinary tract infection

HEMA: Blood dyscrasias

INTEG: Erythema, urticaria, purpura, rash, pruritus, sweating, Stevens-Johnson syndrome

SYST: Angioedema, anaphylaxis

PHARMACOKINETICS

Peak $1\frac{1}{2}$-2 hr, serum protein binding >99%, half-life 7 hr; metabolized by liver (metabolites excreted in urine)

INTERACTIONS

Increase: toxicity—cycloSPORINE, digoxin, lithium, methotrexate, phenytoin, cidofovir, aminoglycosides

Black Box Warning: Increase: GI toxicity—aspirin, NSAIDs

Decrease: effect of—etodolac: antacids

Decrease: effect of—beta blockers, diuretics

Drug/Lab Test

Increase: BUN, creatinine

Decrease: Hgb/Hct, WBC

NURSING CONSIDERATIONS

Assess:

- **Pain:** location, frequency, characteristics; relief after medication
- Blood, renal, liver tests: BUN, creatinine, AST, ALT, Hgb, platelets before treatment, periodically thereafter
- For GI bleeding: black stools, hematemesis
- Audiometric, ophthalmic examination before, during, after treatment
- For eye, ear problems: blurred vision, tinnitus; can indicate toxicity
- For asthma, aspirin hypersensitivity, nasal polyps that may be hypersensitive to etodolac

Evaluate:

- Therapeutic response: decreased pain, stiffness, swelling in joints, ability to move more easily

Teach patient/family:

- To report blurred vision or ringing, roaring in the ears; might indicate toxicity
- Not to break, crush, or chew ext rel tabs
- To report change in urine pattern, weight increase, edema, pain increase in joints, fever, blood in urine; indicates nephrotoxicity

• That therapeutic effects can take up to 1 mo

Black Box Warning: To avoid aspirin, NSAIDs, acetaminophen, alcoholic beverages while taking this medication

⚠ HIGH ALERT

etoposide (Rx)

(e-toe-poe′side)

Toposar, VePesid ♣

etoposide phosphate (Rx)

Etopophos

Func. class.: Antineoplastic—miscellaneous

Chem. class.: Semisynthetic podophyllotoxin

ACTION: Inhibits cells from entering mitosis, depresses DNA/RNA synthesis, cell-cycle–specific S and G_2; binds to a complex of DNA and topoisomerase II leading to DNA strand breaks

USES: Testicular cancer, small-cell lung cancer

Unlabeled uses: Leukemias (ALL, AML), desmoid tumor, gastric/ovarian cancer, bone marrow ablation, Hodgkin's/non-Hodgkin's lymphoma, malignant glioma, neuroblastoma, stem cell transplant preparation, trophoblastic disease

CONTRAINDICATIONS: Pregnancy (D), breastfeeding, hypersensitivity

Precautions: Children, renal/hepatic disease, gout, neutropenia, thrombocytopenia

Black Box Warning: Bone marrow depression, infection, bleeding, requires an experienced clinician

DOSAGE AND ROUTES

Testicular cancer

• **Adult: IV** 100 mg/m²/day on days 1, 2 in combination with bleomycin and Cisplatin (BEP) or 100 mg/m²/day on days 1, 3, 5 or 100 mg/m²/day on days 1, 3, 5, repeat q3-4wk

Renal dose

• **Adult: IV** CCr 45-60 ml/min, reduce dose by 15%; CCr 30-44 ml/min, reduce dose by 20%; CCr <30 ml/min, reduce dose by 25%

Hepatic dose

• **Adult: IV/PO** total bilirubin 1.5-3 mg/dl: reduce dose by 50%; total bilirubin 3-5 mg/dl: reduce dose by 75%; total bilirubin >5 mg/dl: hold

Available forms: Inj 20 mg/ml; 100 mg powder for injection, caps 50 mg

Administer:

• Antiemetic 30-60 min before product and prn to prevent vomiting

• **Urate nephropathy:** Allopurinol, aggressive alkalinization to maintain uric acid levels

• Antispasmodic, EPINEPHrine, corticosteroids, antihistamines for reactions

PO route

• Give without regard to food

• Increase fluid intake to 2-3 L/day to prevent urate deposits, calculi formation

• Refrigerate oral product; do not freeze

IV route

• Do not use acrylic or ABS plastic devices; may crack, leak

Intermittent IV INFUSION route (etoposide)

• Use cytotoxic handling procedures, use Luer-Lok fittings to prevent leakage

• After **diluting** 5-ml vial with 100 mg/250 ml or more D_5W or NaCl to 0.2-0.4 mg/ml, **infuse** over 30-60 min

Y-site compatibilities: Acyclovir, alfentanil, allopurinol, amifostine, amikacin, aminocaproic acid, aminophylline, amiodarone, amphotericin B colloidal, amphotericin B lipid complex, amphotericin B liposome, ampicillin, ampicillin-sulbactam, anidulafungin, atenolol, atracurium, aztreonam, bivalirudin, bleomycin, bumetanide, buprenorphine, butorphanol, calcium chloride/gluconate, CARBOplatin, caspofungin, ceFAZolin, cefotaxime, cefoTEtan, cefOXitin, cefTAZidime, ceftizoxime, cefTRIAXone, cefuroxime, chloramphenicol, chlorproMAZINE, cimetidine, ciprofloxacin, cisatracurium, CISplatin, cladribine, clindamycin, codeine, cyclophosphamide, cycloSPORINE, cytarabine, DACTINomycin, DAPTOmycin, DAUNOrubicin, dexamethasone, dexmedetomidine, dexrazoxane, digoxin, diltiazem, diphenhydrAMINE, DOBUTamine, DOCEtaxel, DOPamine, doxacurium, DOXOrubicin, DOXOrubicin liposomal, doxycycline, droperidol, enalaprilat, ePHEDrine, EPINEPHrine, epirubicin, ertapenem, erythromycin, esmolol, famotidine, fenoldopam, fentaNYL, floxuridine, fluconazole, fludarabine, fluorouracil, foscarnet, fosphenytoin, furosemide, ganciclovir, gatifloxacin, gemcitabine, gentamicin, glycopyrrolate, granisetron, haloperidol, heparin, hydrALAZINE, hydrocortisone, HYDROmorphone, hydrOXYzine, ifosfamide, imipenem-cilastatin, inamrinone, insulin (regular), irinotecan, isoproterenol, ketorolac, labetalol, lansoprazole, leucovorin, levofloxacin, levorphanol, lidocaine, linezolid, LORazepam, magnesium sulfate, mannitol, mechlorethamine, melphalan, meperidine, meropenem, mesna, methohexital, methotrexate, methyldopate, methylPREDNISolone, metoclopramide, metoprolol, metroNIDAZOLE, micafungin, midazolam, milrinone, minocycline, mitoXANtrone, mivacurium, morphine, nafcillin, nalbuphine, naloxone, nesiritide, nitroglycerin, nitroprusside, norepinephrine, NS, octreotide, ofloxacin, ondansetron, oxaliplatin, PACLitaxel, palonosetron, pamidronate, pancuronium, PEMEtrexed, pentamidine, pentazocine, PENTobarbital, PHENobarbital, phenylephrine, piperacillin, piperacillin-tazobactam, polymyxin B, potassium chloride/phosphates, procainamide, prochlorperazine, promethazine, propranolol, quinupristin-dalfopristin, ranitidine, remifentanil, rocuronium, sargramostim, sodium acetate/bicarbonate/phosphates, succinylcholine, SUFentanil, sulfamethoxazole-trimethoprim, tacrolimus, teniposide, theophylline, thiotepa, ticarcillin, ticarcillin-clavulanate, tigecycline, tirofiban, tobramycin, topotecan, trimethobenzamide, vancomycin, vasopressin, vecuronium, verapamil, vinBLAStine, vinCRIStine, vinorelbine, voriconazole, zidovudine, zoledronic acid

Intermittent IV INFUSION route (etoposide phosphate)

- **Reconstitute** each vial with 5 or 10 ml of D_5W, 0.9% NaCl for a concentrations of 20 mg/ml or 10 mg/ml, respectively; may give diluted or undiluted to concentrations of as little as 0.1 mg/ml, **give** over 5-210 min

Y-site compatibilities: Acyclovir, alfentanil, amifostine, amikacin, aminocaproic acid, aminophylline, amiodarone, ampicillin, ampicillin-sulbactam, anidulafungin, atenolol, atracurium, aztreonam, bivalirudin, bleomycin, bumetanide, buprenorphine, butorphanol, calcium acetate/chloride/gluconate, CARBOplatin, carmustine, caspofungin, ceFAZolin, cefonicid, cefoperazone, cefotaxime, cefoTEtan, cefOXitin, cefTAZidime, ceftizoxime, cefTRIAXone, cefuroxime, chloramphenicol, cimetidine, ciprofloxacin, cisatracurium, CISplatin, clindamycin, codeine, cyclophosphamide, cycloSPORINE, cytarabine, dacarbazine, DACTINomycin, DAPTOmycin, DAUNOrubicin, dexamethasone, digoxin, diltiazem, diphenhydrAMINE, DOBUTamine, DOCEtaxel, DOPamine, doripenem, doxacurium, DOXOrubicin, HCL/liposome, doxycycline, enalaprilat, ePHEDrine, EPINEPHrine, epirubicin, ertapenem, erythromycin, esmolol, famotidine, fenoldopam, fentaNYL, floxuridine, fluconazole, fludarabine, fluorouracil, foscarnet, fosphenytoin, furosemide, ganciclovir, gatifloxacin, gemcitabine, gentamicin, glycopyrrolate, granisetron, haloperidol, heparin, hydrALAZINE, hydrocortisone, HYDROmorphone, hydrOXYzine, IDArubicin, ifosfamide, inamrinone, insulin (regular), irinotecan, isoproterenol, ketorolac, labetalol, leucovorin, levofloxacin, levorphanol, lidocaine, linezolid, LORazepam, magnesium sulfate, mannitol, mechlorethamine, meperidine, meropenem, mesna, metaraminol, methotrexate, methyldopate, metoclopramide, metoprolol, metroNIDAZOLE, midazolam, milrinone, minocycline, mitoXANtrone, mivacurium, morphine, nafcillin, nalbuphine, naloxone, nesiritide, netilmicin, nitroglycerin, nitroprusside, norepinephrine, octreotide, ofloxacin, ondansetron, oxaliplatin, PACLitaxel, palonosetron, pamidronate, pancuronium, PEMEtrexed, pentamidine, pentazocine, PENTobarbital, PHENobarbital, phenylephrine, piperacillin, piperacillin-tazobactam, plicamycin, polymyxin B, potassium chloride/phosphates, procainamide, promethazine, propranolol, quiNIDine, quinupristin-dalfopristin, ranitidine, remifentanil, riTUXimab, rocuronium, sodium acetate/bicarbonate/phosphates, streptozocin, succinylcholine, SUFentanil, sulfamethoxazole-trimethoprim, tacrolimus, teniposide, theophylline, thiopental, thiotepa, ticarcillin, ticarcillin-clavulanate, tigecycline, tirofiban, tobramycin, tolazoline, trastuzumab, trimethobenzamide, vancomycin, vasopressin, vecuronium, verapamil, vinBLAStine, vinCRIStine, vinorelbine, voriconazole, zidovudine, zoledronic acid

SIDE EFFECTS

CNS: Headache, *fever,* peripheral neuropathy, paresthesias, confusion, chills, fever

CV: *Hypotension,* MI, dysrhythmias

GI: *Nausea, vomiting, anorexia,* hepatotoxicity, dyspepsia, diarrhea, constipation

GU: Nephrotoxicity

HEMA: Thrombocytopenia, leukopenia, myelosuppression, anemia

INTEG: *Rash, alopecia,* phlebitis at IV site, **Stevens-Johnson syndrome**

RESP: Bronchospasm

SYST: **Anaphylaxis,** secondary malignancy

PHARMACOKINETICS

Half-life ½-2 hr (initial), terminal 5¼ hr, metabolized in liver, excreted in urine, feces, crosses placental barrier, protein binding 95%

INTERACTIONS

Increase: bone marrow depression—other antineoplastics, radiation, immunosuppressives

Increase: adverse reactions—live virus vaccines, toxoids

Increase: effect of etoposide, toxicity—voriconazole, conivaptan, cycloSPORINE, imatinib, nilotinib, etravirine, telithromycin

Increase: risk of bleeding—anticoagulants, NSAIDs, platelet inhibitors, thrombolytics, salicylate

Decrease: etoposide effect—sargramostim, filgrastim, separate by ≥24 hr

Drug/Food

• Decreased oral etoposide—grapefruit juice

Drug/Lab Test

Decrease: platelets, RBC, WBC, neutrophils, Hgb, calcium, phosphate

Increase: uric acid, potassium

NURSING CONSIDERATIONS

Assess:

Black Box Warning: Bone marrow depression: CBC, differential, platelet count weekly; withhold product if WBC is <500 or platelet count is <50,000; notify prescriber, treatment should be delayed

• **Nephrotoxicity:** BUN; serum uric acid; urine CCr; electrolytes before, during therapy; I&O ratio; report fall in urine output to <30 ml/hr; check B/P bid, report any significant decrease

Black Box Warning: Infection: Monitor temperature; fever may indicate beginning infection, treat active infection before treatment

Black Box Warning: Hepatotoxicity: Hepatic studies before, during therapy (bilirubin, AST, ALT, LDH) as needed or monthly

Black Box Warning: Bleeding: hematuria, guaiac stools, bruising or petechiae, mucosa or orifices q8hr

- Effects of alopecia on body image; discuss feelings about body changes
- **Hepatotoxicity:** Jaundice of skin and sclera, dark urine, clay-colored stools, itchy skin, abdominal pain, fever, diarrhea
- B/P q15min during infusion; if systolic reading <90 mm Hg, discontinue infusion, notify prescriber
- Buccal cavity q8hr for dryness, sores or ulceration, white patches, oral pain, bleeding, dysphagia
- **Injection-site reaction:** monitor site closely for infiltration
- Local irritation, pain, burning, discoloration at inj site

⚠ **Symptoms indicating severe allergic reaction:** rash, pruritus, urticaria, purpuric skin lesions, itching, flushing, restlessness, coughing, difficulty breathing

- **Frequency of stools, characteristics:** cramping, acidosis; **signs of dehydration:** rapid respirations, poor skin turgor, decreased urine output, dry skin, restlessness, weakness
- **Geriatric patients:** increased alopecia, GI effects, infection, nephrotoxicity, myelosuppression

Black Box Warning: An experienced clinician knowledgeable in the use of cytotoxic products

Evaluate:
- Therapeutic response: decreased tumor size, spread of malignancy

Teach patient/family:
- To report any changes in breathing or coughing
- That hair may be lost during treatment; that a wig or hairpiece may make patient feel better; that new hair may be different in color, texture
- That metallic taste may occur

Black Box Warning: Infection: To report symptoms of infection (fever, sore throat); to avoid crowds, persons with known infections

- To avoid immunizations
- **Pregnancy:** To notify prescriber if pregnancy is planned or suspected pregnancy (D); to use reliable contraception during and for several mo after therapy; to avoid breastfeeding
- To take as prescribed (PO), not to double dose
- To report signs of infection (flu-like symptoms, fever, fatigue, sore throat)
- To take B/P, hypotension occurs

etravirine (Rx)
(e-tra′veer-een)

Intelence

Func. class.: Antiretroviral

Chem. class.: Nonnucleoside reverse transcriptase inhibitor (NNRTI)

ACTION: Binds directly to reverse transcriptase, thus blocking the RNA- and DNA-dependent DNA polymerase action and causing a disruption of the enzyme's catalytic site

USES: In combination with other antiretroviral agents for HIV infection in treatment-experienced patients with evidence of HIV replication despite ongoing antiretroviral therapy

CONTRAINDICATIONS: Breastfeeding, hypersensitivity

Precautions: Pregnancy (B), children, geriatric patients, impaired hepatic function, antimicrobial resistance, hepatitis, hypercholesterolemia, hypertriglycerides, immune reconstitution syndrome

DOSAGE AND ROUTES
- **Adult/Child/Adolescent ≥6 yr, ≥30 kg: PO** 200 mg bid; Child/Adolescent ≥6 yr, 25 to 29 kg: 150 mg bid; Child/Adolescent ≥6 yr, 20 to 24 kg: 125 mg bid; Child/Adolescent ≥6 yr, 16 to 19 kg:100 mg bid

Available forms: Tabs 25, 100, 200 mg

Administer:
- In combination with other antiretrovirals with food or after a meal

• Tabs may be dispersed in ≥5 ml of water; once dispersed, stir well, give immediately, rinse glass, have patient drink to ensure all medication taken
• Store in cool environment; protect from light

SIDE EFFECTS

CNS: *Headache, insomnia,* amnesia, anxiety, confusion, fatigue, nightmares, peripheral neuropathy, **seizures, stroke,** tremor
CV: **Atrial fibrillation,** hypertension, MI
EENT: Blurred vision
GI: *Nausea, vomiting, diarrhea, anorexia,* abdominal pain, increased AST/ALT, constipation, flatulence, gastritis, GERD, **hematemesis, hepatitis,** hepatomegaly, **pancreatitis**
GU: **Renal failure**
HEMA: **Hemolytic anemia, neutropenia, thrombocytopenia, anemia**
INTEG: *Rash,* erythema multiforme, **angioedema, Stevens-Johnson syndrome**
MS: **Rhabdomyolysis**
OTHER: Diabetes mellitus, gynecomastia, hyperamylasemia, hypercholesterolemia, hyperglycemia, hyperlipidemia
RESP: Dyspnea, **bronchospasm**
SYST: **DRESS**

PHARMACOKINETICS

99.9% plasma protein binding; metabolized by CYP3A4, 2C9, 2C19; half-life 21-61 hr; excreted in feces

INTERACTIONS

• **Do not use concurrently with atazanavir, carBAMazepine, delavirdine, fosamprenavir, fosphenytoin, phenytoin, PHENobarbital, rifapentine, rifampin, tipranavir, rilpivirine**
• Altered effect of cycloSPORINE, tacrolimus, sirolimus
Increase: **myopathy, rhabdomyolysis—HMG-CoA reductase inhibitors**
Increase: etravirine levels—CYP3A4 inhibitors (fluconazole, itraconazole, ketoconazole, lopinavir, posaconazole, ritonavir, voriconazole)
Increase: withdrawal symptoms—methadone
Increase: levels of diazepam, rifampin, voriconazole, warfarin
Decrease: levels of CYP3A4 inducers (amiodarone, atazanavir, clarithromycin, flecainide, fosamprenavir, lidocaine, mexiletine, propafenone, quiNIDine, sildenafil, tadalafil, vardenafil)
Decrease: etravirine levels—darunavir, dexamethasone, disopyramide, efavirenz, nevirapine, ritonavir, saquinavir, tipranavir
Drug/Herb
Decrease: etravirine—St. John's wort

NURSING CONSIDERATIONS

Assess:
• **Symptoms of HIV, possible infections;** increased temperature
⚠ **Fatal hypersensitivity reactions:** fever, rash, nausea, vomiting, fatigue, cough, dyspnea, diarrhea, abdominal discomfort; treatment should be discontinued and not restarted; incidence of rash may be worse in women
• **Blood dyscrasias** (anemia, granulocytopenia): bruising, fatigue, bleeding, poor healing
• **Renal failure:** BUN, serum uric acid, CCr before, during therapy; may be elevated throughout treatment
• **Hepatitis/pancreatitis:** hepatic studies before and during therapy: bilirubin, AST, ALT, amylase, alk phos, creatine phosphokinase, creatinine, monthly
• HIV: monitor viral load, CD4 counts, plasma HIV RNA during treatment; watch for decreasing granulocytes, Hgb; if low, therapy may have to be discontinued and restarted after hematologic recovery; blood transfusions may be required; cholesterol/lipid profile
Evaluate:
• Therapeutic response: increased CD4 count, decreased viral load
Teach patient/family:
• That product is not a cure but will control symptoms; that patient is still infective, may pass AIDS virus to others
• To notify prescriber of sore throat, swollen lymph nodes, malaise, fever; other infections may occur; to stop product and notify prescriber immediately if skin rash,

fever, cough, SOB, GI symptoms occur; to advise all health care providers that allergic reaction has occurred with etravirine
- That follow-up visits must be continued, since serious toxicity may occur; blood counts must be performed
- **To use contraception during treatment; that patient still able to transmit disease**
- About information on medication guide and warning card; discuss points on guide
- That other products may be necessary to prevent other infections
- To take medication after a meal

⚠ HIGH ALERT

everolimus (Rx)

(e-ve-ro′li-mus)

Afinitor, Afinitor Disperz, Zortress

Func. class.: Antineoplastic—miscellaneous

Chem. class.: Immunosuppressant, macrolide

Do not confuse:
everolimus/sirolimus/tacrolimus/temsirolimus

ACTION: Proliferation signal inhibitor that inhibits mammalian target of rapamycin (mTOR); this pathway is dysregulated in cancer

USES: Renal cell cancer in those with failed treatment with SORAfenib or SUNItinib kidney transplant rejection prophylaxis with cycloSPORINE, subependymal giant cell astrocytoma, progressive pancreatic neuroendocrine tumor (PNET) with unresectable locally advanced/metastatic disease, breast cancer hormone receptor positive/HER-2 negative, renal angiomyolipoma, tuberous sclerosis complex, liver transplant rejection prophylaxis

CONTRAINDICATIONS: Breastfeeding; hypersensitivity to this product, Rapamune, Torisel, pregnancy (D)

Precautions: Children, renal/hepatic disease; diabetes mellitus, hyperlipidemia, pleural effusion

Black Box Warning: Immunosuppression, infection, renal artery thrombosis, renal impairment, renal vein thrombosis, neoplastic disease, heart transplant

DOSAGE AND ROUTES

Kidney transplant rejection prophylaxis (Zortress)
- **Adult: PO** 0.75 mg q12hr with cycloSPORINE in combination with basiliximab, corticosteroids, reduced doses of cycloSPORINE

Liver transplant rejection prophylaxis
Adult: PO 1 mg bid starting at least 30 days after transplant in combination with reduced-dose tacrolimus and corticosteroids

Advanced renal cancer (Afinitor)
- **Adult: PO** 10 mg daily as long as clinically beneficial; with strong 3A4 inducers 10 mg daily, then may increase by 5 mg increments to 20 mg daily

Progressive neuroendocrine tumor (PNET) (Afinitor only)
- **Adult: PO** 10 mg daily, reduce dose to 5 mg daily if intolerable adverse reactions occur

Subependymal giant-cell astrocytoma (SEGA) (Afinitor only)
- **Adult/adolescent/child:** 4.5 mg/m^2 daily, then titrate to a target trough of 5-15 ng/ml

Hepatic dose
- **Adult: PO** (Child-Pugh A): Afinitor 7.5 mg/day; (Child-Pugh B) Afinitor: 5 mg/day; Zortress: 0.75 mg/day divided q12hr; (Child-Pugh C) Afinitor 2.5 mg/day

Available forms: Tabs 0.25, 0.5, 0.75 (Zortess); 2.5, 5, 7.5, 10 mg (Afinitor)

Administer:
- Follow procedure for proper handling of antineoplastics
- Swallow tabs whole with a full glass of water; do not chew, crush, or break
- **Afinitor:** take at same time of day; if unable to swallow, consistently with or without food, disperse in 30 ml of water

• **Zortress:** must take consistently with/without food, give at same time of day q12hr with cycloSPORINE
• Store protected from light at room temperature

Afinitor adjustments for toxicity

Noninfectious pneumonitis

• Grade 1, asymptomatic with radiographic findings only: no dosage change
• Grade 2, symptomatic but no interference with activities of daily living (ADL): consider withholding therapy, resume Afinitor at a lower dosage when symptoms improve to ≤ grade 1; discontinue Afinitor if symptoms do not improve within 4 wk
• Grade 3, symptomatic and interfering with ADL and oxygen therapy indicated: hold therapy; consider resuming Afinitor at a lower dosage when symptoms improve to ≤ grade 1; consider discontinuing Afinitor if grade 3 toxicity recurs
• Grade 4, life-threatening and ventilator support indicated: discontinue therapy

Stomatitis

• Grade 1, minimum symptoms and normal diet: no dosage adjustment required
• Grade 2, symptomatic but can eat and swallow modified diet: hold therapy until symptoms improve to ≤ grade 1 and resume Afinitor at the same dosage; if grade 2 toxicity recurs, hold therapy and resume Afinitor at a lower dosage when symptoms improve to ≤ grade 1
• Grade 3, symptomatic and unable to adequately eat or hydrate orally: hold therapy; resume Afinitor at a lower dosage when symptoms improve to ≤ grade 1
• Grade 4, symptomatic and life-threatening: discontinue therapy

Other nonhematologic toxicity (excluding metabolic events)

• **Grade 1:** No dosage adjustment required if toxicity is tolerable
• **Grade 2:** No dosage adjustment required if toxicity is tolerable; if toxicity is intolerable, hold therapy until symptoms improve to ≤ grade 1 and resume Afinitor at the same dosage; if grade 2 toxicity recurs, hold therapy and resume Afinitor at a lower dosage when symptoms improve to ≤ grade 1
• **Grade 3:** Hold therapy; consider resuming Afinitor at a lower dosage when symptoms improve to ≤ grade 1; if grade 3 toxicity recurs, consider discontinuing therapy
• **Grade 4:** Discontinue Afinitor therapy

Metabolic events (hyperglycemia, dyslipidemia)

• **Grade 1 or 2:** No dose adjustment required
• **Grade 3:** Temporarily withhold therapy; resume Afinitor at a lower dosage
• **Grade 4:** Discontinue Afinitor therapy

SIDE EFFECTS

CNS: *Headache, insomnia, paresthesia,* chills, fever, seizure, personality changes, insomnia, dizziness
CV: *Hypertension, CHF, peripheral edema,* chest pain
EENT: Blurred vision, photophobia, eyelid edema, epistaxis, sinusitis, cataracts, conjunctivitis
GI: Nausea, vomiting, diarrhea, constipation, stomatitis, anorexia, abdominal pain, dysgeusia, noninfectious hepatitis
GU: **Renal failure**, UTI, **renal tubular necrosis**
HEMA: **Anemia, leukopenia, thrombocytopenia**
INTEG: *Rash, acne,* leukocytoclastic vasculitis
META: Hyperglycemia, increased creatinine, *hyperlipemia,* hypophosphatemia, weight loss
RESP: **Pleural effusion,** *dyspnea,* noninfectious pneumonitis, pulmonary embolism, pneumonitis, pulmonary alveolar proteinosis
HEMA: **Hemorrhage**

PHARMACOKINETICS

Rapidly absorbed; peak 1-2 hr; protein binding 74%; extensively metabolized by CYP3A4 enzyme system; half-life 30 hr; reduced by high-fat meal; excreted in feces (80%), urine (5%)

INTERACTIONS

Increase: nephrotoxicity—immunosuppressants

Increase: Everolimus effect—CYP3A4 inhibitors (strong, moderate), antifungals, calcium channel blockers, cimetidine, danazol, erythromycin, cycloSPORINE, HIV-protease inhibitors
Decrease: everolimus effect—CYP3A4 inducers, carBAMazepine, PHENobarbital, phenytoin, rifamycin, rifapentine
Decrease: effect of live vaccines

Drug/Herb
- St. John's wort: may decrease effect of everolimus

Drug/Food
- Alters bioavailability; use consistently with/without food; do not use with grapefruit juice

Drug/Lab Test
Increase: bilirubin, calcium, cholesterol, glucose, potassium, lipids, phosphate, triglycerides, uric acid
Decrease: calcium, glucose, potassium, magnesium, phosphate

NURSING CONSIDERATIONS

Assess:
- Lipid profile: cholesterol, triglycerides, lipid-lowering agent may be needed; blood glucose

Black Box Warning: Immunosuppression: CBC with differential during treatment monthly; if leukocytes <3000/mm^3 or platelets <100,000/mm^3, product should be discontinued or reduced; decreased hemoglobulin level may indicate bone marrow suppression

- Hepatic/renal studies: AST, ALT, amylase, bilirubin, creatinine, phosphate, and for hepatotoxicity: dark urine, jaundice, itching, light-colored stools; product should be discontinued

Black Box Warning: Infection: bacterial fungal infections can occur and are more common with combination immunosuppression therapy

- **Renal artery/vein thrombosis (Zortress):** May result in graft loss within 30 days after transplantation
- Obtain everolimus blood levels in kidney transplant, hepatic disease, CYP3A4 inducers, inhibitors

Evaluate:
- Therapeutic response

Teach patient/family:

Black Box Warning: To report fever, rash, severe diarrhea, chills, sore throat, fatigue; serious infections may occur; to report clay-colored stools, cramping (hepatotoxicity)

Black Box Warning: To avoid crowds, persons with known infections to reduce risk for infection

- **Pregnancy:** to notify prescriber if pregnancy is planned or suspected, pregnancy (D)
- To use contraception before, during, and 12 wk after product discontinued; to avoid breastfeeding
- Not to use with grapefruit juice
- To avoid live vaccines; that frequent lab tests are required
- That product may decrease male, female fertility
- That drinking alcohol is not recommended
- To take consistently with or without food
- To report vision changes, weight gain, edema, shortness of breath, impaired wound healing

exemestane (Rx)

(ex-em′eh-stane)

Aromasin

Func. class.: Antineoplastic
Chem. class.: Aromatase inhibitor

Do not confuse:
exemestane/ezetimibe/estramustine

ACTION: Lowers serum estradiol concentrations by irreversibly inhibiting aromatase; many breast cancers have strong estrogen receptors

USES: Advanced breast carcinoma not responsive to other therapy (postmenopausal), estrogen receptor–positive early breast cancer that has received tamoxifen

CONTRAINDICATIONS: Pregnancy (X), breastfeeding, premenopausal women, hypersensitivity

Precautions: Children, geriatric patients, renal/hepatic disease, osteoporosis, vit D deficiency, hepatic/renal disease

DOSAGE AND ROUTES

- **Adult: PO** 25 mg/day after meals; may need 50 mg/day if taken with a potent CYP3A4 inducer

Available forms: Tabs 25 mg

Administer:

- After meals at same time of day
- Store at room temperature

SIDE EFFECTS

CNS: *Headache, depression, insomnia, anxiety, fatigue, hot flashes, diaphoresis,* dizziness, neuropathy

CV: Hypertension, edema, thromboembolism

GI: *Nausea,* vomiting, diarrhea, constipation, abdominal pain, increased appetite

HEMA: *Lymphopenia*

MS: Fracture, bone loss, arthralgia, osteoporosis

RESP: Cough, *dyspnea*

INTEG: Alopecia, hot flashes, sweating

PHARMACOKINETICS

Half-life 24 hr; excreted in feces, urine

INTERACTIONS

Decrease: exemestane action—CYP3A4 inducers, estrogens

Drug/Lab Test

Increase: AST, ALT, alk phos, bilirubin, creatinine

NURSING CONSIDERATIONS

Assess:

- B/P; hypertension may occur
- Bone mineral density, x-ray of thoracic or lumbar spine if bone changes suspected

Evaluate:

- Therapeutic response: decreased tumor size, spread of malignancy

Teach patient/family:

- To report any complaints, side effects to prescriber, to immediately report chest pain
- That hot flashes are reversible after discontinuing treatment
- To use reliable contraception (pregnancy [X]); not to breastfeed
- That vit D, calcium may be used for bone loss

⚠ HIGH ALERT

exenatide (Rx)

(ex-en′a-tide)

Bydureon, Byetta

Func. class.: Antidiabetic

Chem. class.: Incretin mimetic

ACTION: Binds and activates known human GLP-1 receptor, mimics natural physiology for self-regulating glycemic control

USES: Type 2 diabetes mellitus given in combination with metFORMIN, a sulfonylurea, thiazolidinedione, insulin glargine; once-weekly dosing

CONTRAINDICATIONS: Hypersensitivity

Black Box Warning: Medullary thyroid carcinoma, multiple endocrine neoplasia syndrome type 2 (men-2), thyroid cancer

Precautions: Pregnancy (C), geriatric patients, severe renal/hepatic/GI disease, pancreatitis, vit D deficiency

DOSAGE AND ROUTES

- **Adult: SUBCUT** 5 mcg bid 1 hr before morning and evening meal; may increase to 10 mcg bid after 1 mo of therapy; ext rel SUBCUT (Bydureon) 2 mg q7days

Available forms: Inj 5, 10 mcg pen; ext rel powder for susp for inj 2 mg

Administer:

- Store in refrigerator for unopened pen; may store at room temperature after opening for up to 30 days

SUBCUT route (regular release—Byetta)

- May be used as monotherapy or combined with other products
- SUBCUT only, do not give IV/IM
- Pen needles must be purchased separately, compatible; prime before use; inject into thigh, abdomen, upper arm; rotate sites
- Product 1 hr before meals, approximately 6 hr apart; if patient is NPO, may need to hold dose to prevent hypoglycemia
- If added to insulin glargine, insulin, or detemir, a dosage reduction in these products may be required

SUBCUT route (ext rel—Bydureon)

- Give every 7 days (weekly); the dose can be given at any time of day without regard to meals
- Available as a single-dose tray containing a vial of 2 mg, a pre-filled syringe delivering 0.65 ml diluent, a vial connector, and two custom needles (23GX 5/16′) specific to this delivery system (one is a spare needle); do not substitute needles or any other components
- Inject immediately after the white to off-white powder is suspended in the diluent and transferred to the syringe
- Inject subcut into the thigh, abdomen, or upper arm, rotate sites to prevent lipodystrophy

SIDE EFFECTS

CNS: *Headache, dizziness,* feeling jittery, restlessness, weakness

ENDO: Hypoglycemia, thyroid hyperplasia

GI: Nausea, vomiting, diarrhea, dyspepsia, anorexia, gastroesophageal reflux, weight loss, pancreatitis

SYST: Angioedema, anaphylaxis

INTEG: Serious inj-site reactions (cellulitis, abscess, skin necrosis)

PHARMACOKINETICS

Immediate release: Peak 2.1 hr, elimination by glomerular filtration

Ext Rel: Peak 2 wk

INTERACTIONS

- May decrease effect of acetaminophen
- Do not use with erythromycin, metoclopramide

Increase: hypoglycemia—ACE inhibitors, disopyramide, sulfonylureas, androgens, fibric acid derivatives, alcohol

Increase: hyperglycemia—phenothiazines, corticosteroids, anabolic steroids

Decrease: action of digoxin, lovastatin, acetaminophen (elixir)

Decrease: efficacy—niacin, dextrothyroxine, thiazide diuretics, triamterene, estrogens, progestins, oral contraceptives, MAOIs

NURSING CONSIDERATIONS

Assess:

- Fasting blood glucose, A1c levels, postprandial glucose during treatment to determine diabetes control
- **Pancreatitis:** severe abdominal pain, with or without vomiting, product should be discontinued
- **Anaphylaxis, Angioedema:** product should be discontinued immediately
- Renal studies: urinalysis, creatinine
- Hypo/hyperglycemic reaction that can occur soon after meals; for severe hypoglycemia, give IV $D_{50}W$, then IV dextrose solution
- Nausea, vomiting, diarrhea, ability to tolerate product, may cause dehydration

Evaluate:

- Therapeutic response: decrease in polyuria, polydipsia, polyphagia, clear sensorium, improving A1c, weight; absence of dizziness, stable gait

Teach patient/family:

- About the symptoms of hypo/hyperglycemia, what to do about each; to have glucagon emergency kit available; to carry a glucose source (candy, sugar cube) to treat hypoglycemia

- That product must be continued on a daily or weekly basis (ext rel); about consequences of discontinuing product abruptly
- That diabetes is a lifelong illness; product will not cure disease; to carry emergency ID with prescriber and medication information
- To continue weight control, dietary restrictions, exercise, hygiene
- That regular blood glucose monitoring and A1c testing is needed
- To notify prescriber if pregnant or intending to become pregnant (C)
- About the importance of reading "Information for the Patient" and "Pen User Manual;" about self-injection
- **Pancreatitis:** If severe abdominal pain with or without vomiting occurs seek medical attention immediately
- To review injection procedure; to store product in refrigerator, room temperature after first use; discard 30 days after first use; do not freeze; protect from light (Byetta)

ezetimibe (Rx)

(ehz-eh-tim′bee)

Ezetrol ✦, Zetia

Func. class.: Antilipemic; cholesterol absorption inhibitor

ACTION: Inhibits absorption of cholesterol by the small intestine, causes reduced hepatic cholesterol stores

USES: Hypercholesterolemia, homozygous familial hypercholesterolemia (HoFH), homozygous sitosterolemia

CONTRAINDICATIONS: Hypersensitivity, severe hepatic disease

Precautions: Pregnancy (C), breastfeeding, children, hepatic disease

DOSAGE AND ROUTES

- **Adult/adolescent/child >10 yr: PO** 10 mg/day; may be given with HMG-CoA reductase inhibitor at same time; may be given with bile acid sequestrant; give ezetimibe 2 hr before or 4 hr after bile acid sequestrant

Available forms: Tabs 10 mg

Administer:

- Without regard to meals

SIDE EFFECTS

CNS: Fatigue, dizziness, headache

GI: Diarrhea, abdominal pain

MISC: Chest pain

MS: *Myalgias, arthralgias,* back pain, **myopathy, rhabdomyolysis**

RESP: Pharyngitis, sinusitis, cough, *URI*

EENT: Sinusitis, nasopharyngitis

SYST: **Angioedema**

PHARMACOKINETICS

Metabolized in small intestine, liver; excreted in feces 78%, urine 11%; peak 4-12 hr; half-life 22 hr

INTERACTIONS

Increase: action of ezetimibe—fibric acid derivatives, cycloSPORINE

Decrease: action of ezetimibe—antacids, bile acid sequestrants

Drug/Lab Test

Increase: LFTs

NURSING CONSIDERATIONS

Assess:

- **Hypercholestrolemia:** diet history: fat content, lipid levels (triglycerides, LDL, HDL, cholesterol); LFTs at baseline, periodically during treatment
- **Myopathy/rhabdomyolysis: increased CPK, myalgia, muscle cramps, musculoskeletal pain, lethargy, fatigue, fever; more common when combined with statins**

Evaluate:

- Therapeutic response: decreased cholesterol, LDL; increased HDL

Teach patient/family:

- That compliance is needed
- That risk factors should be decreased: high-fat diet, smoking, alcohol consumption, absence of exercise

- To notify prescriber if pregnancy suspected, planned, or if breastfeeding
- To notify prescriber if unexplained weakness, muscle pain present
- To notify prescriber of dietary/herbal supplements

ezogabine

(e-zog′a-been)

Potiga

Func. class.: Anticonvulsant

Controlled Substance Schedule V

ACTION: The exact mechanism of anticonvulsant effects is not fully known; however, studies indicate that the drug enhances transmembrane potassium currents, which may stabilize the resting membrane potential and reduce brain excitability; may also augment GABA-mediated currents

USES: Partial seizures

CONTRAINDICATIONS: Hypersensitivity

Precautions: Suicidal ideation/behavior, prostatic hypertrophy, dementia, psychotic disorders, QT prolongation, congestive heart failure, ventricular hypertrophy, hypokalemia, hypomagnesemia, abrupt discontinuation, renal impairment, hepatic disease, geriatric patients, pregnancy category C, breastfeeding, neonates, infants, children, adolescents

DOSAGE AND ROUTES

- **Adult/geriatric patient ≤65 yr: PO** initially, 100 mg tid, increase by ≤50 mg tid per day at weekly intervals depending on response, up to a maintenance dose of 200-400 mg tid depending on response; max is 400 mg tid (1200 mg/day)
- **Geriatric patient >65 yr: PO** initially, 50 mg tid, increase by ≤50 mg tid per day at weekly intervals depending on response; max 250 mg tid (750 mg/day)

Available forms: Film-coated tabs 50, 200, 300, 400 mg

Administer:

- Tab should be swallowed whole without regard to meals
- Give in 3 equally divided doses

SIDE EFFECTS

CNS: Dizziness, drowsiness, memory impairment, tremor, vertigo, abnormal coordination, disturbance in attention, gait disturbance, aphasia, dysarthria, balance disorder, paresthesias, amnesia, dysphagia, myoclonia, hypokinesia, confusion, anxiety, hallucinations, suicidal thoughts/behaviors, fatigue, asthenia, malaise, euphoria

EENT: Diplopia, blurred vision, retinal pigment change

GI: Nausea, constipation, dyspepsia, xerostomia, constipation, weight gain, appetite stimulation

GU: Urinary retention, hydronephrosis, dysuria, urinary hesitation, hematuria, chromaturia

HEMA: Thrombocytopenia, leukopenia, neutropenia

INTEG: Rash, alopecia, blue skin discoloration

MISC: Influenza, dyspnea, QT prolongation

MS: Muscle spasms, weakness

PHARMACOKINETICS

80% protein bound; extensively distributed in the body; extensively metabolized by glucuronidation and acetylation; inactive N-glucuronides are the primary metabolites; elimination half-lives of ezogabine and its N-acetyl metabolite are 7 hr and 11 hr, respectively; 36% excreted renally as exogabine, 18% as NAMR, 24% as the N-glururonides of ezogabine and NAMR, 14% fecal excretion; rapidly absorbed, peak 0.5-2 hr, bioavailability 60%; high-fat food increases peak concentrations; increased in hepatic/renal disease, geriatric patients, young adult females

INTERACTIONS: Increase: QT prolongation—arsenic trioxide, chloroquine, chlorproMAZINE, mesoridazine thioridazine, clarithromycin, Class IA antiarrhythmics (disopyramide, procainamide, quiNIDine), Class III antiarrhythmics (amiodarone, dofetilide, ibutilide, sotalol), dextromethorphan, dronedarone, droperidol, erythromycin, grepafloxacin, halofantrine, levomethadyl, methadone, pentamidine, pimozide, posaconazole, probucol, propafenone, quiNIDine, saquinavir, sparfloxacin, terfenadine, troleandomycin, ziprasidone

Decrease: effect of phenytoin

Decrease: effect of ezogabine—carBAMazepine

Increase: effect of digoxin

Increase: urinary retention—antimuscarinics, amantadine, H1-blockers

Increase: CNS depression—anxiolytics, sedatives, hypnotics, buprenorphine, butorphanol, dronabinol, mirtazapine, nabilone, nalbuphine, opiate agonists, pentazocine, pregabalin, skeletal muscle relaxants, traMADol, traZODone, ethanol

Drug/Lab Test

Increase: LFTs

NURSING CONSIDERATIONS

Assess:

⚠ **Seizures:** Assess for type, duration, location, activity, presence of aura

⚠ **QT prolongation:** Monitor in those with known QT prolongation, congestive heart failure, ventricular hypertrophy, hypokalemia, hypomagnesemia, and in patients receiving medications known to cause QT prolongation; QT prolongation can occur within 3 hr of dose

⚠ **Abrupt withdrawal:** Withdraw gradually to minimize increased seizure frequency

⚠ **Suicidal thoughts/behaviors:** Assess for any unusual changes in moods or behaviors, including emotional lability or emerging or worsening depression and suicidal ideation

- **Vision changes:** Obtain a baseline eye exam, then periodic eye exams; discontinue if ophthalmic changes occur, unless no other treatment is available

Teach patient/family:

- To avoid driving or operating machinery or performing other tasks that require mental alertness until reaction is known
- To avoid concurrent use of alcohol
- To avoid abruptly discontinuing this product

⚠ **Suicidal thought/behaviors:** Advise patient to notify prescriber immediately of suicidal thought/behaviors

- That skin may turn blue; it is unknown if it is reversible
- To report vision change immediately

RARELY USED

factor IX complex (human) (Rx)

AlphaNine SD, Bebulin, BeneFIX, Mononine, Profilnine SD

Func. class.: Hemostatic

Chem. class.: Factors II, VII, IX, X

USES: Hemophilia B (Christmas disease), factor IX deficiency, anticoagulant reversal, control of bleeding in patients with factor VIII inhibitors, reversal of overdose of anticoagulants in emergencies

CONTRAINDICATIONS: Hypersensitivity to mouse or hamster protein, DIC, mild factor IX deficiency

DOSAGE AND ROUTES

Factor IX complex (human) bleeding in hemophilia B

- **Adult and child: IV** establish 25% of normal factor IX or 60-75 units/kg, then 10-20 units/kg/day 1-2×/wk

Prophylaxis for bleeding in hemophilia B (long term)

- **Adult and child: IV** 25-40 units/kg 2×/wk

Bleeding in hemophilia A/inhibitors of factor VIII (Proplex T, Konyne 80)

- **Adult and child: IV** 75 units/kg, repeat after 12 hr

Oral anticoagulant reversal (factor IX complexer only) (unlabeled)

- **Adult and child: IV** 20-50 units/kg

Factor VII deficiency (use Proplex T only)

- **Adult and child: IV** 0.5 unit/kg × weight (kg) × desired factor IX increase (% of normal); repeat q4-6hr if needed

Factor IX (human) minor to moderate hemorrhage

Use only Alpha-Nine, Alpha-Nine SD

- **Adult and child: IV** dose to increase factor IX level to 20%-30% in one dose

Serious hemorrhage

- **Adult and child: IV** dose to increase factor IX to 30%-50% as daily infusion

Minor hemorrhage (mononine only)

- **Adult and child: IV** dose to increase factor IX to 15%-25% (20-30 units/kg), repeat after 24 hr if needed

Major hemorrhage

- **Adult and child: IV** dose to increase factor IX to 25%-50% (75 units/kg) q18-30hr × ≤10 days

RARELY USED

factor IX Fc fusion protein, recombinant

(fak′tor nine′)

Alprolix

Func. class.: Hemostatic

USES: Hemophilia B, surgical bleeding

CONTRAINDICATIONS: Bleeding disorders

DOSAGE AND ROUTES

Hemophilia B

- Adults, adolescents, children, infants, and neonates: **IV INFUSION** infuse dose ≤10 ml/min dose (IU) = body weight (kg) × desired factor IX increase (IU/dl or % of normal) × reciprocal of recovery (IU/kg per IU/dl) ***or*** IU/dl (or % of normal) = [total dose (IU)/body weight (kg)] × recovery (IU/dl per IU/kg)

Surgical bleeding control, prevention

- Adults, adolescents, children, infants, and neonates: Dose and duration of treatment depend on the severity of the factor IX deficiency, the location and extent of bleeding, and the patient's clinical condition. Refer to hemophilia B for dosage formula

Routine bleeding prophylaxis to prevent/reduce the frequency of bleeding episodes

- Adults, adolescents, children, infants, and neonates: **IV INFUSION** initially, 50 IU/kg every week or 100 IU/kg q10days

famciclovir (Rx)

(fam-cy′clo-veer)

Famvir

Func. class.: Antiviral

Chem. class.: Guanosine nucleoside

ACTION: Inhibits DNA polymerase and viral DNA synthesis by conversion of this guanosine nucleoside to penciclovir

USES: Treatment of acute herpes zoster (shingles), genital herpes; recurrent mucocutaneous herpes simplex virus (HSV) in patients with HIV; initial episodes of herpes genitalis; herpes labialis in the immunocompromised, herpes labialis prophylaxis

Unlabeled uses: Bell's palsy, postherpetic neuralgia prophylaxis

CONTRAINDICATIONS: Hypersensitivity to this product, penciclovir, acyclovir, ganciclovir, valacyclovir, valganciclovir

Precautions: Pregnancy (B), breastfeeding, renal disease

DOSAGE AND ROUTES

Herpes zoster

- **Adult: PO** 500 mg q8hr for 7 days

Renal dose

- **Adult: PO** CCr 40-59 ml/min, 500 mg q12hr; CCr 20-39 ml/min, 500 mg q24hr; CCr <20 ml/min, 250 mg q24hr

Suppression of recurrent herpes simplex virus

- **Adult: PO** 250 mg q12hr up to 1 yr

Renal dose

- **Adult: PO** CCr 20-39 ml/min, 125 mg q12hr × 5 days; CCr <20 ml/min, 125 mg q24hr × 5 days

Recurrent genital herpes

- **Adult: PO** 1000 mg bid on a single day

Renal dose

- **Adult: PO** CCr 40-59 ml/min, 500 mg q12hr × 1 day; CCr 20-39 ml/min, 500 mg as a single dose; CCr <20ml/min, 250 mg as a single dose

Suppression of recurrent genital herpes

- **Adult: PO** 250 mg bid for up to 1 yr

Renal dose

- **Adult: PO** CCr 20-39 ml/min, 125 mg q12hr; CCr <20ml/min, 125 mg q24hr

Herpes genitalis initial episodes

- **Adult: PO** 250 mg tid × 7-10 days

Bell's palsy (unlabeled)

- **Adult: PO** 750 mg tid × 7 days with predniSONE

Varicella-zoster virus (shingles); chickenpox (unlabeled)

- **Adult: PO** 500 mg q8hr × 7 days, preferably within 48 hr of onset

Herpes zoster in HIV (unlabeled)

- **Adult/adolescent: PO** 500 mg tid × 7-10 days

Available forms: Tabs 125, 250, 500 mg

Administer:

- Without regard to meals
- As soon as diagnosed; for herpes zoster within 72 hr

SIDE EFFECTS

CNS: *Headache, fatigue, dizziness,* paresthesia, somnolence, fever

GI: Nausea, vomiting, diarrhea, constipation, abdominal pain, anorexia

GU: Decreased sperm count

INTEG: *Pruritus*

MS: Back pain, arthralgia

RESP: Pharyngitis, sinusitis

PHARMACOKINETICS

Bioavailability 77%, 20% protein binding, 73% excreted via kidneys, terminal plasma half-life 2-3 hr, peak 1 hr

INTERACTIONS

Increase: effect of famciclovir—probenecid

Decrease: effect of zoster vaccine

NURSING CONSIDERATIONS

Assess:

- **Herpes zoster:** number, distribution of lesions; burning, itching, pain, which are

F

early symptoms of herpes infection; assess daily during therapy
- Renal studies: urine CCr; BUN before and during treatment if decreased renal function; dose may have to be lowered; hepatic studies: LFTs
- Bowel pattern before, during treatment; diarrhea may occur
- Posttherapeutic neuralgia during and after treatment

Evaluate:
- Therapeutic response: decreased size, spread of lesions

Teach patient/family:
- How to recognize beginning infection
- How to prevent spread of infection; that this medication does not prevent spread to others; that condoms should be used
- About the reason for medication, expected results
- That women with genital herpes should have yearly Pap smears; that cervical cancer is more likely

famotidine (OTC, Rx)

(fa-moe′ti-deen)

Acid Control ♣, Pepcid, Pepcid AC, Peptic Guard Ulcidine ♣

Func. class.: H_2-histamine receptor antagonist

ACTION: Competitively inhibits histamine at histamine H_2-receptor site, thus decreasing gastric secretion while pepsin remains at a stable level

USES: Short-term treatment of duodenal ulcer, maintenance therapy for duodenal ulcer, Zollinger-Ellison syndrome, multiple endocrine adenomas, gastric ulcers; gastroesophageal reflux disease, heartburn

Unlabeled uses: GI disorders in those taking NSAIDs; urticaria; prevention of stress ulcers, aspiration pneumonitis

CONTRAINDICATIONS: Hypersensitivity

Precautions: Pregnancy (B), breastfeeding, children <12 yr, geriatric patients, severe renal/hepatic disease

DOSAGE AND ROUTES

Short-term treatment of gastric ulcer
- **Adult: PO** 40 mg/day at bedtime × 4-8 wk, then 20 mg/day at bedtime if needed (maintenance); **IV** 20 mg q12hr if unable to take **PO**
- **Child 1-16 yr: PO** 1-2 mg/kg/day in 1-2 divided doses, max 40 mg/day

Pathologic hypersecretory conditions
- **Adult: PO** 20 mg q6hr; may give up to 160 mg q6hr if needed; **IV** 20 mg q6hr if unable to take **PO**

GERD
- **Adult: PO** 20 mg bid ≤6 wk; 40 mg bid ≤2 wk (ulcerative esophagitis)

Heartburn relief/prevention
- **Adult: PO** 10 mg with water or 15 min-1 hr before eating

Renal disease
- **Adult: PO** CCr <50 ml/min, decrease dose by 50% or extend interval to 36-48 hr

Available forms: Tabs 10, 20, 40 mg; powder for oral susp 40 mg/5 ml; inj 10 mg/ml, 20 mg/50 ml

Administer:
- Store in cool environment (oral); IV sol stable for 48 hr at room temperature; do not use discolored sol; discard unused oral sol after 1 mo

PO route
- After shaking oral suspension

Direct IV route
- After diluting 2 ml of product (10 mg/ml) in 0.9% NaCl to total volume of 5-10 ml; inject over 2 min to prevent hypotension

Intermittent IV INFUSION route
- After diluting 20 mg (2 ml) of product in 100 ml of LR, 0.9% NaCl, D_5W, $D_{10}W$; run over 15-30 min

Continuous IV INFUSION route
- *Adults:* Dilute 40 mg of product in 250 ml D_5W, NS; infuse over 24 hr, run at 11 ml/hr, use infusion device

Y-site compatibilities: Acyclovir, alfentanil, allopurinol, amifostine, amikacin, aminocaproic acid, aminophylline, amiodarone, amphotericin B lipid complex, amphotericin B liposome, amsacrine, anakinra, anidulafungin, ascorbic acid injection, atenolol, atracurium, atropine, aztreonam, benztropine, bivalirudin, bleomycin, bumetanide, buprenorphine, butorphanol, calcium chloride/gluconate, CARBOplatin, caspofungin, cefonicid, cefotaxime, cefTAZidime, cefuroxime, chlorproMAZINE, cimetidine, cisatracurium, CISplatin, cladribine, clindamycin, codeine, cyanocobalamin, cyclophosphamide, cycloSPORINE, cytarabine, DACTINomycin, DAPTOmycin, dexamethasone, dexmedetomidine, digoxin, diltiazem, diphenhydrAMINE, DOBUTamine, DOCEtaxel, DOPamine, doripenem, doxacurium, DOXOrubicin, DOXOrubicin liposomal, doxycycline, droperidol, enalaprilat, ePHEDrine, EPINEPHrine, epirubicin, epoetin alfa, eptifibatide, ertapenem, erythromycin, esmolol, etoposide, fenoldopam, fentaNYL, filgrastim, fluconazole, fludarabine, fluorouracil, folic acid, gatifloxacin, gemcitabine, gentamicin, glycopyrrolate, granisetron, heparin, hydrocortisone, HYDROmorphone, hydrOXYzine, IDArubicin, ifosfamide, imipenem-cilastatin, irinotecan, isoproterenol, ketorolac, labetalol, levofloxacin, lidocaine, linezolid, LORazepam, LR, magnesium sulfate, mannitol, mechlorethamine, melphalan, meperidine, metaraminol, methicillin, methotrexate, methoxamine, methyldopate, methylPREDNISolone, metoclopramide, metoprolol, metroNIDAZOLE, miconazole, midazolam, milrinone, mitoXANtrone, morphine, moxalactam, multiple vitamins injection, mycophenolate, nafcillin, nalbuphine, naloxone, nesiritide, netilmicin, niCARdipine, nitroglycerin, nitroprusside, norepinephrine, 0.9% NaCl, octreotide, ondansetron, oxacillin, oxaliplatin, oxytocin, PACLitaxel, palonosetron, pamidronate, pancuronium, papaverine, PEMEtrexed, penicillin G potassium/sodium, pentamidine, pentazocine, PENTobarbital, perphenazine, PHENobarbital, phenylephrine, phytonadione, polymyxin B, potassium chloride/phosphates, procainamide, prochlorperazine, promethazine, propofol, propranolol, protamine, pyridoxine, quiNIDine, ranitidine, remifentanil, Ringer's, ritodrine, riTUXimab, sargramostim, sodium acetate/bicarbonate, succinylcholine, SUFentanil, tacrolimus, teniposide, theophylline, thiamine, thiotepa, ticarcillin, ticarcillin-clavulanate, tigecycline, tirofiban, TNA, tobramycin, tolazoline, TPN, trastuzumab, trimetaphan, urokinase, vancomycin, vasopressin, vecuronium, verapamil, vinCRIStine, vinorelbine, voriconazole, zoledronic acid

SIDE EFFECTS

CNS: *Headache, dizziness,* paresthesia, depression, anxiety, somnolence, insomnia, fever, **seizures in renal disease**

CV: **Dysrhythmias, QT prolongation (impaired renal functioning)**

EENT: Taste change, tinnitus, orbital edema

GI: *Constipation,* nausea, vomiting, anorexia, cramps, abnormal hepatic enzymes, diarrhea

INTEG: Rash, **toxic epidermal necrolysis, Stevens-Johnson syndrome**

MS: Myalgia, arthralgia

RESP: **Pneumonia**

PHARMACOKINETICS

Plasma protein binding 15%-20%, metabolized in liver 30% (active metabolites), 70% excreted by kidneys, half-life $2^1/_2$-$3^1/_2$ hr

PO: Onset 60 min, duration 12 hr, peak 1-3 hr, absorption 50%

IV: Onset 60 min, peak 1-4 hr, duration 12 hr

INTERACTIONS

Decrease: absorption—ketoconazole, itraconazole, cefpodoxime, cefditoren

Decrease: famotidine absorption—antacids

Decrease: effect of—atazanavir, delavirdine

NURSING CONSIDERATIONS

Assess:

- **Ulcers:** epigastric pain, adominal pain, frank or occult blood in emesis, stools
- Intragastric pH, serum creatinine/BUN baseline and periodically
- **For bleeding, hematuria, hematuresis, occult blood in stools; abdominal pain**
- Increase in bulk and fluids in diet to prevent constipation

Evaluate:

- Therapeutic response: decreased abdominal pain

Teach patient/family:

- That product must be continued for prescribed time in prescribed method to be effective; not to double dose
- About possibility of decreased libido; that this is reversible after discontinuing therapy
- To avoid irritating foods, alcohol, aspirin, NSAIDs, extreme-temperature foods that may irritate GI system
- That smoking should be avoided because it diminishes effectiveness of product
- To avoid tasks requiring alertness because dizziness, drowsiness may occur

RARELY USED

fat emulsions (Rx)

Intralipid 10%, Intralipid 20%, Liposyn II 10%, Liposyn II 20%, Liposyn III 10%, Liposyn III 20%

Func. class.: Caloric

Chem. class.: Fatty acid, long chain; nutritional supplement

USES: Increase calorie intake, fatty acid deficiency, prevention

CONTRAINDICATIONS: Hypersensitivity to this product or eggs, soybeans, legumes; hyperlipemia, lipid necrosis, acute pancreatitis accompanied by hyperlipemia, hyperbilirubinemia of the newborn; renal insufficiency, hepatic damage

DOSAGE AND ROUTES

Deficiency

- **Adult and child: IV** 8%-10% of required calorie intake (intralipid)

Adjunct to TPN

- **Adult: IV** 1 ml/min over 15-30 min (10%) or 0.5 ml/min over 15-30 min (20%); may increase to 500 ml over 4-8 hr if no adverse reactions occur; max 2.5 g/kg
- **Child: IV** 0.1 ml/min over 10-15 min (10%) or 0.05 ml/min over 10-15 min (20%); may increase to 1 g/kg over 4 hr if no adverse reactions occur; max 4 g/kg

Prevention of deficiency

- **Adult: IV** 500 ml 2×/wk (10%), given 1 ml/min for 30 min, max 500 ml over 6 hr
- **Child: IV** 5-10 ml/kg/day (10%), given 0.1 ml/min for 30 min, max 100 ml/hr

Available forms: Inj 10% (50, 100, 200, 250, 500 ml), 20% (50, 100, 200, 250, 500 ml)

febuxostat (Rx)

(feb-ux′oh-stat)

Uloric

Func. class.: Antigout drug, antihyperuricemic

Chem. class.: Xanthene oxidase inhibitor

ACTION: Inhibits the enzyme xanthine oxidase, thereby reducing uric acid synthesis; more selective for xanthine oxidase than allopurinol

USES: Chronic gout, hyperuricemia

CONTRAINDICATIONS: Hypersensitivity

Precautions: Pregnancy (C), breastfeeding, children, renal/hepatic/cardiac/neoplastic disease, stroke, MI, organ transplant, Lesch-Nyhan syndrome

DOSAGE AND ROUTES

- **Adult: PO** 40 mg daily, may increase to 80 mg daily if uric acid levels are >6 mg/dl after 2 wk of therapy

Available forms: Tabs 40, 80 mg
Administer:
PO route
• Without regard to meals or antacids; may crush and add to foods or fluids

SIDE EFFECTS
CNS: Weakness, flushing
EENT: Retinopathy, cataracts, epistaxis
GI: *Nausea, vomiting, anorexia,* constipation, diarrhea, dyspepsia, hematemesis, **hepatitis**, hepatomegaly, weight gain/loss, cholecystitis, cholelithiasis, melena
HEMA: **Thrombocytopenia, anemia, pancytopenia, leukopenia, bone marrow suppression**
INTEG: Rash
MISC: Arthralgia, gout flare

PHARMACOKINETICS
Peak 1-1.5 hr; excreted in feces, urine; half-life 5-8 hr; protein binding 99.2%

INTERACTIONS
Increase: toxicity—azaTHIOprine, didanosine, mercaptopurine
Increase: xanthine nephropathy, calculi—rasburicase, antineoplastics
Drug/Lab
Increase: LFTs

NURSING CONSIDERATIONS
Assess:
• **Hyperuricemia:** uric acid levels q2wk; uric acid levels should be ≤6 mg/dl, flares may occur during first 6 wk of treatment
• Hepatic studies before use, then 2, 4 mo and then periodically; assess for fatigue, anorexia, right upper abdominal discomfort, dark urine, jaundice
• CBC, AST, BUN, creatinine before starting treatment, periodically
• **Renal disease:** I&O ratio; increase fluids to 2 L/day to prevent stone formation and toxicity
• For rash, hypersensitivity reactions; discontinue
• **Gout:** joint pain, swelling; may use with NSAIDs for acute gouty attacks and gout flare (first 6 wk)

Evaluate:
• Therapeutic response: decreased pain in joints, decreased stone formation in kidneys, decreased uric acid levels
Teach patient/family:
• That tabs may be crushed
• To take as prescribed; if dose is missed, to take as soon as remembered; not to double dose
• To increase fluid intake to 2 L/day unless contraindicated
• To avoid alcohol, caffeine because they will increase uric acid levels
• To report cardiovascular events to prescriber immediately
• **Gout:** that flares may occur during first 6 wk of treatment

F

felodipine (Rx)
(fe-loe′-di-peen)
Plendil, Renedil ♣
Func. class.: Antihypertensive, calcium channel blocker, antianginal
Chem. class.: Dihydropyridine

Do not confuse:
Plendil/pindolol/Pletal/PriLOSEC/Prinivil/Isordil

ACTION: Inhibits calcium ion influx across cell membrane, resulting in the inhibition of the excitation and contraction of vascular smooth muscle

USES: Essential hypertension alone or with other antihypertensives
Unlabeled uses: Hypertension in adolescents and children, angina pectoris; Prinzmetal's angina (vasospastic)

CONTRAINDICATIONS: Hypersensitivity to this product or dihydropyridines, sick sinus syndrome, 2nd- or 3rd-degree heart block, hypotension <90 mm Hg systolic
Precautions: Pregnancy (C), breastfeeding, children, geriatric patients, CHF, hepatic injury, renal disease, coronary artery disease

DOSAGE AND ROUTES

- **Adult: PO** 5 mg/day initially; usual range 2.5-10 mg/day; max 10 mg/day; do not adjust dosage at intervals of <2 wk
- **Geriatric: PO** 2.5 mg/day

Hepatic disease

- **Adult: PO** 2.5-5 mg, max 10 mg/day

Hypertension in adolescent/child (unlabeled)

- **Adolescent and child: PO** 2.5 mg initially, titrate upward, max 10 mg/day

Available forms: Ext rel tabs 2.5, 5, 10 mg

Administer:

PO route

- Swallow whole; do not break, crush, or chew ext rel products
- Once daily with light meal; avoid grapefruit juice

SIDE EFFECTS

CNS: *Headache,* fatigue, drowsiness, dizziness, anxiety, depression, nervousness, insomnia, light-headedness, paresthesia, tinnitus, psychosis, somnolence, flushing

CV: Dysrhythmia, *edema,* CHF, hypotension, palpitations, MI, pulmonary edema, tachycardia, syncope, AV block, angina

GI: Nausea, vomiting, diarrhea, gastric upset, constipation, increased LFTs, dry mouth

GU: Nocturia, polyuria, sexual dysfunction, decreased libido

HEMA: Anemia

INTEG: Rash, pruritus, peripheral edema

MISC: Flushing, sexual difficulties, cough, nasal congestion, SOB, wheezing, epistaxis, respiratory infection, chest pain, angioedema, gingival hyperplasia, Stevens-Johnson syndrome

PHARMACOKINETICS

Peak plasma levels 2.5-5 hr, highly protein bound >99%, metabolized in liver, 0.5% excreted unchanged in urine, elimination half-life 11-16 hr

INTERACTIONS

Increase: bradycardia, CHF—β-blockers, digoxin, phenytoin, disopyramide

Increase: toxicity, hypotension—nitrates, alcohol, quiNIDine, zileuton, miconazole, diltiazem, delavirdine, quinupristin-dalfopristin, conivaptan, cycloSPORINE, cimetidine, clarithromycin, antiretroviral protease inhibitors, other antihypertensives, MAOIs, ketoconazole, erythromycin, itraconazole, propranolol

Decrease: antihypertensive effects—NSAIDs, carBAMazepine, barbiturates, phenytoin

Drug/Herb

Increase: antihypertensive effect—ginseng, ginkgo, hawthorn

Decrease: antihypertensive effect—ephedra, St. John's wort

Drug/Food

Increase: felodipine level—grapefruit juice

NURSING CONSIDERATIONS

Assess:

- **CHF:** I&O, weight daily; weight gain, crackles, dyspnea, edema, jugular venous distention
- Cardiac status: B/P, pulse, respiration; ECG periodically
- **Angina pain:** location, duration, intensity; ameliorating, aggravating factors

Evaluate:

- Therapeutic response: decreased B/P, decreased anginal attacks, increased activity tolerance

Teach patient/family:

- To avoid hazardous activities until stabilized on product, dizziness no longer a problem
- To avoid OTC products, alcohol unless directed by prescriber; to limit caffeine consumption
- About the importance of complying with all areas of medical regimen: diet, exercise, stress reduction, product therapy
- That tablets may appear in stools but are insignificant
- To report dyspnea, palpitations, irregular heartbeat, swelling of extremities, nausea, vomiting, severe dizziness, severe headache

- To change positions slowly to prevent orthostatic hypotension
- To obtain correct pulse; to contact prescriber if pulse <50 bpm
- Use good oral hygiene to prevent gingival hyperplasia
- Do not stop abruptly
- To avoid grapefruit juice

TREATMENT OF OVERDOSE:
Atropine for AV block, vasopressor for hypotension

fenofibrate (Rx)
(fen-oh-fee′brate)

Antara, Fenoglide ✦, Lipidil EZ ✦, Micro, Lipidil Supra ✦ Lipofen Lofibra, Tricor, Triglide

Func. class.: Antilipemic

Chem. class.: Fibric acid derivative

ACTION: Increases lipolysis and elimination of triglyceride-rich particles from plasma by activating lipoprotein lipase, thereby resulting in changes in triglyceride size and composition of LDL, leading to rapid breakdown of LDL; mobilizes triglycerides from tissue; increases excretion of neutral sterols

USES: Hypercholesterolemia; types IV, V hyperlipidemia that do not respond to other treatment and that increase risk for pancreatitis; Fredrickson type IV, V hypertriglyceridemia

CONTRAINDICATIONS: Hypertensivity, severe renal/hepatic disease, primary biliary cirrhosis, preexisting gallbladder disease, breastfeeding

Precautions: Pregnancy (C), geriatric patients, peptic ulcer, pancreatitis, renal/hepatic disease, diabetes mellitus

DOSAGE AND ROUTES

Hypertriglyceridemia

- **Adult: PO** (Antara) 43-130 mg/day; (Lofibra) 67-200 mg/day; (Tricor) 48-145 mg/day; (Triglide) 50-160 mg/day

Primary hypercholesterolemia/ mixed hyperlipidemia

- **Adult: PO** (Antara) 130 mg/day; (Lofibra) 200 mg/day; (Tricor) 145 mg/day; (Triglide) 160 mg/day

Renal dose (geriatric)

- **Adult: PO** (Tricor) CCr 30-80 ml/min, 48 mg/day; CCr <30 ml/min, contraindicated
- **Adult: PO** CCr 30-80 ml/min, 50 mg/day (Triglide, Liprofen), 30 mg/day (Antara), 40 mg daily (fenoglide), 67 mg/day (Lofibra caps), 54 mg/day (Lofibra tabs); CCr <30 ml/min, contraindicated (Antara, Lipofen, Lofibra, Triglide)

Available forms: Cap: Antara 30, 90 mg; Lipofen 50, 150 mg; **Tab:** Triglide 50, 160 mg; Lofibra 54, 160 mg; Tricor 48, 145 mg; Fenoglide 40, 120 mg

Administer:

- Product with meals (Lipofen, Lofibra); Triglide, Antara without regard to food; may increase q4-8wk; brands are not interchangeable; therapy should be discontinued if there is not adequate response after 2 mo

SIDE EFFECTS

CNS: *Fatigue, weakness,* drowsiness, dizziness, insomnia, depression, vertigo

CV: Angina, hypo/hypertension

GI: *Nausea,* vomiting, dyspepsia, increased liver enzymes, flatulence, hepatomegaly, gastritis, **pancreatitis, cholelithiasis**

GU: Dysuria, urinary frequency

HEMA: Anemia, leukopenia, **thrombosis/pulmonary embolism**

INTEG: *Rash,* urticaria, pruritus, photosensitivity

MISC: Polyphagia, weight gain, infection, flulike syndrome

MS: *Myalgias, arthralgias,* **myopathy, rhabdomyolysis**

RESP: Pharyngitis, bronchitis, cough

PHARMACOKINETICS
Peak 6-8 hr, protein binding 99%, converted to fenofibric acid, metabolized in

liver, excreted in urine (60%), feces (25%), half-life 20 hr

INTERACTIONS

Increase: myopathy—colchicine

Increase: nephrotoxicity—cycloSPORINE

• Avoid use with HMG-CoA reductase inhibitors; rhabdomyolysis may occur

Increase: anticoagulant effects—oral anticoagulants

Increase: effects of—antidiabetics

Decrease: absorption of fenofibrate—bile acid sequestrants

Drug/Herb

Increase: effect—red yeast rice

Drug/Food

Increase: absorption

Drug/Lab Test

Increase: ALT, AST, BUN, CK, creatinine

Decrease: WBC, uric acid, Hgb, paradoxical effect in HDL

NURSING CONSIDERATIONS

Assess:

• **Diet history:** fat content; lipid levels (triglycerides, LDL, HDL, cholesterol), may cause a paradoxical decrease in HDL, LFTs at baseline, periodically during treatment, CPK if muscle pain occurs, CBC, Hct, Hgb; PT with anticoagulant therapy

• **Pancreatitis, cholelithiasis renal failure, rhabdomyolysis** (when combined with HMG Co-A reductase inhibitors), myositis; product should be discontinued

Evaluate:

• Therapeutic response: decreased triglycerides, cholesterol levels

Teach patient/family:

• That compliance is needed; not to consume chipped or broken tabs (Triglide)

• That risk factors should be decreased: high-fat diet, smoking, alcohol consumption, absence of exercise

• To notify prescriber if pregnancy is suspected or planned

• To report GU symptoms: decreased libido, impotence, dysuria, proteinuria, oliguria, hematuria

• To notify prescriber of muscle pain, weakness, fever, fatigue, epigastric pain

⚠ HIGH ALERT

fentaNYL (Rx)

(fen′ta-nill)

RAN-Fentanyl ♣, Sublimaze

fentaNYL transdermal (Rx)

Duragesic

fentaNYL nasal spray (Rx)

Lazanda

fentaNYL SL spray

Subsys

fentaNYL SL

Abstral

fentaNYL buccal

Fentora

fentaNYL lozenge

Actiq

Func. class.: Opioid analgesic

Chem. class.: Synthetic phenylpiperidine

Controlled Substance Schedule II

Do not confuse:

fentaNYL/Sufenta

ACTION: Inhibits ascending pain pathways in CNS, increases pain threshold, alters pain perception by binding to opiate receptors

USES: Controls moderate to severe pain; preoperatively, postoperatively; adjunct to general anesthetic, adjunct to regional anesthesia; **FentaNYL:** anesthesia as premedication, conscious sedation; **Actiq:** breakthrough cancer pain

CONTRAINDICATIONS: Hypersensitivity to opiates, myasthenia gravis

Black Box Warning: Headache, migraine (Actiq, ABSTRAL, Fentora, Lazanda, Onsolis); emergency room use (ABSTRAL, Lazanda); outpatient surgeries (Duragesic TD); opioid-naive patients, respiratory depression

Precautions: Pregnancy (C), breastfeeding, geriatric patients, increased intracranial pressure, seizure disorders, severe respiratory disorders, cardiac dysrhythmias

Black Box Warning: Accidental exposure, ambient temperature increase, fever, skin abrasion (TD patch), substance abuse, surgery, requires an experienced clinician

DOSAGE AND ROUTES

FentaNYL

Anesthetic

- **Adult: IV** 50-100 mcg/kg over 1-2 min

Anesthesia supplement

- **Adult and child >12 yr: IM/IV** 2-20 mcg/kg **IV INFUSION** 0.025-0.25 mcg/kg/min

Induction and maintenance

- **Child 2-12 yr: IV** 2-3 mcg/kg

Preoperatively

- **Adult and child >12 yr: IM/IV** 50-100 mcg q30-60min before surgery

Postoperatively

- **Adult and child >12 yr: IM/IV** 0.05-0.1 mg q1-2hr prn

Moderate/severe pain

- **Adult: IV/IM** 50-100 mcg q1-2hr

Actiq

- **Adult: TRANSMUCOSAL** 200 mcg; redose if needed 15 min after completion of 1st dose; do not give more than 2 doses during titration period, max 4 doses/day

Fentora

- **Adult: BUCCAL/SL** 100 mcg placed above rear molar between upper cheek and gum, a second 100 mcg dose, if needed, may be started 30 min after 1st dose

ABSTRAL

- **Adult: SL** 100 mcg; another dose may be taken 30 min after 1st, max 2 doses per episode of breakthrough pain; ≥2 hr must elapse before treating again; titrate stepwise over consecutive episodes

FentaNYL transdermal

- **Adult:** 25 mcg/hr; may increase until pain relief occurs; apply patch to flat surface on upper torso and wear for 72 hr; apply new patch on different site; may use 12.5 mcg/hr if <60 mg/day morphine equivalent

FentaNYL nasal spray

- **Adult:** 100 mcg (1 spray in 1 nostril), may retreat after ≥2 hr, titrate upward until adequate analgesia; treat a max of 4 episodes daily

FentaNYL SL spray

- **Adult:** 100 mcg sprayed under tongue, titrate stepwise carefully

Available forms: Inj 0.05 mg/ml; lozenges 100, 200, 300, 400, 600, 800, 1200, 1600 mcg; lozenges on a stick 200, 400, 600, 800, 1200, 1600 mcg; buccal tab 100, 200, 400, 600, 800 mcg; SL tab (ABSTRAL) 100, 200, 300, 400, 600, 800 mcg; transdermal: patch 12, 25, 50, 75, 100 mcg/hr; *SL* spray: 100, 200, 400, 600, 800, 1200, 1600 mcg/spray, nasal spray 100, 400 mcg/actuation

Administer:

- By inj (IM, IV); give slowly to prevent rigidity
- Overdose has been fatal when confusing products/dose, recheck both before using
- Must have emergency equipment available, opioid antagonists, O_2; to be used only by those appropriately trained; IV products to be used in OR, ER, ICU

Transmucosal route

- Remove foil just before administration; instruct patient to place product between cheek and lower gum, moving it back and forth and sucking, not chewing (Actiq); place above rear molar (Fentora); place film on the inside of the cheek (Onsolis); all products not used or only partially used should be flushed down the toilet; this product may be used SL

Transdermal route

- q72hr for continuous pain relief; dosage adjusted after at least 2 applications; apply to clean, dry skin and press firmly
- Give short-acting analgesics until patch takes effect (8-24 hr); when reducing dosage or switching to alternative IV treatment, withdraw gradually; serum levels drop gradually, give 1/2 the equianalgesic dose of new analgesic 12-18 hr after removal as ordered

SL spray

- Open blister package with scissors immediately before use; spray contents of unit under tongue; dispose of each used unit after use by placing it into one of the disposable bags provided; seal bag, discard into a trash container out of reach of children

IV route

- IV undiluted by anesthesiologist or diluted with 5 ml or more sterile water or 0.9% NaCl given through Y-tube or 3-way stopcock at 0.1 mg or less/1-2 min. Muscular rigidity may occur with rapid IV administration

Y-site compatibilities: Abciximab, acyclovir, alfentanil, alemtuzumab alprostadil, amikacin, aminocaproic acid, aminophylline, amiodarone, amphotericin B cholesteryl, amphotericin B lipid complex, amphotericin B liposome, anidulafungin, argatroban, ascorbic acid injection, atenolol, atracurium, atropine, azaTHIOprine, aztreonam, benztropine, bivalirudin, bleomycin, bumetanide, buprenorphine, butorphanol, calcium chloride/gluconate, CARBOplatin, caspofungin, ceFAZolin, cefmetazole, cefonicid, cefotaxime, cefoTEtan, cefOXitin, cefTAZidime, ceftizoxime, ceftobiprole, cefTRIAXone, cefuroxime, cephalothin, chloramphenicol, chlorproMAZINE, cimetidine, cisatracurium, CISplatin, clindamycin, cloNIDine, cyanocobalamin, cyclophosphamide, cycloSPORINE, cytarabine, DACTINomycin, DAPTOmycin, dexamethasone, dexmedetomidine, digoxin, diltiazem, diphenhydrAMINE, DOBUTamine, DOCEtaxel, DOPamine, doripenem, doxacurium, doxapram, DOXOrubicin, doxycycline, enalaprilat, ePHEDrine, EPINEPHrine, epirubicin, epoetin alfa, eptifibatide, erythromycin, esmolol, etomidate, etoposide, famotidine, fenoldopam, fluconazole, fludarabine, fluorouracil, folic acid, furosemide, ganciclovir, gatifloxacin, gemcitabine, gentamicin, glycopyrrolate, granisetron, heparin, hydrocortisone, HYDROmorphone, hydrOXYzine, IDArubicin, ifosfamide, imipenem-cilastatin, inamrinone, insulin (regular), irinotecan, isoproterenol, ketorolac, labetalol, lansoprazole, levofloxacin, lidocaine, linezolid, LORazepam, LR, magnesium sulfate, mannitol, mechlorethamine, meperidine, metaraminol, methicillin, methotrexate, methotrimeprazine, methoxamine, methyldopate, methylPREDNISolone, metoclopramide, metoprolol, metroNIDAZOLE, mezlocillin, miconazole, midazolam, milrinone, minocycline, mitoXANtrone, mivacurium, morphine, moxalactam, multiple vitamins injection, mycophenolate, nafcillin, nalbuphine, naloxone, nesiritide, netilmicin, niCARdipine, nitroglycerin, nitroprusside, norepinephrine, octreotide, ondansetron, oxacillin, oxaliplatin, oxytocin, PACLitaxel, palonosetron, pamidronate, pancuronium, papaverine, PEMEtrexed, penicillin G potassium/sodium, pentamidine, pentazocine, PENTobarbital, PHENobarbital, phenylephrine, phytonadione, piperacillin, piperacillin-tazobactam, polymyxin B, potassium chloride, procainamide, prochlorperazine, promethazine, propofol, propranolol, protamine, pyridoxine, quiNIDine, quinupristin-dalfopristin, ranitidine, remifentanil, Ringer's, ritodrine, riTUXimab, rocuronium, sargramostim, scopolamine, sodium acetate/bicarbonate, succinylcholine, SUFentanil, tacrolimus, teniposide, theophylline, thiamine, thiopental, thiotepa, ticarcillin, ticarcillin-clavulanate, tigecycline, tirofiban, TNA, tobramycin, tolazoline, TPN, trastuzumab, trimetaphan, urokinase, vancomycin, vasopressin, vecuronium, verapamil, vinCRIStine, vinorelbine, vitamin B complex/C, voriconazole, zoledronic acid

SIDE EFFECTS

CNS: Dizziness, delirium, euphoria, sedation, confusion, weakness, dizziness
CV: **Bradycardia, arrest,** hypo/hypertension
EENT: Blurred vision, miosis
GI: Nausea, vomiting, constipation
GU: Urinary retention
INTEG: Rash, diaphoresis
MS: Muscle rigidity
RESP: **Respiratory depression, arrest, laryngospasm**

PHARMACOKINETICS

Metabolized by liver, excreted by kidneys, crosses placenta, excreted in breast milk, Half-life: IV: 2-4 hr, Transdermal: 13-22 hr, Transmucosal: 7 hr, Buccal: 4-12 hr, 80% bound to plasma proteins
IM: Onset 7-15 min, peak 30 min, duration 1-2 hr
IV: Onset 1 min, peak 3-5 min, duration ½-1 hr

INTERACTIONS

Black Box Warning: Increase: fentaNYL effect, fetal respiratory depression: CYP3A4 inhibitors (cycloSPORINE, ketoconazole, itraconazole, cimetidine, conivaptan, fluconazole, nefazodone, ranolazine), zafirlukast, zileuton

Increase: fatal reactions—MAOIs
Increase: hypotension—droperidol
Increase: CV depression—diazepam
Increase: fentaNYL effect with other CNS depressants—alcohol, opioids, sedative/hypnotics, antipsychotics, skeletal muscle relaxants, protease inhibitors
Decrease: fentaNYL effect—CYP3A4 inducers (carBAMazepine, phenytoin, PHENobarbital, rifampin)

Drug/Herb

Increase: action of fentaNYL—St. John's wort
Decrease: effect of fentaNYL—echinacea

Drug/Lab Test

Increase: amylase, lipase

NURSING CONSIDERATIONS

Assess:

- VS after parenteral route; note muscle rigidity, drug history, hepatic/renal function tests
- CNS changes: dizziness, drowsiness, hallucinations, euphoria, LOC, pupil reaction
- Allergic reactions: rash, urticaria

Black Box Warning: Respiratory dysfunction: respiratory depression, character, rate, rhythm; notify prescriber if respirations are <10/min

Black Box Warning: Headache/migraine: ABSTRAL, Actiq, Fentora, Lazanda, Onsolis not to be used for this condition; ABSTRAL, Lazanda not to be used in ER; Duragesic TD not to be used for outpatient surgery patients

Black Box Warning: Apnea, respiratory arrest in opioid-naive patients: do not use ABSTRAL, Actiq, Duragesic, Fentora, Lazanda, Onsolis; opioid-tolerant patients are those using ≥60 mg/day oral morphine, ≥30 mg/day oxyCODONE PO, 8 mg/day HYDROmorphone, 25 mcg TD fentaNYL/hr

Evaluate:

- Therapeutic response: induction of anesthesia, relief of breakthrough cancer pain, general pain relief
- Cancer pain, general pain relief

Teach patient/family:

- About CNS changes: physical dependence; not to use with alcohol, other CNS depressants

Black Box Warning: Accidental exposure: Discuss the dangers of children or pets ingesting or coming in contact with product

Transdermal route

Black Box Warning: Ambient temperature: that excessive heat may increase absorption; do not use with heating pads, electric blankets, heat/tanning lamps, saunas, hot tubs, heated waterbeds, when sunbathing

- That excessive perspiration may alter adhesiveness
- To dispose of patch by placing sticky sides together and flushing down toilet
- That patient may need to clip hair before applying to ensure adhesion
- May add first aid tape around the edges if there is a problem with adhesion

RARELY USED

ferric carboxymaltose

(fer′ik car-box-ee-mal′tose)

Injectafer

Func. class. Iron supplement

USES: Iron-deficiency anemia in those intolerant or those who have had poor results with other iron supplements

CONTRAINDICATIONS: Hypersensitivity, iron overload

DOSAGE AND ROUTES

Adults ≥50 kg: **IV** Give 2 doses of 750 mg/dose separated by ≥7 days, max 1500 mg of iron per course, may repeat if iron deficiency anemia recurs

Adults <50 kg: **IV** Give 2 doses of 15 mg/kg/dose separated by ≥7 days, max 1500 mg of iron per course, may repeat if iron-deficiency anemia recurs

Available forms: 750 mg/15 ml solution for injection

ferrous fumarate (Rx)

Femiron, Feostat, Ferrate, Ferretts, Ferrocite Hemocyte, Palafer ♣

ferrous gluconate (Rx)

Fergon

ferrous sulfate (Rx)

Feosol, Fer-Gen-Sol, Fer-In-Sol, FeroSul

ferrous sulfate, dried (Rx)

Feosol, Feratab, Slow Fe, slow-release Iron

carbonyl iron (OTC)

(kar′bo-nil)

ICAR Pediatric, Iron Chews

iron polysaccharide (OTC)

iFerex, Niferex, Nu-Iron

Func. class.: Hematinic

Chem. class.: Iron preparation

ACTION: Replaces iron stores needed for red blood cell development as well as energy and O_2 transport and use; fumarate contains 33% elemental iron; gluconate, 12%; sulfate, 20%; iron, 30%; ferrous sulfate exsiccated

USES: Iron deficiency anemia, prophylaxis for iron deficiency in pregnancy, nutritional supplementation

CONTRAINDICATIONS: Sideroblastic anemia, thalassemia, hemosiderosis/hemochromatosis

Precautions: Pregnancy (B) (ferric gluconate complex), (C) (iron dextran, oral products), anemia (long term), ulcerative colitis/regional enteritis, peptic ulcer disease, hemolytic anemia, cirrhosis, sulfite sensitivity

Black Box Warning: Accidental exposure

DOSAGE AND ROUTES

Fumarate

- **Adult: PO** 200-325 mg tid
- **Child: PO** 3 mg/kg/day (elemental iron) tid-qid
- **Infant: PO** 10-25 mg/day (elemental iron) in 3-4 divided doses, max 15 mg/day

Gluconate

- **Adult: PO** 50-100 mg elemental iron tid
- **Child: PO** 3 mg/kg/day in divided doses

Sulfate

- **Adult: PO** 0.75-1.5 g/day in divided doses tid
- **Child 6-12 yr: PO** 3 mg/kg/day in divided doses

Pregnancy

- **Adult: PO** 300-600 mg/day in divided doses

Iron polysaccharide

- **Adult: PO** 100-200 mg tid
- **Child: PO** 4-6 mg/kg/day in 3 divided doses (severe iron deficiency)

Available forms: Fumarate: tabs 90, 150, 200, 300, 324, 325 mg; chewable tabs 100 mg; ext rel tabs 18 mg; **gluconate:** tabs 225, 240, 324, 325 mg; **sulfate:** tabs 195, 300, 325 mg; elixir 220 mg/5 ml; **dried:** tabs 200 mg; ext rel tabs 160 mg; ext rel caps 160 mg; **iron polysaccharide:** tabs 50 mg; caps 150 mg; sol 100 mg/5 ml

Administer:

PO route

- Swallow tabs whole; do not break, crush, or chew unless labeled as chewable
- Between meals for best absorption; may give with juice; do not give with antacids or milk, delay at least 1 hr; if GI symptoms occur, give after meals even if absorption is decreased; eggs, milk products, chocolate, caffeine interfere with absorption
- Store in tight, light-resistant container
- **Liquid** through plastic straw to avoid discoloration of tooth enamel; dilute thoroughly
- At least 1 hr before bedtime; corrosion may occur in stomach; ferrous gluconate is less irritating to GI tract than ferrous sulfate
- For <6 mo for anemia

SIDE EFFECTS

GI: *Nausea, constipation, epigastric pain, black and red tarry stools,* vomiting, diarrhea

INTEG: Temporarily discolored tooth enamel and eyes

SYST: **Hypersensitivity reactions (Ferrlecit)**

PHARMACOKINETICS

PO: Excreted in feces, urine, skin, breast milk; enters bloodstream; bound to transferrin; crosses placenta

INTERACTIONS

Increase: action of iron preparation—ascorbic acid, chloramphenicol

Decrease: absorption of penicillamine, levodopa, methyldopa, fluoroquinolones, L-thyroxine, tetracycline

Decrease: absorption of iron preparations—antacids, H_2-antagonists, proton pump inhibitors, cholestyramine, vit E

Drug/Food

Decrease: absorption—dairy products, caffeine, eggs

Drug/Lab Test

False positive: occult blood

NURSING CONSIDERATIONS

Assess:

- Blood studies: Hct, Hgb, reticulocytes, bilirubin before treatment, at least monthly; iron studies (iron, TIBC, ferritin)

⚠ **Toxicity: nausea, vomiting, diarrhea (green then tarry stools), hematemesis, pallor, cyanosis, shock, coma**

- Elimination: if constipation occurs, increase water, bulk, activity
- **Nutrition:** amount of iron in diet (meat, dark green leafy vegetables, dried beans, dried fruits, eggs)

- Cause of iron loss or anemia, including salicylates, sulfonamides, antimalarials, quiNIDine

Evaluate:

- Therapeutic response: improvement in Hct, Hgb, reticulocytes; decreased fatigue, weakness

Teach patient/family:

- That iron will turn stools black or dark green, stain teeth
- **Accidental exposure:** to keep out of reach of children, pets; iron poisoning may occur if increased beyond recommended level
- Not to substitute 1 iron salt for another; that elemental iron content differs (e.g., 300 mg ferrous fumarate contains about 100 mg elemental iron; 300 mg ferrous gluconate contains only about 30 mg elemental iron)
- To avoid reclining position for 15-30 min after taking product to avoid esophageal corrosion
- To follow a diet high in iron; to avoid taking iron, dairy products, calcium supplements, and vit C together because they compete for absorption

TREATMENT OF OVERDOSE:

Induce vomiting; give eggs, milk until lavage can be done

fesoterodine (Rx)

(fess′oh-ter-oh-deen)

Toviaz

Func. class.: Overactive bladder product

Chem. class.: Muscarinic receptor antagonist

ACTION: Relaxes smooth muscles in urinary tract by inhibiting acetylcholine at postganglionic sites

USES: Overactive bladder (urinary frequency, urgency), urinary incontinence

CONTRAINDICATIONS: GI obstruction, ileus, pyloric stenosis, urinary retention, gastric retention, hypersensitivity, closed-angle glaucoma

Precautions: Pregnancy (C), breastfeeding, children, renal/hepatic disease, urinary tract obstruction, ambient temperature increase, autonomic neuropathy, constipation, contact lenses, hazardous activity, GERD, gastroparesis, myasthenia gravis, prostatic hypertrophy, toxic megacolon, ulcerative colitis, possible cross-sensitivity with tolterodine

DOSAGE AND ROUTES

- **Adult and geriatric: PO EXT REL** 4 mg/day, may increase to 8 mg/day based on response, max 4 mg/day in those taking potent CYP3A4 inhibitors

Renal dose

- **Adult: PO EXT REL** CCr <30 ml/min, max 4 mg/day in severe renal impairment

Available forms: EXT REL TABS 4, 8 mg

Administer:

- Do not break, crush, or chew ext rel product
- Give without regard to meals
- Store at room temperature; protect from moisture

SIDE EFFECTS

CNS: Insomnia

CV: Chest pain, angina, QT prolongation, peripheral edema

EENT: Xerophthalmia

GI: *Nausea, vomiting,* abdominal pain, constipation, dry mouth

GU: Dysuria, urinary retention, UTI

INTEG: Rash, angioedema

MISC: Peripheral edema, insomnia

MS: Back pain

RESP: Cough, URI

SYST: Infection

PHARMACOKINETICS

Peak 5 hr, rapidly absorbed, protein binding 50%, excreted in urine/feces, half-life 7 hr

INTERACTIONS

Increase: action of fesoterodine—CYP3A4 inhibitors (antiretroviral protease

inhibitors, macrolide antiinfectives, azole antifungals)
Increase: anticholinergic effect—antimuscarinics, anticholinergics
Increase: urinary frequency—diuretics
Drug/Herb
Decrease: fesoterodine—caffeine, green tea, guarana
Drug/Food
Increase: fesoterodine level—grapefruit juice
Decrease: fesoterodine level—cola, coffee, tea

NURSING CONSIDERATIONS

Assess:
- **Urinary patterns:** distention, nocturia, frequency, urgency, incontinence
- **Allergic reactions:** rash; if this occurs, product should be discontinued

Evaluate:
- Therapeutic response: absence of urinary frequency, urgency, incontinence

Teach patient/family:
- Not to drink liquids before bedtime
- About the importance of bladder maintenance
- Not to use new meds, herbs without prescriber approval

fexofenadine (Rx, OTC)

(fex-oh-fi′na-deen)

Allegra

Func. class.: Antihistamine—2nd generation

Chem. class.: Piperidine, peripherally selective

Do not confuse:
Allegra/Viagra

ACTION: Acts on blood vessels, GI, respiratory system by competing with histamine for H_1-receptor site; decreases allergic response by blocking pharmacologic effects of histamine, less sedating

USES: Rhinitis, allergy symptoms, chronic idiopathic urticaria

CONTRAINDICATIONS: Breastfeeding, newborn or premature infants, hypersensitivity
Precautions: Pregnancy (C), children, geriatric patients, respiratory disease, closed-angle glaucoma, prostatic hypertrophy, bladder neck obstruction, asthma, renal failure

F

DOSAGE AND ROUTES

- **Adult and child >12 yr: PO** Rx only, 60 mg bid or 180 mg/day; PO OTC only, 60 mg bid or 180 mg/day (self-treatment of allergic rhinitis)
- **Child 2-11 yr: PO** 30 mg bid; **ORALLY DISINTEGRATING TAB Child 6-11 yr:** 30 mg bid dissolved on tongue

Renal dose
- **Adult and child ≥12 yr: PO** CCr <80 ml/min, 60 mg/day
- **Child 2-11 yr: PO** CCr <80 ml/min, 30 mg daily
- **Child <2 yr: PO** CCr <80 ml/min, 15 mg daily

Available forms: Tabs 30, 60, 180 mg; oral susp 6 mg/ml, orally disintegrating tab 30 mg
Administer:
- Without regard to meals; caps/tabs should not be given with or right before grapefruit, orange, or apple juice
- Store in tight, light-resistant container
- **Orally disintegrating tab:** allow to dissolve, swallow; do not remove from blister pack until time of administration
- **Oral susp:** shake well; use calibrated measuring device

SIDE EFFECTS

CNS: Headache, stimulation, drowsiness, sedation, fatigue, confusion, blurred vision, tinnitus, restlessness, tremors, paradoxical excitation in children or geriatric patients
CV: Hypotension, palpitations, bradycardia, tachycardia, dysrhythmias (rare)
GI: Nausea, diarrhea, abdominal pain, vomiting, constipation

GU: Frequency, dysuria, urinary retention, impotence
HEMA: Hemolytic anemia, thrombocytopenia, leukopenia, agranulocytosis, pancytopenia
INTEG: Rash, eczema, photosensitivity, urticaria
RESP: Thickening of bronchial secretions, dry nose, throat

PHARMACOKINETICS

Well absorbed; onset 1 hr; peak 2-3 hr; duration 12-24 hr; 80% excreted in urine; half-life 14.5 hr, increased in renal disease

INTERACTIONS

Increase: fexofenadine effect—erythromycin, ketoconazole
Decrease: fexofenadine effect—rifampin
Decrease: effect—magnesium-aluminum-containing antacids
Drug/Food
Decrease: absorption of product—apple, orange, grapefruit juice
Drug/Lab Test
False negative: skin allergy tests

NURSING CONSIDERATIONS

Assess:
- **Allergy:** itchy, runny, watery eyes; congested nose; before and during treatment
- I&O ratio: be alert for urinary retention, frequency, dysuria, especially among geriatric patients; product should be discontinued if these occur; serum creatinine/BUN at baseline and periodically during treatment
- Bronchial secretions, lung sounds, increase fluids to 2000 ml/day unless contraindicated to decrease thickness of secretions

Evaluate:
- Therapeutic response: absence of running or congested nose or rashes

Teach patient/family:
- About all aspects of product use; to notify prescriber if confusion, sedation, hypotension occur
- To avoid driving, other hazardous activity if drowsiness occurs
- To avoid alcohol, other CNS depressants
- **Not to exceed recommended dose; that dysrhythmias may occur**

TREATMENT OF OVERDOSE:

Lavage, diazepam, vasopressors, IV phenytoin

fidaxomicin

(fye-dax′oh-mye′sin)

Dificid

Func. class.: Antiinfective-macrolide

ACTION: Bactericidal against *Clostridium difficile;* is a fermentation product obtained from *Dactylosporangium aurantiacum;* inhibits RNA synthesis by inhibiting transcription of bacterial RNA polymerases; may act at the early stages of transcription

USES: Pseudomembraneous colitis *Clostridium difficile*-associated diarrhea

CONTRAINDICATIONS: Hypersensitivity
Precautions: Pregnancy (B), breastfeeding, children

DOSAGE AND ROUTES

- **Adult: PO** 200 mg bid × 10 days

Available forms: Tab 200 mg
Administer:
- Without regard to food
- Store at room temperature

SIDE EFFECTS

GI: Nausea, vomiting, abdominal pain, **GI bleeding**, intestinal obstruction
HEMA: Anemia, **neutropenia**
INTEG: Rash, pruritus
META: Metabolic acidosis, hyperglycemia

PHARMACOKINETICS

Half-life 12 hr, onset <1 hr, peak 1-5 hr, excreted in feces 92%, minimal absorption, substrate of PGP efflux transporter

INTERACTIONS

Increase: fidaxomicin action—cycloSPORINE

Drug/Lab Test

Increase: glucose, LFTs, alk phos

Decrease: sodium bicarbonate, platelets

NURSING CONSIDERATIONS

Assess:

- **Pseudomembraneous colitis:** for diarrhea, abdominal pain, fever, fatigue, anorexia, anemia, elevated WBC and low serum albumin; product may be used in place of vancomycin; monitor CBC with differential and stool culture (*Clostridium difficile*), not to be used for systemic infection, obtain C&S before use, monitor glucose (diabetic patients), monitor fluid, electrolyte depletion

Evaluate:

- Positive therapeutic response: resolution of *Clostridium difficile,* decreased diarrhea

Teach patient/family:

- To report GI bleeding, severe abdominal pain
- To report if pregnancy is planned or suspected or if breastfeeding
- May take without regard to food

⚠ HIGH ALERT

filgrastim (Rx)

(fill-grass′stim)

G-CSF, granulocyte colony stimulator, Neupogen

Func. class.: Biologic modifier

Chem. class.: Granulocyte colony-stimulating factor

ACTION: Stimulates proliferation and differentiation of neutrophils

USES: To decrease infection in patients receiving antineoplastics that are myelosuppressive; to increase WBC in patients with product-induced neutropenia; bone marrow transplantation, acute radiation exposure

Unlabeled uses: Neutropenia with HIV infection, aplastic anemia, ganciclovir-induced neutropenia, zidovudine-induced neutropenia

CONTRAINDICATIONS: Hypersensitivity to proteins of *Escherichia coli*

Precautions: Pregnancy (C), breastfeeding, children, myeloid malignancies, radiation therapy, sepsis, sickle cell disease, chemotherapy, respiratory disease

DOSAGE AND ROUTES

After myelosuppressive chemotherapy

- **Adult and child: IV/SUBCUT** 5 mcg/kg/day in a single dose × up to 14 days; may increase by 5 mcg/kg with each cycle

After myelosuppressive doses of radiation

- **Adult and child >7 mo: SUBCUT** 10 mcg/kg/day, start as soon as possible after receiving ≥2 Gy

After bone marrow transplantation

- **Adult: IV/SUBCUT** 10 mcg/kg/day as **INFUSION (IV)** over 4 hr or 24 hr, begin 24 hr after chemotherapy and 24 hr after bone marrow transplantation

Peripheral blood progenitor cell collection/therapy

- **Adult:** 10 mcg/kg/day as bolus or **CONT INFUSION** × ≥4 days before leukapheresis, continue to last leukapheresis; may alter dose if WBC >100,000 cells/mm^3

Severe neutropenia (chronic), idiopathic/cyclical

- **Adult: SUBCUT** 5 mcg/kg daily

Available forms: Inj 300 mcg/ml, 480 mcg/1.6 ml, 480 mcg/0.8 ml

Administer:

- Given by subcut inj, short IV infusion, or continuous SC or IV infusion
- Avoid use within 24 hr before or after chemotherapy
- Do not shake commercial single-dose vials before withdrawing the dose; if the

vial is shaken and froth or bubbles form, allow the vial to stand undisturbed for a few minutes until the froth or bubbles dissipate
• Before injection, filgrastim may be allowed to reach room temperature for a maximum of 24 hr; any vial or syringe exposed to room temperature for more than 24 hr should be discarded
• Visually inspect for particulate matter and discoloration before use
• Store in refrigerator; do not freeze; may store at room temperature up to 24 hr

SUBCUT route
• **Subcut inj:** no dilution is necessary; inject by rapid subcut inj, taking care not to inject intradermally
• **Subcut continuous infusion:** infuse subcut at a rate not to exceed 2 ml/hr

IV route
• May be diluted with 5% dextrose; do not dilute with NS; product can precipitate
• May be diluted to concentrations 5-15 mcg/ml; should be protected from adsorption to plastic by the addition of albumin to a final albumin concentration of 2 mg/ml; do not dilute filgrastim to a concentration <5 mcg/ml
• **IV infusion:** infuse IV over 15-30 min or as a continuous infusion over 24 hr

Y-site compatibilities: Acyclovir, allopurinol, amikacin, aminophylline, ampicillin, ampicillin/sulbactam, aztreonam, bleomycin, bumetanide, buprenorphine, butorphanol, calcium gluconate, CARBOplatin, carmustine, ceFAZolin, cefoTEtan, cefTAZidime, chlorproMAZINE, cimetidine, CISplatin, cyclophosphamide, cytarabine, dacarbazine, DAUNOrubicin, dexamethasone, diphenhydrAMINE, DOXOrubicin, doxycycline, droperidol, enalaprilat, famotidine, floxuridine, fluconazole, fludarabine, gallium, ganciclovir, granisetron, haloperidol, hydrocortisone, HYDROmorphone, hydrOXYzine, IDArubicin, ifosfamide, leucovorin, LORazepam, mechlorethamine, melphalan, meperidine, mesna, methotrexate, metoclopramide, miconazole, minocycline, mitoXANtrone, morphine, nalbuphine, netilmicin, ondansetron, plicamycin, potassium chloride, promethazine, ranitidine, sodium bicarbonate, streptozocin, ticarcillin, ticarcillin/clavulanate, tobramycin, trimethoprim-sulfamethoxazole, vancomycin, vinBLAStine, vinCRIStine, vinorelbine, zidovudine

SIDE EFFECTS

CNS: Fever, headache
GI: *Nausea,* vomiting, diarrhea, mucositis, anorexia
HEMA: Thrombocytopenia, excessive leukocytosis
INTEG: Alopecia, exacerbation of skin conditions, urticaria, cutaneous vasculitis, allergic reactions
MS: Osteoporosis, skeletal pain
OTHER: Chest pain, hypotension
RESP: Acute respiratory distress syndrome, wheezing, alveolar hemorrhage

PHARMACOKINETICS

SUBCUT: Onset 5-60 min, peak 2-8 hr, duration up to 1 wk
IV: Onset 5-60 min, peak 24 hr, duration up to 1 wk

INTERACTIONS

Increase: adverse reactions—do not use this product concomitantly with antineoplastics, lithium

Drug/Lab Test
Increase: uric acid, LDH, alk phos, WBC

NURSING CONSIDERATIONS

Assess:
• Blood studies: CBC, platelet count before treatment and twice weekly; neutrophil counts drop by 50% if filgrastim is discontinued the next day
• B/P, respirations, pulse before and during therapy
• Bone pain; give mild analgesics
• CBC with differential, platelets
• Respiratory distress syndrome: fever, dyspnea; withhold product if these occur
• Allergic reactions: rash, wheezing, facial edema, dyspnea, may occur within 30 min of use, give antihistamines, bronchodilators and epinephrine if needed

Evaluate:
- Therapeutic response: absence of infection

Teach patient/family:
- About the technique for self-administration: dose, side effects, disposal of containers and needles; provide instruction sheet
- That bone pain is common

finasteride (Rx)

(fin-ass′te-ride)

Propecia, Proscar

Func. class.: Hormone, androgen inhibitor, hair stimulant

Chem. class.: 5-α-Reductase inhibitor

Do not confuse:
finasteride/furosemide
Proscar/ProSom/PROzac

ACTION: Inhibits 5-α-reductase and reduction in DHT; DHT induces androgenic effects by binding to androgen receptors in the cell nuclei of the prostate gland, liver, skin; prevents development of BHP

USES: Symptomatic benign prostatic hyperplasia (Proscar); male-pattern baldness (Propecia)
Unlabeled uses: Hirsutism, prostate cancer prophylaxis

CONTRAINDICATIONS: Pregnancy (X), breastfeeding, children, women who are pregnant or who may become pregnant should not handle tabs, hypersensitivity
Precautions: Large residual urinary volume, severely diminished urinary flow, hepatic function abnormalities

DOSAGE AND ROUTES

BPH
- **Adult: PO** 5 mg/day × 6-12 mo (Proscar)

Male-pattern baldness
- **Adult: PO** 1 mg/day for 3 mo or more for results (Propecia)

Hirsutism (unlabeled)
- **Adult (nonpregnant): PO** 5 mg/day alone or in combination with oral contraceptives

Available forms: Tabs (Propecia) 1 mg, (Proscar) 5 mg

Administer:
- Without regard to meals
- For a minimum of 6 mo; not all patients will respond
- Store <86° F (30° C); protect from light; keep container tightly closed

F

SIDE EFFECTS

GU: Impotence, decreased libido, decreased volume of ejaculate, sexual dysfunction
INTEG: Rash
MISC: Breast tenderness, **secondary malignancy**

PHARMACOKINETICS

Bioavailability 63%; readily absorbed from GI tract; plasma protein binding 90%; metabolized in the liver; excreted in urine (metabolites) 39%, feces (57%); crosses blood-brain barrier; peak 1-2 hr; duration 24 hr

INTERACTIONS

Drug/Lab Test
Decrease: PSA levels

NURSING CONSIDERATIONS

Assess:
- **BPH:** urinary patterns, residual urinary volume, severely diminished urinary flow
- PSA levels and digital rectal exam before initiating therapy and periodically thereafter, PSA levels may be altered by this product
- Hepatic studies before treatment; extensively metabolized in liver

Evaluate:
- Therapeutic response: increased urinary flow; decreased postvoiding dribbling, frequency, nocturia or hair growth within 3-6 mo; regression of prostate size

Teach patient/family:

⚠ That pregnant women or women who may become pregnant should not touch crushed tabs or come into contact with the semen of a patient taking this product; that product may adversely affect developing male fetus

- That volume of ejaculate may be decreased during treatment; that impotence and decreased libido may also occur and may continue after discontinuing treatment
- That Propecia results may not occur for 3 mo
- That Proscar results may not occur for 6-12 mo

fingolimod (Rx)

(fin-gol′i-mod)

Gilenya

Func. class.: Biologic response modifier

Chem. class.: Sphingosine 1-phosphate receptor modulator

ACTION: Binds with high affinity to sphingosine 1-phosphate receptors; blocks lymphocyte egress to lymph nodes, thereby reducing the number of peripheral blood lymphocytes; may reduce lymphocyte migration into the CNS

USES: To reduce frequency of exacerbation, to delay physical disability of relapsing forms of MS

CONTRAINDICATIONS: Hypersensitivity

Precautions: Pregnancy (C), breastfeeding, neonates/infants/children, AIDS, asthma, AV block, bradycardia, cardiac disease, COPD, diabetes mellitus, dysrhythmias, heart failure, hepatic disease, HIV, hypertension, immunosuppression, leukemia, lymphoma, QT prolongation, respiratory insufficiency, sick sinus syndrome, syncope, uveitis

DOSAGE AND ROUTES

- **Adult: PO** 0.5 mg/day

Hepatic dose

- **Adult: PO** Child-Pugh C, total score >10: closely monitor, fingolimod exposure is doubled

Available forms: Caps 0.5 mg

Administer:

PO route

- Watch patient for 6 hr after initial dose or if product not given for >2 wk for development of bradycardia
- Give without regard to food
- Store at room temperature, protect from moisture

SIDE EFFECTS

CNS: Asthenia, depression, fatigue, headache, dizziness, **progressive multifocal leukoencephalopathy,** migraine, paresthesias, **stroke**

CV: **AV block, bradycardia,** chest pain, hypertension, palpitations, **QT prolongation**

EENT: Blurred vision, vision impairment, ocular pain, macular edema

GI: Abdominal pain, anorexia, diarrhea, jaundice, vomiting, weight loss

HEMA: **Leukopenia, lymphopenia, neutropenia**

INTEG: Alopecia, pruritus

MS: Back pain

RESP: Dyspnea, cough

SYST: Infection, influenza, **secondary malignancy**

PHARMACOKINETICS

Protein binding (99.7%), distributed to RBCs (86%), steady state 1-2 mo, metabolized by CYP4F2 and CYP2D6 to a lesser extent, terminal half-life 6-9 days, excreted in urine (81% inactive metabolites), peak 12-16 hr

INTERACTIONS

Increase: risk of heart block, serious bradycardia—β-blockers, calcium channel blockers, digoxin

Increase: immunosuppression—antineoplastics, immunosuppressants, immune-modulating therapies

Increase: fingolimod effect—ketoconazole

Increase: infection risk—live vaccines

Decrease: effect of—inactive vaccines, toxoids
Increase: risk of torsades de pointes—Class Ia/III antidysrhythmics

NURSING CONSIDERATIONS

Assess:

- **Multiple sclerosis:** improving paresthesia, muscle weakness, clonus, muscle spasms, difficulty with moving, difficulty with coordination of balance, speech, swallowing, vision problems, fatigue; prevention of increasing disability
- **Laboratory monitoring:** obtain before initial dose; CBC, LFTs, serum bilirubin, ophthalmologic exam, antibodies to VZV; if there is no history of chickenpox or no vaccination, may give VZV vaccination to antibody-negative patient before giving product, postpone for 1 mo after vaccination; obtain ECG for evidence of bradycardia, AV block
- **Progressive multifocal leukoencephalopathy (PML):** confusion, apathy, dizziness, unstable gait; may be fatal, discontinue product, contact prescriber
- **Bradycardia:** monitor for ≥6 hr after beginning dose, ECG before and after 1st dose, if heart rate <45 bpm or new heart block (2nd degree) occurs, do not use until resolved
- Monitor for QT prolongation

Evaluate:

- Therapeutic response: improved symptoms of multiple sclerosis and prevention of increasing disability

Teach patient/family:

- About use of product and expected results; provide med guide to patient
- That continuing follow-up exams and laboratory tests will be required on a regular basis
- To use contraception during and for 2 mo after conclusion of treatment

Liver dysfunction: report jaundice, nausea, vomiting, anorexia, abdominal pain, fatigue, dark urine red
Cardiac changes: chest pain, palpitations

flecainide (Rx)

(flek-ay′nide)

Tambocor ✦

Func. class.: Antidysrhythmic (Class IC)

ACTION:
Decreases conduction in all parts of the heart, with greatest effect on the His-Purkinje system, which stabilizes cardiac membrane

USES:
Life-threatening ventricular dysrhythmias, sustained ventricular tachycardia, supraventricular tachydysrhythmias, paroxysmal atrial fibrillation/flutter associated with disabling symptoms
Unlabeled uses: Atrial fibrillation, single dose

CONTRAINDICATIONS:
Hypersensitivity, AV bundle branch block, cardiogenic shock
Precautions: Pregnancy (C), breastfeeding, children, geriatric patients, renal/hepatic disease, CHF, respiratory depression, myasthenia gravis, electrolyte abnormalities, atrial fibrillation, sick sinus syndrome, torsades de pointes, MI, bundle branch block, QT prolongation

Black Box Warning: Cardiac arrhythmias, atrial fibrillation

DOSAGE AND ROUTES

PSVT/PAT

- **Adult: PO** 50 mg q12hr; may increase q4days by 50 mg q12hr to desired response, max 300 mg/day

Life-threatening ventricular dysrhythmias

- **Adult: PO** 100 mg q12hr; may increase by 50 mg q12hr q4days, max 400 mg/day

Renal dose

- **Adult: PO** CCr <35 ml/min, 100 mg daily or 50 mg bid initially

Available forms: Tabs 50, 100, 150 mg

Administer:

PO route

- Reduced dosage as soon as dysrhythmia is controlled
- May give with meals for GI upset
- May adjust dose q4days
- Therapeutic trough serum concentrations for adults range from 200 to 1000 ng/ml (average, 500 ng/ml); toxicity is more common with trough serum concentrations >1000 ng/mL; usual therapeutic range in children is 200-500 ng/mL; in some cases, up to 800 ng/mL is required
- Adjust dosage at intervals of ≥4 days (approximate plateau effects) following dosage adjustments; however, longer intervals are needed in patients with renal or hepatic impairment
- Frequent serum drug concentration monitoring is required for patients with severe renal (CrCl <35 ml/min) or hepatic disease and may also be helpful in patients with CHF or in patients with moderate renal disease
- Monitoring of flecainide serum concentrations is strongly recommended in patients receiving amiodarone therapy

SIDE EFFECTS

CNS: *Headache, dizziness,* involuntary movement, confusion, psychosis, restlessness, irritability, paresthesias, ataxia, flushing, somnolence, depression, anxiety, malaise, fatigue, asthenia, tremors

CV: *Hypotension, bradycardia,* angina, PVCs, heart block, cardiovascular collapse, arrest, dysrhythmias, CHF, fatal ventricular tachycardia, palpitations, QT prolongation, torsades de pointes

EENT: Tinnitus, *blurred vision,* hearing loss, corneal deposits, dry eyes

GI: Nausea, vomiting, anorexia, constipation, abdominal pain, flatulence, change in taste, diarrhea

GU: Impotence, decreased libido, polyuria, urinary retention

HEMA: Leukopenia, thrombocytopenia

INTEG: Rash, urticaria, edema, swelling

RESP: Dyspnea, respiratory depression

PHARMACOKINETICS

Peak 3 hr, half-life 12-27 hr, metabolized by liver, excreted unchanged by kidneys (10%), excreted in breast milk

INTERACTIONS

Increase: QT prolongation—class IA/III antidysrhythmics, some phenothiazines, β-agonists, local anesthetics, tricyclics, haloperidol, chloroquine, droperidol, pentamidine; CYP3A4 inhibitors (amiodarone, clarithromycin, erythromycin, telithromycin, troleandomycin), arsenic trioxide, levomethadyl; CYP3A4 substrates (methadone, pimozide, quetiapine, quinidine, risperidone, ziprasidone)

Increase: of both products—propranolol

Increase: CV depressant action—β-blockers, disopyramide, verapamil

Increase: flecainide level—amiodarone, cimetidine, ritonavir

Increase: digoxin level—digoxin

Increase or decrease: effect—urinary, alkalinizing agents, acidifying agents

Drug/Herb

- Do not use with hawthorn

Drug/Lab Test

Increase: CPK

NURSING CONSIDERATIONS

Assess:

Black Box Warning: **CHF, cardiogenic shock:** should not be used in these conditions

Black Box Warning: **Atrial fibrillation:** avoid use, risk of ventricular dysrhythmias

Black Box Warning: **Cardiac dysrhythmias:** discontinue in those with prolonged QRS >180 ms or prolonged PR >300 ms, monitor for QT prolongation, monitor ECG before and during treatment

- **Electrolyte imbalances:** hypo/hyperkalemia before administration; correct electrolytes before use
- CNS effects: dizziness, confusion, psychosis, paresthesias, seizures; product should be discontinued

• **Flecainide level:** Monitor level in those with CHF or renal failure; peak, trough

Evaluate:

• Therapeutic response: decreased dysrhythmias

Teach patient/family:

• To change position slowly from lying or sitting to standing to minimize orthostatic hypotension

• To take as prescribed; not to skip or double dose, take missed dose as soon as remembered (within 6 hr) of next dose

• To avoid hazardous activities that require alertness until response is known

• To carry emergency ID with disorder, medications taken

• To notify all health care providers of treatment, that follow-up will be needed

• To report new or worsening cardiac symptoms (chest pain, trouble breathing, sweating)

TREATMENT OF OVERDOSE:

O_2, artificial ventilation, ECG, DOPamine for circulatory depression, diazepam or thiopental for seizures, treat ventricular dysrhythmias

fluconazole (Rx)

(floo-kon′a-zole)

Diflucan

Func. class.: Antifungal, systemic; azole

Chem class: Triazole

Do not confuse:

Diflucan/Diprivan

ACTION:
Inhibits ergosterol biosynthesis, causes direct damage to fungal membrane phospholipids

USES:
Oropharyngeal candidiasis, chronic mucocutaneous candidiasis; systemic, vaginal, urinary candidiasis; cryptococcal meningitis; prevention of candidiasis in bone marrow transplant in those who receive chemotherapy and/or radiation therapy; cystitis, fungal prophylaxis, peritonitis, pneumonia, pyelonephritis

Unlabeled uses: Prophylaxis, systemic candidiasis in very-low-birthweight premature infants, blastomycosis, chemotherapy-induced neutropenia, coccidioidomycosis cryptococcosis prophylaxis, endocarditis, endophthalmitis, histoplasmosis infectious arthritis, myocarditis, osteomyelitis, pericarditis

CONTRAINDICATIONS:
Hypersensitivity to this product or azoles, pregnancy (D)

Precautions: Breastfeeding, renal/hepatic disease, torsades de pointes

DOSAGE AND ROUTES

Vulvovaginal candidiasis

• **Adult: PO** 150 mg as a single dose

Serious fungal infections

• **Adult: PO/IV** 50-400 mg initially, then 200 mg/day for 4 wk

• **Child:** 6-12 mg/kg/day

Oropharyngeal candidiasis

• **Adult: PO/IV** 200 mg initially, then 100 mg/day for ≥2 wk

• **Child: PO/IV** 6 mg/kg initially, then 3 mg/kg/day for ≥2 wk

Esophageal candidiasis

• **Adult: PO/IV** 200 mg on 1st day, then 100 mg daily × ≥3 wk and for ≥2 wk after resolution of symptoms

• **Child: PO/IV** 6 mg/kg on 1st day, then 3 mg/kg × ≥3 wk and for ≥2 wk after resolution of symptoms

Cryptococcal meningitis

• **Adult: PO/IV** 400 mg on 1st day, then 200 mg daily × 10-12 wk after CSF culture negative

• **Child/infants/neonates ≥14 days: PO/IV** 12 mg/kg on 1st day, then 6-12 mg/kg daily × 10-12 wk after CSF culture negative, max 600 mg/day

• **Neonates 0-14 days: PO/IV** 12 mg/kg on 1st day, then 6-12 mg/kg q72hr × 10-12 wk after CSF culture negative

Prevention of candidiasis in bone marrow transplant

• **Adult: PO/IV** 400 mg/day, those anticipated to have neutrophils <500/mm^3, start several days before anticipated onset of neutropenia and continue for 7 days after rise of neutrophils $>1000/mm^3$

Renal disease

- **Adult: PO/IV** CCr $\leq$50 ml/min, after loading dose, give 50% of usual dose

Available forms: Tabs 50, 100, 150, 200 mg; inj 2 mg/ml; powder for oral susp 10 mg/ml, 40 mg/ml

Administer:

PO route

- Tap bottle to loosen powder, add water in 2 portions, review manufacturer reconstitution instructions
- Shake oral susp before each use, use within 2 wk

Intermittent IV INFUSION route

- After diluting according to package directions; run at $\leq$200 mg/hr; do not use plastic containers in connections; check for bag leaks
- Use infusion pump; check for extravasation and necrosis q2hr
- Do not use if cloudy or precipitated
- Do not admix; do not refrigerate
- Store protected from moisture and light; diluted sol stable 24 hr; do not freeze

Y-site compatibilities: Acyclovir, aldesleukin, alfentanil, allopurinol, amifostine, amikacin, aminocaproic acid, aminophylline, amiodarone, anidulafungin, ascorbic acid injection, atenolol, atracurium, atropine, azaTHIOprine, aztreonam, benztropine, bivalirudin, bleomycin, bumetanide, buprenorphine, butorphanol, calcium chloride, CARBOplatin, caspofungin, ceFAZolin, cefepime, cefmetazole, cefonicid, cefoTEtan, cefOXitin, cefpirome, cefTAZidime, ceftizoxime, ceftobiprole, cephalothin, cephapirin, chlorproMAZINE, cimetidine, cisatracurium, CISplatin, codeine, cyanocobalamin, cyclophosphamide, cycloSPORINE, cytarabine, DACTINomycin, DAPTOmycin, dexamethasone, diltiazem, dimenhyDRINATE, diphenhydrAMINE, DOBUTamine, DOCEtaxel, DOPamine, doripenem, doxacurium, DOXOrubicin, DOXOrubicin liposomal, doxycycline, droperidol, drotrecogin alfa, enalaprilat, ePHEDrine, EPINEPHrine, epirubicin, epoetin alfa, eptifibatide, ertapenem, erythromycin, esmolol, etoposide, famotidine, fenoldopam, fentaNYL, filgrastim, fludarabine, fluorouracil, folic acid, foscarnet, gallium, ganciclovir, gatifloxacin, gemcitabine, gentamicin, glycopyrrolate, granisetron, heparin, hydrocortisone, HYDROmorphone, IDArubicin, ifosfamide, IV immune globulin, inamrinone, indomethacin, insulin (regular), irinotecan, isoproterenol, ketorolac, labetalol, lansoprazole, leucovorin, levofloxacin, lidocaine, linezolid, LORazepam, LR, magnesium sulfate, mannitol, mechlorethamine, melphalan, meperidine, meropenem, metaraminol, methicillin, methotrexate, methoxamine, methyldopate, methylPREDNISolone, metoclopramide, metoprolol, metroNIDAZOLE, mezlocillin, miconazole, midazolam, milrinone, minocycline, mitoXANtrone, morphine, moxalactam, multiple vitamins injection, mycophenolate, nafcillin, nalbuphine, naloxone, nesiritide, nitroglycerin, nitroprusside, norepinephrine, octreotide, ondansetron, oxacillin, oxaliplatin, oxytocin, PACLitaxel, palonosetron, pamidronate, pancuronium, papaverine, PEMEtrexed, penicillin G potassium/sodium, pentazocine, PENTobarbital, PHENobarbital, phenylephrine, phenytoin, phytonadione, piperacillin-tazobactam, polymyxin B, potassium chloride, procainamide, prochlorperazine, promethazine, propofol, propranolol, protamine, pyridoxine, quiNIDine, quinupristin-dalfopristin, ranitidine, remifentanil, Ringer's, ritodrine, riTUXimab, rocuronium, sargramostim, sodium acetate/bicarbonate, succinylcholine, SUFentanil, tacrolimus, temocillin, teniposide, theophylline, thiotepa, ticarcillin-clavulanate, tigecycline, tirofiban, TNA, tobramycin, tolazoline, TPN, trastuzumab, trimetaphan, urokinase, vancomycin, vasopressin, vecuronium, verapamil, vinCRIStine, vinorelbine, voriconazole, zidovudine, zoledronic acid

SIDE EFFECTS

CNS: *Headache,* seizures

CV: **QT prolongation, torsades de pointes**

GI: *Nausea, vomiting,* diarrhea, cramping, flatus, increased AST, ALT, **hepatotoxicity**, abdominal pain, cholestasis

HEMA: **Agranulocytosis, eosinophilia, leukopenia, neutropenia, thrombocytopenia**

INTEG: **Stevens-Johnson syndrome, angioedema, anaphylaxis, exfoliative dermatitis, toxic epidermal necrolysis**

PHARMACOKINETICS

Peak 1-2 hr, bioavailability (PO) >90%, excreted unchanged in urine 80%, metabolized by CYP3A enzyme system at dose >200 mg/day, elimination half-life 30 hr

INTERACTIONS

Increase: hypoglycemia—oral sulfonyl/ureas (glipiZIDE)

Increase: anticoagulation—warfarin

Increase: plasma concentrations—cycloSPORINE, phenytoin, theophylline, rifabutin, tacrolimus, sirolimus, zidovudine, zolpidem

Increase: **myopathy, rhabdomyolysis risk—HMG-CoA reductase inhibitors: lovastatin, simvastatin**

Increase: effect of zidovudine, methadone, SUFentanil, alfentanil, buprenorphine, saquinavir, fentaNYL, ergots

Decrease: effect of oral contraceptives, calcium channel blockers

Decrease: fluconazole effect—proton pump inhibitors

Drug/Lab Test

Increase: alk phos, LFTs

Decrease: WBC, platelets

NURSING CONSIDERATIONS

Assess:

- **Infection:** clearing of CSF and other culture during treatment, obtain C&S baseline and throughout treatment, product may be started as soon as culture is taken
- ⚠ **Hepatotoxicity: increasing AST, ALT, periodically alk phos, bilirubin; for renal status: BUN, creatinine**
- **Skin symptoms: color, lesions, inj-site reactions; if lesions progress, stop product**

Evaluate:

- Therapeutic response: decreasing oral candidiasis, fever, malaise, rash; negative C&S for infection organism

Teach patient/family:

- That long-term therapy may be needed to clear infection, not to add new meds, herbs without prescriber approval
- That medication may be taken with food to reduce GI effects
- **To notify prescriber of nausea, vomiting, diarrhea, jaundice, anorexia, clay-colored stools, dark urine, skin rash, abdominal pain, fever, bruising, bleeding**
- **To use alternative method of contraception while taking this product, pregnancy (D)**

⚠ ***HIGH ALERT***

fludarabine (Rx)

(floo-dar′a-been)

Fludara, Oforta

Func. class.: Antineoplastic, antimetabolite

USES: Chronic lymphocytic leukemia

CONTRAINDICATIONS: Pregnancy (D), breastfeeding, hypersensitivity

Black Box Warning: Hemolytic anemia, bone marrow suppression, coma, seizures, visual disturbances

DOSAGE AND ROUTES

- **Adult: IV** 25 mg/m² over 30 min × 5 days, may repeat q28days; reconstitute with 2 ml of sterile water for inj; dissolution should occur in <15 sec, adjust dose based on toxicity; **PO** 40 mg/m² × 5 days q28days

fludrocortisone (Rx)

(floo-droe-kor′ti-sone)

Func. class.: Corticosteroid, synthetic

Chem. class.: Mineralocorticoid

USES:

Adrenal insufficiency, salt-losing adrenogenital syndrome, Addison's disease

Unlabeled uses: Renal tubular acidosis (type IV), idiopathic orthostatic hypotension

CONTRAINDICATIONS:

Children <2 yr, hypersensitivity

Precautions: Pregnancy (C), breastfeeding, children >2 yr, osteoporosis, CHF, hypertension, diabetes, acute glomerulonephritis, amebiasis, psychoses, Cushing syndrome, fungal infections

DOSAGE AND ROUTES

- **Adult: PO** 100-200 mcg/day
- **Child: PO** 50-100 mcg/day

Idiopathic hypotension (unlabeled)

- **Adult: PO** 50-200 mcg/day

Available forms: Tabs 100 mcg (0.1 mg)

SIDE EFFECTS

CNS: *Flushing, sweating,* headache, paralysis, dizziness, seizures

CV: *Hypertension,* circulatory collapse, thrombophlebitis, embolism, tachycardia, CHF, *edema*

ENDO: Weight gain, adrenal suppression, hyperglycemia

META: *Hypokalemia*

MISC: Hypersensitivity, cataracts, GI ulcers, anaphylaxis, infection

MS: Fractures, osteoporosis, weakness

PHARMACOKINETICS

Peak 1.5 hr, half-life 18-36 hr, metabolized by liver, excreted in urine

INTERACTIONS

Increase: B/P—sodium-containing food or medication

Decrease: fludrocortisone action—barbiturates, rifampin, phenytoin

Decrease: potassium levels—thiazides, potassium-wasting products, loop diuretics, amphotericin B, piperacillin, mezlocillin

Drug/Herb

Increase: hypokalemia—aloe, buckthorn, cascara sagrada, Chinese rhubarb, senna

Increase: corticosteroid effect—aloe, licorice, perilla

Drug/Lab Test

Increase: potassium, sodium

NURSING CONSIDERATIONS

Assess:

- Weight daily; notify prescriber of weekly gain >5 lb
- I&O ratio; be alert for decreasing urinary output, increasing edema
- B/P q4hr, pulse; notify prescriber if chest pain occurs
- Potassium depletion: paresthesias, fatigue, nausea, vomiting, depression, polyuria, dysrhythmias, weakness
- Electrolytes: sodium, potassium, chloride, hypokalemia is common

Administer:

- Titrated dose; use lowest effective dose
- With food or milk to decrease GI symptoms
- Assistance with ambulation in patient with bone tissue disease to prevent fractures

Evaluate:

- Therapeutic response: correction of adrenal insufficiency

Teach patient/family:

- That emergency ID as steroid user should be carried
- Not to discontinue this medication abruptly
- To notify health care provider of muscle cramps, weight gain, edema, nausea, infection, trauma, stress
- Not to breastfeed while taking this medication
- Avoid exposure to disease, trauma

flumazenil (Rx)

(flu-maz′e-nill)

Anexate ✦, Romazicon

Func. class.: Antidote: benzodiazepine receptor antagonist

Chem. class.: Imidazobenzodiazepine derivative

ACTION: Antagonizes actions of benzodiazepines on CNS, competitively inhibits activity at benzodiazepine recognition site on GABA/benzodiazepine receptor complex

USES: Reversal of sedative effects of benzodiazepines

CONTRAINDICATIONS: Hypersensitivity to this product or benzodiazepines, serious cyclic antidepressant overdose, patients given benzodiazepine for control of life-threatening conditions

Precautions: Pregnancy (C), breastfeeding, children, geriatric patients, status epilepticus, head injury, labor/delivery, renal/hepatic disease, hypoventilation, panic disorder, drug and alcohol dependency, ambulatory patients

Black Box Warning: Benzodiazepine dependence, seizures

DOSAGE AND ROUTES

Reversal of conscious sedation or general anesthesia

- **Adult: IV** 0.2 mg given over 15 sec; wait 45 sec, then give 0.2 mg if consciousness does not occur; may be repeated at 60-sec intervals prn (max 3 mg/hr) or 1 mg/5 min
- **Child: IV** 10 mcg (0.01 mg)/kg; cumulative dose of 1 mg or less

Management of suspected benzodiazepine overdose

- **Adult: IV** 0.2 mg given over 30 sec; wait 30 sec, then give 0.3 mg over 30 sec if consciousness does not occur; further doses of 0.5 mg can be given over 30 sec at intervals of 1 min up to cumulative dose of 3 mg
- **Child: IV** 10 mcg (0.01 mg/kg), cumulative dose of <1 mg

Available forms: Inj 0.1 mg/ml

Administer:

- Check airway and IV access before administration
- Use large vein

Direct IV route

- Give undiluted or diluted with 0.9% NaCl, D_5W, LR; give over 15-30 sec into running IV, check for extravasation
- Stable for 24 hr if drawn into a syringe or mixed with other solutions

SIDE EFFECTS

CNS: Dizziness, agitation, emotional lability, confusion, **seizures**, somnolence, panic attacks

CV: Hypertension, palpitations, cutaneous vasodilation, **dysrhythmias**, bradycardia, tachycardia, chest pain

EENT: Abnormal vision, blurred vision, tinnitus

GI: Nausea, vomiting, hiccups

SYST: Headache, inj site pain, increased sweating, fatigue, rigors

PHARMACOKINETICS

Terminal half-life 41-79 min, metabolized in liver, onset 1-2 min

INTERACTIONS

- Toxicity: mixed product overdosage
- Antagonize action of benzodiazepines, zaleplon, zolpidem

NURSING CONSIDERATIONS

Assess:

- Cardiac status using continuous monitoring

Black Box Warning: For seizures; protect patient from injury; most likely among those who are withdrawing from benzodiazepines; flumazenil can precipitate benzodiazepine withdrawal and onset of seizures, seizures are increased in head trauma

• GI symptoms: nausea, vomiting; place patient in side-lying position to prevent aspiration
• **Allergic reactions:** flushing, rash, urticaria, pruritus

Black Box Warning: Seizures/benzodiazepine dependence: do not use in those who have used these products for status epilepticus; use in intensive care setting cautiously, there may be unrecognized benzodiazepine dependence

flunisolide nasal agent
See Appendix B

fluocinolone topical
See Appendix B

fluorometholone ophthalmic
See Appendix B

HIGH ALERT

fluorouracil (Rx)
(flure-oh-yoor′a-sil)

Carac, Efudex, Fluoroplex, 5-FU, Tolak

Func. class.: Antineoplastic, antimetabolite

Chem. class.: Pyrimidine analog

Do not confuse:
fluorouracil/flucytosine
Carac/Kuric

ACTION: Inhibits DNA, RNA synthesis; interferes with cell replication by competitively inhibiting thymidylate production, specific for S phase of cell cycle

USES: **Systemic:** cancer of breast, colon, rectum, stomach, pancreas; **topical:** multiple actinic keratoses, superficial basal cell carcinomas
Unlabeled uses: Anal, biliary tract, cervical, head and neck, hepatocellular, ovarian cancer

CONTRAINDICATIONS: Pregnancy (X), breastfeeding, hypersensitivity, poor nutritional status, serious infections, dihydropyrimidine

Black Box Warning: Bone marrow suppression

Precautions: Children, renal/hepatic disease, angina, stomatitis, diarrhea, sunlight exposure, vaccination, occlusive dressing

Black Box Warning: GI bleeding

DOSAGE AND ROUTES
Doses vary widely, based on actual body weight unless obese, then based on lean body weight

Advanced colorectal cancer
• **Adult: IV bolus** 300-500 mg/m^2/day × 4-5 days q28days or 600-1500 mg/m^2 weekly or every other wk; continuous IV infusion: 300-1000 mg/m^2/day × 4-5 days q4wk or 300 mg/m^2/day indefinitely, high dose 3000-3400 mg/m^2 over 24-72 hr

Breast cancer
• **Adult: IV bolus** 400-600 mg/m^2 on days 1 and 8 of every cycle with cyclophosphamide and methotrexate or 600 mg/m^2 day 1 with cyclophosphamide and methotrexate q21-28days

Pancreatic cancer
• **Adult: IV bolus** 600 mg/m^2 on days 1, 8, 29, 36 with DOXOrubicin and mitoMYcin q8wk or 600 mg/m^2 bolus on days 1, 8, 29, 36 with streptozocin

Actinic/solar keratoses

• **Adult: TOP** 1% cream/sol bid or 2-5% sol for hands

Superficial basal cell carcinoma

• **Adult: TOP** 5% sol or cream 2×/day × 3-12 wk

Available forms: Inj 50 mg/ml; cream 0.5%, 1%, 4%, 5%; sol 2%, 5%

Administer:

• Antiemetic 30-60 min before product to prevent vomiting, for several days thereafter

Topical route

• The 1% strength is used on face; higher strengths are used on other parts of the body

• Wear gloves when applying; may use with a loose dressing; use plastic or wooden applicator, do not use occlusive dressings, may use gauze dressing

IV route

• Prepared in biologic cabinet using gloves, gown, mask; use cytotoxic handling procedures

• Undiluted; may inject through **Y**-tube or 3-way stopcock; give over 1-3 min; may be diluted in NS, D_5W; given as a continuous infusion in plastic containers; given over 2-8 hr; do not refrigerate/freeze; protect from light, discard unused portion, stable for 24 hr at room temperature, do not use discolored, cloudy solution; solution is pale yellow, for crystals, dissolve by warming slowly and shaking, cool to body temperature before use

Y-site compatibilities: Acyclovir, alatrofloxacin, alfentanil, allopurinol, amifostine, amikacin, amphotericin B lipid complex, amphotericin B liposome, ampicillin, ampicillin-sulbactam, anidulafungin, argatroban, atenolol, atracurium, azithromycin, aztreonam, bivalirudin, bleomycin, bumetanide, butorphanol, calcium gluconate, CARBOplatin, ceFAZolin, cefepime, cefotaxime, cefoTEtan, cefOXitin, cefTAZidime, ceftizoxime, cefTRIAXone, cefuroxime, cimetidine, cisatracurium, CISplatin, clindamycin, codeine, cyclophosphamide, cycloSPORINE, DAPTOmycin, dexamethasone, digoxin, DOCEtaxel, DOPamine, doripenem, DOXOrubicin liposomal, enalaprilat, ePHEDrine, ertapenem, erythromycin, esmolol, etoposide phosphate, famotidine, fenoldopam, fentaNYL, fluconazole, fludarabine, foscarnet, fosphenytoin, furosemide, ganciclovir, gatifloxacin, gemcitabine, gentamicin, granisetron, heparin, hydrocortisone, HYDROmorphone, ifosfamide, imipenem-cilastatin, inamrinone, isoproterenol, ketorolac, labetalol, leucovorin, levorphanol, lidocaine, linezolid, magnesium sulfate, mannitol, melphalan, meperidine, meropenem, mesna, methohexital, methotrexate, methylPREDNISolone, metoprolol, metroNIDAZOLE, milrinone, mitoMYcin, mitoXANtrone, morphine sulfate, nalbuphine, naloxone, nesiritide, nitroglycerin, nitroprusside, octreotide, ofloxacin, PACLitaxel, palonosetron, pamidronate, pancuronium, pantoprazole, PEMEtrexed, PENTobarbital, PHENobarbital, phenylephrine, piperacillin, piperacillin-tazobactam, potassium chloride/phosphates, procainamide, propofol, propranolol, ranitidine, remifentanil, riTUXimab, sargramostim, sodium acetate/bicarbonate/phosphates, succinylcholine, SUFentanil, sulfamethoxazole-trimethoprim, teniposide, theophylline, thiopental, thiotepa, ticarcillin, ticarcillin-clavulanate, tigecycline, tirofiban, tobramycin, trastuzumab, vasopressin, vecuronium, vinBLAStine, vinCRIStine, vitamin B complex/C, voriconazole, zidovudine, zoledronic acid

SIDE EFFECTS

Systemic use

CNS: Lethargy, malaise, weakness, acute cerebellar dysfunction

CV: **Myocardial ischemia**, angina

EENT: Light intolerance, lacrimation

GI: *Anorexia, stomatitis,* diarrhea, nausea, vomiting, **hemorrhage**, enteritis, glossitis

HEMA: **Thrombocytopenia, leukopenia, myelosuppression, anemia, agranulocytosis**

INTEG: *Rash,* fever, photosensitivity, **anaphylaxis**

F

PHARMACOKINETICS

Half-life 16 min (IV): metabolized in liver; excreted in urine; crosses blood-brain barrier

INTERACTIONS

Increase: bleeding—anticoagulants, NSAIDs, platelet inhibitors, thrombolytics
Increase: toxicity—metroNIDAZOLE, irinotecan
Increase: toxicity, bone marrow depression—radiation or other antineoplastics, leucovorin
Decrease: antibody response—live virus vaccines
Decrease: effect of phenytoin

Drug/Lab Test

Increase: AST, ALT, LDH, serum bilirubin, Hct, Hgb, WBC, platelets, 5-HIAA
Decrease: albumin

NURSING CONSIDERATIONS

Assess:

Black Box Warning: **Bone marrow suppression monitor daily during IV treatment:** CBC, differential, platelet count daily (IV); withhold product if WBC is <3500/mm^3 or platelet count is <100,000/mm^3; notify prescriber of results; product should be discontinued; nadir of leukopenia within 2 wk, recovery 1 mo, if pretreatment of WBC <2,000/mm^3 or platelets <100,000/mm^3, delay until recovery of counts above this level; nadir usually 9-14 days, recovery 30 days

- **Palmer-planter erythrodysesthesia:** hand/foot tingling changing to pain, redness
- **Infiltration:** monitor frequently for pain, redness, inflammation at site, if present, stop infusion and start at new site, may use ice at site
- Renal studies: BUN, serum uric acid, urine CCr, electrolytes before, during therapy
- Hepatic studies before, during therapy: bilirubin, alk phos, AST, ALT, LDH before, during therapy
- **Bleeding:** hematuria, guaiac, bruising, petechiae, mucosa or orifices q8hr
- Inflammation of mucosa, breaks in skin; buccal cavity q8hr for dryness, sores or ulceration, white patches, oral pain, bleeding, dysphagia
- **Infection:** those with current infections should be treated before receiving 5-FU, the dose reduced or discontinued if infection occurs
- **Toxicity:** hemorrhage, severe vomiting, severe diarrhea, stomatitis, WBC <3500/mm^3, platelets <100,000 notify prescriber
- **Acute cerebellar dysfunction:** dizziness, weakness

Evaluate:

- Therapeutic response: decreased tumor size, spread of malignancy

Teach patient/family:

- To avoid crowds, persons with known infection
- To avoid foods with citric acid, hot or rough texture if stomatitis is present; to drink adequate fluids
- To report stomatitis: any bleeding, white spots, ulcerations in mouth; that patient should examine mouth daily, report symptoms; viscous lidocaine may be used; rinsing of mouth tid-qid with water, club soda; brushing of teeth bid-tid with soft brush or cotton-tipped applicator for stomatitis; use unwaxed dental floss, give ice chips for mucositis
- To report signs of **infection:** fever, sore throat, flulike symptoms
- To report signs of **anemia:** fatigue, headache, faintness, shortness of breath, irritability
- To report **bleeding:** to avoid razors, commercial mouthwash, IM inj if counts are low
- Not to use aspirin products or NSAIDs
- To use contraception during therapy (men and women), pregnancy (X); to avoid breastfeeding (topical use)
- Not to receive vaccinations during therapy
- To use sunscreen or stay out of the sun to prevent photosensitivity
- About hair loss; to explore use of wigs or other products until hair regrowth occurs
- Topical: To apply only to affected areas, being careful around mouth, nose, eyes

FLUoxetine (Rx)

(floo-ox′eh-teen)

PROzac, PROzac Weekly, Sarafem

Func. class.: Antidepressant, SSRI (selective serotonin reuptake inhibitor)

Do not confuse:
PROzac/Proscar/ProSom/PriLOSEC
Sarafem/Serophene

ACTION: Inhibits CNS neuron uptake of serotonin but not of norepinephrine

USES: Major depressive disorder, obsessive-compulsive disorder (OCD), bulimia nervosa, premenstrual dysphoric disorder (PMDD), panic disorder

Unlabeled uses: Alcoholism, anorexia nervosa, borderline personality disorder, obesity, posttraumatic stress disorder, autism, fibromyalgia, orthostatic hypotension, premature ejaculation, social phobia

CONTRAINDICATIONS: Hypersensitivity

Precautions: Pregnancy (C), breastfeeding, geriatric patients, diabetes mellitus, narrow-angle glaucoma, cardiac malformations in infants (exposed to FLUoxetine in utero), osteoporosis, QT prolongation

Black Box Warning: Children, suicidal ideation

DOSAGE AND ROUTES

Depression/obsessive-compulsive disorder

- **Adult: PO** 20 mg/day in AM; after 4 wk, if no clinical improvement is noted, dose may be increased to 20 mg bid in AM, PM, max 80 mg/day; **Del Rel PO** 90 mg/wk
- **Geriatric: PO** 10 mg/day, increase as needed
- **Child 7-17 yr: PO** 10 mg/day, max 20 mg/day

Premenstrual dysphoric disorder (Sarafem)

- **Adult: PO** 20 mg/day, may be taken daily 14 days before menses

Alcoholism (unlabeled)

- **Adult: PO** 20-80 mg/day, give in divided doses if >40 mg/day

Anorexia nervosa (unlabeled)

- **Adult: PO** 10 mg daily, max 60 mg/day

Borderline personality disorder/fibromyalgia/autism/orthostatic hypotension/premature ejaculation/hot flashes (unlabeled)

- **Adult: PO** 20 mg/day, max 80 mg/day

Obesity (unlabeled)

- **Adult: PO** 60 mg/day after titration

Posttraumatic stress disorder (unlabeled)

- **Adult: PO** 10-80 mg/day

Available forms: Caps 10, 20, 40 mg; tabs 10, 20, 60 mg; oral sol 20 mg/5 ml; del rel caps (PROzac Weekly) 90 mg

Administer:

- Without regard to meals
- Crushed if patient is unable to swallow medication whole (tab only)
- Gum, hard candy, frequent sips of water for dry mouth
- Store at room temperature; do not freeze
- **PROzac Weekly** on the same day each wk, swallow whole; do not crush, cut, chew
- **Oral sol:** use oral syringe or calibrated measuring device

SIDE EFFECTS

CNS: *Headache, nervousness, insomnia, drowsiness, anxiety, tremor, dizziness, fatigue, sedation, poor concentrations, abnormal dreams, agitation,* **seizures**, apathy, euphoria, hallucinations, delusions, psychosis, **suicidal ideation, neuroleptic malignant syndrome–like reactions**

CV: *Hot flashes, palpitations,* angina pectoris, hypertension, **tachycardia, 1st-degree AV block, bradycardia, MI, thrombophlebitis,** generalized edema, **torsades de pointes**

EENT: Visual changes, ear/eye pain, photophobia, tinnitus, increased intraocular pressure

F

GI: *Nausea, diarrhea, dry mouth, anorexia, dyspepsia, constipation,* taste changes, flatulence, decreased appetite
GU: *Dysmenorrhea, decreased libido, urinary frequency, UTI,* amenorrhea, cystitis, impotence, urine retention
HEMA: Hemorrhage
INTEG: *Sweating, rash, pruritus,* acne, alopecia, urticaria, angioedema, exfoliative dermatitis, Stevens-Johnson syndrome, toxic epidermal necrolysis
META: Hyponatremia
MS: *Pain,* arthritis, twitching
RESP: *Pharyngitis, cough, dyspnea, bronchitis,* asthma, hyperventilation, pneumonia
SYST: *Asthenia,* serotonin syndrome, flu-like symptoms, neonatal abstinence syndrome

PHARMACOKINETICS

PO: Peak 6-8 hr, metabolized in liver, excreted in urine, terminal half-life 2-3 days, norfluoxetine active metabolite half-life 4-16 days, steady state 28-35 days, protein binding 94%

INTERACTIONS

Increase: serotonin syndrome—SSRIs, SNRIs, serotonin-receptor agonists, selegiline, busPIRone, tryptophan, phenothiazines, haloperidol, loxapine, thiothixene, tricyclics; do not use concurrently
Increase: bleeding risk—platelet inhibitors, thrombolytics, NSAIDs, salicylates, anticoagulants
⚠ Do not use MAOIs with or 14 days before FLUoxetine
Increase: levels or toxicity of carBAMazepine, lithium, digoxin, warfarin, phenytoin, diazepam, vinBLAStine, donepezil, antidiabetics, dorifenacin, paricalcitrol, budesonide, bosentan, thioridazine
Increase: CNS depression—alcohol, antidepressants, opioids, sedatives
Decrease: FLUoxetine effect—cyproheptadine
Drug/Herb
⚠ Do not use together; increased risk of serotonin syndrome: St. John's wort, SAM-e
Increase: CNS effect—hops, kava, lavender, valerian

NURSING CONSIDERATIONS

Assess:

Black Box Warning: Mental status: mood, sensorium, affect, suicidal tendencies (child/young adult), increase in psychiatric symptoms, depression, panic; monitor for seizures, seizure potential increased, sarafem is not approved for children

- **Serotonin syndrome:** symptoms can occur anytime after first dose, nausea/vomiting, sedation, dizziness, diaphoresis, mental changes, elevated B/P; if these occur product should be stopped, notify prescriber
- **Bulimia nervosa:** appetite, weight daily, increase nutritious foods in diet, watch for bingeing and vomiting

⚠ **Allergic reactions/serious skin reactions:** angioedema, exfoliative dermatitis, Stevens-Johnson syndrome, toxic epidermal necrolysis, itching, rash, urticaria; product should be discontinued, may need to give antihistamine

- B/P (lying/standing), pulse q4hr; if systolic B/P drops 20 mm Hg, hold product, notify prescriber; ECG for flattening of T wave, bundle branch, AV block, dysrhythmias in cardiac patients
- **Blood studies:** CBC, leukocytes, differential, cardiac enzymes if patient is receiving long-term therapy; check platelets; bleeding can occur, thyroid function, growth rate (children), weight
- **Hepatic studies:** AST, ALT, bilirubin, creatinine, weight weekly; appetite may decrease with product
- Safety measures, primarily for geriatric patients

Evaluate:

- Therapeutic response: decreased depression, symptoms of OCD

Teach patient/family:

- That therapeutic effect may take 1-4 wk, not to discontinue abruptly, that follow-up will be required

- To use caution when driving, performing other activities requiring alertness because of drowsiness, dizziness, blurred vision
- To avoid alcohol, other CNS depressants
- To notify prescriber if pregnant, planning to become pregnant, or breastfeeding
- To change positions slowly because orthostatic hypotension may occur
- To avoid all OTC products unless approved by prescriber
- To notify prescriber if allergic reactions occur (rash, trouble breathing, itching)

Black Box Warning: That suicidal thoughts/behaviors may occur in young adults, children, usually during early treatment

- To notify prescriber of worsening symptoms, or if insomnia, anxiety, or depression continues
- **Serotonin syndrome:** fever, sweating, diarrhea, poor coordination, nausea/vomiting, sedation, flushing, mental changes

fluPHENAZine decanoate (Rx)

(floo-fen′a-zeen)

Modecate ✦

fluPHENAZine hydrochloride (Rx)

Func. class.: Antipsychotic

Chem. class.: Phenothiazine, piperazine

Do not confuse:
Prolixin/Proloid

ACTION: Depresses cerebral cortex, hypothalamus, limbic system, which control activity and aggression; blocks neurotransmission produced by DOPamine at synapse; exhibits strong α-adrenergic and anticholinergic blocking action; mechanism for antipsychotic effects is unclear

USES: Schizophrenia
Unlabeled use: Agitation

CONTRAINDICATIONS: Hypersensitivity, blood dyscrasias, coma, bone marrow depression

Precautions: Pregnancy (C), breastfeeding, children <12 yr, geriatric patients, seizure disorders, hypertension, cardiac/hepatic disease, abrupt discontinuation; accidental exposure, agranulocytosis, ambient temperature increase, angina, hypersensitivity to benzyl alcohol/parabens/sesame oil/tartrazine dye, QT prolongation, suicidal ideation, renal failure, Parkinson's disease, hypocalcemia, head trauma, prostatic hypertrophy, pulmonary disease, infection, ileus, chemotherapy, breast cancer

Black Box Warning: Increased mortality in elderly patients with dementia-related psychosis

DOSAGE AND ROUTES

Decanoate

- **Adult and child >12 yr: IM/SUBCUT** 12.5-25 mg q1-3wk, may increase slowly, max 100 mg/dose

HCl

- **Adult: PO** 2.5-10 mg in divided doses q6-8hr, max 40 mg/day; **IM** initially 1.25 mg, then 2.5-10 mg in divided doses q6-8hr

Available forms: *Decanoate:* inj 25, 100 ✦ mg/ml; *HCl:* tabs 1, 2.5, 5, 10 mg; inj 2.5 mg/ml; elixir 2.5 mg/5 ml; oral solution 5 mg/ml

Administer:

PO route

- Give with food, milk, or a full glass of water to minimize gastric irritation
- **Oral concentrate:** Give using a calibrated measuring device; dilute just before use with 120-240 ml of water, saline, milk, 7-Up, carbonated orange beverage, or apricot, orange, pineapple, prune, tomato, or V-8 juice; do not mix with beverages containing caffeine (coffee, cola), tannics (tea), or pectinates (apple juice) or with other liquid medications; avoid spilling the solution on the skin and clothing

- **Oral elixir:** Give using a calibrated measuring device; avoid spilling the solution on the skin and clothing

Injectable routes

- Visually inspect for particulate matter and discoloration before use, slight yellow to amber color does not alter potency, markedly discolored solutions should be discarded, protect from light

IM route (fluPHENAZine HCl only)

- No dilution necessary; if irritation occurs, subsequent IM doses may be diluted with NS for injection or 2% procaine
- Inject slowly and deeply into the upper outer quadrant of the gluteal muscle using a dry syringe and needle, aspirate before injection
- Keep patient in a recumbent position ≥30 min following injection to minimize hypotensive effects
- Rotate the site of injection to avoid irritation or sterile abscess formation with repeat use

IM injection (fluPHENAZine decanoate)

- Use a dry syringe and needle of at least 21-G, do not dilute
- Inject slowly and deeply into the upper outer quadrant of the gluteal muscle, aspirate
- Keep patient in a recumbent position for at least 30 min following the initial injection to minimize hypotensive effects; rotate the site of injection to avoid irritation or sterile abscess formation with repeat administration

Subcut injection route (fluPHENAZine decanoate)

- Use a dry syringe and a needle of at least 21-G, do not dilute
- Inject subcut, taking care not to inject intradermally
- Keep patient in a recumbent position for at least 30 min following the initial injection to minimize hypotensive effects. rotate the injection sites

SIDE EFFECTS

CNS: *EPS: pseudoparkinsonism, akathisia, dystonia, tardive dyskinesia, drowsiness, headache,* seizures, neuroleptic malignant syndrome

CV: *Orthostatic hypotension,* hypertension, cardiac arrest, ECG changes, tachycardia

EENT: Blurred vision, glaucoma, dry eyes, nasal congestion

GI: *Dry mouth, nausea, vomiting, anorexia, constipation,* diarrhea, jaundice, weight gain, paralytic ileus, hepatitis, cholecystic jaundice

GU: Urinary retention, urinary frequency, enuresis, impotence, amenorrhea, gynecomastia

HEMA: Anemia, leukopenia, leukocytosis, agranulocytosis, aplastic anemia, thrombocytopenia

INTEG: *Rash,* photosensitivity, dermatitis, hyperpigmentation (long-term use)

RESP: Laryngospasm, dyspnea, respiratory depression

PHARMACOKINETICS

Metabolized by liver, excreted in urine (metabolites), crosses placenta, enters breast milk, protein binding >90%, not dialyzable

PO/IM (HCl): Onset 1 hr, peak 90-120 min, duration 6-8 hr, half-life 15 hr

IM/SUBCUT (decanoate): Onset 1-3 days; peak 1-2 days, duration over 4 wk, single-dose half-life 7-10 days, multiple dose 14.3 days

INTERACTIONS

Increase: QT prolongation, torsades de pointes (at higher doses)—amiodarone, arsenic trioxide, astemizole, dasatinib, disopyramide, dofetilide, droperidol, erythromycin, flecainide, gatifloxacin, ibutilide, levomethadyl, ondansetron, paliperidone, palonosetron, some antidepressants, vorinostat, ziprasidone, haloperidol, phenothiazines, ARIPiprazole, lurasidone

Increase: sedation—other CNS depressants, alcohol, barbiturate anesthetics, haloperidol, metyrosine, risperiDONE

Increase: toxicity—EPINEPHrine

Increase: anticholinergic effects—anticholinergics

Decrease: effects of levodopa, lithium

Decrease: fluPHENAZine effects—smoking, barbiturates

Drug/Lab Test

Increase: LFTs, cardiac enzymes, cholesterol, blood glucose, prolactin, bilirubin, cholinesterase

Decrease: hormones (blood and urine)

False positive: pregnancy tests, PKU urinary steroids, 17-OHCS

NURSING CONSIDERATIONS

Assess:

Black Box Warning: Increased mortality in elderly patients with dementia-related psychosis

⚠ **QT prolongation, torsades de pointes:** ECG for changes

- Bilirubin, CBC, LFTs monthly; ophthalmic exams periodically
- Urinalysis recommended before and during prolonged therapy
- Affect, orientation, LOC, reflexes, gait, coordination, sleep pattern disturbances
- B/P standing and lying; pulse and respirations q4hr during initial treatment; establish baseline before starting treatment; report drops of 30 mm Hg
- Dizziness, faintness, palpitations, tachycardia on rising
- **EPS** including akathisia (inability to sit still, no pattern to movements), tardive dyskinesia (bizarre movements of jaw, mouth, tongue, extremities), pseudoparkinsonism (rigidity, tremors, pill rolling, shuffling gait)
- Constipation, urinary retention daily; if these occur, increase bulk, water in diet
- Supervised ambulation until stabilized on medication; do not involve patient in strenuous exercise; fainting possible; patient should not stand still for long periods

Evaluate:

- Therapeutic response: decrease in emotional excitement, hallucinations, delusions, paranoia, reorganization of patterns of thought, speech

Teach patient/family:

- That orthostatic hypotension occurs often; to rise from sitting or lying position gradually; to avoid hazardous activities until stabilized on medication
- To avoid hot tubs, hot showers, tub baths because hypotension may occur; that in hot weather, heat stroke may occur; to take extra precautions to stay cool

⚠ To avoid abrupt withdrawal of this product or EPS may result; that product should be withdrawn slowly

- To avoid OTC preparations (cough, hay fever, cold) unless approved by prescriber; that serious product interactions may occur; to avoid use with alcohol, CNS depressants; that increased drowsiness may occur
- To use a sunscreen to prevent burns
- About the importance of compliance with product regimen, follow-up, lab, ophthalmic exams
- About EPS and the need for meticulous oral hygiene because oral candidiasis may occur
- To report sore throat, malaise, fever, bleeding, mouth sores; if these occur, CBC should be drawn, product discontinued
- That urine may turn pink to reddish brown

TREATMENT OF OVERDOSE:

Lavage; if orally ingested, provide an airway; *do not induce vomiting*

flurandrenolide topical

See Appendix B

flurbiprofen ophthalmic

See Appendix B

⚠ ***HIGH ALERT***

flutamide (Rx)

(floo′ta-mide)

Euflex ♣

Func. class.: Antineoplastic, hormone

Chem. class.: Antiandrogen

ACTION: Interferes with androgen uptake in the nucleus or androgen activity in target tissues; arrests tumor growth in androgen-sensitive tissue (i.e., prostate gland)

USES:
Metastatic prostatic carcinoma, stage D_2 in combination with LHRH agonistic analogs (leuprolide), B_2-C in combination with goserelin and radiation

CONTRAINDICATIONS:
Pregnancy (D), hypersensitivity

Black Box Warning: Severe hepatic disease

Precautions: G6PD deficiency, hemoglobinopathy, lactase deficiency, polycystic ovary syndrome, tobacco smoking

DOSAGE AND ROUTES
- **Adult: PO** 250 mg q8hr for a daily dosage of 750 mg

Available forms: Caps 125, 250 ✦ mg

Administer:
- Do not break, crush, chew caps
- Give without regard to food with a full glass of water
- Use cytotoxic handling procedures

SIDE EFFECTS
CNS: *Hot flashes,* drowsiness, confusion, depression, anxiety, paresthesia

GI: *Diarrhea, nausea, vomiting,* increased levels in hepatic studies, hepatitis, anorexia, hepatotoxicity, abdominal pain, cholestasis, **hepatic necrosis/failure**

GU: *Decreased libido, impotence, gynecomastia*

HEMA: Hemolytic anemia, leukopenia, thrombocytopenia

INTEG: Irritation at site, rash, photosensitivity

MISC: Edema, neuromuscular and pulmonary symptoms, hypertension, secondary malignancy

PHARMACOKINETICS
Rapidly and completely absorbed; excreted in urine and feces as metabolites; half-life 6 hr, geriatric half-life 8 hr; 94% protein binding, peak 2 hr

INTERACTIONS
Increase: PT—warfarin

Decrease: flutamide action—LHRH analog (leuprolide)

Drug/Lab Test

Increase: LFTs, BUN, creatinine

Decrease: WBC, platelets

NURSING CONSIDERATIONS
Assess:

Black Box Warning: Severe hepatic disease: Monitor before start of therapy and monthly × 4 mo, AST, ALT, alk phos, which may be elevated; if LFTs elevated, product may need to be discontinued; monitor CBC, bilirubin, creatinine periodically

- CNS symptoms, including drowsiness, confusion, depression, anxiety

Evaluate:
- Therapeutic response: decrease in prostatic tumor size, decrease in spread of cancer

Teach patient/family:
- To report side effects: decreased libido, impotence, breast enlargement, hot flashes, diarrhea

Black Box Warning: Hepatotoxicity: to report nausea, vomiting, yellow eyes or skin, dark urine, clay-colored stools; hepatotoxicity may be the cause

- Notify of yellow, green urine discoloration
- Avoid sun exposure, tanning beds
- To use contraception during treatment; pregnancy category (D)
- To use with full glass of water, without regard to food

fluticasone (Rx)
(floo-tic′a-sone)

Flonase, Flovent HFA, Flovent Diskus, Veramyst (nasal spray)

Func. class: Corticosteroids, inhalation; antiasthmatic

ACTION:
Decreases inflammation by inhibiting mast cells, macrophages, and

leukotrienes; antiinflammatory and vasoconstrictor properties

USES: Prevention of chronic asthma during maintenance treatment in those requiring oral corticosteroids; nasal symptoms of seasonal/perennial, allergic/nonallergic rhinitis
Unlabeled uses: COPD

CONTRAINDICATIONS: Hypersensitivity to this product or milk protein, primary treatment in status asthmaticus, acute bronchospasm
Precautions: Pregnancy (C), breastfeeding, active infections, glaucoma, diabetes, immunocompromised patients, Cushing syndrome

DOSAGE AND ROUTES

Prevention of chronic asthma during maintenance treatment in those requiring oral corticosteroids

Flovent HFA

- **Adult and child ≥12 yr: INH** 88-440 mcg bid (in those previously taking bronchodilators alone); **INH** 88-220 mcg bid, max 440 mcg bid (in those previously taking inhaled corticosteroids); **INH** 440 mcg bid, max 880 mcg bid (in those previously taking oral corticosteroids)
- **Child 4-11 yr: INH** 88 mcg bid

Flovent Diskus

- **Adult and child ≥12 yr: INH** 100 mcg bid, max 500 mcg bid (in those previously taking bronchodilators alone); **INH** 100-250 mcg bid, max 500 mcg bid (in those previously taking inhaled corticosteroids); **INH** 500-1000 mcg bid, max 1000 mcg bid (in those previously taking oral corticosteroids)
- **Child 4-11 yr: INH** Initially 50 mcg bid, max 100 mcg bid (in those previously taking bronchodilators alone or inhaled corticosteroids)

Nasal symptoms of seasonal, perennial allergic, nonallergic rhinitis

Flonase

- **Adult:** nasal 2 sprays initially, in each nostril daily or 1 spray bid, when controlled, lower to 1 spray in each nostril daily
- **Adolescent/child >4 yr:** nasal 1 spray in each nostril daily, may increase to 2 sprays in each nostril daily, when controlled lower to 1 spray in each nostril daily

Veramyst

- **Adult/child ≥12 yr:** nasal 2 sprays in each nostril daily
- **Child 2-11 yr:** nasal 1 spray in each nostril daily

Available forms: Oral inhalation aerosol 44, 110, 220 mcg; oral inhalation powder 50, 100, 250 mcg; nasal spray (Veramyst) 27.5 mcg/actuation, (propionate) 50 mcg/actuation, 27.5 mcg/spray (furoate)

Administer:

- Give at 1-min intervals; if a bronchodilator aerosol spray is used, use bronchodilator first, wait 5-15 min, then use fluticasone
- Decrease dose to lowest effective dose after desired effect; decrease dose at 2-4 wk intervals

Inhalation route (aerosol)

- Shake well, prime before 1st use, release 4 sprays into air away from face, prime using 1 spray if not used for ≥7 days; when the counter reads 000, discard; clean mouthpiece daily in warm water, dry; do not share inhaler with others
- Child <4 yr requires a face mask with spacer/VHC device for delivery; allow 3-5 INH per actuation; do not use spacer with Flovent Diskus

Inhalation route: Powder for oral inhalation (Flovent Diskus)

- Fill in the "Pouch opened" and "Use by" dates in the blank lines on the label; the "Use by" date for Flovent Diskus 50 mcg is 6 wk from the date the pouch is opened; the "Use by" date for Diskus 100 mcg and 250 mcg is 2 mo from the date the pouch is opened
- Open the diskus by holding in one hand and using the thumb of the other to push the thumb grip away as far as it will

go until the mouthpiece shows and snaps into place

- Slide the lever away from the patient as far as it will go until it clicks; the number on the dose counter will count down from 1; the diskus is now ready to use
- Before inhaling the dose, have patient breathe out, hold the diskus level and away from mouth, do not breathe out into the mouthpiece
- Instruct the patient to put the mouthpiece to the lips and breathe in through the mouth quickly and deeply through the diskus; remove the diskus from the mouth, hold breath for about 10 sec, and breathe out slowly
- After taking a dose, close the diskus by sliding the thumb grip back as far as it will go; the diskus will click shut; the lever automatically returns to its original position
- The counter displays how many doses are left; the counter number counts down each time the patient uses the diskus; after 55 doses (23 doses from the sample pack), numbers 5 to 0 are red to warn that there are only a few doses left
- After use, patient should rinse mouth with water and spit out the water, not swallow it
- To avoid the spread of infection, do not use the inhaler for more than one person

Intranasal

- Prime before first use
- Shake bottle gently before each use
- Rinse tip after use, dry with tissue
- Blow nose before use

SIDE EFFECTS

CNS: Fatigue, fever, headache, nervousness, dizziness, migraines

EENT: *Pharyngitis*, sinusitis, rhinitis, laryngitis, hoarseness, dry eyes, cataracts, nasal discharge, epistaxis, blurred vision

GI: Diarrhea, abdominal pain, nausea, vomiting, *oral candidiasis*

INTEG: Urticaria, dermatitis

META: Hyperglycemia, growth retardation in children, cushingoid features

MISC: Influenza, eosinophilic conditions, angioedema, Churg-Strauss syndrome, anaphylaxis, adrenal insufficiency (high doses), bone mineral density reduction

MS: Osteoporosis, muscle soreness, joint pain, arthralgia

RESP: *Upper respiratory infection*, dyspnea, cough, bronchitis, bronchospasm

PHARMACOKINETICS

Absorption 30% aerosol, 13.5% powder; protein binding 91%; metabolized in liver after absorption in lung; half-life 7.8 hr; <5% excreted in urine and feces

Oral INH: Onset 24 hr, peak several days, duration 1-2 wk

Intranasal: Onset 12 hr, peak several days

INTERACTIONS

Increase: fluticasone levels—CYP3A4 inhibitors (ketoconazole, itraconazole), darunavir, nelfinavir, ritonavir, amprenavir, fosamprenavir, atazanavir, delavirdine, saquinavir

Increase: cardiac toxicity—isoproterenol (asthma patients)

NURSING CONSIDERATIONS

Assess:

- **Respiratory status:** lung sounds, pulmonary function tests during, for several mo after change from systemic to inhalation corticosteroids
- Withdrawal symptoms from oral corticosteroids: depression, pain in joints, fatigue

⚠ **Adrenal insufficiency:** nausea, weakness, fatigue, hypotension, hypoglycemia, anorexia; may occur when changing from systemic to inhalation corticosteroids; may be life-threatening; adrenal function tests periodically: hypothalamic–pituitary–adrenal axis suppression in long-term treatment

- Growth rate in children; blood glucose, serum potassium for all patients

Evaluate:

- Therapeutic response: decreased severity of asthma, COPD, allergies

Teach patient/family:

- To use bronchodilator 1st, before using inhalation, if taking both

- Not to use for acute asthmatic attack; acute asthma may require oral corticosteroids
- To avoid smoking, smoke-filled rooms, those with URIs, those not immunized against chickenpox or measles
- To rinse mouth after inhaled product to decrease risk of oral candidiasis
- To report immediately cushingoid symptoms: no appetite, nausea, weakness, fatigue, decreased B/P
- How to use, and when it may be empty
- To use medical ID identifying corticosteroid use

fluticasone (topical)

(floo-tic′a-sone)

Cutivate

Func. class.: Corticosteroid, topical

Do not confuse:
fluticasone/mometasone/fludrocortisone

ACTION: Crosses cell membrane to attach to receptors to decrease inflammation, itching; inhibits multiple inflammatory cytokines

USES: Inflammation/itching of corticosteroid-responsive dermatoses on the skin

CONTRAINDICATIONS: Hypersensitivity to this product or milk protein, status asthmaticus, monotherapy in primary infections, Cushing syndrome, rosacea, perioral dermatits, diabetes mellitus

Precautions: Pregnancy (C), children, breastfeeding, skin infections, skin atrophy

DOSAGE AND ROUTES

- Adult: Apply to affected areas bid (cream/ointment) or daily (lotion) × 4 wk

Available forms: Lotion, cream 0.05%, ointment 0.005%

Administer:

Topical route

⚠ Do not use with occlusive dressings

- **Cream/Ointment/Lotion:** Apply sparingly in a thin film and rub gently into the cleansed, affected area, wash hands, use gloves, avoid use on face, groin, underarms
- Reassess treatment after 2 uses

SIDE EFFECTS

INTEG: Burning, pruritus, dermatitis, hypertrichosis, hives, rash, xerosis, irritation, hyperpigmentation, miliaria

META: Hyperglycemia, glycosuria

MISC: HPA axis suppression, Cushing syndrome

PHARMACOKINETICS

Absorption 5% but variable; half life 7 hr

INTERACTIONS

Drug/Lab

Increase: Blood glucose

NURSING CONSIDERATIONS

Assess:

- Skin reactions: burning, pruritus, dermatitis

Evaluate:

- Decreasing itching, inflammation on the skin

Teach patient/family:

Topical route:

⚠ Not to use with occlusive dressings

- **Cream/Ointment/Lotion:** To apply sparingly in a thin film and rub gently into the cleansed, affected area; avoid use on face, groin, underarms; wash hands; use gloves
- To reassess treatment after each use

fluticasone/salmeterol

(floo-tic′a-sone) (sal-mee′ter-ol)

Advair Diskus, Advair HFA

Func. class.: Corticosteroid, long-acting/β_2-adrenergic agonist

ACTION: Decreased inflammation in inhibiting mast cells, macrophages and leukotrienes; anti-inflammatory and vasoconstrictor properties relax bronchial smooth muscles

USES:
Maintenance of asthma (long term), COPD

CONTRAINDICATIONS:
Hypersensitivity, acute asthma/COPD episodes, severe hypersensitivity to milk proteins

Black Box Warning: Asthma-related deaths

Precautions: Pregnancy (C), breastfeeding, active infections, diabetes mellitus, glaucoma, immunosuppression, hyperthyroidism, Cushing syndrome, hypertension, QT prolongation, pheochromocytoma, seizures, MAOIs, other long-acting B_2 agonists, inhaled corticosteroid

DOSAGE AND ROUTES

Asthma maintenance

- **Adult/adolescent ≥12 yr: INH** 1 inhalation of Advair diskus q12hr, or 2 inhalations of Advair HFA q12hr
- **Child 4-11 yr: INH** 1 inhalation of fluticasone 100 mcg/salmeterol 50 mcg (Advair Diskus) q12hr, must be 12 hr apart

COPD

- **Adult: INH** 1 inhalation of Advair 250/50 diskus q12hr, must be 12 hr apart

Available forms: Inhalation 100/50, 250/50, 500/50 mcg fluticasone/salmeterol; aerosol spray 45/21, 115/21, 230/21 mcg fluticasone/salmeterol

Administer:

Oral inhalation route

Powder for oral inhalation (Diskus):

- Most children <4 years of age do not generate sufficient inspiratory flow to activate dry powder inhalers
- Give with the Diskus device: to open and prepare mouthpiece, slide device lever to activate the first dose, do not advance the lever >1 time; holding the Diskus mouthpiece level to, but away from, the mouth, exhale; then put the mouthpiece to the lips and breathe in the dose deeply and slowly; remove the Diskus from the mouth, hold breath for at least 10 sec, and then exhale slowly; close the Diskus, which also resets the dose lever for the next scheduled dose
- Mouth should be rinsed, spit out water
- Discard device after 1 mo or when counter reads 0 (whichever comes first)

HFA aerosol:

- Shake canister; prime the inhaler before first use with 4 test sprays away from face or with 2 test sprays (away from the face) if it has not been used for more than 4 wk, or after dropping; use spacer if unable to coordinate inhalation/activation
- Rinse mouth with water after use, spit out water; clean inhaler mouthpiece at least every day; discard inhaler after 120 sprays or when the counter reads 000

SIDE EFFECTS

CNS: Fever, headache, nervousness, dizziness, migraines, insomnia, tremors, agitation, anxiety, depression, hyperactivity, irritability

EENT: Pharyngitis, sinusitis, rhinitis, laryngitis, hoarseness, dry eyes, cataracts, nasal discharge, epistaxis, hypersalivation, eye edema dysphonia, conjunctivitis

GI: Diarrhea, abdominal pain, nausea, vomiting, oral candidiasis

GU: UTI

INTEG: Urticaria, dermatitis

META: Hyperglycemia, growth retardation in children, cushingoid features

MISC: Influenza, eosinophilic conditions, angioedema, Churg–Strauss syndrome, anaphylaxis, adrenal insufficiency (high doses), reduced bone mineral density, HPA axis suppression

MS: Osteoporosis, muscle soreness, joint pain, decreased growth velocity

RESP: Upper respiratory infection, dyspnea, cough, bronchitis, bronchospasm

PHARMACOKINETICS

Fluticasone: half-life 8 hr, peak 1-2 hr; Salmeterol: half-life 5.5 hr, peak 5 min

INTERACTIONS

Increase: CNS stimulation—theophylline

Increase: fluticasone levels—CYP3A4 inhibitors (ketoconazole, itraconazole), darunavir, nelfinavir, ritonavir, amprenavir, fosamprenavir, atazanavir, delavirdine, saquinavir, MAOIs, linezolid

Increase: tendinitis, tendon rupture—quinolones

Increase: hypokalemia—loop diuretics, thiazides, theophylline

Drug/Lab Test

Increase: LFTs

Decrease: Potassium

NURSING CONSIDERATIONS

Assess:

Respiratory status: Lung status, pulmonary function tests during, for several mo after change from systemic to inhalation corticosteroid

- Withdrawal symptoms from oral corticosteroids: depression, pain in joints, fatigue

Black Box Warning: **Adrenal Insufficiency:** nausea, weakness, fatigue, hypotension, hypoglycemia, anorexia; can occur when changing from systemic to inhalation corticosteroids; may be life threatening; adrenal function tests periodically: hypothalamic–pituitary–adrenal axis suppression in long-term treatment

- Growth rate in children; blood glucose, serum potassium for all patients

Evaluate:

- Therapeutic response: decreased severity of asthma

Teach patient/family:

- To use bronchodilator first, before using inhalation, if taking both; may use spacer or valved chamber
- Not to use for acute asthmatic attack; acute asthma might require oral corticosteroids; may use short-acting B_2 agonists for rescue
- To avoid smoking, smoke-filled rooms, those with URIs, those not immunized against chickenpox or measles
- To rinse mouth after inhaled product to reduce the risk of oral candidiasis; not to swallow

fluvastatin (Rx)

(flu′vah-stay-tin)

Lescol, Lescol XL

Func. class.: Antilipemic

Chem. class.: HMG-CoA reductase inhibitor

F

Do not confuse:

fluvastatin/FLUoxetine

ACTION: Inhibits HMG-CoA reductase enzyme, which reduces cholesterol synthesis

USES: As an adjunct for primary hypercholesterolemia (types Ia, Ib), coronary atherosclerosis in CAD; to reduce the risk for secondary prevention of coronary events in patients with CAD; as an adjunct to diet to reduce LDL, total cholesterol, apo B levels in heterozygous familial hyper-cholesterolemia (LDL-C ≥190 mg/dl) or LDL-C ≥160 mg/dl with history of premature CV disease

CONTRAINDICATIONS: Pregnancy (X), breastfeeding, hypersensitivity, active hepatic disease

Precautions: Previous hepatic disease, alcoholism, severe acute infections, trauma, hypotension, uncontrolled seizure disorders, severe metabolic disorders, electrolyte imbalance, myopathy, rhabdomyolysis

DOSAGE AND ROUTES

- **Adult: PO** 20-40 mg/day in PM initially, usual range 20-80 mg, max 80 mg; may be given in 2 doses (40 mg AM, 40 mg PM); dosage adjustments may be made at ≥ 4-wk intervals or ext rel 80 mg at bedtime

Heterozygous familial hypercholesterolemia

- **Adolescent ≥1 yr postmenarche (10-16 yr): PO** 20 mg daily at bedtime, may increase q6wk, max 40 mg bid (cap) or 80 mg (ext rel)

Available forms: Caps 20, 40 mg; ext rel tab 80 mg

Administer:

- Do not break, crush, or chew ext rel tabs, use at any time of day (tab), in the evening (cap)
- Bile acid sequestrant should be given at least 2 hr before fluvastatin
- Give without regard to food
- Store at room temperature, protected from light

SIDE EFFECTS

CNS: Headache, dizziness, insomnia, confusion

EENT: Lens opacities

GI: *Abdominal pain, cramps, nausea, constipation, diarrhea, dyspepsia, flatus,* hepatic dysfunction, pancreatitis

HEMA: Thrombocytopenia, hemolytic anemia, leukopenia

INTEG: Rash, pruritus

MISC: Fatigue, influenza, photosensitivity

MS: Myalgia, myositis, rhabdomyolysis, *arthritis, arthralgia*

PHARMACOKINETICS

Peak response 3-4 wk, metabolized in liver, >98% protein bound, excreted primarily in feces, enters breast milk, half-life 1.9 hr, steady state 4-5 wk

INTERACTIONS

Increase: effects of warfarin, digoxin, phenytoin, monitor closely

Increase: myopathy—cycloSPORINE, niacin, colchicine, protease inhibitors, fibric acid derivatives, erythromycin

Increase: effects of fluvastatin—alcohol, cimetidine, ranitidine, omeprazole, phenytoin, rifampin

Increase: adverse reactions—fluconazole, itraconazole, ketoconazole

Decrease: fluvastatin effect—cholestyramine, colestipol, separate by ≥4 hr

Drug/Herb

Increase: adverse reactions—red yeast rice

Drug/Lab Test

Increase: LFTs, CK

Decrease: platelets, WBC

NURSING CONSIDERATIONS

Assess:

- **Hypercholesterolemia:** diet history: fats, fasting lipid profile (cholesterol, LDL, HDL, TG) before and q4-6wk, then q3-6mo when stable
- **Hepatotoxicity/pancreatitis:** monitor hepatic studies before, q12wk after dosage change, then q6mo; AST, ALT, LFTs may be increased
- Renal studies in patients with compromised renal system: BUN, I&O ratio, creatinine

⚠ **Myopathy, rhabdomyolysis:** muscle pain, tenderness; obtain baseline CPK if elevated; if these occur, product should be discontinued

Evaluate:

- Therapeutic response: decrease in sLDL, VLDL, total cholesterol; increased HDL, decreased triglycerides, slowing of CAD

Teach patient/family:

- That blood work will be necessary during treatment; to take product as prescribed; that effect may take ≥4 wk
- To report severe GI symptoms, headache, muscle pain, weakness, tenderness
- That previously prescribed regimen will continue: low-cholesterol diet, exercise program, smoking cessation
- To report suspected pregnancy; not to use during pregnancy (X), breastfeeding
- To take without regard to meals; take immediate release product in the evening; separate by ≥4 hr from bile-acid product

fluvoxaMINE (Rx)

(flu-vox′a-meen)

Luvox ♣, Riva-Fluvox ♣

Func. class.: Antidepressant SSRI (selective serotonin reuptake inhibitor)

Do not confuse:

Luvox/Levoxyl/Lasix/Lovenox

FluvoxaMINE/FLUoxetine/FluPHENAZine

ACTION: Inhibits CNS neuron uptake of serotonin but not of norepinephrine

USES:
Obsessive-compulsive disorder, social phobia

Unlabeled uses: Depression, bulimia nervosa, panic disorder, autism, anxiety, posttraumatic stress disorder (PTSD), premenstrual dysphoric disorder (PMDD)

CONTRAINDICATIONS:
Hypersensitivity, MAOIs

Precautions: Pregnancy (C), breastfeeding, geriatric patients, hepatic/cardiac disease, abrupt discontinuation, dehydration, ECT, hyponatremia, hypovolemia, bipolar disorder, seizure disorder

Black Box Warning: Children <8 yr, suicidal ideation

DOSAGE AND ROUTES

Obsessive-compulsive disorder (OCD)

- **Adult: PO** 50 mg at bedtime, increase by 50 mg at 4-7 day intervals, max 300 mg; doses over 100 mg should be divided; **EXT REL** 100 mg at bedtime, may titrate upward by 50 mg/wk, max 300 mg/day
- **Child 12-17 yr: PO** 25 mg at bedtime, increase by 25 mg/day q4-7days, max 300 mg/day; doses over 50 mg should be divided
- **Child 8-11 yr: PO** 25 mg/day at bedtime, may increase q4-7days, max 200 mg/day, divide doses if >50 mg

Social anxiety disorder

- **Adult: PO EXT REL CAP** (Luvox CR) 100 mg at bedtime initially, titrate as needed by 50 mg/wk to 100-300 mg/day; **PO** 50 mg at bedtime, titrate as needed by 50 mg q4-7days to 50-300 mg/day
- **Child/adolescent 12-17 yr: PO** 25 mg at bedtime, titrate by 25-50 mg q4-7days, max 300 mg/day; if total daily dose >50 mg, divide equally

Hepatic dose/geriatric

- **Adult: PO** 25 mg at bedtime, may titrate upward slowly

Bulimia nervosa, depression (unlabeled)

- **Adult: PO** 50 mg at bedtime × 4-7 days, titrate by 25-50 mg/dose q4-7days as needed

Premenstrual dysphoric disorder (unlabeled)

- **Adult: PO** 50 mg/day, may titrate to 100 mg/day

Posttraumatic stress disorder (PTSD) (unlabeled)

- **Adult: PO** 25-50 mg at bedtime × 4-7 days, then titrate by 25-50 mg/dose q4-7days, range 25-300 mg/day single or divided dose × 3-12 wk

Available forms: Tabs 25, 50, 100 mg; ext rel cap 100, 150 mg

Administer:

- With food, milk for GI symptoms
- Store at room temperature; do not freeze
- **Immediate release:** give at bedtime; doses >100 mg/day (or >50 mg/day in those aged 8-17 yr) in 2 divided doses; if doses are not equal, give larger dose at bedtime
- **Ext rel:** give at bedtime; do not break, crush, chew ext rel product

SIDE EFFECTS

CNS: *Headache, drowsiness, dizziness, seizures,* sleep disorders, insomnia, **suicidal ideation (children/adolescents), neuroleptic malignant syndrome–like reactions,** *weakness,* **neuroleptic malignant syndrome, tremors**

CV: Palpitation, chest pain, syncope, nervousness, agitation

GI: *Nausea, anorexia, constipation,* **hepatotoxicity,** *vomiting, diarrhea,* dry mouth, altered taste

GU: *Decreased libido,* anorgasmia, urinary frequency, priapism

INTEG: *Rash, sweating*

MS: **Myalgia**

SYST: **Neonatal abstinence syndrome**

PHARMACOKINETICS

Crosses blood-brain barrier, 77% protein binding, metabolism by the liver, terminal half-life 15.6 hr, peak 2-8 hr

INTERACTIONS

⚠ Fatal reaction—MAOIs

Increase: CNS depression—alcohol, barbiturates, benzodiazepines

Increase: effect of—ramelteon, thioridazine; do not use together

⚠ **Increase:** QT prolongation, death—pimozide, do not use together

Increase: fluvoxaMINE, toxicity levels—tricyclics, cloZAPine, alosetron, tiZANidine; do not use together

Increase: metabolism, decrease effects—smoking

Increase: serotonin syndrome, neuroleptic malignant syndrome: SSRIs, SNRIs, serotonin-receptor agonists, atypical antipsychotics, tramadol

Increase: bleeding risk—anticoagulants, NSAIDs, salicylates, thrombolytics

- Avoid use with clopidogrel

Decrease: metabolism, increase action of propranolol, diazepam, lithium, theophylline, carBAMazepine, warfarin

Drug/Herb

Increase: CNS effect—kava, valerian

Increase: serotonin syndrome—tryptophan, St. John's wort; do not use together

NURSING CONSIDERATIONS

Assess:

- Hepatic studies: AST, ALT, bilirubin
- Mental status: mood, sensorium, affect, **suicidal tendencies;** increase in psychiatric symptoms: depression, panic, obsessive-compulsive symptoms
- Constipation; most likely in geriatric patients
- Growth rate (children), bone density (post-menopausal females), glucose (diabetes)

⚠ For toxicity: nausea, vomiting, diarrhea, syncope, increased pulse, seizures

Evaluate:

- Therapeutic response: decrease in depression

Teach patient/family:

- That therapeutic effects may take 2-3 wk; not to discontinue abruptly
- To use caution when driving, performing other activities requiring alertness because drowsiness, dizziness may occur
- Not to use other CNS depressants, alcohol, barbiturates, benzodiazepines, St. John's wort, kava
- To notify prescriber if pregnancy is suspected, planned
- To notify prescriber of allergic reaction
- To increase bulk in diet if constipation occurs, especially in geriatric patients

Black Box Warning: That suicidal thoughts/behaviors may occur

- To stop taking MAOIs at least 14 days before starting product

TREATMENT OF OVERDOSE:

Activated charcoal, gastric lavage

folic acid (vit B_9) (OTC)

(foe′lik a′sid)

Apo-Folic ♣, Folvite ♣,
Novo-Folacid ♣

Func. class.: Vit B complex group, water-soluble vitamin

ACTION:
Needed for erythropoiesis; increases RBC, WBC, platelet formation with megaloblastic anemias

USES:
Megaloblastic or macrocytic anemia caused by folic acid deficiency; hepatic disease, alcoholism, hemolysis, intestinal obstruction, pregnancy to reduce risk for neural tube defects

Unlabeled uses: Reduce risk for heart disease, stroke, methotrexate toxicity prophylaxis

CONTRAINDICATIONS:
Hypersensitivity

Precautions: Pregnancy (A), anemias other than megaloblastic/macrocytic anemia, vit B_{12} deficiency anemia, uncorrected pernicious anemia

DOSAGE AND ROUTES

RDA

- **Adult and child ≥14 yr: PO** 400 mcg

- **Adult (pregnant/lactating): PO** 600 mcg/day
- **Child 9-13 yr: PO** 300 mcg
- **Child 4-8 yr: PO** 200 mcg
- **Child 1-3 yr: PO** 150 mcg
- **Infant 6 mo-1 yr: PO** 80 mcg
- **Neonate/infant <6 mo: PO** 65 mcg

Megaloblastic/macrocytic anemia due to folic acid or nutritional deficiency

- **Pregnant/lactating: PO** 800-1000 mcg

Therapeutic dose

- **Adult and child: PO/IM/SUBCUT/IV** up to 1 mg/day

Maintenance dose

- **Adult and child >4 yr: PO/IM/SUBCUT/IV** 0.4 mg/day
- **Pregnant and lactating: PO/IM/SUBCUT/IV** 0.8-1 mg/day
- **Child <4 yr: PO/IM/SUBCUT/IV** up to 0.3 mg/day
- **Infant: PO/IM/SUBCUT/IV** up to 0.1 mg/day

Prevention of neural tube defects during pregnancy

- **Adult: PO** 0.6 mg/day

Prevention of megaloblastic anemia during pregnancy

- **Adult: PO/IM/SUBCUT** up to 1 mg/day during pregnancy

Tropical sprue

- **Adult: PO** 3-15 mg/day

Available forms: Tabs 0.1, 0.4, 0.8, 1, 5 mg; inj 5, 10 mg/ml

Administer:

SUBCUT route

- Do not inject intradermally

IM route

- Inject deeply in large muscle mass, aspirate

Direct IV route

- Direct undiluted ≤5 mg/1 min or more

Continuous IV INFUSION route

- May be added to most IV sol or TPN

Y-site compatibilities: Alfentanil, aminophylline, ascorbic acid injection, atracurium, atropine, azaTHIOprine, aztreonam, benztropine, bumetanide, calcium gluconate, ceFAZolin, cefonicid, cefotaxime, cefoTEtan, cefOXitin, cefTAZidime, ceftizoxime, cefTRIAXone, cefuroxime, chloramphenicol, cimetidine, clindamycin, cyanocobalamin, cycloSPORINE, dexamethasone, digoxin, diphenhydrAMINE, DOPamine, enalaprilat, ePHEDrine, EPINEPHrine, epoetin alfa, erythromycin, esmolol, famotidine, fentaNYL, fluconazole, furosemide, ganciclovir, glycopyrrolate, heparin, hydrocortisone, hydrOXYzine, imipenem-cilastatin, indomethacin, insulin (regular), ketorolac, labetalol, lidocaine, LR, magnesium sulfate, mannitol, meperidine, methicillin, methylPREDNISolone, metoclopramide, metoprolol, mezlocillin, midazolam, moxalactam, multiple vitamins injection, naloxone, nitroglycerin, nitroprusside, ondansetron, oxacillin, oxytocin, penicillin G potassium/sodium, PENTobarbital, PHENobarbital, phenylephrine, phytonadione, piperacillin, potassium chloride, procainamide, propranolol, ranitidine, Ringer's, ritodrine, sodium bicarbonate, succinylcholine, SUFentanil, theophylline, ticarcillin, ticarcillin-clavulanate, TPN, trimetaphan, urokinase, vancomycin, vasopressin

SIDE EFFECTS

CNS: Confusion, depression, excitability, irritability

GI: Anorexia, nausea, bitter taste

INTEG: Pruritus, rash, erythema

RESP: **Bronchospasm**

SYST: **Anaphylaxis (rare)**

PHARMACOKINETICS

PO: Peak ½-1 hr, bound to plasma proteins, excreted in breast milk, metabolized by liver, excreted in urine (small amounts)

INTERACTIONS

Increase: need for folic acid—estrogen, hydantoins, carBAMazepine, glucocorticoids

Decrease: folate levels—methotrexate, sulfonamides, sulfaSALAzine, trimethoprim

Decrease: phenytoin levels, fosphenytoin, may increase seizures

NURSING CONSIDERATIONS

Assess:

- **Megaloblastic anemia:** fatigue, dyspnea, weakness
- Hgb, Hct, reticulocyte count
- Nutritional status: bran, yeast, dried beans, nuts, fruits, fresh vegetables, asparagus
- Products currently taken: estrogen, carBAMazepine, glucocorticoids, hydantoins; these products may cause increased folic acid use by body and contribute to a deficiency if taking other neurotoxic products

Evaluate:

- Therapeutic response: increased weight, oriented, well-being; absence of fatigue; increase in reticulocyte count within 5 days of beginning treatment, absence of neural tube defect

Teach patient/family:

- To take product exactly as prescribed; that periodic lab work is required
- To alter nutrition to include high–folic-acid foods: organ meats, vegetables, fruit
- That urine will turn bright yellow
- To notify prescriber of allergic reaction
- To avoid breastfeeding

⚠ HIGH ALERT

fondaparinux (Rx)

(fon-dah-pair′ih-nux)

Arixtra

Func. class.: Anticoagulant, antithrombotic

Chem. class.: Synthetic, selective factor Xa inhibitor

Do not confuse:
Arixtra/Anti-Xa

ACTION: Inhibits factor Xa; neutralization of factor Xa interrupts blood coagulation and thrombin formation

USES: Prevention/treatment of deep venous thrombosis, PE in hip and knee replacement, hip fracture or abdominal surgery

Unlabeled uses: Acute coronary syndrome, acute MI, unstable angina

CONTRAINDICATIONS: Hypersensitivity to this product; hemophilia, leukemia with bleeding, peptic ulcer disease, hemorrhagic stroke, surgery, thrombocytopenic purpura, weight <50 kg, severe renal disease (CCr <30 ml/min), active major bleeding, bacterial endocarditis

Precautions: Pregnancy (B), breastfeeding, children, geriatric patients, alcoholism, hepatic disease (severe), blood dyscrasias, heparin-induced thrombocytopenia, uncontrolled severe hypertension, acute nephritis, mild to moderate renal disease

Black Box Warning: Spinal/epidural anesthesia, lumbar puncture

DOSAGE AND ROUTES

Deep venous thrombosis/PE

- **Adult <50 kg: SUBCUT** 5 mg/day × ≥5 days until INR 2-3; give warfarin within 72 hr of fondaparinux
- **Adult 50-100 kg: SUBCUT** 7.5 mg/day × ≥5 days until INR 2-3; give warfarin within 72 hr of fondaparinux
- **Adult >100 kg: SUBCUT** 10 mg/day × ≥5 days until INR 2-3; give warfarin within 72 hr of fondaparinux

Prevention of deep venous thrombosis

- **Adult: SUBCUT** 2.5 mg/day given 6 hr after surgery; (hemostasis established) continue for 5-9 days; for hip surgery, up to 32 days; for abdominal surgery, up to 24 days

Coronary artery thrombosis prophylaxis/acute coronary syndrome (unlabeled)

- **Adult: SUBCUT** 2.5 mg until hospital discharge or ≤8 days with standard treatment

Renal disease

- **Adult: SUBCUT** CCr 30-50 ml/min, use cautiously; CCr <30 ml/min, do not use

Available forms: Inj 2.5 mg/0.5 ml, 5 mg/0.4 ml, 7.5 mg/0.6 ml, 10 mg/0.8 ml prefilled syringes

Administer:

- Alone; do not mix with other products or solutions; cannot be used interchangeably (unit to unit) with other anticoagulants
- Only after screening patient for bleeding disorders

SUBCUT route

- SUBCUT only; do not give IM; do not give <6 hr after surgery
- Check for discolored sol or sol with particulate; if present, do not give
- Administer 6-8 hr after surgery; administer to recumbent patient, rotate inj sites (left/right anterolateral, left/right posterolateral abdominal wall)
- Wipe surface of inj site with alcohol swab, twist plunger cap and remove, remove rigid needle guard by pulling straight off needle; do not aspirate, do not expel air bubble from surface
- Insert whole length of needle into skinfold held with thumb and forefinger
- When product is injected, a soft click may be felt or heard
- Give at same time each day to maintain steady blood levels; observe inj site
- Avoid all IM inj that may cause bleeding

⚠ Administer only this product when ordered; not interchangeable with heparin

- Store at 77° F (25° C); do not freeze

SIDE EFFECTS

CNS: *Fever*, confusion, headache, dizziness, *insomnia*

GI: *Nausea, vomiting*, diarrhea, dyspepsia, *constipation,* increased AST, ALT

GU: UTI, urinary retention

HEMA: *Anemia,* minor bleeding, purpura, hematoma, **thrombocytopenia, major bleeding (intracranial, cerebral, retroperitoneal hemorrhage), postoperative hemorrhage, heparin-induced thrombocytopenia**

INTEG: Increased wound drainage, bullous eruption, local reaction—*rash,* pruritus, inj-site bleeding

META: Hypokalemia

OTHER: Hypotension, pain, *edema*

PHARMACOKINETICS

Rapidly, completely absorbed; peak steady state 3 hr; distributed primarily in blood; does not bind to plasma proteins except 94% to ATIII; eliminated unchanged in urine within 72 hr with normal renal function; terminal half-life 17-21 hr

INTERACTIONS

Increase: bleeding risk—salicylates, NSAIDs, abciximab, eptifibatide, tirofiban, clopidogrel, dipyridamole, quiNIDine, valproic acid

Drug/Herb

Increase: bleeding risk—feverfew, garlic, ginger, ginkgo, ginseng, green tea, horse chestnut, kava

NURSING CONSIDERATIONS

Assess:

Black Box Warning: Monitor patients who have received epidural/spinal anesthesia or lumbar puncture for neurological impairment, including spinal hematoma, may lead to permanent disability or paralysis

- Blood studies (CBC, anti-Xa, Hgb/Hct, prothrombin time, platelets, occult blood in stools), thrombocytopenia may occur; if platelets <100,000/mm^3, treatment should be discontinued; renal studies: BUN, creatinine
- For bleeding: gums, petechiae, ecchymosis, black tarry stools, hematuria; decreased Hct, notify prescriber
- For risk of hemorrhage if coadministering with other products that may cause bleeding
- For hypersensitivity: rash, fever, chills; notify prescriber

Evaluate:

- Therapeutic response: prevention of DVT

Teach patient/family:
- To use soft-bristle toothbrush to avoid bleeding gums; to use electric razor
- To report any signs of bleeding: gums, under skin, urine, stools
- To avoid OTC products containing aspirin, NSAIDs

formoterol (Rx)
(for-moh′ter-ahl)
Foradil Aerolizer, Oxeze ♣, Perforomist
Func. class.: Bronchodilator
Chem. class.: β-Adrenergic agonist

Do not confuse:
Foradil/Toradol

ACTION: Has β_1 and β_2 action; relaxes bronchial smooth muscle and dilates the trachea and main bronchi by increasing levels of cAMP, which relaxes smooth muscles; causes increased contractility and heart rate by acting on β-receptors in heart

USES: Maintenance, treatment of asthma, COPD; prevention of exercise-induced bronchospasm

CONTRAINDICATIONS: Hypersensitivity to sympathomimetics, monotherapy for asthma, COPD, status asthmaticus
Precautions: Pregnancy (C), geriatric patients, cardiac disorders, hyperthyroidism, diabetes mellitus, prostatic hypertrophy, hypertension, African descent, aneurysm

Black Box Warning: Asthma-related death

DOSAGE AND ROUTES
Maintenance, treatment of asthma
- **Adult and child ≥5 yr:** **INH** AM and PM long-term 1 cap (12 mcg) q12hr using aerolizer inhaler

Maintenance of COPD
- **Adult:** **INH** 12 mcg q12hr

Prevention of exercise-induced bronchospasm
- **Adult and child ≥12 yr:** **INH** prn occasionally 1 cap (12 mcg) ≥15 min before exercise, do not use additional doses for ≥12 hr

Available form: INH powder in cap 12 mcg; nebulizer sol for INH 20 mcg/2 ml

Administer:
Inhalation route
- Place cap in aerolizer inhaler; cap is punctured; do not wash aerolizer inhaler
- Pull off cover, twist mouthpiece to open, push buttons in; make sure the 4 pins are visible; remove cap from blister pack, place cap in chamber; twist to close, press (a click will be heard), release; patient should exhale, place inhaler in mouth, inhale rapidly
- Store at room temperature; protection from heat, moisture

SIDE EFFECTS
CNS: *Tremors, anxiety,* insomnia, headache, dizziness, stimulation
CV: Palpitations, tachycardia, hypertension, chest pain
GI: Nausea, vomiting, xerostomia
RESP: Bronchial irritation, dryness of oropharynx, bronchospasms (overuse), infection, inflammatory reaction (child)

PHARMACOKINETICS
Onset 15 min; peak 1-3 hr; duration 12 hr; metabolized in liver, lungs, GI tract; half-life 10 hr

INTERACTIONS
⚠ **Increase:** serious dysrhythmias—MAOIs, tricyclics
Increase: hypokalemia—loop/thiazide diuretics
Increase: effects of both products—other sympathomimetics, thyroid hormones
Increase: QT prolongation—class IA/III antiarrhythmics, phenothiazines, pimozide, haloperidol, risperiDONE, sertindole, ziprasidone, amoxapine, arsenic trioxide,

chloroquine, clarithromycin, dasatinib, dolasetron, droperidol, erythromycin, halofantrine, halogenated anesthetics, levomethadyl, maprotiline, methadone, some quinolones, ondansetron, paliperidone, palonosetron, pentamidine, probucol, ranolazine, SUNItinib, tricyclics, vorinostat

Decrease: action when used with β-blockers

NURSING CONSIDERATIONS

Assess:

• Respiratory function: B/P, pulse, lung sounds; note sputum color, character; respiratory function tests before, during treatment, be alert for bronchospasm, which may occur with this patient

• Cardiac status: hypertension, palpitations, tachycardia, if CV reactions occur, product may need to be discontinued

• For paresthesias, coldness of extremities; peripheral blood flow may decrease

Evaluate:

• Therapeutic response: ease of breathing

Teach patient/family:

Black Box Warning: Asthma-related death, severe asthma exacerbations; if wheezing worsens and cannot be relieved during an acute asthma attack, immediate medical attention should be sought

• To rinse mouth after use

• About correct use of inhaler/nebulizer (review package insert with patient); to avoid getting aerosol in eyes

• About all aspects of product; to avoid smoking, smoke-filled rooms, persons with respiratory infections; not to swallow caps

TREATMENT OF OVERDOSE:

Administration of β-blocker

fosamprenavir (Rx)

(fos-am-pren′a-veer)

Lexiva

Func. class.: Antiretroviral

Chem. class.: Protease inhibitor

ACTION: A prodrug of amprenavir; inhibits human immunodeficiency virus (HIV) protease, which prevents maturation of the infectious virus

F

USES: HIV-1 infection in combination with antiretrovirals

CONTRAINDICATIONS: Hypersensitivity to protease inhibitors

Precautions: Pregnancy (C), breastfeeding, geriatric patients, hepatic disease, hemolytic anemia, diabetes, sulfa sensitivity, autoimmune disease with immune reconstitution

DOSAGE AND ROUTES

Therapy-naive patients

• **Adult: PO** 1400 mg bid without ritonavir or fosamprenavir 1400 mg/day and with ritonavir 200 mg/day or fosamprenavir 700 mg bid and ritonavir 100 mg bid

• **Child >2 yr-adolescents:** >20 kg: PO 18 mg/kg (max: 700 mg) bid plus ritonavir 3 mg/kg (max: 100 mg) bid; 15 kg to <20 kg: 23 mg/kg bid plus ritonavir 3 mg/kg bid; 11 kg to <15 kg: 30 mg/kg/dose bid plus ritonavir 3 mg/kg/dose bid; <11 kg: 45 mg/kg/dose bid plus ritonavir 7 mg/kg/dose bid

Protease-experienced patients (PI)

• **Adult: PO** 700 mg bid and ritonavir 100 mg bid

• **Child/adolescent ≥20 kg: PO** 18 mg/kg bid with ritonavir 3 mg/kg bid

• **Child/adolescent 15 kg to <20 kg: PO** 23 mg/kg bid with ritonavir 3 mg/kg bid

• **Child/adolescent 11 kg to <15 kg: PO** 30 mg/kg bid with ritonavir 3 mg/kg bid

• **Child/adolescent <11 kg: PO** 45 mg/kg bid with ritonavir 7 mg bid

• **Infant ≥6 mo:** 15 kg to <20 kg: **PO** susp 23 mg/kg bid with ritonavir 3 mg/kg bid
• **Infant ≥6 mo:** 11 kg to <15 kg: **PO** susp 30 mg/kg bid with ritonavir 3 mg/kg bid
• **Infant ≥6 mo:** <11 kg: **PO** susp 45 mg/kg bid with ritonavir 7 mg/kg bid

Combination with efavirenz
• **Adult: PO** add another 100 mg/day of ritonavir for a total of 300 mg/day when all 3 products given

Hepatic dose
• **Adult: PO** (Child-Pugh 5-6) 700 mg bid without ritonavir (treatment-naive patients) or 700 mg bid with ritonavir 100 mg daily (treatment-naive or experienced patients); (Child-Pugh 7-9) 700 mg bid without ritonavir (treatment-naive patients) or 450 mg bid with ritonavir 100 mg daily (treatment-naive or experienced patients); (Child-Pugh 10-15) 350 mg bid without ritonavir (treatment-naive patients) or 300 mg bid with ritonavir 100 mg daily (treatment-naive or experienced patients)

Available forms: Tabs 700 mg (equivalent to 600 mg amprenavir); oral susp 50 mg/ml

Administer:
• **Tab:** without regard to food
• **Oral susp:** give without food (adult), with food (pediatric); if vomiting occurs within 30 min of dose, readminister; shake vigorously before dose, use calibrated device

SIDE EFFECTS

CNS: Headache, fatigue, depression, oral paresthesia
GI: *Nausea, diarrhea, vomiting, abdominal pain*
INTEG: Rash, pruritus
MISC: Redistribution or accumulation of body fat, hyperglycemia, Stevens-Johnson syndrome

PHARMACOKINETICS

Prodrug of amprenavir, peak 1½-4 hr; 90% protein binding; metabolized in liver by CYP3A4; excretion of unchanged product minimal; half-life 7.7 hr

INTERACTIONS

Increase: treatment failure—ritonavir with boceprevir or ritonavir with telaprevir, not recommended
Increase: effect of—warfarin
⚠ **Serious life-threatening reactions:** amiodarone, calcium channel blockers, lidocaine, pimozide, ergots, midazolam, triazolam, flecainide, lovastatin, simvastatin, propafenone
Increase: effect of—ARIPiprazole, rifbutin, ketoconazole, itraconazole, sildenafil, vardenafil
Increase: toxicity—HMG-CoA reductase inhibitors
Decrease: dose of maraviroc with product if used with ritonavir; do not use maraviroc with unboosted fosamprenavir
Decrease: effect of oral contraceptives, methadone
Decrease: fosamprenavir levels—nevirapine, antacids, efavirenz, saquinavir, ranitidine, carBAMazepine, phenytoin, lopinavir/ritonavir, barbiturates, proton-pump inhibitors, H_2-receptor antagonists, dexamethasone; avoid concurrent use

Drug/Herb
• Avoid use with St. John's wort

Drug/Lab Test
Increase: serum glucose, AST, ALT, triglycerides

NURSING CONSIDERATIONS

Assess:
• **HIV:** monitor CD4+ T cell count, plasma HIV RNA, serum cholesterol, serum lipid profile
• Bowel pattern before, during treatment; monitor hydration
• Skin eruptions, rash, urticaria, itching; allergy to sulfonamides; cross-sensitivity may occur
⚠ Stevens-Johnson syndrome; skin reactions, report immediately
• **Immune reconstitution syndrome:** may occur with combination antiretroviral therapy, autoimmune disease may also develop, up to months after treatment starts

Teach patient/family:
- To avoid taking with other medications unless directed by provider
- That product does not cure but does manage symptoms; that product does not prevent transmission of HIV to others
- To use a nonhormonal form of birth control while taking this product
- That if dose is missed, to take as soon as remembered up to 1 hr before next dose; not to double dose
- Not to alter dose or stop therapy without talking to physician
- To advise physician if patient has sulfa allergy
- To report all medications, including herbal supplements, to physician
- That patients receiving phosphodiesterase type 5 inhibitors may be at increased risk for PDE5 inhibitor adverse effects

foscarnet (Rx)
(foss-kar′net)

Foscavir

Func. class.: Antiviral

Chem. class.: Inorganic pyrophosphate organic analog

ACTION: Antiviral activity is produced by selective inhibition at the pyrophosphate binding site on virus-specific DNA polymerases and reverse transcriptases at concentrations that do not affect cellular DNA polymerases

USES: Treatment of CMV retinitis, HSV infections; used with ganciclovir for relapsing patients

CONTRAINDICATIONS: Hypersensitivity, CCr <0.4 ml/min/kg

Precautions: Pregnancy (C), breastfeeding, children, geriatric patients, seizure disorders, severe anemia

Black Box Warning: Renal disease, electrolyte/mineral imbalances

DOSAGE AND ROUTES

Acyclovir-resistant mucocutaneous herpes simplex virus infection (herpes labialis, herpes febrilis, herpes genitalis) in HIV-infected patients
- **Adult/adolescent (unlabeled): IV** 40 mg/kg every 8-12 hr × 2-3 wk or until lesions are healed

Cytomegalovirus (CMV) encephalitis (unlabeled); CMV neurological disease (unlabeled) (including encephalitis) in HIV-infected patients
- **Adult/adolescent: IV** 90 mg/kg every 12 hr or 60 mg/kg every 8 hr × 3 wk (or until symptomatic improvement) with ganciclovir 5 mg/kg IV every 12 hr × 2-3 wk

Encephalitis (unlabeled) caused by human herpesvirus 6 (HHV-6) in immunocompromised patients
- **Adult: IV** 60 mg/kg every 8 hr or 90 mg/kg every 12 hr alone or in combination with ganciclovir 5 mg/kg IV every 12 hr

CMV retinitis or disseminated disease (unlabeled) in HIV-infected patients, recurrent or relapsed CMV retinitis in HIV-infected patients
- **Adult: IV** Induction with 90 mg/kg every 12 hr or 60 mg/kg IV every 8 hr × 14-21 days, depending upon the clinical response

Renal dose
- HSV induction dosage equivalent to 80 mg/kg/day (40 mg/kg IV every 12 hr)
- **Adult: IV** CCr >1.4 ml/min/kg: no change; CCr >1-1.4 ml/min/kg: decrease to 30 mg/kg every 12 hr; CCr >0.8-1 ml/min/kg: decrease to 20 mg/kg every 12 hr; CCr >0.6-0.8 ml/min/kg: decrease to 35 mg/kg every 24 hr; CCr >0.5-0.6 ml/min/kg: decrease to 25 mg/kg every 24 hr; CCr ≥0.4-0.5 ml/min/kg: decrease to 20 mg/kg every 24 hr; CCr <0.4 ml/min/kg: not recommended

HSV induction dosage equivalent to 120 mg/kg/day (40 mg/kg IV every 8 hr)
- **Adult: IV** CCr >1.4 ml/min/kg: no change; CCr >1-1.4 ml/min/kg: decrease to 30 mg/kg every 8 hr; CCr >0.8-1

ml/min/kg: decrease to 35 mg/kg every 12 hr; CCr >0.6-0.8 ml/min/kg: decrease to 25 mg/kg every 12 hr; CCr 0.5-0.6 ml/min/kg: decrease to 40 mg/kg every 24 hr; CCr ≥0.4-0.5 ml/min/kg: decrease to 35 mg/kg every 24 hr; CCr <0.4 ml/min/kg: not recommended

CMV induction dosage equivalent to 180 mg/kg/day (60 mg/kg every 8 hr)

• **Adult: IV** CCr >1.4 ml/min/kg: no change; CCr >1-1.4 ml/min/kg: decrease to 45 mg/kg every 8 hr; CCr >0.8-1 ml/min/kg: decrease to 50 mg/kg every 12 hr; CCr >0.6-0.8 ml/min/kg: decrease to 40 mg/kg every 12 hr; CCr >0.5-0.6 ml/min/kg: decrease to 60 mg/kg every 24 hr; CCr ≥0.4-0.5 ml/min/kg: decrease to 50 mg/kg every 24 hr; CCr <0.4 ml/min/kg: not recommended

CMV induction dosage equivalent to 180 mg/kg/day (90 mg/kg IV every 12 hr)

• **Adult: IV** CCr >1.4 ml/min/kg: no change; CCr >1-1.4 ml/min/kg: decrease to 70 mg/kg every 12 hr; CCr >0.8-1 ml/min/kg: decrease to 50 mg/kg every 12 hr; CCr >0.6-0.8 ml/min/kg: decrease to 80 mg/kg every 24 hr; CCr >0.5-0.6 ml/min/kg: decrease to 60 mg/kg every 24 hr; CCr ≥0.4-0.5 ml/min/kg: decrease to 50 mg/kg every 24 hr; CCr <0.4 ml/min/kg: not recommended

Available forms: Inj 6000 mg/250 ml, 12,000 mg/500 ml (24 mg/ml)

Administer:

• Increased fluids before and during product administration to induce diuresis, minimize renal toxicity

Intermittent IV INFUSION route

• Using infusion device at no more than 1 mg/kg/min; do not give by rapid or bolus IV; give by CVL or peripheral vein; standard 24 mg/ml sol may be used without dilution if using by CVL; dilute the 24 mg/ml sol to 12 mg/ml with D_5W or NS if using peripheral vein

• Manufacturer recommends product not be given with other medications in syringe or admixed

SIDE EFFECTS

CNS: *Fever*, dizziness, *headache*, seizures, *fatigue*, neuropathy, asthenia, encephalopathy, malaise, meningitis, *paresthesia*, depression, *confusion*, *anxiety*

CV: ECG abnormalities, 1st-degree AV block, nonspecific ST-T segment changes, cerebrovascular disorder, cardiomyopathy, cardiac arrest, atrial fibrillation, CHF, sinus tachycardia

GI: *Nausea, vomiting, diarrhea, anorexia,* abdominal pain, pancreatitis

GU: Acute renal failure, decreased CCr, increased serum creatinine, azotemia, diabetes insipidus, renal tubular disorders

HEMA: *Anemia*, granulocytopenia, leukopenia, thrombocytopenia, thrombosis, neutropenia, lymphadenopathy

INTEG: *Rash*, sweating, pruritus, skin discoloration

RESP: *Coughing*, *dyspnea*, pneumonia, pulmonary infiltration, pneumothorax, hemoptysis

SYST: *Hypokalemia, hypocalcemia, hypomagnesemia;* hypophosphatemia

PHARMACOKINETICS

14%-17% protein bound, half-life 18-88 hr in normal renal function, 79%-92% excreted via kidneys

INTERACTIONS

Black Box Warning: Increase: nephrotoxicity—acyclovir, cidofovir, CISplatin, gold compounds, penicillamine, tacrolimus, tenofovir, vancomycin, aminoglycosides, amphotericin B, NSAIDs, lithium, cycloSPORINE

Increase: hypocalcemia—pentamidine

NURSING CONSIDERATIONS

Assess:

Black Box Warning: Renal tubular disorders: I&O ratio, urine pH, serum creatinine at baseline, 3×/wk during initial therapy then 2×/wk thereafter; CCr at baseline, throughout treatment; if CCr <0.4 ml/min/kg, discontinue

• Blood counts q2wk; watch for decreasing granulocytes, Hgb; if low, therapy may have to be discontinued and restarted after hematologic recovery; blood transfusions may be required
• Lesions in HSV
• Electrolytes and minerals (calcium, phosphate, magnesium, potassium); watch closely for tetany during 1st administration
• GI symptoms: nausea, vomiting, diarrhea; severe symptoms may necessitate discontinuing product
⚠ **Blood dyscrasias** (anemia, granulocytopenia): bruising, fatigue, bleeding, poor healing
• **Allergic reactions:** flushing, rash, urticaria, pruritus

CMV retinitis
• Culture should be performed before treatment (blood, urine, throat); a negative culture does not rule out CMV
• Ophthalmic exam should confirm diagnosis
• Close monitoring during therapy for tingling, numbness, paresthesias; if these occur, stop infusion, obtain lab sample for electrolytes

Evaluate:
• Therapeutic response: improvement in CMV retinitis

Teach patient/family:
• To call prescriber if sore throat, swollen lymph nodes, malaise, fever occur, since other infections may occur
• To report perioral tingling, numbness in extremities, and paresthesias
• That serious product interactions may occur if OTC products are ingested; check first with prescriber
• That product is not a cure but will control symptoms

fosinopril (Rx)
(foss′in-oh-pril)
Monopril
Func. class.: Antihypertensive
Chem. class.: Angiotensin-converting enzyme (ACE) inhibitor

Do not confuse:
Monopril/minoxidil//Monurol

F

ACTION: Selectively suppresses renin-angiotensin-aldosterone system; inhibits ACE; prevents conversion of angiotensin I to angiotensin II; results in dilation of arterial, venous vessels

USES: Hypertension, alone or in combination with thiazide diuretics, systolic CHF
Unlabeled uses: Proteinuria in nondiabetic nephropathy

CONTRAINDICATIONS: Breastfeeding, children, hypersensitivity to ACE inhibitors, history of ACE-inhibitor–induced angioedema

Black Box Warning: Pregnancy (D)

Precautions: Geriatric patients, impaired hepatic function, hypovolemia, blood dyscrasias, CHF, COPD, asthma, angioedema, hyperkalemia, renal artery stenosis, renal disease, aortic stenosis, autoimmune disorders, collagen vascular disease, febrile illness

DOSAGE AND ROUTES
CHF
• **Adult: PO** 5-10 mg/day, then up to 40 mg/day increased over several wk; use lower dose for those diuresed before fosinopril

Hypertension
• **Adult: PO** 10 mg/day initially, then 20-40 mg/day divided bid or daily, max 80 mg/day

Available forms: Tabs 10, 20, 40 mg

Administer:
- May be taken without regard to meals
- Store in tight container at ≤86° F (30° C)

SIDE EFFECTS

CNS: *Headache, dizziness,* fatigue, syncope
CV: *Hypotension,* orthostatic hypotension, tachycardia
GI: *Nausea,* constipation, *vomiting,* diarrhea, hepatotoxicity, cholestatic jaundice, fulminant hepatic necrosis, hepatic failure, death
GU: Increased BUN, creatinine, azotemia, renal artery stenosis
HEMA: Decreased Hct, Hgb; eosinophilia, leukopenia, neutropenia, agranulocytosis
META: *Hyperkalemia*
RESP: *Cough*
SYST: Anaphylaxis, angioedema

PHARMACOKINETICS

Peak 3 hr, serum protein binding 99%, half-life 11.5-14 hr, metabolized by liver (metabolites excreted in urine, feces)

INTERACTIONS

Increase: hyperkalemia risk—potassium-sparing diuretics, potassium supplements
Increase: hypotension—diuretics, other antihypertensives, ganglionic blockers, adrenergic blockers, nitrates, acute alcohol ingestion
Increase: toxicity—vasodilators, hydrALAZINE, prazosin, potassium-sparing diuretics, sympathomimetics, digoxin, lithium, NSAIDs
Decrease: absorption—antacids
Decrease: antihypertensive effect—salicylates

Drug/Herb
Increase: antihypertensive effect—hawthorn
Decrease: antihypertensive effect—ephedra

Drug/Lab Test
Increase: AST, ALT, alk phos, glucose, bilirubin, uric acid
False positive: urine acetone
Positive: ANA titer

NURSING CONSIDERATIONS

Assess:
- **Hypertension:** B/P, orthostatic hypotension, syncope
- **Collagen vascular disease:** neutrophils, decreased platelets; obtain WBC with differential baseline and monthly × 6 mo, then q2-3mo × 1 yr; if neutrophils <1000/mm^3, discontinue
- **Pregnancy:** identify pregnancy before starting therapy, pregnancy (D)
- Renal studies: protein, BUN, creatinine; increased levels may indicate nephrotic syndrome
- Baselines of renal, hepatic studies before therapy begins
- Potassium levels, although hyperkalemia rarely occurs
- **CHF:** edema in feet, legs daily; weigh daily
- **Allergic reactions:** rash, fever, pruritus, urticaria; product should be discontinued if antihistamines fail to help
- Supine position for severe hypotension

Evaluate:
- Therapeutic response: decrease in B/P

Teach patient/family:
- Not to discontinue product abruptly; to take at same time of day
- Not to use OTC products (cough, cold, allergy) unless directed by prescriber; not to use salt substitutes containing potassium without consulting prescriber
- About the importance of complying with dosage schedule, even if feeling better
- To rise slowly to sitting or standing position to minimize orthostatic hypotension
- To notify prescriber of mouth sores, sore throat, fever, swelling of hands or feet, irregular heartbeat, chest pain, nonproductive cough
- To report excessive perspiration, dehydration, vomiting, diarrhea; may lead to fall in B/P
- That product may cause dizziness, fainting, light-headedness during first few days of therapy
- That product may cause skin rash or impaired perspiration

• How to take B/P; normal readings for age group

Black Box Warning: To notify prescriber if pregnancy is planned or suspected, pregnancy (D), to use contraception during treatment

TREATMENT OF OVERDOSE:

0.9% NaCl IV infusion, hemodialysis

fosphenytoin (Rx)

(foss-fen′i-toy-in)

Func. class.: Anticonvulsant

Chem. class.: Hydantoin, phosphate phenytoin ester

ACTION: Inhibits spread of seizure activity in motor cortex by altering ion transport; increases AV conduction, prodrug of phenytoin

USES: Generalized tonic-clonic seizures, status epilepticus, partial seizures

CONTRAINDICATIONS: Pregnancy (D), hypersensitivity, bradycardia, SA and AV block, Stokes-Adams syndrome

Precautions: Breastfeeding, allergies, renal/hepatic disease, myocardial insufficiency, hypoalbuminemia, hypothyroidism, Asian patients positive for HLA-B 1502, abrupt discontinuation, agranulocytosis, alcoholism, carBAMazepine/barbiturate hypersensitivity, bone marrow suppression, CAD, geriatric patients, hemolytic anemia, hyponatremia, methemoglobinemia, myasthenia gravis, psychosis, suicidal ideation

Black Box Warning: Rapid IV infusion

DOSAGE AND ROUTES

All doses in PE (phenytoin sodium equivalent)

Status epilepticus

• **Adult and adolescent: IV** 15-20 mg PE/kg

• **Child <12 yr (unlabeled): IV** 15-20 mg PE/kg

Nonemergency/maintenance dosing

• **Adult and adolescent >16 yr: IM/IV** 10-20 mg PE/kg; 4-6 mg PE/kg/day (maintenance); start maintenance 12 hr after loading dose; give in 2-3 divided doses

Available forms: Inj 150 mg (100 mg phenytoin equiv), 750 mg (500 mg phenytoin equiv), 50-mg/ml vials

Administer:

Injectable routes

• Give IM/IV; the dosage, concentration, and infusion rate of fosphenytoin should always be expressed, prescribed, and dispensed in phenytoin sodium equivalents (PE); exercise extreme caution when preparing and administering fosphenytoin; the concentration and dosage should be carefully confirmed; fatal overdoses have occurred in children when the per ml concentration of the product (50 mg PE/mL) was misinterpreted as the total amount of drug in the vial

• Visually inspect for particulate matter and discoloration before use

IV INFUSION route

• Before infusion, dilute in 5% dextrose or 0.9% saline solution to a concentration ranging from 1.5 to 25 mg PE/ml

• Because of the risk of hypotension, do not exceed recommended infusion rates; continuous monitoring of ECG, B/P, and respiratory function is recommended, especially throughout the period where phenytoin concentrations peak (about 10-20 min after the end of the infusion)

• Loading doses should always be followed by maintenance doses of oral or parenteral phenytoin or parenteral fosphenytoin

• **Adult: IV** Infuse at a max rate of 150 mg PE/min

• **Elderly or debilitated adults: IV** Infuse at a max 3 mg PE/kg/min or 150 mg PE/min, whichever is less

• **Child: IV** Infuse at a rate of 0.5-3 mg PE/kg/min or max 150 mg PE/min, whichever is less

• **Infant/neonate: IV** Infuse at a rate max 0.5-3 mg PE/kg/min

F

Y-site compatibilities: Aminocaproic acid, amphotericin B lipid complex, amphotericin B liposome, anidulafungin, atenolol, bivalirudin, bleomycin, CARBOplatin, CISplatin, cyclophosphamide, cytarabine, DACTINomycin, DAPTOmycin, dexmedetomidine, diltiazem, DOCEtaxel, doxacurium, eptifibatide, ertapenem, etoposide, fludarabine, fluorouracil, gatifloxacin, gemcitabine, gemtuzumab, granisetron, ifosfamide, levofloxacin, linezolid, LORazepam, mechlorethamine, meperidine, methotrexate, metroNIDAZOLE, nesiritide, octreotide, oxaliplatin, oxytocin, PACLitaxel, palonosetron, pamidronate, pantoprazole, PEMEtrexed, PHENobarbital, piperacillin-tazobactam, rocuronium, sodium acetate, tacrolimus, teniposide, thiotepa, tigecycline, tirofiban, vinCRIStine, vinorelbine, voriconazole, zoledronic acid

SIDE EFFECTS

CNS: *Drowsiness,* dizziness, insomnia, paresthesias, depression, suicidal tendencies, aggression, headache, confusion, paresthesia, emotional liability, syncope, cerebral edema

CV: Hypo/hypertension, CHF, shock, dysrhythmias

EENT: Nystagmus, diplopia, blurred vision

GI: Nausea, vomiting, diarrhea, constipation, anorexia, weight loss, hepatitis, jaundice, gingival hyperplasia

HEMA: Agranulocytosis, leukopenia, aplastic anemia, thrombocytopenia, megaloblastic anemia

INTEG: Rash, lupus erythematosus, Stevens-Johnson syndrome, hirsutism, hypersensitivity, pruritus

RESP: Bronchospasm, cough

SYST: Hyperglycemia, hypokalemia, SJS/TEN Asian patients positive for HLA-B 1502; drug reaction with eosinophilia and systemic symptoms (DRESS), purple glove syndrome, anaphylaxis

PHARMACOKINETICS

Metabolized by liver, excreted by kidneys, protein binding 95%-99%, rapidly converted to phenytoin

INTERACTIONS

Increase: fosphenytoin level—cimetidine, amiodarone, chloramphenicol, estrogens, H_2 antagonists, phenothiazines, salicylates, sulfonamides, tricyclics, CYP1A2 inhibitors

Decrease: fosphenytoin effects—alcohol (chronic use), antihistamines, antacids, traMADol, antineoplastics, rifampin, folic acid, carBAMazepine, theophylline, CYP1A2 inducers

Decrease: virologic response, resistance—delavirdine, do not use concurrently

Drug/Herb

Increase: anticonvulsant effect—ginkgo

Decrease: anticonvulsant effect—ginseng, valerian

Drug/Lab Test

Increase: glucose, alk phos

Decrease: dexamethasone, metyrapone test serum, PBI, urinary steroids, potassium

NURSING CONSIDERATIONS

Assess:

- Drug level: target level 10-20 mcg/ml, toxic level 30-50 mcg/ml, wait >2 hr after dose before testing, 4 hr after IM dose
- Blood studies: CBC, platelets q2wk until stabilized, then monthly × 12 mo, then q3mo; serum calcium, albumin, phosphorus, potassium
- ⚠ Mental status: mood, sensorium, affect, memory (long, short), **suicidal thoughts/behaviors**
- **Serious skin reactions:** usually occurring within 28 days of treatment; if a rash develops, patient should be evaluated for DRESS
- Seizure activity including type, location, duration, character; provide seizure precaution
- Renal studies: urinalysis, BUN, urine creatinine
- Hepatic studies: ALT, AST, bilirubin, creatinine
- Allergic reaction: red, raised rash; product should be discontinued

• **Toxicity/bone marrow depression:** nausea, vomiting, ataxia, diplopia, cardiovascular collapse, slurred speech, confusion
• Respiratory depression: rate, depth, character of respirations
⚠ **Blood dyscrasias:** fever, sore throat, bruising, rash, jaundice
• Continuous monitoring of ECG, B/P, respiratory function
• Rash; discontinue as soon as rash develops, serious adverse reactions such as **Stevens-Johnson syndrome** can occur

Evaluate:
• Therapeutic response: decrease in severity of seizures

Teach patient/family:
• About the reason for, expected outcomes of treatment
• Not to use machinery or engage in hazardous activity, since drowsiness, dizziness may occur
• To carry emergency ID denoting product use, name of prescriber
• To notify prescriber of rash, bleeding, bruising, slurred speech, jaundice of skin or eyes, joint pain, nausea, vomiting, severe headaches, depression, suicidal thought
• To keep all medical appointments, including those for lab work, physical assessment
• To notify prescriber if pregnancy is planned, suspected
• To use contraception while using this product

frovatriptan (Rx)
(froh-vah-trip′tan)
Frova
Func. class.: Antimigraine agent
Chem. class.: 5-HT_1-Receptor agonist

ACTION: Binds selectively to the vascular 5-HT_{1B}, 5-HT_{1D} receptor subtypes; exerts antimigraine effect; binds to benzodiazepine receptor sites, causes vasoconstriction in cranium

USES: Acute treatment of migraine with/without aura

CONTRAINDICATIONS: Hypersensitivity, angina pectoris, history of MI, documented silent ischemia, Prinzmetal's angina, ischemic heart disease; concurrent ergotamine-containing preparations; uncontrolled hypertension; basilar or hemiplegic migraine; ischemic bowel disease; peripheral vascular disease, severe hepatic disease, prophylactic migraine treatment

Precautions: Pregnancy (C), breastfeeding, children, geriatric patients, postmenopausal women, men >40 yr, risk factors for CAD, hypercholesterolemia, obesity, diabetes, impaired hepatic function, seizure disorder

DOSAGE AND ROUTES
• **Adult: PO** 2.5 mg; a 2nd dose may be taken after ≥2 hr; max 3 tabs (7.5 mg/day)

Available form: Tabs 2.5 mg

Administer:
• Swallow tabs whole; do not break, crush, or chew
• With fluids
• 2 days/wk or less; rebound headache may occur

SIDE EFFECTS
CNS: *Hot/cold sensation*, paresthesia, *dizziness*, headache, fatigue, insomnia, anxiety, somnolence, **seizures**
CV: *Flushing*, chest pain, palpitation
GI: Dry mouth, dyspepsia, abdominal pain, diarrhea, vomiting, nausea
MS: Skeletal pain

PHARMACOKINETICS
Onset of pain relief 2-3 hr, terminal half-life 25-29 hr, protein binding 15%, metabolized liver by CYP1A2

INTERACTIONS
Increase: frovatriptan levels—CYP1A2 inhibitors (cimetidine, ciprofloxacin, erythromycin), estrogen, propranolol, oral contraceptives

Increase: toxicity—SSRIs, other serotonin agonists (dextromethorphan, MAOIs, antidepressants)

NURSING CONSIDERATIONS

Assess:

- **Migraine symptoms:** aura, unable to view light; ingestion of tyramine-containing foods (pickled products, beer, wine, aged cheese), food additives, preservatives, colorings, artificial sweeteners, chocolate, caffeine, which may precipitate these types of headaches
- B/P; signs, symptoms of coronary vasospasms
- For stress level, activity, recreation, coping mechanisms
- Quiet, calm environment with decreased stimulation from noise, bright light, excessive talking

Evaluate:

- Therapeutic response: decrease in frequency, severity of migraine

Teach patient/family:

- To report any side effects to prescriber
- To use contraception while taking product; to inform prescriber if pregnant or planning to become pregnant
- To consult prescriber if breastfeeding

⚠ HIGH ALERT

fulvestrant (Rx)

(full-vess′trant)

Faslodex

Func. class.: Antineoplastic

Chem. class.: Estrogen-receptor antagonist

ACTION:
Inhibits cell division by competitive binding to cytoplasmic estrogen receptors, downregulates estrogen receptors

USES:
Advanced breast carcinoma in estrogen-receptor–positive patients (usually postmenopausal)

Unlabeled uses: Loading dose for metastatic breast cancer

CONTRAINDICATIONS:
Pregnancy (D), breastfeeding, children, hypersensitivity

Precautions: Hepatic disease, jaundice, thrombocytopenia, biliary tract disease, coagulopathy

DOSAGE AND ROUTES

- **Adult: IM** 500 mg as 2-, 5-ml injections on days 1, 15, 29 and monthly thereafter

Available forms: Inj 50 mg/ml

Administer:

IM route

- IM 5 ml give one inj in each buttock slowly, over 1-2 min
- Antiemetic 30-60 min before product to prevent vomiting prn
- Store in refrigerator; protect from light

SIDE EFFECTS

CNS: *Headache,* depression, dizziness, insomnia, paresthesia, anxiety

GI: *Nausea, vomiting,* anorexia, constipation, diarrhea, abdominal pain, hepatitis, hepatic failure, hyperbilirubinemia

HEMA: Anemia

INTEG: *Rash,* sweating, *hot flashes,* inj-site pain

MS: Bone pain, arthritis, back pain

RESP: Pharyngitis, dyspnea, cough

SYST: Angioedema

PHARMACOKINETICS

Half-life 40 days, metabolized by CYP3A4, excretion in feces 90%

INTERACTIONS

Increase: Bleeding—anticoagulants, do not use concurrently

Drug/Lab Test

Increase: LFTs

NURSING CONSIDERATIONS

Assess:

- For anticoagulant use
- For side effects; report to prescriber

Evaluate:

- Therapeutic response: decreased tumor size, spread of malignancy

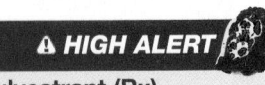

Teach patient/family:
- To report any complaints, side effects to prescriber
- To report vaginal bleeding immediately
- That tumor flare (increase in size of tumor, increased bone pain) may occur, will subside rapidly; that analgesics may be taken for pain
- That premenopausal women must use mechanical birth control because ovulation may be induced; not to breastfeed
- To use contraception to prevent pregnancy; pregnancy category (D)

furosemide (Rx)

(fur-oh′se-mide)

Lasix

Func. class.: Loop diuretic

Chem. class.: Sulfonamide derivative

Do not confuse:
furosemide/torsemide
Lasix/Luvox/Lomotil/Lanoxin/Losec

ACTION: Inhibits reabsorption of sodium and chloride at proximal and distal tubule and in the loop of Henle

USES: Pulmonary edema; edema with CHF, hepatic disease, nephrotic syndrome, ascites, hypertension
Unlabeled uses: Hypercalcemia with malignancy, hypertensive emergency/urgency, pulmonary edema or prevention of hemodynamic effects associated with blood product transfusion, ascites

CONTRAINDICATIONS: Anuria
Precautions: Pregnancy (C), breastfeeding, diabetes mellitus, dehydration, severe renal disease, cirrhosis, ascites, hypersensitivity to sulfonamides/thiazides, infants, hypovolemia, electrolyte depletion, hypersensitivity

DOSAGE AND ROUTES

Edema
- **Adult: PO** 20-80 mg/day in AM; may give another dose after 6 hr up to 600 mg/day; **IM/IV** 20-40 mg; increase by 20 mg q2hr until desired response
- **Child: PO/IM/IV** 1-2 mg/kg; may increase by 1-2 mg/kg q6-8hr up to 6 mg/kg

Antihypercalcemia
- **Adult: IM/IV** 80-100 mg q1-4hr or **PO** 120 mg/day or divided bid
- **Child: IM/IV** 25-50 mg, repeat q4hr if needed

Acute/chronic renal failure
- **Adult: PO** 80 mg/day, increase by 80-120 mg/day to desired response; **IV** 100-200 mg, max 600-800 mg

Hypertensive emergency/urgency (unlabeled)
- **Adult: IV** 40-80 mg

Pulmonary edema/prevention of adverse hemodynamic effects associated with blood product transfusion (unlabeled)
- **Adult: IV** 40 mg injected slowly, then 80 mg injected slowly after 2 hr if needed
- **Child: IM/IV** 1-2 mg/kg q6-12hr
- **Premature neonate >32 wk postconceptional age: IM/IV** 1-2 mg/kg q12-24hr
- **Premature neonate ≤32 wk postconceptional age: IM/IV** max 1 mg/kg, give no more frequently than q24hr

Available forms: Tabs 20, 40, 80 mg; oral sol 8 mg/ml, 10 mg/ml; inj 10 mg/ml

Administer:
- In AM to avoid interference with sleep if using product as diuretic
- Potassium replacement if potassium <3 mg/dl

PO route
- PO with food if nausea occurs; absorption may be decreased slightly; tabs may be crushed

IV route
- Undiluted; may be given through Y-tube or 3-way stopcock; give ≤20 mg/min

Intermittent IV INFUSION route
- May be added to NS or D_5W; if large doses required and given as IV infusion, max 4 mg/min; use infusion pump

Y-site compatibilities: Acyclovir, alfentanil, allopurinol, alprostadil, amifostine, amikacin, aminocaproic acid, aminophylline, amphotericin B cholesteryl/lipid complex/liposome, anidulafungin, argatroban, ascorbic acid, atenolol, atropine, azaTHIOprine, aztreonam, bivalirudin, bleomycin, bumetanide, calcium chloride/gluconate, CARBOplatin, cefamandole, ceFAZolin, cefepime, cefonicid, cefotaxime, cefoTEtan, cefOXitin, cefTAZidime, ceftizoxime, ceftobiprole, cefTRIAXone, cefuroxime, chloramphenicol, CISplatin, cladribine, clindamycin, cyanocobalamin, cyclophosphamide, cycloSPORINE, cytarabine, DACTINomycin, DAPTOmycin, dexamethasone, dexmedetomidine, digoxin, DOCEtaxel, doripenem, doxacurium, DOXOrubicin liposome, enalaprilat, ePHEDrine, EPINEPHrine, etoposide, fentaNYL, fludarabine, fluorouracil, folic acid, foscarnet, gallium nitrate, ganciclovir, granisetron, heparin, hydrocortisone, HYDROmorphone, ifosfamide, imipenem-cilastatin, indomethacin, insulin (regular), isosorbide, kanamycin, leucovorin, lidocaine, linezolid, LORazepam, LR, mannitol, mechlorethamine, melphalan, meropenem, methicillin, methotrexate, methylPREDNISolone, metoprolol, metroNIDAZOLE, mezlocillin, micafungin, miconazole, mitoMYcin, moxalactam, multiple vitamin injection, nafcillin, naloxone, nitroprusside, octreotide, oxacillin, oxaliplatin, oxytocin, PACLitaxel, palonosetron, pamidronate, pantoprazole, PEMEtrexed, penicillin G, PENTobarbital, PHENobarbital, phytonadione, piperacillin, piperacillin-tazobactam, potassium chloride, procainamide, propofol, propranolol, ranitidine, remifentanil, Ringer's, ritodrine, sargramostim, sodium acetate/bicarbonate, succinylcholine, SUFentanil, temocillin, teniposide, theophylline, thiopental, thiotepa, ticarcillin, ticarcillin-clavulanate, tigecycline, tirofiban, TNA, tobramycin, urokinase, vit B/C, voriconazole, zoledronic acid

SIDE EFFECTS

CNS: Headache, fatigue, weakness, vertigo, paresthesias

CV: Orthostatic hypotension, chest pain, ECG changes, circulatory collapse

EENT: Loss of hearing, ear pain, tinnitus, blurred vision

ELECT: *Hypokalemia, hypochloremic alkalosis, hypomagnesemia, hyperuricemia, hypocalcemia, hyponatremia,* metabolic alkalosis

ENDO: *Hyperglycemia*

GI: *Nausea,* diarrhea, dry mouth, vomiting, anorexia, cramps, oral, gastric irritations, pancreatitis

GU: *Polyuria,* renal failure, glycosuria, bladder spasms

HEMA: Thrombocytopenia, agranulocytosis, leukopenia, neutropenia, anemia

INTEG: *Rash, pruritus,* purpura, Stevens-Johnson syndrome, sweating, photosensitivity, urticaria

MS: Cramps, stiffness

SYST: Toxic epidermal necrolysis

PHARMACOKINETICS

PO: Onset 1 hr, peak 1-2 hr, duration 6-8 hr, absorbed 70%

IV: Onset 5 min; peak $^1/_2$ hr; duration 2 hr (metabolized by the liver 30%); excreted in urine, some as unchanged product, and feces; crosses placenta; excreted in breast milk; half-life $^1/_2$-1 hr

INTERACTIONS

Increase: toxicity—lithium, nondepolarizing skeletal muscle relaxants, digoxin, salicylates, aminoglycosides, cisplatin

Increase: hypotensive action of antihypertensives, nitrates

Increase: ototoxicity—aminoglycosides, CISplatin, vancomycin

Increase: effects of anticoagulants, salicylates

Decrease: furosemide effect—probenecid

Drug/Lab Test

Interference: GTT

Increase: LDL

NURSING CONSIDERATIONS

Assess:

- **CHF:** weight, I&O daily to determine fluid loss; effect of product may be decreased if used daily

• **Hypertension:** B/P lying, standing; postural hypotension may occur
• Metabolic alkalosis: drowsiness, restlessness
• **Hypokalemia:** postural hypotension, malaise, fatigue, tachycardia, leg cramps, weakness
• Rashes, temperature elevation daily
• Confusion, especially in geriatric patients; take safety precautions if needed
• **Hearing,** including tinnitus and hearing loss, when giving high doses for extended periods or rapid infusion
• Rate, depth, rhythm of respiration, effect of exertion, lung sounds
• Electrolytes (potassium, sodium, chloride); include BUN, blood glucose, CBC, serum creatinine, blood pH, ABGs, uric acid
• Glucose in urine if patient diabetic
• Allergies to sulfonamides, thiazides

Evaluate:

• Therapeutic response: improvement in edema of feet, legs, sacral area (CHF); increase urine output, decreased B/P; decreased calcium levels (hypercalcemia)

Teach patient/family:

• To discuss the need for a high-potassium diet or potassium replacement with prescriber
• To rise slowly from lying or sitting position because orthostatic hypotension may occur
• To recognize adverse reactions that may occur: muscle cramps, weakness, nausea, dizziness
• About the entire treatment regimen, including exercise, diet, stress relief for hypertension
• To take with food or milk for GI symptoms
• To use sunscreen or protective clothing to prevent photosensitivity
• To take early in the day to prevent sleeplessness
• To avoid OTC medications unless directed by prescriber

TREATMENT OF OVERDOSE:

Lavage if taken orally; monitor electrolytes; administer dextrose in saline; monitor hydration, CV, renal status

F

gabapentin (Rx)

(gab'a-pen-tin)

Gralise, Horizant, Neurontin

Func. class.: Anticonvulsant

Chem. class.: GABA analogue

Do not confuse:
Neurontin/Noroxin/Neoral

ACTION: Mechanism unknown; may increase seizure threshold; structurally similar to GABA; gabapentin binding sites in neocortex, hippocampus

USES: Adjunct treatment of partial seizures, with/without generalization in patients >12 yr; adjunct for partial seizures in children 3-12 yr, postherpetic neuralgia, primary restless leg syndrome in adults

Unlabeled uses: Tremors with multiple sclerosis (MS), neuropathic pain, bipolar disorder, migraine prophylaxis, diabetic neuropathy, nystagmus, pruritus, spasticity, menopause, hot flashes, ALS, MS

CONTRAINDICATIONS: Hypersensitivity to this product

Precautions: Pregnancy (C), breastfeeding, children <3 yr, geriatric patients, renal disease, hemodialysis, suicidal thoughts, depression

DOSAGE AND ROUTES

Adjunctive use in partial seizures with or without secondary generalized tonic-clonic seizures (Neurontin only)

- **Adult and child >12 yr: PO** 900-1800 mg/day in 3 divided doses; may titrate to 1800-2400 mg/day
- **Child 3-12 yr: PO** 10-15 mg/kg/day in 3 divided doses, initially titrate dose upward over approximately 3 days; if >5 yr old, use 25-35 mg/kg/day; if 3-4 yr old, 40 mg/kg/day divided in 3 doses

Postherpetic neuralgia

- **Adult: PO** (Neurontin) 300 mg on day 1, 600 mg/day divided bid on day 2, 900 mg/day divided tid, may titrate to 1800-3600 mg divided tid if needed; **EXT REL** (Gralise only) 300 mg on day 1, 600 mg on day 2, 900 mg on days 3-6, 1200 mg on days 7-10, 1500 mg on days 11-14, 1800 mg on day 15 and thereafter; Horizant only: 600 mg in AM × 3 days, day 4 give 600 mg bid

Moderate to severe restless leg syndrome (RLS) (Horizant only)

- **Adult: PO EXT REL** 600 mg daily with food at about 5 PM; if dose missed, take next day at 5 PM

Renal dose

- **Adult and child >12 yr: PO immediate release:** CCr ≥60 ml/min: no change; CCr >30-59 ml/min: total dose range 400-1400 mg/day given divided bid; CCr >15-29 ml/min: total dose range 200-700 mg/day PO given in a single daily dose; CCr = 15 ml/min: total dose range 100-300 mg/day given in one daily dose as 100, 125, 150, 200, or 300 mg; CCr <15 ml/min: reduce daily dose in proportion to CCr (CCr = 7.5 ml/min should receive half the dose that patients with CCr = 15 ml/min receive)
- **Adult: PO extended-release tablets (Gralise tablets only):** CCr ≥ 60 ml/min: no change; CCr 30-59 ml/min: 600-1800 mg/day as tolerated; CCr <30 ml/min: do not use; **extended-release tablets (Horizant tablets only)** CCr ≥60 ml/min: no change; before discontinuing, reduce the dose to 600 mg daily × 1 wk before discontinuing; CCr 30-59 ml/min: for RLS, start at 300 mg/day, increase to 600 mg/day as needed, for PHN, start at 300 mg in the AM × 3 days, then increase to 300 mg bid, increase to 600 mg bid as needed; for dose tapering before discontinuation, reduce the maintenance dose to daily in the AM × 1 wk before discontinuing; CCr 15-29 ml/min: for RLS, 300 mg/day; for PHN, 300 mg PO on days 1 and 3, then 300 mg daily in the AM, increase dose to 300 mg bid as needed, for dose tapering, if dose is 300 mg bid, reduce dose to 300 mg daily in AM × 1 wk before discontinuation; if the dose is 300 mg daily, no taper is required; CCr <15 ml/min: for RLS and

PHN, 300 mg every other day, for PHN, dose can be increased to 300 mg daily in AM, no dose taper is required before discontinuing

Uremic pruritus in hemodialysis (unlabeled)

• **Adult: PO** 300 mg 3×/wk or 400 mg 2×/wk, at end of hemodialysis ×4 wk

Brachioradical pruritus (unlabeled)

• **Adult: PO** 300-1800 mg/day

ALS (unlabeled)

• **Adult: PO** 1000 mg/day in divided doses × 6 mo

Pendular/congenital nystagmus (unlabeled)

• **Adult: PO** 900 mg/day in divided doses initially, up to 2400 mg/day in divided doses

Spasticity in MS (unlabeled)

• **Adult: PO** 600-1200 mg/day in divided doses

Available forms: Caps 100, 300, 400 mg; tabs 600, 800 mg; Horizant: ext rel tab 300, 600 mg; oral sol 250 mg/5 ml; ext rel tab (Gralise): 300, 600 mg

Administer:

• Do not crush or chew caps, ext rel tabs; caps may be opened and contents put in applesauce or dissolved in juice; scored tabs may be cut in half

• 2 hr apart when giving antacids

• Give without regard to meals immediate release

• Gradually withdraw over 7 days; abrupt withdrawal may precipitate seizures

• Beginning dose at bedtime to minimize daytime drowsiness

• **Oral sol:** measure with calibrated device, refrigerate

• **Ext rel:** give with food at about 5 PM; bioavailability increased with food; swallow whole; do not interchange Gralise with Horizant

• Store at room temperature away from heat and light

SIDE EFFECTS

CNS: *Drowsiness, confusion,* dizziness, fatigue, anxiety, somnolence, ataxia, amnesia, abnormal thinking, unsteady gait, *depression;* children 3-12 yr old, emotional lability, aggression, thought disorder, hyperkinesia, hostility, seizures, suicidal ideation, impaired cognition, euphoria

CV: Vasodilation, peripheral edema, hypotension, hypertension

EENT: Dry mouth, blurred vision, *diplopia,* nystagmus, conjunctivitis; otitis media (child 3-12 yr)

GI: Constipation/diarrhea, weight gain, increased appetite, dental abnormalities, nausea, vomiting; diarrhea (Gralise)

GU: Impotence, bleeding, *UTI*

HEMA: Leukopenia, thrombocytopenia

INTEG: Pruritus, abrasion, Stevens-Johnson syndrome, acne vulgaris

MS: Myalgia, back pain, gout

RESP: *Rhinitis,* pharyngitis, cough, upper respiratory infection (child 3-12 yr)

SYST: Drug reaction with eosinophilia and systemic symptoms (DRESS); dehydration (child 3-12 yr)

PHARMACOKINETICS

Protein binding <3% not metabolized; excreted in urine (unchanged); elimination half-life 5-7 hr; immediate release peak 2 hr, ext rel peak 8 hr (Gralise); 5-7 hr (Horizant)

INTERACTIONS

Increase: CNS depression—alcohol, sedatives, antihistamines, all other CNS depressants

Decrease: gabapentin levels—antacids, sevelamar, cimetidine

Decrease: effect of—HYDROcodone

Drug/Lab Test

False positive: urinary protein using Ames N-multistix SG

NURSING CONSIDERATIONS

Assess:

• **Seizures:** aura, location, duration, frequency, activity at onset

• **Pain:** location, duration, characteristics if using for chronic pain, migraine

⚠ Mental status: mood, sensorium, affect, behavioral changes, **suicidal thoughts/behaviors;** if mental status changes, notify prescriber

- Eye problems, need for ophthalmic exam before, during, after treatment (slit lamp, funduscopy, tonometry)
- WBC, gabapentin level (therapeutic 5.9-21 mcg/ml, toxic >85 mcg/ml), serum creatinine/BUN, weight
- Drug reaction with eosinophilia and systemic symptoms
- **Seizure precautions:** padded side rails; move objects that may harm patient (Gralise)
- Increased fluids, bulk in diet for constipation

Evaluate:

- Therapeutic response: decreased seizure activity; decrease in chronic pain

Teach patient/family:

- To carry emergency ID stating patient's name, products taken, condition, prescriber's name and phone number
- To avoid driving, other activities that require alertness because dizziness, drowsiness may occur
- Not to discontinue medication quickly after long-term use; to taper over ≥1 wk because withdrawal-precipitated seizures may occur; not to double doses if dose is missed; to take if 2 hr or more before next dose
- To notify prescriber if pregnancy planned or suspected; to avoid breastfeeding
- Not to use within 2 hr of antacid, may take regular release without regard to meals; ext rel should be taken with food; to take as directed, doses interval should not be ≥12 hr
- To take ext rel product with food
- To keep oral solution refrigerated

galantamine (Rx)

(gah-lan′tah-meen)

Razadyne, Razadyne ER, Reminyl ✦

Func. class.: Anti-Alzheimer agent

Chem. class.: Centrally acting cholinesterase inhibitor

ACTION: Enhances cholinergic functioning by increasing acetylcholine in cerebral cortex

USES: Mild to moderate dementia of Alzheimer's disease, dementia with Lewy bodies

Unlabeled uses: Vascular dementia, Pick's disease

CONTRAINDICATIONS: Hypersensitivity to this product, GI bleeding, jaundice, renal failure, children

Precautions: Pregnancy (B), geriatric patients, respiratory/renal/hepatic/cardiac disease, seizure disorder, peptic ulcer, asthma, bradycardia, heart block, surgery, urinary tract obstruction, breastfeeding

DOSAGE AND ROUTES

- **Adult: PO** 4 mg bid with morning and evening meals; after 4 wk or more, may increase to 8 mg bid; may increase to 12 mg bid after another 4 wk, usual dose 16-24 mg/day in 2 divided doses; **EXT REL** 8 mg/day in AM; may increase to 16 mg/day after 4 wk and 24 mg/day after another 4 wk

Hepatic dose

- **Adult: PO** Child-Pugh 7-9, max 16 mg/day; Child-Pugh 10-15, avoid use

Renal dose

- **Adult: PO** CCr 10-70 ml/min, max 16 mg/day; CCr <9 ml/min, avoid use

Available forms: Tabs 4, 8, 12 mg; ext rel caps 8, 16, 24 mg; oral sol 4 mg/ml

Administer:

PO route

- With meals; take with morning and evening meal (immediate rel); morning (ext rel)

• Dose increase after minimum of 4 wk at prior dose; if dose is interrupted for ≥3 days, restart at lower dose, titrate to current dose
• Ext rel in AM with food; do not crush, open, or chew
• **Oral sol:** use pipette provided, put in liquid and have patient consume

SIDE EFFECTS

CNS: *Tremors, insomnia,* depression, dizziness, headache, somnolence, fatigue
CV: **Bradycardia,** chest pain, **AV block**
GI: *Nausea, vomiting, anorexia, abdominal distress, flatulence,* diarrhea
GU: Urinary incontinence, bladder outflow obstruction, hematuria
HEMA: Anemia
META: Weight decrease
MS: Asthenia
RESP: Upper respiratory tract infection, rhinitis

PHARMACOKINETICS

Rapidly and completely absorbed; metabolized by CYP2D6, 3A4; excreted via kidneys; clearance is lower in geriatric patients, hepatic disease; clearance is 20% lower in females; elimination half-life 7 hr; 18% protein binding, peak 1 hr

INTERACTIONS

Increase: synergistic effect—cholinomimetics, other cholinesterase inhibitors
Increase: galantamine effect—CYP3A4, CYP2D6 inhibitors (antiretroviral protease inhibitors, ketoconazole, erythromycin, conivaptan, delaviridine, diltiazem, efavirenz, fluconazole, fluvoxaMINE, imatinib, itraconazole, clarithromycin, troleandomycin, nefazodone, niCARdipine, verapamil, voriconazole, zafirlukast)
Increase: GI effects—NSAIDs
Decrease: galantamine effect—CYP3A4, CYP2D6 inducers (bosentan, carBAMazepine, nevirapine, OXcarbazepine, phenytoin, fosphenytoin/rifabutin, rifampin, rifapentine, troglitazone), anticholinergics
Drug/Herb
Decrease: galantamine effect—St. John's wort

NURSING CONSIDERATIONS

Assess:
Alzheimer's disease: mental status: affect, mood, behavioral changes, depression, attention, confusion; neurologic status: long- and short-term memory, cognitive functioning
• Hepatic/renal studies: AST, ALT, alk phos, LDH, bilirubin, CBC; BUN, creatinine
• For severe GI effects: nausea, vomiting, anorexia, weight loss; GU effects: urinary retardation, bladder obstruction
• B/P, heart rate, respiration during initial treatment: bradycardia/AV block may occur
• Fluid status: ensure adequate hydration
• Assistance with ambulation during beginning therapy
Evaluate:
• Therapeutic response: decreased confusion
Teach patient/family:
• To notify all prescribers of use
• About correct procedure for giving oral sol using instruction sheet provided
• To notify prescriber of severe GI effects; hypo/hypertension, slow heart rate
• That product is not a cure but relieves symptoms
• That results may take several wk or mo to occur
• To take with food to minimize side effects

ganciclovir (Rx)

(gan-sye′kloe-vir)
Cytovene, Vitrasert, Zirgan
Func. class.: Antiviral
Chem. class.: Synthetic nucleoside analog

Do not confuse:
Cytovene/Cytosar

ACTION: Inhibits replication of herpesviruses; competitively inhibits human CMV DNA polymerase and is incorporated, resulting in termination of DNA elongation

USES: Cytomegalovirus (CMV) retinitis in immunocompromised persons, including those with AIDS, after indirect ophthalmoscopy confirms diagnosis; prophylaxis for CMV in transplantation; ophthalmic: acute herpes keratitis

Unlabeled uses: CMV pneumonia in organ transplant patients; CMV gastroenteritis, esophagitis, colitis; CMV pneumonitis, congenital CMV disease; Epstein-Barr virus; herpes simplex types 1, 2; varicella-zoster, hepatitis B

CONTRAINDICATIONS: Hypersensitivity to acyclovir, ganciclovir

Black Box Warning: Absolute neutrophil count <500, platelet count <25,000 (intravitreal)

Precautions: Pregnancy (C), breastfeeding, children <6 mo, geriatric patients, preexisting cytopenias, renal function impairment, radiation therapy, hypersensitivity to famciclovir, penciclovir, valacyclovir, valganciclovir

Black Box Warning: Secondary malignancy, bone marrow suppression, anemia, infertility, neutropenia

DOSAGE AND ROUTES

Prevention of CMV

- **Adult/adolescent: IV** 5 mg/kg/dose over 1 hr q12hr × 1-2 wk, then 5 mg/kg/day 7 day/wk, or 6 mg/kg/day × 5 days/wk; **PO** 1000 mg tid starting 10 days posttransplant × 14 wk

Induction treatment

- **Adult: IV** 5 mg/kg/dose given over 1 hr, q12hr × 2-3 wk

Maintenance treatment

- **Adult: IV INFUSION** 5 mg/kg/dose given over 1 hr, daily × 7 days/wk or 6 mg/kg/day × 5 days/wk; **PO** 1000 mg tid with food or 500 mg q3hr while awake for 6 doses; **INTRAVITREAL** 4.5 mg implant

Acute herpes keratitis

- **Adult/adolescent/child ≥2 yr: OPHTH** 1 drop in affected eye 5 times daily

Renal dose

- **Adult: IV** CCr 50-69 ml/min, reduce to 2.5 mg/kg q12hr (induction), 2.5 mg/kg q24hr (maintenance); **PO** 1500 mg/day or 500 mg tid; **IV** CCr 25-49 ml/min, reduce to 2.5 mg/kg (induction); 1.25 mg/kg q24hr (maintenance); **PO** 1000 mg/day or 500 mg bid; **IV** CCr 10-24 ml/min, reduce to 1.25 mg/kg q24hr (induction); 0.625 mg/kg q24hr (maintenance); **PO** 500 mg/day; **IV** CCr <10 ml/min, reduce to 1.25 mg/kg 3×/wk after hemodialysis (induction); 0.625 mg/kg 3×/wk after hemodialysis (maintenance); **PO** 500 mg 3×/wk after hemodialysis

Available forms: Powder for inj 500 mg/vial; caps 250, 500 mg; implant, intraviteral 4.5 mg; ophth gel 0.15% (Zirgan)

Administer:

PO route

- With food and a full glass of water
- Do not open, crush capsules

Intravitreal implant route

- Implanted by surgeon only
- Handle carefully to prevent damage to coating

Intravitreal inj route (unlabeled)

- Reconstitute and dilute IV powder to 2 mg/0.1 ml or 5 mg/0.1 ml, depending on dose; injected using TB syringe

IV route

- Mixed in biologic cabinet using gown, gloves, mask; use cytotoxic handling procedures

Intermittent IV INFUSION route

- IV after reconstituting 500 mg/10 ml sterile water for inj (50 mg/ml); shake; further dilute in 50-250 ml D_5W, 0.9% NaCl, LR, Ringer's and run over 1 hr; use infusion pump, in-line filter, flush line well before and after product
- Do not give by bolus IV, IM, SUBCUT inj
- Use reconstituted sol within 24 hr; do not refrigerate or freeze

Y-site compatibilities: Allopurinol, amphotericin B cholesteryl, CISplatin, cyclophosphamide, DOXOrubicin liposome, enalaprilat, etoposide, filgrastim, fluconazole, gatifloxacin, granisetron, linezolid, melphalan, methotrexate, PACLitaxel, propofol, remifentanil, tacrolimus, teniposide, thiotepa

SIDE EFFECTS

CNS: *Fever,* chills, coma, *confusion*, abnormal thoughts, dizziness, bizarre dreams, *headache*, psychosis, tremors, somnolence, *paresthesia*, *weakness,* **seizures**, peripheral neuropathy
CV: Dysrhythmia, hypo/hypertension
EENT: Retinal detachment in CMV retinitis, ocular hypertension, ocular pain, conjunctival scarring, cataracts
GI: *Abnormal LFTs, nausea, vomiting, anorexia, diarrhea, abdominal pain,* **hemorrhage, perforation, pancreatitis**
GU: **Hematuria,** *increased creatinine,* BUN, infertility, decreased sperm count
HEMA: **Granulocytopenia, thrombocytopenia, irreversible neutropenia, anemia, eosinophilia, pancytopenia**
INTEG: *Rash*, alopecia, *pruritus*, urticaria, pain at site, phlebitis
RESP: Dyspnea

PHARMACOKINETICS

Half-life 3-4½ hr; excreted by kidneys (unchanged); crosses blood-brain barrier, CSF, increased bioavailability with fatty foods

INTERACTIONS

Increase: severe granulocytopenia—zidovudine, antineoplastics, radiation; do not give together
Increase: ganciclovir toxicity—adriamycin, amphotericin B, cycloSPORINE, dapsone, DOXOrubicin, flucytosine, pentamidine, probenecid, trimethoprim-sulfamethoxazole combinations, vinBLAStine, vinCRIStine, other nucleoside analogs, mycophenolate, tenofovir, tacrolimus, aminoglycosides, NSAIDs
Increase: seizures—imipenem/cilastatin
Increase: didanosine effect—didanosine

Drug/Lab Test
Increase: LFTs, creatinine
Decrease: Hgb, WBC, platelets, neutrophils, granulocytes

NURSING CONSIDERATIONS

Assess:

Black Box Warning: Secondary malignancy: avoid direct contact with powder in caps/solution, if skin contact occurs, wash thoroughly with soap and water; do not get in the eyes

- **CMV retinitis:** culture should be completed before starting treatment (urine, blood, throat), ophthalmic exam
- **Infection:** increased temperature, sore throat, chills, fever; report to prescriber

Black Box Warning: Leukopenia/neutropenia/thrombocytopenia: CBC, WBCs, platelets q2days during 2×/day dosing and then q1wk for leukopenia with daily WBC count in patients with prior leukopenia with other nucleoside analogs or for whom leukopenia counts are <1000 cells/mm^3 at start of treatment

- Serum creatinine or CCr ≥q2wk, BUN; LFTs; ophthalmic exam
- For seizures, dysrhythmias

Evaluate:
- Therapeutic response: decreased symptoms or prevention of CMV

Teach patient/family:
- Do not wear contact lenses while using gel
- That product does not cure condition; that regular blood tests, ophthalmologic exams are necessary
- That major toxicities may necessitate discontinuing product

Black Box Warning: To use contraception during treatment and that infertility may occur; to use barrier contraception for 90 days after treatment; may cause reversible infertility at lower doses, irreversible infertility at higher doses

- To take PO with food

⚠ **To report infection:** fever, chills, sore throat; blood dyscrasias: bruising, bleeding, petechiae; to avoid crowds, persons with respiratory infections

⚠ To report itching, redness or eye pain

ganciclovir ophthalmic

See Appendix B

gatifloxacin

(ga-ti-floks′a-sin)

Zymar, Zymaxid

Func. class.: Ophthalmic antiinfective

Chem. class.: Fluoroquinolone

Do not confuse:
gatifloxacin/levofloxacin/moxifloxacin

ACTION: Inhibits DNA gyrase, thereby decreasing bacterial replication

USES: Bacterial conjunctivitis

CONTRAINDICATIONS: Hypersensitivity to this product or fluoroquinolones, infants <1 yr

Precautions: Pregnancy (C), breastfeeding

DOSAGE AND ROUTES

Bacterial conjunctivitis

- **Adult/adolescent/child ≥1 yr: OPHTH SOL** instill 1 drop (0.5% sol) q2hr while awake

Available forms: Ophthalmic solution 0.5%

Administer:

Ophthalmic route

- Commercially available ophthalmic solutions are not for injection subconjunctivally or into the anterior chamber of the eye
- Apply topically to the eye, taking care to avoid contamination, up to 8×/day × 2 days, then 1 drop up to 4×/day × 5 more days; zymaxid: 1 drop into affected eyes q2hr while awake up to 8×/day, then 1 drop 2-4×/day while awake on days 2-7; do not touch the tip of the dropper to the eye, fingertips, or other surface
- Apply pressure to lacrimal sac for 1 min after instillation
- Avoid wearing contact lenses during treatment

SIDE EFFECTS

EENT: Hypersensitivity, irritation, redness, tearing, keratitis, blepharitis, taste changes, ocular discharge/hemorrhage/irritation/pain

CNS: Headache

GI: Taste change

PHARMACOKINETICS

Unknown

NURSING CONSIDERATIONS

Assess:

- **Allergic reaction**: hypersensitivity, discontinue product

Evaluate:

- Decreased ophthalmic infection

Teach patient/family:

Ophthalmic route

- To apply topically to the eye, taking care to avoid contamination; for ophthalmic use only
- Not to touch the tip of the dropper to the eye, fingertips, or other surface
- To apply pressure to lacrimal sac for 1 min after instillation
- To avoid wearing contact lenses during treatment

⚠ HIGH ALERT

gemcitabine (Rx)

(jem-sit′a-been)

Gemzar

Func. class.: Antineoplastic—miscellaneous

Chem. class.: Pyrimidine analog

Do not confuse:
Gemzar/Zinecard

ACTION: Exhibits antitumor activity by killing cells undergoing DNA synthesis (S phase) and blocking G1/S-phase boundary

USES: Adenocarcinoma of the pancreas (nonresectable stage II, III, or metastatic stage IV); in combination with CISplatin for inoperable, advanced, or metastatic non–small-cell lung cancer;

advanced breast cancer in combination with PACLitaxel; with CARBOplatin for ovarian cancer

Unlabeled uses: Bladder cancer, mesothelioma, adjuvant treatment of pancreatic cancer, ovarian cancer single agent, biliary tract cancer, advanced T-cell lymphoma

CONTRAINDICATIONS:
Pregnancy (D), breastfeeding, hypersensitivity

Precautions: Children, geriatric patients, myelosuppression, radiation therapy, renal/hepatic disease, accidental exposure, alcoholism, dental disease, infection

DOSAGE AND ROUTES

Pancreatic carcinoma (nonresectable stage II, III, IV)

• **Adult:** **IV** 1000 mg/m² given over 30 min/wk up to 7 wk, then 1-wk rest period; subsequent cycles should be infused 1×/wk × 3 wk out of every 4 wk depending on hematologic toxicity

Non–small-cell lung cancer

• **Adult:** **IV** (4-wk schedule) 1000 mg/m² given over 30 min on days 1, 8, 15, of each 28-day cycle; give CISplatin **IV** 100 mg/m² on day 1 after gemcitabine; 3-wk schedule: 1250 mg/m² given over 30 min on days 1, 8 of each 21-day cycle; give CISplatin **IV** 100 mg/m² after the infusion of gemcitabine on day 1

Advanced breast cancer

• **Adult:** **IV** 1250 mg/m² over 30 min on days 1 and 8 of 21-day cycle; give with PACLitaxel 175 mg/m² over 3 hr before gemcitabine on day 1

Recurrent ovarian cancer (single agent) (unlabeled)

• **Adult:** **IV** 1 g/m², days 1, 8, 15 of 28-day cycle

Available forms: Lyophilized powder for inj 20 mg/ml (10-, 50-ml vials); solution for inj 1 g/26.3 ml, 2 g/52.26 ml, 200 mg/2.56 ml

Administer:

IV route

• Prepare in biologic cabinet using gown, mask, gloves; use cytotoxic handling procedures

• After reconstituting with 0.9% NaCl 5 ml/200-mg vial of product or 25 ml/1-g vial of product (38 mg/ml) shake; may be further diluted with 0.9% NaCl to concentrations as low as 0.1 mg/ml; discard unused portions, give over 30 min, do not admix

• Diluted solution stable at room temperature for 24 hr, do not refrigerate

• Infusion longer than 60 min increase toxicity

• **Bone marrow depression:** CBC, differential, platelet count before each dose; single agent: absolute granulocyte count >1000 and platelets >100,000, give complete dose; absolute granulocyte count 500-999, platelets 50,000-99,999, give 75%; absolute granulocyte count <500 or platelets <50,000, do not give; combination with PACLitaxel for breast cancer: absolute granulocyte count >1200 and platelets >75,000, give complete dose; absolute granulocyte count 1000-1199 or platelets 50,000-75,000, give 75%; absolute granulocyte 700-999 or platelets ≥50,000, give 50%; granulocyte count <700 or platelet <50,000, do not give; combination with CARBOplatin for ovarian cancer: absolute granulocyte count >1500 and platelet count >100,000, give complete dose; absolute granulocyte count 1000-1499 or platelets 75,000-99,000, give 75%; absolute granulocyte count <1000 or platelets <75,000, do not give

Y-site compatibilities: Alemtuzumab, alfentanil, allopurinol, amifostine, amikacin, aminophylline, ampicillin, anidulafungin, argatroban, aztreonam, bivalirudin, bleomycin, bumetanide, butorphanol, calcium gluconate, caspofungin, cefOXitin, cefTAZidime, ceftizoxime, cefTRIAXone, chlorproMAZINE, cimetidine, ciprofloxacin, CISplatin, clindamycin, cyclophosphamide, cytarabine, DACTINomycin, DAUNOrubicin, diphenhydrAMINE, DOBUTamine, DOCEtaxel, DOPamine, DOXOrubicin, droperidol, enalaprilat, etoposide, famotidine, floxuridine, fluconazole, fludarabine, fluorouracil, gentamicin, granisetron, haloperidol, heparin, hydrocortisone, HYDROmorphone, IDArubicin, ifosfamide, leucovorin, linezolid, LORazepam, mannitol, meperidine, mesna, metoclopramide, metroNIDAZOLE, minocycline, mitoXANtrone, morphine, nalbuphine, ondansetron, PACLitaxel, promethazine, ranitidine, streptozocin, teniposide, thiotepa, ticarcillin, tigecycline, tobramycin, topotecan, trimethoprim/sulfamethoxazole, vancomycin, vinBLAStine, vinCRIStine, vinorelbine, voriconazole, zidovudine, zoledronic acid

SIDE EFFECTS

ENDO: Hyperglycemia
GI: Diarrhea, *nausea, vomiting,* anorexia, constipation, stomatitis, diarrhea, hepatotoxicity
GU: *Proteinuria,* hematuria
HEMA: Leukopenia, anemia, neutropenia, thrombocytopenia
INTEG: Irritation at site, *rash, alopecia*
META: Hypocalcemia, hypokalemia, hypomagnesemia
RESP: Dyspnea, bronchospasm, pneumonitis
OTHER: *Fever,* hemorrhage, infection, flulike symptoms, paresthesia, *peripheral edema,* myalgia, capillary leak syndrome

PHARMACOKINETICS

Half-life 42-379 min, crosses placenta, excretion: renal, 92%-98%

INTERACTIONS

Increase: bleeding—NSAIDs, alcohol, salicylates, anticoagulants
Increase: myelosuppression, diarrhea—other antineoplastics, radiation
Decrease: antibody response—live virus vaccines

Drug/Lab Test
Increase: BUN, AST, ALT, alk phos, bilirubin, creatinine
Decrease: Hgb, WBC, neutrophils, platelets

NURSING CONSIDERATIONS

Assess:
- **Blood dyscrasias:** bruising, bleeding, petechiae
- I&O, nutritional intake; food preferences: list likes, dislikes
- Renal, hepatic studies before and during treatment; may increase AST, ALT, alk phos, bilirubin, BUN, creatinine, calcium, potassium, glucose, magnesium, urine protein
- Buccal cavity for dryness, sores, ulceration, white patches, oral pain, bleeding, dysphagia
- GI symptoms: frequency of stools, cramping
- Signs of dehydration: rapid respirations, poor skin turgor, decreased urine output, dry skin, restlessness, weakness
- Increased fluid intake to 2-3 L/day to prevent dehydration unless contraindicated
- Rinsing of mouth tid-qid with water, club soda; brushing of teeth bid-tid with soft brush or cotton-tipped applicator for stomatitis; use unwaxed dental floss
- Antiemetic agents
- **Capillary leak syndrome:** hemo-concentration, decreased albumin, B/P; discontinue if these occur

Evaluate:
- Therapeutic response: decrease in tumor size; decrease in spread of cancer; symptom relief

Teach patient/family:
- To avoid foods with citric acid or hot or rough texture if stomatitis is present; to drink adequate fluids; to avoid use with NSAIDs, alcohol, salicylates
- To report stomatitis and any bleeding, white spots, ulcerations in mouth; to examine mouth daily, report symptoms
- To report signs of anemia: fatigue, headache, faintness, SOB, irritability; hematuria, dysuria
- To use contraception during therapy and for 4 mo after; pregnancy (D), do not breastfeed
- Not to receive vaccinations during treatment
- About possible hair loss and what can be done
- To report flulike symptoms, swelling of feet/legs
- To report bruising, bleeding: gums, blood in urine, stool, emesis
- To avoid crowds, persons with known upper-respiratory infections

• To avoid use of hard-bristle toothbrush, electric razor
• Infection: to report sore throat, fever, flulike symptoms immediately

gemfibrozil (Rx)

(jem-fi′broe-zil)

Lopid

Func. class.: Antilipemic

Chem. class.: Fibric acid derivative

Do not confuse:
Lopid/Levbid/Slo-bid

ACTION: Inhibits biosynthesis of VLDL, decreases triglycerides, production in the liver increases HDL

USES: Type IIb, IV, V hyperlipidemia as adjunct with diet therapy, hypertriglyceridemia

CONTRAINDICATIONS: Severe renal/hepatic disease, preexisting gallbladder disease, primary biliary cirrhosis, hypersensitivity

Precautions: Pregnancy (C), breastfeeding, renal disease, cholelithiasis

DOSAGE AND ROUTES

• **Adult: PO** 600 mg bid 30 min before AM, PM meal

Hepatic/renal dose

• Avoid use

Available forms: Tabs 600 mg; caps 300 mg ♣

Administer:

PO route

• 30 min before AM, PM meals
• Discontinue product if response does not occur within 3 mo

SIDE EFFECTS

CNS: Fatigue, vertigo, headache, paresthesia, dizziness, somnolence

GI: *Dyspepsia, diarrhea, abdominal pain,* nausea, vomiting

HEMA: Leukopenia, anemia, eosinophilia, thrombocytopenia

INTEG: Rash, urticaria, pruritus

MISC: Taste perversion

MS: Myopathy, rhabdomyolysis

SYST: Angioedema, exfoliative dermatitis

PHARMACOKINETICS

Peak 1-2 hr; plasma protein binding >95%; half-life $1^1/_2$ hr; 70% excreted in urine mostly unchanged; metabolized in liver (minimal)

INTERACTIONS

• Do not use with repaglinide, simvastatin

Increase: hypoglycemic effect—sulfonylureas, repaglinide

Increase: anticoagulant properties—warfarin

Increase: risk of myositis, myalgia, rhabdomyolysis—HMG-CoA reductase inhibitors

Decrease: effect of gemfibrozil—bile acid sequestrants, separate by >2 hr

Drug/Lab Test

Increase: LFTs, CK, bilirubin, alkaline phosphatase

Decrease: Hgb, Hct, WBC, potassium, eosinophils, platelets

NURSING CONSIDERATIONS

Assess:

• **Hyperlipidemia:** diet history: fats, triglycerides, cholesterol; if lipids increase, product should be discontinued; LDL, VLDL baseline and periodically
• **Myopathy, rhabdomyolysis:** For muscle pain, tenderness; obtain baseline CPK; if elevated or if these occur, product should be discontinued; at greater risk if combined with HMG-Co-A reductase inhibitors
• Renal, hepatic studies, CBC, blood glucose if patient is receiving long-term therapy; if LFTs increase, therapy should be discontinued; monitor hematologic and hepatic functions
• Bowel pattern daily; watch for increasing diarrhea (common)

Evaluate:

• Therapeutic response: decreased cholesterol, triglyceride levels; HDL, cholesterol ratios improved

Teach patient/family:
- That compliance is needed for positive results; not to double or skip dose, take missed dose as soon as remembered unless almost time for next dose
- That risk factors should be decreased: high-fat diet, smoking, alcohol consumption, absence of exercise
- To notify prescriber of diarrhea, nausea, vomiting, chills, fever, sore throat, muscle cramps, abdominal cramps, severe flatulence, tendon pain
- To avoid driving, hazardous activities if dizziness, blurred vision occur

gemifloxacin (Rx)

(gem-ah-flox′a-sin)

Factive

Func. class.: Antiinfective

Chem. class.: Fluoroquinolone

ACTION: Inhibits DNA gyrase, which is an enzyme involved in replication, transcription, and repair of bacterial DNA

USES: Acute bacterial exacerbation of chronic bronchitis caused by *Streptococcus pneumoniae, Haemophilus influenzae, Haemophilus parainfluenzae, Moraxella catarrhalis;* community-acquired pneumonia caused by *Streptococcus pneumoniae* including multiproduct-resistant strains, *H. influenzae, M. catarrhalis, Mycoplasma pneumoniae, Chlamydia pneumoniae, Klebsiella pneumoniae*

CONTRAINDICATIONS: Hypersensitivity to quinolones

Precautions: Pregnancy (C), breastfeeding, children, geriatric patients, hypokalemia, hypomagnesemia, renal disease, seizure disorders, excessive exposure to sunlight, psychosis, increased intracranial pressure, history of QT interval prolongation, dysrhythmias, myasthenia gravis, torsades de pointes

Black Box Warning: Tendon pain/rupture, tendinitis, myasthenia gravis

DOSAGE AND ROUTES
- **Adult: PO** 320 mg/day × 5-7 days depending on type of infection

Renal dose
- **Adult: PO** CCr ≤40 ml/min, 160 mg q24hr

Available forms: Tabs 320 mg

Administer:
- 2 hr before or 3 hr after aluminum/magnesium antacids, iron, zinc products, multivitamins, buffered products 2 hr before sucralfate
- Without regard to food

SIDE EFFECTS
CNS: *Dizziness, headache,* somnolence, depression, insomnia, nervousness, confusion, agitation, seizures, pseudotumor cerebri

CV: QT prolongation, vasodilation

EENT: Visual disturbances, retinal detachment

GI: Diarrhea, *nausea,* vomiting, anorexia, flatulence, heartburn, dry mouth; increased AST, ALT; constipation, abdominal pain, pseudomembranous colitis

INTEG: Rash, pruritus, urticaria, *photosensitivity*

MS: Tendinitis, tendon rupture

SYST: Anaphylaxis, Stevens-Johnson syndrome, toxic epidermal necrolysis, exfoliative dermatitis

PHARMACOKINETICS
Rapidly absorbed; bioavailability 71%; peak ½-2 hr; half-life 4-12 hr; excreted in urine as active product, metabolites

INTERACTIONS
Increase: CNS stimulation—NSAIDs

Increase: toxicity of gemifloxacin—probenecid

⚠ **Increase:** QT prolongation—class IA, III antidysrhythmics, tricyclics, amoxapine, maprotiline, phenothiazines, haloperidol, pimozide, risperiDONE, sertindole, ziprasidone, β-blockers, chloroquine, cloZAPine,

dasatinib, dolasetron, droperidol, dronedarone, flecainide, halogenated/local anesthetics, local anesthetics, lapatinib, methadone, erythromycin, telithromycin, troleandomycin, octreotide, ondansetron, palonosetron, pentamidine, propafenone, ranolazine, SUNItinib, tacrolimus, vardenafil, vorinostat
Decrease: absorption antacids containing aluminum, magnesium, sucralfate, zinc, iron; give 2 hr before or 3 hr after meals

NURSING CONSIDERATIONS

Assess:

- Renal, hepatic studies: BUN, creatinine, AST, ALT; I&O ratio, electrolytes
- CNS symptoms: insomnia, vertigo, headache, agitation, confusion

⚠ **Allergic reactions and anaphylaxis:** rash, flushing, urticaria, pruritus, chills, fever, joint pain; may occur a few days after therapy begins; EPINEPHrine and resuscitation equipment should be available for anaphylactic reaction

- **Pseudomembranous colitis:** bowel pattern daily; if severe diarrhea, fever, abdominal pain occur, product should be discontinued
- **QT prolongation:** avoid use of quinolones in patients with known QT prolongation, females and those with ongoing proarrhythmic conditions (TdP) are at a greater risk; monitor ECG and/or holter monitoring if product is used
- **Overgrowth of infection:** perineal itching, fever, malaise, redness, pain, swelling, drainage, rash, diarrhea, change in cough, sputum

Black Box Warning: **Tendon rupture:** tendon pain, inflammation; if present, discontinue use; more common when used with corticosteroids; discontinue immediately if tendon pain, inflammation occurs

- **Toxic psychosis/pseudotumor cerebri:** headache, blurred vision, neck/shoulder pain, nausea, vomiting, dizziness, tinnitus; discontinue immediately

Evaluate

- Therapeutic response: negative C&S, absence of signs, symptoms of infection

Teach patient/family:

- To take with/without food
- That fluids must be increased to 2 L/day to avoid crystallization in kidneys
- That if dizziness or light-headedness occurs, to perform activities with assistance
- To complete full course of product therapy
- To contact prescriber if adverse reactions occur
- To avoid iron- or mineral-containing supplements or aluminum/magnesium antacids, buffered products within 2 hr before and 3 hr after dosing, 2 hr before sucralfate
- That photosensitivity may occur and sunscreen should be used
- To use frequent rinsing of mouth, sugarless candy or gum for dry mouth
- To avoid other medication unless approved by prescriber

gentamicin (Rx)

Cidomycin ✦
(jen-ta-mye′sin)
Func. class.: Antiinfective
Chem. class.: Aminoglycoside

Do not confuse:
gentamicin/kanamycin

ACTION: Interferes with protein synthesis in bacterial cell by binding to 30S ribosomal subunit, thus causing misreading of genetic code; inaccurate peptide sequence forms in protein chain, thereby causing bacterial death

USES: Severe systemic infections of CNS, respiratory, GI, urinary tract, bone, skin, soft tissues caused by susceptible strains of *Pseudomonas aeruginosa, Proteus, Klebsiella, Serratia, Escherichia coli, Enterobacter, Citrobacter, Staphylococcus, Shigella, Salmonella, Acinetobacter, Bacillus anthracis*

Unlabeled uses: Bartonellosis, bronchiectasis, cystic fibrosis, endocarditis prophylaxis, febrile neutropenia, gonorrhea, granuloma inguinale, PID, plaque, surgical infection prophylaxis, tubo-ovarian abscess, tularemia

CONTRAINDICATIONS:
Hypersensitivity to this product, other aminoglycosides

Black Box Warning: Pregnancy (D)

Precautions: Breastfeeding, neonates, geriatric patients, pseudomembranous colitis

Black Box Warning: Renal disease, hearing deficits, myasthenia gravis, Parkinson's disease, infant botulism, neuromuscular disease, tinnitus

DOSAGE AND ROUTES

Severe systemic infections

- **Adult: IV INFUSION** 3-5 mg/kg/day in divided doses q8hr; **IV** (pulse dosing, once-daily dosing) (unlabeled) 5-7 mg/kg; **IM** 3-5 mg/kg/day in divided doses q8hr
- **Child: IM/IV** 2-2.5 mg/kg q8hr; **IV** (pulse dosing, once-daily dosing) (unlabeled) 5 mg/kg
- **Neonate and infant: IM/IV** 2.5 mg/kg q8-12hr
- **Neonate <1 wk: IV** 2.5 mg/kg q12

Renal dose-Regular dosing

- **Adult: IM/IV** CCr 70-100 ml/min, reduce dose by multiplying maintenance dose by 0.85, give q8-12hr; CCr 50-69 ml/min, reduce as above, give q12hr; CCr 25-49 ml/min, reduce as above, give q24hr; CCr <25 ml/min, reduce as above, give based on serum concentrations, give doses after dialysis

Renal dose: extended interval (unlabeled)

- **Adult: IV** CCr 40-59 ml/min 5-7 mg/kg q36hr; CCr 20-39 ml/min 5-7 mg/kg q48hr; CCr <20 ml/min 5-7 mg/kg once, then base on serial levels

Available forms: Inj 10, 40 mg/ml; premixed inj 40, 60, 70, 80, 90, 100, 120/100 ml NS

Administer:

IM route

- IM inj in large muscle mass; rotate inj sites
- Product in evenly spaced doses to maintain blood level

Intermittent IV INFUSION route

- After diluting in 50-200 ml NS, D_5W; decrease vol of diluent in child; maintain 0.1% sol run over $^1/_2$-1 hr (adults) or up to 2 hr (children); flush IV line with NS, D_5W after administration

Y-site compatibilities: Alatrofloxacin, aldesleukin, alemtuzumab, alfentanil, alprostadil, amifostine, amikacin, aminocaproic acid, aminophylline, amiodarone, amsacrine, anidulafungin, argatroban, arsenic trioxide, ascorbic acid injection, asparaginase, atenolol, atracurium, atropine, aztreonam, benztropine, bivalirudin, bleomycin, bumetanide, buprenorphine, butorphanol, calcium chloride/gluconate, carboplatin, carmustine, caspofungin, cefamandole, ceFAZolin, cefepime, cefotaxime, cefOXitin, cefpirome, ceftaroline, cefTAZidime, ceftizoxime, ceftRIAXone, cefuroxime, chlorothiazide, chlorpheniramine, chlorproMAZINE, cimetidine, ciprofloxacin, cisatracurium, CISplatin, clarithromycin, clindamycin, cloxacillin, codeine, colistimethate, cyanocobalamin, cyclophosphamide, cycloSPORINE, cytarabine, DACTINomycin, DAPTOmycin, DAUNOrubicin citrate liposome, DAUNOrubicin hydrochloride, dexmedetomidine, dexrazoxane, digoxin, diltiazem, dimenhyDRINATE, diphenhydrAMINE, DOBUTamine, DOCEtaxel, dolasetron, DOPamine, doripenem, doxacurium, doxapram, DOXOrubicin hydrochloride, doxorubicin hydrochloride liposomal, doxycycline, edetate calcium disodium, edetate disodium, enalaprilat, ePHEDrine, EPINEPHrine, epirubicin, epoetin alfa, eptifibatide, ergonovine, ertapenem, erythromycin lactobionate, esmolol, etoposide, etoposide phosphate, famotidine, fenoldopam, fentaNYL, fluconazole, fludarabine, fluorouracil, foscarnet, gallamine, gallium, gatifloxacin, gemcitabine, glycopyrrolate, granisetron, HYDROmorphone, hydrOXYzine, ifosfamide, imipenem-cilastatin, irinotecan, isoproterenol, ketamine, ketorolac, labetalol, lactated ringer's injection, lansoprazole, lepirudin, leucovorin, levofloxacin, lidocaine, lincomycin, linezolid, LORazepam, magnesium sulfate, mannitol, mechlorethamine, melphalan, meperidine, mephentermine sulfate, meropenem, mesna, metaraminol, methyldopate, methylPREDNISolone sodium succinate, metoclopramide, metoprolol, metroNIDAZOLE, midazolam, milrinone, minocycline, mitoXANtrone, mivacurium, morphine, multiple vitamins injection, mycophenolate mofetil, nafcillin, nalbuphine, nalorphine, naloxone, netilmicin, niCARdipine, nitroglycerin, nitroprusside, norepinephrine, octreotide, ondansetron, oritavancin, oxaliplatin, oxytocin, PACLitaxel (solvent/surfactant), palonosetron, pamidronate, pancuronium, papaverine, penicillin G potassium/sodium, pentazocine, perphenazine, PHENobarbital, phentolamine, phenylephrine, phytonadione, piperacillin, polymyxin B, posaconazole, potassium acetate/chloride, procainamide, prochlorperazine, prochlorperazine, promazine, promethazine, propranolol, protamine, pyridoxine, quiNIDine gluconate, ranitidine, remifentanil, ringer's injection, riTUXimab, rocuronium, sargramostim, sodium acetate/, bicarbonate/citrate, streptomycin, succinylcholine, SUFentanil, tacrolimus, telavancin, temocillin, teniposide, theophylline, thiamine, thiotepa, ticarcillin, ticarcillin-clavulanate, tigecycline, tirofiban, TNA (3-in-1), tobramycin, tolazoline, topotecan, TPN (2-in-1), trastuzumab, trimetaphan, tubocurarine, urokinase, vancomycin, vasopressin, vecuronium, verapamil, vinBLAStine, vinCRIStine, vinorelbine, vitamin B complex with C, voriconazole, zidovudine, zoledronic acid

SIDE EFFECTS

CNS: Confusion, depression, numbness, tremors, **seizures**, muscle twitching, **neurotoxicity**, dizziness, vertigo, **encephalopathy**, fever, headache, lethargy

CV: Hypo/hypertension, palpitations, edema

EENT: **Ototoxicity**, *deafness*, visual disturbances, tinnitus

GI: *Nausea, vomiting, anorexia;* increased ALT, AST, bilirubin; hepatomegaly, **hepatic necrosis**, splenomegaly

GU: **Oliguria, hematuria, renal damage, azotemia, renal failure, nephrotoxicity,** proteinuria

HEMA: **Agranulocytosis, thrombocytopenia, leukopenia**, eosinophilia, anemia

INTEG: *Rash*, burning, urticaria, dermatitis, alopecia, photosensitivity, **anaphylaxis**

MS: Twitching, myasthenia gravis-like symptoms

RESP: **Apnea**

PHARMACOKINETICS

Not metabolized, excreted unchanged in urine, crosses placental barrier

IM: Onset rapid, peak 30-60 min

IV: Onset immediate; peak 30-90 min; plasma half-life 1-2 hr, infants 6-7 hr; duration 6-8 hr

INTERACTIONS

- **Do not use at the same time or physically mix with penicillins**

Black Box Warning: Increase: ototoxicity, neurotoxicity, nephrotoxicity—other aminoglycosides, amphotericin B, polymyxin, vancomycin, ethacrynic acid, furosemide, mannitol, methoxyflurane, CISplatin, cephalosporins, penicillins, cidofovir, acyclovir, foscarnet, cycloSPORINE, tacrolimus, ganciclovir, zoledronic acid, pamidronate

Increase: effects—nondepolarizing neuromuscular blockers, digoxin, entecavir

Drug/Lab Test

Increase: LDH, AST, ALT, bilirubin, BUN, creatinine, eosinophils

Decrease: Hgb, WBC, platelet, granulocytes

NURSING CONSIDERATIONS

Assess:

Black Box Warning: Neuromuscular disease (myasthenia gravis, Parkinson's disease, infant botulism): paresthesias, tetany, positive Chvostek's/Trousseau's signs, confusion (adults), tetany, muscle weakness (infants); correct electrolyte imbalance

- Weight before treatment; calculation of dosage is usually based on ideal body weight but may be calculated on actual body weight

Black Box Warning: Renal disease: I&O ratio, urinalysis daily for proteinuria, cells, casts; report sudden change in urine output; urine pH if product is used for UTI; urine should be kept alkaline; urine for CCr testing, BUN, serum creatinine; lower dosage should be given with renal impairment (CCr <80 ml/min); toxicity is increased in patients with decreased renal function if high doses are given

- VS during infusion; watch for hypotension, change in pulse
- IV site for thrombophlebitis, including pain, redness, swelling q30min, change site if needed; discontinue, apply warm compresses to site
- Serum peak drawn at 30-60 min after IV infusion or 60 min after IM inj and trough level drawn just before next dose; blood level should be 2-4 times bacteriostatic level; peak (5-10 mcg/ml), trough (0.5-2 mcg/ml), depending on type of infection (based on traditional dosing)

Black Box Warning: Hearing deficits: eighth cranial nerve dysfunction by audiometric testing; also ringing, roaring in ears, vertigo; assess hearing before, during, after treatment

- Dehydration: high specific gravity, decrease in skin turgor, dry mucous membranes, dark urine
- **Overgrowth of infection:** fever, malaise, redness, pain, swelling, perineal itching, diarrhea, stomatitis, change in cough or sputum
- C&S before starting treatment to identify infecting organism
- **Vestibular dysfunction:** nausea, vomiting, dizziness, headache; product should be discontinued if severe
- Inj sites for redness, swelling, abscesses; use warm compresses at site
- Adequate fluids of 2-3 L/day unless contraindicated to prevent irritation of tubules
- Supervised ambulation, other safety measures with vestibular dysfunction

Evaluate:

- Therapeutic response: absence of fever, draining wounds, negative C&S after treatment

Teach patient/family:

- To report headache, dizziness, symptoms of overgrowth of infection, renal impairment

Black Box Warning: To report loss of hearing; ringing, roaring in ears; feeling of fullness in head

- To drink adequate fluids
- To avoid hazardous activities until reaction is known

gentamicin (ophthalmic)

(jen-ta-mye′sin)

Gentak, Garamycin

Func. class.: Ophthalmic antiinfective

Chem. class.: Aminoglycoside

Do not confuse:

clindamycin/tobramycin/erythromycin/vancomycin/GenTeal

ACTION: Inhibits protein synthesis, thereby decreasing bacterial replication

USES: External ocular infections

CONTRAINDICATIONS: Hypersensitivity to this product or aminoglycosides

Precautions: Pregnancy (C), breastfeeding, corneal healing, local redness/irritation

DOSAGE AND ROUTES

Ophthalmic (solution)

- **Adult/adolescent/child ≥1 mo: SOL** 1-2 drops in affected eye(s) every 4 hr while awake × 2 days, then every 4 hr; severe infections ≤2 drops every 1 hr
- **Ointment:** apply a small amount (1/2″) to lower conjunctival sac bid or tid

Available forms: Ophthalmic ointment, ophthalmic solution 0.3%

Administer:

Ophthalmic route

- Commercially available ophthalmic solutions are not for injection subconjunctivally or into the anterior chamber of the eye
- Apply topically to the eye, taking care to avoid contamination
- Do not to touch the tip of the dropper to the eye, fingertips, or other surface
- Apply pressure to lacrimal sac for 1 min after instillation
- To apply the ointment, pull down gently on lower eyelid and apply a thin film of the ointment

SIDE EFFECTS

EENT: Burning, hypersensitivity, stinging, blurred vision, hyperemia, corneal ulcers

PHARMACOKINETICS

Unknown

NURSING CONSIDERATIONS

Assess:

- **Allergic reaction**: hypersensitivity, discontinue product

Evaluate:

- Decreased ophthalmic infection

Teach patient/family:

Ophthalmic route

- To apply topically to the eye, taking care to avoid contamination; for ophthalmic use only
- Not to touch the tip of the dropper to the eye, fingertips, or other surface
- To apply pressure to lacrimal sac for 1 min after instillation
- To apply the ointment by pulling down gently on lower eyelid and applying a thin film of the ointment

gentamicin (topical)

(jen-ta-mye′sin)

Func. class.: Topical antiinfective

Chem. class.: Aminoglycoside

Do not confuse:

gentamicin/clindamycin

ACTION: Antibacterial activity results from inhibition of protein synthesis; bactericidal

USES: Superficial infections

CONTRAINDICATIONS: Hypersensitivity to this product or other aminoglycosides

Precautions: Infections, local sensitivity

DOSAGE AND ROUTES

- **Adult/child >1 yr:** apply to affected areas tid-qid

Available forms: Topical cream, ointment 0.1%

Administer:

- For external use only; do not use skin products near the eyes, nose, or mouth
- Wash hands before and after use; wash affected area and gently pat dry
- **Cream/Ointment:** Apply to the cleansed affected area, massage gently into affected areas

SIDE EFFECTS

INTEG: Rash, irritation, erythema, pruritus

PHARMACOKINETICS

Unknown

NURSING CONSIDERATIONS

Assess:

- **Allergic reaction**: hypersensitivity, product may need to be discontinued
- **Infection**: skin infection

G

Evaluate:
- Decreased skin infection

Teach patient/family:
- To use for external use only; do not use skin products near the eyes, nose, or mouth
- To wash hands before and after use; wash affected area and gently pat dry
- **Cream/Ointment:** to apply to the cleansed affected area and massage gently into affected areas

⚠ HIGH ALERT

glatiramer (Rx)

(glah-tear′a-meer)

Copaxone

Func. class.: Multiple sclerosis agent

Chem.. class.: Biological response modifier

ACTION: Unknown; may modify the immune responses responsible for multiple sclerosis (MS)

USES: Reduction of the frequency of relapses in patients with relapsing or remitting MS after first clinical episode with MRI results consistent with MS

CONTRAINDICATIONS: Hypersensitivity to this product or mannitol, IV use

Precautions: Pregnancy (B), breastfeeding, children <18 yr, immune disorders, renal disease, infection, vaccinations, geriatric patients

DOSAGE AND ROUTES

- 20 mg/ml and 40 mg/ml are not interchangeable
- **Adult: SUBCUT** 20 mg/day (20 mg/ml solution); 40 mg (40 mg/ml solution) 3×/wk, give ≥48 hr apart

Available forms: Inj, premixed 20 mg/ml in single-use syringe

Administer:

SUBCUT route
- Refrigerate, allow to warm for 20 min; visually inspect for particulate or cloudiness, if present discard; prefilled syringe contents is for single use; administer SUBCUT into hip, thigh, arm; discard unused portion
- Use SUBCUT route only; do not give IM or IV, do not expel air bubble in prefilled syringe
- Give 40 mg dose on same 3 days of the week, must be 48 hr apart

SIDE EFFECTS

CNS: *Anxiety, hypertonia, tremor, vertigo,* speech disorder, *agitation,* confusion, flushing

CV: *Migraine, palpitations, syncope, tachycardia, vasodilation,* chest pain, hypertension

EENT: *Ear pain, blurred vision*

GI: *Nausea, vomiting, diarrhea, anorexia, gastroenteritis*

GU: *Urinary urgency, dysmenorrhea, vaginal moniliasis*

HEMA: *Ecchymosis, lymphadenopathy*

INTEG: *Pruritus, rash, sweating, urticaria, erythema,* inj-site reaction

META: Edema, weight gain

MS: *Arthralgia, back pain, neck pain,* increased muscle tone

RESP: *Bronchitis, dyspnea, laryngismus, rhinitis*

PHARMACOKINETICS

May be hydrolyzed locally, may reach regional lymph nodes

INTERACTIONS

- **Increase:** serious infection—denosumab, natalizumab, roflumilast
- **Increase:** toxicity—leflunomide

Avoid use with live virus vaccines

Drug/Herb
- **Decrease:** glatiramer effect—echinacea

NURSING CONSIDERATIONS

Assess:
- CNS symptoms: anxiety, confusion, vertigo
- GI status: diarrhea, vomiting, abdominal pain, gastroenteritis

• Cardiac status: tachycardia, palpitations, vasodilation, chest pain

Evaluate:

• Therapeutic response: decreased symptoms of MS

Teach patient/family:

• With written, detailed instructions about product; provide initial and return demonstrations on inj procedure; give information about use and disposal of product, inj-site reaction (hives, rash, irritation, severe pain, flushing, chest pain)

• To notify prescribers of allergic reactions including itching, trouble breathing; chest pain, dizziness, sweating

• That irregular menses, dysmenorrhea, metrorrhagia, breast pain may occur; to use contraception during treatment

• That if pregnancy is suspected or if nursing to notify prescriber

• Not to change dosing or stop taking product without advice of prescriber

• About **immediate postinjection reaction:** flushing, chest pain, palpitations, anxiety, dyspnea, laryngeal constriction, urticaria; does not usually require treatment, may occur months after beginning treatment

• To take as directed; not to stop product or change schedule; teach on self-injection technique

• That the 20 mg/ml and 40 mg/ml are not interchangeable

⚠ HIGH ALERT

glimepiride (Rx)

(glye-me′pi-ride)

Amaryl

glipiZIDE (Rx)

(glip-i′zide)

Glucotrol, Glucotrol XL

Func. class.: Antidiabetic

Chem. class.: Sulfonylurea (2nd generation)

Do not confuse:
glipiZIDE/Glucotrol/glyBURIDE

ACTION: Causes functioning β cells in pancreas to release insulin, leading to drop in blood glucose levels; may improve insulin binding to insulin receptors or increase the number of insulin receptors with prolonged administration; may also reduce basal hepatic glucose secretion; not effective if patient lacks functioning β cells

USES: Type 2 diabetes mellitus

CONTRAINDICATIONS: Hypersensitivity to sulfonylureas/sulfonamides, type 1 diabetes, diabetic ketoacidosis

Precautions: Pregnancy (C), geriatric patients, cardiac disease, severe renal/hepatic disease, G6PD deficiency

DOSAGE AND ROUTES

Glimepiride

• **Adult: PO** 1-2 mg/day with breakfast, then increase by ≤2 mg/day q1-2wk, max 8 mg/day

• **Geriatric: PO** 1 mg/day; may increase if needed

Renal/Hepatic dose

• **Adult: PO** 1 mg/day with breakfast; may titrate upward as needed

GlipiZIDE

• **Adult: PO** 5 mg initially before breakfast, then increase by 2.5-5 mg after several days to desired response; max 40 mg/day in divided doses; **PO** (XL) 5 mg/day with breakfast, may increase to 10 mg/day, max 20 mg/day

• **Geriatric: PO** 2.5 mg/day; may increase if needed

Hepatic disease

• **Adult: PO** 2.5 mg initially, then increase to desired response; max 40 mg/day in divided doses or 15 mg/dose

Available forms: *Glimepiride:* tabs 1, 2, 4 mg; *glipiZIDE:* tabs, scored 5, 10 mg; ext rel tab (XL) 2.5, 5, 10 mg

Administer:

• Do not break, crush, or chew ext rel tabs; may crush tabs and mix with fluids if unable to swallow whole

• **GlipiZIDE:** product 30 min before meals (regular release); with breakfast (ext rel); **Glimepiride:** with breakfast; if patient is NPO, may need to hold dose to prevent hypoglycemia
• Gradual conversion from other oral hypoglycemics to these products is not needed; insulin ≥20 units/day, convert using 25% reduction in insulin dose every day or every other day
• Store in tight, light-resistant container at room temperature

SIDE EFFECTS

CNS: *Headache, weakness, dizziness, drowsiness,* tinnitus, fatigue, vertigo
ENDO: Hypoglycemia
GI: Hepatotoxicity, cholestatic jaundice, nausea, vomiting, diarrhea, heartburn
HEMA: Leukopenia, thrombocytopenia, agranulocytosis, aplastic anemia; increased AST, ALT, alk phos; pancytopenia, hemolytic anemia
INTEG: Rash, allergic reactions, pruritus, urticaria, eczema, photosensitivity, erythema, allergic vasculitis
SYST: Serious hypersensitivity

PHARMACOKINETICS

PO: Completely absorbed by GI route; **glipiZIDE:** onset 1-1½ hr, peak 2-3 hr, duration 12-24 hr, half-life 2-4 hr; **glimepiride:** peak 2-3 hr, half-life 5 hr; metabolized in liver, excreted in urine, 90%-95% plasma-protein bound

INTERACTIONS

• May mask symptoms of hypoglycemia: β-blockers
Increase: action of digoxin, glycosides, cyclosporine
Increase: hypoglycemic effects—insulin, MAOIs, cimetidine, chloramphenicol, guanethidine, methyldopa, NSAIDs, salicylates, probenecid, androgens, anticoagulants, clofibrate, fenfluramine, fluconazole, gemfibrozil, histamine H_2 antagonists, magnesium salts, phenylbutazone, sulfinpyrazone, sulfonamides, tricyclics, urinary acidifiers, clarithromycin, fibric acid derivatives, voriconazole
Decrease: hypoglycemic effect—thiazide diuretics, rifampin, isoniazid, cholestyramine, diazoxide, hydantoins, urinary alkalinizers, charcoal, corticosteroids, colesevelam
Drug/Herb
Increase: antidiabetic effect—garlic, horse chestnut
Decrease: hypoglycemic effect—green tea
Drug/Lab Test
Increase: AST, ALT, LDH, BUN, creatinine

NURSING CONSIDERATIONS

Assess:
• **Hypo/hyperglycemic reaction** that can occur soon after meals; for severe hypoglycemia give IV $D_{50}W$, then IV dextrose solution
• Blood glucose, A1c levels during treatment to determine diabetes control
⚠ Blood dyscrasias: CBC at baseline and throughout treatment; report decreased blood count
Evaluate:
• Therapeutic response: decrease in polyuria, polydipsia, polyphagia; clear sensorium; absence of dizziness; stable gait; improved serum glucose, A1c
Teach patient/family:
• Not to drink alcohol; about disulfiram reaction (nausea, headache, cramps, flushing, hypoglycemia)
• To report bleeding, bruising, weight gain, edema, SOB, weakness, sore throat, swelling in ankles, rash
• To check for symptoms of cholestatic jaundice: dark urine, pruritus, yellow sclera; prescriber should be notified
• About symptoms of hypo/hyperglycemia, what to do about each; to have glucagon emergency kit available; to carry sugar packets
• That product must be continued on daily basis; about consequences of discontinuing product abruptly; to take product in morning to prevent hypoglycemic reactions at night
• To use sunscreen or stay out of the sun, wear protective clothing (photosensitivity)

- To avoid OTC medications unless ordered by prescriber
- That diabetes is a lifelong illness; product will not cure disease
- That all food in diet plan must be eaten to prevent hypoglycemia; to continue weight control, dietary restrictions, exercise, hygiene
- To carry emergency ID with prescriber and medication information
- To test using blood glucose meter while taking this product
- That ext rel tab may appear in stool

TREATMENT OF OVERDOSE:
Glucose 25 g IV via dextrose 50% sol, 50 ml, 1 mg glucagon, oral carbohydrate depending on severity

glucagon
(gloo′ka-gon)
GlucaGen
Func. class.: Antihypoglycemic

ACTION: Increases in blood glucose, relaxation of smooth muscle of the GI tract, and a positive inotropic and chronotropic effect on the heart; increases in blood glucose are secondary to stimulation of glycogenolysis

USES: Hypoglycemia, used to temporarily inhibit movement of GI tract as a diagnostic test

CONTRAINDICATIONS: Hypersensitivity, pheochromocytoma, insulinoma
Precautions: Pregnancy (B), breastfeeding, cardiac disease, adrenal insufficiency

DOSAGE AND ROUTES
Hypoglycemia in those with diabetes mellitus
- **Adult/adolescent/child ≥55 lb (25 kg): IM/IV/SUBCUT (GlucaGen)** 1 mg (1 IU)
- **Child <55 lb (25 kg) or <6-8 yr: IM/IV/SUBCUT** 0.5 mg (0.5 IU) (Glucagon)
- **Adult/adolescent/child ≥44 lb (20 kg): IM/IV/SUBCUT** (Glucagon) 1 mg (1 IU)
- **Child <44 lb (20 kg):** (Glucagon) 0.5 mg (0.5 IU) or 0.02-0.03 mg/kg (IU/kg) max/mg

Severe hypoglycemia
Neonates: IM/IV/SUBCUT 0.2 mg/kg/dose, max 1 mg/dose; cont infusion (unlabeled): 0.5-1 mg/day

Available forms: Powder for injection 1-mg vial

Administer:
- Visually inspect for particulate matter and discoloration before use

Reconstitution: Reconstitute with 1 ml of sterile water for injection or with diluent supplied by the manufacturer; the reconstituted injection should be clear and of water-like consistency (1 mg/ml); discard any unused portion

IM route
- Inject into a large muscle mass; aspirate before injection to avoid injection into a blood vessel

SUBCUT route
- Inject, taking care not to inject intradermally

IV route
- Inject directly into a vein at a rate ≤1 IU/min (mg/min); may be given through line running D_5W or given at the same time as a bolus of dextrose

SIDE EFFECTS
CNS: Dizziness, headache
CV: Hypotension
GI: Nausea, vomiting
SYST: Hypersensitivity

PHARMACOKINETICS
IV: Onset immediate, peak 30 min, duration 1-1½ hr
IM/SUBCUT: Onset 5-10 min, peak 13-20 min, duration 12-30 min

INTERACTIONS
Increase: bleeding risk—anticoagulants
Decrease: effect of insulin, oral antidiabetics
Increase: B/P and heart rate—β-blockers

NURSING CONSIDERATIONS

Assess:

- **Hypoglycemia:** monitor glucose levels before and after product use; use other products to control hypoglycemia if patient is conscious

Evaluate:

- Decreased hypoglycemia

Teach patient/family:

- How to use this product, symptoms of hypoglycemia, instruct patient in use of oral glucose when hypoglycemia occurs, use this product only when patient is unable to swallow
- Not to use outdated product
- Have all patients carry a sugar source at all times

glucarpidase

(glu-car-pie′dase)

Voraxaze

Func. class.: Recombinant bacterial enzyme

ACTION: A recombinant bacterial enzyme that hydrolyzes glutamate residue from methotrexate and provides an alternate nonrenal pathway for methotrexate elimination in patients with renal dysfunction during high-dose methotrexate treatment; as a result of its enzymatic action, converts methotrexate to its inactive metabolites

USES: The treatment of methotrexate toxicity (methotrexate plasma concentrations >1 μmol/l in those with delayed methotrexate clearance due to impaired renal function

Precautions: Pregnancy (C), breastfeeding

DOSAGE AND ROUTES

- **Adult/adolescent/child: IV** 50 units/kg over 5 min; continue to give leucovorin, IV hydration, urinary alkalinization as needed

Available forms: Sol for IV 1000 units

Administer:

IV direct route

- Visually inspect parenteral products for particulate matter and discoloration before administration
- Reconstitution: add 1 ml of sterile saline for injection to vial, roll and tilt the vial gently to mix; do not shake; flush the IV line, then inject as a bolus inj over 5 min; flush the IV line again
- Do not administer to patients who exhibit the expected clearance of methotrexate (plasma methotrexate concentrations within 2 standard deviations of the mean methotrexate excretion curve specific for the dose of methotrexate administered)
- Do not administer to patients with normal or mildly impaired renal function because of the potential risk of subtherapeutic exposure to methotrexate
- Continue to administer leucovorin after glucarpidase, but do not administer leucovorin within 2 hr before or after glucarpidase; for the first 48 hr after glucarpidase administration, administer the same leucovorin dose as given before glucarpidase; after 48 hr after glucarpidase, administer leucovorin based on the measured methotrexate concentrations; do not discontinue therapy with leucovorin based on the determination of a single methotrexate concentration below the leucovorin treatment threshold; continue leucovorin until the methotrexate concentration has been maintained below the leucovorin treatment threshold for a minimum of 3 days; use of a chromatographic method to determine methotrexate concentration is needed for the first 48 hr after glucarpidase receipt
- Continue hydration and alkalinization of the urine as needed
- Store reconstituted solution refrigerated ≤4 hr; discard any unused product, no preservative is present

SIDE EFFECTS

CNS: Paresthesias, headache

CV: Hypo/hypertension

EENT: Throat irritation or tightness

GI: Nausea, vomiting
INTEG: Flushing, hot, burning sensation; rash, hypersensitivity, serious allergic reactions
SYST: Antibody formation

PHARMACOKINETICS

Elimination half-life of 5.6 hr, methotrexate concentrations reduced 97% within 15 min

INTERACTIONS

Decrease: elucarpidase level—PEMEtrexed, PRALAtrexate; avoid concurrent use

NURSING CONSIDERATIONS

Assess:

- Continue monitoring of methotrexate blood levels, renal status (creatinine/BUN) after glucarpidase is given; methotrexate concentrations within 48 hr of glucarpidase are only reliable measure by a chromatographic method; leucovorin receipt is needed until methotrexate level has been maintained below leucovorin treatment threshold for a minimum of 3 days

Evaluate:

- For resolution of methotrexate toxicity

Teach patient/family:

- To immediately report any infusion-related reactions: fever, chills, flushing, feeling hot, rash, hives, itching, throat tightness or breathing problems, tingling, numbness, or headache

⚠ HIGH ALERT

glyBURIDE (Rx)

(glye′byoor-ide)

DiaBeta, Euglucon ✦, Glynase PresTab

Func. class.: Antidiabetic

Chem. class.: Sulfonylurea (2nd generation)

Do not confuse:
glyBURIDE/Glucotrol/glipiZIDE
DiaBeta/Zebeta

ACTION:
Causes functioning β cells in pancreas to release insulin, thereby leading to a drop in blood glucose levels; may improve insulin binding to insulin receptors and increase number of insulin receptors with prolonged administration; may also reduce basal hepatic glucose secretion; not effective if patient lacks functioning β cells

USES:
Type 2 diabetes mellitus
Unlabeled use: Gestational diabetes not controlled by diet

CONTRAINDICATIONS:
Hypersensitivity to sulfonylureas, type 1 diabetes, diabetic ketoacidosis, renal failure
Precautions: Pregnancy (B) Glynase; (C) DiaBeta, geriatric patients, cardiac/thyroid disease, severe renal/hepatic disease, severe hypoglycemic reactions, sulfonamide/sulfonylurea hypersensitivity, G6PD deficiency

DOSAGE AND ROUTES

DiaBeta (nonmicronized)

- **Adult: PO** 1.25-5 mg initially, then increase to desired response at weekly intervals up to 20 mg/day; may be given as a single or divided dose
- **Geriatric: PO** 1.25 mg initially, then increase to desired response; max 20 mg/day, maintenance 1.25-20 mg/day

Glynase PresTab (micronized)

- **Adult: PO** 1.5-3 mg/day initially, may increase by 1.5 mg/wk, max 12 mg/day
- **Geriatric: PO** 0.75-3 mg/day, may increase by 1.5 mg/wk

Gestational diabetes (unlabeled)

- **Adult (pregnant female): PO** 2.5 mg/day titrated up to 20 mg/day (conventional glyBURIDE)

Available forms: Tabs (DiaBeta) 1.25, 2.5, 5 mg (nonmicronized); (Glynase PresTab) 1.5, 3, 6 mg (micronized)
Administer:

- With breakfast as single or divided dose; hold dose if patient NPO to avoid hypoglycemia; take at same time each day

• Gradual conversion from other oral hypoglycemics to product is not needed; insulin ≥20 units/day; convert using 25% reduction in insulin dose every day
• Micronized glyBURIDE/nonmicronized glyBURIDE are not equivalent
• Store in tight container in cool environment

SIDE EFFECTS

CNS: *Headache, weakness,* paresthesia, tinnitus, fatigue, vertigo
EENT: Blurred vision
ENDO: Hypoglycemia
GI: Nausea, fullness, heartburn, hepatotoxicity, cholestatic jaundice, vomiting, diarrhea, hepatic failure
HEMA: Leukopenia, thrombocytopenia, agranulocytosis, aplastic anemia (rare), increased AST, ALT, alk phos
INTEG: Rash, allergic reactions, pruritus, urticaria, eczema, photosensitivity, erythema
MISC: Angioedema
MS: Joint pain, vasculitis

PHARMACOKINETICS

PO: Completely absorbed by GI route; onset 2 hr; peak 2-4 hr; duration 24 hr; half-life 10 hr; metabolized in liver; excreted in urine, feces (metabolites); crosses placenta; 99% plasma-protein bound

INTERACTIONS

Increase: masking symptoms of hypoglycemia—β-blockers
Increase: level—digoxin
Increase: hypoglycemic effects—insulin, MAOIs, oral anticoagulants, chloramphenicol, guanethidine, methyldopa, NSAIDs, salicylates, probenecid, androgens, fenfluramine, fluconazole, gemfibrozil, histamine H_2 antagonists, magnesium salts, phenylbutazone, sulfinpyrazone, sulfonamides, tricyclics, urinary acidifiers, β-blockers, clarithromycin, voriconazole
Increase: LFTs—bosentan; avoid concurrent use
Increase: triglyceride levels—colesevelam
Increase: action of—cycloSPORINE
Decrease: both products' effects—diazoxide
Decrease: glyBURIDE action—thiazide diuretics, rifampin, isoniazid, cholestyramine, hydantoins, urinary alkalinizers, charcoal, corticosteroids, phenothiazines; oral contraceptives, estrogens, thyroid

Drug/Herb

Increase: antidiabetic effect—garlic, horse chestnut
Decrease: hypoglycemic effect—green tea

Drug/Lab Test

Increase: AST, ALT, LDH, BUN, creatinine, alkaline phosphatase
Decrease: Hgb, sodium, glucose, platelets, WBC

NURSING CONSIDERATIONS

Assess:

• Hypo/hyperglycemic reaction that can occur soon after meals; for severe hypoglycemia, give IV $D_{50}W$, then IV dextrose sol
• Blood glucose; A1c levels during treatment
⚠ **Blood dyscrasias:** CBC at baseline, throughout treatment; report decreased blood counts

Evaluate:

• Therapeutic response: decrease in polyuria, polydipsia, polyphagia; clear sensorium; absence of dizziness; stable gait; improved serum glucose, A1c

Teach patient/family:

• To check for symptoms of cholestatic jaundice: dark urine, pruritus, jaundiced sclera; if these occur, notify prescriber
• To use a blood glucose meter for testing while taking this product
• About the symptoms of hypo/hyperglycemia, what to do about each
• That product must be continued on a daily basis; about consequences of discontinuing product abruptly; that in times of stress, infection, surgery, trauma, a higher dose may be needed
• To take product in morning to prevent hypoglycemic reactions at night if taking once a day
• To avoid OTC medications unless ordered by prescriber

• To report bleeding, bruising, weight gain, edema, shortness of breath, weakness, sore throat
• That diabetes is a lifelong illness; that product will not cure disease
• That all food included in diet plan must be eaten to prevent hypoglycemia; to have glucagon emergency kit, sugar packets always available
• To use sunscreen or stay out of the sun, wear protective clothing (photosensitivity)
• To carry an emergency ID with prescriber and medication information

TREATMENT OF OVERDOSE:
Glucose 25 g IV via dextrose 50% sol, 50 ml, 1 mg glucagon, oral carbohydrate depending on severity

golimumab (Rx)
(goal-lim′yu-mab)

Simponi, Simponi Aria

Func. class.: Antirheumatic agent (disease modifying), immunomodulator

Chem. class.: Monoclonal antibody, DMARD, tumor necrosis factor (TNF-α) modifier

ACTION: Monoclonal antibody specific for human tumor necrosis factor (TNF); elevated levels of TNF are found in patients with rheumatoid arthritis

USES: Rheumatoid arthritis (RA), ankylosing spondylitis, psoriatic arthritis, ulcerative colitis

CONTRAINDICATIONS: Hypersensitivity, active infections

Precautions: Pregnancy (B), breastfeeding, children, geriatric patients, CNS demyelinating disease, Guillain-Barré syndrome, CHF, hepatitis B carriers, blood dyscrasias, surgery, MS, neurologic disease, diabetes, immunosuppression

Black Box Warning: Neoplastic disease, TB; fungal, bacterial, viral infections

DOSAGE AND ROUTES
Rheumatoid arthritis
• **Adult: SUBCUT** 50 mg monthly; for RA, give with methotrexate; IV (Simponi Aria only) 2 mg/kg over 30 min, repeat 4 wk later, then q8wk give with methotrexate

Ankylosing spondylitis/psoriatic arthritis
• **Adult: SUBCUT** 50 mg monthly

Ulcerative colitis:
• **Adult: SUBCUT** 200 mg for 1 dose, then 100 mg in 2 wk, maintenance 100 mg q4wk starting at wk 6

Available form: Inj 50 mg/0.5 ml, 100 mg/ml prefilled syringe, SmartJect Auto Injector; inj 50 mg/4 ml single-use vial

Administer:

SUBCUT route
• Refrigerate, do not freeze; allow to warm to room temperature before using
• Visually inspect sol for particulate or discoloration; sol should be clear to slightly opalescent and colorless to slightly yellow; there may be tiny white particles; do not shake; rotate injection sites
• **SmartJect Auto Injector:** allow to reach room temperature for 30 min before use; remove cap, and inject within 5 min of removing cap; do not put cap back on; place open end against the inj site at a 90-degree angle without pushing button; push the injector firmly against the skin; press the button once and release; listen for the first click; wait for the second click or 15 sec, then remove injector; do not rub site
• **Prefilled syringe:** allow to warm to room temperature for 30 min; remove needle cover by pulling straight off; do not twist or recap; inject within 5 min of needle cover removal; hold syringe in one hand like a pencil and use other hand to pinch the skin; inject needle at a 45-degree angle; push plunger down as far as it will go; keep pressure on plunger head and remove needle from skin; remove pressure from plunger head; needle guard will cover needle; do not rub site

IV route (Simponi Aria)
• Calculate number of vials needed; do not shake; dilute total volume of product in NS to yield 100 ml for infusion; slowly add product, mix gently
• Infuse over 30 min, use infusion set with inline, sterile, nonpyrogenic, low-protein binding filter (≤0.22 mm pore size)

SIDE EFFECTS

CNS: Dizziness, paresthesia, CNS demyelinating disorder, weakness
CV: Hypertension, CHF
GI: Hepatitis
HEMA: Agranulocytosis, aplastic anemia, leukopenia, polycythemia, thrombocytopenia, pancytopenia
INTEG: Psoriasis
MISC: Increased cancer risk, antibody development to this drug; risk for infection (TB, invasive fungal infections, other opportunistic infections), may be fatal, inj-site reactions

PHARMACOKINETICS

Terminal half-life 2 wk

INTERACTIONS

• Do not give concurrently with live vaccines; immunizations should be brought up to date before treatment
• Dosage change may be needed: warfarin, cycloSPORINE, theophylline
Increase: infection—abatacept, etanercept, rilonacept, riTUXimab, adalimumab, anakinra, immunosuppressants, inFLIXimab
Drug/Lab Test
Increase: LFTs
Decrease: platelets, WBC

NURSING CONSIDERATIONS

Assess:
• **Pain,** stiffness, ROM, swelling of joints during treatment
• Inj-site pain, swelling; usually occur after 2 inj (4-5 days)

Black Box Warning: TB: obtain TB skin test before starting treatment, treat latent TB before starting therapy

⚠ **Blood dyscrasias:** CBC, differential before and periodically during treatment

Black Box Warning: Infection: fever, flulike symptoms, dyspnea, change in urination, redness/swelling around any wounds; stop treatment if present; some serious infections including sepsis may occur, may be fatal; patients with active infections should not be started on this product; obtain a chest x-ray, fungal serology, TB testing before starting treatment

• LFTs; hepatitis B serology, may reactivate HBV
• **CHF:** B/P, pulse, edema, SOB
• **Psoriasis:** may occur or worsen

Black Box Warning: Neoplastic disease: may occur in those <18 yr, avoid use in those with known malignancies

Evaluate:
• Therapeutic response: decreased inflammation, pain in joints, decreased joint destruction
Teach patient/family:
• About self-administration if appropriate: inj should be made in thigh, abdomen, upper arm; rotate sites at least 1 inch from old site; do not inject in areas that are bruised, red, hard
• That, if medication not taken when due, to inject next dose as soon as remembered and then the following dose as scheduled
• Not to receive any live virus vaccines during treatment

Black Box Warning: To report signs, symptoms of infection, allergic reaction, or lupuslike syndrome

• To notify prescriber if pregnancy is planned or suspected; not to breastfeed

goserelin (Rx)

(goe′se-rel-lin)

Zoladex

Func. class.: Gonadotropin-releasing hormone, antineoplastic (hormone)

Chem. class.: Synthetic decapeptide analog of LHRH

ACTION: Inhibitor of pituitary gonadotropin secretion; initially increases LH and FSH, with increases in testosterone, reduction in sex steroid levels (substitute serum testosterone levels)

USES: Advanced and locally confined prostate cancer stage B2-C (10.8 mg), endometriosis, advanced breast cancer, endometrial thinning (3.6 mg)

CONTRAINDICATIONS: Hypersensitivity; pregnancy D (breast cancer), X (endometriosis); breastfeeding, children, nondiagnosed vaginal bleeding; hypersensitivity to LHRH, LHRH-agonist analogs; 10.8 mg dose contraindicated in women

Precautions: Spinal cord decompression, renal disease, bone mineral density loss, hyperglycemia, diabetes mellitus, CV disease

DOSAGE AND ROUTES

Breast cancer

- **Adult: SUBCUT** 3.6 mg q28days or 10.8 mg q12wk

Endometrial thinning

- **Adult: SUBCUT** 3.6 mg 1-2 depot inj, (usually 1 depot, surgery performed at 4 wk; if 2 depots, surgery performed 2-4 wk after 2nd depot)

Available forms: Depot inj 3.6, 10.8 mg

Administer:

Depot

- SUBCUT using implant, inserted by qualified person into upper subcutaneous tissue in abdominal wall q28days or q12wk (10.8 mg); do not attempt to remove air bubbles from syringe

SIDE EFFECTS

CNS: *Headaches,* spinal cord compression, *anxiety, depression, dizziness, insomnia, lethargy,* hot flashes, emotional lability

CV: Dysrhythmia, cerebrovascular accident, hypertension, chest pain, CHF; MI, sudden cardiac death, stroke (men), *peripheral edema*

ENDO: Gynecomastia, breast tenderness, breast enlargement, *hot flashes;* hyperglycemia, diabetes (men)

GI: *Nausea,* vomiting, constipation, diarrhea, ulcer

GU: *Spotting, breakthrough bleeding, decreased libido,* renal insufficiency, urinary obstruction, urinary tract infection, *impotence*

INTEG: Rash, pain on inj, diaphoresis

MS: Osteoneuralgia

RESP: COPD, URI

PHARMACOKINETICS

Peak 12-15 days, half-life $4^1/_2$ hr, 30% protein bound

INTERACTIONS

Drug/Lab Test

Increase: alk phos, estradiol, FSH, LH, testosterone levels, triglycerides

Decrease: testosterone levels, progesterone

NURSING CONSIDERATIONS

Assess:

- **Reproductive studies:** pelvic ultrasound, pelvic exam, PSA, serum estradiol/testosterone, pregnancy test before therapy
- I&O ratios; palpate bladder for distention in urinary obstruction
- **Cancer metastases:** for relief of bone pain (back pain), change in motor function
- Blood studies: lipid profile, acid phosphatase; calcium; hypercalcemia may occur

Evaluate:

- Therapeutic response: more normal levels of PSA, acid phosphatase, alk phos; testosterone level of <25 ng/dl; thinning of endometrial lining

Teach patient/family:
- To continue with appointments monthly
- That hyperglycemia may occur in diabetic patients
- That gynecomastia and postmenopausal symptoms may occur but will decrease when treatment is discontinued
- That bone pain may increase then decrease, may use analgesics
- To notify prescriber of difficulty urinating, hot flashes
- Not to breastfeed; to use effective nonhormonal contraception; to notify prescriber if menstrual period continues
- To notify prescriber if chest pain, weakness, difficulty breathing occur, may indicate MI or stroke

granisetron (Rx)
(grane-iss′e-tron)

Granisol, Kytril ✤, Sancuso

Func. class.: Antiemetic

Chem. class.: 5-HT_3 receptor antagonist

ACTION: Prevents nausea, vomiting by blocking serotonin peripherally, centrally, and in the small intestine

USES: Prevention of nausea, vomiting associated with cancer chemotherapy, including high-dose CISplatin, radiation

Unlabeled uses: Acute nausea, vomiting after surgery

CONTRAINDICATIONS: Hypersensitivity to this product, benzyl alcohol

Precautions: Pregnancy (B), breastfeeding, children, geriatric patients, ondansetron/palonosetron/dolasetron hypersensitivity, cardiac dysrhythmias, cardiac/hepatic/GI disease, electrolyte imbalances

DOSAGE AND ROUTES

Nausea, vomiting in chemotherapy
- **Adult and child ≥2 yr: IV** 10 mcg/kg over 5 min, 30 min before the start of cancer chemotherapy; **TD** apply 1 patch (3.1 mg/24 hr) to upper outer arm 24-48 hr before chemotherapy, patch may be worn up to 7 days
- **Adult: PO** 1 mg bid, give 1st dose 1 hr before chemotherapy and next dose 12 hr after 1st or 2 mg as a single dose anytime within 1 hr before chemotherapy

Nausea, vomiting in radiation therapy
- **Adult: PO** 2 mg/day 1 hr before radiation

Available forms: Inj 0.1 mg/ml; tab 1 mg; oral sol 2 mg/10 ml; patch TD 3.1 mg/24 hr

Administer:
- Chemotherapy/radiation: given on day of chemotherapy or radiation

PO route
- Give dose 1 hr before chemotherapy/radiation and another 12 hr after 1st dose

Transdermal
- Apply to clean, dry skin on upper arm q24-48 hr before chemotherapy

Direct IV route
- May give undiluted over 30 sec via Y-site

Intermittent IV INFUSION route
- Dilute in 0.9% NaCl for inj or D_5W (20-50 ml); give over 5-15 min 30 min before chemotherapy
- Store at room temperature for 24 hr after dilution

Solution compatibilities: D_5W, 0.9% NaCl

Y-site compatibilities: Acetaminophen, alemtuzumab, alfentanil, allopurinol, amifostine, amikacin, aminophylline, amphotericin B cholesteryl, ampicillin, ampicillin/sulbactam, amsacrine, aztreonam, bleomycin, bumetanide, buprenorphine, butorphanol, calcium gluconate, CARBOplatin, carmustine, ceFAZolin, cefepime, cefonicid, cefotaxime, cefoTEtan, cefOXitin, cefTAZidime, ceftizoxime, cefTRIAXone, cefuroxime, chlorproMAZINE, cimetidine, ciprofloxacin, CISplatin, cladribine, clindamycin, cyclophosphamide, cytarabine, dacarbazine, DACTINomycin, DAUNOrubicin, dexamethasone, diphenhydrAMINE, DOBUTamine, DOPamine, DOXOrubicin, DOXOrubicin liposome, doxycycline, droperidol, enalaprilat, etoposide, famotidine, filgrastim, fluconazole, fluorouracil, floxuridine, fludarabine, furosemide, gallium, ganciclovir, gentamicin, haloperidol, heparin hydrocortisone, HYDROmorphone, hydrOXYzine, IDArubicin, ifosfamide, imipenem-cilastatin, leucovorin, LORazepam, magnesium sulfate, melphalan, meperidine, mesna, methotrexate, methylPREDNISolone, metoclopramide, metroNIDAZOLE, mezlocillin, miconazole, minocycline, mitoMYcin, mitoXANtrone, morphine, nalbuphine, netilmicin, ofloxacin, PACLitaxel, piperacillin, piperacillin/tazobactam, plicamycin, potassium chloride, prochlorperazine, promethazine, propofol, ranitidine, sargramostim, sodium bicarbonate, streptozocin, teniposide, thiotepa, ticarcillin, ticarcillin/clavulanate, tobramycin, trimethoprim-sulfamethoxazole, vancomycin, vinBLAStine, vinCRIStine, vinorelbine, voriconazole, zidovudine, zoledronic acid

Transdermal route

- Apply to dry, clean, intact skin of upper outer arm 24-48 hr before chemotherapy, firmly press on skin, keep on during chemotherapy; can bathe, avoid swimming, whirlpool; remove ≥24 hr after chemotherapy completion; do not cut patch

SIDE EFFECTS

CNS: *Headache, asthenia,* anxiety, dizziness, EPS (rare)

CV: Hypertension, QT prolongation

GI: Diarrhea, *constipation,* increased AST, ALT, *nausea*

HEMA: Leukopenia, anemia, thrombocytopenia

MISC: Rash, bronchospasm

PHARMACOKINETICS

Metabolized in liver to an active metabolite, half-life 10-12 hr, protein binding 65%

INTERACTIONS

Increase: EPS—antipsychotics

Increase: QT prolongation—amoxapine, arsenic, β-blockers, chloroquine, class IA, III antidysrhythmics, cloZAPine, dasatinib, dolasetron, dronedarone, droperidol, erythromycin, flecainide, fluconazole, halogenated/local anesthetics, haloperidol, lapatinib, maprotiline, methadone, octreotide, ondansetron, palonosetron, pentamidine, phenothiazines, pimozide, posaconazole, propafenone, ranolazine, risperiDONE, sertindole, SUNItinib, tacrolimus, telithromycin, tricyclics, troleandomycin, vardenafil, voriconazole, vorinostat, ziprasidone

NURSING CONSIDERATIONS

Assess:

- For absence of nausea, vomiting during chemotherapy
- **Hypersensitivity reaction:** rash, bronchospasm
- **Extrapyramidal symptoms:** grimacing, shuffling gait, tremors, involuntary movements, rare
- **QT prolongation:** monitor ECG in those with heart disease, renal disease, or the elderly

Evaluate:

- Therapeutic response: absence of nausea, vomiting during cancer chemotherapy

Teach patient/family:

- To report diarrhea, constipation, rash, changes in respirations
- That headache requiring an analgesic is common

guaiFENesin (OTC, Rx)
(gwye-fen′e-sin)

Alfen, Altarussin, Balminil ✦, Benylin Chest Congestion Extra Strength ✦, Benylin E ✦, Bismutal ✦, Bronchophan,Calmylin Expectorant ✦, Cough Syrup Expectorant ✦, Diabetic Tussin, Expectorant ✦, Expectorant Syrup ✦, Guiatuss, Jack & Jill ✦, Miltuss EX, Mucinex, Naldecon Senior EX, Organidin NR, Robitussin Guaifenesin, Scot-Tussin Expectorant, Siltussin DAS, Siltussin SA, Vicks Chest Congestion Relief ✦, Vicks DayQuil Mucus Control ✦

Func. class.: Expectorant

ACTION: Increases the volume and reduces the viscosity of secretions in the trachea and bronchi to facilitate secretion removal

USES: Productive and nonproductive cough

CONTRAINDICATIONS: Hypersensitivity; chronic, persistent cough

Precautions: Pregnancy (C), breastfeeding, CHF, asthma, emphysema, fever

DOSAGE AND ROUTES

• **Adult and adolescent: PO** 200-400 mg q4hr; **EXT REL** 600-1200 mg q12hr, max 2.4 g/day

• **Child 6-11 yr: PO** 100-200 mg q4hr; **EXT REL** 600 mg q12hr, max 1.2 g/day

• **Child 2-5 yr: PO** 50-100 mg q4hr; max 600 mg/day; ext rel 300 mg q12hr, max 600 mg/day

Available forms: Tabs 100, 200, 400 mg; oral sol 100 mg/5 ml; ext rel tabs 600, 1200 mg; syrup 100 mg/5 ml; oral granules 50, 100 mg/packet, Caps 200 mg; liquid 100, 200 mg/5 ml

Administer:

• Do not break, crush, chew ext rel tabs

• Store at room temperature

SIDE EFFECTS

CNS: Drowsiness, headache, dizziness

GI: Nausea, anorexia, vomiting, diarrhea

PHARMACOKINETICS

Half-life 1 hr, excreted in urine (metabolites)

NURSING CONSIDERATIONS

Assess:

• **Cough:** type, frequency, character, including sputum; fluids should be increased to 2 L/day

• Increased fluids, room humidification to liquefy secretions

Evaluate:

• Therapeutic response: productive cough, thinner secretions

Teach patient/family:

• To avoid driving, other hazardous activities if drowsiness occurs (rare)

• To avoid smoking, smoke-filled room, perfumes, dust, environmental pollutants, cleansers

• To consult health provider if cough lasts >7 days

halcinonide topical

See Appendix B

haloperidol (Rx)

(hal-oh-pehr′ih-dol)

haloperidol decanoate (Rx)

Haldol Decanoate

haloperidol lactate (Rx)

Haldol

Func. class.: Antipsychotic, neuroleptic
Chem. class.: Butyrophenone

Do not confuse:
haloperidol/Halotestin

ACTION: Depresses cerebral cortex, hypothalamus, limbic system, which control activity and aggression; blocks neurotransmission produced by DOPamine at synapse; exhibits strong α-adrenergic, anticholinergic blocking action; mechanism for antipsychotic effects unclear

USES: Psychotic disorders, control of tics, vocal utterances in Gilles de la Tourette's syndrome, short-term treatment of hyperactive children showing excessive motor activity, prolonged parenteral therapy in chronic schizophrenia, organic mental syndrome with psychotic features, hiccups (short-term), emergency sedation of severely agitated or delirious patients, ADHD
Unlabeled uses: Nausea, vomiting during chemotherapy; hiccups; autism; migraine

CONTRAINDICATIONS: Hypersensitivity, coma, Parkinson's disease
Precautions: Pregnancy (C), breastfeeding, geriatric patients, seizure disorders, hypertension, pulmonary/cardiac/hepatic disease, QT prolongation, torsades de pointes, prostatic hypertrophy, hyperthyroidism, thyrotoxicosis, children, blood dyscrasias, brain damage, bone marrow depression, alcohol and barbiturate withdrawal states, angina, epilepsy, urinary retention, closed-angle glaucoma, CNS depression

Black Box Warning: Increased mortality in elderly patients with dementia-related psychosis

DOSAGE AND ROUTES

Acute psychosis
- **Adult: IM/IV** (lactate) 2-10 mg, may repeat q1hr, convert to **PO** as soon as possible, **PO** should be 150% of total parenteral dose required
- **Child 6-12 yr: IM/IV** (lactate) (unlabeled) 1-3 mg q4-8hr, max 0.15 mg/kg/day, switch to **PO** as soon as possible

Chronic psychosis
- **Adult: IM** (decanoate) 50-100 mg q4wk, max 100 mg for 1st inj
- **Child 3-12 yr: PO/IM** 0.05-0.15 mg/kg/day

Tourette's syndrome
- **Adult and adolescent: PO** 0.5-2 mg bid-tid, increase until desired response occurs
- **Elderly: PO** 0.5-2 mg bid-tid may increase gradually
- **Child 3-12 yr or weighing 15-40 kg: PO** 0.25-0.5 mg/day in 2-3 divided doses, increase by 0.25-0.5 mg q5-7days, max 0.15 mg/kg/day

Nausea and vomiting related to chemotherapy/surgery (unlabeled)
Adult: PO 1-2 mg q4-6hr

Hiccups (Unlabeled)
Adult: PO 0.5-2 mg bid-tid or **SUBCUT** 5-10 mg/day

Autism (unlabeled)
- **Child: PO** 0.04 mg/kg/day or 1-3 mg/day, max 4 mg/day

Available forms: Tabs 0.5, 1, 2, 5, 10, 20 mg; **lactate:** oral sol 2 mg/ml; inj 5 mg/ml, **decanoate:** 50 mg/ml, 100 mg/ml

Administer:
- Reduced dose to geriatric patients
- Antiparkinsonian agent if EPS occurs

H

• Avoid use with CNS depressants

PO route

• Store in tight, light-resistant container

• **Oral liquid:** use calibrated device; do not mix in coffee or tea

• PO with food or milk

• Avoid skin contact with oral suspension or solution—may cause contact dermatitis

IM route

• IM inj into large muscle mass, use 21-G, 2-in needle; give no more than 3 ml/inj site; patient should remain recumbent for 30 min

IV route (lactate) (unlabeled)

• Give undiluted for psychotic episode at 5 mg/min

• Only use lactate for IV

• Closely monitor ECG for QT prolongation

• Switch to oral as soon as possible if needed, give first PO dose within 12-24 hr of last parenteral dose

Y-site compatibilities: Alcohol 10%, dextrose 5%, alemtuzumab, amifostine, aminocaproic acid, amiodarone, amphotericin B liposome (ambisome), amsacrine, anidulafungin, argatroban, arsenic trioxide, asparaginase, atenolol, azithromycin, bleomycin, cangrelor, CARBOplatin, carmustine, caspofungin, ceftaroline, cisatracurium, CISplatin, cladribine, cloNIDine, codeine phosphate, cyclophosphamide, cytarabine, DACTINomycin, DAPTOmycin, DAUNOrubicin liposome, DAUNOrubicin, dexmedetomidine, dexrazoxane, diltiazem, DOCEtaxel, dolasetron, doxacurium, DOXOrubicin, doxorubicin liposomal, epirubicin, eptifibatide, ertapenem, etoposide, etoposide phosphate, fenoldopam, filgrastim, fludarabine, gatifloxacin, gemcitabine, granisetron, HYDROmorphone, IDArubicin, ifosfamide, irinotecan, ketamine, lepirudin, leucovorin, levofloxacin, linezolid, LORazepam, mechlorethamine, melphalan, mesna, methadone, metroNIDAZOLE, milrinone, mitoXANtrone, mivacurium, morphine, moxifloxacin, mycophenolate mofetil, nesiritide, niCARdipine, octreotide, oritavancin, oxaliplatin, PACLitaxel (solvent/surfactant), palonosetron, pamidronate, pancuronium, PEMEtrexed, potassium acetate, propofol, quinupristin-dalfopristin, remifentanil, riTUXimab, rocuronium, sodium acetate, tacrolimus, teniposide, thiotepa, tigecycline, tirofiban, topotecan, TPN (2-in-1), vecuronium, vinBLAStine, vinCRIStine, vinorelbine, voriconazole, zoledronic acid

SIDE EFFECTS

CNS: *EPS: pseudoparkinsonism, akathisia, dystonia, tardive dyskinesia, drowsiness, headache,* seizures, neuroleptic malignant syndrome, confusion

CV: *Orthostatic hypotension,* hypertension, cardiac arrest, ECG changes, tachycardia, QT prolongation, sudden death, torsades de pointes

EENT: Blurred vision, glaucoma, dry eyes

GI: *Dry mouth, nausea, vomiting, anorexia, constipation,* diarrhea, jaundice, weight gain, ileus, hepatitis

GU: Urinary retention, dysuria, urinary frequency, enuresis, impotence, amenorrhea, gynecomastia

INTEG: *Rash,* photosensitivity, dermatitis

RESP: Laryngospasm, dyspnea, respiratory depression

SYST: Risk for death (dementia)

PHARMACOKINETICS

Metabolized by liver; excreted in urine, bile; crosses placenta; enters breast milk; protein binding 92%; terminal half-life 12-36 hr (metabolites)

PO: Onset erratic, peak 2-6 hr, half-life 24 hr

IM: Onset 15-30 min, peak 15-20 min, half-life 21 hr

IM (Decanoate): Peak 4-11 days, half-life 3 wk

INTERACTIONS

Increase: serotonin syndrome, neuroleptic malignant syndrome—SSRIs, SNRIs

Increase: QT prolongation—class IA, III antidysrhythmics, tricyclics, amoxapine, maprotiline, phenothiazines, pimozide, risperiDONE, sertindole, ziprasidone, β-blockers, chloroquine, cloZAPine, dasatinib, dolasetron, droperidol, dronedarone, flecainide, halogenated/local anesthetics, lapatinib, methadone, erythromycin, telithromycin, troleandomycin, octreotide, ondansetron, palonosetron, pentamidine, propafenone, ranolazine, SUNItinib, tacrolimus, vardenafil, vorinostat, usually with IV use

Increase: oversedation—other CNS depressants, alcohol, barbiturate anesthetics

Increase: toxicity—EPINEPHrine, lithium

Increase: both drugs effects—β-adrenergic blockers, alcohol

Increase: anticholinergic effects—anticholinergics

Decrease: effects—lithium, levodopa

Decrease: haloperidol effects—PHENobarbital, carBAMazepine

Drug/Lab Test

Increase: LFTs

NURSING CONSIDERATIONS

Assess:

- Prolactin, CBC, urinalysis, ophthalmic exam before and during prolonged therapy

Black Box Warning: Dementia, affect, orientation, LOC, reflexes, gait, coordination, sleep pattern disturbances, risk for death in dementia-related psychosis

- B/P standing, lying; take pulse, respirations q4hr during initial treatment; establish baseline before starting treatment; report drops of 30 mm Hg
- Dizziness, faintness, palpitations, tachycardia on rising
- **EPS** including akathisia (inability to sit still, no pattern to movements), tardive dyskinesia (bizarre movements of jaw, mouth, tongue, extremities), pseudoparkinsonism (rigidity, tremors, pill rolling, shuffling gait)

⚠ **Neuroleptic malignant syndrome/serotonin syndrome:** hyperthermia, muscle rigidity, altered mental status, increased CPK, seizures, hypo/hypertension, tachycardia; notify prescriber immediately

- Constipation, urinary retention daily; if these occur, increase bulk, water in diet
- **Abrupt discontinuation:** do not withdraw abruptly, taper
- **QT prolongation:** more common with IV use at high doses; monitor ECG in those with CV disease
- Supervised ambulation until patient stabilized on medication; do not involve patient in strenuous exercise program, fainting is possible; patient should not stand still for long periods
- Sips of water, sugarless candy, gum for dry mouth

Evaluate:

- Therapeutic response: decrease in emotional excitement, hallucinations, delusions, paranoia, reorganization of patterns of thought, speech; improvement in specific behaviors

Teach patient/family:

- That orthostatic hypotension occurs often; to rise from sitting or lying position gradually; to remain lying down after IM inj for at least 30 min
- To avoid hazardous activities until stabilized on medication and effects are known
- To avoid abrupt withdrawal of this product because EPS may result; to withdraw slowly
- To avoid OTC preparations (cough, hay fever, cold) unless approved by prescriber, serious product interactions may occur; to avoid use with alcohol, increased drowsiness may occur
- About EPS and necessity of meticulous oral hygiene because oral candidiasis may occur
- To report impaired vision, jaundice, tremors, muscle twitching

TREATMENT OF OVERDOSE:

Activated charcoal, lavage if orally ingested; provide an airway; do not induce vomiting

⚠ HIGH ALERT

heparin (Rx)

(hep′a-rin)

Hepalean ✱, Heparin Leo ✱, Hep-Lock, Hep-Lock U/P, Monoject Prefill

Func. class.: Anticoagulant, antithrombotic

Do not confuse:
heparin/Hespan

ACTION: Prevents conversion of fibrinogen to fibrin and prothrombin to thrombin by enhancing inhibitory effects of antithrombin III

USES: Prevention treatment of deep venous thrombosis, PE, MI, open heart surgery, disseminated intravascular clotting syndrome, atrial fibrillation with embolization, as an anticoagulant in transfusion and dialysis procedures, to maintain patency of indwelling venipuncture devices; diagnosis, treatment of DIC

CONTRAINDICATIONS: Bleeding, hypersensitivity to this product, corn, porcine protein (pork product)

Precautions: Pregnancy (C), children, geriatric patients, alcoholism, hyperlipidemia, diabetes, renal disease, heparin-induced thrombocytopenia (HIT), hemophilia, leukemia with bleeding, peptic ulcer disease, severe thrombocytopenic purpura, severe renal/hepatic disease, blood dyscrasias, severe hypertension, subacute bacterial endocarditis, acute nephritis; benzyl alcohol products in neonates/infants/pregnancy/lactation

DOSAGE AND ROUTES

Deep venous thrombosis/ pulmonary embolism

- **Adult: IV BOL** 80 international units/kg, then maintenance **IV INFUSION** 18 international units/kg/hr; if aPTT <35 (1.2× normal), increase **IV INFUSION** rate by 4 international units/kg/hr and rebolus with 80 international units/kg; if aPTT 35-45 (1.2-1.5× normal), increase **IV INFUSION** by 2 international units/kg/hr and rebolus with 40 international units/kg; if aPTT 46-70 (1.5-2.3× normal), maintain **IV INFUSION;** if aPTT 71-90 (2.3-3× normal), decrease **IV INFUSION** by 2 international units/kg/hr; if aPTT >90 (>3× normal), hold **IV INFUSION** for 1 hr, then decrease rate 3 international units/kg/hr
- **Child/infant/neonate: IV** loading dose 75 international units/kg
- **Child >1 yr:** 20 international units/kg/hr
- **Infant/neonate <1 yr:** 28 international units/kg/hr as initial maintenance dose

Thrombosis prophylaxis (open heart/CV surgery)

- **Adult: IV** ≥150 international units/kg; procedures <60 min, up to 300 international units/kg; procedures >60 min, up to 400 international units/kg based on ACT

Thrombosis prophylaxis (PCI, not receiving abciximab)

- **Adult: IV BOL** weight adjusted with 60-100 international units/kg, maintain ACT within 250-300 sec (HemoTec) or 300-350 sec (Hemochron)
- **Child/infant/neonate: IV BOL** 100-150 international units/kg

Prophylaxis for DVT/PE

- **Adult: SUBCUT** 5000 units q8-12hr

IV catheter occlusion prophylaxis

- **Adult/child: IV** 10-100 units/ml
- **Infant <10 kg: IV** 10 units/ml

Available forms: Sol for inj 10, 100, 1000, 2000, 5000, 7500, 10,000, 20,000 units/ml; premixed 1000 units/500 ml, 2000 units/1000 ml, 12,500 units/250 ml, 25,000 units/250 ml, 25,000 units/500 ml; lock flush preparations 10 units/ml

Administer:

- Cannot be used interchangeably (unit for unit) with LMWHs or heparinoids
- At same time each day to maintain steady blood levels
- Store at room temperature

Heparin Lock route

⚠ Do not mistake heparin sodium inj 10,000 units/ml and Hep-Lock U/P 10 units/ml; they have similar blue labeling; deaths in pediatric patients have occurred when heparin sodium inj vials were confused with heparin flush vials

SUBCUT route

- Give deeply with 25-G 3/8-1/2-in needle; do not massage area or aspirate when giving SUBCUT inj; give in abdomen between pelvic bones, rotate sites; do not pull back on plunger; leave in for 10 sec; apply gentle pressure for 1 min
- Changing needles is not recommended
- Avoid all IM inj that may cause bleeding, hematoma

Direct IV route

- Give loading dose undiluted, over ≥1 min, use before continuous infusion

Continuous IV INFUSION route

- Dilute 25,000 units/250-500 ml 0.9 NaCl or D_5W, (50-100 units) solutions are premixed and ready for use
- When product is added to infusion sol for cont IV, invert container at least 6 times to ensure adequate mixing

Y-site compatibilities: Acetaminophen, acetylcysteine, acyclovir, alcohol 10%, dextrose 5%, alemtuzumab, alfentanil, allopurinol, amifostine, aminocaproic acid, aminophylline, amphotericin B lipid complex, amphotericin B liposome, anidulafungin, argatroban, arsenic trioxide, ascorbic acid injection, asparaginase, atenolol, atropine, azathioprine, azithromycin, aztreonam, benztropine, betamethasone, bivalirudin, bleomycin, bretylium, bumetanide, buprenorphine, butorphanol, caffeine, calcium chloride/gluconate, cangrelor, CARBOplatin, carmustine, cefamandole, ceFAZolin, cefotaxime, cefoTEtan, cefotiam, cefOXitin, ceftaroline, cefTAZidime, ceftizoxime, ceftobiprole, cefTRIAXone, cefuroxime, chloramphenicol succinate, chlordiazePOXIDE, chlorothiazide, chlorpheniramine, cimetidine, CISplatin, cladribine, clindamycin, cloxacillin, codeine, colistimethate, cyanocobalamin, cyclophosphamide, cycloSPORINE, cytarabine, DACTINomycin, DAPTOmycin, DAUNOrubicin citrate liposome, dexamethasone, dexmedetomidine, dexrazoxane, digoxin, DOCEtaxel, DOPamine, doripenem, doxacurium, doxapram, DOXOrubicin liposomal, edetate calcium disodium, edrophonium, enalaprilat, ePHEDrine sulfate, EPINEPHrine, epoetin alfa, eptifibatide, ergonovine, ertapenem, esmolol, estrogens conjugated, ethacrynate, etoposide, etoposide phosphate, famotidine, fenoldopam, fentaNYL, flecainide, fluconazole, fludarabine, fluorouracil, folic acid (as sodium salt), foscarnet, gallamine, gallium, ganciclovir, gemcitabine, gemtuzumab, glycopyrrolate, granisetron, hydrocortisone, HYDROmorphone, ibuprofen lysine, ifosfamide, imipenem-cilastatin, indomethacin, irinotecan, isoproterenol, ketorolac, lactated ringer's injection, lansoprazole, leucovorin, lidocaine, lincomycin, linezolid, lorazepam, magnesium sulfate, mannitol, mechlorethamine, melphalan, mephentermine, meropenem, mesna, metaraminol, methadone, methohexital, methotrexate, methoxamine, methyldopate, methylergonovine, metoclopramide, metoprolol, metroNIDAZOLE, micafungin, midazolam, milrinone, minocycline, mitoMYcin, mivacurium, morphine, moxifloxacin, multiple vitamins injection, nafcillin, nalbuphine, nalorphine, naloxone, neostigmine, nitroglycerin, nitroprusside, norepinephrine, octreotide, ondansetron, oxacillin, oxaliplatin, oxytocin, PACLitaxel (solvent/surfactant), palonosetron, pamidronate, pancuronium, PEMEtrexed, penicillin G potassium, sodium, PENTobarbital, PHENobarbital s, phentolamine, phenylephrine, phytonadione, piperacillin sodium, piperacillin-tazobactam, potassium acetate/chloride, procainamide, prochlorperazine, promazine, propofol, propranolol, pyridostigmine, pyridoxine, ranitidine, remifentanil, ringer's injection, riTUXimab, rocuronium, sargramostim, scopolamine, sodium acetate, bicarbonate/fusidate, succinylcholine, SUFentanil, tacrolimus, theophylline, thiamine, thiopental, thiotepa, ticarcillin,

ticarcillin-clavulanate, tigecycline, tirofiban, tolazoline, topotecan, TPN (2-in-1), tranexamic, trastuzumab, trimetaphan, trimethobenzamide, tubocurarine, urokinase, vasopressin, vecuronium, verapamil, vinBLAStine, vinCRIStine, voriconazole, warfarin, zidovudine, zoledronic acid

SIDE EFFECTS

CNS: *Fever,* chills, headache
GU: Hematuria
HEMA: Hemorrhage, thrombocytopenia, anemia, HIT
INTEG: *Rash,* dermatitis, urticaria, pruritus, alopecia, hematoma, cutaneous necrosis (SUBCUT), inj-site reactions
META: Hyperkalemia, hypoaldosteronism, hyperlipidemia
SYST: Anaphylaxis

PHARMACOKINETICS

Half-life 1-2 hr (dose dependent); excreted in urine; 95% bound to plasma proteins; does not cross placenta or alter breast milk; removed from the system via the lymph and spleen; partially metabolized in kidney, liver; excreted in urine (<50% unchanged)
SUBCUT: Onset 20-60 min, duration 8-12 hr, well absorbed >35,000 international units/24 hr
IV: Peak 5 min, duration 2-6 hr

INTERACTIONS

Increase: heparin action—oral anticoagulants, salicylates, dextran, NSAIDs, platelet inhibitors, cephalosporins, penicillins, ticlopidine, dipyridamole, antineoplastics, clopidogrel, SSRIs, SNRIs, quinidine, valproic acid
Decrease: heparin action—digoxin, tetracyclines, antihistamines, cardiac glycosides, nicotine, nitroglycerin

Drug/Herb

Increase: bleeding risk—arnica, anise, chamomile, clove, dong quai, garlic, ginger, ginkgo, feverfew, green tea, horse chestnut

Drug/Lab Test

Increase: ALT, AST, INR, PT, PTT, potassium
Decrease: platelets

NURSING CONSIDERATIONS

Assess:

⚠ Bleeding, hemorrhage: gums, petechiae, ecchymosis, black tarry stools, hematuria, epistaxis, decrease in Hct, B/P; HIT may occur after product discontinuation

- Blood studies (Hct, occult blood in stools) q3mo
- Partial prothrombin time, which should be 1.5-2.5× control; for continuous IV infusion, check aPTT baseline 6 hr after initiation and 6 hr after any dose change; use aPTT for dosing adjustments; after therapeutic aPTT has been measured 2×, check aPTT daily
- Platelet count q2-3days; thrombocytopenia may occur on 4th day of treatment
- **Hypersensitivity:** rash, chills, fever, itching; report to prescriber

Evaluate:

- Therapeutic response: prevention of DVT and pulmonary emboli, adequate anticoagulation based on aPTT

Teach patient/family:

- To avoid OTC preparations that may cause serious product interactions unless directed by prescriber, notify all health care persons of heparin use
- That product may be held during active bleeding (menstruation), depending on condition
- To use soft-bristle toothbrush to avoid bleeding gums; to avoid contact sports; to use an electric razor, to avoid IM inj
- To carry emergency ID identifying product taken
- **Bleeding:** To report to prescriber any signs of bleeding: gums, under skin, urine, stools
- To report to prescriber any signs of hypersensitivity: rash, chills, fever, itching

TREATMENT OF OVERDOSE:

Withdraw product, protamine 1 mg protamine/100 units heparin

⚠ Nurse Alert

hepatitis B immune globulin (HBIG) (Rx)

HepaGam B, Hyper HEP B S/D, Nabi-HB

Func. class.: Immune globulin

ACTION: Provides passive immunity to hepatitis B

USES: Prevention of hepatitis B virus in exposed patients, including passive immunity in neonates born to HBsAg-positive mother, prevention of hepatitis B recurrence after liver transplant in HBsAg-positive patients

CONTRAINDICATIONS: Hypersensitivity to immune globulins, coagulation disorders

Precautions: Pregnancy (C), breastfeeding, children, geriatric patients, hemophilia, active infection, IgA deficiency, maltose sensitivity

DOSAGE AND ROUTES

Hepatitis B exposure in those at high risk

- **Adult and child: IM** 0.06 ml/kg (usual 3-5 ml) within 7 days of exposure; repeat 28 days after exposure if patient wishes to not receive hepatitis B vaccine

Neonates born to hepatitis B surface-antigen–positive persons

- **Neonate: IM** 0.5 ml within 12 hr of birth

Prevention of hepatitis B infection recurrence after liver transplant

- **Adult: IV** (HepaGam B only) 20,000 international units concurrent with grafting transplanted liver, then 20,000 international units/day on days 1-7, then 20,000 international units q2wk starting on day 14, then 20,000 international units/mo starting with mo 4

Available forms: Inj 1-, 4-, 5-ml vials; neonatal syringe 0.5 ml; HepaGam B sol for inj 312, 1560 units/ml; Hyper HEP B S/D 217 units/ml

Administer:

IM route

- After rotating vial; do not shake
- Only with EPINEPHrine 1:1000 on unit to treat laryngospasm
- In deltoid for better absorption (adult)

IV route (HepaGam B only)

- Calculate volume needed for each 20,000 international unit dose using measured potency of each lot; HBIG potency stamped on label
- Promptly use after vial entered; discard unused product
- Give at 2 ml/min through separate IV line, use infusion pump, decrease to 1 ml/min if infusion-related event occurs, patient becomes uncomfortable
- Do not use HyperHEP B BS/D or Nabi-HB IV

SIDE EFFECTS

CNS: Headache, dizziness, fever, chills

GI: Nausea, vomiting

INTEG: Soreness at inj site, urticaria, erythema, swelling

SYST: Induration, **anaphylaxis, angioedema**

INTERACTIONS

- Do not use within 3 mo of hepatitis B immune globulin, MMR, varicella, or rotavirus vaccines even after discontinuing product

NURSING CONSIDERATIONS

Assess:

- History of allergies, skin conditions (eczema, psoriasis, dermatitis), reactions to vaccinations
- Skin reactions: rash, induration, urticaria
- ⚠ **Anaphylaxis:** inability to breathe, bronchospasm, hypotension, wheezing, diaphoresis, fever, flushing
- Can be used with hepatitis B vaccine in cases of direct contact
- Written record of immunization

Evaluate:

- Prevention of hepatitis B

Teach patient/family:

- That discomfort may occur at site

• To report any rash, wheezing, inability to breathe immediately
• Do not obtain MMR or varicella within 3 mo of this product

homatropine ophthalmic
See Appendix B

hydrALAZINE (Rx)
(hye-dral'a-zeen)
Apresoline ♣
Func. class.: Antihypertensive, direct-acting peripheral vasodilator
Chem. class.: Phthalazine

Do not confuse:
hydrALAZINE/hydrOXYzine
Apresoline/allopurinol

ACTION: Vasodilates arteriolar smooth muscle by direct relaxation; reduction in blood pressure with reflex increases in heart rate, stroke volume, cardiac output

USES: Essential hypertension; hypertensive emergency/urgency
Unlabeled uses: CHF, preeclampsia

CONTRAINDICATIONS: Hypersensitivity to hydrALAZINEs, mitral valvular rheumatic heart disease, CAD
Precautions: Pregnancy (C), breastfeeding, geriatric patients, CVA, advanced renal disease, hepatic disease, SLE, dissecting aortic aneurysm

DOSAGE AND ROUTES
Hypertension
• **Adult: PO** 10 mg qid 2-4 days, then 25 mg for rest of 1st wk, then 50 mg qid individualized to desired response, max 300 mg/day
• **Child: PO** 0.75-1 mg/kg/day in 2-4 divided doses, max 25 mg/dose, increase over 3-4 wk to max 7.5 mg/kg/day or 200 mg, whichever is less

Hypertensive crisis
• **Adult: IV BOL** 10-20 mg q4-6hr, administer **PO** as soon as possible; **IM** 10-50 mg q4-6hr
• **Child: IV BOL** 0.1-0.6 mg/kg q4hr; **IM** 0.1-0.6 mg/kg q4-6hr, max 1.7-3.5 mg/kg/day

CHF (unlabeled)
• **Adult: PO** 10-25 mg tid, max 100 mg tid

Available forms: Inj 20 mg/ml; tabs 10, 25, 50, 100 mg

Administer:
PO route
• Give with meals (PO) to enhance absorption

IM route
• Do not admix, switch to PO as soon as possible
• No dilution needed, inject deeply in large muscle, aspirate

Direct IV route
• IV undiluted; give through Y-tube or 3-way stopcock, give each 10 mg over ≥1 min
• To recumbent patient, keep recumbent for 1 hr after administration

Y-site compatibilities: Alemtuzumab, anidulafungin, argatroban, atenolol, bivalirudin, bleomycin, DACTINomycin, DAPTOmycin, dexrazoxone, diltiazem, DOCEtaxel, etoposide, fludarabine, gatifloxacin, gemcitabine, granisetron, HYDROmorphone, IDArubicin, irinotecan, leucovorin, linezolid, mechlorethamine, metroNIDAZOLE, milrinone, mitoXANtrone, octreotide, oxaliplatin, PACLitaxel, palonosetron, pancuronium, potassium chloride, tacrolimus, teniposide, thiotepa, tirofiban, vecuronium, vinorelbine, vitamin B/C, voriconazole

SIDE EFFECTS
CNS: *Headache, tremors, dizziness, anxiety,* peripheral neuritis, depression, fever, chills
CV: *Palpitations, reflex tachycardia, angina,* shock, rebound hypertension, orthostatic hypotension
GI: *Nausea, vomiting, anorexia, diarrhea,* constipation, paralytic ileus, hepatotoxicity

GU: Urinary retention, glomerulonephritis, hematuria
HEMA: Leukopenia, agranulocytosis, anemia, thrombocytopenia
INTEG: Rash, pruritus, urticaria
MISC: Nasal congestion, muscle cramps, *lupuslike symptoms,* flushing, edema, dyspnea

PHARMACOKINETICS

Half-life 3-7 hr, metabolized by liver, 12%-14% excreted in urine, protein binding 89%
PO: Onset 20-30 min, peak 1-2 hr, duration 2-4 hr
IM: Onset 10-30 min, peak 1 hr, duration 2-6 hr
IV: Onset 5-30 min, peak 10-80 min, duration up to 12 hr

INTERACTIONS

Increase: severe hypotension—MAOIs
Increase: tachycardia, angina—sympathomimetics (EPINEPHrine, norepinephrine)
Increase: hypotension—other antihypertensives, alcohol, thiazide diuretics
Increase: effects of β-blockers (metoprolol, propranolol)
Decrease: hydrALAZINE effects—NSAIDs, estrogens
Drug/Lab Test
Decrease: Hgb, WBC, RBC, platelets, neutrophils
Positive: ANA titer
Drug/Food
Increase: drug absorption; have patient take with food

NURSING CONSIDERATIONS

Assess:
- **Cardiac status:** B/P q5min × 2 hr, then q1hr × 2 hr, then q4hr; pulse, jugular venous distention q4hr
- Electrolytes, blood studies: potassium, sodium, chloride, carbon dioxide, CBC, serum glucose, LE prep, ANA titer before, during treatment; assess for fever, joint pain, rash, sore throat (lupuslike symptoms); notify prescriber
- Weight daily, I&O
- Edema in feet, legs daily, skin turgor, dryness of mucous membranes for hydration status
- Crackles, dyspnea, orthopnea
- IV site for extravasation, rate
- Mental status: affect, mood, behavior, anxiety; check for personality changes

Evaluate:
- Therapeutic response: decreased B/P

Teach patient/family:
- To take with food to increase bioavailability (PO)
- To avoid OTC preparations unless directed by prescriber
- To notify prescriber if chest pain, severe fatigue, fever, muscle or joint pain occurs
- To rise slowly to prevent orthostatic hypotension
- To notify prescriber if pregnancy is suspected

TREATMENT OF OVERDOSE:

Administer vasopressors, volume expanders for shock; if PO, lavage or give activated charcoal, digitalization

H

hydrochlorothiazide (Rx)

(hye-droe-klor-oh-thye′a-zide)
Apo-Hydro ✦, Neo-Codema ✦, Urozide ✦
Func. class.: Thiazide diuretic, antihypertensive
Chem. class.: Sulfonamide derivative

ACTION: Acts on distal tubule and ascending limb of loop of Henle by increasing excretion of water, sodium, chloride, potassium

USES: Edema, hypertension, diuresis, CHF; idiopathic lower extremity edema therapy
Unlabeled uses: Diabetes insipidus, hypercalciuria, nephrolithiasis, premenstrual syndrome, renal calculus

CONTRAINDICATIONS:
Hypersensitivity to thiazides or sulfonamides, pregnancy (D) preeclampsia, anuria, renal decompensation

Precautions: Pregnancy (B), breastfeeding, hypokalemia, renal/hepatic disease, gout, COPD, LE, diabetes mellitus, hyperlipidemia, CCr <30 ml/min, hypomagnesemia

DOSAGE AND ROUTES

Hypertension:

- **Adult/adolescent: PO** 12.5-25 mg/day, may increase to 50 mg/day in 1-2 divided doses, max 100 mg/day
- **Child >6 mo: PO** 1-2 mg/kg/day in divided doses, max 37.5 mg for 6 mo-2 yr; max 37.5 mg/day
- **Child <6 mo: PO** up to 2-3.3 mg/kg/day in divided doses

Renal dose:

- **Adult: PO** CCr <30 ml/min, do not use; not effective

Available forms: Tabs 12.5, 25, 50 mg; caps 12.5 mg

Administer:

PO route

- In AM to avoid interference with sleep if using product as a diuretic; tab may be crushed, mixed with food
- Potassium replacement if potassium <3 mg/dl, replace magnesium if needed
- With food; if nausea occurs, absorption may be decreased slightly

SIDE EFFECTS

CNS: Drowsiness, paresthesia, depression, headache, *dizziness, fatigue, weakness,* fever

CV: Irregular pulse, *orthostatic hypotension,* palpitations, volume depletion, allergic myocarditis

EENT: Blurred vision

ELECT: *Hypokalemia,* hypercalcemia, hyponatremia, hypochloremia, hypomagnesemia

GI: *Nausea, vomiting, anorexia,* constipation, diarrhea, cramps, pancreatitis, GI irritation, hepatitis, jaundice

GU: *Urinary frequency,* polyuria, uremia, glucosuria, hyperuricemia, renal failure, erectile dysfunction

HEMA: Aplastic anemia, hemolytic anemia, leukopenia, agranulocytosis, thrombocytopenia, neutropenia

INTEG: *Rash,* urticaria, purpura, photosensitivity, alopecia, erythema multiforme

META: *Hyperglycemia, hyperuricemia,* increased creatinine, BUN

SYST: Stevens-Johnson syndrome

PHARMACOKINETICS

PO: Onset 2 hr, peak 4 hr, duration 6-12 hr, half-life 6-15 hr, excreted unchanged by kidneys, crosses placenta, enters breast milk

INTERACTIONS

Increase: hyperglycemia, hyperuricemia, hypotension—diazoxide

Increase: hypokalemia—corticosteroids, amphotericin B, piperacillin, ticarcillin

Increase: toxicity—lithium, non-depolarizing skeletal muscle relaxants, cardiac glycosides

Decrease: thiazide effect—NSAIDs

Increase: effects—loop diuretics

Decrease: antidiabetics effects

Decrease: thiazides absorption—cholestyramine, colestipol

Drug/Food

Increase: severe hypokalemia—licorice

Drug/Lab Test

Increase: parathyroid test, uric acid, calcium, glucose, cholesterol, triglycerides

Decrease: potassium, sodium, Hgb, WBC, platelets

NURSING CONSIDERATIONS

Assess:

- Weight, I&O daily to determine fluid loss; effect of product may be decreased if used daily
- **Hypersensitivity to sulfonamides:** rash, discontinue, fatal Stevens-Johnson syndrome may occur

- **Hypertension:** B/P lying, standing; postural hypotension may occur
- Blood studies: BUN, blood glucose, CBC, serum creatinine, blood pH, ABGs, uric acid, electrolytes
- **Signs of metabolic alkalosis:** drowsiness, restlessness
- **Signs of hypokalemia:** postural hypotension, malaise, fatigue, tachycardia, leg cramps, weakness, dehydration
- Confusion, especially in geriatric patients; take safety precautions if needed

Evaluate:

- Therapeutic response: improvement in edema of feet, legs, sacral area daily, decreased B/P

Teach patient/family:

- To rise slowly from lying or sitting position to prevent postural hypotension
- To notify prescriber of muscle weakness, cramps, nausea, dizziness; hypokalemia is common; rash
- That product may be taken with food or milk
- To use sunscreen for photosensitivity
- That blood glucose may be increased in diabetics
- To take early in day at same time of day to avoid nocturia
- To avoid alcohol, OTC meds unless approved by prescriber
- To monitor weight and report prescriber of changes
- To discuss dietary potassium requirements
- That follow-ups and routine lab tests will be required
- How to take B/P, to continue with other medical regimens (weight loss, exercise)

TREATMENT OF OVERDOSE:

Lavage if taken orally; monitor electrolytes; administer dextrose in saline; monitor hydration, CV, renal status

⚠ HIGH ALERT

HYDROcodone (Rx)

(hye-droe-koe′done)

Hycodan ✦, Robidone ✦

HYDROcodone/acetaminophen (Rx)

Anexsia, Co-Gesic, Dolorex Forte, Duocet, Hycet, Lorcet, Lortab, Norco, Verdrocet, Vicodin, Vicodin ES, Vicodin HP, Xodol, Zydone

HYDROcodone/ibuprofen (Rx)

Ibudone, Reprexain, Vicoprofen, Xylon

Func. class.: Antitussive opioid analgesic/nonopioid analgesic

Controlled Substance Schedule II

Do not confuse:
HYDROcodone/hydrocortisone
Hycodan/Vicodin

ACTION: Acts directly on cough center in medulla to suppress cough; binds to opiate receptors in CNS to reduce pain

USES: Mild to moderate pain

CONTRAINDICATIONS: Acne rosacea/vulgaris, Cushing syndrome, measles, perioral dermatitis, varicella, abrupt discontinuation; hypersensitivity to this product, benzyl

Precautions: Pregnancy (C), breastfeeding, neonates, addictive personality, increased intracranial pressure, MI (acute), severe heart disease, respiratory depression, renal/hepatic disease, bowel impaction, urinary retention, viral infection, ulcerative colitis, seizures, sulfite hypersensitivity, psychosis, hypertension, hyperthyroidism

DOSAGE AND ROUTES

Analgesic

• **Adult: PO** 2.5-10 mg q4-6hr prn, max 60 mg/day

Available forms: ***HYDROcodone:*** bulk powder; ***HYDROcodone/acetaminophen:*** 5 mg HYDROcodone/500 mg acetaminophen (Co-Gesic, Lorcet, Lortab 5/500, Vicodin); 7.5 mg HYDROcodone/400 mg acetaminophen (Zydone), 7.5 mg HYDROcodone/500 mg acetaminophen (Lortab 7.5/500), 7.5 mg HYDROcodone/750 mg acetaminophen (Vicodin ES), 5 mg HYDROcodone/325 acetaminophen, 10 mg HYDROcodone/325 acetaminophen (Norco), 10 mg HYDROcodone/500 mg acetaminophen (Lortab 10/500), 10 mg HYDROcodone/650 mg acetaminophen (Lorcet 10/650, Vicodin HP), 10 mg HYDROcodone/660 acetaminophen (Vicodin HP); caps 5 mg HYDROcodone/500 mg acetaminophen (Stagesic, Zydone); ***HYDROcodone/ibuprofen:*** tabs 7.5 mg HYDROcodone/200 mg ibuprofen (Vicoprofen)

Administer:

Check product carefully before using, fatalities have occurred using wrong dose, wrong product

• Do not break, crush, or chew tabs; only scored tabs can be broken

• With antiemetic after meals if nausea or vomiting occurs

Black Box Warning: Do not exceed 4 g acetaminophen with combination product

• Give with food or milk to prevent gastric upset

• Store in light-resistant area at room temperature

SIDE EFFECTS

CNS: *Drowsiness*, dizziness, light-headedness, confusion, headache, sedation, euphoria, dysphoria, weakness, hallucinations, disorientation, mood changes, dependence, seizures

CV: Palpitations, tachycardia, bradycardia, change in B/P, circulatory depression, syncope, cardiac arrest (children)

EENT: Tinnitus, blurred vision, miosis, diplopia

GI: *Nausea, vomiting, anorexia, constipation*, cramps, dry mouth, ulcers

GU: Increased urinary output, dysuria, urinary retention

INTEG: Rash, urticaria, flushing, pruritus

RESP: Respiratory depression; pulmonary edema, bronchopneumonia, respiratory arrest (children)

PHARMACOKINETICS

Onset 10-20 min, duration 4-6 hr, half-life $3^1/_2$-$4^1/_2$ hr, metabolized in liver, excreted in urine, crosses placenta

INTERACTIONS

Increase: CNS depression—alcohol, opioids, sedative/hypnotics, phenothiazines, skeletal muscle relaxants, general anesthetics, tricyclics

Increase: severe reactions—MAOIs

Drug/Herb

Increase: CNS depression—lavender, valerian

Drug/Lab Test

Increase: amylase, lipase

NURSING CONSIDERATIONS

Assess:

• **Pain:** intensity, type, location, other characteristics before, 1 hr after giving product; titrate upward by 25% until pain reduced by half; need for pain medication, physical dependence; opioid is more effective before pain is severe

• **CNS changes:** dizziness, drowsiness, hallucinations, euphoria, LOC, pupil reaction

• B/P, pulse, respirations before, periodically; if respirations <10/min, dose may need to be reduced, oversedation may occur

• Bowel status: constipation; provide fluids, fiber in diet, may need stimulate laxatives

- **Allergic reactions:** rash, urticaria
- Cough and respiratory dysfunction: respiratory depression, character, rate, rhythm

Evaluate:

- Therapeutic response: decrease in pain or cough

Teach patient/family:

- To report any symptoms of CNS changes, allergic reactions
- That physical dependency may result when used for extended periods
- That withdrawal symptoms may occur: nausea, vomiting, cramps, fever, faintness, anorexia
- To avoid driving, other hazardous activities because drowsiness occurs
- To avoid other CNS depressants; they will enhance sedating properties of this product
- To change positions slowly to reduce orthostatic hypotension
- To notify prescriber if pregnancy is planned or suspected
- For dry mouth, use sugarless gum, frequent sips of water
- To notify prescriber of relief of pain

Black Box Warning: Not to exceed 4000 mg in combination product with acetaminophen, check all other products that may contain acetaminophen

TREATMENT OF OVERDOSE:

Naloxone HCl (Narcan) 0.2-0.8 mg IV, O_2, IV fluids, vasopressors

hydrocortisone (Rx)

(hy-dro-kor′tih-sone)

Cortef, Colocort, Cortenema, Cortifoam

hydrocortisone acetate (Rx)

Anucort, Anusol, Cortifoam, Hemril, Proctocort, Rectasol, Rectasol HC

hydrocortisone sodium succinate (Rx)

A-hydroCort, Solu-CORTEF

Func. class.: Corticosteroid

Chem. class.: Short-acting glucocorticoid

Do not confuse:
hydrocortisone/HYDROcodone

ACTION:
Decreases inflammation by suppression of migration of polymorphonuclear leukocytes, fibroblasts, reversal of increased capillary permeability, and lysosomal stabilization

USES:
Severe inflammation, adrenal insufficiency, ulcerative colitis, collagen disorders, asthma, COPD, SLE, Stevens-Johnson syndrome, ulcerative, TB

Unlabeled uses: Carpal tunnel syndrome, Churg-Strauss syndrome, endophthalmitis, mixed connective-tissue disease, multiple myeloma, polyarteritis nodosa, polychondritis, pulmonary edema, temporal arteritis, Wegener's granulomatosis, septic shock

CONTRAINDICATIONS:
Fungal infection, hypersensitivity

Precautions: Pregnancy (C), breastfeeding, children <2 yr, diabetes mellitus, glaucoma, osteoporosis, seizure disorders, ulcerative colitis, CHF, myasthenia gravis, renal disease, esophagitis, peptic ulcer, metastatic carcinoma, psychosis, idiopathic thrombocytopenia (IM), acute glomerulonephritis, amebiasis, nonasthmatic bronchial disease, AIDS, TB, recent MI (associated with left ventricular rupture), Cushing syndrome, hepatic disease, hypothyroidism, coagulopathy, thromboembolism

DOSAGE AND ROUTES

Adrenal insufficiency/inflammation

- **Adult: PO** 20-240 mg daily; in divided doses **IM/IV** 100-500 mg (succinate), may repeat q2-6hr

Shock prevention

- **Adult: IM/IV** (succinate) 50 mg/kg repeated after 4 hr, repeat q24hr as needed

Colitis

- **Adult: PO** 20-240 mg (base)/day in 2-4 divided doses; **ENEMA** 100 mg nightly for 21 days; susp 2-3×/day × 2 wk; foam 1 applicatorful 1-2×/day × 2-3 wk
- **Child: PO** 2-8 mg (base)/kg/day or 60-240 mg (base)/m^2/day in 3-4 divided doses

Available forms: Hydrocortisone: enema 100 mg/60 ml; tabs 5, 10, 20 mg; **Acetate: rectal aerosol foam:** 10%; **Cypionate:** tabs 5, 10, 20 mg; **Succinate:** injection 100, 250, 500, 1000 mg vial

Administer:

- Daily dose in AM for better results
- In one dose in AM to prevent adrenal suppression; avoid SUBCUT administration, may damage tissue
- Do not use acetate or susp for IV

PO route

- With food or milk for GI symptoms

Rectal route

- Tell patient to retain for 1 hr if possible

IM route

- IM inj deep in large muscle mass; rotate sites; avoid deltoid; use 21-G needle

IV route

- **Succinate:** IV in mix-o-vial or reconstitute ≤250 mg/2 ml bacteriostatic water for inj; mix gently; give direct IV over ≥1 min; may be further diluted in 100, 250, 500, or 1000 ml of D_5W, D_5 0.9%, NaCl 0.9% given over ordered rate

Sodium succinate preparations

Y-site compatibilities: Acyclovir, acetaminophen, alemtuzumab, alfentanil, allopurinol, amifostine, amphotericin B cholesteryl, ampicillin, amrinone, amsacrine, atracurium, atropine, aztreonam, betamethasone, calcium gluconate, cefepime, cefmetazole, cephalothin, chlordiazePOXIDE, chlorproMAZINE, cisatracurium, cladribine, cyanocobalamin, cytarabine, dexamethasone, digoxin, diphenhydrAMINE, DOPamine, DOXOrubicin liposome, droperidol, edrophonium, enalaprilat, EPINEPHrine, esmolol, estrogens conjugated, ethacrynate, famotidine, fentaNYL, fentaNYL/droperidol, filgrastim, fludarabine, fluorouracil, foscarnet, furosemide, gallium, granisetron, heparin, hydrALAZINE, insulin (regular), isoproterenol, kanamycin, lidocaine, LORazepam, magnesium sulfate, melphalan, menadiol, meperidine, methicillin, methoxamine, methylergonovine, minocycline, morphine, neostigmine, norepinephrine, ondansetron, oxacillin, oxytocin, PACLitaxel, pancuronium, penicillin G potassium, pentazocine, phytonadione, piperacillin/tazobactam, prednisoLONE, procainamide, prochlorperazine, propofol, propranolol, pyridostigmine, remifentanil, scopolamine, sodium bicarbonate, succinylcholine, tacrolimus, teniposide, theophylline, thiotepa, trimethaphan, trimethobenzamide, vecuronium, vinorelbine, zoledronic acid

SIDE EFFECTS

CNS: *Depression, flushing, sweating,* headache, mood changes, pseudotumor cerebri, euphoria, insomnia, seizures

CV: *Hypertension,* circulatory collapse, thrombophlebitis, embolism, tachycardia, edema, heart failure

EENT: Fungal infections, increased intraocular pressure, blurred vision, cataracts, glaucoma

GI: *Diarrhea, nausea,* abdominal distention, GI hemorrhage, increased appetite, pancreatitis, vomiting

HEMA: Thrombocytopenia

INTEG: Acne, poor wound healing, ecchymosis, petechiae

MISC: Adrenal insufficiency (after stress/withdrawal)
MS: Fractures, osteoporosis, weakness

PHARMACOKINETICS

Metabolized by liver, excreted in urine (17-OHCS, 17-KS), crosses placenta
PO: Peak 1-2 hr, duration 1-1½ days
IM/IV: Onset 20 min, peak 4-8 hr, duration 1-1½ days
IV: Peak 1-2 hr
RECT: Onset 3-5 hr

INTERACTIONS

Increase: GI bleeding risk—salicylates, NSAIDs, acetaminophen
Increase: side effects—alcohol, amphotericin B, digoxin, cycloSPORINE, diuretics
Increase: neurologic reactions—live virus vaccines/toxoids
Decrease/Increase: anticoagulation—oral anticoagulants
Decrease: hydrocortisone action—bosentan, cholestyramine, colestipol, barbiturates, rifampin, phenytoin, theophylline, carBAMazepine
Decrease: anticoagulant effects, anticonvulsants, antidiabetics, calcium supplements, toxoids, vaccines

Drug/Herb
Decrease: hydrocortisone levels—ephedra

Drug/Lab Test
Increase: cholesterol, sodium, blood glucose, uric acid, calcium, glucose
Decrease: calcium, potassium, T_4, T_3, thyroid ^{131}I uptake test, urine 17-OHCS, 17-KS
False negative: skin allergy tests

NURSING CONSIDERATIONS

Assess:

- Potassium, blood glucose, urine glucose while patient receiving long-term therapy; hypokalemia and hyperglycemia; potassium depletion: paresthesias, fatigue, nausea, vomiting, depression, polyuria, dysrhythmias, weakness
- B/P, pulse; notify prescriber of chest pain
- I&O ratio; be alert for decreasing urinary output, increasing edema; weight daily, notify prescriber of weekly gain >5 lb
- **Adrenal insufficiency (cushingoid symptoms):** nausea, anorexia, SOB, moon face, fatigue, dizziness, weakness, joint pain before and during treatment; plasma cortisol levels during long-term therapy (normal level: 138-635 nmol/L SI units when drawn at 8 AM)
- **Infection:** increased temperature, WBC even after withdrawal of medication; product masks infection
- Mental status: affect, mood, behavioral changes, aggression
- **GI effects:** nausea, vomitting, anorexia or appetite stimulation, diarrhea, constipation, abdominal pain, hiccups, gastritis, pancreatitis, GI bleeding/perforation with long-term treatment

Evaluate:

- Therapeutic response: decreased inflammation, GI symptoms

Teach patient/family:

- That emergency ID as corticosteroid user should be carried
- To immediately report abdominal pain, black tarry stools because GI bleeding/perforation can occur
- To notify prescriber if therapeutic response decreases; that dosage adjustment may be needed; about signs of infection
- Not to discontinue abruptly because adrenal crisis can result; that product should be tapered
- That supplemental calcium/vit D may be needed if patient receiving long-term therapy
- That product can mask infection and cause hypo/hyperglycemia (diabetic)
- To avoid OTC products: salicylates, alcohol in cough products, cold preparations unless directed by prescriber
- About cushingoid symptoms of adrenal insufficiency: nausea, anorexia, fatigue, dizziness, dyspnea, weakness, joint pain, moon face
- To avoid live-virus vaccines if using steroids long term

H

hydrocortisone nasal
See Appendix B

hydrocortisone (topical)
(hye-droe-kor′ti-sone)

Ala-Cort, Ala-Scalp, Anusol HC, Cetacort, Cortizone-5, Cortizone-10, Cortizone-10 Dermolate, Procort, Texacort

hydrocortisone acetate
Anusol HC, Cortaid, Cortef, Corticaine, Cortifoam, ProctoCream-HC, ProctoFoam-HC, Tucks, U-cort

hydrocortisone butyrate
Locoid, Locoid Lipocream

hydrocortisone probutate
Pandel

hydrocortisone valerate
Func. class.: Corticosteroid, topical

ACTION: Crosses cell membrane to attach to receptors to decrease inflammation, itching, inhibits multiple inflammatory cytokines

USES: Inflammation/itching in corticosteroid-responsive dermatoses on the skin, rectal area

CONTRAINDICATIONS: Hypersensitivity

Precautions: Pregnancy (C), breastfeeding, children

DOSAGE AND ROUTES
Corticosteroid-responsive dermatoses, inflammation, pruritus

- **Adult/child: TOP** apply to affected area 1 to 4 times per day

Inflammation from proctitis

- **Adult: Rectal** 1 applicator full of foam once or twice a day × 2-3 wk, then every other day as needed; suppository: 1 bid × 2 wk

Available forms:

Hydrocortisone: cream 0.5%, 1%, 2.5%; gel 1%, 2%; lotion 0.25%, 1%, 2%, 2.5%; ointment 0.5%, 1%, 2.5%; rectal cream 1%; rectal ointment 1%; spray 1%; solution 1%, 2.5%; **Hydrocortisone acetate:** cream 0.5%, 1%, 2%, 2.5%; lotion 0.5%; ointment 0.5%, 1%; rectal foam 90 mg/application; suppositories 25 mg, 30 mg; **Hydrocortisone butyrate:** cream 0.1%; ointment 0.1%; lotion; **Hydrocortisone probutate:** cream 0.1%; **Hydrocortisone valerate:** cream 0.2%, ointment 0.2%

Administer:

Topical route

- May be used with dressings

Cream/Ointment/Lotion

- Apply sparingly in a thin film and rub gently

SIDE EFFECTS
CNS: Seizures, increased intracranial pressure, headache

CV: Hypertension

EENT: Cataracts, glaucoma

INTEG: Burning, folliculitis, pruritus, dermatitis, maceration

MISC: Hyperglycemia; glycosuria, HPA suppression

PHARMACOKINETICS
Unknown, minimally absorbed

NURSING CONSIDERATIONS
Assess:

- Skin reactions: burning, pruritus, folliculitis, dermatitis

Evaluate:

- Decreasing itching, inflammation on the skin, rectal area

Teach patient/family:

Topical route

- That product may be used with dressings

Cream/Ointment/Lotion

- To apply sparingly in a thin film and rub gently into the affected area

Gel

• To apply sparingly in a thin film and rub gently

Rectal

• To remove wrapper and insert suppository

⚠ HIGH ALERT

HYDROmorphone (Rx)

(hye-droe-mor′fone)

Dilaudid, Dilaudid HP, Exalgo, Hydromorph Contin ♣

Func. class.: Opiate analgesic

Chem. class.: Semisynthetic phenanthrene

Controlled Substance Schedule II

Do not confuse:
HYDROmorphone/meperidine/morphine
Dilaudid/Demerol

ACTION: Inhibits ascending pain pathways in CNS, increases pain threshold, alters pain perception

USES: Moderate to severe pain

Unlabeled uses: Arthralgia, bone, dental pain, headache, migraine, myalgia

CONTRAINDICATIONS: Hypersensitivity to this product/sulfite, COPD, cor pulmonale, emphysema, GI obstruction, ileus, increased intracranial pressure, obstetric delivery, status asthmaticus

Black Box Warning: Respiratory depression, opioid-naive patients

Precautions: Pregnancy (C), breastfeeding, children <18 yr, addictive personality, renal/hepatic disease, abrupt discontinuation, adrenal insufficiency, angina, asthma, biliary tract disease, bladder obstruction, hypothyroidism, hypovolemia, hypoxemia, IBD, IV use, lactase/paraben deficiency, labor, latex hypersensitivity, myxedema, seizure disorders, sleep apnea

Black Box Warning: Substance abuse, accidental exposure, potential for overdose/poisoning

DOSAGE AND ROUTES

Analgesic

• **Adult: PO** (oral solution) 2.5-10 mg q3-6hr or (tabs) 2-4 mg q4-6hr; **EXT REL** (Exalgo): convert to **EXT REL** by giving total daily dose of immediate release/day, in 1 daily dose, if needed titrate **EXT REL** q3-4days until adequate pain relief; use 25%-50% increase for each titration step, if more than 2 doses of rescue medication needed in 24 hr consider titration; **IV** 0.2-1 mg q2-3hr given over 2-3 min; **IM/SUBCUT** 1-2 mg q4-6hr prn, may be increased (opioid-naive patients may require lower dose); **RECT** 3 mg q6-8hr prn

• **Geriatric: PO** 1-2 mg q4-6hr

• **Child >50 kg (unlabeled): PO** 2-4 mg q3-4hr in opioid-naive patients, titrate; **IV** 0.2-1 mg q2-4hr or 0.3 mg/kg infusion (opioid-naive will require lower dose)

• **Infant >6 mo/child <50 kg (unlabeled): PO** 0.04-0.08 mg/kg q3-4hr in opioid-naive patients, titrate; **IV** 0.015-0.02 mg/kg q2-4hr or 0.006 mg/kg/hr infusion (opioid-naive)

Hepatic disease

• **Adult: Child-Pugh B, or C** (oral liquid, immediate rel tab, supp) give reduced dose based on response, impairment (parental) give 25%-50% of dose (moderate impairment)

Available forms: Powder for inj 250 mg; inj 1, 2, 4, 10 mg/ml; tabs 2, 4, 8 mg; supp 3 mg; oral sol 5 mg/5 ml; ext rel tab 8, 12, 16, 32 mg

Administer:

PO route

• Give with food or milk for GI irritation

• **Ext rel (Exalgo):** discontinue all other ext rel opioids, give q24hr; do not crush, break, chew

- When pain is beginning to return; determine interval by response
- Store in light-resistant area at room temperature

Black Box Warning: Do not use ext rel products in opioid-naive patients or with other ext rel opioids

Extended release

- **Converting from oral opioids:** conversion ratios are approximate; initiate ext rel tabs at 50% of calculated total daily equivalent dose of ext rel, give q24hr; max increase q3-4days, consider titration increases of 25%-50% with each step
- **Converting from transdermal patch (fentaNYL):** initiate ext rel tabs 18 hr after removal of patch; for each 25 mcg/hr dose of transdermal fentaNYL dose is 12 mg q24hr, start dose at 50% of calculated HYDROmorphone ext rel dose q24hr; titrate no more often than q3-4days, consider dose increases of 25%-50% with each step; if more than 2 rescue doses are required in 24 hr, consider titration

SUBCUT route

- Use short 30-G needle; make sure not to inject ID
- Rotate inj sites

IM route

- Rotate sites

IV route

- **Direct,** diluted with 5 ml sterile water or NS; give through Y-connector or 3-way stopcock; give ≤2 mg over 3-5 min
- **IV INFUSION:** Dilute each 0.1-1 mg/ml NS (0.1-1 mg/ml), deliver by opioid syringe infusor; may be diluted in D_5W, D_5/NaCl, 0.45% NaCl, NS for larger amounts, delivery through infusion pump

Y-site compatibilities: Acyclovir, allopurinol, amifostine, amikacin, amsacrine, aztreonam, cefamandole, cefepime, cefoperazone, cefotaxime, cefOXitin, cefTAZidime, ceftizoxime, cefuroxime, chloramphenicol, cisatracurium, CISplatin, cladribine, clindamycin, cyclophosphamide, cytarabine, diltiazem, DOBUTamine, DOPamine, DOXOrubicin, DOXOrubicin liposome, doxycycline, EPINEPHrine, erythromycin lactobionate, famotidine, fentaNYL, filgrastim, fludarabine, foscarnet, furosemide, gentamicin, granisetron, heparin, kanamycin, labetalol, LORazepam, magnesium sulfate, melphalan, methotrexate, metroNIDAZOLE, midazolam, milrinone, morphine, nafcillin, niCARdipine, nitroglycerin, norepinephrine, ondansetron, oxacillin, PACLitaxel, penicillin G potassium, piperacillin, piperacillin/tazobactam, propofol, ranitidine, remifentanil, teniposide, thiotepa, ticarcillin, tobramycin, trimethoprim-sulfamethoxazole, vancomycin, vecuronium, vinorelbine

SIDE EFFECTS

CNS: *Drowsiness, dizziness, confusion, headache, sedation, euphoria,* mood changes, seizures

CV: Palpitations, bradycardia, change in B/P, hypotension, tachycardia, peripheral vasodilation

EENT: Tinnitus, blurred vision, miosis, diplopia

GI: *Nausea, vomiting, anorexia, constipation, cramps,* dry mouth, paralytic ileus

GU: Increased urinary output, dysuria, urinary retention

INTEG: *Rash,* urticaria, bruising, flushing, diaphoresis, pruritus

RESP: Respiratory depression, dyspnea

PHARMACOKINETICS

IM: Onset 15-30 min, peak ½-1 hr, duration 4-5 hr, metabolized by liver, excreted by kidneys, crosses placenta, excreted in breast milk, half-life 2-3 hr

INTERACTIONS

Increase: effects—other CNS depressants (alcohol, opiates, sedative/hypnotics, antipsychotics, skeletal muscle relaxants)

Increase: CNS, respiratory depression—MAOIs

Decrease: HYDROmorphone effects—opiate antagonists

Drug/Herb
Increase: action—chamomile, hops, kava, lavender, St. John's wort, valerian
Drug/Lab Test
Increase: amylase

NURSING CONSIDERATIONS
Assess:

Black Box Warning: Respiratory dysfunction: respiratory depression, character, rate, rhythm; notify prescriber if respirations <10/min

- I&O ratio; check for decreasing output; may indicate urinary retention
- CNS changes: dizziness, drowsiness, hallucinations, euphoria, LOC, pupil reaction
- Bowel function, constipation
- Allergic reactions: rash, urticaria
- Need for pain medication, physical dependence
- **Pain:** control, sedation by scoring on 0-10 scale, ATC dosing is best for pain control
- Assistance with ambulation
- Safety measures: side rails, night-light, call bell within easy reach

Evaluate:
- Therapeutic response: decrease in pain

Teach patient/family:
- To report any symptoms of CNS changes, allergic reactions
- That physical dependency may result when used for extended periods; that withdrawal symptoms may occur: nausea, vomiting, cramps, fever, faintness, anorexia
- To avoid driving, other hazardous activities because drowsiness occurs

Black Box Warning: That extended release products must be taken whole

TREATMENT OF OVERDOSE:
Naloxone (Narcan) 0.2-0.8 mg IV (nontolerant patients), O_2, IV fluids, vasopressors

hydroxychloroquine (Rx)
(hye-drox-ee-klor′oh-kwin)

Apo-Hydroxyquine ✦, Plaquenil
Func. class.: Antimalarial, antirheumatic (DMARDs)
Chem. class.: 4-Aminoquinoline derivative

ACTION:
Impairs complement-dependent antigen–antibody reactions

USES:
Malaria caused by susceptible strains of *Plasmodium vivax, P. malariae, P. ovale, P. falciparum* (some strains); SLE, rheumatoid arthritis
Unlabeled uses: SLE in children

CONTRAINDICATIONS:
Hypersensitivity to this product or chloroquine; retinal field changes

Black Box Warning: Children (long term), ocular disease

Precautions: Pregnancy (C), breastfeeding, blood dyscrasias, severe GI disease, neurologic disease, alcoholism, hepatic disease, G6PD deficiency, psoriasis, eczema

DOSAGE AND ROUTES
Malaria
- **Adult: PO Suppression or prevention:** 400 mg/wk, begin 1-2 wk before travel, continue 4 wk after returning; **treatment:** 800 mg, then 400 mg after 6-8 hr, then 400 mg/day on 2nd and 3rd day, total dose 2 g
- **Child: PO Suppression or prevention:** 6.4 mg/kg (5 mg/kg base) weekly, begin 1-2 wk before travel, continue 4 wk after returning; **treatment:** 10 mg/kg, 6.4 mg/kg (5 mg/kg base) at 6, 18, 24 hr after 1st dose

Lupus erythematosus
- **Adult: PO** 400 mg (310 mg base) daily-bid; length depends on patient response; **maintenance** 200-400 mg/day

• **Child (unlabeled): PO** 5 mg/kg/day, max 400 mg/day; long-term therapy is contraindicated

Rheumatoid arthritis

• **Adult: PO** 400-600 mg/day for 4-12 wk, then 200-300 mg/day after good response

Available forms: Tabs 200 mg

Administer:

PO route

• Tabs may be crushed and mixed with food, fluids
• With food or milk; at same time each day to maintain product level
• For malaria, prophylaxis should be started 2 wk before exposure, continued for 4-6 wk after leaving exposure area
• Store in tight, light-resistant container at room temperature; keep inj in cool environment

SIDE EFFECTS

CNS: Headache, stimulation, fatigue, irritability, seizures, bad dreams, dizziness, confusion, psychosis, decreased reflexes

CV: Hypotension, heart block, asystole with syncope

EENT: *Blurred vision, corneal changes, retinal changes, difficulty focusing,* tinnitus, vertigo, deafness, photophobia, corneal edema

GI: *Nausea, vomiting, anorexia,* diarrhea, cramps

HEMA: Thrombocytopenia, agranulocytosis, leukopenia, aplastic anemia

INTEG: Pruritus, pigmentation changes, skin eruptions, lichen-planus–like eruptions, eczema, exfoliative dermatitis, alopecia, Stevens-Johnson syndrome, photosensitivity

PHARMACOKINETICS

Peak 3 hr; terminal half-life 32-50 days; metabolized in liver; excreted in urine, feces, breast milk; crosses placenta, protein binding 45%

INTERACTIONS

Increase: digoxin, methotrexate levels
Increase: antibody titer—rabies vaccine
Decrease: hydroxychloroquine action—magnesium or aluminum compounds
Decrease: effect of—live virus vaccines, botulinum toxoids

NURSING CONSIDERATIONS

Assess:

• **SLE, malaria symptoms:** before treatment and daily
• **Rheumatoid arthritis:** pain, swelling, ROM, temperature of joints; for decreased reflexes: knee, ankle
• Ophthalmic exam at baseline and q6mo if long-term treatment or product dosage >150 mg/day
• Hepatic studies weekly: AST, ALT, bilirubin if patient receiving long-term treatment
• **Blood dyscrasias:** blood studies: CBC, platelets; WBC, RBC, platelets may be decreased; if severe, product should be discontinued; assess for malaise, fever, bruising, bleeding (rare)
• **ECG** during therapy: watch for depression of T waves, widening of QRS complex
• **Allergic reactions:** pruritus, rash, urticaria
• **Ototoxicity** (tinnitus, vertigo, change in hearing); audiometric testing should be done before, after treatment

⚠ **For toxicity:** blurring vision, difficulty focusing, headache, dizziness, knee, ankle reflexes; product should be discontinued immediately

Evaluate:

• Therapeutic response: decreased symptoms of malaria, SLE, rheumatoid arthritis

Teach patient/family:

• To use sunglasses in bright sunlight to decrease photophobia; to wear protective clothing (photosensitivity)
• That urine may turn rust or brown; that skin may become blue-black
• To report hearing, visual problems, fever, fatigue, bruising, bleeding, which may indicate blood dyscrasias

TREATMENT OF OVERDOSE:

Induce vomiting; gastric lavage; administer barbiturate (ultrashort acting), vasopressor, ammonium chloride; tracheostomy may be necessary

⚠ HIGH ALERT

hydroxyurea (Rx)

(hye-drox′ee-yoo-ree-ah)

Droxia, Hydrea

Func. class.: Antineoplastic, antimetabolite

Chem. class.: Synthetic urea analog

Do not confuse:
hydroxyurea/hydrOXYzine

ACTION: Acts by inhibiting DNA synthesis without interfering with RNA or protein synthesis; incorporates thymidine into DNA, thereby causing direct damage to DNA strands; specific for S phase of cell cycle

USES: Melanoma, chronic myelogenous leukemia, recurrent or metastatic ovarian cancer, squamous cell carcinoma of the head and neck, sickle cell anemia

Unlabeled uses: Psoriasis, acute myelogenous leukemia (AML), astrocytoma, HIV, lung cancer, malignant glioma, polycythemia vera, thrombocytosis

CONTRAINDICATIONS: Pregnancy (D), breastfeeding, hypersensitivity, leukopenia (<2500/mm^3), thrombocytopenia (<100,000/mm^3), anemia (severe)

Precautions: Renal disease (severe), anemia, bone marrow suppression, dental disease, geriatric patients, HIV, hyperkalemia, hyperphosphatemia, hyperuricemia, hypocalcemia, infection, infertility, IM injection, tumor lysis syndrome, vaccinations

Black Box Warning: Requires an experienced clinician, secondary malignancy

DOSAGE AND ROUTES

Ovarian cancer, malignant melanoma

- **Adult: PO** 80 mg/kg as a single dose q3days or 20-30 mg/kg as a single dose daily

Ovarian cancer in combination with radiation

- **Adult: PO** 80 mg/kg as a single dose q3days

Chronic myelogenous leukemia (CML)/acute myelogenous leukemia (unlabeled)

- **Adult: PO** WBC >100,000/mm^3, 50-75 mg/kg/day; WBC <100,000/mm^3, 10-30 mg/kg/day; adjust for WBCs
- **Child: PO** 10-20 mg/kg/day, adjust to hematologic response

Sickle cell anemia

- **Adult: PO** 15 mg/kg/day, may increase by 5 mg/kg/day q12wk, max 35 mg/kg/day

Renal disease

- **Adult:** CCr <59 ml/min use 50% of dose

Available forms: Caps 200, 300, 400, 500 mg

Administer:

- Gloves should be worn when handling bottles or caps, including by caregivers; wash hands immediately and thoroughly
- Do not crush or chew caps; caps can be opened and contents mixed with water
- Antiemetic 30-60 min before product and prn

SIDE EFFECTS

CNS: Headache, confusion, hallucinations, dizziness, seizures

CV: Angina, ischemia

GI: Nausea, vomiting, anorexia, diarrhea, stomatitis, constipation, hepatotoxicity, pancreatitis

GU: Increased BUN, uric acid, creatinine, temporary renal function impairment

HEMA: Leukopenia, anemia, thrombocytopenia, megaloblastic erythropoiesis

INTEG: *Rash*, urticaria, pruritus, dry skin, facial erythema

H

META: Hyperphosphatemia, hyperuricemia, hypocalcemia
MISC: Fever, chills, malaise, secondary cancers, tumor lysis syndrome
RESP: Pulmonary fibrosis, diffuse pulmonary infiltrates

PHARMACOKINETICS

Readily absorbed when taken orally; peak level in 1-4 hr; degraded in liver; excreted in urine; almost totally eliminated within 24 hr; readily crosses blood-brain barrier; eliminated as CO_2; terminal half-life 3.5-4.5 hr

INTERACTIONS

Increase: pancreatitis/hepatotoxicity—didanosine, stavudine
Increase: toxicity—radiation or other antineoplastics
Increase: bleeding risk—NSAIDs, anticoagulants, thrombolytics, salicylates, platelet inhibitors
Increase: uric acid levels—probenecid, sulfinpyrazone

- Do not use with live virus vaccines
- Do not use hematopoietic progenitor cells (sargramostim, filgrastim) 24 hr before or after antineoplastic

Drug/Lab Test
Increase: BUN, creatinine, LFTs, uric acid
False increase: urea, uric acid, lactic acid
Decrease: Hgb, WBC, platelets, phosphate, calcium

NURSING CONSIDERATIONS

Assess:

- **Bone marrow suppression:** determine the hemoglobin concentrations, total leukocyte count, and platelet count at least once a week during entire course; if the WBC is ≤2500/mm^3 or platelets are ≤100,000/mm^3, interrupt Hydrea until the values rise significantly toward normal concentrations; if severe anemia occurs, manage it without interrupting Hydrea receipt; for Droxia, monitor blood counts q2wk and interrupt drug receipt if neutrophils are <2000/mm^3, platelets are <80,000/mm^3, hemoglobin is <4.5 g/dl, or reticulocytes are <80,000/mm^3 when the hemoglobin concentration is <9 g/dl; after recovery, Droxia may be resumed at lower dosage; Droxia therapy requires an experienced clinician knowledgeable in the use of this medication for the treatment of sickle cell anemia
- Renal studies: BUN, serum uric acid, urine CCr, electrolytes before, during therapy
- **Tumor lysis syndrome;** hyperkalemia, hyperphosphatemia, hyperuricemia, hypocalcemia; uric acid nephropathy, acute renal failure, metabolic acidosis can also occur; aggressive alkalinization of urine, allopurinol can prevent this
- I&O ratio; report fall in urine output to <30 ml/hr
- Monitor temperature; fever may indicate beginning infection
- Hepatic studies before, during therapy: bilirubin, alk phos, AST, ALT, LDH; prn or monthly, pancreatitis may also occur
- **Cutaneous vasculitic toxicity and gangrene:** more common in those who are receiving interferon
- **Bleeding:** hematuria, guaiac, bruising or petechiae, mucosa or orifices q8hr
- Buccal cavity for dryness, sores or ulceration, white patches, oral pain, bleeding, dysphagia
- **Pulmonary reactions:** assess for pulmonary fibrosis, fever, dyspnea, diffuse pulmonary infiltrates
- **Symptoms indicating severe allergic reaction:** rash, urticaria, itching, flushing
- **Neurotoxicity:** headaches, hallucinations, seizures, dizziness
- Rinsing of mouth tid-qid with water, club soda; brushing of teeth bid-tid with soft brush or cotton-tipped applicators for stomatitis; use unwaxed dental floss

Black Box Warning: Secondary malignancy: leukemia may occur after extended use

Black Box Warning: Only experienced clinicians should use this product

Evaluate:

- Therapeutic response: decreased tumor size, spread of malignancy

Teach patient/family:
- To report signs of infection: elevated temperature, sore throat, flulike symptoms
- To report signs of anemia: fatigue, headache, faintness, SOB, irritability
- To report bleeding; to avoid use of razors, commercial mouthwash
- To avoid use of aspirin products, ibuprofen (thrombocytopenia)
- To avoid foods with citric acid, hot or rough texture if stomatitis is present
- To report stomatitis: any bleeding, white spots, ulcerations in the mouth; to examine mouth daily, report symptoms
- To notify prescriber if pregnancy is planned or suspected, pregnancy (D)
- To notify prescriber of fever, chills, sore throat, nausea, vomiting, anorexia, diarrhea, bleeding, bruising; may indicate blood dyscrasias; mental status changes, pancreatitis, hepatotoxicity

hydrOXYzine (Rx)

(hye-drox′i-zeen)

Atarax ♣ Vistaril

Func. class.: Antianxiety/antihistamine/sedative/hypnotic, antiemetic

Chem. class.: Piperazine derivative

Do not confuse:
hydrOXYzine/hydrALAZINE
Vistaril/Versed

ACTION: Depresses subcortical levels of CNS, including limbic system, reticular formation; competes with H_1-receptor sites

USES: Anxiety preoperatively, postoperatively to prevent nausea, vomiting; to potentiate opioid analgesics; sedation; pruritus, ethanol withdrawal

Unlabeled uses: Insomnia, allergic rhinitis, generalized anxiety disorder

CONTRAINDICATIONS: Pregnancy 1st trimester, breastfeeding; hypersensitivity to this product or cetirizine; acute asthma

Precautions: Pregnancy (C) (2nd/3rd trimester), geriatric patients, debilitated, renal/hepatic disease, closed-angle glaucoma, COPD, prostatic hypertrophy, asthma

DOSAGE AND ROUTES

Anxiety
- **Adult: PO** 50-100 mg qid, max 400 mg/day; **IM** 50-100 mg q4-6hr
- **Child >6 yr: PO** 50-100 mg/day in divided doses, max 100 mg/day or 2 mg/kg/day
- **Child <6 yr: PO** 50 mg/day in divided doses, max 50 mg/day or 2 mg/kg/day

Alcohol withdrawal
- **Adult: IM** 50-100 mg q4-6hr

Preoperatively/postoperatively (nausea/vomiting)
- **Adult: IM** 25-100 mg q4-6hr
- **Child: IM** 1.1 mg/kg as a single dose

Pruritus
- **Adult: PO** 25 mg tid-qid; **IM** 50-100 mg, then q4-6hr prn, switch to **PO** as soon as feasible
- **Child ≥6 yr: PO** 50-100 mg/day in divided doses; **IM** 0.5-1 mg/kg/dose q4-6hr prn, use **PO** when possible
- **Child <6 yr: PO** 50 mg/day in divided doses

Insomnia (unlabeled)
- **Adult: PO** 50-100 mg 30-60 min before bedtime; **IM** 50 mg 30-60 min before bedtime

Renal dose
- **Adult: PO** CCr <50 ml/min, give 50% of dose

Available forms: Tabs 10, 25, 50 mg; caps 25, 50, 100 mg; oral sol 10 mg/ 5 ml; inj 25, 50 mg/ml; oral susp 25 mg/ 5 ml

Administer:

PO route
- Without regard to meals
- Crushed if patient is unable to swallow medication whole
- Shake oral susp before giving

IM route
- Does not need to be diluted; give by Z-track inj in large muscle to decrease pain, chance of necrosis; never give IV/SUBCUT (HCl)

Additive compatibilities: CISplatin, cyclophosphamide, cytarabine, dimenhyDRINATE, etoposide, lidocaine, mesna, methotrexate, nafcillin

Syringe compatibilities: Atropine, butorphanol, chlorproMAZINE, cimetidine, codeine, diphenhydrAMINE, doxapram, droperidol, fentaNYL, fluPHENAZine, glycopyrrolate, HYDROmorphone, lidocaine, meperidine, metoclopramide, midazolam, morphine, nalbuphine, oxymorphone, pentazocine, perphenazine, procaine, prochlorperazine, scopolamine, SUFentanil

SIDE EFFECTS

CNS: *Dizziness, drowsiness,* confusion, headache, tremors, fatigue, depression, seizures

CV: Hypotension

GI: Dry mouth, increased appetite, nausea, diarrhea, weight gain

PHARMACOKINETICS

PO: Onset 15-60 min, duration 4-6 hr, half-life 3 hr, metabolized by liver, excreted by kidneys

INTERACTIONS

Increase: CNS depressant effect—barbiturates, opioids, analgesics, alcohol, sedative/hypnotics, other CNS depressants

Increase: anticholinergic effects—phenothiazines, quiNIDine, disopyramide, antihistamines, antidepressants, atropine, haloperidol, MAOIs

Drug/Lab Test

False negative: skin allergy testing

False increase: 17-hydroxycorticosteroids

NURSING CONSIDERATIONS

Assess:

- Anticholinergic effects: dry mouth, dizziness, confusion, hypotension, increased sedation; monitor B/P
- Assistance with ambulation during beginning therapy, since drowsiness, dizziness occurs

Evaluate:

- Therapeutic response: decreased anxiety

Teach patient/family:

- To avoid OTC preparations (cold, cough, hay fever) unless approved by prescriber
- To avoid driving, activities that require alertness
- To avoid alcohol, psychotropic medications
- Not to discontinue medication quickly after long-term use
- To rise slowly because fainting may occur

TREATMENT OF OVERDOSE:

Lavage if orally ingested; VS, supportive care; IV norepinephrine for hypotension

hyoscyamine (Rx)

(hye-oh-sye′a-meen)

Anaspaz, Colidrops, Colytrol Pediatric, Cystospaz-M, ED-SPAZ, HyoMax, HyoMax SL, Hyosyne, Levsin SL, NuLev, Oscimin, Spasdel, Symax

Func. class.: Anticholinergic/antispasmodics

Chem. class.: Belladonna alkaloid

ACTION:

Inhibits muscarinic actions of acetylcholine at postganglionic parasympathetic neuroeffector sites; reduces rigidity, tremors, hyperhidrosis of parkinsonism

USES:

Treatment of peptic ulcer disease in combination with other products; other GI disorders, other spastic disorders, IBS, urinary incontinence

CONTRAINDICATIONS:

Hypersensitivity to anticholinergics, closed-angle glaucoma, GI obstruction, myasthenia gravis, paralytic ileus, GI atony, toxic megacolon, prostatic hypertrophy, urinary tract obstruction

Precautions: Pregnancy (C), geriatric patients, hyperthyroidism, dysrhythmias, CHF, ulcerative colitis, hypertension, hiatal hernia, renal/hepatic disease, urinary retention, CAD

DOSAGE AND ROUTES

- **Adult/adolescent/child ≥12 yr: PO/SL** 0.125-0.25 mg q4hr; **EXT REL** 0.375-0.75 mg q12hr
- **Adult: IM/SUBCUT/IV** 0.25-0.5 mg in a single dose or 2-4×/day q6hr
- **Geriatric:** Max 1.5 mg/day in divided doses or max 4 biphasic tabs
- **Child 2-12 yr: PO** SL 0.0625-0.125 q4hr

Available forms: Tabs 0.125, 0.15 mg; ext rel caps 0.375 mg; sol 0.125 mg/ml; elix 0.125 mg/5 ml; sol for inj 0.5 mg/ml; SL tab 0.125 mg; tab, biphasic 0.125, 0.375 mg; orally disintegrating tab 0.125 mg

Administer:

PO route

- Do not break, crush, or chew ext rel caps
- 1/2 hr before meals for better absorption
- Decreased dose to geriatric patients; metabolism may be slowed
- Store in tight container protected from light

IV route

- Use undiluted, inject slowly

SIDE EFFECTS

CNS: *Confusion, stimulation in geriatric patients,* headache, insomnia, dizziness, drowsiness, anxiety, weakness, hallucination

CV: *Palpitations,* tachycardia

EENT: *Blurred vision,* photophobia, mydriasis, cycloplegia, increased ocular tension

GI: *Dry mouth, constipation, paralytic ileus,* heartburn, nausea, vomiting, dysphagia, absence of taste

GU: *Urinary hesitancy, retention,* impotence

INTEG: Urticaria, rash, pruritus, anhidrosis, fever, allergic reactions

PHARMACOKINETICS

PO: Duration 4-6 hr, metabolized by liver, excreted in urine, half-life 3.5 hr

INTERACTIONS

Increase: anticholinergic effect—amantadine, tricyclics, MAOIs, H_1-antihistamines

Decrease: hyoscyamine effect—antacids

Decrease: effect of phenothiazines, levodopa, ketoconazole

NURSING CONSIDERATIONS

Assess:

- VS, cardiac status: checking for dysrhythmias, increased rate, palpitations
- I&O ratio; check for urinary retention or hesitancy
- GI complaints: pain, nausea, vomiting, anorexia
- Increased fluids, bulk, exercise to decrease constipation

Evaluate:

- Therapeutic response: absence of epigastric pain, bleeding, nausea, vomiting

Teach patient/family:

- To avoid driving, other hazardous activities until stabilized on medication
- To avoid alcohol or other CNS depressants; they will enhance sedating properties of this product
- To avoid hot environments because heat stroke may occur; that product suppresses perspiration
- To use sunglasses when outside to prevent photophobia; that product may cause blurred vision
- To notify prescriber if pregnancy is planned or suspected (C)

ibandronate (Rx)

(eye-ban′dro-nate)

Boniva

Func. class.: Bone-resorption inhibitor, electrolyte modifier

Chem. class.: Bisphosphonate

ACTION: Inhibits bone resorption, apparently without inhibiting bone formation and mineralization; absorbs calcium phosphate crystals in bone and may directly block dissolution of hydroxyapatite crystals of bone; more potent than other products

USES: Osteoporosis and prophylaxis

Unlabeled uses: Hypercalcemia of malignancy, osteolytic metastases, Paget's disease, osteoporosis (treatment/prevention) in those taking anastrozole

CONTRAINDICATIONS: Achalasia, esophageal stricture, hypocalcemia, intraarterial administration, renal failure, hypersensitivity to bisphosphonates, inability to stand or sit upright

Precautions: Pregnancy (C), breastfeeding, children, geriatric patients, anemia, chemotherapy, coagulopathy, dental disease, diabetes mellitus, dysphagia, GI/renal disease, GERD, hypertension, infection, multiple myeloma, phosphate hypersensitivity, vit D deficiency

DOSAGE AND ROUTES

Postmenopausal osteoporosis/prophylaxis

- **Adult: PO** 150 mg/mo; **IV BOL** 3 mg q3mo

Paget's disease (unlabeled)

- **Adult: IV** 2 mg as a single dose

Bone metastases (unlabeled)

- **Adult: IV** 6 mg over 1 hr × 3 days, repeat q4wk

Hypercalcemia (unlabeled)

- **Adult: IV INFUSION** 2-4 mg over 2 hr

Renal dose

- **Adult: PO** CCr <30 ml/min, avoid use

Available forms: Tabs 150 mg; sol for inj 1 mg/ml

Administer:

PO route

- Give early AM with a glass of water; if monthly, give on same day of each month
- Store at room temperature

Direct IV route

- Use single-dose prefilled syringe; discard unused portion; give over 15-30 sec; give q3mo; do not use if discolored or contains particulates

SIDE EFFECTS

CNS: Fever, insomnia, dizziness, headache

CV: Hypertension, **atrial fibrillation**

EENT: Ocular pain/inflammation, uveitis

GI: Constipation, nausea, vomiting, diarrhea, dyspepsia

INTEG: Rash, inj-site reaction

META: *Hypomagnesemia, hypophosphatemia, hypocalcemia,* hypercholesterolemia

MS: Bone pain, myalgia, osteonecrosis of the jaw

SYST: **Stevens-Johnson syndrome, erythema multiforme, dermatitis bullous**

PHARMACOKINETICS

Half-life 5-60 hr, 86%-99% protein binding; taken up mainly by bones, primarily in areas of high bone turnover; eliminated primarily by kidneys

INTERACTIONS

Increase: GI irritation—NSAIDs, salicylates

Increase: hypocalcemia—loop diuretics

Decrease: ibandronate effect—calcium/vit D/iron/aluminum/magnesium salts; separate by 1 hr

Drug/Food

- Do not take with food, calcium

Increase: cholesterol

Drug/Lab Test

Decrease: Alk phos, magnesium, calcium, phosphate

Increase: cholesterol

NURSING CONSIDERATIONS

Assess:

- **Anaphylaxis:** swelling of face, lips, mouth, rash, sweating, wheezing, trouble breathing, discontinue immediately, provide supportive treatment
- **Osteoporosis:** before and during treatment; scan for bone mineral density, correct electrolyte imbalances (calcium, magnesium, phosphate) before starting therapy
- Atrial fibrillation
- **Dental health:** before dental extraction, give antiinfectives, osteonecrosis of the jaw may occur
- Blood studies: electrolytes, creatinine/BUN, vit D: correct deficiencies before treatment
- For bone pain; use analgesics; may begin within 24 hr or even years after treatment; pain usually subsides after treatment is discontinued

Evaluate:

- Therapeutic response: increased bone mineral density

Teach patient/family:

- **To report hypercalcemic relapse:** nausea, vomiting, bone pain, thirst, unusual muscle twitching, muscle spasms, severe diarrhea, constipation
- To continue with dietary recommendations, including calcium, vit D
- To obtain an analgesic from provider for bone pain
- That, if nausea, vomiting occur, small, frequent meals may help
- To report vision symptoms: blurred vision, edema, inflammation
- To report if pregnancy is planned or suspected or if planning to breastfeed, pregnancy (C)
- To exercise regularly, stop smoking, decrease alcohol intake
- To take PO first thing in AM at least 60 min before other medications, food, beverages, to take monthly dose on same day
- To sit upright for ≥60 min after PO

⚠ HIGH ALERT

ibrutinib

(eye-broo′ti-nib)

Imbruvica

Func. class.: Antineoplastic-biologic response modifier

Chem. class.: Signal transduction inhibitor (STIs)

ACTION: Irreversible inhibitor of Bruton's tyrosine kinases in B cells responsible for tumor growth

USES: Recurrent mantle cell lymphoma who have received at least 1 prior treatment

CONTRAINDICATIONS: Pregnancy (D), breastfeeding, hypersensitivity

Precautions: Children, geriatric patients, active infections, anticoagulant therapy, bleeding, hepatic/renal disease, neutropenia, surgery

DOSAGE AND ROUTES

- **Adult: PO** 560 mg (4×140 mg caps) daily
- **Dosage adjustment for ≥grade 3 non-hematologic, ≥grade 3 neutropenia with infection or fever, or grade 4 hematologic toxicities:** Interrupt therapy; resume upon recovery to grade 1 or baseline as indicated below:
- **First occurrence:** Resume dosing at original dose (daily dose = 560 mg/day)
- **Second occurrence:** Reduce dose by 1 capsule (daily dose = 420 mg/day)
- **Third occurrence:** Reduce dose by 2 capsules (daily dose = 280 mg/day)
- **Fourth occurrence:** Discontinue

Waldenstrom macroglobulinemia

- **Adult: PO** 420 mg daily until disease progression

Available forms: Caps 140 mg

Administer:

- At same time of day with water, if dose is missed, take as soon as possible on same day, do not double
- Do not open, break, chew cap

SIDE EFFECTS

CNS: Fatigue, fever
CV: Hypertension, atrial fibrillation, peripheral edema
EENT: Sinusitis
GI: Nausea, vomiting, dyspepsia, anorexia, abdominal pain, constipation, stomatitis, diarrhea, GI bleeding
GU: Increased serum creatinine, UTI
HEMA: Neutropenia, thrombocytopenia, anemia, bleeding, epistaxis, transient lymphocytosis
INTEG: Rash, skin infections
MS: Pain, arthralgia, muscle cramps
RESP: Cough, dyspnea
SYST: Secondary malignancy, infection

PHARMACOKINETICS

Protein binding 97.3%; metabolized by CYP3A4/CYP2D6; primarily excreted in feces, small amount in urine; peak 1-2 hr, terminal half-life 4-8 hr

INTERACTIONS

Increase: ibrutinib effect—avoid use with moderate or strong CYP3A4 inhibitors
Decrease: ibrutinib effect—avoid use with moderate or strong CYP3A4 inducers
Drug/Herb
Decrease: SUNItinib concentration—St. John's wort
Drug/Food Test
Increase: plasma concentrations grapefruit juice

NURSING CONSIDERATIONS

Assess:
- **Bleeding:** bruising, grade 3 or higher bleeding events may occur; CBC
- Hepatic/renal function; signs and symptoms infections

Evaluate:
- Therapeutic response: decrease in progression of disease

Teach patient/family:
- To report adverse reactions immediately: SOB bleeding
- About reason for treatment, expected result
- That many adverse reactions may occur: high B/P, bleeding, mouth swelling
- To avoid persons with known upper respiratory infections; that immunosuppression is common
- To avoid grapefruit juice or medications, herbs; there are many interactions
- To report if pregnancy is planned or suspected, pregnancy (D)
- To report bleeding, severe infections, renal toxicity (maintain hydration), development of second malignancies, diarrhea (contact physician if it persists)
- To take with water (avoid food because it increases drug levels) at same time each day; do not open, break, or chew

ibuprofen (OTC, Rx)

(eye-byoo-proe′fen)

Advil, Caldolor, Ibuprohm, Ibutab, Midol, Motrin ✱, Motrin IB, Pamprin IB ✱, Profen, Tab-Profen

ibuprofen lysine (Rx)

NeoProfen

Func.class.: NSAID
Chem. class.: Propionic acid derivative

Do not confuse:
Nuprin/Lupron

ACTION: Inhibits COX-1, COX-2 by blocking arachidonate; analgesic, antiinflammatory, antipyretic

USES: Rheumatoid arthritis, osteoarthritis, primary dysmenorrhea, dental pain, musculoskeletal disorders, fever, migraine, patent ductus arteriosus
Unlabeled uses: Ankylosing spondylitis, bone pain, cystic fibrosis, gouty arthritis, psoriatic arthritis

CONTRAINDICATIONS: Pregnancy (D) 3rd trimester; hypersensitivity to this product, NSAIDs, salicylates; asthma; severe renal/hepatic disease

Black Box Warning: Perioperative pain in CABG

Precautions: Pregnancy (C) 1st and 2nd trimesters, breastfeeding, children, geriatric patients, bleeding disorders, GI disorders, cardiac disorders, hypersensitivity to other antiinflammatory agents, CHF, CCr <25 ml/min

Black Box Warning: GI bleeding, MI, stroke

DOSAGE AND ROUTES

Self-treatment of minor aches/pains

- **Adult/adolescent: PO** (OTC product) 200 mg q4-6hr, may increase to 400 mg q4-6hr if needed, max 1200 mg/day

Analgesic

- **Adult: PO** 200-400 mg q4-6hr, max 3.2 g/day; OTC use max 1200 mg/day
- **Child: PO** 4-10 mg/kg/dose q6-8hr

Moderate to severe pain (hospitalized patients) (Caldolor)

- **Adult: IV** 400-800 mg q6hr as an adjunct to opiate-agonist therapy

Dysmenorrhea

- **Adult: PO** 400 mg q4-6hr, max 1200 mg/day

Antipyretic

- **Child 6 mo-12 yr: PO** 5 mg/kg (temperature <102.5° F or 39.2° C), 10 mg/kg (temperature >102.5° F), may repeat q6-8hr, max 40 mg/kg/day

Antiinflammatory

- **Adult: PO** 400-800 mg tid-qid, max 3.2 g/day
- **Child: PO** 30-40 mg/kg/day in 3-4 divided doses, max 50 mg/kg/day

Patent ductus arteriosus (PDA) (NeoProfen)

- **Premature neonate ≤32 wk gestation who weighs 500-1500 g: IV** 10 mg/kg initially, then, if needed, 2 doses of 5 mg/kg at 24-hr intervals; if oliguria occurs, hold dose

Available forms: Tabs 100, 200, 400, 600, 800 mg; cap, liq gels 200 mg; oral susp 100 mg/5 ml; liq 100 mg/5 ml; chew tabs 100 mg; drops 50 mg/1.25 ml; inj 10 mg/ml (NeoProfen)

Administer:

PO route

- With food, milk, or antacid to decrease GI symptoms; if nausea and vomiting occur or persist, notify prescriber
- Shake susp well before use
- Do not use in pregnancy after 30 wk gestation
- Store at room temperature

IV route

- Patient must be well hydrated before administration
- Dilute to ≤4 mg/ml with 0.9% NaCl, LR, D_5W; infuse over ≥30 min; do not give IM
- Discard unused portion
- Visually inspect for particulate
- **Ibuprofen lysine:** dilute with dextrose or saline to appropriate volume (10 mg/ml of ibuprofen is recommended); give within 30 min of preparation; give via IV port nearest insertion site; give over 15 min
- Check for extravasation; do not give in same line with TPN; interrupt TPN for 15 min before and after product administration

SIDE EFFECTS

CNS: *Headache,* dizziness, drowsiness, fatigue, tremors, confusion, insomnia, anxiety, depression

CV: Tachycardia, peripheral edema, palpitations, dysrhythmias, **CV thrombotic events, MI, stroke**

EENT: Tinnitus, hearing loss, blurred vision

GI: Nausea, *anorexia,* vomiting, diarrhea, jaundice, **hepatitis,** constipation, flatulence, cramps, dry mouth, peptic ulcer, **GI bleeding, ulceration, necrotizing enterocolitis, GI perforation**

GU: **Nephrotoxicity:** dysuria, hematuria, oliguria, azotemia

HEMA: **Blood dyscrasias,** increased bleeding time

INTEG: Purpura, rash, pruritus, sweating, urticaria, **nectrotizing fasciitis,** photosensitivity, photophobia

META: Hyperkalemia, hyperuricemia, hypoglycemia, hyponatremia

SYST: Anaphylaxis, Stevens-Johnson syndrome

PHARMACOKINETICS

PO: Onset 1/2 hr, peak 1-2 hr, half-life 1.8-2 hr, metabolized in liver (inactive metabolites), excreted in urine (inactive metabolites), 90%-99% plasma protein binding, does not enter breast milk, well absorbed

INTERACTIONS

Increase: bleeding risk—valproic acid, thrombolytics, antiplatelets, anticoagulants, salicylates
Increase: blood dyscrasia risk—antineoplastics, radiation
Increase: toxicity—lithium, oral anticoagulants, cycloSPORINE, methotrexate
Increase: GI reactions—aspirin, corticosteroids, NSAIDs, alcohol, tobacco
Increase: hypoglycemia—oral antidiabetics
Decrease: effect of antihypertensives, thiazides, furosemide
Decrease: ibuprofen action—aspirin

Drug/Herb

Increase: bleeding risk—feverfew, garlic, ginger, ginkgo, ginseng *(Panax)*

Drug/Lab Test

Increase: BUN, creatinine, LFTs
Decrease: Hgb/Hct, blood glucose, WBC, platelets

NURSING CONSIDERATIONS

Assess:

- Renal, hepatic, blood studies: BUN, creatinine, AST, ALT, Hgb, stool guaiac, before treatment, periodically thereafter, monitor electrolytes as needed

Black Box Warning: Perioperative pain in CABG: MI and stroke can result for 10-14 days; can be fatal; those taking NSAIDs are at greater risk of MI and stroke, even in first few weeks of therapy

- **Pain:** note type, duration, location, intensity with ROM 1 hr after administration
- Audiometric, ophthalmic exam before, during, after long-term treatment; for eye, ear problems: blurred vision, tinnitus; may indicate toxicity
- **Infection,** may mask symptoms; fever: temperature before and 1 hr after administration
- Cardiac status: edema (peripheral), tachycardia, palpitations; monitor B/P, pulse for character, quality, rhythm, especially in patients with cardiac disease, geriatric patients
- For history of peptic ulcer disorder; asthma, aspirin, hypersensitivity; check closely for hypersensitivity reactions

Black Box Warning: GI bleeding/perforation: chronic use can cause gastritis with or without bleeding, those with a prior history of peptic ulcer disease or GI bleeding, initiate treatment at lower dose; geriatric patients are at greater risk and those who consume >3 alcohol drinks/day

Evaluate:

- Therapeutic response: decreased pain, stiffness in joints; decreased swelling in joints; ability to move more easily; reduction in fever or menstrual cramping

Teach patient/family:

- To use sunscreen, sunglasses, and protective clothing to prevent photosensitivity, photophobia
- To report blurred vision, ringing, roaring in ears (may indicate toxicity); that eye and hearing tests should be done during long-term therapy
- To avoid driving, other hazardous activities if dizziness or drowsiness occurs

▲ **Nephrotoxicity:** to report change in urinary pattern, increased weight, edema, increased pain in joints, fever, blood in urine; monitor fluid status, BUN, creatinine

- That therapeutic antiinflammatory effects may take up to 1 mo

▲ To avoid alcohol, NSAIDs, salicylates; bleeding may occur

- To report use of this product to all health care providers
- **Pregnancy:** notify prescriber if pregnancy (C) is planned or suspected; avoid

during 3rd trimester pregnancy (D) IV after 30 wk

Black Box Warning: MI/Stroke: to report signs/symptoms of MI/stroke immediately and discontinue product

TREATMENT OF OVERDOSE:
Lavage, activated charcoal, induce diuresis

⚠ HIGH ALERT

ibutilide (Rx)
(eye-byoo′tih-lide)

Corvert

Func. class.: Antidysrhythmic (class III)
Chem. class.: Methane sulfonamide

ACTION: Prolongs duration of action potential and effective refractory period

USES: For rapid conversion of atrial fibrillation/flutter, including within 1 wk of coronary artery bypass or valve surgery

CONTRAINDICATIONS: Hypersensitivity

Precautions: Pregnancy (C), breastfeeding, children <18 yr, geriatric patients, sinus node dysfunction, 2nd- or 3rd-degree AV block, electrolyte imbalances, bradycardia, renal/hepatic disease, CHF

Black Box Warning: QT prolongation, torsades de pointes, ventricular arrhythmias, ventricular tachycardia, cardiac dysrhythmias, atrial fibrillation

DOSAGE AND ROUTES
Atrial fibrillation/flutter

- **Adult ≥60 kg:** IV INFUSION 1 vial (1 mg) given over 10 min, may repeat same dose after 10 min
- **Adult <60 kg:** IV INFUSION 0.01 mg/kg given over 10 min, may repeat same dose after 10 min

Available forms: Inj 1 mg/10 ml

Administer:

- Ice compress after stopping infusion for extravasation; tubing should be removed and attempt to aspirate product; elevate affected areas

IV route

- Undiluted or diluted in 50 ml 0.9% NaCl, or D_5W (0.017 mg/ml); give over 10 min
- Solution is stable for 48 hr refrigerated or 24 hr at room temperature
- Do not admix with other sol, products
- Reduce dosage slowly with ECG monitoring
- Stop infusion as soon as arrhythmia is controlled
- Do not use if discolored or particulate is present

SIDE EFFECTS
CNS: *Headache*

CV: *Hypotension, bradycardia,* **sinus arrest, CHF, dysrhythmias, torsades de pointes,** hypertension, extrasystoles, ventricular tachycardia, bundle branch block, AV block, palpitations, supraventricular extrasystoles, syncope, **prolonged QT interval**

GI: Nausea

PHARMACOKINETICS
Elimination half-life 6 hr, metabolized by liver, excreted by kidneys

INTERACTIONS
Increase: prodysrhythmia—phenothiazines, tricyclics, tetracyclics, antidepressants, H_1-receptor antagonists, antihistamines

Increase: masking of cardiotoxicity—digoxin

- **Do not use within 5 hr of ibutilide: class Ia antidysrhythmics (disopyramide, quiNIDine, procainamide), class III agents (amiodarone, sotalol), QT prolongation may occur**

NURSING CONSIDERATIONS

Assess:

Black Box Warning: ECG continuously for ≥4 hr to determine product effectiveness; measure PR, QRS, QT intervals, check for PVCs, other dysrhythmias; discontinue if atrial fibrillation/flutter ceases; continue until QT interval corrected for heart rate (QTc) returned to baseline; if used ≥2 days, anticoagulation must be adequate

- I&O ratio; electrolytes: potassium, sodium, chlorine
- Hepatic studies: AST, ALT, bilirubin, alk phos
- Dehydration or hypovolemia
- Rebound hypertension after 1-2 hr
- Cardiac rate, respiration: rate, rhythm, character, chest pain

Evaluate:

- Therapeutic response: decrease in atrial fibrillation/flutter

Teach patient/family:

- To report side effects immediately
- About reason for medication

icosapent

(eye-koe′sa-pent)

Vascepa

Func. class.: Antilipidemic

Chem. class.: Omega-3 fatty acid ethylester

ACTION: Inhibits hepatic very low density lipoprotein (VLDL) and triglyceride synthesis; enhances clearance of triglycerides from circulating VLDL particles

USES: As adjunct to diet in adults with severe hypertriglyceridemia (≥500 mg/dl)

CONTRAINDICATIONS: Hypersensitivity to icosapent ethyl

Precautions: Hepatic disease, bleeding, breastfeeding, children, fish/shellfish hypersensitivity, thrombolytic/anticoagulation therapy, pregnancy (C)

DOSAGE AND ROUTES

- **Adult: PO** 2 g bid

Available forms: Soft gel cap 1 g

Administer:

- Give with food, swallow whole
- Store at room temperature

SIDE EFFECTS

HEMA: Ecchymosis, epistaxis

MS: Arthralgia

PHARMACOKINETICS

Peak 5 hr, protein binding 99%, half-life 89 hr

INTERACTIONS

Increase: effects of anticoagulants, platelet inhibitors, thrombolytics

Drug/Lab Test

Increase: bleeding time

NURSING CONSIDERATIONS

Assess:

- **Hypertriglyceridemia:** Obtain diet history including fat, cholesterol in diet; cholesterol, triglyceride levels periodically during treatment
- **Liver disease:** Monitor LFTs baseline, periodically in those with liver disease
- **Bleeding:** Monitor for ecchymosis, epistaxis, bleeding time; use cautiously in anticoagulant/thrombolytic therapy
- **Fish/shellfish hypersensitivity:** Identify fish hypersensitivity, use cautiously

Evaluate:

- Therapeutic response: decrease in triglycerides

Teach patient/family:

- That blood work may be necessary during treatment
- To report bleeding if anticoagulants or thrombolytics are used
- Not to break, crush, open, or dissolve caps
- That previously prescribed regimen will continue: low-cholesterol diet, exercise program, smoking cessation

⚠ HIGH ALERT

IDArubicin (Rx)

(eye-dah-roob′ih-sin)

Idamycin PFS

Func. class.: Antineoplastic, antibiotic

Chem. class.: Anthracycline glycoside

Do not confuse:
IDArubicin/DOXOrubicin/DAUNOrubicin/epirubicin
Idamycin/Adriamycin

ACTION:
Non–cell-cycle specific; topoisomerase II inhibitor; vesicant; intercalcalating between DNA base pairs, causing shape change, low free radicals

USES:
Used in combination with other antineoplastics for acute myelocytic leukemia in adults

Unlabeled uses: Breast cancer, liquid tumors, non-Hodgkin's lymphoma, ALL, CML, NHL

CONTRAINDICATIONS:
Pregnancy (D), breastfeeding, hypersensitivity

Black Box Warning: Myelosuppression, bilirubin >5 mg/dl

Precautions: Children, gout, bone marrow depression, preexisting CV disease

Black Box Warning: Renal/hepatic disease, heart failure

DOSAGE AND ROUTES

- **Adult: IV** 8-12 mg/m^2/day × 3 days in combination with cytarabine (induction)
- **Adolescent/child (unlabeled): IV** 10-12 mg/m^2/day × 3 days

Renal/hepatic dose

Black Box Warning: Adult: IV CCr >2.5 mg/dl, reduce dose; bilirubin 2.5-5 mg/dl, reduce dose by 50%; bilirubin >5 mg/dl, do not use

Available forms: Inj 1 mg/ml

Administer:

- Ice compress after stopping infusion for extravasation
- Store at room temperature for 3 days after reconstituting or 7 days refrigerated

Intermittent IV INFUSION route

- Do not give IM/SUBCUT
- Use cytotoxic handling procedures after preparing in biologic cabinet wearing gown, gloves, mask
- Antiemetic 30-60 min before product and 6-10 hr after treatment to prevent vomiting
- After reconstituting 5-mg vial with 5 ml 0.9% NaCl (1 mg/1 ml); give over 10-15 min through Y-tube or 3-way stopcock of infusion of D_5W or NS; discard unused portion; use caution when needle inserted into vial (negative pressure)

- Use a free-flowing IV, do not give IM/SUBCUT
- A vesicant, monitor for necrosis

Y-site compatibilities: Amifostine, amikacin, aztreonam, cimetidine, cladribine, cyclophosphamide, cytarabine, diphenhydrAMINE, droperidol, erythromycin, filgrastim, granisetron, imipenem/CISplatin, magnesium sulfate, mannitol, melphalan, metoclopramide, potassium chloride, ranitidine, sargramostim, thiotepa, vinorelbine

SIDE EFFECTS

CNS: Fever, chills, *headache,* seizures

CV: Dysrhythmias, CHF, pericarditis, myocarditis, peripheral edema, angina, MI, myocardial toxicity

GI: *Nausea, vomiting, abdominal pain, mucositis, diarrhea,* hepatotoxicity

GU: Nephrotoxicity, red urine

HEMA: Thrombocytopenia, leukopenia, anemia

INTEG: Rash, extravasation, dermatitis, *reversible alopecia,* urticaria; thrombophlebitis and tissue necrosis at inj site; radiation recall

SYST: Infection, tumor lysis syndrome

I

PHARMACOKINETICS

Half-life 22 hr; metabolized by liver; crosses placenta; excreted in bile, urine (primarily as metabolites); 97% protein binding

INTERACTIONS

Increase: bleeding risk—anticoagulants, salicylates, NSAIDs, thrombolytics; avoid concurrent use
Decrease: IDArubicin effect—corticosteroids
Increase: CHF, ventricular dysfunction—trastuzumab
Increase: ECG changes (QT prolongation, changes in QRS voltage)—class IA/III antidysrhythmias, some phenothiazines, and other products that increase QT prolongation
Increase: cardiotoxicity—cyclophosphamide
Increase: toxicity—other antineoplastics or radiation
Decrease: antibody response—live virus vaccines

Drug/Lab Test
Decrease: calcium, platelets, neutrophils
Increase: uric acid, phosphate, potassium

NURSING CONSIDERATIONS

Assess:

Black Box Warning: CBC, differential, platelet count weekly; notify prescriber of results, severe myelosuppression can occur

- Renal studies: BUN, serum uric acid, urine CCr, electrolytes before, during therapy

⚠ Tumor lysis syndrome: hyperkalemia, hyperphosphatemia, hyperuricemia, hypocalcemia

- I&O ratio; report fall in urine output to <30 ml/hr
- Monitor temperature; fever may indicate beginning infection

Black Box Warning: Hepatic studies before, during therapy: bilirubin, AST, ALT, alk phos prn or monthly; check for jaundice of skin and sclera, dark urine, clay-colored stools, itchy skin, abdominal pain, fever, diarrhea, do not use if bilirubin >5 mg/dl

Black Box Warning: Cardiac toxicity: CHF, dysrythmias, cardiomyopathy; cardiac studies before and periodically during treatment: ECG, chest x-ray, MUGA; ECG: watch for ST-T wave changes, low QRS and T, possible dysrhythmias (sinus tachycardia, heart block, PVCs)

- **Bleeding:** hematuria, guaiac stools, bruising or petechiae, mucosa or orifices
- Effects of alopecia on body image; discuss feelings about body changes
- Inflammation of mucosa, breaks in skin
- Buccal cavity for dryness, sores, ulceration, white patches, oral pain, bleeding, dysphagia

Black Box Warning: Local irritation, pain, burning at inj site; extravasation (vesicant)

- GI symptoms: frequency of stools, cramping
- Increase fluid intake to 2-3 L/day to prevent urate and calculi formation

Evaluate:

- Therapeutic response: decreased liquid tumor, spread of malignancy

Teach patient/family:

- To report signs of CHF, cardiac toxicity, beginning infection
- That hair may be lost during treatment; that wig or hairpiece may make patient feel better; that new hair may be different in color, texture
- To avoid foods with citric acid, hot or rough texture
- To avoid crowds, persons with upper respiratory illness

- To report any bleeding, white spots, ulcerations in mouth; to examine mouth daily
- That urine may be red-orange for 48 hr
- To report if pregnancy is planned or suspected, pregnancy (D)
- To use contraception during treatment, for ≥4 mo after treatment
- That all body fluids will change color

idelalisib

(eye-del′a-lis′ib)

Zydelig

Func. class.: Antineoplastic-biologic response modifier

Chem. class.: Signal transduction inhibitor (STI)

ACTION: Selective, small-molecule inhibitor of one kinase (expressed in both normal and malignant B-cells). Induces apoptosis and inhibited proliferation, inhibits several cell signaling pathways

USES: Treatment of relapsed chronic lymphocytic leukemia (CLL), in combination with rituximab, in those whom rituximab alone should not be used; non-Hodgkin's lymphoma (NHL), relapsed follicular B-cell non-Hodgkin's lymphoma in those who have received at least 2 prior systemic therapies

CONTRAINDICATIONS: Infusion-related reaction, serious rash, pregnancy (D)

Precautions: Serious allergic reactions, grade 3 or 4 neutropenia, breastfeeding, hyperglycemia/hypoglycemia

Black Box Warning: Serious hepatotoxicity, grade 3 or higher diarrhea or colitis, fatal/serious pneumonitis

DOSAGE AND ROUTES

Treatment of relapsed chronic lymphocytic leukemia (CLL)

- **Adults: PO** 150 mg bid until disease progression or unacceptable toxicity, with 8 doses of rituximab (given as 375 mg/m^2 IV on day 1, then 2 wk later rituximab 500 mg/m^2 IV q2wk × 3 more doses, followed by rituximab 500 mg/m^2 IV q4wk × 4 doses)

Treatment of small lymphocytic lymphoma (SLL) in those who have received at least 2 prior systemic therapies

- **Adults: PO** 150 mg bid until disease progression or unacceptable toxicity

Hepatic dose

- **AST/ALT >3-5 × ULN:** No change; monitor AST/ALT at least every week until ≤1 × ULN
- **AST/ALT >5-20 × ULN:** Hold doses, monitor AST/ALT at least every week, when AST/ALT are ≤1 × ULN, resume at 100 mg bid
- **AST/ALT >20 × ULN:** Permanently discontinue
- **Bilirubin >1.5-3 × ULN:** No change; monitor bilirubin at least every week until ≤1 × ULN
- **Bilirubin >3-10 × ULN:** Hold treatment; monitor bilirubin at least every week; when bilirubin is ≤1 × ULN, resume treatment at 100 mg bid
- **Bilirubin >10 × ULN:** Permanently discontinue

Available forms: Tabs 100, 150 mg

Administer:

- Take without regard to food, do not crush or dissolve tabs
- Do not take 2 doses at the same time, if a dose is missed by <6 hr, take the dose, take next dose at usual time

Therapeutic drug monitoring: dosage adjustments due to treatment-related toxicity

- **Moderate diarrhea (4-6 stools/day over baseline):** Continue current dosing; monitor at least every week until diarrhea is resolved

• **Severe diarrhea (≥7 stools/day over baseline) or diarrhea requiring hospitalization:** Hold treatment, and monitor at least every week for resolution. When diarrhea has resolved, resume with 100 mg bid
• **Life-threatening diarrhea:** Permanently discontinue treatment
• **Neutropenia: ANC 1000-1499 cells/mm^3:** no change; **ANC 500-999 cells/mm^3:** continue current dosing; monitor ANC at least every week; **ANC <500 cells/mm^3:** hold treatment and monitor ANC at least every week, when ANC ≥500 cells/mm^3, resume treatment at 100 mg bid
• **Thrombocytopenia: Platelet count 50,000-75,000 cells/mm^3:** no change; **platelet count 25,000-49,000 cells/mm^3:** continue dose; monitor platelet count at least every week; **platelet count <25,000 cells/mm^3**: hold treatment, monitor platelet count at least every week, when platelet count ≥25,000 cells/mm^3, resume treatment at 100 mg bid
• **Symptomatic pneumonitis (any severity):** Discontinue treatment
• **Other severe or life-threatening toxicities:** Hold until toxicity is resolved; if resuming treatment, reduce the dose to 100 mg bid; permanently discontinue treatment for any recurrence of severe or life-threatening toxicity after rechallenge

SIDE EFFECTS

CNS: Insomnia, fatigue, fever, headache
RESP: Pneumonitis, dyspnea, cough
ENDO: Hypoglycemia, hyperglycemia, hyponatremia
INTEG: Rash
EENT: Sinusitis
GI: Nausea, vomiting, hepatic failure, GI perforation, stomatitis, colitis, diarrhea, anorexia, abdominal pain
HEMA: Thrombocytopenia, neutropenia, anemia
SYST: Serious/fatal rashes

PHARMACOKINETICS

84% protein binding, half-life 8.2 hr, peak 1.5 hr

INTERACTIONS

Avoid use with CYP3A4 inhibitors, inducers, substrates
Drug/lab test
Increase: LFTs

NURSING CONSIDERATIONS

Assess:
• **Hepatic failure:** Increased LFTs generally occurred within the first 12 wk of treatment and were reversible with dose interruption. Monitor LFTs q2wk × 3 mo of treatment, then q4wk for 3 mo, and q1-3 mo thereafter; monitor weekly if AST or ALT are >3 times the upper limit of normal (ULN) or bilirubin >1.5 × ULN. Hepatotoxicity may require treatment interruption, dose reduction, or discontinuation of therapy
• **Severe diarrhea/GI perforation:** Generally responds poorly to antimotility agents. The occurrence of ≥7 stools/day over baseline or hospitalization due to diarrhea may result in interruption of therapy, dose reduction, or permanent discontinuation. Assess for new or worsening abdominal pain, chills, fever, or nausea/vomiting. If intestinal perforation occurs, permanently discontinue treatment
• **Pneumonitis:** Monitor for cough, dyspnea, hypoxia, and bilateral interstitial infiltrates, or a decline in oxygen saturation by >5%. If pneumonitis is suspected, hold therapy. Permanently discontinue treatment for pneumonitis and consider treatment with corticosteroids
Evaluate:
• Therapeutic response
Teach patient/family:
• To report planned or suspected pregnancy (D), use effective contraception during treatment and for at least 1 month after the last dose
• Avoid breastfeeding
• To report new or worsening side effects

⚠ HIGH ALERT

ifosfamide (Rx)
(i-foss′fa-mide)
Ifex
Func. class.: Antineoplastic alkylating agent
Chem. class.: Nitrogen mustard

Do not confuse:
ifosfamide/cyclophosphamide

ACTION: Alkylates DNA, inhibits enzymes that allow synthesis of amino acids in proteins; also responsible for cross-linking DNA strands; activity is not cell-cycle–stage specific

USES: Testicular cancer
Unlabeled uses: Soft-tissue sarcoma, Ewing's sarcoma, non-Hodgkin's lymphoma, lung/pancreatic sarcoma, bladder, breast, cervical, thymic cancer, desmoid tumor, Ewing's sarcoma, rhabdomyosarcoma

CONTRAINDICATIONS: Pregnancy (D), hypersensitivity

Black Box Warning: Bone marrow suppression

Precautions: Breastfeeding, children, renal/hepatic disease, accidental exposure, dehydration, dental disease, infection, IM injection, ocular exposure varicella

Black Box Warning: Coma, hemorrhagic cystitis

DOSAGE AND ROUTES
- **Adult: IV** 1.2-2 g/m^2/day × 5 days, repeat course q3wk, given with mesna, in combination with 1-2 other antineoplastic agents

Renal dose
- **Adult: IV** CCr 31-60 ml/min, give 75% of dose; CCr 10-30 ml/min, give 50% of dose; CCr <10 ml/min, do not give

Available forms: Inj 1-, 3-g vials
Administer:
- Antiemetic 30-60 min before product to prevent vomiting
- Visually inspect parenteral products for particulate matter and discoloration before use
- Store powder at room temperature

IV route
- Give as an intermittent infusion or continuous infusion
- Well hydrate with ≥2 L/day of oral or IV fluids to prevent bladder toxicity
- Must be given in combination with mesna to prevent hemorrhagic cystitis
- Close hematologic monitoring is recommended; WBC count, platelet count, and hemoglobin should be obtained before each use and periodically thereafter
- A urinalysis should be performed before each dose to monitor for hematuria

Reconstitution and further dilution:
- Reconstitute 1 or 3 g with 20 or 60 ml, respectively, of sterile water for injection or bacteriostatic water for injection containing parabens or benzyl alcohol to give IV solutions containing 50 mg/ml
- Solutions may be diluted further to achieve concentrations of 0.6-20 mg/ml in the following solutions: D_5W, NS, LR, or sterile water for injection
- Infuse slowly over at least 30 min
- Diluted and reconstituted solutions must be refrigerated and used within 24 hr

Y-site compatibilities: Acyclovir, alatrofloxacin, alemtuzumab, alfentanil, allopurinol, amifostine, amikacin, aminocaproic acid, aminophylline, amiodarone amphotericin B cholesteryl (amphotec), amphotericin B conventional colloidal, amphotericin B lipid complex (abelcet), amphotericin B liposome (ambisome), ampicillin, ampicillin-sulbactam, anidulafungin, argatroban, arsenic trioxide, atenolol, atracurium, azithromycin, aztreonam, bivalirudin, bleomycin, bumetanide, buprenorphine, butorphanol, calcium chloride/gluconate, CARBOplatin, caspofungin, ceFAZolin, cefoperazone, cefotaxime, cefoTEtan, cefOXitin, cefTAZidime, ceftazidime (L-arginine), ceftizoxime, cefTRIAXone, cefuroxime, chlorproMAZINE, cimetidine, ciprofloxacin, cisatracurium, CISplatin, clindamycin, codeine, cycloSPORINE, cytarabine, DACTINomycin, DAPTOmycin, DAUNOrubicin liposome, dexamethasone phosphate, dexmedetomidine, dexrazoxane, digoxin, diltiazem, diphenhydrAMINE, DOBUTamine, DOCEtaxel, dolasetron, DOPamine, doripenem, doxacurium, DOXOrubicin, DOXOrubicin liposomal, doxycycline, droperidol, enalaprilat, ePHEDrine, EPINEPHrine, epirubicin, ertapenem, erythromycin, esmolol, etoposide, etoposide phosphate, famotidine, fenoldopam, fentaNYL, filgrastim, fluconazole, fludarabine, fluorouracil, foscarnet, fosphenytoin, furosemide, gallium nitrate, ganciclovir, gatifloxacin, gemcitabine, gemtuzumab, gentamicin, granisetron, haloperidol, heparin, hydrocortisone phosphate/succinate, HYDROmorphone, hydrOXYzine, IDArubicin, imipenem-cilastatin, inamrinone, insulin (regular), isoproterenol, ketorolac, labetalol, lansoprazole, lepirudin, leucovorin, levofloxacin, levorphanol, lidocaine, linezolid, LORazepam, magnesium sulfate, mannitol, melphalan, meperidine, meropenem, mesna, methohexital, methylPREDNISolone, metoclopramide, metoprolol, metroNIDAZOLE, midazolam, milrinone, minocycline, mitoMYcin, mitoXANtrone, mivacurium, morphine, moxifloxacin, nalbuphine, naloxone, nesiritide, niCARdipine, nitroglycerin, nitroprusside, norepinephrine, octreotide, ofloxacin, ondansetron, oxaliplatin, PACLitaxel (solvent/surfactant), palonosetron, pamidronate, pancuronium, PEMEtrexed, pentamidine, PENTobarbital, PHENobarbital, phenylephrine, piperacillin, piperacillin-tazobactam, potassium acetate/chloride, procainamide, prochlorperazine, promethazine, propofol, propranolol, quinupristin-dalfopristin, ranitidine, rapacuronium, remifentanil, riTUXimab, rocuronium, sargramostim, sodium acetate/, bicarbonate/phosphates, succinylcholine, SUFentanil, sulfamethoxazole-trimethoprim, tacrolimus, teniposide, theophylline, thiopental s, thiotepa, ticarcillin, ticarcillin -clavulanate, tigecycline, tirofiban, tna (3-in-1), tobramycin, topotecan, tpn (2-in-1), trastuzumab, vancomycin, vasopressin, vecuronium, verapamil, vinBLAStine, vinCRIStine, vinorelbine, voriconazole, zidovudine, zoledronic acid

SIDE EFFECTS

CNS: Facial paresthesia, fever, malaise, somnolence, confusion, depression, hallucinations, dizziness, disorientation, seizures, coma, cranial nerve dysfunction, encephalopathy

GI: Nausea, vomiting, anorexia, hepatotoxicity, stomatitis, dyslipidemia, hyperglycemia, constipation, diarrhea

GU: Hematuria, nephrotoxicity, hemorrhagic cystitis, dysuria, urinary frequency

HEMA: Thrombocytopenia, leukopenia, anemia, retrograde ejaculation

INTEG: Dermatitis, alopecia, pain at inj site, hyperpigmentation

META: Metabolic acidosis

PHARMACOKINETICS

Metabolized by liver, saturation occurs at high doses, excreted in urine, half-life 7-15 hr, depends on dose

INTERACTIONS

Increase: myelosuppression—other antineoplastics, radiation

Increase: toxicity—CYP3A4, a weak P-gp inhibitor, inducers, barbiturates, allopurinol

Increase: bleeding risk—NSAIDs, anticoagulants, salicylates, thrombolytics

Decrease: antibody response—live virus vaccines

Decrease: effect of ifosfamide—CYP3A4 inhibitors

• Do not use within 24 hr of hematopoietic progenitor cells

NURSING CONSIDERATIONS

Assess:

• Hepatic studies before, during therapy (bilirubin, AST, ALT, LDH) monthly or as needed; jaundice of skin and sclera, dark urine, clay-colored stools, itchy skin, abdominal pain, fever, diarrhea

Black Box Warning: CBC, differential, platelet count weekly; withhold product if WBC <2000 or platelet count <50,000; notify prescriber; severe myelosuppression may occur

• Monitor temperature (may indicate beginning infection)

• Blood dyscrasias (anemia, granulocytopenia); bruising, fatigue, bleeding, poor healing

• Allergic reactions: dermatitis, exfoliative dermatitis, pruritus, urticaria

Black Box Warning: I&O ratio; monitor for hematuria; hemorrhagic cystitis can occur; increase fluids to 3 L/day; urinalysis before each dose, not to give at night

Black Box Warning: Neurologic symptoms: hallucinations, confusion, disorientation, coma; product should be discontinued

• Bleeding: hematuria, guaiac, bruising or petechiae, mucosa or orifices

Evaluate:

• Therapeutic response: decrease in size and spread of tumor

Teach patient/family:

• To notify prescriber of sore throat, swollen lymph nodes, malaise, fever; other infections may occur, to discuss encephalopathy, neurotoxicity

• Not to have live virus vaccinations during or for 3 mo-1 yr after treatment

• That hair may be lost during treatment; that wig or hairpiece may make the patient feel better; that new hair may be different in color, texture

• To report signs of anemia: fatigue, headache, faintness, SOB, irritability

• To report bleeding; to avoid use of razors, commercial mouthwash

• To avoid use of aspirin products, NSAIDs, ibuprofen because hemorrhage can occur

• To notify prescriber if pregnancy is planned or suspected, pregnancy (D)

• To use contraceptive measures during therapy; not to breastfeed

• To avoid crowds, persons with infections

• To report confusion, hallucinations, extreme drowsiness, numbness, tingling; to avoid alcohol use for ≥4 mo after treatment

• To avoid driving, hazardous activities until reaction is known

• To use excessive fluids and urinate often to prevent hemorrhagic cystitis

iloperidone (Rx)

(ill-o-pehr′ih-dohn)

Fanapt

Func. class.: Antipsychotic

Chem. class.: Benzisoxazole derivative

ACTION:
Unknown; may be mediated through both DOPamine type 2 (D2) and serotonin type 2 (5-HT2) antagonism, high receptor binding affinity for norepinephrine (alpha 1)

USES:
Schizophrenia

CONTRAINDICATIONS:
Breastfeeding, hypersensitivity

Precautions: Pregnancy (C), children, geriatric patients, renal/hepatic disease, breast cancer, Parkinson's disease, dementia with Lewy bodies, seizure disorder, QT prolongation, bundle branch block, acute MI, ambient temperature increase, AV block, stroke, substance abuse, suicidal ideation, tardive dyskinesia, torsade de pointes, blood dyscrasias, dysphagia

Black Box Warning: Increased mortality in elderly patients with dementia-related psychosis

DOSAGE AND ROUTES

- **Adult: PO** 1 mg bid, may increase to target dose of 6-12 mg bid with daily dose adjustment of max 2 mg bid, titrate slowly; max 24 mg/day in 2 divided doses; reduce dose by 50% in patient who is a poor metabolizer of CYP2D6 or when used with strong CYP2D6/CYP3A4 inhibitors

Available forms: Tabs 1, 2, 4, 6, 8, 10, 12 mg; titration pack

Administer:

- Use without regard to meals
- Reduced dose in geriatric patients
- Anticholinergic agent for EPS
- Avoid use with CNS depressants
- Store in tight, light-resistant container

SIDE EFFECTS

CNS: *EPS, pseudoparkinsonism, akathisia, dystonia, tardive dyskinesia; drowsiness,* seizures, neuroleptic malignant syndrome, dizziness, delirium, depression, paranoia, fatigue, hostility, lethargy, restlessness, vertigo, tremor

CV: Orthostatic hypotension, heart failure, AV block, QT prolongation, tachycardia

EENT: Blurred vision, cataracts, nystagmus, tinnitus

GI: *Nausea,* vomiting, *anorexia, constipation,* jaundice, weight gain/loss, abdominal pain, stomatitis, xerostomia

GU: Hyperprolactinemia, urinary retention/incontinence, testicular pain, renal failure

HEMA: Agranulocytosis, leukopenia, neutropenia

MISC: Renal artery occlusion, hyperglycemia, dyslipidemia

PHARMACOKINETICS

PO: Extensively metabolized by liver to major active metabolite by CYP2D6, CYP3A4; protein binding 95%; peak 2-4 hr; excreted in urine and feces; terminal half-life 18 hr in extensive metabolizers; 33 hr in poor metabolizers

INTERACTIONS

Increase: serotonin syndrome, neuroleptic malignant syndrome—SSRIs, SNRI

Increase: sedation—other CNS depressants, alcohol

Increase: iloperidone effect, decreased clearance—CYP2D6, CYP3A4 inhibitors (delavirdine, indinavir, isoniazid, itraconazole, dalfopristin, ritonavir, tipranavir), reduce dose

Increase: QT prolongation—class IA/III antidysrhythmics, some phenothiazines, β-agonists, local anesthetics, tricyclics, haloperidol, methadone, chloroquine, clarithromycin, droperidol, erythromycin, pentamidine

Decrease: iloperidone action—CYP2D6, CYP3A4 inducers (carBAMazepine, barbiturates, phenytoins, rifampin)

Drug/Lab Test

Increase: prolactin levels, cholesterol, glucose, lipids, triglycerides

Decrease: potassium

NURSING CONSIDERATIONS

Assess:

- AIMS assessment, lipid panel, blood glucose, CBC, glycosylated hemoglobin A1c, LFTs, neurologic function, pregnancy test, serum creatinine, electrolytes, prolactin, thyroid function studies, weight
- Affect, orientation, LOC, reflexes, gait, coordination, sleep-pattern disturbances
- B/P standing and lying; pulse, respirations; q4hr during initial treatment; establish baseline before starting treatment; report drops of 30 mm Hg; watch for ECG changes; QT prolongation may occur; dizziness, faintness, palpitations, tachycardia on rising
- EPS, including akathisia, tardive dyskinesia (bizarre movements of the jaw, mouth, tongue, extremities), pseudoparkinsonism (rigidity, tremors, pill rolling, shuffling gait)

Black Box Warning: Serious reactions in geriatric patients: fatal pneumonia, heart failure, sudden death, not to be used in the elderly with dementia

Black Box Warning: Neuroleptic malignant syndrome: hyperthermia, increased CPK, altered mental status, muscle rigidity

- Constipation, urinary retention daily; if these occur, increase bulk and water in diet
- Weight gain, hyperglycemia, metabolic changes in diabetes
- Supervised ambulation until patient is stabilized on medication; do not involve patient in strenuous exercise program because fainting is possible; patient should not stand still for long periods
- Sips of water, candy, gum for dry mouth

Evaluate:

- Therapeutic response: decrease in emotional excitement, hallucinations, delusions, paranoia; reorganization of patterns of thought, speech

Teach patient/family:

- That orthostatic hypotension may occur; to rise from sitting or lying position gradually
- To avoid hot tubs, hot showers, tub baths because hypotension may occur; that heat stroke may occur in hot weather; to take extra precautions to stay cool
- To avoid abrupt withdrawal of product because EPS may result; that product should be withdrawn slowly, to review symptoms of neuroleptic malignant syndrome
- To avoid OTC preparations (cough, hay fever, cold) unless approved by prescriber because serious product interactions may occur; to avoid use of alcohol because increased drowsiness may occur
- To avoid hazardous activities if drowsy or dizzy
- To comply with product regimen
- To report impaired vision, tremors, muscle twitching
- To use contraception; to inform prescriber if pregnancy is planned or suspected

TREATMENT OF OVERDOSE:

Lavage if orally ingested; provide airway; *do not induce vomiting*

⚠ HIGH ALERT

imatinib (Rx)

(im-ah-tin′ib)

Gleevec

Func. class.: Antineoplastic—miscellaneous

Chem. class.: Protein-tyrosine kinase inhibitor

ACTION:

Inhibits Bcr-Abl tyrosine kinase created in patients with chronic myeloid leukemia (CML), also inhibits tyrosine kinases

USES:

Treatment of CML; Philadelphia-chromosome–positive (Ph+) patients in blast-cell crisis or patients in chronic failure; gastrointestinal stromal tumors (GIST) positive for c-Kit; chronic eosinophilic leukemia, Ph+ acute lymphocytic leukemia, dermatofibrosarcoma protuberans, myelodysplastic syndrome, systemic mastocytosis

Unlabeled uses: Desmoid tumor

CONTRAINDICATIONS:

Pregnancy (D), hypersensitivity

Precautions: Breastfeeding, children, geriatric patients, cardiac/renal/hepatic/dental disease, GI bleeding, bone marrow suppression, infection, thrombocytopenia, neutropenia, immunosuppression

DOSAGE AND ROUTES

For the treatment of Ph+ CML chronic phase as initial therapy

- **Adult: PO** 400 mg/day, continue as long as beneficial; may increase to 600 mg/day in the absence of severe adverse reactions and severe non–leukemia-related neutropenia or thrombocytopenia

• **Adolescent/child >2 yr: PO** 340 mg/m²/day, max 600 mg/day; the daily dose may be given as a single dose or split into 2 doses given once in the morning and once in the evening

Adult with Ph+ CML in chronic phase after the failure of interferon-alfa therapy

• **Adult: PO** 400 mg every day; continue as long as beneficial, may increase to 600 mg/day

Pediatric patients with Ph+ chronic phase CML whose disease has recurred after hematopoietic stem cell transplant or who are resistant to interferon-alfa therapy

• **Adolescent/child >3 yr: PO** 260 mg/m²/day as a single daily dose, or the dose may be divided given once in the morning and once in the evening; may increase to 340 mg/m²/day

Patients with Ph+ CML in accelerated phase or blast crisis

• **Adult: PO** 600 mg every day, continue as long as beneficial, may increase to 800 mg/day (400 mg bid)

Resistant or relapsed Ph+ acute lymphocytic leukemia (ALL)

• **Adult: PO** 600 mg every day, continue as long as beneficial

***Kit* (CD117)-positive unresectable and/or metastatic GIST**

• **Adult: PO** 400-600 mg every day, may increase to 400 mg bid

Adjuvant treatment of *Kit* (CD117)-positive GIST after complete gross resection

• **Adult: PO** 400 mg/day

Hypereosinophilic syndrome (HES) and/or chronic eosinophilic leukemia (CEL) who have the FIPL1L1-PDGFR α-fusion kinase (mutational analysis or FISH demonstration of CHIC2 allele deletion) and for patients with HES and/or CEL who are FIPL1L-PDGFR α-fusion kinase negative or unknown

• **Adult: PO** 400 mg/day in those who are FIPL1L-PDGFR α-fusion kinase negative or unknown; for HES/CEL patients with demonstrated FIP1L1-PDGFR α-fusion kinase, 100 mg/day, may increase to 400 mg

Myelodysplastic syndrome (MDS)/myeloproliferative disease (MPD) associated with the platelet-derived growth factor receptor (PDGFR) gene rearrangements

• **Adult: PO** 400 mg/day

Aggressive systemic mastocytosis (ASM) without D816V c-Kit mutation or with c-Kit mutation status unknown

• **Adult: PO** 400 mg/day in those without the FIP1L1-PDGFR-α c-Kit mutation; if c-Kit status is unknown or not available, give 400 mg/day

Unresectable, recurrent, and/or metastatic dermatofibrosarcoma protuberans (DFSP)

• **Adult: PO** 400 mg bid (800 mg/day)

Renal dose

• **Adult: PO** CCr 40-59 ml/min, max 600 mg/day; CCr 20-39 ml/min, decrease initial dose by 50%, max 400 mg/day; CCr <20 ml/min, use with caution, 100 mg/day

Hepatic dose

• **Adult: PO** Total bilirubin 1.5-3 × ULN and any AST, decrease initial dose to 400 mg/day; total bilirubin >3 × ULN and any AST, decrease initial dose to 300 mg/day

Available forms: Tabs 100, 400 mg

Administer:

• With meal and large glass of water to decrease GI symptoms; doses of 800 mg should be given as 400 mg bid
• Tab may be dispersed in a glass of water or apple juice, use 50 ml of liquid for 100-mg tab, 200 ml liquid for 400-mg tab
• Continue as long as beneficial
• Store at 77° F (25° C)

SIDE EFFECTS

CNS: CNS hemorrhage, headache, dizziness, insomnia, subdural hematoma

CV: Hemorrhage, heart failure, cardiac tamponade, cardiac toxicity

EENT: Blurred vision, conjunctivitis
GI: *Nausea,* hepatotoxicity, vomiting, dyspepsia, GI hemorrhage, *anorexia, abdominal pain,* GI perforation, diarrhea
HEMA: Neutropenia, thrombocytopenia, bleeding, hypereosinophilia
INTEG: *Rash, pruritus,* alopecia, photosensitivity
META: Fluid retention, hypokalemia, edema
MISC: Fatigue, epistaxis, pyrexia, night sweats, increased weight, flulike symptoms, hypothyroidism
MS: Cramps, pain, arthralgia, myalgia
RESP: Cough, dyspnea, nasopharyngitis, pneumonia, upper respiratory tract infection, pleural effusion, edema

PHARMACOKINETICS

Well absorbed (98%); protein binding 95%; metabolized by CYP3A4; excreted in feces, small amount in urine; peak 2-4 hr; duration 24 hr (imatinib), 40 hr (metabolite); half-life 18-40 hr

INTERACTIONS

Increase: hepatotoxicity—acetaminophen
Increase: imatinib concentrations—CYP3A4 inhibitors (ketoconazole, itraconazole, erythromycin, clarithromycin)
Increase: plasma concentrations of simvastatin, calcium channel blockers, ergots
Increase: plasma concentration of warfarin; avoid use with warfarin; use low-molecular-weight anticoagulants instead
Decrease: imatinib concentrations—CYP3A4 inducers (dexamethasone, phenytoin, carBAMazepine, rifampin, PHENobarbital)

Drug/Herb

Decrease: imatinib concentration—St. John's wort

Drug/Lab Test

Increase: bilirubin, amylase, LFTs
Decrease: albumin, calcium, potassium, sodium, phosphate, platelets, neutrophils, leukocytes, lymphocytes

NURSING CONSIDERATIONS

Assess:

- **Bone marrow suppression:** ANC, platelets; during chronic phase, if ANC $<1 \times 10^9$/L and/or platelets $<50 \times 10^9$/L, stop until ANC $>1.5 \times 10^9$/L and platelets $>75 \times 10^9$/L; during accelerated phase/blast crisis, if ANC $<0.5 \times 10^9$/L and/or platelets $<10 \times 10^9$/L, determine whether cytopenia related to biopsy/aspirate; if not, reduce dose by 200 mg; if cytopenia continues, reduce dose by another 100 mg; if cytopenia continues for 4 wk, stop product until ANC $\geq 1 \times 10^9$/L
- **Renal toxicity:** if bilirubin $>3 \times$ IULN, withhold imatinib until bilirubin levels return to $<1.5 \times$ IULN
- **Hepatotoxicity:** monitor LFTs, before treatment monthly; if liver transaminases $>5 \times$ IULN, withhold imatinib until transaminase levels return to $<2.5 \times$ IULN
- Monitor CBC for first mo, biweekly next mo and periodically thereafter; neutropenia (2-3 wk) and thrombocytopenia (3-4 wk) and anemia may occur; may need dosage decrease or discontinuation
- Signs of fluid retention, edema: weigh, monitor lung sounds, assess for edema; some fluid retention is dose dependent

Evaluate:

- Therapeutic response: decrease in leukemic cells or size of tumor

Teach patient/family:

- To report adverse reactions immediately: shortness of breath, swelling of extremities, bleeding
- About reason for treatment, expected results
- That effect on male infertility is unknown
- Not to stop or change dose—to avoid hazardous activities until response is known, dizziness may occur
- To take with food and water; for those unable to swallow tabs, to mix in liquid (30 m for 100 mg) or 200 ml for 400 mg) after dissolved, stir and consume
- To avoid OTC products unless approved by prescriber

- To notify prescriber if pregnancy is planned or suspected, pregnancy (D), do not breastfeed

imipenem/cilastatin (Rx)

(i-me-pen′em sye-la-stat′in)

Primaxin IM, Primaxin IV

Func. class.: Antiinfective—miscellaneous

Chem. class.: Carbapenem

Do not confuse:
imipenem/Omnipen
Primaxin/Premarin

ACTION: Interferes with cell-wall replication of susceptible organisms; osmotically unstable cell-wall swells, bursts from osmotic pressure; addition of cilastatin prevents renal inactivation that occurs with high urinary concentrations of imipenem

USES: Serious infections caused by gram-positive *Streptococcus pneumoniae,* group A β-hemolytic streptococci, *Staphylococcus aureus,* enterococcus; gram-negative *Klebsiella, Proteus, Escherichia coli, Acinetobacter, Serratia, Pseudomonas aeruginosa, Salmonella, Shigella, Haemophilus influenzae, Listeria* sp.

CONTRAINDICATIONS: Hypersensitivity to this product, amide local anesthetics, or carbapenems; AV block, shock (IM)

Precautions: Pregnancy (C), breastfeeding, children, geriatric patients, seizure disorders, renal disease, head trauma; hypersensitivity to cephalosporins, penicillins; pseudomembranous colitis, ulcerative colitis, diabetes mellitus

DOSAGE AND ROUTES

Doses based on imipenem content

Intraabdominal, gynecologic, lower respiratory tract, skin and skin structure, bone and joint infections; septicemia, endocarditis, febrile neutropenia (unlabeled), and polymicrobial infections for fully susceptible organisms including gram-positive or gram-negative aerobes and anaerobes

- **Adult ≥70 kg: IV** 250 mg every 6 hr (mild infections); 500 mg every 6-8 hr (moderate infections); 500 mg every 6 hr (severe life-threatening infections)
- **Adult 60 kg: IV** 250 mg IV every 8 hr (mild infections); 250 mg every 6 hr (moderate or severe life-threatening infections)
- **Adult 50 kg: IV** 125 mg every 6 hr (mild infections); 250 mg every 6 hr (moderate or severe life-threatening infections)
- **Adult 40 kg: IV** 125 mg every 6 hr (mild infections); 250 mg every 6-8 hr (moderate infections); 250 mg every 6 hr (severe life-threatening infections)
- **Adult 30 kg: IV** 125 mg every 8 hr (mild infections); 125 mg every 6 hr or 250 mg every 8 hr (moderate infections); 250 mg every 8 hr (severe life-threatening infections)
- **Adolescent/child/infant ≥3 mo: IV** 15-25 mg/kg every 6 hr
- **Infant 1-3 mo and ≥1500 g: IV** 25 mg/kg every 6 hr
- **Neonate 1-4 wk and ≥1500 g: IV** 25 mg/kg every 8 hr
- **Neonate <7 days and ≥1500 g: IV** 25 mg/kg every 12 hr

Moderately susceptible organisms, primarily some strains of *P. aeruginosa*

- **Adult ≥70 kg: IV** 500 mg every 6 hr (mild infections); 500 mg every 6 hr or 1 g every 8 hr (moderate infections); 1 g every 6-8 hr (life-threatening infections)
- **Adult 60 kg: IV** 500 mg every 8 hr (mild infections); 500 mg every 8 hr or 750 mg every 8 hr (moderate infections); 0.75-1 g every 8 hr (life-threatening infections)
- **Adult 50 kg: IV** 250 mg every 6 hr (mild infections); 250-500 mg every 6 hr (moderate infections); 500 mg every 6 hr or 750 mg every 8 hr (life-threatening infections)

• **Adult 40 kg: IV** 250 mg every 6 hr (mild infections); 250 mg every 6 hr or 500 mg every 8 hr (moderate infections); 500 mg every 6-8 hr (life-threatening infections)

• **Adult 30 kg: IV** 250 mg every 8 hr (mild infections); 250 mg every 6-8 hr; 250 mg every 6 hr or 500 mg every 8 hr (life-threatening infections)

• **Adolescent/child/infant ≥3 mo: IV** 15-25 mg/kg every 6 hr

• **Infant 1-3 mo weighing ≥1500 g: IV** 25 mg/kg every 6 hr

• **Neonate 1-4 wk weighing ≥1500 g: IV** 25 mg/kg every 8 hr

• **Neonate <7 days weighing ≥1500 g: IV** 25 mg/kg every 12 hr

Mild to moderate lower respiratory tract, skin and skin structure, or gynecologic infections

• **Adult/adolescent/child ≥12 yr: IM** 500 or 750 mg every 12 hr, max 1.5 g/day

Mild to moderate intraabdominal infections, including acute gangrenous or perforated appendicitis and appendicitis with peritonitis

• **Adult/adolescent/child ≥12 yr: IM** 750 mg every 12 hr, max 1.5 g/day

Community-acquired pneumonia (CAP) in ICU patients with risk factors for *Pseudomonas* infection

• Imipenem; cilastatin in combination with ciprofloxacin or an aminoglycoside plus a respiratory fluoroquinolone or an advanced macrolide

• **Adult ≥70 kg: IV** 500 mg every 6-8 hr

• **Adult 60 kg: IV** 250 mg every 6 hr

• **Adult 50 kg: IV** 250 mg every 6 hr

• **Adult 40 kg: IV** 250 mg every 6-8 hr

• **Adult 30 kg: IV** 125 mg every 6 hr or 250 mg every 8 hr

Empiric treatment of aspiration pneumonia

• **Adult: IV** 500-1000 mg every 6 hr × 10 days

Renal dose

• **Adult ≥70 kg (reduce normal dose of 1 g/day to): IV CCr 41-70 ml/min,** 250 mg q8hr; **CCr 6-40 ml/min,** 250 mg q12hr; (reduce normal dose of 1.5 g/day to): **CCr 41-70 ml/min,** 250 mg q6hr; **CCr 21-40 ml/min,** 250 mg q8hr; **CCr 6-20 ml/min,** 250 mg q12hr; (reduce normal dose of 2 g/day to): **CCr 41-70 ml/min,** 500 mg q8hr; **CCr 21-40 ml/min,** 250 mg q6hr; **CCr 6-20 ml/min,** 250 mg q12hr

Available forms: Powder for sol inj 250, 500 mg; powder for inj susp 500 mg

Administer:

• After C&S is taken

IM route

• Reconstitute 500 mg/2 ml lidocaine without EPINEPHrine; shake

• Inject deeply in large muscle, aspirate, **product for IM is not for IV use**

IV route

• After reconstitution of 250 or 500 mg with 10 ml of diluent and shake; add to ≥100 ml of same infusion sol

• 250-500 mg over 20-30 min; ≥750 mg over 40-60 min; give through Y-tube or 3-way stopcock; do not give by IV bolus or if cloudy

Y-site compatibilities: Acyclovir, alfentanil, amifostine, amikacin, aminocaproic acid, anidulafungin, argatroban, ascorbic acid, atenolol, atracurium, atropine, benztropine, bivalirudin, bleomycin, bumetanide, buprenorphine, butorphanol, CARBOplatin, carmustine, caspofungin, ceFAZolin, cefotaxime, cefoTEtan, cefOXitin, ceftazidime, cefuroxime, chloramphenicol, cimetidine, cisatracurium, CISplatin, clindamycin, codeine, cyanocobalamin, cyclophosphamide, cycloSPORINE, cytarabine, DACTINomycin, dexamethasone, dexrazoxane, digoxin, diltiazem, diphenhydrAMINE, DOCEtaxel, dolasetron, DOPamine, doxacurium, DOXOrubicin, DOXOrubicin liposomal, doxycycline, enalaprilat, famotidine, fludarabine, foscarnet, granisetron, IDArubicin, insulin (regular), melphalan, methotrexate, ondansetron, propofol, remifentanil, tacrolimus, teniposide, thiotepa, vinorelbine, zidovudine

SIDE EFFECTS

CNS: Fever, somnolence, seizures, confusion, dizziness, weakness, myoclonus, drowsiness

CV: Hypotension, palpitations, tachycardia
GI: *Diarrhea, nausea, vomiting,* pseudomembranous colitis, hepatitis, glossitis, gastroenteritis, abdominal pain, jaundice
GU: Renal toxicity/failure
HEMA: Agranulocytosis, eosinophilia, neutropenia, decreased Hgb, Hct
INTEG: Rash, urticaria, pruritus, pain at inj site, phlebitis, erythema at inj site, erythema multiform
MISC: Hearing loss, tinnitus, electrolyte abnormalities
RESP: Chest discomfort, dyspnea, hyperventilation
SYST: Anaphylaxis, Stevens-Johnson syndrome, toxic epidermal necrolysis, angioedema

PHARMACOKINETICS

IV: Onset immediate, peak 20 min-1 hr, half-life 1 hr, 70%-80% excreted unchanged in urine

INTERACTIONS

Increase: imipenem plasma levels—probenecid
Increase: antagonistic effect—β-lactam antibiotics
Increase: seizure risk—ganciclovir, theophylline, aminophylline, cycloSPORINE
Decrease: effect of valproic acid

Drug/Lab Test
Increase: AST, ALT, LDH, BUN, alk phos, bilirubin, creatinine, potassium, chloride
Decrease: sodium
False positive: direct Coombs' test

NURSING CONSIDERATIONS

Assess:
- Renal studies: creatinine/BUN, electrolytes
- **Infection:** increased temperature, WBC, characteristics of wounds, sputum, urine or stool culture
- Sensitivity to penicillin, other β-lactams—may have sensitivity to this product
- Renal disease: lower dose may be required
- Bowel pattern daily; if severe diarrhea occurs, product should be discontinued; may indicate pseudomembranous colitis

⚠ **Allergic reactions, anaphylaxis:** rash, urticaria, pruritus, wheezing, laryngeal edema; may occur a few days after therapy begins; have EPINEPHrine, antihistamine, emergency equipment available
- **Overgrowth of infection:** perineal itching, fever, malaise, redness, pain, swelling, drainage, rash, diarrhea, change in cough, sputum

Evaluate:
- Therapeutic response: negative C&S; absence of signs and symptoms of infection

Teach patient/family:

⚠ To report severe diarrhea; may indicate pseudomembranous colitis

⚠ To report sore throat, bruising, bleeding, joint pain; may indicate blood dyscrasias (rare)
- To report seizures, immediately

Treatment of anaphylaxis: EPINEPHrine, antihistamines; resuscitate if needed

imipramine (Rx)

(im-ip′ra-meen)

Impril ✦, Novo-Pramine ✦, Tofranil, Tofranil PM

Func. class.: Antidepressant, tricyclic
Chem. class.: Dibenzazepine, tertiary amine

Do not confuse:
imipramine/desipramine

ACTION: Blocks reuptake of norepinephrine, serotonin into nerve endings, thereby increasing action of norepinephrine, serotonin in nerve cells

USES: Depression, enuresis in children
Unlabeled uses: Chronic pain, migraine headaches, cluster headaches as adjunct, incontinence, ADHD, neuralgia, bulimia, neuropathic pain, social phobia

CONTRAINDICATIONS:
Pregnancy (D), hypersensitivity to this product or carBAMazepine; acute MI

Precautions: Breastfeeding, geriatric patients, suicidal patients, severe depression, increased intraocular pressure, closed-angle glaucoma, urinary retention, cardiac/hepatic disease, hyperthyroidism, electroshock therapy, elective surgery, seizure disorders, prostatic hypertrophy, MI, AV block, bundle branch block, ileus, QT prolongation, hypersensitivity to tricyclics

Black Box Warning: Children other than for enuresis; suicidal ideation

DOSAGE AND ROUTES

Depression

- **Adult: PO** 75-100 mg/day in divided doses, may increase by 25-50 mg to 200 mg/day (outpatients), 300 mg/day (inpatients); may give daily dose at bedtime
- **Geriatric: PO** 30-40 mg at bedtime, may increase to 100 mg/day in divided doses
- **Child ≥6 yr (unlabeled): PO** 1.5 mg/kg/day in divided doses, max 2.5 mg/kg/day

Enuresis

- **Child 6-12 yr: PO** 10-25 mg at bedtime, max 50 mg

Social phobia/panic disorder (unlabeled)

- **Adult: PO** 10 mg at bedtime, titrate q2-4days to 100-200 mg/day

Overactive bladder (OAB) (unlabeled)

- **Adult: PO** 10-50 mg daily, may titrate to 150 mg/day

Available forms: Tabs 10, 25, 50 mg; caps 75, 100, 125, 150 mg

Administer:

PO route

- Not to break, crush, or chew caps
- With food or milk for GI symptoms
- Dosage at bedtime if oversedation occurs during day; may take entire dose at bedtime; geriatric patients may not tolerate once-daily dosing
- Sugarless gum, hard candy, or frequent sips of water for dry mouth
- Store in tight container at room temperature; do not freeze

SIDE EFFECTS

CNS: *Dizziness, drowsiness,* confusion, **seizures**, headache, anxiety, tremors, stimulation, weakness, insomnia, nightmares, EPS (geriatric patients), increased psychiatric symptoms, paresthesia, ataxia

CV: *Orthostatic hypotension, ECG changes, tachycardia,* hypertension, palpitations, **dysrhythmias**

EENT: Blurred vision, tinnitus, mydriasis

ENDO: Hyperglycemia, hypo/hyperthyroidism, goiter, SIADH

GI: *Diarrhea, dry mouth,* nausea, vomiting, **paralytic ileus**; increased appetite; cramps, epigastric distress, jaundice, **hepatitis**, stomatitis, constipation, taste change, weight gain

GU: *Retention,* **acute renal failure**, impotence, decreased libido

HEMA: **Agranulocytosis, thrombocytopenia, eosinophilia, leukopenia**

INTEG: Rash, urticaria, sweating, pruritus, photosensitivity; hyperpigmentation (rare)

PHARMACOKINETICS

Steady-state 2-5 days; metabolized to desipramine by liver; excreted in urine, breast milk, feces; crosses placenta; half-life 6-20 hr

INTERACTIONS

⚠ **Hyperpyretic crisis, seizures, hypertensive episode: MAOIs, cloNIDine**

⚠ **Increase: serotonin syndrome, neuroleptic malignant syndrome—SSRIs, SNRIs, serotonin-receptor agonists; avoid concurrent use, linezolid, methylene blue IV**

Increase: QT interval—class IA/III antidysrhythmics, tricyclics, gatifloxacin, levofloxacin, moxifloxacin, ziprasidone

Increase: effects of direct-acting sympathomimetics (EPINEPHrine), alcohol, barbiturates, benzodiazepines, CNS depressants

Decrease: effects of guanethidine, cloNIDine, indirect-acting sympathomimetics (ePHEDrine)

Drug/Herb

Increase: serotonin syndrome—SAM-e, St. John's wort

Drug/Lab Test

Increase: serum bilirubin, alk phos, blood glucose, LFTs

Decrease: 5-HIAA, VMA, urinary catecholamines

NURSING CONSIDERATIONS

Assess:

- B/P (lying, standing), pulse q4hr; if systolic B/P drops 20 mm Hg, hold product, notify prescriber; take vital signs q4hr in patients with CV disease
- Blood studies: CBC, leukocytes, differential, cardiac enzymes, serum imipramine levels (125-250 ng/ml) if patient is receiving long-term therapy
- Hepatic studies: AST, ALT, bilirubin
- Weight weekly; appetite may increase with product

⚠ **QT prolongation:** ECG for flattening of T wave, bundle branch block, AV block, dysrhythmias in cardiac patients

- EPS primarily in geriatric patients: rigidity, dystonia, akathisia

Black Box Warning: Mental status: mood, sensorium, affect, suicidal tendencies especially in children, young adults; increase in psychiatric symptoms: depression, panic

- Urinary retention, constipation; constipation is more likely to occur in children, geriatric patients; increase fluids, bulk in diet

⚠ **Withdrawal symptoms:** headache, nausea, vomiting, muscle pain, weakness, diarrhea, insomnia, restlessness; not usual unless product is discontinued abruptly

- Serotonin syndrome, hypertensive episodes, identify drug interactions before use of product
- Alcohol consumption; if alcohol is consumed, hold dose until morning
- Assistance with ambulation during beginning therapy because drowsiness, dizziness, orthostatic hypotension occurs
- Safety measures, primarily for geriatric patients

Evaluate:

- Therapeutic response: decreased depression, enuresis, pain

Teach patient/family:

- That therapeutic effects may take 2-3 wk
- That product is dispensed in small amounts because of suicide potential, especially at beginning of therapy
- To use caution when driving, performing other activities requiring alertness because of drowsiness, dizziness, blurred vision
- To report urinary retention immediately
- To avoid alcohol, other CNS depressants during treatment
- Not to discontinue medication abruptly after long-term use; may cause nausea, headache, malaise
- To wear sunscreen or large hat because photosensitivity occurs
- To rise slowly, orthostatic hypotension may occur

Black Box Warning: To report suicidal thoughts, behaviors immediately, more common in children, young adults

TREATMENT OF OVERDOSE:

ECG monitoring; lavage, activated charcoal; administer anticonvulsant

immune globulin IM (IMIG/IGIM) (Rx)

Bay Gam 15%, Flebogamma 5%, Flebogamma DIF 5%, Gammagard, GamaSTAN S/D, Gamunex 10%, Privigen 10%, Vivaglobin 10%

immune globulin IV (IGIV, IVIG) (Rx)

Bay Gam 15%, Carimune NF, Flebogamma 5%, Flebogamma 10% DIF, Gammagard S/D, Gammagard Liquid 10%, Gammaked, Gammaplex, Gammar-P IV, Gamunex, Iveegam EN, Octagam, Polygam S/D, Privigen, Vivaglobin

immune globulin SC (SCIG/IGSC)

Bay Gam 15%, Flebogamma 5%, Flebogamma DIF 5%, Gammagard 10%, Gammaked, Gammaplex, Gamunex 10%, Privigen 10%, Vivaglobin, Hizentra

Func. class.: Immune serum
Chem. class.: IgG

ACTION: Provides passive immunity to hepatitis A, measles, varicella, rubella, immune globulin deficiency; contains gamma globulin antibodies (IgG)

USES: Immunodeficiency syndrome; B-cell chronic lymphocytic leukemia; Kawasaki syndrome; bone marrow transplantation; pediatric HIV infection; agammaglobulinemia; hepatitis A, B exposure; measles exposure; measles vaccine complications; purpura; rubella exposure; chickenpox exposure; chronic inflammatory demyelinating polyneuropathy, multifocal motor neuropathy

Unlabeled uses: IV posttransfusion purpura, Guillain-Barré syndrome, refractory pemphigus vulgaris, West Nile virus, meningitis, myasthenia gravis, thrombocytopenia encephalitis, HIV, cytomegalovirus, neonatal jaundice, RSV infection, primary humoral immunodeficiency, refractory pemphigus vulgaris

CONTRAINDICATIONS: Hypersensitivity, coagulopathy, hemophilia, IgA deficiency, thrombocytopenia

Precautions: Pregnancy (C), breastfeeding, children, agammaglobulinemia, bleeding, hypogammaglobulinemia, infection, IV, viral infection

DOSAGE AND ROUTES

Immune globulin IM (IMIG, IGIM)

Hepatitis A prophylaxis

- **Adult/geriatric/adolescent/child/infant (unlabeled): IM** 0.02 ml/kg for those who have not received hepatitis A vaccine and been exposed during the prior 2 wk

Measles prophylaxis (exposed during prior 6 days)

- **Adult: IM** 0.25 ml/kg (immunocompetent)
- **Child (unlabeled): IM** 0.5 ml/kg as a single dose, max 15 ml (immunocompromised)

Varicella prophylaxis

- **Adult: IM** 0.6-1.2 ml/kg as soon as possible and if varicella-zoster immune globulin is not available

Rubella prophylaxis in exposed/susceptible individual who will not consider a therapeutic abortion

- **Adult pregnant women: IM** 0.55 ml/kg

Immunoglobulin deficiency

- **Adult: IM** 1.32 ml/kg, then 0.66 ml/kg ($\geq$100 mg/kg) q3-4wk

Immune globulin IV (IVIG, IGIV)

Primary immunodeficiency

Gammagard S/D

- **Adult/adolescent/child: IV** 300-600 mg/kg q3-4wk

Polygam S/D

- **Adult/adolescent/child: IV** 100 mg/kg/mo; initially 200-400 mg/kg may be used

Gammar-P IV

- **Adult: IV** 200-400 mg/kg q3-4wk
- **Adolescent/child: IV** 200 mg/kg q3-4wk

Gamunex

- **Adult/adolescent/child: IV INFUSION** 300-600 mg/kg (3-6 ml/kg) q3-4wk, initial infusion rate 1 mg/kg/min (max 8 mg/kg/min)

Iveegam EN

- **Adult/adolescent/child: IV** 200 mg/kg monthly, max 800 mg/kg/mo

Carimune NF

- **Adult/adolescent/child: IV** 200 mg/kg/mo

Gamagard liquid/Flebogamma 5%

- **Adult/adolescent/child: IV** 300-600 mg/kg q3-4wk

Privigen

- **Adult/adolescent/child ≥3 yr: IV** 200-800 mg q3wk

Idiopathic thrombocytopenic purpura (ITP)

Carimune NF

- **Adult/child: IV** 400 mg/kg daily × 2-5 days; with acute ITP of childhood, only 2 of 5 days are needed if initial platelets are 30,000-50,000 mcl after 2 doses

Gammagard S/D/Polygam S/D

- **Adult/adolescent/child: IV** 1000 mg/kg as a single dose; may give on alternate days for up to 3 doses

Gamunex

- **Adult/adolescent/child: IV INFUSION** total dose of 2000 mg/kg on 2 consecutive days; initial rate is 1 mg/kg/min (max 8 mg/kg/min); if after 1st dose adequate platelets are observed after 24 hr, may withhold 2nd dose

Privigen

- **Adult/adolescent ≥15 yr: IV** 1 g/kg/day × 2 days

Kawasaki disease

Iveegam EN

- **Child: IV** 400 mg/kg daily × 4 consecutive days or a single dose of 2000 mg/kg over 10 hr, given with aspirin 100 mg/kg/day through 14th day of illness, then 3-5 mg/kg each day thereafter for 5 wk

Gammagard S/D/Polygam S/D

- **Infant/child: IV** 1000 mg/kg as a single dose or 400 mg/kg/day × 4 days beginning within 7 days of fever onset, with aspirin 80-100 mg/kg/day × 4 divided doses

Immune globulin SC (SCIG/IGSC)

- **Adult/child >2 yr: SUBCUT INFUSION** 100-200 mg/kg weekly, **Vivaglobin** brand of SCIG 160 mg IgG/ml, **SUBCUT** inj 15 ml/inj site, given at max of 20 ml/hr

Hizentra

- **Adult/child:** multiply the previous IVIG dose by 1.37, then divide into wk dose based on previous wk treatment

Available forms: IM: Inj 2-, 10-ml vial (Bay Gam); **IV:** 5%, 10% sol (Gamimune N); powder for inj 1-, 3-, 6-, 12-g vials (Carimune NF); 50 mg protein/ml in 2.5-, 5-, 10-g vials (Gammagard S/D); 1-, 2.5-, 5-, 10-g vials (Gammar-P IV); 500 mg, 1-, 2.5-, 5-g vials (Iveegam); 6-, 12-g vials (Panglobulin); 2.5-, 5-, 10-g vials (Polygam S/D); sol for inj 1-, 2.5-, 5-, 10-, 20-g vials (Gamunex); Human sol for inj: Flebogamma 5%, 10% DIF; subcut inj 10, 16, 20% single use

Administer:

- IM ≤3 ml at 1 site; use large muscle mass
- Only with EPINEPHrine 1:1000, resuscitative equipment available
- Only within 2 wk of exposure to hepatitis A
- Store at 36° F-46° F (2° C-8° C)

IV route

- **Gamimune N:** IV undiluted or dilute with D_5W; give 0.01 ml/kg/min; may increase to 0.02-0.04 ml/kg/min
- **Venoglobulin-I:** (50 mg/ml sol) give 0.01-0.02 ml/kg/min; if no adverse reaction within ½ hr, increase to 0.04 ml/kg/min; store at room temperature
- **Gammagard:** reconstitute with sterile water for inj (50 mg protein/ml); give 0.5 ml/kg/hr, may increase to 4 ml/kg/hr; use infusion set provided
- **Gammar-IV:** give 0.01 ml/kg/min (50 mg/ml sol) × 15-30 min, may

increase to 0.02 ml/kg/min, may increase to 0.03-0.06 ml/kg/min

Y-site compatibilities: Fluconazole, sargramostim

SIDE EFFECTS

CNS: Headache, fatigue, malaise
GI: Abdominal pain
HEMA: **Thromboembolism (Vivaglobin)**
INTEG: Pain at inj site, rash, pruritus, chills
MS: Arthralgia, chest pain
SYST: Lymphadenopathy, **anaphylaxis; life-threatening hypoglycemia (Octagam 5, 10%)**

INTERACTIONS

• Do not administer live virus vaccines within 3 mo of this product

Drug/Lab Test

Interference: glucose testing system

NURSING CONSIDERATIONS

Assess:

• **Exposure date:** this product should be given within 6 days of measles, 7 days of hepatitis B, 14 days of hepatitis A

• **Anaphylaxis: diaphoresis, wheezing, chest tightness, hypotension**

Evaluate:

• Prevention of infection, increased platelets

Teach patient/family:

• That passive immunity is temporary

• **About the treatment of anaphylaxis: EPINEPHrine, diphenhydrAMINE, oxygen, vasopressors, corticosteroids**

indacaterol

(in-da-kat′er-ol)

Arcapta Neohaler

Func. class.: β-2 agonist, long-acting respiratory

ACTION:

An agonist at β-2 receptors. These receptors are present in large numbers in the lungs and are located on bronchiolar smooth muscle. Stimulation of β-2 receptors in the lung causes relaxation of bronchial smooth muscle, which produces bronchodilation and an increase in bronchial airflow. These effects may be mediated, in part, by increased activity of adenyl cyclase, an intracellular enzyme responsible for the formation of cyclic-3′,5′-adenosine monophosphate (cAMP); has >24-fold agonist activity at β-2 receptors (primarily in the lung) compared to β-1 receptors (primarily in the heart)

USES:

Bronchitis, chronic obstructive pulmonary disease (COPD), emphysema

CONTRAINDICATIONS:

Acute bronchospasm, acute asthma attack, status asthmaticus, acute respiratory insufficiency, monotherapy of asthma, hypersensitivity

Precautions: Ischemic cardiac disease (coronary artery disease), hypertension, cardiac arrhythmias, tachycardia, QT prolongation, congenital long QT syndrome, torsades de pointes history, hyperthyroidism (thyrotoxicosis, thyroid disease), pheochromocytoma, unusual responsiveness to other sympathomimetic amines, seizure disorder, diabetes mellitus, hypokalemia, milk protein hypersensitivity, severe hepatic disease; not indicated for neonates, infants, children, or adolescents under the age of 18 yr, pregnancy (C), breastfeeding

Black Box Warning: Asthma-related deaths

DOSAGE AND ROUTES

• **Adult: INH** 75 mcg (contents of 1 capsule) inhaled once daily; administer at the same time every day, max 1 dose in 24 hours

Available forms: Powder for inhalation 75 mcg

Administer:

Inhalation route

• For oral inhalation use only; DO NOT swallow the capsules; always use the Neohaler Inhaler; this inhaler should not

be used with any other products; DO NOT use with a spacer
• Use dry hands to remove a capsule from the blister pack immediately before use and place into the capsule chamber of the Neohaler Inhaler; click closed; do not place capsule into the mouthpiece; then, holding the inhaler upright, depress buttons fully once to pierce capsule, a click will be heard; have patient breathe out fully away from inhaler, place inhaler in the mouth with buttons positioned to the left and right (not up and down), close lips around mouthpiece, then breathe deeply, rapidly, and steadily in through the inhaler; a whirring sound should be heard; if no sound is heard, check the chamber because the capsule may be stuck; gently tap the base of the device to loosen capsule, if necessary; after inhalation, patient should hold the breath as long as comfortable while removing inhaler from the mouth; check the chamber to see if any powder remains in the capsule; repeat inhalation steps until no powder remains; most patients empty the capsule in 1 or 2 inhalations; after administration, open chamber and discard empty capsule
• Advise patient that coughing after administration is not problematic; as long as the capsule is empty the full dose has been administered
• The gelatin capsule might break into small pieces that pass through the inhaler screen and reach the mouth; accidental inhalation or ingestion of these pieces is harmless; piercing capsule more than once increases risk of shattering capsule: do not wash inhaler; keep it dry; a clean, dry, lint-free cloth may be used to wipe out the inhaler
• Use the new inhaler provided with each new prescription
• To avoid the spread of infection, do not share inhaler

SIDE EFFECTS

CNS: Headache, tremor
CV: Sinus tachycardia, hypertension, QT prolongation and ST-T wave changes, prolonged QTc (an increase of >60 ms from baseline), nonsustained ventricular tachycardia, supraventricular tachycardia (SVT) episodes, intermittent ectopic atrial rhythm
ENDO: Hyperglycemia
GI: Nausea, dry mouth (xerostomia)
META: Hypokalemia
MS: Muscle cramps/spasm, musculoskeletal pain
RESP: Paradoxical bronchospasm, cough, dyspnea, sputum purulence or volume, wheezing, nasopharyngitis, pneumonia, sinusitis and upper respiratory tract infection

PHARMACOKINETICS:

Protein binding 94%-96%, approximately 1/3 of total drug-related AUC over 24 hours, a hydroxylated derivative, glucuronate and dealkylate metabolites are present; metabolized by CYP3A4, CYP1A1, CYP2D6, UGT1A1; elimination multiphasic with terminal half-life of 45.5-126 hours; excreted renally (2%-6%), fecally (>90%); onset 5 min, peak 15 min, steady-state 12-15 days

INTERACTIONS:

Increase QT prolongation: Class IA/III antiarrhythmics, flecainide, propafenone some antipsychotics (phenothiazines, pimozide, haloperidol risperiDONE, sertindole ziprasidone), amoxapine, arsenic trioxide, astemizole, bepridil, cisapride, citalopram, chloroquine, clarithromycin, dasatinib, dolasetron, dronedarone, droperidol, erythromycin, halofantrine, halogenated anesthetics, levomethadyl, maprotiline, methadone, some quinolones (ofloxacin, gatifloxacin, gemifloxacin, grepafloxacin, levofloxacin, moxifloxacin, sparfloxacin), ondansetron, paliperidone, palonosetron, pentamidine, probucol, propafenone, ranolazine, SUNItinib, terfenadine, thioridazine, tricyclic antidepressants, troleandomycin, vorinostat, tetrabenazine
Increase hypokalemia: Theophylline, aminophylline, corticosteroids

Increase cardiovascular reactions: MAOIs, furazolidone, procarbazine, rasagiline

NURSING CONSIDERATIONS

Assess

Black Box Warning: Asthma-related death; not to be used in asthma

- COPD, emphysema, bronchospasm: monitor pulmonary function tests
- **QT prolongation:** monitor ECG, ejection fraction for QT prolongation
- **Paradoxical bronchospasm:** if paradoxical bronchospasm occurs, discontinue product immediately, use a short-acting β-agonist for rescue therapy, as appropriate

Teach patient/family

- To report dyspnea, wheezing, bronchospasm
- Not to use with other products unless approved by prescriber; there are many interactions

Black Box Warning: Do not use for asthma

indapamide (Rx)

(in-dap′a-mide)

Lozide ♣

Func. class.: Diuretic—thiazide-like, antihypertensive

Chem. class.: Indoline

ACTION: Acts on proximal section of distal renal tubule by inhibiting reabsorption of sodium; may act by direct vasodilation caused by blocking of calcium channels

USES: Edema of CHF, hypertension

CONTRAINDICATIONS: Hypersensitivity to this product or sulfonamides; anuria, hepatic coma

Precautions: Breastfeeding, hypokalemia, dehydration, ascites, hepatic disease, severe renal disease, CCr <30 ml/min (not effective), diabetes mellitus, gout, pregnancy (C), cardiac dysrhythmias

DOSAGE AND ROUTES

Edema

- **Adult: PO** 2.5 mg/day in AM; may be increased to 5 mg/day if needed after 1 wk

Antihypertensive

- **Adult: PO** 1.25 mg/day; may increase to 5 mg/day over 8 wk

Available forms: Tabs 1.25, 2.5 mg

Administer:

- In AM to avoid interference with sleep
- With food if nausea occurs; absorption may be decreased slightly

SIDE EFFECTS

CNS: *Headache, dizziness, fatigue,* weakness, nervousness, agitation, extremity numbness, depression

CV: Orthostatic hypotension, volume depletion, palpitations, dysrhythmias, PVCs, vasculitis

EENT: Blurred vision, nasal congestion, increased intraocular pressure

ELECT: *Hypochloremic alkalosis, hypomagnesemia, hyperuricemia, hypercalcemia, hyponatremia, hypokalemia,* hyperglycemia

GI: *Nausea,* diarrhea, dry mouth, vomiting, anorexia, cramps, constipation, abdominal pain, hypercholesterolemia

GU: *Polyuria,* nocturia, urinary frequency, impotence

HEMA: **Agranulocytosis, anemia**

INTEG: *Rash, pruritus,* **Stevens-Johnson syndrome**

MS: *Cramps*

PHARMACOKINETICS

Well absorbed (PO); widely distributed; metabolized by liver; excreted by kidney (small amounts); onset 1-2 hr; peak 2 hr; duration up to 36 hr; excreted in urine, feces; half-life 14-18 hr

INTERACTIONS

Increase: hyperglycemia—diazoxide
Increase: toxicity of muscle relaxants, steroids, lithium, digoxin
Increase: hypokalemia—corticosteroids, amphotericin B, loop diuretics, thiazide diuretics
Decrease: effects—antidiabetics, antigout agents, anticoagulants
Decrease: absorption—cholestyramine, colestipol
Decrease: hypotensive effect—indomethacin, NSAIDs

Drug/Food

Increase: severe hypokalemia—licorice

Drug/Herb

Increase: antihypertensive effect—hawthorn

Drug/Lab Test

Increase: calcium, parathyroid test, glucose, uric acid

NURSING CONSIDERATIONS

Assess:

- Weight, I&O daily to determine fluid loss; effect of product may be decreased if used daily
- Rate, depth, rhythm of respirations, effect of exertion
- B/P lying, standing; postural hypotension may occur
- Electrolytes: potassium, magnesium, sodium, chloride: include BUN, CBC, serum creatinine, blood pH, ABGs, uric acid, Ca, glucose
- Signs of metabolic alkalosis, hypokalemia
- Rashes, fever daily; allergy to sulfa products
- Confusion, especially in geriatric patients; take safety precautions if needed
- Hydration: skin turgor, thirst, dry mucous membranes

Evaluate:

- Therapeutic response: improvement in edema of feet, legs, sacral area daily; decreased B/P

Teach patient/family:

- To consume diet high in potassium; to rise slowly from lying or sitting position
- To recognize adverse reactions: muscle cramps, weakness, nausea, dizziness
- To take with food, milk for GI symptoms; to take early in day to prevent nocturia; to avoid alcohol
- To notify prescriber if urinary output decreases; to monitor daily weight
- Not to stop product abruptly

TREATMENT OF OVERDOSE:

Lavage if taken orally; monitor electrolytes, administer IV fluids; monitor hydration, CV, renal status

⚠ HIGH ALERT

indinavir (Rx)

(en-den′a-veer)

Crixivan

Func. class.: Antiretroviral
Chem. class.: Protease inhibitor

Do not confuse: indinavir/Denavir

ACTION:

Inhibits human immunodeficiency virus (HIV-1) protease; this prevents the maturation of the virus

USES:

HIV-1 in combination with other antiretrovirals

Unlabeled uses: Prevention of HIV-1 after exposure

CONTRAINDICATIONS:

Hypersensitivity, breastfeeding

Precautions: Pregnancy (C), children, renal/hepatic disease, history of renal stones, diabetes, hypercholesterolemia, hemophilia, autoimmune disease, immune reconstitution syndrome

DOSAGE AND ROUTES

- **Adult: PO** 800 mg q8hr; 600 mg q8hr with delavirdine 400 mg tid; 600 mg q8hr with itraconazole 200 mg bid or ketoconazole

Mild to moderate hepatic impairment

- **Adult: PO** 600 mg q8h

Available forms: Caps 200, 400 mg
Administer:
- Do not break, crush, or chew caps
- With water, 1 hr before or 2 hr after meals; may be given with other liquids or small meal; do not give with high-fat, high-protein meals
- Dosage adjustment will need to be considered when given with other antiretrovirals
- Increase water to 1.5 L/day minimum to prevent nephrolithiasis

SIDE EFFECTS

CNS: *Headache, insomnia,* dizziness, somnolence
GI: *Diarrhea, abdominal pain, nausea, vomiting,* anorexia, dry mouth
GU: Nephrolithiasis
INTEG: Rash
MS: Pain
OTHER: Asthenia, **insulin-resistant hyperglycemia**, hyperlipidemia, **ketoacidosis**, lipodystrophy

PHARMACOKINETICS

Terminal half-life 2 hr; 60% protein binding; metabolized liver; excreted <20% unchanged in urine, 83% in feces

INTERACTIONS

⚠ **Life-threatening dysrhythmias: ergots, midazolam, rifampin, triazolam, amiodarone, pimozide, alfazosin**
Increase: myopathy—statins (atorvastatin, lovastatin, simvastatin)
Increase: indinavir levels—CYP3A4 inhibitors (arepitant, protease inhibitors, azole antifungals, nefazodone, verap amil); phosphodiesterase-5 inhibitors (sildenafil, tadalafil, vardenafil)
Increase: levels of both products—clarithromycin, zidovudine
Increase: levels of isoniazid, oral contraceptives
Decrease: indinavir levels—CYP3A4 inducers (barbiturates, carBAMazepine, nonnucleoside reverse transcriptase inhibitors, phenytoins, rifamycins, modafinil)
Decrease: effect of both products—anticonvulsants
Decrease: effect—CYP3A4 substrates (calcium channel blockers, immunosuppressants, benzodiazepines, azole antifungals, macrolides, SSRIs, statins)
Drug/Herb
Decrease: indinavir levels—St. John's wort; avoid concurrent use
Drug/Food
Decrease: indinavir absorption—grapefruit juice; high-fat, high-protein foods
Drug/Lab Test
Increase: AST, ALT, amylase, total bilirubin

NURSING CONSIDERATIONS

Assess:
- Complaints of lower back, flank pain; indicates kidney stones
- Signs of infection, anemia, presence of other sexually transmitted diseases
- Blood/hepatic studies: ALT, AST; total bilirubin, amylase, blood glucose, serum cholesterol/lipid profile, may be elevated
- Plasma HIV RNA, viral load, CD4 during treatment
- Bowel pattern before, during treatment; if severe abdominal pain with bleeding occurs, product should be discontinued; monitor hydration
- Skin eruptions; rash, urticaria, itching
- Allergies before treatment, reaction of each medication; place allergies on chart

Evaluate:
- Therapeutic response: decreasing viral load, symptoms of HIV

Teach patient/family:
- To take as prescribed; if dose is missed, to take as soon as remembered up to 1 hr before next dose; not to double dose
- That product must be taken in equal intervals around the clock to maintain blood levels for duration of therapy

⚠ **That hyperglycemia may occur; to watch for increased thirst, weight loss, hunger, and dry, itchy skin; to notify prescriber**
- To increase fluids to prevent kidney stones; if stone formation occurs, that treatment may need to be interrupted
- That product does not cure AIDS, only controls symptoms; not to donate blood

indomethacin (Rx)

(in-doe-meth′a-sin)

Indocin, Nu-Indo ♣

Func. class.: Nonsteroidal antiinflammatory product (NSAID), antirheumatic

Chem. class.: Acetic acid derivative

Do not confuse:
Indocin/Endocet/minocin/Vicodin

ACTION: Inhibits prostaglandin synthesis by decreasing enzyme needed for biosynthesis; analgesic, antiinflammatory, antipyretic

USES: RA, ankylosing spondylitis, osteoarthritis, bursitis, tendinitis, acute gouty arthritis; closure of patent ductus arteriosus in premature infants (IV)
Unlabeled uses: Bone pain, headache, heterotopic ossification, juvenile rheumatoid arthritis, pericarditis

CONTRAINDICATIONS: Pregnancy (D) 3rd trimester, aortic coarctation, bleeding salicylate/NSAID hypersensitivity, GI bleeding

Black Box Warning: Perioperative pain in CABG

Precautions: Pregnancy (B) 1st trimester, breastfeeding, children, bleeding disorders, GI disorders, cardiac disorders, depression, renal/hepatic disease, asthma, diabetes, acute bronchospasm, ulcerative colitis, seizures, Parkinson's disease, neonates

Black Box Warning: Stroke, GI bleeding, MI, those taking NSAIDs are at greater risk of MI and stroke, even in first few weeks of therapy

DOSAGE AND ROUTES
Arthritis/antiinflammatory
• **Adult: PO** 25-50 mg bid-tid; max 200 mg/day; **EXT REL** 75 mg/day, may increase to 75 mg bid

Acute gouty arthritis
• **Adult: PO** 50 mg tid; use only for acute attack, then reduce dose

Patent ductus arteriosus
• **Neonates >7 days: IV** Initially, 0.2 mg/kg, then, if necessary, 2 more doses of 0.25 mg/kg at 12-hr intervals if urine output is >1 ml/kg/hr after prior dose or at 24-hr intervals if urine output is <1 ml/kg/hr; hold in cases of oliguria (<0.6 ml/kg/hr) or anuria
• **Neonates 2-7 days: IV** Initially, 0.2 mg/kg, then, if necessary, 2 more doses of 0.2 mg/kg at 12-hr intervals if urine output is >1 ml/kg/hr after prior dose or at 24-hr intervals if urine output is <ml/kg/hr; hold in cases of oliguria (<0.6 ml/kg/hr) or anuria
• **Neonates <2 days: IV** Initially, 0.2 mg/kg, then, if necessary, 1 or 2 doses of 0.1 mg/kg at 12-hr intervals if urine output is >1 ml/kg/hr after prior dose or at 24-hr intervals if urine output is <1 ml/kg/hr; hold in cases of oliguria (<0.6 ml/kg/hr) or anuria
• **Neonates: PO** Doses of 0.3 mg/kg q day × 2 days have been used

Available forms: Caps 25, 50 mg; ext rel caps 75 mg; inj 1-mg vial; supp 50 mg; oral susp 5 mg/ml

Administer:
PO route
• Do not break, crush, or chew sus rel cap or reg caps
• With food to decrease GI symptoms and prevent ulcerations
• Shake susp; do not mix with other liquids
• Store at room temperature

IV route
• After reconstituting 1 mg with 1 or 2 ml NS or sterile water for inj without preservative; to give 1 or 0.5 mg/ml, respectively; do not dilute further
• Infuse over 20-35 min; avoid extravasation
• Do not inject/infuse via umbilical catheter to avoid dramatic shift in cerebral blood flow

SIDE EFFECTS
CNS: Dizziness, drowsiness, fatigue, confusion, insomnia, anxiety, depression, *headache*

CV: Tachycardia, peripheral edema, palpitations, dysrhythmias, hypertension, **CV thrombotic events, MI, stroke**
EENT: Tinnitus, hearing loss, blurred vision
GI: *Nausea,* anorexia, *vomiting,* diarrhea, jaundice, **cholestatic hepatitis,** *constipation,* flatulence, cramps, peptic ulcer, **ulceration, perforation, GI bleeding**
GU: Nephrotoxicity: dysuria, hematuria, oliguria, azotemia
HEMA: Blood dyscrasias, prolonged bleeding
INTEG: Purpura, rash, pruritus, sweating

PHARMACOKINETICS

PO: Onset 30 min; peak 2 hr; duration 4-6 hr; metabolized in liver, kidneys; excreted in urine 60%, feces 33%; crosses placenta; excreted in breast milk; 99% protein binding; half-life 1 hr 1st pass, 2.6-11.2 hr 2nd pass

INTERACTIONS

Increase: hyperkalemia—potassium-sparing diuretics
Increase: toxicity—lithium, methotrexate, cycloSPORINE, probenecid, cidofovir
Increase: effect of—digoxin, phenytoin, aminoglycosides
Increase: bleeding risk—anticoagulants, abciximab, clopidogrel, eptifibatide, plicamycin, ticlopidine, tirofiban, thrombolytics, aspirin, SSRIs, SNRIs
Decrease: effect of—antihypertensives

NURSING CONSIDERATIONS

Assess:

- **Arthritis symptoms:** ROM, pain, swelling before and 2 hr after treatment

Black Box Warning: Cardiac disease, CV, thrombotic events (MI, stroke) before administration, not to be used in perioperative pain in CABG surgery

- Patent ductus arteriosus: respiratory rate, character, heart sounds
- Renal, hepatic, blood studies: BUN, creatinine, AST, ALT, Hgb before treatment, periodically thereafter; if renal function has decreased, do not give subsequent doses
- Eye/ear problems: blurred vision, tinnitus; may indicate toxicity; audiometric, ophthalmic exam before, during, after treatment if patient receiving long-term therapy
- Confusion, mood changes, hallucinations, especially among geriatric patients
- Asthma, nasal polyps, aspirin sensitivity, may develop hypersensitivity to indomethacin

Black Box Warning: GI bleeding/perforation: chronic use can lead to GI bleeding, use cautiously in those with a history of active GI disease

Black Box Warning: MI, stroke: may be greater with longer-term use and those with CV risk factors

Evaluate:

- Therapeutic response: decreased pain, stiffness, swelling in joints; ability to move more easily

Teach patient/family:

- **To report blurred vision, ringing, roaring in ears; may indicate toxicity**
- To avoid driving, other hazardous activities if dizziness, drowsiness occurs
- **To report change in urine pattern, increased weight, edema, increased pain in joints, fever, blood in urine; may indicate nephrotoxicity**
- To report mood changes: anxiety, depression
- That therapeutic antiinflammatory effects may take up to 1 mo
- To avoid alcohol, NSAIDs, salicylates because bleeding may occur
- To report use to all health care providers

Black Box Warning: MI/Stroke: to immediately report and seek medical attention for signs/symptoms of MI/stroke, discontinue product

inFLIXimab (Rx)

(in-fliks′ih-mab)

Remicade

Func. class.: Biologic response modifiers

Chem. class.: Tumor necrosis factor modifiers

Do not confuse: Remicade/Renacidin/inFLIXimab/riTUXimab

ACTION: Monoclonal antibody that neutralizes the activity of tumor necrosis factor-alpha (TNF-α) found in Crohn's disease; decreased infiltration of inflammatory cells

USES: Crohn's disease, fistulizing (moderate to severe); RA, given with methotrexate; plaque psoriasis, ankylosing spondylitis, ulcerative colitis, psoriasis

Unlabeled uses: Psoriatic arthritis, Behçet's syndrome, uveitis, juvenile arthritis

CONTRAINDICATIONS: Hypersensitivity to murines, moderate to severe CHF (NYHA class III/IV)

Precautions: Pregnancy (B), breastfeeding, children, geriatric patients, COPD, hepatotoxicity, hemalologic abnormalities, hepatitis B, Guillain-Barré syndrome, seizures, multiple sclerosis

Black Box Warning: Infection, neoplastic disease, TB

DOSAGE AND ROUTES

Crohn's disease (moderate to severe)/(fistulizing)/ankylosing spondylitis

- **Adult/adolescent/child ≥6 yr:** IV INFUSION 5 mg/kg initially, then at 2 wk, 6 wk, then q8wk; may increase to 10 mg/kg/dose if needed (adults)

Ulcerative colitis/plaque psoriasis

- **Adult/adolescent/child ≥6 yr:** IV INFUSION 5 mg/kg initially and at 2, 4 wk, then 5 mg/kg q8wk

Rheumatoid arthritis

- **Adult:** IV 3 mg/kg initially, then at 2 wk, 6 wk, q8wk thereafter; max 10 mg/kg/dose

Available forms: Powder for inj 100 mg

Administer:

Intermittent IV INFUSION route

- Pretreat with diphenhydrAMINE, acetaminophen, predniSONE if a reaction is infusion related
- Give immediately after reconstitution; reconstitute each vial with 10 ml sterile water for inj; further dilute total dose/250 ml of 0.9% NaCl inj to a total concentration of 0.4-4 mg/ml; use 21-G or smaller needle for reconstitution; direct sterile water at glass wall of vial; gently swirl; do not shake; may foam; allow to stand for 5 min, give within 3 hr
- Give over ≥2 hr, use polyethylene-lined infusion with in-line, sterile, low-protein-bind filter
- Do not admix
- Refrigerated storage; do not freeze

SIDE EFFECTS

CNS: *Headache, dizziness, depression, vertigo, fatigue, anxiety, fever,* seizures, *chills, flulike symptoms,* demyelinating disease

CV: Chest pain, hypo/hypertension, tachycardia, CHF, acute coronary syndrome

GI: *Nausea, vomiting, abdominal pain, stomatitis, constipation, dyspepsia, flatulence*

GU: Dysuria, urinary frequency

HEMA: Anemia, leukopenia, thrombocytopenia, pancytopenia

INTEG: *Rash, dermatitis, urticaria,* dry skin, sweating, flushing, hematoma, pruritus, keratoderma blenorrhagicum

MS: Myalgia, back pain, arthralgia

RESP: URI, pharyngitis, bronchitis, cough, dyspnea, sinusitis

SYST: Anaphylaxis, fatal infections, sepsis, malignancies, immunogenicity, Stevens-Johnson syndrome, toxic epidermal necrolysis

PHARMACOKINETICS
Distributed to vascular compartment, half-life 9.5 days

INTERACTIONS
Increase: infections neutropenia—TNF blockers (abatacept, anakinra, golimumab, rilonacept), avoid concurrent use
• Do not administer live vaccines concurrently

NURSING CONSIDERATIONS
Assess:
• For RA, ROM, pain
• GI symptoms: nausea, vomiting, abdominal pain
• Periodic blood counts (CBC), ANA titer, LFTs
• CV status: B/P, pulse, chest pain
⚠ **Allergic reaction, anaphylaxis:** rash, dermatitis, urticaria, dyspnea, hypotension, fever, chills; discontinue if severe, administer EPINEPHrine, corticosteroids, antihistamines; assess for allergies to murine proteins before starting therapy

Black Box Warning: Fatal infections: discontinue if infection occurs, do not administer to patients with active infection; identify TB before beginning treatment; a TB test should be obtained; if present, TB should be treated before patient receives product; exercise caution when switching from 1 DMARD to another

• Report suspected adverse reactions to the FDA (1-800-FDA-1088)

Black Box Warning: For neoplastic disease in those <18 yr, including hepatosplenic T-cell lymphoma, usually occurs in those with inflammatory bowel disease

Evaluate:
• Therapeutic response: absence of fever, mucus in stools

Teach patient/family:
• Infusion reaction should be reported immediately
• If infection occurs, notify prescriber immediately
• Not to breastfeed while taking this product
• To notify prescriber of GI symptoms, hypersensitivity reactions, heart symptoms
• Not to operate machinery, drive if dizziness, vertigo occur
• To avoid live virus vaccinations; bring up to date before use

insulin, inhaled
(in′su-lin)

Afrezza

Func. class.: Antidiabetic—insulin

I

ACTION: Endogenous insulin regulates carbohydrate, fat, and protein metabolism by the storage of and inhibiting the breakdown of glucose, fat, and amino acids. Insulin decreases glucose concentrations by the uptake of glucose in muscle and adipose tissue, and by inhibiting hepatic glucose production. Insulin also regulates fat metabolism by the storage of fat and inhibiting the mobilization of fat for energy in adipose tissues (lipolysis and free fatty acid oxidation)

USES: Diabetes mellitus types 1 and 2

CONTRAINDICATIONS: Hypersensitivity, lung cancer, asthma, COPD, hypoglycemia, smoking

Precautions: Hepatic disease, renal impairment, renal failure, diabetic ketoacidosis (DKA), hypokalemia, pregnancy C, breastfeeding, child <18 yr

DOSAGE AND ROUTES
• **Adult:** INH: (type 1) the average initial dose is 0.5-0.6 unit/kg/day, usually ≥3 administrations/day; (type 2) the average initial dose is 0.2-0.6 unit/kg/day. When used in combination with oral hypoglycemic agents, may only need a single dose of a longer-acting insulin at a dosage of 10 units or 0.2 unit/kg/day

Available forms: Inhalation 4 units powder

Administer:

• Give by inhalation only; use at beginning of a meal; (blue cartridge = 4 units of regular insulin, green cartridge = 8 units of regular insulin), multiple cartridges may be needed, for single-use only, inhaler should be discarded after 15 days; store unopened cartridge packages in refrigerator, if not refrigerated, use within 10 days

• Sealed (unopened) blister cards and strips must be used within 10 days. Cartridges left over in an opened strip must be used within 3 days. Remove a blister card from the foil package. Tear along a perforation to remove one strip. Press the clear side of the strip to push the cartridge out. To load the cartridge, hold the inhaler level in one hand with the white mouthpiece on the top and purple base on the bottom; open the inhaler by lifting the white mouthpiece to a vertical position. Before placing the cartridge in the inhaler, both the cartridge and the inhaler should be at room temperature for 10 minutes. Hold the cartridge with the cup facing down and line up the cartridge with the opening in the inhaler. The pointed end of the cartridge should line up with the pointed end in the inhaler. The cartridge can be placed into the inhaler; ensure that the cartridge lies flat in the inhaler. Once the cartridge is loaded, keep level

• Remove the purple mouthpiece cover. Hold the inhaler away from the mouth and fully exhale. While keeping the head level, place the mouthpiece in the mouth and tilt the inhaler down toward the chin. Close lips around the mouthpiece to form a seal. Inhale deeply through the inhaler. Have the patient hold his or her breath for as long as comfortable and at the same time remove the inhaler from the mouth. Exhale and continue to breathe normally

SIDE EFFECTS

CNS: Headache, fatigue

GI: Nausea, diarrhea

MISC: Urinary tract infection, weight gain, hypokalemia, peripheral edema

RESP: Cough, throat irritation/pain, productive cough, decreased pulmonary function tests, bronchitis, **acute bronchospasm**

ENDO: Hypoglycemia

INTERACTIONS

Increase: inhaled insulin effect—bronchodilators, other inhaled products, agonists, salicylates, alcohol, fenfluramine, MAOIs

Increase: heart failure, ischemic events—pioglitazone, troglitazone

Increase: hypoglycemia—β-blockers, ACE inhibitors, angiotensin II receptor antagonists, disopyramide, guanethidine, octreotide

Increase or decrease: hypoglycemic effects—clonidine, metoclopramide, tegaserod, testosterone derivatives, or anabolic steroids

Increase: hyperglycemia—niacin (nicotinic acid), bumetanide, furosemide, torsemide

Decrease: hypoglycemic effects—dextrothyroxine, triamterene, thiazide diuretics; thyroid hormones, estrogens, progestins, or oral contraceptives; danazol, corticosteroids, epinephrine

NURSING CONSIDERATIONS

Assess:

• Fasting blood glucose, A1c may be drawn to identify treatment effectiveness

• Urine ketones during illness, insulin requirements may increase during times of stress, trauma, illness, surgery

• Hypoglycemic reaction can occur during peak times (sweating, weakness, dizziness, chills, confusion, headache, nausea, rapid, weak pulse)

• Hyperglycemia: acetone breath, polyuria, fatigue, polydipsia, flushed dry skin, lethargy

Evaluate:

• Therapeutic response: decrease in blood glucose levels

Teach patient/family:

• That blurred vision occurs, not to operate machinery until effect is known, do not change corrective lens for at least 1 month

- To keep all insulin equipment available at all times
- That product does not cure, but controls symptoms
- To carry ID as diabetic
- About the symptoms of hypoglycemia, hyperglycemia, ketoacidosis
- About dosage and how to use product, that the rest of the plan must be followed

⚠ HIGH ALERT

INSULINS

Rapid Acting

insulin glulisine (Rx)
Apidra, Apidra SoloStar

insulin aspart (Rx)
NovoLOG, NovoLOG Flexpen, NovoLOG Pen Fill, NovoMix 30 ♣, Novo Rapid ♣

insulin lispro (Rx)
HumaLOG, Humalog U-200 KwikPen

Short Acting

insulin, regular (OTC)
HumuLIN R, NovoLIN R, ReliOn R

insulin, regular concentrated (Rx)
HumuLIN R U-500

Intermediate Acting

insulin, isophane suspension (NPH) (OTC)
HumuLIN N, NovoLIN ge NPH ♣, NovoLIN N, NovoLIN N Prefilled, ReliOn N

Long Acting

insulin detemir (Rx)
Levemir

insulin glargine (Rx)
Lantus, Toujeo SoloStar

Mixtures

insulin, isophane suspension and regular insulin (Rx)
HumuLIN 70/30, HumuLIN 30/70 ♣, NovoLIN 70/30 Prefilled, ReliOn 70/30

isophane insulin suspension (NPH) and insulin mixtures (Rx)
HumuLIN 50/50

insulin lispro mixture (Rx)
HumaLOG KwikPen Mix 50/50, HumaLOG Mix 25 ♣, HumaLOG Mix 50 ♣, HumaLOG Mix 75/25, HumaLOG Mix 50/50

insulin aspart mixture (Rx)
NovoLOG 70/30, NovoLOG Mix Flexpen Prefilled Syringe 70/30

Func.class.: Antidiabetic, pancreatic hormone
Chem. class.: Modified structures of endogenous human insulin

Do not confuse:
Lantus/lente
NovoLIN 70/30 PenFill/NovoLIN 70/30 Prefilled

ACTION: Decreases blood glucose; by transport of glucose into cells and the conversion of glucose to glycogen, indirectly increases blood pyruvate and lactate, decreases phosphate and potassium; insulin may be human (processed by recombinant DNA technologies)

USES: Type 1 diabetes mellitus, type 2 diabetes mellitus, gestational diabetes; insulin lispro may be used in combination with sulfonylureas in children >3 yr

CONTRAINDICATIONS: Hypersensitivity to protamine; creosol (aspart)

Precautions: Pregnancy (B) lispro, detemir, regular aspart; (C) all others

DOSAGE AND ROUTES

Insulin glulisine

- **Adult/adolescent/child ≥4 yr: SUBCUT** dosage individualized, give within 15 min before or 20 min after starting a meal; **Adult: IV** dilute to 1 unit/ml in infusion systems with 0.9% NaCl, use PVC Viaflex infusion bags and PVC tubing, use dedicated line

Insulin aspart

- **Adult/adolescent/child ≥6 yr: INTERMITTENT SUBCUT** Total daily dose is given as 2-4 inj/day just before beginning of meal; in general, 50%-70% of total daily insulin may be given as insulin aspart, remainder should be intermediate- or long-acting insulin; **CONTINUOUS SUBCUT** used with external insulin pump via cont SUBCUT insulin infusion (CSII), insulin dose should be based on insulin dose from previous regimen

Insulin lispro

- **Adult/adolescent/child ≥3 yr: SUBCUT** 15 min before meals; **CONT SUBCUT INFUSION (external insulin pump):** total daily dose should be based on insulin dose from previous regimen, 50% of total dose can be given as meal-related boluses, remainder as basal infusion

Human regular

- **Adult: SUBCUT** ½-1 hr before meals

Insulin, isophane suspension

- **Adult: SUBCUT** dosage individualized by blood, urine glucose; usual dose 7-26 units; may increase by 2-10 units/day if needed

Insulin detemir

- **Adult/adolescent/child ≥2 yr: SUBCUT** 1-2×/day; if 1×, give with evening meal

Insulin glargine

- **Adult and child ≥6 yr: SUBCUT** 10 international units/day, range 2-100 international units/day

Regular insulin (ketoacidosis)

- **Adult: IV** 5-10 units, then 5-10 units/hr until desired response, then switch to **SUBCUT** dose; **IV/INFUSION** 2-12 units (50 units/500 ml of normal saline)
- **Child: IV** 0.1 units/kg

Replacement

- **Adult and child: SUBCUT** 0.5-1 units/kg/day qid given 30 min before meals
- **Adolescent: SUBCUT** 0.8-1.2 mg/kg/day; this dosage is used during rapid growth

Available forms: ***NPH*** Inj 100 units/ml; ***regular*** inj 100 units/ml, cartridges 100 units/ml; ***insulin analog*** inj 100 units/ml; ***isophane insulin*** inj 100 units/ml, cartridges 100 units/ml; ***insulin lispro*** 100 units/ml, 1.5-ml cartridges, ***insulin lispro*** HumaLOG Pen sol for inj 100 units/ml, Humalog KwikPen 200 U/ml prefilled Pen solution for injection; ***insulin glulisine*** inj 100 units/ml; ***insulin glargine*** inj 100, 300 units/ml; ***insulin detemir*** inj 100 units/ml in 10 vials, 3-ml cartridges; ***insulin aspart*** inj 100 mg/ml (Flexpen, Pen Fill)

Administer:

- Store at room temperature for <1 mo (some insulins); keep away from heat and sunlight; refrigerate all other supply; NPH, premixed insulins are cloudy; regular, rapid-acting analogs, long-acting analogs are clear; do not freeze—IV route, regular only

SUBCUT route

- After warming to room temperature by rotating in palms to prevent injecting cold insulin; use only insulin syringes with markings or syringe matching units/ml; rotate inj sites within one area: abdomen, upper back, thighs, upper arm, buttocks; keep record of sites
- Increased dosages if tolerance occurs
- Premixed insulins, NPH are cloudy suspensions
- Regular human insulin, rapid-acting analogs, long-acting analogs are clear; do not use if cloudy, thick, or discolored

CONT SUBCUT route (insulin infusion CSII)

• Do not mix with other insulins when using a pump

• Insulin lispro 3-ml cartridges to be used in Disetronic H-TRON plus V100 pump using Disetronic rapid infusion sets; infusion set and cartridge adapter should be changed q3days; replace 3-ml cartridge q6days

IV route (insulin glulisine only)

• Dilute to 1 international unit/ml in infusion systems with 0.9% NaCl using PVC viaflex infusion bags and PVC tubing; use dedicated line; do not admix

IV route (regular only)

⚠ When regular insulin is administered IV, monitor glucose, potassium often to prevent fatal hypoglycemia, hypokalemia

• IV direct, undiluted via vein, Y-site, 3-way stopcock; give at ≤50 units/min

• By cont infusion after diluting with IV sol and run at prescribed rate; use IV infusion pump for correct dosing; give reduced dose at serum glucose level of 250 mg/100 ml

Additive compatibilities: Cimetidine, lidocaine, meropenem, ranitidine, verapamil

Y-site compatibilities: Amiodarone, ampicillin, ampicillin/sulbactam, aztreonam, ceFAZolin, cefoTEtan, DOBUTamine, esmolol, famotidine, gentamicin, heparin, heparin/hydrocortisone, imipenem/ cilastatin, indomethacin, magnesium sulfate, meperidine, meropenem, midazolam, morphine, nitroglycerin, oxytocin, PENTobarbital, potassium chloride, propofol, ritodrine, sodium bicarbonate, sodium nitroprusside, tacrolimus, terbutaline, ticarcillin, ticarcillin/clavulanate, tobramycin, vancomycin, vit B/C

SIDE EFFECTS

EENT: Blurred vision, dry mouth

INTEG: Flushing, rash, urticaria, warmth, lipodystrophy, lipohypertrophy, swelling, redness

META: *Hypoglycemia*, rebound hyperglycemia (Somogyi effect 12-72 hr or longer)

MISC: Peripheral edema

SYST: **Anaphylaxis**

PHARMACOKINETICS

Rapid acting

Insulin glulisine: Onset 15-30 min, peak ½-1½ hr, duration 3-4 hr

Insulin aspart: Onset 10-20 min, peak 1-3 hr, duration 3-5 hr

Insulin lispro: Onset 15-30 min, peak ½-1½ hr, duration 3-5 hr

Short acting

Insulin regular: Onset 30 min, peak 2.5-5 hr, duration up to 7 hr

Intermediate acting

Insulin, isophane suspension (NPH): Onset 1.5-4 hr, peak 4-12 hr, duration ≤24 hr

Long acting

Insulin detemir: Onset 0.8-2 hr, peak unknown, duration ≤24 hr (concentration dependent)

Insulin glargine: Onset 1.5 hr, no peak identified, duration ≥24 hr

Mixtures

Insulin, isophane suspension and regular insulin (70/30): Onset 10-20 min, peak 2.4 hr, duration ≤24 hr

Insophane insulin suspension (NPH) and insulin mixtures (50/50): Onset ½-1 hr, peak dual, duration 10-16 hr

INTERACTIONS

Increase: hypoglycemia—salicylate, alcohol, β-blockers, anabolic steroids, phenylbutazone, sulfinpyrazone, guanethidine, oral hypoglycemics, MAOIs, tetracycline

Decrease: hypoglycemia—thiazides, thyroid hormones, oral contraceptives, corticosteroids, estrogens, DOBUTamine, EPINEPHrine

Drug/Lab Test

Increase: VMA

Decrease: potassium, calcium

Interference: LFTs, thyroid function studies

NURSING CONSIDERATIONS

Assess:

• Fasting blood glucose; A1c may be drawn to identify treatment effectiveness q3mo

- Urine ketones during illness; insulin requirements may increase during stress, illness, surgery
- Hypoglycemic reaction that can occur during peak time (sweating, weakness, dizziness, chills, confusion, headache, nausea, rapid weak pulse, fatigue, tachycardia, memory lapses, slurred speech, staggering gait, anxiety, tremors, hunger)
- **Hyperglycemia:** acetone breath; polyuria; fatigue; polydipsia; flushed, dry skin; lethargy

Evaluate:

- Therapeutic response: decrease in polyuria, polydipsia, polyphagia; clear sensorium; absence of dizziness; stable gait

Teach patient/family:

- That blurred vision occurs; not to change corrective lens until vision is stabilized after 1-2 mo
- To keep insulin, equipment available at all times; to carry a glucagon kit, candy, or lump of sugar to treat hypoglycemia
- That product does not cure diabetes but controls symptoms
- To carry emergency ID as diabetic
- To recognize hypoglycemia reaction: headache, tremors, fatigue, weakness
- To recognize hyperglycemia reaction: frequent urination, thirst, fatigue, hunger
- About the dosage, route, mixing instructions, diet restrictions (if any), disease process
- About the symptoms of **ketoacidosis:** nausea; thirst; polyuria; dry mouth; decreased B/P; dry, flushed skin; acetone breath; drowsiness; Kussmaul respirations
- That a plan is necessary for diet, exercise; that all food on diet should be eaten; that exercise routine should not vary
- About blood glucose testing; how to determine glucose level
- To avoid OTC products unless directed by prescriber

TREATMENT OF OVERDOSE:
Glucose 25 g IV, via dextrose 50% sol, 50 ml or glucagon 1 mg

interferon alfacon-1 (Rx)
(in-ter-feer′on al′fa-kon)

Infergen

Func. class.: Recombinant type 1 interferon

ACTION: Induces biologic responses and has antiviral, antiproliferative, and immunomodulatory effects

USES: Chronic hepatitis C infections in those ≥18 yr with compensated liver disease who have anti-HCV antibodies or HCV RNA, may use in combination with ribavirin

CONTRAINDICATIONS: Hypersensitivity to α-interferons or products from *Escherichia coli;* decompensated hepatic disease, autoimmune hepatitis

Precautions: Pregnancy (C), breastfeeding, children <18 yr, geriatric patients, thyroid disorders, myelosuppression, hepatic disease, seizure disorder, alcoholism, hepatitis

Black Box Warning: Cardiac disease, autoimmune disease, infection, depression

DOSAGE AND ROUTES

- **Adult: SUBCUT monotherapy** 9 mcg as single inj 3×/wk × 24 wk; leave ≥48 hr between injections; for patients who did not respond or relapsed after discontinuation, give 15 mcg 3×/wk × 48 wk; **combination: SUBCUT** 15 mcg daily with ribavirin 1000 mg/day PO (<75 kg), 1200 mg/day PO (≥75 kg); give in 2 divided doses for up to 48 wks, use stepwise dose reduction of the interferon dose from 15 mcg to 9 mcg to 6 mcg for serious adverse reactions

Available forms: Inj 9 mcg/0.3 ml, 15 mcg/0.5 ml

Administer:

- Premedicate with acetaminophen or ibuprofen

• Do not shake vial; use 1 dose per vial; discard unused portion; use proper inj sites; rotate sites, discard unused product
• Do not miss doses, give at bedtime for better tolerance

SIDE EFFECTS

CNS: Depression, headache, fatigue, fever, rigors, insomnia, dizziness, agitation, nervousness, anxiety, lability, abnormal thinking
CV: Hypertension, palpitation, tachycardia
EENT: Tinnitus, earache, conjunctivitis, eye pain
GI: Abdominal pain, nausea, diarrhea, anorexia, dyspepsia, vomiting, constipation, flatulence, hemorrhoids, decreased salivation
GU: Dysmenorrhea, vaginitis, menstrual disorders
HEMA: Granulocytopenia, thrombocytopenia, leukopenia, ecchymosis, aplastic anemia
INTEG: Alopecia, pruritus, rash, erythema, dry skin
MISC: Anaphylaxis, angioedema, flulike illness
MS: Back, limb, neck skeletal pain; rigors
RESP: Pharyngitis, upper respiratory infection, cough, sinusitis, rhinitis, respiratory tract congestion, epistaxis, dyspnea, bronchitis

PHARMACOKINETICS

Peak 1-4 hr, peak biologic response 24-36 hr

INTERACTIONS

Increase: hearing loss—eflornithine (systemic), consider serial audiograms
Increase: NRTI, use together cautiously
Increase: myelosuppression—myelosuppressives
Increase: toxicity—aldesleukin, IL-2 eflornithine, theophylline
Decrease: effect of—antiretrovirals (NNRTs, NRTIs, protease inhibitors)

NURSING CONSIDERATIONS

Assess:

Black Box Warning: Past or present history of depression, seizures; use with caution with these disorders

Black Box Warning: Hemolytic anemia: ribavirin may be used with this product and cause hemolytic anemia, cardiac symptoms

• Ophthalmologic status; report periodically
• **Pregnancy:** determine if patient is pregnant before use with ribavirin, pregnancy (X), when used with ribavirin
• CBC, LFTs, ECG, platelet counts, heme concentration, ANC, serum creatinine, albumin, bilirubin, TSH, T_4, triglycerides at baseline and periodically
• Myelosuppression: hold dose if neutrophil count is $<500 \times 10^6$/L or if platelets are $<50 \times 10^9$/L, monitor for infection
• For hypersensitivity: discontinue immediately if hypersensitivity occurs

Evaluate:

• Therapeutic response: decreased chronic hepatitis C signs/symptoms

Teach patient/family:

• With detailed written information about product
• To report signs, symptoms of infection, thyroid/liver dysfunction, changes in behavior
• To report if pregnancy is planned or suspected (C), when combined with ribavirin pregnancy (X)
• To use OTC analgesics to decrease flulike symptoms
• If patient will be self-administering injection, teach all aspects of product use, administration, disposal, provide medication guide

interferon beta-1a (Rx)
(in-ter-feer′on)
Avonex, Rebif

interferon beta-1b (Rx)
Betaseron, Extavia

Func. class.: Multiple sclerosis agent, immune modifier

Chem. class.: Interferon, *Escherichia coli* derivative

ACTION: Antiviral, immunoregulatory; action not clearly understood; biologic response-modifying properties mediated through specific receptors on cells, inducing expression of interferon-induced gene products

USES: Ambulatory patients with relapsing or remitting MS

CONTRAINDICATIONS: Hypersensitivity to natural or recombinant interferon-β or human albumin, hamster protein, rotovirus vaccine

Precautions: Pregnancy (C), breastfeeding, children <18 yr, chronic progressive MS, depression, mental disorders, seizure disorder, latex allergy, autoimmune disorders, bone marrow suppression, hepatotoxicity, cardiac disease, alcoholism, chickenpox, herpes zoster

DOSAGE AND ROUTES

Interferon beta-1a

Remitting or relapsing multiple sclerosis

- **Adult: IM** (Avonex) 30 mcg/wk
- **Adult: SUBCUT** (Rebif) 22 or 44 mcg 3×/wk with each dose 48 hr apart, titrate to full dose over 4-wk period

Interferon beta-1b

Relapsing or remitting multiple sclerosis

- **Adult: SUBCUT** 0.0625 mg every other day for wk 1 and 2, then 0.125 mg every other day for wk 3 and 4, then 0.1875 mg every other day for wk 5 and 6, then 0.25 mg every other day thereafter; higher doses should not be used

Available forms: *beta-1a:* (Avonex) 30 mcg (6.6 million international units/vial) (autoinjector pen); (Rebif) 22 mcg, 44 mcg/0.5 ml; *beta-1b:* powder for inj 0.3 mg (9.6 m international units) kit

Administer:

Interferon beta-1a

- Visually inspect parenteral products for particulate matter and discoloration before use
- Store in refrigerator; do not freeze

IM route

- Premedicate with acetaminophen or ibuprofen and give at bedtime to lessen flulike symptoms
- Interferon-β1a (Avonex) 30 mcg = 6 million IU
- If a dose is missed, give it as soon as possible; continue regular schedule but do not give 2 injections within 2 days; all products are single-use only; do not reuse needles, syringes, prefilled syringes, or autoinjectors
- Rotate injection sites to minimize injection-site reactions
- Do not inject into an area where skin is irritated, reddened, bruised, infected, or scarred
- Check site after 2 hr for redness, edema, or tenderness
- The manufacturer of Avonex offers free training on IM use for patients and health care partners; contact MS ActiveSource for more information (800-456-2255)

Reconstitution and administration of Avonex lyophilized powder for IM route

- Use aseptic technique for preparation of solution
- Sites include the thigh or upper arm
- Slowly add 1.1 ml sterile water for injection, preservative-free (supplied by manufacturer) to the vial; rapid addition of the diluent can cause foaming
- Gently swirl; do not shake; final concentration should be 30 mcg/ml (6 million IU/ml)
- The solution should be clear to slightly yellow without particles; discard if the

reconstituted product contains particulate or is discolored

• Withdraw 1 ml of reconstituted solution into a syringe; attach the sterile needle and inject IM

• A 25-G 1-inch needle for IM may be substituted for the 23-G 1¼-inch needle provided

• **Storage:** Use within 6 hr of reconstitution; store reconstituted solution in refrigerator; *do not freeze;* discard any unused solution; both drug and diluent vials are single-use only

Administration of Avonex prefilled syringe

• Patients may self-inject only if provider determines that it is appropriate, and with medical follow-up, and after proper training in IM injection technique

• The first injection should be performed under the supervision of an appropriately qualified person

• If self-injecting, rotate injection site between thighs; with help from another person, may rotate injection site between thighs and upper arms

• Wash hands before handling the Dose Pack

• Remove prefilled syringe from the refrigerator to warm to room temperature (usually 30 min before use); do not use external heat sources such as hot water to warm the syringe

• Hold the syringe so the cap is facing down and the 0.5 ml mark is at eye level; be sure the amount of liquid in the syringe is the same or very close to the 0.5 ml mark; if the syringe does not contain the correct amount of liquid, do not use it and call the pharmacist

• Hold syringe upright so that the rubber cap faces up; remove the cap by bending it at a 90-degree angle until it snaps free

• Attach the needle by pressing it onto the syringe and turning it clockwise until it locks in place; be careful not to push the plunger while attaching the needle

• Use the alcohol wipe to clean the skin at the injection site you choose; then, pull the protective cover straight off the needle; do not twist the cover off

• Inject intramuscularly at a 90-degree angle into the thigh or upper arm as directed by the provider

• Use gauze pad to apply pressure for a few seconds after the injection

• Dispose of used needles and syringes in a puncture-resistant container and discard appropriately

• Instruct patients to contact the health care provider if a skin reaction occurs that does not resolve in a few days

• A 25-G 1-inch needle for intramuscular injection may be substituted for the 23-G 1¼-inch needle provided by the manufacturer, if deemed appropriate by the physician

• Refer to the Patient Medication Guide for detailed instructions for preparing and giving a dose

• **Storage:** Store refrigerated; if refrigeration is unavailable, may store at 77° F or less for up to 7 days; after removing from refrigerator, do not store product above 25° C; if the product has been exposed to conditions other than recommended, discard the product; do not expose to high temperatures; do not freeze; protect from light

Administration of Avonex prefilled autoinjector

• Patients may self-inject only if their provider determines that it is appropriate, and with medical follow-up, and after proper training in IM technique

• The first injection should be performed under the supervision of provider

• Remove one Administration Dose Pack from the refrigerator to warm to room temperature (about 30 min before use); do not use external heat sources such as hot water to warm the syringe Dose Pack

• Wash hands before handling Dose Pack contents

• Ensure tamper-evident cap has not been removed or is loose; then grasp the cap and bend it at a 90-degree angle until it snaps off; pull off the sterile foil from the needle cover

• Hold the Avonex Pen with the glass syringe tip pointing up; press the needle onto the glass syringe tip; gently turn the needle clockwise until firmly attached; do not remove plastic cover from the needle

• Hold Pen with one hand and, using other hand, hold on to the injector shield (grooved area) tightly and quickly pull up on the injector shield until the injector shield covers the needle all the way; the plastic needle cover will pop off after the injector shield has been fully extended

• When the injector shield is extended the right way, there will be a small blue rectangular area next to the oval medication display window; check the display window and make sure the Avonex is clear and colorless

• Do not use the injection if the liquid is colored, cloudy, or has lumps or particles; air bubbles will not affect the dose

• Do not push down on the injector shield and the blue activation button at the same time until you are ready to give injection

• Avonex Pen should be injected into the upper outer thigh

• Use the alcohol wipe to clean the skin at the injection site and allow it to dry before injection

• Hold Pen at 90-degree angle to the injection site; firmly push the body of the pen down against the thigh to release the safety lock; safety lock is released when blue rectangle area above the oval medication display window is gone, push down on blue activation button with thumb and count to 10, you will hear a click if the injection is given the right way

• After counting to 10, pull the Pen straight out of the skin, use gauze pad to apply pressure for a few seconds

• The circular display window on the Pen is yellow if the full dose is received

• Cover exposed needle with Pen cover; do not hold the Pen cover with your hands while inserting the needle

• Dispose of used needles and syringes in a puncture-resistant container and discard appropriately

• Instruct patients to contact the health care provider if a skin reaction occurs that does not resolve in a few days

• Refer to the Patient Medication Guide for detailed instructions for preparing and giving a dose

• **Storage:** Store at 36°-46° F (2°-8° C); if refrigeration is unavailable, may store at 77° F or less for up to 7 days; after removing from refrigerator, do not store product above 25° C; if the product has been exposed to conditions other than recommended, discard the product and do not use; do not expose to high temperatures; do not freeze; protect from light

Subcutaneous administration

• Give at the same time (preferably late in the afternoon or evening) on the same days of the week at least 48 hours apart

• Do not give on two consecutive days; if a dose is missed, administer the dose as soon as possible, then skip the following day; return to the regular schedule the following week

• Premedication with acetaminophen or ibuprofen can lessen the severity of flulike symptoms

• Interferon-β1a (Rebif) 44 mcg is equivalent to 12 million IU

• Rotate injection sites; appropriate injection sites include thigh, outer surface of upper arm, stomach, or buttocks; do not inject into an area where the skin is irritated, reddened, bruised, or infected

• A Starter Pack containing a lower dose of Rebif syringes is available for the initial titration period; patients and/or their caregivers should be trained and understand appropriate preparation and administration

• The manufacturer offers complimentary services including injection training and reimbursement support; contact MS LifeLines at 877-44-REBIF

Injection (Rebif)

• Interferon-β1a (Rebif) is available in a prefilled syringe with a 29-G needle

• Inject subcutaneously into the outer surface of the upper arm, abdomen, thigh, or buttock, do not inject the area near the navel or waistline; take care not to inject intradermally

• Discard any unused solution; prefilled syringes do not contain preservatives and are single-use only

Interferon beta-1b

SUBCUT route

- The manufacturers of Betaseron and of Extavia offer materials to assist with training on subcut use, call 1-800-788-1467 (Betaseron), 1-888-669-6682 (Extavia)
- Premedication with acetaminophen or ibuprofen and use of product at bedtime can lessen the severity of flulike symptoms
- Visually inspect parenteral products for particulate matter and discoloration before use; do not use if particulate matter is present

Reconstitution

- Add 1.2 ml of 0.54% sodium chloride injection (supplied by the manufacturer) to the vial by using the vial adapter to attach the prefilled syringe that contains the diluent; keep the plunger depressed, and gently swirl, do not shake; if you take your thumb off the plunger, the solution can come back into the syringe before the product is fully reconstituted; if foaming occurs, allow the vial to sit until the foam settles; final concentration (250 mcg interferon-β1b/ml, which corresponds to 8 million IU/ml)
- If not used immediately, store in the refrigerator for up to 3 hr; do not freeze; discard any unused portion after 3 hr

Injection

- Withdraw the desired amount of the reconstituted solution into the syringe by turning the vial and syringe to get the vial on top; pull the plunger back to get the desired amount of product; turn the syringe to point the needle upward, and tap the syringe and release any air bubbles; twist the vial adapter to remove it and the vial
- Choose an injection site on the upper back arm; abdomen; buttock; or front thigh; do not inject within 2 inches of the navel or in a site where the skin is red, bruised, infected, broken, painful, uneven, or scabbed; rotate injection sites to minimize injection-site reactions such as necrosis or localized infection
- Inject subcutaneously; take care not to inject intradermally

SIDE EFFECTS

CNS: *Headache, fever, pain, chills, mental changes, depression,* hypertonia, **suicide attempts, seizures**

CV: *Migraine, palpitations, hypertension,* tachycardia, peripheral vascular disorders

EENT: *Conjunctivitis,* blurred vision

GI: *Diarrhea, constipation, vomiting, abdominal pain*

GU: *Dysmenorrhea, irregular menses, metrorrhagia,* cystitis, breast pain

HEMA: **Decreased lymphocytes, ANC, WBC;** *lymphadenopathy,* anemia

INTEG: *Sweating, inj-site reaction*

MS: *Myalgia,* **myasthenia**

RESP: *Sinusitis,* dyspnea

PHARMACOKINETICS

β-1a: Onset ≤12 hr, peak 16 hr, duration 4 days, half-life 8.6 hr

β-1b: Onset rapid, peak 2-8 hr, duration unknown, half-life 8 min-4.3 hr

INTERACTIONS

Increase: hepatic damage—antiretrovirals (NNRTIs, NRTIs, protease inhibitors)

Increase: myelosuppression—antineoplastics

Decrease: clearance of zidovudine

Drug/Herb

- Change in immunomodulation: astragalus, echinacea, melatonin

Drug/Lab Test

Interference: vaccines, toxoids; avoid concurrent use

Increase: LFTs

NURSING CONSIDERATIONS

Assess:

- Blood, hepatic studies: CBC, differential, platelet counts, BUN, creatinine ALT, urinalysis; if absolute neutrophil count <750/mm^3 or if AST/ALT is 10× normal, discontinue product
- CNS symptoms: headache, fatigue, depression
- GI status: diarrhea or constipation, vomiting, abdominal pain
- Cardiac status: increased B/P, tachycardia

- Mental status: depression, depersonalization, suicidal thoughts, insomnia
- Multiple sclerosis symptoms

Evaluate:

- Therapeutic response: decreased symptoms of multiple sclerosis

Teach patient/family:

- With written, detailed information about product
- That blurred vision, hearing loss, sweating may occur
- That female patients may experience irregular menses, dysmenorrhea or metrorrhagia, breast pain
- To use sunscreen to prevent photosensitivity
- To notify prescriber if pregnancy is suspected
- About injection technique, care of equipment
- To notify prescriber of increased temperature, chills, muscle soreness, fatigue, depression, symptoms of hepatotoxicity

interferon gamma-1b (Rx)

(in-ter-feer′on)

Actimmune

Func. class.: Biologic response modifier

Chem. class.: Lymphokine, interleukin type

ACTION: Species-specific protein synthesized in response to viruses, effects; can mediate killing of *Staphylococcus aureus, Toxoplasma gondii, Leishmania donovani, Listeria monocytogenes, Mycobacterium avium intracellulare;* enhances oxidative metabolism of macrophages, enhances antibody-dependent cellular cytotoxicity

USES: Serious infections associated with chronic granulomatous disease, osteopetrosis

Unlabeled uses: *Mycobacterium avium* complex (MAC)

CONTRAINDICATIONS: Hypersensitivity to interferon-γ, *Escherichia coli*–derived products

Precautions: Pregnancy (C), breastfeeding, children <1 yr, cardiac disease, seizure disorders, CNS disorders, myelosuppression

DOSAGE AND ROUTES

- **Adult: SUBCUT** 50 mcg/m^2 (1.5 million units/m^2) for patients with surface area >0.5 m^2; 1.5 mcg/kg/dose for patients with surface area <0.5 m^2; give Monday, Wednesday, Friday for 3×/wk dosing

Available forms: Inj 100 mcg (2 million units)/single-dose vial

Administer:

- At bedtime to minimize adverse reactions; give acetaminophen for fever, headache
- 50% of dose if severe reactions occur or discontinue treatment until reactions subside
- In right and left deltoid and anterior thigh
- Warm to room temperature before use; do not leave at room temperature >12 hr (unopened vial)
- Store in refrigerator upon receipt; do not freeze; do not shake

SIDE EFFECTS

CNS: *Headache, fatigue,* depression, fever, chills

GI: *Nausea, anorexia,* abdominal pain, weight loss, diarrhea, vomiting, colitis

HEMA: Leukopenia, thrombocytopenia, neutropenia

INTEG: Rash, pain at inj site, Stevens-Johnson syndrome

MS: Myalgia, arthralgia

PHARMACOKINETICS

SUBCUT: Dose absorbed 89%, elimination half-life 5.9 hr, peak 7 hr

INTERACTIONS

Increase: myelosuppression—other myelosuppressive agents

Increase: level of theophylline, aminophylline
Increase: liver toxicity—protease inhibitors, nucleoside reverse transcriptase inhibitors (NRTIs), nonnucleoside reverse transcriptase inhibitors (NNRTIs)

NURSING CONSIDERATIONS

Assess:
- Blood, renal, hepatic studies: CBC, differential, platelet counts, BUN, creatinine, ALT, urinalysis
- CNS symptoms: headache, fatigue, depression

Evaluate:
- Therapeutic response: decreased serious infections; improvement in existing infections and inflammatory conditions

Teach patient/family:
- About the method of administration if family members will be giving medication
- With written, detailed information about product

⚠ HIGH ALERT

ipilimumab

(ip-i-lim′ue-mab)

Yervoy

Func. class.: Antineoplastic; biologic response modifier

ACTION: A recombinant, human monoclonal antibody that binds to the cytotoxic T-lymphocyte–associated antigen 4 (CTLA-4); action is indirect, possibly through T-cell–mediated antitumor immune responses

USES: Treatment of unresectable or metastatic malignant melanoma

CONTRAINDICATIONS Hypersensitivity

Precautions: Pregnancy, breastfeeding, Crohn's disease, hepatitis, immunosuppression, inflammatory bowel disease, iritis, ocular disease, organ transplant, pancreatitis, renal disease, rheumatoid arthritis, sarcoidosis, systemic lupus erythematosus, thyroid disease, ulcerative colitis, uveitis

Black Box Warning: Adrenal insufficiency, diarrhea, Guillain-Barré syndrome, hepatic disease, myasthenia gravis, hypo/hyperthyroidism, hypopituitarism, peripheral neuropathy, serious rash

DOSAGE AND ROUTES

- **Adult/geriatric: IV** 3 mg/kg over 90 min q3wk × 4 doses; permanently discontinue if the full treatment course is not completed within 16 wk from 1st dose or for severe or life-threatening adverse reactions; withhold a dose for any moderate endocrine or immune-mediated adverse reactions; if the moderate adverse reaction completely or partially resolves (Grade 0-1) and if the patient is receiving <7.5 mg predniSONE or equivalent/day, resume at a dose of 3 mg/kg IV q3wk until all 4 planned doses or 16 wk from 1st dose, whichever occurs earlier; if moderate adverse reactions are persistent or if the corticosteroid dose cannot be reduced to 7.5 mg predniSONE or equivalent/day, permanently discontinue

Available forms: Sol for inj 50 mg/10 ml, 200 mg/40 ml

Administer:

Intermittent IV INFUSION route
- Visually inspect parenteral products for particulate matter and discoloration before using whenever sol and container permit; sol may have a pale yellow color and have translucent to white, amorphous particles; discard the vial if sol is cloudy, if there is pronounced discoloration, or if particulate matter is present
- Allow vials to stand at room temperature for 5 min before infusion preparation; withdraw the required volume and transfer into an IV bag; discard partially used vials or empty vials; dilute with 0.9% sodium chloride injection or 5% dextrose injection to a final

concentration (1-2 mg/ml); mix diluted sol by gentle inversion; do not admix
• Give infusion over 90 min through an IV line with a low-protein binding in-line filter, do not give with other products; after each infusion, flush the line with 0.9% sodium chloride injection or 0.5% dextrose injection
• Store once diluted for no more than 24 hr refrigerated or at room temperature

SIDE EFFECTS

CNS: Severe and fatal immune-mediated neuropathies, fatigue, headache, fever
EENT: Uveitis, iritis, episcleritis
ENDO: Severe and fatal immune-mediated endocrinopathies
GI: Severe and fatal immune-mediated enterocolitis, hepatitis, pancreatitis, abdominal pain, nausea, diarrhea, appetite decreased, vomiting, constipation, colitis
INTEG: Severe and fatal immune-mediated dermatitis pruritus, rash, urticaria
MISC: Cough, dyspnea, anemia, eosinophilia, nephritis
SYST: Antibody formation, Stevens-Johnson syndrome, toxic epidermal necrolysis

PHARMACOKINETICS: Steady-state by 3rd dose; terminal half-life 15.4 days

NURSING CONSIDERATIONS

• **Serious skin disorders: Stevens-Johnson syndrome, toxic epidermal necrolysis:** permanently discontinue in these or rash complicated by full-thickness dermal ulceration or necrotic, bullous, or hemorrhagic manifestations like bullous rash; give systemic corticosteroids at a dose of 1-2 mg/kg/day of predniSONE or equivalent; when dermatitis is controlled, taper corticosteroids over a period of at least 1 mo, withhold in patients with moderate to severe reactions; for mild to moderate dermatitis (localized rash and pruritus), give topical or systemic corticosteroids
• **Hepatotoxicity:** LFTs baseline and before each dose to rule out infectious or malignant causes, increase the frequency of liver function test monitoring until resolution, permanently discontinue in patients with Grade 3-5 toxicity, give systemic corticosteroids at a dose of 1-2 mg/kg/day of predniSONE or equivalent
• **Neuropathy:** monitor for motor or sensory neuropathy (unilateral or bilateral weakness, sensory alterations, or paresthesias) before each dose; permanently discontinue if severe neuropathy (interfering with daily activities), such as Guillain-Barré–like syndromes, occur
• **Endocrinopathy:** monitor thyroid function tests at baseline and before each dose; monitor hypophysitis, adrenal insufficiency, adrenal crisis, hypo/hyperthyroidism (fatigue, headache, mental status changes, abdominal pain, unusual bowel habits, hypotension, or nonspecific symptoms that may resemble other causes)

Evaluate:
Decreasing spread of malignant melanoma

Teach patient/family:
• To immediately report allergic reactions, skin rash, severe abdominal pain, yellowing of skin or eyes, tingling of extremities, change in bowel habits
• About the reason for treatment and expected results

ipratropium (Rx)

(i-pra-troe′pee-um)

Atrovent HFA

Func. class.: Anticholinergic, bronchodilator
Chem. class.: Synthetic quaternary ammonium compound

Do not confuse:
Atrovent/Alupent

ACTION: Inhibits interaction of acetylcholine at receptor sites on the bronchial smooth muscle, thereby resulting in decreased cGMP and bronchodilation

USES:
Bronchospasm, COPD; rhinorrhea (nasal spray)

CONTRAINDICATIONS:
Hypersensitivity to this product, atropine, bromide, soybean or peanut products

Precautions: Breastfeeding, children <12 yr, angioedema, heart failure, surgery, acute bronchospasm, bladder obstruction, closed-angle glaucoma, prostatic hypertrophy, urinary retention, pregnancy (B)

DOSAGE AND ROUTES

Bronchospasm in chronic bronchitis/emphysema

- **Adult: INH** 2 sprays (17 mcg/spray) 3-4×/day, max 12 **INH**/24 hr; **SOL** 500 mcg (1 unit dose) given 3-4×/day by nebulizer; nasal spray: 2 sprays (42 mcg/spray) 3-4×/day
- **Child 5-11 yr: INH** 4-8 inhalations q20min as needed for ≤3 hr (asthma, unlabeled); **NEB** 250-500 mcg q20min as needed for ≤3 hr (asthma, unlabeled)

Rhinorrhea perennial rhinitis

- **Adult/child ≥6 yr: INTRANASAL** 2 sprays (43 mcg)/nostril bid or tid
- **Child 5-12 yr: INTRANASAL** 2 sprays (0.03%) in each nostril 3×/day

Available forms: Aerosol 17 mcg/actuation; nasal spray 0.03%, 0.06%; sol for inh 0.0125% ✤, 0.02%

Administer:

- Store at room temperature

Nebulizer route

- Use sol in nebulizer with a mouthpiece rather than a face mask

Intranasal route

- Priming pump initially requires 7 actuations of pump; priming again is not necessary if used regularly, tilt head backward after dose

SIDE EFFECTS

CNS: *Anxiety, dizziness, headache,* nervousness

CV: Palpitation

EENT: Dry mouth, blurred vision, nasal congestion

GI: *Nausea, vomiting, cramps*

INTEG: Rash

RESP: *Cough, worsening of symptoms,* **bronchospasms**

PHARMACOKINETICS
Half-life 2 hr, does not cross blood-brain barrier

INTERACTIONS

Increase: toxicity—other bronchodilators (INH)

Increase: anticholinergic action—phenothiazines, antihistamines, disopyramide

Drug/Herb

Increase: anticholinergic effect—belladonna

Increase: bronchodilator effect—green tea (large amts), guarana

NURSING CONSIDERATIONS

Assess:

- **Palpitations;** if severe, product may have to be changed
- Tolerance over long-term therapy; dose may have to be increased or changed
- **Atropine sensitivity;** patient may also be sensitive to this product
- **Respiratory status:** rate, rhythm, auscultate breath sounds before and after administration
- Hard candy, frequent drinks, sugarless gum to relieve dry mouth

Evaluate:

- Therapeutic response: ability to breathe adequately

Teach patient/family:

- That compliance is necessary with number of inhalations/24 hr or overdose may occur; about spacer device for geriatric patients; that max therapeutic effects may take 2-3 mo
- To shake before using
- About the correct method of inhalation; how to clean equipment daily
- Patients should prime the inhaler before using for the first time by releasing

2 test sprays into the air, away from the face, rinse after use
• Each inhaler has 200 actuations or sprays
• Use spacer to improve drug use if required

irbesartan (Rx)

(er-be-sar′tan)

Avapro

Func. class.: Antihypertensive
Chem. class.: Angiotensin II receptor blocker (Type AT_1)

Do not confuse:
Avapro/Anaprox

ACTION: Blocks the vasoconstrictor and aldosterone-secreting effects of angiotensin II; selectively blocks the binding of angiotensin II to the AT_1 receptor found in tissues

USES: Hypertension, alone or in combination; nephropathy in type 2 diabetic patients; proteinuria
Unlabeled uses: Heart failure

CONTRAINDICATIONS: Hypersensitivity

Black Box Warning: Pregnancy (D) 2nd/3rd trimester

Precautions: Pregnancy (C) 1st trimester, breastfeeding, children <6 yr, geriatric patients, hypersensitivity to ACE inhibitors; hepatic/renal disease; renal artery stenosis, African descent, angioedema

DOSAGES AND ROUTES

Hypertension
• **Adult: PO** 150 mg/day; may be increased to 300 mg/day, volume-depleted patients: start with 75 mg/day

Nephropathy in type 2 diabetic patients
• **Adult: PO** maintenance dose 300 mg/day, start 75 mg/day

Available forms: Tabs 75, 150, 300 mg
Administer:
• Without regard to meals
• May be used with other antihypertensives, diuretic

SIDE EFFECTS

CNS: *Dizziness,* anxiety, *headache, fatigue,* syncope
CV: Hypotension
GI: *Diarrhea, dyspepsia,* hepatitis, cholestasis
HEMA: Thrombocytopenia
MISC: Edema, chest pain, rash, tachycardia, UTI, angioedema, hyperkalemia
RESP: *Cough, upper respiratory tract infection,* sinus disorder, pharyngitis, rhinitis

PHARMACOKINETICS

Peak 1.5-2 hr, extensively metabolized by CYP2C9, half-life 11-15 hr, highly bound to plasma proteins, excreted in urine and feces, protein binding 90%

INTERACTIONS

Increase: hyperkalemia: potassium-sparing diuretics, potassium salt substitutes, ACE inhibitors
Increase: irbesartan level—CYP2C9 inhibitors (amiodarone, delavirdine, fluconazole, FLUoxetine, fluvastatin, fluvoxaMINE, imatinib, sulfonamides, sulfinpyrazone, voriconazole, zafirlukast)
Decrease: antihypertensive effect—NSAIDs

Drug/Herb
Increase: antihypertensive effect—black cohosh, goldenseal, hawthorn, kelp
Increase or decrease: antihypertensive effect—astragalus, cola tree
Decrease: antihypertensive effect—guarana, khat, licorice, yohimbe

NURSING CONSIDERATIONS

Assess:

- **Hypotension:** for severe hypotension, place in supine position and give IV infusion of NS, drug may be continued after B/P is restored
- B/P, pulse q4hr; note rate, rhythm, quality
- Baselines of renal/hepatic studies before therapy begins; periodically monitor LFTs, total/direct bilirubin
- Skin turgor, dryness of mucous membranes for hydration status; edema in feet, legs daily

Evaluate:

- Therapeutic response: decreased B/P

Teach patient/family:

- To comply with dosage schedule, even if feeling better; that max therapeutic effects may take 2-3 mo, to take without regard to food
- That product may cause dizziness, fainting, light-headedness
- To rise slowly to sitting or standing position to minimize orthostatic hypotension
- Do not stop product abruptly

Black Box Warning: To notify prescriber if pregnancy is suspected; discontinue if pregnant; pregnancy (D) 2nd/3rd trimester, (C) 1st trimester

⚠ HIGH ALERT

irinotecan (Rx)

(ear-een-oh-tee′kan)

Camptosar

Func. class.: Antineoplastic

Chem. class.: Camptothecin analog

ACTION: Cytotoxic by producing damage to single-strand DNA during DNA synthesis; binds to topoisomerase I

USES: Metastatic carcinoma of the colon or rectum or 1st-line treatment in combination with 5-FU and leucovorin for metastatic colon or rectal carcinomas

Unlabeled uses: Cervical, gastric, lung, ovarian, pancreatic cancer, malignant glioma, rhabdomyosarcoma

CONTRAINDICATIONS: Pregnancy (D), hypersensitivity

Precautions: Breastfeeding, children, geriatric patients, irradiation, hepatic disease

Black Box Warning: Myelosuppression, diarrhea

DOSAGE AND ROUTES

First-line treatment of colorectal cancer in combination with 5-fluorouracil (5-FU):

Intravenous dosage (with bolus 5-FU/leucovorin)

- **Adult: IV** 125 mg/m^2 over 90 min followed by leucovorin 20 mg/m^2 IV bolus and then 5-FU 500 mg/m^2 IV bolus on days 1, 8, 15, and 22; the next course begins on day 43 or when toxicity has recovered to NCI grade 1 or less

Intravenous dosage (with infusional 5-FU/leucovorin)

- **Adult: IV** 180 mg/m^2 over 90 min followed by leucovorin 200 mg/m^2 IV over 2 hr, then 5-FU bolus and continuous infusion 400 mg/m^2 IV bolus, then 600 mg/m^2 IV infusion over 22 hr on days 1, 15, and 29; leucovorin and 5-FU are given on days 1, 2, 15, 16, 29, and 30; the next course begins on day 43 or when toxicity has recovered to NCI grade 1 or less

Available forms: Inj 20 mg/ml

Administer:

- Use cytotoxic handling precautions

IV route

- Premedicate with antiemetic dexamethasone plus another antiemetic agent, such as a 5-HT_3 blocker, given at least 30 min before use
- Before beginning a course of therapy, the granulocyte count should be ≥1500, the platelet count should be ≥100,000, and treatment-related diarrhea should be fully resolved

Dilution

• Dilute appropriate dose in D_5W (preferred) or NS injection to a final concentration of 0.12-2.8 mg/ml

• Store up to 24 hr at room temperature and room lighting; however, because of possible microbial contamination during preparation, an admixture prepared with D_5W or NS should be used within 6 hr, solutions prepared with D_5W, refrigerated, protected from light must be used within 48 hr; avoid refrigeration if prepared with NS

Intravenous infusion

• Infuse intravenously over 90 min

SIDE EFFECTS

CNS: Fever, headache, chills, dizziness

CV: Vasodilation, edema, thromboembolism

GI: Severe diarrhea, *nausea, vomiting,* anorexia, constipation, cramps, flatus, stomatitis, dyspepsia, hepatotoxicity

HEMA: Leukopenia, anemia, neutropenia

INTEG: Irritation at site, rash, sweating, alopecia

MISC: Edema, asthenia, weight loss, back pain

RESP: Dyspnea, increased cough, rhinitis

PHARMACOKINETICS

Rapidly and completely absorbed, excreted in urine and bile as metabolites, half-life 6-12 hr, bound to plasma proteins 30%-68%, increased risk for toxicity in patients homozygous for UGT1A1 28

INTERACTIONS

Increase: toxicity—fluorouracil

Increase: bleeding risk—NSAIDs, anticoagulants

Increase: irinotecan levels—some CYP3A4 inhibitors (ketoconazole)

Increase: myelosuppression, diarrhea—other antineoplastics, radiation

Increase: lymphocytopenia, hyperglycemia—dexamethasone

Increase: akathisia—prochlorperazine

Increase: dehydration—diuretics

Decrease: irinotecan levels—CYP3A4 inducers (phenytoin, carBAMazepine, PHENobarbital)

Drug/Herb

Decrease: product level—St. John's wort; avoid concurrent use

Drug/Lab Test

Increase: alk phos, LFTs, bilirubin

Decrease: platelets, WBC, neutrophils, Hgb/HcT

NURSING CONSIDERATIONS

Assess:

• CNS symptoms: fever, headache, chills, dizziness

Black Box Warning: CBC, differential, platelet count weekly; use colony-stimulating factor if WBC $<2000/mm^3$ or platelet count $<100,000/mm^3$, Hgb ≤ 9 g/dl, neutrophil $\leq 1000/mm^3$; notify prescriber of results; product should be discontinued

• Buccal cavity for dryness, sores or ulceration, white patches, oral pain, bleeding, dysphagia

Black Box Warning: GI symptoms: frequency of stools; cramping; severe, life-threatening diarrhea may occur with fluid and electrolyte imbalances, treat diarrhea within 24 hr of use with 0.25-1 mg atropine IV; treat diarrhea >24 hr of use with loperamide, diarrhea >24 hr (late diarrhea) can be fatal

• Signs of dehydration: rapid respirations, poor skin turgor, decreased urine output, dry skin, restlessness, weakness

• Bone marrow depression: bruising, bleeding, blood in stools, urine, sputum, emesis

• Increased fluid intake to 2-3 L/day to prevent dehydration unless contraindicated

Evaluate:

• Therapeutic response: decrease in tumor size, spread of cancer

Teach patient/family:

- To avoid foods with citric acid or hot or rough texture if stomatitis is present; to drink adequate fluids
- To report stomatitis; any bleeding, white spots, ulcerations in mouth; to examine mouth daily, report symptoms
- To report signs of anemia: fatigue, headache, faintness, SOB, irritability, infection, rash
- To use contraception during therapy
- To report if pregnancy is planned or suspected pregnancy (D)
- To avoid salicylates, NSAIDs, alcohol because bleeding may occur; to avoid all products unless approved by prescriber
- About alopecia; that, when hair grows back, it will be different texture, thickness
- To avoid vaccinations while taking this product

⚠ To report diarrhea that occurs 24 hr after administration; severe dehydration can occur rapidly

iron dextran (Rx)

DexFerrum, INFeD, Velphoro

Func. class.: Hematinic

Chem. class.: Ferric hydroxide complex with dextran

ACTION:
Iron is carried by transferrin to the bone marrow, where it is incorporated into hemoglobin

USES:
Iron-deficiency anemia

CONTRAINDICATIONS:

Black Box Warning: Hypersensitivity

Precautions: Pregnancy (C), breastfeeding, neonates, infants <4 mo, children, acute renal disease, asthma, rheumatoid arthritis (IV), ankylosing spondylitis, lupus, hypotension, all anemias excluding iron-deficiency anemia, hepatic/cardiac/renal disease

DOSAGE AND ROUTES

- **Adult and child: IM** 0.5 ml as a test dose by Z-track, then no more than the following total dose including test dose per day:
- **Adult/adolescent/child (>15 kg):** Total iron dextran dose in ml = [0.0442 × (Desired Hb − observed Hb) × LBW] + (0.26 × LBW), max of undiluted is 100 mg (2 ml)/day
- **Child (10-15 kg):** Total iron dextran dose in ml = [0.0442 × (Desired Hb − observed Hb) × LBW] + (0.26 × ABW), max of undiluted iron dextran is 100 mg (2 ml)/day
- **Child/Infant >4 mo (5-9.9 kg):** Total iron dextran dose in ml = [0.0442 × (Desired Hb − observed Hb) × LBW] + (0.26 × ABW)
- **Infants >4 mo (<5 kg):** Total iron dextran dose in ml = [0.0442 × (Desired Hb − observed Hb) × LBW] + (0.26 × ABW)

Administer:

- D/C oral iron before parenteral; give only after test dose of 25 mg by preferred route; wait at least 1 hr before giving remaining portion
- Store at room temperature in cool environment
- Recumbent position 30 min after IV inj to prevent orthostatic hypotension

IM route

- IM deeply in large muscle mass; use Z-track method, 19- to 20-G 2- to 3-in needle; ensure needle long enough to place product deep in muscle; change needles after withdrawing product and before injecting to prevent skin, tissue staining

⚠ Only with EPINEPHrine available in case of anaphylactic reaction during dose

IV route

- IV after flushing with 10 ml 0.9% NaCl; give undiluted; may be diluted in 50-250 ml NS for infusion; give ≤1 ml (50 mg) over ≥1 min; flush line after use with 10 ml 0.9% NaCl; patient should remain recumbent for 1/2-1 hr
- IV inj requires single-dose vial without preservative; verify on label that IV use approved

SIDE EFFECTS

CNS: Headache, paresthesia, dizziness, shivering, weakness, seizures
CV: Chest pain, shock, hypotension, tachycardia
GI: *Nausea,* vomiting, metallic taste, abdominal pain
HEMA: Leukocytosis
INTEG: Rash, pruritus, urticaria, fever, sweating, chills, brown skin discoloration, pain at inj site, necrosis, sterile abscesses, phlebitis
OTHER: Anaphylaxis
RESP: Dyspnea

PHARMACOKINETICS

IM: Excreted in feces, urine, bile, breast milk; crosses placenta; most absorbed through lymphatics; can be gradually absorbed over weeks/months from fixed locations

INTERACTIONS

Increase: toxicity—oral iron; do not use
Decrease: reticulocyte response—chloramphenicol
Drug/Lab Test
False increase: serum bilirubin
False decrease: serum calcium
False positive: ^{99m}Tc diphosphate bone scan, iron test (large doses >2 ml)

NURSING CONSIDERATIONS

Assess:
- Observe for 1 hr after test dose
- Blood studies: Hct, Hgb, reticulocytes, transferrin, plasma iron concentrations, ferritin, total iron binding, bilirubin before treatment, at least monthly

Black Box Warning: Allergy: anaphylaxis, rash, pruritus, fever, chills, wheezing; notify prescriber immediately, keep emergency equipment available

- Cardiac status: anginal pain, hypotension, tachycardia
- Nutrition: amount of iron in diet (meat, dark green leafy vegetables, dried beans, dried fruits, eggs)
- Cause of iron loss or anemia, including use of salicylates, sulfonamides
- **Toxicity:** nausea, vomiting, diarrhea, fever, abdominal pain (early symptoms), cyanotic-looking lips, nailbeds, seizures, CV collapse (late symptoms)
- Therapeutic response: increased serum iron levels, Hct, Hgb

Evaluate:
- Therapeutic response: increased serum iron level, increased Hgb, Hct

Teach patient/family:
- That iron poisoning may occur if increased beyond recommended level; not to take oral iron preparation or vitamins containing iron
- That delayed reaction may occur 1-2 days after administration and last 3-4 days (IV), 3-7 days (IM); to report fever, chills, malaise, muscle, joint aches, nausea, vomiting, backache
- To avoid breastfeeding
- That stools may become dark

TREATMENT OF OVERDOSE:

Discontinue product, treat allergic reaction, give diphenhydrAMINE or EPINEPHrine as needed, give iron-chelating product for acute poisoning

iron sucrose (Rx)

Venofer
Func. class.: Hematinic
Chem. class.: Ferric hydroxide complex with dextran

ACTION: Iron is carried by transferrin to the bone marrow, where it is incorporated into hemoglobin

USES: Iron-deficiency anemia, hyperphosphatemia in chronic kidney disease on dialysis
Unlabeled uses: Dystrophic epidermolysis bullosa (DEB)

CONTRAINDICATIONS: Hypersensitivity, all anemias excluding iron-deficiency anemia, iron overload

Precautions: Pregnancy (B), breastfeeding, children, geriatric patients, abdominal pain, anaphylactic shock, arthralgia, chest pain, cough, diarrhea, dizziness, dyspnea, edema, increased LFTs, fever, headache, heart failure, hypo/hypertension, infection, MS pain nausea/vomiting, seizures, weakness

DOSAGE AND ROUTES

- **Adult:** **IV** 5 ml (100 mg of elemental iron) given during dialysis; most will need 1000 mg of elemental iron over 10 sequential dialysis sessions
- **Child ≥2 yr/adolescents:** **IV** 0.5 mg/kg by slow IV inj over 5 min (undiluted) or diluted in 25 ml of 0.9% NaCl, give over 5-60 min, max 100 mg every 2 wk × 12 wk

Hyperphosphatemia in chronic kidney disease

- **Adult:** PO 500 mg tid

Available forms: Inj 20 mg/ml; chew tab 500 mg

Administer:

⚠ Only with EPINEPHrine, Solu-MEDROL available in case of anaphylactic reaction during dose

IV route

- Do not use if particulate is present or if discolored
- Give directly in dialysis line by slow inj or infusion; give by slow inj at 1 ml/min (5 min/vial); infusion dilute each vial exclusively in ≤100 ml 0.9% NaCl, give at 100 mg of iron/15 min; discard unused portions
- Do not use with IV products
- Store at room temperature in cool environment; do not freeze

SIDE EFFECTS

CNS: Headache, dizziness
CV: Chest pain, hypo/hypertension, hypervolemia, heart failure
GI: *Nausea, vomiting, abdominal pain*
INTEG: Rash, pruritus, urticaria, fever, sweating, chills
OTHER: Anaphylaxis, hyperglycemia
RESP: Dyspnea, pneumonia, cough

PHARMACOKINETICS

Excreted in urine, half-life 6 hr

INTERACTIONS

Increase: toxicity—oral iron, dimercaprol, do not use
Decrease: iron sucrose effect—chloramphenicol

Drug/Lab Test

Increase: glucose

NURSING CONSIDERATIONS

Assess:

- Blood studies: Hct, Hgb, reticulocytes, transferrin, plasma iron concentrations, ferritin, total iron binding; bilirubin before treatment, at least monthly
- Allergy, anaphylaxis: rash, pruritus, fever, chills, wheezing; notify prescriber immediately, keep emergency equipment available
- Cardiac status: hypo/hypertension, hypervolemia
- **Toxicity:** nausea, vomiting, diarrhea, fever, abdominal pain (early symptoms), cyanotic-looking lips, nailbeds, seizures, CV collapse (late symptoms)

Evaluate:

- Therapeutic response: increased serum iron levels, Hct, Hgb

Teach patient/family:

- To report itching, rash, chest pain, headache, vertigo, nausea, vomiting, abdominal pain, joint/muscle pain, numbness, tingling
- That iron poisoning may occur if dosage increased beyond recommended level; not to take oral iron preparation

TREATMENT OF OVERDOSE:

Discontinue product, treat allergic reaction, give diphenhydrAMINE or EPINEPHrine as needed, give iron-chelating product for acute poisoning

isoniazid (Rx)

(eye-soe-nye′a-zid)

Isotamine ✦

Func. class.: Antitubercular
Chem. class.: Isonicotinic acid hydrazide

ACTION:

Bactericidal interference with lipid, nucleic acid biosynthesis

USES: Treatment, prevention of TB

CONTRAINDICATIONS: Hypersensitivity

Black Box Warning: Acute hepatic disease

Precautions: Pregnancy (C), renal disease, diabetic retinopathy, cataracts, ocular defects, IV drug users, >35 yr, postpartum, HIV, neuropathy

Black Box Warning: Alcoholism, females (African descent/Hispanic patients)

DOSAGE AND ROUTES

- **Adult/adolescent with/without HIV: PO/IM** 5 mg/kg/day ≤300 mg/day or 15 mg/kg 2-3×/wk, max 900 mg 2-3×/wk
- **Child/infant with HIV: PO/IM** 10-15 mg/kg/day, max 300 mg/day

Available forms: Tabs 100, 300 mg; inj 100 mg/ml; oral sol 10 mg/ml

Administer:

PO route

- PO with meals to decrease GI symptoms; better to take on empty stomach 1 hr before or 2 hr after meals

IM route

- IM deep in large muscle mass; massage; rotate injection site; warm inj to room temperature to dissolve crystals

SIDE EFFECTS

CNS: *Peripheral neuropathy, dizziness,* memory impairment, toxic encephalopathy, seizures, psychosis, slurred speech

EENT: Blurred vision, optic neuritis

GI: *Nausea, vomiting,* epigastric distress, jaundice, fatal hepatitis

HEMA: Agranulocytosis, hemolytic, aplastic anemia, thrombocytopenia, eosinophilia, methemoglobinemia

Hypersensitivity: Fever, skin eruptions, lymphadenopathy, vasculitis

MISC: Dyspnea, B_6 deficiency, pellagra, hyperglycemia, metabolic acidosis, gynecomastia, rheumatic syndrome, SLE-like syndrome

PHARMACOKINETICS

Metabolized in liver, excreted in urine (metabolites),, crosses placenta, excreted in breast milk, half life 1-4 hr

PO: Peak 1-2 hr

IM: Peak 45-60 min

INTERACTIONS

Increase: toxicity—tyramine foods, alcohol, cycloSERINE, ethionamide, rifampin, carBAMazepine, phenytoin, benzodiazepines, meperidine

Increase: serotonin syndrome—SSRIs, SNRIs

Decrease: absorption—aluminum antacids

Decrease: effectiveness of BCG vaccine, ketoconazole

Drug/Food

- Do not give with high-tyramine foods, alcohol

Drug/Lab Test

Increase: LFTs, bilirubin, glucose

Decrease: platelets granulocytes

NURSING CONSIDERATIONS

Assess:

Black Box Warning: Hepatic studies weekly: baseline in all patients, those >35 yr and all women should be monitored periodically; ALT, AST, bilirubin; increased test results may indicate hepatitis; hepatic status: decreased appetite, jaundice, dark urine, fatigue, those with fast acetylation (genetic) may metabolize product more than 5 times faster (black, Asian patients are at greater risk) some Caucasian patients; fatal hepatitis is at greater risk in black/Hispanic patients after birth

- Mental status often: affect, mood, behavioral changes; psychosis may occur
- Paresthesia in hands, feet

Evaluate:

- Therapeutic response: decreased symptoms of TB

Teach patient/family:
- That compliance with dosage schedule, duration is necessary; not to skip or double dose
- That scheduled appointments must be kept or relapse may occur
- ⚠ To avoid alcohol while taking product; may increase risk for hepatic injury
- That, if diabetic, to use blood glucose monitor to obtain correct result
- ⚠ To report weakness, fatigue, loss of appetite, nausea, vomiting, jaundice of skin or eyes, tingling/numbness of hands/feet

Black Box Warning: Fatal hepatitis: to notify prescriber immediately of yellow skin/eyes, dark urine, loss of appetite

isosorbide dinitrate (Rx)
(eye-soe-sor′bide)

Apo-ISDN ✱, Dilatrate-SR, Isochron, IsoDitrate, Isordil

isosorbide mononitrate (Rx)

Apo-ISMN ✱, Imdur

Func. class.: Antianginal, vasodilator
Chem. class.: Nitrate

Do not confuse:
Imdur/Imuran/Inderal/K-Dur

ACTION: Relaxation of vascular smooth muscle, which leads to decreased preload, afterload, which is responsible for decreasing left ventricular end-diastolic pressure, systemic vascular resistance, and reducing cardiac oxygen demand

USES: Treatment, prevention of chronic stable angina pectoris
Unlabeled uses: Diffuse esophageal spasm, heart failure (dinitrate)

CONTRAINDICATIONS: Hypersensitivity to this product or nitrates; severe anemia, closed-angle glaucoma

Precautions: Pregnancy (C), breastfeeding, children, orthostatic hypotension, MI, CHF, severe renal/hepatic disease, increased intracranial pressure, cerebral hemorrhage, acute MI, geriatric patients, GI disease, syncope

DOSAGE AND ROUTES
Dinitrate
- **Adult: PO** 5-20 mg bid-tid initially, maintenance 10-40 mg bid-tid; **SL,** buccal 2.5-5 mg, may repeat q5-10min × 3 doses; **EXT REL** 40-80 mg q8-12hr, max 160 mg/day

Mononitrate
- **Adult: PO** (Monoket) 10-20 mg bid, 7 hr apart; (Imdur) initiate at 30-60 mg/day as a single dose, increase q3days as needed, may increase to 120 mg/day, max 240 mg/day

Available forms: *Dinitrate:* sus rel caps (SR) 40 mg, SR tabs 40 mg; tabs 5, 10, 20, 30, 40 mg; SL tabs 2.5, 5 mg; *mononitrate:* tabs (Monoket) 10, 20 mg; ext rel (Imdur) 30, 60, 120 mg

Administer:
- Do not break, crush, or chew sus rel caps, SL tabs
- After checking expiration date
- PO with 8 oz water on empty stomach
- SL tabs should be placed under the tongue until dissolved; avoid smoking, eating, drinking until dissolved
- **SUS REL cap/tab:** allow dosing interval >18 hr

SIDE EFFECTS
CNS: *Vascular headache, flushing, dizziness,* weakness
CV: *Orthostatic hypotension,* tachycardia, **collapse,** syncope
GI: Nausea, vomiting
INTEG: Pallor, sweating, rash
MISC: Twitching, **hemolytic anemia, methemoglobinemia,** tolerance, xerostomia

PHARMACOKINETICS
Dinitrate
Metabolized by liver, excreted in urine as metabolites (80%-100%)

PO: Onset 15-30 min, duration 4-6 hr, half-life 5-6 hr
SUS REL: Onset ≤4 hr, duration 6-8 hr
SL: Onset 2-5 min, duration 1-4 hr, half-life 2 hr
Mononitrate
SUS REL: Onset 30-60 min, peak 1-4 hr, duration 6-8 hr, half-life 5 hr

INTERACTIONS

⚠ Fatal hypotension: sildenafil, tadalafil, vardenafil, do not use together
Increase: hypotension—β-blockers, diuretics, antihypertensives, alcohol, calcium channel blockers, phenothiazines
Increase: heart rate, B/P—sympathomimetics
Increase: myocardial ischemia—rosiglitazone; avoid concurrent use

NURSING CONSIDERATIONS

Assess:

- **Anginal pain:** duration, time started, activity being performed, character
- **Methemoglobinemia (rare):** Cyanosis of lips, nausea/vomiting, coma, shock, usually caused by high dose of product but may occur with normal dosing
- B/P, pulse, respirations during beginning therapy and periodically thereafter
- Tolerance if taken over long period, to prevent, allow intervals of 12-14 hr/day without product
- Headache, light-headedness, decreased B/P; may indicate a need for decreased dosage, treat headache with OTC analgesics

Evaluate:

- Therapeutic response: decrease or prevention of anginal pain

Teach patient/family:

- To leave tabs in original container
- To avoid alcohol, OTC products unless approved by prescriber
- That product may cause headache; that taking with meals may reduce or eliminate headache; to take no later than 7 PM (last dose)
- To avoid hazardous activities if dizziness occurs
- About the importance of complying with complete medical regimen
- To make position changes slowly to prevent orthostatic hypotension
- Not to use with sildenafil, tadalafil, vardenafil with nitrates, may cause serious drop in B/P
- Not to discontinue abruptly, may cause heart attack
- To use at beginning of angina symptoms, may repeat every 15 min; if no relief, seek medical attention immediately

RARELY USED

ISOtretinoin (Rx)

(eye-soe-tret′i-noyn)

Absorica, Amnesteem, Claravis, Myorisan, Sotret, Zenatane

Func. class.: Antiacne agent, retinoid

USES: Severe recalcitrant nodulocystic acne

CONTRAINDICATIONS: Hypersensitivity to this product, parabens, retinoids, inflamed skin, blood donation

Black Box Warning: Pregnancy (X)

DOSAGE AND ROUTES

- **Adult: PO** 0.5-2 mg/kg/day in 2 divided doses × 15-20 wk; if relapse occurs, repeat after 2 mo off product

itraconazole (Rx)

(it-ra-con′a-zol)

Onmel, Sporanox

Func. class.: Antifungal, systemic
Chem. class.: Triazole derivative

ACTION: Alters cell membranes; inhibits several fungal enzymes

USES: Histoplasmosis, blastomycosis (pulmonary and extrapulmonary), aspergillosis, onychomycosis of toenail/fingernail

Unlabeled uses: Dermatomycosis, histoplasmosis, chromoblastomycosis, coccidioidomycosis, pityriasis versicolor, sebopsoriasis, vaginal candidiasis, cryptococcus, subcutaneous mycoses, dimorphic infections, fungal keratitis, zygomycosis, superficial mycoses (dermatophytoses), chronic mucocutaneous candidiasis

CONTRAINDICATIONS:
Hypersensitivity, fungal meningitis; onychomycosis or dermatomycosis with cardiac dysfunction, in pregnant women

Black Box Warning: Heart failure, ventricular dysfunction, coadministration with other products

Precautions: Pregnancy (C), breastfeeding, children, cardiac/renal/hepatic disease, achlorhydria or hypochlorhydria (product-induced), dialysis, hearing loss, cystic fibrosis neuropathy

DOSAGE AND ROUTES

Dose varies with type of infection

- **Adult: PO** 200 mg/day with food; may increase to 200 mg bid if needed; life-threatening infections may require a loading dose of 200 mg tid × 3 days

Available forms: Caps 100 mg; oral sol 10 mg/ml; tab 200 mg

Administer:

- In the presence of acid products only; do not use alkaline products, antacids within 2 hr of product; may give coffee, tea, acidic fruit juices

PO route

- Swallow caps whole; do not break, crush, or chew caps
- Give caps after full meal to ensure absorption
- Oral sol: patient should swish in mouth vigorously, use on empty stomach
- Oral sol and caps are not interchangeable on mg/mg basis
- Store in tight container at room temperature, do not freeze

SIDE EFFECTS

CNS: *Headache, dizziness,* insomnia, somnolence, depression

CV: Hypertension, CHF

GI: *Nausea, vomiting, anorexia, diarrhea,* cramps, *abdominal pain,* flatulence, **GI bleeding, hepatotoxicity**

GU: Gynecomastia, impotence, decreased libido

INTEG: *Pruritus,* fever, *rash,* **toxic epidermal necrolysis, Stevens-Johnson syndrome**

MISC: *Edema, fatigue,* malaise, hypokalemia, tinnitus, **rhabdomyolysis**

RESP: Rhinitis, sinusitis, upper respiratory infection, pulmonary edema

PHARMACOKINETICS

PO: Peak 3-4 hr; half-life 21 hr, IV 35.4 hr; metabolized in liver; excreted in bile, feces, urine 40%; requires acid pH for absorption; distributed poorly to CSF; 99.8% protein bound; inhibits CYP4503A4

INTERACTIONS

⚠ Life-threatening CV reactions: pimozide, quiNIDine, dofetilide, levomethadyl, dronedarone

Increase: tinnitus, hearing loss—quiNIDine

Increase: hepatotoxicity—other hepatotoxic products

Increase: edema—calcium channel blockers

Increase: severe hypoglycemia—oral hypoglycemics

Increase: sedation—ALPRAZolam, clorazepate, diazepam, estazolam, flurazepam, triazolam, oral midazolam

Increase: levels, toxicity—busPIRone, busulfan, clarithromycin, cycloSPORINE, diazepam, digoxin, felodipine, fentaNYL, atorvastatin, carBAMazepine, disopyramide, indinavir, isradipine, niCARdipine, NiFEdipine, niMODipine, phenytoin, quiNIDine, QUEtiapine, ritonavir, saquinavir, tacrolimus, warfarin

Decrease: itraconazole action—antacids, H_2-receptor antagonists, rifamycins, didanosine, carBAMazepine, isoniazid, proton pump inhibitors

Drug/Food

- Food increases absorption

• Grapefruit juice decreases itraconazole level

Drug/Lab Test

Increase: LFTs, alk phos, bilirubin, triglyceride, GGT

NURSING CONSIDERATIONS

Assess:

• **CHF:** if present, discontinue product
• Type of infection; may begin treatment before obtaining results
• **Infection:** temperature, WBC, sputum at baseline and periodically
• I&O ratio, potassium levels
• Hepatic studies (ALT, AST, bilirubin) if patient receiving long-term therapy
• Allergic reaction: rash, photosensitivity, urticaria, dermatitis

⚠ **Hepatotoxicity:** nausea, vomiting, jaundice, clay-colored stools, fatigue

Evaluate:

• Therapeutic response: decreased fever, malaise, rash, negative C&S for infecting organism

Teach patient/family:

• That long-term therapy may be needed to clear infection (1 wk-6 mo, depending on infection)
• To avoid hazardous activities if dizziness occurs
• To take 2 hr before administration of other products that increase gastric pH (antacids, H_2-blockers, omeprazole, sucralfate, anticholinergics); to avoid grapefruit juice; to notify health care provider of all medications taken; to take after a full meal (caps) or on empty stomach (oral sol)
• About the importance of compliance with product regimen; to use alternative methods of contraception
• To notify prescriber of GI symptoms; signs of hepatic dysfunction (fatigue, jaundice, nausea, anorexia, vomiting, dark urine, pale stools); heart failure (trouble breathing, unusual weight gain, fatigue, swelling); hearing changes

RARELY USED

ivacaftor

(eye′va-kaf′tor)

Kalydeco

Func. class.: Respiratory agent

USES: Cystic fibrosis in those with G551D, G1244E, G1349D, G178R, G5515S, S1255P, S549N, S549R mutation in the CFTR gene

DOSAGE AND ROUTES

• **Adult/adolescent/child ≥6 yr: PO** 150 mg every 12 hr with fat-containing food
• **Child 2-5 yr, ≥14 kg: PO** 75 mg q12hr with fat-containing food
• **Child 2-5 yr, <14 kg: PO** 50 mg q12hr with fat-containing food

⚠ HIGH ALERT

ixabepilone (Rx)

(ix-ab-ep′i-lone)

Ixempra

Func. class.: Antineoplastic—miscellaneous

Chem. class.: Epothilone

ACTION: Microtubule stabilizing agent; microtubules are needed for cell division

USES: Breast cancer

CONTRAINDICATIONS: Pregnancy (D), breastfeeding, hypersensitivity to products with polyoxyethylated castor oil, neutropenia of $<1500/mm^3$, thrombocytopenia

Black Box Warning: Hepatic disease

Precautions: Children, geriatric patients, alcoholism, bone marrow suppression, cardiac dysrhythmias, cardiac/

renal disease, diabetes mellitus, peripheral neuropathy, ventricular dysfunction

DOSAGE AND ROUTES

Breast cancer, metastatic or locally advanced given with capecitabine and resistant to anthracycline, taxane

- **Adult: IV INFUSION** 40 mg/m^2 over 3 hr q3wk plus capecitabine **PO** 2000 mg/m^2/day in 2 divided doses on days 1-14 q21days; in those with BSA >2.2 m^2, dose should be calculated for a BSA of 2.2 m^2

Breast cancer, metastatic or locally advanced resistant/refractory to anthracycline, taxane, capecitabine

- **Adult: IV INFUSION** 40 mg/m^2 over 3 hr q3wk; in those with BSA >2.2 m^2, dose should be calculated for a BSA of 2.2 m^2

Dosage reduction in those taking a strong CYP3A4 inhibitor

- **Adult: IV INFUSION** 20 mg/m^2 over 3 hr q3wk

Available forms: Powder for inj 15, 45 mg

Administer:

- Premedicate with histamine antagonists 1 hr before use, prevents hypersensitivity
- Antiemetic 30-60 min before product and prn

IV route

- Let kit stand at room temperature for 30 min; to reconstitute, withdraw supplied diluent (8 ml for 15-mg vials, 23.5 ml for 45-mg vials); slowly inject sol into vial; gently swirl and invert to mix, final concentration 2 mg/ml; further dilute in LR in DEHP-free bags, final concentration should be between 0.2 and 0.6 mg/ml; after added, mix by manual rotation
- Diluted sol stable for 6 hr at room temperature; infusion must be completed within 6 hr
- Use in-line filter, 0.2-1.2 micron
- Give over 3 hr

SIDE EFFECTS

CNS: *Peripheral neuropathy,* impaired cognition, chills, fatigue, fever, flushing, headache, insomnia, *asthenia*

CV: Bradycardia, *hypotension,* **abnormal ECG,** angina, **atrial flutter, cardiomyopathy,** chest pain, edema, **MI,** vasculitis

GI: *Nausea, vomiting, diarrhea,* abdominal pain, anorexia, colitis, constipation, gastritis, jaundice, GERD, hepatic failure, trismus

GU: **Renal failure**

HEMA: **Neutropenia, thrombocytopenia, anemia,** infections, coagulopathy

INTEG: *Alopecia,* rash, hot flashes

META: Hypokalemia, metabolic acidosis

MS: *Arthralgia, myalgia*

RESP: **Bronchospasm,** cough, dyspnea

SYST: *Hypersensitivity reactions,* **anaphylaxis,** dehydration, **radiation recall reaction**

PHARMACOKINETICS

Metabolized in liver by P45CYP3A4; excreted in feces (65%) and urine (21%); terminal half-life 52 hr

INTERACTIONS

Increase: ixabepilone level—CYP3A4 inhibitors (amiodarone, amprenavir, aprepitant, atazanavir, chloramphenicol, clarithromycin, conivaptan, cycloSPORINE, danazol, darunavir, dalforpistin, delavirdine, diltiazem, erythromycin, estradiol, fluconazole, fluvoxaMINE, fosamprenavir, imatinib, indinavir, isoniazid, itraconazole, ketoconazole, lopinavir, miconazole, nefazodone, nelfinavir, propoxyphene, ritonavir, RU-486, saquinavir, tamoxifen, telithromycin, troleandomycin, verapamil, voriconazole, zafirlukast)

Decrease: ixabepilone levels—CYP3A4 inducers (aminoglutethimide, barbiturates, bexarotene, bosentan, carBAMazepine, dexamethasone, efavirenz, griseofulvin, modafinil, nafcillin, nevirapine, OXcarbazepine, phenytoin, rifamycin, topiramate)

Drug/Herb

- Avoid use with St. John's wort

Drug/Food

- Avoid use with grapefruit products

NURSING CONSIDERATIONS

Assess:

- CBC, differential, platelet count before treatment and weekly; withhold product if WBC is <1500/mm^3 or platelet count is <100,000/mm^3, notify prescriber
- Monitor temperature q4hr (may indicate beginning infection)

Black Box Warning: Liver function tests before, during therapy (bilirubin, AST, ALT, LDH) prn or monthly; check for jaundiced skin and sclera, dark urine, clay-colored stools, itchy skin, abdominal pain, fever, diarrhea

- VS during 1st hr of infusion; check IV site for signs of infiltration

⚠ **Hypersensitivity reactions, anaphylaxis** including hypotension, dyspnea, angioedema, generalized urticaria; discontinue infusion immediately; keep emergency equipment available

- Effects of alopecia on body image; discuss feelings about body changes

Evaluate:

- Therapeutic response: decreased tumor size, spread of malignancy

Teach patient/family:

- To report signs of infection: fever, sore throat, flulike symptoms
- To report signs of anemia: fatigue, headache, faintness, SOB
- To report any complaints or side effects to nurse or prescriber
- That hair may be lost during treatment; that a wig or hairpiece may make patient feel better; that new hair may be different in color, texture
- That pain in muscles and joints 2-5 days after infusion is common
- To use nonhormonal type of contraception
- To avoid receiving vaccinations while receiving product

RARELY USED

ketoconazole (Rx)

(kee-toe-koe′na-zole)

Func. class.: Antifungal

Chem. class.: Imidazole derivative

USES: Systemic candidiasis, chronic mucocandidiasis, oral thrush, candiduria, coccidioidomycosis, histoplasmosis, chromomycosis, paracoccidioidomycosis, blastomycosis; tinea cruris, tinea corporis, tinea versicolor, *Pityrosporum ovale*

CONTRAINDICATIONS: Breastfeeding, hypersensitivity, fungal meningitis

Black Box Warning: Coadministration with other products (ergot derivatives, cisapride, or triazolam) may cause fatal cardiac arrhythmias due to inhibition of CYP3A4 enzyme system

Black Box Warning: Hepatic disease

DOSAGE AND ROUTES

- **Adult: PO** 200-400 mg/day for 1-2 wk (candidiasis), 6 wk (other infections)
- **Child ≥2 yr: PO:** 3.3-6.6 mg/kg/day as a single daily dose

Prostate cancer (unlabeled)

- **Adult: PO** 400 mg tid

ketoconazole (topical)

(kee-toe-koe′na-zole)

Extina, Ketoderm ✤, Ketozole, Nizoral, Nizoral A-D, Xolegel

Func. class.: Topical antifungal

Chem. class.: Imidazole derivative

ACTION: Antifungal activity results from altering cell membrane permeability

USES: Seborrheic dermatitis (immunocompromised), tinea corporis, cruris, pedis, versicolor, dandruff

CONTRAINDICATIONS: Hypersensitivity, sulfite allergy

Precautions: Pregnancy (C), breastfeeding, children

DOSAGE AND ROUTES

Seborrheic dermatitis:

- **Adult/child ≥12 yr: TOP FOAM** apply to affected areas bid × 4 wk
- **GEL** apply to affected areas daily × 2 wk

Tinea corporis, cruris, pedis, versicolor

- **Adult: TOP** cover areas daily × 2 wk

Dandruff:

- **Adult: SHAMPOO** wet hair, lather, massage for 1 min, rinse, repeat 2×/wk spaced by 3 days, for up to 8 wk, then as needed

Available forms: Topical gel, foam, cream 2%; shampoo 1%, 2%

Administer:

Topical route

- For external use only; do not use skin products near the eyes, nose, or mouth, wash hands before and after use
- **Cream/lotion:** Apply to the cleansed affected area, massage gently into affected areas, do not use on skin that is broken or irritated

SIDE EFFECTS

INTEG: Irritation, stinging, pustules, pruritus

NURSING CONSIDERATIONS

Assess allergic reaction:

- Assess for hypersensitivity, product might need to be discontinued

⚠ Assess for sulfite allergy; may be life-threatening

Evaluate:

- Decreased itching scaling

Teach patient/family:

Topical route

- These products are not for intravaginal therapy and are for external use only; do

K

not use skin products near the eyes, nose, or mouth; wash hands before and after use; do not wash affected area for ≥3 hr after application

- **Cream/Ointment/Lotion:** apply a thin film to the cleansed affected area, massage gently
- **Foam Formulations:** do not dispense foam directly onto hands or face; the warmth of the skin will cause the foam to melt; dispense desired amount directly into the cap or onto a cool surface; make sure enough foam is dispensed to cover the affected area(s); if the can feels warm or the foam seems runny, run the can under cold water; to apply, pick up small amounts of the foam with the fingertips and gently massage into the affected areas until the foam disappears
- To continue for prescribed time, tinea corporis/cruris ≥2 wk

ketoprofen (OTC, Rx)

(ke-toe-proe′fen)

Apo-Keto ♣

Func. class.: Nonsteroidal antiinflammatory product (NSAID), antirheumatic

Chem. class.: Propionic acid derivative

ACTION: Inhibits COX-1, COX-2; analgesic, antiinflammatory, antipyretic

USES: Mild to moderate pain, osteoarthritis, rheumatoid arthritis, dysmenorrhea; OTC relief of minor aches, pains

Unlabeled uses: Ankylosing spondylitis, bone pain, gouty arthritis

CONTRAINDICATIONS: Pregnancy (D) 2nd/3rd trimester, hypersensitivity to this product, NSAIDs, salicylates

Black Box Warning: Perioperative pain with CABG

Precautions: Pregnancy (C) 1st trimester, breastfeeding, children, geriatric patients, bleeding, GI/cardiac disorders, hypersensitivity to other antiinflammatory agents; asthma, severe renal/hepatic disease, ulcer disease

Black Box Warning: GI bleeding, MI, stroke

DOSAGE AND ROUTES

Antiinflammatory

- **Adult: PO** 50 mg qid or 75 mg tid, max 300 mg/day or **EXT REL** 200 mg/day

Analgesic

- **Adult: PO** 25-50 mg q6-8hr, max 300 mg/day

Available forms: Caps 50, 75 mg; ext rel cap 200 mg

Administer:

- Do not break, crush, or chew ext rel caps
- Store at room temperature
- Give with antacids, milk, or food for GI upset

SIDE EFFECTS

CNS: Dizziness, drowsiness, fatigue, confusion, insomnia, depression, headache

CV: Tachycardia, peripheral edema, palpitations, hypertension, CV thrombotic events, MI, stroke

EENT: Tinnitus, hearing loss, blurred vision

GI: *Nausea, anorexia, vomiting, diarrhea,* jaundice, hepatitis, constipation, flatulence, cramps, dry mouth, peptic ulcer, GI bleeding

GU: Nephrotoxicity: dysuria, hematuria, azotemia

HEMA: Blood dyscrasias

INTEG: Purpura, rash, pruritus

SYST: Anaphylaxis

PHARMACOKINETICS

PO: Peak 1.2 hr; ext rel 6.8 hr, half-life 2-4 hr; 5.4 hr ext rel, metabolized in liver, urine (metabolites), breast milk; 99% plasma protein binding

INTERACTIONS

Increase: toxicity—cycloSPORINE, lithium, methotrexate, phenytoin, alcohol, cidofovir

Increase: bleeding risk—anticoagulants, clopidogrel, eptifibatide, thrombolytics, ticlopidine, tirofiban, SSRIs

Increase: ketoprofen levels—aspirin, probenecid

Increase: adverse GI reactions—aspirin, corticosteroids, NSAIDs, alcohol

Increase: hematologic toxicity, antineoplastics

Decrease: effect of diuretics, antihypertensives

Drug/Herb

Increase: bleeding risk—feverfew, garlic, ginger, ginkgo

Drug/Lab Test

Increase: BUN, alk phos, AST, ALT, LDH, creatinine, bleeding time

NURSING CONSIDERATIONS

Assess:

- **Pain:** type, location, intensity, ROM before and 1-2 hr after treatment
- Renal, hepatic, blood studies: BUN, creatinine, AST, ALT, Hgb before treatment, periodically thereafter

⚠ Aspirin sensitivity, asthma; these patients may be more likely to develop hypersensitivity to NSAIDs

- Audiometric, ophthalmic exam before, during, after treatment
- For eye/ear problems: blurred vision, tinnitus; may indicate toxicity

Black Box Warning: GI bleeding: blood in sputum, emesis, stools

Black Box Warning: CV thrombotic events: MI, stroke

Evaluate:

- Therapeutic response: decreased pain, stiffness, swelling in joints; ability to move more easily; decreased fever

Teach patient/family:

- To report blurred vision, ringing, roaring in ears; may indicate toxicity
- To avoid driving, other hazardous activities if dizziness, drowsiness occurs, especially in geriatric patients
- To report immediately change in urine pattern, increased weight, edema, increased pain in joints, fever, blood in urine (indicate nephrotoxicity); rash, itching, blurred vision, ringing in ears, flulike symptoms; blood in urine, vomit, or stools (bleeding)
- That therapeutic effects may take up to 1 mo; to take with 8 oz water; to sit upright for ½ hr after administration to prevent GI irritation, not to crush, chew ext rel products
- To avoid aspirin, alcohol, corticosteroids, acetaminophen, other medications, supplements unless approved by prescriber
- To wear sunscreen, protective clothing to prevent photosensitivity
- To report product use to all health care providers
- To report planned or suspected pregnancy (D) (2nd/3rd trimester), (C) (1st trimester); avoid breastfeeding

ketorolac (ophthalmic)

(kee′toe-role-ak)

Acular, Acular LS, Acuvail

Func. class.: Antiinflammatory (ophthalmic)

Chem. class.: Nonsteroidal antiinflammatory drug

ACTION: Inhibits miosis by inhibiting the biosynthesis of ocular prostaglandins; prostaglandins play a role in the miotic response produced during ocular surgery by constricting the iris sphincter independently of cholinergic mechanisms

USES: Pain and inflammation after cataract surgery, refractive surgery, seasonal allergic conjunctivitis

CONTRAINDICATIONS:
Hypersensitivity to this product, NSAIDs, salicylates

Precautions: Bleeding disorders, complicated ocular surgery, corneal denervation, diabetes mellitus, rheumatoid arthritis, dry eye syndrome, pregnancy (C), breastfeeding, children, contact lens

DOSAGE AND ROUTES

Seasonal allergic conjunctivitis (Acular)

- **Adult/child ≥2 yr:** Instill 1 drop into affected eye qid

Inflammation after cataract extraction (Acular)

- **Adult: OPHTH** 1 drop in affected eye qid beginning 24 hr after surgery × 2 wk

Corneal refracture surgery, pain, burning (Acular LS)

- **Adult: OPHTH** 1 drop in affected eye qid × ≤4 days

Incision refraction surgery, pain, photophobia (Acular PF)

- **Adult: OPHTH** 1 drop qid in affected eye × 3 days

Cataract surgery, pain, inflammation (Acuvail)

- **Adult: OPHTH** 1 drop bid in affected eye, starting 1 day before surgery, on the day of surgery, × 2 wk after surgery

Available forms: Ophthalmic solution Acular (0.5%), Acular LS (0.4%), Acuvail (0.45%)

Administer:

- Apply topically to the eye, separate by ≥5 min when using with other ophthalmics
- Remove contact lenses before instillation of solution
- Instruct patient on proper instillation of eye solution
- Do not touch the tip of the dropper to the eye, fingertips, or other surface
- Do not share bottle with other patients

SIDE EFFECTS

CNS: Headache

EENT: Abnormal sensation in eye, conjunctival hyperemia, ocular irritation, ocular pain, ocular pruritus, conjunctival hyperemia, iritis, keratitis, blurred vision, transient burning/stinging

NURSING CONSIDERATIONS

Assess:

- Eyes: for pain, inflammation, burning, redness after cataract surgery

Evaluate:

- Decreased pain and inflammation after cataract surgery, refractive surgery, seasonal allergic conjunctivitis

Teach patient/family:

- To apply topically to the eye
- To remove contact lenses before instillation of solution
- Proper instillation of eye solution
- Not to touch the tip of the dropper to the eye, fingertips, or other surface
- Not to share bottle with other patients

ketorolac (systemic, nasal) (Rx)

(kee-toe′role-ak)

Toradol ✤, Sprix

Func. class.: Nonsteroidal antiinflammatory/nonopioid analgesic

Chem. class.: Acetic acid

Do not confuse:

Ketorolac/Ketalar

ACTION:
Inhibits prostaglandin synthesis by decreasing an enzyme needed for biosynthesis; analgesic, antiinflammatory, antipyretic effects

USES:
Mild to moderate pain (short term)

CONTRAINDICATIONS:
Pregnancy (D) 3rd trimester, hypersensitivity to this product, salicylates, asthma, hepatic disease, peptic ulcer disease, CV bleeding, C-section intracranial bleeding

Black Box Warning: Severe renal disease, L&D, perioperative pain in CABG, before major surgery, epidural/intrathecal administration, GI bleeding, hypovolemia, NSAID hypersensitivity

Precautions: Pregnancy (C), breastfeeding, GI/cardiac disorders, hypersensitivity to other antiinflammatory agents, CCr <25 ml/min

Black Box Warning: Children, geriatric patients, bleeding, MI, stroke

DOSAGE AND ROUTES

For the short-term treatment of moderate pain

Intranasal dosage:

- **Adults ≥50 kg with normal renal function:** 1 spray (15.75 mg/spray) in each nostril (total dose of 31.5 mg) q6-8hr; max 4 doses (8 sprays/126 mg) daily; total systemic therapy max 5 days
- **Adults <50 kg or who have renal impairment, and geriatric patients:** 1 spray (15.75 mg/spray) in one nostril q6-8hr max 4 doses (4 sprays/63 mg)daily; total systemic therapy max 5 days

For the short-term treatment of moderately severe pain

IM/IV (single-dose treatment):

- **Adults/adolescents 17 yr and ≥50 kg and have normal renal function:** 60 mg IM or 30 mg IV
- **Adults/adolescents 17 yr and <50 kg or have renal impairment, and geriatric patients:** 30 mg IM or 15 mg IV
- **Child ≥2 yr/adolescents ≤16 yr:** 1 mg/kg IM; max 30 mg or 0.5 mg/kg IV to a max of 15 mg

IM/IV (multiple-dose treatment):

- **Adults/adolescents 17 yr and weigh ≥50 kg and have normal renal function:** 30 mg IM/IV q6hr; total systemic therapy max 5 days
- **Adults/adolescents 17 yr and weigh <50 kg or have renal impairment, and geriatric patients:** 15 mg IM/IV q6hr; total systemic therapy max 5 days

PO (continuation therapy from IM/IV only):

- **Adults/adolescents 17 yr and weigh ≥50 kg and have normal renal function:** 20 mg initially following IV/IM therapy, then 10 mg q4-6hr; max 40 mg daily; total systemic therapy max 5 days
- **Adults/adolescents 17 yr and weigh <50 kg or have renal impairment, and geriatric patients:** 10 mg initially following IV/IM therapy, then 10 mg q4-6hr; max 40 mg daily; total systemic therapy should not exceed 5 days

Renal dose

- Do not use in advanced renal disease

Available forms: Inj 15, 30 mg/ml (prefilled syringes), 60 mg/2 ml; tab 10 mg; nasal spray 15.75 mg/spray

Administer:

- Not to exceed 5 days
- Store at room temperature, protect from light

IM route

- IM inj deeply and slowly in large muscle mass

Nasal route

- Prime pump before using for the first time, point away from person/pets, pump activator 5 times, no need to reprime
- For single-use only, discard 24 hr after opening if not used
- Do not share with others
- Have patient blow nose, sit upright to spray

IV route

- Give undiluted over ≥15 sec

Solution compatibility: D_5W, 0.9% NaCl, LR, D_5, Plasma-Lyte A

Syringe compatibilities: SUFentanil

Y-site compatibilities: Cisatracurium, remifentanil, SUFentanil

SIDE EFFECTS

CNS: Dizziness, *drowsiness,* tremors, seizures, headache

CV: Hypertension, pallor, edema, CV thrombotic events, MI, stroke

EENT: Tinnitus, hearing loss, blurred vision

GI: Nausea, anorexia, vomiting, diarrhea, constipation, flatulence, cramps, dry mouth, peptic ulcer, **GI bleeding, perforation**, taste change, **hepatic failure**
GU: **Nephrotoxicity: dysuria, hematuria, oliguria**
HEMA: **Blood dyscrasias**, prolonged bleeding
INTEG: Purpura, rash, pruritus, sweating, **angioedema, Stevens-Johnson syndrome, toxic epidermal necrolysis**

PHARMACOKINETICS

Half-life 6 hr, enters breast milk, metabolized by liver, excreted by kidneys
PO: Onset 30-60 min, duration 4-6 hr
IM: Onset 30 min, duration 4-6 hr

INTERACTIONS

Increase: toxicity—methotrexate, lithium, cycloSPORINE, pentoxifylline, probenecid, cidofovir
Increase: bleeding risk—anticoagulants, clopidogrel, eptifibatide, salicylates, ticlopidine, tirofiban, thrombolytics, SSRIs, SNRIs
Increase: renal impairment—ACE inhibitors
⚠ **Increase: ketorolac levels—aspirin, other NSAIDs; contraindicated**
Increase: GI effects—corticosteroids, alcohol, aspirin, NSAIDs
Decrease: effects—antihypertensives, diuretics

Drug/Lab Test
Increase: AST, ALT, LDH, bleeding time

NURSING CONSIDERATIONS

Assess:

- **Aspirin sensitivity, asthma:** patients may be more likely to develop hypersensitivity to NSAIDs; monitor for hypersensitivity
- **Pain:** type, location, intensity, ROM before and 1 hr after treatment

Black Box Warning: Renal, hepatic, blood studies: BUN, creatinine, AST, ALT, Hgb before treatment, periodically thereafter; check for dehydration

Black Box Warning: Bleeding times; check for bruising, bleeding, occult blood in urine

Black Box Warning: Do not use epidurally, intrathecally, alcohol is present in the solution

- Eye/ear problems: blurred vision, tinnitus (may indicate toxicity)

⚠ **Hepatic dysfunction: jaundice, yellow sclera and skin, clay-colored stools**

Black Box Warning: CV thrombotic events: MI, stroke, do not use in perioperative pain in CABG

- Audiometric, ophthalmic exam before, during, after treatment

Evaluate:

- Therapeutic response: decreased pain, stiffness, swelling in joints, ability to move more easily

Teach patient/family:

- To report blurred vision, ringing/roaring in ears (may indicate toxicity)
- To avoid driving, other hazardous activities if dizziness or drowsiness occurs

Black Box Warning: To report change in urine pattern, weight increase, edema; pain increase in joints, fever, blood in urine (indicates nephrotoxicity); bruising, black tarry stools (indicates bleeding); **pruritus, jaundice, nausea, right upper quadrant pain, abdominal pain (hepatotoxicity); to notify prescriber immediately**

- To avoid alcohol, salicylates, other NSAIDs
- To report product use to all health care providers, not to use with other products unless approved by prescriber; use for ≤5 days
- **Nasal:** to discard within 24 hr of opening; may cause irritation, may drink water after dose
- To report if pregnancy is planned or suspected pregnancy (C) systemic; not to breastfeed

ketotifen (ophthalmic)

(kee-toe-tye′fen)

Alaway, Zaditor, ZyrTEC Itchy Eye, Claritin Eye

Func. class.: Antihistamine (ophthalmic)

Chem. class.: Histamine 1 receptor antagonist/mast cell stabilizer

ACTION: A topically active, direct H_1-receptor antagonist and mast cell stabilizer; by reducing these inflammatory mediators, relieves the ocular pruritus associated with allergic conjunctivitis

USES: For the temporary relief of ocular pruritus due to ragweed, pollen, grass, animal hair, animal dander

CONTRAINDICATIONS: Hypersensitivity

Precautions: Pregnancy (C), breastfeeding, children, contact lenses

DOSAGE AND ROUTES

- **Adult/child ≥3 yr:** OPHTH instill 1 drop in affected eye(s) every 8-12 hr

Available forms: Ophthalmic solution 0.025%

Administer:

Ophthalmic route

- For topical ophthalmic use only
- Wash hands before and after use; tilt the head back slightly and pull the lower eyelid down with the index finger; squeeze the prescribed number of drops into the conjunctival sac and gently close eyes for 1-2 min, do not blink
- Do not touch the tip of the dropper to the eye, fingertips, or other surface
- Wait ≥10 min after instilling the ophthalmic solution before inserting contact lenses; contact lenses should not be worn if eye is red
- Do not share ophthalmic drops with others

SIDE EFFECTS

CNS: Headache

EENT: Conjunctival hyperemia, rhinitis, allergic reactions, ocular irritation consisting of burning or stinging, conjunctivitis, eyelid disorder, flu syndrome, keratitis, lacrimation disorder, mydriasis, ocular discharge, ocular pain, pharyngitis, photophobia, pruritus, rash, xerophthalmia (dry eyes)

NURSING CONSIDERATIONS

Assess:

- Eyes: for itching, redness, use of soft or hard contact lens

Evaluate:

- Absence of redness, itching in the eyes

Teach patient/family:

Ophthalmic route

- That product is for topical ophthalmic use only
- To wash hands before and after use; tilt the head back slightly and pull the lower eyelid down with the index finger; squeeze the prescribed number of drops into the conjunctival sac and gently close eyes for 1-2 min; not to blink
- Not to touch the tip of the dropper to the eye, fingertips, or other surface
- To wait ≥10 min after instilling the ophthalmic solution before inserting contact lenses; contact lenses should not be worn if eye is red
- Not to share ophthalmic drops with others
- To remove contact lenses before use because the preservative benzalkonium chloride may be absorbed by soft contact lenses; that product should not be used to treat contact lens-related irritation

K

⚠ HIGH ALERT

labetalol (Rx)

(la-bet′a-lole)

Trandate

Func. class.: Antihypertensive, antianginal

Chem. class.: α-1/β-Blocker

Do not confuse:
Trandate/Tridrate

ACTION: Produces decreases in B/P without reflex tachycardia or significant reduction in heart rate through mixture of α-blocking, β-blocking effects; elevated plasma renins are reduced

USES: Mild to moderate hypertension; treatment of severe hypertension (IV)

Unlabeled uses: Hypertension in patients with pheochromocytoma, hypertension during cloNIDine withdrawal, pediatric hypertension

CONTRAINDICATIONS: Hypersensitivity to β-blockers, cardiogenic shock, heart block (2nd or 3rd degree), sinus bradycardia, CHF, bronchial asthma

Precautions: Pregnancy (C), breastfeeding, geriatric patients, major surgery, diabetes mellitus, thyroid/renal/hepatic disease, COPD, well-compensated heart failure, nonallergic bronchospasm, peripheral vascular disease

Black Box Warning: Abrupt discontinuation

DOSAGE AND ROUTES

Hypertension

• **Adult: PO** 100 mg bid; may be given with diuretic; may increase to 200 mg bid after 2 days; may continue to increase q1-3days; max 2400 mg/day in divided doses

• **Child/adolescent (unlabeled): PO** 1-3 mg/kg/day, titrate to max 10-12 mg/kg/day based on B/P; **IV** 0.2-1 mg/kg over 2 min, max 40 mg/dose; **IV INFUSION** 0.25-3 mg/kg/hr

Hypertensive crisis

• **Adult: IV Intermittent** 20 mg over 2 min; may repeat 20-80 mg over 2 min q10min, 200 mg; **IV Cont INFUSION** after loading dose give 1-2 mg/min until desired response or max 300 mg

Available forms: Tabs 100, 200, 300 mg; inj 5 mg/ml, 20-, 40-ml vials

Administer:

• PO before meals, at bedtime; tab may be crushed or swallowed whole; give with meals to increase absorption

• **Do not discontinue before surgery**

• Store in dry area at room temperature; do not freeze

Direct IV route

• Give undiluted (5 mg/ml) over 2 min

Continuous IV INFUSION route

• Diluted in LR, D_5W, D_5 in 0.2%, 0.9%, 0.33% NaCl, Ringer's inj; infusion is titrated to patient response; 200 mg of product/160 ml sol = 1 mg/ml; 300 mg of product/240 ml sol = 1 mg/ml; 200 mg of product/250 ml sol = 2 mg/3 ml; use infusion pump

• Keep patient recumbent during and for 3 hr after administration; monitor VS q5-15min

Y-site compatibilities: Alemtuzumab, alfentanil, amikacin, aminocaproic acid, aminophylline, amiodarone, anidulafungin, argatroban, arsenic trioxide, ascorbic acid injection, atracurium, atropine, azithromycin, aztreonam, benztropine, bivalirudin, bleomycin, bretylium, bumetanide, buprenorphine, butorphanol, calcium chloride/gluconate, CARBOplatin, carmustine, caspofungin, ceFAZolin, cefotaxime, cefoTEtan, cefOXitin, ceftaroline, cefTAZidime, ceftizoxime, chlorproMAZINE, cimetidine, CISplatin, cloNIDine, cyanocobalamin, cyclophosphamide, cycloSPORINE, cytarabine, DACTINomycin, DAPTOmycin, DAUNOrubicin liposome, dexmedetomidine, dexrazoxane, digoxin, diltiazem, diphenhydrAMINE, DOBUTamine, DOCEtaxel, dolasetron, DOPamine, doripenem, doxacurium, DOXOrubicin,

DOXOrubicin liposomal, doxycycline, enalaprilat, ePHEDrine, EPINEPHrine, epirubicin, epoetin alfa, eptifibatide, ertapenem, erythromycin lactobionate, esmolol, etoposide, etoposide phosphate, famotidine, fenoldopam, fentaNYL, fluconazole, fludarabine, fluorouracil, folic acid, gallium, ganciclovir, gatifloxacin, gemcitabine, gentamicin, glycopyrrolate, granisetron, HYDROmorphone, hydroxyzine, IDArubicin, ifosfamide, imipenem-cilastatin, inamrinone, irinotecan, isoproterenol, lactated Ringer's injection, lepirudin, leucovorin, levofloxacin, lidocaine, linezolid injection, LORazepam, magnesium sulfate, mannitol, mechlorethamine, meperidine, metaraminol, methyldopate, methylPREDNISolone, metoclopramide, metoprolol, metroNIDAZOLE, midazolam, milrinone, minocycline, mitoXANtrone, morphine, moxifloxacin, multiple vitamins injection, mycophenolate, nalbuphine, naloxone, netilmicin, niCARdipine, nitroglycerin, nitroprusside, norepinephrine, octreotide, ondansetron, oxacillin, oxaliplatin, oxytocin, palonosetron, pamidronate, pancuronium, papaverine, PEMEtrexed, pentamidine, pentazocine, PENTobarbital, PHENobarbital, phentolamine, phenylephrine, phytonadione, polymyxin B, potassium acetate/chloride/phosphates, procainamide, prochlorperazine, promethazine, propofol, propranolol, protamine, pyridoxine, quiNIDine, quinupristin-dalfopristin, ranitidine, Ringer's injection, rocuronium, sodium acetate/bicarbonate, succinylcholine, SUFentanil, tacrolimus, telavancin, teniposide, theophylline, thiamine, thiotepa, ticarcillin-clavulanate, tigecycline, tirofiban, tobramycin, tolazoline, urokinase, vancomycin, vasopressin, vecuronium, verapamil, vinBLAStine, VinCRIStine, vinorelbine, voriconazole, zoledronic acid

SIDE EFFECTS

CNS: *Dizziness,* mental changes, drowsiness, *fatigue,* headache, catatonia, depression, anxiety, nightmares, paresthesias, lethargy

CV: *Orthostatic hypotension, bradycardia,* **CHF,** chest pain, **ventricular dysrhythmias,** AV block, scalp tingling

EENT: *Tinnitus,* visual changes; sore throat; double vision; dry, burning eyes, floppy iris syndrome; nasal congestion

ENDO: Hyperkalemia

GI: *Nausea, vomiting, diarrhea,* dyspepsia, taste distortion, **hepatotoxicity**

GU: Impotence, dysuria, ejaculatory failure

HEMA: **Agranulocytosis, thrombocytopenia, purpura** (rare)

INTEG: Rash, alopecia, urticaria, pruritus, fever, **exfoliative dermatitis**

RESP: **Bronchospasm,** dyspnea, wheezing

PHARMACOKINETICS

Half-life 2.5-8 hr, metabolized by liver (metabolites inactive), excreted in urine, crosses placenta, excreted in breast milk, protein binding 50%

PO: Onset 30 min, peak 1-4 hr, duration 8-24 hr

IV: Onset 2-5 min, peak 5-15 min, duration 2-4 hr

L

INTERACTIONS

- **Do not use within 2 wk of MAOIs**

Increase: **myocardial depression—hydantoins, general anesthetics, verapamil, class I antidysrhythmics**

Increase: tremor—tricyclic antidepressants

Increase: hypotension—diuretics, other antihypertensives, cimetidine, nitroglycerin, alcohol, nitrates

Decrease: effects of—sympathomimetics, lidocaine, theophylline, β-blockers, bronchodilators, xanthines

Decrease: antihypertensive effect—NSAIDs, salicylates

Increase or decrease: effects of—antidiabetics

Drug/Herb

Increase: antihypertensive effect—hawthorn

Decrease: antihypertensive effect—ephedra

Drug/Lab Test
Increase: ANA titer, blood glucose, alk phos, LDH, AST, ALT, BUN, potassium, triglyceride, uric acid, serum lipoprotein
False increase: urinary catecholamines

NURSING CONSIDERATIONS

Assess:

- **Hypertension:** B/P during beginning treatment, periodically thereafter; note pulse, rate, rhythm, quality; apical/radial pulse before administration; notify prescriber of any significant changes

⚠ CHF: I&O, weight daily; fluid overload: weight gain, jugular venous distention, edema, crackles in lungs

Black Box Warning: Abrupt discontinuation: product should be tapered to prevent adverse reactions

- Baselines of renal/hepatic studies before therapy begins

Evaluate:

- Therapeutic response: decreased B/P after 1-2 wk

Teach patient/family:

Black Box Warning: Not to discontinue product abruptly; to taper over 2 wk; may cause precipitate angina

- Not to use OTC products containing α-adrenergic stimulants (nasal decongestants, OTC cold preparations) unless directed by prescriber
- To report bradycardia, dizziness, confusion, depression, fever
- To take pulse at home; advise when to notify prescriber
- May mask symptoms of hypoglycemia; monitor blood glucose closely
- To avoid alcohol, smoking, increased sodium intake
- To comply with weight control, dietary adjustments, modified exercise program
- To carry emergency ID to identify product, allergies
- To avoid hazardous activities if dizziness is present
- **To report symptoms of CHF:** difficulty breathing, especially on exertion or when lying down; night cough; swelling of extremities
- To take medication at bedtime for 1 dose to prevent effect of orthostatic hypotension; to rise slowly
- To avoid driving or other hazardous activities until response is known; dizziness, drowsiness, may occur
- To wear support hose

TREATMENT OF OVERDOSE:

Lavage, IV glucagon or atropine for bradycardia, IV theophylline for bronchospasm; digoxin, O_2, diuretic for cardiac failure; hemodialysis useful for removal/hypotension; administer vasopressor

lacosamide (Rx)

(la-koe′sa-mide)

Vimpat

Func. class.: Anticonvulsant
Chem. class.: Functionalized amino acid

Controlled Substance Schedule V

ACTION:

May act through action at sodium channels; exact action is unknown

USES:

Partial seizures

CONTRAINDICATIONS:

Hypersensitivity

Precautions: Pregnancy (C), breastfeeding, children <17 yr, geriatric patients, allergies, cardiac/renal/hepatic disease, acute MI, atrial fibrillation/flutter, AV block, bradycardia, CHD, dehydration, depression, dialysis, hazardous activity, electrolyte imbalance, heart failure, labor, PR prolongation, sick sinus syndrome, substance abuse, suicidal ideation, syncope, torsades de pointes

DOSAGE AND ROUTES

- **Adult and adolescent ≥17 yr: PO** 50 mg bid, may increase weekly by 100 mg bid to 200-400 mg/day; **IV** 50 mg bid, infuse over 30-60 min, may be increased by 100 mg/day weekly up to 200-400 mg/day maintenance

Renal/hepatic dose

• **Adult: PO/IV** max 300 mg/day for mild to moderate hepatic disease or CCr ≤30 ml/min

Available forms: Film-coated tabs 50, 100, 150, 200 mg; IV 20 ml single-use vials (200 mg/20 ml); oral sol 10 mg/ml

Administer:

• Store PO products/IV vials at room temperature; sol is stable for 24 hr when mixed with compatible diluents in glass or PVC bags at room temperature

PO route

• **Tablet:** give without regard to meals
• **Oral sol:** measure with calibrated measuring device

IV route

• May give undiluted or mixed in 0.9% NaCl, D_5W, or LR
• Infuse over 30-60 min, stable for 24 hr at room temperature
• Do not use if discolored or if particulates are present; discard unused portions

SIDE EFFECTS

CNS: Dizziness, syncope, tremor, vertigo, ataxia, drowsiness, fever, hypoesthesia, paresthesias, depression, fatigue, headache, confusion, irritability, psychologic dependence, suicidal ideation, euphoria

CV: Atrial fibrillation/flutter, AV block, bradycardia, myocarditis, orthostatic hypotension, palpitations, PR prolongation

EENT: Diplopia, blurred vision, nystagmus, tinnitus

GI: Nausea, constipation, vomiting, hepatitis, diarrhea, dyspepsia

HEMA: Anemia, neutropenia, agranulocytosis

INTEG: Rash, erythema, inj-site reaction, pruritus, xerostomia

MS: Asthenia, dysarthria, muscle cramps

SYST: Drug reaction with eosinophilia, systemic symptoms (DRESS)

PHARMACOKINETICS

Metabolized by liver; excreted by kidneys, 95%; protein binding <15%

PO: Peak 1-4 hr

IV: Peak 30-60 min; half-life 13 hr; elimination half-life 15-23 hr

INTERACTIONS

⚠ **Increase:** PR prolongation—β-blockers, calcium channel blockers, atazanavir, dronedarone, digoxin, lopinavir, ritonavir

⚠ **Increase:** lacosamide effect—CYP2C19 inhibitors (fluconazole, isoniazid, miconazole)

Drug/Lab Test

Increase: LFTs

NURSING CONSIDERATIONS

Assess:

• **Seizures:** duration, type, intensity precipitating factors
• Renal function: albumin concentration
• CV status: orthostatic hypotension, PR prolongation; monitor cardiac status throughout treatment
• Mental status: mood, sensorium, affect, memory (long, short term), depression, suicidal ideation, psychologic dependence
• Rash, hypersensitivity reactions
• **Pregnancy:** Enroll in UCB Antiepileptic Drugs Registry 1-888-537-7734

Evaluate:

• Therapeutic response: decrease in severity of seizures

Teach patient/family:

• Not to discontinue product abruptly; to taper over 1 week because seizures may occur
• To avoid hazardous activities until stabilized on product
• To carry emergency ID stating product use
• To notify prescriber of suicidal thoughts/behaviors, syncope, cardiac changes
• To notify prescriber if pregnancy is planned or suspected
• That interactions with other medications may occur
• To consult MedGuide for proper use, risks

lactulose (Rx)

(lak′tyoo-lose)

Constulose, Enulose, Generlac, Kristalose

Func. class.: Laxative; ammonia detoxicant (hyperosmotic)

Chem. class.: Lactose synthetic derivative

Do not confuse:
lactulose/lactose

ACTION: Prevents absorption of ammonia in colon by acidifying stool; increases water, softens stool

USES: Chronic constipation, portal-systemic encephalopathy in patients with hepatic disease

CONTRAINDICATIONS: Hypersensitivity, low-galactose diet

Precautions: Pregnancy (B), breastfeeding, geriatric patients, debilitated patients, diabetes mellitus

DOSAGE AND ROUTES

Constipation

- **Adult: PO** 15-30 ml/day (10-20 g), may increase to 60 ml/day prn
- **Child: PO** 7.5 ml/day

Hepatic encephalopathy

- **Adult: PO** 30-45 ml (20-30 g) tid or qid until stools soft; **RETENTION ENEMA** 300 ml (200 g) diluted
- **Child: PO** 40-90 ml/day in 3-4 divided doses
- **Infant: PO** 2.5-10 ml/day in divided doses

Available forms: Oral sol 10 g/15 ml; packets 10, 20 g; rectal sol 10 g/15 ml

Administer:

PO route

- With 8 oz fruit juice, water, milk to increase palatability of oral form; for rapid effect, give on empty stomach
- Increased fluids to 2 L/day; do not give with other laxatives; if diarrhea occurs, reduce dosage
- **Kristalose:** dissolve contents of packet/4 oz water

Rectal route

- **Retention enema** by diluting 300 ml lactose/700 ml of water; administer by rectal balloon catheter

SIDE EFFECTS

GI: *Nausea, vomiting, anorexia, abdominal cramps,* diarrhea, flatulence, distention, belching

META: Hypernatremia

PHARMACOKINETICS

Metabolized in colon, onset 1-2 days, peak unknown, duration unknown

INTERACTIONS

- Do not use with other laxatives (hepatic encephalopathy)

Increase: GI obstruction—NIFEdipine ext-rel tabs

Decrease: lactulose effects—neomycin, other oral antiinfectives, antacids

Drug/Herb

Increase: laxative action—flax, senna

Drug/Lab Test

Increase: blood glucose (diabetic patients)

Decrease: blood ammonia

NURSING CONSIDERATIONS

Assess:

- **Stool:** amount, color, consistency
- **Cause of constipation;** determine whether fluids, bulk, or exercise is missing from lifestyle; use of constipating products
- **Hepatic encephalopathy:** blood ammonia level (30-70 mg/100 ml); may decrease ammonia level by 25%-50%; clearing of confusion, lethargy, restlessness, irritability if portal-systemic encephalopathy, monitor sodium in higher doses
- Blood, urine electrolytes if product used often; may cause diarrhea, hypokalemia, hyponatremia

- I&O ratio to identify fluid loss, replace any loss
- **Cramping, rectal bleeding, nausea, vomiting; if these symptoms occur, product should be discontinued**

Evaluate:

- Therapeutic response: decreased constipation, decreased blood ammonia level, clearing of mental state

Teach patient/family:

- Not to use laxatives long term
- To dilute with water or fruit juice to counteract sweet taste
- To store in cool environment; not to freeze
- To take on an empty stomach for rapid action
- To report diarrhea; may indicate overdose

lamiVUDine 3TC (Rx)

(lam-i-voo′deen)

Epivir, Epivir HBV

Func. class.: Antiretroviral

Chem. class.: Nucleoside reverse transcriptase inhibitor (NRTI)

Do not confuse:
lamiVUDine/lamoTRIgine

ACTION: Inhibits replication of HIV virus by incorporating into cellular DNA by viral reverse transcriptase, thereby terminating cellular DNA chain

USES: HIV-1 infection in combination with at least 2 other antiretrovirals; chronic hepatitis B (Epivir-HBV)

Unlabeled uses: Prophylaxis of HIV: postexposure with indinavir and zidovudine

CONTRAINDICATIONS: Hypersensitivity

Precautions: Pregnancy (C), breastfeeding, children, geriatric patients, granulocyte count $<1000/mm^3$ or Hgb <9.5 g/dl, renal disease, pancreatitis, peripheral neuropathy

Black Box Warning: Severe hepatic dysfunction, lactic acidosis

DOSAGE AND ROUTES

HIV

- **Adult and adolescent >16 yr: PO** 150 mg bid or 300 mg/day
- **Child 3 mo-16 yr: PO** 4 mg/kg bid, max 150 mg bid

Chronic hepatitis B

- **Adult: PO** 100 mg/day
- **Child and adolescent 2-17 yr: PO** 3 mg/kg/day, max 100 mg

Renal dose

- **Adult: PO** CCr 30-49 ml/min: Epivir 150 mg/day; Epivir HBV 100 mg 1st dose, then 50 mg/day; CCr 15-29 ml/min: Epivir 150 mg 1st dose, then 100 mg/day; Epivir HBV 100 mg 1st dose, then 25 mg/day; CCr 5-14 ml/min: Epivir 150 mg 1st dose, then 50 mg/day; Epivir HBV 35 mg 1st dose, then 15 mg/day; CCr <5 ml/min: Epivir 50 mg 1st dose, then 25 mg/day; Epivir HBV 35 mg 1st dose, then 10 mg/day

Available forms: (Epivir) oral sol 10 mg/ml; tabs 150, 300 mg; **(Epivir HBV)** oral sol 5 mg/ml; tabs 100 mg

Administer:

- PO daily or bid, without regard to meals
- Epivir and Epivir HBV are not interchangeable
- With other antiretrovirals only
- Store in cool environment; protect from light

SIDE EFFECTS

CNS: *Fever, headache, malaise, dizziness, insomnia, depression, fatigue, chills,* **seizures**, peripheral neuropathy, paresthesias

EENT: Taste change, hearing loss, photophobia

GI: *Nausea, vomiting, diarrhea,* anorexia, cramps, dyspepsia, **hepatomegaly with steatosis, pancreatitis**

HEMA: **Neutropenia, anemia, thrombocytopenia**

INTEG: *Rash*

MS: *Myalgia, arthralgia, pain*

RESP: *Cough*
SYST: Lactic acidosis, anaphylaxis, Stevens-Johnson syndrome

PHARMACOKINETICS

Rapidly absorbed, distributed to extravascular space, excreted unchanged in urine, protein binding <36%, terminal half-life 5-7 hr

INTERACTIONS

Decrease: both products—zalcitabine; avoid concurrent use
Increase: lamiVUDine level—trimethoprim-sulfamethoxazole, aMILoride, dofetilide, entecavir, metFORMIN, memantine, procainamide, trospium
• Do not use with emtricitabine, duplication
Decrease: lamiVUDine effect—interferons

Drug/Lab Test
Increase: ALT, bilirubin
Decrease: Hgb, neutrophil, platelet count

NURSING CONSIDERATIONS

Assess:
• **HIV:** Test for HIV before starting treatment, blood counts q2wk; watch for neutropenia, thrombocytopenia, Hgb, CD4, viral load; if low, therapy may have to be discontinued and restarted after hematologic recovery; blood transfusions may be required; assess for lessening of symptoms; if HBV is present, a higher dose of Epivir-HBV is needed
• **Hepatitis B:** fatigue, anorexia, pruritus, jaundice during and for several months after discontinuation; AST, ALT, bilirubin; amylase, lipase, triglycerides, periodically during treatment
• **Children for pancreatitis:** abdominal pain, nausea, vomiting, neuropathy

Black Box Warning: Lactic acidosis, severe hepatomegaly with steatosis: obtain baseline LFTs, if elevated, discontinue treatment; discontinue even if LFTs are normal if lactic acidosis, severe hepatomegaly develops, may be fatal

Evaluate:
• Decreasing symptoms of HIV, CD4, viral load

Teach patient/family:
• That GI complaints, insomnia resolve after 3-4 wk of treatment
• That product is not a cure for HIV but will control symptoms; that compliance is necessary; to take as directed; to complete full course of treatment even if feeling better
• To notify prescriber of sore throat, swollen lymph nodes, malaise, fever, peripheral neuropathy; other infections may occur
• That patient is still infective, may pass HIV virus on to others
• That follow-up visits must be continued since serious toxicity may occur; that blood counts must be done
• That other products may be necessary to prevent other infections
• That product may cause fainting or dizziness
• Not to breastfeed, excreted in breast milk

lamoTRIgine (Rx)

(la-moe′tri-geen)

LaMICtal, LaMICtal CD, LaMICtal ODT, LaMICtal XR

Func. class.: Anticonvulsant—miscellaneous
Chem. class.: Phenyltriazine

Do not confuse:
lamoTRIgine/lamiVUDine
LaMICtal/Lomotil/LamISIL

ACTION: Inhibits voltage-sensitive sodium channels, thus decreasing seizures

USES: Adjunct for the treatment of partial, tonic-clonic seizures; children with Lennox-Gastaut syndrome, bipolar disorder
Unlabeled uses: Absence seizures

CONTRAINDICATIONS: Hypersensitivity

Precautions: Pregnancy (C) (cleft lip/palate during 1st trimester), breastfeeding, geriatric patients, cardiac/renal/hepatic disease, severe depression, suicidal, blood dyscrasias, children <16 yr, serious rash

DOSAGE AND ROUTES

Seizures: monotherapy

• **Adult and adolescent ≥16 yr: PO** 50 mg/day while receiving 1 enzyme-inducing AED (carBAMazepine, PHENObarbital, phenytoin, primidone but not valproic acid) wk 1-2, then increase to 100 mg divided bid wk 3-4; maintenance 300-500 mg/day; EXT REL 50 mg/day × 1-2 wk, then 100 mg/day wk 3-4, then 200 mg/day wk 5, then 300 mg/day wk 6, then 400 mg/day wk 7; after wk 7, range is 400-600 mg/day

• **Adolescent <16 yr and child: PO** 0.3 mg/kg/day wk 1-2, then 0.6 mg/kg/day wk 3-4; depends on use of AED; usual dose 4.5-7.5 mg/kg/day, max 300 mg/day

Monotherapy for patients taking valproate

• **Adult and adolescent ≥16 yr receiving lamoTRIgine and valproate without enzyme-inducing drug: PO** (immediate release) stabilize on valproate, target dose of 200 mg/day lamoTRIgine; if patient is not taking lamoTRIgine 200 mg/day, increase dose by 25-50 mg/day q1-2wk to reach 200 mg/day; while maintaining lamoTRIgine 200 mg/day, decrease valproate to 500 mg/day by ≤500 mg/day/wk, maintain valproate at 500 mg/day × 1 wk, then increase lamoTRIgine to 300 mg/day while decreasing valproate 250 mg/day × 1 wk, then discontinue valproate and increase lamoTRIgine by 100 mg/day/wk to maintenance of 500 mg/day

Seizures: multiple therapy with valproate

• **Adult and adolescent ≥16 yr: PO** 25 mg every other day, then 25 mg/day wk 3-4, increase by 25-50 mg q1-2wk, maintenance 100-500 mg/day

• **Adolescent <16 yr and child: PO** 0.1-0.2 mg/kg/day initially, then increase q2wk as needed to 1-5 mg/kg/day or 200 mg/day

Bipolar disorder (escalation regimen for those not taking carBAMazepine, other enzyme-inducing drugs, or valproate)

• **Adult and adolescent ≥16 yr: PO** wk 1-2, 25 mg/day; wk 3-4, 50 mg/day; wk 5, 100 mg/day; wk 6-7, 200 mg/day; for patients taking valproic acid: wk 1-2, 25 mg every other day; wk 3-4, 25 mg/day; wk 5, 50 mg/day; wk 6, 100 mg/day; wk 7, 100 mg/day

Hepatic dose

• **Adult: PO** moderate hepatic impairment or severe without ascites: reduce by 25%; severe hepatic impairment with ascites: reduce by 50%

Absence seizures (unlabeled)

• **Adolescent and child 3-13 yr: PO** 0.5 mg/kg/day in 2 divided doses × 2 wk, then 1 mg/kg/day in 2 divided doses × 2 wk, adjusted q5days

L

Available forms: Tabs 25, 100, 150, 200 mg; PO ext rel 25-50-100, 50-100-200 mg titration kit; PO 25-100 mg starter kit; ext rel 25, 50, 100, 250, 300 mg; chew dispersible tabs 5, 25 mg; oral disintegrating tab 25, 50, 100, 200 mg; oral disintegrating tab 25-50, 50-100 mg, 25-50-100 mg titration kit

Administer:

• Correct starter kit; severe side effects here occurred from incorrect starter kit

• **Orange starter kit:** for those **NOT** taking carBAMazepine, phenytoin, PHENobarbital, primidone, rifampin, valproate

• **Green starter kit:** for those taking carBAMazepine, phenytoin, PHENobarbital, primidone, rifampin but **NOT** valproate

• **Blue starter kit:** for those taking valproate

• Discontinue all products gradually over ≥2 wk; abrupt discontinuation can increase seizures

• All forms may be given without regard to meals

• **Chewable dispersible tab:** may be swallowed whole, chewed, mixed in water or fruit juice; to mix, add to small amount of liquid in glass or spoon; tabs will dissolve in 1 min, then mix in more liquid and swirl and swallow immediately; do not cut tabs in half
• **Orally disintegrating tabs:** place on tongue, move around in mouth, when disintegrated, swallow; examine blister pack before use, do not use if blisters are torn or missing
• **Extended-release tabs:** swallow whole, do not cut, break, chew; without regard to food

SIDE EFFECTS

CNS: *Dizziness,* ataxia, *headache,* fever, insomnia, tremor, depression, anxiety, suicidal ideation, seizures, poor concentration
EENT: Nystagmus, *diplopia, blurred vision*
GI: *Nausea, vomiting, anorexia, abdominal pain,* hepatotoxicity
GU: *Dysmenorrhea*
HEMA: Anemia, DIC, leukopenia, thrombocytopenia
INTEG: Rash (potentially life-threatening), alopecia, photosensitivity
CV: Chest pain, palpitations
MS: Neck pain, myalgias
SYST: Stevens-Johnson syndrome, angioedema, toxic epidermal necrolysis, DRESS

PHARMACOKINETICS

Half-life varies depending on dose; terminal half-life 24 hr, 15 hr with enzyme inducers; rapidly, completely absorbed; metabolized by glucuronic acid conjunction; protein binding 55%; peak 1.4-2.3 hr; crosses placenta; excreted in breast milk

INTERACTIONS

Decrease: metabolic clearance of lamoTRIgine—valproic acid, CYP3A4 inhibitors
Decrease: lamoTRIgine concentration—carBAMazepine, rifamycins, oral contraceptives, acetaminophen, phenytoin, primodone, PHENobarbital, OXcarbazepine, succinimides, estrogen
Drug/Herb
Increase: anticonvulsant effect—ginkgo
Decrease: anticonvulsant effect—ginseng

NURSING CONSIDERATIONS

Assess:
• **Seizure:** duration, type, intensity, halo before seizure
⚠ Rash (Stevens-Johnson syndrome, toxic epidermal necrolysis) in pediatric patients; product should be discontinued at first sign of rash
⚠ **Bipolar disorder:** suicidal thoughts/behaviors
Evaluate:
• Therapeutic response: decrease in severity of seizures or of bipolar symptoms
Teach patient/family:
• To take PO doses divided, with or after meals to decrease adverse effects; not to discontinue product abruptly because seizures may occur
• To avoid hazardous activities until stabilized on product
• To carry emergency ID; to notify prescriber of skin rash, increased seizure activity; to use sunscreen, protective clothing if photosensitivity occurs
• To notify prescriber if pregnant, intending to become pregnant
• To notify prescriber immediately of suicidal thoughts/behaviors
• To notify prescriber if pregnancy is planned or suspected, pregnancy (C), product decreases folate, avoid breastfeeding

lansoprazole (Rx, OTC)

(lan-so-prey′zole)

Prevacid, Prevacid SoluTab

Func. class.: Antiulcer, proton pump inhibitor
Chem. class.: Benzimidazole

Do not confuse:
Prevacid/Pravachol/Prinivil

ACTION: Suppresses gastric secretion by inhibiting hydrogen/potassium ATPase enzyme system in gastric parietal cell; characterized as gastric acid pump inhibitor because it blocks the final step of acid production

USES: Gastroesophageal reflux disease (GERD), severe erosive esophagitis, poorly responsive systemic GERD, pathologic hypersecretory conditions (Zollinger-Ellison syndrome, systemic mastocytosis, multiple endocrine adenomas); possibly effective for treatment of duodenal, gastric ulcers, maintenance of healed duodenal ulcers

Unlabeled uses: GERD (infants/neonates)

CONTRAINDICATIONS: Hypersensitivity

Precautions: Pregnancy (B), breastfeeding, children, hypomagnesemia, osteoporosis

DOSAGE AND ROUTES

Frequent heartburn

- **Adult: PO (OTC)** 15 mg daily up to 14 days

Duodenal ulcer

- **Adult: PO** 15 mg/day before eating for 4 wk, then 15 mg/day to maintain healing of ulcers; associated with **Helicobacter pylori:** 30 mg lansoprazole, 500 mg clarithromycin, 1 g amoxicillin bid × 14 days or 30 mg lansoprazole, 1 g amoxicillin tid × 14 days

Pathologic hypersecretory conditions

- **Adult: PO** 60 mg/day, may give up to 90 mg bid, administer doses of >120 mg/day in divided doses

GERD/esophagitis

- **Adult and adolescent: PO** 15-30 mg/day × 8 wk
- **Child 1-11 yr (>30 kg): PO** 30 mg/day ≤12 wk
- **Child 1-11 yr (≤30 kg): PO** 15 mg/day ≤12 wk
- **Infant (unlabeled): PO** 1-1.74 mg/kg/day; limited data available
- **Neonate (unlabeled): PO** 0.5-1 mg/kg/day

Stress gastric prophylaxis

- **Adult: NG** Use 30 mg oral cap or 30 mg disintegrating tab

Available forms: Del rel caps 15, 30 mg; oral powder; orally disintegrating tabs 15, 30 mg

Administer:

PO route

- Swallow caps whole 30 min before eating; do not crush or chew caps; caps may be opened and contents sprinkled on food

NG route

- **Oral cap:** open cap and pour 1/4 of granules into NG feeding syringe with plunger removed, slowly add water and depress plunger, repeat until all granules used; flush tube with 15 ml water
- Place on tongue, allow to dissolve, use without regard to water
- **Oral syringe:** dissolve 15 mg/4 ml or 30 mg/10 ml water, use extra water in syringe to remove all of the product

NG tube

- **Oral disintegrating tab:** mix 30 mg tab in 10 ml water, give via NG tube, flush tube with 10 ml sterile water, clamp for 60 min

SIDE EFFECTS

CNS: *Headache*

GI: Diarrhea, abdominal pain, vomiting, nausea, *constipation,* flatulence, acid regurgitation, anorexia, irritable colon, microscopic colitis

GU: Hematuria, glycosuria, impotence, kidney calculus, breast enlargement

PHARMACOKINETICS

Absorption after granules leave stomach 80%; plasma half-life 1½-2 hr; protein binding 97%; extensively metabolized in liver; excreted in urine, feces; clearance decreased in geriatric patients, renal/hepatic impairment

INTERACTIONS

Decrease: antiplatelets, effect of—clopidogrel

L

Increase: lansoprazole, toxicity—fluvoxaMINE, voriconazole
Increase: bleeding risk—warfarin
Decrease: lansoprazole absorption—sucralfate
Decrease: absorption of ketoconazole, itraconazole, iron salts, calcium carbonate, atazanavir, ampicillin
Increase: hypomagnesemia—loop/thiazide diuretics
Decrease: lansoprazole effect—antimuscarinics, octreotide, H_2-blockers, misoprostol
Decrease: release of ext rel amphetamine/dextroamphetamine
- Avoid use with dasatinib, delavirdine

Drug/Herb
- Avoid use with red yeast rice, St. John's wort

Drug/Food
- Food decreases rate of absorption, use before food

NURSING CONSIDERATIONS

Assess:
- **GI system:** bowel sounds q8hr, abdomen for pain, swelling, anorexia, blood in stool, emesis
- **Hepatic studies:** AST, ALT, alk phos during treatment
- INR and prothrombin time when taking warfarin
- Magnesium: low magnesium may occur

Evaluate:
- Therapeutic response: absence of epigastric pain, swelling, fullness

Teach patient/family:
- To report severe diarrhea; product may have to be discontinued
- That hypoglycemia may occur if diabetic
- To avoid hazardous activities; that dizziness may occur
- To avoid alcohol, salicylates, ibuprofen; may cause GI irritation
- That if using OTC for heartburn, it may take 1-4 days to see full benefit

RARELY USED

lanthanum (Rx)

(lan′-tha-num)

Fosrenol

Func. class.: Phosphate binder

USES:
End-stage renal disease

CONTRAINDICATIONS:
Hypophosphatemia, hypersensitivity

DOSAGE AND ROUTES
- **Adult: PO** 750-1500 mg/day in divided doses with meals; titrate dose q2-3wk until an acceptable phosphate level is reached; tabs should be chewed completely before swallowing; intact tabs should not be swallowed; maintenance dose 1500-3000 mg/day divided with meals; max 3750 mg/day

RARELY USED

lapatinib (Rx)

(la-pa′tin-ib)

Tykerb

Func. class.: Antineoplastic—miscellaneous

Chem. class.: Biologic response modifier, signal transduction inhibitor (STIs)

USES:
Advanced metastatic breast cancer patients with tumor that overexpresses HER2 protein and who have received previous chemotherapy

CONTRAINDICATIONS:
Pregnancy (D), breastfeeding, hypersensitivity

DOSAGE AND ROUTES

Advanced/metastatic breast cancer with HER2 overexpression who have received previous therapy

- **Adult: PO** 1250 mg (5 tabs)/day 1 hr before or after food on days 1-21 plus capecitabine 2000 mg/m²/day in 2 divided doses on days 1-14 in a repeating 21-day cycle; continue until therapeutic response or toxicity occurs

Metastatic breast cancer with HER2 overexpression for whom hormonal therapy is indicated

- **Adult: PO** 1500 mg (6 tabs) 1 hr before food with letrozole 2.5 mg/day

Hepatic dose

- **Adult: PO** (Child-Pugh C) 750 mg/day (with capecitabine); 1000 mg/day (with letrozole)

latanoprost (ophthalmic)

(lah-tan′oh-prost)

Xalatan

Func. class.: Antiglaucoma agent
Chem. class.: Prostaglandin agonist

Do not confuse:
latanoprost/bimatoprost

ACTION: Increases aqueous humor outflow

USES: Increased intraocular pressure in those who have open-angle glaucoma/ocular hypertension and who do not respond to other IOP-lowering products

CONTRAINDICATIONS: Hypersensitivity to this product, benzalkonium chloride

Precautions: Eye infections, angle-closure glaucoma, renal/hepatic function impairment, children, contact lens

DOSAGE AND ROUTES

- **Adult: OPHTH** Instill 1 drop in each affected eye (conjunctival sac) every night

Available forms: Ophthalmic solution 0.005%

Administer:

Ophthalmic route

- Wash hands before and after use; contact lenses should be removed before using the product, reinsert 15 min after use; contains benzalkonium chloride, which may be absorbed by soft contact lenses
- Tilt the head back slightly and pull the lower eyelid down with the index finger to form a pouch; squeeze the prescribed number of drops into the pouch and gently close the eyes for 1-2 min; do not blink; to avoid contamination, do not touch the tip of the dropper to the eye, fingertips, or other surface
- The solution may be used concomitantly with other topical ophthalmic drug products to lower IOP; if more than one topical ophthalmic drug is being used, the drugs should be administered at least 5 min apart
- Store unopened bottle refrigerated; once opened, it may be stored at room temperature, protected from light, for up to 6 wk

SIDE EFFECTS

EENT: *Conjunctival hyperemia, iris color change, ocular pruritus*, xerophthalmia, visual disturbance, ocular irritation burning, foreign body sensation, ocular pain, blepharitis, cataracts, and superficial punctate keratitis

INTEG: Rash, allergic reactions

MISC: Flulike symptoms

CV: Angina

PHARMACOKINETICS

Ophthalmic: Onset 3-4 hr, peak 8-12 hr; half-life 3 hr

NURSING CONSIDERATIONS

Assess:

- **Intraocular pressure:** in those with ongoing increased IOP

Evaluate:

- Decreasing IOP

L

Teach patient/family:
Ophthalmic route

- To wash hands before and after use; that contact lenses should be removed, reinsert 15 min after use; contains benzalkonium chloride, which may be absorbed by soft contact lenses
- Tilt the head back slightly and pull lower eyelid down to form a pouch; squeeze drops into the pouch and close the eyes for 1-2 min; not to blink; to avoid contamination, do not touch the tip of the dropper to the eye, fingertips, or other surface
- May be used concomitantly with other topical ophthalmic products to lower IOP; if more than one is used, the drugs should be administered at least 5 min apart, do not exceed dose
- To store unopened bottle refrigerated; once opened, it may be stored at room temperature, protected from light, for up to 6 wk

HIGH ALERT

ledipasvir/sofosbuvir

(le-dip′as-vir/soe-fos′bue-veer)

Harvoni

Func. class.: Antiviral antihepatitis agent

ACTION: A combination product with a HCV NS5A inhibitor (ledipasvir) and a nucleotide analog HCV NS5B polymerase inhibitor (sofosbuvir)

USES: Chronic hepatitis C virus (HCV) genotype 1 infection in patients with compensated liver disease

CONTRAINDICATIONS: Hypersensitivity

Precautions: Decompensated hepatic disease, decompensated cirrhosis, severe renal impairment (eGFR <30 ml/min/1.73 m^2), end-stage renal failure requiring dialysis, pregnancy (B), breastfeeding

DOSAGE AND ROUTES

- **Adults with or without cirrhosis who are treatment-naive: PO** One tab (90 mg ledipasvir; 400 mg sofosbuvir) every day with or without food for 12 wk; 8 wk can be considered for those patients with a baseline HCV RNA <6 million IU/ml
- **Adults without cirrhosis who are treatment-experienced: PO** One tablet (90 mg ledipasvir; 400 mg sofosbuvir) every day with or without food for 12 wk
- **Adults with cirrhosis who are treatment-experienced: PO** One tablet (90 mg ledipasvir; 400 mg sofosbuvir) every day with or without food for 24 wk

Available forms: Tab 90/400 mg

Administer:

- Without regard to food

SIDE EFFECTS

CNS: Fatigue, headache, insomnia

GI: Nausea, vomiting, diarrhea

PHARMACOKINETICS

Ledipasvir: >99.8% protein binding, elimination biliary excretion, terminal half-life 47 hr, peak 4-5 hr

Sofosbuvir: 61%-65% protein binding, elimination kidneys 80% recovered in the urine peak 0.8-1 hr

INTERACTIONS

Avoid use with products that increase P-glycoprotein

Drug/lab test:

Increase: bilirubin

NURSING CONSIDERATIONS

Assess:

- **Hepatitis C:** monitor hepatitis C RNA, serum bilirubin, creatinine

Evaluate:

- **Therapeutic response:** hepatitis C RNA reduction

Teach patient/family:

- To report effects to the prescriber

leflunomide (Rx)

(leh-floo′noh-mide)

Arava

Func. class.: Antirheumatic (DMARDs)

Chem. class.: Immune modulator, pyrimidine synthesis inhibitor

ACTION: Inhibits an enzyme involved in pyrimidine synthesis; has antiproliferative, antiinflammatory effect

USES: RA: to reduce disease process and symptoms

Unlabeled uses: Juvenile RA

CONTRAINDICATIONS: Breastfeeding, hypersensitivity

Black Box Warning: Pregnancy (X)

Precautions: Children, renal disorders, vaccinations, infection, alcoholism, immunosuppression, jaundice, lactase deficiency, hepatic disease

Black Box Warning: Hepatic disease (ALT >2 × ULN)

DOSAGE AND ROUTES

Rheumatoid arthritis

- **Adult: PO** Loading dose 100 mg/day × 3 days, maintenance 20 mg/day; may be decreased to 10 mg/day if not well tolerated

Juvenile rheumatoid arthritis (unlabeled)

- **Adolescent and child >40 kg: PO** 20 mg/day
- **Adolescent and child 20-40 kg: PO** 15 mg/day
- **Adolescent and child 10-19.9 kg: PO** 10 mg/day

Available forms: Tabs 10, 20 mg

Administer:

- With food for GI upset, give same time each day, loading dose is recommended
- **Drug elimination:** give cholestyramine 8 g tid × 11 days, check levels

SIDE EFFECTS

CNS: *Headache,* dizziness, insomnia, depression, paresthesia, anxiety, migraine, neuralgia

CV: Palpitations, hypertension, chest pain, angina pectoris, peripheral edema

EENT: Pharyngitis, oral candidiasis, stomatitis, dry mouth, blurred vision

GI: *Nausea, anorexia, vomiting, constipation, flatulence, diarrhea, elevated LFTs,* **hepatotoxicity,** weight loss

HEMA: Anemia, ecchymosis, hyperlipidemia

INTEG: Rash, pruritus, alopecia, acne, hematoma, herpes infections

RESP: Pharyngitis, rhinitis, bronchitis, cough, respiratory infection, pneumonia, sinusitis, **interstitial lung disease**

SYST: Opportunistic/fatal infections, Stevens-Johnson syndrome

PHARMACOKINETICS

Metabolized in liver to active metabolite, half-life of metabolite 2 wk, excreted in urine

INTERACTIONS

Increase: NSAID effect—NSAIDs

Increase: hepatotoxicity—hepatotoxic agents, methotrexate

Increase: leflunomide levels—rifampin

Decrease: antibody response—live virus vaccines

Decrease: leflunomide effect—activated charcoal, cholestyramine, use for overdose

NURSING CONSIDERATIONS

Assess:

- Screen for latent TB before starting treatment; if TB is present, pretreat before using product
- **Interstitial lung disease: increased or worsening cough, SOB, fever; product may need to be discontinued**
- **Arthritic symptoms:** ROM, mobility, swelling of joints at baseline and during treatment

Black Box Warning: Hepatic studies: if ALT elevations are >2× ULN, reduce dose to 10 mg/day, monitor monthly or more frequently

• CBC with differential monthly × 6 mo, then q6-8 wk thereafter; pregnancy test; serum electrolytes
⚠ **Infections:** fatal infections can occur
• B/P, weight; edema can occur

Black Box Warning: Pregnancy (X): determine that patient is not pregnant before treatment; not to be given to women of childbearing potential who are not using reliable contraception

Evaluate:
• Therapeutic response: decreased inflammation, pain in joints
Teach patient/family:
• That product must be continued for prescribed time to be effective, that up to a month may be required for improvement
• To take with food, milk, or antacids to avoid GI upset; to take at same time of day
• To use caution when driving because drowsiness, dizziness may occur
• To take with a full glass of water to enhance absorption, may continue with correct prescribed treatment with other antiinflammatories

Black Box Warning: Not to become pregnant (X) while taking this product; not to breastfeed while taking this product; men should also discontinue product and begin leflunomide removal protocol if pregnancy is planned

• That hair may be lost; review alternatives
• To avoid live virus vaccinations during treatment
• To notify prescriber of weight loss
• Overdose treatment: give cholestyramine 8 g tid × 11 days

⚠ **HIGH ALERT**

letrozole (Rx)
(let′tro-zohl)
Femara
Func. class.: Antineoplastic, nonsteroidal aromatase inhibitor

ACTION: Binds to the heme group of aromatase; inhibits conversion of androgens to estrogens to reduce plasma estrogen levels

USES: Early, advanced, or metastatic breast cancer in postmenopausal women who are hormone receptor positive
Unlabeled uses: Infertility, idiopathic short stature, constitutional delayed puberty

CONTRAINDICATIONS: Pregnancy (D), premenopausal females, hypersensitivity
Precautions: Respiratory/hepatic disease, osteoporosis

DOSAGE AND ROUTES
• **Adult: PO** 2.5 mg/day
Infertility (unlabeled)
• **Adult: PO** 2.5, 5, 7.5 mg/day × 5 days, usually days 3-7 of menstrual cycle
Idiopathic short stature, constitutional delayed puberty (unlabeled)
• **Adolescent and child ≥9 (male): PO** 2.5 mg/day; use with testosterone for delayed puberty
Available forms: Tabs 2.5 mg
Administer:
• Without regard to meals; with small glass of water
• May administer biphosphates to increase bone density

SIDE EFFECTS
CNS: *Headache, lethargy,* somnolence, dizziness, depression, anxiety

CV: Angina, MI, CVA, thromboembolic events, hypertension, peripheral edema
GI: *Nausea, vomiting, anorexia,* constipation, heartburn, diarrhea
GU: Endometrial cancer, vaginal bleeding, endometrial proliferation disorders
INTEG: *Rash, pruritus,* alopecia, sweating
MISC: Hot flashes, night sweats, second malignancies, **anaphylaxis, angioedema**
MS: Arthralgia, arthritis, bone fracture, myalgia, osteoporosis
RESP: Dyspnea, cough

PHARMACOKINETICS

Metabolized in liver, excreted in urine, peak 2 days, terminal half-life 48 hr, steady state 2-6 wk

INTERACTIONS

Decrease: letrozole effect—estrogens, oral contraceptives

NURSING CONSIDERATIONS

Assess:

- Hepatic studies before, during therapy (bilirubin, AST, ALT, LDH) as needed or monthly

Evaluate:

- Therapeutic response: decrease in size of tumor

Teach patient/family:

- To report allergic reactions (rash; hives; difficulty breathing; tightness in chest; swelling of mouth, face, lips, tongue)
- To report vaginal bleeding, diarrhea, chest/bone pain
- To use adequate contraception in perimenopausal, recently postmenopausal women; pregnancy (D)

RARELY USED

leucovorin (Rx)

(loo-koe-vor′in)

Func. class.: Vitamin, folic acid/methotrexate antagonist antidote
Chem. class.: Tetrahydrofolic acid derivative

USES: Megaloblastic or macrocytic anemia caused by folic acid deficiency, overdose of folic acid antagonist, methotrexate/pyrimethamine/trimetrexate/trimethoprim toxicity, pneumocystosis, toxoplasmosis

CONTRAINDICATIONS: Hypersensitivity to this product or folic acid, benzyl alcohol; anemias other than megaloblastic not associated with vit B_{12} deficiency

L

DOSAGE AND ROUTES

Megaloblastic anemia caused by enzyme deficiency

- **Adult and child: PO/IV/IM** up to 6 mg/day

Megaloblastic anemia caused by deficiency of folate

- **Adult and child: IM** ≤1 mg/day until adequate response

Methotrexate toxicity/leucovorin rescue

- **Adult and child: PO/IM/IV Normal elimination** given 6 hr after dose of methotrexate (10 mg/m^2) until methotrexate $<5 \times 10^{-8}$ m, CCr >50% above prior level, or methotrexate level 5×10^{-8} m at 24 hr or $>9 \times 10^{-8}$ m at 48 hr; give leucovorin 100 mg/m^2 q3hr until level drops to $<10^{-8}$ m

Pyrimethamine/trimethoprim toxicity

- **Adult and child: PO/IM** 5-15 mg/day

Advanced colorectal cancer

- **Adult: IV** 200 mg/m^2, then 5-FU 370 mg/m^2 or leucovorin 20 mg/m^2, then 5-FU 425 mg/m^2; give daily × 5 days q4-5wk

⚠ HIGH ALERT

leuprolide (Rx)

(loo-proe′lide)

Eligard, Lupron Depot, Lupron Depot-Ped

Func. class.: Antineoplastic hormone

Chem. class.: Gonadotropin-releasing hormone

Do not confuse:
Lupron/Nuprin/Lopurin

ACTION: Causes initial increase in circulating levels of LH, FSH; continuous administration results in decreased LH, FSH; in men, testosterone is reduced to castrate levels; in premenopausal women, estrogen is reduced to menopausal levels

USES: Metastatic prostate cancer (inj implant), management of endometriosis, central precocious puberty, uterine leiomyomata (fibroids)

Unlabeled uses: Breast cancer, recurrent priapism, benign prostatic hyperplasia

CONTRAINDICATIONS: Pregnancy (X), breastfeeding, hypersensitivity to GnRH or analogs, thromboembolic disorders, undiagnosed vaginal bleeding; Viadur implant or Eligard should not be used in women, children

Precautions: Edema, hepatic disease, CVA, MI, seizures, hypertension, diabetes mellitus, CHF, depression, osteoporosis, spinal cord compression, urinary tract obstruction

DOSAGE AND ROUTES

Prostate cancer

- **Adult: SUBCUT** 1 mg/day; **IM** 7.5 mg/dose monthly; Viadur implant (72 mg) yearly; or **IM** 22.5 mg q3mo; or **IM** 30 mg q4mo; or IM 45 mg q6mo

Endometriosis/fibroids

- **Adult: IM** 3.75 mg monthly for 6 mo or 11.25 mg q3mo for 6 mo or 30 mg q4mo

Central precocious puberty

- **Child: SUBCUT** 50 mcg/kg/day; may increase by 10 mcg/kg/day as needed
- **Child >37.5 kg: IM** 15 mg q4wk
- **Child 25-37.5 kg: IM** 11.25 mg q4wk
- **Child ≤25 kg:** 7.5 mg q4wk

Benign prostatic hyperplasia (BPH) (unlabeled)

- **Adult: SUBCUT** (sol for inj) 1 mg/day, IM (injection susp) 3.75 mg q28day × 24 wk

Available forms: Depot inj: 3.75, 7.5, 11.25, 15, 22.5, 30, 45 mg; Inj: 5 mg/ml (2.8-ml multidose vials)

Administer:

- Store in tight container at room temperature
- **SUBCUT:** No dilution needed if patient self-administering; make sure patient using syringes provided by manufacturer
- **Viadur DUROS Implant:** Insert in inner aspect of arm, remove after 12 mo
- **SUBCUT: Eligard:** bring to room temperature, once mixed, give within 30 min, prepare the 2 syringes for mixing, join the 2 syringes together by pushing in and twisting until secure; mix the product by pushing the contents of both syringes back and forth between syringes until uniform; should be light tan to tan, hold syringes vertically with syringe B on the bottom, draw entire mixed product into syringe B (short, wide syringe) by depressing the syringe A plunger and slightly withdrawing syringe B plunger, uncouple syringe A, while pushing down on syringe A plunger, small air bubbles will remain, hold syringe B upright, remove pink cap, attach needle cartridge to the end of syringe B, remove needle cover, give by subcut

IM route

- **Monthly:** reconstitute single-use vial with 1 ml of diluent; if multiple vials used, withdraw 0.5 ml, inject into each vial (1 ml); withdraw all, inject at 90-degree angle (3.75 mg)
- **3-mo:** reconstitute microspheres using 1.5 ml of diluent, inject into vial; shake, withdraw, inject
- **12-mo:** insert into upper arm; at the end of 12 mo, implant must be removed

SIDE EFFECTS

CNS: Memory impairment, depression, seizures

CV: MI, PE, dysrhythmias, peripheral edema

GI: Nausea, vomiting, anorexia, diarrhea, GI bleeding

GU: Edema, hot flashes, impotence, decreased libido, amenorrhea, vaginal dryness, gynecomastia, profuse vaginal bleeding

INTEG: Alopecia

MS: Bone pain

RESP: Dyspnea, pulmonary fibrosis, interstitial lung disease

PHARMACOKINETICS

IM/SUBCUT: Peak 1-2 mo, duration 1-3 mo; **Implant:** peak 4 hr, duration 12 mo; absorbed rapidly (SUBCUT), slowly (IM depot); half-life 3 hr

INTERACTIONS

Increase: antineoplastic action—flutamide, megestrol

Drug/Herb

- Do not use with black cohosh or chaste tree fruit, may interfere with treatment

NURSING CONSIDERATIONS

Assess:

- **Prostate cancer:** increased bone pain for first 4 wk of treatment; those with metastases in spinal column may exhibit severe back pain
- **Symptoms of endometriosis** (lower abdominal pain)/**fibroids** (pelvic pain, excessive vaginal bleeding, bloating) before, during, after treatment
- **Central precocious puberty (CPP)** diagnosis should have been confirmed by secondary S_4 characteristics in children <9 yr, estradiol/testosterone levels, GnRH test, tomography of head, adrenal steroids, chorionic gonadotropin, wrist x-ray, height, weight
- Hepatic studies before, during therapy (bilirubin, AST, ALT, LDH) monthly, as needed; PSA, calcium, testosterone with prostate cancer; bone mineral density; blood glucose, HbA1c
- Pituitary gonadotropic and gonadal function during therapy and 4-8 wk after therapy decreased
- **Tumor flare:** worsening of signs and symptoms; normal during beginning therapy
- Fatigue, increased pulse, pallor, lethargy; edema in feet, joints; stomach pain

⚠ **Severe allergic reaction:** rash, pruritus, urticaria, purpuric skin lesions, itching, flushing

Evaluate:

- Therapeutic response: decreased tumor size and spread of malignancy; decrease in lesions, pain with endometriosis, fibroids, correction of CPP; increased follicle maturation

Teach patient/family:

- To notify prescriber if menstruation continues; menstruation should stop
- To notify prescriber if pregnancy is planned or suspected (X), avoid breastfeeding
- That bone pain will disappear after 1 wk
- To report any complaints, side effects to nurse, prescriber; hot flashes may occur; record weight, report gain of >2 lb/day
- How to prepare, give; to rotate sites for SUBCUT/IM inj
- To keep accurate records of dose
- **That tumor flare may occur:** increase in size of tumor, increased bone pain, will subside rapidly; may take analgesics for pain
- That voiding problems may increase during beginning of therapy but will decrease in several weeks

levalbuterol (Rx)

(lev-al-byoo′ter-ole)

Xopenex, Xopenex HFA

Func. class.: Bronchodilator, adrenergic β_2-agonist

ACTION: Causes bronchodilation by action on β_2 (pulmonary) receptors by increasing levels of cAMP, which relaxes smooth muscle; produces bronchodilation, CNS, cardiac stimulation as well as increased diuresis and gastric acid secretion

USES:
Treatment or prevention of bronchospasm (reversible obstructive airway disease), asthma

CONTRAINDICATIONS:
Hypersensitivity to sympathomimetics, this product, albuterol

Precautions: Pregnancy (C), breastfeeding, hyperthyroidism, diabetes mellitus, hypertension, prostatic hypertrophy, angle-closure glaucoma, seizures, renal disease, QT prolongation, tachydysrhythmias, severe cardiac disease, hypokalemia, children

DOSAGE AND ROUTES

Bronchospasm

- **Adult/child ≥12 yr: INH** 0.63 mg tid q6-8hr by nebulization, may increase 1.25 mg q8hr
- **Adult/adolescent/child >4 yr:** (HFA, metered dose) 90 mcg (2 **INH**) q4-6hr
- **Child 6-11 yr: INH** 0.31 mg tid by nebulization, max 0.63 mg tid

Asthma, relief

- **Child <4 yr:** (unlabeled) 0.075 mg/kg in Neb Sol q20min × 3 doses, then 0.075-0.15 mg/kg up to 5 mg q1-4hr

Available forms: Sol, inh pediatric 0.31 mg/3 ml; 0.63 mg/3 ml; 1.25 mg/3 ml; 1.25 mg/0.5 ml; 45 mcg per actuation (HFA)

Administer:

- Every 6-8hr; wait ≥1 min between inhalation of aerosols

Inhalation route

- Shake well before use, use a spacer device, prime with 4 test sprays in new canister or when not used for >3 days

Nebulizer route

- Dilute concentrated (1.25 mg/0.5 ml) with normal sterile saline before use

SIDE EFFECTS

CNS: *Tremors, anxiety,* insomnia, *headache,* dizziness, stimulation, *restlessness,* irritability, weakness

CV: Palpitations, tachycardia, hypertension, angina, hypotension, dysrhythmias, QT prolongation

EENT: Dry nose, irritation of nose and throat, rhinitis

GI: Heartburn, nausea, vomiting, diarrhea

INTEG: Rash

META: *Hypokalemia, hyperglycemia*

MS: Muscle cramps

RESP: Cough, dyspnea

SYST: Anaphylaxis, angioedema

PHARMACOKINETICS

Metabolized in the liver and tissues; crosses placenta, breast milk, blood-brain barrier; half-life 3.3-4 hr

INH sol: Onset 10-17 min, peak 1½ hr, duration 5-6 hr; **INH aerosol:** onset 4.5-10.2 min, peak 76-78 min, duration ≤6 hr

INTERACTIONS

Increase: QT prolongation—Class IA, III antidysrhythmics, usually at high doses or hypokalemia

Increase: hypokalemia—loop/thiazide diuretics

Increase: action of aerosol bronchodilators

Increase: levalbuterol action—tricyclics, MAOIs, other adrenergics

Decrease: levalbuterol action—other β-blockers, severe bronchospasm may occur

Drug/Herb

Increase: stimulation—black/green tea, coffee, cola nut, guarana, yerba maté

NURSING CONSIDERATIONS

Assess:

- **Respiratory function:** vital capacity, forced expiratory volume, ABGs, lung sounds, heart rate and rhythm (baseline); character of sputum: color, consistency, amount
- Cardiac status: palpitations, increase/decrease in B/P, dysrhythmias
- ⚠ For evidence of allergic reactions, paradoxic bronchospasm, anaphylaxis, angioedema

Evaluate:

• Therapeutic response: absence of dyspnea, wheezing after 1 hr; improved airway exchange, ABGs

Teach patient/family:

• Not to use OTC medications because excess stimulation may occur

• To avoid getting aerosol in eyes because blurring may result

• To avoid smoking, smoke-filled rooms, persons with respiratory infections

⚠ That paradoxic bronchospasm may occur; to stop product immediately, contact prescriber

• To limit caffeine products such as chocolate, coffee, tea, colas, and herbs such as cola nut, guarana, yerba maté

• To use this product first if using other inhalers; to wait 5 min or more between products; to rinse mouth with water after each dose to prevent dry mouth

TREATMENT OF OVERDOSE:

Administer a β_1-adrenergic blocker

levETIRAcetam (Rx)

(lev-eh-teer-ass′eh-tam)

Keppra, Keppra XR

Func. class.: Anticonvulsant

Do not confuse:

Keppra/Kaletra

ACTION: Unknown; may inhibit nerve impulses by limiting influx of sodium ions across cell membrane in motor cortex

USES: Adjunctive therapy for partial-onset seizures, primary generalized tonic-clonic seizures, myoclonic seizures in juvenile patients

CONTRAINDICATIONS: Hypersensitivity, breastfeeding

Precautions: Pregnancy (C), children, geriatric patients, renal/cardiac disease, psychosis

DOSAGE AND ROUTES

Adjunctive treatment of partial seizures

• **Adult/adolescent ≥16 yr: IV** 500 mg bid, may be titrated by 1000 mg/day q2wk, max 3000 mg/day in divided doses; **EXT REL** 1000 mg/day, may increase q2wk, max 3000 mg/day

• **Adolescent <16 yr/child/infant: PO** 10 mg/kg bid, increase daily dose q2wk by 20 mg/kg to dose of 30 mg/kg bid; if patient unable to tolerate, may reduce dose

Myoclonic seizures/tonic-clonic seizures/partial seizures

• **Adult/adolescent ≥16 yr: PO/IV** 500 mg bid, may increase by 1000 mg/day q2wk, max 3000 mg/day

Renal dose

• **Adult: PO** CCr 50-80 ml/min, 500-1000 mg q12hr or **EXT REL** 1000-2000 mg q24hr, max 2000 mg/day; CCr 30-49 ml/min, 250-750 mg q12hr or **EXT REL** 500-1500 mg q24hr, max 1500 mg/day; CCr <30 ml/min, 250-500 mg q12hr or **EXT REL** 500-1000 mg q24hr, max 1000 mg/day

L

Available forms: Tabs 250, 500, 750, 1000 mg; oral sol 100 mg/ml; sol for inj 100 mg/ml; ext rel tab 500, 750 mg; 1000 mg/100 ml 0.75% NaCl, 1500 mg/100 ml 0.54% NaCl, 500 mg/100 ml 0.82% NaCl

Administer:

PO route

• Extended release product should not be used in dialysis patients

• Swallow tab whole; do not break, crush, or chew

• With food, milk to decrease GI symptoms (rare)

• Store at room temperature (PO)

• **Child:** <20 kg should be given oral solution; use calibrated device

Intermittent IV INFUSION route

• Single-use vials: dilute in 100 ml of 0.9% NaCl, D_5W, LR; give over 15 min, discard unused vial contents, do not use product with particulates or discoloration

• Diluted preparation stable for 24 hr at room temperature in polyvinyl bags

Additive compatibilities: diazepam, LORazepam, valproate

SIDE EFFECTS

CNS: Dizziness, somnolence, asthenia, psychosis, **suicidal ideation**, nonpsychotic behavioral symptoms, headache, ataxia
EENT: Diplopia, conjunctivitis
GI: Nausea, vomiting, anorexia, diarrhea, constipation, **hepatitis**
HEMA: Infection, leukopenia
INTEG: Pruritus, rash
MISC: Infection, abdominal pain, pharyngitis
SYST: **Stevens-Johnson syndrome, toxic epidermal necrolysis**; dehydration (child <4 yr)

PHARMACOKINETICS

Rapidly absorbed; not protein bound; excreted via kidneys 66% unchanged; half-life 6-8 hr, longer in geriatric patients or with renal disease

INTERACTIONS

Increase: sedation—TCAs, antihistamines, benzodiazepines, other CNS depressants, alcohol
• Possible increased carBAMazepine toxicity: carBAMazepine
Decrease: levETIRAcetam absorption—sevelamer; separate by 1 hr before, 3 hr after sevelamer
Drug/Lab Test
Decrease: Hct/Hgb, WBC, RBC

NURSING CONSIDERATIONS

Assess:
• **Seizures:** type, location, duration, character; provide seizure precautions
• Renal studies: urinalysis, BUN, urine creatinine q3mo
• Blood studies: CBC, LFTs
⚠ Mental status: mood, sensorium, affect, behavioral changes, **suicidal thoughts/behaviors;** if mental status changes, notify prescriber
• Assistance with ambulation during early part of treatment; dizziness occurs

Evaluate:
• Therapeutic response: decreased seizure activity; document on patient's chart
Teach patient/family:
• To carry emergency ID stating patient's name, products taken, condition, prescriber's name, phone number
• How to use oral sol; if trouble swallowing, measure oral sol in medicine cup or dropper, do not use teaspoon
• To notify prescriber if pregnant, intending to become pregnant
• To avoid driving, other activities that require alertness, until response is known, drowsiness occurs during first month
• Not to discontinue medication quickly after long-term use because withdrawal seizure may occur
• Not to breastfeed, excreted in breast milk
• To report suicidal thoughts

levobetaxolol ophthalmic

See Appendix B

levobunolol (ophthalmic)

(lee′voe-byoo′no-lahl)

Betagan

Func. class.: Antiglaucoma
Chem. class.: β-Blocker

ACTION: Can decrease aqueous humor and increase outflows

USES: Treatment of chronic open-angle glaucoma and ocular hypertension

CONTRAINDICATIONS: Hypersensitivity, AV block, heart failure, bradycardia, sick sinus syndrome, asthma
Precautions: Abrupt discontinuation, children, pregnancy, breastfeeding, COPD, depression, diabetes mellitus, myasthenia

gravis, hyperthyroidism, pulmonary disease, sulfite sensitivity, angle-closure glaucoma

DOSAGE AND ROUTES

• **Adult:** Instill 1-2 drops in the affected eyes once a day (0.5% solution), bid (0.25% solution)

Available forms: Ophthalmic solution 0.25%, 0.5%

Administer:

• For ophthalmic use only
• Do not touch the tip of the dropper to the eye, fingertips, or other surface to prevent contamination
• Wash hands before and after use; tilt head back slightly and pull the lower eyelid down with the index finger to form a pouch; squeeze the prescribed number of drops into the pouch; close eyes to spread drops; to avoid excessive systemic absorption, apply finger pressure on the lacrimal sac for 1-2 min after use
• If more than one topical ophthalmic drug product is being used, the drugs should be administered at least 5 min apart
• To avoid contamination or the spread of infection, do not use dropper for more than one person
• Decreased intraocular pressure can take several weeks, monitor IOP after a month

SIDE EFFECTS

CNS: Insomnia, headache, dizziness
CV: Palpitations
EENT: Eye stinging/burning, tearing, photophobia
PULM: Bronchospasm

PHARMACOKINETICS

Onset 60 min, peak 2-6 hr, duration 24 hr

INTERACTIONS

Increase: β-blocking effect—oral β-blockers

Increase: Intraocular pressure reduction—topical miotics, dipivefrin, EPINEPHrine, carbonic anhydrase inhibitors; this may be beneficial

Increase: Depression of AV nodal conduction, bradycardia, or hypotension—adenosine, cardiac glycosides, disopyramide, other antiarrhythmics, class 1C antiarrhythmic drugs (flecainide, propafenone, moricizine, encainide, quiNIDine, or drugs that significantly depress AV nodal conduction

Increase: AV block nodal conduction, induce AV block—high doses of procainamide

Increase: Antihypertensive effect—other antihypertensives

NURSING CONSIDERATIONS

Assess:

⚠ **Systemic absorption:** When used in the eye, systemic absorption is common with the same adverse reactions and interactions

• **Glaucoma:** Monitor intraocular pressure

Evaluate:

• Decreasing intraocular pressure

Teach patient/family:

• That product is for ophthalmic use only
• Not to touch the tip of the dropper to the eye, fingertips, or other surface to prevent contamination
• To wash hands before and after use; tilt the head back slightly and pull the lower eyelid down with the index finger to form a pouch; squeeze the prescribed number of drops into the pouch; close eyes to spread drops; to avoid excessive systemic absorption by applying finger pressure on the lacrimal sac for 1-2 min following use
• That if more than one topical ophthalmic drug product is being used, the drugs should be administered at least 5 min apart
• To avoid contamination or the spread of infection by not using dropper for more than one person

L

levocabastine ophthalmic

See Appendix B

levocetirizine (Rx)

(lee-voh-she-teer′ah-zeen)

Xyzal

Func. class.: Antihistamine, low sedating

Chem. class.: H_1 histamine blocker, low sedating

ACTION: Acts on blood vessels, GI, respiratory system by competing with histamine for H_1-receptor site; decreases allergic response by blocking pharmacologic effects of histamine; minimal anticholinergic action

USES: Perennial or seasonal rhinitis, allergy symptoms, chronic idiopathic urticaria

CONTRAINDICATIONS: Breastfeeding; children 6-11 yr with renal disease; end-stage renal disease; dialysis; hypersensitivity to this product, cetirizine, hydrOXYzine

Precautions: Pregnancy (B), driving, renal disease

DOSAGE AND ROUTES

- **Adult and child ≥12 yr: PO** 2.5-5 mg/day in the evening
- **Child 6-11 yr: PO** (oral solution) 2.5 mg/day in the evening
- **Child 2-5 yr: PO** (oral solution) 1.25 mg/day in the evening
- **Geriatric: PO** 2.5-5 mg/day in the evening

Renal dose

- **Adult: PO** CCr 50-80 ml/min, 2.5 mg/day; CCr 30-50 ml/min, 2.5 mg every other day; CCr 10-30 ml/min, 2.5 mg 2×/wk; CCr <10 ml/min, do not use

Available forms: Tabs 5 mg; oral sol 2.5 mg/5 ml

Administer:

- Without regard to meals in the evening; tabs scored, may be broken in half
- Store in tight, light-resistant container

SIDE EFFECTS

CNS: *Drowsiness, fatigue,* asthenia, dizziness

GI: Dry mouth, increase LFTs, **hepatitis**

MISC: Urinary retention

PHARMACOKINETICS

Rapid absorption; peak 0.9 hr; protein binding 91%-92%; half-life 8 hr; excreted in urine 85.4%, feces 12.9%

INTERACTIONS

Increase: CNS depression—alcohol, other CNS depressants

Increase: anticholinergic/sedative effect—MAOIs, phenothiazines, tricyclics

Decrease: clearance of levocetirizine—ritonavir

Drug/Lab Test

False negative: Skin allergy tests

NURSING CONSIDERATIONS

Assess:

- **Allergy symptoms:** pruritus, urticaria, watering eyes at baseline, during treatment
- **Respiratory status:** rate, rhythm, increase in bronchial secretions, wheezing, chest tightness
- Liver function tests, serum creatinine, BUN

Evaluate:

- Therapeutic response: absence of running or congested nose or rashes

Teach patient/family:

- About all aspects of product use; to notify prescriber if confusion, sedation, hypotension occur, not to exceed recommended dose
- To avoid driving, other hazardous activities if drowsiness occurs
- To avoid alcohol, other CNS depressants
- That product not recommended while breastfeeding

TREATMENT OF OVERDOSE:
Administer diazepam, vasopressors, IV phenytoin

levodopa-carbidopa (Rx)

(lee-voe-doe′pa)-(kar-bi-doe′pa)

Apo-Levocarb ✦, Duodopa ✦, Sinemet, Sinemet CR

Func. class.: Antiparkinson agent
Chem. class.: Catecholamine

ACTION: Decarboxylation of levodopa in periphery is inhibited by carbidopa; more levodopa is made available for transport to the brain and for conversion to DOPamine in the brain

USES: Parkinson's disease, parkinsonism resulting from carbon monoxide, chronic manganese intoxication, cerebral arteriosclerosis

Unlabeled uses: Restless leg syndrome

CONTRAINDICATIONS: Hypersensitivity, malignant melanoma, history of malignant melanoma or undiagnosed skin lesions resembling melanoma

Precautions: Pregnancy (C), breastfeeding, diabetes, closed-angle glaucoma, respiratory/cardiac/renal/hepatic disease, MI with dysrhythmias, seizures, peptic ulcer, depression

DOSAGE AND ROUTES

Beginning therapy for those not taking levodopa

- **Adult: PO** 25 mg carbidopa/100 mg levodopa tid, may increase daily or every other day by 1 tab to desired response (8 tabs/day); **EXT REL** tabs (Sinemet CR) 50 mg carbidopa/200 mg levodopa bid; **EXT REL** caps (Rytary) 23.75 mg/95 mg tid × 3 days, then 36.25 mg/145 mg tid on day 4, may increase to 97.5 mg/390 mg tid

For those not taking levodopa ER

- 50 mg carbidopa/200 mg levodopa bid

For those taking levodopa ER

- Begin treatment with 10% more levodopa/day given q4-8hr, may increase or decrease dose q3days

For those taking levodopa <1.5 g/day

- **Adult: PO** 25 mg carbidopa/100 mg levodopa tid-qid, may increase daily to desired response

For those taking levodopa >1.5 g/day

- **Adult: PO** 25 mg carbidopa/250 mg levodopa tid-qid, may increase daily to desired response

Restless leg syndrome (RLS) (unlabeled)

- **Adult: PO** 25 mg carbidopa/100 mg levodopa, 1 tab at bedtime, may repeat if awakening within 2 hr or 50 mg carbidopa/200 mg levodopa sus rel tab 1-2 tabs 1 hr before bedtime

Available forms: Tabs 10 mg carbidopa/100 mg levodopa, 25 mg carbidopa/100 mg levodopa, 25 mg carbidopa/250 mg levodopa; ext rel tab 25 mg/100 mg, 50 mg carbidopa/200 mg levodopa (Sinemet CR); oral disintegrating tab (Parcopa) 10 mg carbidopa/100 mg levodopa, 25 mg carbidopa/100 mg levodopa; 25 mg carbidopa/250 mg levodopa; **EXT REL** caps (Rytary 23.75 mg/95 mg, 36.25 mg/145 mg, 48.75/195 mg, 61.25/245 mg

Administer:

- Pyridoxine (B_6) not effective for reversing Sinemet or Sinemet CR

PO route

- Do not crush or chew **ext rel tabs;** they may be broken in half; adjust dosage to response
- **Oral disintegrating tab** by gently removing from bottle, placing on tongue and swallowing with saliva; after tab dissolves, liquid is not necessary
- With meals if GI symptoms occur; limit protein taken with product
- Only after nonselective MAOIs have been discontinued for 2 wk; if patient has been previously treated with levodopa, discontinue for at least 12 hr before change to carbidopa-levodopa

SIDE EFFECTS

CNS: *Involuntary choreiform movements, hand tremors, fatigue, headache, anxiety, twitching, numbness, weakness, confusion, agitation, insomnia, nightmares,* psychosis, hallucination, hypomania, severe depression, dizziness, impulsive behaviors, neuroleptic malignant syndrome
CV: *Orthostatic hypotension,* tachycardia, hypertension, palpitation
EENT: Blurred vision, diplopia, dilated pupils
GI: *Nausea, vomiting, anorexia, abdominal distress, dry mouth, flatulence, dysphagia,* bitter taste, diarrhea, constipation
HEMA: Hemolytic anemia, leukopenia, agranulocytosis
INTEG: Rash, sweating, alopecia
MISC: Urinary retention, incontinence, weight change, dark urine

PHARMACOKINETICS

PO: Onset 30 min, peak 1-3 hr, excreted in urine (metabolites)
EXT REL: Onset 4-6 hr

INTERACTIONS

Increase: Hypertensive crisis—nonselective MAOIs
Increase: risk for sedation—CNS depressants
Increase: CV reactions—dobutamine, dopamine, epinephrine, isoproterenol, norepinephrine, TCAs
Increase: effects of levodopa—antacids, metoclopramide
Decrease: effects of levodopa—anticholinergics, hydantoins, papaverine, pyridoxine, benzodiazepines, antipsychotics

Drug/Lab Test
Increase: BUN, AST, ALT, bilirubin, alk phos, LDH, serum glucose
Decrease: BUN, creatinine, uric acid
False positive: urine ketones (dipstick), Coombs' test
False negative: urine glucose
False increase: urine protein

Drug/Food
Decrease: absorption of levodopa—protein

NURSING CONSIDERATIONS

Assess:
- **Parkinson's symptoms:** tremors, pill rolling, drooling, akinesia, rigidity, shuffling gait before, during treatment
- B/P, respiration; orthostatic B/P
- Mental status: affect, mood, behavioral changes, depression, complete suicide assessment
- **Toxicity:** muscle twitching, blepharospasm
- Renal, hepatic, hematopoietic tests; also for diabetes, acromegaly if on long-term therapy

Evaluate:
- Therapeutic response: decrease in akathisia/bradykinesis, tremor, rigidity, improved mood

Teach patient/family:
- To change positions slowly to prevent orthostatic hypotension
- To report side effects: twitching, eye spasms because these indicate overdose
- To use product as prescribed; if discontinued abruptly, parkinsonian crisis, neuroleptic malignant syndrome (NMS) may occur; to gradually taper
- That urine, sweat may darken
- To use physical activities to maintain mobility, lessen spasms
- Use with meals to decrease GI upset
- That improvement may not occur for 2-4 mo; about "on-off phenomenon"

levofloxacin (Rx)

(lee-voh-floks′a-sin)

Levaquin

Func. class.: Antiinfective
Chem. class.: Fluoroquinolone

ACTION: Interferes with conversion of intermediate DNA fragments into high-molecular-weight DNA in bacteria; DNA gyrase inhibitor; inhibits topoisomerase IV

USES: Acute sinusitis, acute chronic bronchitis, community-acquired pneumonia, uncomplicated skin infections, UTI, cellulitis, prostatitis, inhalational anthrax (postexposure); acute pyelonephritis caused by *Streptococcus pneumoniae, Streptococcus pyogenes, Haemophilus influenzae, Haemophilis parainfluenzae, Moraxella catarrhalis, Escherichia coli, Serratia marcescens, Klebsiella pneumoniae, Chlamydia pneumoniae, Legionella pneumophilia, Mycoplasma pneumoniae, Enterococcus faecalis, Staphylococcus epidermidis, Staphylococcus pyogenes, Staphylococcus aureus, Bacillus anthracis;* inhalation anthrax in children

Unlabeled uses: Adnexitis, Bartholin abscess, bartholinitis, cervicitis, epididymis, gastroenteritis, *H. pylori* eradication, mastitis, MAC, nongonococcal urethritis, obstetric infections, PID, plague, SARS, shigellosis, TB, typhoid fever, disseminated; otitis media, otitis externa, tonsillitis, pharyngitis, sialadenitis

CONTRAINDICATIONS: Hypersensitivity to quinolones

Precautions: Pregnancy (C), breastfeeding, children, photosensitivity, acute MI, atrial fibrillation, colitis, dehydration, diabetes, QT prolongation, myasthenia gravis, renal disease, seizure disorder, syphilis

Black Box Warning: Tendon pain/rupture, tendinitis

DOSAGE AND ROUTES

Acute bacterial exacerbation of chronic bronchitis

- **Adult: PO/IV** 500 mg q24hr × 7 days

Acute bacterial sinusitis

- **Adult: PO** 500 mg q24hr × 10-14 days or 750 mg q24hr × 5 days

Mild-moderate UTI/acute pyelonephritis

- **Adult: PO/IV** 750 mg q24hr × 5 days or 250 mg q24hr × 10 days

Chronic bacterial prostitis

- **Adult: PO** 500 mg q24hr × 28 days

Postexposure inhalational anthrax

- **Adult/adolescent/child >50 kg: PO/IV** 500 mg q24hr × 60 days
- **Infant >6 mo/child <50 kg: IV** 8 mg/kg q12hr × 60 days, max 250 mg/dose

Pneumonia, community acquired

- **Adult: PO/IV** 500 mg q24hr × 7-14 days or 750 mg q24hr × 5 days

Pneumonia, nosocomial

- **Adult: PO/IV** 750 mg q24hr × 7-14 days

Skin/skin-structure infections, complicated

- **Adult: PO/IV** 750 mg q24hr × 7-14 days

Skin/skin-structure infections, uncomplicated

- **Adult: PO** 500 mg q24hr × 7-10 days

UTI, complicated

- **Adult: PO/IV** 750 mg q24hr × 5 days or 250 mg q24hr × 10 days

UTI, uncomplicated

- **Adult: PO** 250 mg q24hr × 3 days

Plague *(Y. pestis)*

- **Adult: PO/IV** 500 mg q24hr × 10-14 days, with pneumonia 750 mg q24hr
- **Child/adolescent <50 kg: PO/IV** 8 mg/kg (max 250 mg/dose) q12hr × 10-14 days

Otitis media (unlabeled)

- **Adult: PO** 100-200 mg bid-tid × 3-14 days
- **Child 6 mo-14 yr: PO** 10 mg/kg bid × ≥10 days

Renal disease

- **Adult: PO/IV** CCr 20-49 ml/min for 750 mg doses, give 750 mg q48hr; for 500 mg doses, give 500 mg once, then 250 mg q24hr; for 250 mg doses, no adjustment; CCr 10-19 ml/min for 750 mg dose, give 750 mg once, then 500 mg q48hr; for 500 mg dose, give 500 mg once, then 250 mg q48hr; for 250 mg dose, give 250 mg q48hr, except when treating complicated UTI, then no dose adjustment

Available forms: Single-use vials 500, 750 mg; premixed flexible containers 250 mg/50 ml D_5W, 500 mg/100 ml D_5W, 750 mg/150 ml D_5W; tabs 250, 500, 750 mg; oral sol 25 mg/ml

Administer:

- Obtain C&S before treatment and periodically
- PO 2 hr before or after antacids, iron, calcium, zinc, give fluids
- **Oral solution:** Give 1 hr before or 2 hr after food

Intermittent IV INFUSION route

- Discard any unused sol in single-dose vial
- Visually inspect for particulate matter/discoloration before use

IV (single-use vial)

- **500 mg/20 ml vials:** To prepare a dose of 500 mg, withdraw 10 ml from a 20 ml vial and dilute with a compatible IV solution (D_5W, NS) to a total volume of 50 ml; to prepare a 500 mg dosage, withdraw all 20 ml from the vial and dilute with a compatible intravenous solution to a total volume of 100 ml
- **750 mg/30 ml vials:** To prepare a dose of 750 mg, withdraw 30 ml from a 30 ml vial and dilute with a compatible intravenous solution (D_5W, NS) to a total volume of 150 ml
- The concentration of the diluted solution should be 5 mg/ml before administration; solutions contain no preservatives; any unused portions must be discarded
- **Storage:** The diluted solution may be stored for up to 72 hr when stored at or below 25°C (77°F) or for 14 days when stored under refrigeration at 5°C (41°F) in plastic containers; solutions may be frozen for up to 6 mo (−20°C or −4°F) in glass bottles or plastic containers; thaw frozen solutions at room temperature (25°C or 77°F) or in a refrigerator (8°C or 46°F); do not force thaw by microwave or water bath immersion; do not refreeze after initial thawing

Premixed IV solution

- No dilution is necessary

Intermittent IV injection

- Infuse doses of ≤500 mg IV over 60 min and doses of 750 mg IV over 90 min; shorter infusions or bolus inj should be avoided because of the risk of hypotension

Y-site compatibilities: Alemtuzumab, alfentanil, amifostine, amikacin, aminocaproic acid, aminophylline, ampicillin, ampicillin-sulbactam, anidulafungin, argatroban, atenolol, atracurium, aztreonam, bivalirudin, bleomycin, bumetanide, buprenorphine, busulfan, butorphanol, caffeine citrate, calcium gluconate, CARBOplatin, carmustine, caspofungin, cefepime, cefoTEtan, ceftaroline, cefTAZidime, ceftizoxime, cefTRIAXone, cefuroxime, chlorproMAZINE, cimetidine, cisatracurium, CISplatin, clindamycin, codeine, cyclophosphamide, cycloSPORINE, cytarabine, dacarbazine, DACTINomycin, DAPTOmycin, DAUNOrubicin liposomal, dexamethasone, dexrazoxane, digoxin, diltiazem, diphenhydrAMINE, DOBUTamine, DOCEtaxel, dolasetron, DOPamine, doripenem, doxacurium, doxycycline, droperidol, enalaprilat, ePHEDrine, EPINEPHrine, epirubicin, ertapenem, erythromycin, esmolol, etoposide, etoposide phosphate, famotidine, fenoldopam, fentaNYL, filgrastim, floxuridine, fluconazole, fludarabine, foscarnet, fosphenytoin, gallium, gemcitabine, gemtuzumab, gentamicin, granisetron, haloperidol, hydrocortisone, HYDROmorphone, IDArubicin, ifosfamide, imipenem-cilastatin, irinotecan, isoproterenol, labetalol, lepirudin, leucovorin, levorphanol, lidocaine, linezolid, mannitol, mechlorethamine, meperidine, mesna, methylPREDNISolone, metoclopramide, metroNIDAZOLE, midazolam, milrinone, minocycline, mitoMYcin, mitoXANtrone, mivacurium, morphine, mycophenolate mofetil, nalbuphine, naloxone, nesiritide, netilmicin, niCARdipine, octreotide, ondansetron, oxacillin, oxaliplatin, oxytocin, PACLitaxel, palonosetron, pamidronate, pancuronium, PEMEtrexed, penicillin G sodium, pentamidine, phenylephrine, plicamycin, potassium acetate/chloride, promethazine, propranolol, quinupristin-dalfopristin, ranitidine, remifentanil, rocuronium, sargramostim, sodium bicarbonate, succinylcholine, SUFentanil, sulfamethoxazole-trimethoprim, tacrolimus, teniposide, theophylline, thiotepa, ticarcillin, ticarcillin-clavulanate, tigecycline, tirofiban, tobramycin, topotecan, trimethobenzamide, vancomycin, vasopressin, vecuronium, verapamil, vinBLAStine, vinCRIStine, vinorelbine, voriconazole, zidovudine, zoledronic acid

Solution compatibilities: 0.9% NaCl, D_5W, D_5/0.9% NaCl, D_5LR, D_5/0.45% NaCl, sodium lactate, plasma-lyte 56/D_5W

SIDE EFFECTS

CNS: *Headache,* dizziness, *insomnia,* anxiety, **seizures,** *encephalopathy,* paresthesia, **pseudotumor cerebri**

CV: Chest pain, palpitations, vasodilation, **QT prolongation,** hypotension (rapid infusion)

EENT: Dry mouth, visual impairment, tinnitus

GI: *Nausea,* flatulence, *vomiting,* diarrhea, abdominal pain, **pseudomembranous colitis, hepatotoxicity, esophagitis, pancreatitis**

GU: Vaginitis, crystalluria

HEMA: Eosinophilia, **hemolytic anemia,** lymphopenia

INTEG: Rash, pruritus, *photosensitivity,* **epidermal necrolysis,** injection-site reaction, edema

MISC: Hypoglycemia, hypersensitivity, tendinitis, **tendon rupture, rhabdomyolysis**

RESP: Pneumonitis

SYST: Anaphylaxis, multisystem organ failure, Stevens-Johnson syndrome, angioedema, toxic epidermal necrolysis

PHARMACOKINETICS

Excreted in urine unchanged, half-life 6-8 hr, peak 1-2 hr

INTERACTIONS

Black Box Warning: Increase: tendon rupture—corticosteroids

- Do not use with magnesium in same IV line

Increase: QT prolongation products causing a QT prolongation

Increase: levofloxacin levels—probenecid

Increase: CNS stimulation, seizures—NSAIDs, foscarnet, cycloSPORINE

Increase: bleeding risk—warfarin

Decrease: levofloxacin absorption—antacids containing aluminum, magnesium; sucralfate, zinc, iron, calcium

Decrease: clearance of theophylline; toxicity may result

Drug/Lab Test

Increase: PT, INR

Decrease: glucose, lymphocytes

NURSING CONSIDERATIONS

Assess:

- Previous sensitivity reaction to quinolones
- **Signs, symptoms of infection:** characteristics of sputum, WBC >10,000/mm^3, fever; obtain baseline information before, during treatment
- C&S before beginning product therapy to identify if correct treatment initiated

⚠ **Allergic reactions, anaphylaxis:** rash, urticaria, pruritus, chills, fever, joint pain; may occur a few days after therapy begins; EPINEPHrine and resuscitation equipment should be available for anaphylactic reaction

- **Pseudomembranous colitis:** bowel pattern daily; if severe diarrhea, fever occurs, product should be discontinued

⚠ **Overgrowth of infection:** perineal itching, fever, malaise, redness, pain, swelling, drainage, rash, diarrhea, change in cough, sputum

- Renal function (BUN/creatinine)

Black Box Warning: Tendon rupture: discontinue product at first sign of tendon pain or inflammation, usually the Achilles tendon is affected; can occur up to few months after treatment and may require surgical repair; steroids may increase risk

- Increased fluid intake to 2 L/day to prevent crystalluria

Evaluate:

- Therapeutic response: absence of signs, symptoms of infection (WBC <10,000/mm^3, temperature WNL)

Teach patient/family:

- To contact prescriber if vaginal itching; loose, foul-smelling stools; furry tongue occur (may indicate superinfection); to report itching, rash, pruritus, urticaria
- To notify prescriber of diarrhea with blood or pus
- To take product 2 hr before or after antacids, iron, calcium, zinc products
- To complete full course of therapy
- To avoid hazardous activities until response is known
- To use frequent rinsing of mouth, sugarless candy or gum for dry mouth
- To avoid other medication unless approved by prescriber
- To prevent sun exposure or to use sunscreen to prevent phototoxicity
- To monitor glucose (diabetes)

Black Box Warning: To notify prescriber of tendon pain, inflammation; avoid corticosteroids with this product

levofloxacin ophthalmic

See Appendix B

levomilnacipran

(lee′voe-mil-na′si-pran)

Fetzima

Func. class: Antidepressant

Chem. class: Serotonin

ACTION: May potentiate serotonergic, adrenergic activity in the CNS; is a potent inhibitor of adrenal serotonin and norepinephrine reuptake

USES: Major depressive disorder in adults

CONTRAINDICATIONS: Alcohol intoxication, alcoholism, closed angle glaucoma, hepatic disease, hepatitis, jaundice, hypersensitivity

Precautions: Pregnancy (C), breastfeeding, geriatric patients, mania, hypertension, renal/cardiac disease, seizures, increased intraocular pressure, anorexia, bleeding, dehydration, diabetes, hypotension, hypovolemia, orthostatic hypotension, abrupt product withdrawal

Black Box Warning: Children, suicidal ideation

DOSAGE AND ROUTES

- **Adult: PO** 20 mg/day ×2 days, then 40 mg/day; may increase in increments of 40 mg at intervals of at least 2 days, max 120 mg/day; max 80 mg/day (strong CYP3A4 inhibitors therapy)

Renal Dose

- **Adult: PO** CCr 30-59 ml/min max 80 mg/day; 15-29 ml/min, max 40 mg/day; <15 ml/min; avoid use

Available forms: Ext rel caps 20, 40, 80, 120 mg

Administer:

- Swallow cap whole; do not break, crush, or chew; do not sprinkle on food or mix with liquid
- Without regard to food
- Give at the same time each day

SIDE EFFECTS

CNS: Dizziness, agitation, hallucinations, seizures, drowsiness, mania, migraine, paresthesias, serotonin syndrome, suicidal ideation, syncope

CV: Hypertension, palpitations, dysrhythmia, sinus tachycardia

EENT: Teeth grinding, blurred vision

GI: Constipation, diarrhea, nausea, vomiting, anorexia, dry mouth, abdominal pain

GU: Urinary retention

SYST: Serotonin syndrome, Stevens-Johnson syndrome

PHARMACOKINETICS

Peak 6-8 hr metabolized (CYP2D6) in the liver; 22% protein binding, half-life 12 hr

INTERACTIONS

• Do not use with linezolid or methylene blue IV, or within 14 days of MAOIs
• Increase levomilnacipran effect—CYP34A inhibitors
Increase: Serotonin syndrome, SSRIs, serotonin receptor agonists, SNRIs
Increase: bleeding risk—anticoagulants, antiplatelets, salicylates, NSAIDs
Drug/Herb
• Serotonin syndrome: St. John's wort
Increase: CNS depression—kava, valerian

NURSING CONSIDERATIONS

Assess:

Black Box Warning: Hyperthermia, rigidity, rapid fluctuations of vital signs, mental status changes, neuroleptic malignant syndrome-MAOIs coadministration contraindicated within 14 days of MAOI

Black Box Warning: Depression: mood, sensorium, affect, suicidal tendencies, increase in psychiatric symptoms; depression, panic, monitor children weekly face to face during first 4 wk, or dosage change, then every other week for the next 4 wk, then at 12 wk

• B/P lying, standing; pulse q4hr; if systolic B/P drops 20 mm Hg, hold product, notify prescriber; take VS q4hr in patients with CV disease
• **Hepatic studies:** AST ALT, bilirubin
• **Withdrawal symptoms:** headache, nausea, vomiting, muscle pain, weakness; not common unless product is discontinued abruptly

Black Box Warning: Serotonin syndrome: nausea/vomiting, dizziness, facial flush, shivering, sweating

Evaluate:
• Therapeutic response: decreased depression

Teach patient/family:
• About signs and symptoms of bleeding (GI bleeding, nosebleed, ecchymosis, bruising)
• To use with caution when driving and performing other activities requiring alertness because of drowsiness and blurred vision
• To avoid alcohol ingestion, MAOIs, other CNS depressants
• Not to discontinue medication quickly after long term use; may cause headache, malaise; taper

Black Box Warning: That clinical worsening and suicidal risk may occur

• To notify prescriber if pregnancy is planned or suspected or if breastfeeding
• Improvement may occur in 4-8 wk or up to 12 wk (geriatric patients)

levothyroxine (T_4) (Rx)

(lee-voe-thye-rox′een)

Eltroxin ♣, Levothroid, Levoxyl, Synthroid, Tirosint, Unithroid

Func. class.: Thyroid hormone
Chem. class.: Levoisomer of thyroxine

Do not confuse:
Synthroid/Symmetrel

ACTION:
Increases metabolic rate; controls protein synthesis; increases cardiac output, renal blood flow, O_2 consumption, body temperature, blood volume, growth, development at cellular level via action on thyroid hormone receptors

USES:
Hypothyroidism, myxedema coma, thyroid hormone replacement, thyrotoxicosis, congenital hypothyroidism, some types of thyroid cancer, pituitary TSH suppression

CONTRAINDICATIONS:
Adrenal insufficiency, recent MI, thyrotoxicosis, hypersensitivity to beef, alcohol intolerance (inj only)

Black Box Warning: Obesity treatment

L

Precautions: Pregnancy (A), breastfeeding, geriatric patients, angina pectoris, hypertension, ischemia, cardiac disease, diabetes

DOSAGE AND ROUTES

Hypothyroidism

- **Adult ≤50 yr: PO** 1.7 mcg/kg/day, 6-8 wk, average dose 100-200 mcg/day; **IM/IV** 50-100 mcg/day as single dose or 50% of usual oral dosage
- **Adult >50 yr without heart disease or <50 yr with heart disease: PO** 25-50 mcg/day, titrate q6-8wk
- **Adult >50 yr with heart disease: PO** 12.5-25 mcg/day, titrate by 12.5-25 mcg q6-8wk
- **Child >12 yr: PO** 2-3 mcg/kg/day as single dose in AM
- **Child 6-12 yr: PO** 4-5 mcg/kg/day as single dose in AM
- **Child 1-5 yr: PO** 5-6 mcg/kg/day as single dose in AM
- **Child 6-12 mo: PO** 6-8 mcg/kg/day as single dose in AM
- **Child to 6 mo: PO** 8-10 mcg/kg/day as single dose in AM

Myxedema coma

- **Adult: IV** 200-500 mcg, may increase by 100-300 mcg after 24 hr; give oral medication as soon as possible

Subclinical hypothyroidism

- **Adult: PO** 1 mcg/kg/day may be sufficient

Available forms: Powder for inj 100, 200, 500 mcg/vial; tabs 25, 50, 88, 100, 112, 125, 137, 150, 175, 200, 300 mcg; cap (liquid filled) 13, 25, 50, 75, 88, 100, 112, 125, 137, 150 mcg

Administer:

- Store in tight, light-resistant container; sol should be discarded if not used immediately
- Withdrawal of medication 4 wk before RAIU test

PO route

- In AM if possible as single dose to decrease sleeplessness; at same time each day to maintain product level; take on empty stomach
- Only for hormone imbalances; not to be used for obesity, male infertility, menstrual conditions, lethargy
- Lowest dose that relieves symptoms; lower dose to geriatric patients and for those with cardiac diseases
- Crush and mix with water; nonsoy formula or breast milk for infants, children
- Separate antacids, iron, calcium products by 4 hr

Direct IV route

- IV after diluting with provided diluent 500 mcg/5 ml, 200 mcg/2 ml; shake; give through Y-tube or 3-way stopcock; give ≤100 mcg/1 min; do not add to IV infusion
- Considered to be incompatible in syringe with all other products

SIDE EFFECTS

CNS: *Anxiety, insomnia, tremors,* headache, thyroid storm, excitability

CV: *Tachycardia, palpitations, angina, dysrhythmias,* hypertension, cardiac arrest

GI: Nausea, diarrhea, increased or decreased appetite, cramps

MISC: Menstrual irregularities, weight loss, sweating, heat intolerance, fever, alopecia, decreased bone mineral density

PHARMACOKINETICS

Half-life euthyroid 6-7 days, hypothyroid 9-10 days, hyperthyroid 3-4 days, distributed throughout body tissues

PO: Onset 24 hr

INTERACTIONS

Increase: cardiac insufficiency risk—EPINEPHrine products

Increase: effects of anticoagulants, sympathomimetics, tricyclics

Decrease: levothyroxine absorption—bile acid sequestrants, orlistat, ferrous sulfate

Decrease: levothyroxine effect—estrogens, antacids, sucralfate, aluminum, magnesium, calcium, iron, rifampin, rifabutin

Drug/Herb

Decrease: thyroid hormone effect—soy

Drug/Lab Test

Increase: CPK, LDH, AST, blood glucose
Decrease: thyroid function tests

NURSING CONSIDERATIONS

Assess:

- B/P, pulse periodically during treatment
- Weight daily in same clothing, using same scale, at same time of day
- Height, growth rate of child
- T_3, T_4, FTIs, which are decreased; radioimmunoassay of TSH, which is increased; radio uptake, which is increased if patient receiving too low a dose of medication
- Patient may require decreased anticoagulant; check for bleeding, bruising
- Increased nervousness, excitability, irritability, which may indicate too high a dose of medication, usually after 1-3 wk of treatment
- Cardiac status: angina, palpitation, chest pain, change in VS

Evaluate:

- Therapeutic response: absence of depression; increased weight loss, diuresis, pulse, appetite; absence of constipation, peripheral edema, cold intolerance; pale, cool, dry skin; brittle nails, alopecia, coarse hair, menorrhagia, night blindness, paresthesias, syncope, stupor, coma, rosy cheeks

Teach patient/family:

- That hair loss will occur in child, is temporary; that hypothyroid child will show almost immediate behavior/personality change
- To report excitability, irritability, anxiety, which indicate overdose
- Not to switch brands unless approved by prescriber
- That product may be discontinued after giving birth; that thyroid panel should be evaluated after 1-2 mo
- That product is not to be taken to reduce weight
- To avoid OTC preparations with iodine; to read labels; to separate antacids, iron, calcium products by 4 hr
- To avoid iodine-rich food, iodized salt, soybeans, tofu, turnips, high-iodine seafood, some bread
- That product is not a cure but controls symptoms; that treatment is lifelong, full effect may take up to 6 wk

⚠ HIGH ALERT

lidocaine (parenteral) (Rx)

(lye′doe-kane)

LidoPen Auto-Injector, Xylocaine, Xylocard ✦

Func. class.: Antidysrhythmic (Class Ib)
Chem. class.: Aminoacyl amide

ACTION: Increases electrical stimulation threshold of ventricle, His-Purkinje system, which stabilizes cardiac membrane, decreases automaticity

USES: Ventricular tachycardia, ventricular dysrhythmias during cardiac surgery, digoxin toxicity, cardiac catheterization

Unlabeled uses: Attenuation of intracranial pressure increased during intubation/endotracheal tube suctioning

CONTRAINDICATIONS: Hypersensitivity to amides, severe heart block, supraventricular dysrhythmias, Adams-Stokes syndrome, Wolff-Parkinson-White syndrome

Precautions: Pregnancy (B), breastfeeding, children, geriatric patients, renal/hepatic disease, CHF, respiratory depression, malignant hyperthermia, myasthenia gravis, weight <50 kg

DOSAGE AND ROUTES

- **Adult: IV BOL** 50-100 mg (1-1.5 mg/kg) 25-50 mg/min, repeat q3-5min, max 300 mg in 1 hr; begin **IV INFUSION; IV INFUSION** 1-4 mg/min (20-50 mcg/kg/min)

Available forms: IV INFUSION 0.2% (2 mg/ml), 0.4% (4 mg/ml), 0.8% (8 mg/ml); IV 4% (40 mg/ml), 10% (100 mg/ml), 20% (200 mg/ml); **IV dir** 1% (10 mg/ml), 2% (20 mg/ml); **Inj** (to IV admix) 20% (200 mg/ml)

Administer:

- IM inj in deltoid; aspirate to avoid intravascular administration; check IV site daily for infiltration or extravasation

IV route

- Bolus undiluted (1%, 2% only), give ≤50 mg/1 min or dilute 1 g/250-500 ml D_5W; titrate to patient response; use infusion pump; pediatric infusion 120 mg lidocaine/100 ml D_5W; 1-2.5 ml/kg/hr = 20-50 mcg/kg/min; use only 1%, 2% sol for IV bol

Y-site compatibilities: Acetaminophen, alemtuzumab, alfentanil, alteplase, amikacin, aminocaproic acid, aminophylline, amiodarone, amphotericin B lipid/liposome, anidulafungin, argatroban, ascorbic acid injection, atenolol, atropine, atracurium, azithromycin, aztreonam, benztropine, bivalirudin, bleomycin, bumetanide, buprenorphine, butorphanol, calcium chloride/gluconate, CARBOplatin, carmustine, ceFAZolin, cefotaxime, cefoTEtan, cefOXitin, ceftaroline, cefTAZidime, ceftizoxime, cefTRIAXone, cefuroxime, chloramphenicol, chlorproMAZINE, cimetidine, ciprofloxacin, cisatracurium, CISplatin, clarithromycin, clindamycin, cyanocobalamin, cyclophosphamide, cycloSPORINE, cytarabine, DACTINomycin, DAPTOmycin, DAUNOrubicin, dexamethasone, dexmedetomidine, dexrazoxane, digoxin, diltiazem, diphenhydrAMINE, DOBUTamine, DOCEtaxel, dolasetron, DOPamine, doxacurium, DOXOrubicin, DOXOrubicin lipsomal, doxycycline, enalaprilat, EPINEPHrine, epirubicin, epoetin alfa, eptifibatide, ertapenem, erythromycin, esmolol, etomidate, etoposide, etoposide phosphate, famotidine, fenoldopam, fentaNYL, fluconazole, fludarabine, fluorouracil, folic acid, furosemide, gentamicin, granisetron, haloperidol, heparin, hydrocortisone, imipenem/cilastatin, inamrinone, insulin, isoproterenol, ketorolac, labetalol, levofloxacin, linezolid, LORazepam, magnesium sulfate, meperidine, methylPREDNISolone sodium succinate, metoclopramide, metoprolol, metroNIDAZOLE, micafungin, midazolam, morphine, nafcillin, niCARdipine, nitroglycerin, nitroprusside, norepinephrine, ondansetron, palonosetron, penicillin G potassium, phenylephrine, phytonadione, piperacillin/tazobactam, potassium chloride, procainamide, prochlorperazine, promethazine, propofol, propranolol, protamine, quinupristin/dalfopristin, ranitidine, remifentanil, sodium bicarbonate, streptokinase, tacrolimus, theophylline, ticarcillin/clavulanate, tigecycline, tirofiban, tobramycin, vancomycin, vasopressin, verapamil, vitamin B complex with C, voriconazole, warfarin

SIDE EFFECTS

CNS: *Headache, dizziness,* involuntary movement, confusion, tremor, drowsiness, euphoria, seizures, shivering

CV: *Hypotension, bradycardia,* heart block, CV collapse, arrest

EENT: Tinnitus, blurred vision

GI: Nausea, vomiting, anorexia

HEMA: Methemoglobinemia

INTEG: Rash, urticaria, edema, swelling, petechiae, pruritus

MISC: Febrile response, phlebitis at inj site

RESP: Dyspnea, respiratory depression

PHARMACOKINETICS

Half-life 8 min, 1-2 hr (terminal); metabolized in liver; excreted in urine; crosses placenta

IM: Onset 5-15 min, duration 1½ hr

IV: Onset 2 min, duration 20 min

INTERACTIONS

Increase: cardiac depression, toxicity—amiodarone, phenytoin, procainamide, propranolol

Increase: hypotensive effects—MAOIs, antihypertensives

Increase: neuromuscular blockade—neuromuscular blockers, tubocurarine

Increase: lidocaine effects, toxicity—cimetidine, β-blockers, protease inhibitors, ritonavir

Decrease: lidocaine effects—barbiturates, ciprofloxacin, voriconazole

Decrease: effect of—cycloSPORINE
Drug/Lab Test
Increase: CPK

NURSING CONSIDERATIONS

Assess:

⚠ ECG continuously to determine increased PR or QRS segments; if these develop, discontinue or reduce rate; watch for increased ventricular ectopic beats, may have to rebolus; B/P

- **Blood levels:** therapeutic level, 1.5-5 mcg/ml
- I&O ratio, electrolytes (potassium, sodium, chlorine)

⚠ **Malignant hyperthermia:** tachypnea, tachycardia, changes in B/P, increased temperature

- **Respiratory status:** rate, rhythm, lung fields for crackles, watch for respiratory depression; lung fields, bilateral crackles may occur with CHF; increased respiration, pulse; product should be discontinued
- **CNS effects:** dizziness, confusion, psychosis, paresthesias, convulsions; product should be discontinued

Evaluate:

- Therapeutic response: decreased dysrhythmias

Teach patient/family:

- About the use of automatic lidocaine injection device if ordered for personal use
- To report signs of toxicity

TREATMENT OF OVERDOSE:

O_2, artificial ventilation, ECG; administer DOPamine for circulatory depression, diazepam or thiopental for seizures; decrease product if needed

lidocaine ophthalmic

See Appendix B

lidocaine topical

See Appendix B

RARELY USED

linaclotide

(lin′a-kloe′tide)

Linzess

Func. class.: Functional GI disorder agent

Chem. class.: Selective guanylate cyclase C agonist

L

USES:

Irritable bowel syndrome (IBS) with constipation, chronic constipation not associated with IBS

CONTRAINDICATIONS:

Hypersensitivity, urticaria, infection, sinusitis, GI obstruction

Black Box Warning: Children <6 yr, infants, neonates

DOSAGE AND ROUTES

Constipation

- **Adult: PO** 145 mcg/day on empty stomach, AM

Irritable bowel syndrome

- **Adult: PO** 290 mcg/day on empty stomach, AM

⚠ HIGH ALERT

linagliptin

(lin′a-glip′tin)

Tradjenta

Func. class.: Antidiabetic

Chem. class.: Didipeptidyl peptidase-4 inhibitor

ACTION: Slows the inactivation of incretin hormones; concentrations of the active, intact hormones are increased, thereby increasing and prolonging the action of these hormones; incretin hormones are released by the intestine throughout the day, and levels are increased in response to a meal

USES: Type 2 diabetes mellitus

CONTRAINDICATIONS: Hypersensitivity to linagliptin, type 1 diabetes mellitus, diabetic ketoacidosis (DKA)

Precautions: Pregnancy (category B), breastfeeding, adolescents or children <18 yr, debilitated physical condition, malnutrition, uncontrolled adrenal insufficiency, pituitary insufficiency, hypo/hyperthyroidism, diarrhea, gastroparesis, GI obstruction, ileus, female hormonal changes, high fever, severe psychological stress, uncontrolled hypercortisolism

DOSAGE AND ROUTES

- **Adult: PO** 5 mg daily; when used with a sulfonylurea or insulin; a lower dose of the sulfonylurea may be necessary to minimize the risk of hypoglycemia

Available forms: Tab 5 mg

Administer:

- Once daily; may give without regard to food
- Store at room temperature

SIDE EFFECTS

CNS: Headache

EENT: Nasopharyngitis

ENDO: Hypoglycemia, hyperuricemia

GI: Body weight loss, pancreatitis

INTEG: Serious hypersensitivity reactions, urticaria, angioedema, exfoliative dermatitis

MISC: Arthralgia, back pain

RESP: Bronchial hyperreactivity (with bronchospasm), nasopharyngitis, cough

PHARMACOKINETICS

Extensively distributed in the tissues, protein binding is concentration-dependent, a weak to moderate inhibitor of CYP3A4, plasma terminal half life of >100 hr; effective half-life 12 hr, 90% excreted unchanged, 85% excreted via the enterohepatic system (80%) or in urine (5%) within 4 days of dosing, rapidly absorbed, peak in 1.5 hr; bioavailability 30%

INTERACTIONS

Increase: hypoglycemia: sulfonylureas, β-blockers, ACE inhibitors, angiotensin II receptor antagonists, disopyramide, guanethidine, cloNIDine, octreotide, fenfluramine, dexfenfluramine, fibric acid derivatives, monoamine oxidase inhibitors (MAOIs), FLUoxetine, salicylates

Increase: masking of the signs and symptoms of hypoglycemia: reserpine, β-blockers

Increase: need for dosing change: cisapride, metoclopramide, tegaserod, androgens, alcohol, lithium, quinolones

Decrease: hypoglycemic effect—dextrothyroxine, bumetanide, furosemide, ethacrynic acid, torsemide, estrogens, progestins, oral contraceptives, thyroid hormones, glucocorticoids, glucagon, carbonic anhydrase inhibitors, phenytoin, fosphenytoin, or ethotoin; atypical antipsychotics (ARIPiprazole, cloZAPine, OLANZapine, QUEtiapine, risperiDONE, and ziprasidone), phenothiazine, niacin (nicotinic acid), triamterene, thiazide diuretics

Decrease: effect of linagliptin—CYP3A4 inducers (topiramate, rifabutin, pioglitazone, OXcarbazepine, carBAMazepine, nevirapine, modafinil, metyrapone, etravirine, efavirenz, bosentan, barbiturates, aprepitant, fosaprepitant)

Drug/Herb:

Decrease: linagliptin effect—St. John's wort

Drug/Lab Test:
Increase: uric acid

NURSING CONSIDERATIONS

Assess

- Monitor blood glucose, A1c, during treatment to determine diabetes control
- CBC baseline and periodically during treatment, report decreased blood counts

Evaluate:

- Improving blood glucose level, A1c; decreasing polydipsia, polyphagia, polyuria, clear sensorium, absence of dizziness

Teach patient/family:

- About the symptoms of hypo/hyperglycemia and what to do about each; to have glucagon emergency kit available, to carry sugar packets
- That product must be continued on a daily basis, about the consequences of discontinuing product abruptly; to take only as directed
- To avoid OTC products unless approved by prescriber
- That diabetes is a life-long illness, that product will not cure diabetes
- To carry emergency ID with prescriber, condition and medications taken
- To immediately report skin disorders, swelling, difficulty breathing, or severe abdominal pain

lindane (Rx)

(lin′dane)

Hexit ✦

Func. class.: Scabicide, pediculicide
Chem. class.: Chlorinated hydrocarbon (synthetic)

ACTION: Stimulates nervous system of arthropods, resulting in seizures, death

USES: Scabies, lice (head/pubic/body), nits in those intolerant to or who do not respond to other agents

CONTRAINDICATIONS: Hypersensitivity, patients with known seizure disorders, Norwegian (crusted) scabies

Black Box Warning: Premature neonate; inflammation of skin, abrasions, skin breaks; seizure disorder

Precautions: Pregnancy (C), breastfeeding, infants, children <10 yr, avoid contact with eyes

DOSAGE AND ROUTES

Lice

- **Adult and child: CREAM/LOTION** shampoo using 30 ml: work into lather, rub for 5 min, rinse, dry with towel; comb with fine-toothed comb to remove nits; most require 1 oz, max 2 oz

Scabies

- **Adult and child: TOP** apply 1% cream/lotion to skin, from neck to bottom of feet, toes; wash area with soap, water; remove visible crusts; apply to skin surfaces; remove with soap, water in 8-12 hr; repeat after 1 wk prn; most require 1 oz, max 2 oz

Available forms: Lotion, shampoo, cream (1%)

Administer:

- Caregivers should wear gloves less permeable to lindane, thoroughly clean hands after application; avoid natural latex gloves
- **Cream/ointment/lotion:** use for scabies only; skin should be clean without other products on it, wait 1 hr after bathing or showering before application, shake well, apply under fingernails after trimming; toothbrush can be used to apply; after application, wrap toothbrush in paper and throw away; use only a single application, apply as thin layer over all skin from neck down, close bottle containing leftover lotion, throw away
- Do not cover, wash off after 8-12 hr
- Use warm, not hot, water; do not leave on >12hr
- **Shampoo:** for lice only; do not use other hair products before use; shake well; hair should be completely dry; use only enough shampoo to lightly coat hair

L

and scalp, work into hair, do not use water; allow to remain only 4 min, rinse, lather away, towel briskly
- To scalp only; do not apply to face, lips, mouth, eyes, any mucous membrane, anus, or meatus
- Topical corticosteroids as ordered to decrease contact dermatitis; antihistamines
- Lotions of menthol or phenol to control itching
- Topical antibiotics for infection

SIDE EFFECTS

CNS: Seizures, CNS toxicity, stimulation, dizziness
INTEG: *Pruritus, rash, irritation, contact dermatitis*

PHARMACOKINETICS

Onset 3 hr, half-life 18-22 hr

INTERACTIONS

- Oils may increase absorption; if oil-based hair dressing used, shampoo, rinse, dry hair before applying lindane shampoo

NURSING CONSIDERATIONS

Assess:

Black Box Warning: Skin for abrasions, breaks, inflammation; do not use on these areas

- **Infestation:** head, hair for lice, nits before and after treatment; if scabies present, check all skin surfaces; identify source of infection: school, family, sexual contacts
- Isolation until areas on skin, scalp have cleared, treatment completed
- Removal of nits with fine-toothed comb rinsed in vinegar after treatment; use gloves

Evaluate:
- Therapeutic response: decreased crusts, nits, brownish trails on skin, itching papules in skin folds, decreased itching after several weeks

Teach patient/family:
- To wash all inhabitants' clothing using insecticide; that preventive treatment may be required of all persons living in same house using lotion or shampoo to decrease spread of infection; to use rubber gloves when applying product
- That itching may continue for 4-6 wk
- That product must be reapplied if accidently washed off or treatment will be ineffective
- Not to apply to face; if accidental contact with eyes occurs, flush with water
- To remove product after specified time to prevent toxicity
- To treat sexual contacts simultaneously
- To check for CNS toxicity: dizziness, cramps, anxiety, nausea, vomiting, seizures

linezolid (Rx)

(line-zoe′lide)

Zyvox

Func. class.: Broad-spectrum antiinfective
Chem. class.: Oxazolidinone

Do not confuse:
Zyvox/Ziox/Zosyn

ACTION: Inhibits protein synthesis by interfering with translation; binds to bacterial 23S ribosomal RNA of the 50S subunit, thus preventing formation of the bacterial translation process in primarily gram-positive organisms

USES: Vancomycin-resistant *Enterococcus faecium* infections, nosocomial pneumonia caused by *Staphylococcus aureus* or *Streptococcus* pneumonia, uncomplicated or complicated skin and skin-structure infections, community-acquired pneumonia, *Pasteurella multocida,* viridans streptococci, *E. faecium* infections, *S. aureus, S. pyogenes;* can be used for MSSA/MRSA/MDRSP strains

CONTRAINDICATIONS: Hypersensitivity
Precautions: Pregnancy (C), breastfeeding, children, thrombocytopenia,

bone marrow suppression, hypertension, hyperthyroidism, pheochromocytoma, seizure disorder, ulcerative colitis, MI, PKU, renal/GI disease

DOSAGE AND ROUTES

Vancomycin-resistant *Enterococcus faecium* infections

• **Adult/adolescent/child ≥12 yr: IV/PO** 600 mg q12hr × 14-28 days; max 1200 mg/day

• **Child <12 yr/infant/term neonate: IV/PO** 10 mg/kg q8hr × 14-28 days

Nosocomial pneumonia/complicated skin infections/community-acquired pneumonia/concurrent bacterial infection

• **Adult: IV/PO** 600 mg q12hr × 10-14 days; max 1200 mg/day

• **Child: birth-11 yr: PO** 10 mg/kg q8hr × 10-14 days

Uncomplicated skin infections

• **Adult: PO** 400 mg q12hr × 10-14 days; max 1200 mg/day

• **Adolescent: PO** 600 mg q12hr × 10-14 days; max 1200 mg/day

• **Infant preterm <7 days old: PO** 10 mg/kg q12hr × 10-14 days

Available forms: Tabs 600 mg; oral susp 100 mg/5 ml; inj 2 mg/ml

Administer:

PO route

• With/without food

• Store reconstituted oral susp at room temperature, use within 3 wk

Intermittent IV INFUSION route

• Do not use if particulate is present, yellow color is normal

• Premixed sol ready to use (2 mg/ml), give over 30-120 min; do not use IV infusion bag in series connections; do not use with additives in sol; do not use with another product, administer separately, flush line before and after use

Y-site compatibilities: Acyclovir, alfentanil, amikacin, aminophylline, ampicillin, aztreonam, buprenorphine, butorphanol, calcium gluconate, CARBOplatin, ceFAZolin, cefoTEtan, cefOXitin, cefTAZidime, ceftizoxime, cefuroxime, cimetidine, ciprofloxacin, cisatracurium, CISplatin, clindamycin, cyclophosphamide, cycloSPORINE, cytarabine, digoxin, furosemide, ganciclovir, gemcitabine, gentamicin, heparin, HYDROmorphone, ifosfamide, labetalol, leucovorin, levofloxacin, lidocaine, LORazepam, magnesium sulfate, mannitol, meperidine, meropenem, mesna, methotrexate, methylPREDNISolone, metoclopramide, metroNIDAZOLE, midazolam, minocycline, mitoXANtrone, morphine, nalbuphine, naloxone, nitroglycerin, ofloxacin, ondansetron, PACLitaxel, PENTobarbital, PHENObarbital, piperacillin, potassium chloride, prochlorperazine, promethazine, propranolol, ranitidine, remifentanil, SUFentanil, theophylline, ticarcillin, tobramycin, vancomycin, vecuronium, verapamil, vinCRIStine, zidovudine

Solution compatibilities: D_5W, 0.9% NaCl, LR

L

SIDE EFFECTS

CNS: *Headache,* dizziness, insomnia

GI: *Nausea, diarrhea,* **pseudomembranous colitis**, increased ALT/AST, *vomiting,* taste change, tongue-color change

HEMA: Myelosuppression

MISC: Vaginal moniliasis, fungal infection, oral moniliasis, **lactic acidosis, anaphylaxis, angioedema, Stevens-Johnson syndrome**

PHARMACOKINETICS

Peak 1-2 hr, terminal half-life 4-5 hr, rapidly and extensively absorbed, protein binding 31%, metabolized by oxidation of the morpholine ring

INTERACTIONS

⚠ **Do not use with MAOIs (or within 2 wk) or with products that possess MAOI-like action (furazolidone, isoniazid, INH, procarbazine); hypertensive crisis may occur**

⚠ **Increase: hypertensive crisis, seizures, coma—amoxapine, maprotiline, mirtazapine, traZODone, cyclobenzaprine, tricyclics, methyldopa**

Increase: serotonin syndrome—SSRIs, SNRIs, serotonin receptor agonists

Increase: effects of adrenergic agents (DOPamine, EPINEPHrine, pseudoephedrine)

Drug/Herb

• Avoid use with green tea, valerian, ginseng, yohimbine, kava, guarana, St. John's wort

Drug/Food

• Tyramine foods: avoid; increased pressor response

NURSING CONSIDERATIONS

Assess:

• CBC with differential weekly, assess for myelosuppression (anemias, leukopenia, pancytopenia, thrombocytopenia)

• **Serotonin syndrome:** at least 2 wk should elapse between discontinuing linezolid and starting serotonergic agents; assess for increased heart rate, shivering, sweating, dilated pupils, tremor, high B/P, hyperthermia, headache, confusion; if these occur, stop linezolid, administer a serotonin antagonist if needed

• **Lactic acidosis:** repeated nausea/vomiting, unexplained acidosis, low bicarbonate level; notify prescriber immediately

• **Anaphylaxis/angioedema/Stevens-Johnson syndrome:** rash, pruritus, difficulty breathing, fever; have emergency equipment nearby

• CNS symptoms: headache, dizziness

• Hepatic studies: AST, ALT

• **Diabetes mellitus:** monitor those receiving insulin or oral antidiabetics for increased hypoglycemia

⚠ **Pseudomembranous colitis:** diarrhea, abdominal pain, fever, fatigue, anorexia, possible anemia, elevated WBC, low serum albumin; stop product, usually either vancomycin or IV metroNIDAZOLE given

Evaluate:

• Therapeutic response: decreased symptoms of infection, blood cultures negative

Teach patient/family:

• If dizziness occurs, to ambulate, perform activities with assistance

• To complete full course of product therapy

• To contact prescriber if adverse reaction occurs

• To inform prescriber if SSRIs or cold products, decongestants being used

• To inform prescriber of history of hypertension

• To avoid large amounts of high-tyramine foods, drinks; provide list

RARELY USED

liothyronine (T_3) (Rx)

(lye-oh-thye′roe-neen)

Cytomel, Triostat

Func. class.: Thyroid hormone

Chem. class.: Synthetic T_3

USES: Hypothyroidism, myxedema coma, thyroid hormone replacement, congenital hypothyroidism, nontoxic goiter, T_3 suppression test

CONTRAINDICATIONS: Adrenal insufficiency, MI, thyrotoxicosis, untreated hypertension

Black Box Warning: Obesity treatment

DOSAGE AND ROUTES

• **Adult: PO** 25 mcg/day, increase by 12.5-25 mcg q1-2wk until desired response, maintenance dose 25-75 mcg/day, max 100 mcg/day

• **Geriatric: PO** 5 mcg/day, increase by 5 mcg/day q1-2wk, maintenance 25-75 mcg/day

Congenital hypothyroidism

• **Child >3 yr: PO** 50-100 mcg/day

• **Child <3 yr: PO** 5 mcg/day, increase by 5 mcg q3-4days titrated to response, infant maintenance 20 mcg/day; 1-3 yr 50 mcg/day

Myxedema, severe hypothyroidism

• **Adult: PO** 25-50 mcg, then may increase by 5-10 mcg q1-2wk; maintenance dose 50-100 mcg/day

Myxedema coma/precoma

• **Adult: IV** 25-50 mcg initially, 5 mcg in geriatric patients, 10-20 mcg with cardiac disease; give doses q4-12hr

Nontoxic goiter

• **Adult: PO** 5 mcg/day, increase by 12.5-25 mcg q1-2wk; maintenance dose 75 mcg/day

Suppression test

• **Adult: PO** 75-100 mcg/day × 1 wk; radioactive ^{131}I given before and after 1-wk dose

RARELY USED

liotrix (Rx)

(lye′oh-trix)

Thyrolar, T_3/T_4

Func. class.: Thyroid hormone

Chem. class.: Levothyroxine/liothyronine (synthetic T_4, T_3)

USES: Hypothyroidism, thyroid hormone replacement

CONTRAINDICATIONS: Adrenal insufficiency, MI, thyrotoxicosis

Black Box Warning: Obesity treatment

DOSAGE AND ROUTES

• **Adult: PO** single dose of Thyrolar, 1/4 or 1/2 of adult dose, adjust as needed at 2-wk intervals

• **Geriatric: PO** 1/4 tab initially, adjust q6-8wk

⚠ HIGH ALERT

liraglutide (Rx)

(lir′a-gloo′tide)

Saxenda, Victoza

Func. class.: Antidiabetic agent

Chem. class.: Incretin mimetics

ACTION: Improved glycemic control and potential weight loss via activation of the glucagon-like peptide-1 (GLP-1) receptor

USES: Type 2 diabetes mellitus in combination with diet/exercise, obesity

CONTRAINDICATIONS: Hypersensitivity

Black Box Warning: Medullary thyroid carcinoma (MTC), multiple endocrine neoplasia syndrome type 2 (MEN 2), thyroid cancer

Precautions: Breastfeeding, children, geriatric patients, alcoholism, cholelithiasis, ketoacidosis, diarrhea, fever, gastroparesis, hepatic/renal disease, hypoglycemia, infection, surgery, thyroid disease, trauma, vomiting, pancreatitis

DOSAGES AND ROUTES

• **Adult: SUBCUT** 0.6 mg/day × 1 wk, then increase to 1.2 mg/day, max 1.8 mg/day

Available forms: Solution for injection 18 mg/3 ml pre-filled pen

Administer:

SUBCUT route

• Give subcut only, inspect for particulate matter, discoloration; do not use if unusually viscous, cloudy, discolored, or if particles present; give daily anytime, without regard to meals; pen needles must be purchased separately, use Novo Nordisk needle; before first use, prime, see manual for directions; give in thigh, abdomen, or upper arm; lightly pinch fold of skin, insert needle at 90-degree angle (45-degree angle if thin), release skin; aspiration is not needed, give over 6 sec, rotate injection sites

• If dose is missed, resume once-daily dosing at next scheduled dose; if >3 days have elapsed since last dose, reinitiate at 0.6 mg, titrate

• Storage: do not store pen with needle attached; avoid direct heat and sunlight; discard 30 days after first use; after first use may be stored at room temperature or refrigerated; do not freeze

SIDE EFFECTS

CNS: Dizziness, headache
CV: Hypertension
ENDO: Hypoglycemia
EENT: Sinusitis
GI: Abdominal pain, anorexia, constipation, diarrhea, dyspepsia, nausea, vomiting, pancreatitis
INTEG: Angioedema, erythema, injection site reaction, urticaria
MS: Back pain
SYST: Antibody formation, infection, influenza, secondary thyroid malignancy, anaphylaxis, angioedema

INTERACTIONS

Increase: hypoglycemic reactions—angiotensin II receptor antagonists, ACE inhibitors, other antidiabetics, β-blockers, dexfenfluramine, fenfluramine, disopyramide, FLUoxetine, fibric acid derivatives, mecasermin, MAOIs, octreotide, pegvisomant, salicylates
Decrease: liraglutide effect—protease inhibitors, phenothiazines, baclofen, atypical antipsychotics, corticosteroids, cycloSPORINE, tacrolimus, carbonic anhydrase inhibitors, dextrothyroxine, diazoxide, phenytoin, fosphenytoin, ethotoin, isoniazid, INH, niacin, nicotine, estrogens, progestins, oral contraceptives, growth hormones, sympathomimetics
Increase or decrease: hypoglycemic reactions—androgens, bortezomib, quinolones, cloNIDine, alcohol, lithium, pentamidine
Increase or decrease: effects of—atorvastatin, acetaminophen, griseofulvin
Decrease: levels of digoxin

PHARMACOKINETICS

Protein binding (98%); half-life 12-13 hr; binds to albumin, then released into circulation; peak 8-12 hr; body weight significantly affects pharmacokinetics

NURSING CONSIDERATIONS

Assess:

Black Box Warning: Thyroid C-cell tumors; monitor during treatment

- **Hypoglycemic reactions** that may occur soon after meals: hunger, sweating, weakness, dizziness, tremors, restlessness, tachycardia
- Hypersensitivity to this product
- Serum glucose, A1c, CBC during treatment
- **Stress:** those diabetic patients exposed to stress, surgery, fever, infections may require insulin administration temporarily

⚠ **Serious skin reactions:** angioedema; also pancreatitis

Evaluate:

- Therapeutic response: stable and improved serum glucose, A1C, weight loss

Teach patient/family:

- About symptoms of hypo/hyperglycemia, what to do for each; to have glucagon emergency kit available; to carry a carbohydrate source at all times
- About side effects associated with therapy, such as nausea and vomiting; that upward dose titration can be delayed or ignored, depending on tolerance
- That diabetes is a lifelong illness; that product does not cure disease and must be continued on a daily basis
- To carry emergency ID with prescriber's phone number and medications taken
- To continue with other recommendations: diet, exercise, hygiene
- To test blood glucose using a blood glucose meter
- To avoid other medications, herbs, supplements unless approved by prescriber

⚠ To report serious skin effects, abdominal pain with nausea/vomiting

- Provide patient with written instructions if self-administration is ordered

lisdexamfetamine (Rx)

(lis-dex′am-fet′a-meen)

Vyvanse

Func. class.: CNS stimulant

Chem. class.: Amphetamine

Controlled Substance Schedule II

ACTION: Increases release of norepinephrine, DOPamine in cerebral cortex to reticular activating system

USES: Attention-deficit/hyperactivity disorder (ADHD), binge eating disorder

CONTRAINDICATIONS: Breastfeeding, hyperthyroidism, hypertension, glaucoma, severe arteriosclerosis, hypersensitivity to sympathomimetic amines

Black Box Warning: Substance abuse

Precautions: Pregnancy (C), children <6 yr, Gilles de la Tourette's disorder, depression, anorexia nervosa, psychosis, seizure disorder, suicidal ideation, MI, heart failure, alcoholism, aortic stenosis, bipolar disorder, CV disease

DOSAGE AND ROUTES

• **Adult/Child 6-12 yr: PO** 30 mg/day, may increase by 10-20 mg/day at weekly intervals, max 70 mg/day

Available forms: Caps 10, 20, 30, 40, 50, 60, 70 mg

Administer:

• Give daily in AM

• Without regard to meals

• Caps: may take whole or opened and contents dissolved in water

SIDE EFFECTS

CNS: *Hyperactivity, insomnia, restlessness, talkativeness,* dizziness, headache, dysphoria, irritability, CNS tumor, dependence, addiction, mild euphoria, somnolence, lability, psychosis, mania, hallucinations, aggression; movement disorders, psychiatric events (child)

CV: *Palpitations, tachycardia,* hypertension, decrease in heart rate, **dysrhythmias,** MI, **cardiomyopathy**

EENT: Blurred vision, mydriasis, dyplopia

ENDO: Growth inhibition

GI: *Anorexia,* dry mouth, diarrhea, weight loss

GU: Impotence, change in libido

INTEG: Urticaria, **angioedema, Stevens-Johnson syndrome, toxic epidermal necrolysis**

MISC: **Rhabdomyolysis**

PHARMACOKINETICS

Metabolized by liver; urine excretion pH dependent; crosses placenta, breast milk; half-life <1 hr

INTERACTIONS

⚠ **Hypertensive crisis: MAOIs or within 14 days of MAOIs**

Increase: serotonin syndrome, neuroleptic malignant syndrome—SSRIs, SNRIs, serotonin-receptor agonists

Increase: lisdexamfetamine effect—acetaZOLAMIDE, antacids, sodium bicarbonate, urinary alkalinizers

Increase: CNS effect—haloperidol, tricyclics, phenothiazines, modafinil, meperidine, PHENobarbital, phenytoin

Increase: CNS stimulation—melatonin

Decrease: absorption of phenytoin

Decrease: lisdexamfetamine effect—ascorbic acid, ammonium chloride, urinary acidifiers

Decrease: effect of—adrenergic blockers, antidiabetics

Drug/Herb

• **Serotonin syndrome: St. John's wort**

Increase: stimulant effect—khat, melatonin, green tea, guarana

Decrease: stimulant effect—eucalyptus

Drug/Food

Increase: amine effect—caffeine

NURSING CONSIDERATIONS

Assess:

• VS, B/P; product may reverse antihypertensives; check patients with cardiac disease often

• CBC, urinalysis; in diabetes: blood glucose; insulin changes may be required because eating may decrease
• Height, growth rate in children; growth rate may be decreased
• Mental status: mood, sensorium, affect, stimulation, insomnia, irritability
⚠ **Serotonin syndrome, neuroleptic malignant syndrome:** increased heart rate, shivering, sweating, dilated pupils, tremors, high B/P, hyperthermia, headache, confusion; if these occur, stop product, administer serotonin antagonist if needed; at least 2 wk should elapse between discontinuation of serotonergic agents and start of product
• **Tolerance or dependency:** increased amount of product may be used to get same effect; will develop after long-term use
• Overdose: pain, fever, dehydration, insomnia, hyperactivity

Black Box Warning: Before giving this product, identify presence of substance abuse; high potential for abuse

Perform/provide:
• Gum, hard candy, frequent sips of water for dry mouth

Evaluate:
• Therapeutic response: increased CNS stimulation, decreased drowsiness

Teach patient/family:
• **Seizures:** product may decrease seizure threshold; those with a seizure disorder should notify prescriber if seizure occurs
• To report CNS changes, blurred vision, dose may need decreasing
• To decrease caffeine consumption (coffee, tea, cola, chocolate); may increase irritability, stimulation
• To avoid OTC preparations unless approved by prescriber
• To taper product over several weeks; depression, increased sleeping, lethargy may occur
• To avoid alcohol ingestion
• To avoid breastfeeding
• To avoid hazardous activities until stabilized on medication
• To get needed rest; patient will feel more tired at end of day
• To use as part of a comprehensive treatment program

Black Box Warning: Serious CV effects may occur from increasing dose

TREATMENT OF OVERDOSE: Administer fluids, antihypertensive for increased B/P, ammonium chloride for increased excretion, chlorproMAZINE for antagonizing CNS effects

lisinopril (Rx)

(lyse-in′oh-pril)

Prinivil, Zestril

Func. class.: Antihypertensive, angiotensin-converting enzyme 1 (ACE) inhibitor

Chem. class.: Enalaprilat lysine analog

Do not confuse:
lisinopril/RisperDAL/Lipitor
Prinivil/Plendil/Proventil/PriLOSEC
Zestril/Zetia/Zyprexa

ACTION: Selectively suppresses renin-angiotensin-aldosterone system; inhibits ACE, thereby preventing conversion of angiotensin I to angiotensin II

USES: Mild to moderate hypertension, adjunctive therapy of systolic CHF, acute MI

Unlabeled uses: Diabetic nephropathy/retinopathy, proteinuria, post MI

CONTRAINDICATIONS: Hypersensitivity, angioedema

Black Box Warning: Pregnancy (D), 2nd/3rd trimesters

Precautions: Breastfeeding, renal disease, hyperkalemia, renal artery stenosis, CHF, pregnancy (C) 1st trimester, aortic stenosis

DOSAGE AND ROUTES

Hypertension

- **Adult: PO** initially 10 mg, 10-40 mg/day; max 80 mg/day
- **Child ≥6 yr: PO** 0.07 mg/kg/day up to 5 mg/day; titrate q1-2wk up to 0.6 mg/kg/day or 40 mg/day
- **Geriatric: PO** 2.5-5 mg/day, increase q7days

CHF

- **Adult: PO** 5 mg initially with diuretics, range 5-40 mg
- **Acute myocardial infarction in adults who are hemodynamically stable: PO** give 5 mg within 24 hr of onset of symptoms, then 5 mg after 24 hr, 10 mg after 48 hr, then 10 mg daily

Renal dose

- **Adult: PO** CCr <30 ml/min, reduce dose by 50%, initially 5 mg/day, max 40 mg/day; CCr <10 ml/min, 2.5 mg/day, max 40 mg/day

Available forms: Tabs 2.5, 5, 10, 20, 30, 40 mg

Administer:

- Severe hypotension may occur after 1st dose of product; may be prevented by reducing or discontinuing diuretic therapy 3 days before beginning lisinopril therapy
- Without regard to food

SIDE EFFECTS

CNS: *Vertigo,* depression, stroke, insomnia, paresthesias, *headache, fatigue,* asthenia, *dizziness*

CV: Chest pain, *hypotension,* sinus tachycardia

EENT: Blurred vision, nasal congestion

GI: Nausea, vomiting, anorexia, constipation, flatulence, GI irritation, diarrhea, hepatic failure, hepatic necrosis, pancreatitis

GU: Proteinuria, renal insufficiency, sexual dysfunction, impotence

HEMA: Neutropenia, agranulocytosis

INTEG: Rash, pruritus

MISC: Muscle cramps, *hyperkalemia*

RESP: Dry cough, dyspnea

SYST: Angioedema, anaphylaxis, toxic epidermal necrolysis

PHARMACOKINETICS

Onset 1 hr, peak 6-8 hr, duration 24 hr, excreted unchanged in urine, half-life 12 hr

INTERACTIONS

Increase: hyperkalemia—potassium salt substitutes, potassium-sparing diuretics, potassium supplements, cycloSPORINE

Increase: possible toxicity—lithium

Increase: hypotensive effect—diuretics, other antihypertensives, probenecid, phenothiazines, nitrates, acute alcohol ingestion

Increase: hypersensitivity—allopurinol

Decrease: lisinopril effects—aspirin, indomethacin, NSAIDs

Drug/Food

- High-potassium diet (bananas, orange juice, avocados, nuts, spinach) should be avoided; hyperkalemia may occur

Drug/Lab Test

Interference: glucose/insulin tolerance tests, ANA titer

NURSING CONSIDERATIONS

Assess:

⚠ Blood studies, platelets; WBC with differential at baseline, periodically q3mo; if neutrophils <1000/mm³, discontinue treatment (recommended with collagen-vascular disease)

- Baselines of renal, hepatic studies before therapy begins, periodically; LFTs, uric acid, glucose may be increased
- **Angioedema: anaphylaxis, toxic epidermal necrolysis,** facial swelling, dyspnea, tongue swelling (rare)

Black Box Warning: Pregnancy before starting treatment; pregnancy (D)

- **Hypertension:** B/P, pulse q4hr during beginning treatment and periodically thereafter; note rate, rhythm, quality; apical/pedal pulse before administration; notify prescriber of any significant changes
- Electrolytes: potassium, sodium, chlorine

L

• **CHF:** edema in feet, legs daily; weight daily; dyspnea, wet crackles
• Skin turgor, dryness of mucous membranes for hydration status

Evaluate:
• Therapeutic response: decreased B/P, CHF symptoms

Teach patient/family:
• Not to discontinue product abruptly; to taper
• To rise slowly to sitting or standing position to minimize orthostatic hypotension
• To avoid increasing potassium in the diet
• To report dry cough

Black Box Warning: To report if pregnancy is planned or suspected; pregnancy (D) 2nd/3rd trimesters

TREATMENT OF OVERDOSE:
Lavage, IV atropine for bradycardia, IV theophylline for bronchospasm, digoxin, O_2, diuretic for cardiac failure

lithium (Rx)
(li′thee-um)
Carbolith ♣, Lithane ♣, Lithobid ♣
Func. class.: Psychotropic agent—antimanic
Chem. class.: Alkali metal ion salt

ACTION: May alter sodium, potassium ion transport across cell membrane in nerve, muscle cells; may balance biogenic amines of norepinephrine, serotonin in CNS areas involved in emotional responses

USES: Bipolar disorders (manic phase), prevention of bipolar manic-depressive psychosis
Unlabeled Uses: Borderline personality disorder

CONTRAINDICATIONS: Pregnancy (D), breastfeeding, children <12 yr, hepatic disease, brain trauma, organic brain syndrome, schizophrenia, severe cardiac/renal disease, severe dehydration
Precautions: Geriatric patients, thyroid disease, seizure disorders, diabetes mellitus, systemic infection, urinary retention, QT prolongation

Black Box Warning: Lithium level >1.5 mmol/L

DOSAGE AND ROUTES
Bipolar Disorder (mania)
• **Adult: PO** 300-600 mg tid, maintenance 300 mg tid or qid; **EXT REL** 900 mg q12hr; dose should be individualized to maintain blood levels at 1-1.5 mEq/L or 0.6-1.2 mEq/L (maintenance)
• **Geriatric: PO** 300 mg bid, increase q7days by 300 mg to desired dose
• **Child: PO** 15-20 mg/kg/day in 3-4 divided doses; increase as needed; do not exceed adult doses; maintain blood levels at 0.4-0.5 mEq/L

Borderline Personality Disorder (unlabeled)
• **Adult: PO** 900-2400 mg in 3-4 divided doses or **EXT REL** 900-1800 mg in 2 divided doses, maintain levels 0.8-1 mEq/L

Available forms: Caps 150, 300, 600 mg; tabs 300 mg; ext rel tabs 300, 450 mg; syr 300 mg/5 ml (8 mEq/5 ml)

Administer:
• Do not break, crush, chew caps, ext rel tabs
• Reduced dose to geriatric patients
• With meals to avoid GI upset
• Adequate fluids (2-3 L/day) to prevent dehydration during initial treatment, 1-2 L/day during maintenance

SIDE EFFECTS
CNS: *Headache, drowsiness, dizziness,* tremors, twitching, ataxia, **seizure**, slurred speech, restlessness, confusion, stupor, memory loss, clonic movements, fatigue
CV: *Hypotension,* ECG changes, **dysrhythmias, circulatory collapse,** edema, Brugada syndrome, **QT prolongation**

EENT: Tinnitus, blurred vision
ENDO: Hyponatremia, goiter, hyperglycemia, hypo/hyperthyroidism
GI: *Dry mouth, anorexia, nausea, vomiting, diarrhea,* incontinence, abdominal pain, metallic taste
GU: Polyuria, glycosuria, proteinuria, albuminuria, urinary incontinence, polydipsia
HEMA: Leukocytosis
INTEG: Drying of hair, alopecia, rash, pruritus, hyperkeratosis, acneiform lesions, folliculitis
MS: Muscle weakness

PHARMACOKINETICS

PO: Onset rapid, peak ½-3 hr, half-life 18-36 hr depending on age, crosses blood-brain barrier, 80% of filtered lithium reabsorbed by renal tubules, excreted in urine, crosses placenta, enters breast milk, well absorbed by oral method

INTERACTIONS

- Neurotoxicity: haloperidol, thioridazine

Increase: hypothyroid effects—antithyroid agents, calcium iodide, potassium iodide, iodinated glycerol
Increase: effects of neuromuscular blocking agents, phenothiazines
Increase: renal clearance—sodium bicarbonate, acetaZOLAMIDE, mannitol, aminophylline
Increase: masking of lithium toxicity—β-blockers used for lithium tremor
Increase: toxicity—indomethacin, diuretics, NSAIDs, losartan
Increase: lithium effect/toxicity—carBAMazepine, FLUoxetine, methyldopa, thiazide diuretics, probenecid
Decrease: lithium effects—theophyllines, urea, urinary alkalinizers

Drug/Herb

- Avoid use with kava, St. John's wort, valerian

Decrease: lithium levels—black/green tea, guarana

Drug/Food

- Significant changes in sodium intake alter lithium excretion

Drug/Lab Test

Increase: potassium excretion, urine glucose, blood glucose, protein, BUN
Decrease: VMA, T_3, T_4, ^{131}I

NURSING CONSIDERATIONS

Assess:

- **Mental status:** manic symptoms, mood, behavior before, during treatment

Black Box Warning: Lithium toxicity: diarrhea, vomiting, tremor, twitching; serum lithium levels 2×/wk initially, then q2mo (therapeutic level: 0.5-1.5 mEq/L); toxic level >1.5 mcg/L

- Weight daily; check for, report edema in legs, ankles, wrists
- Sodium intake; decreased sodium intake with decreased fluid intake may lead to lithium retention; increased sodium, fluids may decrease lithium retention
- Skin turgor at least daily
- Urine for albuminuria, glycosuria, uric acid during beginning treatment, q2mo thereafter
- Neurologic status: LOC, gait, motor reflexes, hand tremors
- ECG in those >50 yr with CV disease, cardiology consult is recommended in those with risk factor, QT prolongation may occur

Evaluate:

- Therapeutic response: decrease in excitement, manic phase

Teach patient/family:

- About **the symptoms of minor toxicity:** vomiting, diarrhea, poor coordination, fine motor tremors, weakness, lassitude; **major toxicity:** coarse tremors, severe thirst, tinnitus, diluted urine
- To monitor urine specific gravity, emphasize need for follow-up care to determine lithium levels; to monitor lithium levels to ensure effective levels and treatment
- That contraception is necessary because lithium may harm fetus (pregnancy [D]); not to breastfeed
- Not to operate machinery until lithium levels stable

- That beneficial effects may take 1-3 wk
- About products that interact with lithium (provide list); about need for adequate, stable intake of salt and fluids; not to use OTC products unless approved by prescriber

TREATMENT OF OVERDOSE:
Induce emesis or lavage, maintain airway, respiratory function; dialysis for severe intoxication

Iodoxamide ophthalmic
See Appendix B

loperamide (OTC, Rx)
(loe-per′a-mide)

Diamode, Imodium ✤, Imodium A-D

Func. class.: Antidiarrheal

Chem. class.: Piperidine derivative

Do not confuse:
Imodium/Indocin
Loperamide/furosemide

ACTION: Direct action on intestinal muscles to decrease GI peristalsis; reduces volume, increases bulk; electrolytes not lost

USES: Diarrhea (cause undetermined), travelers' diarrhea, chronic diarrhea, to decrease amount of ileostomy discharge

Unlabeled uses: Irritable bowel syndrome, traveler's diarrhea

CONTRAINDICATIONS: Hypersensitivity, pseudomembranous colitis, constipation, dysentery, GI bleeding/obstruction/perforation, ileus, vomiting

Precautions: Pregnancy (C), breastfeeding, children <2 yr, hepatic disease, dehydration, gastroenteritis, toxic megacolon, geriatric patients, severe ulcerative colitis

DOSAGE AND ROUTES
- **Adult: PO** 4 mg, then 2 mg after each loose stool, max 16 mg/day
- **Child 9-11 yr: PO** 2 mg, then 1 mg after each loose stool, max 6 mg/24 hr
- **Child 6-8 yr: PO** 2 mg, then 0.1 mg/kg after each loose stool, max 4 mg/day
- **Child 2-5 yr: PO** 1 mg, then 0.1 mg/kg after each loose stool, max 4 mg/24 hr

Traveler's diarrhea (unlabeled)
- **Adult PO** 4 mg, then 2 mg after each diarrhea stool, max 16 mg/day

Available forms: Caps 2 mg; liq 1 mg/5 ml; tabs 2 mg, chew tabs 2 mg

Administer:
- Do not break, crush, or chew caps
- For 48 hr only
- Do not mix oral sol with other sol

SIDE EFFECTS
CNS: Dizziness, drowsiness, fatigue
GI: *Nausea, dry mouth, vomiting, constipation,* abdominal pain, anorexia, toxic megacolon, bacterial enterocolitis, flatulence
INTEG: Rash
MISC: Hyperglycemia
SYST: Anaphylaxis, angioedema, toxic epidermal necrolysis

PHARMACOKINETICS
PO: Duration 24 hr, half-life 9-14 hr, metabolized in liver, excreted in feces as unchanged product, small amount in urine

INTERACTIONS
Increase: CNS depression—alcohol, antihistamines, analgesics, opioids, sedative/hypnotics

Drug/Herb
Increase: CNS depression—chamomile, hops, kava, valerian

NURSING CONSIDERATIONS
Assess:
- **Stools:** volume, color, characteristics, frequency; bowel pattern before product; rebound constipation
- Electrolytes (potassium, sodium, chlorine) if receiving long-term therapy

• Skin turgor q8hr if dehydration is suspected; fluid replacement
• Response after 48 hr; if no response, product should be discontinued
• **Dehydration, CNS problems in children, those with hepatic disease**
• **Abdominal distention, toxic megacolon; may occur with ulcerative colitis**

Evaluate:
• Therapeutic response: decreased diarrhea (48 hr); decreased chronic diarrhea (10 days)

Teach patient/family:
• To avoid OTC products unless directed by prescriber
• That ileostomy patient may take product for extended time
• If drowsiness occurs, not to operate machinery
• To use hard candy, sips of water for dry mouth

lopinavir/ritonavir

(low-pin′ah-ver/ri-toe′na-veer)

Kaletra

Func. class.: Antiretroviral
Chem. class.: Protease inhibitor

ACTION: Inhibits human immunodeficiency virus (HIV-1) protease and prevents maturation of the infectious virus

USES: HIV-1 in combination with or without other antiretrovirals

CONTRAINDICATIONS: Hypersensitivity to this product or polyoxyethylated castor oil (oral solution), CYP3A4 metabolized products

Precautions: Pregnancy (C), breastfeeding, hepatic disease, pancreatitis, diabetes, hemophilia, AV block, hypercholesterolemia, immune reconstitution syndrome, neonates, cardiomyopathy, congenital long-QT prolongation, hypokalemia, elderly patients, Graves' disease, polymyositis, Guillain-Barré syndrome, children, HBV/HCV coinfection

DOSAGE AND ROUTES

HIV infection in combination with other antiretroviral agents
• **Adult: PO** 400 mg lopinavir/100 mg ritonavir bid or 800 mg lopinavir/200 mg ritonavir per day may be administered to patients with <3 lopinavir resistance–associated substitutions (L10F/I/R/V, K20M/N/R, L24I, L33F, M36I, I47V, G48V, 154L/T/V, V82A/C/F/S/T, and I84V); do not give once-daily dosing with concomitant carBAMazepine, PHENobarbital, or phenytoin; do not give as once-daily dosing with efavirenz, nevirapine, (fos) amprenavir, nelfinavir
• **Pregnant adults: PO** 400 mg lopinavir/100 mg ritonavir bid, may need 600 mg lopinavir/150 mg ritonavir bid in the 2nd/3rd trimesters; once-daily dosing is not recommended; a preferred PI-based regimen for pregnant patients combines twice-daily lopinavir; ritonavir with zidovudine and either lamiVUDine or emtricitabine
• **Adult receiving concomitant efavirenz, nelfinavir, or nevirapine: PO TABS,** 500 mg lopinavir/125 mg ritonavir bid; **CAPS/SOL,** 533 mg lopinavir/133 mg ritonavir bid
• **Adolescent/child/infant >6 mo:** 300 mg lopinavir/75 mg ritonavir/m^2/dose bid. The once-daily regimen is not recommended in pediatric patients; capsules are not recommended for use in patients ≤40 kg; a preferred PI-based regimen for all children combines lopinavir/ritonavir with a dual NRTI; a lopinavir/ritonavir plus dual NRTI regimen is an alternative option in adolescents

Available forms: Oral solution 400 mg lopinavir/100 mg ritonavir/5 ml; tablets 100 mg lopinavir/25 mg ritonavir, 200 mg lopinavir/50 mg ritonavir

Administer:

PO route
• **TAB:** take without regard to food; swallow whole, do not crush, break, chew
• **ORAL SOL:** shake well, use calibrated measuring device
• Drug resistance testing should be done before beginning therapy in antiretroviral-naive patients and before changing therapy for treatment failure

• For adults and adolescents, therapy is recommended in those with a CD4 ≤500/mm³, who is pregnant, who has HIV-associated nephropathy, or who is being treated for hepatitis B (HBV) infection; therapy should be offered to patients at risk of transmitting HIV to sexual partners; treatment in those with a CD4 count >500/mm³ may be considered
• For children, use is recommended in any symptomatic patient; for asymptomatic or mildly symptomatic children ≥5 years, therapy is recommended for those with HIV RNA ≥100,000 copies/ml or CD4 <500/mm³; for asymptomatic or mildly symptomatic children 1-4 yr, therapy is recommended for patients with HIV RNA ≥100,000 copies/ml or CD4 <25%
• For infants <12 mo, therapy is recommended regardless of clinical status, CD4 percentage, or viral load

SIDE EFFECTS

CNS: Paresthesia, headache, seizures, fever, dizziness, insomnia, asthenia, intracranial bleeding, encephalopathy
CV: QT, PR interval prolongation, deep vein thrombosis
EENT: Blurred vision, otitis media, tinnitus
GI: Diarrhea, buccal mucosa ulceration, abdominal pain, nausea, taste perversion, dry mouth, vomiting, anorexia
INTEG: Rash
MISC: Asthenia, angioedema, anaphylaxis, Stevens-Johnson syndrome, increase lipids, lipodystrophy
MS: Pain, rhabdomyolysis, myalgias

PHARMACOKINETICS

Well absorbed, 98% protein binding, hepatic metabolism, peak 4 hr, terminal half-life 6 hr

INTERACTIONS

Increase: Toxicity—amiodarone, avanafil, azole antifungals, benzodiazepines, buPROPion, cloZAPine, desipramine, dihydroergotamine, encainide, ergotamine, flecainide, HMG-CoA reductase inhibitors, interleukins, meperidine, midazolam, pimozide, piroxicam, propafenone, quiNIDine, ranolazine, rivaroxaban, saquinavir, triazolam, zolpidem
Increase: QT prolongation—class 1A/III antidysrhythmics, some phenothiazines, β-agonists, local anesthetics, tricyclics, haloperidol, chloroquine, droperidol, pentamidine, CYP3A4 inhibitors (amiodarone, clarithromycin, erythromycin, telithromycin, troleandomycin), arsenic trioxide, levomethadyl, CYP3A4 substrates (methadone, pimozide, QUEtiapine, quiNIDine, risperiDONE, ziprasidone)
Increase: Ritonavir levels—fluconazole
Increase: Level of both products—clarithromycin, ddI
Increase: Levels of bosentan
Decrease: Ritonavir levels—rifamycins, nevirapine, barbiturates, phenytoin, budesonide, predniSONE
Decrease: Levels of anticoagulants, atovaquone, divalproex, ethinyl estradiol, lamoTRIgine, phenytoin, sulfamethoxazole, theophylline, voriconazole, zidovudine

Drug/Lab Test
Increase: AST, ALT, CPK, cholesterol, GGT, triglycerides, uric acid, glucose
Decrease: Hct, Hgb, RBC, neutrophils, WBC

Drug/Herb
Decrease: Ritonavir levels—St. John's wort; avoid concurrent use
Avoid use with red yeast rice, evening primrose oil

NURSING CONSIDERATIONS

Assess:
• HIV: viral load, CD4 at baseline, throughout therapy; blood glucose, plasma HIV RNA, serum cholesterol/lipid profile; resistance testing before starting therapy and after treatment failure
• Signs of infection, anemia
• Hepatic studies: ALT, AST
• Bowel pattern before, during treatment; if severe abdominal pain with bleeding occurs, discontinue product; monitor hydration
• Skin eruptions; rash
⚠ **Rhabdomyolysis:** Muscle pain, increased CPK, weakness, swelling of

affected muscles; if these occur and if confirmed by CPK, product should be discontinued

QT prolongation: ECG for QT prolongation, ejection fraction; assess for chest pain, palpitations, dyspnea

Serious skin disorders: Stevens–Johnson syndrome, angioedema, anaphylaxis

Evaluate:

- Therapeutic response: improvement in HIV symptoms; improving viral load, CD4+ T cells

Teach patient/family:

- To take as prescribed; if dose is missed, to take as soon as remembered up to 1 hr before next dose; not to double dose
- That product is not a cure for HIV; that opportunistic infections can continue to be acquired
- That redistribution of body fat or accumulation of body fat may occur
- That others can continue to contract HIV from patient
- To avoid OTC, prescription medications, herbs, supplements unless approved by prescriber; not to use St. John's wort because it decreases product's effect
- That regular follow-up exams and blood work will be required

loratadine (OTC, Rx)

(lor-a'ti-deen)

Alavert, Claritin, Claritin Children's, Claritin RediTabs, Clear-Atadine, Dimetapp, Triaminic AllerChews

Func. class.: Antihistamine, 2nd generation

Chem. class.: Selective histamine (H_1)-receptor antagonist

Do not confuse:

loratadine/lovastatin/LORazepam/losartan

ACTION: Binds to peripheral histamine receptors, thereby providing antihistamine action without sedation

USES: Seasonal rhinitis, chronic idiopathic urticaria for those ≥2 yr

CONTRAINDICATIONS: Hypersensitivity, acute asthma attacks, lower respiratory tract disease

Precautions: Pregnancy (B), breastfeeding, increased intraocular pressure, bronchial asthma, hepatic/renal disease

DOSAGE AND ROUTES

- **Adult and child ≥6 yr: PO** 10 mg/day
- **Child 2-5 yr: PO** 5 mg/day

Renal/hepatic dose

- **Adult: PO** CCr <30 ml/min or hepatic disease, 10 mg every other day

Available forms: Tabs 10 mg; rapid-disintegrating tabs 10 mg; orally disintegrating tabs 10 mg; syr 1 mg/ml; susp 5 mg/ml, ext rel tab 10 mg

Administer:

- **Rapid-disintegrating tabs** by placing on tongue, to be swallowed after disintegrated with/without water
- Use within 6 mo of opening pouch and immediately after opening blister pack
- On empty stomach daily

Ext Rel Tab

- Do not break, crush, or chew

SIDE EFFECTS

CNS: Sedation (more common with increased doses), headache, fatigue, restlessness

EENT: Dry mouth

PHARMACOKINETICS

Peak 1.3-2.5 hr, duration 24 hr, metabolized in liver to active metabolites, excreted in urine, active metabolite desloratadine half-life 20 hr

INTERACTIONS

Increase: CNS depressant effects—alcohol, antidepressants, other antihistamines, sedative/hypnotics

Increase: loratadine level—cimetidine, ketoconazole, macrolides (clarithromycin, erythromycin)

Drug/Lab Test

False negative: skin allergy tests (discontinue antihistamine 3 days before testing)

NURSING CONSIDERATIONS

Assess:

- **Allergy:** hives, rash, rhinitis; monitor respiratory status

Evaluate:

- Therapeutic response: absence of running or congested nose, other allergy symptoms

Teach patient/family:

- To avoid driving, other hazardous activities if drowsiness occurs
- To avoid use of other CNS depressants

⚠ HIGH ALERT

LORazepam (Rx)

(lor-a′ze-pam)

Ativan

Func. class.: Sedative, hypnotic; antianxiety

Chem. class.: Benzodiazepine, short acting

Controlled Substance Schedule IV

Do not confuse:
LORazepam/ALPRAZolam/clonazePAM

ACTION: Potentiates the actions of GABA, especially in the limbic system and the reticular formation

USES: Anxiety, irritability with psychiatric or organic disorders, preoperatively; insomnia; adjunct for endoscopic procedures, status epilepticus

Unlabeled uses: Antiemetic before chemotherapy, rectal use, alcohol withdrawal, seizure prophylaxis, agitation, insomnia, sedation maintenance

CONTRAINDICATIONS: Pregnancy (D), breastfeeding, hypersensitivity to benzodiazepines, benzyl alcohol; closed-angle glaucoma, psychosis, history of drug abuse, COPD, sleep apnea

Precautions: Children <12 yr, geriatric patients, debilitated, renal/hepatic disease, addiction, suicidal ideation, abrupt discontinuation

DOSAGE AND ROUTES

Anxiety

- **Adult/adolescent: PO** 2-3 mg/day in divided doses, max 10 mg/day
- **Geriatric: PO** 1-2 mg/day in divided doses or 0.5-1 mg at bedtime

Preoperatively

- **Adult: IM** 50 mcg/kg 2 hr before surgery; **IV** 44 mcg/kg 15-20 min before surgery, max 2 mg 15-20 min before surgery
- **Child ≥12 yr: IV** 0.05 mg/kg, max 4 mg

Status epilepticus

- **Neonate: IV** 0.05 mg/kg
- **Child: IV** 0.1 mg/kg up to 4 mg/dose; **RECT** (unlabeled) 0.05-0.1 mg × 2; wait 7 min before giving 2nd dose

Sedation in mechanically ventilated patients (unlabeled)

- **Adult/Adolescent: Intermittent IV** 0.044 mg/kg q2-4hr, prn, max 4 mg single dose;
- **Adult/Adolescent: IV infusion** 0.5-8 mg/hr titrate, use loading dose of 2-4 mg

Alcohol withdrawal (unlabeled)

- **Adult: PO** 2 mg q6hr × 4 doses, then 1 mg q6hr for 8 doses

Insomnia (unlabeled)

- **Adult: PO** 2-4 mg at bedtime; only minimally effective after 2 wk continuous therapy
- **Geriatric: PO** 0.5-1 mg initially

Available forms: Tabs 0.5, 1, 2 mg; inj 2, 4 mg/ml; concentration oral sol 2 mg/ml

Administer:

PO route

- With food or milk for GI symptoms; crushed if patient is unable to swallow medication whole
- Sugarless gum, hard candy, frequent sips of water for dry mouth
- Give largest dose before bedtime if giving in divided doses

• **Concentrate:** use calibrated dropper; add to food/drink; consume immediately

IM route

• Deep into large muscle mass
• Use this route when IV is not feasible

Direct IV route

• Prepare immediately before use; short stability time
• IV after diluting in equal vol sterile water, 5% dextrose, or 0.9% NaCl for inj; give through Y-tube or 3-way stopcock; give at ≤2 mg/1 min; do not give rapidly
• Do not use in neonates (benzyl alcohol)

Y-site compatibilities: Acetaminophen, acyclovir, albumin, allopurinol, amifostine, amikacin, amoxicillin, amoxicillin/clavulanate, amphotericin B cholesteryl, amsacrine, atenolol, atracurium, bivalirudin, bleomycin, bumetanide, butorphanol, calcium chloride/gluconate, CARBOplatin, ceFAZolin, cefepime, cefotaxime, cefoTEtan, cefOXitin, cefTAZidime, ceftizoxime, ceftobiprole, cefTRIAXone, cefuroxime, chloramphenicol, chlorproMAZINE, cimetidine, ciprofloxacin, cisatracurium, CISplatin, cladribine, clindamycin, cloNIDine, cyclophosphamide, cycloSPORINE, cytarabine, DACTINomycin, DAPTOmycin, dexamethasone, dexmedetomidine, diltiazem, DOBUTamine, DOCEtaxel, DOPamine, doripenem, DOXOrubicin, DOXOrubicin liposomal, droperidol, enalaprilat, ePHEDrine, EPINEPHrine, epirubicin, eptifibatide, erythromycin, esmolol, etomidate, famotidine, fenoldopam, fentaNYL, filgrastim, fluconazole, fludarabine, fosphenytoin, furosemide, ganciclovir, gatifloxacin, gemcitabine, gentamicin, glycopyrrolate, granisetron, haloperidol, heparin, hydrocortisone, HYDROmorphone, hydrOXYzine, ifosfamide, inamrinone, insulin (regular), irinotecan, isoproterenol, ketorolac, labetalol, lidocaine, linezolid, magnesium sulfate, mannitol, mechlorethamine, melphalan, meropenem, metaraminol, methadone, methotrexate, methyldopate, methylPREDNISolone, metoclopramide, metoprolol, metroNIDAZOLE, micafungin, midazolam, milrinone, minocycline, mitoXANtrone, morphine, mycophenolate, nafcillin, nalbuphine, naloxone, nesiritide, niCARdipine, nitroglycerin, nitroprusside, norepinephrine, octreotide, oxaliplatin, oxytocin, PACLitaxel, palonosetron, pamidronate, pancuronium, PEMEtrexed, pentamidine, PENTobarbital, PHENobarbital, piperacillin, piperacillin-tazobactam, polymyxin B, potassium chloride, propofol, ranitidine, remifentanil, tacrolimus, teniposide, theophylline, thiotepa, ticarcillin, ticarcillin-clavulanate, tigecycline, tirofiban, tobramycin, TPN, trastuzumab, trimethobenzamide, trimethoprim-sulfamethoxazole, vancomycin, vasopressin, vecuronium, verapamil, vinCRIStine, vinorelbine, voriconazole, zidovudine

SIDE EFFECTS

CNS: *Dizziness, drowsiness,* confusion, headache, anxiety, tremors, stimulation, fatigue, depression, insomnia, hallucinations, weakness, unsteadiness

CV: *Orthostatic hypotension,* **ECG changes, tachycardia,** hypotension; **apnea, cardiac arrest (IV, rapid)**

EENT: *Blurred vision,* tinnitus, mydriasis

GI: Constipation, dry mouth, nausea, vomiting, anorexia, diarrhea

INTEG: Rash, dermatitis, itching

MISC: Acidosis

PHARMACOKINETICS

Metabolized by liver; excreted by kidneys; crosses placenta, excreted in breast milk; half-life 42 hr (neonates), 10.5 hr (older child), 12 hr (adult), 91% protein bound

PO: Onset 1 hr, peak 2 hr, duration 12-24 hr

IM: Onset 15-30 min, peak 1-1½ hr, duration 6-8 hr

IV: Onset 5 min, peak 1-1½ hr, duration 6-8 hr

INTERACTIONS

Increase: LORazepam effects—CNS depressants, alcohol, disulfiram

Decrease: LORazepam effects—valproic acid, oral contraceptives

L

Drug/Herb
Increase: CNS depression—chamomile, kava, valerian
Drug/Lab Test
Increase: AST, ALT

NURSING CONSIDERATIONS

Assess:

⚠ **Anxiety:** decrease in anxiety; mental status: mood, sensorium, affect, sleeping pattern, drowsiness, dizziness, suicidal tendencies

- Renal/hepatic/blood status if receiving high-dose therapy
- **Physical dependency, withdrawal symptoms:** headache, nausea, vomiting, muscle pain, weakness, tremors, seizures, after long-term, excessive use

Perform/provide:

- Assistance with ambulation during beginning therapy, since drowsiness, dizziness occurs
- Check to confirm that PO medication has been swallowed
- Refrigerate parenteral form

Evaluate:

- Therapeutic response: decreased anxiety, restlessness, insomnia

Teach patient/family:

- That product may be taken with food
- Not to use product for everyday stress or for >4 mo unless directed by prescriber
- Not to take more than prescribed amount; may be habit forming
- To avoid OTC preparations (cough, cold, hay fever) unless approved by prescriber
- To avoid driving, activities that require alertness, since drowsiness may occur
- To avoid alcohol, other psychotropic medications unless directed by prescriber
- Not to discontinue medication abruptly after long-term use
- To rise slowly because fainting may occur, especially among geriatric patients
- That drowsiness may worsen at beginning of treatment
- To notify prescriber if pregnancy is planned or suspected, pregnancy (D), do not breastfeed
- To report suicidal ideation

TREATMENT OF OVERDOSE:

Lavage, VS, supportive care, flumazenil

lorcaserin

(lor-ca-ser′in)

Belviq

Func. class.: Weight-control agent (anorexiant)

Chem. class.: Serotonin 2C ($5\text{-}HT_{2C}$) receptor agonist

Controlled Substance Schedule IV

ACTION:

Decreases food consumption and decreases hunger by selectively activating $5\text{-}HT_{2C}$ receptors

USES:

Obesity management

CONTRAINDICATIONS:

Pregnancy (X), breastfeeding, hypersensitivity, severe renal impairment

Precautions: Children, other organic causes of obesity, anemia, AV block, bradycardia, bundle branch block, depression, dialysis, liver/kidney disease, multiple myeloma, neutropenia, suicidal ideation, Peyronie's disease, pulmonary hypertension, sick sinus syndrome

DOSAGE AND ROUTES

Adult:

- **PO** 10 mg bid; do not exceed recommended dosage

Available forms: Tabs, film-coated 10 mg

Administer:

- For obesity if patient is on weight reduction program that includes dietary changes, exercise
- May give without regard to food

SIDE EFFECTS

CNS: Insomnia, depression, serotonin syndrome, anxiety, suicidal ideation, dizziness, headache, fatigue
CV: Bradycardia, hypertension

GI: Diarrhea, constipation, nausea
HEMA: Neutropenia, leukopenia, lymphopenia
INTEG: Rash
MS: Back pain

PHARMACOKINETICS

70% protein binding, half-life 11 hr

INTERACTIONS

Increase: life-threatening serotonin syndrome or NMS—SSRIs, SNRIs, serotonin-receptor agonists, sibutramine, MAOIs, linezolid, tricyclic antidepressants, buPROPion, lithium, DOPamine antagonist, traMADol
Increase: risk of hypoglycemia with sulfonylureas and insulin
Drug/Herb
Increase: Serotonin syndrome—St. John's wort

NURSING CONSIDERATIONS

Assess:

- Weight weekly; oral hypoglycemic dosage might need to be reduced in diabetic patients
- Monitor blood glucose, CBC with differential, Hct/Hgb, serum prolactin

⚠ Pregnancy (X): do not use in pregnancy

Suicidal Ideation:

⚠ Use caution in psychiatric disorders with emotional lability; assess for depression, suicidal thoughts/behaviors

Evaluate:

- Therapeutic response: decrease in weight

Teach patient/family:

- To avoid hazardous activities until stabilized on medication
- To discuss unpleasant side effects

⚠ To notify prescriber if pregnancy is planned or suspected, pregnancy X

losartan

(lo-zar′tan)

Cozaar

Func. class.: Antihypertensive
Chem. class.: Angiotensin II receptor (type AT_1) antagonist

Do not confuse:
losartan/valsartan
Cozaar/Zocor

ACTION: Blocks the vasoconstrictor and aldosterone-secreting effects of angiotensin II; selectively blocks the binding of angiotensin II to the AT_1 receptor found in tissues

USES: Hypertension, alone or in combination; nephropathy in type 2 diabetes; proteinuria; stroke prophylaxis for hypertensive patients with left ventricular hypertrophy
Unlabeled uses: Heart failure

CONTRAINDICATIONS: Hypersensitivity

Black Box Warning: Pregnancy (D) 2nd/3rd trimesters

Precautions: Pregnancy (C) 1st trimester, breastfeeding, children, geriatric patients; hypersensitivity to ACE inhibitors; hepatic disease, angioedema, renal artery stenosis, African descent, hyperkalemia, hypotension

DOSAGE AND ROUTES

Hypertension

- **Adult: PO** 50 mg/day alone or 25 mg/day in combination with diuretic; maintenance 25-100 mg/day
- **Child ≥6 yr: PO** 0.7 mg/kg/day, max 50 mg/day

Hypertension with left ventricular hypertrophy (benefit does not apply to those of African American descent)

- **Adult: PO** 50 mg/day; add hydrochlorothiazide 12.5 mg/day and/or increase losartan to 100 mg/day, then increase hydrochlorothiazide to 25 mg/day

Nephropathy in type 2 diabetic patients/proteinuria

- **Adult: PO** 50 mg/day, may increase to 100 mg/day

Hepatic dose/volume/depletion

- **Adult: PO** 25 mg/day as starting dose

Available forms: Tabs 25, 50, 100 mg

Administer:

- Without regard to meals

SIDE EFFECTS

CNS: *Dizziness, insomnia,* anxiety, confusion, abnormal dreams, migraine, tremor, vertigo, headache, malaise, depression, fatigue

CV: Angina pectoris, 2nd-degree AV block, cerebrovascular accident, *hypotension,* MI, dysrhythmias

EENT: Blurred vision, burning eyes, conjunctivitis

GI: *Diarrhea, dyspepsia,* anorexia, constipation, dry mouth, flatulence, gastritis, vomiting

GU: Impotence, nocturia, urinary frequency, UTI, renal failure

HEMA: Anemia, thrombocytopenia

INTEG: Alopecia, dermatitis, dry skin, flushing, photosensitivity, rash, pruritus, sweating, angioedema

META: Gout, hyperkalemia, hypoglycemia

MS: Cramps, myalgia, pain, stiffness

RESP: *Cough, upper respiratory infection,* congestion, dyspnea, bronchitis

PHARMACOKINETICS

Peak 1 hr, extensively metabolized, half-life 2 hr, metabolite 6-9 hr, excreted in urine/feces, protein binding 98.7%

INTERACTIONS

Increase: lithium toxicity—lithium

Increase: antihypertensive effect—fluconazole

Increase: hyperkalemia—potassium-sparing diuretics, potassium supplements, ACE inhibitors

Decrease: antihypertensive effect—NSAIDs, PHENobarbital, rifamycin, salicylates

NURSING CONSIDERATIONS

Assess:

- B/P with position changes, pulse before and periodically during treatment; note rate, rhythm, quality
- Baselines of renal, hepatic, electrolyte studies before therapy begins and periodically thereafter
- Skin turgor, dryness of mucous membranes for hydration status

⚠ Angioedema: facial swelling, dyspnea, wheezing; may occur rapidly; tongue swelling (rare)

- **CHF:** jugular venous distention; edema in feet/legs, weight daily
- **Blood dyscrasias:** thrombocytopenia, anemia (rare)

Black Box Warning: Pregnancy before starting treatment; pregnancy (D) 2nd/3rd trimester

Evaluate:

- Therapeutic response: decreased B/P, slowing diabetic neuropathy

Teach patient/family:

- To avoid sunlight or to wear sunscreen if in sunlight; that photosensitivity may occur
- To comply with dosage schedule, even if feeling better; not to discontinue abruptly
- To notify prescriber of mouth sores, fever, swelling of hands or feet, irregular heartbeat, chest pain
- That excessive perspiration, dehydration, vomiting, diarrhea may lead to fall in B/P; to consult prescriber if these occur
- That product may cause dizziness, fainting, light-headedness; to avoid hazardous activities until reaction is known
- To rise slowly to sitting or standing position to minimize orthostatic hypotension

Black Box Warning: To use contraception while taking this product; pregnancy (D) 2nd/3rd trimesters

• To avoid salt substitutes, alcohol, grapefruit juice, OTC products unless approved by prescriber

loteprednol ophthalmic

See Appendix B

lovastatin (Rx)

(loh-vah-stat′in)

Altoprev, Mevacor

Func. class.: Antilipemic

Chem. class.: HMG-CoA reductase inhibitor

Do not confuse:
lovastatin/Lotensin/Leustatin
Mevacor/mivacron

ACTION: Inhibits HMG-CoA reductase enzyme, which reduces cholesterol synthesis

USES: As an adjunct for primary hypercholesterolemia (types IIa, IIb), atherosclerosis; heterozygous familial hypercholesterolemia (adolescents)

CONTRAINDICATIONS: Pregnancy (X), breastfeeding, hypersensitivity, active hepatic disease

Precautions: Children, past hepatic disease, alcoholism, severe acute infections, trauma, hypotension, uncontrolled seizure disorders, severe metabolic disorders, electrolyte imbalances, visual disorder

DOSAGE AND ROUTES

• **Adult: PO** 20 mg/day with evening meal; may increase to 20-80 mg/day in single or divided doses, max 80 mg/day; **EXT REL** 20-60 mg/day at bedtime, max 60 mg/day

Heterozygous familial hypercholesterolemia

• **Adolescent 10-17 yr: PO** 10-40 mg with evening meal

Renal dose

• **Adult: PO** CCr <30 mg/min, max 20 mg/day unless titrated

Available forms: Tabs 10, 20, 40 mg; ext rel tab 20, 40, 60 mg

Administer:

• In evening with meal; if dose is increased, take with breakfast and evening meal
• Altroprev not equivalent to Mevacor
• Do not crush, chew ext rel tab
• Store in cool environment in airtight, light-resistant container

SIDE EFFECTS

CNS: *Dizziness, headache, tremor,* insomnia, paresthesia

EENT: *Blurred vision,* lens opacities

GI: *Flatus, nausea, constipation, diarrhea, dyspepsia, abdominal pain, heartburn,* **hepatic dysfunction,** vomiting, acid regurgitation, dry mouth, dysgeusia

HEMA: **Thrombocytopenia, hemolytic anemia, leukopenia**

INTEG: *Rash, pruritus,* photosensitivity

MS: *Muscle cramps, myalgia,* **myositis, rhabdomyolysis;** leg, shoulder, or localized pain

PHARMACOKINETICS

PO: Peak 2 hr; peak response 4-6 wk, ext rel peak 14 hr; metabolized in liver (metabolites); highly protein bound; excreted in urine 10%, feces 83%; crosses blood-brain barrier, placenta; excreted in breast milk; half-life 1 hr

INTERACTIONS

Increase: myalgia, myositis, rhabdomyolysis—azole antifungals, clarithromycin, clofibrate, cycloSPORINE, danazol, diltiazem, erythromycin, gemfibrozil, niacin, protease inhibitors, quinupristin-dalfopristin, telithromycin, verapamil, avoid concurrent use

Increase: bleeding—warfarin

Increase: lovastatin effects—diltiazem

Decrease: effects of lovastatin—bile acid sequestrants, exonatide, bosentan

Drug/Herb
Decrease: effect—pectin, St. John's wort
Increase: adverse reactions—red yeast rice

Drug/Food
• Possible toxicity: grapefruit juice
Increase: levels of lovastatin with food; must be taken with food
Decrease: absorption—oat bran

Drug/Lab Test
Increase: CK, LFTs

NURSING CONSIDERATIONS

Assess:
• **Diet;** obtain diet history including fat, cholesterol in diet
• Fasting cholesterol, LDL, HDL, triglycerides periodically during treatment
• Hepatic studies at initiation, 6 wk, 12 wk after initiation or change in dose, periodically thereafter; AST, ALT, LFTs may increase
• Renal function in patients with compromised renal system: BUN, creatinine, I&O ratio

Evaluate:
• Therapeutic response: decreased triglycerides, sLDL, total cholesterol; increased HDL; slowing CAD

Teach patient/family:
• To report suspected pregnancy (pregnancy [X]); not to breastfeed
• That blood work, ophthalmic exam will be necessary during treatment
• To report blurred vision, severe GI symptoms, dizziness, headache, muscle pain, weakness
• To use sunscreen or to stay out of the sun to prevent photosensitivity
• That previously prescribed regimen will continue: low-cholesterol diet, exercise program, smoking cessation
• That product should be taken with food, not to crush, chew ext rel product

RARELY USED

loxapine (Rx)
(lox′a-peen)

Adasuve, Loxapac ✱

Func. class.: Antipsychotic, neuroleptic
Chem. class.: Dibenzoxazepine

USES: Schizophrenia, bipolar disorder
Unlabeled uses: Anxiety

CONTRAINDICATIONS: *Hypersensitivity, coma*

Black Box Warning: Acute bronchospasm, asthma, COPD, emphysema

DOSAGE AND ROUTES
• **Adult: PO** 10 mg bid-qid initially, may be rapidly increased depending on severity of condition, maintenance 60-100 mg/day; inhalation powder 10 mg as a single dose in 24 hr
• **Geriatric: PO** 5-10 mg daily-bid, increase q4-7days by 5-10 mg, max 250 mg/day

RARELY USED

lubiprostone (Rx)
(loo-bee-pros′tone)

Amitiza

Func. class.: Gastrointestinal agent—miscellaneous

USES: Chronic idiopathic constipation, constipation-predominant irritable bowel syndrome in women >18 yr, opiate agonist–induced constipation with chronic non-cancer pain

CONTRAINDICATIONS: Hypersensitivity, GI obstruction

DOSAGE AND ROUTES

Chronic idiopathic constipation/opiate agonist–induced constipation
• **Adult: PO** 24 mcg bid with food, water

IBS with constipation (females)
- **Adult and adolescent ≥18 yr: PO** 8 mcg bid with food, water

Hepatic dose
- **Adult: PO For chronic constipation:** 16 mcg bid (Child-Pugh B); 8 mcg bid (Child-Pugh C); **for irritable bowel:** 8 mcg daily (Child-Pugh C), may be increased if tolerated

lucinactant
(loo′sin-ak′tant)

Surfaxin

Func. class.: Synthetic lung surfactant

USES: Prevention of respiratory distress syndrome in premature neonates (RDS)

DOSAGE AND ROUTES
Premature neonate

Intratracheal 5.8 ml/kg birth weight divided in 4 doses; give each dose with neonate in a different position; provide positive pressure ventilation when stable; dosage may be repeated 4 times in first 48 hr

luliconazole topical
See Appendix B

lurasidone (Rx)
(loo-ras′i-done)

Latuda

Func. class.: Atypical antipsychotic
Chem. class.: Benzoisothiazol derivative

ACTION: May modulate central DOPaminergic and serotonergic activity; high affinity for DOPamine-D2 receptors, serotonin 5-HT2A receptors; partial agonist at serotonin 5-HT1A receptor

USES: Schizophrenia, depression associated with bipolar disorder I

CONTRAINDICATIONS: Hypersensitivity

Precautions: Pregnancy (B), breastfeeding, children, geriatric patients, abrupt discontinuation, ambient temperature increase, breast cancer, cardiac disease, dehydration, diabetes, ketoacidosis, driving, operating machinery, dysphagia, heart failure, hematologic/hepatic/renal disease, hypotension, hypovolemia, MI, infertility, obesity, Parkinson's disease, seizures, strenuous exercise, stroke, substance abuse, suicidal ideation, syncope, tardive dyskinesia

Black Box Warning: Dementia: antipsychotics (e.g., as lurasidone) not approved for treatment of dementia-related psychosis in geriatric patients; may increase risk of death in this population

DOSAGE AND ROUTES
Schizophrenia
- **Adult: PO** 40 mg/day, range 40-160 mg/day; for those receiving CYP3A4 inhibitors (max 80 mg/day), do not use with strong CYP3A4 inducers/inhibitors

Bipolar Disorder I
- **Adult: PO** 20 mg daily, max 120 mg/day

Hepatic/renal dose
- **Adult: PO** Child-Pugh class B/C; CCr ≥10 ml/min, ≤50 ml/min, max 40 mg/day

Available forms: Tabs 20, 40, 80, 120 mg

Administer:
- Give with meal of ≥350 calories

SIDE EFFECTS
CNS: Agitation, akathisia, anxiety, dizziness, drowsiness, fatigue, hyperthermia, insomnia, dystonic reactions; **neuroleptic malignant syndrome (rare)**, pseudoparkinsonism, restlessness, **seizures, suicidal ideation**, syncope, tardive dyskinesia, vertigo

CV: Angina, AV block, bradycardia, hypertension, orthostatic hypotension, sinus tachycardia, stroke
EENT: Blurred vision
ENDO: Diabetes mellitus, ketoacidosis, hyperglycemia, hyperprolactinemia
GI: Abdominal pain, diarrhea, dyspepsia, nausea, vomiting, gastritis, weight gain/loss
GU: Amenorrhea, breast enlargement, dysmenorrhea, impotence, dysuria, renal failure
HEMA: Agranulocytosis, anemia, leucopenia, neutropenia
INTEG: Pruritus, rash
MS: Back pain, dysarthria; rhabdomyolysis (rare)
SYST: Angioedema

PHARMACOKINETICS

99% protein binding; excreted 80% in feces, 9% in urine; elimination half-life 18 hr; 9%-19% absorbed; peak 1-3 hr, steady-state 7 days

INTERACTIONS

- Do not use with metoclopramide

Increase: lurasidone effect—strong CYP3A4 inhibitors; do not use concurrently
Increase: serotonin syndrome, neuroleptic malignant syndrome—SSRIs, SNRIs
Increase: sedation—other CNS depressants, alcohol
Decrease: lurasidone effect—CYP3A4 inducers; do not use concurrently

NURSING CONSIDERATIONS

Assess:

- **Schizophrenia:** hallucinations, delusions, agitation, social withdrawal; monitor orientation, behavior, mood before and periodically during therapy
- **Neuroleptic malignant syndrome (rare):** fever, dyspnea, tachycardia, seizures, sweating, hypo/hypertension, muscle stiffness, pallor; report immediately
- **Blood dyscrasias:** CBC periodically; blood dyscrasias may occur
- **Serious cardiac symptoms:** AV block, stroke, bradycardia may occur
- AIMS assessment, thyroid function tests, LFTs, lipid panel, electrolytes
- **EPS:** restlessness, difficulty speaking, loss of balance, pill rolling, masklike face, shuffling gait, rigidity, tremors, muscle spasms; monitor before and periodically during therapy; report tardive dyskinesia immediately

Black Box Warning: Dementia: this product is not approved for geriatric patients with dementia-related psychosis

- Weight gain, hyperglycemia, metabolic changes in diabetes

Evaluate:

- Therapeutic response: decreasing hallucinations, delusions, agitation, social withdrawal

Teach patient/family:

- About reason for treatment, expected results
- That lab work will be needed regularly
- To avoid hazardous activities until response is known
- To avoid OTC products unless approved by prescriber
- To report fast heartbeat, extra beats
- To report EPS symptoms, blood dyscrasias: sore throat, fever, unusual bleeding/bruising

lymphocyte immune globulin (anti-thymocyte, equine) (Rx)

Atgam

Func. class.: Immune globulins—immunosuppressant

ACTION: Produces immunosuppression by inhibiting the function of lymphocytes (T)

USES: Renal organ transplants to prevent rejection, aplastic anemia
Unlabeled uses: Immunosuppressant in liver, bone marrow, heart, and other organ transplants; stem-cell transplant preparations

CONTRAINDICATIONS:
Hypersensitivity to this product or equine/leporine protein; acute illness

Precautions: Pregnancy (C), breastfeeding, children, severe renal/hepatic disease, leukopenia, thrombocytopenia

Black Box Warning: Infection, neoplastic disease

DOSAGE AND ROUTES

Renal allograft rejection

- **Adult/child: IV** 10-15 mg/kg/day × 14 days, then every other day for 14 days if needed up to 21 total

Prevent renal allograft rejection

- **Adult: IV** 15 mg/kg/day × 7-14 days, then every other day × 14 days for total of 21 doses in 28 days

Aplastic anemia

- **Adult: IV** 10-20 mg/kg/day × 8-14 days, then every other day for ≤21 total doses

Available forms: Inj 50 mg equine gamma globulin/ml

Administer:

- Do not infuse <4 hr; usually given over 4-8 hr
- Use 0.2-1 micron in-line filter
- Skin testing must be completed before treatment; use intradermal inj of 0.1 ml of a 1:1000 dilution (5 mcg horse IgG) in 0.9% NaCl; if wheal or rash >10 mm or both, use caution during infusion
- Dilute in saline sol before infusion; invert IV bag so undiluted product does not contact air inside; concentration should not be >4 mg/ml; do not shake
- Keep emergency equipment nearby for severe allergic reaction

SIDE EFFECTS

Renal transplant

CNS: Fever, chills, headache, dizziness, weakness, faintness, seizures

CV: Chest pain, hypo/hypertension, tachycardia

GI: Diarrhea, nausea, vomiting, epigastric pain, GI bleeding

INTEG: Rash, pruritus, urticaria, wheal, injection-site reactions

SYST: Anaphylaxis

Aplastic anemia

CNS: Fever, chills, headache, seizures, light-headedness, encephalitis, postviral encephalopathy

CV: Bradycardia, myocarditis, irregularity

GI: Nausea, LFTs abnormality

HEMA: Thrombocytopenia, leukopenia

MS: Backache

RESP: Dyspnea, pulmonary edema

PHARMACOKINETICS

Onset rapid, half-life 5-7 days

NURSING CONSIDERATIONS

Assess:

- **Infection:** if infection occurs, evaluation will be needed to continue therapy
- Renal studies: BUN, creatinine at least monthly during treatment, for 3 mo after treatment
- Hepatic studies: alk phos, AST, ALT, bilirubin
- CBC with differential

Evaluate:

- Therapeutic response: absence of rejection; hematologic recovery (aplastic anemia)

Teach patient/family:

- To report fever, chills, sore throat, fatigue, since serious infections may occur
- To use contraceptive measures during treatment, for 12 wk after therapy

macitentan
(ma′si-ten′tan)

Opsumit

Func. class.: Antihypertensive

Chem. class.: Vasodilator/endothelin receptor antagonist

ACTION: Prevents the binding of ET-1, to ETA and ETB receptors on human pulmonary arterial smooth muscle

USES: Pulmonary arterial hypertension; WHO Group 1 to delay disease progression

CONTRAINDICATIONS: Pregnancy (X), breastfeeding, hypersensitivity

Precautions: Anemia, hepatic disease, pulmonary edema

DOSAGE AND ROUTES
- **Adult: PO** 10 mg/day

Available forms: Tabs 10 mg

Administer:
- Do not break, crush, chew tabs, without regard to food; if a dose is missed, then take when remember to (do not take more than one tab per day)
- Do not discontinue abruptly

SIDE EFFECTS:
CNS: Headache

GI: Hepatotoxicity

GU: Decreased sperm counts

HEMA: Anemia

RESP: Pharyngitis, pulmonary edema, bronchitis

PHARMACOKINETICS
Rapidly absorbed, peak 2 hr, protein binding 99%, metabolized by CYP3A4, CYP2C19, terminal half-life 15 hr, effective half-life 9 hr

INTERACTIONS
Increase: Macitentan effect CYP3A4 inhibitors

Drug/Herb
- Need for macitentan dosage change: St. John's wort, ephedra (ma huang)

NURSING CONSIDERATIONS
Assess:
- **Pulmonary status:** improvement in breathing, ability to exercise; pulmonary edema that may indicate veno-occlusive disease
- **Blood studies:** CBC with differential; Hct, Hgb may be decreased
- **Liver function tests:** AST, ALT, bilirubin

Black Box Warning: Assess pregnancy status before giving this product; pregnancy (X), do not breastfeed

Evaluate:
- Therapeutic response: decrease in B/P, decreased shortness of breath

Teach patient/family:
- The importance of complying with dosage schedule, even if feeling better

Black Box Warning: To notify if pregnancy is planned or suspected (if pregnant, product will need to be discontinued, pregnancy test done monthly); to use 2 contraception methods while taking this product

- Not to use OTC products including herbs and supplements, unless approved by prescriber
- To report to prescriber immediately: dizziness, faintness, chest pain, palpitations, uneven or rapid heart rate, headache, edema, weight gain
- Do not split, crush, or chew tabs; if a dose is missed, take as soon as remembered (do not take more than one tab per day); there are many drug interactions
- The signs and symptoms of hepatotoxicity

mafenide topical
See Appendix B

MAGNESIUM SALTS
magnesium chloride (Rx)
Mag-64
magnesium citrate (OTC)
magnesium gluconate (OTC)
Magtrate
magnesium oxide (OTC)
Mag-Ox 400, Uro-Mag
magnesium hydroxide (OTC)
Dulcolax, MOM, Phillips' Milk of Magnesia

⚠ HIGH ALERT

magnesium sulfate (OTC, Rx)
Func. class.: Electrolyte; anticonvulsant; saline laxative, antacid

ACTION: Increases osmotic pressure, draws fluid into colon, neutralizes HCl

USES: Constipation, dyspepsia; bowel preparation before surgery or exam; anticonvulsant for preeclampsia, eclampsia (magnesium sulfate); electrolyte; cardiac glycoside-induced arrhythmias, nutritional supplement
Unlabeled uses: *Magnesium sulfate:* persistent pulmonary hypertension of the newborn (PPHN), cardiac arrest, CPR, digitoxin/digoxin toxicity, premature labor, seizure prophylaxis, status asthmaticus, torsades de pointes, ventricular fibrillation/tachycardia

CONTRAINDICATIONS: Hypersensitivity, abdominal pain, nausea/vomiting, obstruction, acute surgical abdomen, rectal bleeding, heart block, myocardial damage
Precautions: Pregnancy (A); (B) (magnesium sulfate), renal/cardiac disease

DOSAGE AND ROUTES
Laxative
- **Adult: PO** (milk of magnesia) 15-60 ml at bedtime
- **Adult and child >12 yr: PO** (magnesium sulfate) 15 g in 8 oz water; **PO** (concentrated milk of magnesia) 5-30 ml; **PO** (magnesium citrate) 5-10 oz at bedtime
- **Child 2-6 yr: PO** (milk of magnesia) 5-15 ml/day

Prevention of magnesium deficiency
- **Adult and child ≥10 yr: PO** (male) 350-400 mg/day; (female) 280-300 mg/day; (breastfeeding) 335-350 mg/day; (pregnancy) 320 mg/day
- **Child 8-10 yr: PO** 170 mg/day
- **Child 4-7 yr: PO** 120 mg/day

Magnesium sulfate deficiency
- **Adult: PO** 200-400 mg in divided doses tid-qid; **IM** 1 g q6hr × 4 doses; **IV** 5 g (severe)
- **Child 6-12 yr: PO** 3-6 mg/kg/day in divided doses tid-qid

Preeclampsia/eclampsia (magnesium sulfate)
- **Adult: IM/IV** 4-5 g IV infusion; with 5 g **IM** in each gluteus, then 5 g q4hr or 4 g **IV INFUSION,** then 1-3 g/hr **CONT INFUSION,** max 40 g/day or 20 g/48 hr in severe renal disease

Persistent pulmonary hypertension of the newborn (PPHN) in mechanically ventilated neonates (unlabeled)
- **Premature infants >33 wk and term neonates:** (magnesium sulfate) 200 mg/kg over 20-30 min, then **CONT IV INFUSION** 20-150 mg/kg/hr to maintain blood magnesium levels at 3.5-5.5 mmol/L

Status asthmaticus (unlabeled)
- **Adult: IV** (magnesium sulfate) 2 g
- **Child: IV INFUSION** (PALS) (magnesium sulfate) 25-50 mg/kg diluted in D_5W, given over 10-20 min, max 2 g/dose

M

Premature labor (unlabeled)

• **Adult: IV INFUSION** (magnesium sulfate) 4-6 g given as a loading dose over 20-30 min, then 2-4 g/hr **CONT INFUSION;** use infusion pump until contractions cease; continue infusion at lowest dose over 12-24 hr; **PO** (magnesium chloride/gluconate/oxide) 648-1200 mg/day elemental magnesium in divided doses

Torsades de pointes/cardiac dysrhythmias with hypomagnesemia (unlabeled)

• **Adult: IV** (magnesium sulfate) use ACLS guidelines or 1-2 g in 50-100 ml D_5W given over 5-20 min in emergent cases or over 5-60 min

Available forms: Chloride: sus rel tabs 535 mg (64 mg Mg); enteric tabs 833 mg (100 mg Mg); **citrate:** oral sol 240-, 296-, 300-ml bottles (77 mEq/100 ml); **gluconate:** tabs 500 mg; liquid 54 mg/5 ml; **oxide:** tabs 400 mg; caps 140 mg; **hydroxide:** liq 400 mg/5 ml; concentration liq 800 mg/5 ml; chew tabs 300, 600 mg; **sulfate:** 500 mg/ml; premixed infusion 1 g/100 ml, 2 g/100 ml, 4 g/50 ml, 4 g/100 ml, 20 g/500 ml, 40 g/1000 ml

Administer:

PO route

• With 8 oz water
• Refrigerate magnesium citrate before giving
• Shake susp before using as antacid at least 2 hr after meals
• Tablets should be chewed thoroughly before patient swallows; give 4 oz of water afterward
• **Laxative:** give on empty stomach

IM route (magnesium sulfate)

• Give deeply in gluteal site

IV route (magnesium sulfate)

• Only when calcium gluconate available for magnesium toxicity

Direct IV route

• Dilute 50% sol to ≤20%, give at ≤150 mg/min

Continuous IV INFUSION route

• May dilute to 20% sol, infuse over 3 hr
• IV at less than 125 mg/kg/hr; circulatory collapse may occur; use INFUSION pump

Y-site compatibilities: Acyclovir, aldesleukin, alemtuzumab, alfentanil, amifostine, amikacin, aminocaproic acid, argatroban, arsenic trioxide, ascorbic acid injection, asparaginase, atenolol, atosiban, atracurium, atropine, azithromycin, aztreonam, benztropine, bivalirudin, bleomycin, bumetanide, buprenorphine, butorphanol, calcium gluconate, cangrelor, CARBOplatin, carmustine, caspofungin, cefotaxime, cefoTEtan, cefOXitin, cefTAZidime, ceftizoxime, cephapirin, chloramphenicol, chlorproMAZINE, cimetidine, cisatracurium, CISplatin, clindamycin, clonidine, codeine, cyanocobalamin, cyclophosphamide, cytarabine, DACTINomycin, DAPTOmycin, DAUNOrubicin liposome, DAUNOrubicin, dexmedetomidine, dexrazoxane, digoxin, diltiazem, dimenhyDRINATE, diphenhydrAMINE, DOBUTamine, DOCEtaxel, dolasetron, DOPamine, doripenem, doxacurium chloride, DOXOrubicin liposomal, doxycycline, enalaprilat, ePHEDrine, EPINEPHrine, epoetin alfa, eptifibatide, ertapenem, esmolol, etoposide, etoposide phosphate, famotidine, fenoldopam, fentaNYL, fluconazole, fludarabine, fluorouracil, folic acid (as sodium salt), foscarnet, gallium, gatifloxacin, gemcitabine, gemtuzumab, gentamicin, glycopyrrolate, granisetron, heparin, HYDROmorphone, hydrOXYzine, IDArubicin, ifosfamide, imipenem-cilastatin, insulin (regular), irinotecan, isoproterenol, kanamycin, ketamine, ketorolac, labetalol, lactated ringer's injection, lepirudin, leucovorin, lidocaine, linezolid, LORazepam, mannitol, mechlorethamine, mesna, metaraminol, methotrexate, methyldopate, metoclopramide, metoprolol, metroNIDAZOLE, micafungin, midazolam, milrinone, minocycline, mitoMYcin, mitoXANtrone, mivacurium, morphine, moxifloxacin, multiple vitamins injection, mycophenolate mofetil, nafcillin, nalbuphine, nesiritide, netilmicin, niCARdipine, nitroglycerin, nitroprusside, norepinephrine, octreotide, ondansetron, oxaliplatin, oxytocin, PACLitaxel, palonosetron, pamidronate, pancuronium, papaverine, PEMEtrexed, penicillin G potassium/sodium, pentazocine, PENTobarbital, PHENobarbital, phentolamine, phenylephrine, piperacillin, piperacillin tazobactam, polymyxin B, potassium acetate/chloride, procainamide, prochlorperazine, promethazine, propranolol, protamine, pyridoxine, quiNIDine, quinupristin-dalfopristin, ranitidine, remifentanil, ringer's injection, riTUXimab, rocuronium, sargramostim, sodium acetate/bicarbonate, succinylcholine, SUFentanil, tacrolimus, telavancin, teniposide, theophylline, thiamine, thiotepa, ticarcillin, ticarcillin-clavulanate, tigecycline, tirofiban, TNA (3-in-1), tobramycin, tolazoline, topotecan, TPN (2-in-1), trastuzumab, urokinase, vancomycin, vasopressin, vecuronium, verapamil, vinBLAStine, vinCRIStine, vinorelbine, vitamin B complex with C, voriconazole, zoledronic acid

SIDE EFFECTS

CNS: Muscle weakness, flushing, sweating, confusion, sedation, depressed reflexes, **flaccid paralysis**, hypothermia
CV: Hypotension, heart block, **circulatory collapse**, vasodilation
GI: *Nausea, vomiting, anorexia, cramps,* diarrhea
HEMA: Prolonged bleeding time
META: Electrolyte, fluid imbalances
RESP: Respiratory depression/paralysis

PHARMACOKINETICS

PO: Onset 1-2 hr
IM: Onset 1 hr, duration 4 hr
IV: Duration 1/2 hr
Excreted by kidney, effective anticonvulsant serum levels 2.5-7.5 mEq/L

INTERACTIONS

Increase: effect of neuromuscular blockers
Increase: hypotension—antihypertensives, calcium channel blockers
Decrease: absorption of tetracyclines, fluoroquinolones, nitrofurantoin
Decrease: effect of digoxin

NURSING CONSIDERATIONS

Assess:

- **Laxative:** cause of constipation; lack of fluids, bulk, exercise; cramping, rectal bleeding, nausea, vomiting; product should be discontinued

⚠ **Eclampsia:** seizure precautions, B/P, ECG (magnesium sulfate); magnesium toxicity: thirst, confusion, decrease in reflexes; I&O ratio; check for decrease in urinary output

Evaluate:

- Therapeutic response: decreased constipation; absence of seizures (eclampsia), normal serum calcium levels

Teach patient/family:

- Not to use laxatives for long-term therapy because bowel tone will be lost
- That chilling improves taste of magnesium citrate
- To shake suspension well
- Not to give at bedtime as a laxative, may interfere with sleep; that MOM is usually given at bedtime
- To give citrus fruit after administering to counteract unpleasant taste
- About reason for product, expected results

M

mannitol (Rx)

(man′i-tole)

Osmitrol, Resectisol

Func. class.: Diuretic, osmotic
Chem. class.: Hexahydric alcohol

ACTION: Acts by increasing osmolarity of glomerular filtrate, which inhibits reabsorption of water and electrolytes and increases urinary output

USES: Edema; promotion of systemic diuresis in cerebral edema; decrease in intraocular/intracranial pressure; improved renal function in acute renal

failure, chemical poisoning, urinary bladder irrigation, kidney transplant
Unlabeled uses: Traumatic brain injury

CONTRAINDICATIONS:
Active intracranial bleeding, hypersensitivity, anuria, severe pulmonary congestion, edema, severe dehydration, progressive heart, renal failure, acute MI, aneurysm, stroke
Precautions: Pregnancy (C), breastfeeding, geriatric patients, dehydration, severe renal disease, CHF, electrolyte imbalances

Black Box Warning: Acute bronchospasm asthma

DOSAGE AND ROUTES

Oliguria, prevention
- **Adult: IV** after initial test dose; if urine output is 30-50 ml/hr × 2 hr, give 20-100 g over a 24-hr period of 15% or 20% sol

Oliguria, treatment
- **Adult: IV** after initial test dose; give balance of 50 g of a 20% sol over 1 hr then 5% via **CONT IV INFUSION** to maintain output at 50 ml/hr
- **Child (unlabeled): IV** 0.5-2 g/kg as 15%-20% sol, run over 30-60 min; maintenance 0.25-0.5 g/kg q4-6hr

Edema
- **Adult: IV** after test dose, use product 10%-20% at a rate of 25-75 ml/hr; give loop diuretics before mannitol
- **Child (unlabeled): IV** 0.5-2 g/kg of 15%-20% mannitol over 2-6 hr

Intraocular pressure
- **Adult: IV** 1.5-2 g/kg of 15%-20% sol over 30-60 min

ICP
- **Adult: IV** 1-2 g/kg, then 0.25-1 g/kg q4hr

Diuresis with drug intoxication
- **Adult and child >12 yr:** 5%-25% sol continuously up to 200 g **IV** while maintaining 100-500 ml urine output/hr

Kidney transplant
- **Adult donor: IV** 12.5 g before nephrectomy, with adequate hydration, may repeat. **Recipient:** 50 g before revascularization

Traumatic brain injury (unlabeled)
- **Adult: IV** 1.4 g/kg before neurosurgery with fluid replacement

Available forms: Inj 5%, 10%, 15%, 20%, 25%; GU irrigation: 5%

Administer:

Intermittent/continuous IV route
- Precipitate may occur with PVC
- Change IV set q24hr
- May warm solution to dissolve crystals
- In 15%-25% sol with filter; rapid infusion may worsen CHF; warm in hot water, shake to dissolve, use in-line filter, do not give as direct injection
- Monitor for infiltration
- **Test dose** with severe oliguria, 0.2 g/kg over 3-5 min; if continued oliguria, give 2nd test dose; if no response, reassess patient

Y-site compatibilities: Acetaminophen, acyclovir, aldesleukin, alemtuzumab, amifostine, amikacin, ampicillin, asparaginase, atropine, aztreonam, bivalirudin, bumetanide, calcium gluconate, caspofungin, ceFAZolin, cefotaxime, cefOXitin, cefTAZidime, ceftizoxime, chloramphenicol, cimetidine, cisatracurium, clindamycin, DAPTOmycin, dexmedetomidine, digoxin, diltiazem, diphenhydrAMINE, DOBUTamine, DOCEtaxel, DOPamine, DOXOrubicin liposome, doxycycline, enalaprilat, EPINEPHrine, ertapenem, esmolol, famotidine, fenoldopam, fentaNYL, fluconazole, fludarabine, gentamicin, granisetron, heparin, HYDROmorphone, hydrOXYzine, IDArubicin, imipenem/cilastatin, insulin, isoproterenol, ketorolac, labetalol, levofloxacin, lidocaine, linezolid, LORazepam, meperidine, metoclopramide, metoprolol, metroNIDAZOLE, micafungin, midazolam, milrinone, morphine, nafcillin, niCARdipine, nitroglycerin, nitroprusside, norepinephrine, ondansetron, oxaliplatin, PACLitaxel, palonosetron, pantoprazole, penicillin G potassium, phenylephrine, piperacillin/tazobactam, potassium chloride, procainamide, prochlorperazine, promethazine, propofol, propranolol, protamine, quinupristin/dalfopristin, ranitidine, remifentanil, sargramostim, sodium bicarbonate, tacrolimus, thiotepa, ticarcillin/clavulanate, tirofiban, tobramycin, trimethoprim/sulfamethoxazole, vancomycin, vasopressin, verapamil, vincristine, vit B complex with C, voriconazole, zoledronic acid

SIDE EFFECTS

CNS: *Dizziness, headache,* **seizures, rebound increased ICP,** confusion

CV: Edema, thrombophlebitis, hypo/hypertension, **tachycardia,** angina-like chest pains, fever, chills, **CHF, circulatory overload,** PVCs

EENT: Loss of hearing, blurred vision, nasal congestion, decreased intraocular pressure

ELECT: Fluid, electrolyte imbalances, *acidosis,* electrolyte loss, dehydration, hypo/hyperkalemia

GI: *Nausea, vomiting,* dry mouth, diarrhea

GU: Marked diuresis, urinary retention, thirst

RESP: Pulmonary congestion, *cough,* dyspnea

INTEG: Injection-site reaction

PHARMACOKINETICS

IV: Onset 1-3 hr for diuresis, ½-1 hr for intraocular pressure, 15 min for cerebrospinal fluid; duration 4-8 hr for intraocular pressure, 3-8 hr for cerebrospinal fluid; excreted in urine; half-life 100 min

INTERACTIONS

Increase: elimination of mannitol—lithium

Increase: excretion of salicylates, barbiturates, imipramine, bromides

Increase: hypokalemia—arsenic trioxide, cardiac glycosides, levomethadyl

Drug/Lab Test

Interference: inorganic phosphorus, ethylene glycol

NURSING CONSIDERATIONS

Assess:

- Weight, I&O daily to determine fluid loss; effect of product may be decreased if used daily; output hourly prn
- B/P lying, standing; postural hypotension may occur
- Electrolytes: potassium, sodium, chloride; include BUN, CBC, serum creatinine, blood pH, ABGs, CVP, PAP
- **Metabolic acidosis:** drowsiness, restlessness
- **Hypokalemia:** postural hypotension, malaise, fatigue, tachycardia, leg cramps, weakness, or hyperkalemia
- Rashes, temperature daily
- Confusion, especially in geriatric patients; take safety precautions if needed
- Hydration including skin turgor, thirst, dry mucous membranes, provide adequate fluids
- Blurred vision, pain in eyes before, during treatment **(increased intraocular pressure);** neurologic checks, intracranial pressure during treatment **(increased intracranial pressure)**

Evaluate:

- Therapeutic response: improvement in edema of feet, legs, sacral area daily if medication being used with CHF; decreased intraocular pressure, prevention of hypokalemia, increased excretion of toxic substances; decreased ICP

Teach patient/family:

- To rise slowly from lying or sitting position
- About the reason for, method of treatment
- To report signs of electrolyte imbalance, confusion, pain at injection site, hearing loss, blurred vision

TREATMENT OF OVERDOSE:

Discontinue infusion; correct fluid, electrolyte imbalances; hemodialysis; monitor hydration, CV status, renal function

M

maraviroc (Rx)
(mah-rav′er-rock)

Selzentry

Func. class.: Antiretroviral

Chem. class.: Fusion inhibitor, CCR5-receptor antagonist

ACTION: Interferes with entry into HIV-1 by inhibiting the fusion of the virus and the cell membrane

USES: CCR5-tropic HIV in combination with other antiretroviral agents for treating experienced patients

CONTRAINDICATIONS: Hypersensitivity, dialysis, renal impairment

Precautions: Pregnancy (B), Asian patients, breastfeeding, renal/hepatic/cardiac disease, electrolyte imbalance, dehydration, immune reconstitution syndrome, infection, MI, orthostatic hypotension, children, geriatric patients, Graves' disease, Guillain-Barré syndrome, polymyositis

Black Box Warning: Hepatitis, fever, serious rash

DOSAGE AND ROUTES

Those not taking any CYP3A inducers/inhibitors

- **Adult/adolescent ≥16 yr: PO** 300 mg bid

Those taking CYP3A4 inhibitors with/without a CYP3A inducer

- **Adult/adolescent ≥16 yr: PO** 150 mg bid

Those taking CYP3A4 inducers without a strong CYP3A inhibitor

- **Adult/adolescent ≥16 yr: PO** 600 mg bid

Renal dose

- **Adult: PO** ≤30 ml/min, reduce dose to 150 mg bid

Available forms: Tabs 150, 300 mg

Administer:

- May give without regard to meals, with 8 oz water; swallow whole; do not crush, chew, break
- Store at room temperature

SIDE EFFECTS

CV: MI, cardiac ischemia, orthostatic hypotension

CNS: Dizziness, depression, viral meningitis, disturbances in consciousness, peripheral neuropathy, paresthesia, dysesthesia, fever

EENT: Gingival hyperplasia, visual changes

GI: Diarrhea, constipation, dyspepsia, pseudomembranous colitis, hepatotoxicity

INTEG: Rash, urticaria, pruritus, folliculitis

MS: Joint pain, leg pain, muscle cramps

RESP: Cough, upper respiratory tract infection, sinusitis, bronchitis, pneumonia, bronchospasm, obstruction, dyspnea

SYST: Herpes virus, lipodystrophy, malignancy

PHARMACOKINETICS

Metabolized by P450 system; CYP3A metabolism; excreted 20% urine, 76% feces; protein binding 76%; terminal half-life 14-18 hr

INTERACTIONS

Increase: maraviroc levels—CYP3A inhibitors (amiodarone, aprepitant, chloramphenicol, clarithromycin, conivaptan, cycloSPORINE, dalfopristin, danazol, diltiazem, erythromycin, estradiol, fluconazole, fluvoxaMINE, imatinib, isoniazid, itraconazole, ketoconazole, miconazole, nefazodone, niCARdipine, propoxyphene, RU-486, tamoxifen, telithromycin, troleandomycin, verapamil, voriconazole, zafirlukast); reduce dose

Decrease: maraviroc levels—CYP3A4 inducers (efavirenz, aminoglutethimide, barbiturates, bexaroten, bosentan, carBAMazepine, dexamethasone, griseofulvin, modafinil, nafcillin, OXcarbazepine, phenytoin, fosphenytoin, rifabutin, rifampin, rifapentine, topiramate, tipranavir); increase dose

Drug/Herb

- Decreased maraviroc effect: St. John's wort

Drug/Food

- High-fat meal decreases absorption 33%

Drug/Lab Test

Increase: AST, ALT, bilirubin, amylase, lipase

NURSING CONSIDERATIONS

Assess:

- **HIV:** CD_4, T-cell count, plasma HIV RNA, CCR5-tropic HIV-1; assess for changes in symptoms, other infections during treatment
- Renal studies: serum creatinine
- Bowel pattern before, during treatment
- **Allergies:** skin eruptions: rash, urticaria, itching; discontinue product

Black Box Warning: Hepatitis/hepatotoxicity: dark urine; abdominal pain, vomiting; yellowing of skin, eyes; hepatomegaly; discontinue product; monitor liver function tests; serious rash, fever, eosinophilia, or elevated IgE before hepatotoxicity may occur

Evaluate:

- Therapeutic response: improvement in CD4, viral load, T-cell count

Teach patient/family:

- To take as prescribed; if dose is missed, to take as soon as remembered up to 1 hr before next dose; not to double dose; that product does not cure condition, should not be shared with others
- That product does not cure infection, just controls symptoms and does not prevent infecting others
- ⚠ To report sore throat, fever, fatigue **(may indicate superinfection);** yellow skin/eyes, abdominal pain, vomiting **(hepatitis);** itching, SOB **(allergic reaction)**
- That product must be taken in equal intervals around the clock to maintain blood levels for duration of therapy
- To avoid all OTC products unless approved by prescriber
- To avoid driving, other hazardous activities until reaction is known; that dizziness may occur
- To make position changes slowly to prevent postural hypotension
- To notify prescriber if pregnancy is planned or suspected; **not to breastfeed**

mebendazole (Rx)

(me-ben′da-zole)

Func. class.: Anthelmintic

Chem. Class.: Carbamate

DISCONTINUED

ACTION: Inhibits glucose uptake, degeneration of cytoplasmic microtubules in the cell; interferes with absorption, secretory function

USES: Pinworms, roundworms, hookworms, whipworms, thread-worms, pork tapeworms, dwarf tapeworms, beef tapeworms, hydatid cysts

CONTRAINDICATIONS: Hypersensitivity

Precautions: Pregnancy (C) (1st trimester), breastfeeding, children <2 yr, Crohn's disease, hepatic disease, inflammatory bowel disease, ulcerative colitis

DOSAGE AND ROUTES

- **Adult and child >2 yr: PO** 100 mg as a single dose (pinworms) or bid ×3 days (whipworms, roundworms, or hookworms); course may be repeated in 3 wk if needed

Available forms: Tabs 100 mg

Administer:

- May be crushed, chewed, swallowed whole, mixed with food
- PO after meals to avoid GI symptoms
- Second course after 3 wk if needed; usually recommended
- Store in tight container

M

SIDE EFFECTS

CNS: Dizziness, fever, headache, seizures (rare)
GI: Transient diarrhea, abdominal pain, nausea, vomiting, constipation, hepatitis
INTEG: Rash

PHARMACOKINETICS

PO: Peak ½-7 hr; excreted in feces primarily (metabolites), small amount in urine (unchanged); highly bound to plasma proteins 95%

INTERACTIONS

Decrease: mebendazole effect—carBAMazepine, hydantoins
Drug/Food
Increase: absorption—high-fat meal

NURSING CONSIDERATIONS

DISCONTINUED

Assess:
- Stools during entire treatment; specimens must be sent to lab while still warm, also 1-3 wk after treatment is completed
- For allergic reaction: rash (rare)
- For diarrhea during expulsion of worms; avoid self-contamination with patient's feces
- For infection in other family members, since infection from person to person is common
- Blood studies: AST, ALT, alk phos, BUN, CBC during treatment

Evaluate:
- Therapeutic response: expulsion of worms and 3 negative stool cultures after completion of treatment

Teach patient/family:
- Proper hygiene after BM, including hand-washing technique; tell patient to avoid putting fingers in mouth; clean fingernails
- That infected person should sleep alone; not to shake bed linen, change bed linen daily, wash in hot water, change and wash undergarments daily
- To clean toilet daily with disinfectant (green soap solution)
- The need for compliance with dosage schedule, duration of treatment
- To wear shoes, wash all fruits and vegetables well before eating; use commercial fruit/vegetable cleaner
- That all members of the family should be treated (pinworms)
- To report jaundice, liver pain

mecasermin (Rx)

(mec-a′sir-men)

Increlex

Func. class.: Biologic response modifier; insulin-like growth factor

ACTION: Stimulates growth; IGF-1 is the principal hormonal mediator of statural growth; GH binds to its receptor in the liver and other tissues

USES: Growth failure in children with severe primary insulin-like growth factor-1 (IGF-1) deficiency (primary IGFD) or with growth hormone (GH) gene deletion who have developed neutralizing antibodies to GH
Unlabeled uses: ALS

CONTRAINDICATIONS: Hypersensitivity, benzyl alcohol, closed epiphyses, active/suspected neoplasia, IV use
Precautions: Pregnancy (C), breastfeeding, children <2 yr, diabetes mellitus, hypothyroidism, lymphoid tissue hypertrophy, increased intracranial pressure, malnutrition, scoliosis, sleep apnea

DOSAGE AND ROUTES

- **Child ≥2 yr: SUBCUT** 0.04-0.08 mg/kg (40-80 mcg/kg) bid; if well tolerated for 1 wk, may increase by 0.04 mg/kg/dose, max 0.12 mg/kg bid

Available forms: Inj 10 mg/ml
Administer:
SUBCUT route
- Give within 20 min of meal or snack; do not give if unable to eat or if vomiting
- Rotate inj site; use sterile, disposable syringe/needles; use small-volume syringe for accurate measurement; if using syringe (units), convert to mg/kg (weight

[kg] × dose [mg/kg] × 1 ml/mg × 100 units/1 ml = units/injection)
• Do not double dose if a dose is missed
• Store in refrigerator before opening, avoid freezing; after opening, stable for 30 days after initial vial entry, store in refrigerator; do not use if particulate matter is present, avoid direct light, do not use after expiration date

SIDE EFFECTS

CNS: Headache, **seizures,** dizziness, cardiac valvulopathy, **increased intracranial pressure**
CV: Cardiac murmur
EENT: Ear pain, otitis media, abnormal tympanometry, papilledema, visual impairment, tonsillar hypertrophy, sinusitis
ENDO: **Hypoglycemia, ketosis, hypothyroidism, hypercholesterolemia, hypertriglyceridemia**
INTEG: Pruritus, urticaria, **anaphylaxis, angioedema**
GI: Vomiting, nausea
HEMA: Thymus hypertrophy, lymphadenopathy
MISC: Bruising, lipohypertrophy, inj-site reaction
MS: Arthralgia, joint pain, slipped upper femoral epiphysis
RESP: Snoring, **apnea**
SYST: **Antibodies to growth hormone, secondary malignancy**

PHARMACOKINETICS

Bioavailability almost 100%, metabolized in liver/kidney, half-life 5.8 hr

INTERACTIONS

Increase: hypoglycemia—antidiabetics, corticosteroids
Decrease: growth suppression possible—psychostimulants

NURSING CONSIDERATIONS

Assess:
• Monitor preprandial glucose at beginning of treatment and until well tolerated
• By funduscopic exam at beginning and periodically during treatment
• **Allergic reactions;** if present, interrupt treatment and notify prescriber
• Growth rate of child at intervals during treatment
• **Serious skin disorders:** angioedema, anaphylaxis

Evaluate:
• Therapeutic response: growth in children

Teach patient/family:
• That treatment may continue for years; that regular assessments are required
• To avoid hazardous activities, driving within 2-3 hr of dosing
• About correct administration, needle disposal, rotation of injection sites

meclizine (OTC, Rx)

(mek′li-zeen)

Antivert, Bonine, Dramamine Less Drowsy Formula

Func. class.: Antiemetic, antihistamine, anticholinergic

Chem. class.: H_1-receptor antagonist, piperazine derivative

ACTION:
Acts centrally by blocking chemoreceptor trigger zone, which in turn acts on vomiting center

USES:
Vertigo, motion sickness

CONTRAINDICATIONS:
Hypersensitivity to cyclizines

Precautions: Pregnancy (B), breastfeeding, children, geriatric patients, closed-angle glaucoma, prostatic hypertrophy, hepatic/renal disease, urinary retention, GI obstruction, contact lenses

DOSAGE AND ROUTES

Vertigo
• **Adult/adolescent: PO** 25-100 mg/day in divided doses

Motion sickness
• **Adult/adolescent: PO** 25-50 mg 1 hr before traveling, repeat dose q24hr prn

Available forms: Tabs 12.5, 25, 50 mg

Administer:

PO route

- May give without regard to food
- **Chew tab:** give without regard to water or may be swallowed whole with water
- Lowest possible dose for geriatric patients; anticholinergic effects

SIDE EFFECTS

CNS: *Drowsiness,* fatigue, restlessness, headache, insomnia

CV: Hypotension

EENT: Dry mouth, blurred vision

GI: Nausea, anorexia, constipation, increased appetite

GU: Urinary retention

SYST: Anaphylaxis

PHARMACOKINETICS

PO: Onset 1 hr, duration 8-24 hr, half-life 6 hr

INTERACTIONS

Increase: sedation—CYP2D6, inhibitors

Increase: anticholinergic effects—other antihistamines, atropine, antidepressants, phenothiazines

Increase: effect of alcohol, opioids, other CNS depressants

Drug/Lab Test

False negative: allergy skin testing (allergen extracts)

NURSING CONSIDERATIONS

Assess:

- **Vertigo/motion sickness:** nausea, vomiting after 1 hr; assess vertigo periodically

⚠ Signs of toxicity of other products, masking of symptoms of disease: brain tumor, intestinal obstruction

- Observe for drowsiness, dizziness, level of consciousness

Evaluate:

- Therapeutic response: absence of dizziness, vomiting

Teach patient/family:

- That a false-negative result may occur with skin testing for allergies; that these procedures should not be scheduled for ≤4 days after discontinuing use
- To avoid hazardous activities, activities requiring alertness because dizziness may occur; to request assistance with ambulation
- To avoid alcohol, other depressants; not to breastfeed, report severe side effects

medroxyPROGESTERone (Rx)

(me-drox′ee-proe-jess′te-rone)

Depo-Provera, Depo-sub Q Provera, Gen-Medroxy ♣, Provera

Func. class.: Antineoplastic, hormone, contraceptive

Chem. class.: Progesterone derivative

Do not confuse:

medroxyPROGESTERone/methylPREDNISolone

Provera/Premarin/Covera

ACTION: Inhibits secretion of pituitary gonadotropins, which prevents follicular maturation and ovulation; antineoplastic action against endometrial cancer

USES: Uterine bleeding (abnormal); secondary amenorrhea; prevention of endometrial changes associated with estrogen replacement therapy (ERT); contraceptive; inoperable, recurrent, metastatic endometrial/renal cancer

Unlabeled uses: Hot flashes; symptoms of menopause; paraphilia (men); hot flashes (men) with prostate cancer

CONTRAINDICATIONS: Pregnancy (X), hypersensitivity, reproductive cancer, genital bleeding (abnormal, undiagnosed), missed abortion, stroke, cerebrovascular disease, cervical cancer, hepatic disease, uterine/vaginal cancer

Black Box Warning: Breast cancer, MI, stroke, thromboembolic disease, thrombophlebitis

Precautions: Breastfeeding, hypertension, asthma, blood dyscrasias, gallbladder disease, CHF, diabetes mellitus, bone disease, depression, migraine headache, seizure disorders, renal/hepatic disease, family history of cancer of breast or reproductive tract, bone mineral density loss, ocular disorders, AIDS/HIV, alcoholism, children, hyperlipidemia

Black Box Warning: Cardiac disease, dementia, osteoporosis

DOSAGE AND ROUTES

Secondary amenorrhea

- **Adult: PO** 5-10 mg/day × 5-10 days

Uterine bleeding

- **Adult: PO** 5-10 mg/day × 5-10 days starting on 16th or 21st day of menstrual cycle

With ERT

- **Adult: PO** 5-10 mg daily × 10-14 or more days/mo (sequential estrogen); 2.5-5 mg daily (continuous estrogen)

Contraceptive

- **Adult: IM** (contraceptive inj) 150 mg q12wk; **SUBCUT** (depot SUBCUT Provera 104 inj) 104 mg q3mo

Endometrial/renal cancer

- **Adult: IM** 400 mg-1 g (using 400 mg/ml depot inj susp) weekly

Hot flashes/symptoms of menopause (unlabeled)

- **Adult (female): PO** 20 mg/day; **IM** 150 mg monthly

Hot flashes (men) in prostate cancer (unlabeled)

- **Adult (male): IM** Depot 150 or 400 mg

Available forms: Tabs 2.5, 5, 10 mg; inj susp, 150, 400 mg/ml; depot-SUBCUT inj: 104 mg/0.65 ml

Administer:

- Store in dark area

PO route

- Give without regard to food

IM route

- Visually inspect particulate matter and discoloration before use

Depo-Provera contraceptive injection suspension

- IM only, *never* IV
- Instruct patient on risks and warnings associated with hormonal contraceptives (see Patient Information)
- The possibility of pregnancy should be excluded before giving the first dose of medroxyPROGESTERone or whenever >14 wk has passed since the last dose
- Do not dilute
- Shake vigorously immediately before administration
- Inject deeply into the gluteal or deltoid muscle; aspirate before injection to avoid injection into a blood vessel

Depo-Provera sterile aqueous suspension, preserved

- IM only, *never* IV
- Instruct patient on risks and warnings associated with progestin use (see Patient Information)
- Shake vigorously immediately before use
- When multidose vials are used, take special care to prevent contamination
- Inject deeply into the gluteal or deltoid muscle; aspirate before injection

M

SUBCUT route

Depo-subQ provera 104 contraceptive injection suspension *only*

- For subcut only, *never* give IM or IV
- Instruct patient on risks and warnings associated with hormonal contraceptives (see Patient Information)
- Shake vigorously for at least 1 min before use
- Inject the entire contents of the prefilled syringe subcut into the anterior thigh or abdomen, avoiding bony areas and the umbilicus; gently grasp and squeeze a large area of skin in the chosen injection area, ensuring that the skin is pulled away from the body; insert the needle at a 45-degree angle; inject until the syringe is empty; this usually requires 5-7 sec; following use, press lightly on the injection site with a clean cotton pad for a few seconds; do not rub the area

SIDE EFFECTS

CNS: Dizziness, headache, migraines, depression, fatigue, nervousness

CV: Hypotension, thrombophlebitis, edema, **thromboembolism, stroke, PE, MI**
EENT: Diplopia
GI: *Nausea,* vomiting, anorexia, cramps, increased weight, **cholestatic jaundice,** abdominal pain
GU: Amenorrhea, cervical erosion, breakthrough bleeding, dysmenorrhea, vaginal candidiasis, breast changes, *gynecomastia, testicular atrophy, impotence,* endometriosis, **spontaneous abortion,** vaginitis, libido increased/decreased
INTEG: Rash, urticaria, acne, hirsutism, alopecia, oily skin, seborrhea, purpura, melasma, photosensitivity, injection-site reaction
META: Hyperglycemia
MS: Decreased bone density
SYST: **Angioedema, anaphylaxis**

PHARMACOKINETICS

PO: Duration 3-5 days; **IM** duration 3-4 months; excreted in urine and feces; metabolized in liver

INTERACTIONS

Decrease: medroxyPROGESTERone action—aminoglutethimide, carBAMazepine, phenytoins, PHENobarbital, rifampin
Decrease: bone mineral density—anticoagulants, corticosteroids

Drug/Lab Test

Increase: LFTs, HDL, triglycerides, coagulation tests
Decrease: GTT

NURSING CONSIDERATIONS

Assess:

- Pelvic exam, Pap smear before treatment, periodically
- ⚠ **Severe allergic reaction, angioedema;** have EPINEPHrine and rescusitative equipment available
- Weight daily; notify prescriber of weekly weight gain >5 lb; bone mineral density
- B/P at beginning of treatment and periodically
- I&O ratio; be alert for decreasing urinary output, increasing edema
- Hepatic studies: ALT, AST, bilirubin periodically during long-term therapy
- Edema, hypertension, cardiac symptoms, jaundice
- Mental status: affect, mood, behavioral changes, depression

Black Box Warning: This product should not be given to those with breast cancer, MI, stroke, thromboembolic disorders

- **Bone mineral density loss:** in those taking anticoagulants, corticosteroids with Depo-Provera or Depo-sub Q Provera

Black Box Warning: Use of product shown to increase dementia in women ≥65 yr old; use may increase osteoporosis in long-term treatment; those who smoke also at greater risk; adequate calcium and vit D should be taken

Evaluate:

- Therapeutic response: decreased abnormal uterine bleeding, absence of amenorrhea

Teach patient/family:

- To avoid sunlight or to use sunscreen; photosensitivity can occur
- ⚠ To report breast lumps, vaginal bleeding, edema, jaundice, dark urine, clay-colored stools, dyspnea, headache, blurred vision, abdominal pain, sudden change in speech/coordination, numbness or stiffness in legs, chest pain; males to report impotence, gynecomastia
- To report suspected pregnancy (X); fertility returns 6-12 mo after discontinuing

Black Box Warning: Long-term use decreases bone density; exercise, calcium supplements can help lessen osteoporosis

⚠ HIGH ALERT

megestrol (Rx)

(me-jess′trole)

Megace, Megace ES

Func. class.: Antineoplastic hormone

Chem. class.: Progestin

Do not confuse:
Megace/Reglan

ACTION: Affects endometrium with antiluteinizing effect; thought to bring about cell death, stimulates appetite by unknown action

USES: Breast, endometrial cancer; cachexia, anorexia, weight loss with AIDS

Unlabeled uses: Hot flashes in women (menopause), unexplained weight loss in geriatric patients, endometriosis, endometrial cancer, breast cancer (metastatic)

CONTRAINDICATIONS: Pregnancy (D) tabs, (X) susp; hypersensitivity

Precautions: Diabetes, thrombosis, adrenal insufficiency

DOSAGE AND ROUTES

Endometrial/ovarian carcinoma

- **Adult: PO** 40-320 mg/day in divided doses

Breast carcinoma

- **Adult: PO** 40 mg qid or 160 mg/day

Cachexia (AIDS)

- **Adult: PO** 800 mg/day (oral susp) or 625 mg/day (ES)

Hot flashes (unlabeled)

- **Adult: PO** 20 mg bid

Metastatic endometrial cancer

- **Adult: PO** 40-320 mg/day in divided doses × ≥2 mo

Available forms: Tabs 20, 40 mg; oral susp 40, 125 mg/ml

Administer:

- Oral susp for AIDS patients; shake well
- Tablets for carcinoma
- Without regard to food
- Store in tight container at room temperature

SIDE EFFECTS

CNS: Mood swings, insomnia, fever, lethargy, depression

CV: **Thrombophlebitis, thromboembolism**, hypertension

ENDO: Adrenal insufficiency

GI: Nausea, vomiting, diarrhea, abdominal cramps, weight gain, flatus, indigestion

GU: Gynecomastia, fluid retention, hypercalcemia, vaginal bleeding, discharge, impotence, decreased libido, menstruation disorders

INTEG: Alopecia, rash, pruritus, purpura, itching, sweating

META: Hyperglycemia

MISC: Tumor flare

RESP: Dyspnea

PHARMACOKINETICS

PO: Half-life 13-105 hr; metabolized in liver; excreted in feces, urine, breast milk; food increases bioavailability of oral sol

INTERACTIONS

- **Do not use with dofetilide**

Decrease: megestrol effect—antidiabetics

Drug/Lab Test

Increase: glucose

NURSING CONSIDERATIONS

Assess:

- PSA levels in men (prostate cancer); blood glucose, LFTs, serum calcium, weight
- Effects of alopecia on body image; feelings about body changes
- Frequency of stools, characteristics: cramping, acidosis, signs of dehydration (rapid respirations, poor skin turgor, decreased urine output, dry skin, restlessness, weakness)
- Anorexia, nausea, vomiting, constipation, weakness, loss of muscle tone

⚠ **Thrombophlebitis: Homans' sign, edema; pain in calf, thigh; notify prescriber immediately**

M

Evaluate:
- Therapeutic response: decreased tumor size, spread of malignancy; weight gain in AIDS patients; resolved dysfunctional uterine bleeding

Teach patient/family:
- To report vaginal bleeding
- That nonhormonal contraception should be used during and for 4 mo after treatment; pregnancy (D) tabs, (X) susp
- That gynecomastia, alopecia can occur; reversible after discontinuing treatment

⚠ To recognize signs of fluid retention, thromboemboli; to report these immediately
- To monitor blood glucose if diabetic

⚠ HIGH ALERT

melphalan (Rx)
(mel′fa-lan)

Alkeran

Func. class.: Antineoplastic, alkylating agent

Chem. class.: Nitrogen mustard

Do not confuse:
melphalan/Myleran

ACTION: Responsible for cross-linking DNA strands, thereby leading to cell death; activity is not cell-cycle–phase specific

USES: Multiple myeloma, advanced ovarian cancer

Unlabeled uses: Breast, testicular, prostate carcinoma; osteogenic sarcoma, amyloidosis, chronic myelogenous leukemia, non-Hodgkin's lymphoma, pediatric rhabdomyosarcoma, stem cell transplant, bone marrow ablation, AML, myelodysplastic syndrome

CONTRAINDICATIONS: Pregnancy (D), breastfeeding

Black Box Warning: Hypersensitivity to this product

Precautions: Children, radiation therapy, infections, renal disease

Black Box Warning: Bone marrow depression, secondary malignancy, radiation therapy; requires an experienced clinician

DOSAGE AND ROUTES

Multiple myeloma
- **Adult: PO** 6 mg daily × 2-3 wk, adjust dose based on blood counts or 10 mg daily × 7-10 days
- **Adult: IV INFUSION** 16 mg/m^2, reduce with renal insufficiency, give over 15-20 min, give at 2-wk intervals × 4 doses, then at 4-wk intervals

Ovarian carcinoma
- **Adult: PO** 200 mcg/kg/day × 5 days q4-5wk

Available forms: Tabs 2 mg, powder for inj 50 mg

Administer:
- Antiemetic 30-60 min before product to prevent vomiting

PO route
- Give on empty stomach
- Protect from light; store refrigerated

Intermittent IV INFUSION route
- Use gloves during administration; if skin exposure occurs, wash immediately with soap and water; use cytotoxic handling procedures
- Give after reconstituting with 10 ml diluent provided (5 mg/ml); shake, dilute dose with 0.9% NaCl (≤0.45 mg/ml); give within 1 hr, run over ≥15-20 min; degrading of product occurs rapidly; make sure infusion is completed in time specified

Y-site compatibilities: Acyclovir, amikacin, aminophylline, ampicillin, aztreonam, bleomycin, bumetanide, buprenorphine, butorphanol, calcium gluconate, CARBOplatin, carmustine, ceFAZolin, cefepime, cefoperazone, cefotaxime, cefoTEtan, cefTAZidime, ceftizoxime, cefTRIAXone, cefuroxime, cimetidine, CISplatin, clindamycin, cyclophosphamide, cytarabine, dacarbazine,

DACTINomycin, DAUNOrubicin, dexamethasone, diphenhy-drAMINE, DOXOrubicin, doxycycline, droperidol, enalaprilat, etoposide, famotidine, floxuridine, fluconazole, flu-darabine, fluorouracil, furosemide, gallium, ganciclovir, gentamicin, grani-setron, haloperidol, heparin, hydrocortisone, hydrocortisone sodium phosphate, HYDROmorphone, hydrOXYzine, IDArubicin, ifosfamide, imipenem-cilastatin, LORazepam, mannitol, mechlorethamine, meperidine, mesna, methotrexate, methylPREDNISolone, metoclopramide, metroNIDAZOLE, miconazole, minocycline, mitoMYcin, mitoXANtrone, morphine, nalbuphine, netilmicin, ondansetron, pentostatin, piperacillin, plicamycin, potassium chloride, prochlorperazine, promethazine, ranitidine, sodium bicarbonate, streptozocin, teniposide, thiotepa, ticarcillin, ticarcillin/clavulanate, tobramycin, trimethoprim-sulfamethoxazole, vancomycin, vinBLAStine, vinCRIStine, vinorelbine, zidovudine

SIDE EFFECTS

GI: *Nausea, vomiting,* stomatitis, diarrhea, hepatotoxicity
GU: Amenorrhea, hyperuricemia, gonadal suppression, hyperuricemia
HEMA: Thrombocytopenia, neutropenia, leukopenia, anemia
INTEG: Rash, urticaria, alopecia, pruritus, necrosis, extravasation
RESP: Fibrosis, dysplasia, dyspnea, pneumonitis
SYST: Anaphylaxis, allergic reactions, secondary malignancies, edema

PHARMACOKINETICS

Metabolized in liver, excreted in urine, half-life 2 hr, protein binding ≤30%-90%

INTERACTIONS

- Avoid administration of sargramostim, GM-CSF, filgrastim, G-CSF 24 hr before or 24 hr after product

Increase: toxicity—antineoplastics, radiation
Increase: pulmonary toxicity—carmustine
Increase: renal failure risk—cycloSPORINE
Increase: enterocolitis risk—nalidixic acid
Increase: bleeding risk—NSAIDs, anticoagulants, salicylates, thrombolytics, platelet inhibitors
Decrease: antibody response—live virus vaccines

Drug/Lab Test
Decrease: Hgb, RBC, WBC, platelets
False-positive: Direct Coombs' test

NURSING CONSIDERATIONS

Assess:

Black Box Warning: Bone marrow depression: Full nadir 2-3 wk; CBC, differential, platelet count weekly; notify prescriber, withhold product if WBC is <3000/mm³ or platelet count is <100,000/mm³; notify prescriber; recovery usually occurs in 6 wk

M

- Renal studies: BUN, serum uric acid before, during therapy
- I&O ratio; report fall in urine output to 30 ml/hr
- **Infection:** fever, cough, temperature, chills, sore throat; notify prescriber
- Hepatic studies before, during therapy (bilirubin, AST, ALT, LDH) as needed; jaundiced skin and sclera, dark urine, clay-colored stools, itchy skin, abdominal pain, fever, diarrhea
- **Bleeding:** hematuria, guaiac, bruising or petechiae, mucosa or orifices q8hr
- Buccal cavity q8hr for dryness, sores, ulceration, white patches, oral pain, bleeding, dysphagia
- Local irritation, pain, burning, discoloration at inj site
- **Hyperuricemia:** joint pain, edema, increased uric acid, increase fluids to >2 L unless contraindicated, monitor uric acid levels

⚠ **Severe allergic reaction:** rash, pruritus, urticaria, purpuric skin lesions, itching, flushing; assess allergy to chlorambucil; cross-sensitivity may occur

- Increase fluid intake to 2-3 L/day to prevent urate deposits, calculi formation
- Rinsing of mouth tid-qid with water, club soda; brushing of teeth bid-tid with soft brush or cotton-tipped applicators for stomatitis; use unwaxed dental floss

Evaluate:

- Therapeutic response: decreased tumor size, spread of malignancy

Teach patient/family:

- That usually sterility, amenorrhea occur; reversible after discontinuing treatment
- To avoid foods with citric acid, hot or rough texture
- To report any bleeding, white spots, or ulcerations in mouth to prescriber; to examine mouth daily
- To report signs of infection: fever, sore throat, flulike symptoms
- To report suspected pregnancy; to use contraception during treatment; pregnancy (D)
- To report signs of anemia: fatigue, headache, faintness, SOB, irritability, nausea/vomiting, dehydration, decreased urine output
- To avoid use of aspirin products, NSAIDs, alcohol

memantine (Rx)

(me-man′teen)

Ebixa ♣, Namenda, Namenda XR

Func. class.: Anti-Alzheimer agent

Chem. class.: NMDA receptor antagonist

ACTION: Antagonist action of CNS NMDA receptors that may contribute to the symptoms of Alzheimer's disease

USES: Moderate to severe dementia in Alzheimer's disease

Unlabeled uses: Vascular dementia, acquired pendular nystagmus

CONTRAINDICATIONS: Children, hypersensitivity

Precautions: Pregnancy (B), breastfeeding, renal disease, GU conditions that raise urine pH, seizures, severe hepatic disease, renal failure

DOSAGE AND ROUTES

- **Adult: PO** 5 mg/day, may increase dose in 5-mg increments ≥1 wk intervals over a 3-wk period; recommended target dose as 10 mg bid; at wk 4; ext rel 7 mg daily, increased by 7 mg ≥1 wk up to target dose of 28 mg daily

Available forms: Tabs 5, 10 mg; tab titration pak 5, 10 mg; oral sol 2 mg/ml (10 mg/5 ml); cap ext rel 7, 14, 21, 28 mg

Administer:

- Can be taken without regard to meals
- Twice a day if dose >5 mg
- Dosage adjusted to response no more than q1wk
- **Ext rel caps:** do not crush, chew, divide; swallow whole or open and sprinkle on applesauce
- When switching from immediate release product, begin the ext rel the day after the last dose of immediate release product. Those on 10 mg bid should be switched to ext rel 28 mg daily
- **Oral sol** using device provided; remove dosing syringe, green cap, plastic tube from plastic; attach tube to green cap; open cap by pushing down on cap, turning counterclockwise; remove unscrewed cap; remove seal from bottle, discard; insert plastic tube fully into bottle, screw green cap tightly onto bottle by turning cap clockwise; keeping bottle upright on table, remove lid; with plunger fully depressed, insert tip of syringe into cap; while holding syringe, gently pull up on plunger; remove syringe; invert syringe, slowly press plunger to level that removes large air bubbles; keep plunger in inverted position; few small air bubbles may be present

SIDE EFFECTS

CNS: *Dizziness, confusion,* somnolence, headache, hallucinations, **stroke,** insomnia, depression, anxiety

CV: Hypertension, **heart failure, CHF**

GI: Vomiting, constipation

HEMA: Anemia

INTEG: Rash
MISC: Back pain, fatigue, pain, influenza-like symptoms
RESP: Coughing, dyspnea

PHARMACOKINETICS

Rapidly absorbed PO, 44% protein binding, very little metabolism, 57%-82% excreted unchanged in urine, terminal elimination half-life 60-80 hr

INTERACTIONS

Increase/decrease: both products: hydrochlorothiazide, triamterene, cimetidine, quiNIDine, ranitidine, nicotine
Increase: effect—levodopa, some ergots
Decrease: clearance of memantine—products that make urine alkaline (sodium bicarbonate, carbonic anhydrase inhibitors)
• Use cautiously with amantadine, dextromethorphan, ketamine; reaction unknown
Drug/Lab Test
Increase: alkaline phosphatase

NURSING CONSIDERATIONS

Assess:
• **Alzheimer's dementia:** affect, mood, behavioral changes; hallucinations, confusion, attention, orientation, memory; monitor serum creatinine
• Provide assistance with ambulation during beginning therapy; dizziness may occur
Evaluate:
• Therapeutic response: decrease in confusion, improved mood, maintenance of function, even with no improvement in symptoms
Teach patient/family:
• To report side effects: restlessness, psychosis, visual hallucinations, stupor, LOC; may indicate overdose
• To use product exactly as prescribed; that product not a cure; to avoid alcohol, nicotine
• To use oral sol dispenser
• To avoid OTC, herbal products unless approved by prescriber

⚠ HIGH ALERT

meperidine (Rx)

(me-per′i-deen)

Demerol, Meperitab

Func. class.: Opioid analgesic
Chem. class.: Phenylpiperidine derivative

Controlled Substance Schedule II

Do not confuse:
meperidine/HYDROmorphone/meprobamate/morphine
Demerol/Dilaudid/Desyrel/Demulen

ACTION: Depresses pain impulse transmission at the spinal cord level by interacting with opioid receptors

USES: Moderate to severe pain preoperatively, postoperatively, general anesthesia maintenance, sedation induction
Unlabeled uses: Obstetric/regional analgesic, acute severe headache/migraine, shaking chills induced by IV amphotericin B or postoperative shivering

CONTRAINDICATIONS: Hypersensitivity, severe respiratory insufficiency, MAOI therapy
Precautions: Pregnancy (C), breastfeeding, children, geriatric patients, addictive personality, increased intracranial pressure, respiratory depression, renal/hepatic disease, seizure disorder, abrupt discontinuation, chronic pain, cardiac disease, adrenal insufficiency, alcoholism, angina, anticoagulant therapy, asthma, atrial flutter, biliary tract disease, bladder obstruction, cardiac dysrhythmias, COPD, CNS depression, coagulopathy, constipation, cor pulmonale, dehydration, diarrhea, driving, epidural use, geriatric patients, GI obstruction, head trauma, heart failure, hypotension, hypothyroidism, ileus, IBS, IM/intrathecal/IV use, labor, myxedema, thrombocytopenia

M

DOSAGE AND ROUTES

Moderate to severe pain

- **Adult: PO/SUBCUT/IM** 50-150 mg q3-4hr prn
- **Child: PO/SUBCUT/IM** 1-1.8 mg/kg q3-4hr prn, max single dose 150 mg

Labor analgesia

- **Adult: SUBCUT/IM** 50-100 mg given when contractions regularly spaced, repeat q1-3hr prn

Preoperatively

- **Adult: IM/SUBCUT** 50-100 mg 30-90 min before surgery
- **Child: IM/SUBCUT** 1-2.2 mg/kg 30-90 min before surgery, max 100 mg

Shaking chills (unlabeled)

- **Adult: IV** 25-50 mg as a single dose
- **Child/adolescent: IV** 0.35-1 mg/kg, max adult dose

Renal dose

- Avoid or modify dose

Available forms: Inj 10, 25, 50, 75, 100 mg/ml; tabs 50, 100 mg; oral sol 50 mg/5 ml

Administer:

PO route

- May give with food or milk to decrease GI irritation
- **Oral liquid:** dilute in 4 oz water
- Store in light-resistant container at room temperature

IM/SUBCUT route

- Patient should remain recumbent for 1 hr after IM/SUBCUT route
- With antiemetic for nausea, vomiting
- When pain beginning to return; determine dosage interval by patient response
- In gradually decreasing dose after long-term use; withdrawal symptoms may occur
- Inject IM into large muscle mass; IM preferred route for multiple inj

Direct IV route

- Dilute to concentration of 10 mg/ml with sterile water for inj or NS
- Inject slowly ≤25 mg/min
- Have emergency equipment and opiate antagonist on hand

Continuous IV INFUSION route

- Dilute to concentration of 1 mg/ml
- Infuse using infusion pump

Syringe compatibilities: Acetaminophen, butorphanol, chlorproMAZINE, cimetidine, dimenhyDRINATE, diphenhydrAMINE, droperidol, fentaNYL, glycopyrrolate, hydrOXYzine, ketamine, metoclopramide, midazolam, ondansetron, pentazocine, perphenazine, prochlorperazine, promazine, ranitidine, scopolamine

Y-site compatibilities: Abelcet, acetaminophen, amifostine, amikacin, anidulafungin, atenolol, aztreonam, bumetanide, ceFAZolin, cefotaxime, cefOXitin, cefTAZidime, ceftizoxime, cefTRIAXone, cefuroxime, cisatracurium, cladribine, clindamycin, diltiazem, diphenhydrAMINE, DOBUTamine, DOPamine, DOXOrubicin HCL, doxycycline, droperidol, erythromycin, famotidine, filgrastim, fluconazole, fludarabine, gallium, gentamicin, granisetron, hydrocortisone, insulin (regular), kanamycin, labetalol, lidocaine, methyldopate, melphalan, metoclopramide, metoprolol, metroNIDAZOLE, ondansetron, oxytocin, PACLitaxel, penicillin G potassium, piperacillin, potassium chloride, propofol, propranolol, ranitidine, remifentanil, sargramostim, teniposide, thiotepa, ticarcillin, ticarcillin/clavulanate, tobramycin, vancomycin, verapamil, vinorelbine

Continuous intrathecal INFUSION route

- Use controlled infusion device; implantable controlled microinfusion device used for highly concentrated infusion; monitor for several days after implantation
- Filling of infusion reservoir should only be done by those fully qualified
- To prevent pain, depletion of reservoir should be avoided

SIDE EFFECTS

CNS: *Drowsiness, dizziness, confusion, headache, sedation, euphoria,* increased intracranial pressure, seizures, serotonin syndrome

CV: Palpitations, bradycardia, hypotension, change in B/P, tachycardia (IV)

EENT: Tinnitus, blurred vision, miosis, diplopia, depressed corneal reflex
GI: Nausea, vomiting, anorexia, constipation, cramps, biliary spasm, paralytic ileus
GU: Urinary retention, dysuria
INTEG: Rash, urticaria, bruising, flushing, diaphoresis, pruritus
RESP: Respiratory depression
SYST: Anaphylaxis

PHARMACOKINETICS

Metabolized by liver (to active/inactive metabolites), excreted by kidneys; crosses placenta, excreted in breast milk; half-life 3-4 hr; toxic by-product accumulation can result from regular use or renal disease; protein binding 65%-75%
PO: Onset 15 min, peak 1.5 hr, duration 2-4 hr, absorption 50%
SUBCUT/IM: Onset 10 min, peak 30-60 min, duration 2-4 hr, well absorbed
IV: Onset immediate, peak 5-7 min, duration 2 hr

INTERACTIONS

⚠ **May cause fatal reaction: MAOIs, procarbazine**
Increase: serotonin syndrome, neuroleptic malignant syndrome, SSRIs, SNRIs, serotonin-receptor agonists
Increase: effects with other CNS depressants, alcohol, opioids, sedative/hypnotics, antipsychotics, skeletal muscle relaxants
Increase: adverse reactions—protease inhibitor antiretrovirals
Decrease: meperidine effect—phenytoin
Drug/Herb
Increase: CNS depression—St. John's wort
Drug/Lab Test
Increase: amylase, lipase

NURSING CONSIDERATIONS

Assess:
- **Pain:** location, type, character; give product before pain becomes extreme; reassess after 60 min (IM, SUBCUT, PO) and 5-10 min (IV)
- Renal function before initiating therapy; poor renal function can lead to accumulation of toxic metabolite and seizures
- I&O ratio; check for decreasing output; may indicate urinary retention
- For constipation; increase fluids, bulk in diet; give stimulant laxatives if needed
- CNS changes: dizziness, drowsiness, hallucinations, euphoria, LOC, pupil reactions with chronic or high-dose use
- Allergic reactions: rash, urticaria

⚠ **Respiratory dysfunction: depression, character, rate, rhythm; notify prescriber if respirations are <12/min**
- CNS stimulation: with chronic or high doses

Evaluate:
- Therapeutic response: decrease in pain

Teach patient/family:
- To report any symptoms of CNS changes, allergic reactions
- That physical dependency may result from extended use; use should be short-term only
- That drowsiness, dizziness may occur
- That withdrawal symptoms may occur: nausea, vomiting, cramps, fever, faintness, anorexia
- To make position changes slowly; orthostatic hypotension can occur
- To avoid OTC medications, alcohol unless directed by prescriber

TREATMENT OF OVERDOSE:

Naloxone (Narcan) 0.2-0.8 mg IV, caution in physically dependent patients, O_2, IV fluids, vasopressors

⚠ **HIGH ALERT**

mercaptopurine (6-MP) (Rx)

(mer-kap-toe-pyoor′een)

Purinethol, Purixan

Func. class.: Antineoplastic-antimetabolite

Chem. class.: Purine analog

ACTION: Inhibits purine metabolism at multiple sites, which inhibits DNA and

RNA synthesis; specific for S phase of cell cycle

USES:
Acute lymphocytic leukemia
Unlabeled uses: Ulcerative colitis, Crohn's disease

CONTRAINDICATIONS:
Pregnancy (D), breastfeeding, patients with prior product resistance, hypersensitivity
Precautions: Renal/hepatic disease, tumor lysis syndrome, dental disease, herpes, radiation therapy, leukopenia, thrombocytopenia, anemia, requires an experienced clinician, secondary malignancy, infection, hypocalcemia, hyperuricemia, hyperphosphatemia, hyperkalemia

DOSAGE AND ROUTES
Acute lymphocytic leukemia
- **Adult: PO** 2.5-5 mg/kg/day or 80-100 mg/m^2/day, maintenance 1.5-2.5 mg/kg/day
- **Child: PO** 2.5-5 mg/kg/day, maintenance 1.5-2.5 mg/kg/day or 70-100 mg/m^2/day

Crohn's disease/ulcerative colitis (unlabeled)
- **Adult: PO** 1.5-2 mg/kg/day

Available forms: Tabs 50 mg; susp 2000 mg/100 ml
Administer:
- Store in tightly closed container in cool environment
- Give product after evening meal, before bedtime, on an empty stomach
- **Suspension:** Shake well, wash syringe with warm, soapy water, rinse, move plunger up and down several times, use only after dry; after opening, use within 6 wk

SIDE EFFECTS
CNS: Weakness
GI: *Nausea, vomiting, anorexia, diarrhea, stomatitis,* hepatotoxicity (high doses), jaundice, gastritis, pancreatitis
GU: Renal failure, hyperuricemia, oliguria, crystalluria, hematuria
HEMA: Thrombocytopenia, leukopenia, myelosuppression, anemia
INTEG: *Rash,* dry skin, urticaria, alopecia

PHARMACOKINETICS
Incompletely absorbed when taken orally, metabolized in liver, excreted in urine, peak 1-2 hr, terminal half-life 47 min (adult), 21 min (child)

INTERACTIONS
Increase: effects of mercaptopurine—allopurinol, avoid use or decrease dose
Increase: effects—radiation or other antineoplastics, immunosuppressants
Increase: bone marrow depression—azaTHIOprine, sulfamethoxazole-trimethoprim, avoid concurrent use
Increase: anticoagulant action—anticoagulants, NSAIDs, thrombolytics, platelet inhibitors, salicylates
Decrease: antibodies—live virus vaccines
Decrease: TPMT, rapid bone marrow suppression—balzalazide, olsalazine, mesalamine, sulfaSALAzine, use cautiously

NURSING CONSIDERATIONS
Assess:
- ⚠ **Bone marrow suppression:** CBC, differential, platelet count weekly; withhold product at first sign of abnormally large decrease in blood counts, unless bone marrow aplasia is the goal
- **Thiopurine methyltransferase (TPMT) deficiency:** individuals are prone to rapid bone marrow suppression; dosage reduction may be required in homozygous-TPMT-deficient persons
- **Tumor lysis syndrome:** monitor for increased potassium, uric acid, phosphate, decreased urine output, calcium
- Renal studies: BUN, serum uric acid, urine CCr, electrolytes before, during therapy
- I&O ratio; report fall in urine output to $<$30 ml/hr
- Monitor temperature; fever may indicate beginning infection; no rectal temperature
- **Hepatotoxicity:** Hepatic studies before, during therapy: bilirubin, alk phos, AST, ALT, weekly during beginning therapy,

hepatic encephalopathy, toxic hepatitis, ascites can be fatal

- **Bleeding:** hematuria, guaiac, bruising, petechiae, mucosa or orifices, avoid IM inj if platelets are low; blood transfusions may be needed
- **Stomatitis:** buccal cavity for dryness, sores, ulceration, white patches, oral pain, bleeding, dysphagia
- Increase fluid intake to 2-3 L/day to prevent urate deposits, calculi formation, unless contraindicated
- Rinsing of mouth tid-qid with water, club soda; brushing of teeth bid-tid with soft brush or cotton-tipped applicators for stomatitis; use unwaxed dental floss

Evaluate:

- Therapeutic response: decreased size of tumor, spread of malignancy

Teach patient/family:

- To avoid foods with citric acid, hot or rough texture for stomatitis; to report stomatitis: any bleeding, white spots, ulcerations in mouth; to examine mouth daily, report symptoms
- **Pregnancy:** that contraceptive measures recommended during therapy (D); to avoid breastfeeding
- To drink 10-12 8-oz glasses of fluid/day
- To notify prescriber of fever, chills, sore throat, nausea, vomiting, anorexia, diarrhea, bleeding, bruising, all of which may indicate blood dyscrasias/infection
- To report signs of infection: fever, sore throat, flulike symptoms
- To report signs of anemia: fatigue, headache, faintness, SOB, irritability
- To report bleeding; to avoid use of razors, commercial mouthwash
- To avoid use of aspirin products, NSAIDs
- To take entire dose at one time

meropenem (Rx)

(mer-oh-pen′em)

Merrem

Func. class.: Antiinfective—miscellaneous

Chem. class.: Carbapenem

ACTION: Bactericidal; interferes with cell-wall replication of susceptible organisms

USES: *Acinetobacter* sp., *Aeromonas hydrophila, Bacteroides distasonis, Bacteroides fragilis, Bacteroides ovatus, Bacteroides thetaiotaomicron, Bacteroides uniformis, Bacteroides ureolyticus, Bacteroides vulgatus, Campylobacter jejuni, Citrobacter diversus, Citrobacter freundii, Clostridium difficile, Clostridium perfringens, Enterobacter cloacae, Enterococcus faecalis, Escherichia coli, Eubacterium lentum, Fusobacterium* sp., *Haemophilus influenzae* (beta-lactamase negative), *Haemophilus influenzae* (beta-lactamase positive), *Hafnia alvei, Klebsiella oxytoca, Klebsiella pneumoniae, Moraxella catarrhalis, Morganella morganii, Neisseria meningitidis, Pasteurella multocida, Peptostreptococcus* sp., *Porphyromonas asaccharolytica, Prevotella bivia, Prevotella intermedia, Prevotella melaninogenica, Propionibacterium acnes, Proteus mirabilis, Proteus vulgaris, Pseudomonas aeruginosa, Salmonella* sp., *Serratia marcescens, Shigella* sp., *Staphylococcus aureus* (MSSA), *Staphylococcus epidermidis, Streptococcus agalactiae* (group B streptococci), *Streptococcus pneumoniae, Streptococcus pyogenes* (group A beta-hemolytic streptococci), *Viridans streptococci, Yersinia enterocolitica;* appendicitis, bacteremia, intraabdominal infections, meningitis, peritonitis, skin/skin structure infections

Unlabeled uses: Febrile, neutropenic, community-acquired pneumonia

M

CONTRAINDICATIONS:
Hypersensitivity to this product, carbapenems, hypersensitivity to cephalosporins, penicillins

Precautions: Pregnancy (B), breastfeeding, geriatric patients, renal disease, seizure disorder, gram-negative infection, hypersensitivity to pneumonia

DOSAGE AND ROUTES

Intraabdominal infections (complicated appendicitis, peritonitis)

- **Adult/child/adolescent >50 kg: IV** 1 g q8hr or adult 500 mg q6hr
- **Infant ≥3 mo/child/adolescent ≤50 kg: IV** 20 mg/kg q8hr
- **Term neonates/infants <3 mo (unlabeled): IV** 30 mg/kg/dose q8hr

Extended dose (3-hr infusion) (unlabeled)

- **Adult: IV** 1 g over 3 hr, q8hr

Complicated skin and skin structure infections

- **Adult/adolescents/child >50 kg: IV** 500 mg q8hr over 15-30 min
- **Infants ≥3 mo/children/adolescents ≤50 kg: IV** 10 mg/kg q8hr over 15-30 min

Bacterial meningitis

- **Adult/child/adolescent >50 g: IV** 2 g q8hr
- **Infant/child/adolescent ≤50 kg: IV** 40 mg/kg q8hr

Renal disease

- **Adult: IV** CCr 26-50 ml/min, give dose q12hr; CCr 10-25 ml/min, give 1/2 dose q12hr; CCr <10 ml/min, give 1/2 dose q24hr

Febrile neutropenia (unlabeled)

- **Adult: IV** 1 g q8hr

Community-acquired pneumonia (CAP) (unlabeled)

- **Adult: IV** 1 g q8hr with ciprofloxacin/levaquin or with aminoglycoside plus fluoroquinolone

Available forms: Powder for inj 500 mg, 1 g

Administer:

- After C&S is taken

Direct IV route

- Reconstitute 500-mg or 1-g vials with 10, 20 ml of sterile water for inj, respectively; shake to dissolve; let stand until clear (average concentration 50 mg/ml); reconstituted sol may be stored for 3 hr at room temperature or for 13 hr refrigerated; inject up to 1 g in 5-20 ml over 3-5 min

Intermittent IV INFUSION route

- Vials may be directly reconstituted with compatible infusion fluid (NS, D_5W) to 2.5-50 mg/ml; vials with NS can be stored 2 hr at room temperature or for ≤18 hr refrigerated, (D_5W solutions) may be stored for up to 1 hr at room temperature or ≤15 hr refrigerated; infuse over 15-30 min

Continuous IV INFUSION (unlabeled)

- **3 g/day continuous IV infusion:** Constitute a 1-g vial according to manufacturer recommendations; further dilute in 50 ml or 250 ml of NS and run over 8 hr; for continuous infusion, administer a new infusion bag q8hr
- **4 g/day continuous IV infusion:** Constitute a 1-g vial according to manufacturer recommendations; further dilute in 100 ml of NS and administer over 6 hr; for continuous infusion, administer a new infusion bag q6hr
- **3 g/day IV continuous infusion in ambulatory infusion pump with freezer packs:** Reconstitute 1-g vial according to manufacturer recommendations by adding 20 ml of NS into each vial; add 3 g (60 ml) to a 100 ml medication cassette reservoir and bring the final volume to 100 ml (final concentration, 30 mg/ml) run over 24 hr

Y-site compatibilities: Alemtuzumab, aminocaproic acid, aminophylline, anidulafungin, argatroban, atenolol, atropine, azithromycin, bivalirudin, bleomycin, CARBOplatin, carmustine, caspofungin, cimetidine, CISplatin, cyclophosphamide, cycloSPORINE, cytarabine, DACTINomycin, DAPTOmycin, dexamethasone, dexmedetomidine, dexrazoxane, digoxin, diltiazem, diphenhydrAMINE, DOCEtaxel, doxacurium, DOXOrubicin liposomal, enalaprilat, eptifibatide, etoposide, etoposide phosphate, fluconazole, fludarabine, fluorouracil, foscarnet, furosemide, gallium, gatifloxacin, gemcitabine, gemtuzumab, gentamicin, granisetron, heparin sodium, HYDROmorphone, ifosfamide, insulin, regular, irinotecan, lepirudin, leucovorin, linezolid injection, LORazepam, mechlorethamine, methotrexate, metoclopramide, metroNIDAZOLE, milrinone, mitoXANtrone, morphine, nesiritide, norepinephrine, octreotide, oxaliplatin, oxytocin, PACLitaxel, palonosetron, pamidronate, pancuronium, PEMEtrexed, PHENobarbital, potassium acetate/chloride, rocuronium, teniposide, thiotepa, tigecycline, tirofiban, TNA (3-in-1) total nutrient admixture, vancomycin, vasopressin, vecuronium, vinBLAStine, vinCRIStine, vinorelbine, voriconazole, zoledronic acid

SIDE EFFECTS

CNS: **Seizures,** dizziness, weakness, *headache,* insomnia, agitation, confusion, drowsiness
CV: Hypotension, tachycardia
ENDO: Hypoglycemia
GI: Diarrhea, nausea, vomiting, **pseudomembranous colitis, hepatitis,** glossitis, jaundice
INTEG: *Rash,* urticaria, *pruritus,* pain at inj site, phlebitis, erythema at inj site
RESP: Dyspnea, hyperventilation
SYST: **Anaphylaxis, Stevens-Johnson syndrome, angioedema**

PHARMACOKINETICS

IV: Onset immediate, peak dose dependent, half-life 1 hr, excreted unchanged in urine (70%)

INTERACTIONS

Increase: meropenem plasma levels—probenecid
Decrease: effect of valproic acid
Drug/Lab Test
Increase: AST, ALT, LDH, BUN, alk phos, bilirubin, creatinine
Decrease: prothrombin time
False positive: direct Coombs' test

NURSING CONSIDERATIONS

Assess:

- Sensitivity to carbapenem antibiotics, penicillins, cephalosporins
- Renal disease: lower dose may be required; monitor serum creatinine/BUN before, during therapy
- **Pseudomembranous colitis:** bowel pattern daily; if severe diarrhea, fever, abdominal pain, fatigue occurs, product should be discontinued
- **Infection:** temperature, sputum, characteristics of wound before, during, and after treatment
- ⚠ **Allergic reactions, anaphylaxis:** rash, laryngeal edema, wheezing, urticaria, pruritus; may occur immediately or several days after therapy begins; identify if there has been hypersensitivity to penicillins, cephalosporins, beta-lactams, cross-sensitivity may occur
- **Seizures:** may occur in those with brain lesions, seizure disorder, bacterial meningitis, or renal disease; stop product, notify prescriber if seizures occur
- Overgrowth of infection: perineal itching, fever, malaise, redness, pain, swelling, drainage, rash, diarrhea, change in cough, sputum

Evaluate:

- Therapeutic response: negative C&S; absence of symptoms and signs of infection

Teach patient/family:

- **Pseudomembranous colitis:** to report severe diarrhea
- To report sore throat, bruising, bleeding, joint pain; may indicate blood dyscrasias (rare)
- To report overgrowth of infection: black, furry tongue; vaginal itching; foul-smelling stools; seizures
- To avoid breastfeeding; product is excreted in breast milk

TREATMENT OF ANAPHYLAXIS:

EPINEPHrine, antihistamines; resuscitate if necessary

mesalamine, 5-ASA (Rx)

(mez-al′a-meen)

Apriso, Asacol, Asacol HD, Canasa, Delzicol, Lialda, Pentasa, Rowasa ✤

Func. class.: GI antiinflammatory

Chem. class.: 5-Aminosalicylic acid

Do not confuse:
Asacol/Ansaid/Os-Cal

ACTION: May diminish inflammation by blocking cyclooxygenase, inhibiting prostaglandin production in colon; local action only

USES: Mild to moderate active distal ulcerative colitis, proctitis

Unlabeled uses: Crohn's disease

CONTRAINDICATIONS: Hypersensitivity to this product or salicylates, 5-aminosalicylates

Precautions: Pregnancy (B), breastfeeding, children, geriatric patients, renal disease, sulfite sensitivity, pyloric stenosis, GI obstruction

DOSAGE AND ROUTES

Treatment of ulcerative colitis

- **Adult: RECT** 60 ml (4 g) at bedtime, retained for 8 hr × 3-6 wk; **DEL REL TAB (Lialda)** 2.4-4.8 g/day × 8 wk; **DEL REL TAB (Asacol)** 1.6 g × 6 wk; **CONTROLLED REL CAP (Pentasa)** 1 g qid up to 8 wk; **RECT SUPP** 500 mg bid retained for 1-3 hr × 3-6 wk until remission, may increase tid if needed; del rel cap (Delzicol) 800 mg tid × 6 wk

Maintenance of remission

- **Adult: PO** (del rel tab: Asacol) 800 mg bid or 400 mg qid; **PO** (del rel cap: Apriso) 1500 mg (4 caps) each AM; **PO** (del rel tab: Lialda) 2.4 g (2 tabs) daily with meal; del rel cap (Delzicol) 800 mg bid

Available forms: Rectal susp 4 g/60 ml (Rowasa); ext rel tab 500 mg; ext rel cap 250, 500 mg (Pentasa); 0.375 g (Apriso); del rel tab 400 mg (Asacol), 800 mg (Asacol HD); del rel tab (Lialda) 1.2 g; rectal supp 1000 mg (Canasa); del rel cap (Delzicol) 400 mg

Administer:

PO route

- Swallow tabs whole; do not break, crush, or chew tabs
- **Lialda:** take with meal
- **Apriso caps:** take without regard to meals in AM
- **Delzicol caps:** give ≥1 hr before a meal or 2 hr after a meal

Rectal suspension

- Product should be given at bedtime, retained until morning (8 hr); empty bowel before insertion, shake well

Rectal suppository

- Moisten before insertion; suppository should be retained for 1-3 hr

SIDE EFFECTS

CNS: *Headache, fever, dizziness,* insomnia, asthenia, weakness, fatigue

CV: Pericarditis, myocarditis, chest pain, palpitations

EENT: Sore throat, cough, pharyngitis, rhinitis

GI: *Cramps, gas, nausea, diarrhea,* rectal pain, constipation

GU: Nephrotoxicity, interstitial nephritis

INTEG: *Rash, itching,* acne

SYST: *Flulike symptoms, malaise,* back pain, peripheral edema, leg and joint pain, arthralgia, dysmenorrhea, anaphylaxis, acute intolerance syndrome

PHARMACOKINETICS

RECT: Primarily excreted in feces but some in urine as metabolite; half-life 1 hr, metabolite half-life 5-10 hr

INTERACTIONS

- Do not give H_2 blockers with Apriso

Increase: nephrotoxicity—NSAIDs

Increase: action, adverse reactions of azaTHIOprine, mercaptopurine

Decrease: mesalamine absorption—lactulose, antacids

Decrease: effect of—warfarin

Drug/Lab Test

Increase: AST, ALT, alk phos, LDH, GGTP, amylase, lipase

NURSING CONSIDERATIONS

Assess:

- **Allergy to salicylates, sulfonamides;** if allergic reactions occur, discontinue product
- Renal studies: BUN, creatinine before, periodically during treatment; renal toxicity may occur
- **Bowel disorders:** cramps, gas, nausea, diarrhea, rectal pain; if severe, product should be discontinued

Evaluate:

- Therapeutic response: absence of pain, bleeding from GI tract, decrease in number of diarrhea stools

Teach patient/family:

- That usual course of therapy is 3-6 wk
- To shake bottle well (rectal susp)
- About method of rectal administration
- To inform prescriber of GI symptoms
- To report abdominal cramping, pain, diarrhea with blood, headache, fever, rash, chest pain; product should be discontinued

⚠ HIGH ALERT

metFORMIN (Rx)

(met-for′min)

Fortamet, Glucophage, Glucophage XR, Glumetza, Riomet

Func. class.: Antidiabetic, oral

Chem. class.: Biguanide

ACTION: Inhibits hepatic glucose production and increases sensitivity of peripheral tissue to insulin

USES: Type 2 diabetes mellitus

Unlabeled uses: Precocious puberty or early-normal onset of puberty to delay menarche; polycystic ovary syndrome, infertility

CONTRAINDICATIONS: Creatinine ≥1.5 mg/ml (males); diabetic ketoacidosis, metabolic acidosis, renal failure, radiographic contrast use

Precautions: Pregnancy (B), breastfeeding, geriatric patients, previous hypersensitivity, thyroid disease, CHF, type 1 diabetes mellitus, hepatic disease; creatinine ≥1.4 (females); alcoholism; cardiopulmonary disease; acidemia; acute MI; cardiogenic shock; renal disease, heart failure

Black Box Warning: History of lactic acidosis

DOSAGE AND ROUTES

Type 2 diabetes mellitus

- **Adult: PO** 500 mg bid or 850 mg/day initially, then 500 mg weekly or 850 mg q2wk up to 2000 mg/day in divided doses with morning meal, with dosage increased every other wk, max 2550 mg/day, **EXT REL** (Glucophage XR) 500 mg daily with evening meal, may increase by 500 mg per wk, max 2000 mg/day; (Glumetza) 1000 mg daily with food, preferably with PM meal, may increase by 500 mg per wk, max 2000 mg daily; (Fortamet) 500-1000 mg daily with PM meal, may increase by 500 mg per wk, max 2550 mg daily; regular rel or oral sol 2000-2500 mg/day for ext rel tab, depending on formulation
- **Geriatric: PO** Use lowest effective dose

To delay early menarche and to prolong pubertal growth with early onset of puberty (unlabeled)

- **Child 8-9 yr: PO** 825 mg/day with PM meal

To delay clinical puberty and early menarche in precocious puberty (unlabeled)

- **Child >6 yr: PO** 425 mg/day with PM meal

Polycystic ovary syndrome/infertility related to hyperinsulinemia secondary to polycystic ovary syndrome (unlabeled)

- **Adult (female): PO** 500 mg tid

M

Available forms: Tabs 500, 850, 1000 mg; ext rel tab 500, 850, 1000 mg; oral sol 500 mg/5 ml

Administer:

PO route

- **Immediate rel product:** twice a day given with meals to decrease GI upset, and provide the best absorption; immediate rel tabs crushed, mixed with meal, fluids for patients with difficulty swallowing
- **Ext rel product** may also be taken as single dose; titrate slowly to therapeutic response, side effect tolerance
- Ext rel tabs: do not chew, break, crush

SIDE EFFECTS

CNS: *Headache, weakness, dizziness, drowsiness,* tinnitus, fatigue, vertigo, *agitation*

ENDO: Lactic acidosis, hypoglycemia

GI: *Nausea, vomiting, diarrhea,* heartburn, anorexia, metallic taste

HEMA: Thrombocytopenia, decreased vit B_{12} levels

INTEG: Rash

PHARMACOKINETICS

Excreted by kidneys unchanged 35%-50%, half-life 6 hr, peak 2-3 hr (immediate release); 7 hr (ext release); $2^1/_2$ hr (solution)

INTERACTIONS

- Do not give with radiologic contrast media; may cause renal failure
- Do not use with dofetilide; may cause lactic acidosis

Increase: digoxin levels—digoxin

Increase: metFORMIN level—cimetidine, digoxin, morphine, procainamide, quiNIDine, ranitidine, triamterene, vancomycin

Increase: hyperglycemia—calcium channel blockers, corticosteroids, estrogens, oral contraceptives, phenothiazines, sympathomimetics, diuretics, phenytoin, β-blockers

Drug/Herb

Increase: hyperglycemia—glucosamine

Increase: hypoglycemia—garlic, green tea, horse chestnut

Drug/Lab Test

Decrease: vit B_{12}

NURSING CONSIDERATIONS

Assess:

- **Hypoglycemic reactions** (sweating, weakness, dizziness, anxiety, tremors, hunger); hyperglycemic reactions soon after meals; these occur rarely with product, may occur when product combined with sulfonylureas
- CBC (baseline, q3mo) during treatment; check LFTs periodically, AST, LDH, renal studies: BUN, creatinine during treatment; glucose, A1c; folic acid, vit B_{12} q1-2yr
- **Surgery:** product should be discontinued temporarily for surgical procedures when patient is NPO or if contrast media is used, resume when patient is eating

Black Box Warning: **Lactic acidosis:** malaise, myalgia, abdominal distress; risk increases with age, poor renal function; monitor electrolytes, lactate, pyruvate, blood pH, ketones, glucose; suspect in any diabetic patient with metabolic acidosis, with ketoacidosis; immediately stop product if hypoxemia or significant renal dysfunction occurs

Perform/provide:

- Conversion from other oral hypoglycemic agents; change may be made without gradual dosage change; monitor serum glucose, urine ketones tid during conversion
- Store in tight container in cool environment

Evaluate:

- Therapeutic response: decrease in polyuria, polydipsia, polyphagia; clear sensorium; absence of dizziness; stable gait; blood glucose, A1c at normal level

Teach patient/family:

Black Box Warning: **Lactic acidosis:** hyperventilation, fatigue, malaise, chills, myalgia, somnolence; to notify prescriber immediately; stop product

- To regularly self-monitor blood glucose with blood-glucose meter
- About signs, symptoms of hypo/hyperglycemia; what to do about each (rare)
- That product must be continued on daily basis; about consequences of discontinuing product abruptly
- To avoid OTC medications, alcohol unless approved by prescriber
- That diabetes is a lifelong illness; that product is not a cure, only controls symptoms
- To carry emergency ID and glucagon emergency kit
- That Glucophage XR tab may appear in stool
- To take with meals; not to break, crush, chew ext rel product

⚠ HIGH ALERT

methadone (Rx)

(meth'a-done)

Dolophine, Metadol ♣, Methadose

Func. class.: Opioid analgesic

Chem. class.: Synthetic diphenylheptane derivative

Controlled Substance Schedule II

Do not confuse:
methadone/methylphenidate

ACTION: Depresses pain impulse transmission at the spinal cord level by interacting with opioid receptors; produces CNS depression

USES: Severe pain, opioid withdrawal
Unlabeled uses: Bone pain

CONTRAINDICATIONS: Hypersensitivity to this product or chlorobutanol (inj); asthma, ileus

Black Box Warning: Respiratory depression

Precautions: Pregnancy (C), breastfeeding, children <18 yr, geriatric patients, addictive personality, increased intracranial pressure, MI (acute), severe heart disease, respiratory depression, pulmonary/renal/hepatic disease, respiratory insufficiency, torsades de pointes, COPD, seizures

Black Box Warning: QT prolongation, pain, substance abuse, potential for overdose, poisoning, accidental exposure

DOSAGE AND ROUTES

Severe pain

- **Adult: PO** 2.5 mg q8-12hr in opioid-naive, titrate; **IV/IM/SUBCUT** 2.5-10 mg q8-12hr in opioid-naive

Opioid withdrawal

- **Adult including pregnant woman:** 20-30 mg initially unless low opioid tolerance expected; additional 5-10 mg q2-4hr as needed after initial dose; if symptoms continue, may give for ≤5 days

Renal/hepatic disease

- **Adult:** may need to be modified

Available forms: Inj 10 mg/ml; tabs 5, 10 mg; oral sol 5, 10 mg/5 ml; 10 mg/ml (concentrate); dispersible tabs 40 mg

Administer:

PO route

- When using during a methadone maintenance program, use only PO according to NATA guidelines

IM route

- Rotating inj sites, give deep in large muscle mass (IM)

SUBCUT route

- Pain and induration may occur at site

SIDE EFFECTS

CNS: *Drowsiness, dizziness, confusion, headache, sedation,* euphoria, **seizures**

CV: Palpitations, bradycardia, change in B/P, **cardiac arrest, shock,** hypotension, **torsades de pointes, QT prolongation**

EENT: Tinnitus, blurred vision, miosis, diplopia

M

GI: *Nausea, vomiting, anorexia, constipation, cramps,* biliary tract spasm
GU: Increased urinary output, dysuria, urinary retention, impotence
INTEG: *Rash,* urticaria, bruising, flushing, diaphoresis, pruritus
RESP: Respiratory depression, respiratory arrest

PHARMACOKINETICS

Metabolized by liver; excreted by kidneys; crosses placenta; excreted in breast milk; half-life 2-3 hr, extended interval with continued dosing; 90% bound to plasma proteins
PO: Onset 30-60 min, peak 1-1.5 hr, duration 6-8 hr, cumulative 22-48 hr; PO half as active as INJ
SUBCUT/IM: Onset 10-20 min, peak $1^1/_2$-2 hr, duration 4-6 hr, cumulative 22-48 hr

INTERACTIONS

⚠ Unpredictable reactions: MAOIs; do not use together
- Do not use within 2 wk of selegiline

Increase: effects with other CNS depressants—alcohol, opiates, sedative/hypnotics, antipsychotics, skeletal muscle relaxants
Increase: toxicity—CYP3A4 inhibitors (aprepitant, antiretroviral protease inhibitors, clarithromycin, danazol, delavirdine, diltiazem, erythromycin, fluconazole, FLUoxetine, fluroxamine, imatinib, ketoconazole, mibefradil, nefazodone, telithromycin, voriconazole)
Increase: QT prolongation—class IA antiarrhythmics (disopyramide, procainamide, quiNIDine), class III antiarrhythmics (amiodarone, dofetilide, ibutilide, sotalol), astemizole, arsenic trioxide, cisapride, chloroquine, clarithromycin, levomethadye, pentamidine, some phenothiazines, pimozide, terfenadine
Decrease: analgesia—rifampin, phenytoin, nalbuphine, pentazine
Decrease: methadone effect—CYP3A4 inducers (barbiturates, bosentan, carBAMazepine, efavirenz, phenytoins, nevirapine, rifabutin, rifampin), withdrawal symptoms may occur

Drug/Food
- Avoid use with grapefruit juice

Drug/Herb
- Avoid use with St. John's wort; withdrawal may result

Increase: CNS depression—chamomile, hops, kava, valerian

Drug/Lab Test
Increase: amylase, lipase

NURSING CONSIDERATIONS

Assess:
- **Pain:** type, location, intensity, grimacing before, $1^1/_2$-2 hr after administration; use pain scoring
- I&O ratio; check for decreasing output; may indicate urinary retention
- CNS changes: dizziness, drowsiness, hallucinations, euphoria, LOC, pupil reaction
- Allergic reactions: rash, urticaria

Black Box Warning: Respiratory dysfunction: respiratory depression, character, rate, rhythm; notify prescriber if respirations are <10/min

Black Box Warning: QT prolongation: may be dose related or use with other products that increase QT

Black Box Warning: Accidental exposure: make sure product is not accessible to children, pets

Black Box Warning: Overdose, poisoning: advise persons involved in correct use

Black Box Warning: Substance abuse: may occur but has less psychological dependence than other opiate agonists

- Opioid detoxification: no analgesia occurs, only prevention of withdrawal symptoms

Black Box Warning: B/P, pulse, ECG; hypotension, palpitations may occur

- Bowel changes, bulk, fluids, laxatives should be used for constipation

Evaluate:

- Therapeutic response: decrease in pain, successful opioid withdrawal

Teach patient/family:

- To report any symptoms of CNS changes, allergic reactions
- That physical dependency may result from extended use

⚠ That withdrawal symptoms may occur: nausea, vomiting, cramps, fever, faintness, anorexia

- To maintain proper hydration; to avoid alcohol use
- To avoid use with other products without approval of prescriber; many drug interactions

TREATMENT OF OVERDOSE:
Naloxone (Narcan) 0.2-0.8 mg IV, O_2, IV fluids, vasopressors

methimazole (Rx)
(meth-im′a-zole)

Tapazole

Func. class.: Thyroid hormone antagonist (antithyroid)

Chem. class.: Thioamide

Do not confuse:
methimazole/metoprolol/minoxidil

Action: Inhibits synthesis of thyroid hormones by decreasing iodine use in manufacture of thyroglobin and iodothyronine; does not affect circulatory T_4, T_3

USES: Hyperthyroidism, preparation for thyroidectomy

CONTRAINDICATIONS: Pregnancy (D), breastfeeding, hypersensitivity

Precautions: Infection, bone marrow suppression, hepatic disease, bleeding disorders

DOSAGE AND ROUTES
Hyperthyroidism

- **Adult: PO** 15 mg/day (mild hyperthyroidism); 30-40 mg/day (moderate to severe); 60 mg/day (severe); maintenance 5-15 mg/day; may be divided
- **Child: PO** 0.4 mg/kg/day in divided doses q8hr; continue until euthyroid; maintenance dose 0.2 mg/kg/day in divided doses q8hr, max 30 mg/24 hr; may be divided

Preparation for thyroidectomy

- **Adult and child: PO** same as above; iodine may be added × 10 days before surgery

Thyrotoxic crisis

- **Adult and child: PO** same as hyperthyroidism with iodine and propranolol

Available forms: Tabs 5, 10, 20 mg

Administer:

- With meals to decrease GI upset
- At same time each day to maintain product level
- Lowest dose that relieves symptoms; discontinue before RAIU

M

SIDE EFFECTS
CNS: *Drowsiness, headache, vertigo, fever,* paresthesias, neuritis

ENDO: *Enlarged thyroid*

GI: *Nausea, diarrhea, vomiting,* **jaundice, hepatitis,** loss of taste

GU: **Nephritis**

HEMA: **Agranulocytosis, leukopenia, thrombocytopenia, hypothrombinemia, lymphadenopathy,** bleeding, vasculitis

INTEG: *Rash, urticaria, pruritus, alopecia, hyperpigmentation,* lupuslike syndrome

MS: Myalgia, arthralgia, nocturnal muscle cramps

PHARMACOKINETICS
Onset rapid; peak 30-60 min; half-life 5-13 hr; excreted in urine, breast milk; crosses placenta

INTERACTIONS
Increase: bone marrow depression—radiation, antineoplastic agents

Increase: response to digoxin

Decrease: effectiveness—amiodarone, potassium iodide
Decrease: anticoagulant effect—warfarin
Drug/Lab Test
Increase: PT, AST, ALT, alk phos

NURSING CONSIDERATIONS
Assess:
- **Hyperthyroidism:** palpitation, nervousness, loss of hair, insomnia, heat intolerance, weight loss, diarrhea
- **Hypothyroidism:** constipation, dry skin, weakness, fatigue, headache, intolerance to cold, weight gain; adjustment may be needed
- Pulse, B/P, temperature
- I&O ratio; check for edema: puffy hands, feet, periorbits; these indicate hypothyroidism
- Weight daily; same clothing, scale, time of day
- T_3, T_4, which are increased; serum TSH, which is decreased; free thyroxine index, which is increased if dosage too low; discontinue product 3-4 wk before RAIU

⚠ **Blood dyscrasias:** CBC, leukopenia, thrombocytopenia, agranulocytosis; if these occur, product should be discontinued and other treatment initiated; may occur at higher doses
- **Hypersensitivity:** rash, enlarged cervical lymph nodes; product may have to be discontinued
- **Hypoprothrombinemia:** bleeding, petechiae, ecchymosis
- **Clinical response:** after 3 wk should include increased weight; decreased T_4, pulse

⚠ **Bone marrow suppression:** sore throat, fever, fatigue
- Increased fluids to 3-4 L/day unless contraindicated

Evaluate:
- Therapeutic response: weight gain, decreased pulse, decreased T_4, B/P

Teach patient/family:
- Not to breastfeed
- To take pulse daily
- To report redness, swelling, sore throat, mouth lesions, fever, which indicate blood dyscrasias
- To keep graph of weight, pulse, mood
- To avoid OTC products, seafood that contains iodine, other iodine products
- Not to discontinue product abruptly because thyroid crisis may occur; stress patient response
- That response may take several months if thyroid is large
- **Symptoms and signs of overdose:** periorbital edema, cold intolerance, mental depression
- **Symptoms of inadequate dose:** tachycardia, diarrhea, fever, irritability
- To take medication as prescribed; not to skip or double dose

⚠ HIGH ALERT

methotrexate (Rx)
(meth-oh-trex′ate)

Rheumatrex, Trexall

Func. class.: Antineoplastic-antimetabolite (vesicant)

Chem. class.: Folic acid antagonist

Do not confuse:
methotrexate/metolazone/mitoXANtrone

ACTION: Inhibits an enzyme that reduces folic acid, which is needed for nucleic acid synthesis in all cells; specific to S phase of cell cycle; immunosuppressive

USES: Acute lymphocytic leukemia; in combination for breast, lung, head, neck carcinoma; lymphoma, sarcoma, gestational choriocarcinoma, hydatidiform mole, psoriasis, RA, mycosis fungoides, osteosarcoma
Unlabeled uses: Burkitt's lymphoma, bladder or ovarian cancer, carcinomatous meningitis, desmoid tumor, fibromatosis, asthma, active Crohn's disease, ulcerative colitis, GVHD prophylaxis, ectopic pregnancy, pregnancy termination, psoriatic arthritis, pruritus due to cholestasis or primary biliary cirrhosis, SLE, sarcoidosis

CONTRAINDICATIONS: Hypersensitivity, leukopenia ($<3500/mm^3$), thrombocytopenia (<100,000/mm^3), anemia; psoriatic patients with severe renal disease, alcoholism, AIDS

Black Box Warning: Pregnancy (X), hepatic disease

Precautions: Breastfeeding, children

Black Box Warning: Renal disease, ascites, diarrhea, exfoliative dermatitis, infection, intrathecal administration, lymphoma, pleural effusion, pulmonary disease, radiation therapy, stomatitis, tumor lysis syndrome, renal impairment

DOSAGE AND ROUTES

Acute lymphocytic leukemia

- **Adult and child: PO/IM/IV** 3.3 mg/m^2/day × 4-6 wk or until remission, then 30 mg/m^2 **PO/IM** weekly in 2 divided doses or 2.5 mg/kg **IV** × q2 wk

Choriocarcinoma

- **Adult and child: PO/IM** 15-30 mg/day × 5 days, then off 1 wk; may repeat

Meningeal leukemia

- **Adult:** 12 mg/m^2 **INTRATHECALLY** q2-5days until CSF is normal, then 1 additional dose, max 15 mg
- **Child ≥3 yr:** Intrathecally 12 mg q2-5days
- **Child 2-3 yr:** 10 mg q2-5days
- **Child 1-2 yr:** 8 mg q2-5days

Osteosarcoma

- **Adult and child: IV** 12 g/m^2 given over 4 hr, then leucovorin rescue

Mycosis fungoides

- **Adult: PO** 5-50 mg weekly or 15-37.5 mg twice weekly; **IV/IM** 50 mg weekly or 15-37.5 mg twice weekly

Psoriasis

- **Adult: PO/IM/IV** 10-25 mg/wk or 2.5 mg **PO** q12hr × 3 doses/wk, may increase to 25 mg/wk, max 30 mg/wk

Breast cancer

- **Adult: IV** 40-60 mg/m^2 on day 1 of every 21-28 days with other antineoplastics

Epidermal head/neck cancer

- **Adult/child: IV** 40 mg/m^2 on days 1 and 15, q21days alone or in combination with bleomycin, CISplatin
- **Adult: PO** 25-50 mg/m^2 q7days
- **Child: PO** 7.5-30 mg/m^2 q7-14days

Rheumatoid arthritis

- **Adult: PO** 7.5 mg/wk or in divided doses of 2.5 mg q12hr × 3 doses once a wk; max 20 mg/wk

Polyarticular-course juvenile RA

- **Child: PO/IM** 10 mg/m^2/wk

Burkitt's lymphoma (stages I, II, III)

- **Adult/adolescent/child: IV** 200 mg/m^2 days 8 and 15 q21days with bleomycin, cyclophosphamide, vinCRIStine, dexamethasone

Bladder cancer (unlabeled)

- **Adult: IV** 30 mg/m^2 on days 1, 15, 22 q28days in combination with vinBLAStine, DOXOrubicin, CISplatin (MVAC) regimen

Active Crohn's disease/ulcerative colitis (unlabeled)

- **Adult: IM** 25 mg/wk; **SUBCUT** 15 mg/kg/wk × 16 wk

GVHD prophylaxis (unlabeled)

- **Adult and child: IV** 15 mg/m^2 on day 1 after transplant, then 10 mg/m^2 on days 3, 6, 11

Ectopic pregnancy (unlabeled)

- **Adult: IM** 50 mg/m^2 may be used in combination with mifepristone

Pregnancy termination before 63rd day of pregnancy (unlabeled)

- **Adult: IM** 50 mg/m^2, then intravaginal misoprostol 5-7 days later

Psoriatic arthritis (unlabeled)

- **Adult: PO** 5-7.5 mg weekly

Available forms: Tabs 2.5, 5, 7.5, 10, 15 mg; inj 25 mg/ml (2, 4, 8, 10, 20, 40 ml vials); 25 mg/ml (2-, 10-ml vials with benzyl alcohol); powder for inj 1 g

Administer:

- Using chemotherapeutic handling
- Antiemetic 30-60 min before product
- Allopurinol or sodium bicarbonate to reduce uric acid levels, alkalinization of urine (pH >7.5), adequate fluids
- Store in tightly closed container in cool environment; store injection, powder for inj in dark, dry area

Direct IV route

- After reconstituting to 5 mg/2ml of sterile water for inj; give through Y-tube or 3-way stopcock

M

Intermittent/Continuous IV INFUSION route

- Further dilute in D_5W, D_5NS, NS, before infusion check patency of vein; flush with 5-10 ml of D_5W, NS; infuse at 4-20 mg/hr or prescribed rate

⚠ **Leucovorin rescue:** leucovorin calcium within 24-48 hr of product to prevent tissue damage; check agency policy; continue until methotrexate level $<10^{-8}$ m

IV INFUSION intermediate or high dose (500 mg/m^2 over <4 hr or >1 g/m^2 over >4 hr): confirm WBC >1500/mm^3, neutrophils >200/mm^3, platelets >75,000/mm^3, serum bilirubin <1.2 mg/dl, serum creatinine WNL, SGPT <450 U, creatinine clearance >60 ml/min

⚠ Give sodium bicarbonate tabs or IV fluids to prevent precipitation of product at high doses; urine pH should be >7; may need to reduce dosage if BUN 20-30 mg/dl or creatinine is 1.2-2 mg/dl; stop product if BUN >30 mg/dl or creatinine >2 mg/dl

Additive compatibilities: Cephalothin, cyclophosphamide, cytarabine, fluorouracil, hydrOXYzine, mercaptopurine, ondansetron, sodium bicarbonate, vinCRIStine

Solution compatibilities: Amino acids, 4.25%/D_{25}, D_5W, sodium bicarbonate 0.05 mol/L, sodium chloride 0.9%

Y-site compatibilities: Acyclovir, alemtuzumab, alfentanil, allopurinol, amifostine, aminophylline, amphotericin B cholesteryl, asparaginase, aztreonam, bleomycin, cefepime, cefTRIAXone, cimetidine, CISplatin, cyclophosphamide, cytarabine, DAUNOrubicin, dexchlorpheniramine, diphenhydrAMINE, doripenem, DOXOrubicin, DOXOrubicin liposome, etoposide, famotidine, filgrastim, fludarabine, fluorouracil, furosemide, gallium, ganciclovir, graniset-ron, heparin, HYDROmorphone, imipenem-cilastatin, leucovorin, LORazepam, melphalan, mesna, methylPREDNISolone, metoclopramide, mitoMYcin, morphine, ondansetron, oxacillin, PACLitaxel, piperacillin/tazobactam, prochlorperazine, ranitidine, sargramostim, teniposide, thiotepa, vinBLAStine, vinCRIStine, vinorelbine, zoledronic acid

Intrathecal route

Black Box Warning: Use preservative-free sol, reconstitute with NS; dose should be drawn into 5- to 10-ml syringe after LP, vol of CSF should be withdrawn equal to vol of methotrexate; allow CSF to flow into syringe and mix, inject over 15-30 sec with bevel of needle upward

SIDE EFFECTS

CNS: Dizziness, seizures, leukoencephalopathy, headache, confusion, encephalopathy, hemiparesis, malaise, fatigue, chills, fever; arachnoiditis (intrathecal)

EENT: Blurred vision, optic neuropathy

GI: *Nausea, vomiting, anorexia, diarrhea, ulcerative stomatitis,* hepatotoxicity, cramps, ulcer, gastritis, GI hemorrhage, abdominal pain, hematemesis, hepatic fibrosis, acute toxicity

GU: Urinary retention, renal failure, menstrual irregularities, defective spermatogenesis, hematuria, azotemia, uric acid nephropathy

HEMA: Leukopenia, thrombocytopenia, myelosuppression, anemia

INTEG: *Rash, alopecia,* dry skin, urticaria, photosensitivity, folliculitis, vasculitis, petechiae, ecchymosis, acne, alopecia, severe fatal skin reaction

RESP: Methotrexate-induced lung disease

SYST: Sudden death, *Pneumocystis jiroveci,* tumor lysis syndrome, secondary malignancy

PHARMACOKINETICS

Not metabolized; excreted in urine (unchanged); crosses placenta, blood-brain barrier; 50% plasma protein bound; terminal half-life 10-12 hr

PO: Readily absorbed

PO/IM/IV: Onset, duration unknown

IT: Onset, peak, duration unknown

INTERACTIONS

Do not use with proton pump inhibitors

Increase: toxicity—salicylates, sulfa

products, other antineoplastics, radiation, alcohol, probenecid, NSAIDs, phenylbutazone, theophylline, penicillins

Increase: hypoprothrombinemia—oral anticoagulants

Increase: hepatitis—acitretin; avoid concurrent use

Decrease: effect of oral digoxin, vaccines, phenytoin, fosphenytoin

Decrease: antibody response—live-virus vaccines

Decrease: effect of methotrexate—folic acid supplements, asparaginase

NURSING CONSIDERATIONS

Assess:

- Make sure product is taken weekly in RA, JRA

Black Box Warning: **Infection:** those with active infections should be treated for infection before product use; monitor temperature, fever may indicate beginning of infection

- Make sure drug–drug interacting products are discontinued before therapy, and do not resume until methotrexate level is safe

⚠ CBC, differential, platelet count weekly; avoid use until WBC is >1500/mm^3 or platelet count is >75,000/mm^3, neutrophils >200/mm^3; notify prescriber; WBC, platelet nadirs occur on day 7; monitor

Black Box Warning: **Renal disease:** avoid use in renal failure, BUN, serum uric acid, urine CCr, electrolytes before, during therapy; I&O ratio; report fall in urine output to <30 ml/hr

- Bleeding time, coagulation time during treatment; bleeding: hematuria, guaiac, bruising, or petechiae in mucosa or orifices
- Effects of alopecia on body image; discuss feelings about body changes

Black Box Warning: **Pulmonary toxicity:** those with ascites or pleural effusion at greater risk for toxicity; fluid should be removed before treatment; monitor plasma methotrexate levels

Black Box Warning: **Tumor lysis syndrome:** hyperkalemia, hyperphosphatemia, hyperuricemia, hypocalcemia, decreased urine output; use aggressive hydration, allopurinol to correct severe electrolyte imbalances, renal toxicity

Black Box Warning: **Hepatotoxicity:** jaundiced skin and sclera, dark urine, clay-colored stools, pruritus, abdominal pain, fever, diarrhea, hepatic studies before and during therapy: bilirubin, alk phos, AST, ALT; liver biopsy should be done before start of therapy (psoriasis)

- Monitor methotrexate levels, adjust leucovorin dose based on level
- Buccal cavity for dryness, sores, ulceration, white patches, oral pain, bleeding, dysphagia

Black Box Warning: **Serious skin reaction:** Stevens-Johnson syndrome, exfoliate dermatitis, skin necrosis, erythema multiform may occur within days of receiving product by any route; product should be discontinued

- **Strokelike encephalopathy:** common in high-dose therapy; assess for confusion, hemiparesis, seizures, coma; usually transient
- **Rheumatoid arthritis:** ROM, pain, joint swelling before, during treatment
- **Psoriasis:** skin lesions before, during treatment
- Increased fluid intake to 2-3 L/day to prevent urate deposits, calculi formation unless contraindicated
- Rinsing of mouth tid-qid with water, club soda; brushing of teeth bid-tid with soft brush or cotton-tipped applicators for stomatitis; use unwaxed dental floss

M

Evaluate:

- Therapeutic response: decreased tumor size, spread of malignancy; decreased joint inflammation, pain in RA

Teach patient/family:

Black Box Warning: To report any complaints, side effects to nurse or prescriber: black tarry stools, chills, fever, sore throat, bleeding, bruising, cough, SOB, dark or bloody urine, seizures

- That hair may be lost during treatment; that wig or hairpiece may make patient feel better; that new hair may be different in color, texture (alopecia rare)
- To avoid foods with citric acid, hot or rough texture if stomatitis is present
- To report stomatitis and any bleeding, white spots, ulcerations in mouth to prescriber; to examine mouth daily; to report symptoms to nurse; to use good oral hygiene

Black Box Warning: That contraceptive measures are recommended during therapy and for at least 8 wk after cessation of therapy for women and men; to discontinue breastfeeding; that toxicity to infant may occur; pregnancy (X)

- To drink 10-12 glasses of fluid/day
- To avoid alcohol, salicylates, live vaccines
- To avoid use of razors, commercial mouthwash
- To use sunblock to prevent burns
- To use good dental care to prevent overgrowth of infection in the mouth
- How to use this product with leucovorin rescue
- To continue leucovorin until told it is safe to stop
- To report CNS symptoms, vision changes
- To report fever, other symptoms of infection
- To report decreased urine output

HIGH ALERT

methyldopa/ methyldopate (Rx)

(meth-ill-doe′pa)

Func. class.: Antihypertensive

Chem. class.: Centrally acting α-adrenergic inhibitor

Do not confuse:

methyldopa/L-dopa/levodopa

ACTION: Stimulates central inhibitory α-adrenergic receptors or acts as false transmitter, resulting in reduction of arterial pressure

USES: Hypertension, hypertensive crisis

CONTRAINDICATIONS: Active hepatic disease, hypersensitivity, MAOI therapy

Precautions: Pregnancy (B), geriatric patients, cardiac disease, autoimmune disease, depression, dialysis, hemolytic anemia, Parkinson's disease, pheochromocytoma, sulfite hypersensitivity

DOSAGE AND ROUTES

- **Adult: PO** 250-500 mg bid or tid, then adjusted q2days as needed, 0.5-2 g/day in 2-4 divided doses (maintenance), max 3 g/day; **IV** 250-500 mg in 100 ml D_5W q6hr, run over 30-60 min, max 1 g q6hr; switch to oral as soon as possible
- **Child: PO** 10 mg/kg/day in 2-4 divided doses, max 65 mg/kg or 3 g/day, whichever is less; **IV** 20-40 mg/kg/day in 4 divided doses, max 65 mg/kg or 3 g, whichever is less

Renal dose

- **Adult: PO** CCr 10-50 ml/min dose q8-12hr; CCr <10 ml/min dose q12-24hr

Available forms: *Methyldopa:* tabs 250, 500 mg; *methyldopate:* inj 50 mg/ml

Administer:

PO route

- Increase in dose should be done in the evening to minimize drowsiness

Intermittent IV INFUSION route

- After diluting with 100 ml D_5W; run over $^1/_2$-1 hr

Y-site compatibilities: Alemtuzumab, alfentanil, amikacin, aminophylline, anidulafungin, ascorbic acid, atenolol, atracurium, atropine, aztreonam, benztropine, bivalirudin, bleomycin, bumetanide, buprenorphine, butorphanol, calcium chloride/gluconate, caspofungin, cefamandole, ceFAZolin, cefmetazole, cefonicid, cefotaxime, cefoTEtan, cefOXitin, cefTAZidime, ceftizoxime, cefTRIAXone, cefuroxime, cephalothin, chlorproMAZINE, cimetidine, clindamycin, cyanocobalamin, cycloSPORINE, DACTINomycin, DAPTOmycin, dexamethasone, digoxin, diltiazem, diphenhydrAMINE, DOCEtaxel, DOPamine, doxycycline, enalaprilat, ePHEDrine, EPINEPHrine, epoetin alfa, ertapenem, erythromycin, esmolol, etoposide, etoposide phosphate, famotidine, fenoldopam, fentaNYL, fluconazole, fludarabine, gatifloxacin, gemcitabine, gentamicin, glycopyrrolate, granisetron, heparin, hydrocortisone, HYDROmorphone, hydrOXYzine, IDArubicin, insulin (regular), irinotecan, isoproterenol, labetalol, lidocaine, linezolid, LORazepam, magnesium sulfate, mannitol, mechlorethamine, meperidine, metaraminol, methicillin, methoxamine, methylPREDNISolone, metoclopramide, metoprolol, metroNIDAZOLE, mezlocillin, miconazole, midazolam, milrinone, minocycline, mitoXANtrone, morphine, moxalactam, multiple vitamins, mycophenolate mofetil, nafcillin, nalbuphine, naloxone, netilmicin, nitroglycerin, nitroprusside, norepinephrine, octreotide, ondansetron, oxacillin, oxaliplatin, oxytocin, PACLitaxel, palonosetron, pamidronate, pancuronium, pantoprazole, papaverine, PEMEtrexed, penicillin G potassium/sodium, pentazocine, phentolamine, phenylephrine, phytonadione, piperacillin, polymyxin B, potassium chloride, procainamide, prochlorperazine, promethazine, propranolol, protamine, pyridoxine, quiNIDine, ranitidine, ritodrine, sodium bicarbonate, succinylcholine, SUFentanil, tacrolimus, teniposide, theophylline, thiamine, thiotepa, ticarcillin, ticarcillin-clavulanate, tigecycline, tirofiban, tobramycin, tolazoline, trimetaphan, urokinase, vancomycin, vasopressin, vecuronium, verapamil, vinorelbine, voriconazole, zoledronic acid

SIDE EFFECTS

CNS: *Drowsiness, weakness, dizziness, sedation, headache,* depression, psychosis, paresthesias, parkinsonism, Bell's palsy, nightmares, **drug fever**

CV: Bradycardia, **myocarditis,** orthostatic hypotension, angina, edema, weight gain, **CHF,** paradoxic pressor response (IV)

EENT: Nasal congestion

ENDO: Breast enlargement, gynecomastia, amenorrhea

GI: Nausea, vomiting, diarrhea, constipation, **hepatic dysfunction,** sore or "black" tongue, **pancreatitis,** colitis, flatulence

GU: Impotence, failure to ejaculate

HEMA: **Leukopenia, thrombocytopenia, hemolytic anemia, granulocytopenia,** positive Coombs' test

INTEG: Rash, **toxic epidermal necrolysis,** lupuslike syndrome

M

PHARMACOKINETICS

PO: Onset 4-6 hr, duration 24-48 hr

IV: Onset 4-6 hr, duration 10-16 hr

Metabolized by liver, excreted in urine, half-life 2 hr

INTERACTIONS

- **Lithium toxicity: lithium**

⚠ **Increase: pressor effect—sympathomimetic amines, MAOIs; do not use concurrently with MAOIs**

Increase: hypotension, CNS toxicity—levodopa

Increase: hypotension—diuretics, other antihypertensives

Increase: psychosis—haloperidol

Increase: CNS depression—alcohol, antihistamines, antidepressants, analgesics, sedative/hypnotics
Increase: B/P—phenothiazines, β-blockers, amphetamines, NSAIDs, tricyclics, barbiturates
Increase: hypoglycemia—TOLBUTamide
Decrease: methyldopa absorption—iron

Drug/Lab Test
Increase: creatinine, LFTs
Decrease: platelets, WBC, Hgb/HcT
Interference: urinary uric acid, serum creatinine, AST
False increase: urinary catecholamines

NURSING CONSIDERATIONS

Assess:
- Blood studies: neutrophils, decreased platelets, CBC
- **Hemolytic anemia:** Direct Coombs' test before, after 6, 12 mo of therapy; a positive test may indicate hemolytic anemia; usually reverses within weeks to months after discontinuing treatment; monitor Hgb/HcT and RBC; do not start therapy in those with hemolytic anemia
- Baselines of renal, hepatic studies before therapy begins
- **Drug-induced hepatitis/drug fever:** Usually subsides within 3 months of discontinuing therapy
- **Hypertension:** B/P when beginning treatment, periodically thereafter; report significant changes
- **Allergic reaction:** rash, fever, pruritus, urticaria; product should be discontinued if antihistamines fail to help
- CNS symptoms, especially in geriatric patients; depression, change in mental status
- **CHF:** edema, dyspnea, wet crackles, B/P
- Renal symptoms: polyuria, oliguria, urinary frequency; I&O ratio, weight; report weight gain >5 lb
- **Product tolerance:** may occur within 3 mo of starting treatment; a dosage change and other products may be needed

Evaluate:
- Therapeutic response: decrease in B/P

Teach patient/family:
- To avoid hazardous activities
- Not to discontinue product abruptly because withdrawal symptoms may occur: anxiety, increased B/P, headache, insomnia, increased pulse, tremors, nausea, sweating
- To rise slowly to sitting or standing position to minimize orthostatic hypotension
- To notify prescriber of mouth sores, sore throat, fever, swelling of hands or feet, irregular heartbeat, chest pain, signs of angioedema
- That excessive perspiration, dehydration, vomiting, diarrhea may lead to fall in B/P; to consult prescriber
- That dizziness, fainting, lightheadedness may occur during first few days of therapy
- Not to use OTC (cough, cold, allergy) products unless directed by prescriber; that compliance is necessary; not to skip or stop product unless directed by prescriber
- That product may cause skin rash or impaired perspiration

TREATMENT OF OVERDOSE:

Gastric evacuation, sympathomimetics may be indicated; if severe, hemodialysis

methylergonovine (Rx)

(meth-ill-er-goe-noe′veen)

Func. class.: Oxytocic
Chem. class.: Ergot alkaloid

ACTION: Stimulates uterine, vascular, and smooth muscle, thereby causing contractions; decreases bleeding; arterial vasoconstriction

USES: Prevention, treatment of hemorrhage postpartum or postabortion, uterine contractions

CONTRAINDICATIONS: Pregnancy (other than obstetric delivery/

abortion), hypertension, preeclampsia, eclampsia, elective induction of labor, hypersensitivity to ergot preparations
Precautions: Severe renal/hepatic disease, jaundice, diabetes mellitus, seizure disorders, sepsis, CAD, last stage of labor

DOSAGE AND ROUTES

- **Adult: PO** 200 mcg tid-qid × ≤7 days; **IM/IV** 200 mcg q2-4hr × 1-5 doses

Available forms: Inj 200 mcg/ml; tabs 200 mcg

Administer:

PO route

- Do not exceed dosage limits
- Store tabs at room temperature
- Give with water
- **Only during 4th stage of labor; not to be used to augment labor**

IM route

- Protect from light
- IM in deep muscle mass; rotate inj sites for additional doses, aspirate

Direct IV route

- Undiluted through Y-tube or 3-way stopcock; give ≤0.2 mg/min or diluted in 5 ml 0.9% NaCl given through Y-site
- With crash cart available on unit; IV route used only in emergencies
- Refrigerated storage of ampules; protect from light; give only if solution is clear; colorless

Y-site compatibilities: Heparin, hydrocortisone sodium succinate, potassium chloride, vit B/C

SIDE EFFECTS

CNS: *Headache, dizziness,* **seizures, hallucinations; stroke (IV)**
CV: **Hypotension,** chest pain, palpitation, **hypertension, dysrhythmias, CVA (IV)**
EENT: Tinnitus
GI: *Nausea, vomiting*
GU: Cramping
INTEG: Sweating, rash, allergic reactions
MS: Leg cramps
RESP: Dyspnea

PHARMACOKINETICS

Metabolized in liver, excreted in urine
PO: Onset 5-15 min, duration 3 hr
IM: Onset 2-5 min, duration 3 hr
IV: Onset immediate, duration 45 min-3 hr

INTERACTIONS

Increase: vasoconstriction—DOPamine, ergots, anesthetics (regional), vasopressors, nicotine
Increase: ergot toxicity—CYP3A4 inhibitors, do not use together

NURSING CONSIDERATIONS

Assess:

- B/P, pulse, character and amount of vaginal bleeding; watch for indications of hemorrhage
- Uterine relaxation; observe for severe cramping

⚠ **Ergot toxicity: tinnitus, hypertension, palpitations, chest pain, nausea, vomiting, weakness; cold, numb extremities**

Evaluate:

- Therapeutic response: absence of hemorrhage

Teach patient/family:

- **To report increased blood loss, severe abdominal cramps, fever, or foul-smelling lochia**

methylnaltrexone (Rx)

(meth-il-nal-trex′one)

Relistor

Func. class.: Opioid antagonist

ACTION: Peripheral μ-opioid receptor antagonist that reduces constipation associated with opiate agonists

USES: Treatment of opioid-induced constipation in patients with advanced illness who are receiving palliative care when response to laxative therapy has been insufficient
Unlabeled uses: Pruritus; nausea, vomiting related to morphine; urinary retention from opioids

CONTRAINDICATIONS:
Hypersensitivity, GI obstruction, IV route

Precautions: Pregnancy (B), breastfeeding, children, geriatric patients, renal disease, diarrhea, driving, operating machinery, neoplastic disease, Crohn's disease, peptic ulcer, ulcerative colitis

DOSAGE AND ROUTES

Opiate-agonist–induced constipation

- **Adult >114 kg: SUBCUT** 0.15 mg/kg every other day prn
- **Adult 62-114 kg: SUBCUT** 12 mg every other day prn, max 12 mg/24 hr
- **Adult 38-<62 kg: SUBCUT** 8 mg every other day prn, max 8 mg/24 hr
- **Adult <38 kg: SUBCUT** 0.15 mg/kg every other day prn, max 0.15 mg/kg/24 hr

Renal dose

- **Adult: SUBCUT** CCr <30 ml/min, reduce normal adult dose by 50%

Available forms: Sol for inj 12 mg/0.6 ml, 8 mg/0.4 ml

Administer:

- SUBCUT only; oral dose investigational, not currently available
- Do not give IV; IV dosing for urinary retention investigational
- Store at 59° F-86° F (15° C-30° C); do not freeze
- Store away from light

SUBCUT route

- Inspect sol before use; should be clear, colorless to pale yellow aqueous sol; do not use if particulate matter or discoloration are present
- Withdraw needed amount of sol into sterile syringe; if immediate administration is impossible, syringe may be kept at room temperature for ≤24 hr; syringe does not need to be kept away from light during the 24-hr period; immediately discard any unused portion in vial; no preservatives are present
- Administer into upper arm, abdomen, or thigh ≤1×/24 hr; rotate inj sites; do not inject same spot each time; do not inject into areas where skin is tender, bruised, red, or hard; avoid areas with scars or stretch marks
- If using with retractable needle, slowly push down on plunger past resistance point until the syringe is empty and click is heard

SIDE EFFECTS

CNS: Dizziness

GI: Nausea, vomiting, diarrhea, flatulence, abdominal pain, GI perforation

INTEG: Hyperhidrosis

PHARMACOKINETICS

Terminal half-life 8 hr, protein binding 11%-15.3%; renal impairment has marked effect on renal excretion of methylnaltrexone; dose adjustment is required for patients with CCr <30 ml/min; renal clearance decreased and total systemic exposure increased in patients with severe renal impairment who receive single SUBCUT dose of 0.3 mg/kg

SUBCUT: Peak 30 min

NURSING CONSIDERATIONS

Assess:

- Serum creatinine
- **Opioid-induced constipation:** stool characteristics, bowel sounds during treatment

Evaluate:

- Therapeutic response: decreasing constipation

Teach patient/family:

- That, after 30 min, to remain near toilet facilities because bowel relaxation occurs; not to use more than 1 dose in 24 hr
- To notify prescriber of abdominal pain, continuous or severe diarrhea, nausea, vomiting
- To avoid use in pregnancy unless absolutely necessary; avoid in breastfeeding

methylphenidate (Rx)

(meth-ill-fen′i-date)

Biphentin ✦, Concerta, Daytrana, Metadate CD, Metadate ER, Methylin, Quillivant XR, Ritalin, Ritalin LA, Ritalin SR

Func. class.: Cerebral stimulant
Chem. class.: Piperidine derivative

Controlled Substance Schedule II

Do not confuse:
methylphenidate/methadone

ACTION: Increases release of norepinephrine, DOPamine in cerebral cortex to reticular activating system; exact action not known

USES: Attention deficit disorder (ADD), attention-deficit/hyperactivity disorder (ADHD); narcolepsy (except Concerta, Metadate CD, Ritalin LA)

CONTRAINDICATIONS: Children <6 yr, hypersensitivity, anxiety, history of Gilles de la Tourette's syndrome; glaucoma, anorexia nervosa, tartrazine dye hypersensitivity

Precautions: Pregnancy (C), breastfeeding, hypertension, depression, seizures

Black Box Warning: Substance abuse

DOSAGE AND ROUTES

Attention-deficit/hyperactivity disorder (ADHD) initial treatment, not currently on methylphenidate

Regular release: Ritalin, Methylin, Methylin oral sol, Methylin chew tabs

- **Adult: PO** 20-30 mg/day, range 10-60 mg/day in 2-3 divided doses, 30-45 min before meals
- **Child ≥6 yr: PO** 5 mg bid initially, increase 5-10 mg/day weekly, usual dose 0.3-2 mg/kg/day, max 60 mg/day

Extended release: Ritalin SR, Metadate ER, Methylin ER

- **Adult/adolescent/child ≥6 yr: PO** max 20-30 mg tid

Extended-release once-daily tabs: Concerta

- **Adult: PO** 18-36 mg/day initially, then adjust by 18 mg/wk, max 72 mg/day
- **Adolescent: PO** 18 mg/day initially, then adjust by 18 mg/wk, max 72 mg/day
- **Child ≥6 yr: PO** 18 mg/day initially, then adjust by 18 mg/wk, max 54 mg/day

Extended-release once-daily capsules: Ritalin LA

- **Adult/adolescent/child ≥6 yr: PO** 10-20 mg daily in AM initially, adjust by 10 mg/wk, max 60 mg/day

Extended-release once-daily capsules: Metadate CD

- **Adult/adolescent/child ≥6 yr: PO** 20 mg/day in AM, adjust by 10-20 mg/wk, max 60 mg/day

Transdermal: Daytrana

- **Adolescent/child ≥6 yr: TD** wk 1: 10 mg/day (9-hr patch); wk 2: 15 mg/day (9-hr patch); wk 3: 20 mg/day (9-hr patch); wk 4: 30 mg/day (9-hr patch)

Conversion to once-daily treatment from other forms for ADHD

Extended-release once-daily capsules: Metadate CD

- **Adult/adolescent/child ≥6 yr: PO** give no more than total daily dose of other forms, may adjust by 20 mg/wk, max 60 mg/day

Extended-release once-daily capsules: Ritalin LA

- **Adult/adolescent/child ≥6 yr: PO** give no more than total daily dose of other forms, may adjust by 10 mg/wk, max 60 mg/day

Extended-release once-daily tablets: Concerta

- **Adult/adolescent/child ≥6 yr (currently on 10-15 mg/day): PO** 18 mg every AM initially, adjust by 18 mg/wk, max 72 mg/day (adult); max 72 mg/day,

2 mg/kg/day (adolescent); 54 mg/day (child) mg/day

• **Adult/adolescent/child ≥6 yr (currently receiving 20-30 mg/day): PO** 36 mg every AM, adjust by 18 mg/wk, max 72 mg/day (adult); 72 mg/day, 2 mg/kg/day (adolescent); 54 mg/day (child)

• **Adult/adolescent/child ≥6 yr (currently receiving 30-45 mg/day): PO** 54 mg every AM, adjust by 18 mg/wk, max 72 mg/day (adult); 72 mg/day, 2 mg/kg/day (adolescent); 54 mg/day (child)

• **Adult/adolescent/child ≥6 yr (currently receiving 40-60 mg/day): PO** 72 mg every AM, 72 mg/day

Extended-release once-daily suspension: Quillivant XR

• **Adolescents/child ≥6 yr: PO** give 20 mg in AM, increase in 10-20 mg increments weekly

Narcolepsy

Immediate release: Ritalin, Methylin oral sol, Methylin chew tabs

• **Adult: PO** 20-30 mg/day, range 10-60 mg/day in 2-3 divided doses

• **Child ≥6 yr: PO** 5 mg bid, may increase by 5-10 mg/wk, max 60 mg/day

Extended-release tabs: Ritalin SR, Metadate ER

• **Adult/adolescent/child ≥6 yr: PO** max 20 mg tid

Poststroke depression; major depression (unlabeled)

• **Adult and geriatric: PO** (immediate rel tabs) 2.5 mg morning/noon, may increase by 2.5-5 mg q2-3days

Available forms: Tabs 5, 10, 20 mg; ext rel tabs 10, 20, mg; ext rel tabs (Concerta) 18, 27, 36, 54 mg; ext rel caps 10, 20, 30, 40 mg; oral sol 5 mg, 10 mg/ml; chew tabs (Methylin) 2.5, 5, 10 mg; transdermal patch 12.5 cm^2 (10 mg), 18.75 cm^2 (15 mg), 25 cm^2 (20 mg), 37.5 cm^2 (30 mg); ext rel oral susp 300 mg/60 ml, 600 mg/120 ml, 750 mg/150 ml, 900 mg/180 ml

Administer:

PO route

• Do not crush, chew ext rel product; caps may be opened, beads sprinkled over spoonful of applesauce; give without regard to meals

• Gum, hard candy, frequent sips of water for dry mouth

• Give immediate rel dose 30-45 min before meals

• **Chew tab** with adequate water to prevent choking; contains phenylalanine

• Avoid metadate CD on day of surgery

Extended release oral suspension (Quillivant XR)

• Shake bottle well; use calibrated dosing dispenser provided; give in AM without regard to meals; reconstitute as per manufacturer

Transdermal route

• Place on clean, dry area of hip; avoid waist; remove 9 hr after application; fold after removal; flush down toilet

• If patch falls off, apply new patch to different site; total wear time should be 9 hr

SIDE EFFECTS

CNS: *Hyperactivity, insomnia, restlessness, talkativeness,* dizziness, drowsiness, toxic psychosis, headache, akathisia, dyskinesia, masking or worsening of Tourette's syndrome, seizures, hallucinations, malignant neuroleptic syndrome, aggression; cerebral vasculitis, hemorrhage, stroke (rare)

CV: *Palpitations, tachycardia,* B/P changes, angina, dysrhythmias

ENDO: Growth retardation

GI: Nausea, anorexia, dry mouth, weight loss, abdominal pain

HEMA: Leukopenia, anemia, thrombocytopenic purpura

INTEG: Exfoliative dermatitis, urticaria, rash, erythema multiforme, hypersensitivity reactions; patch: permanent loss of skin color

MISC: Fever, arthralgia, scalp hair loss, rhabdomyolysis

PHARMACOKINETICS

PO: Varies with formulation, metabolized by liver, excreted by kidneys, half-life 3-4 hr

INTERACTIONS

• **Hypertensive crisis:** MAOIs or within 14 days of MAOIs, vasopressors

Increase: effects of tricyclics, SSRIs, anticonvulsants, SNRIs, CNS stimulants

Decrease: effect of antihypertensives

Drug/Herb

Increase: CNS stimulation—cola nut, guarana, horsetail, yerba maté, yohimbe

Drug/Food

Increase: stimulation—caffeine

NURSING CONSIDERATIONS

Assess:

• **ADHD:** attention span, decreased hyperactivity

> **Black Box Warning:** Substance abuse: there is a high potential for abuse; use caution in those with history of substance abuse

• VS, B/P; may reverse antihypertensives; check patients with cardiac disease more often for increased B/P

• CBC with differential, platelets, LFTs, urinalysis; in diabetes: blood glucose, urine glucose; insulin changes may have to be made because eating will decrease

• Height, growth rate q3mo in children; growth rate may be decreased, but normal growth will resume when product is discontinued

• Mental status: mood, sensorium, affect, stimulation, insomnia, aggressiveness

⚠ **Withdrawal symptoms:** headache, nausea, vomiting, muscle pain, weakness, usually not associated with drug holidays

• Appetite, sleep, speech patterns

• **Narcolepsy:** identify frequency, length of narcoleptic episodes

Evaluate:

• Therapeutic response: decreased hyperactivity (ADHD); increased ability to stay awake (narcolepsy)

Teach patient/family:

• To decrease caffeine consumption (coffee, tea, cola, chocolate), may increase irritability, stimulation; not to use guarana, yerba maté, cola nut

• To avoid OTC preparations unless approved by prescriber

• To taper off product over several weeks because depression, increased sleeping, lethargy will occur

• To avoid driving, hazardous activities if dizziness, blurred vision occur

• To avoid alcohol

• To avoid hazardous activities until stabilized on medication

• To get needed rest; patients will feel more tired at end of day

• That shell of Concerta tab may appear in stools

• To take regular tab at least 6 hr before sleep, 10 hr for ext rel, use dosing syringe to measure liquid; not to use household teaspoon

• **Transdermal:** after tray is opened, use within 2 mo; do not store patches without protective patch; notify prescriber if skin irritation or rash occurs

TREATMENT OF OVERDOSE:

Administer fluids; hemodialysis or peritoneal dialysis; antihypertensive for increased B/P; administer short-acting barbiturate before lavage

methylPREDNISolone (Rx)

(meth-il-pred-niss′oh-lone)

A-Methapred, Depo-Medrol, Medrol, Solu-MEDROL

Func. class.: Corticosteroid, synthetic

Chem. class.: Glucocorticoid, immediate acting

Do not confuse:

methylPREDNISolone/predniSONE/medroxyPROGESTERone/methylTESTOSTERone

ACTION:

Decreases inflammation by suppression of migration of polymorphonuclear leukocytes, fibroblasts; reversal of increased capillary permeability and lysosomal stabilization

USES:
Severe inflammation, shock, adrenal insufficiency, collagen disorders, management of acute spinal cord injury, multiple sclerosis

Unlabeled uses: Multiple myeloma, bronchospasm prophylaxis, airway-obstructing hemangioma, noncardiogenic pulmonary edema, idiopathic pulmonary fibrosis, carpal tunnel syndrome, temporal arteritis, Churg-Strauss syndrome, mixed connective-tissue disease, polyarteritis nodosa, relapsing polychondritis, polymyalgia rheumatica, vasculitis, Wegener's granulomatosis, *Pneumocystis jiroveci* pneumonia in AIDS patients, acute spinal cord injury, severe acute respiratory syndrome (SARS), acute interstitial nephritis

CONTRAINDICATIONS:
Hypersensitivity, intrathecal use, neonates

Precautions: Pregnancy (C), breastfeeding, diabetes mellitus, glaucoma, osteoporosis, seizure disorders, ulcerative colitis, CHF, myasthenia gravis, renal disease, esophagitis, peptic ulcer, tartrazine, benzyl alcohol, corticosteroid hypersensitivity, viral infection, TB, traumatic brain injury, Cushing syndrome, measles, varicella, fungal infections

DOSAGE AND ROUTES

Adrenal insufficiency/inflammation

- **Adult: PO** 4-48 mg in 4 divided doses; **IM** 10-120 mg (acetate); **IM/IV** 10-40 mg (succinate); **INTRAARTICULAR** 4-80 mg (acetate)
- **Child: IV** 0.5-1.7 mg/kg in 3-4 divided doses (succinate)

Multiple sclerosis

- **Adult: PO** 160 mg/day × 1 wk, then 64 mg every other day × 30 days

Multiple myeloma/temporal arteritis/Churg-Strauss syndrome/mixed connective-tissue disease/polyarteritis nodosa/relapsing polychondritis/polymyalgia rheumatica/vasculitis/Wegener's granulomatosis (unlabeled)

- **Adult: PO** 4-48 mg/day in 4 divided doses; **IM** 10-120 mg (acetate); **IV** 10-40 mg over several min (sodium succinate)
- **Child: PO/IM** 0.5-1.7 mg/kg or 5-25 mg/m^2/day in divided doses q6-12hr

Bronchospasm prophylaxis (unlabeled)

- **Adult and adolescent: PO/IV** 40-80 mg/day in 1-2 divided doses
- **Child: PO/IV** 1 mg/kg in 2 divided doses (max 60 mg)

Airway-obstructing hemangioma (unlabeled)

- **Child: PO** 0.5-1.7 mg/kg or 5-25 mg/m^2/day in divided doses q6-12hr

Idiopathic pulmonary fibrosis (unlabeled)

- **Adult: IV** 1-2 g/wk or every other week

Carpal tunnel syndrome (unlabeled)

- **Adult: INJ** (local) 40-80 mg as a single inj

Available forms: Tabs 2, 4, 8, 16, 32 mg; inj 20, 40, 80 mg/ml acetate; inj 40, 125, 500, 1000, 2000 mg/vial succinate

Administer:

- Titrated dose; use lowest effective dose

PO route

- With food or milk to decrease GI symptoms (PO)
- Once-a-day dose should be given in AM to coincide with body's normal cortisol secretion

IM route

- IM inj deep in large muscle mass; rotate sites; avoid deltoid; use 21-G needle; after shaking suspension (parenteral); inj-site reaction may occur (induration, pain at site, atrophy)
- In one dose in AM to prevent adrenal suppression; avoid SUBCUT administration; may damage tissue

⚠ Do not give Solu-MEDROL intrathecally

IV route

- Use only Solu-MEDROL; never use acetate product

Direct IV route

- Use only methylPREDNISolone sodium succinate (Solu-MEDROL) IV; never use methylPREDNISolone acetate suspension IV
- After diluting with diluent provided; agitate slowly; give ≤500 mg/≥1 min

directly over 3-15 min; doses ≥2 mg/kg or 250 mg should be given by intermittent IV infusion unless potential benefits outweigh risks

Intermittent/continuous INFUSION route

- Dilute further in D_5W, NS, D_5NS; haze may form; give over 15-60 min; large dose (≥500 mg) should be given over 30-60 min

Y-site compatibilities: Acetaminophen, acyclovir, amifostine, amphotericin B cholesteryl, amrinone, aztreonam, cefepime, CISplatin, cladribine, cyclophosphamide, cytarabine, DOPamine, DOXOrubicin, enalaprilat, famotidine, fludarabine, grani-setron, heparin, melphalan, meperidine, methotrexate, metroNIDAZOLE, midazolam, morphine, piperacillin/tazobactam, remifentanil, sodium bicarbonate, tacrolimus, teniposide, theophylline, thiotepa

SIDE EFFECTS

CNS: Depression, flushing, sweating, headache, mood changes

CV: Hypertension, **circulatory collapse, thrombophlebitis, embolism**, tachycardia

EENT: Fungal infections, increased intraocular pressure, blurred vision, cataracts

GI: Diarrhea, nausea, abdominal distention, **GI hemorrhage**, increased appetite, pancreatitis

HEMA: **Thrombocytopenia**

INTEG: Acne, poor wound healing, ecchymosis, petechiae

MS: Fractures, osteoporosis, weakness

PHARMACOKINETICS

Half-life >3½ hr (plasma), 18-36 hr (tissue); crosses placenta, enters breast milk in small amounts; metabolized in liver; excreted by kidneys (unchanged)

PO: Peak 1-2 hr, duration 1½ days, well absorbed

IM: Peak 4-8 days, duration 1-4 wk, well absorbed

Intraarticular: Peak 1 wk

INTERACTIONS

Increase: side effects—amphotericin B, diuretics

Increase: methylPREDNISolone action—oral contraceptives, estrogens

Increase: adrenal suppression—CYP3A4 inhibitors (aprepitant, antiretroviral protease inhibitors, clarithromycin, danazol, delavirdine, diltiazem, erythromycin, fluconazole, FLUoxetine, fluvoxaMINE, imatinib, ketoconazole, mibefradil, nefazodone, telithromycin, voriconazole)

Decrease: methylPREDNISolone effect—CYP3A4 inducers (barbiturates, bosentan, carBAMazepine, efavirenz, phenytoins, nevirapine, rifabutin, rifampin)

Decrease: effects of antidiabetics, vaccines, somatrem

Drug/Herb

- Avoid use with St. John's wort

Drug/Food

- **Do not use with grapefruit juice; level of methylPREDNISolone will be increased**

Drug/Lab Test

Increase: cholesterol, blood glucose

Decrease: calcium, potassium, T_4, T_3, thyroid ^{131}I uptake test, urine 17-OHCS, 17-KS

False negative: skin allergy tests

NURSING CONSIDERATIONS

Assess:

- **Potassium depletion:** parethesias, fatigue, nausea, vomiting, depression, polyuria, dysrhythmias, weakness
- Edema, hypertension, cardiac symptoms
- Mental status: affect, mood, behavioral changes, aggression
- Potassium, blood glucose, urine glucose while receiving long-term therapy; hypokalemia and hyperglycemia
- Joint mobility, pain, edema if product given intraarticularly
- B/P q4hr, pulse; notify prescriber of chest pain, crackles
- I&O ratio; be alert for decreasing urinary output, increasing edema; weight daily; notify prescriber of weekly gain >5 lb

M

⚠ **Adrenal insufficiency:** weight loss, nausea, vomiting, confusion, anxiety, hypotension, weakness; plasma cortisol levels during long-term therapy (normal level: 138-635 nmol/L SI units when drawn at 8 AM)
- Growth in children receiving long-term treatment
- **Infection:** increased temperature, WBC, even after withdrawal of product; product masks infection

Evaluate:
- Therapeutic response: ease of respirations, decreased inflammation; decreased symptoms of adrenal insufficiency

Teach patient/family:
- To increase intake of potassium, calcium, protein
- To carry emergency ID as corticosteroid user
- To notify prescriber if therapeutic response decreases; that dosage adjustment may be needed

⚠ Not to discontinue abruptly because adrenal crisis can result
- To take PO with food, milk to decrease GI symptoms
- To avoid OTC products: salicylates, alcohol in cough products, cold preparations unless directed by prescriber; to avoid vaccinations because immunosuppression occurs
- **Adrenal insufficiency:** nausea, anorexia, fatigue, dizziness, dyspnea, weakness, joint pain
- **Cushingoid symptoms:** buffalo hump, moon face, rapid weight gain, excess sweating
- **Infection:** to avoid persons with known infections; corticosteroids can mask symptoms of infection

metipranolol ophthalmic
See Appendix B

metoclopramide (Rx)
(met-oh-kloe-pra′mide)

Apo-Metoclop ✤, Metozolv ODT, Reglan

Func. class.: Cholinergic, antiemetic
Chem. class.: Central dopamine receptor antagonist

Do not confuse:
metoclopramide/metolazone
Reglan/Megace/Renagel

ACTION: Enhances response to acetylcholine of tissue in upper GI tract, which causes the contraction of gastric muscle; relaxes pyloric, duodenal segments; increases peristalsis without stimulating secretions; blocks dopamine in chemoreceptor trigger zone of CNS

USES: Prevention of nausea, vomiting induced by chemotherapy, radiation, delayed gastric emptying, gastroesophageal reflux

Unlabeled uses: Hiccups, migraines, breastfeeding induction, lung cancer

CONTRAINDICATIONS: Hypersensitivity to this product, procaine, or procainamide; seizure disorder, pheochromocytoma, breast cancer (prolactin dependent), GI obstruction

Precautions: Pregnancy (B), breastfeeding, GI hemorrhage, CHF, Parkinson's disease·

Black Box Warning: Tardive dyskinesia

DOSAGE AND ROUTES
Nausea/vomiting (chemotherapy)
- **Adult:** **IV** 1-2 mg/kg 30 min before administration of chemotherapy, then q2hr × 2 doses, then q3hr × 3 doses

- **Child (unlabeled): IV** 1-2 mg/kg/dose

Facilitate small-bowel intubation for radiologic exams

- **Adult and child >14 yr: IV** 10 mg over 1-2 min
- **Child <6 yr: IV** 0.1 mg/kg
- **Child 6-14 yr: IV** 2.5-5 mg

Diabetic gastroparesis

- **Adult: PO** 10 mg 30 min before meals, at bedtime × 2-8 wk
- **Geriatric: PO** 5 mg 30 min before meals, at bedtime, increase to 10 mg if needed

Gastroesophageal reflux

- **Adult: PO** 10-15 mg qid 30 min before meals and at bedtime
- **Child: PO** 0.4-0.8 mg/kg/day in 4 divided doses

Renal dose

- **Adult:** CCr <40 ml/min 50% of dose

Lactation induction (unlabeled)

- **Adult: PO** 10 mg bid-tid, may increase to 20-45 mg/day in divided doses

Non–small-cell lung cancer (NSCLC) radiation sensitizer (unlabeled)

- **Adult: IV** (Sensamide IV) 2 mg/kg given 1 hr before radiation therapy 3×/wk

Hiccups (unlabeled)

- **Adult: PO/IM/IV** 10 mg q6hr

Available forms: Tabs 5, 10 mg; syr 5 mg/5 ml; inj 5 mg/ml; oral sol 5 mg/5 ml; orally disintegrating tab 5, 10 mg

Administer:

PO route

- ½-1 hr before meals for better absorption
- Gum, hard candy, frequent rinsing of mouth for dry oral cavity
- **Oral disintegrating:** place on tongue, allow to dissolve, swallow, remove from bottle immediately before use

IM route

- Give for postoperative nausea, vomiting before end of surgery

Direct IV route

- DiphenhydrAMINE IV or benztropine IM for EPS
- Undiluted if dose ≤10 mg; give over 2 min

Intermittent IV INFUSION route

- >10 mg may be diluted in ≥50 ml D_5W, NaCl, Ringer's, LR, given over ≥15 min
- Protect from light with aluminum foil during infusion
- Discard open ampules

Y-site compatibilities: Acetaminophen, alfentanil, amifostine, amikacin, aminophylline, ascorbic acid, atracurium, atropine, azaTHIOprine, aztreonam, bivalirudin, bleomycin, bumetanide, buprenorphine, butorphanol, calcium chloride/gluconate, CARBOplatin, caspofungin, ceFAZolin, cefonicid, cefoperazone, cefotaxime, cefoTEtan, cefOXitin, cefTAZidime, ceftizoxime, cefTRIAXone, cefuroxime, chloramphenicol, chlorproMAZINE, cimetidine, ciprofloxacin, cisatracurium, CISplatin, cladribine, clindamycin, cyanocobalamin, cyclophosphamide, cycloSPORINE, cytarabine, DACTINomycin, DAPTOmycin, dexamethasone, dexmedetomidine, digoxin, diltiazem, diphenhydrAMINE, DOBUTamine, DOCEtaxel, DOPamine, doripenem, doxapram, DOXOrubicin hydrochloride, doxycycline, droperidol, enalaprilat, ePHEDrine, EPINEPHrine, epirubicin, epoetin alfa, ertapenem, erythromycin, esmolol, etoposide, etoposide phosphate, famotidine, fenoldopam, fentaNYL, filgrastim, fluconazole, fludarabine, folic acid, foscarnet, gallium nitrate, gemcitabine, gentamicin, glycopyrrolate, granisetron, heparin, hydrocortisone, HYDROmorphone, IDArubicin, ifosfamide, imipenem/cilastatin, indomethacin, insulin, isoproterenol, ketorolac, labetalol, leucovorin, levofloxacin, lidocaine, linezolid, LORazepam, magnesium sulfate, mannitol, mechlorethamine, melphalan, meperidine, meropenem, metaraminol, methadone, methotrexate, methoxamine, methyldopate, methylPREDNISolone, metoprolol, metroNIDAZOLE, miconazole, midazolam, milrinone, minocycline, mitoMYcin, morphine, moxalactam, multiple vitamins, nafcillin, nalbuphine, naloxone, nesiritide,

M

nitroglycerin, nitroprusside, norepinephrine, octreotide, ondansetron, oxaliplatin, oxytocin, PACLitaxel, palonosetron, pantoprazole, papaverine, PEMEtrexed, penicillin G, pentamidine, pentazocine, PENTobarbital, PHENobarbital, phentolamine, phenylephrine, phytonadione, piperacillin/tazobactam, potassium chloride, procainamide, prochlorperazine, promethazine, propranolol, protamine, pyridoxine, quinupristin/dalfopristin, ranitidine, remi-fentanil, riTUXimab, rocuronium, sargramostim, sodium acetate/bicarbonate, succinylcholine, SUFentanil, tacrolimus, teniposide, theophylline, thiamine, thiotepa, ticarcillin/clavulanate, tigecycline, tirofiban, tobramycin, tolazoline, topotecan, trastuzumab, trimethaphan, urokinase, vancomycin, vasopressin, vecuronium, verapamil, vinBLAStine, vinCRIStine, vinorelbine, voriconazole, zidovudine

SIDE EFFECTS

CNS: *Sedation, fatigue, restlessness, headache, sleeplessness, dystonia,* dizziness, drowsiness, suicidal ideation, seizures, EPS, neuroleptic malignant syndrome; tardive dyskinesia (>3 mo, high doses)

CV: Hypotension, supraventricular tachycardia

GI: Dry mouth, constipation, nausea, anorexia, vomiting, diarrhea

GU: Decreased libido, prolactin secretion, amenorrhea, galactorrhea

HEMA: Neutropenia, leukopenia, agranulocytosis

INTEG: Urticaria, rash

PHARMACOKINETICS

Metabolized by liver, excreted in urine, half-life $2^1/_2$-6 hr

PO: Onset $^1/_2$-1 hr, duration 1-2 hr

IM: Onset 10-15 min, duration 1-2 hr

IV: Onset 1-3 min, duration 1-2 hr

INTERACTIONS

- Avoid use with MAOIs

Increase: sedation—alcohol, other CNS depressants

Increase: risk for EPS—haloperidol, phenothiazines

Decrease: action of metoclopramide—anticholinergics, opiates

Drug/Lab Test

Increase: prolactin, aldosterone, thyrotropin

NURSING CONSIDERATIONS

Assess:

Black Box Warning: EPS, tardive dyskinesia; more likely to occur in treatment >3 mo, geriatric patients and may be irreversible; assess for involuntary movements often

- **Neuroleptic malignant syndrome:** hyperthermia, change in B/P, pulse, tachycardia, sweating, rigidity, altered consciousness (rare)
- Mental status: depression, anxiety, irritability
- GI complaints: nausea, vomiting, anorexia, constipation

Evaluate:

- Therapeutic response: absence of nausea, vomiting, anorexia, fullness

Teach patient/family:

- To avoid driving, other hazardous activities until stabilized on product
- To avoid alcohol, other CNS depressants that will enhance sedating properties of this product

metolazone (Rx)

(me-tole′a-zone)

Zaroxolyn

Func. class.: Diuretic, antihypertensive

Chem. class.: Thiazide-like quinazoline derivative

Do not confuse:
metolazone/methotrexate/metoclopramide

ACTION: Acts on distal tubule by increasing excretion of water, sodium, chloride, potassium, magnesium, bicarbonate; decreases GFR

USES:
Edema, hypertension

Unlabeled uses: Heart failure, nephrotic syndrome

CONTRAINDICATIONS:
Pregnancy (D) (preeclampsia, intrauterine growth retardation), hypersensitivity to thiazides, sulfonamides; anuria, coma, hepatic encephalopathy

Precautions: Pregnancy (B), breastfeeding, geriatric patients, hypokalemia, renal/hepatic disease, gout, COPD, lupus erythematosus, diabetes mellitus, hypotension, history of pancreatitis; hypersensitivity to sulfonamides, thiazides; electrolyte imbalance

DOSAGE AND ROUTES

Edema

- **Adult: PO** 5-10 mg/day; max 20 mg/day

Hypertension

- **Adult: PO** 2.5-5 mg/day
- **Child: PO** 0.2-0.4 mg/kg/day in divided doses q12-24hr

Available forms: Tabs 2.5, 5, 10 mg

Administer:

- In AM to avoid interference with sleep if using product as diuretic
- Potassium replacement if potassium <3 mg/dl
- With food if nausea occurs; absorption may be decreased slightly

SIDE EFFECTS

CNS: Anxiety, depression, *headache, dizziness, fatigue, weakness*

CV: *Orthostatic hypotension,* palpitations, volume depletion, hypotension, chest pain

EENT: Blurred vision

ELECT: *Hypokalemia,* hypercalcemia, hyponatremia

GI: *Nausea, vomiting, anorexia,* constipation, diarrhea, cramps, pancreatitis, GI irritation, dry mouth, jaundice, **hepatitis**

GU: *Urinary frequency,* polyuria, **uremia, glucosuria,** nocturia, impotence

HEMA: **Aplastic anemia, hemolytic anemia, leukopenia, agranulocytosis, neutropenia**

INTEG: *Rash,* urticaria, purpura, photosensitivity, fever, dry skin, **toxic epidermal necrolysis, Stevens-Johnson syndrome**

META: *Hyperglycemia,* increased creatinine, BUN

MS: Muscle cramps, joint pain, swelling

PHARMACOKINETICS
Protein binding 33%, peak 8 hr, duration 12-24 hr, excreted unchanged by kidneys, crosses placenta, enters breast milk, half-life 14 hr

INTERACTIONS

Increase: hyperglycemia—antidiabetics

Increase: hypokalemia—mezlocillin, piperacillin, amphotericin B, glucocorticoids, digoxin, stimulant laxatives

Increase: hypotension—alcohol (large amounts), nitrates, antihypertensives, barbiturates, opioids

Increase: toxicity—lithium

Increase: metolazone effects—loop diuretics

Decrease: action of metolazone—NSAIDs, salicylates

Drug/Food

Increase: severe hypokalemia—licorice

Drug/Herb

Decrease: antihypertensive effect—ephedra (Ma huang)

Increase: antihypertensive effect—hawthorn

Drug/Lab Test

Increase: calcium, cholesterol, glucose, triglycerides

Decrease: potassium, sodium, chloride, magnesium

NURSING CONSIDERATIONS

Assess:

- Weight, I&O daily to determine fluid loss; effect of product may be decreased if used daily
- **CHF:** improvement in edema of feet, legs, sacral area daily if product being used

M

• **Hypertension:** B/P lying, standing; postural hypotension may occur
• Electrolytes: potassium, magnesium, sodium, chloride; include BUN, blood glucose, CBC, serum creatinine, blood pH, ABGs, uric acid, calcium
• **Hypokalemia:** postural hypotension, malaise, fatigue, tachycardia, leg cramps, weakness
• Rashes, fever daily
• Confusion, especially among geriatric patients; take safety precautions if needed

Black Box Warning: Hepatic encephalopathy: do not use in hepatic coma or precoma; fluctuations in electrolytes can occur rapidly and precipitate hepatic coma; use caution in patients with impaired hepatic function

Evaluate:
• Therapeutic response: decreased edema, B/P

Teach patient/family:
• To increase fluid intake to 2-3 L/day unless contraindicated; to rise slowly from lying or sitting position
• To notify prescriber of muscle weakness, cramps, nausea, dizziness
• That product may be taken with food or milk
• To use sunscreen for photosensitivity
• That blood glucose may be increased in diabetics
• To take early in day to avoid nocturia
• To avoid alcohol
• To avoid sodium foods; to increase potassium foods in diet
• Not to stop product abruptly

TREATMENT OF OVERDOSE:
Lavage if taken orally; monitor electrolytes; administer dextrose in saline; monitor hydration, CV, renal status

metoprolol (Rx)
(meh-toe′proe-lole)
Lopressor, Nu-Metop ♣, Toprol-XL
Func. class.: Antihypertensive, antianginal
Chem. class.: β_1-Blocker

Do not confuse:
metoprolol/misoprostol

ACTION: Lowers B/P by β-blocking effects; reduces elevated renin plasma levels; blocks β_2-adrenergic receptors in bronchial, vascular smooth muscle only at high doses; negative chronotropic effect

USES: Mild to moderate hypertension, acute MI to reduce cardiovascular mortality, angina pectoris, NYHA class II, III heart failure, cardiomyopathy
Unlabeled uses: Migraine prevention, heart rate control for atrial fibrillation/flutter without accessory pathway, essential tremor, unstable angina

CONTRAINDICATIONS: Hypersensitivity to β-blockers, cardiogenic shock, heart block (2nd, 3rd degree), sinus bradycardia, pheochromocytoma, sick sinus syndrome
Precautions: Pregnancy (C), breastfeeding, geriatric patients, major surgery, diabetes mellitus, thyroid/renal/hepatic disease, COPD, CAD, nonallergic bronchospasm, bronchial asthma, CVA, children, depression, vasospastic angina

Black Box Warning: Abrupt discontinuation

DOSAGE AND ROUTES
Hypertension
• **Adult: PO** 50 mg bid or 100 mg/day; may give up to 100-450 mg in divided doses; **EXT REL** 25-100 mg daily, titrate at weekly intervals; max 400 mg/day

• **Geriatric: PO** 25 mg/day initially, increase weekly as needed
• **Child and adolescent 6-16 yr: PO ER** 1 mg/kg up to 50 mg daily

Myocardial infarction
• **Adult: IV BOL** (early treatment) 5 mg q2min × 3, then 50 mg **PO** 15 min after last dose and q6hr × 48 hr; (late treatment) **PO** maintenance 50-100 mg bid for 1-3 yr

Heart failure (NYHA class II/III)
• **Adult: PO EXT REL** 25 mg daily × 2 wk (class II); 12.5 mg daily (class III)

Angina
• **Adult: PO** 100 mg/day as a single dose or in 2 divided doses, increase weekly prn or 100 mg **EXT REL** daily, max 400 mg/day ext rel

Migraine prevention (unlabeled)
• **Adult: PO** 25-100 mg bid; 50-200 mg daily (XL)

Heart rate control for atrial fibrillation/flutter without accessory pathway (unlabeled)
• **Adult: IV BOL** (acute setting) 2.5-5 mg over 2 min, may repeat dose × 3; **PO** (nonacute setting) 25-100 mg bid

Essential tremor (unlabeled)
• **Adult: PO** 50 mg/day, may increase, max 300 mg/day in divided doses; **EXT REL** 100 mg/day, max 400 mg/day

Available forms: Tabs 25, 50, 100 mg; inj 1 mg/ml; ext rel tab (succinate) (XL) 25, 50, 100, 200 mg; ext rel tabs, tartrate: 100 mg

Administer:

PO route
• Do not break, crush, or chew ext rel tabs
• Regular release tab after meals, at bedtime; tab may be crushed or swallowed whole; take at same time each day
• Store in dry area at room temperature; do not freeze

Direct IV route
• IV, undiluted, give over 1 min × 3 doses at 2- to 5-min intervals; start **PO** 15 min after last IV dose

Y-site compatibilities: Abciximab, acyclovir, alemtuzumab, alfentanil, alteplase, amikacin, aminophylline, amiodarone, amphotericin B liposome, anidulafungin, argatroban, ascorbic acid, atracurium, atropine, azaTHIOprine, aztreonam, benztropine, bivalirudin, bleomycin, bumetanide, buprenorphine, butorphanol, calcium chloride/gluconate, CARBOplatin, caspofungin, ceFAZolin, cefonicid, cefoperazone, cefotaxime, cefoTEtan, cefOXitin, cefTAZidime, ceftizoxime, cefTRIAXone, cefuroxime, chloramphenicol, chlorproMAZINE, cimetidine, CISplatin, clindamycin, cyanocobalamin, cyclophosphamide, cycloSPORINE, cytarabine, DACTINomycin, DAPTOmycin, dexamethasone, dexmedetomidine, digoxin, diltiazem, diphenhydrAMINE, DOBUTamine, DOCEtaxel, DOPamine, doxacurium, DOXOrubicin, doxycycline, enalaprilat, ePHEDrine, EPINEPHrine, epirubicin, epoetin alfa, eptifibatide, esmolol, etoposide, etoposide phosphate, famotidine, fenoldopam, fentaNYL, fluconazole, fludarabine, fluorouracil, folic acid, furosemide, ganciclovir, gemcitabine, gentamicin, glycopyrrolate, granisetron, heparin, hydrocortisone, HYDROmorphone, IDArubicin, ifosfamide, imipenem/cilastatin, indomethacin, insulin, isoproterenol, ketorolac, labetalol, linezolid, LORazepam, magnesium sulfate, mannitol, mechlorethamine, meperidine, metaraminol, methotrexate, methoxamine, methyldopate, methylPREDNISolone, metoclopramide, metroNIDAZOLE, midazolam, milrinone, mitoXANtrone, morphine, multivitamins, nafcillin, nalbuphine, naloxone, nitroprusside, norepinephrine, octreotide, ondansetron, oxacillin, oxaliplatin, oxytocin, PACLitaxel, palonosetron, pancuronium, papaverine, PEMEtrexed, penicillin G, pentamidine, pentazocine, PENTobarbital, PHENobarbital, phentolamine, phenylephrine, phytonadione, piperacillin/tazobactam, potassium chloride, procainamide, prochlorperazine, promethazine, propranolol, protamine, pyridoxime, quinupristin/dalfopristin, ranitidine, rocuronium, sodium bicarbonate, succinylcholine, SUFentanil, tacrolimus, teniposide,

M

theophylline, thiamine, thiotepa, ticarcillin/clavulanate, tigecycline, tirofiban, tobramycin, tolazoline, trimetaphan, urokinase, vancomycin, vasopressin, vecuronium, verapamil, vinCRIStine, vinorelbine, voriconazole

SIDE EFFECTS

CNS: *Insomnia, dizziness,* mental changes, hallucinations, depression, anxiety, headaches, nightmares, confusion, fatigue

CV: *Hypotension,* bradycardia, CHF, *palpitations,* dysrhythmias, cardiac arrest, AV block, pulmonary/peripheral edema, chest pain

EENT: Sore throat; dry, burning eyes

GI: *Nausea, vomiting,* colitis, cramps, *diarrhea,* constipation, flatulence, dry mouth, *hiccups*

GU: Impotence

HEMA: Agranulocytosis, eosinophilia, thrombocytopenia, purpura

INTEG: Rash, purpura, alopecia, dry skin, urticaria, pruritus

RESP: Bronchospasm, dyspnea, wheezing

PHARMACOKINETICS

Half-life 3-4 hr, metabolized in liver (metabolites), excreted in urine, crosses placenta, enters breast milk

PO: Peak 2-4 hr, duration 13-19 hr

PO-ER: Peak 6-12 hr, duration 24 hr

IV: Onset immediate, peak 20 min, duration 6-8 hr

INTERACTIONS

- Do not use with MAOIs

Increase: hypotension, bradycardia—reserpine, hydrALAZINE, methyldopa, prazosin, amphetamines, EPINEPHrine, H_2-antagonists, calcium channel blockers

Increase: hypoglycemic effects—insulin, oral antidiabetics

Increase: metoprolol level—cimetidine

Increase: effects of benzodiazepines

Decrease: antihypertensive effect—salicylates, NSAIDs

Decrease: metoprolol level—barbiturates

Decrease: effects of—xanthines

Drug/Food

Increase: absorption with food

Drug/Lab Test

Increase: BUN, potassium, ANA titer, serum lipoprotein, triglycerides, uric acid, alk phos, LDH, AST, ALT

NURSING CONSIDERATIONS

Assess:

Black Box Warning: Abrupt withdrawal: may cause MI, ventricular dysrhythmias, myocardial ischemia; taper dose over 7-14 days

- **Hypertension/angina:** ECG directly when giving IV during initial treatment
- I&O, weight daily; check for CHF (weight gain, jugular venous distention, crackles, edema, dyspnea)
- Monitor B/P during initial treatment, periodically thereafter; pulse q4hr; note rate, rhythm, quality; apical/radial pulse before administration; notify prescriber of any significant changes or pulse <60 bpm
- Baselines of renal, hepatic studies before therapy begins

Evaluate:

- Therapeutic response: decreased B/P after 1-2 wk, decreased anginal pain

Teach patient/family:

- To take immediately after meals; to take medication at bedtime to prevent effect of orthostatic hypotension

Black Box Warning: Not to discontinue product abruptly; to taper over 2 wk; may cause angina

- Not to use OTC products containing α-adrenergic stimulants (nasal decongestants, OTC cold preparations) unless directed by prescriber; to avoid alcohol, smoking, sodium intake
- To report bradycardia, dizziness, confusion, depression, fever, sore throat, SOB, decreased vision to prescriber
- To take pulse, B/P at home; when to notify prescriber

- To comply with weight control, dietary adjustments, modified exercise program
- To carry emergency ID to identify product, allergies
- To monitor blood glucose closely if diabetic
- To avoid hazardous activities if dizziness is present
- To report symptoms of CHF: difficult breathing, especially on exertion or when lying down; night cough; swelling of extremities
- To wear support hose to minimize effects of orthostatic hypotension
- To report Raynaud's symptoms

TREATMENT OF OVERDOSE:
Lavage, IV atropine for bradycardia, IV theophylline for bronchospasm, digoxin, O_2, diuretic for cardiac failure, hemodialysis, administer vasopressor

metroNIDAZOLE (Rx)
(me-troe-ni′da-zole)

Flagyl, Flagyl ER, Flagyl IV, Flagyl IV RTU, Florazone ER ✤, Novo-Nidazol ✤

Func. class.: Antiinfective—miscellaneous

Chem. class.: Nitroimidazole derivative

ACTION:
Direct-acting amebicide/trichomonacide binds and disrupts DNA structure, thereby inhibiting bacterial nucleic acid synthesis

USES:
Intestinal amebiasis, amebic abscess, trichomoniasis, refractory trichomoniasis, bacterial anaerobic infections, giardiasis, septicemia, endocarditis; bone, joint, lower respiratory tract infections; rosacea

Unlabeled uses: Crohn's disease, urethritis, amebiasis due to *Dientamoeba fragilis, Entamoeba polecki,* giardiasis, pruritus; gastric ulcer, dyspepsia *(H. pylori),* pseudomembranous colitis, guinea worm disease, periodontitis

CONTRAINDICATIONS:
Pregnancy 1st trimester, breastfeeding, hypersensitivity to this product

Precautions: Pregnancy (B) 2nd/3rd trimesters, geriatric patients, *Candida* infections, heart failure, fungal infection, dental disease, bone marrow suppression, hematologic disease, GI/renal/hepatic disease, contracted visual or color fields, blood dyscrasias, CNS disorders

Black Box Warning: Secondary malignancy

DOSAGE AND ROUTES
Trichomoniasis
- **Adult: PO** 500 mg bid × 7 days or 2 g as single dose; do not repeat treatment for 4-6 wk
- **Child ≥45 kg (unlabeled): PO** 2 g once
- **Child <45 kg (unlabeled): PO** 15 mg/kg/day in 3 divided doses × 7-10 days
- **Infant (unlabeled): PO** 15 mg/kg/day divided in 3 doses × 7 days

Amebic hepatic abscess
- **Adult: PO** 750 mg tid × 7-10 days
- **Child: PO** 35-50 mg/kg/day in 3 divided doses × 7-10 days

Intestinal amebiasis
- **Adult: PO** 750 mg tid × 7-10 days
- **Child: PO** 35-50 mg/kg/day in 3 divided doses × 7-10 days, then oral iodoquinol

Anaerobic bacterial infections
- **Adult: IV INFUSION** 15 mg/kg over 1 hr, then 7.5 mg/kg **IV** or **PO** q6hr, not to exceed 4 g/day; 1st maintenance dose should be administered 6 hr after loading dose

Bacterial vaginosis
- **Adult: PO** regular rel 500 mg bid or 250 mg tid × 7 days; ext rel 750 mg/day × 7 days

Persistent urethritis (unlabeled)
- **Adult and adolescent: PO** 2 g as single dose with azithromycin

***Dientamoeba fragilis* (unlabeled)**
- **Child: PO** 250 mg tid × 7 days

***Entamoeba polecki* (unlabeled)**
- **Adult: PO** 750 mg tid × 10 days, then diloxanide furoate (500 mg tid × 10 days

M

• **Child: PO** 30-50 mg/kg/day in 3 divided doses × 5-10 days

Crohn's disease (unlabeled)

• **Adult: PO** 250 mg tid-qid

Giardiasis (unlabeled)

• **Adult: PO** 250 mg tid × 5-7 days

• **Child: PO** 15 mg/kg/day in 3 divided doses × 5 days

Antibiotic-associated pseudomembranous colitis (unlabeled)

• **Adult: PO** 500 mg/day × 10-14 days; **IV** 500 mg q8hr

• **Child: PO/IV** 30 mg/kg/day (max 2 g) divided q6hr × 10 days

Available forms: Tabs 250, 500 mg; ext rel tab (ER) 750 mg; caps 375 mg; injection solution 5 mg/ml

Administer:

• Store in light-resistant container; do not refrigerate

PO route

• Do not break, crush, or chew ext rel product, give on empty stomach

• PO with or after meals to avoid GI symptoms, metallic taste; crush tabs if needed

IV route

Intermittent INFUSION ([Flagyl] IV RTU)

• Prediluted, ready to use; infusion over 30-60 min

• Lyophilized vials: dilute with 4.4 ml sterile water, 0.9% NaCl; must be diluted further with ≤8 mg/ml with 0.9% NaCl, D_5W, or LR; must neutralize with 5 mEq $NaCO_3$/500 mg; CO_2 gas will be generated and may require venting; run over ≥1 hr; primary IV must be discontinued; may be given as cont infusion; do not use aluminum products; IV may require venting

• Do not use aluminum needles or other products to prepare product

Y-site compatibilities: Acyclovir, alemtuzumab, alfentanil, allopurinol, amifostine, amikacin, aminophylline, amiodarone, ampicillin, ampicillin/sulbactam, anidulafungin, atracurium, bivalirudin, bumetanide, buprenorphine, busulfan, butorphanol, calcium acetate/chloride/gluconate, CARBOplatin, ceFAZolin, cefepime, cefoperazone, cefotaxime, cefoTEtan, cefTRIAXone, cefuroxime, chloramphenicol, chlorproMAZINE, cimetidine, ciprofloxacin, cisatracurium, CISplatin, clindamycin, codeine, cyclophosphamide, cycloSPORINE, cytarabine, DACTINomycin, dexamethasone, dexmedetomidine, dexrazoxane, digoxin, diltiazem, dimenhyDRINATE, diphenhydrAMINE, DOBUTamine, DOCEtaxel, DOPamine, doripenem, doxacurium, doxapram, DOXOrubicin, DOXOrubicin liposome, doxycycline, droperidol, enalaprilat, ePHEDrine, EPINEPHrine, epirubicin, eptifibatide, ertapenem, erythromycin, esmolol, etoposide, etoposide phosphate, famotidine, fenoldopam, fentaNYL, fluconazole, fludarabine, fluorouracil, foscarnet, fosphenytoin, furosemide, gemcitabine, gentamicin, glycopyrrolate, granisetron, haloperidol, heparin, hydrALAZINE, hydrocortisone, HYDROmorphone, IDArubicin, ifosfamide, imipenem/cilastatin, inamrinone, insulin, isoproterenol, ketorolac, labetalol, leucovorin, levofloxacin, lidocaine, linezolid, LORazepam, magnesium sulfate, mannitol, mechlorethamine, melphalan, meperidine, meropenem, mesna, metaraminol, methotrexate, methyldopate, methylPREDNISolone, metoclopramide, metoprolol, midazolam, milrinone, mitoXANtrone, morphine, nafcillin, nalbuphine, naloxone, nesiritide, niCARdipine, nitroglycerin, nitroprusside, norepinephrine, octreotide, ondansetron, oxaliplatin, oxytocin, PACLitaxel, palonosetron, pancuronium, pentamidine, pentazocine, PENTobarbital, perphenazine, PHENobarbital, phentolamine, phenylephrine, piperacillin/tazobactam, potassium chloride/phosphates, prochlorperazine, promethazine, propranolol, ranitidine, remifentanil, riTUXimab, rocuronium, sargramostim, sodium acetate/bicarbonate/phosphates, streptozocin, succinylcholine, SUFentanil, tacrolimus, teniposide, theophylline, thiopental, thiotepa, ticarcillin/clavulanate, tigecycline, tirofiban, tobramycin, trastuzumab, trimethobenzamide, trimethoprim/sulfamethoxazole, vancomycin, vasopressin, vecuronium, verapamil, vinCRIStine, vinorelbine, voriconazole, zidovudine, zoledronic acid

SIDE EFFECTS

CNS: *Headache, dizziness,* confusion, irritability, restlessness, ataxia, depression, fatigue, drowsiness, insomnia, paresthesia, peripheral neuropathy, **seizures,** incoordination, depression, encephalopathy, **aseptic meningitis**
CV: Flattening of T waves
EENT: Blurred vision, sore throat, retinal edema, dry mouth, metallic taste, furry tongue, glossitis, stomatitis, photophobia, optic neuritis
GI: *Nausea, vomiting, diarrhea,* epigastric distress, *anorexia,* constipation, *abdominal cramps,* **pseudomembranous colitis,** xerostomia, metallic taste, abdominal pain, **pancreatitis**
GU: Darkened urine, vaginal dryness, polyuria, **albuminuria,** dysuria, cystitis, decreased libido, **nephrotoxicity,** incontinence, dyspareunia, candidiasis, increased urinary frequency
HEMA: **Leukopenia, bone marrow, depression, aplasia, thrombocytopenia**
INTEG: Rash, pruritus, urticaria, flushing, **Stevens-Johnson syndrome, phlebitis at injection site, toxic epidermal necrolysis**

PHARMACOKINETICS

Crosses placenta, enters breast milk, metabolized by liver 30%-60%, excreted in urine (60%-80%), half-life 6-8 hr
PO: Peak 2 hr, absorbed 80%-85%
IV: Onset immediate, peak end of infusion

INTERACTIONS

- Avoid use with zalcitabine, bortezomib, norfloxacin, disulfiram
- **Do not use with amprenavir**

Decrease: metroNIDAZOLE half-life—barbiturates
Decrease: metroNIDAZOLE—cholestyramine
Increase: disulfiram reaction—alcohol, oral ritonavir, any product with alcohol
Increase: busulfan toxicity—busulfan; avoid concurrent use
Increase: metroNIDAZOLE level, toxicity—cimetidine
Increase: lithium, CYP3A4 substrates
Increase: action of warfarin, phenytoin, lithium, fosphenytoin
Increase: leukopenia—azaTHIOprine, fluorouracil

Drug/Lab Test
Altered: AST, ALT, LDH
Decrease: WBC, neutrophils
False decrease: triglycerides

NURSING CONSIDERATIONS

Assess:

- **Infection:** WBC, wound symptoms, fever, skin or vaginal secretions; start treatment after C&S; for opportunistic fungal infections; superinfection: fever, monilial growth, fatigue, malaise
- Stools during entire treatment; should be clear at end of therapy; stools should be free of parasites for 1 yr before patient considered cured (amebiasis)
- Vision by ophthalmic exam during, after therapy; vision problems often occur
- ⚠ **Neurotoxicity: peripheral neuropathy, seizures, dizziness, uncoordination, pruritus, joint pain; product may be discontinued**
- **Allergic reaction:** fever, rash, itching, chills; product should be discontinued if these occur
- Renal, reproductive dysfunction: dysuria, polyuria, impotence, dyspareunia, decreased libido, I&O; weight daily

Black Box Warning: Secondary malignancy: use only when indicated; avoid unnecessary use

Evaluate:

- Therapeutic response: decreased symptoms of infection

Teach patient/family:

- That urine may turn dark reddish brown; that product may cause metallic taste
- About proper hygiene after bowel movement; handwashing technique
- To notify physician about numbness or tingling of extremities

M

- To avoid hazardous activities because dizziness can occur
- About need for compliance with dosage schedule, duration of treatment
- To use condoms if treatment for trichomoniasis or cross-contamination may occur; to notify prescriber if pregnant or planning to become pregnant; that treatment of both partners is necessary for trichomoniasis
- To use frequent sips of water, sugarless gum, candy for dry mouth
- Not to drink alcohol or use preparations containing alcohol during use or for 48 hr after use of product; disulfiram-like reaction can occur
- To notify if pregnancy is planned or suspected, pregnancy (B) 2nd/3rd trimester in trichomoniasis

metroNIDAZOLE (topical, vaginal)

(met-roe-ni′da-zole)

MetroCream, MetroGel, MetroGel Vaginal, MetroLotion, Noritate, Rosasol ✤, Rosadan, Vandazole

Func. class.: Antiprotozoal, antibacterial

Chem. class.: Nitroimidazole

ACTION: Antibacterial and antiprotozoal activity may result from interacting with DNA

USES: Acne rosacea, bacterial vaginosis

CONTRAINDICATIONS: Hypersensitivity to this product or nitroimidazoles, parabens

Precautions: Hepatic disease, blood dyscrasias; CNS conditions (vaginal), children

DOSAGE AND ROUTES

Acne rosacea

- **Adult: TOP** apply to affected areas bid (0.75%) daily (1%); adjust therapy based on response

Bacterial vaginosis

- **Adult: VAG** 1 applicatorful daily × 5 days

Available forms: Topical cream 0.75%, 1%; gel 0.75%, 1%; lotion 0.75%; vaginal gel 0.75%

Administer:

Topical route

- Topical skin products are not for intravaginal therapy and are for external use only; do not use skin products near the eyes, nose, or mouth
- Wash hands before and after use; wash affected area and gently pat dry
- **Cream/Gel/Lotion:** Apply a thin film to the cleansed affected area; massage gently into affected areas

Intravaginal route

- Only use dosage formulations specified for intravaginal use; intravaginal dosage forms are not for topical therapy; do not ingest
- Avoid vaginal intercourse during treatment
- **Cream:** Use applicator(s) supplied by the manufacturer

SIDE EFFECTS

GU: Vaginitis, cervicitis; nausea, vomiting, cramping

INTEG: Redness, burning, dermatitis, rash, pruritus

INTERACTIONS

- MetroNIDAZOLE may increase warfarin anticoagulant effect
- Caution with drinking alcohol or using disulfiram while using metroNIDAZOLE products(vaginal gel)
- Possible lithium toxicity (vaginal gel)

NURSING CONSIDERATIONS

Assess:

- **Allergic reaction:** assess for hypersensitivity; product may need to be discontinued
- **Infection:** assess for number of lesions and severity of acne rosacea, itching in vaginosis

Evaluate:

- Decreased severity of acne rosacea, infection in vaginosis

Teach patient/family:
- That topical skin products are not for intravaginal therapy and are for external use only; not to use skin products near the eyes, nose, or mouth
- To wash hands before and after use; to wash affected area and gently pat dry
- **Cream/Gel/Lotion:** to apply a thin film to the cleansed affected area and massage gently into affected areas
- **Intravaginal route:** to use only dosage formulations specified for intravaginal use; not to ingest intravaginal dosage forms because these are not for topical therapy; to avoid vaginal intercourse during treatment
- **Cream:** to use applicator(s) supplied by the manufacturer

micafungin (Rx)
(my-ca-fun′gin)

Mycamine

Func. class.: Antifungal, systemic
Chem. class.: Echinocandin

ACTION: Inhibits an essential component of fungal cell walls; causes direct damage to fungal cell wall

USES: Treatment of esophageal candidiasis; prophylaxis for *Candida* infections in patients undergoing hematopoietic stem-cell transplantation (HSCT); susceptible *Candida* sp.: *C. albicans, C. glabrata, C. krusei, C. parapsilosis, C. tropicalis*
Unlabeled uses: *Aspergillus* sp., pediatrics to prevent candidiasis, endocarditis, endophthalmitis, infectious arthritis, myocarditis, osteomyelitis, pericarditis, pneumonia, sinusitis, tracheobronchitis, prophylaxis of HIV-related esophageal candidiasis

CONTRAINDICATIONS: Hypersensitivity to this product or other echinocandins
Precautions: Pregnancy (C), breastfeeding, children, geriatric patients, severe hepatic disease, renal impairment, hemolytic anemia

DOSAGE AND ROUTES
Esophageal candidiasis
- **Adult: IV INFUSION** 150 mg/day given over 1 hr

Candidemia/acute disseminated candidiasis, abscess/peritonitis
- **Adult: IV** 100 mg/day over 1 hr

Prophylaxis for *Candida* infections
- **Adult: IV INFUSION** 50 mg/day given over 1 hr
- **Adolescent/child/infant ≥6 mo (unlabeled): IV INFUSION** 1 mg/kg/day, max 50 mg/day

***Aspergillus* sp. (unlabeled)**
- **Adult: IV INFUSION** 100-150 mg/day × ≥30 days

Available forms: Powder for inj 50 mg, in single-dose vials 50-, 100-mg vial
Administer:
- Do not use if cloudy or precipitated; do not admix; by IV infusion only; product diluted, solution protected from light
- Store at room temperature, away from light, do not freeze; discard unused sol

IV route
- Flush line before and after use with 0.9% NaCl
- **For *Candida* prevention:** reconstitute with provided diluent 0.9% NaCl without bacteriostatic product; 50-mg vial/5 ml (10 mg/ml), swirl to dissolve, do not shake; further dilute with 100 ml 0.9% NaCl only; run over 1 hr
- **For *Candida* infection:** reconstitute with provided diluent 50 mg/5 ml (10 mg/ml); further dilute 3 reconstituted vials in 100 ml 0.9% NaCl, run over 1 hr

Y-site compatibilities: Aminophylline, bumetanide, calcium chloride/gluconate, cycloSPORINE, DOPamine, eptifibatide, esmolol, fenoldopam, furosemide, heparin, HYDROmorphone, lidocaine, LORazepam, magnesium sulfate, milrinone, nitroglycerin, nitroprusside, norepinephrine, phenylephrine, potassium chloride, potassium phosphate, tacrolimus, vasopressin

M

SIDE EFFECTS

CNS: Seizures, dizziness, *headache, somnolence,* fever, anxiety
CV: Flushing, hypertension, phlebitis, tachycardia, atrial fibrillation
GI: Abdominal pain, *nausea, anorexia, vomiting, diarrhea, hyperbilirubinemia,* hepatitis
GU: Renal failure
HEMA: Neutropenia, thrombocytopenia, leukopenia, coagulopathy, anemia, hemolytic anemia
INTEG: *Rash, pruritus, inj-site pain*
META: Hypokalemia, hypocalcemia, hypomagnesemia
MS: *Rigors*

PHARMACOKINETICS

Metabolized in liver; excreted in feces, urine; terminal half-life 14-17.2 hr; protein binding 99%

INTERACTIONS

Increase: plasma concentrations—itraconazole, sirolimus, NIFEdipine; may need dosage reduction

Drug/Lab Test

Increase: ALT/AST, alk phos, bilirubin, potassium, sodium
Decrease: blood glucose

NURSING CONSIDERATIONS

Assess:

- **Infection,** clearing of cultures during treatment; obtain culture at baseline and during treatment; product may be started as soon as culture is taken (esophageal candidiasis); monitor cultures during HSCT for prevention of *Candida* infections
- CBC (RBC, Hct, Hgb), differential, platelet count periodically; notify prescriber of results
- Renal studies: BUN, urine CCr, electrolytes before and during therapy
- Hepatic studies before and during treatment: bilirubin, AST, ALT, alk phos as needed
- **Bleeding:** hematuria, heme-positive stools, bruising, or petechiae, mucosa or orifices; blood dyscrasias can occur
- **For hypersensitivity:** rash, pruritus, facial swelling, phlebitis
- For hemolytic anemia
- **GI symptoms:** frequency of stools, cramping; if severe diarrhea occurs, electrolytes may need to be given

Evaluate:

- Therapeutic response: prevention of *Candida* infection with HSCT or decreased symptoms of *Candida* infection, negative culture

Teach patient/family:

- To notify prescriber if pregnancy is suspected or planned
- To avoid breastfeeding while taking this product
- To inform prescriber of kidney or liver disease
- To report bleeding, facial swelling, wheezing, difficulty breathing, itching, rash, hives, increasing warmth, flushing
- To report signs of infection: increased temperature, sore throat, flulike symptoms
- To notify prescriber of nausea, vomiting, diarrhea, jaundice, anorexia, clay-colored stools, dark urine; heptatotoxicity may occur

miconazole

(mi-kon′a-zole)

Oravig

miconazole nitrate

Desenex, Femizol-M, Fungoid, Lotrimin AF, Micatin, Micozole ✱, Monistat-1, Monistat-3, Monistat-7, M-Zole 3, Vagistat-3

Func. class.: Antifungal
Chem. class.: Imidazole

Do not confuse: miconazole/clotrimazole/metroNIDAZOLE

ACTION: Antifungal activity results from disruption of cell membrane permeability

USES: Treatment of topical fungal infection, vulvovaginal candidiasis; athlete's foot (tinea pedis), jock itch (tinea cruris), and ringworm (tinea corporis)

CONTRAINDICATIONS: Hypersensitivity to this product or imidazoles; pregnancy first trimester (vaginal)
Precautions: Breastfeeding, children

DOSAGE AND ROUTES

Oropharyngeal candidiasis (thrush)

- **Adult/adolescent ≥16 yr: BUCCAL** apply 1 tab (50 mg) to upper gum region, just above incisor daily × 14 days

Tinea corporis, cruris, pedis; cutaneous candidiasis

- **Adult/child >2 yr: TOP** apply bid × 2-4 wk

Tinea versicolor

- **Adult/child >2 yr: TOP** use bid × 2 wk, apply sparingly every day

Vulvovaginal candidiasis

- **Adult/child ≥12 yr: VAG** 1 applicatorful of Monistat-7 (100 mg) or 1 supp (100 mg) at bedtime × 7 days, repeat if needed, or Monistat-3 (200 mg) × 3 days or a 1200 mg supp × 1 day

Available forms: Topical cream, ointment, solution, lotion, powder, aerosol, powder 2%; aerosol spray 2%; vag cream 2, 4%; vag supp 100, 200, 1200 mg; buccal tab 50 mg

Administer:

Transmucosal use (adhesive buccal tablet)

- Apply tab in the morning after brushing the teeth, use dry hands
- Place the rounded surface of the tab against the upper gum just above the incisor tooth, hold in place with slight pressure over the upper lip for 30 sec to assure adhesion
- Although the tab is rounded on one side for comfort, the flat side may also be applied to the gum
- The tab will gradually dissolve
- Administration of subsequent tab should be made to alternate sides of the mouth
- Before applying the next tab, clear away any remaining tab material
- Do not crush, chew, or swallow; food and drink can be taken normally; avoid chewing gum
- If tab does not adhere or falls off within the first 6 hr, the same tab should be repositioned immediately; if the tab still does not adhere, a new tab should be used
- If the tab falls off or is swallowed after it was in place for 6 hr or more, a new tab should not be applied until the next regularly scheduled dose

Topical route

- Topical skin products are not for intravaginal therapy and are for external use only; do not use skin products near the eyes, nose, or mouth
- Wash hands before and after use; wash affected area and gently pat dry
- **Cream/ointment/lotion/solution:** apply a thin film to the cleansed affected area; massage gently into affected areas
- **Solution formulations:** apply a thin film to the cleansed affected area; massage gently into affected areas; if using a solution-soaked pledget, patient may use more than 1 pledget per application as needed to treat affected areas, but each pledget should be used only once and then discarded
- **Intravaginal route:** only use dosage formulations specified for intravaginal use; intravaginal dosage forms are not for topical therapy; do not ingest
- **Suppository:** unwrap vaginal ovule (suppository) before insertion; use applicator(s) supplied by the manufacturer
- **Cream:** use applicator(s) supplied by the manufacturer

SIDE EFFECTS

CNS: Headache
GI: Diarrhea, nausea
GU: Pruritus, irritation, vaginal burning
INTEG: Burning, dermatitis, rash

NURSING CONSIDERATIONS

Assess:

Allergic reaction:

- Assess for hypersensitivity; product may need to be discontinued

Infection:
- Assess for severity of infection

Evaluate:
- Decreasing severity of infection

Teach patient/family:

Topical route
- That topical skin products are not for intravaginal therapy and are for external use only; not to use skin products near the eyes, nose, or mouth
- To wash hands before and after use; wash affected area and gently pat dry
- **Cream/ointment/lotion/solution:** to apply a thin film to the cleansed affected area and massage gently into affected areas
- **Solution formulations:** to shake well before use, apply a thin film to the cleansed affected area, and massage gently into affected areas

Intravaginal route
- To only use dosage formulations specified for intravaginal use; not to ingest intravaginal dosage forms; not to use tampons, douches, spermicides; not to engage in sexual activity; product may damage condoms, diaphragms, cervical caps
- **Suppository:** to unwrap vaginal ovule (suppository) before inserting; to use applicator(s) supplied by the manufacturer
- **Cream:** to use applicator(s) supplied by the manufacturer

HIGH ALERT

midazolam (Rx)

(mid′ay-zoe-lam)

Func. class.: Sedative, hypnotic, antianxiety

Chem. class.: Benzodiazepine, short-acting

Controlled Substance Schedule IV

ACTION:
Depresses subcortical levels in CNS; may act on limbic system, reticular formation; may potentiate γ-aminobutyric acid (GABA) by binding to specific benzodiazepine receptors

USES:
Preoperative sedation, general anesthesia induction, sedation for diagnostic endoscopic procedures, intubation, anxiety

Unlabeled uses: Refractory status epilepticus, alcohol withdrawal, agitation

CONTRAINDICATIONS:
Pregnancy (D), hypersensitivity to benzodiazepines, acute closed-angle glaucoma, epidural/intrathecal use

Precautions: Breastfeeding, children, geriatric patients, COPD, CHF, chronic renal failure, chills, debilitated, hepatic disease, shock, coma, alcohol intoxication, status asthmaticus

Black Box Warning: Neonates (contains benzyl alcohol), IV administration, respiratory depression/insufficiency, specialized care setting, experienced clinician

DOSAGE AND ROUTES

Preoperative sedation/amnesia induction
- **Adult and child ≥12 yr: IM** 0.07-0.08 mg/kg ½-1 hr before general anesthesia
- **Child 6 yr-12 yr: IV** 0.025-0.05 mg/kg; total dose of 0.4 mg/kg may be necessary
- **Child 6 mo-5 yr: IV** 0.05-0.1 mg/kg; total dose of 0.6 mg/kg may be necessary

Induction of general anesthesia
- **Adult >55 yr:** (ASA I/II) **IV** 150-300 mcg/kg over 30 sec; (ASA III/IV) limit dose to 250 mcg/kg (nonpremedicated) or 150 mcg/kg (premedicated)
- **Adult <55 yr: IV** 200-350 mcg/kg over 20-30 sec; if patient has not received premedication, may repeat by giving 20% of original dose; if patient has received premedication, reduce dose by 50 mcg/kg
- **Child:** no safe and effective dose established; however, doses of 50-200 mcg/kg **IV** have been used

Continuous infusion for mechanical ventilation (critical care)
- **Adult: IV** 0.01-0.05 mg/kg over several min; repeat at 10- to 15-min intervals until adequate sedation, then 0.02-0.10 mg/kg/hr maintenance; adjust as needed

• **Child:** IV 0.05-0.2 mg/kg over 2-3 min then 0.06-0.12 mg/kg/hr by cont infusion; adjust as needed
• **Neonate:** IV 0.03 mg/kg/hr, titrate using lowest dose

Status epilepticus (unlabeled)
• **Child and infant >2 mo:** IV 0.15 mg/kg then **CONT IV** 1 mcg/kg/min, titrate upward q5min until seizures controlled

Alcohol withdrawal (unlabeled)
• **Adult:** IV 1-5 mg q1-2hr (mild-moderate symptoms); **CONT IV INFUSION** 1-20 mg q1-2hr (delirium tremens)

Available forms: Inj 1, 5 mg/ml, 25 mg/5 ml, 50 mg/10 ml; syr 2 mg/ml

Administer:
• Store at room temperature; protect from light

PO route
• Remove cap of press-in bottle adaptor, push adaptor into neck of bottle; close with cap; remove cap, insert tip of dispenser, insert into adaptor; turn upside-down, withdraw correct dose; place in mouth

IM route
• IM deep into large muscle mass

IV route
• May be given diluted or undiluted
• After diluting with D_5W or 0.9% NaCl to 0.25 mg/ml; give over 2 min (conscious sedation) or over 30 sec (anesthesia induction)

Y-site compatibilities: Abciximab, acetaminophen, alemtuzumab, alfentamil, amikacin, amiodarone, anidulafungin, argatroban, atracurium, atropine, aztreonam, benzotropine, calcium gluconate, ceFAZolin, cefotaxime, cefOXitine, cefTRIAXone, cimetidine, ciprofloxacin, CISplatin, clindamycin, cloNIDine, cyanocobalamin, cycloSPORINE, DACTINomycin, digoxin, diltiazem, diphenhydrAMINE, DOCEtaxal, DOPamine, doxycyclin, enalaprilat, EPINEPHrine, erythromycin, esmolol, etomidate, etoposide, famotidine, fentaNYL, fluconazole, folic acid, gatifloxacin, gemcitabine, gentamicin, glycopyrrolate, granisetron, heparin, hetastarch, HYDROmorphone, hydrOXYzine, inamrinone, isoproterenol, labetalol, lactated Ringer's, levofloxacin, lidocaine, linezolid, LORazepam, magnesium, mannitol, meperdine, methadone, methyldopa, methylPREDNISolone, metoclopromide, metomolol, metroNIDAZOLE, milrinone, morphine, nalbuphine, naloxone, niCARdipine, nitroglycerin, nitroprusside, norepinephrine, ondansetron, oxacillin, oxytocin, PACLitaxel, palonasetron, pancuronium, papaverin, phytonadione, piperacillin, potassium chloride, propanolol, protamine, pyridoxine, ranitidine, remifentanil, sodium nitroprusside, succinylcholine, SUFentanil, teniposide, theophylline, thiotepa, ticarcillin, tobramycin, vancomycin, vasopressin, vecuronium, verapamil, voriconazole, zoledronic acid

SIDE EFFECTS

CNS: Retrograde amnesia, euphoria, confusion, headache, anxiety, insomnia, slurred speech, paresthesia, tremors, weakness, chills, agitation, paradoxic reactions

CV: Hypotension, PVCs, tachycardia, bigeminy, nodal rhythm, **cardiac arrest**

EENT: Blurred vision, nystagmus, diplopia, loss of balance

GI: *Nausea, vomiting,* increased salivation, hiccups

INTEG: Urticaria; pain, swelling, pruritus at inj site; rash

RESP: Coughing, **apnea, bronchospasm, laryngospasm**, dyspnea, **respiratory depression**

PHARMACOKINETICS

Protein binding 97%; half-life 1-5 hr, metabolized in liver; by CYP3A4 to metabolites excreted in urine; crosses placenta, blood-brain barrier

PO: Onset 10-30 min

IM: Onset 15 min, peak 1/2-1 hr, duration 2-3 hr

IV: Onset 1.5-5 min, onset of anesthesia 1 1/2-2 1/2 min, duration 2 hr

INTERACTIONS

Increase: hypotension—antihypertensives, opiates, alcohol, nitrates

M

Increase: extended half-life—CYP3A4 inhibitors (cimetidine, erythromycin, ranitidine)
Increase: respiratory depression—other CNS depressants, alcohol, barbiturates, opiate analgesics, verapamil, ritonavir, indinavir, fluvoxaMINE, protease inhibitors
Decrease: midazolam metabolism—CYP3A4 inducers (azole antifungals, theophylline)
Drug/Herb
Increase: sedation—kava, valerian
Decrease: midazolam effect—St. John's wort
Drug/Food
Increase: (PO) midazolam effect—grapefruit juice

NURSING CONSIDERATIONS

Assess:

- B/P, pulse, respirations during IV; emergency equipment should be nearby
- Inj site for redness, pain, swelling
- Degree of amnesia in geriatric patients; may be increased
- Anterograde amnesia
- Vital signs for recovery period in obese patients; half-life may be extended

Black Box Warning: **Respiratory depression insufficiency:** apnea, respiratory depression that may be increased in geriatric patients

- Assistance with ambulation until drowsy period ends
- Immediate availability of resuscitation equipment, O_2 to support airway; do not give by rapid bolus

Evaluate:

- Therapeutic response: induction of sedation, general anesthesia

Teach patient/family:

- That amnesia occurs; that events may not be remembered

TREATMENT OF OVERDOSE:

Flumazenil, O_2

miglitol (Rx)

(mig′lih-tol)

Glyset

Func. class.: Oral hypoglycemic
Chem. class.: α-Glucosidase inhibitor

ACTION:
Delays digestion and absorption of ingested carbohydrates, which results in a smaller rise in blood glucose after meals; does not increase insulin production

USES:
Type 2 diabetes mellitus
Unlabeled uses: Type 1 diabetes mellitus

CONTRAINDICATIONS:
Hypersensitivity, diabetic ketoacidosis, cirrhosis, inflammatory bowel disease, colonic ulceration, partial intestinal obstruction, chronic intestinal disease, ileus
Precautions: Pregnancy (B), breastfeeding, children, diarrhea, hiatal hernia, hypoglycemia, renal disease, type 1 diabetes, vomiting

DOSAGE AND ROUTES

- **Adult: PO** 25 mg tid initially, with 1st bite of meal; maintenance dose may be increased to 50 mg tid; may be increased to 100 mg tid if needed with dosage adjustment at 4- to 8-wk intervals

Available forms: Tabs 25, 50, 100 mg
Administer:

- Tid with first bite of each meal
- Store in tight container at room temperature

SIDE EFFECTS

GI: *Abdominal pain, diarrhea, flatulence,* hepatotoxicity
HEMA: Low iron
INTEG: Rash
RESP: Pneumatosis cystoides, intestinalis

PHARMACOKINETICS

Peak 2-3 hr, not metabolized, excreted in urine as unchanged product, half-life 2 hr

INTERACTIONS

Decrease: levels of digoxin, propranolol, ranitidine

Decrease: miglitol levels—digestive enzymes, intestinal adsorbents; do not use together

Drug/Food

Increase: diarrhea—carbohydrates

NURSING CONSIDERATIONS

Assess:

- **Hypo/hyperglycemia;** even though product does not cause hypoglycemia, if patient receiving sulfonylureas or insulin, hypoglycemia may be additive (rare)
- Blood glucose levels, hemoglobin, A1c, LFTs; if hypoglycemia occurs with monotherapy, treat with glucose

Evaluate:

- Therapeutic response: decreased signs, symptoms of diabetes mellitus (polyuria, polydipsia, polyphagia; clear sensorium, absence of dizziness; stable gait); improved blood glucose, A1c

Teach patient/family:

- About the symptoms of hypo/hyperglycemia; what to do about each; that, during periods of stress, infection, or surgery, insulin may be required
- That medication must be taken as prescribed; about consequences of discontinuing medication abruptly
- To avoid OTC medications unless approved by health care provider
- That diabetes is lifelong; that product is not a cure
- To carry ID for emergency purposes
- That diet and exercise regimen must be followed
- About GI side effects

⚠ HIGH ALERT

milrinone (Rx)

(mill′rih-nohn)

Func. class.: Inotropic/vasodilator agent with phosphodiesterase activity

Chem. class.: Bipyridine derivative

ACTION: Positive inotropic agent; increases contractility of cardiac muscle with vasodilator properties; reduces preload and afterload by direct relaxation on vascular smooth muscle

USES: Short-term management of advanced heart failure that has not responded to other medication

Unlabeled uses: Adolescents, children, infants

CONTRAINDICATIONS: Hypersensitivity to this product, severe aortic disease, severe pulmonic valvular disease, acute MI

Precautions: Pregnancy (C), breastfeeding, children, geriatric patients, renal/hepatic disease, atrial flutter/fibrillation

DOSAGE AND ROUTES

- **Adult: IV BOL** 50 mcg/kg given over 10 min; start infusion of 0.375-0.75 mcg/kg/min
- **Adolescent/child/infant (unlabeled): IV** 50 mcg/kg over 10-60 min, then 0.5-0.75 mcg/kg/min

Renal dose

- **Adult: IV** CCr 41-50 ml/min, 0.43 mcg/kg/min, titrate up; CCr 31-40 ml/min, 0.38 mcg/kg/min, titrate up; CCr 21-30 ml/min, 0.33 mcg/kg/min, titrate up; CCr 11-20 ml/min, 0.28 mcg/kg/min; CCr 6-10 ml/min, 0.23 mcg/kg/min; CCr $\leq$5 ml/min, 0.20 mcg/kg/min; max for all doses 0.75 mcg/kg/min

Available forms: Inj 1 mg/ml; premixed inj 200 mcg/ml in D_5W

Administer:

- Potassium supplements if ordered for potassium levels <3 mg/dl

M

Direct IV route
- Give IV loading dose undiluted over 10 min, use infusion device

Continuous IV route
- Dilute 20-mg vial with 80, 113, 180 ml of 0.45% NaCl, 0.9% NaCl, or D_5W to a concentration of 200, 150, 100 mcg/ml, respectively
- Titrate rate based on hemodynamic and clinical response, use infusion device
- Precipitation will form when furosemide is injected into line with milrinone

Y-site compatibilities: Acyclovir, alfentanil, allopurinol, amifostine, amikacin, aminocaproic acid, aminophylline, amiodarone, amphotericin B liposome, ampicillin, ampicillin-sulbactam, anidulafungin, argatroban, atenolol, atracurium, aztreonam, bivalirudin, bleomycin, bumetanide, buprenorphine, busulfan, butorphanol, calcium chloride/gluconate, CARBOplatin, caspofungin, ceFAZolin, cefepime, cefotaxime, cefoTEtan, cefOXitin, cefTAZidime, ceftizoxime, cefTRIAXone, cefuroxime, chloramphenicol, chlorproMAZINE, cimetidine, ciprofloxacin, cisatracurium, CISplatin, clindamycin, cyclophosphamide, cycloSPORINE, cytarabine, DACTINomycin, DAPTOmycin, dexamethasone, digoxin, diltiazem, DOBUTamine, DOCEtaxel, DOPamine, doripenem, doxacurium, DOXOrubicin, doxycycline, droperidol, enalaprilat, ePHEDrine, EPINEPHrine, epirubicin, eptifibatide, ertapenem, erythromycin, etoposide, famotidine, fenoldopam, fentaNYL, fluconazole, fludarabine, fluorouracil, gallium, ganciclovir, gatifloxacin, gemcitabine, gentamicin, glycopyrrolate, granisetron, haloperidol, heparin, hydrALAZINE, hydrocortisone, HYDROmorphone, IDArubicin, ifosfamide, insulin (regular), irinotecan, isoproterenol, ketorolac, labetalol, levofloxacin, linezolid, LORazepam, magnesium sulfate, mannitol, mechlorethamine, melphalan, meperidine, meropenem, methohexital, methotrexate, methyldopate, methylPREDNISolone, metoclopramide, metoprolol, metroNIDAZOLE, micafungin, midazolam, mitoXANtrone, morphine, mycophenolate, nafcillin, nalbuphine, naloxone, nesiritide, niCARdipine, nitroglycerin, nitroprusside, norepinephrine, octreotide, oxacillin, oxaliplatin, oxytocin, PACLitaxel, palonosetron, pamidronate, pancuronium, PEMEtrexed, pentamidine, pentazocine, PENTobarbital, PHENobarbital, phenylephrine, piperacillin, piperacillin-tazobactam, polymyxin B, potassium chloride/phosphates, prochlorperazine, promethazine, propofol, propranolol, quiNIDine, quinupristin-dalfopristin, ranitidine, remifentanil, rocuronium, sodium acetate/bicarbonate/phosphates, streptozocin, succinylcholine, SUFentanil, sulfamethoxazole-trimethoprim, tacrolimus, teniposide, theophylline, thiopental, thiotepa, ticarcillin, ticarcillin-clavulanate, tigecycline, tirofiban, tobramycin, torsemide, vancomycin, vasopressin, vecuronium, verapamil, vinCRIStine, vinorelbine, voriconazole, zidovudine, zoledronic acid

SIDE EFFECTS

CV: **Dysrhythmias,** hypotension, chest pain, *PVCs*

GI: Nausea, vomiting, anorexia, abdominal pain, **hepatotoxicity, jaundice**

HEMA: **Thrombocytopenia**

MISC: Headache, hypokalemia, tremor, inj site reactions

PHARMACOKINETICS

IV: Onset 2-5 min, peak 10 min, duration variable; terminal half-life 2.3 hr; metabolized in liver; excreted in urine as product (83%), metabolites (12%)

INTERACTIONS

Increase: effects of antihypertensives, diuretics

NURSING CONSIDERATIONS

Assess:

⚠ **ECG continuously during IV; ventricular dysrhythmia can occur**

- B/P, pulse q5min during infusion; if B/P drops 30 mm Hg, stop infusion, call prescriber

- Electrolytes: potassium, sodium, chloride, calcium; renal studies: BUN, creatinine; blood studies: platelet count
- ALT, AST, bilirubin daily
- I&O ratio, weight daily; diuresis should increase with continuing therapy
- If platelets are <150,000/mm³, product is usually discontinued and another product started

Evaluate:

- Therapeutic response: increased cardiac output, decreased PCWP, adequate CVP; decreased dyspnea, fatigue, edema, ECG

Teach patient/family:

- To report angina immediately during infusion
- To report headache, which can be treated with analgesics

TREATMENT OF OVERDOSE:
Discontinue product, support circulation

minocycline (Rx)
(min-oh-sye′kleen)

Arestin, Dynacin, Minocin, Solodyn

Func. class.: Broad-spectrum antiinfective

Chem. class.: Tetracycline

ACTION: Inhibits protein synthesis, phosphorylation in microorganisms by binding to ribosomal subunits, reversibly binding to ribosomal subunits; bacteriostatic

USES: Syphilis, *Chlamydia trachomatis*, gonorrhea, lymphogranuloma venereum, rickettsial infections, inflammatory acne, *Neisseria meningitidis, Neisseria gonorrhoeae, Treponema pallidum, Chlamydia trachomatis, Ureaplasma urealyticum, Mycoplasma pneumoniae, Nocardia*, periodontitis, methicillin-resistant *S. aureus* (MRSA) infection, nonnodular moderate to severe acne vulgaris, *Rickettsia* sp.

Unlabeled uses: Rheumatoid arthritis, bullous pemphigoid, dental infection, prostatis, pleural effusion

CONTRAINDICATIONS: Pregnancy (D), children <8 yr, hypersensitivity to tetracyclines

Precautions: Hepatic disease, breastfeeding

DOSAGE AND ROUTES

- **Adult: PO/IV** 200 mg, then 100 mg q12hr, max 400 mg/24 hr **IV; SUBGINGIVAL** inserted into periodontal pocket
- **Child >8 yr: PO/IV** 4 mg/kg, then 4 mg/kg/day **PO** in divided doses q12hr

Rickettsial infections

- **Adult: PO/IV** 200 mg, then 100 mg q12hr
- **Child ≥8 yr/adolescent: PO/IV** 4 mg/kg, then 2 mg/kg q12hr, max adult dose

Gonorrhea

- **Adult: PO** 200 mg, then 100 mg q12hr × ≥4 days

Syphilis

- **Adult: PO** 200 mg, then 100 mg q12hr × 10-15 days

Uncomplicated gonococcal urethritis in men

- **Adult: PO** 100 mg q12hr × 5 days

Acne vulgaris (Solodyn only)

- **Adult/adolescent/child ≥12 yr:** ext rel 1 mg/kg/day × 12 wk or those weighing 126-136 kg—135 mg/day; 111-125 kg—115 mg/day; 97-110 kg—105 mg/day; 85-96 kg—90 mg/day; 72-84 kg—80 mg/day; 60-71 kg—65 mg/day; 50-59 kg—55 mg/day; 45-49 kg—45 mg/day

Acne vulgaris (all except Solodyn)

- **Adult/adolescent/child ≥12 yr:** ext rel 1 mg/kg × 12 wk or 91-136 kg, 135 mg/day; 60-90 kg, 90 mg/day; 45-59 kg, 45 mg/day

Rheumatoid arthritis (unlabeled)

- **Adult: PO** 100 mg bid for ≤48 wk

Bullous pemphigus (unlabeled)

- **Adult: PO** 50 mg/day; may increase to 100 mg/day after 1-2 wk

Available forms: Caps 50, 75, 100 mg; powder for inj 100 mg; caps, pellet filled 50, 100 mg; tabs 50, 75, 100 mg; ext rel tabs 45, 55, 65, 80, 90, 105, 115, 135 mg

Administer:

- After C&S obtained
- Store in airtight, light-resistant container at room temperature

M

PO route

- With full glass of water; with food for GI symptoms
- 2 hr before or after laxative or ferrous products; 3 hr after antacid

IV route

- After diluting 100 mg/5 ml sterile water for inj; further dilute in 500-1000 ml of NaCl, dextrose sol, LR, Ringer's sol; run 100 mg/6 hr

Y-site compatibilities: Alfentanil, amikacin, atracurium, benztropine, buprenorphine, butorphanol, calcium chloride, CARBOplatin, caspofungin, cefonicid, chlorproMAZINE, cimetidine, cisatracurium, codeine, cyclophosphamide, cycloSPORINE, cytarabine, DACTINomycin, dexmedetomidine, diltiazem, diphenhydrAMINE, DOBUTamine, DOCEtaxel, doxacurium, doxycycline, enalaprilat, ePHEDrine, EPINEPHrine, eptifibatide, etoposide, fenoldopam, fentaNYL, filgrastim, fludarabine, gatafloxacin, gemcitabine, gentamicin, glycopyrrolate, granisetron, heparin, hetastarch, IDArubicin, ifosfamide, inamrinone, isoproterenol, labetalol, levofloxacin, lidocaine, linezolid, LORazepam, magnesium sulfate, mannitol, melphalan, metaraminol, methotrexate, methyldopa, metoclopramide, metoprolol, midazolam, mitoXANtrone, nalbuphine, naloxone, perphenazine, potassium chloride, remifentanil, sargramostim, teniposide, vinorelbine, vit B/C

SIDE EFFECTS

CNS: *Dizziness*, fever, lightheadedness, vertigo, **seizures, increased intracranial pressure**

CV: Pericarditis

EENT: Dysphagia, glossitis, decreased calcification of deciduous teeth, permanent discoloration of teeth, oral candidiasis

GI: *Nausea,* abdominal pain, *vomiting, diarrhea,* anorexia, enterocolitis, **hepatotoxicity,** flatulence, abdominal cramps, epigastric burning, stomatitis, **pseudomembranous colitis**

GU: *Increased BUN,* polyuria, polydipsia, **renal failure, nephrotoxicity**

HEMA: **Eosinophilia, neutropenia, thrombocytopenia, hemolytic anemia, pancytopenia**

INTEG: *Rash, urticaria, photosensitivity, increased pigmentation,* **exfoliative dermatitis,** pruritus, blue-gray color of skin, mucous membranes

MS: Myalgia, arthritis, bone discoloration, joint stiffness

SYST: **Angioedema, Stevens-Johnson syndrome**

PHARMACOKINETICS

PO: Peak 1-4 hr, half-life 11-22 hr; excreted in urine, feces, breast milk; crosses placenta

INTERACTIONS

Increase: effect of warfarin, digoxin, insulin, oral anticoagulants, theophylline, neuromuscular blockers

Increase: chance of pseudomotor cerebri—retinoids; do not use concurrently

Decrease: effect of minocycline—antacids, sodium bicarbonate, alkali products, iron, kaolin/pectin, cimetidine, quinapril, sucralfate

Decrease: effect of barbiturates, carBAMazepine, phenytoin, penicillins, oral contraceptives, calcium

Drug/Lab Test

False negative: urine glucose with Clinistix or Tes-Tape

NURSING CONSIDERATIONS

Assess:

⚠ **Pseudomembranous colitis: diarrhea, abdominal cramps, fever; may start up to 2 mo after treatment ends**

- I&O ratio
- Age and tooth development
- Blood tests: PT, CBC, AST, ALT, BUN, creatinine
- Signs of anemia: Hct, Hgb, fatigue

⚠ **Allergic reactions: rash, itching, pruritus, angioedema**

- Nausea, vomiting, diarrhea; administer antiemetic, antacids as ordered

⚠ **Overgrowth of infection: fever, malaise, redness, pain, swelling, drainage,** perineal itching, diarrhea; changes in cough or sputum; black, furry tongue

Evaluate:

- Therapeutic response: decreased temperature, absence of lesions, negative C&S

Teach patient/family:

- To avoid sunlight, wear protective clothing; sunscreen does not seem to decrease photosensitivity
- That all prescribed medication must be taken to prevent superinfection; not to use outdated product because Fanconi's syndrome may occur
- To avoid taking antacids, iron, cimetidine; use 2 hr before, 6 hr after this product; absorption may be decreased
- That teeth discoloration, joint or muscle pain may occur

minoxidil (Rx, OTC)

(mi-nox′i-dill)

Rogaine (topical)

Func. class.: Antihypertensive

Chem. class.: Vasodilator, peripheral

Do not confuse:

minoxidil/Monopril

ACTION: Directly relaxes arteriolar smooth muscle, causing vasodilation; reduces peripheral vascular resistance, decreases B/P

USES: Severe hypertension unresponsive to other therapy (use with diuretic and β-blocker); topically to treat alopecia

Unlabeled uses: Scleroderma renal crisis (SRC) to control hypertension, anal fissures

CONTRAINDICATIONS: Dissecting aortic aneurysm, hypersensitivity, pheochromocytoma

Black Box Warning: Acute MI

Precautions: Pregnancy (C), breastfeeding, children, geriatric patients, renal disease, CVD

Black Box Warning: CAD, CHF, cardiac disease, cardiac tamponade, edema, hypotension, orthostatic hypotension, pericardial effusion

DOSAGE AND ROUTES

Severe hypertension

- **Adult: PO** 5 mg/day in 1-2 divided doses; max 100 mg/day; usual range 10-40 mg/day divided in 1-2 doses
- **Geriatric: PO** 2.5 mg/day, may be increased gradually
- **Child <12 yr: PO** (initial) 0.1-0.2 mg/kg/day; (effective range) 0.25-1 mg/kg/day; (max) 50 mg/day

Alopecia

- **Adult: TOP** 1 ml bid, rub into scalp daily, max 2 ml/day

Renal dose

- **Adult: PO** CCr 10-15 ml/min extend interval to q24hr; CCr <10 ml/min not recommended

Anal fissures (unlabeled)

- **Adult/adolescent: TOP** (0.5% minoxidil in white paraffin base) 0.5 g each compounded minoxidil and lignocaine ointment q8hr

Scleroderma renal crisis (unlabeled)

- **Adult: PO** 5 mg/day in 1-2 divided doses, increase after 3 days by 10-20 mg/day to reach desired B/P, max 100 mg/day

Available forms: Tabs 2.5, 10 mg; topical 2%, 5% sol; topical foam 5%

Administer:

- Store protected from light and heat

PO route

- Without regard to meals
- With β-blocker and/or diuretic for hypertension

Topical route

- 1 ml no matter how much balding has occurred; increasing dosage does not speed growth

SIDE EFFECTS

Systemic

CNS: Headache, fatigue

CV: *Severe rebound hypertension on withdrawal in children,* tachycardia,

M

angina, increased T wave, **CHF, pulmonary edema, pericardial effusion**, edema, sodium, water retention, *hypotension*
GI: Nausea, vomiting
GU: Breast tenderness
HEMA: Hct, Hgb; erythrocyte count may decrease initially, leukopenia
INTEG: Pruritus, **Stevens-Johnson syndrome**, rash, hirsutism, contact dermatitis

PHARMACOKINETICS

PO: Onset 30 min, peak 2-3 hr, duration 48-120 hr; half-life 4.2 hr; metabolized in liver; metabolites excreted in urine, feces; protein binding minimal

INTERACTIONS

Increase: hypotension—antihypertensives, MAOIs
Decrease: antihypertensive effect—NSAIDs, salicylates, estrogens

Drug/Herb

Increase: antihypertensive effect—hawthorn

Drug/Lab Test

Increase: renal studies
Decrease: Hgb/Hct/RBC

NURSING CONSIDERATIONS

Assess:

⚠ **Monitor closely; usually given with β-blocker to prevent tachycardia and increased myocardial workload; usually given with diuretic to prevent serious fluid accumulation; patient should be hospitalized during beginning treatment**

- Nausea, edema in feet, legs daily
- Skin turgor, dryness of mucous membranes for hydration status
- Crackles, dyspnea, orthopnea
- Electrolytes: potassium, sodium, chloride, CO_2
- Renal studies: catecholamines, BUN, creatinine
- Hepatic studies: AST, ALT, alk phos
- B/P, pulse
- Weight daily, I&O

Evaluate:

- Therapeutic response: decreased B/P, increased hair growth

Teach patient/family:

- That body hair will increase but is reversible after discontinuing treatment
- Not to discontinue product abruptly
- To report pitting edema, dizziness, weight gain >5 lb, SOB, bruising or bleeding, heart rate >20 beats/min over normal, severe indigestion, dizziness, lightheadedness, panting, new or aggravated symptoms of angina
- To take product exactly as prescribed because serious side effects may occur

Topical

- That for topical use, treatment must continue for the long term, or new hair will be lost
- Not to use except on scalp; use on clean, dry scalp before styling aids; wash hands after each use

TREATMENT OF OVERDOSE:

Administer normal saline IV, vasopressors

mipomersen

(mye′poe-mer-sen)

Kynamro

Func. class.: Antilipemics
Chem. class.: Antisense oligonucleotide

ACTION: Inhibits synthesis of the principal apolipoprotein of LDL, VLDL, binds to messenger ribonucleic acid (mRNA)

USES: Decreasing LDL, total cholesterol, apolipoprotein B, non-high density lipoprotein cholesterol to reduce LDL, total cholesterol, apolipoprotein B, non-high density lipoprotein cholesterol (homozygous familial hypercholesterolemia)

CONTRAINDICATIONS:

Black Box Warning: Hepatic disease

Precautions: Pregnancy (B), breastfeeding, dialysis, alcohol ingestion, geriatric patients, proteinuria, renal disease, low density lipoprotein apheresis

DOSAGE AND ROUTES

Homozygous familial hypercholesterolemia

- **Adult: SUBCUT** 200 mg weekly

Renal/hepatic dose

- **Adult: SUBCUT** do not use in severe renal, hepatic disease

Available forms: Solution for injection 200 mg/ml

Administer:

- Give on the same day weekly; if a dose is missed, give ≥3 days from the next weekly dose
- Monitor ALT, AST, alkaline phosphatase, and total bilirubin before start of therapy; monitor lipid levels ≥q3-4mo for the first year
- Monitor LDL-C level after 6 mo
- Dose adjustments for elevated transaminases during treatment
- ALT or AST ≥3× and <5× ULN: confirm elevation with a repeat test within 1 wk; if confirmed, withhold product; obtain other tests if not already obtained (total bilirubin, alkaline phosphatase, INR) to identify the probable cause; if resuming product after transaminases resolve to <3× ULN, consider monitor liver-related tests more frequently
- ALT or AST ≥5× ULN: withhold, obtain additional liver-related tests if not already obtained (total bilirubin, alkaline phosphatase, INR), and identify the probable cause; if resuming product after transaminases resolve to <3× ULN, monitor liver-related tests more frequently

SIDE EFFECTS

CNS: Fatigue, headache, fever
CV: Hypertension, palpitations
GI: Abdominal pain, vomiting
GU: Glomerulonephritis, proteinuria
MS: Musculoskeletal pain
SYST: Angioedema

PHARMACOKINETICS

Half-life 1-2 mo protein binding >90%

INTERACTIONS

Increase: hepatotoxicity risk—acetaminophen, methotrexate, tetracyclines, tamoxifen

NURSING CONSIDERATIONS

Assess:

- Determine if the LDL-C reduction achieved is sufficient to warrant the potential risk of liver toxicity
- Assess geriatric patients: increased risk for hypertension, peripheral edema, hepatic steatosis
- Hypercholesterolemia: diet history: fat content, lipid levels (triglycerides, LDL, HDL, cholesterol); LFTs are at baseline, periodically during treatment

Evaluate:

- Therapeutic response: decreasing LDL, total cholesterol, apolipoprotein B, non-high density lipoprotein cholesterol

Teach patient/family:

- That compliance is needed
- That risk factors should be decreased: high fat diet, smoking, alcohol consumption, absence of exercise
- To notify prescriber if pregnancy is suspected, planned, or if breastfeeding
- To notify prescriber of dietary/herbal supplements

mirabegron

(mir′a-beg′ron)

Myrbetriq

Func. class.: Bladder antispasmodic
Chem. class.: β_3-Adrenergic receptor agonist

ACTION: Relaxes smooth muscles in urinary tract

USES: Overactive bladder (urinary frequency, urgency), urinary incontinence

CONTRAINDICATIONS: Hypersensitivity

Precautions: Pregnancy (C), breastfeeding, children, kidney/liver disease, bladder obstruction, dialysis, hypertension

DOSAGE AND ROUTES

• **Adult: PO** 25 mg/day, may increase to 50 mg/day if needed

Hepatic/renal dose

⚠ **PO** Child–Pugh B or (CCr 15-29 ml/min, max 25 mg/day; Child–Pugh C or CCr <15 ml/min, not recommended

Available forms: Tabs ext rel 25, 50 mg

Administer:

• Give whole; take with liquids; do not crush, chew, or break ext rel product; use without regard to meals

SIDE EFFECTS

CNS: Fatigue, dizziness, headache

CV: Hypertension

EENT: Xerophthalmia, blurred vision

GI: Nausea, vomiting, anorexia, abdominal pain, constipation, diarrhea, dyspepsia

GU: Dysuria, urinary retention, frequency, UTI, bladder discomfort

INTEG: Rash, pruritus

MISC: Arthralgia, back pain

RESP: Pharyngitis

SYST: Stevens–Johnson syndrome

PHARMACOKINETICS

71% protein binding, excretion 25% unchanged in urine, terminal half-life 50 hr, peak 3.5 hr

INTERACTIONS

Increase: mirabegron effect—CYP3A4 inhibitors

Increase: effect of CYP2D6 substrates

Increase: effect of digoxin, warfarin, desipramine, thioridazine, flecainide, propafenone

Increase: risk of urinary retention with antimuscarinic agents (e.g., atropine, scopolamine)

NURSING CONSIDERATIONS

Assess:

• Urinary patterns: distention, nocturia, frequency, urgency, incontinence

• LFTs at baseline, periodically

• Monitor B/P

Evaluate:

• Decreasing dysuria, frequency, nocturia, incontinence

Teach patient/family:

• To avoid hazardous activities; dizziness can occur

• Not to drink liquids before bedtime

• About the importance of bladder maintenance

mirtazapine (Rx)

(mer-ta′za-peen)

Remeron, Remeron Soltab

Func. class.: Antidepressant

Chem. class.: Tetracyclic

ACTION:

Blocks reuptake of norepinephrine and serotonin into nerve endings, thereby increasing action of norepinephrine and serotonin in nerve cells; antagonist of central α_2-receptors; blocks histamine receptors

USES:

Depression; dysthymic disorder; bipolar disorder: depressed, agitated depression

Unlabeled uses: Resting tremor, benign familial tremor, levodopa-induced dyskinesias, pruritus

CONTRAINDICATIONS:

Hypersensitivity to tricyclics, recovery phase of MI, agranulocytosis, jaundice

Precautions: Pregnancy (C), geriatric patients, suicidal patients, severe depression, increased intraocular pressure, closed-angle glaucoma, urinary retention, cardiac/renal/hepatic disease, hypo/hyperthyroidism, electroshock therapy, elective surgery, seizure disorder, bone marrow suppression, thrombocytopenia

Black Box Warning: Suicidal ideation, children

DOSAGE AND ROUTES

• **Adult: PO** 15 mg/day at bedtime, maintenance to continue for 6 mo, titrate up to

45 mg/day; **ORALLY DISINTEGRATING** tabs: open blister pack, place tab on tongue, allow to disintegrate, swallow

- **Geriatric: PO** 7.5 mg at bedtime, increase by 7.5 mg q1-2wk to desired dose, max 45 mg/day

Resting tremor/benign familial tremor/levodopa-induced dyskinesias (unlabeled)

- **Adult: PO** titrate up to 30 mg at bedtime

Pruritus (unlabeled)

- **Adult: PO** 15-30 mg/day

Available forms: Tabs 7.5, 15, 30, 45 mg; orally disintegrating tab (Soltab) 15, 30, 45 mg

Administer:

- Increased fluids, bulk in diet for constipation, especially for geriatric patients
- Without regard to meals
- Dosage at bedtime if oversedation occurs during day; may take entire dose at bedtime; geriatric patients may not tolerate once-daily dosing
- Gum, hard candy, or frequent sips of water for dry mouth
- Store in tight container at room temperature; do not freeze
- **Orally disintegrating tab:** no water needed; allow to dissolve on tongue, do not split; contains phenylalanine

SIDE EFFECTS

CNS: *Dizziness, drowsiness,* confusion, headache, anxiety, tremors, stimulation, weakness, nightmares, EPS (geriatric patients), increased psychiatric symptoms, **seizures,** abnormal dreams

CV: *Orthostatic hypotension, ECG changes,* tachycardia, **hypertension,** palpitations

EENT: *Blurred vision,* tinnitus, mydriasis

GI: *Diarrhea, dry mouth,* nausea, vomiting, **paralytic ileus,** increased appetite, cramps, epigastric distress, constipation, **jaundice, hepatitis,** stomatitis, weight gain

GU: *Urinary retention,* **acute renal failure,** urinary frequency

HEMA: **Agranulocytosis, thrombocytopenia, eosinophilia, leukopenia**

INTEG: Rash, urticaria, sweating, pruritus, photosensitivity

MS: Back pain, myalgia

RESP: Cough

SYST: Flulike symptoms, increased lipid levels

PHARMACOKINETICS

PO: Peak 2 hr, metabolized by CYP1A2, 2D6, 3A4 in liver; excreted in urine, feces; crosses placenta; half-life 20-40 hr, protein binding 85%

INTERACTIONS

⚠ **Increase: hyperpyretic crisis, seizures, hypertensive episode—MAOIs**

Increase: CNS depression—alcohol, barbiturates, benzodiazepines, other CNS depressants

Increase: serotonin syndrome—SSRIs, SNRIs, serotonin-receptor agonists, fenfluramine, dexfenfluramine, sibutramine, nefazodone

Decrease: effects of cloNIDine, indirect-acting sympathomimetics (ePHEDrine)

Drug/Herb

- **Serotonin syndrome: St. John's wort**

Increase: CNS depression—kava

Drug/Lab Test

Increase: serum bilirubin, blood glucose, alk phos

Decrease: VMA, 5-HIAA

False increase: urinary catecholamines

NURSING CONSIDERATIONS

Assess:

- B/P (lying, standing), pulse q4hr; if systolic B/P drops 20 mm Hg, hold product, notify prescriber; vital signs q4hr in patients with CV disease
- Blood studies: CBC, leukocytes, differential, cardiac enzymes, lipid profile, blood glucose, LFTs, serum creatinine/BUN if patient is receiving long-term therapy
- Weight weekly; appetite may increase with product
- **ECG for flattening of T wave, bundle branch block, AV block, dysrhythmias in cardiac patients**

M

Black Box Warning: Mental status: mood, sensorium, affect, suicidal tendencies (especially among adolescents, young adults), increase in psychiatric symptoms: depression, panic; EPS primarily in geriatric patients: rigidity, dystonia, akathisia

⚠ **Serotonin syndrome:** hyperthermia, hypertension, myoclonus, rigidity, delirium, coma; if using other serotonergic products

- Alcohol consumption; if alcohol consumed, hold dose until morning
- Assistance with ambulation during beginning therapy, since drowsiness, dizziness occurs

Evaluate:

- Therapeutic response: decreased depression

Teach patient/family:

- That therapeutic effects may take 2-3 wk; to take at bedtime; that there is decreased sedation with increased doses; not to discontinue abruptly
- To use caution when driving, performing other activities requiring alertness because of drowsiness, dizziness, blurred vision
- To avoid alcohol, other CNS depressants
- About how to take orally disintegrating tabs; dissolve on tongue, swallow
- Not to use within 14 days of MAOIs

Black Box Warning: To notify prescriber of suicidal thoughts, behavior

TREATMENT OF OVERDOSE:
ECG monitoring, lavage, activated charcoal; administer anticonvulsant, IV fluids

misoprostol (Rx)
(mye-soe-prost′ole)

Cytotec

Func. class.: Gastric mucosa protectant, antiulcer

Chem. class.: Prostaglandin E_1 analog

Do not confuse:
misoprostol/metoprolol
Cytotec/Cytoxan

ACTION:
Inhibits gastric acid secretion; may protect gastric mucosa; can increase bicarbonate, mucous production

USES:
Prevention of NSAID-induced gastric ulcers

Unlabeled uses: Pregnancy termination, postpartum hemorrhage, cervical ripening/labor induction (vaginal), active duodenal/gastric ulcer, kidney transplant rejection prophylaxis

CONTRAINDICATIONS:
Hypersensitivity to this product or prostaglandins

Black Box Warning: Pregnancy (X), females

Precautions: Breastfeeding, children, geriatric patients, renal/CV disease, abnormal fetal position, cardiac/renal/inflammatory bowel disease, C-section, dehydration, diarrhea, fever, ectopic pregnancy, fetal distress, sepsis, vaginal bleeding

DOSAGE AND ROUTES

- **Adult: PO** 200 mcg qid with food for duration of NSAID therapy, with last dose given at bedtime; if 200 mcg is not tolerated, 100 mcg may be given

Active duodenal/gastric ulcer (unlabeled)

- **Adult: PO** 100-200 mcg qid with meals at bedtime × 4-8 wk

Pregnancy termination before 63rd day (unlabeled)

- **Adult: INTRAVAGINALLY** 800 mcg 5-7 days after methotrexate IM

Cervical ripening induction for term pregnancy (unlabeled)

- **Adult: INTRAVAGINALLY** 25 mcg q3-6hr

Available forms: Tabs 100, 200 mcg

Administer:

- PO with meals for prolonged product effect; avoid use of magnesium antacids
- Store at room temperature

SIDE EFFECTS

GI: *Diarrhea,* nausea, vomiting, flatulence, constipation, dyspepsia, abdominal pain
GU: Spotting, cramps, hypermenorrhea, menstrual disorders

PHARMACOKINETICS

PO: Peak 12 min, plasma steady-state achieved within 2 days, excreted in urine

INTERACTIONS

Drug/Food
Decrease: maximum concentrations when taken with food

NURSING CONSIDERATIONS

Assess:
• **NSAID-induced ulcer prophylaxis:** monitor GI symptoms (hematemesis, occult or frank blood in stools, gastric aspirate, cramping, severe diarrhea)

Black Box Warning: Pregnancy (X): Obtain a negative pregnancy test; miscarriages are common

Evaluate:
• Therapeutic response: absence of pain or GI complaints; prevention of ulcers
Teach patient/family:
• To take only as directed; to read patient information leaflet

Black Box Warning: Not to take if pregnant (can cause miscarriage) (X); not to become pregnant while taking product; if pregnancy occurs during therapy, discontinue product, notify prescriber; not to breastfeed

• Not to give product to anyone else or to take for more than 4 wk unless directed by prescriber
• To avoid OTC preparations: aspirin, cough, cold products; condition may worsen

⚠ HIGH ALERT

mitoMYcin (Rx)

(mye-toe-mye′sin)

Mitosol

Func. class.: Antineoplastic, antibiotic

Do not confuse:
mitoMYcin/mithramycin/mitotane/mitoXANtrone

ACTION: Inhibits DNA synthesis, primarily; derived from *Streptomyces caespitosus;* appears to cause cross-linking of DNA; vesicant

USES: Pancreatic, stomach, colorectal, bladder cancer
Unlabeled uses: Palliative treatment of anal, bladder, head, neck, colon, breast, biliary, cervical, lung malignancies; bone marrow ablation, desmoid tumor, mesothelioma, stem cell transplant preparation

CONTRAINDICATIONS: Pregnancy (D) 1st trimester, breastfeeding, hypersensitivity, as single agent, coagulation disorders

Black Box Warning: Thrombocytopenia

Precautions: Accidental exposure, acute bronchospasm, anemia, children, dental disease/work, extravasation, females, infection, radiation therapy, surgery, vaccines, renal/respiratory disease

Black Box Warning: Bone marrow suppression, hemolytic-uremic syndrome

DOSAGE AND ROUTES

• **Adult: IV** 20 mg/m^2 q6-8wk
Available forms: Inj 5, 20, 40 mg/vial
Administer:
Direct IV route
• Use port or central line if possible
• Antiemetic 30-60 min before product to prevent vomiting

M

- IV after diluting 5 mg/10 ml, 20 mg/ 40 ml, 40 mg/80 ml (0.5 mg/ml) sterile water for inj; shake, allow to stand, give through Y-tube or 3-way stopcock; give slow IV push or infuse over 15-30 min; color of reconstituted sol is gray
- Avoid excessive heat; store reconstituted product in refrigerator; discard after 2 wk; store unreconstituted product at room temperature

Y-site compatibilities: Amifostine, amphotericin B lipid complex, amphotericin B liposome, anidulafungin, argatroban, atenolol, bivalirudin, bleomycin, caspofungin, CISplatin, cyclophosphamide, DACTINomycin, dolasteron, DOXOrubicin, droperidol, epirubicin, ertapenem, fluorouracil, furosemide, granisetron, heparin, leucovorin, melphalan, methotrexate, metoclopramide, nesiritide, octreotide, ondansetron, oxaliplatin, PACLitaxel, palonosetron, PEMEtrexed, riTUXimab, teniposide, thiotepa, tigecycline, tirofiban, trastuzumab, vinBLAStine, vinCRIStine, voriconazole, zoledronic acid

SIDE EFFECTS

CNS: Fever, headache, confusion, drowsiness, syncope, fatigue
EENT: Blurred vision
GI: *Nausea, vomiting, anorexia, stomatitis,* hepatotoxicity, diarrhea
GU: Urinary retention, renal failure, edema
HEMA: Thrombocytopenia, leukopenia, anemia
INTEG: *Rash,* alopecia, extravasation, nail discoloration
MISC: Hemolytic uremic syndrome, CHF
RESP: Fibrosis, pulmonary infiltrate, dyspnea

PHARMACOKINETICS

Half-life 1 hr, metabolized in liver, 10% excreted in urine (unchanged)

INTERACTIONS

Increase: toxicity—other antineoplastics, radiation
Increase: bleeding risk—NSAIDs, anticoagulants
- Avoid use with vaccines

Drug/Herb
- Avoid use with black cohosh

NURSING CONSIDERATIONS

Assess:

Black Box Warning: Bone marrow suppression: CBC, differential, platelet count weekly; withhold product if WBC is $<4000/mm^3$, serum creatinine >1.7 mg/dl, or platelet count is $<100,000/mm^3$; notify prescriber; bleeding: hematuria, guaiac, bruising, petechiae, mucosa, or orifices

Black Box Warning: Fatal hemolytic-uremic syndrome: hypertension, thrombocytopenia, microangiopathic hemolytic anemia; occurs in those receiving long-term therapy

- Renal studies: BUN, serum uric acid, urine CCr, electrolytes before, during therapy, adjust dose based on renal function
- I&O ratio; report fall in urine output to <30 ml/hr
- Monitor temperature q4hr; fever may indicate beginning infection
- Hepatic studies before, during therapy: bilirubin, AST, ALT, alk phos as needed or monthly; check for jaundiced skin and sclera, dark urine, clay-colored stools, itchy skin, abdominal pain, fever, diarrhea

⚠ **Pulmonary fibrosis:** bronchospasm, dyspnea, crackles, unproductive cough; chest pain, tachypnea, fatigue, increased pulse, pallor, lethargy; pulmonary function tests; chest x-ray before, during therapy; chest x-ray should be obtained q2wk during treatment

- Effects of alopecia on body image; discuss feelings about body changes
- Buccal cavity q8hr for dryness, sores, ulceration, white patches, oral pain, bleeding, dysphagia
- Local irritation, pain, burning at inj site

• GI symptoms: frequency of stools, cramping
• Adequate fluids 2-3 L/day unless contraindicated
• Rinsing of mouth tid-qid with water; brushing of teeth with baking soda bid-tid with soft brush or cotton-tipped applicators for stomatitis; use unwaxed dental floss

Evaluate:

• Therapeutic response: decreased tumor size, spread of malignancy

Teach patient/family:

• That hair may be lost during treatment; that wig or hairpiece may make patient feel better; that new hair may be different in color, texture
• To avoid foods with citric acid, hot or rough texture
• To report any bleeding, white spots, ulcerations in mouth; to examine mouth daily
• To report sign of IV-site reaction, redness, inflammation, burning, pain
• To avoid crowds, persons with infections if granulocyte count is low
• **Infection:** report fever, flulike symptoms, sore throat
• To immediately report urine retention, absence of urine, dyspnea, bleeding, jaundice, signs of pulmonary toxicity
• To report if pregnancy is planned or suspected; pregnancy (D) 1st trimester, do not breastfeed

⚠ HIGH ALERT

mitoXANtrone (Rx)

(mye-toe-zan′trone)

Func. class.: Antineoplastic, antiinfective, immunomodulator

Chem. class.: Synthetic anthraquinone

Do not confuse:
mitoXANtrone/mitoMYcin/mithramycin/mitotane

ACTION: DNA reactive agent; cytocidal effect on both proliferating and nonproliferating cells; topoisomerase II inhibitor (vesicant)

USES: Acute myelogenous leukemia (adult), relapsed leukemia; used with steroids to treat bone pain (advanced prostate cancer), multiple sclerosis (MS)

Unlabeled uses: Liver malignancies, non-Hodgkin's lymphoma, breast cancer, ALL, bone marrow ablation, CLL, hepatocellular cancer, ovarian cancer, pleural effusion, stem cell transplant preparation

CONTRAINDICATIONS: Pregnancy (D), hypersensitivity

Precautions: Breastfeeding, children; myelosuppression, renal/cardiac/hepatic disease; gout

Black Box Warning: Secondary malignancy, neutropenia, intrathecal administration, extravasation, heart failure

DOSAGE AND ROUTES

M

Acute myelogenous leukemia/induction

• **Adult: IV INFUSION** 12 mg/m^2/day on days 1-3 and 100 mg/m^2 cytarabine × 7 days as continuous 24-hr infusion

Consolidation

• **Adult: IV** 12 mg/m^2 given as short 5- to 15-min infusion for 2 days with cytarabine × 5 days

Advanced prostate cancer

• **Adult: IV** 12-14 mg/m^2 as single dose or short infusion q21days

Multiple sclerosis, relapsing

• **Adult: IV INFUSION** 12 mg/m^2 as 5- to 15-min infusion q3mo, cumulative lifetime dose 140 mg/m^2

Available forms: Inj 2, 10, 12.5, 15 mg/ml

Administer:

• Other medications by oral route if possible; avoid IM, SUBCUT, IV routes
• Antiemetic 30-60 min before product to prevent vomiting

Direct IV route

• IV after diluting with ≥50 ml NS or D_5W; give over 3-5 min into running IV of

D_5W or NS; check for extravasation; do not give IM, SUBCUT, or intraarterially

Intermittent IV INFUSION route

- May be diluted further in D_5W, NS, run over 15-30 min

Continuous IV INFUSION route

- Give over 24 hr

Y-site compatibilities: Acyclovir, alemtuzumab, alfentanil, allopurinol, amikacin, aminocaproic acid, aminophylline, amiodarone, anidulafungin, argatroban, arsenic trioxide, atracurium, bivalirudin, bleomycin, bretylium, bumetanide, buprenorphine, butorphanol, calcium chloride, calcium gluconate, CARBOplatin, carmustine, caspofungin, cefoTEtan, ceftizoxime, chloramphenicol, chlorproMAZINE, cimetidine, ciprofloxacin, cisatracurium, CISplatin, cladribine, codeine, cyclophosphamide, cycloSPORINE, cytarabine, DACTINomycin, DAPTOmycin, DAUNOrubicin citrate liposome, dexmedetomidine, dexrazoxane, diltiazem, diphenhydrAMINE, DOBUTamine, DOCEtaxel, dolasetron, DOPamine, doxacurium, doxycycline, droperidol, enalaprilat, ePHEDrine, EPINEPHrine, erythromycin, esmolol, etoposide, etoposide phosphate, famotidine, fenoldopam, fentaNYL, filgrastim, fluconazole, fludarabine, fluorouracil, ganciclovir, gatifloxacin, gemcitabine, gentamicin, glycopyrrolate, granisetron, haloperidol, hydrALAZINE, hydrocortisone sodium succinate, HYDROmorphone, hydrOXYzine, ifosfamide, imipenem-cilastatin, inamrinone, insulin regular, irinotecan, isoproterenol, ketorolac, labetalol, leucovorin, levofloxacin, levorphanol, lidocaine, linezolid, LORazepam, magnesium sulfate, mannitol, melphalan, meperidine, meropenem, mesna, metaraminol, methohexital, methotrexate, methyldopate, metoclopramide, metoprolol, metroNIDAZOLE, midazolam, milrinone, minocycline, mivacurium, morphine sulfate, nalbuphine, naloxone, nesiritide, niCARdipine, nitroglycerin, norepinephrine, octreotide, ondansetron, oxaliplatin, palonosetron, pamidronate, pancuronium, pentamidine, pentazocine, PENTObarbital, PHENObarbital, phentolamine, phenylephrine, polymyxin b, potassium acetate, potassium chloride, procainamide, prochlorperazine, promethazine hydrochloride, propranolol, quiNIDine gluconate, quinupristin-dalfopristin, ranitidine, remifentanil, riTUXimab, rocuronium, sargramostim, sodium acetate, sodium bicarbonate, succinylcholine, SUFentanil, sulfamethoxazole-trimethoprim, tacrolimus, teniposide, theophylline, thiopental, thiotepa, tigecycline, tirofiban, tobramycin, tolazoline, trastuzumab, trimethobenzamide, vancomycin, vasopressin, vecuronium, verapamil, vinCRIStine, vinorelbine, zidovudine, zoledronic acid

SIDE EFFECTS

CNS: Headache, seizures, fatigue
CV: CHF, cardiopathy, dysrhythmias
EENT: Conjunctivitis, blue/green sclera, blurred vision
GI: *Nausea, vomiting, diarrhea, anorexia, mucositis,* hepatotoxicity, abdominal pain, constipation, jaundice
GU: Amenorrhea, menstrual disorders
HEMA: Thrombocytopenia, leukopenia, myelosuppression, anemia, secondary leukemia
INTEG: *Rash, necrosis at inj site,* dermatitis, thrombophlebitis at inj site, alopecia
MISC: Fever, hyperuricemia, infections
RESP: Cough, dyspnea
SYST: Tumor lysis syndrome, sepsis

PHARMACOKINETICS

Protein binding 78%; excreted via renal, hepatobiliary systems; half-life 23-215 hr

INTERACTIONS

Increase: bone marrow depression toxicity—radiation, other antineoplastics
Increase: adverse reactions—live virus vaccines, trastuzumab
Increase: bleeding risk—NSAIDs, anticoagulants

Increase: mitoXANtrone effects of—digoxin, phenytoin

Drug/Lab Test

Increase: LFTs, uric acid

Decrease: HcT/Hgb, platelets, WBC

NURSING CONSIDERATIONS

Assess:

- CBC, differential, platelet count weekly; withhold product if WBC is $<1500/mm^3$; leukopenia, neutropenia, thrombocytopenia are expected, leukocyte nadir 10-14 days, recovers in 2-3 wk
- **Hepatotoxicity:** hepatic studies before, during therapy: bilirubin, AST, ALT, alk phos prn or monthly; dose reduction needed with hepatic disease; jaundiced skin and sclera, dark urine, clay-colored stools, itchy skin, abdominal pain, fever, diarrhea
- Renal studies: BUN, serum uric acid, urine CCr, electrolytes before, during therapy
- Bleeding, hematuria, guaiac, bruising or petechiae, mucosa or orifices q8hr

Black Box Warning: ECG, ECHO, chest x-ray, MUGA, RAI angiography; assess ejection fraction before and during treatment; cardiotoxic may develop during treatment or months to years after treatment; use vigilant cardiac monitoring in MS

Black Box Warning: Secondary acute myelogenous leukemia (AML) that can develop after taking this product

Black Box Warning: Multiple sclerosis: obtain MUGA, LVEF baselines; repeat LVEF if symptoms of CHF occur or if cumulative dose is >100 mg/m^2; do not administer to patients who have received lifetime dose of ≥140 mg/m^2 or if LVEF $<50\%$ or significant LVEF

- Obtain pregnancy test for all women of childbearing age, even if birth control is used, pregnancy (D)
- Rinsing of mouth tid-qid with water, club soda; brushing of teeth bid-qid with soft brush or cotton-tipped applicators for stomatitis; use unwaxed dental floss
- Provide increased fluids to 2-3 L/day unless contraindicated

Evaluate:

- Therapeutic response: decreased tumor size, spread of malignancy

Teach patient/family:

- To immediately report bleeding, dyspnea, possible infections, seizure, jaundice, fever, cough, or dyspnea
- To avoid hot foods or those with citric acid, rough texture
- To report any bleeding, white spots, ulcerations in mouth; to examine mouth daily
- To avoid crowds, persons with infections
- That sclera, urine may turn blue or green; that hair loss may occur

Black Box Warning: To notify prescriber if pregnancy is suspected or planned; to use effective contraception

M

modafinil (Rx)

(mo-daf′i-nil)

Alertec ✦, Provigil

Func. class.: CNS stimulant

Chem. class.: Racemic compound

Controlled Substance IV

ACTION: Similar action as that of sympathomimetics; does not alter release of DOPamine, norepinephrine

USES: Narcolepsy, shift-work sleep disturbance, obstructive sleep apnea

Unlabeled uses: Fatigue in MS, ADHD, symptoms of major depression

CONTRAINDICATIONS: Hypersensitivity, ischemic heart disease, left ventricular hypertrophy, chest pain, dysrhythmias

Precautions: Pregnancy (C), breastfeeding, child <16 yr, geriatric patients, unstable angina, history of MI, severe hepatic disease

DOSAGE AND ROUTES

To improve wakefulness with daytime sleepiness

- **Adult and adolescent ≥16 yr: PO** 200 mg daily

Hepatic dose (severe hepatic disease)

- **Adult: PO** 100 mg daily

Multiple sclerosis/fatigue (unlabeled)

- **Adult/geriatric/adolescents ≥6 yr: PO** 200-400 mg daily in the AM

Major depression symptoms (unlabeled)

- **Adult: PO** 100 mg/day, max 400 mg/day

Available forms: Tabs 100, 200 mg

Administer:

- Give 1 hr before start of shift work or in AM for those with narcolepsy or sleep apnea
- Store at room temperature

SIDE EFFECTS

CNS: *Headache,* anxiety, cataplexy, depression, dizziness, insomnia, amnesia, confusion, ataxia, tremors, paresthesia, dyskinesia, suicidal ideation

CV: Dysrhythmias, hypo/hypertension, chest pain, vasodilation

EENT: Change in vision, *rhinitis,* pharyngitis, epistaxis

GI: Nausea, vomiting, changes in LFTs, anorexia, diarrhea, thirst, mouth ulcers

GU: Ejaculation disorder, urinary retention, albuminuria

HEMA: Eosinophilia

INTEG: Rash, dry skin, herpes simplex, Stevens-Johnson syndrome

MISC: Infection, hyperglycemia, neck pain

RESP: *Dyspnea*, lung changes

PHARMACOKINETICS

Absorbed rapidly, 60% protein binding, metabolized by the liver (90%), half-life 15 hr, peak 2-4 hr

INTERACTIONS

Increase: altered levels of CYP3A4 inhibitors (azole antibiotics some SSRIs), reaction difficult to predict

Increase: levels of CYP2C19 substrates (diazepam, phenytoin some tricyclics)

Decrease: effects of—cycloSPORINE, hormonal contraceptives, theophylline, estrogens

Delayed effect modafinil by 1 hr: methylphenidate

Altered: levels of CYP3A4 inducers (carBAMazepine, phenytoin, rifampin, cycloSPORINE, theophylline)

Drug/Herb

Increase: stimulation—cola nut, guarana, yerba maté, coffee, tea

Drug/Lab Test

Increase: LFTs, glucose, eosinophils

NURSING CONSIDERATIONS

Assess:

- Narcolepsy, shift work, history of sleep apnea
- Depression, suicidal ideation
- Monitor B/P in those with hypertension

Evaluate:

- Ability to stay awake

Teach patient/family:

- To take only as directed; that product may be taken with/without food
- To use other form of contraception during and for ≥30 days after discontinuing medication if using hormonal birth control; to notify prescriber if pregnancy is planned or suspected or if breastfeeding
- To notify prescriber of allergic reaction, tremors, confusion
- To avoid all OTC medications unless approved by prescriber
- To avoid hazardous activities until drug effect is known

moexipril (Rx)

(moe-ex′ih-prill)

Univasc

Func. class.: Antihypertensive

Chem. class.: Angiotensin-converting enzyme inhibitor

ACTION: Selectively suppresses renin-angiotensin-aldosterone system; inhibits

ACE; prevents conversion of angiotensin I to angiotensin II; results in dilation of arterial, venous vessels

USES:
Hypertension, alone or in combination with thiazide diuretics

CONTRAINDICATIONS:
Breastfeeding, children, hypersensitivity, heart block, bilateral renal stenosis, history of angioedema

Black Box Warning: Pregnancy (D)

Precautions: Dialysis patients, hypovolemia, leukemia, scleroderma, lupus erythematosus, blood dyscrasias, CHF, diabetes mellitus, thyroid/renal disease, COPD, asthma, potassium-sparing diuretics

DOSAGE AND ROUTES
• **Adult: PO** 7.5 mg 1 hr before meals initially; may be increased or divided depending on B/P response; maintenance dosage 7.5-30 mg/day in 1-2 divided doses 1 hr before meals

Renal dose

• Adult: PO CCr <40 ml/min, 3.75 mg/day; titrate to desired dose; max 15 mg/day

Available forms: Tabs 7.5, 15 mg

Administer:

• 1 hr before meals

• Do not use with potassium-sparing diuretics, sympathomimetics, potassium supplements

• Storage in tight container at ≤86° F (30° C)

SIDE EFFECTS
CNS: Fever, chills, fatigue, headache

CV: Hypotension, postural hypotension

GI: Loss of taste, **hepatic failure/necrosis, hepatitis**

GU: Impotence, dysuria, nocturia, proteinuria, **nephrotic syndrome**, acute reversible renal failure, polyuria, oliguria, frequency

HEMA: **Neutropenia**

INTEG: Rash, photosensitivity

META: Hypokalemia, hyperkalemia, hyponatremia

MS: Myalgia

RESP: **Bronchospasm**, dyspnea, dry cough, pneumonitis

SYST: **Angioedema, anaphylaxis**

PHARMACOKINETICS
Peak 1.5 hr, metabolized by liver (metabolites); excreted in feces (52%), urine; crosses placenta, excreted in breast milk, protein binding 50%-70%, half-life 2-10 hr

INTERACTIONS
• Do not use with potassium-sparing diuretics, sympathomimetics, potassium supplements

Increase: hypotension—diuretics, other antihypertensives, ganglionic blockers, adrenergic blockers, phenothiazines

Increase: toxicity—digoxin, lithium

Increase: hyperkalemia—cycloSPORINE, potassium-sparing diuretics

Increase: myelosuppression—azaTHIOprine

Decrease: antihypertensive effect—NSAIDs

Drug/Herb

Increase: antihypertensive effect—hawthorn

Decrease: antihypertensive effect—yohimbe

Drug/Lab Test

False positive: urine acetone

NURSING CONSIDERATIONS
Assess:

• Blood tests: neutrophils, decreased platelets

• Renal studies: protein, BUN, creatinine; watch for increased levels that may indicate nephrotic syndrome

• Baselines of renal, hepatic studies before therapy begins

• Potassium levels, although hyperkalemia rarely occurs

• Edema in feet, legs daily

• **Allergic reaction:** rash, fever, pruritus, urticaria; product should be discontinued if antihistamines fail to help

- **Symptoms of CHF;** edema, dyspnea, wet crackles, B/P, difficulty breathing
- Renal symptoms: polyuria, oliguria, frequency

Evaluate:
- Therapeutic response: decrease in B/P with hypertension

Teach patient/family:
- To take 1 hr before meals
- Not to discontinue product abruptly
- Not to use OTC (cough, cold, allergy) products unless directed by prescriber
- To comply with dosage schedule even if feeling better
- To rise slowly to sitting or standing position to minimize orthostatic hypotension
- To notify prescriber of mouth sores, sore throat, fever, swelling of hands or feet, irregular heartbeat, chest pain, signs of angioedema
- That excessive perspiration, dehydration, vomiting, diarrhea may lead to fall in B/P; to consult prescriber if these occur
- That dizziness, fainting, lightheadedness may occur during 1st few days of therapy
- That skin rash or impaired perspiration may occur
- How to take B/P

Black Box Warning: Notify prescriber if pregnancy is planned or suspected

TREATMENT OF OVERDOSE:
0.9% NaCl IV inf, hemodialysis

montelukast (Rx)
(mon-teh-loo′kast)

Singulair

Func. class.: Bronchodilator

Chem. class.: Leukotriene receptor antagonist, cysteinyl

ACTION: Inhibits leukotriene (LTD_4) formation; leukotrienes exert their effects by increasing neutrophil, eosinophil migration; aggregation of neutrophils, monocytes; smooth muscle contraction, capillary permeability; these actions further lead to bronchoconstriction, inflammation, edema

USES: Chronic asthma in adults and children, seasonal allergic rhinitis, bronchospasm prophylaxis

CONTRAINDICATIONS: Hypersensitivity

Precautions: Pregnancy (B), breastfeeding, children <6 yr, acute attacks of asthma, alcohol consumption, severe hepatic disease, corticosteroid withdrawal, phenylketonuria, suicidal ideation, depression

DOSAGE AND ROUTES
- **Adult and child ≥15 yr: PO** 10 mg/day in PM
- **Child 6-14 yr: PO** 5-mg chew tab/day in PM
- **Child 2-5 yr: PO** (chew tab/granules) 4 mg/day

Asthma
- **Child 12-23 mo: PO** 1 packet (4 mg) granules taken in PM

Exercise-induced bronchoconstriction
- **Adult/child ≥6 yr: PO** 10 mg 2 hr before exercise; do not take another dose within 24 hr

Available forms: Tabs 10 mg; chew tabs 4, 5 mg; oral granules 4 mg/packet

Administer:

PO route
- In PM daily for all uses except exercise-induced bronchoconstriction; then take 2 hr before exercise
- Granules directly in mouth or mixed with spoonful of soft food (carrots, applesauce, ice cream, rice)
- Do not open granules packet until ready to use; mix whole dose; give within 15 min

SIDE EFFECTS
CNS: *Dizziness, fatigue, headache,* behavior changes, hallucinations, **seizures,**

agitation, anxiety, depression, fever, drowsiness, **suicidal ideation, memory impairment, hostility, somnambulism**
GI: *Abdominal pain,* dyspepsia, nausea, vomiting, diarrhea, **pancreatitis**
HEMA: **Thrombocytopenia**
INTEG: Rash, pruritus, erythema
MS: Asthenia, myalgia, muscle cramps
RESP: *Influenza, cough,* nasal congestion
SYST: **Anaphylaxis, angioedema, Churg-Strauss syndrome, Stevens-Johnson syndrome, toxic epidermal necrolysis**

PHARMACOKINETICS

Rapidly absorbed; peak 3-4 hr, chew tab (5 mg) 2-2.5 hr; half-life 2.7-5.5 hr, extended in hepatic disease; protein binding 99%; metabolized by liver; excreted via bile

INTERACTIONS

Increase: adverse reactions of CYP2C8 substrates
Decrease: montelukast levels—barbiturates, rifabutin, rifapentine, carBAMazepine, fosphenytoin, phenytoin, rifampin
Drug/Herb
Increase: stimulation—black, green tea, guarana
Drug/Lab Test
Increase: ALT, AST

NURSING CONSIDERATIONS

Assess:

⚠ **Churg-Strauss syndrome:** rare adult patients carefully for symptoms: eosinophilia, vasculitic rash, worsening pulmonary symptoms, cardiac complications, neuropathy

- Allergic reactions: rash, urticaria; product should be discontinued

⚠ For behavior changes and suicidal ideation, other neuropsychiatric reactions

- **Severe hepatic disease:** use cautiously

Evaluate:

- Therapeutic response: ability to breathe more easily

Teach patient/family:

- To check OTC medications, current prescription medications for ePHEDrine, which will increase stimulation; to avoid alcohol
- To avoid hazardous activities; dizziness may occur
- That product is not to be used for acute asthma attacks
- If aspirin sensitivity is known, not to take NSAIDs while taking this product
- To continue to use inhaled β-agonists if exercise-induced asthma occurs
- **Granules:** to give directly in mouth or mixed in a spoonful of room temperature soft food (use only applesauce, carrots, rice, or ice cream); use within 15 min of opening packets; discard unused portions

⚠ HIGH ALERT

morphine (Rx)

(mor′feen)

Astramorph PF, AVINza, Depo Dur, Infumorph PF, Kadian, M.O.S. ✦, MS Contin, MSIR ✦, Oramorph SR

Func. class.: Opioid analgesic
Chem. class.: Alkaloid

Controlled Substance Schedule II

Do not confuse:
morphine/HYDROmorphone
MS Contin/OxyCONTIN

ACTION: Depresses pain impulse transmission at the spinal cord level by interacting with opioid receptors

USES: Moderate to severe pain
Unlabeled uses: Agitation, bone/dental pain, dyspnea in end-stage cancer or pulmonary disease, sedation induction, rapid-sequence intubation

CONTRAINDICATIONS: Hypersensitivity, addiction (opioid/alcohol), hemorrhage, bronchial asthma, increased intracranial pressure, paralytic ileus, hypovolemia, shock, MAOI therapy

Black Box Warning: Respiratory depression

Precautions: Pregnancy (C), breastfeeding, children <18 yr, geriatric patients, addictive personality, acute MI, severe heart disease, renal/hepatic disease, bowel impaction, abrupt discontinuation, seizures

Black Box Warning: Accidental exposure, epidural/intrathecal/IM/subcut administration, opioid-naive patients, substance abuse

DOSAGE AND ROUTES

Acute moderate to severe pain

PO regular-release route

- **Adult ≥50 kg:** initially, 10-30 mg every 3-4 hr as needed
- **Adult <50 kg/geriatric patients:** might require lower doses and/or extended dosing intervals; doses should be titrated carefully
- **Child/infant ≥6 mo:** 0.2-0.5 mg/kg every 4-6 hr as needed
- **Infants <6 mo/neonate: PO** 0.1 mg/kg every 3-4 hr

IV/IM/SUBCUT route

- **Adult ≥50 kg:** 2.5-15 mg every 2-6 hr as needed, titrate; or a loading dose of 0.05-0.1 mg/kg IV, followed by 0.8-10 mg/hr IV, titrate
- **Adult <50 kg/geriatric patients:** might require lower doses and/or extended dosing intervals 0.1 mg/kg every 3-4 hr, titrate
- **Child/infant ≥6 mo:** 0.05-0.2 mg/kg every 2-4 hr, titrate to relief; max initial dose 15 mg/dose, avoid IM when possible
- **Infants <6 mo/neonate:** 0.03-0.05 mg/kg every 3-8 hr, titrate to relief, avoid IM when possible

Epidural (morphine sulfate injection, but *not* DepoDur)

- **Adult:** initially, 5 mg in the lumbar region; if pain relief does not occur in 1 hr, give 1-2 mg epidurally; max 10 mg/24 hr; **continuous epidural infusion** 2-4 mg/24 hr; may give another 1-2 mg

Intrathecal route (morphine sulfate injection, but *not* DepoDur)

- Do not inject >2 ml of the 0.5 mg/ml or 1 ml of the 1 mg/ml ampule
- **Adult:** 0.2-1 mg in the lumbar area as a single dose or to establish dosage for continuous intrathecal infusion; repeated injections are not recommended

Rectal route

- **Adult: PR** 10-20 mg every 4 hr, as needed
- **Child:** Individualize

Chronic moderate and severe pain:

Do not use extended-release cap or tab as PRN analgesics, for acute pain, or if the pain is mild or not expected to persist for an extended period of time; use for postoperative pain only if the patient is receiving chronic opioid therapy before surgery or if the postoperative pain is expected to be moderate to severe and expected to persist for an extended period of time; do not use controlled-release tablets (MS Contin) immediately after surgery (for the first 24 hr) in patients not previously taking the drug

Do not use in opioid-naïve patients: 90 mg, 120 mg morphine biphasic-release capsules (AVINza); 100 mg, 130 mg, 150 mg, 200 mg morphine extended-release capsules (Kadian), 100 mg, 200 mg morphine control-release tablets (MS Contin); patients considered opioid tolerant are those who are taking at least 60 mg/day oral morphine, 30 mg/day oral oxyCODONE, 8 mg/day oral HYDROmorphone, or an equal dose of another opioid, for 1 wk or longer

PO (extended-release tab [MS Contin, Oramorph SR] or caps [Kadian, AVINza]) in opiate agonist naive patients

- **Adult:** 15-30 mg every 12 hr (tabs); 10 mg bid or 20 mg daily (Kadian); or 30 mg daily (AVINza), titrate; AVINza should be adjusted in increments ≤30 mg every 4 days; Kadian should be increased ≤20 mg every 1-2 days, taper gradually; to discontinue, gradually decrease AVINza and Kadian every 2-4 days
- **Child (unlabeled):** 0.3-0.6 mg/kg every 12 hr (tabs)

IV/SUBCUT route (opiate)

- **Adult: IV** 2-10 mg loading dose, then 0.8-10 mg/hour IV, titrate; maintenance 0.8-80 mg/hour IV
- **Children/infants ≥6 mo: IV** initially, 0.04-0.07 mg/kg/hr (range: 0.025-2.6 mg/kg/hr)
- **Subcut infusion** 0.025-1.79 mg/kg/hour
- Infants <6 mo/neonate: **IV** 0.01 mg/kg/hour initially; infusion rates max 0.015-0.02 mg/kg/hour IV

Breakthrough pain in patients receiving long-acting or continuous-infusion morphine

PO (regular-release) route

- **Adult/child:** the dose is usually 1/4 to 1/3 the 8- to 12-hour extended-release dose every 4-6 hr as needed
- **Adult/child:** For PCA, intermittent dosage is usually 25%-30% of the hourly rate IV/SC every 6-15 min as needed; intermittent IV injection dosage is 25%-30% of the hourly rate given IV/SC every 1-2 hr as needed

Available forms: HCL: suppositories 10, 20, 30 mg; syrup 1, 5, 10, 20, 50 mg/ml; tabs 10, 20, 40, 60 mg; **Sulfate:** caps ext rel microgranules 10, 15, 30, 60, 100, 200 mg; cap ext rel pellets (Avinza): 30, 45, 60, 75, 90, 120 mg; caps ext rel pellets (Kadian) 10, 20, 30, 40, 50, 60, 70, 80, 100, 130, 150, 200 mg; drops: 20, 50 mg/ml; injection epidural: 0.5, 1, 10, 15 mg/ml; injection (preservative): 0.5, 1, 2, 10, 15, 25, 50 mg/ml; injection (Corpuject/prefilled syringes): 2, 4, 8, 10, 15 mg/ml; oral solution 2 mg/5 ml, 10 mg/ml; suppositories 5, 10, 20, 30 mg; syrup 1, 5, 10 mg/ml; tab 5, 10, 15, 25, 30, 50 mg; tabs ext rel 15, 30, 60, 100, 200 mg

Administer:

PO route

- Give with food or milk to minimize GI effects
- Begin with immediate-release products and titrate to correct dose and convert to a sustained-release product
- **Immediate-release cap:** may swallow whole, or cap may be opened and contents sprinkled on cool food (pudding or applesauce) or added to juice; give immediately or delivered via gastric or NG tube by either adding to or following with liquid
- **Extended-release and controlled-release tabs:** swallow whole; do not crush, break, dissolve, or chew
- The use of MS Contin 100-mg or 200-mg tabs should be limited to opioid-tolerant patients requiring oral doses equivalent to ≥200 mg/day; use of the 100-mg or 200-mg tablet is only recommended for patients who have already been titrated to a stable analgesic regimen using lower strengths of MS Contin or other opioids
- **Sustained-release caps:** swallow; do not chew, crush, or dissolve; caps may be opened and contents sprinkled on applesauce (at room temperature or cooler) immediately before ingestion; do not chew, crush, or dissolve the pellets/beads inside the cap; the applesauce should be swallowed without chewing; if the pellets/beads are chewed, an immediate release of a potentially fatal morphine dose may be delivered; rinse mouth to ensure all the pellets/beads have been swallowed; do not separate applesauce into separate doses; the entire portion should be taken; discard unused portion
- **Kadian caps:** may be given through a 16-F gastrostomy tube; flush with water, and sprinkle the cap contents into 10 ml of water; using a funnel and a swirling motion, pour the pellets and water into the tube; rinse the beaker with 10 ml of water, and pour the water into the funnel; repeat until no pellets remain in the beaker; do not administer AVINza tabs through a gastrostomy tube; *do not* administer Kadian or AVINza through a nasogastric tube
- Avoid concurrent administration of AVINza with prescription or nonprescription medications that contain alcohol; consumption of alcohol while taking the extended-release capsules can result in the rapid release and absorption of a potentially fatal dose of morphine

M

- AVINza ≥90 mg or Kadian 100 mg, 130 mg, 150 mg, or 200 mg caps are given only to opioid-tolerant patients

Oral liquid

- Check dose before use because many concentrations of oral solution are available; may be diluted in fruit juice; protect from light

Injectable administration

- Visually inspect for particulate matter, discoloration before use; do not use if a precipitate is present after shaking; do not use the Duramorph solution if a precipitate is present or if the color is darker than pale yellow

SUBCUT route

- Inject, taking care not to inject intradermally
- **Continuous SC infusion:** morphine is not approved by the FDA for subcut use; dilute to an appropriate concentration in D_5W; give using a portable, controlled, subcut device; adjust rate based on patient response and tolerance; max subcut rate is 2 ml/hour/site

Intrathecal/epidural route

⚠ Morphine sulfate injection is not interchangeable with morphine sulfate extended-release liposome injection (DepoDur); DepoDur is only for epidural administration

⚠ Do not use Infumorph (10 mg/ml or 25 mg/ml) for single-dose neuraxial injection because lower doses can be more reliably administered with Duramorph (0.5 mg/ml or 1 mg/ml

Rectal route

- Moisten the suppository with water before insertion; if suppository is too soft, chill in the refrigerator for 30 min or run cold water over it before removing the wrapper

IV route

- Before use, an opiate antagonist and emergency facilities should be available

⚠ Do not use the highly concentrated morphine injections (i.e., 10-25 mg/ml) for IV, IM, or SC administration of single doses; these injection solutions are intended for use via continuous, controlled microinfusion devices

- **Direct IV route:** dilute dose with ≥5 ml of sterile water for injection or NS injection; inject 2.5-15 mg directly into a vein or into the tubing of a freely flowing IV solution over 4-5 min; do not give rapidly
- **Continuous IV infusion:** dilute in 5% dextrose; use a controlled-infusion device; adjust dosage and rate based on patient response
- **Patient-controlled analgesia (PCA):** a compatible patient-controlled infusion device must be used; dilute solutions to obtain a concentration of 1 or 10 mg/ml for ease in calculations and programming of PCA pumps; adjust dosage and rate based on patient response; consult the patient-controlled infusion device manual for directions on rate of infusion

Y-site compatibilities: Acetaminophen, aldesleukin, allopurinol, amifostine, amikacin, aminophylline, amiodarone, amsacrine, atenolol, atracurium, aztreonam, bumetanide, calcium chloride, cefamandole, ceFAZolin, cefotaxime, cefoTEtan, cefOXitin, cefTAZidime, ceftizoxime, cefTRIAXone, cefuroxime, cephalothin, chloramphenicol, cisatracurium, cladribine, clindamycin, cyclophosphamide, cytarabine, dexamethasone, digoxin, diltiazem, DOBUTamine, DOPamine, doxycycline, enalaprilat, EPINEPHrine, erythromycin, esmolol, etomidate, famotidine, fentaNYL, filgrastim, fluconazole, fludarabine, foscarnet, gentamicin, granisetron, heparin, hydrocortisone, HYDROmorphone, kanamycin, labetalol, lidocaine, LORazepam, magnesium sulfate, melphalan, meropenem, methotrexate, methyldopate, methylPREDNISolone, metoclopramide, metoprolol, metroNIDAZOLE, midazolam, milrinone, nafcillin, niCARdipine, nitroglycerin, norepinephrine, ondansetron, oxacillin, oxytocin, PACLitaxel, pancuronium, penicillin G potassium, piperacillin, piperacillin/tazobactam, potassium chloride, propranolol, ranitidine, remifentanil, sodium bicarbonate, teniposide, thiotepa, ticarcillin, ticarcillin/clavulanate, tigecycline, tobramycin, vancomycin, vecuronium, vinorelbine, vit B/C, warfarin, zidovudine, zoledronic acid

SIDE EFFECTS

CNS: Drowsiness, dizziness, confusion, headache, sedation, euphoria, insomnia, **seizures**
CV: Palpitations, **bradycardia**, change in B/P, **shock, cardiac arrest**, chest pain, hypo/hypertension, edema, **tachycardia**
EENT: Blurred vision, miosis, diplopia
ENDO: Gynecomastia
GI: Nausea, vomiting, anorexia, constipation, cramps, biliary tract pressure
GU: Urinary retention, impotence, gonadal suppression
HEMA: **Thrombocytopenia**
INTEG: Rash, urticaria, bruising, flushing, diaphoresis, pruritus
RESP: **Respiratory depression, respiratory arrest, apnea**

PHARMACOKINETICS

PO: Onset variable, peak 60 min, duration 4-5 hr
IM: Onset $1/2$ hr, peak 30-60 min, duration 4-5 hr
SUBCUT: Onset 15-20 min, peak 50-90 min, duration 4-5 hr
IV: Peak 20 min, duration 4-5 hr
RECT: Peak $1/2$-1 hr, duration 3-7 hr
Intrathecal: Onset rapid, duration ≤24 hr
Metabolized by liver, crosses placenta; excreted in urine, breast milk; half-life IM 3-4 hr; AVINza 24 hr; Kadian 11-13 hr

INTERACTIONS

- **Unpredictable reaction, avoid use: MAOIs**

Increase: effects with other CNS depressants—alcohol, opiates, sedative/hypnotics, antipsychotics, skeletal muscle relaxants
Decrease: morphine action—rifampin
Drug/Herb
Increase: CNS depression—chamomile, hops, kava, St. John's wort, valerian
Drug/Lab Test
Increase: amylase

NURSING CONSIDERATIONS

Assess:

- **Pain:** location, type, character; give dose before pain becomes severe
- Bowel status; constipation common, use stimulant laxative if needed
- I&O ratio; check for decreasing output; may indicate urinary retention; monitor serum sodium
- B/P, pulse, respirations (character, depth, rate)
- CNS changes: dizziness, drowsiness, hallucinations, euphoria, LOC, pupil reaction
- **Abrupt discontinuation: gradually taper to prevent withdrawal symptoms; decrease by 50% q1-2days; avoid use of narcotic antagonists**
- Allergic reactions: rash, urticaria

Black Box Warning: Accidental exposure: if Duramorph or Infumorph gets on skin, remove contaminated clothing, rinse affected area with water

- **Respiratory dysfunction: depression, character, rate, rhythm; notify prescriber if respirations are <12/min; accidental overdose has occurred with high-potency oral sols**
- Gradual withdrawal after long-term use

Evaluate:

- Therapeutic response; decrease in pain intensity

Teach patient/family:

- To change position slowly; orthostatic hypotension may occur
- To report any symptoms of CNS changes, allergic reactions
- That physical dependency may result from long-term use
- To avoid use of alcohol, CNS depressants
- That withdrawal symptoms may occur: nausea, vomiting, cramps, fever, faintness, anorexia

TREATMENT OF OVERDOSE:

Naloxone (Narcan) 0.2-0.8 mg IV, (caution with opioid-tolerant individuals) O_2, IV fluids, vasopressors

moxifloxacin (Rx)

Avelox, Avelox IV

Func. class.: Antiinfective

Chem. class.: Fluoroquinolone

ACTION: Interferes with conversion of intermediate DNA fragments into high-molecular-weight DNA in bacteria; DNA gyrase inhibitor

USES: Acute bacterial sinusitis: *Streptococcus pneumoniae, Haemophilus influenzae, Moraxella catarrhalis;* acute bacterial exacerbation of chronic bronchitis: *S. pneumoniae, H. influenzae, Haemophilus parainfluenzae, Klebsiella pneumoniae, Staphylococcus aureus, M. catarrhalis;* community-acquired pneumonia: *S. pneumoniae, H. influenzae, Mycoplasma pneumoniae, Chlamydia pneumoniae, M. catarrhalis;* uncomplicated skin/skin-structure infections: *S. aureus, Streptococcus pyogenes;* complicated intraabdominal infections including polymicrobial infections: *E. coli, Bacterioides fragilis, S. anginosus, S. constellatus, Enterococcus faecalis, Proteus mirabilis, Clostridium perfringens, Bacteroides thetaiotaomicron, Peptostreptococcus* sp; complicated skin, skin-structure infections caused by methicillin-susceptible: *S. aureus, E. coli, K. pneumoniae, Enterobacter cloacae*

Unlabeled uses: Anthrax treatment/prophylaxis, gastroenteritis, MAC, nongonococcal urethritis, shigellosis, surgical infection prophylaxis, TB

CONTRAINDICATIONS: Hypersensitivity to quinolones

Precautions: Pregnancy (C), breastfeeding, children, hepatic/cardiac/renal/GI disease, epilepsy, uncorrected hypokalemia, prolonged QT interval; patients receiving class IA, III antidysrhythmics; seizure disorder, pseudomembranous colitis, diabetes mellitus

Black Box Warning: Tendon pain, rupture; tendinitis, myasthenia gravis

DOSAGE AND ROUTES

Acute bacterial sinusitis

- **Adult: PO/IV** 400 mg q24hr × 10 days

Acute bacterial exacerbation of chronic bronchitis

- **Adult: PO/IV** 400 mg q24hr × 5 days

Community-acquired pneumonia

- **Adult: PO/IV** 400 mg q24hr × 7-14 days

Uncomplicated skin/skin-structure infections

- **Adult: PO/IV** 400 mg q24hr × 7 days

Complicated intraabdominal infections

- **Adult: IV** 400 mg/day × 5-14 days

Complicated skin, skin-structure infections

- **Adult: PO/IV** 400 mg/day × 7-21 days

Available forms: Tabs 400 mg; inj premix 400 mg/250 ml

Administer:

PO route

- 4 hr before or 8 hr after antacids, zinc, iron, calcium
- Without regard to food
- Store at room temperature

IV route

- Discontinue primary IV while administering moxifloxacin, give over 60 min
- Do not give SUBCUT, IM
- Available as premixed sol; may be diluted at ratios from 1:10 to 10:1; do not refrigerate; give by direct infusion or through Y-type infusion set; do not add other medications to sol or infusion through same IV line at same time
- Flush line with compatible sol before and after use
- Do not admix

Solution compatibilities: 0.9% NaCl, D_5, D_{10}, LR, sterile water for inj

SIDE EFFECTS

CNS: *Headache,* dizziness, fatigue, insomnia, depression, *restlessness,* seizures, confusion, increased intracranial pressure, peripheral neuropathy, pseudotumor cerebri, fever

CV: Prolonged QT interval, dysrhythmias, torsades de pointes, tachycardia
EENT: Blurred vision, tinnitus, taste changes
GI: *Nausea, diarrhea,* increased ALT, AST, flatulence, heartburn, *vomiting,* oral candidiasis, dysphagia, pseudomembranous colitis, abdominal pain, dyspepsia, constipation, gastroenteritis, xerostomia
GU: Renal failure
INTEG: *Rash,* pruritus, urticaria, photosensitivity, flushing, fever, chills, injection-site reactions
MISC: Candidiasis vaginitis
MS: Tremor, arthralgia, tendinitis, tendon rupture, myalgia
SYST: Anaphylaxis, Stevens-Johnson syndrome, angioedema, toxic epidermal necrolysis

PHARMACOKINETICS

Excreted in urine as active product, metabolites; parent product excreted in urine (20%), feces (25%); terminal half-life PO 12-16 hr, IV 8-15 hr

INTERACTIONS

Increase: QT prolongation—drugs that interval QT
Increase: moxifloxacin serum levels—probenecid
Increase: warfarin, cycloSPORINE effect
Increase: seizure risk—NSAIDs

Black Box Warning: Increase: tendon rupture—corticosteroids

Decrease: moxifloxacin absorption—magnesium antacids, aluminum hydroxide, zinc, iron, sucralfate, calcium, enteral feeding, didanosine
Drug/Lab Test
Increase: glucose, amylase, lipids, triglycerides, uric acid, LDH
Decrease: potassium

NURSING CONSIDERATIONS

Assess:
- CNS symptoms: headache, dizziness, fatigue, insomnia, depression, seizures
- Renal, hepatic studies: BUN, creatinine, AST, ALT, electrolytes
- I&O ratio, urine pH <5.5 is ideal

⚠ **Allergic reactions, Stevens-Johnson syndrome, toxic epidermal necrolysis, anaphylaxis:** fever, flushing, rash, urticaria, pruritus, sore throat, fatigue, ulcers, other lesions; keep EPINEPHrine, emergency equipment nearby for anaphylaxis

Black Box Warning: Tendon pain, rupture, tendinitis; if tendon becomes inflamed, product should be discontinued; more common in Achilles tendon

⚠ **Cardiac status:** prolonged QT or use of products that increase QT prolongation
⚠ **Pseudomembranous colitis:** assess for diarrhea, abdominal pain, fever, fatigue, anorexia; possible anemia, elevated WBC, low serum albumin; stop product; usually either vancomycin or IV metroNIDAZOLE given
- Increased fluids to 3 L/day to avoid crystallization in kidneys

Evaluate:
- Therapeutic response: decreased pain, C&S; absence of infection

Teach patient/family:

Black Box Warning: To notify prescriber of tendon pain, inflammation; stop drug

- Not to take any products containing magnesium or calcium (such as antacids), iron, or aluminum with this product or 4 hr before or 8 hr after
- That photosensitivity may occur; to avoid sunlight or use sunscreen to prevent burns
- To use frequent rinsing of mouth, sugarless candy or gum for dry mouth
- To take as prescribed; not to double or miss doses
- If dizziness occurs, to ambulate, perform activities with assistance
- To complete full course of product therapy
- To contact prescriber if abnormal heart rhythm or seizures occur

M

moxifloxacin (ophthalmic)

(mocks-ih-floks′a-sin)

Vigamox, Moxeza

Func. class.: Ophthalmic antiinfective

Chem. class.: Fluoroquinolone

Do not confuse: ciprofloxacin/gatifloxacin/levofloxacin

ACTION: Inhibits DNA gyrase, thereby decreasing bacterial replication

USES: Bacterial conjunctivitis (aerobic gram-positive/negative organisms), *Chlamydia trachomatis*

CONTRAINDICATIONS: Hypersensitivity to this product or fluoroquinolones

Precautions: Pregnancy (C), breastfeeding

DOSAGE AND ROUTES

Bacterial conjunctivitis

- **Adult/adolescent/child ≥1 yr: ophthalmic SOL** 1 drop in affected eye(s) bid (Moxeza) or tid (Vigamox) × 7 days

Available forms: Ophthalmic solution 0.5%

Administer:

Ophthalmic route

- Commercially available ophthalmic solutions are not for injection subconjunctivally or into the anterior chamber of the eye
- Apply topically to the eye, taking care to avoid contamination
- Do not touch the tip of the dropper to the eye, fingertips, or other surface
- Apply pressure to lacrimal sac for 1 min after instillation
- Avoid wearing contact lenses during treatment

SIDE EFFECTS

EENT: Hypersensitivity, pruritus, blurred vision, tearing

PHARMACOKINETICS

Half-life 13 hr

NURSING CONSIDERATIONS

Assess:

- **Allergic reaction:** assess for hypersensitivity, discontinue product

Evaluate:

- Decreased ophthalmic infection

Teach patient/family:

Ophthalmic route

- To apply topically to the eye, taking care to avoid contamination
- That product is for ophthalmic use only
- Not to touch the tip of the dropper to the eye, fingertips, or other surface
- To apply pressure to lacrimal sac for 1 min after installation
- To avoid wearing contact lenses during treatment

mupirocin (topical, nasal)

(myoo-pihr′oh-sin)

Bactroban, Centany

Func. class.: Topical antiinfective

ACTION: Antibacterial activity results from inhibition of protein synthesis; bacteriostatic at low concentration, bactericidal at high concentration

USES: Impetigo, skin lesions *(Staphylococcus aureus/Streptococcus pyogenes);* nasal: methicillin-resistant *S. aureus*

CONTRAINDICATIONS: Hypersensitivity to this product

Precautions: Open wounds, burns, severe kidney disease, children, pregnancy (B), breastfeeding

DOSAGE AND ROUTES

Impetigo

- **Adult/child: TOP** apply to affected area tid × 1-2 wk

Skin lesions

• **Adult/child: TOP** apply to affected area tid × 10 days

Methicillin-resistant *S. aureus* in the nose

• **Adult/child ≥12 yr: NASAL** divide ointment in single use tube in half; use in each nostril bid × 5 days

Available forms: Topical cream, ointment 2%; intranasal ointment 2%

Administer:

Topical route

• Do not use skin products near the eyes, nose, or mouth
• Wash hands before and after use; wash affected area and gently pat dry
• May cover treated areas with gauze dressing

Cream/ointment

• Apply a thin film to the cleansed affected area; massage gently into affected areas, do not use near eyes, mouth
• **Nasal:** Close nostrils by squeezing and releasing and gently massaging over 1 min

SIDE EFFECTS

CNS: Headache
EENT: Burning, pharyngitis, rhinitis (nasal)
GI: Taste change, nausea
INTEG: Burning, rash, pruritus

INTERACTIONS

Decrease: Effect of other nasal products

NURSING CONSIDERATIONS

Assess:

• **Allergic reaction:** assess for hypersensitivity; product may need to be discontinued
• **Infection:** assess for number of lesions, severity in impetigo, other skin disorders

Evaluate:

• Decreased lesions in impetigo, other skin disorders

Teach patient/family:

Topical route

• Not to use skin products near the eyes, nose, or mouth
• To wash hands before and after use and to wash affected area and gently pat dry
• **Cream/Ointment:** to apply a thin film to the cleansed affected area; to cover treated areas with gauze dressing if desired
• **Nasal:** to close nostrils by squeezing and releasing and gently massaging over 1 min

mycophenolate mofetil (Rx)

(mye-koe-phen′oh-late)

CellCept, Myfortic

Func. class.: Immunosuppressant

ACTION:
Inhibits inflammatory responses that are mediated by the immune system

USES:
Prophylaxis for organ rejection in allogenic cardiac, hepatic, renal transplants

Unlabeled uses: Refractory uveitis, second-line therapy for Churg-Strauss syndrome, diffuse proliferative lupus nephritis (in combination), rheumatoid arthritis, psoriasis, GVHD, kidney disease, myasthenia gravis, atopic dermatitis

CONTRAINDICATIONS:
Hypersensitivity to this product or mycophenolic acid

Black Box Warning: Pregnancy (D)

Precautions: Breastfeeding, lymphomas, neutropenia, renal disease, accidental exposure, anemia

Black Box Warning: Infection, neoplastic disease

DOSAGE AND ROUTES

Renal transplant

To prevent organ rejection

• **Adult: PO** mycophenolate mofetil 1 g or 720 mg mycophenolate sodium; 1 g or 720 mg bid given to renal transplant

M

patients in combination with corticosteroids, cycloSPORINE

• **Child: PO** 600 mg bid (suspension) or **PO** cap 750 mg bid body surface area (BSA) of 1.25 to 1.5 m^2 or 1 g bid BSA >1.5 m^2

Renal dose

• **Adult: PO/IV** GFR <25 ml/min, max 2 g/day

Cardiac transplant

To prevent organ rejection

• **Adult: PO/IV** 1.5 g bid, **IV** can be started ≤24 hr after transplant, switch to **PO** when able

Hepatic transplant

To prevent organ rejection

• **Adult: PO** 1.5 g bid; **IV** 1 g over ≥2 hr

Refractory acute kidney transplant rejection (unlabeled)

• **Adult: PO** 1.5 g (Mofetil) bid

Rheumatoid arthritis (unlabeled)

• **Adult: PO** 250 mg-2 g/day (Mofetil)

GVHD (unlabeled)

• **Adult: PO** 2 g/day (Mofetil) with cycloSPORINE and prednisoLONE

Diffuse proliferative lupus nephritis (unlabeled)

• **Adult: PO** 1 g/day (Mofetil)

Uveitis (unlabeled)

• **Adult: PO** 1 g (Mofetil) bid × 6-41 mo

Atopic dermatitis (unlabeled)

• **Adult: PO** 1 g (Mofetil) bid × 4 wk, then 500 mg bid × 4 wk

• **Adolescent/child ≥2 yr: PO** 30-50 mg/kg/day (Mofetil) in 2 divided doses

Available forms: Caps 250 mg; tabs 500 mg; inj (powder) 500 mg/20-ml vial; powder for oral susp 200 mg/ml; ext rel tab (Myfortic) 180, 360 mg

Administer:

• May be given in combination with corticosteroids, cycloSPORINE

• Del rel tab, cap, oral susp, tab are not interchangeable

PO route

• Do not break, crush, or chew tabs; do not open caps

• Give at same time each day

• Avoid inhalation or direct contact with skin, mucous membranes; teratogenic in animals

• **Oral susp:** tap closed bottle several times to loosen powder; use 94 ml of water in graduated cylinder; add 1/2 total amount of water for constitution and shake the closed bottle; add remaining water and shake again; remove child-resistant cap; push adapter into neck of bottle; close tightly

• Give alone for better absorption

Intermittent IV INFUSION route

• Reconstitute each vial with 14 ml D_5W; shake gently; further dilute to 6 mg/ml; dilute 1 g/140 ml D_5W, 1.5 g/210 ml D_5W; give by slow IV infusion ≥2 hr; never give by bolus or rapid IV inj

• Do not give with other medications or sol

Y-site compatibilities: Alemtuzumab, alfentanil, amikacin, anidulafungin, argatroban, bivalirudin, caspofungin, cefepime, DAPTOmycin, DOPamine, norepinephrine, octreotide, oxytocin, tacrolimus, tigecycline, tirofiban, vancomycin, zoledronic acid

SIDE EFFECTS

CNS: *Tremor, dizziness, insomnia, headache, fever,* anxiety, pain, progressive multifocal leukoencephalopathy, asthenia, paresthesia

CV: *Hypertension, chest pain,* hypotension, edema

GI: *Diarrhea, constipation, nausea, vomiting,* stomatitis, GI bleeding, abdominal pain, anorexia, dyspepsia

GU: *UTI, hematuria,* renal tubular necrosis, polyomavirus-associated nephropathy

HEMA: Leukopenia, thrombocytopenia, anemia, pancytopenia, pure red cell aplasia, neutropenia

INTEG: *Rash*

META: *Peripheral edema, hypercholesterolemia, hypophosphatemia, edema, hyperkalemia, hypokalemia, hyperglycemia,* hypocalcemia, hypomagnesemia

MS: Arthralgia, muscle wasting, back pain, weakness

RESP: *Dyspnea, respiratory infection, increased cough, pharyngitis, bronchitis, pneumonia,* plural effusion, pulmonary fibrosis

SYST: Lymphoma, *nonmelanoma skin carcinoma,* sepsis

PHARMACOKINETICS

Rapidly and completely absorbed; metabolized to active metabolite (MPA); excreted in urine, feces; protein binding (MPA) 97%; half-life (MPA) 17.9 hr

INTERACTIONS

Increase: bone marrow suppression—azaTHIOprine
- Increased bleeding risk: anticoagulants, NSAIDs, thrombolytics, salicylates

Increase: toxicity—acyclovir, ganciclovir, valacyclovir

Increase: effects of phenytoin, theophylline

Increase: mycophenolate levels—probenecid, immunosuppressives, salicylates

Decrease: mycophenolate levels—antacids (magnesium, aluminum), cholestyramine, cycloSPORINE, rifamycin

Decrease: protein binding of phenytoin, theophylline

Decrease: effect of live attenuated vaccines, oral contraceptives

Drug/Herb

Interference with immunosuppression: astragalus, echinacea, melatonin

Drug/Food

Decrease: absorption if taken with food

Drug/Lab Test

Increase: serum creatitine, BUN
- Abnormal LFTs

NURSING CONSIDERATIONS

Assess:

⚠ **Progressive multifocal leukoencephalopathy,** may be fatal; ataxia, confusion, apathy, hemiparesis, visual problems, weakness; side effects should be reported to FDA
- Blood studies: CBC during treatment monthly
- Hepatic studies: alk phos, AST, ALT, bilirubin
- Renal studies: BUN, CCr, electrolytes

Black Box Warning: Pregnancy test within 1 wk before initiation of treatment; confirm negative pregnancy test

Evaluate:
- Therapeutic response: absence of graft rejection

Teach patient/family:
- To report fever, rash, severe diarrhea, chills, sore throat, fatigue because serious infections may occur
- To reduce risk of infection by avoiding crowds
- About the need for repeated lab tests

Black Box Warning: To use 2 forms of contraception before, during, and for 6 wk after therapy

- To take at same time each day

M

RARELY USED

nabumetone (Rx)

(na-byoo′me-tone)

Relafen

Func. class.: Nonsteroidal antiinflammatory

Chem. class.: Acetic acid derivative

USES: Osteoarthritis, rheumatoid arthritis, acute or chronic treatment

CONTRAINDICATIONS: Hypersensitivity to this product or aspirin, NSAIDs

Black Box Warning: Perioperative pain with CABG surgery

DOSAGE AND ROUTES

- **Adult: PO** 1 g as single dose or divided bid; max 2 g/day if needed

Renal dose

- **Adult: PO** CCr 31-49 ml/min, 750 mg daily, max 1500 mg/day; CCr <30 ml/min 500 mg daily, max 1000 mg/day

nadolol (Rx)

(nay-doe′lole)

Corgard, Syn-Nadol ✦

Func. class.: Antihypertensive, antianginal

Chem. class.: β-Adrenergic receptor blocker

Do not confuse:

Corgard/Cognex/Coreg

Nadolol/Mandol

ACTION: Long-acting, nonselective β-adrenergic receptor blocking agent, blocks β_1 in the heart and β_2 in the lungs, uterus, and circulatory system; mechanism is similar to that of propranolol

USES: Chronic stable angina pectoris, mild to moderate hypertension

Unlabeled uses: Tachydysrhythmias, anxiety, tremors, esophageal varices (rebleeding only), prophylaxis of migraine headaches, portal hypertension, atrial fibrillation

CONTRAINDICATIONS: Hypersensitivity to this product, cardiac failure, cardiogenic shock, 2nd/3rd-degree heart block, bronchospastic disease, sinus bradycardia, CHF, COPD

Precautions: Pregnancy (C), breastfeeding, diabetes mellitus, renal disease, hyperthyroidism, peripheral vascular disease, myasthenia gravis, major surgery, nonallergic bronchospasm

Black Box Warning: Abrupt discontinuation

DOSAGE AND ROUTES

- **Adult: PO** 40 mg/day, increase by 40-80 mg q2-14days; maintenance 40-240 mg/day for angina, 40-320 mg/day for hypertension
- **Geriatric: PO** 20 mg/day, may increase by 20 mg until desired dose

Renal dose

- **Adult: PO** CCr 31-50 ml/min, give q24-36hr; CCr 10-30 ml/min, give q24-48hr; CCr <10 ml/min, give q40-60hr

Migraine prevention (unlabeled)

- **Adult: PO** 40-240 mg/day × 2-18 mo

Available forms: Tabs 20, 40, 80 mg

Administer:

- With 8 oz water, check apical pulse before use, if <50 bpm, withhold; notify prescriber
- Give without regard to food
- Tabs may be crushed and mixed with food
- Discontinue other antihypertensives gradually

SIDE EFFECTS

CNS: Depression, *dizziness, fatigue,* lethargy, paresthesias, headache, *weakness,* insomnia, memory loss, nightmares

CV: *Bradycardia, hypotension,* CHF, palpitations, **AV block**, chest pain, peripheral ischemia, flushing, edema, vasodilation, conduction disturbances
EENT: Blurred vision, dry eyes, nasal congestion
ENDO: Hyperglycemia, hypoglycemia
GI: Nausea, vomiting, diarrhea, colitis, constipation, cramps, dry mouth, flatulence, hepatomegaly, **pancreatitis**, taste distortion
GU: *Impotence,* decreased libido
HEMA: **Agranulocytosis, thrombocytopenia**
INTEG: Rash, pruritus, fever, alopecia
RESP: Dyspnea, respiratory dysfunction, **bronchospasm**, cough, wheezing, **pulmonary edema**, pharyngitis, **laryngospasm**

PHARMACOKINETICS

PO: Onset variable, peak 3-4 hr, duration 10-24 hr; half-life 20-24 hr; not metabolized; excreted in urine (unchanged), bile, breast milk; protein binding 30%

INTERACTIONS

- **Do not use with MAOIs; bradycardia may occur**
- Peripheral ischemia: ergots

Increase: bradycardia—digoxin
Increase: hypotension, bradycardia—cloNIDine, EPINEPHrine
Increase: hypotensive effects—other hypotensive agents, phenothiazines
Decrease: β-blocking effect—thyroid hormones
Decrease: antihypertensive effect—NSAIDs

Drug/Lab Test

Increase: serum potassium, serum uric acid, ALT, AST, alk phos, LDH, blood glucose, cholesterol, ANA, triglycerides

NURSING CONSIDERATIONS

Assess:

- B/P, pulse, respirations during beginning therapy and periodically thereafter; orthostatic hypotension may occur
- Weight daily; report gain of 5 lb
- I&O ratio, CCr if kidney damage diagnosed; crackles, jugular venous distention, fatigue, dyspnea
- **Pain:** duration, time started, activity being performed, character
- **Hypertension:** check that prescriptions have been filled
- **Angina:** monitor frequency of angina, alleviating factors; duration, time started, activity being performed, character
- Headache, light-headedness, decreased B/P; may indicate a need for decreased dosage

Black Box Warning: Abrupt discontinuation: can result in MI, myocardial ischemia, ventricular dysrhythmias, severe hypertension; withdraw slowly by tapering

Evaluate:

- Therapeutic response: decreased B/P, heart rate, symptoms of angina

Teach patient/family:

- That product may mask signs of hypoglycemia or alter blood glucose in diabetics
- To avoid OTC products unless prescriber approves, to take as prescribed, at same time each day, do not double, take missed dose as soon as remembered if before 8 hr before next dose
- To avoid hazardous activities if dizziness occurs
- **Hypertension:** to comply with complete medical regimen; to report weight gain of >5 lb, swelling, unusual bruising, bleeding
- To rise slowly to prevent orthostatic hypotension
- About how and when to check B/P, pulse; to hold dose, contact prescriber if pulse ≤60 bpm, systolic B/P <90 mm Hg; to take missed dose as soon as possible if less than 8 hr

Black Box Warning: Not to discontinue abruptly; may cause life-threatening cardiac changes

N

nafcillin (Rx)

(naf-sill′in)

Func. class.: Antiinfective, broad-spectrum

Chem. class.: Penicillinase-resistant penicillin

ACTION: Bacteriocidal, interferes with cell-wall replication of susceptible organisms; cell lysis mediated by cell wall autolytic enzymes

USES: Effective for gram-positive cocci *(Staphylococcus aureus, Streptococcus viridans, Streptococcus pneumoniae)*, infections caused by penicillinase-producing *Staphylococcus*

CONTRAINDICATIONS: Hypersensitivity to penicillins or corn

Precautions: Pregnancy (B), breastfeeding, neonates; hypersensitivity to cephalosporins or carbapenems; GI disease, asthma, electrolyte imbalances, hepatic/renal disease, pseudomembranous colitis

DOSAGE AND ROUTES

- **Adult: IV** 500-2000 mg q4hr; IM 500 mg q6-8hr, max 12 g/day
- **Child and infant >1 mo: IV** 150-200 mg/kg/day in divided doses
- **Neonates >7 days (weight >2000 g): IV** 25 mg/kg q6hr
- **Neonates ≤7 days (weight <2000 g): IV** 25 mg/kg q8hr

Available forms: Powder for inj 1 g, premixed or Add-Vantage vials

Administer:

- Product after C&S has been drawn, begin therapy while waiting for results

IM route

- Reconstitute vials: add 1.7 (1.8 nafcil), 3, 4, or 6.4 ml (6.6 ml NaCl) (sterile water for inj, 0.9% NaCl, bacteriostatic water for inj with benzyl alcohol or parabens) to vials with 1 g, 2 g of nafcillin, respectively (250 mg/ml)
- No further dilution needed; after reconstitution, inject in deep muscle mass

IV route

- Reconstitute vials: add 1.7 (1.8 nafcil), 3, 4, or 6.4 ml (6.6 ml NaCl) sterile water for inj, 0.9% NaCl, bacteriostatic water for inj with benzyl alcohol or parabens to vials with 1 g, 2 g of nafcillin, respectively (250 mg/ml); pharmacy bulk pack reconstitute 10 g/93 ml sterile water inj or 0.9% NaCl (100 mg/ml)
- **Nallpen piggyback units:** reconstitute 1 or 2 g with 50-100 ml or 99 ml, respectively, of sterile water for inj, 0.45% NaCl, 0.9% NaCl
- **Unipen piggyback units:** reconstitute according to manufacturer

Direct Intermittent IV INJ route

- Further dilute reconstituted sol in 15-30 ml sterile water inj, 0.45% NaCl, 0.9% NaCl; inj slowly over 5-10 min into tubing of free-flowing compatible IV solution

Intermittent IV INFUSION route

- Vials, further dilute reconstituted sol to 2-40 mg/ml for peripheral vein infusion ≤20 mg/ml (preferred); piggyback unit, no further dilution needed; infuse ≥30-60 min, make sure entire dose is given before ≥10% of sol is inactivated
- Extravasation management: stop infusion and disconnect, leave needle/cannula in place, gently aspirate extravasated solution, do not flush line, use hyaluronidase, remove cannula/needle, apply dry cold compresses, elevate extremity

Y-site compatibilities: Acyclovir, alfentanil, amikacin, aminophylline, amphotericin B lipid complex (Abelcet), anidulafungin, argatroban, ascorbic acid injection, atenolol, atracurium, atropine, aztreonam, benztropine, bivalirudin, bleomycin, bretylium, bumetanide, buprenorphine, butorphanol, calcium chloride/gluconate, CARBOplatin, carmustine, cefamandole, ceFAZolin, cefoperazone, cefotaxime, cefoTEtan, cef OXitin, cefTAZidime, ceftizoxime, cefTRIAXone, cefuroxime, chlorproMAZINE, cimetidine, CISplatin, clindamycin, cyanocobalamin, cyclophosphamide, cycloSPORINE, DACTINomycin,

DAPTOmycin, DAUNOrubicin liposome, dexamethasone, digoxin, DOBUTamine, DOCEtaxel, DOPamine, DOXOrubicin liposomal, enalaprilat, EPHEDrine, EPINEPHrine, epoetin alfa, erythromycin, etoposide, etoposide phosphate, famotidine, fenoldopam, fentaNYL, fluconazole, fludarabine, foscarnet, furosemide, gallium, ganciclovir, gatifloxacin, gemtuzumab, gentamicin, glycopyrrolate, granisetron, heparin, hydrocortisone, HYDROmorphone, imipenem-cilastatin, indomethacin, isoproterenol, ketorolac, lactated Ringer's, lepirudin, leucovorin, lidocaine, linezolid injection, LORazepam, magnesium sulfate, mannitol, methyldopate, methylPREDNISolone, metoclopramide, metoprolol, metroNIDAZOLE, milrinone, morphine, multiple vitamins injection, naloxone, niCARdipine, nitroglycerin, nitroprusside, norepinephrine, octreotide, ondansetron, oxacillin, oxaliplatin, oxytocin, PACLitaxel (solvent/surfactant), pamidronate, pancuronium, pantoprazole, PEMEtrexed, penicillin G potassium/sodium, PENTobarbital, perphenazine, PHENobarbital, phentolamine, phenylephrine, phytonadione, piperacillin, polymyxin B, potassium acetate/chloride, procainamide, prochlorperazine, propofol, propranolol, ranitidine, Ringer's injection, sodium bicarbonate, SUFentanil, tacrolimus, teniposide, theophylline, thiamine, thiotepa, ticarcillin, ticarcillin-clavulanate, tigecycline, tirofiban, TNA (3-in-1), tobramycin, tolazoline, TPN (2-in-1), urokinase, vasopressin, vinBLAStine, voriconazole, zidovudine, zoledronic acid

SIDE EFFECTS

CNS: Lethargy, hallucinations, anxiety, depression, twitching, **coma, seizures**

GI: *Nausea, vomiting, diarrhea,* increased AST, ALT, abdominal pain, glossitis, **pseudomembranous colitis**

GU: Oliguria, **proteinuria, hematuria,** vaginitis, moniliasis, **glomerulonephritis, interstitial nephritis**

HEMA: Anemia, increased bleeding time, **bone marrow depression, neutropenia, agranulocytosis**

INTEG: Tissue necrosis, extravasation injury at inj site, **rash, pruritus, exfoliative dermatitis**

SYST: Anaphylaxis, serum sickness, Stevens-Johnson syndrome

PHARMACOKINETICS

Half-life 30-90 min; metabolized by liver; excreted in bile, urine; 70%-90% protein bound; peak 30-120 min (PO); peak 30-60 min (IM)

INTERACTIONS

- Avoid use with tetracyclines

Increase: nafcillin concentrations—probenecid

Decrease: effect of cycloSPORINE—warfarin

Decrease: nafcillin effect—chloramphenicol, macrolides, sulfonamides, tetracyclines, aminoglycosides

Drug/Food

Decrease: absorption—food, carbonated drinks, citrus fruit juices

Decrease: Hgb/HcT, neutrophils

Drug/Lab Test

False positive: urine glucose, urine protein

Decrease: potassium

NURSING CONSIDERATIONS

Assess:

- I&O ratio; report hematuria, oliguria, high doses are nephrotoxic
- **Pseudomembranous colitis: assess for diarrhea, abdominal pain, fever, fatigue, anorexia; possible anemia, elevated WBC, low serum albumin; stop product; usually either vancomycin or IV metroNIDAZOLE given**
- Hepatic studies: AST, ALT
- Blood studies: CBC with differential bleeding time, electrolytes

⚠ **Renal studies: urinalysis, BUN, creatinine; abnormal urinalysis may indicate nephrotoxicity**

- C&S before product therapy; product may be given as soon as culture is taken
- Respiratory status: rate, character, wheezing, tightness in chest

⚠ **Allergies before initiation of treatment; monitor for anaphylaxis, dyspnea, rash,**

laryngeal edema; stop product; keep emergency equipment nearby; skin eruptions after administration of penicillin to 1 wk after discontinuing product; cross-sensitivity with cephalosporins may occur
- Differential WBC 2× per wk in patients receiving long-term therapy
- IV site: for redness, swelling, pain at site

Evaluate:
- Therapeutic response: absence of fever, draining wounds

Teach patient/family:

⚠ To report sore throat, fever, fatigue (may indicate superinfection); CNS reactions; pseudomembraneous colitis (diarrhea, fever, abdominal pain, fatigue)
- To wear or carry emergency ID if allergic to penicillins
- To avoid use with other products unless approved by prescriber

TREATMENT OF ANAPHYLAXIS: Withdraw product; maintain airway; administer EPINEPHrine, aminophylline, O_2, IV corticosteroids

⚠ *HIGH ALERT*

nalbuphine (Rx)

(nal′byoo-feen)

Nubain ✦

Func. class.: Opioid analgesic

Chem. class.: Synthetic opioid agonist, antagonist

ACTION: Depresses pain impulse transmission at the spinal cord level by interacting with opioid receptors

USES: Moderate to severe pain, supplement to anesthesia

CONTRAINDICATIONS: Hypersensitivity to this product or parabens, addiction (opiate)

Precautions: Pregnancy (B), breastfeeding, addictive personality, increased intracranial pressure, MI (acute), severe heart disease, respiratory depression, renal/hepatic disease, bowel impaction, abrupt discontinuation

DOSAGE AND ROUTES

Analgesic
- **Adult: SUBCUT/IM/IV** 10 mg q3-6hr prn (based on 70-kg body weight), max 160 mg/day (IV/IM/SUBCUT); max 20 mg/dose if opiate naïve (IV/IM/SUBCUT)

Balanced anesthesia adjunct
- **Adult: IV** 0.3-3 mg/kg given over 10-15 min; may give 0.25-0.5 mg/kg as needed for maintenance

Available forms: Inj 10, 20 mg/ml

Administer:
- With antiemetic if nausea, vomiting occur
- When pain beginning to return; determine dosage interval by response
- Store in light-resistant area at room temperature

IM route
- IM deep in large muscle mass, rotate inj sites, protect from light

Direct IV route
- Undiluted ≤10 mg over 3-5 min into free-flowing IV line of D_5W, NS, or LR

Syringe compatibilities: Atropine, cimetidine, diphenhydrAMINE, droperidol, glycopyrrolate, hydrOXYzine, lidocaine, midazolam, prochlorperazine, ranitidine, scopolamine, trimethobenzamide

Y-site compatibilities: Amifostine, aztreonam, cisatracurium, cladribine, filgrastim, fludarabine, granisetron, melphalan, PACLitaxel, propofol, remifentanil, teniposide, thiotepa, vinorelbine

SIDE EFFECTS

CNS: *Drowsiness, dizziness, confusion, headache, sedation, euphoria,* dysphoria (high doses), hallucinations, dreaming, tolerance, physical, psychologic dependency

CV: Bradycardia, change in B/P, cardiac arrest

EENT: Blurred vision, miosis, diplopia

GI: *Nausea, vomiting, anorexia, constipation, cramps,* abdominal pain, dyspepsia, xerostomia, bitter taste

GU: Urinary urgency
INTEG: *Rash,* urticaria, flushing, diaphoresis, pruritus
RESP: **Respiratory depression/arrest,** pulmonary edema

PHARMACOKINETICS

SUBCUT/IM/IV: Peak 30 min, onset 2-15 min, IV 2-3 min, duration 3-6 hr, metabolized by liver, excreted by kidneys, half-life 3-6 hr

INTERACTIONS

Increase: effects with other CNS depressants—alcohol, opiates, sedative/hypnotics, antipsychotics, skeletal muscle relaxants
Increase: severe reactions—MAOIs
Drug/Herb
Increase: CNS depression, kava, valerian, hops, chamomile

NURSING CONSIDERATIONS

Assess:

- **Pain:** type, location, intensity before and 30-60 min after administration; titrate upward with 25%-50% until 50% of pain reduced; need for pain medication by pain sedation scoring, physical dependency
- Bowel status; constipation is common; may need laxative or stool softener

⚠ **Withdrawal reactions in opiate-dependent individuals: PE, vascular occlusion; abscesses, ulcerations, nausea, vomiting, seizures; low potential for dependence**

- **CNS changes:** dizziness, drowsiness, hallucinations, euphoria, LOC, pupil reaction
- Allergic reactions: rash, urticaria
- **Respiratory dysfunction: respiratory depression,** character, rate, rhythm; notify prescriber if respirations are <10/min

Evaluate:

- Therapeutic response: decrease in pain without respiratory depression

Teach patient/family:

- To report any symptoms of CNS changes, allergic reactions
- That physical dependency may result from long-term use; low potential for dependency
- **That withdrawal symptoms may occur: nausea, vomiting, cramps, fever, faintness, anorexia, profuse sweating, twitching; without treatment symptoms resolve in 5-14 days, chronic abstinence syndrome may last 2-6 mo**
- To avoid CNS depressants, alcohol
- To avoid driving, operating machinery if drowsiness occurs

TREATMENT OF OVERDOSE:

Naloxone (Narcan) 0.2-0.8 mg IV, O_2, IV fluids, vasopressors

naloxone (Rx)

(nal-oks′one)

Evzio, Narcan

Func. class.: Opioid antagonist, antidote

Chem. class.: Thebaine derivative

Do not confuse:
naloxone/naltrexone

N

ACTION:

Competes with opioids at opiate receptor sites

USES:

Respiratory depression induced by opioids, opiate agonist overdose
Unlabeled uses: IBS, opiate agonist dependence, opiate agonist-induced constipation, pruritus, urinary retention, coma, nausea, vomiting

CONTRAINDICATIONS:

Hypersensitivity
Precautions: Pregnancy (B), breastfeeding, children, neonates, CV disease, opioid dependency, seizure disorder, drug dependency, hepatic disease

DOSAGE AND ROUTES

Opioid-induced respiratory depression (known for suspected opiate agonist overdose)

- **Adult: IV/SUBCUT/IM** 0.4-2 mg, repeat q2-3min if needed, max 10 mg; **IV** infusion loading dose 0.005 mg/kg, then 0.0025 mg/kg/hr

- **Child <5 yr or ≤20 kg: IV/INTRAOSSEOUS** 0.01 mg/kg slowly followed by 0.1 mg/kg if needed; IV infusion (PALS) 0.04-0.16 mg/kg/hr, titrate
- **Adult/Adolescent/Child: Nasal** 1 spray, may repeat q2-3min if needed

Postoperative opioid-induced respiratory depression

- **Adult: IV** 0.1-0.2 mg q2-3min prn
- **Child: IV** 0.005-0.01 mg/kg q2-3min prn

Diagnosis of opiate-agonist dependence (unlabeled)

- **Adult: IM** 0.16 mg; if no withdrawal symptoms after 20-30 min, give 0.24 mg **IV**

Nausea/vomiting from continuous morphine infusion/urinary retention (unlabeled)

- **Adult: IV** 0.2 mg

Available forms: Inj 0.4, 1 mg/ml; nasal spray 4 mg/0.1 ml

Administer:

- Only with resuscitative equipment, O_2 nearby
- Only sol prepared within 24 hr
- Dark storage at room temperature
- Double-check dose, those taking opioids longer term are sensitive to this product

Direct IV route

- Undiluted (suspected opioid overdose) with sterile water for inj; give ≤0.4 mg over 15 sec

Continuous IV INFUSION route

- Dilute 2 mg/500 ml 0.9% NaCl or D_5W (4 mcg/ml), titrate to response

Y-site compatibilities: Acyclovir, alfentanil, amikacin, aminocaproic acid, aminophylline, anidulafungin, ascorbic acid, atenolol, atracurium, atropine, azaTHIOprine, aztreonam, benztropine, bivalirudin, bleomycin, bumetanide, buprenorphine, butorphanol, calcium chloride/gluconate, CARBOplatin, caspofungin, cefamandole, ceFAZolin, cefmetazole, cefonicid, cefoperazone, cefotaxime, cefoTEtan, cefOXitin, cefTAZidime, ceftizoxime, cefTRIAXone, cefuroxime, cephalothin, cephapirin, chloramphenicol, chlorproMAZINE, cimetidine, CIS platin, clindamycin, cyanocobalamin, cyclophosphamide, cycloSPORINE, cytarabine, DACTINomycin, DAPTOmycin, dexamethasone, digoxin, diltiazem, diphenhydrAMINE, DOBUTamine, DOCE taxel, DOPamine, doxacurium, DOXOrubicin, doxycycline, enalaprilat, ePHEDrine, EPINEPHrine, epirubicin, epoetin alfa, eptifibatide, ertapenem, erythromycin, esmolol, etoposide, etoposide phosphate, famotidine, fenoldopam, fentaNYL, fluconazole, fludarabine, fluorouracil, folic acid, furosemide, ganciclovir, gatifloxacin, gemcitabine, gentamicin, glycopyrrolate, granisetron, heparin, hydrocortisone, hydrOXYzine, IDArubicin, ifosfamide, imipenem-cilastatin, inamrinone, indomethacin, insulin (regular), irinotecan, isoproterenol, ketorolac, labetalol, levofloxacin, lidocaine, linezolid, LORazepam, mannitol, mechloreth amine, meperidine, metaraminol, methicillin, methotrexate, methoxamine, methyldopate, methylPREDNISolone, metoclopramide, metoprolol, metroNIDAZOLE, mezlocillin, miconazole, midazolam, milrinone, minocycline, mitoXANtrone, morphine, moxalactam, multiple vitamins, mycophenolate, nafcillin, nalbuphine, nesiritide, netilmicin, nitroglycerin, nitroprusside, norepinephrine, octreotide, ondansetron, oxacillin, oxaliplatin, oxytocin, PACLitaxel, palonosetron, pamidronate, pancuronium, papaverine, PEMEtrexed, penicillin G potassium/sodium, pentamidine, pentazocine, PENTobarbital, PHENobarbital, phentolamine, phenylephrine, phytonadione, piperacillin, piperacillin-tazobactam, polymyxin B, potassium chloride, procainamide, prochlorperazine, promethazine, propofol, propranolol, protamine, pyridoxine, quiNIDine, quinupristin-dalfopristin, ranitidine, ritodrine, rocuronium, sodium acetate/bicarbonate, succinylcholine, SUFentanil, tacrolimus, teniposide, theophylline, thiamine, ticarcillin, ticarcillin-clavulanate, tigecycline, tirofiban, tobramycin, tolazoline, trimetaphan, urokinase, vancomycin, vasopressin, vecuronium, verapamil, vinCRIStine, vinorelbine, voriconazole, zoledronic acid

SIDE EFFECTS

CNS: Nervousness, **seizures**, tremor, opioid withdrawal symptoms
CV: Rapid pulse, increased systolic B/P (high doses), **ventricular tachycardia, fibrillation, hypo/hypertension, cardiac arrest, sinus tachycardia**
GI: Nausea, vomiting
RESP: **Pulmonary edema, dyspnea**

PHARMACOKINETICS

Well absorbed IM, SUBCUT; metabolized by liver, crosses placenta; excreted in urine, breast milk; half-life 30-81 min
IM/SUBCUT: Onset 2-5 min, duration 45-60 min
IV: Onset 1 min, duration 45 min

INTERACTIONS

Increase: **seizures—traMADol overdose**
Decrease: effect of opioid analgesics

NURSING CONSIDERATIONS

Assess:
- **Withdrawal: cramping, hypertension, anxiety, vomiting, signs of withdrawal in drug-dependent individuals may occur ≤2 hr after administration**
- VS q3-5min
- ABGs including Po_2, Pco_2
- Cardiac status: tachycardia, hypertension; monitor ECG
- **Respiratory dysfunction: respiratory depression, character, rate, rhythm; if respirations are <10/min, administer naloxone; probably due to opioid overdose; monitor LOC**
- **Pain:** duration, intensity, location before and after administration; may be used for respiratory depression

Evaluate:
- Therapeutic response: reversal of respiratory depression; LOC—alert

Teach patient/family:
- When patient is lucid, about reasons for, expected results of product

naltrexone (Rx)

(nal-trex′one)

ReVia, Vivitrol

Func. class.: Opioid antagonist
Chem. class.: Thebaine derivative

Do not confuse:
naloxone/naltrexone

ACTION: Competes with opioids at opioid-receptor sites

USES: Blockage of opioid analgesics; used for treatment of opiate addiction, alcoholism, opiate agonist overdose
Unlabeled uses: Nicotine withdrawal, opiate-agonist withdrawal, pruritus

CONTRAINDICATIONS: Hypersensitivity, opioid dependence

Black Box Warning: Hepatic failure, hepatitis

Precautions: Pregnancy (B), breastfeeding, children, renal disease, depression, suicidal ideation, coagulopathy, respiratory depression, IV use

Black Box Warning: Hepatic disease

DOSAGE AND ROUTES

Adjunct in opiate-agonist dependence
- **Adult:** **PO** 25 mg; if no withdrawal symptoms in 1 hr, then 25 mg additionally; if no withdrawal symptoms, then 50-150 mg/day or in divided doses

Adjunct in alcoholism treatment
- **Adult:** **PO** 50 mg/day with food × 12 wk; **IM** (Vivitrol) 380 mg q4wk

Pruritus (unlabeled)
- **Adult:** **PO** 50 mg/day × 7 days to 4 wk

Nicotine withdrawal (unlabeled)
- **Adult:** **PO** 50 mg/day

Ultrarapid opiate detoxification (unlabeled)
• **Adult: PO** 50 mg before sedation with midazolam

Available forms: Tabs 50 mg; powder for inj 380 mg

Administer:

PO route
• Give with food or after meals, antacid to prevent nausea, vomiting
• Store in tight container

IM route
• Do not give until opioid-free for 7-10 days to prevent opioid withdrawal (relapse only)
• IM deep in gluteal, alternate inj sites; use supplied needle to prevent inj-site reaction; aspirate before inj
• Only if resuscitative equipment is nearby
• Not to use IV or SUBCUT

SIDE EFFECTS

CNS: *Stimulation, drowsiness,* dizziness, confusion, seizures, headache, flushing, hallucinations, nervousness, irritability, suicidal ideation, syncope, anxiety
CV: Rapid pulse, pulmonary edema, hypertension, DVT
EENT: Tinnitus, hearing loss, blurred vision
GI: *Nausea, vomiting, diarrhea, heartburn,* hepatotoxicity, constipation, abdominal pain
GU: Delayed ejaculation, impotence
INTEG: *Rash,* urticaria, bruising, oily skin, acne, pruritus, inj-site reactions
MISC: Increased thirst, chills, fever
MS: Joint and muscle pain
RESP: Wheezing, hyperpnea, nasal congestion, rhinorrhea, sneezing, sore throat, pneumonia

PHARMACOKINETICS

Metabolized by liver, excreted by kidneys; crosses placenta, excreted in breast milk; half-life 4 hr; IM half-life 5-10 days; extensive first-pass metabolism; protein binding 21%-28%
PO: Onset 15-30 min, peak 1 hr
IM: Peak 2-3 days, duration >1 month

INTERACTIONS

Increase: lethargy—phenothiazines
Increase: hepatotoxicity—disulfiram
Increase: bleeding risk—anticoagulants

NURSING CONSIDERATIONS

Assess:

Black Box Warning: Hepatic status: LFTs, jaundice, hepatitis, hepatic failure

• ABGs including Po_2, Pco_2, LFTs, VS q3-5min
• Signs of withdrawal in drug-dependent individuals, use naltrexone challenge to test opioid dependence; must be free of opioids for 7-10 days before using this product, or withdrawal symptoms can occur
• Cardiac status: tachycardia, hypertension
• **Respiratory dysfunction: respiratory depression,** character, rate, rhythm; if respirations <10/min, respiratory stimulant should be administered
• Mental status: depression, suicidal ideation

Evaluate:
• Therapeutic response: blocking opiate ingestion; successful nicotine, alcohol withdrawal

Teach patient/family:
• That patient must be drug-free to start treatment
⚠ That using opioid while taking this product could prove fatal because high dose is needed to overcome this antagonist; not to self-dose with OTC products unless approved by prescriber
• To carry emergency ID stating product used
• That, if surgery is needed, all involved should be aware of this product
• To use caution while driving or performing other hazardous tasks until effect is known
⚠ That suicidal thoughts/behaviors may occur; to report these immediately

naphazoline (ophthalmic)

(na-faz′oh-leen)

Advanced Eye Relief, Redness Maximum Relief, Ak-Con, All Clear, Clear Eyes, Naphcon Forte ♣, VasoClear

Func. class.: Ophthalmic vasoconstrictor

Chem. class.: Sympathomimetic

ACTION: Acts on the blood vessels in the eye to produce vasoconstriction

USES: Ocular congestion, irritation, itching of the eye

CONTRAINDICATIONS: Hypersensitivity, acute angle-closure glaucoma, 0.1% solution in children/infants

Precautions: Hyperthyroidism, diabetes mellitus, hypertension, cardiac conditions

DOSAGE AND ROUTES

• **Adult: OPHTH** instill 1-2 drops in affected eye in the conjunctival sac every 3-4 hr, up to qid

Available forms: ophthalmic solution 0.012%, 0.1%, 0.02%

Administer:

• Store at room temperature; keep tightly closed

SIDE EFFECTS

CNS: Headache

EENT: Blurred vision, irritation, photophobia, dilation, stinging, elevated IOP, keratitis

PHARMACOKINETICS

Onset 10 min, duration up to 6 hr

INTERACTIONS

Increase: Systemic effects—β-blockers

• Do not use within 14 days of MAOIs

NURSING CONSIDERATIONS

Assess:

• Ocular itching, congestion, irritation: should show improvement quickly; avoid using more than 3 days; long-term use or exceeding dosage can lead to rebound congestion; report eye pain, blurred vision

Evaluate:

• Decreasing ocular itching, congestion, irritation

Teach patient/family:

• Method for instilling drops

• **To notify prescriber of eye pain, blurred vision**

• That ocular itching, congestion, irritation should show improvement quickly

• To avoid using longer than 3 days; that long-term use or exceeding dosage can lead to rebound congestion

• To wait for at least 15 min before wearing contact lenses

naproxen (Rx, OTC)

Aleve, Anaprox, Anaprox DS, Apo-Napro-Na ♣, Midol Extended Relief, Naprelan, Novo-Naprox ♣, Novo-Naprox Sodium ♣, Nu-Naprox ♣, TH Naproxen

Func. class.: Nonsteroidal antiinflammatory, nonopioid analgesic

Chem. class.: Propionic acid derivative

Do not confuse:

Naprosyn/Natacyn/Naprelan

ACTION: Inhibits COX-1, COX-2 by blocking arachidonate; analgesic, antiinflammatory, antipyretic

USES: Osteoarthritis; rheumatoid, gouty arthritis; primary dysmenorrhea; ankylosing spondylitis, bursitis, tendinitis, myalgia, dental pain, juvenile rheumatoid arthritis

N

Unlabeled uses: Bone pain, migraine/migraine prophylaxis, heterotropic ossification

CONTRAINDICATIONS:
Pregnancy (D) 3rd trimester, hypersensitivity to NSAIDs, salicylates

Black Box Warning: Perioperative pain in CABG surgery

Precautions: Pregnancy (C) breastfeeding, children <2 yr, geriatric patients, bleeding disorders, GI disorders, cardiac disorders, hypersensitivity to other antiinflammatory agents, CCr <30 ml/min, asthma, renal failure, hepatic disease

Black Box Warning: MI, GI bleeding, stroke

DOSAGE AND ROUTES
200 mg base = 220 mg naproxen sodium

Antiinflammatory/analgesic/antidysmenorrheal

- **Adult: PO** 250-500 mg bid, max 1500 mg/day; **DEL REL** 375-500 mg bid
- **Child ≥2 yr: PO** 7 mg/kg q12hr

Antigout

- **Adult: PO** 750 mg, then 250 mg q8hr

OTC use

- **Adult: PO** 220 mg q8-12hr or 440 mg, then 220 mg q12hr; max 660 mg/24hr taken ≤10 days
- **Geriatric >65 yr: PO** max 220 mg q12hr

Available forms: Naproxen: tabs 250, 375, 500 mg; del rel tabs (EC-Naprosyn, Naprosyn-E) 250 ♣, 375, 500 mg; oral susp 125 mg/5 ml; ext rel tabs (CR) 375, 500, 750 mg; **naproxen sodium:** tabs 220, 275, 550 mg tab, ext rel 220 mg

Administer:

- Store at room temperature
- With food to decrease GI symptoms; take on empty stomach to facilitate absorption; give with full glass of liquid
- Do not crush, break, or chew ext rel tabs
- OTC for ≤10 days unless approved by prescriber
- Adequately hydrate in those taking angiotensin receptor blockers/angiotensin-converting enzyme inhibitors
- **Oral susp:** shake well; use measuring cup provided or other calibrated device

SIDE EFFECTS
CNS: Dizziness, drowsiness, fatigue, tremors, confusion, insomnia, anxiety, depression

CV: Tachycardia, peripheral edema, palpitations, dysrhythmias, **MI, stroke**

EENT: Tinnitus, hearing loss, blurred vision

GI: Nausea, anorexia, vomiting, diarrhea, jaundice, **hepatitis,** constipation, flatulence, cramps, peptic ulcer, **GI ulceration, bleeding, perforation**

GU: Nephrotoxicity: dysuria, hematuria, oliguria, azotemia

HEMA: Blood dyscrasias

INTEG: Purpura, rash, pruritus, sweating

SYST: Anaphylaxis, Stevens-Johnson syndrome

PHARMACOKINETICS
PO: Peak 2-4 hr, half-life 12-17 hr; metabolized in liver; excreted in urine (metabolites), breast milk; 99% protein binding

INTERACTIONS
- **Do not use with adefovir, cidofovir; nephrotoxicity is increased**

Increase: renal impairment—ACE inhibitors

⚠ **Increase: toxicity risk—methotrexate, lithium, antineoplastics, probenecid, radiation treatment**

Increase: bleeding risk—oral anticoagulants, thrombolytic agents, eptifibatide, tirofiban, clopidogrel, ticlopidine, plicamycin, SSRIs, SNRIs, tricyclics

Increase: GI side effects risk—aspirin, corticosteroids, alcohol, NSAIDs

Decrease: effect of antihypertensives, diuretics

Decrease: absorption of naproxen—antacids, sucralfate, cholestyramine

Drug/Herb

• Bleeding risk: feverfew, garlic, ginger, ginkgo, ginseng *(Panax)*

Drug/Lab Test

Increase: BUN, alk phos, LFTs, potassium, glucose, cholesterol

Decrease: potassium, sodium

False increase: 5-HIAA, 17KS

NURSING CONSIDERATIONS

Assess:

Black Box Warning: Cardiac status: CV thrombotic events, MI, stroke; may be fatal; not to be used with CABG

Black Box Warning: GI status: ulceration, bleeding, perforation; may be fatal; obtain stool guaiac

• **Pain:** frequency, characteristics, intensity; relief before and 1-2 hr after product

• **Arthritis:** range of motion, pain, swelling before and 1-2 hr after use

• **Fever:** before, 1 hr after use

⚠ Asthma, aspirin hypersensitivity or nasal polyps, increased risk of hypersensitivity

• **Renal, hepatic blood studies:** BUN, creatinine, AST, ALT, Hgb, LDH, blood glucose, Hct, WBC, platelets, CCr before treatment, periodically thereafter during long-term therapy

• Audiometric, ophthalmic exam before, during, after treatment; if taking long term, eye, ear problems: blurred vision, tinnitus (may indicate toxicity)

Evaluate:

• Therapeutic response: decreased pain, stiffness, swelling in joints; ability to move more easily

Teach patient/family:

• To report blurred vision, ringing, roaring in ears (may indicate toxicity)

• To avoid driving, other hazardous activities if dizziness or drowsiness occurs

⚠ To report change in urine pattern, weight increase, edema (face, lower extremities), pain increase in joints, fever, blood in urine (indicates nephrotoxicity); black stools, flu-like symptoms, signs of MI, stroke

• That therapeutic effects may take up to 1 mo in arthritis

• To avoid ASA, alcohol, steroids, or other OTC medications without prescriber approval

• To report use to all health care providers

• To notify prescriber if pregnancy is planned or suspected, pregnancy (C); to avoid breastfeeding

naratriptan (Rx)

(nair′ah-trip-tan)

Amerge

Func. class.: Antimigraine agent

Chem. class.: 5-HT_1 receptor agonist

Do not confuse:

Amerge/Altace/Amaryl

N

ACTION: Binds selectively to the vascular 5-HT_1 B/D receptor subtype; exerts antimigraine effect; causes vasoconstriction in cranial arteries

USES: Acute treatment of migraine with/without aura

CONTRAINDICATIONS: Hypersensitivity, angina pectoris, history of MI, documented silent ischemia, ischemic heart disease, concurrent ergotamine-containing preparations, uncontrolled hypertension, CV syndromes, hemiplegic or basilar migraines, severe renal disease (CCr <15 ml/min); severe hepatic disease (Child-Pugh grade C)

Precautions: Pregnancy (C), breastfeeding, children, geriatric patients, postmenopausal women, men >40 yr, CAD risk, hypercholesterolemia, obesity, diabetes, impaired renal/hepatic function, peripheral vascular disease overuse

DOSAGE AND ROUTES

• **Adult: PO** 1 or 2.5 mg with fluids; if headache returns, repeat 1× after 4 hr; max 5 mg/24 hr

Hepatic/renal dose

• **Adult: PO** CCr 15-39 ml/min or mild to moderate hepatic disease max 2.5 mg/24 hr

Available forms: Tabs 1, 2.5 mg

Administer:

• With fluids as soon as symptoms appear; may take another dose after 4 hr; do not take >5 mg during any 24-hr period

SIDE EFFECTS

CNS: Dizziness, sedation, fatigue

CV: Increased B/P, palpitations, tachydysrhythmias, PR, QTc prolongation, ST/T wave changes, PVCs, atrial flutter/fibrillation, coronary vasospasm

EENT: EENT infections, photophobia

GI: *Nausea, vomiting*

MISC: Temperature change sensations; tightness, pressure sensations

MS: *Weakness, neck stiffness,* myalgia

PHARMACOKINETICS

Onset 2-3 hr; peak 2-3 hr; 28%-31% protein binding; half-life 6 hr; metabolized in liver (metabolite); excreted in urine, feces; may be excreted in breast milk

INTERACTIONS

Increase: serotonin syndrome, neuroleptic malignant syndrome—SSRIs (FLUoxetine, fluvoxaMINE, PARoxetine, sertraline), SNRIs, serotonin receptor agonists, sibutramine

Increase: vasospastic effects—ergot, ergot derivatives, other 5-HT_1 agonists

Increase: adverse reactions risk—MAOIs; do not use together

Drug/Herb

• Serotonin syndrome: SAM-e, St. John's wort

NURSING CONSIDERATIONS

Assess:

• **Migraine symptoms:** aura, duration, effect on lifestyle, aggravating/alleviating factors

⚠ **Serotonin syndrome, neuroleptic malignant syndrome:** increased heart rate, shivering sweating, dilated pupils, tremors, high B/P, hyperthermia, headache, confusion; if these occur, stop product, administer serotonin antagonist if needed; at least 2 wk should elapse between discontinuation of serotonergic agents and start of product

⚠ Cardiac status: ECG, increased B/P, dysrhythmias, monitor for PR, QT prolongation, ST-T wave changes, PVCs in those with cardiac disease

• Stress level, activity, recreation, coping mechanisms

• Neurologic status: LOC blurred vision, nausea, vomiting, tingling in extremities preceding headache

• Quiet, calm environment with decreased stimulation (noise, bright light, excessive talking)

Evaluate:

• Therapeutic response: decrease in frequency, severity of headache

Teach patient/family:

⚠ To report pain, tightness in chest, neck, throat, or jaw; to notify prescriber immediately if sudden, severe abdominal pain occurs

• Not to use if another 5-HT_1 agonist or ergot preparation has been used during past 24 hr; to avoid using >2 days/wk because rebound headache may occur

• To notify prescriber if pregnancy is planned or suspected; to avoid breastfeeding

natalizumab (Rx)

(na-ta-liz′u-mab)

Tysabri

Func. class.: Biologic response modifier, immunoglobulins, monoclonal antibody

ACTION:

Biologic-response-modifying properties mediated through specific receptors on cells; may be secondary to blockade of the interaction of inflammatory cells with vascular endothelial cells

USES:
Ambulatory patients with relapsing/remitting MS who have not responded to other treatment; those with moderate to severe Crohn's disease

CONTRAINDICATIONS:
Hypersensitivity, immunocompromised individuals (HIV, AIDS, leukemia, lymphoma, transplants), PML, murine (mouse) protein allergy

Black Box Warning: Progressive multifocal leukoencephalopathy

Precautions: Pregnancy (C), breastfeeding, geriatric patients, chronic progressive MS, depression, mental disorders, diabetes, TB, active infections, hepatotoxicity

DOSAGE AND ROUTES
- **Adult: IV INFUSION** 300 mg q4wk; give over 1 hr q4wk; observe during and for 1 hr after infusion
- **Adolescent and child ≥11 yr (unlabeled): IV INFUSION** pediatric Crohn's disease activity index (PCDAI) >30, 3 mg/kg q4wk

Available forms: Single-use vial, 300 mg/100 ml 0.9% NaCl

Administer:
- Acetaminophen for fever, headache
- Only after being enrolled in the TOUCH Prescribing Program

Intermittent IV INFUSION route
- Use only clear, colorless solution, without particulates
- Withdraw 15 ml from the vial using aseptic technique: inj concentration into 100 ml 0.9% NaCl; do not use other diluents; mix completely; do not shake; infusion immediately or refrigerate for ≤8 hr; warm to room temperature before using; flush with 0.9% NaCl before, after infusion; do not admix or use in same line with other agents
- Withhold product at first sign of PML
- Prescribers must be registered in the TOUCH Prescribing Program (1-800-456-2255)
- Store sol in refrigerator; do not freeze or shake; protect from light

SIDE EFFECTS
CNS: *Headache, fatigue,* rigors, syncope, tremors, *depression,* **progressive multifocal leukoencephalopathy (PML), suicidal ideation,** anxiety

CV: Chest discomfort, hypo/hypertension, tachycardia

GI: *Abdominal discomfort,* abnormal LFT, gastroentritis, **severe hepatic injury**

GU: Amenorrhea, *UTI, irregular menses,* vaginitis, urinary frequency

INTEG: *Rash,* dermatitis, pruritus, **skin melanoma,** infusion-related reactions

MS: *Arthralgia,* myalgia

RESP: *Lower respiratory tract infection,* dyspnea

SYST: **Anaphylaxis, angioedema**

PHARMACOKINETICS
Half-life approximately 11 days

INTERACTIONS
- Do not use with vaccines

Increase: infection—immunosuppressants, antineoplastics, immunomodulators, tumor necrosis factors

N

NURSING CONSIDERATIONS
Assess:

Black Box Warning: Progressive multifocal leukoencephalopathy (weakness, paralysis, vision loss, impaired speech, cognitive deterioration; obtain gadolinium-enhanced MRI scan of the brain, possibly cerebrospinal fluid for JC viral DNA; signs, symptoms of PML (decreased cognition, vision; ataxia, dysphagia), incidences increase with number of doses, over 2 yr immunosuppressants and anti-JC virus antibody; consider testing for the anti-JC virus and periodically retest

- **Infection:** report serious opportunistic infections to the manufacturer; those with Crohn's disease and chronic oral corticosteroids may be at greater risk of infection
- Blood, renal, hepatic studies: CBC, differential, platelet counts, BUN, creatinine, ALT, urinalysis, antibody testing

- CNS symptoms: headache, fatigue, depression, rigors, tremors
- GI status: abdominal discomfort, gastroenteritis, severe hepatic injury, abnormal LFTs
- Mental status: depression, depersonalization, suicidal thoughts, insomnia
- **MS symptoms;** product should only be used by patients who have not responded to other treatments

⚠ **Anaphylaxis:** SOB, hives; swelling, tightness in throat, chest pain; usually within 2 hr of infusion

Evaluate:

- Therapeutic response: decreased symptoms of MS, Crohn's disease

Teach patient/family:

- Provide patient or family member with written, detailed information about product (med guide)
- That female patients may experience irregular menses, amenorrhea; may worsen over several days; to notify prescriber if pregnancy is suspected; to avoid breastfeeding while taking this product; if pregnant, call the Tysabri Pregnancy Exposure Registry (1-800-456-2255)

⚠ To notify prescriber of possible infection: sore throat, cough, increased temperature, infusion-site reactions

- That continuing follow-up will be needed at 3, 6 mo after first dose, then every 6 mo
- To inform all prescribers of product use

natamycin ophthalmic

See Appendix B

nebivolol (Rx)

(ne-biv′oh-lol)

Bystolic

Func. class.: Antihypertensive

Chem. class.: β_1-blocker

ACTION: Competitively blocks stimulation of β-adrenergic receptors within vascular smooth muscle; decreases rate of SA node discharge; increases recovery time; slows conduction of AV node, thereby resulting in decreased heart rate (negative chronotropic effect), which decreases O_2 consumption in myocardium due to β_1-receptor antagonism; decreases renin-aldosterone-angiotensin system at high doses; inhibits β_2-receptors in bronchial system at high doses

USES: Hypertension alone or in combination

Unlabeled uses: Heart failure

CONTRAINDICATIONS: Cardiogenic shock, acute heart failure, severe hepatic disease, severe bradycardia, sick sinus syndrome, AV heart block; hypersensitivity to product, β-blockers

Precautions: Pregnancy (C), breastfeeding, children, major surgery, peripheral vascular disease, diabetes mellitus, thyrotoxicosis disease, COPD, asthma, well-compensated heart failure, renal/hepatic disease, abrupt discontinuation, acute bronchospasm

DOSAGE AND ROUTES

Hypertension

- **Adult: PO** 5 mg/day, may be increased to desired response q2wk; max 40 mg/day
- **Geriatric: PO** max 40 mg/day

Renal/hepatic dose

- **Adult: PO** CCr <30 ml/min, 2.5 mg/day; may increase cautiously; (Child-Pugh class B) 2.5 mg daily, use dose escalation cautiously

Heart failure (unlabeled)

- **Adult: PO** 1.25 mg titrated to max 10 mg/day

Available forms: Tabs 2.5, 5, 10, 20 mg

Administer:

PO route

- Without regard to meals; tab may be crushed or swallowed whole; give with food to prevent GI upset
- Taper over 1-2 wk when discontinuing, minimize physical exertion, if angina recurs, give nebivolol
- Store protected from light, moisture; place in cool environment

SIDE EFFECTS

CNS: *Insomnia, fatigue, dizziness, mental changes,* drowsiness, *headache*
CV: **Bradycardia, MI,** AV heart block, edema
GI: *Nausea, diarrhea,* vomiting, abdominal pain
GU: *Impotence*
HEMA: **Thrombocytopenia**
INTEG: Rash, pruritus, vasculitis, urticaria, psoriasis, **angioedema**
MISC: **Renal failure, pulmonary edema,** hyperuricemia, hypercholesterolemia, withdrawal symptoms
RESP: **Bronchospasm,** dyspnea

PHARMACOKINETICS

Peak 1.5-4 hr; half-life 12 hr; metabolized in liver by CYP2D6; 38% excreted in urine, 44% in feces

INTERACTIONS

⚠ **Do not give with other β-blockers, mefloquine**
Increase: nebivolol action—CYP2D6 inhibitors (amiodarone, buPROPion, chloroquine, chlorpheniramine, chlorproMAZINE, cinacalcet, diphenhydrAMINE, DULoxetine, FLUoxetine, haloperidol, imatinib, PARoxetine, promethazine, propoxyphene, quiNIDine, quiNINE, ritonavir, terbinafine, thioridazine), cimetidine, calcium channel blockers (nondihydropyridine)
Decrease: nebivolol action—CYP2D6 inducers (rifampin), sildenafil

Drug/Herb

- May increase nebivolol effect—hawthorn
- May decrease nebivolol effect—ephedra

Drug/Lab Test

Increase: serum lipoprotein levels, BUN, potassium, triglycerides, uric acid, LDH, AST, ALT, alk phos
Decrease: platelets

NURSING CONSIDERATIONS

Assess:

- **Hypertension:** B/P during beginning treatment, periodically thereafter; apical/radial pulse before administration; notify prescriber of any significant changes (pulse <50 bpm); **signs of CHF** (dyspnea, crackles, weight gain, jugular venous distention)
- Blood glucose in diabetics
- Baselines of renal, hepatic function tests before therapy begins and periodically, **do not use in Child-Pugh class >B**
- Edema in feet, legs daily: monitor I&O

Evaluate:

- Therapeutic response: decreased B/P after 1-2 wk; decreased dysrhythmias

Teach patient/family:

⚠ **Not to discontinue product abruptly because severe cardiac reactions may occur; to taper over 2 wk; not to double dose; if dose is missed, to take as soon as remembered up to 4 hr before next dose**

- That product may mask signs of hypoglycemia or alter blood glucose levels
- Not to use OTC products containing α-adrenergic stimulants (nasal decongestants, OTC cold preparations) unless directed by prescriber
- To report low pulse, dizziness, confusion, depression, fever
- To take pulse, B/P at home; advise patient when to notify prescriber
- To comply with weight control, dietary adjustments, modified exercise program
- To carry emergency ID to identify product, allergies
- To avoid hazardous activities if dizziness, drowsiness present
- **To report symptoms of CHF:** difficulty breathing, especially on exertion or when lying down, night cough, swelling of extremities
- To continue with required lifestyle changes (exercise, diet, weight loss, stress reduction)

TREATMENT OF OVERDOSE:

Lavage, IV atropine for bradycardia, IV theophylline for bronchospasm, digoxin, O_2, diuretic for cardiac failure, IV glucose for hypoglycemia, IV diazepam (or phenytoin) for seizures, IV fluids, IV pressors

nelfinavir (Rx)

(nell-fin′a-ver)

Viracept

Func. class.: Antiretroviral

Chem. class.: Protease inhibitor

ACTION:
Inhibits human immunodeficiency virus (HIV-1) protease, which prevents maturation of the infectious virus

Uses: HIV-1 in combination with other antiretrovirals

CONTRAINDICATIONS:
Hypersensitivity to protease inhibitors

Precautions: Pregnancy (B), breastfeeding, renal/hepatic disease, hemophilia, PKU, pancreatitis, diabetes, infection, immune reconstitution syndrome

DOSAGE AND ROUTES
HIV infection

- **Adult and child >13 yr: PO** 750 mg tid or 1250 mg bid, max 2500 mg/day
- **Child 2-13 yr: PO** 25-35 mg/kg tid, max 2500 mg/day

Prevention of HIV infection after exposure (unlabeled)

- **Adult: PO** 1250 mg bid with 2 other antiretroviral agents × 4 wk

Available forms: Tabs 250, 625 mg; powder, oral 50 mg/g/scoop

Administer:

PO route

- Do not mix with juice or acidic fluids
- **Oral powder:** mixed with fluids if desired; stable mixed for 6 hr; may use in child unable to take tabs; do not mix with water in original bottle
- **Tabs** may be crushed and dispersed in water or mixed with food; consume immediately

SIDE EFFECTS
CNS: Headache, asthenia, poor concentration, seizures, suicidal ideation

CV: Bleeding

ENDO: Hyperglycemia, hyperlipidemia

GI: *Diarrhea,* anorexia, dyspepsia, *nausea, flatulence,* hepatitis, pancreatitis

HEMA: Anemia, leukopenia, thrombocytopenia, Hgb abnormalities

INTEG: *Rash,* dermatitis, anaphylaxis

MS: Pain, arthralgia, myalgia, myopathy

Other: Hypoglycemia, redistribution/accumulation of body fat, immune reconstitution syndrome

PHARMACOKINETICS
Half-life 3½-5 hr, excreted in feces (87%), peak 2-4 hr, 98% protein binding; metabolized by CYP3A4 enzyme system; potent inhibitor of CYP3A4

INTERACTIONS
Drug/Herb

⚠ **Increase:** serious dysrhythmias: amiodarone, ergots, lovastatin, midazolam, pimozide, quiNIDine, simvastatin, triazolam, salmeterol

Increase: effect of—atorvastatin, azithromycin, rifabutin, indinavir, saquinavir, cycloSPORINE, tacrolimus, sirolimus, sildenafil, alfentanil, alosetron, buprenorphine, busPIRone, bortezomib, calcium channel blockers, cilostazol, disopyramide, dofetilide, DOCEtaxel, donepezil, ethosuximide, fentaNYL, galantamine, gefitinib, levomethadyl, systemic lidocaine, PACLitaxel, sibutramine, SUFentanil, vinca alkaloids, ziprasidone, zonisamide, traZODone, tricyclic antidepressants, sildenafil

Increase: nelfinavir levels—ketoconazole, indinavir, ritonavir; delavirdine, other HIV protease inhibitors

Decrease: nelfinavir levels—rifamycins, nevirapine, PHENobarbital, phenytoin, carBAMazepine

Decrease: effect of—didanosine, methadone, oral contraceptives, phenytoin

Drug/Herb

⚠ **Decrease:** antiretroviral effect—St. John's wort; do not use concurrently

Drug/Food

Increase: absorption with food

Drug/Lab Test
Increase: AST, ALT, alk phos, total bilirubin, CPK, LDH, lipids, uric acid
Decrease: WBC, platelets

NURSING CONSIDERATIONS
Assess:
- Resistance testing at initiation, with failure of treatment
- Signs of infection, anemia
- Hepatic studies: ALT, AST
- Bowel pattern before, during treatment; if severe abdominal pain with bleeding occurs, product should be discontinued; monitor hydration

⚠ **Immune reconstitution syndrome:** occurs with combination therapy, including MAC, CMV, PCP TB requiring treatment

⚠ **Anaphylaxis, hypersensitivity reaction:** wheezing, flushing; swelling of lips, tongue, throat, skin eruptions, rash, urticaria, itching
- **HIV:** serum lipid profile, plasma HIV RNA, blood glucose, viral load, CD4 cell counts at baseline and throughout treatment

Teach patient/family:
- To avoid taking with other medications unless directed by prescriber
- **Diarrhea** is most common side effect; may use loperamide to control
- That product does not cure but does manage symptoms; that product does not prevent transmission of HIV to others
- To use a nonhormonal form of birth control while taking this product if using contraceptives
- If dose is missed, to take as soon as remembered up to 1 hr before next dose; not to double dose
- To take with food
- To report symptoms of hyperglycemia, bleeding, abdominal pain; yellowing of skin, eyes
- **Phenylketonuria:** powder contains phenylalanine

RARELY USED

neomycin (Rx)
(nee-oh-mye′sin)
Func. class.: Antiinfective—aminoglycoside

USES: Severe systemic infections of CNS, respiratory, GI, urinary tract, eye, bone, skin, soft tissues; hepatic coma, preoperatively to sterilize bowel, infectious diarrhea caused by enteropathogenic *E. coli, Enterobacter* sp., *Escherichia coli, Klebsiella* sp. May be effective for *Acinetobacter* sp., *Bacillus anthracis, Citrobacter* sp., *Haemophilus influenzae* (beta-lactamase negative), *Haemophilus influenzae* (beta-lactamase positive), *Neisseria* sp., *Proteus mirabilis, Proteus vulgaris, Providencia* sp., *Salmonella* sp., *Serratia* sp., *Shigella* sp., *Staphylococcus aureus* (MSSA), *Staphylococcus epidermidis*

CONTRAINDICATIONS: Infants, children, bowel obstruction (oral use), severe renal disease, hypersensitivity, GI disease

Precautions: Dehydration, geriatric patients, respiratory insufficiency

Black Box Warning: Hearing impairment, neuromuscular disease, renal disease

DOSAGE AND ROUTES
Hepatic encephalopathy
- **Adult: PO** 4-12 g/day in divided doses q6hr × 5-6 days
- **Child: PO** 50-100 mg/kg/day in divided doses q6hr × 5-6 days

Preoperative intestinal antisepsis
- **Adult: PO** 1 g/hr × 4 hr, then 1 g q4hr for remaining 24 hr

N

nepafenac ophthalmic

See Appendix B

HIGH ALERT

nesiritide (Rx)

(neh-seer′ih-tide)

Natrecor

Func. class.: Vasodilator

Chem. class.: Human B-type natriuretic peptide

ACTION: Uses DNA technology; human B-type natriuretic peptide binds to the receptor in vascular smooth muscle and endothelial cells, thereby leading to smooth muscle relaxation

USES: Acutely decompensated CHF

CONTRAINDICATIONS: Hypersensitivity to this product or *Escherichia coli* protein; cardiogenic shock or B/P <90 mm Hg as primary therapy

Precautions: Pregnancy (C); breastfeeding; children; mitral stenosis; significant valvular stenosis, restriction, or obstructive cardiomyopathy, or any condition dependent on venous return; renal disease; constrictive pericarditis

DOSAGE AND ROUTES

- **Adult: IV BOL** 2 mcg/kg, then **CONT IV INFUSION** 0.01 mcg/kg/min

Available forms: Powder for inj, 1.5-mg single-use vial

Administer:

IV route

- Do not give through a central catheter containing other products; administer other products through separate catheter or central line heparin-coated catheter because nesiritide binds to heparin
- Reconstitute one 1.5-mg vial/5 ml of diluent from prefilled 250-ml plastic IV bag with diluent of choice (preservative free D_5, 0.9% NaCl, $D_5/{}^1/_2$ NaCl, D_5/0.2% NaCl); do not shake vial; roll gently; use only clear sol
- Withdraw all contents of reconstituted vial and add to 250-ml plastic IV bag (6 mcg/ml), invert bag several times
- Use within 24 hr of reconstituting
- Prime IV fluid with infusion of 5 ml before connecting to patient's vascular access port and before bolus dose or IV infusion

Direct IV route

- Prime tubing with 5 ml infusion sol; calculate dose based on patient's weight, 0.33 × patient weight (kg) = bolus vol (ml) (6 mcg/ml); withdraw prescribed bolus dose (volume) from prepared infusion bag; give over 1 min through IV port

Intermittent IV INFUSION route

- After bolus dose, use infusion, give at 0.1 ml/kg/hr (0.01 mcg/kg/min)

Y-site compatibilities: Acyclovir, alfentanil, allopurinol, amifostine, aminocaproic acid, aminophylline, amiodarone, amphotericin B colloidal, amphotericin B lipid complex, amphotericin B liposome, anidulafungin, argatroban, atenolol, atracurium, azithromycin, aztreonam, bivalirudin, bleomycin, buprenorphine, busulfan, butorphanol, calcium acetate/chloride/gluconate, CARBOplatin, carmustine, ceFAZolin, cefotaxime, cefoTEtan, cefOXitin, cefTAZidime, ceftizoxime, cefTRIAXone, cefuroxime, chloramphenicol, cimetidine, ciprofloxacin, cisatracurium, CISplatin, clindamycin, cyclophosphamide, cycloSPORINE, cytarabine, dacarbazine, DACTINomycin, DAUNOrubicin, digoxin, diltiazem, diphenhydrAMINE, DOCEtaxel, dolasetron, doxacurium, DOXOrubicin, doxycycline, droperidol, ePHEDrine, epirubicin, ertapenem, erythromycin, esmolol, etoposide, etoposide phosphate, famotidine, fenoldopam, fentaNYL, filgrastim, fluconazole, fludarabine, fluorouracil, foscarnet, fosphenytoin, ganciclovir, gatifloxacin, gemcitabine, gemtuzumab, glycopyrrolate, granisetron, haloperidol, hydrocortisone, HYDROmorphone, hydrOXYzine, IDArubicin, ifosfamide, imipenem-cilastatin, irinotecan, ketorolac, leucovorin, levofloxacin, lidocaine, linezolid, LORazepam, magnesium sulfate, mannitol, mechlorethamine, melphalan, meropenem, mesna, metaraminol, methohexital, methotrexate, methylPREDNISolone, metoclopramide, metroNIDAZOLE, midazolam, milrinone, minocycline, mitoMYcin, mitoXANtrone, mivacurium, moxifloxacin, mycophenolate, nalbuphine, naloxone, niCARdipine, nitroglycerin, nitroprusside, octreotide, ondansetron, oxaliplatin, oxytocin, PACLitaxel, palonosetron, pamidronate, pancuronium, PEMEtrexed, pentamidine, PENTobarbital, PHENobarbital, phentolamine, phenylephrine, polymyxin B sulfate, potassium chloride/phosphates, prochlorperazine, propranolol, quiNIDine, quinupristin-dalfopristin, ranitidine, remifentanil, rocuronium, sodium acetate/bicarbonate/phosphates, streptozocin, succinylcholine, SUFentanil, tacrolimus, teniposide, theophylline, thiotepa, ticarcillin, tigecycline, tirofiban, tolazoline, topotecan, torsemide, trimethobenzamide, vancomycin, vasopressin, vecuronium, verap-amil, vinBLAStine, vinCRIStine, vinorelbine, zidovudine, zoledronic acid

SIDE EFFECTS

CNS: Headache, insomnia, dizziness, anxiety, confusion, paresthesia, tremor

CV: *Hypotension,* tachycardia, dysrhythmias, bradycardia, **ventricular tachycardia, ventricular extrasystoles, atrial fibrillation**

GI: Vomiting, nausea

INTEG: Rash, sweating, pruritus, inj-site reaction

MISC: Abdominal pain, back pain

RESP: Increased cough, hemoptysis, **apnea**

PHARMACOKINETICS

Half-life 18 min

INTERACTIONS

Increase: hypotension—ACE inhibitors, antihypertensives, IV nitrates

NURSING CONSIDERATIONS

Assess:

- PCWP, RAP, cardiac index, MPAP, respiratory rate, CUP, B/P, pulse during treatment until stable
- Daily serum creatinine, BUN
- **CHF:** weight gain, dyspnea, crackles, I&O ratios, peripheral edema

Evaluate:

- Therapeutic response: improvement in CHF with improved PCWP, RAP, MPAP
- **Allergic reactions to peptides: rash, pruritus, wheezing, discontinue immediately, keep emergency equipment available**

Teach patient/family:

- About purpose of medication, expected results; to report pain at IV site
- To report dizziness, blurred vision, lightheadedness, sweating, allergic reaction

nevirapine (Rx)

(ne-veer′a-peen)

Viramune, Viramune XR

Func. class.: Antiretroviral

Chem. class.: Nonnucleoside reverse transcriptase inhibitor (NNRTI)

N

Do not confuse:
nevirapine/nelfinavir
Viramune/Viracept

ACTION: Binds directly to reverse transcriptase and blocks RNA, DNA, thus causing a disruption of the enzyme's site

USES: HIV-1 in combination with other highly active antiretroviral therapy (HAART)

CONTRAINDICATIONS:

Black Box Warning: Hypersensitivity, hepatic disease

Precautions: Pregnancy (B), breastfeeding, children, renal disease, Hispanic patients

Black Box Warning: Females, hepatitis

DOSAGE AND ROUTES

Treatment of HIV infection in combination with other antiretrovirals

- **Adult and adolescent: PO** 200 mg/day × 2 wk, then 200 mg bid in combination; **EXT REL** tab (adults not currently taking immediate rel nevirapine) 200 mg/day (immediate rel tab) × 14 days with other antiretrovirals; if rash develops during lead-in periods and persists beyond 14 days, do not use ext rel tab; if no consistent rash present, then give 400 mg/day ext rel tab with other antiretrovirals; if interrupted >7 days, restart 14 day lead-in dosing; for adults switched from immediate rel tab, give 400 mg/day ext rel tab
- **Child/adolescent ≥6 yr: PO EXT REL** not currently taking immediate release 150 mg/m^2 (immediate release) daily (max 200 mg/day) × 14 days, then BSA 0.58-0.83 m^2 200 mg/day; BSA 0.84-1.16 m^2 300 mg/day
- **Child/infant/neonate ≥15 days old: PO** 150 mg/m^2/day × 14 days, then 150 mg/m^2 bid, max 400 mg/day

Perinatal transmission prophylaxis (unlabeled)

- **Females with no previous antiretroviral therapy: PO** 200 mg as a single dose at onset of labor with zidovudine 2 mg/kg over 1 hr followed by zidovudine 1 mg/kg/hr until delivery
- **Neonate ≥34 wk gestation: PO** Nevirapine 12 mg (>2 kg) or 8 mg (1.5-2 kg) × 3 doses; 1st dose 48 hr after birth, 2nd dose 48 hr after 1st dose, 3rd dose 96 hr after 2nd dose and **PO** zidovudine

Hepatic Dose

- **Adult: PO** do not use with Child-Pugh grade B or C

Available forms: Tabs 200 mg; oral susp 50 mg/5 ml; ext rel 400 mg

Administer:

- Do not initiate treatment in females when CD4 counts >250 cells/mm^3 or in males when >400 cells/mm^3 unless benefits outweigh risks
- Without regard to meals
- Use in combination with at least 1 other antiretroviral
- **Oral susp** should be shaken before giving

SIDE EFFECTS

CNS: *Paresthesia, headache, fever, peripheral neuropathy*
GI: *Diarrhea,* abdominal pain, *nausea, stomatitis,* hepatotoxicity, hepatic failure
HEMA: Neutropenia, anemia, thrombocytopenia
INTEG: *Rash,* toxic epidermal necrolysis
MISC: Stevens-Johnson syndrome, anaphylaxis
MS: Pain, myalgia, rhabdomyolysis

PHARMACOKINETICS

Rapidly absorbed, peak 4 hr, 60% bound to plasma proteins, metabolized by liver; metabolized by hepatic P450 enzyme system, excreted 91% in urine, terminal half-life 25-30 hr, 50% removed by peritoneal dialysis; with hepatic disease and in Hispanic patients, African American patients, slower rate of clearance

INTERACTIONS

Increase: nevirapine levels—cimetidine, macrolide antiinfectives
Decrease: effects of protease inhibitors, oral contraceptives, ketoconazole, methadone, itraconazole
Decrease: nevirapine levels—rifamycins, anticonvulsants, clonazePAM, diazepam, warfarin

Drug/Herb
Decrease: action of antiretroviral—St. John's wort; do not use concurrently

Drug/Lab Test
Increase: ALT, AST, GGT, bilirubin, Hgb
Decrease: neutrophil count

NURSING CONSIDERATIONS

Assess:

- Resistance testing before therapy and when therapy fails

⚠ Signs of infection, anemia, hepatotoxicity, immune reconstitution syndrome; hepatitis B or C, liver toxicity may occur
• **HIV:** blood studies during treatment: ALT, AST, viral load, CD4, plasma HIV RNA, renal studies; if LFTs elevated significantly, product should be withheld; glucose levels in diabetic patients, if treatment is interrupted by >1 wk, restart at initial dose
⚠ **Rhabdomyolysis:** pain, tenderness, weakness, edema; product should be discontinued
• Bowel pattern before, during treatment; if severe abdominal pain with bleeding occurs, product should be discontinued; monitor hydration
⚠ **Stevens-Johnson syndrome, toxic epidermal necrolysis,** allergies before treatment, reaction to each medication; skin eruptions; rash, urticaria, itching; if rash is severe or systemic symptoms occur, discontinue immediately

Evaluate:
• Therapeutic response: absence of AIDS-defining symptoms, improvement in quality of life; decreased viral load, increase in CD4 count

Teach patient/family:
⚠ To report any right quadrant pain, yellowing of eyes or skin, dark urine, nausea, anorexia, muscle pain or tenderness, rash immediately
• That product may be taken with food, antacids
• To take as prescribed; if dose is missed, to take as soon as remembered up to 1 hr before next dose; not to double dose
• That product is not a cure, does not prevent transmission; controls symptoms of HIV
• To avoid OTC agents unless approved by prescriber
• To use a nonhormonal form of contraception during treatment in those using contraceptives

RARELY USED

niacin (OTC, Rx)
(nye′a-sin)
Equaline Niacin, Niaspan, Ni-Odan ✤, Slo-Niacin

niacinamide (OTC, Rx)
Func. class.: Vit B_3, antihyperlipidemic
Chem. class.: Water-soluble vitamin

USES: Pellagra, hyperlipidemias (types 4, 5), peripheral vascular disease that presents a risk for pancreatitis

CONTRAINDICATIONS: Breastfeeding, hypersensitivity, peptic ulcer, hepatic disease, hemorrhage, severe hypotension

DOSAGE AND ROUTES

Niacin deficiency
• **Adult: PO** 100-500 mg/day in divided doses; **IM/SUBCUT** 5-100 mg ≥5×/day; **IV** 25-100 mg bid or tid
• **Child: PO** ≤300 mg/day in divided doses

Adjunct in hyperlipidemia
• **Adult: PO** 250 mg after evening meal; may increase dose at 1-4 wk intervals to 1-2 g tid, max 6 g/day; **EXT REL** 500 mg at bedtime × 4 wk, then 1000 mg at bedtime for wk 5-8; do not increase by >500 mg q4wk, max 2000 mg/day

Pellagra
• **Adult: PO** 300-500 mg/day in divided doses; **IM** 50-100 mg 5×/day or **IV** 25-100 mg bid by slow **IV INFUSION**
• **Child: PO** 100-300 mg/day in divided doses; **IV** ≤300 mg/day by slow **IV/INFUSION**

Peripheral vascular disease
• **Adult: PO** 250-800 mg/day in 3-5 divided doses

N

niCARdipine (Rx)

(nye-card′i-peen)

Cardene, Cardene IV, Cardene SR

Func. class.: Calcium channel blocker, antianginal, antihypertensive

Chem. class.: Dihydropyridine

Do not confuse:

niCARdipine/NIFEdipine
Cardene/Cardizem
Cardene SR/Cardizem SR

ACTION: Inhibits calcium ion influx across cell membrane during cardiac depolarization; produces relaxation of coronary vascular smooth muscle, peripheral vascular smooth muscle; dilates coronary vascular arteries; increases myocardial oxygen delivery in patients with vasospastic angina

USES: Chronic stable angina pectoris, hypertension

CONTRAINDICATIONS: Sick sinus syndrome, 2nd-/3rd-degree heart block; hypersensitivity to this product or dihydropyridine; advanced aortic stenosis

Precautions: Pregnancy (C), breastfeeding, children, geriatric patients, CHF, hypotension, hepatic injury, renal disease

DOSAGE AND ROUTES

Hypertension

- **Adult: PO** 20 mg tid initially; may increase after 3 days (range 20-40 mg tid) or 30 mg bid **SUS REL;** may increase to 60 mg bid or **IV** 5 mg/hr; may increase by 2.5 mg/hr q15min; max 15 mg/hr

Angina

- **Adult: PO** 20 mg tid; may be adjusted q3days; may use 20-40 mg tid

Renal dose

- **Adult: PO** adjust based on response

Hepatic dose

- **Adult: PO** 20 mg bid

Available forms: Caps 20, 30 mg; sus rel caps 30, 45, 60 mg; inj 2.5 mg/ml, premixed 20 mg/200 ml, 40 mg/200 ml

Administer:

PO route

- Do not break, crush, chew, or open sus rel cap
- Without regard to meals

IV route

Continuous IV INFUSION

- Dilute each 25 mg/240 ml of compatible sol (0.1 mg/ml), give slowly, titrate to patient response, change IV site q12hr
- Stable at room temperature for 24 hr

Solution compatibilities: D_5W, D_5/0.45% NaCl, D_5/0.9% NaCl

Y-site compatibilities: Alemtuzumab, amikacin, aminophylline, aztreonam, bivalirudin, butorphanol, calcium gluconate, CARBOplatin, caspofungin, ceFAZolin, ceftizoxime, chloramphenicol, cimetidine, CISplatin, clindamycin, cytarabine, DAPTOmycin, dexmedetomidine, diltiazem, DOBUTamine, DOCEtaxel, DOPamine, DOXOrubicin hydrochloride, enalaprilat, EPINEPHrine, epirubicin, erythromycin, esmolol, famotidine, fenoldopam, fentaNYL, gentamicin, hydrocortisone, HYDROmorphone, labetalol, lidocaine, linezolid, LORazepam, magnesium sulfate, mechlorethamine, methylPREDNISolone, metroNIDAZOLE, midazolam, milrinone, morphine, nafcillin, nesiritide, nitroglycerin, nitroprusside, norepinephrine, octreotide, oxaliplatin, oxytocin, palonosetron, penicillin G potassium, potassium chloride/phosphate, quinupristin/dalfopristin, ranitidine, rocuronium, tacrolimus, tirofiban, tobramycin, trimethoprim/sulfamethoxazole, vancomycin, vasopressin, vecuronium, vinCRIStine, voriconazole, zoledronic acid

SIDE EFFECTS

CNS: *Headache, dizziness,* anxiety, depression, confusion, paresthesia, somnolence, ***flushing***

CV: Edema, bradycardia, hypotension, palpitations, **pulmonary edema,** chest pain, tachycardia, increased angina, **arrhythmias, CHF**
GI: Nausea, vomiting, gastric upset, constipation, **hepatitis,** abdominal cramps, dry mouth, sore throat
GU: Nocturia, polyuria
INTEG: Rash, infusion-site discomfort, **Stevens-Johnson syndrome**
OTHER: Blurred vision, flushing, sweating, SOB, impotence

PHARMACOKINETICS

Metabolized by liver, excreted in urine 60%, feces 35%, half-life 2-5 hr
PO: Onset 20 min, peak 1-2 hr, duration 8 hr
PO-SR: Onset unknown, duration 10-12 hr
Onset
IV: 1 min, peak 45 min

INTERACTIONS

Increase: effects of digoxin, neuromuscular blocking agents, theophylline, other antihypertensives, nitrates, alcohol, quiNIDine
Increase: niCARdipine effects—cimetidine
Increase: toxicity risk—cycloSPORINE, prazosin, carBAMazepine, quiNIDine, propranolol
Decrease: antihypertensive effect—NSAIDs, rifampin
Drug/Herb
Increase: effect—ginkgo, ginseng, hawthorn
Decrease: effect—ephedra, melatonin, St. John's wort, yohimbe
Drug/Food
Increase: hypotensive effect—grapefruit juice
Increase: LFTs
Drug/Lab Test
Decrease: potassium (IV), phosphate, platelets

NURSING CONSIDERATIONS

Assess:

⚠ **Cardiac status: B/P often, pulse, respiration, ECG during long-term treatment**
- **Anginal pain:** intensity, location, duration; alleviating, precipitating factors
- Potassium, renal, hepatic studies periodically

⚠ **CHF: weight gain, crackles, jugular venous distention, dyspnea, I&O**
- **Allergic reactions (Stevens-Johnson syndrome): if rash is severe and joint aches, mouth lesions, discontinue immediately**
- **Hypertension:** decreasing B/P; assess salt in diet, smoking, exercise, weight, monitor B/P often

Evaluate:
- Therapeutic response: decreased anginal pain, decreased B/P

Teach patient/family:
- To avoid hazardous activities until stabilized on product, dizziness is no longer a problem
- To limit caffeine consumption; to avoid alcohol products; to take without regard to food, avoid high-fat foods; to swallow sus rel product whole
- To avoid OTC products, grapefruit juice unless directed by prescriber
- **Hypertension:** comply in all areas of medical regimen: diet, exercise, stress reduction, product therapy

⚠ **To notify prescriber of irregular heartbeat, SOB, swelling of feet and hands, pronounced dizziness, constipation, nausea, hypotension, change in severity/pattern/incidence of angina**

TREATMENT OF OVERDOSE:

Defibrillation, β-agonists, IV calcium, diuretics, atropine for AV block, vasopressor for hypotension

N

nicotine
(nik′o-teen)

nicotine chewing gum
Thrive, Nicorette

nicotine inhaler (OTC, Rx)
Nicotrol

nicotine lozenge (OTC)
Commit, Nicorette

nicotine nasal spray (Rx)
Nicotrol NS

nicotine transdermal (OTC, Rx)
Nicoderm CQ

Func. class.: Smoking deterrent
Chem. class.: Ganglionic cholinergic agonist

ACTION: Agonist at nicotinic receptors in peripheral, central nervous systems; acts at sympathetic ganglia, on chemoreceptors of aorta, carotid bodies; also affects adrenalin-releasing catecholamines

USES: Deter cigarette smoking
Unlabeled uses: Gilles de la Tourette's syndrome, ulcerative colitis

CONTRAINDICATIONS: Pregnancy (D) (transdermal, inhaler); hypersensitivity, immediate post-MI recovery period, severe angina pectoris
Precautions: Pregnancy (C) (gum); breastfeeding, vasospastic disease, dysrhythmias, diabetes mellitus, hyperthyroidism, pheochromocytoma, esophagitis, peptic ulcer, coronary/renal/hepatic disease; MRI (patch); soy hypersensitivity (mint lozenge)

DOSAGE AND ROUTES
Nicotine chewing gum
- **Adult:** chew 1 piece of gum (2 mg nicotine) whenever urge to smoke occurs; dose varies; usually 20 mg/day during first mo, max 24 pieces/day, max 3 mo

Nicotine inhaler
- **Adult: INH** 6 cartridges/day for first 3-6 wk, max 16 cartridges/day × 12 wk

Nicotine lozenge
- **Adult:** if cigarette is desired >30 min after awakening, start with 2-mg lozenge; if <30 min after awakening, start with 4-mg lozenge, then again q1-2hr, max 20 lozenges/day or 5 lozenges/6 hr × 6 wk, then 1 lozenge q2-4hr × 2 wk, then 1 lozenge q4-8hr × 2 wk, then discontinue

Nicotine nasal spray
- **Adult:** 1 spray in each nostril 1-2×/hr, max 5×/hr or 40×/day, max 3 mo

Nicotine transdermal/inhaler system
- **Nicoderm:** 21 mg/day × 4-8 wk; 14 mg/day × 2-4 wk; 7 mg/day × 2-4 wk
- **Nicotrol:** 15 mg/day × 12 wk; 10 mg/day × 2 wk; 5 mg/day × 2 wk
- **Nicotrol inhaler:** delivers 30% of nicotine that smoker receives from an actual cigarette

Gilles de la Tourette's syndrome (unlabeled)
- **Adult and child: chewing gum** 2 mg chewed × 30 min bid for 1-6 mo; **TRANSDERMAL** 7- or 10-mg patch daily × 2 days

Available forms: Transdermal patch (Habitrol ♣, Nicoderm, nicotine transdermal system) delivering 7, 14, 21 mg/day; (Nicoderm) 5, 10, 15 mg/day; **nicotine inhaler** 4 mg delivered; **nasal spray** 0.5 mg nicotine/actuation; **gum** 2, 4 mg/piece; **lozenge** 2 mg, 4 mg

Administer:
- **Gum:** chew gum slowly for 30 min to promote buccal absorption of product; do not chew >45 min
- Begin product withdrawal after 3 mo of use; do not exceed 6 mo
- **Transdermal patch:** 1 × day to nonhairy, clean, dry area of skin on upper body or upper outer arm; rotate sites to prevent skin irritation

- **Inhaler:** puffing on mouthpiece delivers nicotine through mouth

SIDE EFFECTS

CNS: Dizziness, vertigo, insomnia, headache, confusion, seizures, depression, euphoria, numbness, tinnitus, strange dreams

CV: Dysrhythmias, tachycardia, palpitations, edema, flushing, hypertension

EENT: Jaw ache, irritation in buccal cavity

GI: *Nausea, vomiting, anorexia, indigestion,* diarrhea, abdominal pain, constipation, eructation, irritation

RESP: Breathing difficulty, cough, hoarseness, sneezing, wheezing, bronchial spasm

PHARMACOKINETICS

Onset 15-30 min, metabolized in liver, excreted in urine, half-life 2-3 hr, 30-120 hr (terminal)

INTERACTIONS

Increase: vasoconstriction—ergots, bromocriptine, cabergoline

Increase: effect of—adenosine

Increase: B/P—buPROPion

Decrease: effect of—α-blockers, insulin

Decrease: nicotine clearance—cimetidine

Drug/Food

- Avoid use of gum with acidic foods (colas, coffee) and for 15 min after

NURSING CONSIDERATIONS

Assess:

- **Smoking:** number of cigarettes smoked, years used; **withdrawal:** headache, cravings, restlessness, irritation, drowsiness, insomnia, sore throat, increased appetite
- **Adverse reaction:** irritation of buccal cavity, dislike of taste, jaw ache

Evaluate:

- Therapeutic response: decrease in urge to smoke, decreased need for gum after 3-6 mo

Teach patient/family:

- **Gum:** about all aspects of product use; give package insert to patient and explain
- That gum will not stick to dentures, dental appliances
- That gum is as toxic as cigarettes; that it is to be used only to deter smoking, call prescriber immediately, stop use if difficulty breathing or rash occur
- To avoid use during pregnancy
- **Transdermal patch:** that patch is as toxic as cigarettes; to be used only to deter smoking
- Not to use during pregnancy because birth defects may occur; not to breastfeed
- To keep used and unused system out of reach of children and pets
- To stop smoking immediately when beginning patch treatment
- To apply promptly after removing from protective patch because system may lose strength
- **Nasal spray:** to tilt head back; not to swallow or inhale during administration; after smoking is stopped, to use spray up to 8 wk, then discontinue over 6 wk by tapering
- **Lozenges:** to allow to dissolve; to avoid swallowing
- **Inhalation:** to use by inhaler for 20 min

N

NIFEdipine (Rx)

(nye-fed′i-peen)

Adalat CC, Adalat XL ♣, Afeditab CR, Procardia, Procardia XL

Func. class.: Calcium channel blocker, antianginal, antihypertensive

Chem. class.: Dihydropyridine

Do not confuse:

NIFEdipine/niCARdipine/niMODipine

ACTION: Inhibits calcium ion influx across cell membrane during cardiac depolarization; relaxes coronary vascular smooth muscle; dilates coronary arteries; increases myocardial oxygen delivery in patients with vasospastic angina; dilates peripheral arteries

USES: Chronic stable angina pectoris, variant angina, hypertension

Unlabeled uses: Migraines, migraine prophylaxis; preterm labor, chronic/ acute hypertension (pediatrics), diabetic nephropathy, proteinuria, hiccups

CONTRAINDICATIONS:

Hypersensitivity to this product or dihydropyridine; cardiogenic shock

Precautions: Pregnancy (C), breastfeeding, children, hypotension, sick sinus syndrome, 2nd-/3rd-degree heart block, hypotension <90 mm Hg systolic, hepatic injury, renal disease, acute MI, aortic stenosis, GERD, heart failure

DOSAGE AND ROUTES

- **Adult: PO** Immediate release 10 mg tid, increase in 10-mg increments q7-14days, max 180 mg/24 hr or single dose of 30 mg; **SUS REL** 30-60 mg/day, may increase q7-14days, max 90 mg/day

Hypertension

- **Adult: PO EXT REL** 30-60 mg daily, titrate upward as needed, max 90 mg/day (Adalat CC), 120 mg/day (Procardia XL)
- **Child/adolescent (unlabeled): PO EXT REL** 0.25-0.5 mg/kg/day, max 3 mg/kg/day

Acute hypertensive episodes in pediatric patients (unlabeled)

- **Adolescent/child/infant: PO** 0.2-0.5 mg/kg/dose up to 10 mg (total dose)

Migraine prophylaxis (unlabeled)

- **Adult: PO** 30-180 mg/day

Preterm labor (unlabeled)

- **Pregnant female: PO** Immediate release (Procardia, Adalat) 30-mg loading dose, then 10-20 mg q4-6hr; use in monitored settings

Hiccups (unlabeled)

- **Adult:** 10-20 mg tid

Available forms: Caps 10, 20 mg; ext rel tabs (CC, XL) 30, 60, 90 mg

Administer:

- Do not break, crush, or chew ext rel tabs, do not use immediate release caps within 7 days of MI, coronary syndrome
- Without regard to meals; avoid grapefruit juice
- Protect caps from direct light, keep in dry area, do not freeze

SIDE EFFECTS

CNS: *Headache,* fatigue, drowsiness, *dizziness,* anxiety, depression, weakness, insomnia, light-headedness, paresthesia, tinnitus, blurred vision, nervousness, tremor, *flushing*

CV: **Dysrhythmias**, edema, hypotension, palpitations, tachycardia

GI: Nausea, vomiting, diarrhea, gastric upset, constipation, increased LFTs, dry mouth, flatulence, gingival hyperplasia

GU: *Nocturia, polyuria*

HEMA: Bruising, bleeding, petechiae

INTEG: Rash, pruritus, flushing, hair loss, **Stevens-Johnson syndrome, toxic epidermal necrolysis, exfoliative dermatitis**

MISC: Sexual difficulties, cough, fever, chills

PHARMACOKINETICS

Metabolized by liver; excreted in urine 60%-80% (metabolites), feces 15%; protein binding 92%-98%, half-life 2-5 hr, well absorbed

PO: Onset 20 min, duration 6-8 hr

PO-ER: Duration 24 hr

PO-CC, PA, XL: Peak 6 hr, duration 24 hr

INTERACTIONS

⚠ **Contraindicated with strong CYP3A4 inducers**

Increase: level of digoxin, phenytoin, cycloSPORINE, prazosin, carBAMazepine

⚠ **Increase: NIFEdipine, toxicity—cimetidine, ranitidine**

Increase: effects of β-blockers, antihypertensives

Decrease: antihypertensive effect—NSAIDs

Decrease: effects of quiNIDine

Decrease: NIFEdipine level—smoking

Drug/Herb

Increase: effect—ginkgo biloba, ginseng, hawthorn

Decrease: effect—ephedra, melatonin, St. John's wort, yohimbe

Drug/Food

Increase: NIFEdipine level—grapefruit juice

Drug/Lab Test
Increase: CPK, LDH, AST
Positive: ANA, direct Coombs' test

NURSING CONSIDERATIONS

Assess:

- **Anginal pain:** location, intensity, duration, character, alleviating, aggravating factors
- Cardiac status: B/P, pulse, respiration, ECG at baseline and periodically, in those taking antihypertensives, β-blockers, monitor B/P often
- Potassium, renal, hepatic studies periodically during treatment
- For bruising, petechiae, bleeding
- **GI obstruction:** Ext rel products have been associated with rare reports of obstruction in those with strictures and no known GI disease
- **Serious skin disorders:** rash that starts suddenly, fever, cutaneous lesions that may have pustules present; discontinue product

Evaluate:

- Therapeutic response: decreased anginal pain, B/P, activity tolerance

Teach patient/family:

- To avoid hazardous activities until stabilized on product, dizziness is no longer a problem
- To limit caffeine consumption; to avoid alcohol products
- To avoid OTC products unless directed by prescriber without regard to meals, Adelat CC should be taken on empty stomach
- That empty tab shells may appear in stools and is not significant
- **Hypertension:** to comply with all areas of medical regimen: diet, exercise, stress reduction, product therapy
- To change position slowly because orthostatic hypotension is common
- ⚠ To notify prescriber of dyspnea, edema of extremities, nausea, vomiting, severe ataxia, severe rash; changes in pattern, frequency, severity of angina
- To increase fluid intake to prevent constipation
- To check for gingival hyperplasia and report promptly
- Not to discontinue abruptly; to gradually taper

TREATMENT OF OVERDOSE:

Defibrillation, atropine for AV block, vasopressor for hypotension

⚠ HIGH ALERT

nilotinib (Rx)

(nye-loe′ti-nib)

Tasigna

Func. class.: Antineoplastic—miscellaneous

Chem. class.: Protein-tyrosine kinase inhibitor

ACTION: Inhibits BCR-ABL tyrosine kinase created in patients with chronic myeloid leukemia (CML)

USES: Chronic phase/accelerated phase Philadelphia-chromosome–positive CML that is resistant or intolerant to imatinib

CONTRAINDICATIONS: Pregnancy (D), breastfeeding, hypersensitivity

Black Box Warning: Hypokalemia, hypomagnesemia, QT prolongation

Precautions: Children, females, geriatric patients, active infections, anemia, cardiac disease, bone marrow suppression, cholestasis, diabetes, gelatin hypersensitivity, infertility, galactose-free diet, lactase deficiency, neutropenia, pancreatitis, thrombocytopenia

Black Box Warning: Hepatic disease

DOSAGE AND ROUTES

- **Adult: PO** 400 mg q12hr, continue until disease progression or unacceptable toxicity

Adjustment after discontinuation of a strong CYP3A4 inducer

- **Adult: PO** reduce to 400 mg/bid

N

For those taking a strong CYP3A4 inhibitor

- **Adult: PO** reduce dose to 300 mg/day

QT prolongation

- **QTcF >480 msec:** withhold dose

Myelosuppression

- **ANC 1 × 10^9/L or platelets <50 × 10^9/L:** withhold dose

Hepatic dose

- **Adult: PO** (Child-Pugh A/B/C) newly diagnosed CML 200 mg bid, then escalation to 300 mg bid initially

Available forms: Caps 150, 200 mg

Administer:

- Do not break, crush, or chew caps; if whole capsule cannot be swallowed, disperse capsule contents in 1 tsp. applesauce
- Without regard to meals; separate doses by 12 hr; make-up dose should not be taken if dose is missed
- Store at 59° F-86° F (15° C- 30° C)

SIDE EFFECTS

CNS: Headache, dizziness, fatigue, fever, flushing, paresthesia

CV: QT prolongation, palpitations, torsades de pointes, AV block

GI: *Nausea,* hepatotoxicity, vomiting, dyspepsia, *anorexia, abdominal pain,* constipation, pancreatitis, diarrhea, xerostomia

HEMA: Neutropenia, thrombocytopenia, anemia, pancytopenia

INTEG: *Rash,* alopecia, erythema

META: Hyperamylasemia, hyperbilirubinemia, hyperglycemia, hyperkalemia, hypocalcemia, hyponatremia, hypomagnesemia

MISC: Diaphoresis, anxiety

MS: Arthralgia, myalgia, back or bone pain, muscle cramps

RESP: Cough, dyspnea

SYST: Bleeding, tumor lysis syndrome

PHARMACOKINETICS

Protein binding 98%, metabolized by CYP3A4, plasma levels 3 hr, elimination half-life 17 hr

INTERACTIONS

- Product interactions are numerous
- Do not use with phenothiazines, pimozide, ziprasidone

⚠ **Increase:** QT prolongation—class IA/III antidysrhythmics, some phenothiazines, β agonists, local anesthetics, tricyclics, haloperidol, chloroquine, droperidol, pentamidine; CYP3A4 inhibitors (amiodarone, clarithromycin, erythromycin, telithromycin, troleandomycin), arsenic trioxide, levomethadyl; CYP3A4 substrates (methadone, pimozide, QUEtiapine, quiNIDine, risperiDONE, zipra sidone)

⚠ **Increase:** hepatotoxicity—acetaminophen

Increase: concentrations—ketoconazole, itraconazole, erythromycin, clarithromycin

Increase: plasma concentrations of simvastatin, calcium channel blockers

Increase: plasma concentration of warfarin; avoid use with warfarin, use low-molecular-weight anticoagulants instead

Decrease: concentrations—dexamethasone, phenytoin, carBAMazepine, rifampin, PHENobarbital

Drug/Herb

Decrease: concentration—St. John's wort

Drug/Food

Increase: plasma concentrations—grapefruit juice

NURSING CONSIDERATIONS

Assess:

- **Tumor lysis syndrome:** maintain hydration, correct uric acid before use with this product

Black Box Warning: QT prolongation can occur; monitor ECG, left ventricular ejection fraction (LVEF) at baseline periodically; hypertension, assess for chest pain, palpitations, dyspnea

Black Box Warning: Hepatotoxicity: monitor LFTs before treatment and monthly; if liver transaminases >5 × IULN, withhold until transaminase levels return to <2.5 × IULN

- **Myelosuppression:** Monitor CBC ×2 mo, then monthly, differential, platelet count; for bleeding: epistaxis, rectal, gingival, upper GI, genital and wound bleeding; **tumor-related hemorrhage may occur rapidly**
- ANC and platelets; if ANC <1 ×10⁹/L and/or platelets <50 ×10⁹/L, stop until ANC >1.5 ×10⁹/L and platelets >75 ×10⁹/L
- **Electrolytes:** calcium, potassium, magnesium, sodium; lipase, phosphate; hypokalemia, hypomagnesemia should be corrected before use
- AST/ALT/Bilirubin/Lipase/Amylase if increased to grade 3, withhold product, resume at 400 mg daily when levels return to grade 1 or below

Evaluate:

- Therapeutic response: decrease in progression of disease

Teach patient/family:

- To report adverse reactions immediately: SOB, bleeding
- About reason for treatment, expected results
- That many adverse reactions may occur
- To avoid persons with known upper respiratory tract infections; immunosuppression is common
- To watch for signs, symptoms of low potassium or magnesium

nisoldipine (Rx)

(nye-sole′dih-peen)

Sular

Func. class.: Calcium channel blocker, antihypertensive

Chem. class.: Dihydropyridine

Do not confuse:

nisoldipine/NIFEdipine/niMODipine

ACTION:
Inhibits calcium ion influx across the cell membrane, thereby resulting in the dilation of peripheral arteries

USES:
Essential hypertension, alone or in combination with other antihypertensives

Unlabeled uses: Variant (Prinzmetal's) angina, stable angina pectoris

CONTRAINDICATIONS:
Hypersensitivity to this product or dihydropyridines; sick sinus syndrome; 2nd-/3rd-degree heart block; aortic stenosis

Precautions: Pregnancy (C), breastfeeding, children, geriatric patients, CHF, hypotension <90 mm Hg systolic, hepatic injury, renal disease, acute MI, unstable angina, CAD, cardiogenic shock

DOSAGE AND ROUTES

Hypertension

- **Adult: PO** 17 mg/day initially, may increase by 8.5 mg/wk, usual dose 17-34 mg/day, max 34 mg/day
- **Geriatric/hepatic dose: PO** 8.5 mg/day, increase based on patient response

Variant (Prinzmetal's) angina/stable angina pectoris (unlabeled)

- **Adult: PO** 17-34 mg/day, max 34 mg/day

Hepatic dose

- **Adult: PO** 8.5 mg/day

Available forms: Ext rel tabs 8.5, 17, 20, 25.5, 30, 34, 40 mg

Administer:

PO route

- Swallow whole; do not break, crush, or chew
- Once daily as whole tablet; avoid high-fat foods, grapefruit juice

SIDE EFFECTS

CNS: Headache, fatigue, drowsiness, dizziness, anxiety, depression, nervousness, insomnia, lightheadedness, paresthesia, tinnitus, psychosis, somnolence, ataxia, confusion, malaise, migraine, flushing

CV: Dysrhythmia, edema, **CHF**, hypotension, palpitations, **MI, pulmonary edema,** tachycardia, syncope, AV block, angina, chest pain, ECG abnormalities

N

GI: Nausea, vomiting, diarrhea, gastric upset, constipation, increased LFTs, dry mouth, dyspepsia, dysphagia, flatulence
GU: Nocturia, hematuria, dysuria
HEMA: Anemia, leukopenia, petechiae
INTEG: Rash, pruritus
MISC: Sexual difficulties, cough, nasal congestion, SOB, wheezing, epistaxis, dyspnea, gingival hyperplasia, chills, fever, gout, sweating

PHARMACOKINETICS

Metabolized by liver, excreted in urine, peak 6-12 hr, protein binding 99%, half-life 7-12 hr

INTERACTIONS

Increase: effects of β-blockers, antihypertensives, digoxin
Increase: nisoldipine level—CYP3A4 inhibitors, cimetidine, ranitidine, azole antifungals
Decrease: nisoldipine effect—CYP3A4 inducers, hydantoins
Drug/Herb
Increase: B/P—ephedra, melatonin
Decrease: B/P—hawthorn
Decrease: nisoldipine effect—St. John's wort, ginseng, ginkgo biloba
Drug/Food
Increase: nisoldipine level—high-fat foods
Increase: hypotensive effect—grapefruit juice

NURSING CONSIDERATIONS

Assess:
- Cardiac status: B/P, pulse, respiration, ECG before treatment and periodically
- **CHF:** weight gain, jugular venous distention, edema, crackles, I&O ratios
- **Angina:** frequency, severity of attacks, if angina worsens, report immediately

Evaluate:
- Therapeutic response: decreased B/P

Teach patient/family:
- To avoid hazardous activities until stabilized on product, dizziness is no longer a problem
- To report nausea, dizziness, swelling, SOB, palpitations, severe headache
- To avoid OTC products unless directed by prescriber; to avoid grapefruit juice
- About the importance of complying with all areas of the medical regimen: diet, exercise, stress reduction, product therapy
- To rise slowly to prevent orthostatic hypotension
- If dose is missed, to take as soon as remembered; not to double dose
- How to perform B/P monitoring at home

TREATMENT OF OVERDOSE:

Defibrillation, atropine for AV block, vasopressor for hypotension

RARELY USED

nitazoxanide (Rx)

(nye-taz-ox′a-nide)

Alinia

Func. class.: Antiprotozoal

USES: Diarrhea caused by *Cryptosporidium parvum* or *Giardia lamblia*

CONTRAINDICATIONS: Hypersensitivity

DOSAGE AND ROUTES

- **Adult: PO** 500 mg q12hr × 3 days
- **Child 4-11 yr: PO** 10 ml (200 mg) q12hr × 3 days
- **Child 12-47 mo: PO** 5 ml (100 mg) q12hr × 3 days

nitrofurantoin (Rx)

(nye-troe-fyoor′an-toyn)

Furadantin, Macrobid, Macrodantin, Novo-Furantoin ✦

Func. class.: Urinary tract antiinfective

Chem. class.: Synthetic nitrofuran derivative

ACTION: Inhibits bacterial acetyl-CoA inteference with carbohydrate metabolism

USES: Urinary tract infections caused by *Escherichia coli, Klebsiella, Pseudomonas, Proteus vulgaris, Proteus morganii, Serratia, Citrobacter, Staphylococcus aureus, Staphylococcus epidermidis, Enterococcus, Salmonella, Shigella*

CONTRAINDICATIONS: Infants <1 mo, hypersensitivity, anuria, severe renal disease CCr <60 ml/min, at term pregnancy (38-42 wk), labor, delivery, cholestatic jaundice due to nitrofurantoin therapy

Precautions: Pregnancy (B), breastfeeding, geriatric patients, G6PD deficiency, GI disease, diabetes

DOSAGE AND ROUTES

Active infections

- **Adult: PO** 50-100 mg qid after meals
- **Child: PO** 5-7 mg/kg/day in 4 divided doses

Chronic suppression

- **Adult: PO** 50-100 mg q PM
- **Child: PO** 1-2 mg/kg/day in PM or 0.5-1 mg/kg q12hr if dose not well tolerated

Available forms: Caps 25, 50, 100 mg; susp 25 mg/5 ml; macrocrystal caps (Macrodantin) 25, 50, 100 mg; Macrobid cap 100 mg (25 macrocrystals, 75 monohydrate)

Administer:

PO route

- Give with meals
- Do not break, crush, chew, or open tabs, caps, store in original container
- Two daily doses if urine output is high or if patient diabetic
- Use calibrated device to measure liquid product; may mix water, fruit juice; rinse mouth after liquid product; staining of teeth may occur

SIDE EFFECTS

CNS: *Dizziness, headache,* drowsiness, peripheral neuropathy, chills, confusion, vertigo

CV: **Bundle branch block,** chest pain

GI: *Nausea, vomiting, abdominal pain, diarrhea,* **cholestatic jaundice,** loss of appetite, **pseudomembranous colitis, hepatitis, pancreatitis**

HEMA: **Anemia, agranulocytosis, hemolytic anemia, leukopenia, thrombocytopenia**

INTEG: Pruritus, rash, urticaria, angioedema, alopecia, tooth staining, **exfoliative dermatitis, Stevens-Johnson syndrome**

MS: Arthralgia, myalgia, numbness, peripheral neuropathy

RESP: Cough, dyspnea, **pneumonitis, pulmonary fibrosis or infiltrate**

SYST: **Superinfection,** SLE-like syndrome

PHARMACOKINETICS

PO: Half-life 20-60 min; crosses blood-brain barrier, placenta; enters breast milk; excreted as inactive metabolites in liver, unchanged in urine; protein binding 60%-90%

INTERACTIONS

Increase: antagonistic effect—norfloxacin

Increase: levels of nitrofurantoin—probenecid

Decrease: absorption of magnesium trisilicate antacid

Drug/Lab Test

Increase: BUN, alk phos, bilirubin, creatinine, blood glucose

N

NURSING CONSIDERATIONS

Assess:

- Blood count during chronic therapy, LFTs, pulmonary function tests
- **Urinary tract infection:** burning, pain on urination; fever; cloudy, foul-smelling urine; I&O ratio: C&S before treatment, after completion; serum creatinine, BUN
- **Pseudomembraneous colitis:** diarrhea with mucus, abdominal pain, fever, fatigue, anorexia; may be treated with vancomycin or metroNIDAZOLE
- CNS symptoms: insomnia, vertigo, headache, drowsiness, seizures

⚠ **Hepatotoxicity:** yellowing of skin or eyes, dark urine, clay-colored stools; monitor AST, ALT

⚠ **Pulmonary fibrosis, pneumonitis:** dyspnea, tachypnea, persistent cough

⚠ **Serious skin disorders:** fever, flushing, rash, urticaria, pruritus

- **Peripheral neuropathy:** paresthesias (more common in diabetes mellitus, electrolyte imbalances, vit B deficiency, debilitated patients)

Evaluate:

- Therapeutic response: decreased dysuria, fever; negative C&S

Teach patient/family:

- To notify prescriber of continued symptoms of UTI, fever, myalgias, arthralgias, numbness or tingling of extremities
- To take with food or milk; to avoid alcohol
- To protect susp from freezing; shake well before taking
- That product may cause drowsiness; to seek aid with walking, other activities; not to drive or operate machinery while taking medication
- That diabetics should monitor blood glucose levels
- That product may turn urine rust-yellow to brown

⚠ **Pseudomembranous colitis:** fever; diarrhea with mucus, pus, or blood; report immediately

⚠ HIGH ALERT

nitroglycerin (Rx)

(nye-troe-gli′ser-in)

extended release caps (Rx)

Nitro-Time, Nitrogard SR ✱

topical ointment (Rx)

Nitro-Bid

rectal ointment

Rectiv

SL (Rx)

Nitrostat

translingual spray (Rx)

Nitrolingual, NitroMist

transdermal (Rx)

Minitran, Nitro-Dur

Func. class.: Coronary vasodilator, antianginal

Chem. class.: Nitrate

Do not confuse:
Nitro-Bid/Nicobid

ACTION: Decreases preload and afterload, which are responsible for decreasing left ventricular end-diastolic pressure, systemic vascular resistance; dilates coronary arteries, improves blood flow through coronary vasculature, dilates arterial and venous beds systemically

USES: Chronic stable angina pectoris, prophylaxis of angina pain, CHF, acute MI, controlled hypotension for surgical procedures, anal fissures

Unlabeled uses: Pulmonary hypertension, hemorrhoids, retained placenta

CONTRAINDICATIONS: Hypersensitivity to this product or nitrites; severe anemia, increased intracranial

pressure, cerebral hemorrhage, closed-angle glaucoma, cardiac tamponade, cardiomyopathy, constrictive pericarditis
Precautions: Pregnancy (C), breastfeeding, children, postural hypotension, severe renal/hepatic disease, acute MI, abrupt discontinuation, hyperthyroidism

DOSAGE AND ROUTES

• **Adult: SL** Dissolve tab under tongue when pain begins; may repeat q5min until relief occurs; take ≤3 tabs/15 min; use 1 tab prophylactically 5-10 min before activities; **SUS CAP** q6-12hr on empty stomach; **TOP** 1-2 in q8hr, increase to 4 in q4hr as needed; **IV** 5 mcg/min, then increase by 5 mcg/min q3-5min; if no response after 20 mcg/min, increase by 10-20 mcg/min until desired response; **TRANS PATCH** apply a patch daily to a site free of hair; remove patch at bedtime to provide 10-12 hr nitrate-free interval to avoid tolerance
• **Child: IV** Initially 0.25-0.5 mcg/kg/min, titrate to patient response, usual dose 1-3 mcg/kg/min transmucosal

Anal fissures (Rectiv)
• **Adult: Rectal** Apply 1 inch of 0.4% ointment q12hr × 3 wk

Available forms: Translingual aero 0.4 mg/metered spray; sus rel tabs 2.5, 6.5, 9 mg; SL tabs 0.3, 0.4, 0.6 mg; topical oint 2%; trans syst 0.1, 0.2, 0.3, 0.4, 0.6, 0.8 mg/hr; inj sol 25 mg/250 ml, 50 mg/250 ml, 50 mg/500 ml, 100 mg/250 ml, 200 mg/500 ml; rectal ointment 0.4% (Rectiv)

Administer:
• **Topical ointment** should be measured on papers supplied; use paper to spread on nonhairy area of chest, abdomen, thigh skin; thin layer spread over 2-3 inches; do not rub

PO route
• Swallow sus rel products whole; do not break, crush, or chew
• With 8 oz water on empty stomach (oral tablet) 1 hr before or 2 hr after meals
• **SL:** should be dissolved under tongue, not swallowed
• **Aerosol** sprayed under tongue **(nitrolingual)**, not inhaled; prime before 1st-time use or if product has not been used in >6 wk; press valve head with forefinger

Transdermal route
• Apply new TD patch daily; remove after 12-14 hr to prevent tolerance

Rectal route
• Cover finger with plastic wrap, disposable glove, or finger cot; lay finger alongside 1-inch dosing line on carton; squeeze tube until equal to 1-inch dosing line; insert covered finger gently into anal canal no further than 1st finger joint and apply to sides; wash hands thoroughly; if too painful, apply directly to outside of anus

Continuous IV INFUSION route
• Diluted in D_5, D_5W, 0.9% NaCl for infusion to 200-400 mcg/ml, depending on patient's fluid status; common dilution 50 mg/250 ml, use controlled infusion device; use glass infusion bottles, non–polyvinyl-chloride infusion tubing; titrate to patient response; do not use filters

N

Y-site compatibilities: Acyclovir, alfentanil, amikacin, aminocaproic acid, aminophylline, amiodarone, amphotericin B cholesteryl, amphotericin B lipid complex, amphotericin B liposome, anidulafungin, argatroban, ascorbic acid, atenolol, atracurium, atropine, azaTHIOprine, aztreonam, benztropine, bivalirudin, bleomycin, bumetanide, buprenorphine, butorphanol, calcium chloride/gluconate, CARBOplatin, caspofungin, cefamandole, ceFAZolin, cefmetazole, cefonicid, cefoperazone, cefotaxime, cefoTEtan, cefOXitin, cefTAZidime, ceftizoxime, cefTRIAXone, cefuroxime, cephalothin, cephapirin, chloramphenicol, chlorproMAZINE, cimetidine, cisatracurium, CISplatin, clindamycin, cloNIDine, cyanocobalamin, cyclophosphamide, cycloSPORINE, cytarabine, DACTINomycin, dexamethasone, digoxin, diltiazem, diphenhydrAMINE, DOBUTamine, DOCEtaxel, DOPamine, doxacurium, DOXOrubicin, doxycycline, drotrecogin alfa, enalaprilat, ePHEDrine, EPINEPHrine, epirubicin, epoetin alfa, eptifibatide, ertapenem, erythromycin, esmolol, etoposide, famotidine, fenoldopam, fentaNYL, fluconazole, fludarabine, fluorouracil, folic acid, ganciclovir, gati floxacin, gemcitabine, gemtuzumab, gentamicin, glycopyrrolate, granisetron, heparin, hydrocortisone, HYDROmorphone, hydrOXYzine, IDArubicin, ifosfamide, imipenem-cilastatin, indomethacin, insulin (regular), irinotecan, isoproterenol, ketorolac, labetalol, lidocaine, linezolid, LORazepam, magnesium sulfate, mannitol, mechlorethamine, meperidine, metaraminol, methicillin, methotrexate, methoxamine, methyldopate, methylPREDNISolone, metoclopramide, metroNIDAZOLE, mezlocillin, micafungin, miconazole, midazolam, milrinone, minocycline, mitoXANtrone, morphine, moxalactam, mycophenolate, nafcillin, nalbuphine, naloxone, nesiritide, netilmicin, niCARdipine, nitroprusside, norepinephrine, octreotide, ondansetron, oxacillin, oxaliplatin, oxytocin, PACLitaxel, palonosetron, pamidronate, pancuronium, pantoprazole, papaverine, PEMEtrexed, penicillin G potassium/ sodium, pentamidine, pentazocine, PENTobarbital, PHENobarbital, phentolamine, phenylephrine, phytonadione, piperacillin, piperacillin-tazobactam, polymyxin B, potassium chloride, procainamide, prochlorperazine, promethazine, propofol, propranolol, protamine, pyridoxine, quiNIDine, quinupristin-dalfopristin, ranitidine, remifentanil, ritodrine, rocuronium, sodium bicarbonate, succinylcholine, SUFentanil, tacrolimus, teniposide, theophylline, thiamine, thiopental, thiotepa, ticarcillin, ticarcillin-clavulanate, tigecycline, tirofiban, tobramycin, tolazoline, trimetaphan, urokinase, vancomycin, vasopressin, vecuronium, verapamil, vinCRIStine, vinorelbine, voriconazole, warfarin, zoledronic acid

SIDE EFFECTS

CNS: *Headache, flushing, dizziness*
CV: *Postural hypotension,* tachycardia, **collapse,** syncope, palpitations
GI: Nausea, vomiting
INTEG: Pallor, sweating, rash

PHARMACOKINETICS

Metabolized by liver, excreted in urine, half-life 1-4 min
SUS REL: Onset 20-45 min, duration 3-8 hr
SL: Onset 1-3 min, duration 30 min
TRANSDERMAL: Onset 30 min-1 hr, duration 12-24 hr
AEROSOL: Onset 2 min, duration 30-60 min
TOPICAL OINT: Onset 30-60 min, duration 2-12 hr
IV: Onset 1-2 min, duration 3-5 min

INTERACTIONS

- **Severe hypotension, CV collapse: alcohol**

Increase: effects of β-blockers, diuretics, antihypertensives, calcium channel blockers
Increase: fatal hypotension—sildenafil, tadalafil, vardenafil; do not use together
Increase: nitrate level—aspirin
Decrease: heparin—IV nitroglycerin

Drug/Lab Test
Increase: urine catecholamine, urine VMA
False increase: cholesterol

NURSING CONSIDERATIONS

Assess:

- **Pain:** duration, time started, activity being performed, character
- Orthostatic B/P, pulse before and after administration
- Tolerance if taken over long period
- Headache, lightheadedness, decreased B/P; may indicate a need for decreased dosage

Evaluate:

- Therapeutic response: decrease, prevention of anginal pain

Teach patient/family:

- To place buccal tab between lip and gum above incisors or between cheek and gum
- To keep tabs in original container; to replace q6mo because effectiveness is lost; to keep away from heat, moisture, light

- That if 3 SL tabs in 15 min do not relieve pain, to seek immediate medical attention
- To avoid alcohol
- That product may cause headache; that tolerance usually develops; to use nonopioid analgesic
- That product may be taken before stressful activity: exercise, sexual activity
- That SL may sting when product comes in contact with mucous membranes
- To avoid hazardous activities if dizziness occurs
- To comply with complete medical regimen
- To make position changes slowly to prevent fainting

⚠ Never to use erectile dysfunction products (sildenafil, tadalafil, vardenafil); may cause severe hypotension, death

⚠ HIGH ALERT

nitroprusside (Rx)

(nye-troe-pruss′ide)

Nitropress

Func. class.: Antihypertensive, vasodilator

ACTION: Directly relaxes arteriolar, venous smooth muscle, thereby resulting in reduction in cardiac preload and afterload

USES: Hypertensive crisis/urgency/induction; to decrease bleeding by creating hypotension during surgery; acute CHF

Unlabeled uses: Postoperative hypertension, mitral regurgitation

CONTRAINDICATIONS: Hypersensitivity, hypertension (compensatory) due to aortic coarctation or AV shunting, acute CHF associated with reduced peripheral vascular resistance, AV shunt, Leber's disease, toxic amblyopia

Black Box Warning: Cyanide toxicity, do not use in hypothyroidism

Precautions: Anemia, increased intracranial pressure, pregnancy (C), breastfeeding, children, geriatric patients, hypovolemia, electrolyte imbalances, renal/hepatic disease, hypothyroidism

Black Box Warning: Hypotension

DOSAGE AND ROUTES

- **Adult and child: IV INFUSION** 0.25-10 mcg/kg/min; max 10 mcg/kg/min × 10 min

Renal dose

- **Adult: IV INFUSION** CCr <60 ml/min, maintain doses <3 mcg/kg/min to reduce thiocyanate accumulation

Available forms: Inj 50 mg/2 ml

Administer:

- Antidote is sodium thiosulfate

Continuous IV INFUSION route

- Depending on B/P reading q15min
- Reconstitute 50 mg/2-3 ml of D_5W, further dilute in 250, 500, or 1000 ml of D_5W to 200, 100, 50 mcg/ml, respectively; use infusion pump only; wrap bottle with aluminum foil to protect from light; observe for color change in infusion; discard if highly discolored (blue, green, dark red); titrate to patient response, protect from light

Y-site compatibilities: Alfentanil, alprostadil, amikacin, aminocaproic acid, aminophylline, amphotericin B lipid compex, amphotericin B liposome, anidulafungin, argatroban, atenolol, atropine, aztreonam, benztropine, bivalirudin, bleomycin, bumetanide, buprenorphine, butorphanol, calcium chloride/gluconate, CARBOplatin, cefamandole, ceFAZolin, cefmetazole, cefonicid, cefoperazone, cefotaxime, cefoTEtan, ce fOXitin, cefTAZidime, ceftizoxime, cef TRIAXone, cefuroxime, cephalothin, chloramphenicol, cimetidine, CISplatin, clindamycin, cyanocobalamin, cyclophosphamide, cycloSPORINE, cytarabine, DACTINomycin, DAPTOmycin, dexamethasone, digoxin, diltiazem, DOCEtaxel, DOPamine, doxacurium, DOXOrubicin, doxycycline, enalaprilat, ePHEDrine,

N

EPINEPHrine, epirubicin, epoetin alfa, eptifibatide, ertapenem, esmolol, etoposide, famotidine, fenoldopam, fentaNYL, fluconazole, fludarabine, fluorouracil, folic acid, furosemide, ganciclovir, gatifloxacin, gemcitabine, gemtuzumab, gentamicin, glycopyrrolate, granisetron, heparin, hydrocortisone, HYDROmorphone, IDArubicin, ifosfamide, inamrinone, indomethacin, insulin (regular), isoproterenol, ketorolac, labetalol, lidocaine, linezolid, LORazepam, magnesium sulfate, mannitol, mechlorethamine, meperidine, metaraminol, methicillin, methoxamine, methyldopate, methylPREDNISolone, metoclopramide, metoprolol, metroNIDAZOLE, mezlocillin, micafungin, miconazole, midazolam, milrinone, minocycline, morphine, moxalactam, multiple vitamins injection, nafcillin, nalbuphine, naloxone, nesiritide, netilmicin, niCARdipine, nitroglycerin, norepinephrine, octreotide, ondansetron, oxacillin, oxaliplatin, oxytocin, PACLitaxel, palonosetron, pamidronate, pancuronium, pantoprazole, penicillin G potassium/sodium, pentamidine, PENTobarbital, PHENobarbital, phentolamine, phenylephrine, phytonadione, piperacillin, piperacillin-tazobactam, polymyxin B, potassium chloride/phosphates, procainamide, propofol, propranolol, protamine, pyridoxine, ranitidine, ritodrine, rocuronium, sodium acetate/bicarbonate, succinylcholine, SUFentanil, tacrolimus, teniposide, theophylline, thiamine, ticarcillin, ticarcillin-clavulanate, tigecycline, tirofiban, tobramycin, tolazoline, trimetaphan, urokinase, vancomycin, vasopressin, vecuronium, verapamil, vinCRIStine, zoledronic acid

SIDE EFFECTS

CNS: *Dizziness, headache,* agitation, twitching, decreased reflexes, *restlessness*

CV: *Bradycardia,* ECG changes, tachycardia, *hypotension*

GI: Nausea, vomiting, abdominal pain

INTEG: Pain, irritation at inj site, sweating

MISC: Cyanide, thiocyanate toxicity, flushing, hypothyroidism

PHARMACOKINETICS

IV: Onset 1-2 min, duration 1-10 min, half-life 2 min; metabolized in liver, excreted in urine

INTERACTIONS

Increase: severe hypotension—ganglionic blockers, volatile liquid anesthetics, halothane, enflurane, circulatory depressants

Drug/Herb

Increase: antihypertensive effect—hawthorn

NURSING CONSIDERATIONS

Assess:

- Electrolytes: potassium, sodium, chloride, CO_2, CBC, serum glucose, serum methemoglobin if pulmonary O_2 levels are decreased; use IV 1-2 mg/kg methylene blue given over several min for methemoglobinemia, ABGs
- Renal studies: catecholamines, BUN, creatinine
- Hepatic studies: AST, ALT, alk phos

Black Box Warning: Hypotension: B/P by direct means if possible; check ECG continuously; pulse, jugular venous distention; PCWP; rebound hypertension may occur after nitroprusside is discontinued, give only with emergency equipment nearby, rapid decrease in B/P may occur

- Weight daily, I&O

⚠ **Thiocyanate, lactate, cyanide toxicity:** obtain levels daily if infusion >3 mcg/kg/min; thiocyanate toxicity occurs at plasma levels of 50-100 mcg/ml; thiocyanate toxicity includes confusion, weakness, seizures, hyperreflexia, psychosis, tinnitus, coma

- Nausea, vomiting, diarrhea
- Edema in feet, legs daily; skin turgor, dryness of mucous membranes for hydration status
- Crackles, dyspnea, orthopnea q30min
- For decrease in bicarbonate, P_{CO_2} blood pH, acidosis

⚠ Nurse Alert

Evaluate:

- Therapeutic response: decreased B/P, decreasing symptoms of cardiogenic shock or cardiac pump failure

Teach patient/family:

- To report headache, dizziness, loss of hearing, blurred vision, dyspnea, faintness, pain at IV site
- About the reason for giving product and expected results

nizatidine (OTC, Rx)

(ni-za′ti-deen)

Axid, Axid AR

Func. class.: H_2-receptor antagonist

Chem. class.: Substituted thiazole

ACTION: Blocks H_2-receptors, thereby reducing gastric acid output

USES: Benign gastric and duodenal ulceration, prevention of duodenal ulcer recurrence, symptomatic relief of gastroesophageal reflux, heartburn prevention

CONTRAINDICATIONS: Hypersensitivity

Precautions: Pregnancy (B), breastfeeding, renal/hepatic impairment (reduce dose in renal impairment)

DOSAGE AND ROUTES

Gastric and duodenal ulcer

- **Adult: PO** 300 mg at night or 150 mg bid for 4-8 wk; maintenance 150 mg at night

Prophylaxis of duodenal ulcer

- **Adult: PO** 150 mg/day at bedtime

Gastroesophageal reflux

- **Adult and child ≥12 yr: PO** 150 mg bid × ≤12 wk, max 300 mg/day

Heartburn prevention

- **Adult: PO** 75 mg before eating bid

Renal dose

- **Adult: PO** CCr 20-50 ml/min, give 150 mg every other day; CCr <20 ml/min, give 150 mg q72hr

Available forms: Caps 150, 300 mg; tabs 75 mg

Administer:

- With meals for prolonged product effect; antacids 1 hr before or 1 hr after product; at bedtime if taken daily

SIDE EFFECTS

CNS: Headache, somnolence, confusion, abnormal dreams, dizziness

CV: **Cardiac dysrhythmias, cardiac arrest**

ENDO: Gynecomastia

GI: Elevated hepatic enzymes, **hepatitis,** jaundice, nausea

HEMA: **Thrombocytopenia, agranulocytosis, aplastic anemia**

INTEG: Pruritus, sweating, urticaria, **exfoliative dermatitis**

METAB: Hyperuricemia

MS: Myalgia

RESP: **Bronchospasm, laryngeal edema, pneumonia**

PHARMACOKINETICS

Partially metabolized by liver, excreted by kidneys, plasma half-life 1-2.8 hr, 70% absorbed orally, small amount (0.1% of plasma concentration) enters breast milk, 35% bound to plasma proteins

N

INTERACTIONS

Increase: GI obstruction risk—NIFEdipine (ext rel tabs)

Increase: effect of—mefloquine

Decrease: effect of—ketoconazole, itraconazole, atazanavir, cefditoren, cefpodoxime, delavirdine, gefitinib, raltegravir

Drug/Lab Test

Increase: ALT, AST, serum creatinine

False negative: allergy skin tests

NURSING CONSIDERATIONS

Assess:

- **GI pain:** epigastric, abdominal, character, alleviating factors, hematemesis, occult blood in stool, heartburn, GERD
- ⚠ **Agranulocytosis: CBC with differential if patient receiving long-term therapy**

Evaluate:

- Decreased GI pain, heartburn, GERD; resolution of gastric, duodenal ulcers

Teach patient/family:
- That gynecomastia, impotence may occur, are reversible
- To avoid driving or other hazardous activities until stabilized on product; that dizziness may occur
- To avoid black pepper, caffeine, alcohol, harsh spices, extremes in temperature of food
- To avoid OTC preparations: aspirin, cough, cold preparations

TREATMENT OF OVERDOSE:
Symptomatic and supportive therapy is recommended; activated charcoal, emesis, or lavage may reduce absorption

⚠ HIGH ALERT

norepinephrine (Rx)
(nor-ep-i-nef′rin)

Levophed

Func. class.: Adrenergic
Chem. class.: Catecholamine

Do not confuse:
norepinephrine/EPINEPHrine

ACTION: Causes increased contractility and heart rate by acting on β-receptors in heart; also acts on α-receptors, thereby causing vasoconstriction in blood vessels; B/P is elevated, coronary blood flow improves, and cardiac output increases

USES: Acute hypotension, shock

CONTRAINDICATIONS: Hypersensitivity to this product or cyclopropane/halothane anesthesia, sulfites; ventricular fibrillation, tachydysrhythmias, pheochromocytoma, hypotension, hypovolemia

Precautions: Pregnancy (C), breastfeeding, geriatric patients, arterial embolism, peripheral vascular disease, hypertension, hyperthyroidism, cardiac disease

Black Box Warning: Extravasation

DOSAGE AND ROUTES
- **Adult: IV INFUSION** 0.5-1 mcg/min titrated to B/P; maintenance 2-4 mcg/min; max 30 mcg/min
- **Child: IV INFUSION** 0.1 mcg/kg/min titrated to B/P; max 2 mcg/kg/min

Available forms: Inj 1 mg/ml

Administer:
- Plasma expanders for hypovolemia

Continuous IV INFUSION route
- Dilute with 500-1000 ml D_5W or D_5/0.9% NaCl; average dilution 4 mg/1000 ml diluent (4 mcg base/ml); give as infusion 2-3 ml/min; titrate to response
- Store reconstituted sol in refrigerator ≤24 hr, protect from light, store unopened product at room temperature, do not use discolored sol

Y-site compatibilities: Alemtuzumab, alfentanil, amikacin, amiodarone, anidulafungin, argatroban, ascorbic acid, atenolol, atracurium, atropine, aztreonam, benztropine, bivalirudin, bleomycin, bumetanide, buprenorphine, butorphanol, calcium chloride/gluconate, CARBOplatin, caspo fungin, cefamandole, ceFAZolin, cefmetazole, cefonicid, cefoperazone, cefotaxime, cefoTEtan, cefOXitin, cefTAZidime, ceftizoxime, ceftobiprole, cef TRIAXone, cefuroxime, cephalothin, chloramphenicol, chlorproMAZINE, cimetidine, cisatracurium, CISplatin, clindamycin, cloNIDine, cyanocobalamin, cyclophosphamide, cycloSPORINE, cytarabine, DAPTOmycin, dexamethasone, digoxin, diltiazem, diphen hydrAMINE, DOBUTamine, DOCEtaxel, DOPamine, doripenem, doxycycline, enalaprilat, ePHEDrine, EPINEPHrine, epirubicin, epoetin alfa, ertapenem, erythromycin, esmolol, etoposide, famotidine, fenoldopam, fentaNYL, fluconazole, fludarabine, gatifloxacin, gemcitabine, gentamicin, glycopyrrolate, granisetron, heparin, hydrocortisone, HYDROmorphone, hydrOXYzine, IDArubicin, ifosfamide, imipenem-cilastatin, irinotecan, isoproterenol, ketorolac, labetalol, lidocaine, linezolid, LORazepam, magnesium sulfate, mannitol, mechlorethamine, meperidine, meropenem, metaraminol, methicillin, methotrexate, methoxamine, methyldopate, methylPREDNISolone, metoclopramide, metoprolol, metroNIDAZOLE, mezlocillin, micafungin, miconazole, midazolam, milrinone, minocycline, mitoXANtrone, morphine, moxalactam, multiple vitamins injection, mycophenolate, nafcillin, nalbuphine, naloxone, netilmicin, niCARdipine, nitroglycerin, nitroprusside, octreotide, ondansetron, oxacillin, oxaliplatin, oxytocin, PACLitaxel, palonosetron, pamidronate, pancuronium, papaverine, PEMEtrexed, penicillin G potassium/ sodium, pentamidine, pentazocine, phenylephrine, phytonadione, piperacillin, piperacillin-tazobactam, polymyxin B, potassium chloride, procainamide, prochlorperazine, promethazine, propofol, propranolol, protamine, pyridoxine, quiNIDine, ranitidine, remifentanil, ritodrine, succinylcholine, SUFentanil, tacrolimus, teniposide, theophylline, thiamine, thiotepa, ticarcillin, ticarcillin-clavulanate, tigecycline, tirofiban, tobramycin, tolazoline, trimetaphan, urokinase, vancomycin, vasopressin, vecuronium, verapamil, vinCRIStine, vinorelbine, vitamin B complex with C, voriconazole, zoledronic acid

SIDE EFFECTS

CNS: *Headache,* anxiety, dizziness, insomnia, restlessness, tremor, **cerebral hemorrhage**

CV: *Palpitations, tachycardia, hypertension, ectopic beats, angina*

GI: *Nausea, vomiting*

GU: Decreased urine output

INTEG: **Necrosis, tissue sloughing with extravasation, gangrene**

RESP: Dyspnea

SYST: **Anaphylaxis**

PHARMACOKINETICS

IV: Onset 1-2 min; metabolized in liver; excreted in urine (inactive metabolites); crosses placenta

INTERACTIONS

Increase: dysrhythmias—general anesthetics

- **Incompatible with alkaline solutions: sodium, bicarbonate**
- **Severe hypertension: guanethidine**

⚠ **Do not use within 2 wk of MAOIs, antihistamines, ergots, methyldopa, oxytocics, tricyclics, guanethidine because hypertensive crisis may result**

Increase: B/P—oxytocics

Increase: pressor effect—tricyclics, MAOIs

Decrease: norepinephrine action—α-blockers

NURSING CONSIDERATIONS

Assess:

- I&O ratio; notify prescriber if output <30 ml/hr
- B/P, pulse q2-3min after parenteral route, ECG during administration continuously; if B/P increases, product is decreased, CVP or PWP during infusion if possible
- Paresthesias and coldness of extremities; peripheral blood flow may decrease

Black Box Warning: Extravasation: inj site: tissue sloughing

- **Sulfite sensitivity, which may be life-threatening**

Evaluate:

- Therapeutic response: increased B/P with stabilization, adequate tissue perfusion

Teach patient/family:

- About the reason for product administration; to report dyspnea, dizziness, chest pain

TREATMENT OF OVERDOSE:

Administer fluids, electrolyte replacement

N

norethindrone (Rx)

(nor-eth-in′drone)

Aygestin, Camila, Deblitane, Errin ♣, Heather, Jencycla, Jolivette, Lyza, Micronor, Nora-BE, Norlyroc, Nor-QD, Sharobel

Func. class.: Progestogen

ACTION: Inhibits the secretion of pituitary gonadotropins, which prevents follicular maturation and ovulation; stimulates growth of mammary tissue; antineoplastic action against endometrial cancer

USES: Uterine bleeding (abnormal), amenorrhea, endometriosis, contraception

CONTRAINDICATIONS: Pregnancy (X), breast cancer, hypersensitivity, thromboembolic disorders, reproductive cancer, genital bleeding (abnormal, undiagnosed), liver tumors, hepatic disease

Precautions: Breastfeeding, hypertension, asthma, blood dyscrasias, CHF, diabetes mellitus, depression, migraine headache, seizure disorders, bone/gallbladder/renal/hepatic disease, family history of breast or reproductive tract cancer, smoking, HIV

DOSAGE AND ROUTES

Amenorrhea, abnormal uterine bleeding (Aygestin)

- **Adult: PO** 2.5-10 mg/day on days 5-25 of menstrual cycle

Endometriosis (Aygestin)

- **Adult: PO** 5 mg/day × 2 wk, then increased by 2.5 mg/day × 2 wk up to 15 mg/day, may continue for 6-9 mo

Contraception

- **Adult: PO** 0.35 mg on 1st day of menses, then 0.35 mg/day

Available forms: Tabs (Aygestin) 5 mg; tabs 0.35 mg

Administer:

- Titrated dose; use lowest effective dose
- One dose in AM; do not interrupt between pill packs; give at roughly same time of day
- Without regard to meals
- Store in dark area

SIDE EFFECTS

CNS: *Dizziness, headache,* migraines, depression, fatigue

CV: Hypotension, thrombophlebitis, edema, thromboembolism, CVA, stroke, PE, MI

EENT: Diplopia

GI: *Nausea,* vomiting, anorexia, cramps, increased weight, cholestatic jaundice

GU: Amenorrhea, cervical erosion, breakthrough bleeding, dysmenorrhea, vaginal candidiasis, breast changes, (gynecomastia, testicular atrophy, impotence), endometriosis, spontaneous abortion, *breast tenderness*

INTEG: Rash, urticaria, acne, hirsutism, alopecia, oily skin, seborrhea, purpura, melasma

META: Hyperglycemia

PHARMACOKINETICS

Excreted in urine, feces; metabolized in liver, half-life 5-14 hr

INTERACTIONS

Decrease: progestin effect—barbiturates, carBAMazepine, fosphenytoin, phenytoin, rifampin

Drug/Herb

Decrease: contraception—St. John's wort

Drug/Food

Increase: caffeine level—caffeine

Drug/Lab Test

Increase: LDL

Decrease: GTT, HDL, alk phos

NURSING CONSIDERATIONS

Assess:

- Weight daily: notify prescriber of weekly weight gain >5 lb
- B/P at beginning of treatment and periodically
- I&O ratio; be alert for decreasing urinary output, increasing edema
- Hepatic studies: ALT, AST, bilirubin periodically during long-term therapy

- Edema, hypertension, cardiac symptoms, jaundice, thromboembolism
- Mental status: affect, mood, behavioral changes, depression
- Hypercalcemia
- Breast exam, pap smear

Evaluate:

- Therapeutic response: decreased abnormal uterine bleeding, absence of amenorrhea

Teach patient/family:

- About cushingoid symptoms

⚠ To report breast lumps, vaginal bleeding, amenorrhea, edema, jaundice, dark urine, clay-colored stools, dyspnea, headache, blurred vision, abdominal pain, numbness or stiffness in legs, chest pain; impotence or gynecomastia (men)

- To take at same time of day; not to interrupt between pill packs
- To report suspected pregnancy immediately, to wait ≥3 mo after stopping product to become pregnant, pregnancy (X); to use backup contraception methods for 48 hr if treatment is not begun on the first day of menstruation
- To avoid smoking; CV reactions may occur
- That product does not protect against HIV, STDs
- That product may mask onset of menopause

nortriptyline (Rx)

(nor-trip′ti-leen)

Arentyl ♣, Pamelor

Func. class.: Antidepressant, tricyclic

Chem. class.: Dibenzocycloheptene—secondary amine

Do not confuse:

nortriptyline/amitriptyline

ACTION: Blocks reuptake of norepinephrine and serotonin into nerve endings, thereby increasing action of norepinephrine and serotonin in nerve cells

USES: Major depression

Unlabeled uses: Chronic pain management, PMDD, social phobia, panic disorder, enuresis, migraine prophylaxis

CONTRAINDICATIONS: Hypersensitivity to tricyclics, recovery phase of MI, seizure disorders, prostatic hypertrophy

Precautions: Breastfeeding, suicidal patients, severe depression, increased intraocular pressure, closed-angle glaucoma, urinary retention, cardiac/hepatic disease, hyperthyroidism, electroshock therapy, elective surgery, pregnancy (C), carBAMazepine hypersensitivity

Black Box Warning: Children, suicidal ideation

DOSAGE AND ROUTES

- **Adult: PO** 25 mg tid or qid; may increase to 150 mg/day; may give daily dose at bedtime
- **Adolescent: PO** 1-3 mg/kg/day in 3-4 divided doses or daily at bedtime, max 150 mg/day
- **Child 6-12 yr (unlabeled): PO** 1-3 mg/kg/day in 3-4 divided doses, max 150 mg/day
- **Geriatric: PO** 10-25 mg at bedtime, increase by 10-25 mg at weekly intervals to desired dose; usual maintenance 75 mg/day, max 150 mg/day

Available forms: Caps 10, 25, 50, 75 mg; sol 10 mg/5 ml

Administer:

- Store in tight, light-resistant container at room temperature
- Increased fluids, bulk in diet if constipation occurs
- Without regard to meals
- Dosage at bedtime for oversedation during day; may take entire dose at bedtime; geriatric patients may not tolerate once-daily dosing
- Gum, hard candy, frequent sips of water for dry mouth
- **Oral solution:** with fruit juice, water, or milk to disguise taste

N

SIDE EFFECTS

CNS: *Dizziness, drowsiness,* confusion, headache, anxiety, tremors, stimulation, weakness, insomnia, nightmares, EPS (geriatric patients), increased psychiatric symptoms, seizures

CV: *Orthostatic hypotension,* ECG changes, *tachycardia,* hypertension, palpitations, dysrhythmias

EENT: *Blurred vision,* tinnitus, mydriasis, dry eyes

ENDO: SIADH, hyponatremia, hypothyroidism

GI: *Constipation, dry mouth,* nausea, vomiting, paralytic ileus, increased appetite, cramps, epigastric distress, jaundice, hepatitis, stomatitis, weight gain

GU: *Urinary retention,* acute renal failure, sexual dysfunction

HEMA: Agranulocytosis, thrombocytopenia, eosinophilia, leukopenia

INTEG: Rash, urticaria, sweating, pruritus, photosensitivity

SYST: Serotonin syndrome

PHARMACOKINETICS

PO: Steady-state 4-19 days; metabolized by liver; excreted by kidneys; crosses placenta; excreted in breast milk; half-life 18-28 hr, protein binding 93%-95%

INTERACTIONS

⚠ **Increase:** QT prolongation—class IA/III antidysrhythmics, some phenothiazines, β agonists, local anesthetics, tricyclics, haloperidol, chloroquine, droperidol, pentamidine; CYP3A4 inhibitors (amiodarone, clarithromycin, erythromycin, telithromycin, troleandomycin), arsenic trioxide, levomethadyl; CYP3A4 substrates (methadone, pimozide, QUEtiapine, quiNIDine, risperiDONE, ziprasidone)

• Heavy smoking: decreased product effect

⚠ Hyperpyretic crisis, seizures, hypertensive episode: MAOI

Increase: effects of direct-acting sympathomimetics (EPINEPHrine), alcohol, barbiturates, benzodiazepines, CNS depressants, products increasing QT interval, other anticholinergics

⚠ **Increase:** serotonin syndrome, neuroleptic malignant syndrome—SSRIs, SNRIs, serotonin receptor agonists, linezolid; methylene blue (IV)

Decrease: effects of guanethidine, cloNIDine, indirect-acting sympathomimetics (ePHEDrine)

Drug/Herb

Increase: CNS effect—kava, valerian

Decrease: nortriptyline level—St. John's wort

Drug/Lab Test

Increase: serum bilirubin, blood glucose, alk phos

Decrease: VMA, 5-HIAA

False increase: urinary catecholamines

NURSING CONSIDERATIONS

Assess:

Black Box Warning: **Suicidal thoughts/behaviors in children/young adults:** not approved for children, monitor for suicidal ideation in depression, adolescents, young adults

• Monitor for glaucoma exacerbation and paralytic ileus

• B/P (lying, standing), pulse q4hr; if systolic B/P drops 20 mm Hg, hold product, notify prescriber; VS q4hr in patients with CV disease

• Blood studies: thyroid function tests, LFTs, serum nortriptyline level/target 50-150 mg/ml if patient is receiving long-term therapy

• Weight weekly; appetite may increase with product

⚠ **PR, QT prolongation:** ECG for flattening of T wave, bundle branch block, AV block, QT prolongation, dysrhythmias in cardiac patients; assess for chest pain, palpitations, dyspnea

• EPS primarily in geriatric patients: rigidity, dystonia, akathisia, preferred tricyclic in geriatric patients

• Mental status changes: mood, sensorium, affect, suicidal tendencies, increase in psychiatric symptoms, depression, panic

• Urinary retention, constipation; constipation is more likely to occur in children

⚠ **Withdrawal symptoms:** headache, nausea, vomiting, muscle pain, weakness; do not usually occur unless product was discontinued abruptly
- Alcohol intake; if alcohol is consumed, hold dose until AM
- **Serotonin syndrome, neuroleptic malignant syndrome:** assess for increased heart rate, shivering, sweating, dilated pupils, tremors, high B/P, hyperthermia, headache, confusion; if these occur, stop product, administer serotonin antagonist if needed **(rare)**
- Assistance with ambulation during beginning therapy because drowsiness/dizziness occurs; safety measures including side rails, primarily for geriatric patients

Evaluate:
- Therapeutic response: decreased depression

Teach patient/family:
- That therapeutic effects may take 2-3 wk; only small quantities may be dispersed
- To use caution when driving, during other activities requiring alertness because of drowsiness, dizziness, blurred vision
- To avoid alcohol ingestion, other CNS depressants; to avoid MAOIs within 14 days
- Not to discontinue medication quickly after long-term use; may cause nausea, headache, malaise
- To wear sunscreen or large hat because photosensitivity occurs

⚠ To immediately report urinary retention, worsening depression, suicidal thoughts/behaviors

TREATMENT OF OVERDOSE:
ECG monitoring; lavage, activated charcoal; administer anticonvulsant

nystatin (Rx)
(nye-stat′in)

Bio-Statin, Mycostatin, Nadostine ✦, Nilstat, Nyamyc

Func. class.: Antifungal

Chem. class.: Amphoteric polyene

ACTION:
Interferes with fungal DNA replication; binds sterols in fungal cell membrane, which increases permeability, leaking of cell nutrients

USES:
Candida species causing oral, intestinal infections

CONTRAINDICATIONS:
Hypersensitivity

Precautions: Pregnancy (C)

DOSAGE AND ROUTES
Oral infection
- **Adult/adolescent/child: SUSP** 400,000-600,000 units qid; use 1/2 dose in each side of mouth; swish and swallow; use for at least 48 hr after symptoms resolved
- **Infant: SUSP** 200,000 units qid (100,000 units in each side of mouth)
- **Newborn and premature infant: SUSP** 100,000 units qid
- **Adult/child: TROCHES** 200,000-400,000 units qid × ≤2 wk

GI infection
- **Adult: PO** 500,000-1,000,000 units tid

Cutaneous candidiasis
- **Adult/child: Top cream/ointment** apply to affected area bid; **powder** apply to affected area bid-tid

Available forms: Tabs 500,000 units; oral caps 500,000, 1,000,000 units, bulk powder; suspension 100,000 mg/ml

Administer:
- Store at room temperature for oral susp; tabs in tight, light-resistant containers at room temperature

N

PO route

• Oral susp dose by placing ½ in each cheek, then swallow; do not mix with food

• Topical dose after cleansing area; mouth may be swabbed; very moist lesions best treated with topical powder

SIDE EFFECTS

GI: Nausea, vomiting, anorexia, diarrhea, cramps

INTEG: Rash, urticaria (rare)

PHARMACOKINETICS

PO: Little absorption, excreted in feces

NURSING CONSIDERATIONS

Assess:

• **Allergic reaction:** rash, urticaria, irritated oral mucous membranes; product may have to be discontinued

• Obtain culture, histologic tests to confirm organism

• Predisposing factors: antibiotic therapy, pregnancy, diabetes mellitus, sexual partner infection (vaginal infections)

Evaluate:

• Therapeutic response: culture negative for *Candida*

Teach patient/family:

• That long-term therapy may be needed to clear infection; to complete entire course of medication

• To avoid commercial mouthwashes for mouth infection

• To shake susp before measuring each dose

• To notify prescriber of irritation; product may have to be discontinued

nystatin topical

See Appendix B

⚠ HIGH ALERT

obinutuzumab

(oh′bi-nue-tooz′ue-mab)

Gazyva

Func. class.: Antineoplastic; biologic response modifier

ACTION: A recombinant, human monoclonal antibody that binds to the gastric B-lymphocyte-associated antibody; action is indirect, possible through T-cell-mediated anti-tumor responses

USES: Chronic lymphocytic leukemia, previously untreated in combination

CONTRAINDICATIONS: Hypersensitivity

Precautions: Pregnancy (C), breastfeeding, cardiac disease, children, human antichimeric antibody (HACA), human antimurine antibody (HAMA), infection, infusion-related reactions, neutropenia, pulmonary disease, thrombocytopenia, tumor lysis syndrome, vaccination

Black Box Warning: Hepatitis, progressive multifocal leukoencephalopathy

DOSAGE AND ROUTES

• **Adult: IV cycle 1** 100 mg over 4 hr (day 1); then 900 mg (50 mg/hr, increased by 50 mg/hr q30min, to max 400 mg/hr) (day 2); then 1000 mg (100 mg/hr, increased by 100 mg/hr q30min to max 400 mg/hr (day 8, day 115); **cycle 2-6** 1000 mg (100 mg/hr increased by 100 mg/hr q30min to max 400 mg/hr (day 1 repeat q28days)

Available forms: Sol for inj 1000 mg/40 ml

Administer:

IV intermittent INFUSION route

• Due to the risk of hypotension, consider withholding antihypertensive medications for 12 hr before, during, and for the 1st hr after use until blood pressure is stable

• Single-use vials do not contain preservatives

• Do not mix with other products

• Give antimicrobial prophylaxis to neutropenic patients throughout treatment; consider antiviral and antifungal prophylaxis as needed

• **Premedication for cycle 1, days 1 and 2:** acetaminophen 650-1000 mg, and diphenhydrAMINE 50 mg at least 30 min before infusion, dexamethasone 20 mg IV or methylPREDNISolone 80 mg IV at least 1 hr before infusion

• **Premedication for cycle 1, days 8 and 15 and cycles 2-6, day 1:** acetaminophen 650-1000 mg at least 30 min before infusion; those with any infusion-related reaction with the previous infusion should also receive diphenhydrAMINE 50 mg at least 30 min before the infusion; if the patient had a grade 3 infusion-related reaction with the previous dose or has a lymphocyte count $>25 \times 10^9$/L, additionally administer dexamethasone 20 mg IV or methylPREDNISolone 80 mg IV at least 1 hr before infusion

• Use in a facility to adequately monitor and treat infusion reactions

• Visually inspect parenteral products for particulate matter and discoloration before use

• Prepare all doses in 0.9% NaCl; do not admix; use a final concentration of 0.4-4 mg/mL; give as an IV infusion only

Reconstitution: Cycle 1, days 1 and 2:

• Withdraw 4 mL (100 mg) from the vial and dilute into 100 mL 0.9% NaCL use on day 1; mix by gentle inversion; do not shake, use immediately

• Withdraw the remaining 36 mL (900 mg) and dilute into 250 mL 0.9% NaCl for use on day 2, mix by gentle inversion; do not shake

Cycle 1, days 8 and 15; cycles 2-6:

• Withdraw 40 mL (1000 mg) from the vial and dilute into 250 mL 0.9% NaCl; mix by gentle inversion; do not shake

• Store following reconstitution: store at 2° C-8° C (36° F-46° F) for up to 24 hr;

O

do not freeze; allow to come to room temperature before administration; use a dedicated line, protect from light

- ***Day 1 (100 mg dose):*** give at initial rate of 25 mg/hr over 4 hr; do not increase the infusion rate
- ***Day 2 (900 mg dose):*** give at 50 mg/hr ×30 min; if no hypersensitivity or infusion-related events occur, increase the rate by 50 mg/hr q30min to a max rate of 400 mg/hr; if a grade 1-2 infusion-related reaction occurs, temporarily interrupt or reduce rate; the infusion may be resumed at a reduced rate upon improvement; if the reaction does not recur, the rate may be increased for the current cycle and dose; if a grade 3 hypersensitivity or infusion-related event develops, the infusion should be temporarily interrupted; upon improvement, the infusion can be resumed at half the rate at the time that the reaction occurred; if the reaction does not recur, the rate may be increased; if a grade 4 hypersensitivity or infusion-related event develops, discontinue the infusion and do not resume
- ***Subsequent infusions (1000 mg dose):*** give at rate of 100 mg/hr for 30 min; if no hypersensitivity or infusion-related events occur, increase the infusion rate by 100 mg/hr q30min, max rate of 400 mg/hr; if a grade 1-2 infusion-related reaction occurs, the infusion should be temporarily interrupted or the rate reduced; the infusion may be resumed at a reduced rate upon improvement; if the reaction does not recur, the rate may be increased for the current cycle and dose; if a grade 3 hypersensitivity or infusion-related event develops, temporarily interrupt; upon improvement, resume at half the rate being used at the time that the reaction occurred; if the reaction does not recur, the rate may be increased for the current cycle and dose; if a grade 4 hypersensitivity or infusion-related event develops, discontinue the infusion and do not resume

SIDE EFFECTS

CNS: Headache, fever, chills, flushing
CV: Cardiac arrest, MI, sinus tachycardia, hypertension
GI: Constipation, decreased appetite, diarrhea, hepatitis/hepatic failure, nausea, vomiting
HEMA: Neutropenia, thrombocytopenia, lymphopenia, leukopenia
META: Lower potassium/sodium/calcium, aluminum, higher potassium/uric acid
RESP: Wheezing, dyspnea
SYST: Tumor lysis syndrome

PHARMACOKINETICS

Terminal half-life 28.4 days

INTERACTIONS

Increase: adverse reactions—abciximab, belimumab, clozapine, pimecrolimus, avoid concurrent use
Increase: infection—denosumab, natalizumab, live virus vaccines
Increase: hypotension—antihypertensives
Increase: thrombocytopenia—chlorambucil
Increase: hematologic toxicity—leflunomide
Increase: immunosuppression—tofacitinib, avoid concurrent use

Drug/Herb

Decrease: obinutuzumab—echinacea

NURSING CONSIDERATIONS

Assess:

Black Box Warning: Hepatitis B: reactivation of HBV in those who are HBsAg positive, HBsAg negative, and core antibody anti-HBc positive; may result in fulminant hepatitis, hepatic failure, or death, screen high-risk patients before use, monitor carriers for active HBV infection during and for several months after therapy completion, discontinue treatment of any other antineoplastics if infection is reactivated

Black Box Warning: Progressive multifocal leukoencephalopathy (PML): notify prescriber any new, worsening neurological signs/symptoms (ataxia, visual changes, confusion)

- **Tumor lysis syndrome:** can occur within 24 hr of 1st infusion; those with high tumor burden or lymphocyte count >25 × 10^9/L are at increased risk; monitor serum creatinine, potassium, calcium, uric acid, phosphate closely
- **Severe/life-threatening infusion reactions:** 2/3 have a reaction to 1st dose; consider withholding antihypertensives for 12 hr before, during, and after 1st hr of infusion

Evaluate:
- Decreased disease progression

Teach patient/family:
- About the reason for treatment and expected results

Black Box Warning: **Hepatitis B:** to report yellow skin, eyes, fatigue, dark urine, that continuing follow-up will be needed

Black Box Warning: **Progressive multifocal leukoencephalopathy (PML):** to report confusion, visual changes, dizziness

octreotide (Rx)

(ok-tree′oh-tide)

SandoSTATIN, SandoSTATIN LAR Depot

Func. class.: Growth hormone, antidiarrheal

Chem. class.: Synthetic octapeptide

ACTION: A potent growth hormone similar to somatostatin

USES: **SandoSTATIN:** acromegaly, improves symptoms of carcinoid tumors, vasoactive intestinal peptide tumors (VIPomas); **LAR Depot:** long-term maintenance of acromegaly, carcinoid tumors, VIPomas

Unlabeled uses: GI fistula, variceal bleeding, diarrheal conditions, pancreatic fistula, irritable bowel syndrome, dumping syndrome, short bowel syndrome, insulinoma, hepatorenal syndrome

CONTRAINDICATIONS: Hypersensitivity

Precautions: Pregnancy (B), breastfeeding, children, geriatric patients, diabetes mellitus, hypothyroidism, renal disease

DOSAGE AND ROUTES

Acromegaly
- **Adult: SUBCUT/IV** (SandoSTATIN) 50-100 mcg bid-tid, adjust q2wk based on growth hormone levels or **IM** (SandoSTATIN LAR) 20 mg q4wk × 3 mo, adjust based on growth hormone levels

VIPomas
- **Adult: SUBCUT/IV** (SandoSTATIN) 200-300 mcg/day in 2-4 doses for 2 wk, or **IM** (SandoSTATIN LAR) 20 mg q4wk × 2 mo, adjust dose

Flushing/diarrhea in carcinoid tumors
- **Adult: SUBCUT/IV** (SandoSTATIN) 100-600 mcg/day in 2-4 doses for 2 wk, titrated to patient response or **IM** (SandoSTATIN LAR) 20 mg q4wk × 2 mo, adjust dose

GI fistula
- **Adult: SUBCUT** (SandoSTATIN) 50-200 mcg q8hr

Antidiarrheal in AIDS patients (unlabeled)
- **Adult: SUBCUT** (SandoSTATIN) 50 mcg q8hr prn, increase to 500 mcg q8hr

Irritable bowel syndrome (unlabeled)
- **Adult: SUBCUT** (SandoSTATIN) 100 mcg in single dose, up to 125 mcg bid

Dumping syndrome (unlabeled)
- **Adult: SUBCUT** (SandoSTATIN) 50-150 mcg/day

O

Chemotherapy-induced diarrhea (unlabeled)
• **Adult: SUBCUT** 0.1-0.5 mg or IV 0.15-2.4 mg/24 hr
Variceal bleeding (unlabeled)
• **Adult: IV** (SandoSTATIN) 25-50 mcg/hr **CONT IV INFUSION** for 18 hr-5 days
Available forms: Inj (SandoSTATIN) 0.05, 0.1, 0.2, 0.5, 1 mg/ml; inj powder for susp (LAR depot) 10, 20, 30 mg/5 ml
Administer:
• Store in refrigerator for unopened amps, vials or at room temperature for 2 wk; protect from light; do not use discolored or cloudy sol
• Do not use if discolored or particulates are present
IM route
• Reconstitute with diluent provided; give in gluteal region, rotate injection sites
SUBCUT route
• Rotate inj site; use hip, thigh, abdomen
• Avoid using medication that is cold; allow to reach room temperature; do not use LAR depot, do not use if discolored or if particulates are present
IV route
• **IV direct:** give over 3 min; during an emergency carcinoid crisis, give rapid bolus
• **Intermittent IV infusion:** dilute in 50-200 ml D_5W, 0.9% NaCl; give over 15-30 min
• Solution is stable for 24 hr

Y-site compatibilities: Acyclovir, alfentanil, allopurinol, amifostine, amikacin, aminocaproic acid, aminophylline, amiodarone, amphotericin B colloidal, amphotericin B lipid complex, amphotericin B liposome, ampicillin, ampicillin-sulbactam, anidulafungin, argatroban, arsenic trioxide, atenolol, atracurium, azithromycin, aztreonam, bivalirudin, bleomycin, bumetanide, buprenorphine, busulfan, butorphanol, calcium chloride/gluconate, capreomycin, CARBOplatin, carmustine, caspofungin, ceFAZolin, cefepime, cefotaxime, cefoTEtan, cefOXitin, cefTAZidime, ceftizoxime, cefTRIAXone, cefuroxime, chloramphenicol, chlorproMAZINE, cimetidine, ciprofloxacin, cisatracurium, CISplatin, clindamycin, cyclophosphamide, cycloSPORINE, cytarabine, dacarbazine, DACTINomycin, DAPTOmycin, DAUNOrubicin, DAUNOrubicin liposome, dexamethasone, digoxin, diltiazem, diphenhydrAMINE, DOBUTamine, DOCEtaxel, dolasetron, DOPamine, DOXOrubicin, DOXOrubicin liposomal, doxycycline, droperidol, enalaprilat, ePHEDrine, EPINEPHrine, epirubicin, eptifibatide, ertapenem, erythromycin, esmolol, etoposide, famotidine, fenoldopam, fentaNYL, fluconazole, fludarabine, fluorouracil, foscarnet, fosphenytoin, furosemide, gallium nitrate, ganciclovir, gatifloxacin, gemcitabine, gentamicin, glycopyrrolate, granisetron, haloperidol, heparin, hydrALAZINE, hydrocortisone, HYDROmorphone, hydrOXYzine, IDArubicin, ifosfamide, imipenem-cilastatin, insulin (regular), irinotecan, isoproterenol, ketorolac, labetalol, lansoprazole, leucovorin, levofloxacin, lidocaine, linezolid, LORazepam, magnesium sulfate, mannitol, mechlorethamine, melphalan, meperidine, meropenem, mesna, methohexital, methotrexate, methyldopate, methylPREDNISolone, metoclopramide, metoprolol, metroNIDAZOLE, midazolam, milrinone, minocycline, mitoMYcin, mitoXANtrone, mivacurium, morphine, moxifloxacin, mycophenolate, nafcillin, nalbuphine, naloxone, nesiritide, niCARdipine, nitroglycerin, nitroprusside, norepinephrine, ondansetron, oxaliplatin, PACLitaxel, palonosetron, pamidronate, pancuronium, PEMEtrexed, pentamidine, pentazocine, PENTobarbital, PHENobarbital, phenylephrine, piperacillin, piperacillin-tazobactam, polymyxin B, potassium acetate/chloride/phosphates, procainamide, prochlorperazine, promethazine, propranolol, quiNIDine, quinupristin-dalfopristin, ranitidine, remifentanil, rocuronium, sodium acetate/bicarbonate/phosphates, streptozocin, succinylcholine, SUFentanil, sulfamethoxazole-trimethoprim, tacrolimus, teniposide, thiopental, thiotepa, ticarcillin, ticarcillin-clavulanate, tigecycline, tirofiban, tobramycin, topotecan, vancomycin, vasopressin, vecuronium, verapamil, vinBLAStine, vinCRIStine, vinorelbine, voriconazole, zidovudine, zoledronic acid

SIDE EFFECTS

CNS: *Headache, dizziness, fatigue, weakness,* depression, anxiety, tremors, seizure, paranoia
CV: *Sinus bradycardia, conduction abnormalities,* dysrhythmias, chest pain, SOB, thrombophlebitis, ischemia, CHF, hypertension, palpitations, QT prolongation, ST- or T-wave changes
ENDO: *Hypo/hyperglycemia, ketosis, hypothyroidism,* galactorrhea, diabetes insipidus
GI: *Diarrhea, nausea, abdominal pain, vomiting, flatulence, distention, constipation,* hepatitis, increased LFTs, GI bleeding, pancreatitis, cholelithiasis, ileus
GU: UTI
HEMA: Hematoma of inj site, bruise
INTEG: Rash, urticaria, pain; inflammation at inj site
MS: *Joint and muscle pain*

PHARMACOKINETICS

Absorbed rapidly, completely; peak 1/2 hr (subcut/IV), 2-3 wk (IM); half-life 1.7 hr, duration 12 hr, excreted unchanged in urine

INTERACTIONS

⚠ **Increase:** QT prolongation—class IA/III antidysrhythmics, some phenothiazines, β agonists, local anesthetics, tricyclics, haloperidol, chloroquine, droperidol, pentamidine; CYP3A4 inhibitors (amiodarone, clarithromycin, erythromycin, telithromycin, troleandomycin), arsenic trioxide, levomethadyl; CYP3A4 substrates (methadone, pimozide, QUEtiapine, quiNIDine, risperiDONE, ziprasidone)
Increase: effect of β-blockers, reduction of dose may be required
Decrease: effect of insulin, oral antidiabetics, monitor blood glucose
Decrease: excretion of CYP3A4 metabolized products, reduction of dose may be required
Decrease: effect of bromocriptine
Decrease: effect of—cycloSPORINE

Drug/Food

Decrease: absorption of dietary fat, vit B_{12} levels

Drug/Lab Test

Increase: glucose
Decrease: T_4, thyroid function tests, vit B_{12}, glucose

NURSING CONSIDERATIONS

Assess:

- Growth hormone antibodies, IGF-1 at 1- to 4-hr intervals for 8-12 hr after dose **(acromegaly)**; 5-HIAA, plasma serotonin; blood glucose, serotonin levels **(carcinoid tumors)**, plasma substance P, plasma vasoactive intestinal peptide **(VIP) (VIPoma)**
- Thyroid function tests: T_3, T_4, T_7, TSH to identify hypothyroidism
- Fecal fat, serum carotene, somatomedin-C q14days, glucose; plasma serotonin levels (carcinoid tumors); plasma vasoactive intestinal peptide levels (VIPoma); serum growth hormone, serum IGF-1 baseline and periodically, diabetes to monitor blood glucose
- **Allergic reaction:** rash, itching, fever, nausea, wheezing
- ⚠ **Cardiac status:** bradycardia, conduction abnormalities, dysrhythmias; monitor ECG for QT prolongation, low voltage, axis shifts, early repolarization, R/S transition, early wave progression
- Gall bladder disease, pancreatitis: monitor closely

Evaluate:

- Therapeutic response: relief of diarrhea in patients with AIDS; improved symptoms of carcinoid or VIP tumors; decreasing symptoms of acromegaly

Teach patient/family:

- That regular assessments are required; diabetics to monitor blood glucose

O

• About SUBCUT inj if patient or other persons will be giving inj

⚠ That product may cause dizziness, drowsiness, weakness; to avoid hazardous activities if these occur; to report abdominal pain immediately

• That pregnancy may occur in acromegaly because fertility may be restored

• That in diabetes, to monitor glucose regularly

ofloxacin (Rx)

(o-flox′a-sin)

Func. class.: Antiinfective

Chem. class.: Fluoroquinolone

ACTION: Interferes with conversion of intermediate DNA fragments into high-molecular-weight DNA in bacteria; inhibits DNA gyrase

USES: Treatment of lower respiratory tract infections (pneumonia, bronchitis), genitourinary infections (prostatitis, UTIs) caused by *Escherichia coli, Klebsiella pneumoniae, Chlamydia trachomatis,* skin and skin-structure infections; otitis media, PID

Unlabeled uses: Leprosy, anthrax, epididymitis, meningococcal infection, prophylaxis, mycobacterium avium complex (MAC), plague, proctitis, traveler's diarrhea, typhoid fever, TB

CONTRAINDICATIONS: QT prolongation, hypersensitivity to quinolones

Precautions: Pregnancy (C), breastfeeding, children, geriatric patients, renal disease, seizure disorders, excessive sunlight, hypokalemia, colitis

Black Box Warning: Tendon pain/rupture, tendinitis, myasthenia gravis

DOSAGE AND ROUTES

Lower respiratory tract infections/ skin and skin-structure infections

• **Adult: PO** 400 mg q12hr × 10 days

Prostatitis from *E. coli*

• **Adult: PO** 300 mg q12hr × 6 wk

Urinary tract infection

• **Adult: PO** 200 mg q12hr × 3-7 days depending on organism 10 days (complicated)

Pelvic inflammatory disease

• **Adult: PO** 400 mg q12hr with metronidazole × 10-14 days

Traveler's diarrhea (unlabeled)

• **Adult: PO** 200 mg bid × 3 days

Epididymitis (unlabeled)

• **Adult: PO** 300 mg bid × 10 days

Spontaneous bacterial peritonitis (unlabeled)

• **Adult: PO** 400 mg bid

Renal dose

• **Adult: PO** CCr 20-50 ml/min, give q24hr; CCr <20 ml/min, give 50% of dose q24hr

Hepatic dose

• **Adult (Child-Pugh class C): PO** max 400 mg/day

Available forms: Tabs 200, 300, 400 mg

Administer:

PO route

• 2 hr before or 2 hr after antacids, calcium, iron, zinc products, without regard to food, maintain hydration

• Store at room temperature, protect from light

SIDE EFFECTS

CNS: *Dizziness, headache, fatigue, somnolence,* depression, insomnia, lethargy, malaise, seizures, vertigo

CV: QT prolongation, dysrhythmias, chest pain

EENT: Visual disturbances, pharyngitis

GI: *Diarrhea, nausea, vomiting,* anorexia, flatulence, heartburn, dry mouth, increased AST, ALT, abdominal pain, constipation, pseudomembranous colitis, abnormal taste, xerostomia

HEMA: Blood dyscrasias

INTEG: Rash, pruritus, photosensitivity

MS: Tendinitis, tendon rupture, rhabdomyolysis

SYST: Anaphylaxis, Stevens-Johnson syndrome, toxic epidermal necrolysis

PHARMACOKINETICS

PO: Peak 1-2 hr; half-life 4-8 hr; steady-state 2 days; excreted in urine as active product, metabolites; 90%-95% bioavailability

INTERACTIONS

Black Box Warning: Increase: tendon rupture/tendinitis—corticosteroids

• May alter blood glucose levels: antidiabetics

• Possible theophylline toxicity: theophylline

⚠ **Increase:** QT prolongation—class IA/III antidysrhythmics, some phenothiazines, β-agonists, local anesthetics, tricyclics, haloperidol, methadone, chloroquine, clarithromycin, droperidol, erythromycin, pentamidine

Increase: CNS stimulation, seizures—NSAIDs

Increase: anticoagulation—warfarin

Decrease: ofloxacin—sevelamer

Decrease: absorption—antacids with aluminum, magnesium, iron products, sucralfate, zinc products; separate by 2 hr

Drug/Lab Test

Increase: INR

NURSING CONSIDERATIONS

Assess:

Black Box Warning: Tendon rupture/tendinitis: more common in lung, heart, kidney transplants or geriatric patients; assess for pain or inflammation

• Blood studies: BUN, creatinine, AST, ALT, CBC, blood glucose, INR (warfarin use)

• **CNS symptoms:** insomnia, vertigo, headache, agitation, confusion

Black Box Warning: Myasthenia gravis: product may increase weakness, avoid use

• For overgrowth of infection in long-term treatment

• **Allergic reactions:** rash, flushing, urticaria, pruritus, stop product if these occur

Evaluate:

• Therapeutic response: urine culture, absence of symptoms of infection

Teach patient/family:

• That if dizziness or light-headedness occur, to ambulate, perform activities with assistance

• To complete full course of therapy; take with plenty of fluids

• To avoid iron- or mineral-containing supplements within 2 hr before or after dose; take without regard to meals

• That allergic reactions usually occur after first dose but may occur later; stop product

• To avoid sun exposure; photosensitivity can occur

• To avoid use with other products unless approved by prescriber

• To notify prescriber immediately if tingling, pain in extremities occur

ofloxacin ophthalmic

See Appendix B

OLANZapine (Rx)

(oh-lanz′a-peen)

Zyprexa, Zyprexa Relprevv, Zyprexa Zydis

Func. class.: Antipsychotic, neuroleptic

Chem. class.: Thienobenzodiazepine

Do not confuse:

OLANZapine/osalazine

Zyprexa/CeleXA/Zyrtec

ACTION: May mediate antipsychotic activity by both DOPamine and serotonin type 2 (5-HT2) antagonists; may antagonize muscarinic receptors, histaminic (H_1)- and α-adrenergic receptors

USES:
Schizophrenia, acute manic episodes with bipolar disorder, acute agitation

Unlabeled uses: Acute psychosis

CONTRAINDICATIONS:
Hypersensitivity

Precautions: Pregnancy (C), breastfeeding, geriatric patients, hypertension, cardiac/renal/hepatic disease, diabetes, agranulocytosis, abrupt discontinuation, Asian patients, closed-angle glaucoma, coma, leukopenia, QT prolongation, tardive dyskinesia, torsades de pointes, suicidal ideation, stroke history, TIA

Black Box Warning: Increased mortality in elderly patients with dementia-related psychosis, postinjection delirium/sedation syndrome

DOSAGE AND ROUTES

Schizophrenia

- **Adult: PO** 5-10 mg/day initially, may increase dosage by 5 mg at ≥1 wk intervals, max 20 mg/day; **ORALLY DISINTEGRATING** tabs: open blister pack, place tab on tongue, let disintegrate, swallow; **ext rel inj** (Zyprexa Relprevv) **IM** 150-300 mg q2wk or 405 mg q4wk
- **Geriatric: PO** 5 mg, may increase cautiously at 1-wk intervals, max 20 mg/day
- **Adolescent: PO** 2.5 or 5 mg/day, target 10 mg/day, max 20 mg
- **Child 6-12 yr (unlabeled): PO** 2.5 mg daily, may increase to 5 mg/day after 4-7 days

Bipolar mania

- **Adult: PO** 10-15 mg/day, may increase dose after >24 hr by 5 mg, max 20 mg/day
- **Adolescent: PO** 2.5 or 5 mg/day, target 10 mg/day, max 20 mg/day

Agitation associated with schizophrenia, bipolar I mania

- **Adult: IM** (reg rel) 10 mg once
- **Geriatric: IM** (reg rel) 2.5-5 mg once

Severe behavioral disturbances in geriatric patients (unlabeled)

- **Adult: PO** 2.5-5 mg/day; **acute psychosis PO** 5-10 mg every night

Obsessive compulsive disorder (unlabeled)

- **Adult: PO** 5 mg daily, may increase as needed

Tourette syndrome (unlabeled)

- **Adult: PO** 5 mg daily titrate to 20 mg daily × 6-8 wk

Available forms: Tab 2.5, 5, 7.5, 10, 15, 20 mg; **orally disintegrating tabs** 5, 10, 15, 20 mg (Zyprexia Zydis); **powder for inj** 10 mg; **ext rel powder for susp for inj** 210, 300, 405 mg (Zyprexa Relprevv)

Administer:

- Decreased dose in geriatric patients

PO route

- With full glass of water, milk, food to decrease GI upset
- Store in tight, light-resistant container
- **Orally disintegrating tabs:** open blister pack; place tab on tongue until dissolved; swallow; no water needed; do not break, crush, chew

IM route (Zyprexa Intramuscular)

- Dissolve contents of vials with 2.1 ml sterile water for inj (5 mg/ml); use immediately
- Do not use IV or SUBCUT
- Inject slowly, deep into muscle mass

IM route (Zyprexa Relprevv)

Black Box Warning: Available only through restricted distribution program due to postinjection delirium/sedation syndrome; given at a facility with emergency services; continuous observation

- Use deep IM gluteal inj only
- Use only diluent provided in kit; give q2-4wk using 19-G, 1.5-inch needle in kit; for obese patients, use 19-G, 2-inch or larger needle

SIDE EFFECTS

CNS: EPS: (pseudoparkinsonism, akathisia, dystonia, tardive dyskinesia), seizures, headache, neuroleptic malignant syndrome (rare), agitation, nervousness, hostility, *dizziness,* hypertonia, *tremor,* euphoria, confusion, *drowsiness,* fatigue, *abnormal gait, insomnia, fever*

CV: Hypotension, tachycardia, chest pain, **heart failure, sudden death (geriatric patients, IM)**, orthostatic hypotension, peripheral edema
ENDO: Increased prolactin levels, hypo/hyperglycemia
GI: *Dry mouth, nausea, vomiting, appetite, dyspepsia,* anorexia, *constipation,* abdominal pain, *weight gain,* jaundice, **hepatitis**
GU: Urinary retention, urinary frequency, enuresis, impotence, amenorrhea, gynecomastia, breast engorgement, premenstrual syndrome
HEMA: **Neutropenia**
INTEG: Rash
MISC: Peripheral edema, accidental injury, hypertonia, hyperlipidemia
MS: *Joint pain,* twitching
RESP: *Cough, pharyngitis;* **fatal pneumonia (geriatric patients, IM)**

PHARMACOKINETICS

Well absorbed (60%), metabolized by liver, glucuronidation/oxidation by CYP1A2 and CYP2D6; excreted in urine (57%), feces (30%); 93% bound to plasma proteins; half-life 21-54 hr, extended in geriatric patients; clearance decreased in women, increased in smokers, peak PO 6 hr, IM 15-45 min

INTERACTIONS

⚠ **Increase:** **serotonin syndrome, neuroleptic malignant syndrome—SSRIs, SNRIs**
Increase: sedation—other CNS depressants, alcohol, barbiturate anesthetics, antihistamines, sedatives/hypnotics, antidepressants
Increase: OLANZapine levels—CYP1A2 inhibitors (fluvoxaMINE)
Increase: hypotension—antihypertensives, alcohol, diazepam
Increase: anticholinergic effects—anticholinergics
Decrease: OLANZapine levels—CYP1A2 inducers: carBAMazepine, omeprazole, rifampin
Decrease: antiparkinson activity—levodopa, bromocriptine, other DOPamine agonists

Drug/Lab Test
Increase: LFTs, prolactin, CPK

NURSING CONSIDERATIONS

Assess:

Black Box Warning: Postinjection delirium/sedation syndrome (Zyprexa Relprevv); monitor continuously for ≥3 hr after injection; patient must be accompanied when leaving: sedation, coma, delirium, EPS, slurred speech, altered gait, aggression, dizziness, weakness, hypertension, seizures; before leaving, confirm that patient is alert, oriented, and free of any other symptoms

- Mental status: orientation, mood, behavior, presence of hallucinations and type before initial administration, monthly; EPS, including akathisia (inability to sit still, no pattern to movements), tardive dyskinesia (bizarre movements of jaw, mouth, tongue, extremities), pseudoparkinsonism (rigidity, tremors, pill rolling, shuffling gait)
- I&O ratio; palpate bladder if low urinary output occurs, urinary retention may be cause, especially in geriatric patients
- Bilirubin, CBC, LFTs
- Urinalysis recommended before, during prolonged therapy
- Affect, orientation, LOC, reflexes, gait, coordination, sleep pattern disturbances
- B/P sitting, standing, lying: take pulse, respirations q4hr during initial treatment; establish baseline before starting treatment; report drops of 30 mm Hg; obtain baseline ECG
- Dizziness, faintness, palpitations, tachycardia on rising

⚠ **Geriatric patients for serious reactions: fatal pneumonia, heart failure, stroke leading to death (IM)**

⚠ **Neuroleptic malignant syndrome: hyperpyrexia, muscle rigidity, increased CPK, altered mental status, for acute dystonia (check chewing, swallowing, eyes, pill rolling)**

- Constipation, urinary retention daily; increase bulk, water in diet

O

• Weight gain, hyperglycemia, metabolic changes in diabetic patients
• Supervised ambulation until patient stabilized on medication; do not involve patient in strenuous exercise program because fainting is possible; patient should not stand still for long periods

Evaluate:
• Therapeutic response: decrease in emotional excitement, hallucinations, delusion, paranoia, reorganization of patterns of thought, speech

Teach patient/family:

Black Box Warning: About postinjection delirium/sedation syndrome: teach about all symptoms

• To use good oral hygiene; frequent rinsing of mouth; sugarless gum, candy, ice chips for dry mouth
• To avoid hazardous activities until product response is determined
• That orthostatic hypotension occurs often; to rise from sitting or lying position gradually
• To avoid hot tubs, hot showers, tub baths because hypotension may occur
• To avoid abrupt withdrawal of this product because EPS may result; product should be withdrawn slowly
• To avoid OTC preparations (cough, hay fever, cold) unless approved by prescriber because serious product interactions may occur; to avoid use with alcohol, CNS depressants because increased drowsiness may occur
• That in hot weather, heat stroke may occur; to take extra precautions to stay cool

TREATMENT OF OVERDOSE:
Lavage if orally ingested; provide airway; do not induce vomiting or use EPINEPHrine

RARELY USED

olaparib
(oh-lap′a-rib)
Lynparza
Func. class.: Antineoplastic-PARP

USES: Treatment of deleterious or suspected deleterious germline BRCA-mutated advanced ovarian cancer in patients who have not responded successfully to ≥3 prior courses of chemotherapy, as monotherapy

CONTRAINDICATIONS: Hypersensitivity

DOSAGE AND ROUTES
• **Adult females: PO** 400 mg bid, until disease progression or unacceptable toxicity. Avoid use of concomitant strong and moderate CYP3A4 inhibitors if possible

olmesartan (Rx)
(ol-meh-sar′tan)
Benicar
Func. class.: Antihypertensive
Chem. class.: Angiotensin II receptor (type AT_1) antagonist

Do not confuse:
Benicar/Mevacor

ACTION: Blocks the vasoconstrictor and aldosterone-secreting effects of angiotensin II; selectively blocks the binding of angiotensin II to the AT_1 receptor found in tissues

USES: Hypertension, alone or in combination with other antihypertensives

CONTRAINDICATIONS: Hypersensitivity, pregnancy (D)
Precautions: Breastfeeding, children, geriatric patients, hepatic disease, CHF,

renal artery stenosis, African descent, hyperkalemia

DOSAGE AND ROUTES

- **Adult: PO** single agent 20 mg/day initially in patients who are not volume depleted; may be increased to 40 mg/day if needed after 2 wk
- **Child ≥6 yr/adolescents ≤16 yr weighing ≥35 kg: PO** 20 mg/day; may increase to max 40 mg/day after 2 wk
- **Child ≥6 yr/adolescents ≤16 yr weighing 20-<35 kg: PO** 10 mg daily; may increase to max 20 mg/day after 2 wk

Available forms: Tabs 5, 20, 40 mg

Administer:

- Without regard to meals
- Compounded suspension may be made in the pharmacy, refrigerate, shake well before use

SIDE EFFECTS

CNS: *Dizziness,* fatigue, *headache,* insomnia, syncope

CV: Chest pain, peripheral edema, tachycardia, *hypotension*

EENT: Sinusitis, rhinitis, pharyngitis

GI: *Diarrhea,* abdominal pain

META: Hyperkalemia

MS: Arthralgia, pain, rhabdomyolysis

RESP: *Upper respiratory infection,* bronchitis

SYST: Angioedema

PHARMACOKINETICS

Peak 1-2 hr; excreted in urine, feces; half-life 13 hr; protein binding 99%

INTERACTIONS

Increase: antihypertensive effects—other antihypertensives, diuretics

Increase: hyperkalemia—potassium supplements, potassium-sparing diuretics, ACE inhibitors

Increase: effect of lithium, antioxidants

Decrease: antihypertensive effect—NSAIDs, colesevelan

Drug/Herb

Increase: antihypertensive effect—hawthorn

Decrease: antihypertensive effect—ephedra

NURSING CONSIDERATIONS

Assess:

> **Black Box Warning: Pregnancy;** product can cause fetal death when given during pregnancy (D) 2nd/3rd trimesters

- Response, adverse reactions, especially in renal disease; monitor renal function
- **Hypertension:** B/P, pulse q4hr; note rate, rhythm, quality; electrolytes: sodium, potassium, chloride; baselines for renal, hepatic studies before therapy begins
- **Hypotension:** place supine; may occur with hyponatremia or those with volume depletion; more common in those taking a diuretic also

Evaluate:

- Therapeutic response: decreased B/P

Teach patient/family:

- To comply with dosage schedule, even if feeling better
- To notify prescriber of mouth sores, fever, swelling of hands or feet, irregular heartbeat, chest pain
- That excessive perspiration, dehydration, vomiting, diarrhea may lead to fall in B/P; to consult prescriber if these occur; to maintain adequate hydration
- That product may cause dizziness, fainting, lightheadedness; to avoid hazardous activities
- To rise slowly to sitting or standing position to minimize orthostatic hypotension

> **Black Box Warning:** To notify prescriber immediately if pregnant; not to use during breastfeeding

- To avoid all OTC medications unless approved by prescriber
- That blood glucose may increase and antidiabetic product may need dosage change
- To inform all health care providers of medication use
- To use proper technique for obtaining B/P, acceptable parameters

O

olopatadine nasal agent
See Appendix B

olopatadine ophthalmic
See Appendix B

olsalazine (Rx)
(ohl-sal′ah-zeen)

Dipentum

Func. class.: Antiinflammatory

Chem. class.: Salicylate derivative

Do not confuse:
olsalazine/OLANZapine

ACTION: Bioconverted to 5-aminosalicylic acid, which decreases inflammation

USES: Maintenance of remission of ulcerative colitis in patients intolerant to sulfasalazine

CONTRAINDICATIONS: Hypersensitivity to this product or salicylates

Precautions: Pregnancy (C), breastfeeding, children <14 yr; impaired renal/hepatic function; severe allergy; bronchial asthma

DOSAGE AND ROUTES
- **Adult: PO** 500 mg bid, max 3 g/day

Available forms: Caps 250 mg

Administer:
- Total daily dose evenly spaced to minimize GI intolerance; give with food
- Store in tight, light-resistant container at room temperature

SIDE EFFECTS
CNS: Headache, hallucinations, depression, vertigo, fatigue, dizziness

GI: Nausea, vomiting, abdominal pain, hepatitis, diarrhea, bloating, pancreatitis

HEMA: Leukopenia, neutropenia, thrombocytopenia, agranulocytosis, anemia

INTEG: Rash, dermatitis, urticaria

PHARMACOKINETICS
Partially absorbed, peak $1^1/_2$ hr, half-life 30-90 min (rectal), 2-15 hr (PO), excreted in urine as 5-aminosalicylic acid and metabolites, crosses placenta

INTERACTIONS
Increase: azaTHIOprine toxicity—azaTHIOprine

Increase: myelosuppression—mercaptopurine, thioguanine

Increase: PT, INR—warfarin

Drug/Lab Test

Increase: AST, ALT

NURSING CONSIDERATIONS
Assess:
- **Colitis:** bowel pattern, number of stools, consistency, frequency, pain, mucus before treatment and periodically
- ⚠ **Blood dyscrasias:** skin rash, fever, sore throat, bruising, bleeding, fatigue, joint pain (rare); CBC before treatment and periodically
- **Allergic reaction:** rash, dermatitis, urticaria, pruritus, dyspnea, bronchospasm; allergy to salicylates
- BUN, creatinine in those with renal disease; LFTs (liver disease)

Evaluate:
- Therapeutic response: absence of fever, mucus in stools, decreased diarrhea, abdominal pain

Teach patient/family:
- To report diarrhea, rash, bleeding, bruising, fever, hallucinations
- That product may cause dizziness; to avoid hazardous activities until reaction is known
- To take even if feeling better; to take as directed; to take missed dose when remembered, but not to double

RARELY USED

omacetaxine
(oh′ma-set-ax′een)

Synribo

Func. class.: Antineoplastic-miscellaneous

Chem. class.: Cephalotaxine ester (derived from the Evergreen tree: *Cephalotaxus harringtonia*)

USES: Chronic or accelerated phase chronic myelogenous leukemia (CML) with resistance or/and intolerance to 2 or more tyrosine kinase inhibitors

CONTRAINDICATIONS: Pregnancy (D), breastfeeding, hypersensitivity

DOSAGE AND ROUTES

• Adult: **SUBCUT** 1.25 mg/m^2 bid × 14 days every 28 days

⚠ ***Grade 4 neutropenia (absolute neutrophil count [ANC] <0.5 × 10^9/L) or grade 3 thrombocytopenia (platelet count <50 × 10^9/L):*** Do not start the next cycle until the ANC is ≥1 × 10^9/L and platelets are ≥50 × 10^9/L; when therapy is resumed, reduce the number of dosing days by 2 days/cycle (initial cycles, from 14 to 12 days; maintenance cycles, from 7 to 5 days)

omalizumab (Rx)
(oh-mah-lye-zoo′mab)

Xolair

Func. class.: Antiasthmatic

Chem. class.: Monoclonal antibody

ACTION: Recombinant DNA-derived humanized IgG murine monoclonal antibody that selectively binds to IgE to limit the release of mediators in the allergic response

USES: Moderate to severe persistent asthma

Unlabeled uses: Seasonal allergic rhinitis, food allergy

CONTRAINDICATIONS: Hypersensitivity to hamster protein

Black Box Warning: Hypersensitivity to this product

Precautions: Pregnancy (B), breastfeeding, children <12 yr, acute attacks of asthma, lymphoma, nephrotic disease, bronchospasm, neoplastic disease, status asthmaticus

DOSAGE AND ROUTES

• **Adult/adolescent/child ≥12 yr: SUBCUT** 150-375 mg × 2-4 wk; divide inj into 2 sites if dose >150 mg; dose is adjusted based on IgE levels, significant changes in body weight

Available forms: Powder for inj, lyophilized 202.5 mg (150 mg/1.2 ml after reconstitution)

Administer:

SUBCUT route

• Reconstitute using 1.4 ml sterile water for inj (150 mg/1.2 ml or 125 mg/ml); gently swirl to dissolve; allow vial to stand and q5min gently swirl for 5-10 sec to dissolve; some vials may take ≥20 min; do not use if contents do not dissolve within 40 min; should be clear or slightly opalescent; use large-bore needle to withdraw medication; replace needle with small-bore needle

• Given q2-4wk; product is viscous; if >150 mg is given, divide into 2 sites; inj may take 5-10 sec to administer

SIDE EFFECTS

CV: Heart failure, cardiomyopathy, hypotension

HEMA: Serious systemic eosinophilia

INTEG: Pruritus, dermatitis, inj-site reactions, rash

MISC: Earache, dizziness, fatigue, pain, malignancies, viral infections, anaphylaxis, thrombocytopenia, headache

MS: Arthralgia, fracture, leg, arm pain

RESP: Sinusitis, upper respiratory infections, pharyngitis, pulmonary hypertension, bronchospasm

PHARMACOKINETICS

Slowly absorbed, peak 7-8 days, half-life 26 days, degradation by liver, excretion in bile

INTERACTIONS

- Use cautiously with live virus vaccines

Drug/Lab Test

Increase: IgE

NURSING CONSIDERATIONS

Assess:

- **Asthma:** respiratory rate, rhythm, depth; auscultate lung fields bilaterally; notify prescriber of abnormalities; monitor pulmonary function tests; serum IgE (may increase and continue for 1 yr)
- **Inj-site reactions:** inflammation, edema, redness, warmth at site; may occur within 60 min of inj; may decrease with repeated dosing

Black Box Warning: Anaphylaxis, allergic reactions: rash, urticaria, inability to breathe, edema of throat; product should be discontinued; have emergency equipment available; observe for 2 hr; reaction can occur ≤24 hr

Evaluate:

- Therapeutic response: ability to breathe more easily

Teach patient/family:

- That improvement will not be immediate
- Not to stop taking or decrease current asthma medications unless instructed by prescriber
- To avoid live virus vaccines while taking this product

Black Box Warning: To report signs of allergic reaction immediately, can be life-threatening

omeprazole (OTC, Rx)

(oh-mep′ray-zole)

Losec ✦, PriLOSEC, PriLOSEC OTC

Func. class.: Antiulcer, proton pump inhibitor

Chem. class.: Benzimidazole

Do not confuse:

PriLOSEC/Prinivil/PROzac/predniSONE

ACTION: Suppresses gastric secretion by inhibiting hydrogen/potassium ATPase enzyme system in gastric parietal cells; characterized as gastric acid pump inhibitor because it blocks the final step of acid production

USES: Gastroesophageal reflux disease (GERD), severe erosive esophagitis, poorly responsive systemic GERD, pathologic hypersecretory conditions (Zollinger-Ellison syndrome, systemic mastocytosis, multiple endocrine adenomas); treatment of active duodenal ulcers with/without antiinfectives for *Helicobacter pylori*

Unlabeled uses: NSAID-induced ulcer prophylaxis, stress gastritis prophylaxis

CONTRAINDICATIONS: Hypersensitivity

Precautions: Pregnancy (C), breastfeeding, children

DOSAGE AND ROUTES

Active duodenal ulcers

- **Adult: PO** 20 mg/day × 4-8 wk; associated with *H. pylori* 40 mg q AM and clarithromycin 500 mg tid on days 1-14, then 20 mg/day on days 15-28

Severe erosive esophagitis/poorly responsive GERD

- **Adult: PO** (del rel cap/del rel susp) 20 mg/day × 4-8 wk

Pathologic hypersecretory conditions
- **Adult: PO** 60 mg/day; may increase to 120 mg tid; daily doses >80 mg should be divided

Gastric ulcer
- **Adult: PO** 40 mg/day 4-8 wk
- **Geriatric: PO** ≤20 mg/day

Heartburn (OTC)
- **Adult: PO** 1 del rel tab (20 mg)/day before AM meal with glass of water × 14 days

Available forms: Del rel caps 10, 20, 40 mg; del rel tabs 20 mg; granules for oral susp 2.5, 10 mg (del rel)

Administer:
- Swallow caps whole; do not crush or chew; caps may be opened and sprinkled over applesauce
- Before eating, usually in the AM, separate with other medications
- **Oral susp powder:** give on empty stomach ≥1 hr before food; if there is NG or enteral feeding tube, do not feed 3 hr before or 1 hr after giving product: contents of packet should be mixed with 1-2 tbsp water; add 20 ml water for NG tube; for oral, stir well, drink, add more water, and drink

SIDE EFFECTS
CNS: *Headache, dizziness, asthenia*
GI: *Diarrhea, abdominal pain, vomiting, nausea, constipation, flatulence, acid regurgitation,* abdominal swelling, anorexia, irritable colon, esophageal candidiasis, dry mouth, hepatic failure
INTEG: *Rash,* dry skin, urticaria, pruritus, alopecia
MISC: *Back pain,* fever, fatigue, malaise
RESP: *Upper respiratory infections, cough,* epistaxis, pneumonia

PHARMACOKINETICS
Bioavailabity 30%-40%; peak ½-3½ hr; half-life ½-1 hr; protein binding 95%; eliminated in urine as metabolites and in feces; in geriatric patients, elimination rate decreased, bioavailability increased; metabolized by CYP2C19 enzyme system

INTERACTIONS
Increase: bleeding—warfarin
Increase: serum levels of diazepam, phenytoin, flurazepam, triazolam, cycloSPORINE, disulfiram, digoxin
Decrease: effect of iron salts, ketoconazole, cyanocobalamin, calcium carbonate, ampicillin, indinavir, gefitinib

Drug/Lab Test
Increase: alk phos, AST, ALT, bilirubin, gastrin

NURSING CONSIDERATIONS
Assess:
- **GI system:** bowel sounds q8hr, abdomen for pain, swelling, anorexia, blood in stools
- **Electrolyte imbalances:** hyponatremia; hypomagnesemia in patients using product (3 mo-1 yr); if hypomagnesemia occurs, use of magnesium supplements may be sufficient; if severe, discontinue product
- **Hepatic enzymes:** AST, ALT, alk phos during treatment; **blood studies:** CBC, differential during treatment, blood dyscrasias may occur; vit B_{12} in long-term treatment

Evaluate:
- Therapeutic response: absence of epigastric pain, swelling, fullness, bleeding: decreased GERD, esophagitis symptoms

Teach patient/family:
- To report severe diarrhea; black, tarry stools; abdominal cramps/pain; or continuing headache; product may have to be discontinued
- That, if diabetic, hypoglycemia may occur
- To avoid hazardous activities because dizziness may occur
- To avoid alcohol, salicylates, NSAIDs; may cause GI irritation
- To take as directed, even if feeling better; to take missed dose as soon as remembered; not to double; PriLOSEC OTC takes up to 4 days for full effect

O

ondansetron (Rx)

(on-dan-seh'tron)

Zofran, Zofran ODT, Zuplenz

Func. class.: Antiemetic

Chem. class.: 5-HT_3 receptor antagonist

Do not confuse:
Zofran/Zantac

ACTION: Prevents nausea, vomiting by blocking serotonin peripherally, centrally, and in the small intestine

USES: Prevention of nausea, vomiting associated with cancer chemotherapy, radiotherapy; prevention of postoperative nausea, vomiting

Unlabeled uses: Pruritus (rectal use), alcoholism, hyperemesis gravidarum

CONTRAINDICATIONS: Hypersensitivity; phenylketonuric hypersensitivity (oral disintegrating tab), torsades de pointes

Precautions: Pregnancy (B), breastfeeding, children, geriatric patients, granisetron hypersensitivity, QT prolongation, torsades de pointes

DOSAGE AND ROUTES

Prevention of nausea/vomiting (cancer chemotherapy)

- **Adult and child 4-18 yr: IV** 0.15 mg/kg infused over 15 min given 30 min before start of cancer chemotherapy, max 16 mg/dose; 0.15 mg/kg given 4 hr and 8 hr after 1st dose or 16 mg as single dose; dilute in 50 ml of D_5 or 0.9% NaCl before giving; **RECT** (unlabeled) 16 mg/day 2 hr before chemotherapy; **PO** 8 mg 1/2 hr before chemotherapy, repeat 4, 8 hr after 1st dose
- **Child ≥4 yr: PO** 4 mg tid, first dose 1/2 hr before chemotherapy

Prevention of nausea/vomiting (radiotherapy)

- **Adult: PO** 8 mg tid, may repeat q8hr

Prevention of postoperative nausea/vomiting

- **Adult: IV/IM** 4 mg undiluted over >30 sec before induction of anesthesia
- **Child 2-12 yr: IV** 0.1 mg/kg (≤40 kg); **IV** 4 mg (≥40 kg), give over ≥30 sec

Hepatic dose

- **Adult: PO/IM/IV** max dose 8 mg/day

Hyperemesis gravidarum (unlabeled)

- **Adult: PO/IV** 4-8 mg bid-tid

Pruritus (unlabeled)

- **Adult: PO** 8 mg bid

Alcoholism (unlabeled)

- **Adult: PO** 4 mcg/kg bid

Available forms: Inj 2 mg/ml, 32 mg/50 ml (premixed); tabs 4, 8 mg; oral sol 4 mg/5 ml; oral disintegrating tabs 4, 8 mg; oral dissolving film 4, 8 mg

Administer:

PO route

- **Oral disintegrating tab:** do not push through foil; gently remove; immediately place on tongue to dissolve; swallow with saliva
- **Oral dissolving film:** fold pouch along dotted line to expose tear notch; while folded, tear and remove film; place film on tongue until dissolved; swallow after dissolved; to reach desired dose, administer successive films, allowing each to dissolve before using another

IM route

- Visually inspect for particulate or discoloration
- May give 4 mg undiluted IM; inject deeply in large muscle mass; aspirate

Direct IV route

- Check for discoloration or particulate; if particulate is present, shake to dissolve
- After diluting single dose in 50 ml NS or D_5W, 0.45% NaCl or NS; give over 15 min
- Do not use IV 32 mg/dose in chemotherapy nausea/vomiting due to QT prolongation, max 16 mg/dose (adult)
- Store at room temperature for 48 hr after dilution

Y-site compatibilities: Aldesleukin, amifostine, amikacin, aztreonam, bleomycin, CARBOplatin, carmustine, ceFAZolin, cefmetazole, cefotaxime, cefOXitin, cefTAZidime, ceftizoxime, cefuroxime, chlorproMAZINE, cimetidine, cisatracurium, CISplatin, cladribine, clindamycin, cyclophosphamide, cytarabine, dacarbazine, DACTINomycin, DAUNOrubicin, dexamethasone, diphenhydrAMINE, DOPamine, DOXOrubicin, DOXOrubicin liposome, doxycycline, droperidol, etoposide, famotidine, filgrastim, floxuridine, fluconazole, fludarabine, gallium, gentamicin, haloperidol, heparin, hydrocortisone, HYDROmorphone, hydrOXYzine, ifosfamide, imipenem-cilastatin, magnesium sulfate, mannitol, mechlorethamine, melphalan, meperidine, mesna, methotrexate, metoclopramide, miconazole, mitoMYcin, mitoXANtrone, morphine, PACLitaxel, pentostatin, piperacillin/tazobactam, potassium chloride, prochlorperazine, promethazine, ranitidine, remifentanil, streptozocin, teniposide, thiotepa, ticarcillin, ticarcillin-clavulanate, vancomycin, vinBLAStine, vinCRIStine, vinorelbine, zidovudine

SIDE EFFECTS

CNS: *Headache, dizziness, drowsiness, fatigue, EPS*

GI: *Diarrhea, constipation,* abdominal pain, dry mouth

MISC: Rash, bronchospasm (rare), *musculoskeletal pain, wound problems, shivering, fever, hypoxia, urinary retention*

PHARMACOKINETICS

IV: Mean elimination half-life 3.5-4.7 hr, plasma protein binding 70%-76%, extensively metabolized in the liver, excreted 45%-60% in urine

INTERACTIONS

Increase: unconsciousness, hypotension—apomorphine, do not use together

Increase: QT prolongation—other products that prolong QT

Decrease: ondansetron effect—rifampin, carBAMazepine, phenytoin

Drug/Lab Test

Increase: LFTs

NURSING CONSIDERATIONS

Assess:

- Absence of nausea, vomiting during chemotherapy
- Hypersensitivity reaction: rash, bronchospasm (rare)
- **EPS:** shuffling gait, tremors, grimacing, rigidity periodically
- **QT prolongation:** monitoring ECG in those with cardiac disease or receiving other products that increase QT

Evaluate:

- Therapeutic response: absence of nausea, vomiting during cancer chemotherapy

Teach patient/family:

- To report diarrhea, constipation, rash, changes in respirations, or discomfort at insertion site
- Headache requiring analgesic is common

oritavancin

(or-it′a-van′sin)

Orbactiv

Func. class.: Antiinfective agents

Chem. class.: Glycopeptides

ACTION:

Inhibits bacterial cell-wall biosynthesis by preventing transglycosylation (polymerization) by binding to precursors, as well as by preventing cross-linking by binding to the peptide bridging segments of the cell wall, also disrupts the bacterial cell membrane integrity, resulting in depolarization, increased permeability, and eventual cell death

USES:

Enterococcus faecalis, Enterococcus faecium, Staphylococcus aureus (MRSA), *Staphylococcus aureus* (MSSA), *Streptococcus agalactiae* (group B streptococci), *Streptococcus anginosus, Streptococcus constellatus, Streptococcus dysgalactiae, Streptococcus intermedius, Streptococcus pyogenes* (group A β-hemolytic streptococci); treatment of acute bacterial skin and skin structure infections (ABSSSI) due to gram-positive organisms, including cellulitis/erysipelas, major cutaneous abscesses, and wound infections

CONTRAINDICATIONS: Hypersensitivity

Precautions: Anticoagulant therapy, antimicrobial resistance, breastfeeding, colitis, diarrhea, inflammatory bowel disease, infusion reactions, pregnancy, pseudomembranous colitis, vancomycin hypersensitivity, viral infection

DOSAGE AND ROUTES

• **Adults: IV** 1200 mg once

Available forms: Powder for injection: 400 mg

Administer:

• Visually inspect for particulate matter and discoloration beforehand, the reconstituted solution is clear, colorless to pale yellow

• **Reconstitution:** Reconstitute each 400-mg vial with 40 ml sterile water for injection. Three vials are necessary for a single dose, gently swirl until dissolved

• **Dilution**: Withdraw and discard 120 ml from a 1000-ml intravenous bag of D_5W, transfer 40 ml solution from each of the 3 reconstituted vials to the D_5W IV bag (1.2 mg/mg)

• **Storage:** Refrigerate or store at room temperature. The combined storage time (from reconstitution to dilution) and 3-hour infusion time should not exceed 6 hr at room temperature or 12 hr if refrigerated

Intermittent IV INFUSION

• Infuse over 3 hr, do not infuse with other medications or electrolytes, do not use saline-based solution

SIDE EFFECTS

CNS: Dizziness, flushing, headache

CV: Sinus tachycardia, phlebitis

GI: Nausea, vomiting, diarrhea

HEMA: Anemia, eosinophilia

MS: Myalgia, osteomyelitis

INTEG: Rash, vasculitis, pruritus, angioedema, infusion-related reaction

MISC: Wheezing, bronchospasm

PHARMACOKINETICS

85% protein binding, terminal half-life 245 hr

INTERACTIONS

Increase: toxicity—products metabolized by CYP2D6 CYP3A4

Drug/lab test

Increase: LFTs

NURSING CONSIDERATIONS

Assess:

• CBC and differential

• For diarrhea, bloody stools, cramping

Evaluate:

• Therapeutic response: resolution of infection

Teach patient/family:

• Reason for product, expected result

• Used only once to resolve infection

orlistat (Rx, OTC)

(or′lih-stat)

Alli, Xenical

Func. class.: Weight-control agent

Chem. class.: Lipase inhibitor

Do not confuse: Xenical/Xeloda

ACTION: Inhibits the absorption of dietary fats

USES: Obesity management

CONTRAINDICATIONS: Hypersensitivity, chronic m alabsorption syndrome, cholestasis

Precautions: Pregnancy (X), children, hypothyroidism, other organic causes of obesity, anorexia nervosa, bulimia, nephrolithiasis, GI disease, diabetes, fat-soluble vitamin deficiency, breastfeeding

DOSAGE AND ROUTES

• **Adult: PO** (Alli) 60 mg, (Xenical) 120 mg tid with each main meal containing fat, max 360 mg/day

Available forms: Caps (Alli) 60 mg, (Xenical) 120 mg

Administer:

- For obesity only if patient on weight-reduction program that includes dietary changes, exercise; patient should be on a diet with 30% of calories from fat; omit dose of orlistat if meal contains no fat

SIDE EFFECTS

CNS: *Insomnia,* depression, anxiety, dizziness, headache, fatigue

GI: *Oily spotting, flatus with discharge, fecal urgency, fatty/oily stool, oily evacuation, fecal incontinence, frequent defecation,* nausea, vomiting, abdominal pain, infectious diarrhea, rectal pain, tooth disorder, hypovitaminosis, hepatic failure, hepatitis, pancreatitis

GU: UTI, vaginitis, menstrual irregularity

INTEG: Dry skin, rash

MS: Back pain, arthritis, myalgia, tendinitis

RESP: Influenza, URI

PHARMACOKINETICS

Minimal absorption, peak 8 hr, 99% protein binding, excretion in feces, half-life 1-2 hr

INTERACTIONS

Increase: lipid-lowering effect—pravastatin

Increase: effects of warfarin

Decrease: absorption—fat-soluble vitamins (A, D, E, K), cycloSPORINE

NURSING CONSIDERATIONS

Assess:

- **Weight status:** before starting therapy, obtain testing to rule out physiologic reactions for weight, obtain thyroid testing, BMI, glucose; weight weekly; diabetic patients may need reduction in oral hypoglycemics
- For misuse in certain populations (anorexia nervosa, bulimia)

⚠ **Hepatotoxicity/pancreatitis:** jaundice, weakness, abdominal pain (rare)

Evaluate:

- Therapeutic response: decrease in weight

Teach patient/family:

- That 60-mg cap can be obtained OTC; 60 mg tid is highest OTC dose
- That safety and effectiveness beyond 2 yr have not been determined
- To read patient information sheet; to discuss unpleasant GI side effects
- To take multivitamin containing fat-soluble vitamins 2 hr before or after orlistat; that psyllium taken with each dose or at bedtime may decrease GI symptoms
- To avoid hazardous activities until stabilized on medication; to discuss unpleasant side effects
- To notify prescriber if pregnancy is planned or suspected pregnancy (X); if breastfeeding take proper fat-soluble vitamins

⚠ **Hepatotoxicity/pancreatitis:** yellowing of skin, eyes; dark urine; weakness; abdominal pain

oseltamivir (Rx)

(oss-el-tam′ih-veer)

Tamiflu

Func. class.: Antiviral

Chem. class.: Neuramidase inhibitor

O

ACTION:
Inhibits influenza virus neuraminidase with possible alteration of virus particle aggregation and release

USES:
Prevention and treatment of influenza type A or B

Unlabeled uses: Avian flu (H5N1), avian influenzae A (H5N1), swine flu (H1N1), encephalitis

CONTRAINDICATIONS:
Hypersensitivity

Precautions: Pregnancy (C), neonates, breastfeeding, infants, children, geriatric patients, renal/hepatic/pulmonary/cardiac disease, psychosis, viral infection

DOSAGE AND ROUTES

Treatment of influenza

- **Adult/child >40 kg: PO** 75 mg bid × 5 days, begin treatment within 2 days of onset of symptoms

• **Child 23-40 kg and ≥1 yr: PO** 60 mg bid
• **Child 15-23 kg and ≥1 yr: PO** 45 mg bid
• **Child ≤15 kg and ≥1 yr: PO** 30 mg bid
• **Neonates ≥14 days, infants: PO** 3 mg/kg/dose bid × 5 days

Prevention of influenza

• **Adult/child ≥13 yr: PO** 75 mg/day × ≥10 days; begin treatment within 2 days of contact, max use 6 wk

Renal dose

• **Adult: PO** Treatment: CCr 10-30 ml/min, 30 mg/day × 5 days; CCr 30-60 ml/min, 30 mg bid × 5 days; Prophylaxis: CCr 10-30 ml/min, 30 mg every other day; CCr 30-60 ml/min, 30 mg daily

H1N1 influenzae A virus (swine flu) (unlabeled)

• **Adult/adolescent/child >40 kg: PO** 75 mg bid × 5 days
• **Adolescent/child 24-40 kg: PO** 60 mg bid × 5 days
• **Child >1 yr and 15-23 kg: PO** 45 mg bid × 5 days
• **Child >1 yr and ≤15 kg: PO** 30 mg bid × 5 days

Available forms: Caps 30, 45, 75 mg; powder for oral susp 6 mg/ml

Administer:

• Within 2 days of symptoms of influenza; continue for 5 days
• At least 4 hr before bedtime to prevent insomnia
• Without regard to food; give with food for GI upset
• Take with full glass of water
• Store in tight, dry container
• **Oral susp:** 6 mg/ml concentration, take care to administer correct dose; loosen powder from side of bottle, add 55 ml, shake well (6 mg/ml), remove child-resistant cap, push bottle adapter into neck of bottle, close tightly with child-resistant cap to ensure sealing, use within 17 days of preparation when refrigerated or within 10 days at room temperature, write expiration date on bottle, shake well before use, use oral syringe provided but only with markings for 30, 45, 60 mg, confirm that dosing instructions are in same units as syringe provided

SIDE EFFECTS

CNS: *Headache, dizziness,* fatigue, *insomnia,* seizures, delirium, self-injury (children)
ENDO: Hyperglycemia
GI: *Nausea, vomiting,* diarrhea, abdominal pain
INTEG: Toxic epidermal necrolysis, Stevens-Johnson syndrome, erythema multiforme
RESP: Cough

PHARMACOKINETICS

Rapidly absorbed, protein binding 40%-45%, converted to oseltamivir carboxylate (active form), active forms half-life 1-3 hr, metabolite 6-10 hr, excreted in urine (99%), protein binding 3%

INTERACTIONS

• Avoid use with H1N1 virus vaccine, intranasal influenzae vaccine

NURSING CONSIDERATIONS

Assess:

• Bowel pattern before, during treatment
• **Influenza:** fever, fatigue, sore throat, headache, muscle soreness, aches

Evaluate:

• Therapeutic response: absence of fever, malaise, cough, dyspnea in infection

Teach patient/family:

• About aspects of product therapy
• To avoid hazardous activities if dizziness occurs
• To take as soon as symptoms appear; to take full course even if feeling better
• To take missed dose as soon as remembered if within 2 hr of next dose
⚠ To stop immediately; to report to prescriber skin rash, delirium, psychosis, hallucinations (child)
• That this product should not be substituted for flu shot
• Will not treat the common cold
• To avoid other products unless approved by prescriber

⚠ HIGH ALERT

oxaliplatin (Rx)
(ox-al-i′plat-in)
Eloxatin
Func. class.: Antineoplastic
Chem. class.: 3rd-generation platinum analog

ACTION:
Forms crosslinks, thereby inhibiting DNA replication and transcription; not specific to cell cycle

USES:
Metastatic carcinoma of the colon or rectum in combination with 5-FU/leucovorin

Unlabeled uses: Relapsed or refractory non-Hodgkin's lymphoma; advanced ovarian cancer; breast, head/neck, testicular, pancreatic, gastric cancer; mesothelioma

CONTRAINDICATIONS:
Pregnancy (D), breastfeeding, radiation therapy or chemotherapy within 1 mo, thrombocytopenia, smallpox vaccination

Black Box Warning: Hypersensitivity to this product or other platinum products

Precautions: Children, geriatric patients, pneumococcus vaccination, renal disease

DOSAGE AND ROUTES
Dosage protocols may vary

Colorectal cancer

• **Adult: IV INFUSION** *Day 1:* oxaliplatin 85 mg/m^2 in 250-500 ml D_5W and leucovorin 200 mg/m^2 in D_5W; give both over 2 hr at the same time in separate bags using a Y-line, followed by 5-FU 400 mg/m^2 **IV BOL** over 2-4 min, then 5-FU 600 mg/m^2 **IV INFUSION** in 500 ml D_5W as a 22-hr **CONT INFUSION;** *day 2:* leucovorin 200 mg/m^2 **IV INFUSION** over 2 hr, then 5-FU 400 mg/m^2 **IV BOL** over 2-4 min, then 5-FU 600 mg/m^2 **IV INFUSION** in 500 ml D_5W as a 22-hr **CONT INFUSION;** repeat cycle q2wk

Renal dose

• **Adult: IV** CCr <30 ml/min, reduce starting dose to 65 mg/m^2

Advanced ovarian cancer (unlabeled)

• **Adult: IV** 130 mg/m^2 q3wk as a single agent in those previously treated

Advanced breast cancer (unlabeled)

• **Adult: IV** 130 mg/m^2 on day 1 plus 5-fluorouracil (1000 mg/m^2 **CONT IV INFUSION** days 1-4) q3wk

Pancreatic cancer (unlabeled)

• **Adult: IV** 100 mg/m^2 on day 2, with gemcitabine 1000 mg/m^2 on day 1, repeat q2wk; 625 mg/m^2 bid throughout treatment or fluorouracil 200 mg/m^2/day throughout treatment

Gastric cancer (unlabeled)

• **Adult: IV** 130 mg/m^2 over 2 hr on day 1 with epirubic 50 mg/m^2 and capecitabine

Available forms: Powder for inj 50, 100-mg single-use vials (5 mg/ml); solution for inj 50 mg/10 ml, 100 mg/20 ml, 200 mg/40 ml

Administer:

Intermittent IV INFUSION route

• Premedicate with antiemetics including $5HT_3$ blockers, with or without dexamethasone; prehydration not needed

• Do not reconstitute or dilute with sodium chloride or any chloride-containing sol; do not use aluminum equipment during any preparation or administration; will degrade platinum; do not refrigerate unopened powder or sol; do not freeze; protect from light

• Use cytotoxic handling procedures; prepare in biologic cabinet using gown, gloves, mask; do not allow product to come in contact with skin; use soap and water if contact occurs

• EPINEPHrine, antihistamines, corticosteroids for hypersensitivity reaction

• **Lyophilized powder:** reconstitute vial 50 mg/10 ml or 100 mg/20 ml sterile water for inj or D_5W; after reconstitution, sol may be stored for ≤24 hr in refrigerator; after dilution in 250-500 ml D_5W, may store ≤24 hr in refrigerator or 6 hr at room temperature; infuse over 2 hr

- **Aqueous solution:** dilute in 250-500 ml of D_5W; after dilution, may store ≤24 hr refrigerator, 6 hr at room temperature, infuse over 2 hr

Y-site compatibilities: Alfentanil, amifostine, amikacin, aminocaproic acid, amiodarone, amphotericin B colloidal, amphotericin B lipid complex, amphotericin B liposome, ampicillin, ampicillin-sulbactam, anidulafungin, atenolol, atracurium, azithromycin, aztreonam, bivalirudin, bleomycin, bumetanide, buprenorphine, butorphanol, calcium chloride/gluconate, CARBOplatin, caspofungin, ceFAZolin, cefotaxime, cefoTEtan, cefOXitin, cefTAZidime, ceftizoxime, cefTRIAXone, cefuroxime, chloramphenicol, chlorproMAZINE, cimetidine, ciprofloxacin, cisatracurium, CISplatin, clindamycin, cyclophosphamide, cycloSPORINE, cytarabine, dacarbazine, DACTINomycin, DAPTOmycin, DAUNOrubicin, dexamethasone, digoxin, diltiazem, diphenhydrAMINE, DOBUTamine, DOCEtaxel, dolasetron, DOPamine, doxacurium, DOXOrubicin, doxycycline, droperidol, enalaprilat, ePHEDrine, EPINEPHrine, epirubicin, ertapenem, erythromycin, esmolol, etoposide, famotidine, fenoldopam, fentaNYL, fluconazole, fludarabine, foscarnet, fosphenytoin, furosemide, gatifloxacin, gemcitabine, gemtuzumab, gentamicin, glycopyrrolate, granisetron, haloperidol, heparin, hydrALAZINE, hydrocortisone, HYDROmorphone, hydrOXYzine, IDArubicin, ifosfamide, imipenem-cilastatin, inamrinone, insulin (regular), irinotecan, isoproterenol, ketorolac, labetalol, leucovorin, levofloxacin, levorphanol, lidocaine, linezolid, LORazepam, magnesium sulfate, mannitol, meperidine, meropenem, mesna, metaraminol, methyldopate, methylPREDNISolone, metoclopramide, metoprolol, metroNIDAZOLE, midazolam, milrinone, minocycline, mitoMYcin, mitoXANtrone, mivacurium, morphine, nafcillin, nalbuphine, naloxone, nesiritide, niCARdipine, nitroglycerin, nitroprusside, norepinephrine, octreotide, ondansetron, PACLitaxel, palonosetron, pancuronium, PEMEtrexed, pentamidine, pentazocine, phenylephrine, piperacillin, polymyxin B, potassium chloride/phosphates, procainamide, prochlorperazine, promethazine, propranolol, quiNIDine, quinupristin-dalfopristin, ranitidine, rocuronium, sodium acetate/phosphates, succinylcholine, SUFentanil, sulfamethoxazole-trimethoprim, tacrolimus, teniposide, theophylline, thiotepa, ticarcillin, ticarcillin-clavulanate, tigecycline, tirofiban, tobramycin, tolazoline, topotecan, trimethobenzamide, vancomycin, vasopressin, vecuronium, verapamil, vinBLAStine, vinCRIStine, vinorelbine, voriconazole, zidovudine, zoledronic acid

SIDE EFFECTS

CNS: Peripheral neuropathy, fatigue, headache, dizziness, insomnia
CV: Cardiac abnormalities, thromboembolism
EENT: *Decreased visual acuity, tinnitus, hearing loss*
GI: *Severe nausea, vomiting, diarrhea, weight loss,* stomatitis, anorexia, gastroesophageal reflux, constipation, dyspepsia, mucositis, flatulence
GU: Hematuria, dysuria, creatinine
HEMA: Thrombocytopenia, leukopenia, pancytopenia, neutropenia, anemia, hemolytic uremic syndrome
INTEG: *Alopecia,* rash, flushing, extravasation, redness, swelling, pain at inj site
META: Hypokalemia
RESP: Fibrosis, dyspnea, cough, rhinitis, URI, pharyngitis
SYST: Anaphylaxis, angioedema

PHARMACOKINETICS

Metabolized in liver, excreted in urine; after administration, 15% of platinum in systemic circulation, 85% either in tissues or being eliminated in urine; half-life 390 hr; protein binding >90%

INTERACTIONS

Increase: bleeding risk—NSAIDs, alcohol, anticoagulants, platelet inhibitors, thrombolytics, salicylates
Increase: oxaliplatin toxicity—tannins

Increase: myelosuppression—myelosuppressive agents, radiation
Increase: nephrotoxicity—aminoglycosides, loop diuretics
Decrease: antibody response—live virus vaccines

Drug/Lab Test
Increase: ALT, AST, bilirubin, creatinine
Decrease: potassium, neutrophils, WBC, platelets

NURSING CONSIDERATIONS

Assess:

⚠ **Bone marrow depression:** CBC, differential, platelet count each cycle; withhold product if WBC is <4000 or platelet count is <100,000; notify prescriber of results

- Renal/hepatic studies: BUN, creatinine, serum uric acid, urine CCr before, electrolytes during therapy; dose should not be given if BUN >19 mg/dl; creatinine <1.5 mg/dl; I&O ratio; report fall in urine output of <30 ml/hr; LFTs

Black Box Warning: Anaphylaxis: wheezing, tachycardia, facial swelling, fainting; discontinue product, report to prescriber; resuscitation equipment should be nearby

⚠ **Pulmonary fibrosis:** cough, crackles, dyspnea, pulmonary infiltrate; discontinue immediately, death may occur

- Monitor temperature; may indicate beginning infection
- Hepatic studies before each cycle (bilirubin, AST, ALT, LDH) as needed or monthly
- **Bleeding:** hematuria, guaiac, bruising or petechiae, mucosa or orifices; obtain prescription for viscous lidocaine (Xylocaine)
- Effects of alopecia on body image; discuss feelings about body changes
- Edema in feet, joint pain, stomach pain, shaking
- Comprehensive oral hygiene
- All medications PO if possible; avoid IM inj when platelets <100,000/mm^3
- Increase fluid intake to 2-3 L/day to prevent urate deposits, calculi formation; elimination of product
- Blankets, hat, gloves for cold prevention

Evaluate:

- Therapeutic response: decreased tumor size, spread of malignancy

Teach patient/family:

⚠ To report signs of **infection:** increased temperature, sore throat, flulike symptoms

- To report signs of **anemia:** fatigue, headache, faintness, SOB, irritability
- To report **bleeding;** to avoid use of razors, commercial mouthwash
- To avoid aspirin, ibuprofen, NSAIDs, alcohol; may cause GI bleeding

⚠ To report any changes in breathing, coughing

- That hair may be lost during treatment; that a wig or hairpiece may make patient feel better; that new hair may be different in color, texture
- To report numbness, tingling in face or extremities, poor hearing, or joint pain or swelling
- Not to receive vaccines during treatment

⚠ To use contraception during treatment and for 4 mo after; that product may cause infertility, pregnancy (D)

- **Dysesthesias:** to avoid contact with cold (air, ice, liquid)

⚠ HIGH ALERT

oxazepam (Rx)

(ox-ay′ze-pam)

Func. class.: Sedative/hypnotic; antianxiety

Chem. class.: Benzodiazepine, short acting

Controlled Substance Schedule IV

ACTION: Potentiates the actions of GABA, especially in the limbic system and the reticular formation

USES:
Anxiety, alcohol withdrawal
Unlabeled uses: Insomnia

CONTRAINDICATIONS:
Pregnancy (D), breastfeeding, children <6 yr, hypersensitivity to benzodiazepines, closed-angle glaucoma, psychosis
Precautions: Geriatric patients, debilitated, renal/hepatic disease, depression, suicidal ideation, dementia, sleep apnea, seizure disorder, respiratory depression

DOSAGE AND ROUTES
Anxiety
- **Adult: PO** 10-15 mg tid-qid, max 120 mg/day
- **Geriatric: PO** 10 mg daily-bid, max 60 mg/day tid

Alcohol withdrawal
- **Adult: PO** 15-30 mg tid-qid

Available forms: Caps 10, 15, 30 mg
Administer:
- Without regard to food

SIDE EFFECTS
CNS: *Dizziness, drowsiness,* confusion, headache, anxiety, tremors, fatigue, depression, insomnia, hallucinations, paradoxical excitement, transient amnesia
CV: *Orthostatic hypotension,* ECG changes, tachycardia, hypotension
EENT: *Blurred vision,* tinnitus, mydriasis
GI: Nausea, vomiting, anorexia
HEMA: Leukopenia
INTEG: Rash, dermatitis, itching
SYST: Dependence

PHARMACOKINETICS
Peak 2-4 hr; metabolized by liver; excreted by kidneys; half-life 5-15 hr; crosses placenta, breast milk; protein binding 97%

INTERACTIONS
Increase: oxazepam effects—CNS depressants, alcohol, disulfiram, oral contraceptives
Decrease: oxazepam effects—oral contraceptives, phenytoin, theophylline, valproic acid
Decrease: effects of levodopa
Drug/Herb
Increase: CNS depression—kava, melatonin, valerian
Drug/Lab Test
Increase: AST, ALT, serum bilirubin
Decrease: WBC

NURSING CONSIDERATIONS
Assess:
- B/P (lying, standing), pulse; if systolic B/P drops 20 mm Hg, hold product, notify prescriber
- ⚠ Mental status: mood, sensorium, affect, sleeping pattern, drowsiness, dizziness, **suicidal thoughts/behaviors**
- ⚠ **Physical dependency, withdrawal symptoms:** headache, nausea, vomiting, muscle pain, weakness, tremors, seizures (long-term use)

Evaluate:
- Therapeutic response: decreased anxiety, restlessness, insomnia

Teach patient/family:
- That product may be taken without regard to food
- That medication not to be used for everyday stress or used >4 mo unless directed by prescriber; not to take more than prescribed dose because product may be habit forming
- To avoid OTC preparations (cough, cold, hay fever) unless approved by prescriber
- To avoid driving, activities that require alertness because drowsiness may occur
- To avoid alcohol, other psychotropic products unless directed by prescriber
- Not to discontinue product abruptly after long-term use
- To rise slowly because fainting may occur, especially among geriatric patients
- That drowsiness may worsen at beginning of treatment
- To notify prescriber if pregnancy is planned or suspected pregnancy (D)

OXcarbazepine (Rx)
(ox′kar-baz′uh-peen)

Trileptal, Oxtellar XR

Func. class.: Anticonvulsant

Chem. class.: CarBAMazepine analog

ACTION: May inhibit nerve impulses by limiting influx of sodium ions across cell membrane in motor cortex

USES: Partial seizures

Unlabeled uses: Trigeminal neuralgia, atypical panic disorder, bipolar disorder

CONTRAINDICATIONS: Hypersensitivity

Precautions: Pregnancy (C), breastfeeding, children <4 yr, hypersensitivity to carBAMazepine, renal disease, fluid restriction, hyponatremia, abrupt discontinuation, suicidal ideation

DOSAGE AND ROUTES

Seizures, adjunctive therapy

- **Adult: PO** 300 mg bid, may be increased by 600 mg/day in divided doses bid at weekly intervals; maintenance 1200 mg/day; ext rel; 600 mg daily × 1 wk, increase weekly in 600 mg/day increments to 1200-2400 mg daily
- **Child 4-16 yr: PO** 8-10 mg/kg/day divided bid; dose determined by weight, increase by 5 mg/kg/day q3days, max doses weight dependent

Conversion to monotherapy for partial seizures

- **Adult: PO** 300 mg bid with reduction in other anticonvulsants; increase OXcarbazepine by 600 mg/day each week over 2-4 wk; withdraw other anticonvulsants over 3-6 wk; max 2400 mg/day

Initiation of monotherapy for partial seizures

- **Adult: PO** 300 mg bid, increase by 300 mg/day q3days to 1200 mg in divided doses bid, max 2400 mg/day

Renal dose

- **Adult: PO** CCr <30 ml/min, 150 mg bid, increase slowly

Bipolar disorder/trigeminal neuralgia (unlabeled)

- **Adult: PO** 300 mg bid, may increase by ≤600 mg/day

Available forms: Film-coated tabs 150, 300, 600 mg; oral susp 300 mg/5 ml; ext rel tab 150, 300, 600 mg

Administer:

PO route

- Without regard to meals
- **Oral susp:** shake well, use calibrated oral syringe provided, use or discard within 7 days of opening
- **Ext rel:** do not crush, break, or chew
- Store at room temperature

SIDE EFFECTS

CNS: *Headache, dizziness, confusion, fatigue,* feeling abnormal, ataxia, abnormal gait, tremors, anxiety, agitation, **worsening of seizures, suicidal thoughts/behaviors**

CV: *Hypotension,* chest pain, edema, bradycardia, syncope

EENT: *Blurred vision, diplopia, nystagmus,* rhinitis, sinusitis

ENDO: Hypothyroidism, hot flashes

GI: *Nausea, constipation, diarrhea,* anorexia, vomiting, abdominal pain, gastritis

GU: Urinary frequency, hematuria, menses change

INTEG: Purpura, rash, acne

META: Hyponatremia

RESP: Flulike symptoms

SYST: **Angioedema, anaphylaxis, Stevens-Johnson syndrome, toxic epidermal necrolysis, drug reaction with eosinophilia and systemic symptoms (DRESS)**

PHARMACOKINETICS

PO: Onset unknown; peak 4-6 hr; metabolized by liver to active metabolite; terminal half-life 7-9 hr metabolite; inhibits P450 CYP2C19, induces CYP3A4/5, 95% renal extraction

O

INTERACTIONS

⚠ Contraindicated: MAOIs, ranolazine, nisoldipine

Increase: CNS depression—alcohol

Decrease: effects—felodipine, oral contraceptive, carBAMazepine

Decrease: OXcarbazepine levels—carBAMazepine, PHENobarbital, phenytoin, valproic acid, verapamil

Drug/Herb

Increase: anticonvulsant effect—ginkgo

Decrease: anticonvulsant effect—ginseng, santonica

Drug/Lab Test

Decrease: sodium

NURSING CONSIDERATIONS

Assess:

- Description of seizures: frequency, duration, aura
- Hyponatremia: headache, nausea, confusion, usually within the first 3 mo of treatment, but may occur ≤1 yr, if this product is being used with other products that decrease sodium, monitor sodium levels
- Electrolyte: sodium; T_4; phenytoin (when given together)

⚠ **Serious reactions:** angioedema, anaphylaxis, Stevens-Johnson syndrome

- CNS/mental status: mood, sensorium, affect, behavioral changes, confusion, suicidal thoughts/behaviors; if mental status changes, notify prescriber
- Eye problems: need for ophthalmic exams before, during, after treatment (slit lamp, funduscopy, tonometry)
- **Pregnancy:** lack of seizure control due to MHD, a metabolite of OXcarbazepine, monitor seizure control
- May monitor target serum level 12-30 mcg/ml to identify compliance/toxicity

Evaluate:

- Therapeutic response: decreased seizure activity

Teach patient/family:

- To avoid driving, other activities that require alertness
- To take twice a day at same intervals
- Not to discontinue medication quickly after long-term use, seizures may increase
- To inform prescriber if hypersensitive to carBAMazepine; multisystem hypersensitivity may occur; to report fever, other allergic symptoms
- To avoid use of alcohol while taking product
- To use alternative contraception if using hormonal method; to report if pregnancy is planned or suspected (C)
- To report skin rashes immediately, serious skin reactions can occur
- To report suicidal thoughts/behavior immediately

TREATMENT OF OVERDOSE:

Activated charcoal; give 0.9% NaCl (hypotensive state), atropine (bradycardia); use benzodiazepines, barbiturates for seizures

oxybutynin (Rx, OTC)

(ox-i-byoo′ti-nin)

Ditropan ✱, Ditropan XL, Gelnique, Oxytrol ✱, Oxytrol Transdermal, Uromax ✱

Func. class.: Anticholinergic

Chem. class.: Synthetic tertiary amine

Do not confuse:

Ditropan/diazepam

ACTION:

Relaxes smooth muscles in urinary tract by inhibiting acetylcholine at postganglionic sites

USES:

Antispasmodic for neurogenic bladder, overactive bladder in females (OTC)

CONTRAINDICATIONS:

Hypersensitivity, GI obstruction, urinary retention, glaucoma, severe colitis, myasthenia gravis, unstable CV disease

Precautions: Pregnancy (B), breastfeeding, children <12 yr, geriatric patients, suspected glaucoma, cardiac disease, dementia

DOSAGE AND ROUTES

- **Adult: PO** 5 mg bid-tid, max 5 mg qid; **EXT REL** 5-10 mg/day, may increase by 5 mg, max 30 mg/day; **TD** apply 1 patch to abdomen, hip, buttock 2×/wk (q3-4 days); **GEL** apply contents of 1 packet to abdomen, upper arms, shoulders, thighs daily
- **Geriatric: PO** 2.5-5 mg bid-tid, increase by 2.5 mg q several days
- **Child >6 yr: PO** 5 mg bid, max 5 mg tid; **EXT REL** 5 mg/day, max 20 mg/day
- **Child 1-5 yr: PO** 0.2 mg/kg/dose bid-tid

Available forms: Syr 5 mg/5 ml; tabs 5 mg; ext rel tabs 5, 10, 15 mg; TD 3.9 mg/day; top gel 10% (Gelnique)

Administer:

PO route

- Do not crush, break, or chew ext rel tabs
- Without regard to meals

Topical route

- Wash hands; apply to clean, dry, intact skin on abdomen, upper arms/shoulders, thighs; avoid navel, rotate sites
- Squeeze contents into palm of hand or directly on site, rub gently
- Do not bathe, exercise, swim for 1 hr after application
- Allow to dry before putting on clothing
- Do not be near flame, fire, or smoke until gel has dried
- Delivers 100 mg

Transdermal route

- Apply to clean, dry, intact skin on abdomen, hip, buttock; use firm pressure; not affected by showering/bathing; rotate sites
- Delivers 3.9 mg/day

SIDE EFFECTS

CNS: *Anxiety, restlessness, dizziness, somnolence, insomnia, nervousness,* **seizures**, headache, *drowsiness,* confusion

CV: *Palpitations, sinus tachycardia,* hypertension, peripheral edema, **QT prolongation**

EENT: *Blurred vision, dry eyes,* increased intraocular tension, *dry mouth,* throat

GI: *Nausea, vomiting, anorexia,* abdominal pain, *constipation, dyspepsia,* diarrhea, taste perversion, GERD

GU: Dysuria, impotence, *urinary retention, hesitancy*

MISC: Hyperthermia, anaphylaxis, angioedema

PHARMACOKINETICS

Onset ½-1 hr, peak 3-6 hr, duration 6-10 hr; metabolized by liver, excreted in urine; terminal half-life 2-3 hr

INTERACTIONS

- Altered pharmacokinetic parameters: CYP3A4 inhibitors

Increase: CNS depression—benzodiazepines, sedatives, hypnotics, opioids

Increase: levels of atenolol, digoxin, nitrofurantoin

Increase: anticholinergic effects—antihistamines, amantidine, other anticholinergics

Increase or decrease: levels of phenothiazines

Decrease: levels of acetaminophen, haloperidol, levodopa

Decrease: effects of oxybutynin—CYP3A4 inducers

O

NURSING CONSIDERATIONS

Assess:

- **Urinary patterns:** distention, nocturia, frequency, urgency, incontinence, I&O ratios; cystometry to diagnose dysfunction, urinary tract infections should be treated

⚠ **Allergic reactions: rash, urticaria; if these occur, product should be discontinued; angioedema**

⚠ **QT prolongation: ECG for QT prolongation, ejection fraction; assess for chest pain, palpitations, dyspnea**

- CNS effects: confusion, anxiety; anticholinergic effects in geriatric patients

Evaluate:

- Urinary status: dysuria, frequency, nocturia, incontinence

Teach patient/family:

- To avoid hazardous activities because dizziness, blurred vision may occur

- To avoid OTC medications with alcohol, other CNS depressants
- To avoid hot weather, strenuous activity because product decreases perspiration
- About the correct application of each product form
- **Transdermal:** change patch 2×/wk; do not use same site within 7 days; dispose of and use container not accessible to pets/children
- To open patch immediately before using
- Do not use during MRI, remove
- **Topical gel:** rotate sites
- Apply to clean, dry skin on abdomen, upper arm/shoulders/thighs
- Gel is flammable

⚠ HIGH ALERT

oxyCODONE (Rx)

(ox-i-koe′done)

Oxecta, Oxy-CONTIN, Oxy IR ✱, Roxicodone, Supeudol ✱

oxyCODONE/aspirin (Rx)

Endodan, Percodan

oxyCODONE/ acetaminophen (Rx)

Endocet, Oxycet, Percocet, Primalev, Roxicet, Roxilox, Tylox, Xartemis

oxyCODONE/ibuprofen (Rx)

Func. class.: Opiate analgesic
Chem. class.: Semisynthetic derivative

Controlled Substance Schedule II

Do not confuse:
Percodan/Decadron
Roxicet/Roxanol
Tylox/Xanax/Trimox/Wymox
OxyCODONE/HYDROcodone
OxyCODONE/OxyCONTIN
Roxicodone/roxanol

ACTION: Inhibits ascending pain pathways in CNS, increases pain threshold, alters pain perception

USES: Moderate to severe pain
Unlabeled uses: Postherpetic neuralgic (cont rel)

CONTRAINDICATIONS: Hypersensitivity, addiction (opiate), asthma, ileus

Black Box Warning: Respiratory depression

Precautions: Pregnancy (B), breastfeeding, child <18 yr, addictive personality, increased intracranial pressure, MI (acute), severe heart disease, renal/hepatic disease, bowel impaction

Black Box Warning: Opioid-naive patients, substance abuse, accidental exposure, potential for overdose/poisoning, status asthmaticus

DOSAGE AND ROUTES

- **Adult: PO** 10-30 mg q4hr (5-15 mg q4-6hr for opiate-naive patients) Concentration sol is extremely concentrated; do not use interchangeably; **CONT REL** 10 mg q12hr for opiate-naive patients

Available forms: OxyCODONE: cont rel tabs (OxyCONTIN) 10, 15, 20, 30, 40, 80, 160 mg; immediate rel tabs 5, 7.5, 10, 15, 20, 30 mg; immediate rel caps 5 mg; oral sol 5 mg/5 ml, 20 mg/ml; **oxyCODONE with acetaminophen:** 2.5 mg/325 mg, 5 mg/325 mg, 7.5 mg/325 mg, 7.5 mg/300 mg, 10 mg/325 mg, oral sol 5 mg/325 mg/5 ml; **oxyCODONE with aspirin:** 4.88/325 mg; **oxyCODONE with ibuprofen:** 5 mg/400 mg

Administer:
- Store in light-resistant area at room temperature
- OxyCODONE should be titrated from the initial recommended dosage to the dosage required to relieve pain
- There is no maximum dosage of oxyCODONE; however, careful titration is required until tolerance develops to some of the side effects (drowsiness, respiratory depression)

Oral solid formulations

Immediate-release tablets route

- May be administered with food or milk to minimize GI irritation
- **Oxecta brand tablets:** swallow whole; do not crush or dissolve; owing to nature of this formulation, do not presoak, lick, or otherwise wet tablet before administering dose; administer 1 tablet at a time; allow patient to swallow each tablet separately with sufficient liquid to ensure prompt and complete transit through the esophagus; do not use this brand for administration via nasogastric, gastric, or other feeding tubes because it can obstruct feeding tubes

Oral solid formulations

Controlled-release tablets route (OxyCONTIN):

- Administer whole; do not crush, chew, or break in half; taking chewed, broken, or crushed controlled-release tablets could lead to the rapid release and absorption of a potentially toxic dose of oxyCODONE
- **OxyCONTIN brand tablets:** owing to hydro-gelling nature of the 2010 reformulation, do not presoak, lick, or otherwise wet tablet before administering dose; administer 1 tablet at a time; allow patient to swallow each tablet separately with sufficient liquid to ensure prompt and complete transit through the esophagus
- **OxyCODONE controlled-release (OxyCONTIN)** 60-mg and 80-mg tablets are for use only in opioid-tolerant patients
- May be administered without food

Oral liquid formulations

Oral concentrate solution route

- **OxyFAST** is a highly concentrated sol (20 mg oxyCODONE/ml), and care should be taken in dispensing and administering this medication; for ease of administration, the sol may be added to 30 ml of a liquid or semisolid food; if the medication is placed in liquid or food, the patient needs to consume it immediately; do not store diluted oxyCODONE for future use

SIDE EFFECTS

CNS: *Drowsiness, dizziness, confusion, headache, sedation, euphoria,* fatigue, abnormal dreams/thoughts, hallucinations

CV: Palpitations, bradycardia, change in B/P

EENT: Tinnitus, blurred vision, miosis, diplopia

GI: *Nausea, vomiting, anorexia, constipation, cramps,* gastritis, dyspepsia, biliary spasms

GU: Increased urinary output, dysuria, urinary retention

INTEG: *Rash,* urticaria, bruising, flushing, diaphoresis, pruritus

RESP: **Respiratory depression**

PHARMACOKINETICS

PO: Onset 15-30 min, peak 1 hr, duration reg rel 2-6 hr, cont rel 12 hr, metabolized by liver, excreted in urine, crosses placenta, excreted in breast milk, half-life 3-5 hr, protein binding 45%

INTERACTIONS

Increase: effects with other CNS depressants—alcohol, opioids, sedative/hypnotics, antipsychotics, skeletal muscle relaxants

Increase: oxyCODONE level: CYP3A4 inhibitors

Increase: toxicity—cimetidine, MAOIs

Drug/Herb

Increase: sedative effect—kava, St. John's wort, valerian

Drug/Lab Test

Increase: amylase, lipase

NURSING CONSIDERATIONS

Assess:

- **Pain:** intensity, location, type, characteristics; need for pain medication by pain/sedation scoring; physical dependence
- I&O ratio; check for decreasing output; may indicate urinary retention
- **CNS changes:** dizziness, drowsiness, hallucinations, euphoria, LOC, pupil reaction
- **Allergic reactions:** rash, urticaria

O

Black Box Warning: Respiratory dysfunction: respiratory depression, character, rate, rhythm; notify prescriber if respirations are <10/min; B/P, pulse

- **Bowel status:** constipation; stimulant laxative may be needed with fluids, fiber

Black Box Warning: Substance abuse: assess for substance abuse in patient/family/friends before prescribing: monitor for abuse

Black Box Warning: Accidental exposure: dispose of properly away from pets, children

- Assistance with ambulation
- Safety measures: night-light, call bell within easy reach

Evaluate:

- Therapeutic response: decrease in pain without dependence

Teach patient/family:

- To report any symptoms of CNS changes, allergic reactions
- That physical dependency may result from extended use
- That withdrawal symptoms may occur after long-term use: nausea, vomiting, cramps, fever, faintness, anorexia
- To avoid CNS depressants, alcohol
- To avoid driving, operating machinery if drowsiness occurs

TREATMENT OF OVERDOSE:

Naloxone (Narcan) 0.2-0.8 mg IV, O_2, IV fluids, vasopressors, caution with patients physically dependent on opioids

oxymetazoline nasal agent

See Appendix B

oxymetazoline ophthalmic

See Appendix B

⚠ HIGH ALERT

oxymorphone (Rx)

(ox-i-mor′fone)

Opana, Opana ER

Func. class.: Opiate analgesic

Chem. class.: Semisynthetic phenanthrene derivative

Controlled Substance Schedule II

Do not confuse:
oxymorphones/oxyCODONE

ACTION: Inhibits ascending pain pathways in CNS, increases pain threshold, alters pain perception

USES: Moderate to severe pain

CONTRAINDICATIONS: Hypersensitivity, addiction (opiate), asthma, hepatic disease, ileus, intrathecal use, surgery

Black Box Warning: Respiratory depression

Precautions: Pregnancy (B) (short-term), breastfeeding, children <18 yr, addictive personality, increased intracranial pressure, MI (acute), severe heart disease, respiratory depression, renal/hepatic disease, bowel impaction

Black Box Warning: Alcoholism, opioid-naive patients, substance abuse

DOSAGE AND ROUTES

- **Adult: IM/SUBCUT** 1 mg q4-6hr prn; **IV** 0.5 mg q4-6hr prn; *opiate naive* **PO** (immediate release only) 5-20 mg q4-6hr prn; *opiate naive* **PO-ER** 5 mg q12hr in those requiring around-the-clock dosing

Labor analgesia

- **Adult: IM** 0.5-1 mg

Available forms: Inj 1, 1.5 mg/ml; ER tab, crush resistant 5, 7.5, 10, 15, 20, 30, 40 mg; tabs 5, 10 mg

Administer:
- 1 hr before or 2 hr after food (PO)
- With antiemetic for nausea, vomiting
- Do not break, crush, chew ER product
- When pain is beginning to return; determine interval by response
- Store in light-resistant area at room temperature

CONTROLLED REL
- **Opiate naive:** start with lowest dose, titrate upward 5-10 mg q12hr q3-7days to therapeutic response
- When converting from immediate rel to ext rel, give ½ daily dose of ext rel product q12hr

SUBCUT route
- Rotate inj sites
- Do not use if respirations are <12/min

IV route
- Give undiluted over 2-3 min, may be diluted in NS solution

Syringe compatibilities: Glycopyrrolate, hydrOXYzine, ranitidine

SIDE EFFECTS

CNS: *Drowsiness, dizziness, confusion, headache,* hallucinations, increased intracranial pressure, *sedation,* seizures, *euphoria (geriatric patients)*
CV: Palpitations, bradycardia, change in B/P, hypotension
EENT: Tinnitus, blurred vision, miosis, diplopia
GI: *Nausea, vomiting, anorexia, constipation, cramps*
GU: Dysuria, urinary retention
INTEG: *Rash,* urticaria, bruising, flushing, diaphoresis, pruritus
RESP: Respiratory depression

PHARMACOKINETICS

Metabolized by liver, excreted in urine, crosses placenta, half life: PO: 7-9 hr, ext rel: 9-11 hr
PO: Peak 1 hr (fasting)
SUBCUT/IM: Onset 10-15 min, peak 1½ hr, duration 3-6 hr
IV: Onset 5-10 min, peak 15-30 min, duration 3-6 hr

INTERACTIONS

⚠ **Increase:** effects with other CNS depressants—alcohol, opiates, sedative/hypnotics, antipsychotics, skeletal muscle relaxants
⚠ **Increase:** unpredictable effects/reactions—MAOIs

Drug/Herb
Increase: sedative effect—kava, St. John's wort, valerian

Drug/Lab Test
Increase: amylase

NURSING CONSIDERATIONS

Assess:
- **Pain:** location, intensity, type, other characteristics before and 1 hr after (IM) IV 30 min; need for pain medication, physical dependence, give 25%-50% until pain reduction of 50% on pain rating scale, repeat dose may be given at time of peak if previous dose does not control pain and respiratory depression has not occurred; give short-acting opioids for breakthrough pain if patient receiving controlled rel product
- I&O ratio for decreasing output; may indicate urinary retention
- **Bowel status:** constipation; may need stimulative laxative, increased fluids, fiber
- **CNS changes:** dizziness, drowsiness, hallucinations, euphoria, LOC, pupil reaction
- **Allergic reactions:** rash, urticaria

Black Box Warning: **Respiratory dysfunction:** respiratory depression, character, rate, rhythm; notify prescriber if respirations are <10/min

Black Box Warning: **Accidental exposure:** dispose of properly, away from children/pets

Black Box Warning: **Overdose/poisoning:** avoid alcohol ingestion, do not crush, chew, snort, or inject tabs, high abuse potential

Black Box Warning: Opioid-naive patients: ext rel tabs are not to be used immediately postop (12-24 hr after surgery) in these patients

Evaluate:

- Therapeutic response: decrease in pain

Teach patient/family:

- To report any symptoms of CNS changes, allergic reactions
- That physical dependency may result from extended use
- That withdrawal symptoms may occur: nausea, vomiting, cramps, fever, faintness, anorexia
- Not to drive or operate machinery if drowsiness occurs

⚠ Not to use other CNS depressants, alcohol

- To make position changes slowly to prevent orthostatic hypotension

TREATMENT OF OVERDOSE:

Naloxone (Narcan) 0.2-0.8 mg IV, (caution with patients physically dependent on opioids) O_2, IV fluids, vasopressors

⚠ HIGH ALERT

oxytocin (Rx)

(ox-i-toe′sin)

Pitocin

Func. class.: Hormone

Chem. class.: Oxytocic, uterine-active agent

ACTION: Acts directly on myofibrils, thereby producing uterine contraction; stimulates milk ejection by the breast; vasoactive antidiuretic effect

USES: Stimulation, induction of labor; missed or incomplete abortion; postpartum bleeding

CONTRAINDICATIONS: Hypersensitivity, serum toxemia, cephalopelvic disproportion, fetal distress, hypertonic uterus, prolapsed umbilical cord, active genital herpes

Precautions: Cervical/uterine surgery, uterine sepsis, primipara >35 yr, 1st/2nd stage of labor

Black Box Warning: Elective induction of labor

DOSAGE AND ROUTES

Postpartum hemorrhage

- **Adult: IV** 10-40 units in 1000 ml nonhydrating diluent infused at 20-40 mU/min
- **Adult: IM** 3-10 units after delivery of placenta

Contraction stress test (CST)

- **Adult: IV** 0.5 mU/min, increase q20min until 3 contractions within 10 min

Stimulation of labor

- **Adult: IV** 0.5-2 mU/min, increase by 1-2 mU q15-60min until contractions occur, then decrease dose

Incomplete abortion

- **Adult: IV INFUSION** 10 units/500 ml D_5W or 0.9% NaCl at 10-20 mU/min, max 30 units/12 hr

Available forms: Inj 10 units/ml

Administer:

IV route

- Use infusion pump

Labor induction

- After diluting 10 units/1000 ml of 0.9% NS or D_5 NS run at 1-2 mU/min at 15- to 30-min intervals to begin normal labor; dilute 10-40 mU/min; titrate to control postpartum bleeding; dilute 10 units/500 ml sol; run 10 units-20 mU/ml; administer by only 1 route at a time; use infusion pump; rotate infusion to provide mixing; do not shake

Control of postpartum bleeding

- Dilute 10-40 units/1000 ml of sol; run at 10-20 mU/min; adjust rate as needed
- With crash cart available on unit (magnesium sulfate at bedside)

Incomplete, inevitable, elective abortion

- Dilute 10 units/500 ml compatible IV sol

Y-site compatibilities: Heparin, hydrocortisone, insulin (regular), meperidine, morphine, potassium chloride, vit B/C, warfarin

SIDE EFFECTS

CNS: Seizures, tetanic contractions
CV: Hypo/hypertension, dysrhythmias, increased pulse, bradycardia, tachycardia, PVC
FETUS: Dysrhythmias, jaundice, hypoxia, intracranial hemorrhage
GI: Anorexia, nausea, vomiting, constipation
GU: Abruptio placentae, decreased uterine blood flow
HEMA: Increased hyperbilirubinemia
INTEG: Rash
RESP: Asphyxia
SYST: Water intoxication of mother

PHARMACOKINETICS

IM: Onset 3-7 min, duration 1 hr, half-life 12-17 min
IV: Onset 1 min, duration 30 min, half-life 12-17 min

INTERACTIONS

- Hypertension: vasopressors

Drug/Herb

- Hypertension: ephedra

NURSING CONSIDERATIONS

Assess:

- I&O ratio
- B/P, pulse; watch for changes that may indicate hemorrhage
- Respiratory rate, rhythm, depth; notify prescriber of abnormalities
- Length, intensity, duration of contraction; notify prescriber of contractions lasting >1 min or absence of contractions; turn patient on her side; discontinue oxytocin
- FHTs, fetal distress; watch for acceleration, deceleration; notify prescriber if problems occur; fetal presentation, pelvic dimensions; turn patient on left side if FHT change in rate, give O_2

⚠ **Water intoxication;** confusion, anuria, drowsiness, headache

Evaluate:

- Therapeutic response: stimulation of labor, control of postpartum bleeding

Teach patient/family:

- To report increased blood loss, abdominal cramps, fever, foul-smelling lochia
- That contractions will be similar to menstrual cramps, gradually increasing in intensity

Black Box Warning: Elective induction of labor: use only for induction when medically necessary

O

⚠ *HIGH ALERT*

PACLitaxel (Rx)

(pa-kli-tax′el)

PACLitaxel nanoparticle albumin-bound (Rx)

Abraxane

Func. class.: Antineoplastic—miscellaneous

Chem. class.: Taxane

Do not confuse:
PACLitaxel/PARoxetine/Paxil

ACTION: Inhibits reorganization of microtubule network needed for interphase and mitotic cellular functions; causes abnormal bundles of microtubules during cell cycle and multiple esters of microtubules during mitosis

USES: **Taxol:** metastatic carcinoma of the ovary, breast; AIDS-related Kaposi's sarcoma (2nd-line), non–small-cell lung cancer (1st-line), adjuvant treatment for node-positive breast cancer

Unlabeled uses: Advanced head, neck, small-cell lung cancer; non-Hodgkin's lymphoma, adenocarcinoma of the upper GI tract, hormone-refractory prostate cancer, bladder cancer

CONTRAINDICATIONS: Pregnancy (D); hypersensitivity to PACLitaxel or other products with polyoxyethylated castor oil, albumin

Black Box Warning: Neutropenia of <1500/mm^3

Precautions: Breastfeeding, children, females, geriatric patients, cardiovascular/hepatic/renal disease, CNS disorder, bone marrow suppression, dental disease/work, extravasation, herpes, infection, infertility, jaundice, ocular exposure, radiation therapy, thrombocytopenia, vaccination

Black Box Warning: Taxane hypersensitivity, requires a specialized care setting, requires an experienced clinician

DOSAGE AND ROUTES

PACLitaxel

Ovarian carcinoma

- **Adult: IV INFUSION** 135 mg/m^2 given over 24 hr q3wk, then CISplatin 75 mg/m^2; or (refractory or metastatic) 175 mg/m^2 over 3 hr q3wk; or 175 mg/m^2 over 3 hr

Advanced ovarian carcinoma

- **Adult: IV/INFUSION** 175 mg/m^2 with CISplatin 75 mg/m^2 using a 3-hr regimen q3wk

Breast carcinoma

- **Adult: IV INFUSION** 175 mg/m^2 over 3 hr q3wk × 4 courses

AIDS-related Kaposi's sarcoma

- **Adult: IV INFUSION** 135 mg/m^2 over 3 hr q3wk or 100 mg/m^2 over 3 hr q2wk

1st-line non–small-cell lung cancer

- **Adult: IV INFUSION** 135 mg/m^2/24 hr infusion with CISplatin 75 mg/m^2 × 3 wk

Hepatic dose

- **Adult:** for 135 mg/m^2 24-hr IV INFUSION AST/ALT 2-10 × ULN, total bilirubin ≤1.5 mg/dl: 100 mg/m^2; AST/ALT <10 × ULN, total bilirubin 1.6-7.5 mg/dl: 50 mg/m^2; AST/ALT ≥10 × ULN or total bilirubin >7.5 mg/dl; avoid use; for 175/m^2 3-hr IV INFUSION AST/ALT <10 × ULN, total bilirubin 1.26-2 × ULN: 135 mg/m^2; AST/ALT <10 × ULN, total bilirubin 2.01-5 × ULN: 90 mg/m^2; AST/ALT ≥10 × ULN or total bilirubin >5 × ULN: avoid use

Bladder cancer (unlabeled)

- **Adult: IV** 225 mg/m^2 over 3 hr with CARBOplatin

Head/neck cancer (unlabeled)

- **Adult: IV** 40-45 mg/m^2 with CARBOplatin over 24 hr or 175-300 mg/m^2 over 3 hr

Stem cell transplant/bone marrow ablation (unlabeled)

- **Adult: IV** 250-775 mg/m^2 over 24 hr in combination with other chemotherapy

PACLitaxel protein-bound particles

- **Adult: IV** 260 mg/m^2 q3wk

Available forms: Inj 6 mg/ml, 30 mg/5-ml vial, 100 mg/16.7-ml vial, 150 mg/25-ml vial, 300 mg/50-ml vial; powder for inj, lyophilized 100 mg in single-use vials (Abraxane)

Administer:

Black Box Warning: CBC, differential, platelet count before treatment and weekly; withhold product if WBC is <1500/mm^3 or platelet count is <100,000/mm^3; notify prescriber

- If CISplatin is given, use after taxane
- Confirmation that dexamethasone was given 12 hr and 6 hr before infusion begins
- Store prepared sol up to 27 hr in refrigerator

Continuous IV INFUSION route

- After premedicating with dexamethasone 20 mg PO 12 hr and 6 hr before PACLitaxel, diphenhydrAMINE 50 mg IV $^1/_2$-1 hr before PACLitaxel and cimetidine 300 mg or ranitidine 50 mg IV $^1/_2$-1 hr before PACLitaxel
- For extravasation if given by regular IV, not port

PACLitaxel

- After diluting in 0.9% NaCl, D_5, D_5 and 0.9% NaCl, D_5LR (0.3-1.2 mg/ml), chemo dispensing pin or similiar devices with spikes should not be used in vials of Taxol; use in-line filter ≤0.22 micron; give as 3-hr or 24-hr infusion
- Using only glass bottles, polypropylene, polyolefin bags, and administration sets; do not use PVC infusion bags or sets

Y-site compatibilities: Acyclovir, amikacin, aminophylline, ampicillin/sulbactam, bleomycin, butorphanol, calcium chloride, CARBOplatin, cefepime, cefoTEtan, cefTAZidime, cefTRIAXone, cimetidine, CISplatin, cladribine, cyclophosphamide, cytarabine, dacarbazine, dexamethasone, diphenhydrAMINE, DOXOrubicin, droperidol, etoposide, famotidine, floxuridine, fluconazole, fluorouracil, furosemide, ganciclovir, gentamicin, granisetron, haloperidol, heparin, hydrocortisone, HYDROmorphone, ifosfamide, LORazepam, magnesium sulfate, mannitol, meperidine, mesna, methotrexate, metoclopramide, morphine, nalbuphine, ondansetron, pentostatin, potassium chloride, prochlorperazine, propofol, ranitidine, sodium bicarbonate, thiotepa, vancomycin, vinBLAStine, vinCRIStine, zidovudine

Abraxane

Intermittent IV INFUSION route

- Reconstitute vial by injecting 20 ml of 0.9% NaCl; slowly inject 20 ml of 0.9% NaCl over at least 1 min to direct sol flow on wall of vial; do not inject 0.9% NaCl directly onto lyophilized cake (foaming will occur); allow vial to sit for at least 5 min to ensure proper wetting of lyophilized cake; gently swirl or invert vial slowly for ≥2 min until completely dissolved
- Calculate dose by dosing vol/ml = total dose (mg) ÷ 5 (mg/ml)

SIDE EFFECTS

CNS: *Peripheral neuropathy*

CV: Bradycardia, *hypotension,* abnormal ECG, **supraventricular tachycardia (SVT)**

GI: *Nausea, vomiting, diarrhea, mucositis, stomatitis, increased bilirubin, alk phos, AST*

HEMA: **Neutropenia, leukopenia, thrombocytopenia, anemia, bleeding, infections**

INTEG: *Alopecia,* **tissue necrosis,** generalized urticaria, *flushing*

MS: *Arthralgia, myalgia*

RESP: **Pulmonary embolism,** dyspnea

SYST: *Hypersensitivity reactions,* **anaphylaxis, Stevens-Johnson syndrome, toxic epidermal necrolysis, angioedema**

PHARMACOKINETICS

89%-98% of product serum protein bound, metabolized in liver, excreted in bile and urine; terminal half-life 5.3-17.4 hr

INTERACTIONS

Increase: myelosuppression—other antineoplastics, radiation

Increase: DOXOrubicin levels—DOXOrubicin

P

⚠ **Increase:** toxicity, decrease metabolism—ketoconazole; avoid concurrent use
Increase: bleeding risk—NSAIDs, anticoagulants
Decrease: PACLitaxel metabolism—verapamil, diazepam, cycloSPORINE, teniposide, etoposide, quiNIDine, dexamethasone, vinCRIStine, testosterone
Decrease: PACLitaxel levels—CYP2C8, CYP2C9 inducers
Decrease: immune response—live virus vaccines

Drug/Lab Test
Increase: AST/ALT, alk phos, triglycerides
Decrease: neutrophils, platelets, WBC, Hgb

NURSING CONSIDERATIONS

Assess:

Black Box Warning: Requires a specialized care setting such as a hospital or facility with management of complications; should be used by a clinician experienced in cytotoxic agents

- **Cardiovascular status:** ECG continuously in CV conditions; monitor for hypotension, sinus bradycardia/tachycardia
- **Peripheral neuropathy:** paresthesias, numbness; during infusion, use ice packs on extremities to lessen continued neuropathy; may use acupuncture for some relief; use of ice on extremities when infusing
- **Arthralgia, myalgia:** may begin 2-3 days after infusion and continue for 4-5 days; may use analgesics
- **Nausea, vomiting:** premedicate with antiemetics; nausea and vomiting occur often
- Hepatic studies before, during therapy (bilirubin, AST, ALT, LDH) prn or monthly, check for jaundiced skin and sclera, dark urine, clay-colored stool, itchy skin, abdominal pain, fever, diarrhea
- VS during 1st hr of infusion, check IV site for signs of infiltration

⚠ **Hypersensitivity reactions, anaphylaxis:** hypotension, dyspnea, angioedema, generalized urticaria; discontinue infusion immediately; keep emergency equipment available, monitor continuously during first 30-60 min, then periodically

- **Flush:** for mild to moderate flush, may continue diphenhydrAMINE for ≤48 hr
- Effects of alopecia on body image; discuss feelings about body changes

Evaluate:

- Therapeutic response: decreased tumor size, spread of malignancy

Teach patient/family:

- To report signs of infection: fever, sore throat, flulike symptoms
- To report signs of anemia: fatigue, headache, faintness, SOB, irritability
- To report bleeding; to avoid use of razors, commercial mouthwash; to use soft-bristle toothbrush; to use viscous xylocaine or compounded formula for stomatitis
- To avoid use of aspirin, ibuprofen
- To avoid crowds, persons with known infections
- That hair may be lost during treatment; that a wig or hairpiece may make patient feel better; that new hair may be different in color, texture
- That pain in muscles and joints 2-5 days after infusion is common
- To notify prescriber if pregnancy is planned or suspected, pregnancy (D); do not breastfeed
- To avoid receiving vaccinations while taking product

⚠ HIGH ALERT

palbociclib

(pal-boe-sye′klib)

Ibrance

Func. class.: Antineoplastic
Chem. class.: Signal transduction inhibitor

ACTION: Inhibits progression of the cell cycle from G_1 into S phase, decreased proliferation of ER-positive breast cancer cell lines. When combined with antiestrogen therapy (letrozole), decreases retinoblastoma protein (Rb) phosphorylation, reducing E2F expression and signaling, and increasing growth arrest

USES:
Treatment of estrogen receptor (ER)–positive, HER2-negative advanced breast cancer in postmenopausal women, in combination with letrozole as initial endocrine-based therapy

CONTRAINDICATIONS:
Hypersensitivity

Precautions: Breastfeeding, children, fungal/viral infection, infants, infertility, neutropenia, pregnancy, testicular failure, thromboembolic disease

DOSAGE AND ROUTES
- **Adult females: PO** 125 mg daily with food × 21 days, followed by 7 days off, repeat q28 days with letrozole 2.5 mg daily, given continuously through each 28-day cycle until progressive disease or unacceptable toxicity occurs

Available forms: Caps 75, 100, 125 mg

Administer:

Treatment-related hepatotoxicity:
- Grade 1 or 2 hepatotoxicity: No dosage change
- Grade ≥3 hepatotoxicity (AST or ALT >5 × ULN or total bilirubin >3 × ULN) that persists despite medical treatment: Hold until toxicity resolves to grade ≤2 (AST or ALT ≤5 × ULN or total bilirubin ≤3 × ULN), resume treatment at the next lower dose level if not considered a safety risk for the patient; discontinue if grade ≥3 toxicity occurs at a dose of 75 mg/day

Treatment-related nephrotoxicity:
- Grade 1 or 2 nephrotoxicity: No change
- Grade ≥3 nephrotoxicity (CCr >3 × baseline or >4 mg/dl, or requiring hospitalization or dialysis) that persists despite medical treatment: Hold therapy. When toxicity resolves to grade ≤2 (CCr <3 × baseline or <4 mg/dl), resume at the next lower dose level if not considered a safety risk for the patient, discontinue if grade ≥3 toxicity occurs at a dose of 75 mg/day

Other dosage adjustments
- **Strong CYP3A4 inhibitors:** Avoid concomitant use. If a strong CYP3A4 inhibitor is needed, consider reducing the dose to 75 mg daily, if the strong CYP3A4 inhibitor is discontinued, increase the dose upward to the previously tolerated/recommended dose after a washout period of 3-5 half-lives of the inhibitor
- **Strong CYP3A4 inducers:** Avoid use

SIDE EFFECTS
CNS: Weakness, fever, fatigue

EENT: Stomatitis, oral ulceration, glossitis, pharyngitis, sinusitis, epistaxis

GI: Vomiting, nausea, anorexia, diarrhea,

HEMA: Thrombocytopenia, neutropenia, leukopenia, lymphopenia, anemia

MISC: Peripheral neuropathy, alopecia, infection, pulmonary embolism, thromboembolism

PHARMACOKINETICS
85% protein bound, elimination half-life was 24-34 hr, metabolized by CYP3A, peak 6-12 hr

INTERACTIONS
Avoid use with CYp3A inhibitors and inducers

Drug/Herb: Avoid use with St. John's wort

Drug/Food: Avoid use with grapefruit juice

NURSING CONSIDERATIONS
Assess:

Pregnancy: Product can cause fetal harm, identify if the patient is pregnant or if pregnancy is planned

Pulmonary embolism/thromboembolic events: Dyspnea/shortness of breath, chest pain, arm or leg swelling, sudden numbness or weakness, severe headache or confusion, or problems with vision, speech, or balance

Blood dyscrasias: CBC/differential

Evaluate: Therapeutic response: Decreased progression of disease

Teach patient/family:
- Identify if pregnancy is planned or suspected. Discuss the need for contraception

P

due to possible fetal harm, avoid breastfeeding
- Laboratory testing will be needed during treatment
- **Pulmonary/thromboembolic events:** Instruct to seek medical attention if dyspnea/shortness of breath, chest pain, arm or leg swelling, sudden numbness or weakness, severe headache or confusion, or problems with vision, speech, or balance develop

paliperidone (Rx)

(pal-ee-per′i-done)

Invega, Invega Sustenna

Func. class.: Antipsychotic

Chem. class.: Benzisoxazole derivative

Do not confuse:
Invega/Iveegam
paliperidone/risperiDONE

ACTION: Mediated through both DOPamine type 2 (D_2) and serotonin type 2 ($5\text{-}HT_2$) antagonism

USES: Schizophrenia, schizoaffective disorder

Unlabeled uses: Agitation

CONTRAINDICATIONS: Breastfeeding, geriatric patients, seizure disorders, AV block, QT prolongation, torsades de pointes; hypersensitivity to this product, risperidone

Precautions: Pregnancy (C), children, renal/hepatic disease, obesity, Parkinson's disease, suicidal ideation, diabetes mellitus, hematological disease

Black Box Warning: Dementia-related psychosis (mortality)

DOSAGE AND ROUTES
- **Adult: PO** 6 mg/day, max 12 mg/day; **IM** 234 mg on day 1, then 156 mg 1 wk later; after 2nd dose, give 117 mg each mo; range 39-234 mg, dosage change may be needed when used with CYP3A4 inducers
- **Child/adolescent ≥12 yr and ≥51 kg: PO** 3 mg daily, may increase if needed by 3 mg/day in intervals of >5 days, up to max 12 mg/day; <51 kg max 6 mg/day

Renal dose
- **Adult: PO** CCr 50-79 ml/min, 3 mg/day, max 6 mg/day; **EXT REL/IM** 156 mg on day 1, 117 mg 1 wk later, then 78 mg each mo; CCr 10-49 ml/min, 1.5 mg/day, max 3 mg/day; IM not recommended

Available forms: Ext rel tabs 1.5, 3, 6, 9 mg; ext rel susp for inj 39 mg/0.25 ml, 78 mg/0.5 ml, 117 mg/0.75 ml, 156 mg/ml, 234 mg/1.5 ml

Administer:
- Avoid use with CNS depressants

PO route
- Do not break, crush, or chew ext rel tabs; use plenty of water
- Without regard for food
- Reduced dose for geriatric patients

IM route
- Use for IM only; do not use IV or subcut; inj kits contain prefilled syringe and 2 safety needles; for single use only; shake for 10 sec; **deltoid inj:** ≥90 kg, use 1.5-inch, 22-G needle; <90 kg, use 1-inch, 23-G needle; alternate injections between deltoid muscles; **gluteal inj:** use 1.5-inch, 22-G needle; attach needle to Luer connection in clockwise motion; pull needle sheath away using straight pull; bring syringe with attached needle upright to de-aerate, de-aerate, inject; after inj, use finger, thumb, or flat surface to activate needle protection system until click heard; use deltoid × 2 doses

SIDE EFFECTS

CNS: *EPS, pseudoparkinsonism, akathisia, dystonia, tardive dyskinesia; drowsiness, insomnia, agitation, anxiety, headache,* seizures, neuroleptic malignant syndrome, dizziness

CV: Orthostatic hypotension, tachycardia; heart failure, QT prolongation, heart block, dysrhythmias

EENT: Blurred vision, cough

ENDO: Hyperinsulinemia, weight gain, hyperglycemia, dyslipidemia, diabetes mellitus

GI: *Nausea,* vomiting, *anorexia, constipation,* weight gain in adolescents, xerostomia
GU: Priapism, menstrual irregularities
HEMA: **Agranulocytosis**

PHARMACOKINETICS

Peak 24 hr; elimination half-life 23 hr; excreted 80% urine, 11% feces, protein binding >74%

INTERACTIONS

Increase: sedation—other CNS depressants, alcohol, sedative/hypnotics, opiates
Increase: EPS—other antipsychotics
⚠ **Increase:** **QT prolongation—class IA, III antidysrhythmics, azole antifungals, tricyclics (high doses), some phenothiazines, β-blockers, chloroquine, pimozide, droperidol, some antipsychotics, abarelix, alfuzosin, amoxapine, apomorphine, dasatinib, dolasetron, flecainide, halogenated anesthetics**
Increase: **neurotoxicity—lithium**
Increase: **serotonin syndrome, neuroleptic malignant syndrome—SSRIs, SNRIs**
Decrease: effect of paliperidone—carBAMazepine, other CYP3A4 inducers
Decrease: levodopa effect—levodopa
Drug/Lab Test
Increase: prolactin levels

NURSING CONSIDERATIONS

Assess:

Black Box Warning: Mental status: mood, behavior, confusion, orientation, suicidal thoughts/behaviors; dementia, especially in geriatric patients before initial administration and periodically

⚠ **QT prolongation:** **ECG for QT prolongation, ejection fraction; chest pain, palpitations, dyspnea**
- AIMS assessment, blood glucose, CBC, glycosylated hemoglobulin A1c (HbA1c), LFTs, neurologic function, pregnancy testing, serum creatinine/electrolytes/lipid profile/prolactin, thyroid function tests, weight
- Swallowing of PO medication; check for hoarding, giving of medication to others
- Affect, orientation, LOC, reflexes, gait, coordination, sleep pattern disturbances
- B/P (standing, lying), pulse, respirations; q4hr during initial treatment; establish baseline before starting treatment; report drops of 30 mm Hg; watch for ECG changes
- **Hyperprolactinemia:** sexual dysfunction, decreased menstruation, breast pain
- Dizziness, faintness, palpitations, tachycardia on rising
- **EPS:** akathisia, tardive dyskinesia (bizarre movements of jaw, mouth, tongue, extremities), pseudoparkinsonism (rigidity, tremors, pill rolling, shuffling gait)

⚠ **Serotonin syndrome, neuroleptic malignant syndrome:** **hyperthermia, increased CPK, altered mental status, muscle rigidity, fever, seizures, discontinue**
- Constipation, urinary retention daily; if these occur, increase bulk and water in diet; monitor for weight gain, especially among adolescents
- Supervised ambulation until patient is stabilized on medication; do not involve patient in strenuous exercise program because fainting is possible; patient should not stand still for a long time
- Increased fluids to prevent constipation
- Sips of water, candy, gum for dry mouth

Evaluate:
- Therapeutic response: decrease in emotional excitement, hallucinations, delusions, paranoia; reorganization of patterns of thought, speech

Teach patient/family:
- That orthostatic hypotension may occur; to rise gradually from sitting or lying position
- To avoid hot tubs, hot showers, tub baths because hypotension may occur
- To avoid abrupt withdrawal of this product because EPS may result; that product should be withdrawn slowly
- To avoid OTC preparations (cough, hay fever, cold) unless approved by prescriber because serious product interactions may

occur; to avoid alcohol because increased drowsiness may occur
- To avoid hazardous activities if drowsy or dizzy
- About compliance with product regimen; that nonabsorbable tab shell is expelled in stool
- To report impaired vision, tremors, muscle twitching
- That heat stroke may occur in hot weather; to take extra precautions to stay cool
- To use contraception; to inform prescriber if pregnancy is planned or suspected; do not breastfeed

Black Box Warning: To notify prescriber of suicidal thoughts/behaviors, other changes in behavior; identify dementia in the elderly

TREATMENT OF OVERDOSE:
Lavage if orally ingested; provide airway; *do not induce vomiting*

palonosetron (Rx)
(pa-lone-o′se-tron)

Aloxi

Func. class.: Antiemetic

Chem. class.: 5-HT_3 receptor antagonist

ACTION: Prevents nausea, vomiting by blocking serotonin peripherally, centrally, and in the small intestine at the 5-HT_3 receptor

USES: Prevention of nausea, vomiting associated with cancer chemotherapy, postoperative nausea/vomiting

CONTRAINDICATIONS: Hypersensitivity

Precautions: Pregnancy (B), breastfeeding, children, geriatric patients, hypokalemia, hypomagnesium, patients taking diuretics

DOSAGE AND ROUTES
- **Adult: IV** 0.25 mg as single dose over 30 sec ½ hr before chemotherapy, max 25 mg **IV** over q7days

Postoperative nausea/vomiting prophylaxis for ≤24 hr after surgery
- **Adult: IV** 0.075 mg given over 10 sec immediately before induction

Available forms: Inj 0.25 mg/5 ml

Administer:

Direct IV route
- **Chemotherapy nausea/vomiting:** give as single dose over 30 sec
- **Postoperative nausea/vomiting:** give over 10 sec immediately before anesthesia induction

Syringe compatibilities: Dexamethasone

Y-site compatibilities: Alemtuzumab, alfentanil, amifostine, amikacin, aminocaproic acid, aminophylline, amiodarone, amphotericin B liposome, ampicillin, ampicillin/sulbactam, atracurium, atropine, azithromycin, aztreonam, bivalirudin, bleomycin, bumetanide, buprenorphine, busulfan, butorphanol, calcium acetate/chloride/gluconate, CARBOplatin, carmustine, caspofungin, ceFAZolin, cefepime, cefotaxime, cefoTEtan, cefOXitin, cefTAZidime, ceftizoxime, cefTRIAXone, cefuroxime, chloramphenicol, chlorproMAZINE, cimetidine, ciprofloxacin, cisatracurium, CISplatin, clindamycin, cyclophosphamide, cycloSPORINE, cytarabine, dacarbazine, DACTINomycin, dantrolene, DAPTOmycin, DAUNOrubicin, dexamethasone, dexmedetomidine, dexrazoxane, digoxin, diltiazem, diphenhydrAMINE, DOBUTamine, DOCEtaxel, DOPamine, doxacurium, DOXOrubicin hydrochloride, droperidol, enalaprilat, ePHEDrine, EPINEPHrine, epirubicin, eptifibatide, erythromycin, esmolol, etoposide, etoposide phosphate, famotidine, fenoldopam, fentaNYL, fluconazole, fludarabine, fluorouracil, foscarnet, fosphenytoin, furosemide, gemcitabine, gentamicin, glycopyrrolate, haloperidol, heparin, hydrALAZINE, hydrocortisone, HYDROmorphone, IDArubicin, ifosfamide, inamrinone, insulin, irinotecan, isoproterenol, ketorolac, labetalol, leucovorin, levofloxacin, lidocaine, linezolid, LORazepam, magnesium sulfate, mannitol, mechlorethamine, melphalan, meperidine, meropenem, mesna, metaraminol, methotrexate, methyldopate, metoclopramide, metoprolol, metroNIDAZOLE, midazolam, milrinone, mitoMYcin, mitoXANtrone, mivacurium, morphine, nalbuphine, naloxone, neostigmine, nesiritide, niCARdipine, nitroglycerin, nitroprusside, norepinephrine, octreotide, oxaliplatin, oxytocin, PACLitaxel, pamidronate, pancuronium, pentazocine, PHENobarbital, phentolamine, phenylephrine, piperacillin/tazobactam, potassium acetate/chloride/phosphates, procainamide, prochlorperazine, promethazine, propranolol, quinupristin/dalfopristin, ranitidine, remifentanil, rocuronium, sodium acetate/bicarbonate/phosphates, streptozocin, succinylcholine, SUFentanil, tacrolimus, teniposide, theophylline, thiotepa, ticarcillin/clavulanate, tigecycline, tirofiban, tobramycin, topotecan, trimethobenzamide, trimethoprim/sulfamethoxazole, vancomycin, vasopressin, vecuronium, verapamil, vinBLAStine, vinCRIStine, vinorelbine, zidovudine

SIDE EFFECTS

CNS: *Headache, dizziness, drowsiness, fatigue, insomnia*

GI: *Diarrhea, constipation,* abdominal pain

MISC: Weakness, hyperkalemia, anxiety, rash, bronchospasm (rare), arthralgia, *fever, urinary retention*

PHARMACOKINETICS

62% protein bound; metabolized by liver; unchanged product and metabolites excreted by kidney; terminal elimination half-life 40 hr

INTERACTIONS

• Possible QT prolongation: class 1A antidysrhythmics (disopyramide, procainamide, quiNIDine), class III antidysrhythmics (amiodarone, dofetilide, ibutilide, sotalol), chloroquine, clarithromycin, droperidol, erythromycin, haloperidol, levomethadyl, methadone, pentamidine, some phenothiazines, diuretics (except potassium sparing)

Increase: hypotension, severe—apomorphine

Drug/Lab

Increase: potassium

NURSING CONSIDERATIONS

Assess:

• For agents that cause QT prolongation, even if manufacturer has removed QT prolongation from warnings
• Absence of nausea, vomiting during chemotherapy
• **Hypersensitivity reaction:** rash, bronchospasm (rare)
• Cardiac disease: check ECG before use
• Hyperkalemia: monitor potassium baseline and periodically

Evaluate:

• Therapeutic response: absence of nausea, vomiting during cancer chemotherapy, postoperatively

Teach patient/family:

• To report diarrhea, constipation, rash, changes in respirations, or discomfort at insertion site
• To avoid alcohol, barbiturates
• Use other antiemetics if nausea occurs

P

pamidronate (Rx)

(pam-i-drone′ate)

Aredia

Func. class.: Bone-resorption inhibitor, electrolyte modifier

Chem. class.: Bisphosphonate

Do not confuse:

Aredia/Adriamycin

ACTION: Inhibits bone resorption, apparently without inhibiting bone formation and mineralization; adsorbs calcium phosphate crystals in bone and may directly block the dissolution of hydroxyapatite crystals of bone

USES:
Moderate to severe Paget's disease, hypercalcemia, osteolytic bone metastases in breast cancer, patients with multiple myeloma

Unlabeled uses: Postmenopausal osteoporosis and prevention, osteoporosis prophylaxis, ankylosing spondylitis, osteogenesis imperfecta, hyperparathyroidism

CONTRAINDICATIONS:
Pregnancy (D), hypersensitivity to bisphosphonates

Precautions: Children, nursing mothers, renal dysfunction, poor dentition

DOSAGE AND ROUTES

Hypercalcemia of malignancy

• **Adult: IV INFUSION** 60-90 mg as single dose for moderate hypercalcemia; 90 mg for severe hypercalcemia over 2-24 hr; dose should be diluted in 1000 ml 0.45% NaCl, 0.9% NaCl, or D_5W; wait 7 days before 2nd course

Osteolytic lesions

• **Adult: IV** 90 mg/500 ml of D_5W, 0.45% NaCl, or 0.9% NaCl given over 4 hr each mo (multiple myeloma) or over 2 hr q3-4wk (breast carcinoma)

Paget's disease

• **Adult: IV INFUSION** 30 mg/day given over 4 hr × 3 days

Severe osteogenesis imperfecta (unlabeled)

• **Child: IV** 1.5-3 mg/kg/cycle, cycle dose is divided in 3, administered via slow IV over 4 hr/day × 3 days

Hypercalcemia (hyperparathyroidism) (unlabeled)

• **Adult: IV** 15-60 mg as a single dose

Corticosteroid-induced osteoporosis (unlabeled)

• **Adult: IV** 30 mg q3mo × 1 yr

Ankylosing spondylitis (unlabeled)

• **Adult: IV INFUSION** 60 mg over 4 hr; 6-hr infusion for 1st dose

Osteoporosis prophylaxis in Crohn's disease (unlabeled)

• **Adult: IV INFUSION** 30 mg over 1 hr q3mo × 1 yr

Available forms: Powder for inj 30, 90 mg/vial; inj 3, 6, 9 mg/ml

Administer:

IV route

• After reconstituting by adding 10 ml sterile water for inj to each vial (30 mg/10 ml or 90 mg/10 ml, depending on vial used); add to 1000 ml of sterile 0.45%, 0.9% NaCl, D_5W, run over 2-24 hr **(hypercalcemia);** dilute reconstituted sol in 500 ml of 0.9% NaCl, 0.45% NaCl, or D_5W, give over 4 hr **(multiple myeloma, Paget's disease);** dilute reconstituted sol in 250 ml of 0.9% NaCl, 0.45% NaCl, or D_5W; give over 2 hr **(osteolytic bone metastases of breast cancer)**

• Do not mix with calcium-containing infusion sol such as Ringer's sol

• Store infusion sol up to 24 hr at room temperature

• Reconstituted sol with sterile water may be refrigerated for ≤24 hr

Y-site compatibilities: Acyclovir, alfentanil, allopurinol, amifostine, amikacin, aminocaproic acid, aminophylline, amphotericin B lipid complex, amphotericin B liposome, ampicillin, anidulafungin, atenolol, atracurium, azithromycin, aztreonam, bivalirudin, bleomycin, bumetanide, buprenorphine, butorphanol, CARBOplatin, carmustine, ceFAZolin, cefepime, cefoperazone, cefotaxime, cefoTEtan, cefOXitin, cefTAZidime, ceftizoxime, cefTRIAXone, cefuroxime, chloramphenicol, chlorproMAZINE, cimetidine, ciprofloxacin, cisatracurium, CISplatin, clindamycin, cyclophosphamide, cycloSPORINE, cytarabine, dacarbazine, DAPTOmycin, dexamethasone, dexmedetomidine, dexrazoxane, digoxin, diltiazem, diphenhydrAMINE, DOBUTamine, DOCEtaxel, dolasetron, DOPamine, doxacurium, DOXOrubicin, doxycycline, droperidol, enalaprilat, ePHEDrine, EPINEPHrine, epirubicin, ertapenem, erythromycin, esmolol, etoposide, famotidine, fenoldopam, fentaNYL, fluconazole, fludarabine, fluorouracil, foscarnet, fosphenytoin, furosemide, gallium, ganciclovir, gatifloxacin, gemcitabine, gentamicin, glycopyrrolate, granisetron, haloperidol, heparin, hetastarch 6%, hydrALAZINE, hydrocortisone, HYDROmorphone, hydrOXYzine, ifosfamide, imipenem-cilastatin, inamrinone, insulin (regular), isoproterenol, ketorolac, labetalol, levofloxacin, levorphanol, lidocaine, linezolid, LORazepam, magnesium sulfate, mannitol, mechlorethamine, melphalan, meperidine, meropenem, mesna, metaraminol, methotrexate, methyldopate, methylPREDNISolone, metoclopramide, metoprolol, metroNIDAZOLE, midazolam, milrinone, minocycline, mitoXANtrone, mivacurium, morphine, mycophenolate, nafcillin, nalbuphine, naloxone, nesiritide, niCARdipine, nitroglycerin, nitroprusside, norepinephrine, octreotide, ondansetron, oxytocin, PACLitaxel, palonosetron, pancuronium, PEMEtrexed, pentamidine, pentazocine, PENTobarbital, PHENobarbital, phenylephrine, piperacillin, polymyxin B, potassium chloride/phosphates, procainamide, prochlorperazine, promethazine, propranolol, quiNIDine, quinupristin-dalfopristin, ranitidine, remifentanil, rocuronium, sodium acetate/bicarbonate/phosphates, succinylcholine, SUFentanil, sulfamethoxazole-trimethoprim, teniposide, theophylline, thiopental, thiotepa, ticarcillin, ticarcillin-clavulanate, tigecycline, tirofiban, tobramycin, tolazoline, topotecan, trimethobenzamide, vancomycin, vasopressin, vecuronium, verapamil, vinBLAStine, vinCRIStine, vinorelbine, voriconazole, zidovudine

SIDE EFFECTS

CNS: *Fever,* fatigue
CV: Hypertension, **atrial fibrillation**
EENT: Ocular pain, inflammation, vision impairment
GI: Abdominal pain, anorexia, constipation, nausea, vomiting, dyspepsia
GU: **Renal failure**
HEMA: **Thrombocytopenia, anemia, leukopenia**
INTEG: Redness, swelling, induration, pain on palpation at site of catheter insertion
META: *Hypokalemia, hypomagnesemia, hypophosphatemia, hypocalcemia,* hypothyroidism
MS: Severe bone pain, myalgia, osteonecrosis of the jaw
RESP: Coughing, dyspnea, upper respiratory tract infection
SYST: **Angioedema, anaphylaxis**

PHARMACOKINETICS

Rapidly cleared from circulation and taken up mainly by bones, primarily in areas of high bone turnover; eliminated primarily by kidneys; half-life 21-35 hr, terminal half-life in bone is 300 days

INTERACTIONS

Increase: hypokalemia—loop diuretics
Increase: **nephrotoxicity—aminoglycosides, NSAIDs, vancomycin, radiopaque contrast agents, cycloSPORINE, tacrolimus**
Increase: effect of entecavir
Decrease: pamidronate effect—calcium, vit D

Drug/Lab Test
Increase: creatinine
Decrease: potassium, magnesium, phosphate, calcium, WBC, platelets

NURSING CONSIDERATIONS

Assess:

- **Hypocalcemia:** nausea, vomiting, constipation, thirst, dysrhythmias, hypocalcemia, paresthesia, twitching, laryngospasm, Chvostek's sign, Trousseau's sign; **hypercalcemia:** thirst, nausea, vomiting, dysrhythmias
- Dehydration/hypovolemia: should be corrected during treatment of hypercalcemia, before therapy, maintain adequate urine output
- Monitor WBCs, platelets, electrolytes, creatinine, BUN, Hgb/Hct before beginning treatment
- **Dental health:** cover with antiinfectives for dental extractions
- Temperature may be elevated during the first 3 days after a dose; risk of fever increases as dose increases
- **Renal disease: max 90-mg single dose, longer infusions >2 hr may increase risk for renal toxicity**
- Bone pain; use analgesics

P

• I&O, check for fluid overload edema, crackles, increased B/P; BUN, creatinine

Evaluate:

• Therapeutic response: decreased calcium levels

Teach patient/family

• To notify prescriber if pregnancy is planned or suspected, pregnancy (D)

• To report hypercalcemic relapse: nausea, vomiting, bone pain, thirst; unusual muscle twitching, muscle spasms; severe diarrhea, constipation

• To continue with dietary recommendations, including calcium and vit D

• To obtain analgesic from provider for bone pain

• That, if nausea, vomiting occur, small, frequent meals may help

• To report ocular symptoms to prescriber: blurred vision, edema, inflammation

pancrelipase (Rx)

(pan-kre-li′pase)

Creon, DMH ✱, Pancrease ✱, Pancreaze, Pancrecarb MS, Pertzye, Ultrase MT, Ultresa, Viokase, Zenpep

Func. class.: Digestant

Chem. class.: Pancreatic enzyme—bovine/porcine

ACTION: Pancreatic enzyme needed for the breakdown of substances released from the pancreas

USES: Exocrine pancreatic secretion insufficiency, cystic fibrosis (digestive aid), steatorrhea, pancreatic enzyme deficiency

CONTRAINDICATIONS: Allergy to pork

Precautions: Pregnancy (B), ileus, pancreatitis, Crohn's disease, diabetes mellitus

DOSAGE AND ROUTES

Many products listed above are not interchangeable

• **Adult/adolescent/child ≥4 yr (del rel caps: Creon Caps, Zenpap Caps, Pancreaze Caps): PO** 500 lipase units/kg/meal, titrate based on patient response, max 2500 lipase units/kg/meal

• **Child 1-4 yr: PO** 1000 lipase units/kg/meal, titrate based on patient response, max 2500 lipase units/kg/meal

Available forms: Tabs (Viokase) 10, 20; cap, del rel 4, 8, 16 (Pancrecarb MS), 12, 18, 20 (Ultrase MT), Ultrase; cap 3000, 4200, 5000, 6000, 8000, 10,500, 12,000, 15,000, 16,000, 16,800, 24,000, 25,000 units

Administer:

• After antacid or cimetidine; decreased pH inactivates product

• Low-fat diet for GI symptoms

• Have patient sit up during administration; give with meals

• Do not crush, chew del rel products, caps

• Viokase is not interchangeable with other products

• Store in tight container at room temperature

SIDE EFFECTS

ENDO: Hypo/hyperglycemia

GI: Anorexia, nausea, vomiting, diarrhea, cramping, bloating

GU: Hyperuricuria, hyperuricemia

INTERACTIONS

Decrease: absorption—cimetidine, antacids, oral iron

Decrease: effect of acarbose, miglitol

NURSING CONSIDERATIONS

Assess:

• Appropriate height, weight development before and periodically; may be delayed

• I&O ratio; watch for increasing urinary output

• Fecal fat, nitrogen, PT during treatment

• **Diabetes mellitus:** for polyuria, polydipsia, polyphagia; monitor glucose level more frequently

• Pork sensitivity; cross-sensitivity may occur

• Adequate hydration

Evaluate:

- Therapeutic response: improved digestion of carbohydrates, protein, fat; absence of steatorrhea

Teach patient/family:

- To notify prescriber of allergic reactions, abdominal pain, cramping, or blood in urine
- To always take with food; not to crush, chew del rel product, caps
- To store at room temperature, away from moisture

⚠ HIGH ALERT

pancuronium (Rx)

(pan-kyoo-roe′nee-um)

Func. class.: Neuromuscular blocker (nondepolarizing)

Chem. class.: Synthetic curariform

ACTION: Inhibits transmission of nerve impulses by binding with cholinergic receptor sites, antagonizing action of acetylcholine

USES: Facilitation of endotracheal intubation, skeletal muscle relaxation during mechanical ventilation, surgery, or general anesthesia

CONTRAINDICATIONS: Hypersensitivity to bromide ion

Precautions: Pregnancy (C), breastfeeding, children <2 yr, neuromuscular/cardiac/renal/hepatic disease, electrolyte imbalances, dehydration, previous anaphylactic reactions (other neuromuscular blockers)

Black Box Warning: Respiratory insufficiency

DOSAGE AND ROUTES

- **Adult/child/infant >1 mo: IV** 0.04-0.1 mg/kg initially or 0.05 mg/kg after initial dose of succinylcholine; maintenance 0.01 mg/kg 60-100 min after initial dose, then 0.01 mg/kg q25-60min as needed; for obese patients, use ideal body weight
- **Neonate <1 mo: IV** test dose 0.02 mg/kg, then 0.03 mg/kg/dose initially, repeat 2× as needed at 5-10 min intervals; maintenance 0.03-0.09 mg/kg/dose q30min-4 hr as needed

Available forms: Inj 1, 2 mg/ml

Administer:

Direct IV route

- May be given undiluted over 1-2 min (1 mg/ml [10-ml vial], 2 mg/ml [2-, 5-ml vial])

Intermittent IV INFUSION route

- Add 100 mg of product to 250 ml D_5W, NS, LR (0.4 mg/ml)
- Store in refrigerator; do not store in plastic; use only fresh sol
- Reassurance if communication is difficult during recovery from neuromuscular blockade
- Frequent (q2hr) instillation of artificial tears, covering of eyes to prevent drying of cornea

Additive compatibilities: Verapamil, ciprofloxacin

Y-site compatibilities: Aminophylline, ceFAZolin, cefuroxime, cimetidine, DOBUTamine, DOPamine, EPINEPHrine, esmolol, fenoldopam, fentaNYL, fluconazole, gentamicin, heparin, hydrocortisone, isoproterenol, levofloxacin, LORazepam, midazolam, morphine, nitroglycerin, ranitidine, trimethoprim-sulfamethoxazole, vancomycin

SIDE EFFECTS

CV: Bradycardia; tachycardia; increased, decreased B/P; ventricular extrasystoles, edema, hypertension

EENT: Increased secretions

INTEG: Rash, flushing, pruritus, urticaria, sweating, salivation

MS: Weakness to prolonged skeletal muscle relaxation

RESP: **Prolonged apnea, bronchospasm, cyanosis, respiratory depression, dyspnea**

SYST: **Anaphylaxis**

P

PHARMACOKINETICS

IV: Onset 3-5 min, dose dependent, peak 3-5 min; metabolized (small amounts), excreted in urine (unchanged), crosses placenta

INTERACTIONS

• Dysrhythmias: theophylline

Increase: neuromuscular blockade—aminoglycosides, clindamycin, enflurane, isoflurane, lincomycin, lithium, local anesthetics, opioid analgesics, polymyxin antiinfectives, quiNIDine, thiazides

Drug/Lab Test

Decrease: cholinesterase

NURSING CONSIDERATIONS

Assess:

• **Respiratory recovery:** decreased paralysis of face, diaphragm, leg, arm, rest of body; allow to recover fully before neurologic assessment

• Electrolyte imbalances (K, Mg); may lead to increased action of product

• VS (B/P, pulse, respirations, airway) until fully recovered; rate, depth, pattern of respirations, strength of hand grip

• I&O ratio; check for urinary retention, frequency, hesitancy

⚠ **Allergic reactions, anaphylaxis:** rash, fever, respiratory distress, pruritus; product should be discontinued

Evaluate:

• Therapeutic response: paralysis of jaw, eyelid, head, neck, rest of body

TREATMENT OF OVERDOSE:

Neostigmine, atropine, monitor VS; may require mechanical ventilation

⚠ HIGH ALERT

panitumumab (Rx)

(pan-i-tue′moo-mab)

Vectibix

Func. class.: Antineoplastic—miscellaneous

Chem. class.: Multikinase inhibitor, signal transduction inhibitor

ACTION: Decreases growth and survival of cancer cells by competitive inhibition of EGF receptor

USES: EGFR expressing metastatic colorectal cancer; not beneficial with KRAS mutations in codon 12 or 13

CONTRAINDICATIONS: Hypersensitivity

Precautions: Pregnancy (C), breastfeeding, children, hepatic disease, acute bronchospasm, diarrhea, hamster protein allergy, hypomagnesemia, hypotension, pulmonary fibrosis, sepsis, KRAS mutations, soft tissue toxicities

Black Box Warning: Exfoliative dermatitis, infusion-related reactions

DOSAGE AND ROUTES

• **Adult: IV INFUSION** 6 mg/kg over 60 min every 2 wk; doses >1000 mg over 90 min

Available forms: Sol for inj 20 mg/ml (100 mg/5 ml, 400 mg/20 ml)

Administer:

Intermittent IV INFUSION route

• Give in hospital or clinic setting with full resuscitation equipment

• Only as IV infusion using controlled IV infusion pump; do not give IV push or bolus; use low-protein binding 0.2- or 0.22-micron in-line filter; flush line with 0.9% NaCl before and after administration

- Give over 60 min through a peripheral line or indwelling catheter; infuse doses of >1000 mg over 90 min
- Dilute in 100 ml of 0.9% NaCl; dilute doses >1000 mg in 150 ml of 0.9% NaCl; mix by inverting; do not exceed 10 mg/ml; use within 6 hr if stored at room temperature; can be stored between 2° C and 8° C for up to 24 hr
- **Dosage adjustment for infusion/dermatologic reaction;** Grade 1 or 2: reduce infusion by 50%; Grade 3 or 4: terminate, permanently discontinue depending on severity/resistance
- Store unopened vials in refrigerator; do not shake; protect from direct sunlight; do not freeze

SIDE EFFECTS

CNS: Fatigue
CV: Peripheral edema
EENT: Ocular irritation, ocular toxicity
GI: *Nausea, diarrhea, vomiting,* anorexia, mouth ulceration, abdominal pain, constipation
HEMA: Thrombophlebitis
INTEG: *Rash,* pruritus, exfoliative dermatitis, skin fissure, angioedema, severe/fatal INFUSION reactions
META: Hypocalcemia, hypomagnesemia, antibody formation
RESP: Bronchospasm, cough, dyspnea, hypoxia, pulmonary fibrosis/embolism, pneumonitis, wheezing, interstitial lung disease

PHARMACOKINETICS

Bioavailability 38%-49%; elimination half-life 7.5 days; peak 3 hr; high-fat meal decreases bioavailability; plasma protein binding 99.5%; metabolized in liver; oxidative metabolism by CYP3A4, glucuronidation by UGT1A9; 77% excreted in feces

INTERACTIONS

- Do not use in combination with other antineoplastics

NURSING CONSIDERATIONS

Assess:

Black Box Warning: **Serious skin disorders:** fever, sore throat, fatigue, then lesions in mouth, lips; withhold product, notify prescriber

- Serum electrolytes periodically (calcium, magnesium)
- **Infection:** increased temperature

Black Box Warning: **Infusion reactions:** bronchospasm, fever, chills, hypotension; may require discontinuation, have emergency equipment available

- **Ocular toxicity:** ocular irritation, hyperemia
- **Pulmonary fibrosis:** dyspnea, cough, wheezing; may require discontinuation

Evaluate:

- Therapeutic response: decrease in colon carcinoma progression

Teach patient/family:

⚠ To report adverse reactions immediately: difficulty breathing, mouth sores, skin rash, ocular toxicity
- About reason for treatment, expected results, adverse reactions
- To use contraception while taking product, for 6 mo after treatment; not to breastfeed for ≥2 mo after stopping treatment, enroll in Amgen Pregnancy Surveillance Program (1-800-772-6436)
- To avoid the sun, use sunscreen while taking product

P

pantoprazole (Rx)

(pan-toe-pray′zole)

Panto ✦, Pantoloc ✦, Protonix, Prontonix IV, Tecta

Func. class.: Proton pump inhibitor
Chem. class.: Benzimidazole

ACTION: Suppresses gastric secretion by inhibiting hydrogen/potassium ATPase enzyme system in gastric parietal cell; characterized as gastric acid pump inhibitor because it blocks the final step of acid production

USES: Gastroesophageal reflux disease (GERD), severe erosive esophagitis; maintenance of long-term pathologic hypersecretory conditions, including Zollinger-Ellison syndrome

Unlabeled uses: Duodenal/gastric ulcer, NSAID ulcer prophylaxis, *Helicobacter pylori*-associated ulcer, dyspepsia

CONTRAINDICATIONS: Hypersensitivity to this product or benzimidazole

Precautions: Pregnancy (C), breastfeeding, children, proton pump hypersensitivity

DOSAGE AND ROUTES

GERD

• **Adult: PO** 40 mg/day × 8 wk, may repeat course

Erosive esophagitis

• **Adult: IV** 40 mg/day × 7-10 day; **PO** 40 mg/day × 8 wk; may repeat **PO** course

Pathologic hypersecretory conditions

• **Adult: PO** 40 mg bid; **IV** 80 mg q12hr, max 240 mg/day

Duodenal ulcer/gastric ulcer/ NSAID ulcer prophylaxis (unlabeled)

• **Adult: PO** 40 mg/day

***H. pylori*–associated ulcers (unlabeled)**

• **Adult: PO** 40 mg bid; may be used with other products

Available forms: Del rel tabs 20, 40 mg; powder for inj 40 mg/vial; del rel granules for susp 40 mg

Administer:

PO route

• Swallow del rel tabs whole; do not break, crush, or chew; take del rel tabs at same time of day

• May take with/without food

• **Suspension:** give in apple juice 30 min before a meal or sprinkled on 1 tbsp of applesauce

• **NG tube:** empty contents of packet of granules into barrel of a 60-ml catheter tip syringe (plunger removed) connected to ≥16F NG tube; add 10 ml apple juice and tap or shake barrel of syringe to empty into the tube; add another 10 ml of apple juice; rinse with additional apple juice until syringe is clear

IV route

• Use of Protonix IV vials with spiked IV system adaptors is not recommended

• Visually inspect for particulate matter and discoloration before use

• Give as an IV infusion over 15 min either through a dedicated line or a Y-site; a 2-min slow-injection regimen is also approved; do not give fast IV push

• When using a Y-site, immediately stop use if a precipitation or discoloration occurs

• **Reconstitution of vial**: use 40-mg vial/10 ml NS; do not freeze

• **Two-minute slow IV infusion injection:** dilute one or two 40-mg vials with 10 ml NS per vial to 4 mg/ml; store ≤24 hr at room temperature before use; infuse slowly over ≥2 min; do not give with other IV fluids or medications; flush line with D_5W, NS, or LR before and after each dose

• **Fifteen-minute IV infusion:** dilute each 40-mg dose with 10 ml NS; the reconstituted vial should be further admixed with 100 ml (for one vial) or 80 ml (for 2 vials) of D_5W, NS, or LR (to 0.4 mg/ml or 0.8 mg/ml, respectively); store ≤6 at room temperature before further dilution; the admixed solution (0.4 mg/ml or 0.8 mg/ml) may be stored at room temperature and must be used within 24 hr from the time of initial reconstitution; infuse over 15 min at 7 ml/min; do not administer with other IV fluids or medications; flush IV line with D_5W, NS, or LR before and after each dose

Y-site compatibilities: Acyclovir, allopurinol, amifostine, amikacin, aminocaproic acid, aminophylline, amoxicillin-clavulanate, amphotericin B liposome, ampicillin, ampicillin-sulbactam, anidulafungin, azithromycin, bleomycin, bumetanide, calcium gluconate, CARBOplatin, carmustine, ceFAZolin, cefOXitin, cefTAZidime, ceftizoxime, cefTRIAXone, cefuroxime, clindamycin, cyclophosphamide, cycloSPORINE, cytarabine, dextrose 3.3% in sodium chloride 0.3%, digoxin, dimenhyDRINATE, DOCEtaxel, DOPamine, doripenem, doxycycline, enalaprilat, EPINEPHrine, ertapenem, fluorouracil, foscarnet, fosphenytoin, furosemide, ganciclovir, gentamicin, granisetron, heparin, hydrocortisone HYDROmorphone, imipenem-cilastatin, inamrinone, insulin (regular), irinotecan, isoproterenol, magnesium, mannitol, mesna, methohexital, methyldopate, metoclopramide, nafcillin, nitroglycerin, nitroprusside, ofloxacin, oxytocin, PACLitaxel, pentazocine, PENTobarbital, phenylephrine, piperacillin-tazobactam, potassium chloride, procainamide, rifampin, sodium bicarbonate, succinylcholine, SUFentanil, sulfamethoxazole-trimethoprim, teniposide, theophylline, thiopental, ticarcillin, ticarcillin-clavulanate, tigecycline, tirofiban, tobramycin, traMADol, vasopressin, zidovudine

SIDE EFFECTS

CNS: *Headache,* insomnia, asthenia, fatigue, malaise, insomnia, somnolence
GI: *Diarrhea, abdominal pain,* flatulence, pancreatitis, weight changes
INTEG: *Rash*
META: Hyperglycemia, weight gain/loss, hyponatremia, hypomagnesemia
MS: Rhabdomyolysis, myalgia
RESP: Pneumonia
SYST: Stevens-Johnson syndrome, toxic epidermal necrolysis, anaphylaxis, angioedema

PHARMACOKINETICS

Peak 2.4 hr, duration >24 hr, half-life 1.5 hr, protein binding 97%, eliminated in urine as metabolites and in feces; in geriatric patients, elimination rate decreased; some Asian patients (15%-20%) may be poor metabolizers

INTERACTIONS

Increase: pantoprazole serum levels—diazepam, phenytoin, flurazepam, triazolam, clarithromycin
Increase: bleeding—warfarin
Decrease: absorption of these products—sucralfate, calcium carbonate, vit B_{12}, ketoconazole, itraconazole, atazanavir, ampicillin, iron salts
Decrease: clopidogrel effect
Drug/Herb
Decrease: effect of pantoprazole—St. John's wort

NURSING CONSIDERATIONS

Assess:
- **GI system:** bowel sounds q8hr; abdomen for pain, swelling; anorexia
- **Hepatic studies:** AST, ALT, alk phos during treatment
- For vit B_{12} deficiency in patients receiving long-term therapy
- ⚠ **Serious skin reactions:** toxic epidermal necrolysis, Stevens-Johnson syndrome, exfoliative dermatitis: fever, sore throat, fatigue, thin ulcers; lesions in the mouth, lips
- **Electrolyte imbalances:** hyponatremia; hypomagnesemia in patients using product 3 mo to 1 year; if hypomagnesemia occurs, use of magnesium supplements may be sufficient; if severe, discontinuation of product may be required
- ⚠ **Rhabdomyolysis, myalgia:** muscle pain, increased CPK; weakness, swelling of affected muscles

Evaluate:
- Therapeutic response: absence of epigastric pain, swelling, fullness

Teach patient/family:
- To report severe diarrhea; black, tarry stools; abdominal pain; product may have to be discontinued
- That hyperglycemia may occur in diabetic patients
- To avoid alcohol, salicylates, NSAIDs; may cause GI irritation
- To notify prescriber if pregnant or planning to become pregnant; not to breastfeed
- To continue taking even if feeling better

P

paricalcitol (Rx)

(par-ih-cal′sih-tol)

Zemplar

Func. class.: Vit D analog

Chem. class.: Fat-soluble vitamin

ACTION: Reduces parathyroid hormone (PTH) levels; suppresses PTH levels in patients with chronic renal failure with absence of hypercalcemia/hyperphosphatemia; serum PO_4, calcium, CaXP may increase

USES: Hyperparathyroidism in chronic renal failure

Unlabeled uses: Renal osteodystrophy

CONTRAINDICATIONS: Hypersensitivity, hypercalcemia

Precautions: Pregnancy (C), breastfeeding, children, geriatric patients, CV disease, renal calculi

DOSAGE AND ROUTES

- **Adult: IV BOL** 0.04-0.1 mcg/kg (2.8-7 mcg) no more than every other day during dialysis; may increase by 2-4 mcg q2-4wk until target serum intact PTH (1.5-3× nonuremic upper limit of normal) achieved; **PO** 1 mcg/day or 2 mcg 3×/wk (IPTH ≤500 pg/ml); 2 mcg/day or 4 mcg 3×/wk (IPTH >500 pg/ml)

Available forms: Inj 2, 5 mcg/ml; caps 1, 2, 4 mcg

Administer:

PO route

- Daily or 3×/wk; may give without regard to food

IV route

- By IV bolus only

SIDE EFFECTS

CNS: Lightheadedness

CV: Palpitations

GI: Nausea, vomiting, anorexia, dry mouth

OTHER: Pneumonia, edema, chills, fever, flu, sepsis

PHARMACOKINETICS

Crosses placenta, enters breast milk

INTERACTIONS

Decrease: paricalcitol effect—cholestyramine, colestipol, mineral oil, orlistat, corticosteroids, barbiturates, hydantoins, CYP3A4 enzymes (nevirapine, rifampin, bosentan)

Increase: calcium levels—thiazide diuretics, calcium products, vit D supplements

Increase: effect of cardiac glycosides

Altered: paricalcitol effect—CYP3A4 inhibitors (amiodarone, protease inhibitors, systemic azole antifungals, chloramphenicol, clarithromycin, delavirdine, erythromycin)

NURSING CONSIDERATIONS

Assess:

- **Hypocalcemia:** twitching, dysrhythmias, Chvostek's/Trousseau signs, paresthesia, laryngospasm, prolonged QTc/ST interval
- Serum calcium, serum intact parathyroid hormone concentrations (iPTH), phosphate 2×/wk during initial therapy; after dose is established, take calcium and phosphorus monthly

Evaluate:

- Decreased hypoparathyroidism with chronic renal disease, normal serum calcium, phosphate, iPTH

Teach patient/family:

- To report weakness, lethargy, headache, anorexia, loss of weight
- To report nausea, vomiting, palpitations
- To adhere to dietary regimen of calcium supplementation/phosphorus restriction
- To avoid excessive use of aluminum compounds, antacids
- Not to breastfeed
- Not to take mineral oil, antacids (magnesium) while taking vit D

PARoxetine (Rx)

(par-ox′e-teen)

Paxil, Paxil CR, Pexeva

Func. class.: Antidepressant, SSRI

Chem. class.: Phenylpiperidine derivative

Do not confuse:
PARoxetine/PACLitaxel
Paxil/PACLitaxel/Taxol

ACTION: Inhibits CNS neuron uptake of serotonin but not of norepinephrine or DOPamine

USES: Major depressive disorder, obsessive-compulsive disorder, panic disorder, generalized anxiety disorder, posttraumatic stress disorder, premenstrual disorders, social anxiety disorder

Unlabeled uses: Premature ejaculation, hot flashes, menopause

CONTRAINDICATIONS: Pregnancy (D), hypersensitivity, MAOI use, alcohol use

Precautions: Breastfeeding, geriatric patients, seizure history; patients with history of mania, renal/hepatic disease

Black Box Warning: Children, suicidal ideation

DOSAGE AND ROUTES

Generalized anxiety disorder

- **Adult: PO** 20 mg/day in AM, range 20-50 mg/day

Posttraumatic stress disorder

- **Adult: PO** 20 mg/day, range 20-60 mg/day

Depression

- **Adult: PO** 20 mg/day in AM; after 4 wk, if no clinical improvement is noted, dose may be increased by 10 mg/day each wk to desired response, max 50 mg/day or **CONT REL** 25 mg/day, may increase by 12.5 mg/day/wk up to 62.5 mg/day
- **Geriatric: PO** 10 mg/day, increase by 10 mg to desired dose, max 40 mg/day

Obsessive-compulsive disorder

- **Adult: PO** 40 mg/day in AM, start with 20 mg/day, increase in 10-mg/day increments, max 60 mg/day

Panic disorder

- **Adult: PO** start with 10 mg/day, increase in 10-mg/day increments to 40 mg/day, max 60 mg/day or **CONT REL** 12.5 mg/day, max 75 mg/day

Premenstrual disorders

- **Adult: CONT REL** 12.5 mg/day in AM

Renal dose

- **Adult: PO** CCr 30-60 ml/min, lower doses may be needed; CCr <30 ml/min, 10 mg/day initially, regular rel, max 40 mg/day; **CONT REL** 12.5 mg/day initially, max 50 mg/day

Hepatic dose

- **Adult: PO** 10 mg/day initially, max 40 mg **regular rel**; 12.5 mg/day initially, max 50 mg/day **(cont rel)**

Menopause symptoms/hot flashes (unlabeled)

- **Adult: PO (CONT REL)** 12.5 mg/day, may increase to 25 mg/day after 1 wk

Premature ejaculation (unlabeled)

- **Adult: PO** 20 mg/day

Available forms: Tabs 10, 20, 30, 40 mg; oral susp 10 mg/5 ml; cont rel tab 12.5, 25, 37.5 mg

Administer:

- Do not substitute Pexeva with Paxil, Paxil CR, or generic PARoxetine
- Store at room temperature; do not freeze
- Increased fluids, bulk in diet for constipation, urinary retention
- With food, milk for GI symptoms
- Crushed if patient is unable to swallow medication whole (regular rel only)
- Gum, hard candy, frequent sips of water for dry mouth
- Avoid use with other CNS depressants
- **Oral susp:** shake, measure with oral syringe or calibrated measuring device
- **Cont rel tab:** do not cut, chew, crush; do not give concurrently with antacids

SIDE EFFECTS

CNS: *Headache,* nervousness, insomnia, *drowsiness, anxiety, tremors, dizziness,* fatigue, *sedation,* abnormal dreams, agitation, apathy, euphoria, hallucinations, delusions, psychosis, seizures, neuroleptic-malignant-syndrome–like reactions, restless leg syndrome

CV: Vasodilation, postural hypotension, palpitations, bleeding

EENT: Visual changes

GI: *Nausea, diarrhea, dry mouth,* anorexia, dyspepsia, *constipation,* cramps, vomiting, taste changes, flatulence, decreased appetite

GU: Dysmenorrhea, decreased libido, urinary frequency, UTI, amenorrhea, cystitis, impotence; decreased sperm quality, decreased fertility, *abnormal ejaculation (male)*

INTEG: *Sweating,* rash

MS: Pain, arthritis, myalgia, myopathy, myosthenia

RESP: Infection, pharyngitis, nasal congestion, sinus headache, sinusitis, cough, dyspnea, yawning

SYST: Asthenia, fever, abrupt withdrawal syndrome

PHARMACOKINETICS

PO: Peak 5.2 hr, ext rel peak 6-10 hr; metabolized in liver by CYP2D6 enzyme system, unchanged products and metabolites excreted in feces and urine; half-life 21 hr (reg rel); 15-20 hr (cont rel); protein binding 95%

INTERACTIONS

⚠ **Increase:** serotonin syndrome—SSRIs, SNRIs, atypical psychotics, serotonin-receptor agonists, tricyclics, amphetamines, methylphenidate, traMADol

Decrease: level of digoxin

⚠ Do not use with MAOIs, pimozide, thioridazine; potentially fatal reactions can occur

Increase: bleeding—NSAIDs, thrombolytics, salicylates, platelet inhibitors, anticoagulants

Increase: PARoxetine plasma levels—cimetidine

Increase: agitation—L-tryptophan

Increase: side effects—highly protein-bound products

Increase: theophylline levels—theophylline

Increase: toxicity—CYP2D6 inhibitors (aprepitant, delavirdine, imatinib, nefazodone)

Decrease: PARoxetine levels—PHENobarbital and phenytoin

Drug/Herb

- Avoid use with St. John's wort, kava
- Possible serotonin syndrome: St. John's wort
- Hypertensive crisis: ephedra

NURSING CONSIDERATIONS

Assess:

Black Box Warning: **Depression/OCD/anxiety/panic attacks:** mental status: mood, sensorium, affect, suicidal tendencies (especially in child/young adult), increase in psychiatric symptoms, decreasing obsessive thoughts, compulsive behaviors, restrict amount available

- **Postural hypotension:** B/P (lying/standing), pulse q4hr; if systolic B/P drops 20 mm Hg, hold product, notify prescriber; take vital signs q4hr for patients with CV disease
- Hepatic/renal studies: AST, ALT, bilirubin, creatinine
- Weight weekly; appetite may decrease with product, constipation
- ECG for flattening of T wave, bundle branch or AV block, dysrhythmias in cardiac patients
- EPS, primarily in geriatric patients: rigidity, dystonia, akathisia
- **Renal status:** BUN, creatinine, urinary retention
- **Withdrawal symptoms:** headache, nausea, vomiting, muscle pain, weakness; not usual unless product discontinued abruptly, taper over 1-2 wk
- Alcohol intake; if alcohol is consumed, hold dose until morning

⚠ **Serotonin, neuroleptic malignant syndrome:** hallucinations, coma, headache, agitation, shivering, sweating, tachycardia, diarrhea, tremors, hypertension, hyperthermia, rigidity, delirium, coma, myoclonus, agitation, nausea, vomiting

Evaluate:

• Therapeutic response: decreased depression

Teach patient/family:

• That therapeutic effect may take 1-4 wk

• To use caution when driving, performing other activities requiring alertness because of drowsiness, dizziness, blurred vision

• Not to discontinue medication quickly after long-term use; may cause nausea, headache, malaise (abrupt withdrawal syndrome)

Black Box Warning: That depression may worsen, suicidal thoughts/behaviors; children/adolescents, young adults, to notify prescriber

• To avoid alcohol ingestion, OTC products unless approved by prescriber

• To report bleeding, headache, nausea, anxiety, or if depression continues

• To discuss sexual side effects: impotence, possible male infertility while taking product

TREATMENT OF OVERDOSE:

Gastric lavage, airway; for seizures, give diazepam, symptomatic treatment

⚠ HIGH ALERT

pazopanib

(paz-oh′pa-nib)

Votrient

Func. class.: Antineoplastic biologic response modifiers/multikinase angiogenesis inhibitor

Chem. class.: Kinase inhibitor

ACTION:

Targets vascular endothelial growth factor receptors; a multikinase angiogenesis inhibitor

USES:

Advanced renal cell carcinoma; soft-tissue sarcoma patients who have received prior chemotherapy

Unlabeled uses: Breast, ovarian cancer

CONTRAINDICATIONS:

Pregnancy (D), hypothyroidism, QT prolongation, MI, wound dehiscence, hypertension

Precautions: Breastfeeding, children, cardiac/renal/hepatic/dental disease, GI bleeding

Black Box Warning: Hepatic disease

DOSAGE AND ROUTES

• **Adult: PO** 800 mg/day without food (1 hr before, 2 hr after a meal), may decrease to 400 mg/day if not tolerated (renal cell cancer); or adjust in 200-mg increments based on toxicity (soft-tissue sarcoma)

Available forms: Tabs 200 mg

Administer:

• Give on an empty stomach (1 hr before or 2 hr after a meal); separate doses by ~24 hr

• Do not crush tablets owing to the potential for an increased rate of absorption, which can affect systemic exposure; only intact, whole tablets should be used

• If a dose is missed, it should not be taken if it is <12 hr until the next dose

• Store at 77°F (25°C)

SIDE EFFECTS

CNS: **Intracranial bleeding**, headache

CV: **Heart failure**, hypertension, **hypertensive crisis**, chest pain, **MI**, **QT prolongation**, **torsades de pointes**

GI: Nausea, **hepatotoxicity**, vomiting, dyspepsia, **GI hemorrhage**, anorexia, abdominal pain, **GI perforation**, **pancreatitis**, diarrhea; **hepatotoxicity (geriatric)**

HEMA: **Neutropenia**, **thrombocytopenia**, **bleeding**

INTEG: Rash, alopecia

MISC: Fatigue, epistaxis, pyrexia, hot sweats, increased weight, flulike symptoms, hypothyroidism, **hand–foot syndrome**, retinal tear/detachment

PHARMACOKINETICS

Protein binding 99%, peak 2-4 hr, duration 24 hr, half-life 31 hr

INTERACTIONS

Increase: QT prolongation—class IA/III antidysrhythmics, some phenothiazines, β-agonists, local anesthetics, tricyclics, haloperidol, chloroquine, droperidol, pentamidine; CYP3A4 inhibitors (amiodarone, clarithromycin, erythromycin, telithromycin, troleandomycin), arsenic trioxide, levomethadyl; CYP3A4 substrates (methadone, pimozide, QUEtiapine, quiNIDine, risperiDONE, ziprasidone)

Increase: pazopanib concentrations—CYP3A4 inhibitors (ketoconazole, itraconazole, erythromycin, clarithromycin)

Increase: plasma concentrations of simvastatin, calcium-channel blockers, ergots

Increase: plasma concentration of warfarin; avoid use with warfarin; use low-molecular-weight anticoagulants instead

Decrease: pazopanib concentrations—CYP3A4 inducers (dexamethasone, phenytoin, carBAMazepine, rifampin, PHENobarbital)

Drug/Food

Increase: pazopanib effect—grapefruit juice; avoid use while taking product

Drug/Herb

Decrease: pazopanib concentration—St. John's wort

NURSING CONSIDERATIONS

Assess:

Black Box Warning: Hepatic disease: fatal hepatotoxicity can occur; obtain LFTs baseline and at least every 2 wk × 2 mo, then monthly

⚠ **Fatal bleeding:** from GI, respiratory, GU tracts, permanently discontinue in those with severe bleeding

⚠ **Palmar-plantar erythrodysesthesia (hand-foot syndrome):** more common in those previously treated; reddening swelling, numbness, desquamation on palms and soles

⚠ **GI perforation/fistula:** discontinue if this occurs, assess for pain in epigastric area, dyspepsia, flatulence, fever, chills

⚠ **Hypertension/hypertensive crisis:** hypertension usually occurs in the first cycle; in those with preexisting hypertension, do not start treatment until B/P is controlled; monitor B/P every wk × 6 wk, then at start of each cycle or more often if needed, temporarily or permanently discontinue for severe uncontrolled hypertension

Evaluate:

- Therapeutic response: decreased in size, spread of tumor

Teach patient/family:

- To report adverse reactions immediately: bleeding
- About reason for treatment, expected results
- That effect on male fertility is unknown

⚠ **HIGH ALERT**

pegfilgrastim (Rx)

(peg-fill-grass′stim)

Neulasta

Func. class.: Hematopoietic agent

Chem. class.: Granulocyte colony-stimulating factor

ACTION: Stimulates proliferation and differentiation of neutrophils

USES: To decrease infection in patients receiving antineoplastics that are myelosuppressive; to increase WBC count in patients with product-induced neutropenia

CONTRAINDICATIONS: Hypersensitivity to proteins of *Escherichia coli*, filgrastim

Precautions: Pregnancy (C), breastfeeding, children <45 kg, adolescents, myeloid malignancies, sickle cell disease, leukocytosis, splenic rupture, ARDS, allergic-type reactions, peripheral blood stem cell (PBSC) mobilization

DOSAGE AND ROUTES

• **Adult: SUBCUT** 6 mg per chemotherapy cycle

Available forms: Sol for inj 6 mg/0.6 ml

Administer:

SUBCUT route

• Using single-use vials; after dose is withdrawn, do not reenter vial
• Do not use 6-mg fixed dose in infants, children, or others <45 kg
• Inspect sol for discoloration, particulates; if present, do not use
• Do not administer during the period 14 days before and 24 hr after cytotoxic chemotherapy
• Store in refrigerator; do not freeze; may store at room temperature up to 6 hr; avoid shaking, protect from light

SIDE EFFECTS

CNS: Fever, fatigue, headache, dizziness, insomnia, peripheral edema

GI: *Nausea,* vomiting, diarrhea, mucositis, anorexia, constipation, dyspepsia, abdominal pain, stomatitis, splenic rupture

HEMA: Leukocytosis, granulocytopenia, sickle cell crisis, hemoglobin S disease with crisis

INTEG: Alopecia

MISC: Chest pain, hyperuricemia, anaphylaxis, influenza-like illness, angioedema, antibody formation

MS: Skeletal pain

RESP: Respiratory distress syndrome

PHARMACOKINETICS

Half-life: 15-80 hr; 20-38 hr (children)

INTERACTIONS

• Do not use product concomitantly, 2 wk before, or 24 hr after administration of cytotoxic chemotherapy

Increase: release of neutrophils—lithium

Drug/Lab Test

Increase: uric acid, LDH, alk phos

NURSING CONSIDERATIONS

Assess:

⚠ **Allergic reactions, anaphylaxis:** rash, urticaria; discontinue product, have emergency equipment nearby

⚠ **ARDS:** dyspnea, fever, tachypnea, occasionally confusion; obtain ABGs, chest x-ray; product may need to be discontinued

• **Bone pain;** give mild analgesics
• Blood studies: CBC with differential, platelet count before treatment, 2× weekly; neutrophil counts may be increased for 2 days after therapy
• B/P, respirations, pulse before and during therapy

Evaluate:

• Therapeutic response: absence of infection

Teach patient/family:

• How to perform the technique for self-administration if product to be given at home: dose, side effects, disposal of containers and needles; provide instruction sheet
• To notify prescriber immediately of allergic reaction, trouble breathing, abdominal pain

⚠ HIGH ALERT

peginterferon alfa-2a (Rx)

(peg-in-ter-feer′on)

Pegasys

peginterferon alfa-2b (Rx)

PegIntron, SYLATRON

Func. class.: Immunomodulator

ACTION: Stimulates genes to modulate many biologic effects, including the inhibition of viral replication; inhibits ion cell proliferation, immunomodulation; stimulates effector proteins; decreases leukocyte, platelet counts

USES: Chronic hepatitis C infections in adults with compensated liver disease; chronic hepatitis B in adults who are HBe AG positive, HBe AG negative; HCV patients coinfected with HIV; nonresponders or relapsers with chronic hepatitis C, malignant melanoma

Unlabeled uses: Adenovirus, coronavirus, encephalomyocarditis virus, herpes simplex types 1 and 2, hepatitis D, acute hepatitis C, HIV, HPV, polio virus, rhinovirus, varicella-zoster, variola, vesicular stomatitis

CONTRAINDICATIONS:

Neonates, infants, sepsis; hypersensitivity to interferons, benzyl alcohol, *Escherichia coli* protein

Precautions: Pregnancy (C), breastfeeding, children <18 yr, geriatric patients, thyroid disorders, myelosuppression, renal/hepatic disease, suicidal/homicidal ideation, preexisting ophthalmologic disorders, pancreatitis, hemodialysis

Black Box Warning: Cardiac disease, depression, autoimmune disease, infection, use with ribavirin

DOSAGE AND ROUTES

Pegasys

• **Adult: SUBCUT** 180 mcg weekly × 48 wk; if poorly tolerated, reduce dose to 135 mcg weekly; in some cases, reduction to 90 mcg may be needed

Peg-Intron (chronic hepatitis C with compensated liver disease)

• **Adult >105 kg: SUBCUT** 1.5 mcg/kg/wk plus ribavirin 600 mg in AM and 800 mg in PM plus a HCV NS3/4A protease inhibitor; **86-105 kg:** 150 mcg/0.5 ml (0.5 ml of 150 mcg vial or Redipen) per wk plus ribavirin 1200 mg/day in 2 divided doses plus a HCV NS3/4A protease inhibitor; **81-85 kg:** 120 mcg/0.5 ml (0.5 ml of 120 mcg vial or Redipen) per wk plus ribavirin 1200 mg/day in 2 divided doses plus a HCV NS3/4A protease inhibitor; **76-80 kg:** 120 mcg/0.5 ml (0.5 ml of 120 mcg vial or Redipen) per wk plus ribavirin 400 mg in AM and 600 mg in PM plus a HCV NS3/4A protease inhibitor; **66-75 kg:** 96 mcg/0.4 ml (0.4 ml of 120 mcg vial or Redipen) per wk plus ribavirin 400 mg in AM and 600 mg in PM plus a HCV NS3/4A protease inhibitor; **61-65 kg:** 96 mcg/0.4 ml (0.4 ml of 120 mcg vial or Redipen) per wk plus ribavirin 800 mg/day in 2 divided doses plus a HCV NS3/4A protease inhibitor; **51-60 kg:** 80 mcg/0.5 ml (0.5 ml of 80 mcg vial or Redipen) per wk plus ribavirin 800 mg/day in 2 divided doses plus a HCV NS3/4A protease inhibitor; **40-50 kg:** 64 mcg/0.4 ml (0.4 ml of 80 mcg vial or Redipen) per wk plus ribavirin 800 mg/day in 2 divided doses plus a HCV NS3/4A protease inhibitor; **<40 kg:** 50 mcg/0.5 ml (0.5 ml of 50 mcg vial or Redipen) per wk plus ribavirin 800 mg/day in 2 divided doses plus a HCV NS3/4A protease inhibitor

Malignant melanoma (SYLATRON only)

• **Adult: SUBCUT** 6 mcg/kg/wk × 8 wk then 3 mcg/kg/wk × ≤5 yr, premedicate with acetaminophen 500-1000 mg 30 min before first dose, prn for subsequent doses

Available forms: Pegasys: inj 180 mcg/0.5 ml; **Pegintron:** 50, 80, 120, 150 mcg/0.5 ml; **SYLATRON** 296, 444, 888 mcg powder for inj

Administer:

• In evening to reduce discomfort, to allow patient to sleep through some side effects

• Continue pediatric dose in those who turn 18 yr

Interferon alfa-2a

• Use prefilled syringes; store in refrigerator

Interferon alfa-2b

SUBCUT/IM route

• Reconstitute with 1 ml of provided diluent/10-, 18-, or 50-million unit vials, swirl; sol for inj vials do not need reconstitution

SIDE EFFECTS

CNS: *Headache, insomnia, dizziness,* anxiety, hostility, lability, nervousness, depression, fatigue, poor concentration, pyrexia, suicidal ideation, homicidal

ideation, relapse of drug addiction, emotional lability, mania, psychosis
CV: Ischemic CV events
ENDO: Hypothyroidism, diabetes
GI: *Abdominal pain, nausea, diarrhea, anorexia, vomiting,* dry mouth, **fatal colitis, fatal pancreatitis**
HEMA: **Thrombocytopenia**, neutropenia, anemia, lymphopenia
INTEG: *Alopecia, pruritus, rash,* dermatitis
MISC: Blurred vision, inj-site reaction, rigors
MS: *Back pain,* myalgia, arthralgia
RESP: Cough, dyspnea

PHARMACOKINETICS

Half-life 15-80 hr, large variability in other pharmacokinetics

INTERACTIONS

- Use caution when giving with theophylline, myelosuppressive agents

Increase: hepatic damage-NNRTIs, NRTIs, protein inhibitors

Drug/Lab Test

Increase: triglycerides, ALT
Decrease: Hgb, platelets, WBCs, neutrophils
Abnormal: thyroid function test

NURSING CONSIDERATIONS

Assess:

- **Neuropsychiatric symptoms:** severe depression with suicidal ideation; monitor q3wk then 8 wk, then q6mo
- B/P, blood glucose, ophthalmic exam, pulmonary function
- ALT, HCV viral load; patients who show no reduction in ALT, HCV unlikely to show benefit of treatment after 6 mo
- Platelet counts, heme concentration, ANC, serum creatinine concentration, albumin, bilirubin, TSH, T_4, AFP

⚠ **Myelosuppression:** hold dose if neutrophil count is $<500 \times 10^6$/L or if platelets are $<50 \times 10^9$/L

- **Hypersensitivity:** discontinue immediately if hypersensitivity occurs
- **Infection:** vital signs, increased WBCs, fever; product may need to be discontinued

⚠ **Colitis/pancreatitis:** may be fatal; diarrhea, fever, nausea, vomiting, severe abdominal pain; if these occur, product should be discontinued

Evaluate:

- Therapeutic response: decreased chronic hepatitis C signs, symptoms; undetectable viral load

Teach patient/family:

- Provide patient or family member with written, detailed information about product
- Use 2 forms of effective contraception throughout treatment and for 6 mo after treatment (men and women) (combination therapy with ribavirin)
- To avoid driving, other hazardous activity if dizziness, confusion, fatigue, somnolence occur
- To use puncture-resistant container for disposal of needles/syringes if using at home

⚠ To report suicidal/homicidal ideation, visual changes, bleeding/bruising, pulmonary symptoms

pegloticase (Rx)

(peg-loe′ti-kase)

Krystexxa

Func. class.: Antigout agent
Chem. class.: Pegylated, recombinant, mammalian urate oxidase enzyme

ACTION: Lowers plasma uric acid concentration by converting uric acid to allantoin, which is readily excreted by the kidneys

USES: Chronic gout in patients experiencing treatment failure

CONTRAINDICATIONS: Hypersensitivity, G6PD deficiency

Precautions: Pregnancy (C), breastfeeding, children/infants/neonates, African-American patients, heart failure

Black Box Warning: Requires specialized setting, experienced clinician

P

DOSAGE AND ROUTES

• **Adult: IV INFUSION** 8 mg over 2 hr q2wk

Available forms: Sol for inj 8 mg/ml

Administer:

Intermittent IV INFUSION route

• ***Reconstitute:*** visually inspect for particulate matter, discoloration whenever sol/container permits; use aseptic technique; withdraw 8 mg (1 ml) of product/250 ml 0.9% NaCl or 0.45% NaCl; invert several times to mix, do not shake; discard remaining product in vial

• ***Premedicate:*** with antihistamines and corticosteroids in all patients and acetaminophen if deemed necessary to prevent anaphylaxis, infusion site reactions

• ***Infusion:*** if refrigerated, allow to come to room temperature; do not warm artificially; give over 120 min; do not give IV push or bolus; use infusion by gravity feed, syringe-type pump, or infusion pump; given in a specialized setting by those who can manage anaphylaxis or inj-site reactions; monitor during and for 1 hr after infusion; if reaction occurs, slow or stop infusion, may be restarted at a slower rate; do not admix

• Store diluted product in refrigerator or at room temperature for up to 4 hr; refrigerator is preferred; protect from light; do not freeze; use within 4 hr of preparation

SIDE EFFECTS

CNS: Dizziness, fatigue, fever

CV: *Chest pain,* heart failure, hypotension

GI: *Nausea,* vomiting, diarrhea, constipation

GU: Nephrolithiasis

HEMA: Anemia

INTEG: Ecchymosis, *erythema, pruritus, urticaria*

MS: Back pain, arthralgia, muscle spasm

SYST: Antibody formation, infection, anaphylaxis, infusion-related reactions

RESP: *Dyspnea,* upper respiratory infection

PHARMACOKINETICS

Remains primarily in intravascular space after administration, elimination half-life 2 wk, mean nadir uric acid concentration 24-72 hr

INTERACTIONS

Do not use with urate-lowering agents (allopurinol, probenecid, febuxostat, sulfinpyrazone)

NURSING CONSIDERATIONS

Assess:

• **Gout:** pain in big toe, feet, knees, redness, swelling, tenderness lasting a few days to weeks; intake of alcohol, purines, if patient is overweight or taking diuretics

• Obtain uric acid levels at baseline, before administration; 2 consecutive uric acid levels of >6 mg/dl may indicate therapy failure; greater chance of anaphylaxis; infection-related reactions

Black Box Warning: Specialized care setting: use only in facility where emergency equipment is available, anaphylaxis may occur

Black Box Warning: Infusion reactions: monitor for reactions for ≥1 hr after use

Evaluate:

• Therapeutic response: decrease uric acid levels; relief of pain, swelling, redness in toes, feet, knees

Teach patient/family:

• About reason for infusion, expected results

• To notify prescriber during infusion of allergic reactions or redness, swelling, pain at infusion site

• That continuing follow-up exams and uric acid levels will be needed

⚠ HIGH ALERT

PEMEtrexed (Rx)

(pem-ah-trex′ed)

Alimta

Func. class.: Antineoplastic-antimetabolite

Chem. class.: Folic acid antagonist

ACTION: Inhibits multiple enzymes that reduce folic acid, which is needed for cell replication

USES: Malignant pleural mesothelioma in combination with CISplatin; non–small-cell lung cancer as single agent; nonsquamous, non–small-cell lung cancer (1st-line treatment)

Unlabeled uses: Bladder, breast, colorectal, gastric, head/neck, pancreatic, renal cancers

CONTRAINDICATIONS: Pregnancy (D), hypersensitivity, ANC <1500 cells/mm³, CCr <45 ml/min, thrombocytopenia (<100,000/mm³), anemia

Precautions: Breastfeeding, children, renal/hepatic disease

DOSAGE AND ROUTES

• **Adult: IV INFUSION** 500-600 mg/m² given over 10 min on day 1 of 21-day cycle with CISplatin 75 mg/m² infused over 2 hr beginning ½ hr after end of PEMEtrexed infusion

Renal dose

• **Adult: IV INFUSION** CCr <45 ml/min, not recommended

Available forms: Inj, single-use vials, 100, 500 mg

Administer:

• Store at 77° F, excursions permitted at 59° F to 86° F, not light sensitive, discard unused portions

• Vit B_{12} and low-dose folic acid as prophylactic measure to treat related hematologic, GI toxicity; 400-1000 mcg/day × 7 days before 1st dose and × 21 days after last dose, vit B_{12} 1 mg IM 1 wk before 1st dose and q 3 cycles (9 wk) thereafter

• Premedicate with corticosteroid (dexamethasone) given PO bid day before, day of, and day after administration of PEMEtrexed

Intermittent IV INFUSION route

• Use cytotoxic handling procedures

• Reconstitute 500-mg vial/20 ml 0.9% NaCl inj (preservative free) = 25 mg/ml, swirl until dissolved, further dilute with 100 ml 0.9% NaCl inj (preservative free), give as IV infusion over 10 mg

• Use only 0.9% NaCl inj (preservative free) for reconstitution, dilution

• Do not begin a new cycle unless neutrophils (ANC) are ≥1500 cells/mm³, platelets are ≥100,000 cells/mm³, CCr is ≥45 ml/min

• **Platelet nadir <50,000/mm³ regardless of the ANC:** if necessary, delay until platelet count recovery, reduce PEMEtrexed and CISplatin by 50%; if grade 3/4 toxicity occurs after 2 reductions, discontinue both products

• **ANC nadir <500/mm³ when platelet nadir is ≥50,000/mm³:** if necessary, delay until ANC recovery, reduce PEMEtrexed and CISplatin by 75%; if grade 3/4 toxicity occurs after 2 reductions, discontinue both products

• **CTC Grade 3/4 nonhematologic toxicity including diarrhea requiring hospitalization and excluding neurotoxicity, mucositis, and grade 3 transaminase elevations:** withhold therapy until pretherapy value or condition, reduce by 75% both products; if grade 3 or 4 toxicity occurs after 2 reductions, discontinue both products

• **CTC grade 3/4 mucositis:** withhold therapy until pretherapy condition, reduce 50% of PEMEtrexed; if grade 3 or 4 mucositis occurs after 2 dosage reductions, discontinue both products

• **CTC grade 2 neurotoxicity:** withhold therapy until pretherapy value or condition, reduce dose of CISplatin by 50%

• **CTC grade 3/4 neurotoxicity:** discontinue both products

P

Y-site compatibilities: Acyclovir sodium, alfentanil, allopurinol, amifostine, amikacin, aminocaproic acid, aminophylline, amiodarone, amphotericin B lipid complex, amphotericin B liposome, ampicillin, ampicillin-sulbactam, atenolol, atracurium, azithromycin, aztreonam, bivalirudin, bleomycin, bumetanide, buprenorphine, butorphanol, CARBOplatin, carmustine, ceftizoxime, cefTRIAXone, cefuroxime, cimetidine, cisatracurium, CISplatin, clindamycin, cyclophosphamide, cycloSPORINE, cytarabine, DACTINomycin, DAPTOmycin, dexamethasone, digoxin, diltiazem, diphenhydrAMINE, DOCEtaxel, dolasetron, DOPamine, doxacurium, enalaprilat, ePHEDrine, EPINEPHrine, eptifibatide, ertapenem, esmolol, etoposide, famotidine, fenoldopam, fentaNYL, fluconazole, fludarabine, fluorouracil, foscarnet, fosphenytoin, furosemide, ganciclovir, gatifloxacin, glycopyrrolate, granisetron, haloperidol, heparin, hydrocortisone, HYDROmorphone, hydrOXYzine, ifosfamide, imipenem-cilastatin, insulin (regular), isoproterenol, ketorolac, labetalol, leucovorin, levofloxacin, lidocaine, linezolid, LORazepam, magnesium, mannitol, meperidine, meropenem, mesna, methyldopate, methylPREDNISolone, metoclopramide, metoprolol, midazolam, milrinone, mitoMYcin, mivacurium, morphine, moxifloxacin, nafcillin, naloxone, nesiritide, nitroglycerin, norepinephrine, octreotide, oxaliplatin, PACLitaxel, pamidronate, pancuronium, PENTobarbital, PHENobarbital, piperacillin-tazobactam, polymyxin B, potassium chloride/phosphates, procainamide, promethazine, propranolol, ranitidine, remifentanil, rocuronium, sodium acetate/bicarbonate/phosphates, succinylcholine, SUFentanil, sulfamethoxazole-trimethoprim, tacrolimus, theophylline, thiopental, thiotepa, ticarcillin, ticarcillin-clavulanate, tigecycline, tirofiban, trimethobenzamide, vancomycin, vecuronium, verapamil, vinBLAStine, vinCRIStine, vinorelbine, zidovudine, zoledronic acid

SIDE EFFECTS

CNS: *Fatigue, fever, mood alteration, neuropathy*

CV: Thrombosis/embolism, *chest pain,* arrhythmia exacerbation

GI: *Nausea, vomiting, anorexia, diarrhea, ulcerative stomatitis, constipation, dysphagia, dehydration*

GU: Renal failure, creatinine elevation

HEMA: Neutropenia, leukopenia, thrombocytopenia, myelosuppression, anemia

INTEG: *Rash, desquamation*

RESP: *Dyspnea*

SYST: Infection with/without neutropenia, radiation recall reaction, toxic epidermal necrolysis, Stevens-Johnson syndrome, anaphylaxis

PHARMACOKINETICS

Not metabolized; excreted in urine (unchanged 70%-90%); not known if excreted in breast milk; half-life 3.5 hr, 81% protein binding

INTERACTIONS

Increase: bleeding risk—NSAIDs, anticoagulants, platelet inhibitors, salicylates, thrombolytics

Decrease: clearance of PEMEtrexed—nephrotoxic products

NURSING CONSIDERATIONS

Assess:

⚠ Previous radiation treatments; radiation recall reactions have occurred (erythema, exfoliative dermatitis, pain, burning)

⚠ **Bone marrow depression:** CBC, differential, platelet count; monitor for nadir, recovery; new cycle should not begin if ANC <1500 cells/mm^3, platelets <100,000 cells/mm^3, CCr <45 ml/min

- Renal studies: BUN, serum uric acid, urine CCr, electrolytes before, during therapy
- I&O ratio; report fall in urine output to <30 ml/hr
- Monitor temperature q4hr; fever may indicate beginning infection; no rectal temperature

⚠ Neurotoxicity: CTC grade 2: withhold until resolution to at least pretherapy value/condition, reduce CISplatin by 50%; CTC grade 3-4: immediately discontinue product and CISplatin if given in combination
• **Mucositis:** CTC 3/4: withhold until resolution to at least pretherapy value/condition, reduce dose by 50%; if grade 3/4 occurs after 2 dosage reductions, discontinue product and CISplatin
• **Bleeding:** bleeding time, coagulation time during treatment; bleeding: hematuria, guaiac, bruising or petechiae, mucosa or orifices q8hr
• Buccal cavity q8hr for dryness, sores, ulceration, white patches, oral pain, bleeding, dysphagia
⚠ Severe allergic reaction/toxic epidermal necrolysis: rash, urticaria, itching, flushing
• Rinsing of mouth tid-qid with water, club soda; brushing of teeth bid-tid with soft brush or cotton-tipped applicators for stomatitis; use unwaxed dental floss

Evaluate:
• Therapeutic response: decreased spread of malignancy

Teach patient/family:
• To report any complaints, side effects to nurse or prescriber: black, tarry stools, chills, fever, sore throat, bleeding, bruising, cough, SOB, dark or bloody urine
• To avoid foods with citric acid, hot or rough texture if stomatitis is present
• To report stomatitis: any bleeding, white spots, ulcerations in mouth to prescriber; to examine mouth daily; to report symptoms to nurse; to use good oral hygiene
• That contraceptive measures recommended during therapy, for ≤8 wk after cessation of therapy; to discontinue breastfeeding because toxicity to infant may occur
• To avoid alcohol, salicylates, live vaccines
• To avoid use of razors, commercial mouthwash
• To eat foods high in folic acid; to take supplements as prescribed

⚠ HIGH ALERT

pembrolizumab
(pem′broe-liz′ue-mab)
Keytruda
Func. class.: Antineoplastics, biologic response modifiers
Chem. class.: Monoclonal antibodies

ACTION: A human monoclonal antibody that binds to the programmed death receptor-1 (PD-1) found on T-cells and blocks the interaction of PD-1 with its ligands, PD-L1 and PD-L2, on the tumor cell

USES: Treatment of unresectable or metastatic malignant melanoma in those who have disease progression after ipilimumab or in BRAF V600 mutation–positive patients who have disease progression after ipilimumab and a BRAF inhibitor

CONTRAINDICATIONS: Hypersensitivity, pregnancy (D), breastfeeding
Precautions: Immune-mediated colitis, immune-mediated hepatitis, immune-mediated hyperthyroidism/hypothyroidism; immune-mediated nephritis, acute interstitial nephritis, and renal failure; immune-mediated pneumonitis, adrenocortical insufficiency, arthritis, exfoliative dermatitis, hemolytic anemia, hypophysitis, myasthenia syndrome, myositis, optic neuritis, pancreatitis, partial seizures after inflammatory foci identified in brain parenchyma, rhabdomyolysis, uveitis, incidence of abortion/stillbirths

DOSAGE AND ROUTES
• **Adults: IV** INFUSION: 2 mg/kg over 30 min q3wk until disease progression
Available forms: Powder for injection 50 mg
Administer:
IV INFUSION route
• Add 2.3 ml of sterile water for injection, 50-mg vial (25 mg/ml); inject sterile

P

water along the walls of the vial and not directly on the powder
- Gently swirl and allow up to 5 min for bubbles to clear, do not shake, solution will be a clear to slightly opalescent, colorless to slightly yellow
- Add the required amount of product to a bag of normal saline (0.9% sodium chloride injection) to a final diluted concentration between 1 and 10 mg/ml; mix by gentle inversion
- Discard any unused solution left in the vial
- **Storage after reconstitution and dilution:** Store at room temperature up to 4 hr or refrigerate up to 24 hr (includes reconstitution, dilution, and administration time). If refrigerated, allow the diluted solution to warm to room temperature before use, give over 30 min
- Use a sterile, nonpyrogenic, low-protein binding 0.2- to 5-micron in-line or add-on filter
- Do not use with other drugs through the same infusion line
- **Grade 2 or 3 toxicity:** Withhold and give corticosteroids; resume when the adverse event recovers to grade ≤1. Permanently discontinue if there is no recovery within 12 wk, if the corticosteroid dose cannot be reduced to ≤10 mg/day of prednisone (or equivalent) within 12 wk, or for recurrent severe or grade 3 colitis
- **Grade 4 toxicity:** Permanently discontinue, give corticosteroids

Hepatitis:
- **Grade 2 toxicity (AST or ALT >3-5 × upper limit of normal [ULN] or total bilirubin >1.5-3 × ULN):** Withhold and give corticosteroids; resume when adverse event recovers to grade 1 or less. Permanently discontinue if there is no recovery within 12 wks or if the corticosteroid dose cannot be reduced to ≤10 mg/day of prednisone (or equivalent) within 12 wks
- **Grade 3 or 4 toxicity (AST or ALT >5 × ULN or total bilirubin >3 × ULN):** Permanently discontinue, give corticosteroids
- **Liver metastases and grade 2 elevated transaminase levels at baseline:** Permanently discontinue if AST/ALT levels increase by ≥50% over baseline and transaminase level elevations persist for at least 1 wk

SIDE EFFECTS

CNS: Seizures, myasthenia, headache, fever, insomnia, chills, dizziness, fatigue
ENDO: Hyponatremia, hypothyroidism/hyperthyroidism, hyperglycemia, hypocalcemia
EENT: Optic neuritis
GI: Nausea, vomiting, abdominal pain, pancreatitis, colitis, diarrhea, hepatitis, constipation
GU: Interstitial nephritis, renal failure
RESP: Cough, dyspnea, pneumonitis
INTEG: Rash, pruritus, skin discoloration
MS: Myalgia, rhabdomyolysis
SYST: Exfoliative dermatitis

INTERACTIONS

None known

Drug/lab test

Increase: LFTs, renal function studies

NURSING CONSIDERATIONS

Assess:
- For hyperthyroidism/hypothyroidism, renal function studies baseline, periodically during therapy, temporarily withheld or permanently discontinued
- For pneumonitis (new or worsening cough, chest pain, shortness of breath), confirm with radiographic imaging
- Liver function tests and hepatitis (e.g., jaundice, severe nausea/vomiting, easy bleeding or bruising, withhold and give corticosteroids if grade 2 hepatitis (AST or ALT >3-5 × ULN or total bilirubin >1.5-3 × ULN)

Evaluate:
- Therapeutic response: Decreased progression of multiple myeloma

Teach patient/family:
- To use highly effective contraceptive methods during and for 4 months after treatment, to contact their health care provider if pregnancy is suspected or confirmed (pregnancy D)

penciclovir topical

See Appendix B

PENICILLINS

penicillin G benzathine (Rx)

(pen-i-sill′in)

Bicillin L-A

penicillin G potassium (Rx)

Pfizerpen

penicillin G procaine (Rx)

penicillin V (Rx)

Apo-Pen-VK ♣, Penicillin VK

Func. class.: Broad-spectrum antiinfective

Chem. class.: Natural penicillin

ACTION: Interferes with cell-wall replication of susceptible organisms; lysis is mediated by cell-wall autolytic enzymes, results in cell death

USES: Respiratory infections, scarlet fever, erysipelas, otitis media, pneumonia, skin and soft-tissue infections, gonorrhea; effective for gram-positive cocci *(Staphylococcus, Streptococcus pyogenes, S. viridans, S. faecalis, S. bovis, S. pneumoniae)*, gram-negative cocci *(Neisseria gonorrhoeae)*, gram-positive bacilli *(Actinomyces, Bacillus anthracis, Clostridium perfringens, C. tetani, Corynebacterium diphtheriae, Listeria monocytogenes)*, gram-negative bacilli *(Escherichia coli, Proteus mirabilis, Salmonella, Shigella, Enterobacter, Streptobacillus moniliformis)*, spirochetes *(Treponema pallidum)*

CONTRAINDICATIONS: Hypersensitivity to penicillins, corn

Precautions: Pregnancy (B), breastfeeding; hypersensitivity to cephalosporins, carbapenem, sulfites; severe renal disease, GI disease, asthma

DOSAGE AND ROUTES

Penicillin G benzathine

Early syphilis

- **Adult: IM** 2.4 million units in single dose

Congenital syphilis

- **Child <2 yr: IM** 50,000 units/kg in single dose, max 2.4 million units as single inj

Prophylaxis of rheumatic fever, glomerulonephritis

- **Adult: IM** 1.2 million units in single dose
- **Child >27 kg: IM** 900,000-1.2 million units as single dose
- **Child ≤27 kg: IM** 300,000-600,000 units as single dose

Upper respiratory infections (group A streptococcal)

- **Adult: IM** 1.2 million units as single dose
- **Child >27 kg: IM** 900,000-1.2 million units as single dose
- **Child <27 kg: IM** 300,000-600,000 units as single dose

Available forms: Inj 600,000 units/ml

Penicillin G

Pneumococcal/streptococcal infections (serious)

- **Adult: IM/IV** 5-24 million units in divided doses q4-6hr
- **Child <12 yr: IV** 150,000-300,000 units/kg/day in 4-6 divided doses; max 24 million units/day

Renal dose

- CCr <10 ml/min, give full loading dose then 1/2 of loading dose q8-10hr

Available forms: Powder for inj 1, 5, 20 million units/vial; inj 1, 2, 3 million units/50 ml

Penicillin G procaine

Moderate to severe pneumococcal infections

- **Adult/child: IM** 600,000-1 million units as single dose or divided bid doses/day for 10 days to 2 wk

P

Pneumococcal pneumonia
• **Adult/child >12 yr: IM** 600,000-1 million units/day × 7-10 days
Moderately severe group A streptococcal/staphylococcal pneumonia
• **Adult/adolescent/child ≥60 lbs: IM** 600,000-1 million units/day
• **Adolescent/child <60 lbs: IM** 300,000 units/day
Available forms: Inj 600,000, 1,200,000 units/unit dose

Penicillin V

Pneumococcal/staphylococcal infections
• **Adult/adolescents/child >12 yr: PO** 250-500 mg q6hr
• **Child <12 yr: PO** 25-50 mg/kg/day in divided doses q6-8hr; max 2 g/day
Streptococcal infections
• **Adult/adolescent/child ≥12 yr: PO** 125-250 mg q6-8hr × 10 days
• **Child <12 yr and >27 kg: PO** 500 mg q8 or 12 hr × 10 days
• **Child <12 yr and ≤27 kg: PO** 250 mg q8hr or q12hr or 40 mg/kg/day in 3 divided doses × 10 days
Prevention of recurrence of rheumatic fever/chorea
• **Adult: PO** 125-250 mg bid continuously
Vincent's gingivitis/pharyngitis
• **Adult: PO** 250-500 mg q6-8hr
Renal dose
• Dosage reduction indicated with renal impairment (CCr <50 ml/min) based on clinical response, degree of impairment
Available forms: Tabs 250, 500 mg; powder for oral sol 125, 250 mg/5 ml
Administer:
• Store in dry, tight container; oral susp refrigerated 2 wk
Penicillin G benzathine
• No dilution needed, shake well, deep IM inj in large muscle mass; avoid intravascular inj; aspirate; do not give IV
Penicillin G
• Penicillin G sodium or potassium can be given IM or IV, vials containing 10 or 20 million units not for IM use

Intermittent IV INFUSION route
• Vials/bulk packages: dilute according to manufacturer's directions
• Frozen bags: thaw at room temperature, do not force thaw, no reconstitution needed
• Final concentration (100,000-500,000 units/ml—adults; 50,000 units/ml—neonate/infant)
• Total daily dose divided q4-6hr and given over 1-2 hr (adult), 15 min (infant/neonate)

Penicillin G potassium
Y-site compatibilities: Acyclovir, amiodarone, cyclophosphamide, diltiazem, enalaprilat, esmolol, fluconazole, foscarnet, heparin, HYDROmorphone, labetalol, magnesium sulfate, meperidine, morphine, perphenazine, potassium chloride, tacrolimus, theophylline, verapamil, vit B/C
Penicillin G procaine
• No dilution needed; give deep IM inj; avoid intravascular inj; aspirate; do not give IV
Penicillin V
• Orally on empty stomach for best absorption
• Oral susp: tap bottle to loosen, add 1/2 total amount of water, shake, add remaining water, shake; final concentration (125 or 250 mg/ml) store in refrigerator after reconstitution, discard after 14 days

SIDE EFFECTS

CNS: Lethargy, hallucinations, anxiety, depression, twitching, coma, seizures, hyperreflexia
GI: *Nausea, vomiting, diarrhea,* increased AST, ALT, abdominal pain, glossitis, colitis, pseudomembranous colitis
GU: Oliguria, proteinuria, hematuria, *vaginitis, moniliasis,* glomerulonephritis, renal tubular damage
HEMA: Anemia, increased bleeding time, bone marrow depression, granulocytopenia, hemolytic anemia
META: Hypo/hyperkalemia, alkalosis, hypernatremia
MISC: Anaphylaxis, serum sickness, Stevens-Johnson syndrome, *local pain,* tenderness and fever with IM inj

PHARMACOKINETICS

Penicillin G benzathine:

IM: Very slow absorption; time to peak 12-24 hr; duration 21-28 days; excreted in urine, feces, breast milk; crosses placenta

Penicillin G:

IV: Peak immediate

IM: Peak $^1/_4$-$^1/_2$ hr

PO: Peak 1 hr, duration 6 hr

Excreted in urine unchanged, excreted in breast milk, crosses placenta, half-life 30-60 min

Penicillin G procaine:

IM: Peak 1-4 hr, duration 15 hr, excreted in urine

Penicillin V:

PO: Peak 30-60 min, half-life 30 min, excreted in urine, breast milk

INTERACTIONS

Increase: penicillin effect—aspirin, probenecid

Increase: effect of heparin, methotrexate

Decrease: effect of oral contraceptives, typhoid vaccine

Decrease: antimicrobial effect of penicillin—tetracyclines

Drug/Lab Test

False positive: urine glucose, urine protein

NURSING CONSIDERATIONS

Assess:

- **Infection:** temperature; characteristics of sputum; wounds; urine; stools before, during, after treatment; C&S before therapy; product may be given as soon as culture is taken
- I&O ratio; report hematuria, oliguria because penicillin in high doses is nephrotoxic; renal tests: urinalysis, protein, blood

⚠ Any patient with compromised renal system because product is excreted slowly with poor renal system function; toxicity may occur rapidly

- Hepatic studies: AST, ALT
- Blood studies: WBC, RBC, Hct, Hgb, bleeding time

⚠ **Pseudomembranous colitis:** diarrhea, mucus, pus; bowel pattern before, during treatment

- Respiratory status: rate, character, wheezing, tightness in chest

⚠ Allergies before initiation of treatment, reaction of each medication; because of prolonged action, allergic reaction may be prolonged and severe; watch for anaphylaxis: rash, dyspnea, pruritus, laryngeal edema; skin eruptions after administration of penicillin to 1 wk after discontinuing product

- EPINEPHrine, suction, tracheostomy set, endotracheal intubation equipment
- Adequate fluid intake (2 L) during diarrhea episodes
- Scratch test to assess allergy after securing order from prescriber; usually done when penicillin is only product of choice

Evaluate:

- Therapeutic response: resolution of infection

Teach patient/family:

- To report sore throat, fever, fatigue; may indicate superinfection; CNS effects: depression, hallucinations, seizures
- To wear or carry emergency ID if allergic to penicillins
- To report diarrhea, with blood, pus, mucus to prevent dehydration
- To shake susp well before each dose; to store in refrigerator for up to 2 wk
- To use all medication prescribed
- To use additional contraception if using any of these products

TREATMENT OF ANAPHYLAXIS: Withdraw product; maintain airway; administer EPINEPHrine, aminophylline, O_2, IV corticosteroids

pentamidine (Rx)

(pen-tam′i-deen)

NebuPent, Pentam 300

Func. class.: Antiprotozoal

Chem. class.: Aromatic diamide derivative

ACTION: Interferes with DNA/RNA synthesis in protozoa

P

USES:
Treatment/prevention of *Pneumocystis jiroveci* infections

Unlabeled uses: *Leishmania/Trypanosoma* infections

CONTRAINDICATIONS:
Hypersensitivity

Precautions: Pregnancy (C), breastfeeding, children, blood dyscrasias, cardiac/renal/hepatic disease, diabetes mellitus, hypocalcemia, hypo/hypertension, anemia

DOSAGE AND ROUTES

- **Adult and child ≥4 mo: IV/IM** 4 mg/kg/day × 2-3 wk; **NEB** 300 mg via specific nebulizer given q4wk for prevention

Available forms: Inj, aerosol 300 mg/vial; sol for aerosol 60 mg/vial ✱

Administer:

- Store in refrigerator protected from light

Inhalation route

- Through nebulizer, using Raspirgard II jet nebulizer; mix contents in 6 ml of sterile water; do not use low pressure (<20 psi); flow rate should be 5-7 L/min (40-50 psi) air or O_2 source over 30-45 min until chamber is empty

IM route

- 300 mg diluted in 3 ml sterile water; give deep IM by Z-track; if painful by this route, rotate inj site

Intermittent IV INFUSION route

- Reconstitute 300 mg/3-5 ml of sterile water for inj, D_5W, withdraw dose and further dilute in 50-250 ml D_5W, give over 1-2 hr with patient lying down; check B/P often

Y-site compatibilities: Alfentanil, atracurium, atropine, benztropine, buprenorphine, calcium gluconate, CARBOplatin, caspofungin, chlorproMAZINE, cimetidine, CISplatin, cyclophosphamide, cycloSPORINE, cytarabine, DACTINomycin, diltiazem, gatifloxacin, zidovudine

SIDE EFFECTS

CNS: Disorientation, hallucinations, *dizziness,* confusion, drowsiness

CV: Hypotension, ventricular tachycardia, QT prolongation, dysrhythmias

GI: *Nausea, vomiting, anorexia;* increased AST, ALT; acute pancreatitis, metallic taste

GU: Acute renal failure, increased serum creatinine, renal toxicity, decreased urination

HEMA: Anemia, leukopenia, thrombocytopenia

INTEG: Sterile abscess, pain at inj site, pruritus, urticaria, *rash*

META: *Hyperkalemia,* hypocalcemia, hypoglycemia, hypomagnesemia

MISC: Fatigue, fever, chills, night sweats, anaphylaxis, Stevens-Johnson syndrome

RESP: Cough, SOB, bronchospasm (with aerosol), sore throat

PHARMACOKINETICS

IV: Peak 1 hr

IM: Peak 30 min

Excreted unchanged in urine (66%); half-life 9-12 hr (IM), 6 hr (IV)

INTERACTIONS

- Nephrotoxicity: aminoglycosides, amphotericin B, CISplatin, NSAIDs, vancomycin

⚠ Fatal dysrhythmias: erythromycin IV

Increase: QT prolongation—class IA/III antidysrhythmics, some phenothiazines, β-agonists, local anesthetics, tricyclics, haloperidol, chloroquine, droperidol, pentamidine; CYP3A4 inhibitors (amiodarone, clarithromycin, erythromycin, telithromycin, troleandomycin, arsenic trioxide, levomethadyl); CYP3A4 substrates (methadone, pimozide, QUEtiapine, quiNIDine, risperiDONE, ziprasidone)

Increase: myelosuppression—antineoplastics, radiation

Drug/Lab Test

Decrease: WBC, platelets, Hbg, Hct

Increase: BUN, creatinine

NURSING CONSIDERATIONS

Assess:

- Blood tests, blood glucose, CBC, platelets, calcium, magnesium
- I&O ratio; report hematuria, oliguria

- ECG for cardiac dysrhythmias; patient should be lying down when receiving product; severe hypotension may develop; monitor B/P during administration and until B/P stable
- Hepatic studies: AST, ALT
- Renal studies: urinalysis, BUN, creatinine; nephrotoxicity may occur; any patient with compromised renal system; product is excreted slowly with poor renal system function; toxicity may occur rapidly
- Signs of infection, anemia
- Bowel pattern before, during treatment
- Sterile abscess, pain at inj site
- Respiratory status: rate, character, wheezing, dyspnea
- Dizziness, confusion, hallucination
- Allergies before treatment, reaction of each medication; place allergies on chart in bright red letters; notify all people giving products
- Diabetic patients, hypoglycemia may occur, then hyperglycemia with prolonged therapy

Evaluate:

- Therapeutic response: resolution of AIDS-related PCP

Teach patient/family:

- To report sore throat, fever, fatigue (may indicate superinfection)
- To maintain adequate fluid intake
- IM injection is painful
- Complete entire course of medication

HIGH ALERT

pentazocine (Rx)

(pen-taz′oh-seen)

Talwin, Talwin NX

Func. class.: Opiate analgesic, antagonist

Chem. class.: Synthetic benzomorphan

Controlled Substance Schedule IV

ACTION: Inhibits ascending pain pathways in CNS, increases pain threshold, alters pain perception

USES: Moderate to severe pain

CONTRAINDICATIONS: Hypersensitivity to this product or sulfites; addiction (opiate)

Precautions: Pregnancy (C), breastfeeding, children <18 yr, addictive personality, increased intracranial pressure, MI (acute), severe heart disease, respiratory depression, renal/hepatic disease, seizure disorder, head trauma, bowel impaction, geriatric patients

DOSAGE AND ROUTES

- **Adult: IV/IM/SUBCUT** 30 mg q3-4hr prn, max 360 mg/day

Labor

- **Adult: IM** 30 mg as a single dose; **IV** 20 mg q2-3hr when contractions are regular, max 2-3 times

Renal dose

- **Adult:** CCr 10-50 ml/min, reduce dose by 25%; CCr <10 ml/min, reduce dose by 50%

Available forms: Inj 30 mg/ml

Administer:

- Store in light-resistant area at room temperature
- With antiemetic if nausea, vomiting occur
- When pain is beginning to return; determine dosage interval by patient response

IM/SUBCUT route

• Give IM deeply into large muscle mass, rotate sites; SUBCUT may cause necrosis with repeated inj

Direct IV route

• Undiluted or diluted in 5 mg/ml of sterile water for inj; give ≤5 mg over 1 min

Syringe compatibilities: Atropine, benzquinamide, butorphanol, chlorproMAZINE, cimetidine, dimenhyDRINATE, diphenhydrAMINE, droperidol, fentaNYL, HYDROmorphone, hydrOXYzine, meperidine, metoclopramide, morphine, perphenazine, prochlorperazine, promazine, promethazine, ranitidine, scopolamine

Y-site compatibilities: Heparin, hydrocortisone, potassium chloride, vit B/C

SIDE EFFECTS

CNS: *Drowsiness, dizziness, confusion, headache, sedation, euphoria,* hallucinations, dreaming, insomnia, lightheadedness

CV: Palpitations, bradycardia, change in B/P, tachycardia, increased B/P (high doses), hypotension, syncope, flushing

EENT: Tinnitus, blurred vision, miosis, diplopia

GI: *Nausea,* vomiting, anorexia, constipation, *cramps,* dry mouth

GU: Increased urinary output, dysuria, urinary retention

HEMA: Eosinophilia, decreased WBC

INTEG: *Rash,* urticaria, bruising, flushing, diaphoresis, pruritus, severe irritation at inj sites, Stevens-Johnson syndrome

RESP: Respiratory depression

PHARMACOKINETICS

Metabolized by liver, excreted by kidneys, crosses placenta, half-life 2-3 hr, extensive first-pass metabolism with <20% entering circulation

IM/SUBCUT: Onset 15-30 min, peak 1-2 hr, duration 2-4 hr

IV: Onset 2-3 min, duration 4-6 hr

INTERACTIONS

⚠ Unpredictable reactions: MAOIs

Increase: effects—CNS depressants; alcohol, sedative/hypnotics, antipsychotics, skeletal muscle relaxants

Decrease: effects—opiates

Drug/Lab Test

Increase: amylase

NURSING CONSIDERATIONS

Assess:

• **Pain:** intensity, duration, location before and 1 hr after SUBCUT/IM dose or 30 min after IV dose

• I&O ratio; check for decreasing output; may indicate urinary retention

• Bowel status: constipation; may need stimulant laxatives/stool softeners

• **Withdrawal symptoms** in opiate-dependent patients

• Abscesses, ulcerations, WBC count

• CNS changes: dizziness, drowsiness, hallucinations, euphoria, LOC, pupil reaction

• Allergic reactions: rash, urticaria

• **Respiratory depression:** character, rate, rhythm; notify prescriber if respirations are <10/min

• Need for pain medication, physical dependence

• Assistance with ambulation

• Safety measures: night-light, call bell within easy reach

Evaluate:

• Therapeutic response: decrease in pain

Teach patient/family:

• To report any symptoms of CNS changes, allergic reactions

• That physical dependency may result from extended use

• That withdrawal symptoms may occur: nausea, vomiting, cramps, fever, faintness, anorexia

• To avoid CNS depressants, alcohol

• To avoid driving, operating machinery if drowsiness occurs

• To use good oral hygiene, frequent rinsing of mouth to decrease dry mouth; to avoid gum, candy if drowsy

TREATMENT OF OVERDOSE:

Naloxone (Narcan) 0.2-0.8 mg IV, O_2, IV fluids, vasopressors

peramivir

(per-am′i-vir)

Rapivab

Func. class.: Antiviral

ACTION: Competitively binds to the active site of the influenza virus, inhibits the activity of strains of influenza A and B viruses

USES: Treatment of uncomplicated acute influenza (seasonal influenza A virus infection or seasonal influenza B virus infection)

Unlabeled uses: Treatment of H1N1 influenza A virus (swine influenza) infection in pediatric patients requiring hospitalization

CONTRAINDICATIONS: Hypersensitivity

Precautions: Breastfeeding, children, dialysis, infants, infection, pregnancy, psychosis, renal impairment

DOSAGE AND ROUTES

Influenzae

- **Adults: IV** 600 mg as a single dose infused over 15-30 min, give within 48 hr of onset of influenza symptoms

Available forms: Solution for injection 200 mg/20 ml

Administer:

- For IV use only, do not give IM, visually inspect parenteral products for particulate matter and discoloration
- **Dilute** the 10 mg/ml to a max volume of 100 ml, use only 0.9% or 0.45% NaCl, 5% dextrose, or LR
- **Storage of diluted solution:** Use immediately or refrigerate up to 24 hr. Refrigerated solution should be allowed to reach room temperature before administration. Discard any unused diluted solution after 24 hr
- Give over 15-30 min, do not mix or coadminister with other IV products

SIDE EFFECTS

CNS: delirium, psychosis, hallucinations, insomnia

GI: Constipation, diarrhea, vomiting

MISC: Rash, **Stevens-Johnson syndrome**

PHARMACOKINETICS

Protein binding <30%

INTERACTIONS

Avoid use with intranasal influenza vaccines, H1N1 vaccines

NURSING CONSIDERATIONS

Assess:

- Hypersensitivity reactions/Stevens-Johnson syndrome

Neuropsychiatric reactions: Delirium, psychosis, hallucinations

Evaluate:

- Therapeutic response: absence of developing influenza A or B

Teach patient/family:

- That product is only for use within 48 hr of infection

perindopril (Rx)

(per-in′doe-pril)

Aceon, Coversyl ✦

Func. class.: Antihypertensive

Chem. class.: Angiotensin-converting enzyme inhibitor

ACTION: Selectively suppresses the renin-angiotensin-aldosterone system; inhibits ACE; prevents the conversion of angiotensin I to angiotensin II and the dilation of arterial and venous vessels

USES: Hypertension, MI prophylaxis

Unlabeled uses: Heart failure, MI

CONTRAINDICATIONS: Hypersensitivity, history of angioedema

Black Box Warning: Pregnancy (D)

P

Precautions: Breastfeeding, renal disease, hyperkalemia, hepatic failure, dehydration, bilateral renal artery stenosis, cough, severe CHF, aortic stenosis, African descent

DOSAGE AND ROUTES

Hypertension

• **Adult: PO** 4 mg/day, may increase or decrease to desired response, range 4-8 mg/day; may give in 2 divided doses or as single dose, max 16 mg/day

Patients on diuretics

• **Adult: PO** 2-4 mg/day in 1-2 divided doses, range 4-8 mg/day

Stable CAD

• **Adult: PO** 4 mg/day × 2 wk, then increase as tolerated to 8 mg/day

Renal dose

• **Adult: PO** CCr 16-29 ml/min, 2 mg every other day; CCr 30-59 ml/min, 2 mg/day; CCr ≤15 ml/min 2 mg on dialysis days only

Available forms: Tabs scored 2, 4, 8 mg

Administer:

• As single dose or in 2 divided doses, without regard to meals

SIDE EFFECTS

CNS: *Insomnia, dizziness,* paresthesias, *headache,* fatigue, anxiety, depression

CV: *Hypotension,* chest pain, tachycardia, dysrhythmias, syncope, cardiac arrest

EENT: *Tinnitus;* visual changes; sore throat; double vision; dry, burning eyes

GI: Nausea, vomiting, colitis, cramps, diarrhea, constipation, flatulence, dry mouth, loss of taste, liver failure

GU: Proteinuria, renal failure, increased frequency of polyuria or oliguria

HEMA: Agranulocytosis, neutropenia, bone marrow suppression

INTEG: Rash, purpura, alopecia, hyperhidrosis

META: *Hyperkalemia*

RESP: Dyspnea, *dry cough,* crackles

SYST: Angioedema

PHARMACOKINETICS

Bioavailability 75%; peak 1 hr parent product, 3-7 hr prodrug; protein binding 68%; metabolized by liver (active metabolite perindoprilat); half-life 0.8-10 hr; excreted in urine

INTERACTIONS

Increase: effects of neuromuscular blocking agents, antihypertensives, lithium

Increase: antihypertensive effect—diuretics, NSAIDs

Increase: hypersensitivity—allopurinol

Increase: severe hypotension—diuretics, other antihypertensives

Increase: hyperkalemia—salt substitutes, potassium-sparing diuretics, potassium supplements, angiotensin II receptor antagonists

Decrease: effects of NSAIDs

Decrease: antihypertensive effect—NSAIDs, salicylates

Drug/Herb

Increase: antihypertensive effect—hawthorn

Decrease: antihypertensive effect—ephedra

Drug/Lab Test

Increase: ALT, alk phos, cholesterol, uric acid

Decrease: Hgb/Hct

Interference: glucose/insulin tolerance tests

NURSING CONSIDERATIONS

Assess:

• **Hypertension:** B/P, pulse q4hr; note rate, rhythm, quality

• Electrolytes: K, Na, Cl during 1st 2 wk of therapy

• Baselines of renal, hepatic studies before therapy begins, 1 wk into therapy

• Skin turgor, dryness of mucous membranes for hydration status, dry mouth

• **CHF:** edema, dyspnea, wet crackles

• **Angioedema:** facial swelling, urticaria; product should be discontinued, may be more common in African Americans

Evaluate:

• Therapeutic response: decreased B/P

Teach patient/family:

- Not to use OTC (cough, cold, allergy) products unless directed by prescriber; to avoid salt substitutes
- To avoid sunlight or to wear sunscreen for photosensitivity
- To comply with dosage schedule, even if feeling better
- To notify prescriber of mouth sores, sore throat, fever, swelling of hands or feet, irregular heartbeat, chest pains, signs of angioedema
- That excessive perspiration, dehydration, vomiting, diarrhea may lead to fall in B/P; to consult prescriber if these occur
- That product may cause dizziness, fainting; that lightheadedness may occur during 1st few days of therapy; to avoid hazardous activities
- That product may cause skin rash or impaired perspiration; that angioedema may occur and to discontinue product if it occurs
- Not to discontinue product abruptly
- To rise slowly to sitting or standing position to minimize orthostatic hypotension
- To report persistent, sustained cough
- To avoid potassium supplements, salt substitutes

Black Box Warning: To notify prescriber if pregnancy is planned or suspected; pregnancy (D)

TREATMENT OF OVERDOSE:

Lavage, IV atropine for bradycardia, IV theophylline for bronchospasm, digoxin, O_2, diuretic for cardiac failure

pertuzumab

(per-too′zoo-mab)

Perjeta

Func. class.: Antineoplastic biologic-response modifier

Chem. class.: Monoclonal antibody, antineoplastic

ACTION: Blocks liquid-dependent action of human epidermal growth factor-2 (HER2), inhibiting signal pathways

USES: First-line treatment of (HER2) positive metastatic breast cancer with trastuzumab and DOCEtaxel

CONTRAINDICATIONS:

Black Box Warning: Pregnancy (category D)

Precautions: Breastfeeding, children, infants, neonates, cardiac arrhythmias, MI, cardiac disease, heart failure, hypertension, infusion-related reactions

DOSAGE AND ROUTES

- **Adult: IV** 840 mg over 60 min, then after 3 wk 420 mg over 30-60 min every 3 wk; give with trastuzumab 8 mg/kg IV over 90 min, then after 3 wk 6 mg/kg over 30-90 min every 3 wk and DOCEtaxel 75 mg/m^2 IV every 3 wk; dosage may be escalated to 100 mg/m^2

Available forms: Solution for inj 420 mg/14 ml (single-use vials)

Administer:

- Visually inspect for particulate matter and discoloration

Dilution and preparation

- Withdraw the calculated dose from the vial and add to 250 ml 0.9% sodium chloride to PVC or non-PVC polyolefin infusion bag; do not dilute with dextrose 5% solution
- Dilute in normal saline only; do not mix or dilute with other drugs or dextrose solutions
- Mix the diluted solution by gentle inversion; do not shake

IV infusion

- Administer the diluted solution immediately
- Do not administer as an IV push or bolus
- Give the first dose of 840 mg over 60 min and subsequent 420 mg doses over 30–60 min
- If the diluted solution is not used immediately, store at 2°-8° C for up to 24 hr

Delayed or missed doses

- If time since previous dose is <6 wk, give 420 mg IV (do not wait for next scheduled dose)
- If time since previous dose is ≥6 wk, give 840 mg IV over 60 min, followed 3 wk later by 420 mg IV over 30–60 min repeated every 3 wk
- If DOCEtaxel is discontinued, this product and trastuzumab may continue

SIDE EFFECTS

CNS: Headache, fever, *peripheral neuropathy,* chills, *fatigue*, asthenia
CV: Heart failure
EENT: Lacrimation, stomatitis
GI: *Nausea*, vomiting, diarrhea, dysgeusia
HEMA: Anemia, neutropenia
MS: Myalgia
RESP: Upper respiratory infection
SYST: Anaphylaxis, infection, antibody formation

PHARMACOKINETICS

Median half-life 18 days

NURSING CONSIDERATIONS

Assess:

HER2 overexpression: Testing should be done to identify HER2 overexpression before using this product

Decreased left ventricular ejection fraction (LVEF): ⚠ Can occur and is increased in those with a history of prior anthracycline use or radiotherapy to the chest; evaluate LVEF at baseline and every 3 mo; withhold therapy ×3 wk if LVEF is <40% or LVEF is 40%-45% with a 10% or greater absolute decrease from baseline; resume therapy if the LVEF is recovered to >45% or to 40%-45% with <10% absolute decrease at reassessment; if the LVEF has not improved or has declined further, consider permanently discontinuing pertuzumab and trastuzumab after a risk/benefit assessment

Infusion-related reactions/hypersensitivity: ⚠ Assess anaphylactoid reaction, acute infusion reaction, cytokine-release syndrome 60 min after the first infusion, 30 min after other infusions; monitor for pyrexia, chills, fatigue, headache, asthenia, hypersensitivity, and vomiting; if a significant reaction occurs, slow or interrupt the infusion; permanent discontinuation may be needed in severe reactions

Black Box Warning: Pregnancy: Determine if pregnancy is planned or suspected; patients who become pregnant during therapy should report exposure to the Genentech Adverse Event line at 1-888-835-2555 and enroll in the MOTHER pregnancy registry at 1-800-690-6720

Neutropenia: ⚠ Can occur, but occurs more commonly when trastuzumab is also used

Upper respiratory infection:

- Monitor for dyspnea, shortness of breath, fever

Evaluate:

- Decreased size, spread of tumor

Teach patient/family:

Black Box Warning: Counsel women of childbearing age on the need for contraception during and for 6 mo after therapy; advise patients who suspect pregnancy to contact their health care provider immediately; discontinue breastfeeding

RARELY USED

phentolamine (Rx)

(fen-tole′a-meen)

Func. class.: Antihypertensive

Chem. class.: α-Adrenergic blocker

USES: Hypertension; pheochromocytoma; prevention/treatment of dermal necrosis following extravasation of norepinephrine, DOPamine, EPINEPHrine

CONTRAINDICATIONS: Hypersensitivity, MI, coronary insufficiency, angina, hypotension

DOSAGE AND ROUTES

Treatment of hypertensive episodes in pheochromocytoma

- **Adult: IM/IV**5 mg, repeat if necessary
- **Child: IV** 0.05-0.1 mg/kg/dose, repeat if necessary; max 5 mg

Diagnosis of pheochromocytoma

- **Adult: IV** 5 mg
- **Child: IV** 0.05 mg/kg; if negative, repeat with 0.1 mg/kg IV

Treatment of necrosis

- **Adult:** 5-10 mg/10 ml **NS** injected into area of norepinephrine extravasation within 12 hr
- **Child:** 0.1-0.2 mg/kg, max 5 mg

Prevention of necrosis

- **Adult:** 10 mg/L of norepinephrine-containing sol
- **Child: IV** 0.1-0.2 mg/kg, max 5 mg

phenylephrine nasal agent

See Appendix B

phenylephrine ophthalmic

See Appendix B

phenytoin (Rx)

(fen′i-toh-in)

Dilantin, Dilantin Infatabs, Phenytek

Func. class.: Anticonvulsant; antidysrhythmic (IB)

Chem. class.: Hydantoin

ACTION: Inhibits spread of seizure activity in motor cortex by altering ion transport; increases AV conduction

USES: Generalized tonic-clonic seizures; status epilepticus; nonepileptic seizures associated with Reye's syndrome or after head trauma; complex partial seizures

Unlabeled uses: Migraines, diabetic neuropathy, neuropathic pain, paroxysmal atrial tachycardia, ventricular tachycardia

CONTRAINDICATIONS: Pregnancy (D), hypersensitivity, psychiatric condition, bradycardia, SA and AV block, Stokes-Adams syndrome

Precautions: Geriatric patients, allergies, renal/hepatic disease, petit mal seizures, hypotension, myocardial insufficiency, Asian patients positive for HLA-B1502, hepatic failure, acute intermittent porphyria

Black Box Warning: IV use

DOSAGE AND ROUTES

Seizures

- **Adult: PO** 15-20 mg/kg (ext rel) in 3-4 divided doses given q2hr or 400 mg, then 300 mg q2hr × 2 doses; maintenance 4-7 mg/kg/day; **IV** 15-20 mg/kg, max 25-50 mg/min, then 100 mg q6-8hr
- **Child: PO** 5 mg/kg/day in 2-3 divided doses, maintenance 4-8 mg/kg/day in 2-3 divided doses, max 300 mg/day; **IV** 15-20 mg/kg at 1-3 mg/kg/min

Status epilepticus

- **Adult: IV** 15-20 mg/kg, max 25-50 mg/min, may give 100 mg q6-8hr thereafter
- **Child: IV** 15-20 mg/kg, max in divided doses 1-3 mg/kg/min

Ventricular dysrhythmias

- **Adult: PO** loading dose 1 g divided over 24 hr, then 500 mg/day × 2 days; **IV** 250 mg over 5 min until dysrhythmias subside or until 1 g is given or 100 mg q15min until dysrhythmias subside or until 1 g is given
- **Child: PO** 3-8 mg/kg or 250 mg/m^2/day as single dose or 2 divided doses; **IV** 3-8 mg/kg over several min or 250 mg/m^2/day as single dose or 2 divided doses

Renal/hepatic dose

- Do not use loading dose if CCr <10 ml/min or hepatic failure

P

Neuropathic pain/diabetic neuropathy (unlabeled)
- **Adult: PO** 300 mg/day in divided doses

Migraine prophylaxis (unlabeled)
- **Adult: PO** 200-400 mg/day

Available forms: Susp 25 mg/5 ml; chewable tabs 50 mg; inj 50 mg/ml; ext rel caps 100, 200, 300 mg; prompt rel caps 100 mg

Administer:

PO route
- Do not interchange chewable product with caps, not equivalent; only ext rel caps to be used for once-a-day dosing
- **Oral susp:** shake well before each dose given via G tube/NG tube; dilute susp before administration; flush tube with 20 ml water after dose; hold tube feedings 1 hr before and 1 hr after dose
- Allow 7-10 days between dosage changes
- Divided PO doses with or after meals to decrease adverse effects
- 2 hr before or after antacid, enteral feeding

Direct IV route

Black Box Warning: Give undiluted at ≤50 mg/min (adult) 1-3 mg/kg/min; 0.5-1 mg/kg/min (neonates), monitor for CV reactions

Intermittent IV INFUSION route

Black Box Warning: Dilute dose in NS to ≤6.7 mg/ml; complete infusion within 1 hr of preparation; use 0.22- or 0.55-micron in-line particulate final filter between IV catheter and tubing; flush IV line or catheter with NS before and after use; give at ≤50 mg/min (adult), 0.5-1 mg/kg/min (child, infant, neonate)

Additive compatibilities: Do not admix

SIDE EFFECTS

CNS: Dizziness, insomnia, paresthesias, depression, suicidal tendencies, aggression, headache, confusion, slurred speech, peripheral neuropathy

CV: Hypotension, ventricular fibrillation, bradycardia, cardiac arrest

EENT: Nystagmus, diplopia, blurred vision

ENDO: Diabetes insipidus

GI: Nausea, vomiting, constipation, anorexia, weight loss, hepatitis, jaundice, gingival hyperplasia, abdominal pain

GU: Nephritis, urine discoloration, sexual dysfunction

HEMA: Agranulocytosis, leukopenia, aplastic anemia, thrombocytopenia, megaloblastic anemia

INTEG: Rash, lupus erythematosus, Stevens-Johnson syndrome, hirsutism, toxic epidermal necrolysis

SYST: Hypocalcemia, purple glove syndrome (IV), DRESS, anaphylaxis, exacerbates myasthenia gravis

PHARMACOKINETICS

Metabolized by liver, excreted by kidneys, protein binding 90%-95%, half-life 7-42 hr, dose dependent

PO: Onset 2-24 hr, peak 1½-2½ hr, duration 6-12 hr

PO-ER: Onset 2-24 hr, peak 4-12 hr, duration 12-36 hr

IV: Onset 1-2 hr, duration 12-24 hr

INTERACTIONS

- Do not use with delavirdine, decreased response, resistance

Increase: phenytoin effect—benzodiazepines, cimetidine, tricyclics, salicylates, valproate, cycloSERINE, diazepam, chloramphenicol, disulfiram, alcohol, amiodarone, sulfonamides, FLUoxetine, gabapentin, H_2 antagonists, azole antifungals, estrogens, succinamides, phenothiazines, methylphenidate, felbamate, traZODone

Decrease: phenytoin effects—alcohol (chronic use), antacids, barbiturates, carBAMazepine, rifampin, calcium (high dose), folic acid

Drug/Food

Enteral tube feeding: may decrease absorption of oral product; do not use enteral feedings 2 hr before or 2 hr after dose

Drug/Lab Test
Increase: glucose, alk phos, GGT
Decrease: dexamethasone, metyrapone test serum, PBI, urinary steroids

NURSING CONSIDERATIONS

Assess:

⚠ **Phenytoin hypersensitivity syndrome** 3-12 wk after start of treatment: rash, temperature, lymphadenopathy; may cause hepatotoxicity, renal failure, rhabdomyolysis

⚠ **Serious skin disorders:** for beginning rash that may lead to Stevens-Johnson syndrome or toxic epidermal necrolysis; phenytoin should not be used again; may occur more often among Asian patients with HLA-B 1502

⚠ **Purple glove syndrome** with IV use

- Phenytoin level: toxic level 30-50 mcg/ml, therapeutic level: 7.5-20 mcg/ml; wait ≥1 wk to draw levels
- **Seizures:** duration, type, intensity, precipitating factors; obtain EEG periodically; monitor therapeutic level
- Blood studies: CBC, platelets q2wk until stabilized, then monthly × 12, then q3mo; discontinue product if neutrophils <1600/mm^3; renal function: albumin concentration; folic acid levels, LFTs

⚠ Mental status: mood, sensorium, affect, memory (long, short), suicidal thoughts/behaviors

- Monitor EKG, B/P, respiratory function during IV loading dose; verify potency of IV access port before IV infusion
- Monitor EEG function and serum levels periodically
- **Blood dyscrasias:** fever, sore throat, bruising, rash, jaundice

Evaluate:

- Therapeutic response; decrease in severity of seizures, ventricular dysrhythmias

Teach patient/family:

- That, if diabetic, blood glucose should be monitored
- That urine may turn pink
- Not to discontinue product abruptly because seizures may occur
- **Oral hygiene:** about the proper brushing of teeth using a soft toothbrush, flossing to prevent gingival hyperplasia; about the need to see dentist frequently
- To avoid hazardous activities until stabilized on product
- To carry emergency ID stating product use
- That heavy use of alcohol may diminish effect of product; to avoid OTC medications
- Not to change brands or forms once stabilized on therapy because brands may vary
- Not to use antacids within 2 hr of product
- To use nonhormonal contraception; to notify prescriber if pregnancy is planned or suspected, pregnancy (D)
- To notify prescriber of unusual bleeding, bruising, petechiae (bleeding), clay-colored stools, abdominal pain, dark urine, yellowing of skin or eyes (hepatotoxicity); slurred speech, headache, drowsiness
- To report suicidal thoughts/behaviors immediately

phosphate/biphosphate (OTC)

Fleet Enema, Phospho-Soda
Func. class.: Laxative, saline

ACTION: Increases water absorption in the small intestine by osmotic action; laxative effect occurs by increased peristalsis and water retention

USES: Constipation, bowel or rectal preparation for surgery, exam

CONTRAINDICATIONS: Hypersensitivity, rectal fissures, abdominal pain, nausea, vomiting, appendicitis, acute surgical abdomen, ulcerated hemorrhoids, sodium-restricted diet, renal failure, hyperphosphatemia, hypocalcemia, hypokalemia, hypernatremia, Addison's disease, CHF, ascites, bowel perforation, megacolon, imperforate anus

Black Box Warning: GI obstruction, renal failure

Precautions: Pregnancy (C)

Black Box Warning: Colitis, geriatric hypovolemia, renal disease

DOSAGE AND ROUTES

- **Adult: PO** 20-30 ml (Phospho-Soda)
- **Child: PO** 5-15 ml (Phospho-Soda)
- **Adult and child >12 yr: RECT** 1 enema (118 ml)
- **Child 2-12 yr: RECT** 1/2 enema (59 ml)

Available forms: Enema 7 g phosphate/19 g biphosphate/118 ml; oral sol 18 g phosphate/48 g biphosphate/100 ml

Administer:

- Alone for better absorption; do not take within 1-2 hr of other products

SIDE EFFECTS

CV: Dysrhythmias, cardiac arrest, hypotension, widening QRS complex

GI: *Nausea, cramps,* diarrhea

META: Electrolyte, fluid imbalances

PHARMACOKINETICS

Onset 30 min-3 hr, excreted in feces

NURSING CONSIDERATIONS

Assess:

- **Stools:** color, amount, consistency; bowel pattern, bowel sounds, flatulence, distention, fever, dietary patterns, exercise; cramping, rectal bleeding, nausea, vomiting; if these occur, product should be discontinued
- Blood, urine electrolytes if product used often

Evaluate:

- Therapeutic response: decrease in constipation

Teach patient/family:

- Not to use laxatives for long-term therapy because bowel tone will be lost
- That normal bowel movements do not always occur daily
- Not to use in presence of abdominal pain, nausea, vomiting
- To notify prescriber if constipation unrelieved or if symptoms of electrolyte imbalance occur: muscle cramps, pain, weakness, dizziness, excessive thirst
- To maintain fluid consumption

physostigmine ophthalmic

See Appendix B

phytonadione (Rx)

(fye-toe-na-dye′one)

Mephyton, Vit K

Func. class.: Vit K_1, fat-soluble vitamin

ACTION:
Needed for adequate blood clotting (factors II, VII, IX, X)

USES:
Vit K malabsorption, hypoprothrombinemia, prevention of hypoprothrombinemia caused by oral anticoagulants, prevention of hemorrhagic disease of the newborn

CONTRAINDICATIONS:
Hypersensitivity, severe hepatic disease, last few weeks of pregnancy

Precautions: Pregnancy (C), neonates, hepatic disease

Black Box Warning: IV use

DOSAGE AND ROUTES

Hypoprothrombinemia caused by vit K malabsorption

- **Adult: PO/IM** 2.5-25 mg, may repeat or increase to 50 mg
- **Child: PO** 2.5-5 mg
- **Infant: PO/IM** 2 mg

Prevention of hemorrhagic disease of the newborn

- **Neonate: IM** 0.5-1 mg within 1 hr after birth, repeat after 2-3 wk if required

Hypoprothrombinemia caused by oral anticoagulants

- **Adult and child: PO/SUBCUT/IM** 1-10 mg, may repeat 12-48 hr after **PO** dose or 6-8 hr after **SUBCUT/IM** dose based on INR

Available forms: Tabs 5 mg; inj 10 mg/ml, 1 mg/0.5 ml

Administer:

- Store in tight, light-resistant container (PO)

Intermittent IV INFUSION route

- After diluting with ≥10 ml D_5NS; give max 1 mg/min

⚠ IV only when other routes not possible (deaths have occurred)

Y-site compatibilities: Alfentanil, amikacin, aminophylline, ascorbic acid, atracurium, atropine, azaTHIOprine, aztreonam, bumetanide, buprenorphine, butorphanol, calcium chloride/gluconate, ceFAZolin, cefonicid, cefoperazone, cefotaxime, cefoTEtan, cefOXitin, cefTAZidime, ceftizoxime, cefTRIAXone, cefuroxime, chloramphenicol, chlorproMAZINE, cimetidine, clindamycin, cyanocobalamin, cycloSPORINE, dexamethasone, digoxin, diphenhydrAMINE, DOPamine, doxycycline, enalaprilat, ePHEDrine, EPINEPHrine, epoetin alfa, erythromycin, esmolol, famotidine, fentaNYL, fluconazole, folic acid, furosemide, ganciclovir, gentamicin, glycopyrrolate, heparin, hydrocortisone, imipenem/cilastatin, indomethacin, insulin, isoproterenol, ketorolac, labetalol, lidocaine, mannitol, meperidine, metaraminol, methoxamine, methyldopate, metoclopramide, metoprolol, metroNIDAZOLE, midazolam, morphine, multivitamins, nafcillin, nalbuphine, naloxone, nitroglycerin, nitroprusside, norepinephrine, ondansetron, oxacillin, oxytocin, papaverine, penicillin G potassium, pentamidine, pentazocine, PENTobarbital, PHENobarbital, phentolamine, phenylephrine, potassium chloride, procainamide, prochlorperazine, propranolol, pyridoxime, ranitidine, sodium bicarbonate, succinylcholine, SUFentanil, theophylline, thiamine, ticarcillin/clavulanate, tobramycin, tolazoline, trimetaphan, urokinase, vancomycin, vasopressin, verapamil, vit B with C

SIDE EFFECTS

CNS: Headache, **brain damage** (large doses)

GI: Nausea, decreased LFTs

HEMA: **Hemolytic anemia, hemoglobinuria, hyperbilirubinemia**

INTEG: Rash, urticaria

RESP: **Bronchospasm**, dyspnea, feeling of chest constriction, **respiratory arrest**

PHARMACOKINETICS

PO/INJ: Metabolized, crosses placenta

INTERACTIONS

Decrease: action of phytonadione—bile acid sequestrants, sucralfate, antiinfectives, salicylates, mineral oil

Decrease: action of warfarin—large dose of product

NURSING CONSIDERATIONS

Assess:

- **Bleeding:** emesis, stools, urine; pressure on all venipuncture sites; avoid all inj if possible
- PT during treatment (2-sec deviation from control time, bleeding time, clotting time); monitor for bleeding, pulse, and B/P

Evaluate:

- Therapeutic response: prevention of hemorrhagic disease of the newborn, resolution of hypoprothrombinemia

Teach patient/family:

- Not to take other supplements, OTC products, prescription products unless directed by prescriber
- About the necessary foods for associated diet
- To avoid IM inj; to use soft toothbrush; not to floss; to use electric razor until coagulation defect corrected
- To report symptoms of bleeding
- About the importance of frequent lab tests to monitor coagulation factors
- To notify all health care providers of use of this product
- To carry emergency ID describing condition and products used

P

pilocarpine ophthalmic

See Appendix B

pimecrolimus topical

See Appendix B

HIGH ALERT

pioglitazone (Rx)

(pie-oh-glye′ta-zone)

Actos

Func. class.: Antidiabetic, oral

Chem. class.: Thiazolidinedione

ACTION: Specifically targets insulin resistance; an insulin sensitizer; regulates the transcription of a number of insulin-responsive genes

USES: Type 2 diabetes mellitus

CONTRAINDICATIONS: Breastfeeding, children, hypersensitivity to thiazolidinedione, diabetic ketoacidosis

Black Box Warning: NYHA Class III/IV heart failure

Precautions: Pregnancy (C), geriatric patients, geriatric patients with CV disease, renal/hepatic/thyroid disease, edema, polycystic ovary syndrome, bladder cancer, osteoporosis, pulmonary disease, secondary malignancy

DOSAGE AND ROUTES

Monotherapy

• **Adult: PO** 15 or 30 mg/day, may increase to 45 mg/day; with strong CYP2C8, max 15 mg/day; with NYHA class I/II heart failure, max 15 mg/day

Combination therapy

• **Adult: PO** 15 or 30 mg/day with a sulfonylurea, metFORMIN, or insulin; decrease sulfonylurea dose if hypoglycemia occurs; decrease insulin dose by 10%-25% if hypoglycemia occurs or if plasma glucose is <100 mg/dl, max 45 mg/day

Hepatic dose

• Do not use in active hepatic disease or if ALT >2.5 times ULN

Available forms: Tabs 15, 30, 45 mg

Administer:

• Once a day; without regard to meals
• Tabs crushed and mixed with food or fluids for patients with difficulty swallowing

SIDE EFFECTS

CNS: *Headache*

CV: MI, heart failure, death (geriatric patients)

ENDO: Hypo/hyperglycemia

MISC: *Sinusitis, upper respiratory tract infection, pharyngitis,* hepatotoxicity, edema, weight gain, anemia, macular edema; risk of bladder cancer (use >1 yr), peripheral/pulmonary edema

MS: Rhabdomyolysis, fractures (females), myalgia

PHARMACOKINETICS

Maximal reduction in FBS after 12 wk; half-life 3-7 hr, terminal 16-24 hr; protein binding >99%

INTERACTIONS

Decrease: effect of atorvastatin

Decrease: effect of oral contraceptives; use alternative contraceptive method

Decrease: pioglitazone effect—CYP2C8 inducers (ketoconazole, fluconazole, itraconazole, miconazole, voriconazole)

Drug/Herb

Increase: hypoglycemia—garlic, green tea, horse chestnut

Drug/Lab Test

Increase: CPK, LFTs, HDL, cholesterol

Decrease: glucose, Hct/Hgb

NURSING CONSIDERATIONS

Assess:

Black Box Warning: Heart failure: do not use in NYHA Class III/IV; excessive/rapid weight gain >5 lb, dyspnea, edema; may need to be reduced or discontinued

• **Bladder cancer:** avoid use in a history of bladder cancer; use of pioglitazone >1 yr has shown an increase in bladder cancer
• **Hypoglycemic reactions:** sweating, weakness, dizziness, anxiety, tremors, hunger; hyperglycemic reactions soon after meals (rare); may occur more often with insulin or other antidiabetics
• **Hepatic disease:** check LFTs periodically: AST, LDH; do not start treatment in active heart disease or if ALT >2.5× upper limit of normal; if treatment has already begun, follow closely with continuing ALT levels; if ALT increases to >3× upper limit of normal, recheck ALT as soon as possible; if ALT remains >3× upper limit of normal, discontinue
• FBS, glycosylated HbA1c, plasma lipids/lipoproteins, B/P, body weight during treatment
• CBC with differential before and during therapy; more necessary in those with anemia, Hct/Hgb (may be decreased in first few months of treatment)

Evaluate:
• Therapeutic response: decrease in polyuria, polydipsia, polyphagia; clear sensorium; absence of dizziness; stable gait; blood glucose A1c improvement

Teach patient/family:
• To self-monitor using a blood glucose meter
• About the symptoms of hypo/hyperglycemia; what to do about each
• That product must be continued on daily basis; about the consequences of discontinuing product abruptly
• To avoid OTC medications or herbal preparations unless approved by prescriber
• That diabetes is a lifelong illness; that product is not a cure, it only controls symptoms
• To notify prescriber if oral contraceptives are used, effect may be decreased; not to use product if breastfeeding
• To report symptoms of hepatic dysfunction: nausea, vomiting, abdominal pain, fatigue, anorexia, dark urine, jaundice
• To report weight gain, edema
• That lab work, eye exams will be needed periodically

piperacillin/tazobactam (Rx)

(pip′er-ah-sill′in/ta-zoe-bak′tam)

Tazocin ✤, Zosyn

Func. class.: Antiinfective, broad spectrum

Chem. class.: Extended-spectrum penicillin, β-lactamase inhibitor

ACTION: Interferes with cell-wall replication of susceptible organisms; tazobactam is a β-lactamase inhibitor that protects piperacillin from enzymatic degradation

USES: Moderate to severe infections: piperacillin-resistant, β-lactamase–producing strains causing infections in respiratory, skin, urinary tract, bone, gonorrhea, pneumonia; effective for resistant *Staphylococcus aureus,* resistant *Escherichia coli, Bacteroides fragilis, Bacteroides ovatus, Bacteroides thetaiotaomicron, Bacteroides vulgatus, Haemophilus influenzae*

Unlabeled uses: Endocarditis

P

CONTRAINDICATIONS: Hypersensitivity to penicillins; neonates; carbapenem allergy

Precautions: Pregnancy (B), breastfeeding, renal insufficiency in neonates, hypersensitivity to cephalosporins, seizures, GI disease, electrolyte imbalances, biliary obstruction

DOSAGE AND ROUTES

Nosocomial pneumonia
• **Adult: IV** 4.5 g q6hr or 3.375 g q4hr with an aminoglycoside or antipseudomonal fluoroquinolone × 1-2 wk

Appendicitis/peritonitis
• **Adults/adolescents/child ≥40 kg (88 lb): IV**3.375 g q6hr × 7-10 days
• **Child ≥9 mo and <40 kg: IV** 100 mg/kg (piperacillin)/kg q8hr × 7-10 days

• **Infant 2 mo to <9 mo: IV** 80 mg/kg (piperacillin) q8hr × 7-10 days

Renal dose

• **Adult: IV** CCr 20-40 ml/min, give 3.375 g q6hr (nosocomial pneumonia); give 2.25 g q6hr (all other indications); CCr <20 ml/min, give 2.25 g q6hr (nosocomial pneumonia); give 2.25 g q8hr (all other indications)

Available forms: Powder for inj 2 g piperacillin/0.25 g tazobactam, 3 g piperacillin/0.375 g tazobactam, 4 g piperacillin/0.5 g tazobactam, 36 g piperacillin/4.5 g tazobactam

Administer:

• Separate aminoglycoside from piperacillin to avoid inactivation

• Product after C&S is complete

Intermittent IV INFUSION route

• Reconstitute each 1 g of product/5 ml 0.9% NaCl for inj or sterile water for inj, dextrose 5%; shake well; further dilute in ≥50 ml compatible IV sol, run as int infusion over ≥30 min

ADD-Vantage IV solution:

Reconstitution:

• Reconstitute with 0.9% sodium chloride or D_5W in the appropriate flexible diluent container provided; for 500-mg vials, use at least a 100 ml diluent container and for 750 mg and 1-g vials, use only the 250-ml diluent container

• Remove the protective covers from the top of the vial and vial port; remove vial cap (do not access with a syringe) and vial port cover; screw the vial into the vial port until it will go no further to assure a seal; once vial is sealed to the port, do not remove; to activate the contents of the vial, squeeze the bottom of the diluent container gently to inflate the portion of the container surrounding the end of the drug vial; with the other hand, push the drug vial down into the container telescoping walls of the container and grasp the inner cap of the vial through the walls of the container; pull the inner cap from the drug vial; verify the rubber stopper has been pulled out, allowing the drug and diluent to mix; mix the container contents thoroughly

• *Storage after reconstitution:* the admixture solution may be stored for up to 24 hr at room temperature; do not refrigerate or freeze after reconstitution

• Do not use in series connections with flexible containers

Premixed Galaxy IV solution:

• Thaw frozen containers at room temperature (20-25°C or 68-77°F) or under refrigeration (2-8°C or 36-46°F); do not force thaw by immersion in water baths or by microwaving; check for leaks by squeezing bag firmly

• Do not admix

• Contents of the solution may precipitate in the frozen state and should dissolve with little or no agitation once the solution has reached room temperature

• ***Storage:*** the thawed solution is stable for 24 hr at room temperature or for 14 days under refrigeration; do not refreeze thawed product

• Do not use plastic containers in series connections as this could result in an embolism due to residual air being drawn from the primary container before administration of the fluid from the secondary container is complete

IV INFUSION:

• Infuse IV over at least 30 min; ambulatory intravenous infusion pumps can be used; the solution is stable for up to 12 hr at room temperature

Y-site compatibilities: Alfentanil, allopurinol, amifostine, amikacin, aminocaproic acid, aminophylline, amphotericin B lipid complex, amphotericin B liposome, anidulafungin, argatroban, atenolol, aztreonam, bivalirudin, bleomycin, bumetanide, buprenorphine, busulfan, butorphanol, calcium acetate/chloride/gluconate, CARBOplatin, carmustine, cefepime, chloramphenicol, cimetidine, clindamycin, cyclophosphamide, cycloSPORINE, cytarabine, DACTINomycin, DAPTOmycin, dexamethasone, dexrazoxane, diazepam, digoxin, diphenhydrAMINE, DOCEtaxel, DOPamine, doxacurium, enalaprilat, ePHEDrine, EPINEPHrine, eptifibatide, erythromycin, esmolol, etoposide, fenoldopam, fentaNYL, floxuridine, fluconazole, fludarabine, fluorouracil, foscarnet, fosphenytoin, furosemide, gallium, granisetron, heparin, hydrocortisone, HYDROmorphone, ifosfamide, isoproterenol, ketorolac, lansoprazole, lepirudin, leucovorin, lidocaine, linezolid, LORazepam, magnesium sulfate, mannitol, mechlorethamine, melphalan, meperidine, mesna, metaraminol, methotrexate, methylPREDNISolone, metoclopramide, metoprolol, metroNIDAZOLE, milrinone, morphine, naloxone, nitroglycerin, nitroprusside, norepinephrine, octreotide, ondansetron, oxytocin, PACLitaxel, palonosetron, pamidronate, pancuronium, PEMEtrexed, PENTobarbital, PHENobarbital, phentolamine, phenylephrine, plicamycin, potassium chloride/phosphates, procainamide, ranitidine, remifentanil, riTUXimab, sargramostim, sodium acetate/bicarbonate/phosphates, uccinylcholine, SUFentanil, sulfamethoxazole-trimethoprim, tacrolimus, telavancin, teniposide, theophylline, thiotepa, tigecycline, tirofiban, trimethobenzamide, vasopressin, vinBLAStine, vinCRIStine, voriconazole, zidovudine, zoledronic acid

SIDE EFFECTS

CNS: Lethargy, hallucinations, anxiety, depression, twitching, insomnia, headache, fever, dizziness, **seizures**, vertigo

CV: **Cardiac toxicity**, edema

GI: *Nausea, vomiting, diarrhea;* increased AST, ALT; abdominal pain, glossitis, **pseudomembranous colitis**, constipation, **pancreatitis**

GU: **Oliguria, proteinuria, hematuria,** *vaginitis, moniliasis,* **glomerulonephritis, renal failure**

HEMA: Anemia, increased bleeding time, **bone marrow depression, agranulocytosis, hemolytic anemia**

INTEG: Rash, pruritus, **exfoliative dermatitis**

META: Hypokalemia, hypernatremia

SYST: **Serum sickness, anaphylaxis, Stevens-Johnson syndrome**

PHARMACOKINETICS

Half-life 0.7-1.2 hr; excreted in urine, bile, breast milk; crosses placenta; 33% bound to plasma proteins

IV: Peak completion of IV

INTERACTIONS

Increase: effect of neuromuscular blockers, oral anticoagulants, methotrexate

Increase: piperacillin concentrations—aspirin, probenecid

Decrease: antimicrobial effect of piperacillin—tetracyclines, aminoglycosides IV

Drug/Lab Test

Increase: eosinophilia, neutropenia, leukopenia, serum creatinine, PTT, AST, ALT, alk phos, bilirubin, BUN, electrolytes

Decrease: Hct, Hgb, electrolytes

False positive: urine glucose, urine protein, Coombs' test

NURSING CONSIDERATIONS

Assess:

- **Infection:** temperature, stools, urine, sputum, wounds
- I&O ratio; report hematuria, oliguria because penicillin in high doses is nephrotoxic; maintain hydration unless contraindicated
- Hepatic studies: AST, ALT before treatment and periodically thereafter
- Blood studies: WBC, RBC, Hct, Hgb, bleeding time before treatment and periodically thereafter; serum potassium
- Renal studies: urinalysis, protein, blood, BUN, creatinine before treatment and periodically thereafter
- C&S before product therapy; product may be given as soon as culture is taken
- **Pseudomembranous colitis: diarrhea, bloody stools, fever, abdominal cramps; may occur ≤2 mo after treatment; bowel pattern before and during treatment**
- Skin eruptions after administration of penicillin to 1 wk after discontinuing product
- Respiratory status: rate, character, wheezing, tightness in chest
- **Anaphylaxis: wheezing, laryngeal edema, rash, itching; discontinue product, have emergency equipment nearby**
- Adequate intake of fluids (2 L) during diarrhea episodes

P

Evaluate:

- Therapeutic response: absence of fever, purulent drainage, redness, inflammation; culture shows decreased organisms

Teach patient/family:

- That culture may be taken after completed course of medication
- To report sore throat, fever, fatigue (superinfection); CNS effects (anxiety, depression, hallucinations, seizures); **pseudomembranous colitis:** fever, diarrhea with blood, pus, mucus
- To wear or carry emergency ID if allergic to penicillins
- To notify nurse of diarrhea

TREATMENT OF OVERDOSE:

Withdraw product, maintain airway, administer EPINEPHrine, aminophylline, O_2, IV corticosteroids for anaphylaxis

pirbuterol (Rx)

(peer-byoo′ter-ole)

Maxair

Func. class.: Bronchodilator

Chem. class.: β-Adrenergic agonist

ACTION: Causes bronchodilation with little effect on heart rate by action on β-receptors, causing increased cAMP and relaxation of smooth muscle

USES: Reversible bronchospasm (prevention, treatment) including asthma; may be given with theophylline or steroids

CONTRAINDICATIONS: Hypersensitivity to sympathomimetics, tachycardia

Precautions: Pregnancy (C), breastfeeding, cardiac disorders, hyperthyroidism, hypertension, diabetes mellitus, prostatic hypertrophy

DOSAGE AND ROUTES

- **Adult and child >12 yr:** INH 1-2 inhalations (0.4 mg) q4-6hr; max 12 INH/day

Available forms: Aerosol delivery 0.2 mg pirbuterol/actuation

Administer:

- Store in light-resistant container; do not expose to temperatures over 86° F (30° C)
- After shaking; exhale; place mouthpiece in mouth; inhale slowly; hold breath; remove; exhale slowly
- Gum, sips of water for dry mouth

SIDE EFFECTS

CNS: Tremors, anxiety, insomnia, headache, dizziness, stimulation, restlessness, hallucinations, drowsiness, irritability

CV: Palpitations, tachycardia, hypertension, angina, hypotension, dysrhythmias

EENT: Dry nose and mouth, irritation of nose, throat

GI: Gastritis, nausea, vomiting, anorexia

MS: Muscle cramps

RESP: Paradoxical bronchospasm, dyspnea, coughing

PHARMACOKINETICS

INH: Onset 3 min, peak ½-1 hr, duration 5 hr, terminal half-life 2 hr

INTERACTIONS

⚠ Hypertensive crisis: MAOIs

Increase: action of other aerosol bronchodilators

Increase: pirbuterol action—tricyclics, antihistamines, levothyroxine

Decrease: pirbuterol action—β-blockers

Drug/Herb

Increase: action of both—cola nut, guarana, yerba maté

Increase: effect—green tea (large amounts), guarana

NURSING CONSIDERATIONS

Assess:

- Respiratory function: vital capacity, forced expiratory volume, ABGs, B/P, lung sounds, pulse, characteristics of sputum

⚠ Paradoxical bronchospasm, that can occur rapidly, hold product, notify prescriber

- Fluid intake >2 L/day to liquefy thick secretions

Evaluate:

- Therapeutic response: absence of dyspnea, wheezing over 1 hr

⚠ Nurse Alert

Teach patient/family:
- Not to use OTC medications; extra stimulation may occur
- Use of inhaler; review package insert with patient
- To avoid getting aerosol in eyes
- Actuator is for Maxair autoinhaler; do not use with other inhaler canister
- About all aspects of product; avoid smoking, smoke-filled rooms, persons with respiratory infections
- To keep fluid intake >2 L/day to liquefy thick secretions

TREATMENT OF OVERDOSE:
Administer a β-adrenergic blocker

RARELY USED

pirfenidone
(pir-fen′i-done)
Esbriet
Func. class.: Respiratory agent

USES: Pulmonary fibrosis

CONTRAINDICATIONS: Hypersensitivity

DOSAGE AND ROUTES
- **Adults: PO** Titrate over 2 wk to a maintenance dose of 801 mg tid. Give 267 mg tid on days 1-7, 534 mg tid on days 8-14, and 801 mg tid from day 15 onward

Available forms: Cap 267 mg

pitavastatin (Rx)
(pit′a-va-stat′-in)
Livalo
Func. class.: Antilipidemic
Chem. class.: HMG-CoA reductase inhibitor

Do not confuse:
pitavastatin/pravastatin

ACTION: Inhibits HMG-CoA reductase enzyme, which reduces cholesterol synthesis; high doses lead to plaque regression

USES: As an adjunct for primary hypercholesterolemia (types Ia, Ib), dysbetalipoproteinemia, elevated triglyceride levels, prevention of CV disease by reduction of heart risk in those with mildly elevated cholesterol
Unlabeled Uses: Atherosclerosis

CONTRAINDICATIONS: Pregnancy (X), breastfeeding, hypersensitivity, active hepatic disease, cholestasis
Precautions: Past hepatic disease, alcoholism, severe acute infections, trauma, severe metabolic disorders, electrolyte imbalance, seizures, surgery, organ transplant, endocrine disease, females, hypotension, renal disease

DOSAGE AND ROUTES
- **Adult: PO** 2 mg/day, usual range 1-4, max 4 mg/day

Renal dose
- **Adult: PO** CCr 30-<60 ml/min, 1 mg daily, max 2 mg daily; CCr <30 ml/min on hemodialysis, 1 mg daily, max 2 mg daily; CCr <30 ml/min, not recommended

Atherosclerosis (unlabeled)
- **Adult: PO** 4 mg/day

Available forms: Tabs 1, 2, 4 mg
Administer:
- Total daily dose any time of day without regard to meals
- Store in cool environment in tight container protected from light

SIDE EFFECTS
CNS: Headache
GI: Constipation, diarrhea
INTEG: Rash, pruritus, alopecia
MS: Arthralgia, myalgia, **rhabdomyolysis**
RESP: Pharyngitis

PHARMACOKINETICS
Peak 1 hr; metabolized in liver, excreted in urine, feces; half-life 12 hr; protein binding 99%; concentrations lower in healthy African Americans

P

INTERACTIONS

Increase: risk for possible rhabdomyolysis—azole antifungals, cycloSPORINE, erythromycin, niacin, gemfibrozil, clofibrate
Increase: levels of pitavastatin—erythromycin
Drug/Herb
Increase: pitavastatin—red yeast rice
Drug/Lab Test
Increase: bilirubin, alk phos, ALT, AST
Interference: thyroid function tests

NURSING CONSIDERATIONS

Assess:

- **Diet;** obtain diet history including fat, cholesterol in diet
- Cholesterol, triglyceride levels periodically during treatment; check lipid panel 6 wk after changing dose
- Hepatic studies at 12 wk after starting treatment, then q6mo; if AST >3× normal, reduce or discontinue; AST, ALT, LFTs may be increased
- Renal studies in patients with compromised renal system: BUN, I&O ratio, creatinine

⚠ **Rhabdomyolysis:** muscle pain, tenderness; obtain CPK baseline; if markedly increased, product may need to be discontinued

Evaluate:

- Therapeutic response: decrease in cholesterol to desired level after 6 wk

Teach patient/family:

- That blood work will be necessary during treatment
- To report blurred vision, severe GI symptoms, headache, muscle pain, weakness, tenderness
- That previously prescribed regimen will continue: low-cholesterol diet, exercise program, smoking cessation
- Not to take product if pregnant (X) or if pregnancy is planned or suspected (notify prescriber); to avoid breastfeeding

plasma protein fraction (Rx)

Plasmanate

Func. class.: Hematological agent
Chem. class.: Plasma volume expander

USES: Hypovolemic shock, hypoproteinemia, ARDS, preoperative cardiopulmonary bypass, acute hepatic failure, nephrotic syndrome, cardiogenic shock

CONTRAINDICATIONS: Hypersensitivity to this product or albumin; CHF, severe anemia, renal insufficiency, hyponatremia, cardiopulmonary bypass

DOSAGE AND ROUTES

Hypovolemia

- **Adult: IV INFUSION** 250-500 ml (12.5-25 g protein), max 10 ml/min
- **Child: IV INFUSION** 10-30 ml/kg at max 5-10 ml/min

Hypoproteinemia

- **Adult: IV INFUSION** 1000-1500 ml/day, max 8 ml/min

plerixafor (Rx)

(pler-ix′a-fore)

Mozobil

Func. class.: Biologic modifier
Chem. class.: Colony-stimulating factor

USES: For peripheral blood stem cell (PBSC) mobilization for collection and autologous transplant in patients with non-Hodgkin's lymphoma, multiple myeloma; used with a granulocyte colony-stimulating factor (G-CSF)

CONTRAINDICATIONS: Hypersensitivity, breastfeeding, pregnancy (D)

DOSAGE AND ROUTES

- **Adult: SUBCUT** 0.24 mg/kg daily about 11 hr before initiation of apheresis, give for up to 4 consecutive days; give filgrastim 10 mcg/kg; **SUBCUT** daily each AM beginning 4 days before the 1st evening dose of plerixafor and on each day of apheresis; give filgrastim before procedure

pomalidomide

(pom–a-lid′oh-mide)

Pomalyst

Func. class.: Antineoplastic, biologic response modifier, hormone

Chem. class.: TNF modifier

ACTION: Inhibits growth of tumor cells and induces apoptosis, can be used in those resistant to lenalidomide

USES: Multiple myeloma in those who have received ≥2 treatments including lenalidomide and bortezomib and disease has progressed within 60 days of completion of the treatment or in BRAF V600 mutation-positive patients who have disease progression following ipilimumab and a BRAF inhibitor

CONTRAINDICATIONS: Breastfeeding, hypersensitivity

Black Box Warning: Pregnancy (X)

Precautions: Children, geriatric patients, accidental exposure, bone marrow suppression, uterine bleeding, dental disease, fungal/viral infections, smoking

Black Box Warning: Thrombocytopenia

DOSAGE AND ROUTES

- **Adult: PO** 4 mg on days 1-21

Hepatic/renal dose:

- Adult: PO bilirubin >2 mg/dl and AST/ALT >3× ULN or CCr >3 mg/dl, do not use

Available forms: Tabs 1, 2, 3, 4 mg

Administer:

- With or without dexamethasone, may use dexamethasone 40 mg on days 1, 8, 15, 22 of each cycle, if >75 yr, decrease dexamethasone to 20 mg/dose

SIDE EFFECTS

CNS: Dizziness, fatigue, fever, headache, peripheral neuropathy

CV: Chest pain

GI: Constipation, diarrhea, nausea/vomiting, **hepatic failure**

HEMA: **Leukopenia, neutropenia, thrombocytopenia, pancytopenia**

META: Hypokalemia

MS: Arthralgia, back pain

RESP: Cough, dyspnea, **pulmonary embolism**, epistaxis

SYST: **Secondary malignancy, angioedema**

PHARMACOKINETICS

12%-44% protein binding

INTERACTIONS

Increase: pomalidomide effect—CYP3A4 inhibitors (amprenavir, boceprevir, delavirdine, ketoconazole, indinavir, itraconazole, dalfopristin/quinupristin, ritonavir, tipranavir, fluconazole, isoniazid, miconazole); P-gb inhibitors; avoid using together

Decrease: pomalidomide effect—CYP3A4 inducers (rifampin, rifapentine, rifabutin, primidone, phenytoin, PHENobarbital, nevirapine, nafcillin, modafinil, griseofulvin, etravirine, efavirenz, barbiturates, bexarotene, bosentan, carBAMazepine, enzalutamide, dexamethasone); avoid using together

Drug/Herb

- Decreased pomalidomide effect—St. John's wort, avoid using together

Drug/Smoking

Decrease: pomalidomide effect—cigarettes

NURSING CONSIDERATIONS

Assess:

Black Box Warning: Blood studies: Hct, Hgb, thrombolytic disease may occur

Black Box Warning: For pregnancy before treatment, pregnancy (X)

P

Evaluate:
- Therapeutic response: decreased growth of tumor cells

Team patient/family:
- To avoid driving or hazardous activity during beginning of treatment

Black Box Warning: Advise patient to use adequate contraception, pregnancy (X)

posaconazole (Rx)

(poe′sa-kon′a-zole)

Noxafil, Posanol ✦

Func. class.: Antifungal—systemic

Chem. class.: Triazole derivative

ACTION: Inhibits a portion of cell-wall synthesis; alters cell membranes and inhibits several fungal enzymes

USES: Prevention of aspergillus, candida infection, oropharyngeal candidiasis in immunocompromised patients, chemotherapy-induced neutropenia, mucocutaneous candidiasis

Unlabeled uses: Aspergillosis, cellulitis, coccidioidomycosis, endocarditis, endophthalmitis, esophageal candidiasis, febrile neutropenia, fungal keratitis, fusariosis, histoplasmosis, infectious arthritis, myocarditis, osteomyelitis, pericarditis, sinusitis, tracheobronchitis

CONTRAINDICATIONS: Hypersensitivity to this product or other systemic antifungals or azoles; fungal meningitis, onchomycosis or dermatomycosis in cardiac dysfunction; use with ergots, sirolimus, CYP3A4 substrates

Precautions: Pregnancy (C), breastfeeding, children, cardiac/hepatic/renal disease

DOSAGE AND ROUTES

- **Adult, adolescent: PO** 600 mg/day in 2-4 divided doses

Oropharyngeal Candidiasis
- **Adult: PO** 100 mg bid × 1 day, then 100 mg/day × 13 days

Oropharyngeal candidiasis resistant to fluconazole or itraconazole

Adult/Child ≥13 yr: PO 400 mg bid

Available forms: Oral susp 200 mg/5 ml

Administer:

PO route
- **Oral susp:** shake well; use calibrated measuring device; take only with full meal or liquid nutritional supplements such as Ensure; rinse measuring device after each use
- Store in tight container in refrigerator; do not freeze

SIDE EFFECTS

CNS: *Headache, dizziness,* insomnia, fever, rigors, weakness, anxiety

CV: Hypo/hypertension, tachycardia, anemia, QT prolongation, torsades de pointes

GI: *Nausea, vomiting, anorexia, diarrhea,* cramps, abdominal pain, flatulence, GI bleeding, hepatotoxicity

GU: Gynecomastia, impotence, decreased libido

INTEG: *Pruritus,* fever, *rash,* toxic epidermal necrolysis

MISC: *Edema, fatigue,* malaise, hypokalemia, tinnitus, rhabdomyolysis, hypokalemia

PHARMACOKINETICS

Well absorbed, enhanced by food, protein binding 98%-99%, peak 3-5 hr, half-life 35 hr, metabolized in liver, excreted in feces (77% unchanged)

INTERACTIONS

- Do not use with lovastatin, atorvastatin

⚠ **Increase:** QT prolongation—class IA/III antidysrhythmics, some phenothiazines, β agonists, local anesthetics, tricyclics, haloperidol, chloroquine, droperidol, pentamidine; CYP3A4 inhibitors (amiodarone, clarithromycin, erythromycin, telithromycin, troleandomycin), arsenic trioxide, levomethadyl; CYP3A4 substrates (methadone, pimozide, QUEtiapine, quiNIDine, risperiDONE, ziprasidone)

Increase: tinnitus, hearing loss—quiNIDine

Increase: hepatotoxicity—other hepatotoxic products

Increase: severe hypoglycemia—oral hypoglycemics
Increase: sedation—triazolam, oral midazolam
Increase: levels, toxicity—busPIRone, busulfan, calcium-channel blockers, clarithromycin, cycloSPORINE, diazepam, digoxin, felodipine, HMG-CoA reductase inhibitors, indinavir, isradipine, midazolam, niCARdipine, NIFEdipine, niMODipine, phenytoin, quiNIDine, ritonavir, saquinavir, sirolimus, tacrolimus, vinca alkaloids, warfarin
Decrease: posaconazole level—cimetidine, phenytoin
Decrease: posaconazole action—antacids, H_2-receptor antagonists, rifamycin, didanosine

Drug/Food
- Food increases absorption

NURSING CONSIDERATIONS

Assess:

⚠ **Infection:** type of, may begin treatment before obtaining results; temperature, WBC, sputum at baseline and periodically, break-through infections may occur when used with fosamprenavir
- I&O ratio, electrolytes; correct electrolyte imbalances before starting treatment
- For allergic reaction: rash, photosensitivity, urticaria, dermatitis

⚠ **Rhabdomyolysis:** muscle pain, increased CPK; weakness, swelling of affected muscles; if these occur and if confirmed by CPK, product should be discontinued

⚠ **Hepatotoxicity:** nausea, vomiting, jaundice, clay-colored stools, fatigue; hepatic studies (ALT, AST, bilirubin) if patient receiving long-term therapy

⚠ **QT prolongation:** ECG for QT prolongation, ejection fraction; assess for chest pain, palpitations, dyspnea

Evaluate:
- Therapeutic response: decreased symptoms of fungal infection, negative C&S for infecting organism

Teach patient/family:
- That long-term therapy may be needed to clear infection (1 wk-6 mo, depending on infection)
- To avoid hazardous activities if dizziness occurs
- To take 2 hr before administration of other products that increase gastric pH (antacids, H_2-blockers, omeprazole, sucralfate, anticholinergics); to notify health care provider of all medications taken (many interactions)
- About the importance of compliance with product regimen; to use alternative method of contraception
- To notify prescriber of GI symptoms, signs of hepatic dysfunction (fatigue, nausea, anorexia, vomiting, dark urine, pale stools)
- To take during or within 20 min of eating

potassium acetate
potassium bicarbonate (OTC, Rx)
K Effervescent, Klor-Con EF, K-Vescent
potassium bicarbonate and potassium chloride (OTC, Rx)
Neo-K ✱
potassium bicarbonate and potassium citrate (OTC, Rx)

⚠ **HIGH ALERT**

potassium chloride (OTC, Rx)
Epiklor, Klor-Con, K-Tab, Micro-K, Odan K-20 ✱

potassium gluconate (OTC, Rx)
Func. class.: Electrolyte, mineral replacement
Chem. class.: Potassium

ACTION: Needed for the adequate transmission of nerve impulses and

P

cardiac contraction, renal function, intracellular ion maintenance

USES:
Prevention and treatment of hypokalemia

CONTRAINDICATIONS:
Renal disease (severe), severe hemolytic disease, Addison's disease, hyperkalemia, acute dehydration, extensive tissue breakdown

Precautions: Pregnancy (C), cardiac disease, potassium-sparing diuretic therapy, systemic acidosis

DOSAGE AND ROUTES

Hypokalemia (prevention) (bicarbonate, chloride, gluconate)

- **Adult: PO** 20 mEq/day in 1-2 divided doses
- **Child: PO** 1-2 mEq/kg/day in 1-2 divided doses

Hypokalemia, digoxin toxicity (acetate, chloride)

- **Adult:** serum potassium concentration >2.5 mEq/L: **IV** max 10 mEq/1 hr with 24-hr max dose 200 mEq, initial dose of 20-40 mEq has been recommended; **PO** 40-100 mEq/day in 2-4 divided doses
- **Child: IV** 0.25-0.5 mEq/kg/dose at 0.25-0.5 mEq/kg/hr; **PO** 2-5 mEq/day in divided doses

Available forms: Tabs for sol 6.5, 25 mEq; ext rel caps 8, 10 mEq; powder for sol 3.3, 5, 6.7, 10, 13.3 mEq/5 ml; tabs 2, 4, 5, 13.4 mEq; ext rel tabs 6.7, 8, 10 mEq; elix 6.7 mEq/5 ml; oral sol 2.375 mEq/5 ml; inj for prep of IV 1.5, 2, 2.4, 3, 3.2, 4.4, 4.7 mEq/ml

Administer:

PO route

- Do not break, crush, or chew ext rel tabs, caps, or enteric products
- With or after meals; dissolve effervescent tabs, powder in 8 oz cold water or juice; do not give IM, SUBCUT
- Caps with full glass of liquid

IV route

- Through large-bore needle to decrease vein inflammation; check for extravasation; in large vein, avoid scalp vein in child (IV)

Potassium acetate

Additive compatibilities: Metoclopramide

Y-site compatibilities: Ciprofloxacin

Potassium chloride

- **Potassium chloride** must be diluted; concentrated potassium injections fatal

Continuous IV INFUSION route

- Concentration max 80 mcg/L for peripheral line; 120 mEq/L for central line
- Dehydrated patients should receive 1 L of potassium-free hydrating solution, then infuse 10 mEq/hr; in severe hypokalemia, rate may be 40 mEq/hr

Y-site compatibilities: Acyclovir, aldesleukin, allopurinol, amifostine, aminophylline, amiodarone, ampicillin, amrinone, atropine, aztreonam, betamethasone, calcium gluconate, cephalothin, cephapirin, chlordiazePOXIDE, chlorproMAZINE, ciprofloxacin, cladribine, cyanocobalamin, dexamethasone, digoxin, diltiazem, diphenhydrAMINE, DOBUTamine, DOPamine, droperidol, edrophonium, enalaprilat, EPINEPHrine, esmolol, estrogens, ethacrynate, famotidine, fentaNYL, filgrastim, fludarabine, fluorouracil, furosemide, gallium, granisetron, heparin, hydrALAZINE, IDArubicin, indomethacin, insulin (regular), isoproterenol, kanamycin, labetalol, lidocaine, LORazepam, magnesium sulfate, melphalan, meperidine, methicillin, methoxamine, methylergonovine, midazolam, minocycline, morphine, neostigmine, norepinephrine, ondansetron, oxacillin, oxytocin, PACLitaxel, penicillin G potassium, pentazocine, phytonadione, piperacillin/tazobactam, prednisoLONE, procainamide, prochlorperazine, propofol, propranolol, pyridostigmine, remifentanil, sargramostim, scopolamine, sodium bicarbonate, succinylcholine, tacrolimus, teniposide, theophylline, thiotepa, trimethaphan, trimethoenzamide, vinorelbine, warfarin, zidovudine

SIDE EFFECTS

CNS: Confusion

CV: Bradycardia, cardiac depression, dysrhythmias, arrest; peaking T waves,

lowered R, depressed RST, prolonged P-R interval, widened QRS complex
GI: *Nausea, vomiting, cramps,* pain, *diarrhea,* ulceration of small bowel
GU: Oliguria
INTEG: Cold extremities, rash

PHARMACOKINETICS

PO: Excreted by kidneys and in feces; onset of action ≈30 min
IV: Immediate onset of action

INTERACTIONS

Increase: hyperkalemia—potassium phosphate IV; products containing calcium or magnesium; potassium-sparing diuretic or other potassium products; ACE inhibitors

NURSING CONSIDERATIONS

Assess:

- **Hyperkalemia:** indicates toxicity; fatigue, muscle weakness, confusion, dyspnea, palpitation; ECG for peaking T waves, lowered R, depressed RST, prolonged P-R interval, widening QRS complex, hyperkalemia; product should be reduced or discontinued, administer sodium bicarbonate (metabolic acidosis)
- Potassium level during treatment (3.5-5 mg/dl is normal level)
- Determine hydration status, I&O ratio; watch for decreased urinary output; notify prescriber immediately
- Cardiac status: rate, rhythm, CVP, PWP, PAWP if being monitored directly

Evaluate:

- Therapeutic response: absence of fatigue, muscle weakness; decreased thirst, urinary output; cardiac changes

Teach patient/family:

- To add potassium-rich foods to diet: bananas, orange juice, avocados, whole grains, broccoli, carrots, prunes, cocoa after product is discontinued
- To avoid OTC products: antacids, salt substitutes, analgesics, vitamin preparations unless specifically directed by prescriber; to avoid licorice in large amounts because it may cause hypokalemia, sodium retention
- To report hyperkalemia symptoms (lethargy, confusion, diarrhea, nausea, vomiting, fainting, decreased output) or continued hypokalemia symptoms (fatigue, weakness, polyuria, polydipsia, cardiac changes)
- To dissolve powder or tablet completely in ≥120 ml water or juice
- About the importance of regular follow-up visits
- That potassium levels will need to be monitored periodically

potassium iodide (Rx)

Lugol's, SSKI, Pima, ThyroSafe, ThyroShield
Func. class.: Thyroid hormone antagonist
Chem. class.: Iodine product

ACTION: Inhibits secretion of thyroid hormone, fosters colloid accumulation in thyroid follicles, decreases vascularity of gland

USES: Preparation for thyroidectomy, thyrotoxic crisis, neonatal thyrotoxicosis, radiation protectant, thyroid storm
Unlabeled uses: Erythema multiforme, erythema nodosum leprosum (ENL), sporotrichosis, thyroid involution induction

CONTRAINDICATIONS: Pregnancy (D), pulmonary edema, pulmonary TB, bronchitis, hypersensitivity to iodine
Precautions: Breastfeeding, children

DOSAGE AND ROUTES

Hyperthyroidism/thyrotoxicosis

- **Adult and child: PO** (SSKI) 250 mg tid × 10-14 days preoperatively

Preparation for thyroidectomy

- **Adult and child: PO** 3-5 gtt strong iodine sol tid or 1-5 drops SSKI in water tid after meals for 10 days before surgery

P

Radiation exposure (radioactive iodine)

- **Adult: PO** 130 mg/day (distribution by government/public health officials or OTC purchase)
- **Child ≥3 yr: PO** 65 mg daily
- **Child/infant >1 mo-3 yr: PO** 32 mg/day
- **Neonate: PO** 16 mg/day

Available forms: Oral sol (Lugol's solution) iodine 5%/potassium iodide 10%; oral sol (SSKI) 1 g/ml (ThyroShield) 65 mg/ml; syrup (PIMA) 325 mg/5 ml; tabs 65, 130 mg

Administer:

- Products are not interchangeable
- Strong iodine solution after diluting with water or juice to improve taste
- Through straw to prevent tooth discoloration
- With meals to decrease GI upset
- At same time each day to maintain product level
- At lowest dose that relieves symptoms; discontinue before RAIU

SIDE EFFECTS

CNS: Headache, confusion, paresthesias
EENT: Metallic taste, stomatitis, salivation, periorbital edema, sore teeth and gums, cold symptoms
ENDO: Hypothyroidism, hyperthyroid adenoma
GI: *Nausea, diarrhea, vomiting,* small-bowel lesions, upper gastric pain, metallic taste
INTEG: Rash, urticaria, angioneurotic edema, acne, mucosal hemorrhage, fever
MS: Myalgia, arthralgia, weakness

PHARMACOKINETICS

PO: Onset 24-48 hr, peak 10-15 days after continuous therapy, uptake by thyroid gland or excreted in urine, crosses placenta

INTERACTIONS

Increase: hypothyroidism—lithium, other antithyroid agents
Increase: hyperkalemia—angiotensin II receptor antagonist, ACE inhibitors, potassium salts, potassium-sparing diuretics

NURSING CONSIDERATIONS

Assess:

- Pulse, B/P, temperature; serum potassium
- I&O ratio; check for edema: puffy hands, feet, periorbit; indicate hypothyroidism
- Weight daily; same clothing, scale, time of day
- T_3, T_4, which is increased; serum TSH, which is decreased; free thyroxine index, which is increased if dosage is too low; discontinue product 3-4 wk before RAIU

⚠ Overdose: peripheral edema, heat intolerance, diaphoresis, palpitations, dysrhythmias, severe tachycardia, fever, delirium, CNS irritability

- **Hypersensitivity:** rash; enlarged cervical lymph nodes may indicate product should be discontinued
- **Hypoprothrombinemia:** bleeding, petechiae, ecchymosis
- Clinical response: after 3 wk should include increased weight, pulse; decreased T_4
- Fluids to 3-4 L/day unless contraindicated

Evaluate:

- Therapeutic response: weight gain; decreased pulse, T_4, size of thyroid gland

Teach patient/family:

- To abstain from breastfeeding after delivery
- To keep graph of weight, pulse, mood
- To avoid OTC products that contain iodine
- That seafood, other iodine products may be restricted
- Not to discontinue product abruptly; that thyroid crisis may occur as part of stress response
- That response may take several mo if thyroid is large
- To discontinue product, notify prescriber of fever, rash, metallic taste, swelling of throat; burning of mouth, throat; sore gums, teeth; severe GI distress, enlargement of thyroid, cold symptoms

pramipexole (Rx)

(pra-mi-pex′ol)

Mirapex, Mirapex ER

Func. class.: Antiparkinson agent

Chem. class.: DOPamine-receptor agonist, non-ergot

ACTION: Selective agonist for D_2 receptors (presynaptic/postsynaptic sites); binding at D_3 receptor contributes to antiparkinson effects

USES: Idiopathic Parkinson's disease, restless leg syndrome

CONTRAINDICATIONS: Hypersensitivity

Precautions: Pregnancy (C), cardiac/renal disease, MI with dysrhythmias, affective disorders, psychosis, preexisting dyskinesias, history of falling asleep during daily activities, rapid dose reduction

DOSAGE AND ROUTES

Parkinson's disease

- **Adult: PO** 0.125 mg tid; increase gradually by 0.125 mg/dose at 5- to 7-day intervals until total daily dose of 4.5 mg/day reached; ER 0.375 mg daily initially, then up to 0.75 mg/day; may increase by 0.75 mg/day no more than q5-7days as needed, max 4.5 mg/day

Restless leg syndrome

- **Adult: PO** 0.125 mg 2-3 hr before bedtime, increase gradually, max 0.5 mg/day

Renal dose

- **Adult: PO CCr 35-59 ml/min, 0.125 mg bid, may increase q5-7days to 1.5 mg bid if required; CCr 15-34 ml/min, 0.125 mg/day, increase q5-7days to 1.5 mg/day**

Available forms: Tabs 0.125, 0.25, 0.5, 1, 1.5 mg; ER tab 0.375, 0.75, 1.5, 3.0, 4.5 mg

Administer:

- Adjust dosage to patient response, titrate slowly, taper when discontinuing
- With meals to minimize GI symptoms
- Do not crush, chew, or break ext rel product

SIDE EFFECTS

CNS: *Agitation, insomnia,* psychosis, hallucinations, depression, dizziness, headache, confusion, amnesia, dream disorder, asthenia, dyskinesia, hypersomnolence, **sudden sleep onset,** impulse control disorders

CV: *Orthostatic hypotension,* edema, syncope, tachycardia, increased B/P, heart rate, **heart failure**

EENT: Blurred vision, retinal/vision deterioration

ENDO: Antidiuretic hormone secretion (SIADH)

GI: *Nausea, anorexia,* constipation, dysphagia, dry mouth

GU: Impotence, urinary frequency

HEMA: Hemolytic anemia, leukopenia, agranulocytosis

INTEG: Pruritus

PHARMACOKINETICS

Minimally metabolized, peak 2 hr, half-life 8 hr, 8.5-12 hr in geriatric patients

INTERACTIONS

Increase: pramipexole levels—levodopa, cimetidine, ranitidine, diltiazem, triamterene, verapamil, quiNIDine

Decrease: pramipexole levels—DOPamine antagonists, phenothiazines, metoclopramide, butyrophenones

NURSING CONSIDERATIONS

Assess:

- **Parkinson's disease:** involuntary movements: bradykinesia, tremors, staggering gait, muscle rigidity, drooling
- B/P, ECG, respiration during initial treatment; hypo/hypertension should be reported
- Mental status: affect, mood, behavioral changes, depression; complete suicide assessment, worsening of symptoms of restless leg syndrome, impulse control disorders

⚠ **Sleep attacks: may fall asleep during activities without warning; may need to discontinue medication**

- Assistance with ambulation during beginning therapy
- Testing for diabetes mellitus, acromegaly if patient receiving long-term therapy

Evaluate:

- Therapeutic response: movement disorder improves

Teach patient/family:

- That therapeutic effects may take several weeks to a few months
- To change positions slowly to prevent orthostatic hypotension
- To use product exactly as prescribed; if product is discontinued abruptly, parkinsonian crisis may occur; to avoid alcohol, OTC sleeping products
- To notify prescriber if pregnancy is planned or suspected
- To notify prescriber of impulse control disorders: shopping

⚠ HIGH ALERT

pramlintide (Rx)

(pram′lin-tide)

Symlin

Func. class.: Antidiabetic

Chem. class.: Synthetic human amylin analog

ACTION: Modulates and slows stomach emptying, prevents postprandial rise in plasma glucagon, decreases appetite, leads to decreased caloric intake and weight loss

USES: As an adjunct prandial to insulin therapy for uncontrolled type 1 or type 2 diabetes

CONTRAINDICATIONS: Hypersensitivity to this product or cresol; gastroparesis

Black Box Warning: Hypoglycemia

Precautions: Pregnancy (C), breastfeeding

DOSAGE AND ROUTES

Type 1 diabetes

- **Adult: SUBCUT** 15 mcg before each meal (≥30 g carbohydrate), titrate up in 15-mcg increments to target dose of 60 mcg/dose; each dose titration should occur after no nausea for 3 days

Type 2 diabetes

- **Adult: SUBCUT** 60 mcg before each meal (≥30 g CHO), titrate up to 120 mcg **SUBCUT** with each meal after no nausea for 3-7 days

Available forms: PEN 60, 120 (1000 mcg/ml solution for j-injection)

Administer:

- Store at room temperature for ≤30 days; keep away from heat and sunlight; refrigerate all other supply
- Premeal insulin should be decreased by 50% when starting and adjusted to therapeutic dose to prevent hypoglycemia

SUBCUT route

- Rotate injection sites, allow solution to warm to room temperature before use
- Take immediately before mealtime or if 30 g of carbohydrates will be consumed
- Do not use if a meal is skipped
- Do not use if discolored; do not give in arm; absorption is variable

SIDE EFFECTS

CNS: *Headache,* fatigue, dizziness, confusion

EENT: Blurred vision

GI: *Nausea, vomiting, anorexia,* abdominal pain

INTEG: Inj-site reactions, diaphoresis

META: Hypoglycemia

MS: Arthralgia

RESP: *Cough,* pharyngitis

SYST: *Systemic allergy*

PHARMACOKINETICS

Bioavailability 30%-40%, not extensively bound to blood cells or albumin, 40% bound in plasma, half-life 48 min, metabolized by kidneys, peak 20 min, duration 3 hr

INTERACTIONS

- Do not use with erythromycin, metoclopramide

Increase: effect of acetaminophen

Increase: pramlintide action—antimuscarinics, α-glucosidase inhibitors, diphenoxylate, loperamide, octreotide, opiate agonist, tricyclics

Increase: hypoglycemia—ACE inhibitors, disopyramide, anabolic steroids, androgens, fibric acid derivatives, alcohol, corticosteroids, insulin

Increase: hyperglycemia—phenothiazines

Decrease: hypoglycemia—niacin, dextrothyroxine, thiazide diuretics, triamterene, estrogens, progestins, oral contraceptives, MAOIs

NURSING CONSIDERATIONS

Assess:

- Fasting blood glucose, 2 hr postprandiol (80-150 mg/dl, normal fasting level; 70-130 mg/dl, normal 2 hr level); A1c may also be drawn to identify treatment effectiveness; also monitor weight, appetite
- **Hypoglycemic reaction:** sweating; weakness; dizziness; chills; confusion; headache; nausea; rapid, weak pulse; fatigue; tachycardia; memory lapses; slurred speech; staggering gait; anxiety; tremors; hunger
- **Hyperglycemia:** acetone breath; polyuria; fatigue; polydipsia; flushed, dry skin; lethargy

Evaluate:

- Therapeutic response: decrease in polyuria, polydipsia, polyphagia; clear sensorium; absence of dizziness; stable gait; improving blood glucose, A1c

Teach patient/family:

- That product does not cure diabetes but rather controls symptoms
- To carry emergency ID as diabetic
- To recognize hypoglycemia reaction: headache, fatigue, weakness, fast pulse
- About the dosage, route, mixing instructions, diet restrictions, disease process
- To carry a glucose source (candy or lump sugar, glucose tabs) to treat hypoglycemia
- About the symptoms of ketoacidosis: nausea; thirst; polyuria; dry mouth; decreased B/P; dry, flushed skin; acetone breath; drowsiness; Kussmaul respirations
- That a plan is necessary for diet, exercise; that all food on diet should be eaten; that exercise routine should not vary
- About blood glucose testing; how to determine glucose level
- To avoid OTC products, alcohol unless directed by prescriber
- Not to operate machinery or drive until effect is known
- About how to use pen

TREATMENT OF OVERDOSE:

Glucose 25 g IV or 50 ml dextrose 50% sol or 1 mg glucagon SUBCUT

pramoxine topical

See Appendix B

⚠ HIGH ALERT

prasugrel (Rx)

(pra′soo-grel)

Effient

Func. class.: Platelet aggregation inhibitor

Chem. class.: ADP receptor antagonist

P

ACTION:
Inhibits ADP-induced platelet aggregation

USES:
Reducing the risk of stroke, MI, vascular death, peripheral arterial disease in high-risk patients

CONTRAINDICATIONS:
Hypersensitivity, stroke, TIA

Black Box Warning: Active bleeding

Precautions: Pregnancy (B), breastfeeding, children, geriatric patients, hepatic disease, increased bleeding risk, neutropenia, agranulocytosis, renal disease, surgery, trauma, thrombotic thrombocytopenic purpura, Asian patients, weight <60 kg, CABG, abrupt discontinuation

DOSAGE AND ROUTES

- **Adult/geriatric <75 yr and ≥60 kg:** **PO** 60-mg loading dose, then 10 mg daily with aspirin (75-325 mg/day)
- **Adult/geriatric <75 yr and <60 kg:** **PO** 60 mg loading dose, then 5 mg daily
- Geriatric **>75 yr:** not recommended

Available forms: Tabs 5, 10 mg

Administer:

- With food to decrease gastric symptoms
- Do not break tablets
- Do not discontinue therapy abruptly

SIDE EFFECTS

CNS: Headache, dizziness

CV: Edema, atrial fibrillation, bradycardia, chest pain, hypo/hypertension

GI: Nausea, vomiting, diarrhea

HEMA: Epistaxis, leukopenia, thrombocytopenia, neutropenia, anaphylaxis, angioedema, anemia

INTEG: Rash, hypercholesterolemia

MISC: Fatigue, intracranial hemorrhage, secondary malignancy, angioedema

MS: Back pain

PHARMACOKINETICS

Rapidly absorbed; peak 30 min; metabolized by liver (CYP3A4; CYP2B6); excreted in urine, feces; half-life 7 hr

INTERACTIONS

Increase: bleeding risk—anticoagulants, aspirin, NSAIDs, abciximab, eptifibatide, tirofiban, thrombolytics, ticlopidine, SSRIs, treprostinil, rifampin

NURSING CONSIDERATIONS

Assess:

⚠ **Thrombotic/thrombocytic purpura:** fever, thrombocytopenia, neurolytic anemia

- Hepatic studies: AST, ALT, bilirubin, creatinine with long-term therapy
- Blood studies: CBC, differential, Hct, Hgb, PT, cholesterol with long-term therapy

Black Box Warning: Bleeding: may be fatal, decreased B/P in those who have had CABG may be the first indication; bleeding should be controlled while continuing product; may use transfusion; do not use within 1 wk of CABG; may use lower doses in those <60 kg

Evaluate:

- Therapeutic response: absence of stroke, MI

Teach patient/family:

- That blood work will be necessary during treatment
- To report any unusual bruising, bleeding to prescriber; that it may take longer to stop bleeding
- To take with food or just after eating to minimize GI discomfort
- To report diarrhea, skin rashes, subcutaneous bleeding, chills, fever, sore throat
- To tell all health care providers that prasugrel is being used; that product may be held before surgery

pravastatin (Rx)

(pra′va-sta-tin)

Pravachol

Func. class.: Antilipemic

Chem. class.: HMG-CoA reductase enzyme

Do not confuse:

Pravachol/Prevacid/propranolol

ACTION: Inhibits HMG-CoA reductase enzyme, which reduces cholesterol synthesis

USES: As an adjunct for primary hypercholesterolemia (types IIa, IIb, III, IV), to reduce the risk for recurrent MI, atherosclerosis, primary/secondary CV events, stroke, TIAs

CONTRAINDICATIONS: Pregnancy (X), breastfeeding, hypersensitivity, active hepatic disease

Precautions: Past hepatic disease, alcoholism, severe acute infections, trauma, severe metabolic disorders, electrolyte imbalances, renal disease

DOSAGE AND ROUTES

- **Adult: PO** 40 mg/day at bedtime (range 10-80 mg/day); start at 10 mg/day if patient also taking immunosuppressants
- **Adolescent 14-18 yr: PO** 40 mg/day
- **Child 8-13 yr: PO** 20 mg/day
- **Geriatric/renal/hepatic disease: PO** 10 mg/day initially

Renal dose

- **Adult: PO** 10-20 mg daily at bedtime, increase at 4-wk intervals

Available forms: Tabs 10, 20, 40, 80 mg

Administer:

- Without regard to meals, at bedtime
- Give 4 hr after bile acid sequestrants
- Store in cool environment in tight container protected from light

SIDE EFFECTS

CNS: Headache, dizziness, fatigue, confusion

CV: Chest pain

EENT: Lens opacities

GI: Nausea, constipation, diarrhea, flatus, abdominal pain, heartburn, hepatic dysfunction, pancreatitis, hepatitis

GU: Renal failure (myoglobinuria)

INTEG: Rash, pruritus

MS: Muscle cramps, myalgia, myositis, rhabdomyolysis

RESP: Common cold, rhinitis, cough

PHARMACOKINETICS

Peak 1-1½ hr; metabolized by liver; protein binding 50%; excreted in urine 20%, feces 70%, breast milk; crosses placenta; half-life 1.25-2.25 hr

INTERACTIONS

Increase: myopathy, rhabdomyolysis risk—erythromycin, niacin, cycloSPORINE, gemfibrozil, clofibrate, clarithromycin, itraconazole, protease inhibitors

Decrease: bioavailability of pravastatin—bile acid sequestrants

Drug/Herb

Increase: adverse reactions—red yeast rice

Increase: hepatotoxicity—eucalyptus

Decrease: effect—St. John's wort

Drug/Lab Test

Increase: CK, LFTs

Altered: thyroid function tests

NURSING CONSIDERATIONS

Assess:

- Fasting lipid profile: LDL, HDL, triglycerides, cholesterol at baseline, q12wk, then q6mo when stable; obtain diet history
- Hepatic studies: baseline, q12wk, then q6mo for remainder of yr; AST, ALT, LFTs may increase
- Renal studies of patients with compromised renal systems: BUN, I&O ratio, creatinine

⚠ **Rhabdomyolysis:** muscle tenderness, pain; obtain CPK at baseline and if these occur, therapy should be discontinued

Evaluate:

- Therapeutic response: decrease in LDL total cholesterol, triglycerides; increase in HDL

Teach patient/family:

- That blood work will be necessary during treatment

⚠ To report blurred vision, severe GI symptoms, dizziness, headache, muscle pain, weakness, fever

- That regimen will continue: low-cholesterol diet, exercise program

⚠ To report suspected, planned pregnancy; not to use product during pregnancy, pregnancy category (X); not to breastfeed

- **Hepatic disease:** to notify prescriber of lack of appetite, yellow sclera/skin, dark urine, abdominal pain, weakness

P

prazosin (Rx)

(pray′zoe-sin)

Minipress

Func. class.: Antihypertensive

Chem. class.: α_1-Adrenergic blocker, peripheral

ACTION: Blocks α-mediated vasoconstriction of adrenergic receptors, thereby inducing peripheral vasodilation

USES: Hypertension

Unlabeled uses: Benign prostatic hypertrophy to decrease urine outflow obstruction, heart failure, hypertensive urgency, Raynaud's phenomenon, posttraumatic stress disorder (PTSD), scorpion venom poisoning

CONTRAINDICATIONS: Hypersensitivity

Precautions: Pregnancy (C), breastfeeding, children, geriatric patients, prostate cancer, ocular surgery, orthostatic hypotension

DOSAGE AND ROUTES

Hypertension

- **Adult: PO** 1 mg bid or tid increasing to 20 mg/day in divided doses, if required; usual range 6-15 mg/day, max 1 mg initially; max 20 mg/day, some may require 40 mg/day
- **Child (unlabeled): PO** 5 mcg/kg q6hr; max 400 mcg/kg/day or 15 mg/day

Benign prostatic hyperplasia (unlabeled)

- **Adult: PO** 2 mg bid

Raynaud's phenomenon (unlabeled)

- **Adult: PO** 0.5-3 mg bid

CHF (unlabeled)

- **Adult: PO** 1 mg bid-tid, may gradually increase to max 20 mg/day
- **Child: PO** 5 mcg/kg q6hr, may gradually increase to 25 mcg/kg q6hr

Hypertensive urgency (unlabeled)

- **Adult: PO** 10-20 mg, may repeat after 30 min

Post-traumatic Stress Disorder (unlabeled)

Adult: PO up to 15 mg/day

Adolescents ≥15 yr: PO 1 mg at bedtime, then titrated to 1.5-4 mg at bedtime (to relieve nightmares)

Available forms: Caps 1, 2, 5 mg

Administer:

- 1st dose at bedtime to avoid fainting
- Without regard to meals
- Store at room temperature

SIDE EFFECTS

CNS: *Dizziness, headache, drowsiness,* anxiety, depression, vertigo, *weakness,* fatigue, syncope

CV: *Palpitations, orthostatic hypotension,* tachycardia, edema, rebound hypertension

EENT: Blurred vision, epistaxis, tinnitus, dry mouth, red sclera

GI: *Nausea,* vomiting, diarrhea, constipation, abdominal pain, pancreatitis

GU: Urinary frequency, incontinence, impotence, priapism; water, sodium retention

PHARMACOKINETICS

Onset 2 hr, peak 2-4 hr, duration 6-12 hr, half-life 2-4 hr; metabolized in liver, excreted via bile, feces (>90%), urine (<10%); protein binding 97%

INTERACTIONS

Increase: hypotensive effects—β-blockers, nitroglycerin, alcohol, phosphodiesterase inhibitors (vardenafil, tadalafil, sildenafil); diuretics, other antihypertensives, MAOIs

Decrease: antihypertensive effect—NSAIDs

Increase: antihypertensive effect—hawthorn

Drug/Lab Test

Increase: urinary norepinephrine, VMA

NURSING CONSIDERATIONS

Assess:

- **Hypertension/CHF:** B/P (sitting, standing) during initial treatment, periodically thereafter; pulse, jugular venous distention

- BUN, uric acid if patient receiving long-term therapy
- Weight daily, I&O; edema in feet, legs daily
- **Benign prostatic hypertrophy (unlabeled):** urinary patterns, frequency, stream, dribbling; flow before, during, and after therapy

Evaluate:
- Therapeutic response: decreased B/P

Teach patient/family:
- That fainting occasionally occurs after 1st dose; to take 1st dose at bedtime; not to drive or operate machinery for 4 hr after 1st dose; that full effect may take 4-6 wk
- To change positions slowly to prevent orthostatic hypotension
- To avoid OTC medications, alcohol unless approved by prescriber
- Not to discontinue abruptly

TREATMENT OF OVERDOSE:
Administer volume expanders or vasopressors, discontinue product, place patient in supine position

prednisoLONE (Rx)
(pred-niss′oh-lone)

Flo-Pred, Orapred, Prelone

Func. class.: Corticosteroid, synthetic

Chem. class.: Glucocorticoid, immediate acting

Do not confuse:
prednisoLONE/predniSONE

ACTION: Decreases inflammation by the suppression of migration of polymorphonuclear leukocytes, fibroblasts; reversal to increase capillary permeability and lysosomal stabilization

USES: Severe inflammation, immunosuppression, neoplasms, asthma

CONTRAINDICATIONS: Hypersensitivity, fungal infections, viral infection, varicella

Precautions: Pregnancy (C), breastfeeding, children, diabetes mellitus, glaucoma, osteoporosis, seizure disorders, ulcerative colitis, CHF, myasthenia gravis, abrupt discontinuation, children, acute MI, GI ulcers, hypertension, hepatitis, psychosis, thromboembolism, peptic ulcer disease, renal disease, Cushing syndrome

DOSAGE AND ROUTES
Primary (Addison's disease)/secondary adrenocortical insufficiency or for the treatment of congenital adrenal hyperplasia
- **Adults: PO** 5-60 mg **PO** per day as a single dose or divided doses
- **Infants, children, and adolescents: PO** 0.14-2 mg/kg or 4-60 mg/m^2 per day in 3-4 divided doses

Nonsuppurative thyroiditis
- **Adults: PO** 5-60 mg/day as a single dose or in divided doses
- **Infants, children, and adolescents: PO** 0.14-2 mg/kg or 4-60 mg/m^2 **PO** per day given in 3-4 divided doses

Management of symptomatic sarcoidosis; or treatment of hypercalcemia associated with sarcoidosis or with various cancers
- **Adults: PO** 5-60 mg/day as a single dose or divided doses
- **Infants, children, and adolescents: PO** 0.14-2 mg/kg or 4-60 mg/m^2 per day in 3-4 divided doses

Adjunct in rheumatic disorders (ankylosing spondylitis, gout with gouty arthritis, juvenile rheumatoid arthritis (JRA)/juvenile idiopathic arthritis (JIA), post-traumatic osteoarthritis psoriatic arthritis, rheumatoid arthritis) or acute episodes or exacerbation of nonrheumatic inflammation (acute and subacute bursitis, epicondylitis, and acute non-specific tenosynovitis)
- **Adults: PO** 5-60 mg/day as a single dose or in divided doses
- **Infants, children, and adolescents: PO** 0.14-2 mg/kg or 4-60 mg/m^2 per day in 3-4 divided doses

P

Adjunct in carpal tunnel syndrome (unlabeled)

- **Adults: PO** 20 mg/day × 2 wk, then 10 mg/day for an additional 2 wk relief

For maintenance therapy in selected cases of acute rheumatic carditis, systemic dermatomyositis (polymyositis), systemic lupus erythematosus (SLE); (Unlabeled): temporal arteritis, Churg-Strauss syndrome, mixed connective tissue disease, polyarteritis nodosa, relapsing polychondritis, polymyalgia rheumatica, vasculitis, or Wegener's granulomatosis:

- **Adults: PO** 5-60 mg per day as a single dose or in divided doses
- **Infants, children, and adolescents:** 0.14-2 mg/kg or 4-60 mg/m^2 **PO** per day given in 3-4 divided doses

Corticosteroid-responsive respiratory disorders (airway-obstructing hemangioma in infants (unlabeled), aspiration pneumonitis, berylliosis, chronic obstructive pulmonary disease (COPD), laryngotracheobronchitis (croup), Loeffler's syndrome, noncardiogenic pulmonary edema (unlabeled)

- **Adults: PO** 5-60 mg/day as a single dose or in divided doses
- **Infants, children, and adolescents: PO** 0.14-2 mg/kg or 4-60 mg/m^2 per day given in 3-4 divided doses

Asthma; bronchospasm prophylaxis (unlabeled)

- **Adults and adolescents: PO** 40-80 mg **PO** per day in 1-2 divided doses until the peak expiratory flow (PEF) reaches 70% of predicted or personal best; total course of treatment is 3-10 days
- **Children: PO** 1 mg/kg (up to 60 mg) per day in 2 divided doses until PEF reaches 70% of predicted or personal best; if a patient is given systemic corticosteroids, continue **PO** corticosteroids for a total course of 3-10 days; tapering is not necessary for courses <1 wk

Acute asthma exacerbation on an outpatient basis

- **Adults and adolescents: PO** 40-60 mg **PO** per day as a single dose or in 2 divided doses for 3-10 days
- **Children 5-12 yr: PO** 1-2 mg/kg (up to 60 mg) **PO** per day in 2 divided doses for 3-10 days
- **Infants and children ≤4 yr: PO** 1-2 mg/kg (up to 30 mg) **PO** per day in 2 divided doses for 3-10 days

Long-term prevention of symptoms in severe persistent asthma

- **Adults, adolescents, and children ≥12 yr: PO** 7.5-60 mg once daily in the morning or every other day
- **Infants and children ≤11 yr: PO** 0.25-2 mg/kg **PO** daily given as a single dose each morning or every other day

Hematologic disorders with thrombocytopenia (immune thrombocytopenia/idiopathic thrombocytopenic purpura (ITP), or secondary thrombocytopenia)

- **Adults: PO** 5-60 mg/day as a single dose or in divided doses
- **Children and adolescents (unlabeled): PO** 0.14-2 mg/kg or 4-60 mg/m^2 per day in 3-4 divided doses

Available forms: Tabs 5 mg; oral dissolving tab 10, 15, 30 mg; oral sol 5 mg/5 ml, 10 mg/5 ml, 15 mg/5 ml, 25 mg/5 ml; syrup 5 mg/5 ml

Administer:

- **Oral sol:** use calibrated measuring device
- **Orally disintegrating tabs:** place on tongue; allow to dissolve, swallow or swallow whole; do not cut, split

SIDE EFFECTS

CNS: *Depression,* headache, mood changes

CV: *Hypertension,* circulatory collapse, thrombophlebitis, embolism, tachycardia

EENT: Fungal infections, increased intraocular pressure, blurred vision

GI: *Diarrhea, nausea, abdominal distention,* GI hemorrhage, increased appetite, pancreatitis

INTEG: Acne, poor wound healing, ecchymosis, petechiae, sweating
MS: Fractures, osteoporosis, weakness, arthralgia, myopathy, **tendon rupture**

PHARMACOKINETICS

PO: Peak 1-2 hr, duration 2 days

INTERACTIONS

Increase: tendon rupture—quinolones
Increase: side effects—alcohol, salicylates, indomethacin, amphotericin B, digitalis, cycloSPORINE, diuretics
Increase: prednisoLONE action—salicylates, estrogens, indomethacin, oral contraceptives, ketoconazole, macrolide antibiotics
Increase: prednisoLONE effect—CYP3A4 inhibitors
Increase: **toxicity—azole antifungals, cycloSPORINE, NSAIDs**
Decrease: prednisoLONE action—cholestyramine, colestipol, barbiturates, rifampin, ePHEDrine, phenytoin, theophylline
Decrease: effects of anticoagulants, anticonvulsants, antidiabetics, ambenonium, neostigmine, isoniazid, toxoids, vaccines, anticholinesterases, salicylates, somatrem
Decrease: prednisoLONE effect—CYP3A4 inducers

Drug/Lab Test

Increase: cholesterol, sodium, blood glucose, uric acid, calcium, urine glucose
Decrease: calcium, potassium, T_4, T_3, thyroid ^{131}I uptake test, urine 17-OHCS, 17-KS, PBI
False negative: skin allergy tests

NURSING CONSIDERATIONS

Assess:

- Potassium, blood glucose, urine glucose while patient receiving long-term therapy; hypokalemia, hyperglycemia
- Weight daily; notify prescriber if weekly gain of >5 lb
- B/P q4hr, pulse; notify prescriber if chest pain occurs
- I&O ratio; be alert for decreasing urinary output, increasing edema
- Plasma cortisol levels with long-term therapy; normal level: 138-635 nmol/L SI units when drawn at 8 AM
- **Infection:** increased temperature, WBC, even after withdrawal of medication; product masks infection
- **Potassium depletion:** paresthesias, fatigue, nausea, vomiting, depression, polyuria, dysrhythmias, weakness
- Edema, hypertension, cardiac symptoms
- Mental status: affect, mood, behavioral changes, aggression
- **Adrenal insufficiency: nausea, vomiting, lethargy, restlessness, confusion, weight loss, hypotension before, during treatment; HPA suppression may be precipitated by abrupt withdrawal**

Evaluate:

- Therapeutic response: ease of respirations, decreased inflammation

Teach patient/family:

- That emergency ID as steroid user should be carried
- To notify prescriber if therapeutic response decreases; that dosage adjustment may be needed
- Not to discontinue abruptly; that adrenal crisis can result; to take product exactly as prescribed
- To avoid OTC products: salicylates, cough products with alcohol, cold preparations unless directed by prescriber
- About cushingoid symptoms
- **About the symptoms of adrenal insufficiency: nausea, anorexia, fatigue, dizziness, dyspnea, weakness, joint pain**

P

prednisoLONE ophthalmic (Rx)

See Appendix B

predniSONE (Rx)

(pred′ni-sone)

Rayos, Winpred ✦

Func. class.: Corticosteroid

Chem. class.: Intermediate-acting glucocorticoid

Do not confuse:
predniSONE/methylPREDNISolone/prednisoLONE/PriLOSEC

ACTION: Decreases inflammation by increasing capillary permeability and lysosomal stabilization, minimal mineralocorticoid activity

USES: Severe inflammation, neoplasms, multiple sclerosis, collagen disorders, dermatologic disorders, pulmonary fibrosis, asthma

Unlabeled uses: Adjunct for refractory seizures, infantile spasms, acute interstitial nephritis, amyloidosis, autoimmune hepatitis, Behçet's syndrome, Bell's palsy, carpal tunnel syndrome, Churg-Strauss syndrome, dermatomyositis, Duchenne muscular dystrophy, endophthalmitis, Lennox-Gastaut syndrome, lupus nephritis, mixed connective-tissue disease, pericarditis, pneumonia, polyarteritis nodosa, polychondritis, polymyositis, rheumatic carditis, temporal arteritis, TB, Wegener's granulomatosis

CONTRAINDICATIONS: Fungal infections, hypersensitivity

Precautions: Pregnancy (C), diabetes mellitus, glaucoma, osteoporosis, seizure disorders, ulcerative colitis, CHF, myasthenia gravis, renal disease, esophagitis, peptic ulcer, cataracts, coagulopathy, abrupt discontinuation, children, corticosteroid hypertensitivity, Cushing syndrome, diabetes mellitus, ulcerative colitis, thromboembolism, geriatric patients, acute MI

DOSAGE AND ROUTES

- **Adult: PO** 5-60 mg/day or divided bid-qid
- **Child: PO** 0.05-2 mg/kg/day divided 1-4×/day

Nephrotic syndrome

- **Child: PO** 2 mg/kg/day in divided doses, until urine is protein-free for 3 consecutive days, then 1-1.5 mg/kg/day every other day × 4 wk

Multiple sclerosis

- **Adult: PO** 200 mg/day × 1 wk, then 80 mg every other day × 1 mo

Asthma

- **Adult/adolescent: PO** 40-80 mg/day in 1-2 divided doses until PEF is 70% of predicted or best
- **Child: PO** 1 mg/kg (max 60 mg)/day in 2 divided doses until PEF is 70% of predicted or personal best

Available forms: Tabs 1, 2.5, 5, 10, 20, 50 mg; oral sol 5 mg/5 ml; syr 5 mg/5 ml, del rel tab 1, 2, 5 mg

Administer:

- For long-term use, alternate-day therapy recommended to decrease adverse reactions; give in AM to coincide with normal cortisol secretion
- Titrated dose; use lowest effective dose
- With food or milk to decrease GI symptoms
- **Oral sol:** use calibrated measuring device
- **Del rel tab:** swallow whole; do not break, crush, chew; give once a day

SIDE EFFECTS

CNS: Depression, flushing, sweating, headache, mood changes

CV: Hypertension, thrombophlebitis, embolism, tachycardia, fluid retention

EENT: Fungal infections, increased intraocular pressure, blurred vision

GI: Diarrhea, nausea, abdominal distention, GI hemorrhage, increased appetite, pancreatitis

INTEG: Acne, poor wound healing, ecchymosis, petechiae
META: Hyperglycemia
MS: Fractures, osteoporosis, weakness

PHARMACOKINETICS

PO: Well absorbed PO, peak 1-2 hr, duration; del rel peak 6-6½ hr; 1-1½ days, half-life 3½-4 hr, crosses placenta, enters breast milk, metabolized by liver after conversion, excreted in urine

INTERACTIONS

Increase: tendon rupture quinolones
Increase: side effects—alcohol, salicylates, NSAIDs, amphotericin B, digoxin, cycloSPORINE, diuretics
Increase: predniSONE action—salicylates, estrogens, NSAIDs, oral contraceptives, ketoconazole, macrolide antiinfectives
Increase: predniSONE effect—CYP3A4 inhibitors
Decrease: predniSONE effect—CYP3A4 inducers
Decrease: predniSONE action—cholestyramine, colestipol, barbiturates, rifampin, phenytoin, theophylline
Decrease: effects of anticoagulants, anticonvulsants, antidiabetics, ambenonium, neostigmine, isoniazid, toxoids, vaccines, anticholinesterases, salicylates, somatrem

Drug/Herb

Decrease: predniSONE effect—ephedra (ma huang)

Drug/Lab Test

Increase: cholesterol, sodium, blood glucose, uric acid, calcium, urine glucose
Decrease: calcium, potassium, T_4, T_3, thyroid ^{131}I uptake test, urine 17-OHCS, 17-KS, PBI
False negative: skin allergy tests

NURSING CONSIDERATIONS

Assess:

- **Adrenal insufficiency:** nausea, vomiting, anorexia, confusion, hypotension, weight loss before, during treatment; HPA suppression may be precipitated by abrupt withdrawal
- Potassium, blood glucose, urine glucose while patient receiving long-term therapy; hypokalemia and hyperglycemia; plasma cortisol with long-term therapy, normal: 138-635 nmol/L SI units drawn at 8 AM
- Weight daily; notify prescriber of weekly gain of >5 lb
- B/P, pulse; notify prescriber of chest pain; monitor for crackles, dyspnea if edema is present; hypertension, cardiac symptoms
- I&O ratio; be alert for decreasing urinary output, increasing edema
- **Infection:** increased temperature, WBC, even after withdrawal of medication; product masks infection
- Potassium depletion: paresthesias, fatigue, nausea, vomiting, depression, polyuria, dysrhythmias, weakness
- Mental status: affect, mood, behavioral changes, aggression

Evaluate:

- Therapeutic response: ease of respirations, decreased inflammation

Teach patient/family:

- That emergency ID as corticosteroid user should be carried; provide information about product being taken and condition
- To notify prescriber if therapeutic response decreases; that dosage adjustment may be needed
- To avoid vaccinations

⚠ Not to discontinue abruptly because adrenal crisis can result

- To avoid OTC products: salicylates, cough products with alcohol, cold preparations unless directed by prescriber
- **Cushingoid symptoms:** moon face, weight gain; symptoms of adrenal insufficiency: nausea, anorexia, fatigue, dizziness, dyspnea, weakness, joint pain
- That product causes immunosuppression; to report any symptoms of infection (fever, sore throat, cough)
- To notify prescriber if pregnancy is planned or suspected; cleft palate, stillbirth, abortion reported

pregabalin (Rx)

(pre-gab′a-lin)

Lyrica

Func. class.: Anticonvulsant

Chem. class.: γ-Aminobutyric acid (GABA) analog

Controlled Substance Schedule V

ACTION: Binds to high-voltage–gated calcium channels in CNS tissues; this may lead to anticonvulsant action similar to the inhibitory neurotransmitter GABA; anxiolytic, analgesics, and antiepileptic properties

USES: Neuropathic pain associated with spinal cord injury/diabetic peripheral neuropathy, partial-onset seizures, postherpetic neuralgia, fibromyalgia

Unlabeled uses: Moderate pain, social anxiety disorder

CONTRAINDICATIONS: Hypersensitivity to this product or gabapentin, abrupt discontinuation

Precautions: Pregnancy (C), breastfeeding, children <12 yr, geriatric patients, renal disease, PR interval prolongation, creatine kinase elevations, CHF (class III, IV), decreased platelets, substance abuse, dependence, glaucoma, myopathy, angioedema history, suicidal behavior

DOSAGE AND ROUTES

Diabetic peripheral neuropathic pain

- **ADULT: PO/ORAL SOL** 50 mg tid, may increase to 300 mg/day (max) within 1 wk, adjust in patients with renal disease

Partial-onset seizures

- **ADULT: PO/ORAL SOL** 75 mg bid or 50 mg tid; may increase to 600 mg/day (max)

Postherpetic neuralgia

- **Adult: PO/ORAL SOL** 150 mg/day in 2-3 divided doses, may increase to 300 mg/day in 2-3 divided doses; if higher dose is required after 2-4 wk, may increase to 600 mg/day in 2-3 divided doses

Fibromyalgia spinal cord injury, pain

- **Adult: PO/ORAL SOL** 75 mg bid, may increase to 150 mg bid within 1 wk and 225 mg bid after 1 wk

Renal dose

- **Adult: PO** CCr 30-60 ml/min, 75-300 mg/day in 2-3 divided doses; CCr 15-30 ml/min, 25-150 mg/day in 1-2 divided doses; CCr <15 ml/min, 25-75 mg/day as a single dose

Social phobia (unlabeled)

- **Adult: PO** 150-600 mg/day in 3 divided doses

Available forms: Caps 25, 50, 75, 100, 150, 200, 225, 300 mg; oral sol 20 mg/ml

Administer:

- Do not crush or chew caps; caps may be opened and contents put in applesauce or dissolved in juice
- Give without regard to meals
- Gradually withdraw over 7 days; abrupt withdrawal may precipitate seizures
- **Oral sol:** should be written in mg and calculated to mL

SIDE EFFECTS

CNS: Dizziness, fatigue, confusion, euphoria, incoordination, nervousness, neuropathy, tremor, vertigo, somnolence, ataxia, amnesia, abnormal thinking, suicidal ideation, drowsiness

EENT: Dry mouth, blurred vision, nystagmus, amblyopia, sinusitis

GI: Constipation, flatulence, abdominal pain, weight gain, nausea, vomiting, increased appetite

GU: Gynecomastia

HEMA: Ecchymosis, thrombocytopenia

MS: Back pain, rhabdomyolysis, myopathy

OTHER: Pruritus, orgasm/erectile dysfunction, peripheral edema, angioedema

RESP: Dyspnea

PHARMACOKINETICS

Well absorbed, peak 1.5 hr; 90% recovered in urine unchanged; negligible metabolism; not bound to plasma proteins; half-life 6 hr

INTERACTIONS

Increase: weight gain/fluid retention—thiazolidinedione; avoid use if possible

Increase: CNS depression—anxiolytics, sedatives, hypnotics, barbiturates, general anesthetics, opiate agonists, phenothiazines, sedating H_1 blockers, thiazolidinediones, tricyclics, alcohol

Drug/Lab Test

Increase: creatine kinase

Decrease: platelets

NURSING CONSIDERATIONS

Assess:

- **Seizures:** aura, location, duration, activity at onset, use seizure precaution
- **Pain:** location, duration, characteristics if using for diabetic neuropathy
- Renal studies: urinalysis, BUN, urine creatinine q3mo, creatine kinase; if markedly increased, discontinue product
- ⚠ Mental status: mood, sensorium, affect, behavioral changes, suicidal thoughts/behaviors; if mental status changes, notify prescriber
- **Angioedema/hypersensitivity:** monitor for blisters, hives, rash, dyspnea, wheezing; angioedema; if these occur, discontinue; cross-hypersensitivity with this product and gabapentin may occur
- **Rhabdomyolysis and creatinine kinase elevations:** monitor for muscle pain, tenderness, weakness accompanied by malaise or fever; product should be discontinued

Evaluate:

- Therapeutic response: decreased seizure activity; decrease in neuropathic pain

Teach patient/family:

- To carry emergency ID stating patient's name, products taken, condition, prescriber's name and phone number
- To avoid driving, other activities that require alertness because dizziness, drowsiness may occur
- Not to discontinue medication quickly after long-term use, to taper over ≥1 wk; that withdrawal-precipitated seizures may occur; not to double doses if dose is missed, to take if 2 hr or more before next dose
- To notify prescriber if pregnancy planned or suspected; to avoid breastfeeding
- To report muscle pain, tenderness, weakness when accompanied by fever, malaise, suicidal thoughts/behaviors
- To avoid alcohol, live virus vaccines

TREATMENT OF OVERDOSE:

Lavage, VS, hemodialysis

primaquine (Rx)

(prim′a-kween)

Func. class.: Antimalarial

Chem. class.: Synthetic 8-aminoquinolone

ACTION:

Unknown; thought to destroy exoerythrocytic forms by gametocidal action

USES:

Malaria caused by *Plasmodium vivax;* in combination with clindamycin for *Pneumocystis jiroveci* pneumonia

P

CONTRAINDICATIONS:

Lupus erythematosus, rheumatoid arthritis; hypersensitivity to this product or idoquinol

Precautions: Pregnancy (C), breastfeeding, methemoglobin reductase deficiency

Black Box Warning: Bone marrow suppression, hemolytic anemia, G6PD deficiency

DOSAGE AND ROUTES

- **Adult: PO** 15-30 mg (base)/day × 2 wk or 45 mg (base)/wk × 8 wk; 26.3-mg tab is 15-mg base
- **Child: PO** 0.5 mg/kg (0.3 mg/base/day) daily × 2 wk

Available forms: Tabs 26.3 mg

Administer:

PO route

- Before or after meals at same time each day to maintain product level; take with food to decrease GI upset

SIDE EFFECTS

CNS: Headache, dizziness

CV: Hypertension, dysrhythmias

EENT: *Blurred vision, difficulty focusing*

GI: *Nausea, vomiting, anorexia,* cramps

HEMA: Agranulocytosis, granulocytopenia, leukopenia, hemolytic anemia, leukocytosis, mild anemia, methemoglobinemia

INTEG: Pruritus, skin eruptions, pallor, weakness

PHARMACOKINETICS

PO: Metabolized by liver (metabolites), half-life 3.7-9.6 hr

INTERACTIONS

- Toxicity: quinacrine

Decrease: effect of carBAMazepine, PHENobarbital, phenytoins, rifamycins, nafcillin

Drug/Food

Increase: primaquine effect—food

Decrease: primaquine effect—grapefruit juice

Drug/Lab Test

Increase: WBC

Decrease: WBC, RBC, Hgb

NURSING CONSIDERATIONS

Assess:

- Ophthalmic test if patient receiving long-term treatment or product dosage of >150 mg/day
- Hepatic studies weekly: AST, ALT, bilirubin if patient receiving long-term therapy
- Blood studies: CBC; blood dyscrasias occur
- Allergic reactions: pruritus, rash, urticaria
- Blood dyscrasias: malaise, fever, bruising, bleeding (rare)
- Renal status: dark urine, hematuria, decreased output

⚠ **Hemolytic reaction:** chills, fever, chest pain, cyanosis; product should be discontinued immediately; hemolytic anemia may be severe in patients of Asian, Mediterranean descent

Evaluate:

- Therapeutic response: decreased symptoms of malaria

Teach patient/family:

- To report visual problems, fever, fatigue, dark urine, bruising, bleeding; may indicate blood dyscrasias
- To complete full course of therapy
- That an eye exam will be needed q4-6mo if using product for an extended period of time

RARELY USED

primidone (Rx)

(pri′mi-done)

Mysoline, Sertan ✦

Func. class.: Anticonvulsant

Chem. class.: Barbiturate derivative

USES: Generalized tonic-clonic (grand mal), complex seizures

CONTRAINDICATIONS: Pregnancy (D), breastfeeding, hypersensitivity to this product or barbiturates, porphyria

DOSAGE AND ROUTES

- **Adult and child >8 yr: PO** 125-250 mg at bedtime, increase by 125-250 mg/day q3-7days, usual dose 750-1500 mg/day in 3-4 divided doses, max 2 g/day in divided doses
- **Child <8 yr: PO** 50-125 mg at bedtime, increase by 50-125 mg/day q3-7days, usual dose 10-25 mg/kg/day in 3-4 divided doses
- **Neonate: PO** 12-20 mg/kg/day in 2-4 divided doses, start at lower dose and titrate

Benign familial tremor/essential tremor (unlabeled)

- **Adult: PO** 50-62.5 mg, increase as tolerated up to 750 mg/day in 3 divided doses

Renal dose

- **Adult: PO** CCr 10-50 ml/min, increase interval between doses to 8-12 hr; CCr <10 ml/min, increase interval to 12-24 hr

probenecid (Rx)

(proe-ben′e-sid)

Func. class.: Uricosuric, antigout agent

Chem. class.: Sulfonamide derivative

ACTION: Inhibits tubular reabsorption of urates, with increased excretion of uric acids

USES: Hyperuricemia in gout, gouty arthritis, adjunct to penicillin treatment

CONTRAINDICATIONS: Hypersensitivity, severe renal/hepatic disease, CCr <50 mg/min, history of uric acid calculus

Precautions: Pregnancy (C), children <2 yr, sulfonamide hypersensitivity, pepticular

DOSAGE AND ROUTES

Adjunct to penicillin

- **Adult/adolescent >15 yr, >50 kg (110 lb): PO** 500 mg qid

Gout/gouty arthritis

- **Adult: PO** 250 mg bid for 1 wk, then 500 mg bid, max 2 g/day; maintenance 500 mg/day × 6 mo

Adjunct in penicillin treatment

- **Adult and adolescent >50 kg: PO** 500 mg qid
- **Child <50 kg: PO** 25 mg/kg, then 40 mg/kg in divided doses qid

Renal dose

- Avoid use if CCr <50 ml/min

Available forms: Tabs 500 mg

Administer:

- After meals or with milk if GI symptoms occur
- Increase fluid intake to 2-3 L/day to prevent urinary calculi

SIDE EFFECTS

CNS: Drowsiness, headache, flushing

CV: Bradycardia

GI: *Gastric irritation, nausea, vomiting, anorexia,* hepatic necrosis

GU: Glycosuria, thirst, frequency, nephrotic syndrome

INTEG: Rash, dermatitis, pruritus, fever

META: *Acidosis, hypokalemia, hyperchloremia,* hyperglycemia

RESP: Apnea, irregular respirations

PHARMACOKINETICS

Peak 2-4 hr, duration 8 hr, half-life 5-8 hr; metabolized by liver; excreted in urine

INTERACTIONS

Increase: effect of acyclovir, barbiturates, allopurinol, benzodiazepines, dyphylline, zidovudine, cephalosporins, penicillins, sulfonamides

Increase: toxicity—sulfa products, dapsone, clofibrate, indomethacin, rifampin, naproxen, methotrexate

Decrease: action of probenecid—salicylates

Drug/Lab Test

Increase: theophylline levels

NURSING CONSIDERATIONS

Assess:

- Uric acid levels (3-7 mg/dl); mobility, joint pain, swelling, maintain fluid intake at 2-3 L/day
- Respiratory rate, rhythm, depth; notify prescriber of abnormalities
- Electrolytes; CO_2 before, during treatment
- Urine pH, output, glucose during beginning treatment, poor effect in GFR <30 ml/min

⚠ For CNS symptoms: confusion, twitching, hyperreflexia, stimulation, headache; may indicate overdose

Evaluate:

- Therapeutic response: absence of pain, stiffness in joints

Teach patient/family:

- To avoid OTC preparations (aspirin) unless directed by prescriber; to increase water intake, avoid alcohol, caffeine

⚠ HIGH ALERT

procainamide (Rx)

(proe-kane-ah′mide)

Func. class.: Antidysrhythmic (class IA)

Chem. class.: Procaine HCl amide analog

ACTION: Depresses excitability of cardiac muscle to electrical stimulation and slows conduction velocity in atrium, bundle of His, and ventricle; increases refractory period

USES: Life-threatening ventricular dysrhythmias

Unlabeled uses: Atrial fibrillation/flutter, paroxysmal atrial tachycardia, PSVT, Wolff-Parkinson-White (WPW) syndrome

CONTRAINDICATIONS: Hypersensitivity, severe heart block, torsades de pointes

Black Box Warning: Lupus erythematosus

Precautions: Pregnancy (C), breastfeeding, children, renal/hepatic disease, CHF, respiratory depression, cytopenia, dysrhythmia associated with digoxin toxicity, myasthenia gravis, digoxin toxicity

Black Box Warning: Bone marrow failure, cardiac arrhythmias

DOSAGE AND ROUTES

Ventricular tachycardia during CPR

- **Adult: IV** loading dose 20 mg/min; either ventricular tachycardia resolves or patient becomes hypotensive; QRS complex is widened by 50% of original width or total is 17 mg/kg (1.2 g for a 70-kg patient); may give up to 50 mg/min in urgent situations; maintenance: 1-4 mg/min **CONT IV INFUSION; IM** 50 mg/kg/day in divided doses q3-6hr
- **Child: IV** PALS 15 mg/kg over 30-60 min

Renal dose

- **Adult: IV** CCr 35-59 ml/min, give 70% maintenance dose; CCr 15-34 ml/min, give 40%-60% maintenance dose; CCr <15 ml/min, individualize dose

Available forms: Inj 100, 500 mg/ml

Administer:

IM route

- IM inj in deltoid; aspirate to avoid intravascular administration; use only when unable to use IV

Direct IV route

- Dilute each 100 mg/10 ml of 0.9% NaCl; give at max 50 mg/min

Intermittent IV INFUSION route

- Dilute 0.2-1 g/50-500 ml of D_5W (2-4 mg/ml); give over 30-60 min at max 25-50 mg/min; use infusion pump

Y-site compatibilities: Alfentanil, amikacin, aminocaproic acid, aminophylline, amiodarone, amphotericin B lipid complex, amphotericin B liposome, anidulafungin, ascorbic acid, atenolol, atracurium, atropine, aztreonam, benztropine, bivalirudin, bleomycin, bumetanide, buprenorphine, butorphanol, calcium chloride/gluconate, caspofungin, ceFAZolin, cefmetazole, cefonicid, cefoperazone, cefotaxime, cefoTEtan, cefOXitin, cefTAZidime, cefTRIAXone, cefuroxime, cephalothin, chlorproMAZINE, cimetidine, cisatracurium, CISplatin, clindamycin, cyanocobalamin, cyclophosphamide, cycloSPORINE, cytarabine, DACTINomycin, DAPTOmycin, dexamethasone, digoxin, diphenhydrAMINE, DOBUTamine, DOCEtaxel, DOPamine, doxacurium, DOXOrubicin, doxycycline, enalaprilat, ePHEDrine, EPINEPHrine, epirubicin, epoetin alfa, eptifibatide, ertapenem, erythromycin, esmolol, etoposide, etoposide phosphate, famotidine, fenoldopam, fentaNYL, fluconazole, fludarabine, fluorouracil, folic acid, furosemide, gatifloxacin, gemcitabine, gentamicin, glycopyrrolate, granisetron, heparin, hydrocortisone, HYDROmorphone, IDArubicin, ifosfamide, indomethacin, insulin (regular), irinotecan, isoproterenol, ketorolac, labetalol, lidocaine, linezolid, LORazepam, magnesium sulfate, mannitol, mechlorethamine, meperidine, metaraminol, methicillin, methotrexate, methoxamine, methyldopate, methylPREDNISolone, metoclopramide, metoprolol, mezlocillin, miconazole, midazolam, mitoXANtrone, morphine, moxalactam, multivitamins, mycophenolate, nafcillin, nalbuphine, naloxone, netilmicin, nitroglycerin, nitroprusside, norepinephrine, octreotide, ondansetron, oxacillin, oxaliplatin, oxytocin, PACLitaxel, palonosetron, pamidronate, pancuronium, pantoprazole, papaverine, PEMEtrexed, penicillin G potassium/sodium, pentamidine, pentazocine, PENTobarbital, PHENobarbital, phenylephrine, phytonadione, piperacillin, piperacillin-tazobactam, polymyxin B, potassium chloride, prochlorperazine, promethazine, propranolol, protamine, pyridoxine, quiNIDine, quinupristin-dalfopristin, ranitidine, remifentanil, ritodrine, rocuronium, sodium bicarbonate, succinylcholine, SUFentanil, tacrolimus, teniposide, theophylline, thiamine, thiotepa, ticarcillin, ticarcillin-clavulanate, tigecycline, tirofiban, tobramycin, tolazoline, trimetaphan, urokinase, vancomycin, vasopressin, vecuronium, verapamil, vinCRIStine, vinorelbine, vitamin B complex/C, voriconazole, zoledronic acid

SIDE EFFECTS

CNS: *Headache, dizziness,* confusion, psychosis, restlessness, irritability, weakness, depression

CV: *Hypotension,* **heart block, cardiovascular collapse, arrest, torsades de pointes**

GI: Nausea, vomiting, anorexia, diarrhea, hepatomegaly, pain, bitter taste

HEMA: SLE syndrome, **agranulocytosis, thrombocytopenia, neutropenia, hemolytic anemia**

INTEG: Rash, urticaria, edema, swelling (rare), pruritus, flushing, **angioedema**

SYST: SLE

PHARMACOKINETICS

Metabolized in liver to active metabolites, excreted unchanged by kidneys (60%), protein binding 15%

IM: Peak 10-60 min, half-life 3 hr

INTERACTIONS

Increase: effects of neuromuscular blockers

Increase: procainamide effects—cimetidine, quiNIDine, trimethoprim, β-blockers, ranitidine

Increase: **toxicity—other antidysrhythmics, thioridazine, quinolones**

Drug/Lab Test

Increase: ALT, AST, alk phos, LDH, bilirubin

NURSING CONSIDERATIONS

Assess:

Black Box Warning: Cardiac dysrhythmias: ECG continuously if using IV to determine increased PR or QRS segments; discontinue immediately; watch for increased ventricular ectopic beats, maximum need to rebolus

• Therapeutic blood levels, 4-10 mcg/ml or NAPA levels 10-20 mcg/ml

Black Box Warning: Bone marrow suppression: CBC q2wk × 3 mo; leukocyte, neutrophil, platelet counts may be decreased, treatment may need to be discontinued

• I&O ratio; electrolytes (K, Na, Cl), weight weekly, report gain of >2 lb

⚠ **Toxicity:** confusion, drowsiness, nausea, vomiting, tachydysrhythmias, oliguria

• ANA titer; during long-term treatment, watch for lupuslike symptoms

• Cardiac rate, rhythm, character, B/P continuously for fluctuations

• Respiratory status: rate, rhythm, character, lung fields; bilateral crackles may occur in CHF patient; watch for respiratory depression

⚠ CNS effects: dizziness, confusion, psychosis, paresthesias, seizures; product should be discontinued

Evaluate:

• Therapeutic response: decreased dysrhythmias

Teach patient/family:

• That wax matrix may appear in stools

P

• Not to discontinue without provider's approval

Black Box Warning: To notify prescriber immediately if lupuslike symptoms appear (joint pain, butterfly rash, fever, chills, dyspnea)

Black Box Warning: To notify prescriber of leukopenia (sore mouth, gums, throat) or thrombocytopenia (bleeding, bruising)

• How to take pulse and when to report to prescriber
• To avoid driving, other hazardous activities until product effect is known

TREATMENT OF OVERDOSE:
O_2, artificial ventilation, ECG, administer DOPamine for circulatory depression, diazepam or thiopental for seizures, isoproterenol

HIGH ALERT

procarbazine (Rx)
(proe-kar′ba-zeen)

Matulane

Func. class.: Antineoplastic, alkylating agent

Chem. class.: Hydrazine derivative

ACTION:
Inhibits DNA, RNA, protein synthesis; has multiple sites of action; nonvesicant

USES:
Lymphoma, Hodgkin's disease, cancers resistant to other therapy

Unlabeled uses: Brain, lung malignancies; other lymphomas; multiple myeloma, malignant melanoma, polycythemia vera

CONTRAINDICATIONS:
Pregnancy (D), breastfeeding, hypersensitivity, thrombocytopenia, bone marrow depression

Precautions: Cardiac/renal/hepatic disease, radiation therapy, seizure disorder, anemia, bipolar disorder, Parkinson's disease

Black Box Warning: Requires a specialized care setting and an experienced clinician

DOSAGE AND ROUTES
• **Adult: PO** 2-4 mg/kg/day for 1st wk; maintain dosage of 4-6 mg/kg/day until platelets, WBC fall; after recovery, 1-2 mg/kg/day
• **Child: PO** 50 mg/m^2/day for 7 days, then 100 mg/m^2 until desired response, leukopenia, or thrombocytopenia occurs; 50 mg/m^2/day maintenance after bone marrow recovery

Available forms: Caps 50 mg

Administer:
• In divided doses and at bedtime to minimize nausea and vomiting
• Nonphenothiazine antiemetic 30-60 min before product and 4-10 hr after treatment to prevent vomiting

SIDE EFFECTS
CNS: Headache, dizziness, insomnia, hallucinations, confusion, coma, pain, chills, fever, sweating, paresthesias, seizures, peripheral neuropathy

EENT: Retinal hemorrhage, nystagmus, photophobia, diplopia, dry eyes

GI: *Nausea, vomiting,* anorexia, diarrhea, constipation, dry mouth, stomatitis, elevated hepatic enzymes

GU: Azoospermia, cessation of menses

HEMA: Thrombocytopenia, anemia, leukopenia, myelosuppression, bleeding tendencies, purpura, petechiae, epistaxis, hemolysis

INTEG: *Rash,* pruritus, dermatitis, alopecia, herpes, hyperpigmentation

MS: Arthralgias, myalgias

RESP: Cough, pneumonitis, hemoptysis

SYST: Secondary malignancy

PHARMACOKINETICS
Half-life 1 hr; concentrates in liver, kidney, skin; metabolized in liver, excreted in urine

INTERACTIONS
⚠ **Increase:** hypotension—meperidine; do not use together

Increase: neuroleptic malignant syndrome, seizures, hyperpyrexia—alcohol, MAOIs, tricyclics, sympathomimetic products, SSRIs, SNRIs
Increase: hypertension—guanethidine, levodopa, methyldopa, reserpine, caffeine
⚠ Life-threatening hypertension: sympathomimetics
Increase: bleeding risk—NSAIDs, anticoagulants, platelet inhibitors, thrombolytics
Increase: CNS depression—barbiturates, antihistamines, opioids, hypotensive agents, phenothiazines

Drug/Food

- Hypertensive crisis: tyramine foods

NURSING CONSIDERATIONS

Assess:

- **Bone marrow suppression:** CBC, differential, platelet count weekly; withhold product if WBC is $<4000/mm^3$ or platelet count is $<100,000/mm^3$; notify prescriber
- **Hepatic/renal disease:** can cause accumulation of drug, increased toxicity; renal studies: BUN; serum uric acid; urine CCr; electrolytes before, during therapy; I&O ratio, report fall in urine output to <30 ml/hr; hepatic studies before, during therapy: bilirubin, AST, ALT, alk phos, LDH prn or monthly
- Monitor temperature; fever may indicate beginning infection

Black Box Warning: To be used only in a specialized care setting with emergency equipment

Black Box Warning: To be given only by an experienced clinician knowledgeable in cytotoxic products

- CNS changes: confusion, paresthesias, neuropathies; product should be discontinued

⚠ Tyramine foods in diet; hypertensive crisis can occur
⚠ **Toxicity:** facial flushing, epistaxis, increased PT, thrombocytopenia; product should be discontinued

- **Bleeding:** hematuria, guaiac stools, bruising or petechiae, mucosa or orifices q8hr
- Effects of alopecia on body image; discuss feelings about body changes
- Jaundiced skin, sclera; dark urine, clay-colored stools, itchy skin, abdominal pain, fever, diarrhea
- Buccal cavity for dryness, sores or ulceration, white patches, oral pain, bleeding, dysphagia
- GI symptoms: frequency of stools, cramping
- **Acidosis, signs of dehydration:** rapid respirations, poor skin turgor, decreased urine output, dry skin, restlessness, weakness

Evaluate:

- Therapeutic response: decreasing malignancy

Teach patient/family:

- To report any complaints, side effects to nurse or prescriber: CNS changes, diarrhea, cough, SOB, fever, chills, sore throat, bleeding, bruising, vomiting blood; black, tarry stools
- That hair may be lost during treatment and wig or hairpiece may make patient feel better; that new hair may be different in color, texture
- To avoid sunlight or UV exposure; to wear sunscreen or protective clothing
- To avoid foods with citric acid, hot or rough texture
- To report any bleeding, white spots, ulcerations in mouth to prescriber; to examine mouth daily
- To avoid driving, activities requiring alertness because dizziness may occur
- To use effective contraception; to avoid breastfeeding; that product may cause infertility
- To avoid the ingestion of alcohol, caffeine, tyramine-containing foods; that cold, hay fever, and weight-reducing products may cause serious product interactions; to avoid smoking
- To avoid crowds, persons with infections if granulocytes are low
- To avoid vaccines

P

prochlorperazine (Rx)

(proe-klor-pair′a-zeen)

Compro

Func. class.: Antiemetic, antipsychotic

Chem. class.: Phenothiazine, piperazine derivative

Do not confuse:
prochlorperazine/chlorproMAZINE

ACTION: Decreases DOPamine neurotransmission by increasing DOPamine turnover through the blockade of the D_2 somatodendritic autoreceptor in the mesolimbic system

USES: Nausea, vomiting, psychotic disorders

Unlabeled uses: Migraine

CONTRAINDICATIONS: Hypersensitivity to phenothiazines, coma; infants, neonates, children <2 yr or <20 lb; surgery

Precautions: Pregnancy (C), breastfeeding, geriatric patients, seizure, encephalopathy, glaucoma, hepatic disease, Parkinson's disease, BPH

Black Box Warning: Increased mortality in elderly patients with dementia-related psychosis

DOSAGE AND ROUTES

Postoperative nausea/vomiting

- **Adult: IM** 5-10 mg 1-2 hr before anesthesia; may repeat after 30 min; **IV** 5-10 mg 15-30 min before anesthesia; **IV INFUSION** 20 mg/L D_5W or **NS** 15-30 min before anesthesia, max 40 mg/day

Severe nausea/vomiting

- **Adult: PO** 5-10 mg tid-qid; **SUS REL** 15 mg/day in AM or 10 mg q12hr; **RECT** 25 mg/bid; **IM** 5-10 mg q3-4hr prn, max 40 mg/day
- **Child 18-39 kg: PO** 2.5 mg tid or 5 mg bid; **IM** 0.132 mg/kg q3-4hr prn, max 15 mg/day
- **Child 14-17 kg: PO/RECT** 2.5 mg bid-tid; **IM** 0.132 mg/kg q3-4hr prn, max 10 mg/day
- **Child 9-13 kg: PO/RECT** 2.5 mg/day-bid; **IM** 0.132 mg/kg q3-4hr prn, max 7.5 mg/day

Antipsychotic

- **Adult and child ≥12 yr: PO** 5-10 mg tid-qid; may increase q2-3days, max 150 mg/day; **IM** 10-20 mg q2-4hr up to 4 doses, then 10-20 mg q4-6hr
- **Child 2-12 yr: PO** 2.5 mg bid-tid; **IM** 0.132 mg/kg change to oral ASAP

Antianxiety

- **Adult and child ≥12 yr: PO** 5 mg tid-qid, max 20 mg/day
- **Child 2-12 yr: IM** 0.132 mg/kg change to oral ASAP

Available forms: Tabs 5, 10, 25 mg; supp 25 mg

Administer:

- Avoid other CNS depressants

IM route

- IM inj in large muscle mass; aspirate to avoid IV administration
- Keep patient recumbent for ½ hr

Direct IV route

- No dilution needed; inject directly in a vein ≤5 mg/min; do not give as bolus

Intermittent IV INFUSION route

- May dilute 20 mg/L NaCl and give as infusion 15-30 min before anesthesia induction

Y-site compatibilities: Amsacrine, calcium gluconate, cisatracurium, CISplatin, cladribine, cyclophosphamide, cytarabine, DOXOrubicin, DOXOrubicin liposome, fluconazole, granisetron, heparin, hydrocortisone, melphalan, methotrexate, ondansetron, PACLitaxel, potassium chloride, propofol, remifentanil, sargramostim, SUFentanil, teniposide, thiotepa, vinorelbine, vit B/C

SIDE EFFECTS

CNS: Neuroleptic malignant syndrome, *extrapyramidal reactions, tardive dyskinesia, euphoria,* depression, *drowsiness,* restlessness, tremor, dizziness, headache

CV: Circulatory failure, tachycardia, hypotension, ECG changes
EENT: Blurred vision
GI: Nausea, vomiting, anorexia, dry mouth, diarrhea, constipation, weight loss, metallic taste, cramps
HEMA: Agranulocytosis
MISC: Impotence
RESP: Respiratory depression

PHARMACOKINETICS

Metabolized by liver; excreted in urine, breast milk; crosses placenta; 91%-99% protein binding
IM: Onset 10-20 min, duration 4-6 hr; children: 12 hr
PO: Onset 30-40 min, duration 3-4 hr
RECT: Onset 60 min, duration 3-4 hr

INTERACTIONS

Increase: anticholinergic action—anticholinergics, antiparkinson products, antidepressants
Increase: CNS depression—CNS depressants
Increase: serotonin syndrome, neuroleptic malignant syndrome—SSRIs, SNRIs
Decrease: prochlorperazine effect—barbiturates, antacids, lithium
Drug/Herb
Increase: CNS depression—chamomile, hops, kava, St. John's wort, valerian
Increase: EPS—kava
Drug/Lab Test
Increase: LFTs, cardiac enzymes, cholesterol, blood glucose, prolactin, bilirubin, PBI, ^{131}I, alk phos, leukocytes, granulocytes, platelets
Decrease: hormones (blood and urine)
False positive: pregnancy tests, urine bilirubin
False negative: urinary steroids, 17-OHCS, pregnancy tests

NURSING CONSIDERATIONS

Assess:
- **EPS:** abnormal movement, tardive dyskinesia, akathisia
- VS, B/P; check patients with cardiac disease more often

⚠ **Neuroleptic malignant syndrome:** seizures, hypo/hypertension, fever, tachycardia, dyspnea, fatigue, muscle stiffness, loss of bladder control; notify prescriber immediately

⚠ CBC, LFTs during course of treatment; blood dyscrasias, hepatotoxicity may occur

- Respiratory status before, during, after administration of emetic; check rate, rhythm, character; respiratory depression can occur rapidly among geriatric or debilitated patients

Evaluate:
- Therapeutic response: absence of nausea, vomiting; reduced anxiety, agitation, excitability

Teach patient/family:
- To avoid hazardous activities, activities requiring alertness because dizziness may occur
- To avoid alcohol
- Not to double or skip doses
- That urine may be pink to reddish brown
- That suppositories may contain coconut/palm oil
- To report dark urine, clay-colored stools, bleeding, bruising, rash, blurred vision
- To avoid sun; wear sunscreen, protective clothing

P

progesterone (Rx)

(proe-jess′ter-one)

Crinone, Endometrin, Prochieve, Prometrium

Func. class.: Progestogen

Chem. class.: Progesterone derivative

ACTION:
Inhibits secretion of pituitary gonadotropins, which prevents follicular maturation, ovulation; stimulates growth of mammary tissue; antineoplastic action against endometrial cancer

USES:
Contraception, amenorrhea, premenstrual syndrome, abnormal uterine bleeding, endometrial hyperplasia

prevention, assisted reproductive technology (ART) gel

Unlabeled uses: Corpus luteum insufficiency, early pregnancy failure, PMS, preterm delivery prophylaxis

CONTRAINDICATIONS:

Pregnancy (B), ectopic pregnancy; hypersensitivity to this product, peanuts, or peanut oil; thromboembolic disorders, reproductive cancer, genital bleeding (abnormal, undiagnosed), cerebral hemorrhage, PID, STDs, thrombophlebitis

Black Box Warning: Breast cancer

Precautions: Breastfeeding, hypertension, asthma, blood dyscrasias, CHF, diabetes mellitus, bone disease, depression, migraine headache, seizure disorders, gallbladder/renal/hepatic disease, family history of breast/reproductive tract cancer

Black Box Warning: Cardiac disease, dementia

DOSAGE AND ROUTES

Infertility

- **Adult: VAG** 90 mg/day (micronized gel); 100 mg 2-3 times/day starting day after oocyte retrieval and for ≤10 wk total (insert)

Amenorrhea/functional uterine bleeding

- **Adult: IM** 5-10 mg/day × 6-8 doses

Endometrial hyperplasia prevention

- **Adult: PO** 200 mg/day × 12 days

Assisted reproductive therapy

- **Adult: GEL** 90 mg (8%) vaginally daily for supplementation; 90 mg (8%) vaginally bid for replacement; if pregnancy occurs, continue × 10-12 wk

Corpus luteum insufficiency (unlabeled)

- **Adult: VAG INSERT** 90-100 mg bid-tid starting at oocyte retrieval and continuing up to 10-12 wk gestation

Available forms: Inj 50 mg/ml; vag gel 4%, 8%; caps 100, 200 mg; vag insert 100 mg; vag supp 25, 100, 200, 500 mg; compounding kit 25, 50, 100, 200, 400 mg

Administer:

PO route

- Do not break, crush, or chew caps
- Titrated dose; use lowest effective dose
- In 1 dose in AM
- With food or milk to decrease GI symptoms
- Start progesterone 14 days after estrogen dose if given concomitantly

Vaginal route

- Wait at least 6 hr after any vaginal treatment before using vaginal gel

IM route

- Shake vial, inject deeply into large muscle, aspirate
- Check for particulate matter and discoloration before injecting

SIDE EFFECTS

CNS: *Dizziness, headache,* migraines, depression, *fatigue,* mood swings, dementia, drowsiness

CV: Hypotension, thrombophlebitis, edema, thromboembolism, stroke, pulmonary embolism, MI

EENT: Diplopia, retinal thrombosis

GI: *Nausea,* vomiting, anorexia, cramps, increased weight, cholestatic jaundice, *constipation,* abdominal pain

GU: Amenorrhea, cervical erosion, breakthrough bleeding, dysmenorrhea, vaginal candidiasis, nocturia, breast changes, *gynecomastia, testicular atrophy, impotence,* endometriosis, spontaneous abortion, breast pain, ectopic pregnancy

INTEG: Rash, urticaria, acne, hirsutism, alopecia, oily skin, seborrhea, purpura, melasma

META: Hyperglycemia

SYST: Angioedema, anaphylaxis

PHARMACOKINETICS

Excreted in urine, feces; metabolized in liver

IM/RECT/VAG: Duration 24 hr

INTERACTIONS

Increase: progesterone effect—CYP3A4 inhibitors (ketoconazole, cimetidine,

clarithromycin, danazol, diltiazem, erythromycin, fluconazole, itraconazole, troleandomycin, verapamil, voriconazole)
Decrease: progesterone effect—barbiturates, phenytoin

Drug/Lab Test

Increase: alk phos, nitrogen (urine), pregnanediol, amino acids, factors VII, VIII, IX, X
Decrease: GTT, HDL

NURSING CONSIDERATIONS

Assess:

- **Abnormal uterine bleeding:** vaginal bleeding; obtain pad count, patient menstrual history, breast exam, cervical cytology
- Weight daily; notify prescriber of weekly weight gain of >5 lb
- B/P at beginning of treatment and periodically
- I&O ratio; be alert for decreasing urinary output, increasing edema
- Hepatic studies: ALT, AST, bilirubin periodically during long-term therapy
- Edema, hypertension, cardiac symptoms, jaundice, thromboembolism
- Mental status: affect, mood, behavioral changes, depression
- Hypercalcemia

Evaluate:

- Therapeutic response: decreased abnormal uterine bleeding, absence of amenorrhea

Teach patient/family:

⚠ To report breast lumps, vaginal bleeding, edema, jaundice, dark urine, clay-colored stools, dyspnea, headache, blurred vision, abdominal pain, numbness or stiffness in legs, chest pain

- To avoid gel with other vaginal products; if to be used together, to separate by ≥6 hr; for vaginal route, on proper insertion technique
- To report suspected pregnancy
- To monitor blood glucose if diabetic
- To avoid activities requiring mental alertness until effects are realized; can cause dizziness

⚠ HIGH ALERT

promethazine (Rx)

(proe-meth'a-zeen)

Promethegan

Func. class.: Antihistamine, H_1-receptor antagonist, antiemetic
Chem. class.: Phenothiazine derivative

ACTION: Acts on blood vessels, GI, respiratory system by competing with histamine for H_1-receptor sites; decreases allergic response by blocking histamine

USES: Motion sickness, rhinitis, allergy symptoms, sedation, nausea, preoperative and postoperative sedation
Unlabeled uses: Allergic rhinitis, acute peripheral vestibular nystagmus, hyperemesis gravidarum

CONTRAINDICATIONS: Hypersensitivity, breastfeeding, agranulocytosis, bone marrow suppression, coma, jaundice, Reye's syndrome

Black Box Warning: Infants, neonates, children, intraarterial/SUBCUT administration, extravasation

Precautions: Pregnancy (C), cardiac/renal/hepatic disease, asthma, seizure disorder, prostatic hypertrophy, bladder obstruction, glaucoma, COPD, GI obstruction, ileus, CNS depression, diabetes, sleep apnea, urinary retention

Black Box Warning: IV use

DOSAGE AND ROUTES

Nausea/vomiting

- **Adult: PO/IM/IV/RECT** 12.5-25 mg; q4-6hr prn
- **Child >2 yr: PO/IM/IV/RECT** 0.25-0.5 mg/kg q4-6hr prn

Motion sickness

- **Adult: PO** 25 mg bid, give ½-1 hr before departure, then q8-12hr prn

P

- **Child ≥2 yr: PO/IM/RECT** 12.5-25 mg bid, give ½-1 hr before departure, then q8-12hr prn

Sedation

- **Adult: PO/IM** 25-50 mg at bedtime
- **Child ≥2 yr: PO/IM/RECT** 12.5-25 mg at bedtime

Sedation (preoperative/ postoperative)

- **Adult: PO/IM/IV** 25-50 mg
- **Child >2 yr: PO/IM/IV** 0.5-1.1 mg/kg

Allergy/rhinitis (unlabeled)

- **Adult: PO** 12.5 mg qid or 25 mg at bedtime
- **Child ≥2 yr: PO** 6.25-12.5 mg tid or 25 mg at bedtime

Hyperemesis gravidarum (unlabeled)

- **Pregnant females: PO/RECT/IM/IV** 12.5-25 mg q4hr

Nystagmus (unlabeled)

- **Adult: PO** 12.5-25 mg q4-6hr for ≤48 hr

Available forms: Tabs 12.5, 25, 50 mg; supp 12.5, 25, 50 mg; inj 25, 50 mg/ml

Administer:

- Avoid use with other CNS depressants

PO route

- With meals for GI symptoms; absorption may slightly decrease
- When used for motion sickness, 30 min-1 hr before travel

IM route

- IM inj deep in large muscle; rotate site

Direct IV route

Black Box Warning: Check for extravasation: burning, pain, swelling at IV site; can cause tissue necrosis

- Do not use if precipitate is present
- Rapid administration may cause transient decrease in B/P
- After diluting each 25-50 mg/9 ml of NaCl for inj; give ≤25 mg/2 min

Y-site compatibilities: Alfentanil, amifostine, amikacin, aminocaproic acid, amsacrine, anidulafungin, ascorbic acid, atenolol, atracurium, atropine, aztreonam, benztropine, bivalirudin, bleomycin, bumetanide, buprenorphine, butorphanol, calcium chloride/gluconate, CARBOplatin, caspofungin, chlorproMAZINE, cimetidine, ciprofloxacin, cisatracurium, CISplatin, cladribine, codeine, cyanocobalamin, cyclophosphamide, cycloSPORINE, cytarabine, DACTINomycin, DAPTOmycin, dexmedetomidine, digoxin, diltiazem, diphenhydrAMINE, DOBUTamine, DOCEtaxel, DOPamine, doxacurium, DOXOrubicin, doxycycline, enalaprilat, ePHEDrine, EPINEPHrine, epirubicin, epoetin, eptifibatide, erythromycin, esmolol, etoposide, famotidine, fenoldopam, fentaNYL, filgrastim, fluconazole, fludarabine, gemcitabine, gentamicin, glycopyrrolate, granisetron, HYDROmorphone, hydrOXYzine, IDArubicin, ifosfamide, insulin (regular), irinotecan, isoproterenol, labetalol, levofloxacin, lidocaine, linezolid, LORazepam, magnesium sulfate, mannitol, mechlorethamine, melphalan, meperidine, metaraminol, methoxamine, methyldopate, metoclopramide, metoprolol, metroNIDAZOLE, miconazole, midazolam, milrinone, mitoXANtrone, morphine, mycophenolate, nalbuphine, naloxone, netilmicin, nitroglycerin, norepinephrine, octreotide, ondansetron, oxaliplatin, oxytocin, PACLitaxel, palonosetron, pamidronate, pancuronium, PEMEtrexed, pentamidine, pentazocine, phenylephrine, polymyxin B, procainamide, prochlorperazine, propranolol, protamine, pyridoxine, quiNIDine, quinupristin-dalfopristin, ranitidine, remifentanil, Ringer's, ritodrine, riTUXimab, rocuronium, sargramostim, sodium acetate, succinylcholine, SUFentanil, tacrolimus, teniposide, theophylline, thiamine, thiotepa, tigecycline, tirofiban, TNA, tobramycin, tolazoline, trastuzumab, trimetaphan, vancomycin, vasopressin, vecuronium, verapamil, vinCRIStine, vinorelbine, voriconazole

SIDE EFFECTS

CNS: *Dizziness, drowsiness,* poor coordination, fatigue, anxiety, euphoria, confusion, paresthesia, neuritis, EPS, neuroleptic malignant syndrome

CV: Hypo/hypertension, palpitations, tachycardia

EENT: Blurred vision, dilated pupils, tinnitus, nasal stuffiness; dry nose, throat, mouth; photosensitivity
GI: *Constipation,* dry mouth, nausea, vomiting, anorexia, diarrhea
GU: *Urinary retention,* dysuria, frequency
HEMA: **Thrombocytopenia, agranulocytosis, hemolytic anemia**
INTEG: Rash, urticaria, photosensitivity
RESP: Increased thick secretions, wheezing, chest tightness; **apnea in neonates, infants, young children**

PHARMACOKINETICS

Metabolized in liver; excreted by kidneys, GI tract (inactive metabolites)
PO: Onset 20 min, duration 4-12 hr
IV: Onset 3-5 min

INTERACTIONS

Increase: CNS depression—barbiturates, opioids, hypnotics, tricyclics, alcohol
Increase: promethazine effect—MAOIs
Decrease: oral anticoagulants effect—heparin
Drug/Lab Test
False negative: skin allergy test
False positive: urine pregnancy test
Interference: blood grouping (ABO), GTT

NURSING CONSIDERATIONS

Assess:

Black Box Warning: Not to be used in children <2 yr, fatal respiratory depression may occur; use cautiously in children >2 yr, seizures, paradoxical CNS stimulation may occur

- **Antiemetic/motion sickness:** nausea, vomiting before, after dose
- I&O ratio; be alert for urinary retention, frequency, dysuria; product should be discontinued
- ⚠ **CBC with differential, LFTs during long-term therapy; blood dyscrasias, jaundice may occur**
- Respiratory status: rate, rhythm, increase in bronchial secretions, wheezing, chest tightness
- Cardiac status: palpitations, increased pulse, hypo/hypertension, B/P in those receiving IV doses
- **Neuroleptic malignant syndrome: fever, confusion, diaphoresis, rigid muscles, elevated CPK, encephalopathy; discontinue product, notify prescriber**
- Hard candy, gum, frequent rinsing of mouth for dryness

Evaluate:

- Therapeutic response: absence of running, congested nose; rashes; absence of motion sickness, nausea; sedation

Teach patient/family:

- That product may cause photosensitivity; to avoid prolonged exposure to sunlight
- To notify prescriber of confusion, sedation, hypotension, jaundice, fever
- To avoid driving, other hazardous activity if drowsy
- To avoid concurrent use of alcohol or other CNS depressants
- That product may reduce sweating; that there is a risk of heat stroke
- How to use frequent sips of water, gum to decrease dry mouth

⚠ ***HIGH ALERT***

propafenone (Rx)

(pro-paff'e-nown)

Rythmol, Rythmol SR

Func. class.: Antidysrhythmic (class IC)

ACTION:
Slows conduction velocity; reduces membrane responsiveness; inhibits automaticity; increases ratio of effective refractory period to action potential duration; β-blocking activity

USES:
Sustained ventricular tachycardia, atrial fibrillation (single dose), paroxysmal supraventricular tachycardia (PSVT) prophylaxis, supraventricular dysrhythmias
Unlabeled uses: Wolff-Parkinson-White (WPW) syndrome

CONTRAINDICATIONS:
2nd/3rd-degree AV block, right bundle branch block, cardiogenic shock, hypersensitivity, bradycardia, uncontrolled CHF, sick-sinus syndrome, marked hypotension, bronchospastic disorders, electrolyte imbalance, Brugada syndrome

Precautions: Pregnancy (C), breastfeeding, children, geriatric patients, CHF, hypo/hyperkalemia, nonallergic bronchospasm, renal/hepatic disease, hematologic disorders, myasthenia gravis, COPD

Black Box Warning: Recent MI, cardiac arrhythmias, QT prolongation, torsades de pointes

DOSAGE AND ROUTES

PSVT

- **Adult: PO** 150 mg q8hr; allow 3-4 day interval before increasing dose, max 900 mg/day

Atrial fibrillation

- **Adult: PO** 450 or 600 mg as single dose; SR 225 mg q12hr, may increase to 325 q12hr, max 425 mg q12hr

Available forms: Tabs 150, 225, 300 mg; SR cap 225, 325, 425 mg

Administer:

- Do not break, crush, or chew tabs; swallow whole
- To hospitalized patients because heart monitoring is required
- After hypo/hyperkalemia is corrected
- With dosage adjustment q3-4days
- Without regard to meals

SIDE EFFECTS

CNS: Headache, dizziness, abnormal dreams, syncope, confusion, seizures, insomnia, tremor, anxiety, fatigue

CV: Supraventricular dysrhythmia, ventricular dysrhythmia, bradycardia, prodysrhythmia, palpitations, AV block, intraventricular conduction delay, AV dissociation, hypotension, chest pain, asystole

EENT: Blurred vision, altered taste, tinnitus

GI: *Nausea, vomiting,* constipation, dyspepsia, cholestasis, abnormal hepatic studies, dry mouth, diarrhea, anorexia

HEMA: Leukopenia, agranulocytosis, granulocytopenia, thrombocytopenia, anemia, bruising

INTEG: Rash

RESP: Dyspnea

PHARMACOKINETICS

Peak 3-8 hr, half-life 2-10 hr, poor metabolizers 10-32 hr; metabolized in liver; excreted in urine (metabolite)

INTERACTIONS

Increase: propafenone effects—CYP1A2, CYP2D6, CYP3A4 inhibitors (protease inhibitors, quiNINE, PARoxetine, saquinavir, erythromycin, azole antifungals, sertraline, tricyclics)

Increase: QT prolongation—other class IA/IC antidysrhythmics, arsenic trioxide, chloroquine, clarithromycin, droperidol, erythromycin, haloperidol, levomethadyl, methadone, pentamidine, chlorproMAZINE, mesoridazine, thioridazine

Increase: anticoagulation—warfarin

Increase: CNS effects—local anesthetics

Increase: digoxin level—digoxin

Increase: β-blocker effect—propranolol, metoprolol

Increase: cycloSPORINE levels—cycloSPORINE

Decrease: propafenone effect—rifampin, cimetidine, quiNIDine

Drug/Food

Increase: propafenone effect—grapefruit juice

Drug/Herb

Decrease: propafenone effect—St. John's wort

Drug/Lab Test

Increase: CPK

NURSING CONSIDERATIONS

Assess:

- GI status: bowel pattern, number of stools

Black Box Warning: QT/PR prolongation: ECG or Holter monitor before and during therapy

Black Box Warning: CHF: dyspnea, jugular venous distention, crackles, edema in extremities, I&O ratio; check for decreasing output; daily weight

- CBC, ANA titer, LFTs
- Chest x-ray, pulmonary function test during treatment
- Lung fields; bilateral crackles, dyspnea, peripheral edema, weight gain; jugular venous distention may occur in patient with CHF

⚠ **Toxicity:** fine tremors, dizziness, hypotension, drowsiness, abnormal heart rate

Evaluate:

- Therapeutic response: absence of ventricular dysrhythmias; decreasing recurrence of PAF, PSVT

Teach patient/family:

- To avoid hazardous activities until response is known
- To report fever, chills, sore throat, bleeding, SOB, chest pain, palpitations, blurred vision
- To take tab with food, not to use with grapefruit juice or St. John's wort
- To carry emergency ID identifying medication and prescriber
- To avoid abrupt discontinuation of product; to take as prescribed; not to miss, double doses

TREATMENT OF OVERDOSE:

O_2, artificial ventilation, defibrillation ECG; administer DOPamine for circulatory depression, diazepam or thiopental for seizures, isoproterenol

proparacaine ophthalmic

See Appendix B

⚠ HIGH ALERT

propofol (Rx)

(pro′poh-fole)

Diprivan

Func. class.: Hypnotic

Chem. class.: Phenol derivative

ACTION: Produces dose-dependent CNS depression by activation of GABA receptor

USES: Induction or maintenance of anesthesia as part of balanced anesthetic technique; sedation in mechanically ventilated patients

CONTRAINDICATIONS: Hypersensitivity to this product or soybean oil, egg, benzyl alcohol (some products)

Precautions: Pregnancy (B), breastfeeding, children, geriatric patients, respiratory depression, severe respiratory disorders, cardiac dysrhythmias, labor and delivery, renal disease, hyperlipidemia

DOSAGE AND ROUTES

Anesthesia

- **Adult <55 yr and ASA I/II IV (Diprivan or generic): IV** 40 mg q10sec until induction onset, maintenance 100-200 mcg/kg/min or **IV BOL** 20-50 mg prn, allow 3-5 min between adjustments; Fresenius Propoven 1% **IV** 20-40 mg q10sec until induction, then 3-6 mg/kg/hr
- **Child ≥3 yr or ASA I or II: IV induction:** 2.5-3.5 mg/kg over 20-30 sec when not premedicated or lightly premedicated
- **Child 2 mo-16 yr maintenance: IV** 125-300 mcg/kg/min, lower dose for ASA III or **IV**

ICU sedation

- **Adult: IV** 5 mcg/kg/min over 5 min; may increase by 5-10 mcg/kg/min over 5-10 min until desired response (Diprivan or generic): 0.3-4 mg/kg/hr, max 4 mg/kg/hr (Fresenius Propoven)

Available forms: Inj 10 mg/ml in 20-ml ampule, vials, syringes

P

Administer:

IV route

- Shake well before use; dilution is not necessary but, if diluted, use only D_5W to ≥2 mg/ml; give over 3-5 min, titrate to needed level of sedation; use only glass containers when mixing, not stable in plastic; use aseptic technique when transferring from original container
- Only with resuscitative equipment available; only by qualified persons trained in anesthesia
- Store in light-resistant area at room temperature, use within 6 hr of opening
- If transferred from original container to another container, complete infusion within 12 hr (Diprivan), 6 hr (generic propofol)

Y-site compatibilities: Acyclovir, alfentanil, aminophylline, ampicillin, aztreonam, bumetanide, buprenorphine, butorphanol, calcium gluconate, CARBOplatin, ceFAZolin, cefoperazone, cefotaxime, cefoTEtan, cefOXitin, ceftizoxime, cefTRIAXone, cefuroxime, chlorproMAZINE, cimetidine, CISplatin, clindamycin, cyclophosphamide, cycloSPORINE, cytarabine, dexamethasone, diphenhydrAMINE, DOBUTamine, DOPamine, doxycycline, droperidol, enalaprilat, ePHEDrine, EPINEPHrine, esmolol, famotidine, fentaNYL, fluconazole, fluorouracil, furosemide, ganciclovir, glycopyrrolate, granisetron, haloperidol, heparin, hydrocortisone, HYDROmorphone, hydrOXYzine, ifosfamide, imipenem/cilastatin, inamrinone, regular insulin, isoproterenol, ketamine, labetalol, levorphanol, lidocaine, LORazepam, magnesium sulfate, mannitol, meperidine, mezlocillin, miconazole, morphine, nafcillin, nalbuphine, naloxone, nitroglycerin, norepinephrine, ofloxacin, PACLitaxel, PENTobarbital, PHENobarbital, piperacillin, potassium chloride, prochlorperazine, propranolol, ranitidine, scopolamine, sodium bicarbonate, sodium nitroprusside, succinylcholine, SUFentanil, thiopental ticarcillin, ticarcillin/clavulanate, vecuronium, verapamil

Solution compatibilities: if given together via Y-site: D_5W, D_5LR, LR, $D_5/0.45\%$ NaCl, $D_5/0.2\%$ NaCl

SIDE EFFECTS

CNS: Involuntary movement, headache, jerking, fever, dizziness, shivering, tremor, confusion, somnolence, paresthesia, agitation, abnormal dreams, euphoria fatigue, **increased intracranial pressure, impaired cerebral flow, seizures**

CV: *Bradycardia, hypotension,* hypertension, PVC, PAC, tachycardia, abnormal ECG, ST segment depression, **asystole, bradydysrhythmias**

EENT: Blurred vision, tinnitus, eye pain, strange taste, diplopia

GI: *Nausea, vomiting, abdominal cramping,* dry mouth, swallowing, hypersalivation, **pancreatitis**

GU: Urine retention, green urine, cloudy urine, oliguria

INTEG: *Flushing, phlebitis, hives, burning/stinging at inj site,* rash, pain of extremities

MS: Myalgia

RESP: **Apnea,** *cough, hiccups,* dyspnea, hypoventilation, sneezing, wheezing, tachypnea, hypoxia, respiratory acidosis

SYST: **Propofol infusion syndrome**

PHARMACOKINETICS

Onset 15-30 sec, rapid distribution, half-life 1-8 min, terminal half-life 3-12 hr; 70% excreted in urine; metabolized in liver by conjugation to inactive metabolites, 95%-99% protein binding

INTERACTIONS

- **Do not use within 10 days of MAOIs**

Increase: CNS depression—alcohol, opioids, sedative/hypnotics, antipsychotics, skeletal muscle relaxants, inhalational anesthetics

Drug/Herb

Increase: propofol effect—St. John's wort

NURSING CONSIDERATIONS

Assess:

- Inj site: phlebitis, burning, stinging

- **ECG** for changes: PVC, PAC, ST segment changes; monitor VS
- **Neurologic excitatory symptoms:** movement, tremors, dizziness, LOC, pupil reaction
- Allergic reactions: hives

⚠ **Respiratory dysfunction:** respiratory depression, character, rate, rhythm; notify prescriber if respirations are <10/min

- **Propofol infusion syndrome:** rhabdomyolysis, renal failure, hyperkalemia, metabolic acidosis, cardiac dysrhythmias, heart failure usually between 35 and 93 hr after infusion begun at >5 mg/kg/hr for >58 hr

Evaluate:

- Therapeutic response: induction of anesthesia

Teach patient/family:

- That product will cause dizziness, drowsiness, sedation; to avoid hazardous activities until drug effect wears off

TREATMENT OF OVERDOSE:

Discontinue product; administer vasopressor agents or anticholinergics, artificial ventilation

⚠ HIGH ALERT

propranolol (Rx)

(proe-pran′oh-lole)

Inderal, Inderal LA, InnoPran XL

Func. class.: Antihypertensive, antianginal, antidysrhythmic (class II)

Chem. class.: β-Adrenergic blocker

Do not confuse:

propranolol/Pravachol

Inderal/Toradol/Inderide/Adderall/Imuran

ACTION: Nonselective β-blocker with negative inotropic, chronotropic, dromotropic properties

USES: Chronic stable angina pectoris, hypertension, supraventricular dysrhythmias, migraine prophylaxis, pheochromocytoma, cyanotic spells related to hypertrophic subaortic stenosis, essential tremor, acute MI

Unlabeled uses: Anxiety, prevention of variceal bleeding caused by portal hypertension, akathisia induced by antipsychotics, portal hypertension, sclerodermal renal crisis, unstable angina, infantile capillary hemangioma, lithium-induced tremor

CONTRAINDICATIONS: Hypersensitivity to this product; cardiogenic shock, AV heart block; bronchospastic disease; sinus bradycardia; bronchospasm; asthma

Precautions: Pregnancy (C), breastfeeding, children, diabetes mellitus, hyperthyroidism, COPD, renal/hepatic disease, myasthenia gravis, peripheral vascular disease, hypotension, cardiac failure, Raynaud's disease, sick sinus syndrome, vasospastic angina, smoking, Wolff-Parkinson-White syndrome, thyrotoxicosis

Black Box Warning: Abrupt discontinuation

DOSAGE AND ROUTES

Dysrhythmias

- **Adult: PO** 10-30 mg tid-qid; **IV BOL** 1-3 mg give 1 mg/min; may repeat after 2 min, may repeat q4hr thereafter
- **Child: PO** 1 mg/kg/day in 2 divided doses; **IV** 0.01-0.1 mg/kg over 5 min

Hypertension

- **Adult: PO** 40 mg bid or 80 mg/day (ext rel) initially; usual dose 120-240 mg/day bid-tid or 120-160 mg/day (ext rel)
- **Child: PO** 0.5-1 mg/kg/day divided q6-12hr

Angina

- **Adult: PO** 10-20 mg bid-qid, increase at 3-7 day intervals up to 160-320 mg/day or 80 mg daily

MI prophylaxis

- **Adult: PO** 180-240 mg/day tid-qid starting 5 days to 2 wk after MI

Pheochromocytoma

- **Adult: PO** 60 mg/day × 3 days preoperatively in divided doses or 30 mg/day in divided doses (inoperable tumor)

Migraine

- **Adult: PO** 80 mg/day (ext rel) or in divided doses; may increase to 160-240 mg/day in divided doses
- **Child >35 kg (unlabeled): PO** 20-40 mg tid
- **Child ≤35 kg (unlabeled): PO** 10-20 mg tid

Essential tremor

- **Adult: PO** 40 mg bid; usual dose 120 mg/day

Acute MI

- **Adult: PO** 180-320 mg/day in 3-4 divided doses; IV 0.1 mg/kg in 3 divided doses at 2-3 min intervals

Anxiety (unlabeled)

- **Adult: PO** 10-80 mg given 1 hr before anxiety-producing event

Scleroderma renal crisis (unlabeled)

- **Adult: PO** 40 mg bid, may increase q3-7days, max 160-480 mg/day

Esophageal varices (portal hypertension) (unlabeled)

- **Adult: PO** 40 mg bid, titrate to heart rate reduction of 25%

Infantile capillary hemangioma (unlabeled)

- **Infant: PO** 2-3 mg/kg/day

Available forms: Ext rel caps 60, 80, 120, 160 mg; tabs 10, 20, 40, 60, 80, 90 mg; inj 1 mg/ml; oral sol 4 mg/ml, 8 mg/ml

Administer:

PO route

- Do not break, crush, chew, or open ext rel cap
- Do not use ext rel cap for essential tremor, MI, cardiac dysrhythmias; do not use InnoPran XL in hypertropic subaortic stenosis, migraine, angina pectoris
- Ext rel caps should be taken daily; InnoPran XL should be taken at bedtime
- May mix oral sol with liquid or semisolid food; rinse container to get entire dose
- With 8 oz water with food; food enhances bioavailability
- Do not give with aluminum-containing antacid; may decrease GI absorption

Direct IV route

- IV undiluted or diluted 10 ml D_5W for inj; give ≤1 mg/min

Intermittent IV INFUSION route

- May be diluted in 50 ml NaCl and run 1 mg over 10-15 min

Y-site compatibilities: Acyclovir, alfentanil, alteplase, amikacin, aminocaproic acid, aminophylline, anidulafungin, ascorbic acid, atracurium, atropine, azaTHIOprine, aztreonam, benztropine, bivalirudin, bleomycin, bumetanide, buprenorphine, butorphanol, calcium chloride/gluconate, CARBOplatin, carmustine, caspofungin, cefamandole, ceFAZolin, cefmetazole, cefonicid, cefoperazone, cefotaxime, cefoTEtan, cefOXitin, cefTAZidime, ceftizoxime, cefTRIAXone, cefuroxime, cephalothin, cephapirin, chloramphenicol, chlorproMAZINE, cimetidine, CISplatin, clindamycin, cyanocobalamin, cyclophosphamide, cycloSPORINE, cytarabine, DACTINomycin, DAPTOmycin, dexamethasone, digoxin, diltiazem, diphenhydrAMINE, DOBUTamine, DOCEtaxel, DOPamine, doxacurium, DOXOrubicin, doxycycline, enalaprilat, ePHEDrine, EPINEPHrine, epirubicin, epoetin alfa, eptifibatide, ertapenem, erythromycin, esmolol, etoposide, etoposide phosphate, famotidine, fenoldopam, fentaNYL, fluconazole, fludarabine, fluorouracil, folic acid, furosemide, ganciclovir, gatifloxacin, gemcitabine, gemtuzumab, gentamicin, glycopyrrolate, granisetron, heparin, hydrocortisone, HYDROmorphone, hydrOXYzine, IDArubicin, ifosfamide, imipenem-cilastatin, inamrinone, irinotecan, isoproterenol, ketorolac, labetalol, levofloxacin, lidocaine, linezolid, LORazepam, magnesium, mannitol, mechlorethamine, meperidine, metaraminol, methicillin, methotrexate, methoxamine, methyldopate, methylPREDNISolone, metoclopramide, metoprolol, metroNIDAZOLE, mezlocillin, miconazole, midazolam, milrinone, minocycline, mitoXANtrone, morphine, moxalactam, multiple vitamins, mycophenolate, nafcillin, nalbuphine, naloxone, nesiritide, netilmicin, nitroglycerin, nitroprusside, norepinephrine, octreotide, ondansetron, oxacillin, oxaliplatin, oxytocin, palonosetron, pamidronate, pancuronium, papaverine, PEMEtrexed, penicillin G potassium/sodium, pentamidine, pentazocine, PENTobarbital, PHENobarbital, phenylephrine, phytonadione, piperacillin, polymyxin B, potassium chloride, procainamide, prochlorperazine, promethazine, propofol, protamine, pyridoxine, quiNIDine, quinupristin-dalfopristin, ranitidine, ritodrine, rocuronium, sodium acetate/bicarbonate, succinylcholine, SUFentanil, tacrolimus, teniposide, theophylline, thiamine, thiotepa, ticarcillin, ticarcillin-clavulanate, tigecycline, tirofiban, tobramycin, tolazoline, trimetaphan, urokinase, vancomycin, vasopressin, vecuronium, verapamil, vinCRIStine, vinorelbine, vitamin B complex/C, voriconazole, zoledronic acid

SIDE EFFECTS

CNS: Depression, hallucinations, *dizziness, fatigue,* lethargy, paresthesias, bizarre dreams, disorientation

CV: **Bradycardia,** hypotension, **CHF,** palpitations, AV block, peripheral vascular insufficiency, vasodilation, cold extremities, **pulmonary edema, dysrhythmias**

EENT: Sore throat, **laryngospasm,** blurred vision, dry eyes

GI: Nausea, vomiting, diarrhea, colitis, constipation, cramps, dry mouth, hepatomegaly, gastric pain, acute pancreatitis

GU: Impotence, decreased libido, UTIs

HEMA: **Agranulocytosis, thrombocytopenia**

INTEG: Rash, pruritus, fever, **Stevens-Johnson syndrome, toxic epidermal necrolysis**

META: Hyperglycemia, hypoglycemia

MISC: Facial swelling, weight change, Raynaud's phenomenon

MS: Joint pain, arthralgia, muscle cramps, pain

RESP: Dyspnea, respiratory dysfunction, *bronchospasm,* cough

PHARMACOKINETICS

Metabolized by liver; crosses placenta, blood-brain barrier; excreted in breast milk; protein binding 90%

PO: Onset 30 min, peak 1-1½ hr, duration 12 hr, half-life 3-8 hr

PO-ER: Peak 6 hr, duration 24 hr, half-life 8-11 hr

IV: Onset 2 min, peak 1 min, duration 2-4 hr

INTERACTIONS

Increase: toxicity—phenothiazines

Increase: propranolol level—propafenone

Increase: effect of calcium channel blockers, neuromuscular blocker

Increase: negative inotropic effects—disopyramide

Increase: β-blocking effect—cimetidine

Increase: hypotension—quiNIDine, haloperidol, prazosin

Decrease: β-blocking effects—barbiturates

Decrease: propranolol levels—smoking

Drug/Herb

- Avoid use with feverfew

Increase: antihypertensive effect—hawthorn

Decrease: antihypertensive effect—ma huang

Drug/Lab Test

Increase: serum potassium, serum uric acid, ALT, AST, alk phos, LDH

Decrease: blood glucose

Interference: glaucoma testing

NURSING CONSIDERATIONS

Assess:

Black Box Warning: Abrupt withdrawal: taper over a few weeks, do not discontinue abruptly; dysrhythmias, angina, myocardial ischemia, or MI may occur, taper over at least a few weeks

- B/P, pulse, respirations during beginning therapy; notify prescriber if pulse <50 bpm or systolic B/P <90 mm Hg

⚠ ECG continuously if using as antidysrhythmic IV, PCWP (pulmonary capillary wedge pressure), CVP (central venous pressure)
- Hepatic enzymes: AST, ALT, bilirubin; blood glucose (diabetes mellitus)
- Angina pain: duration, time started, activity being performed, character
- Tolerance with long-term use
- Headache, lightheadedness, decreased B/P; may indicate need for decreased dosage; may aggravate symptoms of arterial insufficiency
- **Fluid overload:** weight daily; report gain of >5 lb

⚠ I&O ratio, CCr if kidney damage is diagnosed; fatigue, weight gain, jugular distention, dyspnea, peripheral edema, crackles

Evaluate:
- Therapeutic response: decreased B/P, dysrhythmias

Teach patient/family:

⚠ Not to discontinue abruptly; may precipitate life-threatening dysrhythmias, exacerbation of angina, MI; to take product at same time each day, either with or without food consistently; to decrease dosage over 2 wk
- To avoid OTC products unless approved by prescriber; to avoid alcohol
- To avoid hazardous activities if dizzy
- About the importance of compliance with complete medical regimen; to monitor blood glucose, may mask symptoms of hypoglycemia
- To make position changes slowly to prevent fainting
- That sensitivity to cold may occur
- How to take pulse, B/P; to withhold product if <50 bpm or systolic B/P <90 mm Hg

⚠ HIGH ALERT

propylthiouracil (Rx)

(proe-pill-thye-oh-yoor′a-sill)

Propyl-Thyracil ♣

Func. class.: Thyroid hormone antagonist (antithyroid)

Chem. class.: Thioamide

ACTION: Blocks synthesis peripherally of T_3, T_4 (triiodothyronine, thyroxine), inhibits organification of iodine

USES: Preparation for thyroidectomy, thyrotoxic crisis, hyperthyroidism, thyroid storm

CONTRAINDICATIONS: Pregnancy (D), breastfeeding, hypersensitivity, agranulocytosis, hepatitis, jaundice

Precautions: Infants, bone marrow depression, fever

Black Box Warning: Hepatic disease

DOSAGE AND ROUTES

Thyrotoxic crisis
- **Adult and child: PO** 200-400 mg q4hr for 1st 24 hr

Preparation for thyroidectomy
- **Adult: PO** 600-1200 mg/day
- **Child: PO** 10 mg/kg/day in divided doses

Hyperthyroidism
- **Adult: PO** 100 mg tid increasing to 300 mg q8hr if condition is severe; continue to euthyroid state, then 100 mg daily tid
- **Child >6 yr: PO** 50 mg/day divided q8hr, titrate based on TSH/free T_4 levels
- **Neonate (unlabeled): PO** 5-10 mg/kg/day in divided doses q8hr

Available forms: Tabs 50 mg

Administer:
- With meals to decrease GI upset
- At same time each day to maintain product level
- At lowest dose that relieves symptoms

SIDE EFFECTS

CNS: *Drowsiness, headache, vertigo, fever,* paresthesias, neuritis
GI: *Nausea, diarrhea, vomiting,* jaundice, hepatitis, loss of taste, liver failure, death
GU: Nephritis
HEMA: Agranulocytosis, leukopenia, thrombocytopenia, hypothrombinemia, lymphadenopathy, bleeding, vasculitis, periarteritis
INTEG: *Rash, urticaria, pruritus, alopecia, hyperpigmentation,* lupuslike syndrome
MS: Myalgia, arthralgia, nocturnal muscle cramps, osteoporosis

PHARMACOKINETICS

Onset up to 3 wk, peak 6-10 wk, duration 1 wk to 1 mo, half-life 1-2 hr; excreted in urine, bile, breast milk; crosses placenta; concentration in thyroid gland

INTERACTIONS

- Bone marrow suppression: radiation, antineoplastics
- Agranulocytosis: phenothiazines

Increase: effects—potassium/sodium iodide, lithium
Decrease: anticoagulant effect—heparin, oral anticoagulants

Drug/Lab Test
Increase: PT, AST, ALT, alk phos

NURSING CONSIDERATIONS

Assess:

- **Hyperthyroidism:** weight loss, nervousness, insomnia, fever, diaphoresis, tremors; **hypothyroidism:** constipation, dry skin, weakness, headache; monitor T_3, T_4, which are increased; serum TSH, which is decreased; free thyroxine index, which is increased if dosage is too low; discontinue product 3-4 wk before RAIU
- Pulse, B/P, temperature
- I&O ratio; check for edema: puffy hands, feet, periorbits; indicates hypothyroidism
- Weight daily; same clothing, scale, time of day
- ⚠ **Blood dyscrasias:** CBC with differential; leukopenia, thrombocytopenia, agranulocytosis
- ⚠ **Overdose:** peripheral edema, heat intolerance, diaphoresis, palpitations, dysrhythmias, severe tachycardia, increased temperature, delirium, CNS irritability
- ⚠ **Hypersensitivity:** rash, enlarged cervical lymph nodes; product may have to be discontinued
- **Hypoprothrombinemia:** bleeding, petechiae, ecchymosis
- Clinical response: after 3 wk should include increased weight, pulse; decreased T_4
- **Bone marrow suppression:** sore throat, fever, fatigue

Black Box Warning: Hepatotoxicity: LFTs before, during treatment; jaundice, nausea, vomiting, abdominal pain, anorexia, diarrhea, fatigue

- Fluids to 3-4 L/day unless contraindicated

Evaluate:

- Therapeutic response: weight gain, decreased pulse, decreased T_4, decreased B/P

Teach patient/family:

- To abstain from breastfeeding after delivery
- To take pulse daily
- To report redness, swelling, sore throat, mouth lesions, which indicate blood dyscrasias; to report symptoms of hepatic dysfunction
- To keep graph of weight, pulse, mood
- To avoid OTC products that contain iodine
- That seafood, other iodine products may be restricted
- Not to discontinue product abruptly because thyroid crisis may occur; about stress response
- That response may take several months if thyroid is large
- About the symptoms/signs of overdose: periorbital edema, cold intolerance, mental depression

P

- About the symptoms of an inadequate dose: tachycardia, diarrhea, fever, irritability
- To take medication as prescribed; not to skip or double dose; that missed doses should be taken when remembered up to 1 hr before next dose
- To carry emergency ID listing condition, medication

protamine (Rx)

(proe′ta-meen)

Func. class.: Heparin antagonist

Chem. class.: Low-molecular-weight protein

ACTION: Binds heparin, thereby making it ineffective

USES: Heparin, LMWH toxicity, hemorrhage

CONTRAINDICATIONS: Hypersensitivity

Precautions: Pregnancy (C), breastfeeding, fish allergy, diabetes, previous exposure to protamine, insulins, heparin rebound or bleeding

DOSAGE AND ROUTES

Heparin overdose

- **Adult and child: IV** 1 mg of protamine/100 units heparin given; administer slowly over 1-3 min; max 50 mg/10 min

Enoxaparin overdose

- **Adult: IV** 1 mg protamine/1 mg enoxaparin

Dalteparin/tinzaparin overdose

- **Adult: IV** 1 mg protamine/100 anti-Xa unit

Available forms: Inj 10 mg/ml

Administer:

- Store at 36° F-46° F (2° C-8° C)

Direct IV route

- After reconstituting 50 mg/5 ml sterile bacteriostatic water for inj; shake, give ≤20 mg over 1-3 min

Y-site compatibilities: Alfentanil, amikacin, aminophylline, ascorbic acid, atracurium, atropine, azaTHIOprine, aztreonam, benztropine, bumetanide, buprenorphine, butorphanol, calcium chloride/gluconate, cefTAZidime, chlorproMAZINE, cimetidine, clindamycin, cyanocobalamin, cycloSPORINE, digoxin, diphenhydrAMINE, DOBUTamine, DOPamine, doxycycline, enalaprilat, ePHEDrine, EPINEPHrine, epoetin alfa, erythromycin, esmolol, famotidine, fentaNYL, fluconazole, ganciclovir, gentamicin, glycopyrrolate, hydrOXYzine, imipenem-cilastatin, inamrinone, iohexol, iopamidol, iothalamate, isoproterenol, labetalol, lidocaine, magnesium, mannitol, meperidine, metaraminol, methoxamine, methyldopate, metoclopramide, metoprolol, miconazole, midazolam, minocycline, morphine, multiple vitamins, nalbuphine, naloxone, netilmicin, nitroglycerin, nitroprusside, norepinephrine, ondansetron, oxytocin, papaverine, pentazocine, phenylephrine, polymyxin B, potassium chloride, procainamide, prochlorperazine, promethazine, propranolol, pyridoxine, quiNIDine, ranitidine, Ringer's, ritodrine, sodium bicarbonate, succinylcholine, SUFentanil, theophylline, thiamine, tobramycin, tolazoline, trimetaphan, urokinase, vancomycin, vasopressin, verapamil

SIDE EFFECTS

CNS: Lassitude, flushing

CV: Hypotension, bradycardia, circulatory collapse, capillary leak

GI: Nausea, vomiting, anorexia

HEMA: Bleeding

INTEG: *Rash,* dermatitis, urticaria

RESP: Dyspnea, pulmonary edema, severe respiratory distress, bronchospasm

SYST: Anaphylaxis, angioedema

PHARMACOKINETICS

IV: Onset 5 min, duration 2 hr

NURSING CONSIDERATIONS

Assess:

⚠ **Hypersensitivity:** urticaria, cough, wheezing, have emergency equipment nearby; **allergy to fish;** use with caution; men who have had vasectomies may be more prone to hypersensitivity

- Blood studies (Hct, platelets, occult blood in stools) q3mo
- Coagulation tests (aPTT, ACT) 15 min after dose, then again after several hours
- VS, B/P, pulse after 30 min, then 3 hr after dose
- Skin rash, urticaria, dermatitis

Evaluate:
- Therapeutic response: reversal of heparin overdose

Teach patient/family:
- Not to take if allergic to fish

pseudoephedrine (OTC, Rx)

(soo-doh-eh-fed′rin)

Elix Sure Cold, Eltor ✦, Nasofed, Sudafed, Sudafed 24 Hour, Sudogest

Func. class.: Adrenergic

Chem. class.: Substituted phenylethylamine

ACTION: Primary activity through α-effects on respiratory mucosal membranes reducing congestion hyperemia, edema; minimal bronchodilation secondary to β-effects

USES: Nasal decongestant, adjunct for otitis media; with antihistamines

CONTRAINDICATIONS: Hypersensitivity to sympathomimetics, closed-angle glaucoma

Precautions: Pregnancy (C), breastfeeding, cardiac disorders, hyperthyroidism, diabetes mellitus, prostatic hypertrophy, hypertension

DOSAGE AND ROUTES
- **Adult and child >12 yr: PO** 60 mg q6hr; **EXT REL** 120 mg q12hr or 240 mg q24hr
- **Geriatric: PO** 30-60 mg q6hr prn
- **Child 6-12 yr: PO** 30 mg q6hr, max 120 mg/day
- **Child 2-6 yr: PO** 15 mg q6hr, max 60 mg/day

Available forms: Ext rel caps 120, 240 mg; oral sol 15 mg, 30 mg/5 ml; tabs 30, 60 mg; ext rel tabs 120, 240 mg

Administer:
- Avoid taking at or near bedtime; stimulation can occur

SIDE EFFECTS
CNS: *Tremors, anxiety,* stimulation, insomnia, headache, dizziness, hallucinations, **seizures** (geriatric patients)

CV: Palpitations, tachycardia, hypertension, chest pain, **dysrhythmias, CV collapse**

EENT: Dry nose; irritation of nose and throat

GI: *Anorexia, nausea, vomiting,* dry mouth, ischemic colitis

GU: Dysuria

PHARMACOKINETICS
PO: Onset 15-30 min; duration 4-6 hr, 8-12 hr (ext rel); metabolized in liver; excreted in feces and breast milk; terminal half-life 9-16 hr

INTERACTIONS
⚠ **Do not use with MAOIs or tricyclics; hypertensive crisis may occur**

Increase: effect of this product—urinary alkalizers, adrenergics, β-blockers, phenothiazines, tricyclics

Decrease: effect of this product—urinary acidifiers

NURSING CONSIDERATIONS
Assess:
- Nasal congestion: auscultate lung sounds; check for tenacious bronchial secretions
- B/P, pulse throughout treatment
- CNS side effects in geriatric patients: excitation, seizures, hallucinations

Evaluate:
- Therapeutic response: decreased nasal congestion

Teach patient/family:
- About the reason for product administration

P

- Ext rel: do not divide, crush, chew, or dissolve
- Do not use within 14 days of MAOIs
- Not to use continuously or to take more than recommended dose because rebound congestion may occur

⚠ **To notify prescriber immediately of anxiety; slow or fast heart rate; dyspnea; seizures**

- To check with prescriber before using other products because product interactions may occur
- To avoid taking near bedtime because stimulation can occur
- **Not to use if stimulation, restlessness, tremors occur**
- **That use in children may cause excessive agitation**

psyllium (OTC, Rx)

(sill′ee-um)

Hydrocil, Leader Fiber Laxative, Metamucil, Natural Fiber, Natural Vegetable Fiber, Reguloid, Wal-Mucil

Func. class.: Bulk laxative

Chem. class.: Psyllium colloid

ACTION: Bulk-forming laxative

USES: Chronic constipation, ulcerative colitis

Unlabeled uses: Diarrhea, diverticulosis, irritable bowel syndrome, hypercholesterolemia

CONTRAINDICATIONS: Hypersensitivity, intestinal obstruction, abdominal pain, nausea, vomiting, fecal impaction

Precautions: Pregnancy (C)

DOSAGE AND ROUTES

- **Adult: PO** 1-2 tsp in 8 oz water bid or tid, then 8 oz water or 1 premeasured packet in 8 oz water bid or tid, then 8 oz water
- **Child >6 yr: PO** 1 tsp in 4 oz water at bedtime

Available forms: Chew pieces 1.7, 3.4 g/piece; effervescent powder 3.4, 3.7 g/packet; powder 3.3, 3.4, 3.5, 4.94 g/tsp; wafers 3.4 g/wafer

Administer:

PO route

- Alone for better absorption, separate from other products by 1-2 hr
- In morning or evening (oral dose)
- Immediately after mixing with water or will congeal
- With 8 oz water or juice followed by another 8 oz of fluid

SIDE EFFECTS

GI: *Nausea, vomiting, anorexia, diarrhea,* cramps, intestinal esophageal blockage

PHARMACOKINETICS

Onset 12-72 hr, excreted in feces, not absorbed in GI tract

INTERACTIONS

Decrease: absorption of cardiac glycosides, oral anticoagulants, salicylates

Drug/Herb

Increase: laxative effect—flax, senna

NURSING CONSIDERATIONS

Assess:

- Blood, urine electrolytes if used often
- I&O ratio to identify fluid loss
- **Constipation:** cause of constipation; fluids, bulk, exercise missing; bowel sounds, distention, usual bowel function; color, consistency, amount
- Cramping, rectal bleeding, nausea, vomiting; product should be discontinued

Evaluate:

- Therapeutic response: decrease in constipation, decreased diarrhea with colitis

Teach patient/family:

- To maintain adequate fluid consumption
- That normal bowel movements do not always occur daily
- Not to use in presence of abdominal pain, nausea, vomiting

• To notify prescriber if constipation unrelieved or if symptoms of electrolyte imbalance occur: muscle cramps, pain, weakness, dizziness, excessive thirst

pyridostigmine (Rx)

(peer-id-oh-stig′meen)

Mestinon, Mestinon SR, Regonol

Func. class.: Cholinergic; anticholinesterase

Chem. class.: Tertiary amine carbamate

ACTION: Inhibits destruction of acetylcholine, which increases concentration at sites where acetylcholine is released; this facilitates the transmission of impulses across the myoneural junction

USES: Nondepolarizing muscle relaxant antagonist, myasthenia gravis, pretreatment for nerve gas exposure (military only)

CONTRAINDICATIONS: Bradycardia; hypotension; obstruction of intestine, renal system; bromide, benzyl alcohol sensitivity; adrenal insufficiency; cholinesterase inhibitor toxicity

Precautions: Pregnancy (C), seizure disorders, bronchial asthma, coronary occlusion, hyperthyroidism, dysrhythmias, peptic ulcer, megacolon, poor GI motility

DOSAGE AND ROUTES

Myasthenia gravis

• **Adult: PO** 600 mg/day in 5-6 divided doses, max 1.5 g/day; **IM/IV** 2 mg or 1/30 of **PO** dose; **SUS REL** 180-540 mg/day or bid at intervals of ≥6 hr

• **Child: PO** 7 mg/kg/day in 5-6 divided doses; **IM/IV** 0.05-0.15 mg/kg/dose

Nondepolarizing neuromuscular blocker antagonist

• **Adult:** 0.6-1.2 mg **IV** atropine, then 0.1-0.25 mg/kg/dose

• **Child: IV** 0.1-0.25 mg/kg/dose

Nerve gas exposure prophylaxis (military)

• **Adult: PO** 30 mg q8hr if threat of exposure to Soman gas is anticipated; start several hours before exposure and discontinue upon exposure; after product is discontinued, give antidotes (atropine, pralidoxime)

Available forms: Tabs 60 mg; ext rel tabs 180 mg; syr 60 mg/5 ml; inj 5 mg/ml

Administer:

• Only with atropine sulfate available for cholinergic crisis

• Only after all other cholinergics have been discontinued

• Increased doses for tolerance as ordered

• Larger doses after exercise or fatigue as ordered

• Do not break, crush, or chew sus rel tabs

PO route

• On empty stomach for better absorption

Direct IV route

• Undiluted (5 mg/ml), give through Y-tube or 3-way stopcock, give ≤0.5 mg/min (myasthenia gravis); 5 mg/min (reversal of nondepolarizing neuromuscular blockers)

Y-site compatibilities: Heparin, hydrocortisone, potassium chloride, vit B/C

SIDE EFFECTS

CNS: Dizziness, headache, sweating, weakness, **seizures**, incoordination, **paralysis**, drowsiness, LOC

CV: Tachycardia, dysrhythmias, bradycardia, AV block, hypotension, ECG changes, **cardiac arrest**, syncope

EENT: Miosis, blurred vision, lacrimation, visual changes

GI: *Nausea, diarrhea, vomiting, cramps, increased salivary and gastric secretions, peristalsis*

GU: Urinary frequency, incontinence, urgency

INTEG: Rash, urticaria, flushing

P

RESP: Respiratory depression, bronchospasm, constriction, laryngospasm, respiratory arrest
SYST: Cholinergic crisis

PHARMACOKINETICS

Metabolized in liver, excreted in urine (unchanged)
PO: Onset 20-30 min, duration 3-6 hr
PO-EXT REL: Onset 30-60 min, duration 6-12 hr
IM/IV/SUBCUT: Onset 2-15 min, duration $2^1/_2$-4 hr

INTERACTIONS

Increase: action—succinylcholine
Decrease: action—gallamine, metocurine, pancuronium, tubocurarine, atropine
Decrease: pyridostigmine action—aminoglycosides, anesthetics, procainamide, quiNIDine, mecamylamine, polymyxin, magnesium, corticosteroids, antidysrhythmics, quinolones

NURSING CONSIDERATIONS

Assess:

- **Myasthenia gravis:** fatigue, ptosis, diplopia, difficulty swallowing, SOB, hand/gait before, after product; improvement should be seen after 1 hr
- VS, respiration q8hr
- I&O ratio; check for urinary retention or incontinence
- **Toxicity:** bradycardia, hypotension, bronchospasm, headache, dizziness, seizures, respiratory depression; product should be discontinued if toxicity occurs

Evaluate:

- Therapeutic response: increased muscle strength, hand grasp, improved gait, absence of labored breathing (if severe); reversal of nondepolarizing neuromuscular blockers; prevention of nerve gas toxicity

Teach patient/family:

- **Myasthenia gravis:** that product is not a cure, only relieves symptoms
- To wear emergency ID specifying myasthenia gravis, products taken
- To avoid driving, other hazardous activities until effect is known
- To report muscle weakness (cholinergic crisis or underdosage), bradycardia
- Not to drink alcohol
- To take with food to decrease gastric side effects

TREATMENT OF OVERDOSE:

Discontinue product, atropine 1-4 mg IV

pyridoxine (vit B_6) (Rx, OTC)

(peer-i-dox′een)

Equaline Vitamin B6, Neuro-K, Walgreens Finest B-6, Walgreens Gold Seal Vitamin B6

Func. class.: Vit B_6, water soluble

ACTION: Needed for fat, protein, carbohydrate metabolism; enhances glycogen release from liver and muscle tissue; needed as coenzyme for metabolic transformations of a variety of amino acids

USES: Vit B_6 deficiency of inborn errors of metabolism, seizures, isoniazid therapy, oral contraceptives, alcoholic polyneuritis
Unlabeled uses: Palmar-plantar erythrodysesthesia syndrome

CONTRAINDICATIONS: Hypersensitivity
Precautions: Pregnancy (A), breastfeeding, children, Parkinson's disease; patients taking levodopa should avoid supplemental vitamins with >5 mg pyridoxine

DOSAGE AND ROUTES

RDA

- **Adult: PO** (male) 1.7-2 mg; (female) 1.4-1.6 mg
- **Child 9-13 yr: PO** 1 mg/day
- **Child 4-8 yr: PO** 0.6 mg/day
- **Child 1-3 yr: PO** 0.5 mg/day
- **Infant 7-12 mo: PO** 0.3 mg/day

Vit B_6 deficiency
- **Adult: PO** 5-25 mg/day × 3 wk
- **Child: PO** 10 mg until desired response

Pyridoxine deficiency neuritis/ seizure (not drug induced)
- **Adult: PO** *without neuritis* 2.5-10 mg/day after corrected 2-5 mg/day; *with neuritis* 100-200 mg/day × 3wk, then 2-5 mg/day
- **Child: PO** *without neuritis* 5-25 mg/ day × 3wk, then 1.5-2.5 mg/day in a multivitamin; *with neuritis:* 10-50 mg/ day × 3wk, then 1-2 mg/day
- **Neonate with seizures: IM/IV** 50-100 mg as single dose

Deficiency caused by isoniazid, cycloSERINE, hydrALAZINE, penicillamine
- **Adult: PO** 100-300 mg/day
- **Child: PO** 10-50 mg/day

Prevention of deficiency caused by isoniazid, cycloSERINE, hydrALAZINE, penicillamine
- **Adult: PO** 25-100 mg/day
- **Child: PO** 1-2 mg/kg/day

Palmar-plantar erythrodysesthesia syndrome (unlabeled)
- **Adult: PO** 50-150 mg/day

Available forms: Tabs 10, 25, 50, 100 mg; ext rel tabs 100 mg; inj 100 mg/ml; ext rel caps 150 mg

Administer:

PO route
- Do not break, crush, or chew ext rel tabs/caps

IM route
- Rotate sites; burning or stinging at site may occur
- Z-track to minimize pain

IV route
- Undiluted or added to most IV sol; give ≤50 mg/1 min if undiluted

Syringe compatibilities: Doxapram

SIDE EFFECTS
CNS: Paresthesia, flushing, warmth, lethargy (rare with normal renal function)
INTEG: Pain at inj site

PHARMACOKINETICS
PO/INJ: Half-life 2-3 wk, metabolized in liver, excreted in urine

INTERACTIONS
Decrease: effects of levodopa
Decrease: effects of pyridoxine—oral contraceptives, isoniazid, cycloSERINE, hydrALAZINE, penicillamine, chloramphenicol, immunosuppressants

NURSING CONSIDERATIONS
Assess:
- **Pyridoxine deficiency:** seizures, irritability, cheilitis, conjunctivitis, anemia, confusion, red tongue, weakness, fatigue before and during treatment; monitor pyridoxine levels
- Nutritional status: yeast, liver, legumes, bananas, green vegetables, whole grains
- Blood studies: Hct, Hgb

Evaluate:
- Therapeutic response: absence of nausea, vomiting, anorexia, skin lesions, glossitis, stomatitis, edema, seizures, restlessness, paresthesia

Teach patient/family:
- To avoid vitamin supplements unless directed by prescriber
- To increase meat, bananas, potatoes, lima beans, whole grain cereals in diet
- To take as directed; to continue with follow-up exams, blood work

P

pyrimethamine (Rx)
(peer-i-meth′a-meen)
Daraprim
Func. class.: Antimalarial, antiprotozoal
Chem. class.: Folic acid antagonist

ACTION:
Inhibits folic acid metabolism in parasite, prevents transmission by stopping growth of fertilized gametes

USES:
Malaria prophylaxis, *Plasmodium vivax, Pneumocystis jiroveci*

Unlabeled uses: Isosporiasis, pneumocystis pneumonia prophylaxis, toxoplasmic encephalitis prophylaxis

CONTRAINDICATIONS:
Hypersensitivity, chloroquine-resistant malaria, megaloblastic anemia caused by folate deficiency

Precautions: Pregnancy (C), breastfeeding, geriatric patients, blood dyscrasias, seizure disorder, G6PD disease, renal/hepatic disease

DOSAGE AND ROUTES

Prophylaxis of malaria

Begin 2 wk before entering endemic area, continue for 6-10 wk after return

- **Adult/child >10 yr: PO** 25 mg/wk
- **Child 4-10 yr: PO** 12.5 mg/wk
- **Child <4 yr: PO** 6.25 mg/wk

Malaria treatment

- **Adult/adolescent/child >10 yr: PO** 25 mg daily × 2 days with a sulfonamide
- **Child 4-10 yr: PO** 25 mg/day × 2 days

Toxoplasmosis

- **Adult: PO** 50-75 mg, then reduce by about 50% for 4-5 wk with 1-4 g sulfadoxine × 1-3 wk, then reduce by 50% for 4-5 wk
- **Child: PO** 1 mg/kg/day in 2 divided doses or 2 mg/kg/day × 3 days, then 1 mg/kg/day or divided twice daily × 4 wk, max 25 mg/day

Toxoplasmosis in AIDS patients

- **Adult: PO** 100-200 mg/day × 1-2 days, then 50-100 mg/day × 3-6 wk, then 25-50 mg/day for life (given with clindamycin or sulfADIAZINE)

Isosporiasis (unlabeled)

- **Adult: PO** 75 mg/day with leucovorin 10 mg/day × 14 days

Available forms: Tabs 25 mg; combo tabs 500 mg sulfadoxine/25 mg pyrimethamine

Administer:

PO route

- Leucovorin IM 3-9 mg/day × 3 days if folic acid deficiency occurs
- Before or after meals at same time each day to maintain product level, decrease GI symptoms
- Store in tight, light-resistant container
- **Extemporaneous susp:** tabs may be crushed and mixed with 25 ml distilled water, sucrose-containing solution (1 mg/ml); shake well; stable for 5-7 days at room temperature if mixed with sucrose-containing solutions

SIDE EFFECTS

CNS: Stimulation, irritability, seizures, tremors, ataxia, fatigue, fever

CV: Dysrhythmias

GI: *Nausea, vomiting, cramps, anorexia,* diarrhea, atrophic glossitis, gastritis

HEMA: Thrombocytopenia, leukopenia, pancytopenia, megaloblastic anemia, decreased folic acid, agranulocytosis

INTEG: Skin eruptions, photosensitivity, Stevens-Johnson syndrome

RESP: Respiratory failure

PHARMACOKINETICS

PO: Peak 2 hr, half-life 96 hr, half-life accelerated to 23 hr in AIDS patients, metabolized in liver, highly protein bound, excreted in urine (metabolites)

INTERACTIONS

- Synergistic action: folic acid

Increase: Megaloblastic anemia risk, agranulocytosis, thrombocytopenia—zidovudine

Increase: bone marrow suppression—bone marrow depressants, folate antagonists, radiation therapy

NURSING CONSIDERATIONS

Assess:

- Folic acid level; megaloblastic anemia occurs

⚠ **Blood dyscrasias:** blood studies, CBC, platelets; 2×/wk if dosage is increased

⚠ **Toxicity:** vomiting, anorexia, seizure, blood dyscrasia, glossitis; product should be discontinued immediately

- **Serious skin disorders:** Stevens-Johnson syndrome (swelling of face, lips, throat, fever)

Evaluate:

• Therapeutic response: decreased symptoms of malaria, toxoplasmosis

Teach patient/family:

• To report visual problems, fever, fatigue, bruising, bleeding, sore throat; may indicate **blood dyscrasias**

TREATMENT OF OVERDOSE:

Gastric lavage, short-acting barbiturate, leucovorin, respiratory support if needed

P

QUEtiapine (Rx)

(kwe-tie′a-peen)

Seroquel, Seroquel XR

Func. class.: Antipsychotic, atypical

Chem. class.: Dibenzothiazepine

ACTION: Functions as an antagonist at multiple neurotransmitter receptors in the brain, including $5HT_{1A}$, $5HT_2$, dopamine D_1, D_2, H_1, and adrenergic α_1, α_2 receptors

USES: Bipolar disorder, bipolar I disorder, depression, mania, schizophrenia

Unlabeled uses: Agitation, dementia, OCD, acute psychosis

CONTRAINDICATIONS: Hypersensitivity, breastfeeding

Precautions: Pregnancy (C), geriatric patients, hepatic/cardiac disease, breast cancer, long-term use, seizures, QT prolongation, brain tumor, hematologic disease, torsades de pointes, cataracts, dehydration, abrupt discontinuation

Black Box Warning: Children, suicidal ideation, increased mortality in elderly patients with dementia-related psychosis

DOSAGE AND ROUTES

Bipolar I disorder

- **Adult: PO** (monotherapy or adjunct to lithium, divalproex), (not at increased risk for hypotension) 50 mg bid on day 1, 100 mg on day 2 in 2 divided doses as tolerated to 400 mg/day on day 4, range 400-800 mg/day; ext rel give in evening 300 mg daily day 1, then 600 mg daily day 2, then adjusted as tolerated
- **Geriatric, debilitated, or at risk for hypotension: PO** 25 mg bid, titrate upward slowly; ext rel 50 mg in evening, max 800 mg/day
- **Child ≥10 yr/adolescents: PO** 25 mg bid day 1, 50 mg bid day 2, 100 mg bid day 3, 150 mg bid day 4, 200 mg bid beginning day 5 dose adjusted, max 600 mg/day; ext rel 50 mg day 1, 100 mg day 2, 200 mg day 3, 300 mg day 4, 400 mg day 5, give in evening

Schizophrenia

- **Adult: PO** (not at risk for hypotension) 25 mg bid on day 1, increase by 25-50 mg divided 2 to 3× on day 2 and day 3 to a target of 300-400 mg/day in divided doses by day 4, further dosage adjustment can be made in 25-50 mg bid increments, max 800 mg/day; (XR) 300 mg/day in PM, range 400-800 mg/day, max 800 mg/day
- **Adolescents 13-17 yr: PO** 25 mg bid on day 1, 50 mg bid on day 2, 100 mg bid on day 3, 150 mg bid on day 4, 200 mg on day 5; ext rel 50 mg on day 1, then 100 mg on day 2, 200 mg on day 3, 300 mg on day 4, 400 mg on day 5
- **Geriatric: PO EXT REL** 50 mg/day may increase in 50 mg/day increments

Depressive disorder (inadequate response to antidepressants alone)

- **Adult: PO EXT REL** 50 mg/day in PM on days 1, 2; on day 3, give 150 mg in PM
- **Geriatric, debilitated or at risk for hypotension: PO EXT REL** 50 mg on day 1 and 2, may increase by 50 mg/day based on response

Obsessive compulsive disorder (unlabeled)

- **Adult: PO** 50 mg daily, increase on response, continue for 1-2 yr before tapering by 10-25% q1-2mo

Available forms: Tabs 25, 50, 100, 200, 300, 400 mg; ext rel tab 50, 150, 200, 300, 400 mg

Administer:

- Reduced dose to geriatric patients
- Avoid use of CNS depressants
- Store in tight, light-resistant container
- **Immediate release:** without regard to meals
- **Ext rel:** without food or with light meal ≤300 calories; swallow whole; do not split, crush, chew; can switch from

immediate release to extended release by giving total daily dose daily

SIDE EFFECTS

CNS: EPS, pseudoparkinsonism, akathisia, dystonia, tardive dyskinesia; *drowsiness,* insomnia, agitation, anxiety, *headache,* seizures, neuroleptic malignant syndrome, *dizziness,* dystonia, restless legs
CV: Orthostatic hypotension, tachycardia, QT prolongation, CV disease, Parkinson's disease, cardiomyopathy, myocarditis
ENDO: SIADH, hyperglycemia
GI: *Nausea, anorexia, constipation,* abdominal pain, dry mouth
HEMA: Leukopenia, agranulocytosis
INTEG: Rash
META: Hyponatremia
MISC: Asthenia, back pain, fever, ear pain
MS: Rhabdomyolysis
RESP: Rhinitis
SYST: Stevens-Johnson syndrome, anaphylaxis

PHARMACOKINETICS

Extensively metabolized by liver, half-life ≥6 hr, peak 1½ hr, ext rel 6 hr, inhibits P450 CYP3A4 enzyme system, 83% protein binding, excretion: <1% unchanged urine

INTERACTIONS

⚠ **Increase:** QT prolongation—class IA/III antidysrhythmics, some phenothiazines, β-agonists, local anesthetics, tricyclics, haloperidol, methadone, chloroquine, clarithromycin, droperidol, erythromycin, pentamidine
Increase: CNS depression—alcohol, opioid analgesics, sedative/hypnotics, antihistamines
Increase: hypotension—alcohol, antihypertensives
Increase: QUEtiapine clearance, decrease QUEtiapine effect—phenytoin, thioridazine, barbiturates, glucocorticoids, carBAMazepine, rifampin
Increase: neurotoxicity—lithium
Increase: QUEtiapine action—fluconazole, itraconazole, ketoconazole (CYP3A4 inhibitors)
Increase: effects of erythromycin
Decrease: QUEtiapine clearance—cimetidine
Decrease: effects of DOPamine agonists, levodopa, LORazepam

Drug/Lab Test
Increase: cholesterol, triglycerides, LFTs, glucose
Decrease: thyroid tests, WBC

NURSING CONSIDERATIONS

Assess:

⚠ CV status: QT prolongation, tachycardia, orthostatic B/P

Black Box Warning: Mental status before initial administration, AIMS assessment; affect, orientation, LOC, reflexes, gait, coordination, sleep pattern disturbances; suicidal thoughts/behaviors (child/young adult); dementia (geriatric patients)

Black Box Warning: Not to be used in child <10 yr (imm rel) or <18 yr (ext rel)

Black Box Warning: Suicide: restrict amount of product given; usually suicidal thoughts/behaviors occur early during treatment and among children/adolescents/young adults

- Baseline blood glucose, LFTs, neurologic function, ophthalmologic exam, weight, monitor glucose often in diabetes mellitus, thyroid function tests, serum electrolytes/creatinine/lipid profile/prolactin
- B/P standing, lying; pulse, respirations; determine q4hr during initial treatment; establish baseline before starting treatment; report drops of 30 mm Hg; watch for ECG changes
- Dizziness, faintness, palpitations, tachycardia on rising
- **EPS:** including akathisia (inability to sit still, no pattern to movements), tardive dyskinesia (bizarre movements of jaw, mouth, tongue, extremities), pseudoparkinsonism (rigidity, tremors, pill rolling, shuffling gait)

⚠ Neuroleptic malignant syndrome: hyperthermia, increased CPK, altered mental status, muscle rigidity, seizures, tachycardia, diaphoresis, hypo/hypertension, fatigue; notify prescriber immediately if symptoms occur

- Constipation, urinary retention daily; if these occur, increase bulk, water in diet
- Supervised ambulation until patient stabilized on medication; do not involve patient in strenuous exercise program because fainting possible; patient should not stand still for long period of time

Evaluate:

- Therapeutic response: decrease in emotional excitement, hallucinations, delusions, paranoia; reorganization of patterns of thought, speech

Teach patient/family:

- Not to become overheated, drink plenty of fluids
- To rise slowly to prevent orthostatic hypotension
- To take medication only as prescribed; not to crush, chew ext rel product; not to use with alcohol; to take regular tabs without regard to food, ext rel without food, not to use other products unless approved by prescriber; not to stop abruptly
- That follow-up is necessary, including LFTs, blood glucose, neurologic, cholesterol profile, weight
- If drowsiness occurs, to avoid hazardous activities such as driving; not to stand quickly, may be worse during first few days of dose change
- To avoid use of OTC meds unless directed by prescriber
- To notify prescriber if pregnancy planned, suspected; not to breastfeed
- To notify prescriber immediately of fever, difficulty breathing, fatigue, sore throat, rash, bleeding

Black Box Warning: Suicide: Thoughts/behaviors, primarily among children/adolescents/young adults

- To have eye exam before treatment and q6mo, cataracts may occur

quinapril (Rx)

(kwin′a-pril)

Accupril

Func. class.: Antihypertensive

Chem. class.: Angiotensin-converting enzyme (ACE) inhibitor

Do not confuse:
Accupril/Aciphex

ACTION: Selectively suppresses renin-angiotensin-aldosterone system; inhibits ACE, prevents conversion of angiotensin I to angiotensin II; results in dilation of arterial, venous vessels

USES: Hypertension, alone or in combination with thiazide diuretics; systolic CHF

CONTRAINDICATIONS: Children, hypersensitivity to ACE inhibitors, angioedema

Black Box Warning: Pregnancy (D)

Precautions: Breastfeeding, geriatric patients, impaired renal/hepatic function, dialysis patients, hypovolemia, blood dyscrasias, bilateral renal stenosis, cough, hyperkalemia, aortic stenosis, African descent

DOSAGE AND ROUTES

Hypertension

- **Adult: PO** 10-20 mg/day initially, then 20-80 mg/day divided bid or daily (monotherapy); start at 5 mg/day (with diuretics), titrate ≥2 wk
- **Geriatric: PO** 10 mg/day, titrate to desired response (monotherapy); start at 2.5 mg/day (with diuretics)

Congestive heart failure

- **Adult: PO** 5 mg bid, may increase weekly until 20-40 mg/day in 2 divided doses

Renal dose

- **Adult: PO** CCr 61-89 ml/min 10 mg daily (hypertension), 5 mg bid (heart failure); CCr 30-60 ml/min, 5 mg/day initially; CCr 10-29 ml/min, 2.5 mg/day initially

Available forms: Tabs 5, 10, 20, 40 mg

Administer:

- Tabs may be crushed if necessary
- Store in airtight container at room temperature
- Do not use with high-fat meal, decreases absorption

SIDE EFFECTS

CNS: *Headache, dizziness, fatigue,* somnolence, depression, malaise, nervousness, vertigo, syncope

CV: *Hypotension,* postural hypotension, syncope, palpitations, *angina pectoris,* MI, tachycardia, vasodilation, chest pain

GI: *Nausea,* diarrhea, constipation, *vomiting,* gastritis, GI hemorrhage, dry mouth

GU: Increased BUN, creatinine; decreased libido, impotence

INTEG: Angioedema, rash, sweating, photosensitivity, pruritus

META: Hyperkalemia

MISC: Back pain, amblyopia

MS: Myalgia

RESP: *Cough,* pharyngitis, dyspnea

PHARMACOKINETICS

Bioavailability ≥60%, onset <1 hr, peak 1-2 hr, duration 24 hr, protein binding 97%, half-life 2 hr, metabolized by liver (active metabolites quinaprilat), metabolites excreted in urine (60%)/feces (37%)

INTERACTIONS

Increase: hyperkalemia—vasodilators, hydrALAZINE, prazosin, potassium-sparing diuretics, sympathomimetics, potassium supplements, ACE/angiotensin II receptor antagonists; aliskiren (diabetic patients)

Increase: hypotension—diuretics, other antihypertensives, ganglionic blockers, adrenergic blockers, phenothiazines, nitrates, acute alcohol ingestion

Increase: toxicity of lithium

Decrease: absorption of tetracycline, quinolone antibiotics

Decrease: hypotensive effect of quinapril—NSAIDs

Drug/Herb

- Cough: capsaicin
- **Decrease:** antihypertensive effect—ma huang

Drug/Food

- **Hyperkalemia:** do not use with potassium-containing salt substitutes, read label carefully

Drug/Lab Test

Increase: potassium, creatinine, BUN, LFTs

NURSING CONSIDERATIONS

Assess:

⚠ **Collagen-vascular disease:** blood studies: neutrophils, decreased platelets; WBC with differential at baseline, periodically, q3mo; if neutrophils <1000/mm³, discontinue treatment

- **Hypertension:** B/P, orthostatic hypotension, syncope, monitor B/P before giving and after 2 hr; African American patients are more resistant to antihypertension effect
- Renal studies: protein, BUN, creatinine; watch for increased levels; may indicate nephrotic syndrome
- Baselines of hepatic studies before therapy, periodically; increased LFTs; uric acid, glucose may be increased
- Potassium levels; hyperkalemia rare
- **CHF:** edema in feet, legs daily; weight daily

⚠ **Allergic reactions:** rash, fever, pruritus, urticaria, swelling of eyes/face/throat/neck, SOB, difficulty breathing; product should be discontinued; angioedema is more common in African American patients

Black Box Warning: For pregnancy (D), 2nd/3rd trimester, if pregnancy is suspected, discontinue use

Q

Evaluate:
- Therapeutic response: decrease in B/P

Teach patient/family:
- Not to discontinue product abruptly
- Not to use OTC products (cough, cold, allergy); not to use salt substitutes containing potassium unless directed by prescriber, avoid high-fat meal at same time as product
- To comply with dosage schedule, even if feeling better
- To rise slowly to sitting or standing position to minimize orthostatic hypotension, to report excessive perspiration, dehydration, vomiting, diarrhea; may lead to fall in B/P; maintain adequate hydration
- To notify prescriber of mouth sores, sore throat, fever, swelling of hands/feet, irregular heartbeat, chest pain, persistent dry cough
- That product may cause dizziness, fainting, lightheadedness; may occur during first few days of therapy
- That product may cause skin rash, impaired taste perception
- How to take B/P, normal readings for age group

Black Box Warning: Pregnancy: to report if pregnancy planned, suspected; pregnancy category (D) 2nd/3rd trimester; do not breastfeed

TREATMENT OF OVERDOSE:
0.9% NaCl IV infusion

HIGH ALERT

quiNIDine gluconate (Rx)
(kwin′i-deen)

quiNIDine sulfate (Rx)
Func. class.: Antidysrhythmic (Class IA)
Chem. class.: Quinine dextroisomer

Do not confuse:
quiNIDine/quiNINE

ACTION: Prolongs duration of action potential and effective refractory period, thus decreasing myocardial excitability; anticholinergic properties

USES: Atrial fibrillation, PAT, ventricular tachycardia, atrial flutter, Wolff-Parkinson-White syndrome; PVST, malaria/IV quiNIDine gluconate
Unlabeled uses: Singultus (hiccups)

CONTRAINDICATIONS: Hypersensitivity, idiosyncratic response, digoxin toxicity, blood dyscrasias, myasthenia gravis, AV block
Precautions: Pregnancy (C), breastfeeding, children, geriatric patients, electrolyte imbalance, renal/hepatic disease, CHF, respiratory depression, bradycardia, hypotension, syncope

Black Box Warning: Cardiac arrhythmias, MI

DOSAGE AND ROUTES
QuiNIDine gluconate
- **Adult: PO** (ext rel) 324-648 mg q8-12hr; **IM** 600 mg, then 400 mg q2hr; **IV** give 16 mg/min

Severe *Plasmodium falciparum*
Malaria
- **Adult: IV** 10 mg/kg/dose over 1-2 hr, then IV Infusion of 0.02 mg/kg/min for ≥24 hr

QuiNIDine sulfate
PVST/WPW/atrial fibrillation/flutter
- **Adult: PO** 200-300 mg q6-8hr × 5-8 doses; may increase daily until sinus rhythm restored; max 4 g/day given only after digitalization; maintenance 200-300 mg tid-qid or **EXT REL** 300-600 mg q8-12hr

Hiccups (unlabeled)
- **Adult: PO** 200 mg qid

Available forms: *Gluconate:* ext rel tabs 324 mg; inj gluconate 80 mg/ml; *sulfate:* tabs 200, 300 mg; sus rel tabs 300 mg
Administer:
- AV node blocker (digoxin) before starting quinidine to avoid increased ventricular rate

PO route

- Do not break, crush, chew ext rel products
- With full glass of water on empty stomach; if GI upset occurs, may take with food
- **Sus rel forms not interchangeable**
- Do not use with grapefruit juice

IM route

- IM inj in deltoid; aspirate to avoid intravascular administration

Intermittent IV INFUSION route

- After diluting 800 mg/50 ml D_5W (16 mg/ml); give ≤1 mg/min, use infusion pump; quiNIDine absorbed by PVC tubing, minimize length

Y-site compatibilities: Alfentanil, amikacin, anidulafungin, argatroban, arsenic trioxide, ascorbic acid, asparaginase, atenolol, atracurium, atropine, benztropine, bleomycin, bumetanide, buprenorphine, butorphanol, calcium gluconate, caspofungin, chlorproMAZINE, cimetidine, CISplatin, cyanocobalamin, cycloSPORINE, DACTINomycin, digoxin, diltiazem, diphenhydrAMINE, DOBUTamine, DOCEtaxel, DOPamine, doxycycline, enalaprilat, ePHEDrine, EPINEPHrine, epoetin alfa, erythromycin, esmolol, etoposide, famotidine, fenoldopam, fentaNYL, fluconazole, fludarabine, gatifloxacin, gemcitabine, gentamicin, glycopyrrolate, granisetron, HYDROmorphone, IDArubicin, imipenem-cilastatin, irinotecan, isoproterenol, labetalol, lidocaine, linezolid, LORazepam, magnesium sulfate, mannitol, mechlorethamine, meperidine, metaraminol, methoxamine, methyldopate, metoclopramide, metoprolol, metroNIDAZOLE, miconazole, milrinone, mitoXANtrone, morphine, multiple vitamins, mycophenolate, nalbuphine, naloxone, nesiritide, netilmicin, nitroglycerin, norepinephrine, octreotide, ondansetron, oxaliplatin, PACLitaxel, palonosetron, pamidronate, pancuronium, papaverine, pentamidine, pentazocine, phenylephrine, phytonadione, polymyxin B, potassium chloride, procainamide, prochlorperazine, promethazine, propranolol, protamine, pyridoxine, ranitidine, ritodrine, succinylcholine, SUFentanil, tacrolimus, teniposide, theophylline, thiamine, thiotepa, tirofiban, tobramycin, tolazoline, trimetaphan, urokinase, vancomycin, vasopressin, verapamil, vinorelbine, voriconazole, zoledronic acid

SIDE EFFECTS

CNS: *Headache, dizziness,* involuntary movement, confusion, psychosis, restlessness, irritability, syncope, excitement, depression, ataxia

CV: **Hypotension,** *bradycardia,* PVCs, **heart block, CV collapse, arrest,** torsades de pointes, widening QRS complex, **ventricular tachycardia**

EENT: Cinchonism: tinnitus, blurred vision, hearing loss, mydriasis, disturbed color vision

GI: Nausea, vomiting, anorexia, abdominal pain, *diarrhea,* **hepatotoxicity**

HEMA: **Thrombocytopenia,** hemolytic anemia, **agranulocytosis,** hypoprothrombinemia

INTEG: Rash, urticaria, **angioedema,** swelling, photosensitivity, flushing with severe pruritus

RESP: Dyspnea, **respiratory depression**

PHARMACOKINETICS

PO: (sulfate) peak 1-6 hr, duration 6-8 hr, (Sulfate ER) peak 4 hr, duration 8-12 hr; (gluconate PO) peak 3-4 hr, duration 6-8 hr, half-life 6-7 hr (prolonged in geriatric patients, cirrhosis, CHF), metabolized in liver, excreted unchanged (10%-50%) by kidneys, protein bound (80%-90%)

INTERACTIONS

- Additive vagolytic effect: anticholinergic blockers

Increase: cardiac depression: other antidysrhythmics, phenothiazines, reserpine

Increase: effects of neuromuscular blockers, digoxin, warfarin, tricyclics, propranolol

Increase: **QT prolongation—macrolides, quinolones, tricyclics procainamide, antipsychotics**

Increase: quiNIDine effects—cimetidine, sodium bicarbonate, carbonic anhydrase

Q

inhibitors, antacids, hydroxide suspensions, amiodarone, verapamil, NIFEdipine, protease inhibitors

Decrease: quiNIDine effects—barbiturates, phenytoin, rifampin, sucralfate, cholinergics

Drug/Herb

Increase: quiNIDine effect—hawthorn, licorice

Drug/Food

• Delayed absorption, decreased metabolism: grapefruit juice

Drug/Lab Test

Decrease: platelets, Hgb, granulocytes

NURSING CONSIDERATIONS

Assess:

⚠ ECG B/P, pulse continuously during IV, baseline, and periodically (PO) to determine increased PR or QRS segments, QT interval; discontinue product or reduce dose

• Blood levels (therapeutic level 2-7 mcg/ml), CBC, LFTs

⚠ **For cinchonism:** tinnitus, headache, nausea, dizziness, fever, vertigo, tremors; may lead to hearing loss

• **Cardiac toxicity:** asystole, ventricular dysrhythmias, widening QRS, torsades de pointes

• CNS effects: dizziness, confusion, psychosis, paresthesias, seizures; product should be discontinued

• **Hepatotoxicity:** monitor LFTs for first 1-2 mo of treatment

Evaluate:

• Therapeutic response: decreased dysrhythmias

Teach patient/family:

• That if dizziness, drowsiness occurs, to avoid driving or hazardous activities

• To use sunglasses; product may cause sensitivity to light

• To carry emergency ID stating disease, medication use

• How to take pulse; when to notify prescriber

• To avoid all products unless approved by prescriber

• Not to crush, chew ext rel product

• Not to use grapefruit juice with this product

• **QuiNIDine toxicity:** visual changes, nausea, headache, ringing in the ears; report immediately

• To report signs of cinchonism, diarrhea, anorexia, decreased B/P

RABEprazole (Rx)

(rah-bep′rah-zole)

Aciphex, Aciphex Sprinkle, Pariet ✤

Func. class.: Antiulcer, proton pump inhibitor

Chem. class.: Benzimidazole

Do not confuse:
Aciphex/Aricept/Accupril
RABEprazole/ARIPiprazole

ACTION: Suppresses gastric secretion by inhibiting hydrogen/potassium ATPase enzyme system in the gastric parietal cells; characterized as a gastric acid pump inhibitor because it blocks the final step of acid production

USES: Gastroesophageal reflux disease (GERD), severe erosive esophagitis, poorly responsive systemic GERD, pathologic hypersecretory conditions (Zollinger-Ellison syndrome, systemic mastocytosis, multiple endocrine adenomas); treatment of active duodenal ulcers with/without antiinfectives for *Helicobacter pylori;* daytime, nighttime heartburn
Unlabeled uses: Gastric ulcer, heartburn, *H. pylori* eradication in children

CONTRAINDICATIONS: Hypersensitivity to this product or proton pump inhibitors (PPIs)
Precautions: Pregnancy (C), breastfeeding, children, Asian patients, diarrhea, geriatric patients, gastric cancer, hepatic/GI disease, IBS, osteoporosis, pseudomembranous colitis, ulcerative colitis, vit B_{12} deficiency

DOSAGE AND ROUTES

Healing of duodenal ulcers
- **Adult: PO** 20 mg/day × ≤4 wk; to be taken after breakfast

Healing of erosive esophagitis or ulcerative GERD
- **Adult: PO** 20 mg/day × 4-8 wk; may use an additional course
- **Adolescent and child ≥12 yr: PO** 20 mg/day up to 8 wk
- **Child 1-11 yr (≥15 kg): PO** (sprinkle) 10 mg daily up to 12 wk
- **Child 1-11 yr (<15 kg):** 5 mg daily up to 12 wk; may increase to 10 mg daily if needed

***H. pylori* eradication**
- **Adult: PO** 20 mg bid × 7 days with amoxicillin 1 g bid × 7 days with clarithromycin 500 mg bid × 7 days

Pathologic hypersecretory conditions
- **Adult: PO** 60 mg/day; may increase to 120 mg in 2 divided doses

Gastric ulcer (unlabeled)
- **Adult: PO** 20 mg/day after AM meal × 3-6 wk

Dyspepsia/heartburn (unlabeled)
- **Adult: PO** 20 mg/day × ≤14 days

Available forms: Del rel tabs 20 mg; del rel caps 5, 10 mg
Administer:
- **PO:** Do not break, crush, chew del rel tab; after breakfast daily with full glass of water, without regard to food

SIDE EFFECTS

CNS: *Headache, dizziness, asthenia*
CV: Chest pain, angina, tachycardia, bradycardia, palpitations, peripheral edema
EENT: Tinnitus, taste perversion
GI: *Diarrhea, abdominal pain, vomiting, nausea, constipation, flatulence, acid regurgitation,* abdominal swelling, anorexia, irritable colon, esophageal candidiasis, dry mouth; **pseudomembranous colitis (rare)**
GU: UTI, urinary frequency, increased creatinine, **proteinuria, hematuria,** testicular pain, glycosuria
HEMA: **Pancytopenia, thrombocytopenia, neutropenia, leukocytosis,** anemia
INTEG: *Rash,* dry skin, urticaria, pruritus, alopecia
META: Hypoglycemia, increased hepatic enzymes, weight gain
MISC: *Back pain,* fever, fatigue, malaise, **Stevens-Johnson syndrome**
RESP: *Upper respiratory tract infections, cough,* epistaxis, **pneumonia**

R

PHARMACOKINETICS

Eliminated in urine as metabolites and in feces, terminal half-life 1-2 hr, metabolized by CYP2C19 enzyme system, protein binding 96.3%

INTERACTIONS

Increase: bleeding risk—warfarin, clopidogrel
Increase: serum levels of RABEprazole—benzodiazepines, phenytoin, clarithromycin, antacids, other proton pump inhibitors, H_2 blockers
Increase: levels of—digoxin, nelfinavir/omeprazole
Decrease: levels of RABEprazole—sucralfate, calcium carbonate, vit B_{12}
Decrease: levels of ketoconazole, itraconazole, iron salts, atazanavir/ritonavir, ampicillin

Drug/Herb
Decrease: RABEprazole—St. John's wort

Drug/Lab Test
Decrease: magnesium

NURSING CONSIDERATIONS

Assess:

• GI system: bowel sounds, abdomen for pain, swelling, anorexia, emesis/stool for occult blood
• **Pseudomembranous colitis:** may occur with most antibiotic therapy; watery diarrhea, abdominal pain, fever
• **Vit B_{12} deficiency/cyanocobalamin/hypomagnesemia:** may occur after 3-12 mo of treatment; use magnesium, vit B_{12}, cyanocobalamin supplement; if severe, discontinuing of product may be needed
• Hepatic studies: AST, ALT, alk phos during treatment; CBC with differential periodically
⚠ Serious skin reactions: Stevens-Johnson syndrome
• CBC with differential before, periodically during treatment; blood dyscrasias may occur (rare)
• Obtain susceptibility testing if *H. pylori* treatment is ineffective, another anti-infective may be needed

Evaluate:

• Therapeutic response: absence of epigastric pain, swelling, fullness; decreased symptoms of GERD after 4-8 wk

Teach patient/family:

• To report severe diarrhea or black, tarry stools; product may have to be discontinued
• That hypoglycemia may occur if patient is diabetic
• To avoid hazardous activities because dizziness, drowsiness may occur
• To avoid alcohol, salicylates, NSAIDs because they may cause GI irritation; to avoid other OTC, herbal products unless approved by prescriber
• To use as directed for length of time prescribed; to take missed dose when remembered; not to double dose, take del rel tab whole, do not cut, break; cap should be opened and sprinkled on food (applesauce)
• To notify prescriber if pregnancy planned, suspected

RARELY USED

radioactive iodine (sodium iodide) ^{131}I (Rx)

Func. class.: Antithyroid
Chem. class.: Radiopharmaceutical

USES:

High dose: Thyroid cancer, hyperthyroidism
Low dose: Visualization to determine thyroid cancer, diagnostic aid for thyroid function studies

CONTRAINDICATIONS:

Pregnancy (X), breastfeeding, age <30 yr, recent MI, large nodular goiter, vomiting/diarrhea, acute hyperthyroidism, use of thyroid products

DOSAGE AND ROUTES

Thyroid cancer

• **Adult: PO** 50-150 mCi; may repeat, depending on clinical status

⚠ Nurse Alert

Hyperthyroidism

• **Adult: PO** 4-10 mCi, depending on serum thyroxine level

Available forms: Caps 1-50, 0.8-100 mCi; oral sol 7.05 mCi/ml, 3.5-150 mCi/vial; concentrated oral solution 1000 mCi/ml

raloxifene (Rx)

(ral-ox′ih-feen)

Evista

Func. class.: Bone resorption inhibitor

Chem. class.: Hormone modifier, selective estrogen receptor modulator (SERM)

ACTION: Tissue-selective estrogen agonist/antagonist; agonist activity in bone and on lipid metabolism; antagonist activity on breast and uterus; reduces resorption of bone and decreases bone turnover

USES: Prevention, treatment of osteoporosis in postmenopausal women; breast cancer prophylaxis in postmenopausal women with osteoporosis or in postmenopausal women at high risk for developing the disease

Unlabeled uses: Uterine leiomyomata in postmenopausal women with osteoporosis or in postmenopausal women who are at high risk for developing the disease

CONTRAINDICATIONS: Pregnancy (X), breastfeeding, hypersensitivity

Black Box Warning: Women with active or history of venous thromboembolic events

Precautions: CV/hepatic disease, cervical/uterine cancer, elevated triglycerides, pulmonary embolism

Black Box Warning: Stroke

DOSAGE AND ROUTES

• **Adult postmenopausal women: PO** 60 mg/day, max 60 mg/day

Available forms: Tabs 60 mg

Administer:

• PO: without regard to meals, vit D
• Add calcium supplement if inadequate
• Do not use during immobilization or prolonged bedrest

SIDE EFFECTS

CNS: Insomnia, depression, migraines

CV: Hot flashes, peripheral edema, **thromboembolism, stroke**

EENT: Retinal vein occlusion (rare)

GI: *Nausea,* vomiting, diarrhea, dyspepsia, abdominal pain

GU: Vaginitis, leukorrhea, cystitis, *hot flashes,* vaginal bleeding

INTEG: Rash, sweating

META: Weight gain, peripheral edema

MS: Arthralgia, myalgia, *leg cramps,* arthritis

RESP: Sinusitis, pharyngitis, increased cough, pneumonia, laryngitis, bronchitis, **pulmonary embolism**, flulike symptoms

PHARMACOKINETICS

Duration 24 hr, elimination half-life 28-32 hr; excreted in feces, breast milk; highly bound to plasma proteins

INTERACTIONS

• Administer cautiously with other highly protein-bound products, ibuprofen, diazepam, naproxen, systemic estrogens

Decrease: action of anticoagulants, dessicated thyroid, levothyroxine, liotrix

Decrease: action of raloxifene—ampicillin, cholestyramine

Drug/Food

Decrease: raloxifene—soy

Drug/Lab Test

Increase: apolipoprotein A-1, hormone-binding globulin

Decrease: total cholesterol, LDL, lipoprotein, apolipoprotein B, serum calcium, albumin, total protein

R

NURSING CONSIDERATIONS

Assess:

Black Box Warning: History of stroke, TIA, thrombosis, atrial fibrillation, hypertension, smoking; venous thrombosis may occur; avoid prolonged sitting; discontinue 3 days before surgery, other immobilization

- Bone density test at baseline, throughout treatment, bone-specific alk phos, osteocalcin

Evaluate:

- Therapeutic response: prevention, treatment of osteoporosis in postmenopausal women; prevention of breast cancer in postmenopausal women with osteoporosis or in those who are at high risk for developing the disease

Teach patient/family:

Black Box Warning: To discontinue product 72 hr before prolonged bedrest; to avoid staying in one position for long periods, to report possible blood clots immediately usually during first few months of therapy

- To take calcium supplements, vit D if intake is inadequate
- To increase exercise using weights
- To stop smoking; to decrease alcohol consumption
- That product does not help to control hot flashes

⚠ To report fever, acute migraine, insomnia, emotional distress; urinary tract infection, vaginal burning/itching; swelling, warmth, pain in calves

⚠ To notify prescriber if pregnancy planned, suspected, pregnancy (X); to avoid breastfeeding

- Provide product package insert and discuss with patient

raltegravir (Rx)

(ral-teg′ra-vir)

Isentress

Func. class.: Antiretroviral

Chem. class.: HIV integrase strand transfer inhibitor (ISTIs)

ACTION:
Inhibits catalytic activity of HIV integrase, which is an HIV-encoded enzyme needed for replication

USES:
HIV in combination with other antiretrovirals

CONTRAINDICATIONS:
Breastfeeding, hypersensitivity

Precautions: Pregnancy (C), children, geriatric patients, hepatic disease, immune reconstitution syndrome, hepatitis, antimicrobial resistance, lactase deficiency

DOSAGE AND ROUTES

- **Adult and adolescent ≥16 yr: PO** 400 mg bid; if using with rifampin, give 800 mg bid

Available forms: Tabs 400 mg; chew tabs 25, 100 mg, granules for oral suspension 100mg

Administer:

PO route

- Do not break, crush, chew tabs
- May give without regard to meals, with 8 oz of water
- Store at room temperature

Oral suspension:

- Open foil, use 5 ml of water in provided measuring cup, close swirl, do not turn upside down, use oral syringe to administer, use within 30 min, discard any remaining suspension

SIDE EFFECTS

CNS: *Fatigue,* fever, *dizziness, headache,* asthenia, suicidal ideation

CV: MI

GI: *Nausea,* vomiting, diarrhea, abdominal pain, asthenia, gastritis, **hepatitis**
GU: Oliguria, proteinuria, hematuria, glomerulonephritis, acute renal failure, renal tubular necrosis
HEMA: Anemia, neutropenia
INTEG: Rash, urticaria, pruritus, pain or phlebitis at IV site, unusual sweating, alopecia
META: Hyperamylasia, hyperglycemia
MS: Myopathy, **rhabdomyolysis**
SYST: Immune reconstitution syndrome

PHARMACOKINETICS

Max absorption 3 hr if taken on an empty stomach; terminal half-life 9 hr; metabolized in the liver by uridine diphosphate glucuronosyltransferase (UGT A1A enzyme system); excreted in feces 51%, urine 32%

INTERACTIONS

Increase: raltegravir effect—proton pump inhibitors, H_2 blockers; UGT1A1 inhibitors (atazanavir)
⚠ **Increase: rhabdomyolysis, myopathy, elevated CPK—fibric acid derivatives, HMG-CoA reductase inhibitors**
Decrease: raltegravir levels—rifampin, efavirenz, tenofovir, tipranavir/ritonavir

Drug/Lab Test

Increase: AST, ALT, GGT, total bilirubin, alk phos, amylase/lipase, CK, serum glucose, total/HDL/LDL cholesterol
Decrease: Hgb, platelets, ANC

NURSING CONSIDERATIONS

Assess:

- **HIV infection:** CD4, T-cell count, plasma HIV RNA, viral load; resistance testing before therapy, at treatment failure

⚠ **Rhabdomyolysis: Assess for calf pain, increased CPK, product should be discontinued**

- Skin eruptions: rash, urticaria, itching
- **Suicidal thoughts/behaviors: monitor for depression; more common in those with mental illness**
- **Immune reconstitution syndrome, usually during initial phase of treatment, may give antiinfective before starting**
- Monitor total/HDL/LDL cholesterol baseline and periodically; all may be elevated

Evaluate:

- Therapeutic response: improvement in CD4 counts, T-cell counts

Teach patient/family:

- To take as prescribed; if dose missed, to take as soon as remembered up to 1 hr before next dose; not to double dose; not to share with others
- That sexual partners need to be told that patient has HIV; that product does not cure infection, just controls symptoms; does not prevent infecting others

⚠ **To report sore throat, fever, fatigue (may indicate superinfection)**

- That product must be taken in equal intervals 2×/day to maintain blood levels for duration of therapy

⚠ To notify prescriber immediately of suicidal thoughts/behaviors

- To notify prescriber if pregnancy planned, suspected; to avoid breastfeeding
- To continue with follow-up exams, blood work

⚠ HIGH ALERT

ramelteon (Rx)

(rah-mel′tee-on)

Rozerem

Func. class.: Sedative/hypnotic, antianxiety
Chem. class.: Melatonin receptor agonist

ACTION: Binds selectively to melatonin receptors (MT_1, MT_2); thought to be involved in circadian rhythms and in the normal sleep/wake cycle

USES: Insomnia (difficulty with sleep onset)

CONTRAINDICATIONS: Breastfeeding, children, infants, hypersensitivity
Precautions: Pregnancy (C), hepatic

R

disease, alcoholism, COPD, seizure disorder, sleep apnea, suicidal ideation, angioedema, depression, sleep-related behaviors (sleepwalking), schizophrenia, bipolar disorder; alcohol intoxication, hepatic encephalopathy

DOSAGE AND ROUTES

• **Adult: PO** 8 mg within 30 min of bedtime

Hepatic dose

• Do not use with severe hepatic disease; use with caution for mild to moderate hepatic disease

Available forms: Tabs 8 mg

Administer:

• Within 30 min of bedtime for sleeplessness; on empty stomach for fast onset

• Do not break tabs, swallow whole

• Store in tight container in cool environment

SIDE EFFECTS

CNS: Dizziness, somnolence, fatigue, headache, insomnia, depression, complex sleep-related reactions (sleep driving, sleep eating), suicidal thoughts/behaviors

GI: Nausea, diarrhea, dysgeusia, vomiting

MISC: Myalgia, arthralgia, decreased blood cortisol, influenza, upper RI

SYST: Severe allergic reactions, angioedema

PHARMACOKINETICS

Absorbed rapidly; peak ½-1½ hr; protein binding 82%; rapid first-pass metabolism via liver; 84% excreted in urine, 4% in feces; half-life 2-5 hr metabolite

INTERACTIONS

⚠ Possible toxicity: antiretroviral protease inhibitors

⚠ **Increase:** ramelteon effect, toxicity—alcohol; CYP1A2 inhibitors, azole antifungals (ketoconazole, fluconazole), fluvoxaMINE, anxiolytics, sedatives, hypnotics, barbiturates, ciprofloxacin, strong CYP2C9 inhibitors, strong CYP3A4 inhibitors

Decrease: effect of ramelteon—strong CYP inducer (rifampin)

Drug/Food

• Prolonged absorption, sleep onset reduced: high-fat/heavy meal

Drug/Lab

Increase: protein level

Decrease: testosterone level

NURSING CONSIDERATIONS

Assess:

⚠ **Severe hypersensitive reactions:** Assess for angioedema (facial swelling), product should be discontinued

• **Sleep characteristics:** type of sleep problem: falling asleep, staying asleep; complex sleep disorders (sleep walking/driving/eating) after taking product

• Mental status: mood, sensorium, affect, memory (long, short term), suicidal ideation

• LFTs: before treatment, periodically

Evaluate:

• Therapeutic response: ability to sleep at night, decreased amount of early morning awakening

Teach patient/family:

• To avoid driving, other activities requiring alertness until product stabilized; drowsiness may continue the next day

• To avoid alcohol ingestion, CNS depressants

• About alternative measures to improve sleep: reading, exercise several hr before bedtime, warm bath, warm milk, TV, self-hypnosis, deep breathing

• To report if pregnancy is planned or suspected (C); to avoid breastfeeding

• To take product immediately before going to bed

• Not to ingest a high-fat/heavy meal before taking product

⚠ To report cessation of menses, galactorrhea (women), decreased libido, infertility, worsening of insomnia, behavioral changes, severe allergic reactions, suicidal thoughts/behaviors, if insomnia gets worse

• Med guide should be given to patient and reviewed

ramipril (Rx)

(ra-mi′pril)

Altace

Func. class.: Antihypertensive

Chem. class.: Angiotensin-converting enzyme inhibitor (ACE)

Do not confuse:
ramipril/enalapril
Altace/alteplase

ACTION: Selectively suppresses renin-angiotensin-aldosterone system; inhibits ACE, prevents conversion of angiotensin I to angiotensin II; results in dilation of arterial, venous vessels

USES: Hypertension, alone or in combination with thiazide diuretics; CHF (post-MI), reduction in risk for MI, stroke, death from CV disorders

Unlabeled uses: Proteinuria due to diabetic nephropathy

CONTRAINDICATIONS: Breastfeeding, children, hypersensitivity to ACE inhibitors, history of ACE-inhibitor–induced angioedema

Black Box Warning: Pregnancy (D) 2nd/3rd trimesters

Precautions: Geriatric patients, impaired renal/hepatic function, dialysis patients, hypovolemia, blood dyscrasias, CHF, renal artery stenosis, cough, African descent, aortic stenosis

DOSAGE AND ROUTES

Hypertension

- **Adult: PO** 2.5 mg/day initially, then 2.5-20 mg/day divided bid or daily

CHF post-MI

- **Adult: PO** 1.25-2.5 mg bid; may increase to 5 mg bid

Reduction in risk for MI, stroke, death

- **Adult: PO** 2.5 mg/day × 7 days, then 5 mg/day × 21 days, then may increase to 10 mg/day

Renal dose

- **Adult: PO** CCr <40 ml/min, reduce by 50%, titrate upward to max 5 mg/day

Proteinuria due to diabetic nephropathy (unlabeled)

- **Adult: PO** 2.5 mg/day up to 20 mg/day

Available forms: Caps 1.25, 2.5, 5, 10 mg; tabs 1.25, 2.5, 5, 10 mg

Administer:

- Without regard to meals
- Caps can be opened, added to food; mixture is stable for 24 hr at room temperature, 48 hr refrigerated
- Store in tight container at ≤86° F (30° C)

SIDE EFFECTS

CNS: *Headache, dizziness,* anxiety, insomnia, paresthesia, *fatigue,* depression, malaise, vertigo, syncope

CV: *Hypotension,* chest pain, palpitations, angina, syncope, dysrhythmia, **heart failure, MI**

EENT: Hearing loss

GI: *Nausea,* constipation, vomiting, dyspepsia, dysphagia, anorexia, diarrhea, abdominal pain, **hepatitis, hepatic failure, pancreatitis, hepatic necrosis**

GU: **Proteinuria,** increased BUN, creatinine, impotence

HEMA: Decreased Hct, Hgb, **eosinophilia, leukopenia, pancytopenia, thrombocytopenia, agranulocytosis (rare)**

INTEG: Rash, sweating, photosensitivity, pruritus

META: *Hyperkalemia*, hyperglycemia

MISC: **Angioedema, toxic epidermal necrolysis, anaphylaxis, Stevens-Johnson syndrome**

MS: Arthralgia, arthritis, myalgia

RESP: *Cough,* dyspnea

PHARMACOKINETICS

Bioavailability >50%-60%, onset 1-2 hr, peak 1-3 hr, duration 24 hr, protein binding 73%, half-life 13-17 hr, metabolized by liver (metabolites excreted in urine, feces)

INTERACTIONS

Do not use with AlisKiren in moderate-severe renal disease

R

Increase: hyperkalemia—potassium-sparing diuretics, potassium supplement, angiotensin II receptor agonists
Increase: hypotension—diuretics, other antihypertensives, ganglionic blockers, adrenergic blockers, nitrates, acute alcohol ingestion
⚠ **Increase:** toxicity—vasodilators, hydrALAZINE, prazosin, potassium-sparing diuretics, sympathomimetics, potassium supplements
Increase: serum levels of lithium
Decrease: absorption—antacids
Decrease: antihypertensive effect—indomethacin, NSAIDs, salicylates

Drug/Herb
Increase: antihypertensive effect—hawthorn
Decrease: antihypertensive effect—ephedra

Drug/Food
Increase: hyperkalemia—potassium salt substitutes, avoid use

Drug/Lab Test
Increase: LFTs, BUN, creatinine, glucose, potassium
Decrease: RBC, Hgb, platelets

NURSING CONSIDERATIONS

Assess:

⚠ **Collagen-vascular disease (SLE, scleroderma):** neutrophils, decreased platelets; WBC with differential at baseline, periodically; if neutrophils <1000/mm^3, discontinue treatment
- **Hypertension:** monitor B/P baseline and regularly, orthostatic hypotension, syncope
- **Renal disease:** protein, BUN, creatinine, potassium, sodium at baseline, periodically; increased levels may indicate nephrotic syndrome; renal symptoms: polyuria, oliguria, urinary frequency, dysuria
- **CHF:** edema in feet, legs daily; weight daily

⚠ **Serious allergic reactions:** angioedema, Stevens-Johnson syndrome, rash, fever, pruritus, urticaria; product should be discontinued if antihistamines fail to help
- Monitor electrolytes baseline and periodically; potassium may be increased

Evaluate:
- Therapeutic response: decrease in B/P; CHF

Teach patient/family:
- Not to discontinue product abruptly; to comply with dosage schedule, even if feeling better
- Not to use OTC products (cough, cold, allergy) unless directed by prescriber; not to use salt substitutes containing potassium without consulting prescriber
- To rise slowly to sitting or standing position to minimize orthostatic hypotension

⚠ To notify prescriber of mouth sores, sore throat, fever, swelling of hands or feet, irregular heartbeat, chest pain
- To report excessive perspiration, dehydration, vomiting, diarrhea; may lead to fall in B/P; to maintain hydration
- That product may cause dizziness, fainting, lightheadedness; that these may occur during first few days of therapy; to avoid hazardous activities until response is known
- That product may cause skin rash, impaired perspiration
- How to take B/P, normal readings for age group

Black Box Warning: To inform prescriber if pregnancy planned, suspected, pregnancy (D); not to breastfeed

TREATMENT OF OVERDOSE:
0.9% NaCl IV infusion, hemodialysis

ranibizumab (Rx)
(ran-ih-biz′oo-mab)
Lucentis
Func. class.: Ophthalmic
Chem. class.: Selective vascular endothelial growth factor antagonist

ACTION: Binds to receptor-binding site of active forms of vascular endothelial growth factor A (VEGF-A) that causes angiogenesis and cell proliferation

USES:
Macular degeneration (neovascular) (wet), macular edema after retinal vein occlusion (RVO), diabetic macular edema

CONTRAINDICATIONS:
Hypersensitivity, ocular infections

Precautions: Pregnancy (C), breastfeeding, children, retinal detachment, increased intraocular pressure

DOSAGE AND ROUTES

Macular degeneration/macular edema after retinal vein occlusion (RVO)

- **Adult: INTRAVITREAL** 0.5 mg (0.05 ml) of 10 mg/ml product monthly or 0.5 mg monthly ×4 mo, then 0.5 mg q3mo

Diabetic macular edema

- **Adults: INTRAVITREAL** 0.3 mg of 6 mg/ml product q28day

Available forms: Sol for inj 6 mg/ml, 10 mg/ml

Administer:

- By ophthalmologist via intravitreal injection using adequate anesthesia; use 19-gauge filter
- Store in refrigerator; do not freeze
- Protect from light

SIDE EFFECTS

CNS: Dizziness, headache, peripheral neuropathy

EENT: Blepharitis, cataract, conjunctival hemorrhage/hyperemia, detachment of retinal pigment epithelium, dry/irritation/pain in eye, visual impairment, vitreous floaters, ocular infection

GI: Constipation, nausea

MISC: Hypertension, UTI, **thromboembolism, nonocular bleeding**, anemia, arthralgia

RESP: Bronchitis, cough, sinusitis, URI

INTEG: Impaired wound healing

PHARMACOKINETICS

Elimination half-life 9 days, peak 1 day

INTERACTIONS

Increase: severe inflammation—verteporfin photodynamic therapy (PDT)

NURSING CONSIDERATIONS

Assess:

- **Eye changes:** redness; sensitivity to light, vision change; increased intraocular pressure change; report infection to ophthalmologist immediately, complete procedure with anesthesia and antibiotic before use, check perfusion of optic nerve after use
- **Hypersensitivity:** monitor for inflammation

Evaluate:

- Therapeutic response: prevention of increasing macular degeneration

Teach patient/family:

- That, if eye becomes red, sensitive to light, painful, or if there is a change in vision, to seek immediate care from ophthalmologist
- About reason for treatment, expected results

ranitidine (Rx, OTC)

(ra-nit′i-deen)

Acid Reducer ✦, Nu-Ranit ✦, Zantac, Zantac C ✦

Func. class.: H_2-Histamine receptor antagonist

Do not confuse:
ranitidine/amantadine/rimantadine
Zantac/Xanax/Zofran/ZyrTEC

ACTION:
Inhibits histamine at H_2-receptor site in parietal cells, which inhibits gastric acid secretion

USES:
Duodenal ulcer, Zollinger-Ellison syndrome, gastric ulcers, hypersecretory conditions, gastroesophageal reflux disease, stress ulcers, erosive esophagitis (maintenance), active duodenal ulcers with *Helicobacter pylori* in combination with clarithromycin,

systemic mastocytosis, multiple endocrine adenoma syndrome, heartburn

Unlabeled uses: Prevention of aspiration pneumonitis, upper GI bleeding, angioedema, gastritis, urticaria, NSAID-induced ulcer prophylaxis

CONTRAINDICATIONS: Hypersensitivity

Precautions: Pregnancy (B), breastfeeding, child <12 yr, renal/hepatic disease

DOSAGE AND ROUTES

Duodenal ulcer

- **Adult: PO** 150 mg bid or 300 mg/day after PM meal or at bedtime; maintenance 150 mg at bedtime
- **Infant and child: PO** 2-4 mg/kg bid, max 300 mg/day

Zollinger-Ellison syndrome

- **Adult: PO** 150 mg bid, may increase if needed

Gastric ulcer

- **Adult: PO** 150 mg bid × 6 wk, then 150 mg at bedtime
- **Infant and child: PO** 2-4 mg/kg bid, max 300 mg/day

GERD

- **Adult: PO** 150 mg bid

Erosive esophagitis

- **Adult: PO** 150 mg qid for up to 12 wk
- **Child ≥1 mo: PO** 5-10 mg/kg/day in 2-3 divided doses

Renal dose

- **Adult:** CCr <50 ml/min, give 50% of dose or extend dosing interval

NSAID-induced ulcer prophylaxis (unlabeled)

- **Adult: PO** 150 mg bid

Stress gastritis prophylaxis (unlabeled)

- **Adult: IM/INT IV INFUSION** 50 mg q6-8hr

Severe, acute urticaria/angioedema (unlabeled)

- **Adult: INT IV INFUSION** 50 mg with H_1-blocker

Available forms: Tabs 75, 150, 300 mg; sol for inj 25 mg/ml; caps 150, 300 mg; syr 15 mg/ml

Administer:

PO route

- Antacids 1 hr before or 1 hr after ranitidine
- Without regard to meals
- Store at room temperature

IM route

- No dilution needed; inject in large muscle mass, aspirate

Direct IV route

- Dilute to max 2.5 mg/ml (50 mg/20 ml) using 0.9% NaCl (nonpreserved) or D_5W, give dose over ≥5 min (max 4 mg/ml)

Intermittent IV INFUSION route

- Dilute to max 0.5 mg/ml with D_5W, NS, give over 15-20 min (5-7 ml/min); premixed ready-to-use bags as 1 mg/ml (50 mg/50 ml), infusion over 15-20 min

Continuous 24 hr IV INFUSION route

- **Adult:** dilute 150 mg/250 ml of D_5W or NS; run over 24 hr (6.25 mg/hr or as directed); use infusion device; use within 48 hr; *Zollinger-Ellison syndrome:* dilute in D_5W, NS; max concentration 2.5 mg/ml, use infusion device

Y-site compatibilities: Acyclovir, aldesleukin, alemtuzumab, alfentanil, allopurinol, amifostine, amikacin, aminophylline, amphotericin B liposome, amsacrine, anikinra, anidulafungin, ascorbic acid, atracurium, atropine, aztreonam, bivalirudin, bumetanide, buprenorphine, butorphanol, calcium chloride/gluconate, CARBOplatin, ceFAZolin, cefepime, cefonicid, cefoperazone, cefotaxime, cefoTEtan, cefOXitin, cefTAZidime, ceftizoxime, cefTRIAXone, cefuroxime, chloramphenicol, chlorproMAZINE, cimetidine, ciprofloxacin, cisatracurium, CISplatin, clindamycin, cyanocobalamin, cyclophosphamide, cycloSPORINE, cytarabine, DACTINomycin, DAPTOmycin, dexamethasone, dexmedetomidine, digoxin, diltiazem, DOBUTamine, DOCEtaxel, DOPamine, doripenem, doxacurium, doxapram, DOXOrubicin, DOXOrubicin liposome, doxycycline, enalaprilat, ePHEDrine, EPINEPHrine, epirubicin, epoetin alfa, ertapenem, erythromycin, esmolol, etoposide, etoposide phosphate, famotidine, fenoldopam, fentaNYL, filgrastim, fluconazole, fludarabine, fluorouracil, folic acid, foscarnet, furosemide, ganciclovir, gemcitabine, gentamicin, glycopyrrolate, granisetron, heparin, hydrocortisone, HYDROmorphone, IDArubicin, ifosfamide, imipenem/cilastatin, inamrinone, indomethacin, isoproterenol, ketorolac, labetalol, levofloxacin, lidocaine, linezolid, LORazepam, magnesium sulfate, mannitol, mechlorethamine, melphalan, meperidine, metaraminol, methotrexate, methoxamine, methyldopate, methylPREDNISolone, metoclopramide, metoprolol, metroNIDAZOLE, midazolam, milrinone, mitoXANtrone, morphine, multivitamin, nalbuphine, naloxone, nesiritide, niCARdipine, nitroglycerin, nitroprusside, norepinephrine, octreotide, ondansetron, oxacillin, oxaliplatin, oxytocin, PACLitaxel, palonosetron, pancuronium, papaverine, PEMEtrexed, penicillin G, pentamidine, pentazocine, PENTobarbital, PHENobarbital, phentolamine, phenylephrine, phytonadione, piperacillin/tazobactam, potassium chloride, procainamide, prochlorperazine, promethazine, propofol, propranolol, protamine, pyrdoxime, remifentanil, riTUXimab, rocuronium, sargramostim, sodium acetate/bicarbonate, succinylcholine, SUFentanil, tacrolimus, teniposide, theophylline, thiamine, thiopental, thiotepa, ticarcillin/clavulanate, tigecycline, tirofiban, tobramycin, tolazoline, trastuzumab, trimethaphan, urokinase, vancomycin, vecuronium, vinCRIStine, vinorelbine, warfarin, zidovudine, zoledronic acid

SIDE EFFECTS

CNS: Headache, sleeplessness, dizziness, confusion, agitation, depression, hallucination (geriatric patients)

CV: Tachycardia, bradycardia, PVCs

EENT: Blurred vision, increased ocular pressure

GI: Constipation, abdominal pain, diarrhea, nausea, vomiting, **hepatotoxicity**

GU: Impotence, **acute interstitial nephritis (rare)**

INTEG: Urticaria, rash, fever

RESP: **Pneumonia**

SYST: **Anaphylaxis (rare)**

PHARMACOKINETICS

PO: Peak 2-3 hr; duration 8-12 hr; metabolized by liver; excreted in urine (30% unchanged, PO), breast milk; half-life 2-3 hr; protein binding 15%

INTERACTIONS

Increase: effect of pramipexole, procainamide, trospium, triazolam, calcium channel blockers, memantine, saquinavir, adefovir

⚠ **Increase: GI obstruction risk—NIFEdipine ext rel products**

Increase: toxicity—sulfonylureas, procainamide, benzodiazepines, calcium channel blockers

Decrease: absorption of ranitidine—antacids, anticholinergics

Decrease: effects of cephalosporins, iron salts, ketoconazole, itraconazole

Increase: GI obstruction risk—NIFEdipine ext rel products

Drug/Lab Test

Increase: AST, ALT, creatinine

False positive: urine protein (Multistix)

NURSING CONSIDERATIONS

Assess:

- **GI complaints:** nausea, vomiting, diarrhea, cramps, abdominal discomfort, jaundice; report immediately
- I&O ratio, BUN, creatinine, LFTs, serum, stool guaiac before, periodically during therapy

Evaluate:

- Therapeutic response: decreased abdominal pain, heartburn

Teach patient/family:

- To avoid driving, other hazardous activities until stabilized on product
- That product must be continued for prescribed time to be effective
- To notify prescriber if pregnancy planned, suspected; to avoid breastfeeding
- Not to take maximum OTC daily dose for >2 wk
- To take once-daily dose before bedtime

R

ranolazine (Rx)

(ruh-no′luh-zeen)

Ranexa

Func. class: Antianginal

ACTION: Antianginal, antiischemic; unknown, may work by inhibiting portal fatty-acid oxidation

USES: Chronic stable angina pectoris; use in patients who have not responded to other treatment options; should be used in combination with other antianginals such as amlodipine, β-blockers, nitrates

Unlabeled uses: Unstable angina

CONTRAINDICATIONS: Preexisting QT prolongation, hepatic disease (Child-Pugh class A, B, C), hypersensitivity, hypokalemia, renal failure, torsades de pointes, ventricular dysrhythmia, ventricular tachycardia, hepatic cirrhosis

Precautions: Pregnancy (C), breastfeeding, children, geriatric patients, hypotension, renal disease, females at risk for torsades de pointes

DOSAGE AND ROUTES

- **Adult: PO** 500 mg bid, increased to 1000 mg bid based on response; max 1000 mg bid

Available forms: Ext rel tabs 500, 1000 mg

Administer:

- **Ext rel tabs:** do not break, crush, chew tabs; take product as prescribed; do not double or skip dose
- Without regard to meals, bid; do not use with grapefruit juice

SIDE EFFECTS

CNS: *Headache, dizziness,* hallucinations

CV: Palpitations, QT prolongation, orthostatic hypotension

EENT: Tinnitus

GI: Nausea, vomiting, constipation, dry mouth

MISC: Peripheral edema

RESP: Dyspnea

PHARMACOKINETICS

Absorption varied; peak 2-5 hr; half-life 7 hr; extensively metabolized by the liver (CYP3A and less by CYP2D6); excreted in urine (75%), feces (25%); protein binding 62%

INTERACTIONS

Increase: ranolazine action—diltiazem, ketoconazole, macrolide antibiotics, dofetilide, PARoxetine, protease inhibitors, quiNIDine, sotalol, thioridazine, verapamil, ziprasidone

Increase: action of digoxin, simvastatin

Increase: ranolazine absorption, toxicity—antiretroviral protease inhibitors

⚠ **Increase:** QT prolongation and torsades de pointes—class IA/III antidysrythmics, arsenic trioxide, chloroquine, droperidol, haloperidol, levomethadyl, methadone, pentamidine, chlorproMAZINE, mesoridazine, thioridazine, pimozide; CYP3A4 inhibitors (ketoconazole, fluconazole, itraconazole, IV miconazole, voriconazole, diltiazem, verapamil)

Drug/Food

- Do not use with grapefruit, grapefruit juice

NURSING CONSIDERATIONS

Assess:

- **Angina:** characteristics of pain (intensity, location, duration, alleviating/precipitating factors)

⚠ **QT prolongation:** ECG for QT prolongation, ejection fraction; assess for chest pain, palpitations, dyspnea

- Cardiac status: B/P, pulse, respirations
- LFTs, serum creatinine/BUN, magnesium, potassium before treatment, periodically

Evaluate:

- Therapeutic response: decreased anginal pain

Teach patient/family:

- To avoid hazardous activities until stabilized on product, dizziness no longer a problem

⚠ To avoid OTC drugs, grapefruit juice, products prolonging QTc (quiNIDine, dofetilide, sotalol, erythromycin, thioridazine, ziprasidone or protease inhibitors, diltiazem, ketoconazole, macrolide antibiotics, verapamil) unless directed by prescriber; to notify prescriber of palpitations, fainting
• To comply with all areas of medical regimen
• To take as directed; not to skip dose, double doses
• Not to chew or crush; not to use with grapefruit juice
• To notify all health care providers of product use
• To notify prescriber of palpitations, dizziness, edema, dyspnea
• For acute angina, take other products prescribed; this product does not decrease acute attack

rasagiline (Rx)

(ra-sa′ji-leen)

Azilect

Func. class.: Antiparkinson agent
Chem. class.: MAOI, type B

ACTION: Inhibits MAOI type B at recommended doses; may increase DOPamine levels

USES: Idiopathic Parkinson's disease monotherapy or with levodopa

CONTRAINDICATIONS: Breastfeeding; hypersensitivity to this product, MAOIs; pheochromocytoma
Precautions: Pregnancy (C), children, psychiatric disorders, moderate to severe hepatic disorders

DOSAGE AND ROUTES

Monotherapy
• **Adult: PO** 1 mg/day
Adjunctive therapy
• **Adult: PO** 0.5 mg/day, may increase 1 mg/day; change of levodopa dose for adjunct therapy; reduced levodopa dose may be needed
Hepatic dose
• **Adult: PO** 0.5 mg for mild hepatic disease
Concomitant ciprofloxacin, other CYP1A2 inhibitors
• **Adult: PO** 0.5 mg; plasma concentrations of rasagiline may double
Available forms: Tabs 0.5, 1 mg
Administer:
⚠ With meals to prevent nausea; continuing therapy usually reduces or eliminates nausea; do not give with foods/liquids containing large amounts of tyramine
• Reduce dose of carbidopa/levodopa cautiously
• Renal failure: in dialysis, increase dose slowly

SIDE EFFECTS

CNS: Drowsiness, hallucinations, depression, headache, malaise, paresthesia, vertigo, syncope
CV: Angina, **hypertensive crisis** (ingestion of tyramine products), orthostatic hypotension
GI: *Nausea*, diarrhea, dry mouth, dyspepsia
GU: Impotence, decreased libido
HEMA: Leukopenia
INTEG: Alopecia, skin cancers
MISC: Conjunctivitis, fever, flu syndrome, neck pain, allergic reaction, alopecia
MS: Arthralgia, arthritis, dyskinesia
RESP: Rhinitis

R

PHARMACOKINETICS

Onset, peak, duration unknown; well absorbed; protein binding >88%-94%; metabolized by CYP1A2 in liver; excreted by kidneys, half-life 3 hr

INTERACTIONS

⚠ Do not give with meperidine, other analgesics because serious reactions (including coma and death) may occur; do not give with sympathomimetics
Increase: levels of rasagiline up to 2-fold—ciprofloxacin, CYP1A2 inhibitors (atazanavir, mexiletine, taurine)

Increase: severe CNS toxicity with antidepressants (tricyclics, SSRIs, SNRIs, mirtazapine, cyclobenzaprine)

⚠ **Increase:** hypertensive crisis—MAOIs

Drug/Herb

- Do not give with St. John's wort, yohimbe

Drug/Food

- Do not give with foods/liquids that have large amounts of tyramine

Drug/Lab Test

Increase: LFTs

Decrease: WBCs

NURSING CONSIDERATIONS

Assess:

- **Parkinson's symptoms:** tremors, ataxia, muscle weakness and rigidity at baseline, periodically; increased dyskinesia, postural hypotension if used in combination with levodopa
- Mental status: hallucinations, confusion, notify prescriber

⚠ **Hypertensive crisis:** severe headache, blurred vision, seizures, chest pain, difficulty thinking, nausea, vomiting, signs of stroke; any unexplained severe headache should be considered to be hypertensive crisis

⚠ **Melanoma:** periodic skin exams by a dermatologist

- Cardiac status: B/P, ECG periodically, orthostatic hypotension during 2 months of treatment during beginning treatment

⚠ **Tyramine products:** foods, other medications may lead to hypertensive crisis (tachycardia, bradycardia, chest pain, nausea, vomiting, sweating, dilated pupils)

- Drowsiness, daytime sleepiness or falling asleep, may need to be discontinued
- Skin should be checked periodically for possible skin cancer

Evaluate:

- Therapeutic response: improved symptoms in patients with Parkinson's disease

Teach patient/family:

- To change positions slowly to prevent orthostatic hypotension
- To avoid hazardous activities until stabilized on product; that dizziness can occur
- To rinse mouth frequently; to use sugarless gum to alleviate dry mouth
- To take as prescribed; not to miss dose or double doses; to take missed dose as soon as remembered if several hours before next dose

⚠ To prevent hypertensive crisis by avoiding high-tyramine foods (>150 mg)

- To report signs of hypertensive crisis
- To avoid CNS depressants, alcohol
- To notify all providers of product use; to avoid elective surgery, other procedures involving CNS depressants

rasburicase (Rx)

(rass-burr′i-case)

Elitek, Fasturtec ✦

Func. class.: Enzyme

Chem. class.: Recombinant urate-oxidase enzyme

ACTION: Catalyzes enzymatic oxidation of uric acid into an inactive and soluble metabolite (allantoin)

USES: To reduce uric acid levels in children with leukemia, lymphoma, solid tumor malignancies who are receiving chemotherapy

CONTRAINDICATIONS: Hypersensitivity

Black Box Warning: G6PD deficiency (Mediterranean, African descent), hemolytic reactions, methemoglobinemia reactions to product

Precautions: Pregnancy (C), breastfeeding, children <2 yr, anemia

Black Box Warning: Acute bronchospasm, angina, angioedema, atony, African American and Mediterranean patients, hypotension, urticaria

DOSAGE AND ROUTES

• **Adult/adolescent/infant: IV INFUSION** 0.2 mg/kg as single daily dose × 5 days

Available forms: Powder for inj 1.5, 7.5 mg/vial

Administer:

Intermittent IV INFUSION route

• Reconstitute with diluent provided, add 1 ml of diluent/each vial, swirl, withdraw amount needed, mix with NS to final volume of 50 ml, use within 24 hr, give over 30 min, do not use filter, use different line; if not possible, flush with ≥15 ml of saline before, after use

• Chemotherapy started 4-24 hr after 1st dose

SIDE EFFECTS

CNS: *Headache,* fever

CV: Chest pain, hypotension

GI: *Nausea, vomiting, anorexia, diarrhea, abdominal pain, constipation, dyspepsia, mucositis*

HEMA: **Neutropenia with fever, hemolysis, methemoglobinemia**

INTEG: *Rash*

MISC: Edema

RESP: **Bronchospasm,** wheezing, dyspnea

SYST: **Anaphylaxis, hemolysis, methemoglobinemia, sepsis**

PHARMACOKINETICS

Elimination half-life 16-21 hr

INTERACTIONS

⚠ **Increase:** toxicity—allopurinol

NURSING CONSIDERATIONS

Assess:

• Blood studies: BUN, serum uric acid, urine creatinine clearance, electrolytes, CBC with differential before, during therapy

• Monitor temperature; fever may indicate beginning infection; no rectal temperatures

⚠ **Anaphylaxis:** dyspnea, urticaria, flushing, wheezing, swelling of lips, tongue, throat; have emergency equipment nearby

⚠ **G6PD deficiency, hemolytic reactions, methemoglobinemia;** these patients should not be given this product; screen patients who are at higher risk for these disorders

• GI symptoms: frequency of stools, cramping; if severe diarrhea occurs, fluid, electrolytes may need to be given

Evaluate:

• Therapeutic response: decreased uric acid levels in children when antineoplastics causing high uric acid levels used

Teach patient/family:

• About the reason for therapy, expected results

⚠ To report trouble breathing, jaundice, chest pain

⚠ HIGH ALERT

regorafenib

(re′goe-raf′e-nib)

Stivarga

Func. class.: Antineoplastic biologic-response modifier; multikinase inhibitor

Chem. class.: Signal transduction inhibitor (STI)

ACTION:
Inhibits tyrosine kinase in patients with colorectal cancer

USES:
Metastatic colorectal cancer in those who have received fluoropyrimidine, oxaliplatin, irinotecan-based chemotherapy, an anti-VEGF therapy; and an anti-EGFR therapy if *KRAS* wild type

CONTRAINDICATIONS:
Pregnancy (D)

Precautions: Breastfeeding, children, geriatric patients, cardiac/renal/hepatic/dental disease, fistula, GI bleeding or perforation, bone marrow suppression, infection, wound dehiscence, thrombocytopenia, neutropenia, immunosuppression

Black Box Warning: Hepatic disease

DOSAGE AND ROUTES

• **Adult: PO** 160 mg/day with a low-fat breakfast × 21 days of a 28-day cycle, cycles may be repeated

Available forms: Tabs 40 mg

Administer:

• Store at 77°F (25°C)

• Give at the same time each day with a low-fat breakfast that contains less than 30% fat such as 2 slices of white toast with 1 tbsp of low-fat margarine and 1 tbsp of jelly, and 8 oz of skim milk; or 1 cup of cereal, 8 oz of skim milk, 1 slice of toast with jam, apple juice, and 1 cup of coffee or tea

• Swallow tablets whole

• If a dose is missed, take as soon as possible that day; do not take 2 doses on the same day

⚠ **Hand–foot skin reaction:** Reduce to 120 mg (grade 2 palmar–plantar erythrodysesthesia); hold if grade 2 toxicity does not improve in ≤7 days or recurs; hold for ≥7 days in grade 3 toxicity; reduce to 80 mg for recurrent grade 2 toxicity; discontinue if 80 mg is not tolerated

⚠ **Hypertension:** Hold in grade 2 hypertension

Other severe toxicity (except hepatotoxicity)

⚠ Hold until toxicity resolves in grade 3 or 4 toxicity; consider the risk/benefits of continuing therapy in grade 4 toxicity, reduce dosage to 120 mg; if grade 3 or 4 toxicity recurs, hold until toxicity resolves, then reduce to 80 mg; discontinue in those who do not tolerate 80-mg dose

⚠ **Hepatic dose:** Baseline mild (Child-Pugh class A) or moderate (Child-Pugh class B): no change; baseline severe hepatic impairment (Child-Pugh class C): use not recommended; AST/ALT elevations during therapy: For grade 3 AST/AST level elevations, hold dose; if therapy is continued, reduce to 120 mg after levels recover; discontinue in those with AST/ALT >203 ULN; AST/ ALT >33 ULN and bilirubin >23 ULN; recurrence of AST/ALT >53 ULN despite a reduction to 120 mg

SIDE EFFECTS

CNS: Headache, tremor

CV: Hypertensive crisis, MI

EENT: Blurred vision, conjunctivitis

GI: Hepatotoxicity, GI hemorrhage, diarrhea, GI perforation, xerostomia

HEMA: Neutropenia, thrombocytopenia, bleeding

INTEG: Rash, alopecia

META: Hypokalemia

MISC: Fatigue, decreased weight, hand–foot syndrome, hypothyroidism

PHARMACOKINETICS

Protein binding 99%, metabolized by CYP3A4, UGT1A0, half-life 14-58 hr

INTERACTIONS

Increase: regorafenib concentrations—CYP3A4 inhibitors (ketoconazole, itraconazole, erythromycin, clarithromycin)

Increase: plasma concentrations of simvastatin, calcium channel blockers, ergots

Increase: plasma concentration of warfarin; avoid use with warfarin; use low-molecular-weight anticoagulants instead

Decrease: regorafenib concentrations—CYP3A4 inducers (dexamethasone, phenytoin, carBAMazepine, rifampin, PHENobarbital)

Drug/Food

Increase: regorafenib effect—grapefruit juice; avoid use while taking product

Drug/Herb

Decrease: imatinib concentration—St. John's wort

NURSING CONSIDERATIONS

Assess:

Black Box Warning: Hepatic disease: fatal hepatotoxicity can occur; obtain LFTs baseline and at least every 2 wk × 2 mo, then monthly

⚠ **Fatal bleeding:** From GI, respiratory, GU tracts; permanently discontinue in those with severe bleeding

⚠ **Palmar–plantar erythrodysesthesia (hand–foot syndrome):** More common in those previously treated; reddening swelling, numbness, desquamation on palms, soles

⚠ **GI perforation/fistula:** Discontinue if this occurs; assess for pain in epigastric area, dyspepsia, flatulence, fever, chills

⚠ **Hypertension/hypertensive crisis:** Hypertension usually occurs in the first cycle in those with preexisting hypertension; do not start treatment until B/P is controlled; monitor B/P every wk × 6 wk, then at start of each cycle or more often if needed; temporarily or permanently discontinue for severe uncontrolled hypertension

Evaluate:

- Therapeutic response: decrease in spread or size of tumor

Teach patient/family:

- To report adverse reactions immediately: bleeding, rash
- About reason for treatment, expected results
- That effect on male fertility is unknown

⚠ ***HIGH ALERT***

remifentanil (Rx)

(rem-ih-fin′ta-nill)

Ultiva

Func. class.: Opiate agonist analgesic

Chem. class.: μ-Opioid agonist

Controlled Substance Schedule II

ACTION: Inhibits ascending pain pathways in limbic system, thalamus, midbrain, hypothalamus

USES: In combination with other products for general anesthesia to provide analgesia

CONTRAINDICATIONS: Hypersensitivity

Precautions: Pregnancy (C), breastfeeding, children <12 yr, geriatric patients, increased intracranial pressure, acute MI, severe heart disease, GI/renal/hepatic disease, asthma, respiratory conditions, seizure disorders, bradyarrhythmias

DOSAGE AND ROUTES

- **Adult:** induction **IV** 0.5-1 mcg/kg/min with hypnotic or volative agent; maintenance with isoflurane (0.4-1.5 MAC) or propofol (100-200 mcg/kg/min); **CONT INFUSION** 0.025-0.2 mcg/kg/min
- **Child 1-12 yr: CONT IV INFUSION** 0.25 mcg/kg/min with isoflurane
- **Full-term neonate and infant up to 2 mo: CONT IV INFUSION** 0.4 mcg/kg/min with nitrous oxide

Available forms: Powder for inj lyophilized 1, 2, 5 mg

Administer:

- Add 1 ml diluent per mg remifentanil
- Shake well; further dilute to a final concentration of 20, 25, 50, or 250 mcg/mg
- Store in light-resistant area at room temperature
- Interruption of infusion results in rapid reversal (no residual opioid effect within 5-10 min)

Direct IV route

- To be used only during maintenance of general anesthesia; inject into tubing close to venous cannula; give to nonintubated patients over 30-60 sec

Continuous IV INFUSION route

- Use infusion device, max 16 hr; do not use same tubing as blood, do not admix

Y-site compatibilities: Acyclovir, alfentanil, amikacin, aminophylline, ampicillin, ampicillin/sulbactam, aztreonam, bumetanide, buprenorphine, butorphanol, calcium gluconate, ceFAZolin, cefepine, cefotaxime, cefoTEtan, cefOXitin, cefTAZidime, ceftizoxime, cefTRIAXone, cefuroxime, cimetidine, ciprofloxacin, cisatracurium, clindamycin, dexamethasone, digoxin, diltiazem, diphenhydrAMINE, DOBUTamine, DOPamine, doxacurium, doxycycline, droperidol, enalaprilat, EPINEPHrine, esmolol, famotidine, fentaNYL, fluconazole, furosemide, ganciclovir, gatifloxacin, gentamicin,

R

haloperidol, heparin, hydrocortisone sodium succinate, HYDROmorphone, hydrOXYzine, imipenem-cilastatin, inamrinone, isoproterenol, ketorolac, lidocaine, LORazepam, magnesium sulfate, mannitol, meperidine, methylPREDNISolone sodium succinate, metoclopramide, metroNIDAZOLE, midazolam, morphine, nalbuphine, nitroglycerin, norepinephrine, ondansetron, phenylephrine, piperacillin, potassium chloride, procainamide, prochlorperazine, promethazine, ranitidine, SUFentanil, theophylline, thiopental, ticarcillin/clavulanale, tobramycin, vancomycin, zidovudine

Solution compatibilities: D_5, 0.45% NaCl, LR, D_5 LR, 0.9% NaCl

SIDE EFFECTS

CNS: Drowsiness, *dizziness,* confusion, *headache,* sedation, euphoria, delirium, agitation, anxiety

CV: Palpitations, *bradycardia,* change in B/P, facial flushing, syncope, asystole

EENT: Tinnitus, blurred vision, miosis, diplopia

GI: *Nausea, vomiting,* anorexia, constipation, cramps, dry mouth

GU: Urinary retention, dysuria

INTEG: Rash, urticaria, bruising, flushing, diaphoresis, pruritus

MS: Rigidity

RESP: Respiratory depression, apnea

PHARMACOKINETICS

70% protein binding, terminal half-life 3-10 min, excreted in urine; onset: 1-3 min

INTERACTIONS

Increase: respiratory depression, hypotension, profound sedation: alcohol, sedatives, hypnotics, other CNS depressants; antihistamines, phenothiazines, MAOIs

Drug/Herb

Increase: CNS depression—kava

NURSING CONSIDERATIONS

Assess:

- I&O ratio; check for decreasing output; may indicate urinary retention, especially in geriatric patients
- CNS changes; dizziness, drowsiness, hallucinations, euphoria, LOC, pupil reaction
- GI status: nausea, vomiting, anorexia, constipation
- Allergic reactions: rash, urticaria
- **Respiratory dysfunction:** respiratory depression, character, rate, rhythm; notify prescriber if respirations <12/min; CV status; bradycardia, syncope

Evaluate:

- Therapeutic response: maintenance of anesthesia

Teach patient/family:

- To call for assistance when ambulating or smoking; that drowsiness, dizziness may occur
- To make position changes slowly to prevent orthostatic hypotension

⚠ HIGH ALERT

repaglinide (Rx)

(re-pag′lih′nide)

Gluconorm ✱, Prandin

Func. class.: Antidiabetic

Chem. class.: Meglitinide

Do not confuse:
Prandin/Avandia

ACTION: Causes functioning β-cells in pancreas to release insulin, thereby leading to a drop in blood glucose levels; closes ATP-dependent potassium channels in the β-cell membrane; this leads to the opening of calcium channels; increased calcium influx induces insulin secretion

USES: Type 2 diabetes mellitus

CONTRAINDICATIONS: Hypersensitivity to meglitinides; diabetic ketoacidosis, type 1 diabetes

Precautions: Pregnancy (C), breastfeeding, children, geriatric patients, thyroid/cardiac disease, severe renal/hepatic disease, severe hypoglycemic reactions

DOSAGE AND ROUTES

• **Adult: PO** 0.5-4 mg with each meal, max 16 mg/day; adjust at weekly intervals; oral-hypoglycemic–naive patients or patients with A1c <8% should start with 0.5 mg with each meal

Renal/hepatic dose

• **Adult: PO** CCr 20-39 ml/min, 0.5 mg/day; titrate upward cautiously

Available forms: Tabs 0.5, 1, 2 mg

Administer:

• Up to 15-30 min before meals; 2, 3, or 4×/day preprandially
• Skip dose if meal skipped; add dose if meal added
• Store in tight container at room temperature

SIDE EFFECTS

CNS: *Headache, weakness,* paresthesia
CV: Angina
EENT: Tinnitus, sinusitis
ENDO: **Hypoglycemia**
GI: Nausea, vomiting, diarrhea, constipation, dyspepsia, **pancreatitis**
HEMA: **Hemolytic anemia, leukopenia**
INTEG: Rash, allergic reactions
MISC: Chest pain, UTI, allergy
MS: Back pains, arthralgia
RESP: URI, sinusitis, rhinitis, bronchitis

PHARMACOKINETICS

Completely absorbed by GI route; onset 30 min; peak 1 hr; duration <4 hr; half-life 1 hr; metabolized in liver by CYP3A4; excreted in urine, feces (metabolites); crosses placenta; 98% protein bound

INTERACTIONS

⚠ **Do not use with gemfibrozil, isophane insulin (NPH)**

Increase: repaglinide effect—CYP3A4, OATP101, CYP2C9 inhibitors

Increase: in both—levonorgestrel/ethinyl estradiol

Increase: repaglinide metabolism—CYP3A4 inducers: rifampin, barbiturates, carBAMazepine

Increase: repaglinide effect—NSAIDs, salicylates, sulfonamides, chloramphenicol, MAOIs, coumarins, β-blockers, probenecid, gemfibrozil, simvastatin, fenofibrate, deferasirox

Decrease: repaglinide metabolism—CYP3A4 inhibitors: antifungals (ketoconazole, miconazole), erythromycin, macrolides

Decrease: repaglinide action—calcium channel blockers, corticosteroids, oral contraceptives, thiazide diuretics, thyroid preparations, estrogens, phenothiazines, phenytoin, rifampin, isoniazid, PHENobarbital, sympathomimetics

Drug/Herb

Increase: antidiabetic effect—garlic, chromium, horse chestnut

Drug/Food

Decrease: repaglinide level; give before meals

Decrease: repaglinide metabolism—grapefruit juice

Drug/Lab Test

Increase/decrease: glucose

NURSING CONSIDERATIONS

Assess:

⚠ **Hypo/hyperglycemic reaction, which can occur soon after meals: dizziness, weakness, headache, tremors, anxiety, tachycardia, hunger, sweating, abdominal pain, A1c, fasting, postprandial glucose during treatment**

Evaluate:

• Therapeutic response: decrease in polyuria, polydipsia, polyphagia; clear sensorium; absence of dizziness; stable gait; blood glucose, A1c improvement

Teach family/patient:

• About technique for blood glucose monitoring; how to use blood glucose meter
• About the symptoms of hypo/hyperglycemia, what to do about each
• That product must be continued on daily basis; about the consequences of discontinuing product abruptly
• To avoid OTC medications unless ordered by prescriber
• That diabetes is a lifelong illness; that product will not cure disease
• That all food included in diet plan must be eaten to prevent hypoglycemia;

R

that if a meal is omitted, dose should be omitted; to have glucagon emergency kit available; to take repaglinide 15-30 min before meals 2, 3, or 4×/day; to carry emergency ID

TREATMENT OF OVERDOSE:
Glucose 25 g IV via dextrose 50% solution, 50 ml or 1 mg glucagon

retapamulin (topical)
(re-te-pam′you-lin)

Altabax

Func. class.: Topical antiinfective

Chem. class.: Pleuromutilin

ACTION: Antibacterial activity results from inhibition of protein synthesis

USES: For the treatment of impetigo

CONTRAINDICATIONS: Hypersensitivity to this product

Precautions: Children

DOSAGE AND ROUTES
- **Adult/child ≥9 mo: TOP** apply to affected area bid × 5 days

Available forms: Topical ointment 1%

Administer:

Topical route
- Do not use skin products near the eyes, nose, or mouth
- Wash hands before and after use
- **Ointment:** Apply a thin film to the cleansed, affected area and massage gently into affected areas

SIDE EFFECTS
INTEG: Pruritus, irritation, headache, diarrhea, nausea

NURSING CONSIDERATIONS
Assess:

Allergic reaction
- Hypersensitivity, product may need to be discontinued

Infection
- Number of lesions, severity of impetigo

Evaluate:
- Decreased lesions, infusion in impetigo

Teach patient/family:

Topical route
- Not to use skin products near the eyes, nose, or mouth
- To wash hands before and after use
- **Ointment:** to apply a thin film to the cleansed, affected area

Rh_o(D) immune globulin standard dose IM (Rx)
HyperRHO SD, RhoGAM Ultra-Filtered Plus

Rh_o(D) immune globulin microdose IM (Rx)
HyperRHO S/D mini-Dose, MICRhoGAM Ultra-Filtered Plus, mini-Gamulin R, Rho(D) immune globulin microdose (IM, IV) Rhophylac

Rh_o(D) immune globulin IV (Rx)
Rhophylac, WinRho SDF

Func. class.: Immune globulins

ACTION: Suppresses immune response of nonsensitized Rh_0(D or D^u)-negative patients who are exposed to Rh_0(D or D^u)-positive blood

USES: Prevention of isoimmunization in Rh-negative women given Rh-positive blood after abortions, miscarriages, amniocentesis; chronic idiopathic thrombocytopenia purpura (Rhophylac)

CONTRAINDICATIONS: Previous immunization with this product, Rh_0(O)-positive/D^u-positive patient

Black Box Warning: Hemolysis

Precautions: Pregnancy (C)

Black Box Warning: Requires a specialized setting

DOSAGE AND ROUTES

To reduce risk of Rh isoimmunization antepartum/ suppression of Rh isoimmunization postpartum following delivery of full-term infant

- **Adult and adolescent ≥16 yr: IM** ([HyperRHO S/D] full dose only) 300 mcg (1500 international units) at 28 wk gestation, repeat within 72 hr of delivery of confirmed Rho(D)-positive infant; dose not needed after delivery if delivery within 3 wk of last dose and no fetal maternal hemorrhage of >15 ml of RBC; **IM** (RhoGam only) 300 mcg (1500 international units) at 26-28 wk gestation, repeat within 72 hr even if status of Rho unknown or if 72 hr have passed; **IM/IV** (WinRho SDF only) 300 mcg (1500 international units) at 28 wk gestation; if given earlier during pregnancy, give at 12-wk intervals during pregnancy, 120-mcg (600 international units) dose; IM/IV should be given as soon as possible and preferably within 72 hr of delivery of confirmed Rho(D)-positive infant and even if status unknown; give ≤28 days after delivery

Known or suspected massive fetomaternal hemorrhage (>15 ml of fetal RBC or >30 ml of fetal whole blood)

- **Adult and adolescent ≥16 yr: IM** ([HyperRHO S/D] full dose only) 300 mcg (1500 international units) per every 15 ml of fetal blood cells or 30 ml of whole blood; multiple syringes may be injected IM at same time in different sites, give within 72 hr of exposure, repeat dose within 72 hr of delivery; **IM** (RhoGAM only) 300 mcg (1500 international units) for every 15 ml of fetal blood cells or 30 ml of whole blood, give total dose within 72 hr of exposure; **IM/IV** (WinRho SDF only) if large fetomaternal hemorrhage suspected, give **IV** 9 mcg (45 international units) or **IM** 12 mcg (60 international units) for every ml of fetal whole blood, give **IV** 600 mcg (3000 international units) q8hr or **IM** 1200 mcg (6000 international units) q12hr until total dose given, total dose should be given within 72 hr of exposure

Threatened abortion at any stage of pregnancy

- **Adult and adolescent ≥16 yr: IM** ([HyperRHO S/D] full dose only) 300 mcg (1500 international units) as soon as possible; if given at 13-18 wk gestation, give another 300 mcg (1500 international units) at 26-28 wk gestation; repeat dose within 72 hr of delivery; **IM** (RhoGam only) 300 mcg (1500 international units) as soon as possible and within 72 hr of exposure; **IM/IV** (Rhophylac only) 300 mcg (1500 international units) as soon as possible and within 72 hr; **IM/IV** (WinRho SDF only) 300 mcg (1500 international units) as soon as possible and within 72 hr, repeat dose at 12-wk intervals during pregnancy and give 120 mcg (600 international units) as soon as possible after delivery and within 72 hr

After spontaneous abortion, induced termination of pregnancy, or ectopic pregnancy that occurs at ≤12 wk gestation

- **Adult and adolescent ≥16 yr: IM** (HyperRHO Minidose, MICRhoGAM only) 50 mcg (250 international units) as soon as possible, give within 3 hr of spontaneous or surgical removal, if possible within 72 hr

After spontaneous abortion, induced termination of pregnancy, or ruptured tubal pregnancy that occurs at ≥13 wk

- **Adult and adolescent ≥16 yr: IM** ([HyperRHO SD] full dose, RhoGAM only) 300 mcg (1500 international units) as soon as possible and within 72 hr of event

R

After spontaneous abortion, induced termination of pregnancy, amniocentesis, chorionic villus sampling, abdominal trauma, ruptured tubal pregnancy, or percutaneous umbilical cord sampling at ≤34 wk gestation

• **Adult and adolescent ≥16 yr: IM/IV** (WinRho SDF only) 300 mcg (1500 international units) within 72 hr, repeat at 12-wk intervals during pregnancy, give 120 mcg (600 international units) as soon as possible and preferably within 72 hr of delivery

Available forms: BayRho-D sol for inj 300 mcg/ml (HyperRHO S/D sol for inj), MICRhoGAM Ultra Filtered Plus Solution for inj 50 mcg/ml; RhoGam Ultra Filtered Plus Solution for inj 50 mcg; Rhophylac Pre-Filled Syringes Solution for inj 300 mcg/2 ml; WinRho SDF liquid for inj

Administer:

• Store in refrigerator

• HyperRHO SD, MICRhoGAM, RhoGAM given by IM only; do not give IV

• Rhophylac can be given IM or IV

• Inspect for particulate matter; do not use if particulate matter present

• Reconstitute/dilution: no reconstitution or dilution needed for HyperRHO SD; Rhophylac, MICRhoGAM, RhoGAM, or liquid formulation of WinRho SDF

IM route

• Use aseptic technique, observe for 20 min after administration

• Bring Rhophylac to room temperature before use

• Inject into deltoid muscle of upper arm or anterolateral portion of upper thigh; do not inject into gluteal muscle

• If dose calculated requires multiple vials or syringes, use different sites at same time

IV route

• Use aseptic technique

• WinRho SDF: remove entire contents of vial to obtain calculated dose; if partial vial required for dosage calculation, withdraw entire vial contents to ensure correct calculation; infuse correct calculated dose over 3-5 min; do not infuse with other fluids, products

• Rhophylac: bring to room temperature; infuse by slow IV; observe for 20 min

SIDE EFFECTS

CNS: Lethargy

CV: Hypo/hypertension

INTEG: Irritation at inj site, fever

MISC: Infection, ARDs, anaphylaxis, pulmonary edema, DIC

MS: Myalgia, arthralgia

INTERACTIONS

Decrease: antibody response—live virus vaccines (measles, mumps, rubella)

NURSING CONSIDERATIONS

Assess:

⚠ Allergies, reactions to immunizations; previous immunization with product

⚠ **Intravascular hemolysis:** back pain, chills, hemoglobinuria, renal insufficiency; usually when WinRho SDF is given in those with immune thrombocytopenia purpura

• Type, crossmatch mother and newborn's cord blood; if mother Rh_0(D)-negative, D^u-negative and newborn Rh_0(D)-positive, product should be given

Evaluate:

• Rh_0(D) sensitivity in transfusion error, prevention of erythroblastosis fetalis for normal vision

Teach patient/family:

• How product works; that product must be given after subsequent deliveries if subsequent babies are Rh-positive

⚠ To report immediately: shaking, fever, chills, dark urine, swelling of hands or feet, back pain, SOB (intravascular hemolysis)

riboflavin (vit B_2) (OTC)

(rye′boh-flay-vin)

Func. class.: Vit B_2, water soluble

ACTION: Needed for respiratory reactions by catalyzing proteins

USES: Vit B_2 deficiency or polyneuritis; cheilosis adjunct with thiamine

Unlabeled uses: Migraine prophylaxis

DOSAGE AND ROUTES

Deficiency

- **Adult: PO** 5-30 mg/day
- **Child ≥12 yr: PO** 3-10 mg/day, then 0.6 mg/1000 calories ingested

RDA

- **Adult: PO** (males) 1.3 mg, (females) 1.1 mg

Migraine prophylaxis (unlabeled)

- **Adult: PO** 400 mg/day × 3 mo

Available forms: Tabs 5, 10, 25, 50, 100, 250 mg

Administer:

- With food for better absorption
- Store in airtight, light-resistant container

SIDE EFFECTS

GU: Yellow discoloration of urine

Precautions: Pregnancy (A)

PHARMACOKINETICS

Half-life 65-85 min, 60% protein bound, unused amounts excreted in urine (unchanged)

INTERACTIONS

Increase: riboflavin need—alcohol, probenecid, tricyclics, phenothiazines

Decrease: action of tetracyclines

Drug/Lab Test

- May cause false elevations of urinary catecholamines

NURSING CONSIDERATIONS

Assess:

- Nutritional status: liver, eggs, dairy products, yeast, whole grains, green vegetables

Evaluate:

- Therapeutic response: absence of headache, GI problems, cheilosis, skin lesions, depression; burning, itchy eyes; anemia

Teach patient/family:

- That urine may turn bright yellow
- About the addition of needed foods rich in riboflavin
- To avoid alcohol

rifabutin (Rx)

(riff′a-byoo-ten)

Mycobutin

Func. class.: Antimycobacterial agent

Chem. class.: Rifamycin S derivative

Do not confuse:
rifabutin/rifampin/rifapentine

ACTION: Inhibits DNA-dependent RNA polymerase in susceptible strains of *Escherichia coli* and *Bacillus subtilis;* mechanism of action against *Mycobacterium avium* unknown

USES: Prevention of *M. avium* complex (MAC) in patients with advanced HIV infection

Unlabeled uses: *Helicobacter pylori* that has not responded to other treatment

CONTRAINDICATIONS: Hypersensitivity, active TB, WBC $<1000/mm^3$ or platelet count $<50,000/mm^3$

Precautions: Pregnancy (B), breastfeeding, children, hepatic disease, blood dyscrasias

DOSAGE AND ROUTES

- **Adult: PO** 300 mg/day (may take as 150 mg bid); max 600 mg/day

R

Renal dose

• **Adult: PO** CCr <30 ml/min, reduce by 50%

Available forms: Caps 150 mg

Administer:

• With food if GI upset occurs; better to take on empty stomach 1 hr before or 2 hr after meals; high-fat foods slow absorption; may take in 2 divided doses, may open capsule, mix with applesauce if unable to swallow whole cap

• Antiemetic if vomiting occurs

• After C&S completed; monthly to detect resistance

SIDE EFFECTS

CNS: *Headache,* fatigue, anxiety, confusion, insomnia

GI: *Nausea, vomiting, anorexia, diarrhea,* heartburn, hepatitis, discolored saliva, pseudomembranous colitis

GU: *Discolored urine*

HEMA: Hemolytic anemia, eosinophilia, thrombocytopenia, leukopenia

INTEG: *Rash*

MISC: Flulike symptoms, shortness of breath, chest pressure

MS: Asthenia, arthralgia, myalgia

PHARMACOKINETICS

53% absorbed, peak 2-3 hr, duration >24 hr, half-life 45 hr, metabolized in liver (active/inactive metabolites), excreted in urine primarily as metabolites

INTERACTIONS

Increase: levels of rifabutin: ritonavir

Decrease: action of amprenavir, anticoagulants, β-blockers, barbiturates, busPIRone, clofibrate, corticosteroids, cycloSPORINE, dapsone, delavirdine, disopyramide, doxycycline, efavirenz, estrogens, fluconazole, indinavir, ketoconazole, losartan, nelfinavir, nevirapine, oral contraceptives, phenytoin, quiNIDine, saquinavir, sulfonylureas, theophylline, tricyclic antidepressants, zidovudine, zolpidem

Drug/Food

• High-fat diet decreases absorption

Drug/Lab Test

Interference: folate level, vit B_{12}, BSP, gallbladder studies

NURSING CONSIDERATIONS

Assess:

⚠ **Acute TB:** chest x-ray, sputum culture, blood culture, biopsy of lymph nodes, PPD; product should not be given for active TB

• CBC for neutropenia, thrombocytopenia, eosinophilia

⚠ **Pseudomembranous colitis:** diarrhea, abdominal pain/cramping, fever, bloody stools

• Signs of anemia: Hct, Hgb, fatigue

• Hepatic studies weekly: ALT, AST, bilirubin

• Renal status before, each mo: BUN, creatinine, output, specific gravity, urinalysis

• Hepatic status: decreased appetite, jaundice, dark urine, fatigue

Evaluate:

• Therapeutic response: not used for active TB because of risk for development of resistance to rifampin; culture negative

Teach patient/family:

⚠ That patients using oral contraceptives should consider using nonhormonal methods of birth control, may decrease effect; to notify prescriber if pregnancy planned, suspected

• That compliance with dosage schedule, duration necessary

• That scheduled appointments must be kept because relapse may occur

• That urine, feces, saliva, sputum, sweat, tears may be colored red-orange; that soft contact lenses may be permanently stained

⚠ To report flulike symptoms: excessive fatigue, anorexia, vomiting, sore throat; unusual bleeding, yellowish discoloration of skin, eyes; myositis: muscle or bone pain; diarrhea, fever, abdominal cramping, bloody stools

rifampin (Rx)

(rif′am-pin)

Rifadin, Rofact ✦

Func. class.: Antitubercular

Chem. class.: Rifamycin B derivative

Do not confuse:
rifampin/rifabutin/rifaximin

ACTION: Inhibits DNA-dependent polymerase, decreases tubercle bacilli replication

USES: Pulmonary TB, meningococcal carriers (prevention)

Unlabeled uses: Endocarditis, *Haemophilus influenzae type B prophylaxis,* Hansen's disease, *Mycobacterium avium* complex (MAC), orthopedic-device–related infection, pruritus

CONTRAINDICATIONS: Hypersensitivity to this product, rifamycins; active *Neisseria meningitidis* infection

Precautions: Pregnancy (C), breastfeeding, children <5 yr, hepatic disease, blood dyscrasias

DOSAGE AND ROUTES

Tuberculosis

- **Adult: PO/IV** Max 600 mg/day as single dose 1 hr before meals or 2 hr after meals or 10 mg/kg/day 5 days/wk or 2-3×/wk
- **Child >5 yr: PO/IV** 10-20 mg/kg/day as single dose 1 hr before meals or 2 hr after meals, max 600 mg/day with other antituberculars
- **6-mo regimen:** 2 mo treatment of isoniazid, rifampin, pyrazinamide, and possibly streptomycin or ethambutol, then rifampin and isoniazid 3-4 mo
- **9-mo regimen:** rifampin and isoniazid supplemented with pyrazinamide, streptomycin, or ethambutol

Meningococcal carriers

- **Adult: PO/IV** 600 mg bid × 2 days, max 600 mg/dose
- **Child >5 yr: PO/IV** 10-20 mg/kg × 2 days, max 600 mg/dose
- **Infant 3 mo-1 yr:** 5 mg/kg **PO** bid × 2 days

Prevention of *H. influenzae* type B infection (unlabeled)

- **Adult: PO** 600 mg/day × 4 days
- **Child: PO** 20 mg/kg/day × 4 days

MAC (unlabeled)

- **Adult: PO/IV** 600 mg/day used with ≥3 other active microbials
- **Child: PO/IV** 10-20 mg/kg/day used with ≥3 other active microbials

Endocarditis with prosthetic valves (unlabeled)

- **Adult: PO** 300 mg q8hr with gentamicin and vancomycin
- **Child: PO** 20 mg/kg/day in 2 divided doses with gentamicin and vancomycin, max 900 mg/day

Available forms: Caps 150, 300 mg; powder for inj 600 mg/vial

Administer:

- After C&S completed; monthly to detect resistance
- Do not give IM, SUBCUT

PO route

- On empty stomach, 1 hr before or 2 hr after meals with full glass of water; give with other products for TB
- Antiemetic if vomiting occurs
- Capsules may be opened, mixed with applesauce or jelly

Intermittent IV INFUSION route

- After diluting each 600 mg/10 ml of sterile water for inj (60 mg/ml), swirl, withdraw dose, and dilute in 100 ml or 500 ml of D_5W given as infusion over 3 hr; if diluted in 100 ml, give over ½ hr; do not admix with other sol or products

Y-site compatibilities: amiodarone, bumetanide, midazolam, pantoprazole, vancomycin

SIDE EFFECTS

CNS: Headache, fatigue, anxiety, drowsiness, confusion

EENT: Visual disturbances

GI: *Nausea, vomiting, anorexia, diarrhea,* **pseudomembranous colitis,**

heartburn, sore mouth and tongue, pancreatitis, increased LFTs
GU: Hematuria, acute renal failure, hemoglobinuria
HEMA: Hemolytic anemia, eosinophilia, thrombocytopenia, leukopenia
INTEG: Rash, pruritus, urticaria
MISC: Flulike symptoms, menstrual disturbances, edema, SOB, Stevens-Johnson syndrome, toxic epidermal necrolysis, angioedema, anaphylaxis
MS: Ataxia, weakness

PHARMACOKINETICS

PO: Peak 1-4 hr, half-life 1-5 hr, metabolized in liver (active/inactive metabolites), excreted in urine as free product (30% crosses placenta) and in breast milk

INTERACTIONS

⚠ Do not use with protease inhibitors
Increase: hepatotoxicity—isoniazid
Decrease: action of acetaminophen, alcohol, anticoagulants, antidiabetics, β-blockers, barbiturates, benzodiazepines, chloramphenicol, clofibrate, corticosteroids, cycloSPORINE, dapsone, digoxin, doxycycline, haloperidol, hormones, imidazole antifungals, NIFEdipine, oral contraceptives, phenytoin, protease inhibitors, theophylline, verapamil, zidovudine
Increase: LFTs
Decrease: Hgb

Drug/Lab Test

Increase: alk phosphatase, ALT, AST, uric acid, bilirubin, eosinophils
Interference: folate level, vit B_{12}

NURSING CONSIDERATIONS

Assess:

- **Infection:** sputum culture, lung sounds, characteristics of sputum
- Signs of anemia: Hct, Hgb, fatigue
- Hepatic function monthly: ALT, AST, bilirubin, decreased appetite, jaundice, dark urine, fatigue
- Renal status before, each mo: BUN, creatinine, output, specific gravity, urinalysis

⚠ **Serious skin reactions:** fever, sore throat, fatigue, ulcers; lesions in mouth, lips, rash; can be fatal

⚠ **Pseudomembranous colitis:** diarrhea, fever, abdominal pain/cramping, bloody stools; product should be discontinued, prescriber notified

Evaluate:

- Therapeutic response: decreased symptoms of TB, culture negative

Teach patient/family:

- That compliance with dosage schedule, duration necessary
- That scheduled appointments must be kept because relapse may occur
- To avoid alcohol because hepatotoxicity may occur
- That urine, feces, saliva, sputum, sweat, tears may be colored red-orange; that soft contact lenses may be permanently stained

⚠ To report flulike symptoms: excessive fatigue, anorexia, vomiting, sore throat; unusual bleeding; yellowish discoloration of skin, eyes; diarrhea with pus, mucous, blood

- To use nonhormonal form of birth control; to notify prescriber if pregnancy planned, suspected; not to breastfeed

rifapentine (Rx)

(riff′ah-pen-teen)

Priftin

Func. class.: Antitubercular
Chem. class.: Rifamycin derivative

Do not confuse:
rifapentine/rifampin/rifabutin

ACTION: Inhibits DNA-dependent polymerase, decreases tubercle bacilli replication

USES: Pulmonary TB; must be used with at least one other antitubercular agent

CONTRAINDICATIONS: Hypersensitivity to rifamycins, porphyria
Precautions: Pregnancy (C), breastfeeding, children <12 yr, geriatric patients, hepatic disease, blood dyscrasias, HIV

DOSAGE AND ROUTES

Intensive phase

• **Adult/Adolescent >12 yr: PO** 600 mg (four 150-mg tabs) 2×/wk with an interval of 72 hr between doses × 2 mo; must be given with at least 1 other antitubercular agent

Continuation phase

• **Adult/Adolescent >12 yr: PO** 600 mg weekly × 4 mo in combination with isoniazid or other appropriate antitubercular product

Available forms: Tabs 150 mg

Administer:

• May give with food for GI upset; use other products for TB

• Antiemetic if vomiting occurs

• After C&S completed; monthly to detect resistance

SIDE EFFECTS

CNS: Headache, fatigue, anxiety, dizziness

EENT: Visual disturbances

GI: *Nausea, vomiting, anorexia, diarrhea,* bilirubinemia, hepatitis, increased ALT, AST, *heartburn,* pancreatitis, pseudomembranous colitis

GU: Hematuria, pyuria, proteinuria, urinary casts, urine discoloration

HEMA: Thrombocytopenia, leukopenia, neutropenia, lymphopenia, anemia, leukocytosis, purpura, hematoma

INTEG: Rash, pruritus, urticaria, acne

MISC: Increased B/P

MS: Gout, arthrosis

PHARMACOKINETICS

Peak 5-6 hr; half-life 13 hr; metabolized in liver (active/inactive metabolites); excreted in urine, feces, breast milk; protein binding 97%; steady-state 10 days; CYP450 3A4, 2C8/9 inducer

INTERACTIONS

⚠ Do not use with protease inhibitors

Decrease: action of amitriptyline, anticoagulants, antidiabetics, barbiturates, β-blockers, chloramphenicol, clarithromycin, clofibrate, corticosteroids, cycloSPORINE, dapsone, delavirdine, diazepam, digoxin, diltiazem, disopyramide, doxycycline, fentaNYL, fluconazole, haloperidol, indinavir, itraconazole, ketoconazole, methadone, mexiletine, nelfinavir, NIFEdipine, nortriptyline, oral contraceptives, phenothiazines, phenytoin, progestins, quiNIDine, quiNINE, ritonavir, saquinavir, sildenafil, tacrolimus, theophylline, thyroid preparations, tocainide, verapamil, warfarin, zidovudine

Drug/Food

Increase: absorption with food

Drug/Lab Test

Increase: LFTs, platelets

Decrease: Hgb, WBC

Interference: folate level, vit B_{12}

NURSING CONSIDERATIONS

Assess:

• Baselines of CBC, AST, ALT, bilirubin, platelets

• **Infection:** sputum culture, lung sounds

• Signs of anemia: Hct, Hgb, fatigue

• Hepatic studies monthly: ALT, AST, bilirubin; decreased appetite, jaundice, dark urine, fatigue

• Renal status monthly: BUN, creatinine, output, specific gravity, urinalysis

⚠ **Pseudomembranous colitis:** diarrhea, fever, abdominal pain/cramping, bloody diarrhea; discontinue if present, notify prescriber

Evaluate:

• Therapeutic response: decreased symptoms of TB, culture negative

Teach patient/family:

• That compliance with dosage schedule, duration necessary

• That scheduled appointments must be kept because relapse may occur

• That urine, feces, saliva, sputum, sweat, tears may be colored red-orange; that soft contact lenses, dentures may be permanently stained

⚠ To use alternative method of contraception; that oral contraceptive action may be decreased; to notify prescriber if pregnancy planned, suspected; to avoid breastfeeding

⚠ To report flulike symptoms: excessive fatigue, anorexia, vomiting, sore throat;

R

unusual bleeding, yellowish discoloration of skin, eyes; diarrhea with pus, mucus, blood

rifaximin (Rx)

(rif-ax′i-min)

Xifaxan

Func. class.: Antiinfective—miscellaneous

Chem. class.: Analog of rifampin

Do not confuse:
rifaximin/rifampin

ACTION: Binds to bacterial-DNA–dependent RNA polymerase, thereby inhibiting bacterial RNA synthesis

USES: Traveler's diarrhea in those ≥12 yr caused by *E. coli,* hepatic encephalopathy

Unlabeled uses: Crohn's disease, diverticulitis, irritable bowel syndrome

CONTRAINDICATIONS: Hypersensitivity to product, rifamycins; diarrhea with fever, blood in stool

Precautions: Pregnancy (C), breastfeeding, children, geriatric patients

DOSAGE AND ROUTES

Traveler's diarrhea

- **Adult and child ≥12 yr: PO** 200 mg tid × 3 days without regard to meals

Hepatic encephalopathy

- **Adult: PO** 550 mg bid

Crohn's disease (unlabeled)

- **Adult: PO** 200 mg tid × 16 wk

Diverticulitis (unlabeled)

- **Adult: PO** 400 mg bid with mesalamine 800 mg tid × 7 days, then 7 days/mo

Irritable bowel syndrome (unlabeled)

- **Adult: PO** 550 mg tid × 14 day

Available forms: Tabs 200, 550 mg

Administer:

- Without regard to food

SIDE EFFECTS

CNS: Abnormal dreams, dizziness, insomnia, *headache,* fatigue, depression

CV: Hypotension, chest pain, peripheral edema, ascites

GI: *Abdominal pain, constipation, defecation urgency, flatulence, nausea, rectal tenesmus,* vomiting, ascites, pseudomembranous colitis

GU: Proteinuria, polyuria, increased urinary frequency

MISC: *Pyrexia,* motion sickness, tinnitus, rash, photosensitivity, exfoliative dermatitis

MS: Arthralgia, muscle pain, myalgia

RESP: Dyspnea, cough, pharyngitis

PHARMACOKINETICS

Low systemic absorption, half-life 1.8-4.5 hr, excreted in feces, peak 1-4 hr

INTERACTIONS

Increase: effect of—afatinib

Drug/Lab Test

Increase: LFTs, potassium

Decrease: blood glucose, sodium

NURSING CONSIDERATIONS

Assess:

- GI symptoms: amount, character of diarrhea; abdominal pain, nausea, vomiting, blood in stool; do not use in those with blood in stool, increased temperature with diarrhea

⚠ Overgrowth of infection, pseudomembranous colitis

Evaluate:

- Therapeutic response: absence of infection

Teach patient/family:

⚠ To discontinue rifaximin, notify prescriber if diarrhea persists >24-48 hr, if diarrhea worsens, or if blood in stools and fever present

- To avoid hazardous activities if dizziness occurs
- To notify prescriber if pregnancy planned, suspected
- That headache, rash, insomnia, abnormal dreams, tinnitus may occur

- To take without regard to food
- To take as directed, consume all of the product prescribed

rilpivirine

Edurant

Func. class.: Antiretroviral

Chem. class.: Nonnucleoside transcriptase inhibitors (NNTIs)

ACTION: Inhibits HIV-1 reverse transcriptase; unlike nucleoside reverse transcriptase inhibitors (NRTIs), it does not compete for binding nor does it require phosphorylation to be active; binds directly to a site on reverse transcriptase causing disruption of the enzyme's active site thereby blocking RNA-dependent and DNA-dependent DNA polymerase activities

USES: HIV in combination with other antiretrovirals

CONTRAINDICATIONS: Hypersensitivity

Precautions: Pregnancy (B), breastfeeding, neonates, infants, children, adolescents <18 yr, immune reconstitution syndrome, antimicrobial resistance, pancreatitis, coinfection hepatitis B or C and HIV, hepatic disease, depression, suicidal ideation, QT prolongation, torsades de pointes, hyperlipidemia, hypertriglyceridemia, hypercholesterolemia, immune reconstitution syndrome

DOSAGE AND ROUTES

Antiretroviral treatment-naive adults (HIV) with other antiretroviral agents

- **Adults: PO** 25 mg/day with a meal

Available forms: Tab 25 mg

Administer:

- Give with other antiretroviral agents; in antiretroviral treatment-naive adults, rilpivirine is used as an alternative to efavirenz in NNRTI-based treatment regimens; potential rilpivirine-based treatment regimens combine rilpivirine with either tenofovir plus emtricitabine or lamiVUDine; or abacavir plus emtricitabine or lamiVUDine; or zidovudine plus emtricitabine or lamiVUDine
- Give with a meal
- Store at room temperature away from heat and moisture

SIDE EFFECTS

CNS: Depressed mood, dysphoria, major depression, mood alteration, negative thoughts, **suicide attempts**, fatigue, headache, dizziness, drowsiness

GI: Nausea, vomiting, abdominal pain, diarrhea, cholecystitis, cholelithiasis, decreased appetite, elevated hepatic enzymes, hyperbilirubinemia, hypercholesterolemia

GU: **Glomerulonephritis membranous/glomerulonephritis mesangioproliferative**

PHARMACOKINETICS: Protein binding (99.7%) to albumin; metabolism via oxidation CYP3A; terminal elimination half-life 50 hr, excretion feces (85%), 25% excreted unchanged; urine (6.1%); peak 4-5 hr; increased effect 40% (food), decreased effect 50% (high protein drink)

INTERACTIONS:

Increase: rilpivirine effect—CYP3A4 inhibitors (delavirdine, efavirenz, darunavir, tipranavir, atazanavir, fosamprenavir, indinavir, nelfinavir, aldesleukin IL-2, amiodarone aprepitant, basiliximab, boceprevir, bromocriptine, chloramphenicol, clarithromycin, conivaptan danazol, dalfopristin, dasatinib, diltiazem, dronedarone, erythromycin, ethinyl estradiol, fluconazole, FLUoxetine, fluvoxaMINE, fosaprepitant, imatinib, isoniazid, itraconazole, ketoconazole, lanreotide, lapatinib, miconazole, nefazodone, niCARdipine, octreotide, posaconazole, quiNINE, ranolazine, rifaximin, tamoxifen, telaprevir, telithromycin, troleandomycin, verapamil, voriconazole, zafirlukast)

⚠ **Increase:** QT prolongation—class IA/III antidysrhythmics, some phenothiazines, β-agonists, local anesthetics, tricyclics, chloroquine, droperidol, haloperidol, pentamidine; CYP3A4 inhibitors (amiodarone, clarithromycin, erythromycin, telithromycin, troleandomycin, arsenic trioxide, levomethadyl); CYP3A4 substrates (methadone, pimozide, QUEtiapine, quiNIDine, risperiDONE, ziprasidone, lopinavir, saquinavir, fluconazole, posaconazole, dasatinib, dronedarone, lapatinib, octreotide, ranolazine, citalopram, abarelix, alfuzosin, amoxapine, apomorphine, artemether, lumefantrine, asenapine, ofloxacin, ciprofloxacin, cloZAPine, cyclobenzaprine, dolasetron, eribulin, flecainide, gatifloxacin, gemifloxacin, halogenated anesthetics, iloperidone, levofloxacin, maprotiline, mefloquine, moxifloxacin, nilotinib, norfloxacin, OLANZapine, ondansetron, paliperidone, palonosetron, QUEtiapine)

Increase: rilpivirine adverse reactions, fungal infections—fluconazole, voriconazole

Decrease: rilpivirine effect, treatment failure—CYP3A4 inducers (phenytoin, fosphenytoin, barbiturates, OXcarbazepine, carBAMazepine, rifabutin, rifampin, rifapentine, dexamethasone), efavirenz, nevirapine, ritonavir; aminoglutethimide, bexarotene, bosentan, griseofulvin, metyrapone, modafinil, flutamide, nafcillin, pioglitazone, primidone, topiramate); proton pump inhibitors (PPIs)

Decrease: rilpivirine effect, treatment failure—H2 receptor antagonists (cimetidine, famotidine, nizatidine, ranitidine), give 12 hr before or 4 hr after rilpivirine

Decrease: rilpivirine effect—antacids, use >2 hr before or 4 hr after rilpivirine

Drug/Food

Increase: adverse reactions—grapefruit juice

NURSING CONSIDERATIONS

Assess:

- **HIV:** Assess symptoms of HIV including opportunistic infections before and during treatment; some may be life-threatening; monitor plasma HIV RNA, CD4+, CD8+ cell counts, serum β-2 microglobulin, serum ICD+24 antigen levels; treatment failures occur more frequently in those with baseline HIV-1 RNA concentrations >100,000 copies/ml than in patients with concentrations <100,000 copies/ml; monitor serum cholesterol, lipid panel
- Antiretroviral drug resistance testing before initiation of therapy in antiretroviral treatment-naive patients
- For adults and adolescents, initiation of antiretroviral therapy is recommended in any patient with a history of an AIDS-defining infection; with a CD4 ≤500/mm^3; who is pregnant; who has HIV-associated nephropathy; or who is being treated for hepatitis B (HBV) infection

⚠ **Suicidal thoughts/behaviors:** Assess frequently for suicidal ideation; report any increase in depressive symptoms

- **Hepatic disease:** Monitor for elevated hepatic enzymes (>2.5 × ULN); grade 3 and 4 may be higher in patients co-infected with hepatitis B or C

Teach patient/family:

- That product is not a cure but controls symptoms, that continuing use is required
- That product must be taken in combination with other prescribed products
- To report if pregnancy is suspected immediately, do not breastfeed
- To advise prescriber of all products that are used
- To report mood changes and depression

RARELY USED

riluzole (Rx)

(rill'you-zole)

Rilutek

Func. class.: ALS agent

Chem. class.: Benzathiazole

USES: Amyotropic lateral sclerosis (ALS)

CONTRAINDICATIONS: Hypersensitivity

DOSAGE AND ROUTES

• **Adult: PO** 50 mg q12hr; take 1 hr before or 2 hr after meals

rimexolone ophthalmic

See Appendix B

riociguat

(rye'oh-sig'ue-at)

Adempas

Func. class.: Antihypertensive/vasodilator

Chem. class.: Guanylate cyclase stimulator

ACTION: Guanylate cyclase stimulator, also a vasoconstrictor

USES: WHO group I pulmonary arterial hypertension and WHO group IV persistent/recurrent chronic thromboembolic pulmonary hypertension

CONTRAINDICATIONS: Breastfeeding hypersensitivity

Black Box Warning: Pregnancy (X)

Precautions: Hypotension, hypovolemia, pulmonary edema, tobacco smoking

DOSAGE AND ROUTES

• **Adult: PO** 1 mg tid; may start at 0.5 mg tid if needed; if systolic B/P remains >95 mmHg increase by 0.5 mg tid; increase no sooner than 2 wk, max 2.5 mg tid

Renal/hepatic dose

• **Adult:** Not recommended in CCr <15 ml/min or Child-Pugh C

Available forms: Tabs 0.5, 1, 1.5, 2, 2.5 mg

Administer:

• tid without regard to food
• Do not discontinue abruptly
• If dose is missed, take at next scheduled dose; if stopped for ≥3 days, begin with initial dose

SIDE EFFECTS

CNS: Dizziness

CV: Hypotension, peripheral edema, palpitations

EENT: Sinusitis, rhinitis

GI: Constipation, gastritis, gastroesophageal reflux, nausea, vomiting

GU: Decreased sperm counts

HEMA: Anemia, bleeding, nosebleeds

RESP: Pulmonary edema

PHARMACOKINETICS

95% protein binding, peak 1.5 hr, metabolized by P-gb, CYP1A1, CYP3A4, CYP3A, CYP2C8, CYP2J2, terminal half-life 15 hr, half-life 12 hr

INTERACTIONS

• Do not use with nitrates, nitric oxide donors, phosphodiesterase-5 inhibitors

• Decreased riociguat effect: tobacco smoking

Increase: riociguat—CYP3A4 inhibitors (amprenavir, aprepitant, atazanavir, clarithromycin, conivaptan, cycloSPORINE, dalfopristin, danazol, darunavir, erythromycin, estradiol, imatinib, itraconazole, ketoconazole, nefazodone, nelfinavir, propoxyphene, quinupristin, ritonavir, RU-486, saquinavir, tamoxifen, telithromycin, troleandomycin, zafirlukast)

Drug/Herb

• Need for dosage change: St. John's wort, ephedra (ma huang)

R

NURSING CONSIDERATIONS

Assess:

• Pulmonary status: improvement in breathing, ability to exercise; pulmonary edema may indicate venoocclusive disease

Black Box Warning: Assess pregnancy status before giving this product; pregnancy (X)

Evaluate:

• Therapeutic response: decrease in B/P; decreased shortness of breath

Teach patient/family:

• The importance of complying with dosage schedule even if feeling better

Black Box Warning: To notify if pregnancy is planned or suspected (if pregnant, product will need to be discontinued, pregnancy test done monthly); to use 2 contraception methods while taking this product

• Not to use OTC products including herbs, supplements unless approved by prescriber

risedronate (Rx)

(rih-sed′roh-nate)

Actonel, Atelvia

Func. class.: Bone resorption inhibitor

Chem. class.: Bisphosphonate

Do not confuse:

Actonel/Actos

ACTION: Inhibits bone resorption, absorbs calcium phosphate crystal in bone, and may directly block dissolution of hydroxyapatite crystals of bone

USES: Paget's disease; prevention, treatment of osteoporosis in postmenopausal women; glucocorticoid-induced osteoporosis; osteoporosis in men

Unlabeled uses: Osteolytic metastases

CONTRAINDICATIONS: Hypersensitivity to bisphosphonates, inability to stand or sit upright for ≥30 min, esophageal stricture, achalasia, hypocalcemia

Precautions: Pregnancy (C), breastfeeding, children, renal disease, active upper GI disorders, dental disease, hyperparathyroidism, infection, vit D deficiency, coagulopathy, chemotherapy, asthma

DOSAGE AND ROUTES

Paget's disease

• **Adult: PO** 30 mg/day × 2 mo; patients with Paget's disease should receive calcium and vit D if dietary intake lacking; if relapse occurs, retreatment advised

Treatment/prevention of postmenopausal osteoporosis

• **Adult: PO** 5 mg/day or 35 mg/wk or 75 mg/day × 2 consecutive days 2× monthly or 150 mg/mo

Glucocorticoid osteoporosis

• **Adult: PO** 5 mg/day

Osteoporosis in men

• **Adult: PO** 35 mg/wk

Osteolytic metastases (unlabeled)

• **Adult: PO** 30 mg/day × 6 mo

Renal dose

• **Adult: PO** CCr <30 ml/min, avoid use

Available forms: Tabs 5, 30, 35, 150 mg; tab, weekly 35 mg

Administer:

• For 2 mo to be effective for Paget's disease

• With a full glass of water; patient should be in upright position for ½ hr; swallow whole; do not crush, break, chew, give del rel tablet in AM after breakfast, only use with food (del rel)

• Supplemental calcium and vit D for Paget's disease if instructed by prescriber

• Give daily ≥30 min before meals or give weekly

• Store in cool environment, out of direct sunlight

SIDE EFFECTS

CNS: Dizziness, headache, depression

CV: *Chest pain,* hypertension, atrial fibrillation

GI: *Abdominal pain, diarrhea, nausea,* constipation, esophagitis
MISC: Rash, UTI, pharyngitis, hypocalcemia, hypophosphatemia, increase PTH
MS: **Osteonecrosis of the jaw,** severe muscle/joint/bone pain, fractures
SYST: **Angioedema**

PHARMACOKINETICS

Rapidly cleared from circulation, taken up mainly by bones (50%), eliminated primarily through kidneys, absorption decreased by food, terminal half-life 230 hr

INTERACTIONS

Increase: GI irritation—NSAIDs, salicylates
Decrease: absorption of risedronate—aluminum, calcium, iron, magnesium salts, antacids
Decrease: absorption of del rel risedronate-H2 antagonists, proton pump inhibitors, do not use together

Drug/Food

Decrease: bioavailability—take ½ hr before food or drinks other than water

Drug/Lab Test

Decrease: calcium, phosphorus

NURSING CONSIDERATIONS

Assess:

- **Paget's disease:** headache, bone pain, increased head circumference
- **Osteoporosis:** in men or postmenopausal women; bone density study before and periodically during treatment
- Phosphate, alk phos, calcium; creatinine, BUN (renal disease)
- **Hypocalcemia:** paresthesia, twitching, laryngospasm, Chvostek's/Trousseau's signs

⚠ **Serious skin reactions:** angioedema

- **Dental health:** assess dental health, provide antiinfectives for dental extraction; cover with antiinfectives before dental extraction

⚠ For atrial fibrillation

Evaluate:

- Therapeutic response: increased bone mass, absence of fractures

Teach patient/family:

- To sit upright for ½ hr after dose to prevent irritation
- To notify prescriber immediately if difficulty swallowing, severe heartburn, or pain in chest
- To comply with diet, vitamin/mineral supplements
- To notify prescriber if pregnancy is suspected or if breastfeeding
- To maintain good oral hygiene
- To notify all health care providers of use
- That musculoskeletal pain may occur within a few days/mo after starting but usually resolves; use acetaminophen
- To exercise regularly; to avoid alcohol, tobacco

risperiDONE (Rx)

(ris-pehr′ih-dohn)

RisperDAL, RisperDAL Consta, RisperDAL M-TAB

Func. class.: Antipsychotic
Chem. class.: Benzisoxazole derivative

Do not confuse:
RisperDAL/reserpine

ACTION: Unknown; may be mediated through both dopamine type 2 (D_2) and serotonin type 2 ($5\text{-}HT_2$) antagonism

USES: Irritability associated with autism, bipolar disorder, mania, schizophrenia
Unlabeled uses: Acute psychosis, agitation, ADHD, dementia, psychotic depression, Tourette's syndrome

CONTRAINDICATIONS: Hypersensitivity, breastfeeding
Precautions: Pregnancy (C), children, geriatric patients, cardiac/renal/hepatic disease, breast cancer, Parkinson's disease, CNS depression, brain tumor, dehydration, diabetes, hematologic disease, seizure disorders, abrupt discontinuation, suicidal ideation, phenylketonuria

R

Black Box Warning: Increased mortality in elderly patients with dementia-related psychosis

DOSAGE AND ROUTES

- **Adult: PO** 2 mg/day as single dose or in 2 divided doses, adjust dose at intervals of ≥24 hr and 1-2 mg/day as tolerated to 4-8 mg/day; **IM** establish dosing with **PO** before **IM** 25 mg q2wk, may increase to max 50 mg q2wk
- **Adolescent: PO** 0.5 mg/day in AM or PM, adjust dose at intervals of ≥24 hr and 0.5-1 mg/day as tolerated to 3 mg/day
- **Geriatric: PO** 0.5 mg daily-bid, increase by 1 mg/wk; **IM** 25 mg q2wk

Hepatic/renal dose

- **Adult: PO** 0.5 mg bid, increase by 0.5 mg bid, increase to 1.5 mg bid at intervals ≥1 wk

Available forms: Tabs 0.25, 0.5, 1, 2, 3, 4 mg; oral sol 1 mg/ml; orally disintegrating tabs 0.25, 0.5, 1, 2, 3, 4 mg; long-acting inj kit (Risperdal Consta) 12.5, 25, 37.5, 50 mg

Administer:

- Reduced dose in geriatric patients
- Anticholinergic agent on order from prescriber, to be used for EPS
- Avoid use with CNS depressants
- Conventional tabs: give without regard to meals
- **Oral disintegrating tab** (Risperdal M-TAB): do not open blister pack until ready to use; tear at perforation; bend corner where indicated; peel back foil; do not push tab through foil; remove from pack and place product on patient's tongue; tab disintegrates in seconds and can be swallowed with/without liquids, do not split or chew
- **Oral sol:** May dilute 3-4 oz of beverage, measure dose using calibrated pipette; not compatible with tea, cola; compatible with water, coffee, orange juice, low-fat milk

IM route

Preparation

- Only suspend in the diluent provided and with the supplied needle
- Before admixing, allow to come to room temperature for 30 min
- Remove colored cap from the vial without removing the gray rubber stopper; wipe top of stopper with an alcohol wipe
- Peel back the blister pouch and remove the Vial Access Device by holding between the white Luer cap and the skirt; do not touch the spike tip at any time
- Place the vial on a hard surface and hold the base; orient the Vial Access Device vertically over the vial so that the spike tip is at the center of the vial's rubber stopper
- With a straight downward push, press the spike tip of the Vial Access Device through the center of the vial's rubber stopper until the device securely snaps onto the vial top; improper placement of the Vial Access Device on the vial could result in leakage of the diluent upon transfer
- Hold the base of the vial and swab the syringe connection point (blue circle) of the Vial Access Device with an alcohol wipe and allow to dry before attaching the syringe
- Avoid over-tightening or syringe component parts might loosen from the syringe body
- While holding the white collar of the syringe, insert and press the syringe tip into the blue circle of the Vial Access Device and twist in a clockwise motion to secure the connection of the syringe to the Vial Access Device; hold the skirt of the Vial Access Device during attachment to prevent it from spinning; keep the syringe and the Vial Access Device aligned
- Inject the entire contents of the syringe containing the diluent into the vial
- Holding the plunger down with the thumb, shake the vial vigorously for a minimum of 10 sec; suspension should appear uniform, thick, and milky colored, and all the powder is dispersed in

liquid; the microspheres will be visible in liquid, but no dry microspheres remain
- Invert completely and slowly withdraw the contents of the suspension from the vial into the syringe; tear the section of the vial label at the perforation and apply the detached label to the syringe
- While holding the white collar of the syringe, unscrew the syringe from the Vial Access Device, then discard both the vial and the Vial Access Device appropriately
- Select the appropriate color-coded needle provided with the kit; two distinct needles are provided: the needle with the yellow hub and print is for injection into the gluteal muscle (2-inch needle), and the needle with the green hub and print is for deltoid muscles (1-inch needle); they are not interchangeable; do not use the needle intended for gluteal injection for deltoid injection, and vice versa
- Peel the blister pouch of the Needle-Pro safety device open halfway; grasp the transparent needle sheath using the plastic peel pouch; to prevent contamination, do not touch the orange Needle-Pro safety device's Luer connector; while holding the white collar of the syringe, attach the Luer connection of the orange Needle-Pro safety device to the syringe with an easy clockwise twisting motion
- While holding the white collar of the syringe, grasp the transparent needle sheath and seat the needle firmly on the orange Needle-Pro safety device with a push and a clockwise twist; seating the needle will secure the connection between the needle and the orange Needle-Pro safety device
- While holding the white collar of the syringe, pull the transparent needle sheath straight away from the needle; do not twist the sheath because this can loosen the Luer connection
- Resuspension is necessary before administration, because settling occurs after reconstitution; resuspend the microspheres in the syringe by shaking vigorously
- Refer to the Instructions for Use section of the product labeling for detailed visual aids that accompany the written instructions

Administration
- Only for IM; do not give IV
- Resuspension is necessary before administration, because settling occurs after reconstitution; resuspend the microspheres in the syringe by shaking vigorously
- Remove any air bubbles by tapping the syringe and slowly depressing the plunger with the needle in an upright position
- Inject the entire contents of the syringe into the upper outer quadrant of the gluteal area or the deltoid muscle; inject immediately after reconstitution to avoid settling; gluteal injections should be alternated between the two buttocks
- After the injection is complete, press the needle into the orange Needle-Pro safety device by gently pressing the orange Needle-Pro safety device against a flat surface with one hand; as the orange Needle-Pro safety device is pressed, the needle firmly engages into the orange Needle-Pro safety device
- Visually confirm full engagement of the needle into the Needle-Pro safety device, then appropriately discard both the used and unused needle provided in the dose pack
- Do not store the vial after reconstitution or the suspension will settle
- Do not combine 2 different dosage strengths of RisperDAL Consta in a single administration
- The dose pack device is for single use only; do not reprocess for subsequent reuse because the integrity of the device may be compromised, leading to a deterioration in performance

Stability after reconstitution
- Once in suspension, the product may remain at room temperature, but it must be used within 6 hr; always resuspend before administration if not used immediately

SIDE EFFECTS

CNS: *EPS, pseudoparkinsonism, akathisia, dystonia, tardive dyskinesia; drowsiness, insomnia, agitation, anxiety, headache,* seizures, neuroleptic

R

malignant syndrome, dizziness, suicidal ideation, head titubation (shaking)
CV: Orthostatic hypotension, tachycardia; heart failure, sudden death (geriatric patients), AV block
EENT: Blurred vision, tinnitus
GI: *Nausea,* vomiting, *anorexia, constipation,* jaundice, weight gain
GU: Hyperprolactinemia, gynecomastia, dysuria
HEMA: Neutropenia, granulocytopenia
MISC: Renal artery occlusion; hyperprolactinemia (child)
MS: Rhabdomyolysis
RESP: Rhinitis; sinusitis, upper respiratory infection, cough

PHARMACOKINETICS

PO: Extensively metabolized by liver to major active metabolite, plasma protein binding 90%, peak 1-2 hr, excreted 90% in urine, terminal half-life 3-24 hr

INTERACTIONS

Increase: seizures—traMADol
⚠ **Increase:** possible death in dementia-related psychosis: furosemide
Increase: sedation—other CNS depressants, alcohol
⚠ **Increase:** serotonin syndrome, neuroleptic malignant syndrome—CYP2D6 inhibitors (SSRIs, SNRIs)
Increase: EPS—other antipsychotics
Increase: risperiDONE excretion—carBAMazepine
⚠ **Increase:** QT prolongation—class IA/III antidysrhythmics, some phenothiazines, β-agonists, local anesthetics, tricyclics, haloperidol, methadone, chloroquine, clarithromycin, droperidol, erythromycin, pentamidine, thioridazine, ziprasidone
Increase: risperiDONE levels: acetylcholinesterase, inhibitors, CYP2D6 inhibitors, SSRIs, valproic acid, verapamil
Decrease: risperiDONE action—CYP2D6 inducers (carBAMazepine, barbiturates, phenytoins, rifampin)
Decrease: levodopa effect—levodopa

Drug/Herb
Decrease: risperiDONE effect—echinacea

Drug/Lab Test
Increase: prolactin levels, blood, glucose, lipids

NURSING CONSIDERATIONS

Assess:

⚠ **Suicidal thoughts/behaviors:** often when depression is lessened; mental status before initial administration
• Thyroid function test, blood glucose, serum electrolytes/prolactin/lipid profile, bilirubin, creatinine, weight, pregnancy test, CBC, LFTs, AIMS assessment, baseline and periodically
• Affect, orientation, LOC, reflexes, gait, coordination, sleep pattern disturbances
⚠ **QT prolongation:** B/P standing, lying; pulse, respirations; take these q4hr during initial treatment; establish baseline before starting treatment; report drops of 30 mm Hg; watch for ECG changes
• Dizziness, faintness, palpitations, tachycardia on rising
• **EPS:** akathisia, tardive dyskinesia (bizarre movements of the jaw, mouth, tongue, extremities), pseudoparkinsonism (rigidity, tremors, pill rolling, shuffling gait)
⚠ **Serious reactions in geriatric patient:** fatal pneumonia, heart failure, sudden death, dementia
⚠ **Neuroleptic malignant syndrome:** hyperthermia, increased CPK, altered mental status, muscle rigidity, seizures, change in B/P, fatigue, tachycardia
• Constipation, urinary retention daily; if these occur, increase bulk, water in diet
• Decreased stimuli by dimming lights, avoiding loud noises
• Supervised ambulation until patient stabilized on medication; do not involve patient in strenuous exercise program because fainting is possible; patient should not stand still for a long time
• Increased fluids to prevent constipation
• Store in tight, light-resistant container (PO); unopened vials in refrigerator, protect from light; do not freeze

Evaluate:

- Therapeutic response: decrease in emotional excitement, hallucinations, delusions, paranoia; reorganization of patterns of thought, speech

Teach patient/family:

- That orthostatic hypotension may occur; to rise from sitting or lying position gradually
- To avoid abrupt withdrawal of product because EPS may result; product should be withdrawn slowly
- To avoid OTC preparations (cough, hay fever, cold) unless approved by prescriber; that serious product interactions may occur; to avoid use of alcohol because increased drowsiness may occur
- To avoid hazardous activities if drowsy or dizzy
- To comply with product regimen
- To report impaired vision, tremors, muscle twitching
- That heat stroke may occur in hot weather; to take extra precautions to stay cool; to avoid hot tubs, hot showers, tub baths
- To use contraception; to inform prescriber if pregnancy is planned or suspected; not to breastfeed
- To notify provider of suicidal thoughts/behaviors

TREATMENT OF OVERDOSE:

Lavage if orally ingested; provide airway; *do not induce vomiting*

ritonavir (Rx)

(ri-toe′na-veer)

Norvir

Func. class.: Antiretroviral

Chem. class.: Protease inhibitor

Do not confuse:

ritonavir/Retrovir

ACTION:

Inhibits human immunodeficiency virus (HIV-1) protease and prevents maturation of the infectious virus

USES:

HIV-1 in combination with at least 2 other antiretrovirals

CONTRAINDICATIONS:

Hypersensitivity

Black Box Warning: Coadministration with other drugs

Precautions: Pregnancy (B), breastfeeding, hepatic disease, pancreatitis, diabetes, hemophilia, AV block, hypercholesterolemia, immune reconstitution syndrome, neonates, cardiomyopathy, immune reconstitution syndrome, infants 1-6 mo (overdose)

DOSAGE AND ROUTES

- **Adult and adolescent >16 yr: PO** 600 mg bid; if nausea occurs, begin at ½ dose and gradually increase, max 1200 mg/day in divided doses
- **Adolescent ≤16 yr and child, infant: PO** 400 mg/m² bid up to 1200 mg/day in divided doses, may start lower and escalate

Available forms: Caps 100 mg; oral sol 80 mg/ml; tab 100 mg

Administer:

Tablet/capsule

- Take with food, swallow whole; do not crush, break, chew
- When switching from cap to tab, more GI symptoms may occur, will lessen over time
- Use dosage titration to minimize side effects
- Store caps in refrigerator
- **Oral sol:** shake well, use calibrated measuring device
- Mix liquid formulation with chocolate milk or liquid nutritional supplement to improve taste
- **Overdose:** infants, children, 43.2% alcohol, 26.57% propylene glycol oral sol, calculate total amount of alcohol, propylene glycol from all products given

SIDE EFFECTS

CNS: *Paresthesia, headache,* **seizures,** fever, dizziness, insomnia, asthenia, **intracranial bleeding**

R

CV: QT, PR interval prolongation
GI: *Diarrhea,* buccal mucosa ulceration, *abdominal pain, nausea, taste perversion,* dry mouth, *vomiting, anorexia*
INTEG: Rash
MISC: Asthenia, angioedema, anaphylaxis, Stevens-Johnson syndrome, increase lipids, lipodystrophy, toxic epidermal necrolysis
MS: Pain, rhabdomyolysis, myalgia

PHARMACOKINETICS

Well absorbed, 98% protein binding, hepatic metabolism, peak 2-4 hr, terminal half-life 3-5 hr

INTERACTIONS

Black Box Warning: Increase: toxicity—amiodarone, astemizole, azole antifungals, benzodiazepines, buPROPion, CISapride, cloZAPine, desipramine, dihydroergotamine, encainide, ergotamine, flecainide, HMG-CoA reductase inhibitors, interleukins, meperidine, midazolam, pimozide, piroxicam, propafenone, propoxyphene, quiNIDine, ranolazine, saquinavir, terfenadine, triazolam, zolpidem; CYP2D6 inhibitors

Black Box Warning: Increase: QT prolongation—class 1A/III antidysrhythmics, some phenothiazines, β-agonists, local anesthetics, tricyclics, haloperidol, chloroquine, droperidol, pentamidine, CYP3A4 inhibitors (amiodarone, clarithromycin, dasatinib, erythromycin, telithromycin, troleandomycin), arsenic trioxide, levomethadyl, CYP3A4 substrates (methadone, pimozide, QUEtiapine, quiNIDine, risperiDONE, ziprasidone)

Increase: ritonavir levels—fluconazole
Increase: level of both products—clarithromycin, ddI
Increase: levels of—bosentan
Decrease: ritonavir levels—rifamycins, nevirapine, barbiturates, phenytoin
Decrease: levels of anticoagulants, atovaquone, divalproex, ethinyl estradiol, lamotrigine, phenytoin, sulfamethoxazole, theophylline, voriconazole, zidovudine

Drug/Herb
Decrease: ritonavir levels—St. John's wort; avoid concurrent use
- Avoid use with red yeast rice

Drug/Lab Test
Increase: AST, ALT, K, CK, cholesterol, GGT, triglycerides, uric acid
Decrease: Hct, Hgb, RBC, neutrophils, WBC

NURSING CONSIDERATIONS

Assess:
- **HIV:** viral load, CD4 at baseline, throughout therapy; blood glucose, plasma HIV RNA, serum cholesterol/lipid profile; resistance testing before starting therapy and after treatment failure
- **Immune reconstitution syndrome:** may occur with combination therapy; may develop inflammatory response with opportunistic infection (MAC, Graves' disease, Guillain-Barré Syndrome, TB, PCP); may occur during initial treatment or months after
- Signs of infection, anemia
- Hepatic studies: ALT, AST, in those with hepatic disease, monitor q3mo
- Bowel pattern before, during treatment; if severe abdominal pain with bleeding occurs, discontinue product; monitor hydration
- Skin eruptions; rash

⚠ **Rhabdomyolysis:** muscle pain, increased CPK, weakness, swelling of affected muscles; if these occur and if confirmed by CPK, product should be discontinued

⚠ **QT prolongation:** ECG for QT prolongation, ejection fraction; assess for chest pain, palpitations, dyspnea

⚠ **Serious skin disorders:** Stevens-Johnson syndrome, angioedema, anaphylaxis, toxic epidermal necrolysis

Evaluate:
- Therapeutic response: improvement in HIV symptoms; improving viral load, CD4+ T cells

Teach patient/family:
- To take as prescribed; if dose is missed, to take as soon as remembered up to 1 hr before next dose; not to double dose
- That product not a cure for HIV; that opportunistic infections may continue to be acquired
- That redistribution of body fat or accumulation of body fat may occur
- That others may continue to contract HIV from patient
- To avoid OTC, prescription medications, herbs, supplements unless approved by prescriber; not to use St. John's wort because it decreases product's effect
- That regular follow-up exams and blood work will be required

⚠ HIGH ALERT

riTUXimab (Rx)

(rih-tuks′ih-mab)

Rituxan

Func. class.: Antineoplastic—miscellaneous; DMARDs

Chem. class.: Murine/human monoclonal antibody

ACTION: Directed against the CD20 antigen that is found on malignant B lymphocytes; CD20 regulates a portion of cell-cycle initiation/differentiation

USES: Non-Hodgkin's lymphoma (CD20+, B-cell), bulky disease (tumors >10 cm), rheumatoid arthritis, Wegener's granulomatosis, microscopic polyangitis

Unlabeled uses: Acquired blood factor deficiency, acute lymphocytic leukemia (ALL), Burkitt's lymphoma, chronic lymphocytic leukemia (CLL), hemolytic anemia, human herpesvirus 8, mantle cell lymphoma (MCL), multicentric Castleman's disease, peripheral blood stem cell (PBSC) mobilization, refractory pemphigus vulgaris, relapsing/remitting MS, ITP with dexamethasone, steroid refractory chronic graft-versus-host disease

CONTRAINDICATIONS: Hypersensitivity, murine proteins

Precautions: Pregnancy (C), breastfeeding, children, geriatric patients, pulmonary/cardiac/renal conditions

Black Box Warning: Exfoliative dermatitis, infusion-related reactions, progressive multifocal leukoencephalopathy

DOSAGE AND ROUTES

Relapsed or refractory low-grade or follicular, CD20+, B-cell non-Hodgkin's lymphoma (NHL)
- **Adult:** IV 375 mg/m² every wk × 4 doses, may re-treat with 4 more doses of 375 mg/m²/wk

First-line treatment of follicular, CD20+, B-cell NHL in combination with chemotherapy
- **Adult:** IV 375 mg/m² on day 1 of each cycle for up to 8 cycles; may be given with cyclophosphamide IV 750 mg/m² on day 1, vinCRIStine IV 1.4 mg/m² (max 2 mg) on day 1, and predniSONE 40 mg/m²/day PO on days 1-5

Single-agent maintenance therapy in patients with follicular, CD20+, B-cell NHL (complete or partial response following first-line treatment with riTUXimab in combination with chemotherapy)
- **Adult:** IV 375 mg/m² IV every 8 wk × 12 doses as maintenance therapy starting 8 wk after the completion of induction chemotherapy with 8 doses of riTUXimab with 6-8 cycles of cyclophosphamide, vinCRIStine, and predniSONE 4-6 cycles of cyclophosphamide, DOXOrubicin, vinCRIStine, and predniSONE

Component of the Zevalin (ibritumomab tiuxetan) regimen
- **Adult:** IV As a required component of the ibritumomab regimen; riTUXimab 250 mg/m² given within 4 hr before administration of Yttrium-90 ibritumomab that may occur on day 7, 8, or 9

R

First-line treatment of diffuse large B-cell, CD20+ NHL in combination with CHOP or other anthracycline-based chemotherapy regimen

• **Adult 18-59 yr: IV** 375 mg/m² on day 1 of each cycle for up to 8 infusions

Single-agent maintenance therapy in patients with low-grade, CD20+, B-cell NHL with nonprogressing disease (stable disease or better) following first-line treatment with cyclophosphamide, vinCRIStine, and predniSONE (CVP)

• **Adult: IV** 375 mg/m² weekly × 4 wk repeated every 6 mo × 2 yr (total of 16 doses) as maintenance therapy starting 4 wk after the completion of first-line chemotherapy with 6-8 cycles of cyclophosphamide, vinCRIStine, and predniSONE (CVP)

Available forms: Inj 10 mg/ml (100 mg/10 ml, 500 mg/50 ml)

Administer:

Rheumatoid arthritis:

• Give methylPREDNISolone 100 mg or similar product 30 min before infusion to decrease reactions

Intermittent IV INFUSION route

• Hold antihypertensives 12 hr before administration

• After diluting to final concentration of 1-4 mg/ml; use 0.9% NaCl, D_5W, gently invert bag to mix; do not mix with other products; give 50 mg/hr initially; if no reaction, increase rate by 50 mg/hr to max 400 mg/hr

• Store vials at 36° F-40° F; protect vials from direct sunlight; infusion sol is stable at 36° F-46° F × 24 hr and at room temperature for another 12 hr

Y-site compatibilities: Amcyclovir, amifostine, amikacin, aminophylline, ampicillin, ampicillin/sulbactam, aztreonam, bleomycin, bumetanide, buprenorphine, busulfan, butorphanol, calcium gluconate, CARBOplatin, carmustine, ceFAZolin, cefoperazone, cefotaxime, cefoTEtan, cefOXitin, cefTAZidime, ceftizoxime, cefTRIAXone, cefuroxime, chlorproMAZINE, cimetidine, CISplatin, clindamycin, cyclophosphamide, cytarabine, DACTINomycin, DAUNOrubicin hydrochloride, dexamethasone, dexrazoxane, digoxin, diphenhydrAMINE, DOBUTamine, DOCEtaxel, DOPamine, DOXOrubicin liposome, doxycycline, droperidol, enalaprilat, etoposide phosphate, famotidine, fentaNYL, filgrastim, floxuridine, fluconazole, fludarabine, fluorouracil, ganciclovir, gemcitabine, gentamicin, granisetron, haloperidol, heparin, hydrocortisone, HYDROmorphone, IDArubicin, ifosfamide, imipenem/cilastatin, irinotecan, leucovorin, levorphanol, LORazepam, magnesium sulfate, mannitol, meperidine, mesna, methotrexate, methylPREDNISolone, metoclopramide, metroNIDAZOLE, mitoMYcin, mitoXANtrone, morphine, nalbuphine, netilmicin, PACLitaxel, pentamidine, piperacillin/tazobactam, plicamycin, potassium chloride, prochlorperazine, promethazine, ranitidine, sargramostim, streptozocin, teniposide, theophylline, thiotepa, ticarcillin/clavulanate, tobramycin, trimethoprim/sulfamethoxazole, trimethobenzamide, vinBLAStine, vincCRIStine, vinorelbine, zidovudine

SIDE EFFECTS

CNS: Life-threatening brain infection (progressive multifocal leukoencephalopathy)

CV: Cardiac dysrhythmias, heart failure, hypertension, MI, supraventricular tachycardia, angina

GI: *Nausea, vomiting, anorexia,* GI obstruction/perforation

GU: Renal failure

HEMA: Leukopenia, neutropenia, thrombocytopenia, anemia

INTEG: *Irritation at site, rash,* fatal mucocutaneous infections (rare)

MISC: *Fever,* chills, asthenia, *headache,* angioedema, hypotension, myalgia, bronchospasm, ARDs

SYST: Toxic epidermal necrolysis, tumor lysis syndrome, Stevens-Johnson syndrome, exfoliative dermatitis

PHARMACOKINETICS

Half-life varies, binds to CD20 sites or lymphoma cells

INTERACTIONS

Increase: hypotension—antihypertensives, separate by 12 hr

Increase: nephrotoxicity—CISplatin, avoid concurrent use; if used, monitor renal status

Increase: bleeding—anticoagulants

- Avoid with vaccines, toxoids

NURSING CONSIDERATIONS

Assess:

Black Box Warning: Fatal infusion reaction: hypoxia, pulmonary infiltrates, ARDS, MI, ventricular fibrillation, cardiogenic shock; most fatal reactions occur with 1st infusion; potentially fatal

Black Box Warning: Severe mucocutaneous reactions: Stevens-Johnson syndrome, lichenoid dermatitis, toxic epidermal lysis; occur 1-13 wk after product given, discontinue treatment immediately

Black Box Warning: Tumor lysis syndrome: acute renal failure requiring hemodialysis, hyperkalemia, hypocalcemia, hyperuricemia, hyperphosphatemia; allopurinol and adequate hydration may be needed

Black Box Warning: Multifocal leukoencephalopathy: confusion, dizziness, lethargy, hemiparesis; monitor periodically

- CBC, differential, platelet count weekly; withhold product if WBC is $<3500/mm^3$ or platelet count $<100,000/mm^3$; notify prescriber of results; product should be discontinued
- ECG, serum creatinine/BUN, electrolytes, uric acid
- GI symptoms: frequency of stools, abdominal pain, perforation/obstruction may occur
- **Infection:** fever, increased temperature, flulike symptoms in those with Wegener's granulomatosis and microscopic polyangiitis in those using DMARDs

Evaluate:

- Therapeutic response: prevention of increasing cancer progression

Teach patient/family:

- To avoid use with vaccines, toxoids
- To use contraception during, for up to 12 mo after therapy
- ⚠ To report to prescriber possible infection (cough, fever, chills, sore throat), renal issues (painful urination, back/side pain), bleeding (gums, stools, urine, bruising, emesis, fatigue)
- To avoid OTC products
- To avoid crowds, those with known infections
- To maintain fluid intake

⚠ HIGH ALERT

rivaroxaban

Xarelto

Func. class.: Anticoagulant

Chem. class.: Factor Xa inhibitor

ACTION:
A novel, oral anticoagulant that selectively and potently inhibits coagulation factor Xa

USES:
For deep venous thrombosis (DVT) prophylaxis/treatment, pulmonary embolism (PE), in patients undergoing knee or hip replacement surgery; for stroke prophylaxis and systemic embolism prophylaxis in patients with nonvalvular atrial fibrillation

CONTRAINDICATIONS

Severe hypersensitivity

Black Box Warning: Active bleeding

Precautions Pregnancy (C), breastfeeding, neonates, infants, children, adolescents, geriatric patients, moderate or severe hepatic disease (Child-Pugh Class B or C), hepatic disease associated with coagulopathy, creatinine clearance <30 ml/min for use as DVT prophylaxis and

R

<15 ml/min for stroke and systemic embolism prophylaxis in nonvalvular atrial fibrillation, dental procedures, aneurysm, diabetes retinopathy, diverticulitis, endocarditis, GI bleeding, hypertension, obstetric delivery, peptic ulcer disease, stroke, surgery

Black Box Warning: Abrupt discontinuation, epidermal/spinal anesthesia

Patients, especially those with dental disease, should be instructed in proper oral hygiene, including caution in use of regular toothbrushes, dental floss, toothpicks

DOSAGE AND ROUTES

DVT prophylaxis, which may lead to pulmonary embolism (PE) (knee or hip replacement)

• **Adult: PO** 10 mg/day × 12 days after knee replacement surgery or × 35 days after hip replacement; administer the initial dose ≥6-10 hr after surgery once hemostasis has been established

DVT/PE treatment/reduction of risk

• **Adult: PO** 15 mg bid with food × 21 days, then 20 mg daily for a total of 6 mo, may continue after 6 mo to reduce risk

Stroke prophylaxis and systemic embolism prophylaxis (with nonvalvular atrial fibrillation)

• Unless pathological bleeding occurs, do not discontinue rivaroxaban in the absence of alternative anticoagulation

• **Adult: PO** 20 mg/day with evening meal (CrCl >50 ml/min)

Converting from warfarin to rivaroxaban

• Discontinue warfarin and start rivaroxaban when INR is <3

Converting from another anticoagulant other than warfarin to rivaroxaban

• Start rivaroxaban 0-2 hr before the next scheduled evening administration of anticoagulant (omit that dose of anticoagulant); for continuous infusion of unfractionated heparin, stop the infusion and initiate rivaroxaban simultaneously

Converting from rivaroxaban to another anticoagulant with rapid onset (not warfarin)

• Discontinue rivaroxaban and give the first dose of the other anticoagulant (oral or parenteral) at the time that the next dose of rivaroxaban would have been administered

Hepatic Dose

• **Adult: PO** Child-Pugh class B or C: avoid use

Renal Dose

• **Adult: PO** (nonvalvular atrial fibrillation) CCr 15-50 ml/min 15 mg daily; CCr <15 ml/min avoid use; (treatment/prophylaxis of DVT/pulmonary embolism) CCr <30 ml/min avoid use

Available forms: Tabs 10, 15, 20 mg

Administer:

⚠ **For DVT prophylaxis:** give daily without regard to food; give initial dose ≥6-10 hr after surgery when hemostasis has been established

⚠ **For stroke/systemic embolism prophylaxis:** give daily with evening meal

• If dose is not given at correct time, give as soon as possible on the same day

• 15-, 20-mg tabs should be taken with food; for those unable to swallow whole, tabs may be crushed, mixed with applesauce; immediately following administration, instruct to eat; crushed tabs are stable in applesauce for up to 4 hr

• 10-mg tab can be taken without regard to food

Nasogastric (NG) tube or gastric feeding tube:

• Confirm gastric placement of tube

• Crush 15- or 20-mg tab, suspend in 50 ml of water, and administer via NG or gastric feeding tube

• To minimize reduced absorption, avoid administration distal to the stomach

• Enteral feeding should immediately follow administration of a crushed dose

• Crushed tabs are stable in water for up to 4 hr

Missed doses

• Patients receiving 15 mg twice daily should take their missed dose immediately to ensure intake of 30 mg per day; two 15-mg tabs may be taken at once followed by the regular 15 mg twice daily dose the next day

- For patients receiving once-daily dosing, take the missed dose as soon as it is remembered
- Store at room temperature

SIDE EFFECTS

GI: Increased hepatic enzymes, hyperbilirubinemia, jaundice, nausea, cholestasis, cytolytic hepatitis

HEMA: Bleeding, intracranial bleeding, epidural hematoma, GI bleeding, retinal hemorrhage, adrenal bleeding, retroperitoneal hemorrhage, cerebral hemorrhage, subdural hematoma, epidural hematoma, hemiparesis, thrombocytopenia

INTEG: Pruritus, blister, hypersensitivity, anaphylactic reaction, anaphylactic shock

SYST: Stevens-Johnson syndrome

PHARMACOKINETICS

Bioavailability 80%-100%, protein binding (92%-95%) albumin, excreted in urine 66% (36% unchanged, 30% metabolites), 28% in feces (7% unchanged, 21% metabolites), unchanged drug excreted in urine (via active tubular secretion, glomerular filtration); terminal elimination half-life 5-9 hr, peak 2-4 hr; increased effect in hepatic/renal disease, Japanese patients, increased terminal half-life in geriatric patients

INTERACTIONS

Increase: rivaroxaban effect, possible bleeding—ketoconazole itraconazole, ritonavir, lopinavir/ritonavir; conivaptan, clarithromycin, erythromycin, salicylates, NSAIDs, other anticoagulants, thrombolytics, platelet inhibitors, niCARdipine, fluconazole

Decrease: rivaroxaban effect—carBAMazepine, phenytoin, rifampin

Increase: rivaroxaban effect in renal impairment—telithromycin, darunavir, mifepristone, nelfinavir, pantoprazole, posaconazole, saquinavir, tamoxifen, lapatinib, azithromycin, diltiazem, verapamil, quiNIDine, ranolazine, dronedarone, amiodarone, felodipine

Drug/Herb:

Decrease: rivaroxaban effect—St. John's wort

Drug/Food:

Increase: rivaroxaban effect in renal disease—grapefruit juice

NURSING CONSIDERATIONS

Assess:

Black Box Warning: **Bleeding:** monitor for bleeding, including bleeding during dental procedures (easy bruising, blood in urine, stools, emesis, sputum, epistaxis); there is no specific antidote

Black Box Warning: **Abrupt discontinuation:** avoid abrupt discontinuation unless an alternative anticoagulant in those with atrial fibrillation; discontinuing puts patients at an increased risk of thrombotic events; if product must be discontinued for reasons other than pathological bleeding, consider administering another anticoagulant

- **Pregnancy/breastfeeding:** pregnancy (C); identify if pregnancy is suspected or planned; pregnancy-related hemorrhage may occur and anticoagulation cannot be monitored with standard laboratory testing; breastfeeding should be discontinued before beginning use of this product

Black Box Warning: **Epidural/spinal anesthesia:** epidural or spinal hematomas that result in long-term or permanent paralysis may occur in patients who have received anticoagulants and are receiving neuraxial anesthesia or undergoing spinal puncture; epidural catheter should not be removed <18 hr after the last dose of rivaroxaban; do not administer the next rivaroxaban dose <6 hr after the catheter removal; delay rivaroxaban administration for 24 hr if traumatic puncture occurs; monitor for neuro changes

• **Hepatic/renal disease:** increase in effect of product in hepatic disease (Child-Pugh class B or C), hepatic disease with coagulopathy; renal failure/severe renal impairment (creatinine clearance <30 ml/min in DVT prophylaxis and <15 ml/min for stroke or systemic embolism prophylaxis in nonvalvular atrial fibrillation); product should be discontinued in acute renal failure; reduce dose in those with atrial fibrillation and CrCl 15-50 ml/min; monitor renal function periodically (creatinine clearance, BUN)

Evaluate:

• Prevention of DVT, stroke, and systemic embolism

Teach patient/family:

• To report if pregnancy is planned or suspected; not to breastfeed

Black Box Warning: To report bleeding (bruising, blood in urine, stools, sputum, emesis, heavy menstrual flow); use soft toothbrush, electric shaver

• To inform all health care providers of use, report to prescriber all products used, to take only as directed

Black Box Warning: To avoid abrupt discontinuation without another blood thinner

• To report numbness of extremities, weakness, tingling, contact prescriber immediately (neuraxial anesthesia, spinal puncture)

rivastigmine (Rx)

(riv-as-tig′mine)

Exelon, Exelon Patch

Func. class.: Anti-Alzheimer agent

Chem. class.: Cholinesterase inhibitor

ACTION: Potent, selective inhibitor of brain acetylcholinesterase (AChE) and butyrylcholinesterase (BChE)

USES: Mild to severe Alzheimer's dementia, mild to moderate Parkinson's disease dementia (PDD)

Unlabeled uses: Vascular dementia, dementia with Lewy bodies, Pick's disease

CONTRAINDICATIONS: Hypersensitivity to this product, other carbamates

Precautions: Pregnancy (B), breastfeeding, children, respiratory/cardiac/renal/hepatic disease, seizure disorder, peptic ulcer, urinary obstruction, asthma, increased intracranial pressure, surgery, GI bleeding, jaundice

DOSAGE AND ROUTES

• **Adult: PO** 1.5 mg bid with food; after ≥4 wk, may increase to 3 mg bid; may increase to 4.5 mg bid and thereafter 6 mg bid, max 12 mg/day; **TRANSDERMAL** apply 4.6 mg/24 hr/day, after ≥4 wk may increase to 9.5 mg/24 hr/day; max 13.3 mg/24 hr; for those using 6-12 mg/day PO and switching to transdermal use one 9.5 mg/24 hr daily, for those using <6 mg/day PO and switching to transdermal use one 4.6 mg/24 hr daily

Available forms: Caps 1.5, 3, 4.5, 6 mg; transdermal patch 4.6, 9.5, 13.3 mg/24 hr

Administer:

• With meals; take with morning and evening meal even though absorption may be decreased

• Discontinue treatment for several doses; restart at same or next lower dosage level if adverse reactions cause intolerance

• If treatment is interrupted for more than several days, treatment should be initiated with lowest daily dose and titrated as indicated previously

Transdermal route

• Once a day to hairless, clean, dry skin, not in an area that clothing will rub; rotate sites daily; do not apply to same site more than once q14days; remove liner; apply firmly; may be used during bathing, swimming; avoid saunas, excess sunlight; or external heat such as saunas; each 5-cm^2 patch contains 9 mg base, rate of 4.6 mg/24 hr, each 10-cm^2 patch 18 mg base, rate of 9.5 mg/24 hr

SIDE EFFECTS

CV: **QT prolongation, AV block, cardiac arrest**, angina, MI, palpitations

CNS: *Tremors, confusion, insomnia,* psychosis, hallucination, depression, dizziness, headache, anxiety, somnolence, fatigue, syncope, EPS, exacerbation of Parkinson's disease

GI: *Nausea, vomiting, anorexia, abdominal distress, flatulence,* diarrhea, constipation, dyspepsia, colitis, eructation, fecal incontinence, **GI bleeding/obstruction**, GERD, gastritis, **pancreatitis**

MISC: Urinary tract infection, asthenia, increased sweating, hypertension, flulike symptoms, weight change

PHARMACOKINETICS

Rapidly and completely absorbed; peak 1 hr, metabolized to decarbamylated metabolite; half-life 1.5 hr; excreted via kidneys (metabolites); clearance lowered in geriatric patients, hepatic disease and increased with nicotine use; 40% protein binding

INTERACTIONS

Increase: synergistic effect—cholinergic agonists, other cholinesterase inhibitors

Increase: metabolism—nicotine

Increase: GI effects—NSAIDs

Decrease: rivastigmine effect—anticholinergics, sedating H_1 blockers, tricyclics, phenothiazines

NURSING CONSIDERATIONS

Assess:

- Hepatic studies: AST, ALT, alk phos, LDH, bilirubin, CBC
- **Severe GI effects:** nausea, vomiting, anorexia, weight loss, diarrhea, GI bleeding
- B/P, heart rate, respiration during initial treatment; hypo/hypertension should be reported
- **Cognitive/mental status:** affect, mood, behavioral changes, depression, insomnia; complete suicide assessment
- Assistance with ambulation during beginning therapy; dizziness may occur

Evaluate:

- Therapeutic response: improved mood/cognition

Teach patient/family:

- How to apply **transdermal** product, to fold in half and throw away, not to get in eyes, to wash hands after application; not to use heating pad, sauna, tanning bed
- To notify prescriber of severe GI effects
- That product may cause dizziness, anorexia, weight loss
- That effect may take weeks or months; not to discontinue abruptly
- To notify prescriber if pregnancy is planned or suspected
- To give with food in AM, PM
- To report nausea, vomiting, diarrhea
- To inform prescriber to all products taken

rizatriptan (Rx)

(rye-zah-trip′tan)

Maxalt, Maxalt-MLT

Func. class.: Migraine agent

Chem. class.: 5-HT_{1D} receptor agonist, abortive agent-triptan

R

ACTION:
Binds selectively to the vascular 5-$HT_{1B/1D}$ receptor subtype; exerts antimigraine effect; causes vasoconstriction of the cranial arteries

USES:
Acute treatment of migraine

CONTRAINDICATIONS:
Angina pectoris, history of MI, documented silent ischemia, Prinzmetal's angina,

ischemic heart disease, concurrent ergotamine-containing preparations, uncontrolled hypertension, hypersensitivity, basilar or hemiplegic migraine

Precautions: Pregnancy (C), breastfeeding, children, geriatric patients, postmenopausal women, men >40 yr, risk factors for CAD, hypercholesterolemia, obesity, diabetes, impaired renal/hepatic function

DOSAGE AND ROUTES

• **Adult: PO** 5-10 mg single dose, redosing separated by ≥2 hr, max 30 mg/24 hr; use 5 mg for patient receiving propranolol, max 15 mg/24 hr

Available forms: Tabs (Maxalt) 5, 10 mg; orally disintegrating tabs (Maxalt-MLT) 5, 10 mg

Administer:

• **Orally disintegrating tab:** do not open blister until use; peel blister open with dry hands; place tab on patient's tongue, where it will dissolve, and have patient swallow with saliva (contains phenylalanine)

• Not to be used for more than 3-4 times per month

SIDE EFFECTS

CNS: *Dizziness, drowsiness, headache, fatigue,* warm/cold sensations, flushing

CV: MI, ventricular fibrillation, ventricular tachycardia, coronary artery vasospasm, palpitations, hypertension, peripheral vascular ischemia, ECG changes

ENDO: Hot flashes, mild increase in growth hormone

GI: *Nausea,* dry mouth, diarrhea, abdominal pain, ischemic colitis

RESP: Chest tightness, pressure, dyspnea

PHARMACOKINETICS

Onset of pain relief 10 min-2 hr; peak 1-1½ hr; duration 14-16 hr; 14% plasma protein binding; metabolized in liver (metabolite); excreted in urine (82%), feces (12%); half-life 2-3 hr

INTERACTIONS

⚠ Weakness, hyperreflexia, incoordination: SSRIs

Increase: levels of sibutramine

Increase: rizatriptan action—cimetidine, oral contraceptives, MAOIs, nonselective MAOI (type A and B), isocarboxazide, pargyline, phenelzine, propranolol, tranylcypromine

Increase: vasospastic effects—ergot, ergot derivatives, other 5-HT receptor agonists

Drug/Herb

⚠ Serotonin syndrome: St. John's wort

NURSING CONSIDERATIONS

Assess:

• **Migraine symptoms:** visual disturbances, aura, intensity, nausea, vomiting, photophobia

• Stress level, activity, recreation, coping mechanisms

• Neurologic status: LOC, blurring vision, nausea, vomiting, tingling in extremities preceding headache

• **Ingestion of tyramine foods** (pickled products, beer, wine, aged cheese), food additives, preservatives, colorings, artificial sweeteners, chocolate, caffeine, which may precipitate these types of headaches

• Renal status: urine output

• Quiet, calm environment with decreased stimulation: noise, bright light, excessive talking

Evaluate:

• Therapeutic response: decrease in frequency, severity of headache

Teach patient/family:

• **About use of orally disintegrating tab:** instruct patient not to open blister until use, to peel blister open with dry hands, to place tab on tongue, where it will dissolve, and to swallow with saliva (contains phenylalanine)

• To report any side effects to prescriber

• To use alternative contraception while taking product if oral contraceptives are being used

• That product does not prevent or reduce number of migraines; if 1st dose does not relieve pain, do not use more; notify prescriber

---

⚠ Nurse Alert

roflumilast

Daliresp

Func. class.: Respiratory anti-inflammatory agent

Chem. class.: Phosphodiesterase-4 (PDE4) inhibitor

ACTION: Roflumilast (and the active metabolite roflumilast N-oxide) selectively inhibit phosphodiesterase-4 (PDE4); not a bronchodilator; inhibition of the PDE4 enzyme blocks the hydrolyses and inactivation of cyclic adenosine monophosphate (cAMP), resulting in intracellular cAMP accumulation; decreases inflammatory activity, PDE4 inhibition may affect migration and actions of proinflammatory cells (neutrophils, other leukocytes, T-lymphocytes, monocytes, macrophages, fibroblasts)

USES: For the prevention of COPD exacerbations in patients with severe COPD associated with chronic bronchitis and a history of exacerbations

CONTRAINDICATIONS: *Moderate to severe hepatic disease* (Child-Pugh B or C)

Precautions: Pregnancy (C), breastfeeding, neonates, infants, children, adolescents, acute bronchospasm, anxiety, insomnia, depression, suicidal ideation or behavior

DOSAGE AND ROUTES

• **Adult: PO** 500 mcg/day

Available forms: Tabs 500 mcg

Administer:

PO route

• Give without regard to meals
• Store at room temperature

SIDE EFFECTS

CNS: Insomnia, anxiety, depression, headache, dizziness, tremors, suicidal ideation

EENT: Rhinitis, sinusitis

GI: *Weight loss, diarrhea, nausea,* anorexia, abdominal pain, dyspepsia, gastritis, vomiting

GU: Urinary tract infection

MS: Back pain, muscle cramps/spasm

SYST: Infections, influenza

PHARMACOKINETICS

80% absolute bioavailability; protein binding 99% (roflumilast); 97% (N-oxide metabolite); low penetration across the blood–brain barrier; extensively metabolized (liver); metabolism by CYP3A4 and CYP1A2 produces (active metabolite N-oxide); half-life parent drug 17 hr, metabolite 30; steady-state 4 days (parent drug), 6 days (metabolite); 70% excreted in urine; parent drug peak 1 hr (range, 0.5-2 hr), metabolite peak 8 hr (range, 4-13 hr); contraindicated in moderate to severe hepatic impairment; use with caution in patients with mild hepatic

INTERACTIONS

Increase: roflumilast effect—CYP3A4/CYP1A2 inhibitors (enoxacin, cimetidine, delavirdine, indinavir, isoniazid, itraconazole, dalfopristin, quinupristin, tipranavir)

Increase: roflumilast effect—oral contraceptives (gestodene and ethinyl estradiol)

Decrease: roflumilast effect—CYP3A4 inducers (rifampin, barbiturates, carBAMazepine, phenytoin, erythromycin, ketoconazole, fluvoxaMINE, alcohol, etravirine, ritonavir, bexarotene, rifabutin, OXcarbazepine, nevirapine, modafinil, metyrapone, PHENobarbital, bosentan, dexamethasone)

Altered effect of: fosamprenavir

Drug/Herb

Decrease: roflumilast effect—St. John's wort

NURSING CONSIDERATIONS

Assess:

• Lung sounds and respiratory function baseline and periodically thereafter

R

⚠ Behavioral changes including mood, depression, suicidal thoughts/behaviors
- Liver function tests baseline and periodically thereafter; if increases in liver function studies occur, product should be discontinued
- Weight; weight loss is common

Evaluate:
- Decreasing exacerbations in COPD

Teach patient/family:
- To take product as directed; not to skip or double doses; to take missed doses as soon as remembered unless almost time for next dose
- Not to use OTC or other products without prescriber approval; not to discontinue other respiratory products unless approved by prescriber
- Not to be used for acute bronchospasm but may be continued during acute asthma attacks

⚠ **Suicidal thoughts/behaviors:** To notify prescriber of worsening depression or suicidal thoughts/behaviors

romiPLOStim (Rx)

(roe-mi-ploe′stim)

Nplate

Func. class.: Hematopoietin

Chem. class.: Thrombopoietin receptor agonist

ACTION: Thrombopoietin-like fusion protein produced by DNA recombinant technology

USES: Chronic idiopathic thrombocytopenic purpura in patients who have had an insufficient response to corticosteroids, immunoglobulins, or splenectomy

CONTRAINDICATIONS: Hypersensitivity to this product or mannitol

Precautions: Pregnancy (C), breastfeeding, children, malignancies, bleeding, bone marrow suppression

DOSAGE AND ROUTES

Thrombocytopenia in chronic idiopathic thrombocytopenic purpura (ITP) with insufficient response to corticosteroids, immunoglobulins, splenectomy

- **Adult: SUBCUT** 1 mcg/kg q wk (based on actual body weight); increase the weekly dosage by 1 mcg/kg until platelet count $\geq$50,000/mm^3; 10 mcg/kg/wk max; use the lowest dosage needed to achieve and maintain a platelet count $\geq$50,000/mm^3; monitor CBC, including platelet counts, weekly until a stable platelet count is achieved with platelets $\geq$50,000/mm^3 $\geq$4 wk without dosage adjustment; then monitor the CBC, including platelet counts, monthly; once a stable dosage is achieved, if the platelet count falls to $<$50,000/mm^3, increase the dosage by 1 mcg/kg/wk; if the platelet count increases to $>$200,000/mm^3 for 2 consecutive weeks, reduce the dosage by 1 mcg/kg; if the platelet count is $>$400,000/mm^3, temporarily stop romiPLOStim and continue to monitor the platelet count every wk; once the platelets are $<$200,000/mm^3, restart, but reduce the previous dosage by 1 mcg/kg/wk; romiPLOStim may be administered concomitantly with other medical ITP therapies; if platelet counts exceed 50,000/mm^3, other medical ITP therapies may be reduced or discontinued; discontinue romiPLOStim if the platelet count does not increase to avoid important bleeding after 4 wk of therapy at max dosage of 10 mcg/kg

Available forms: Inj vials 250, 500 mcg

Administer:
- Refrigerated storage of vials; do not freeze; protect from light; diluted sol is stable refrigerated or at room temperature for 24 hr

SUBCUT route
- Use syringe with 0.01-ml graduations
- Discard any unused portion in vial; do not pool unused portions from vials

- Dilute 250 mcg/0.72 preservative-free sterile water for inj; 500 mcg/1.2 preservative-free sterile water for inj; final concentration 500 mcg/ml
- Gently swirl until dissolved; do not shake
- Do not use if discolored or if particulate matter is present
- Inject into outer aspect of upper arm or abdomen except for 2 inches around navel or front aspect of middle thigh; do not use areas that are bruised, scratched, or scarred
- Rotate inj sites

SIDE EFFECTS

CNS: *Dizziness, insomnia, headache,* fatigue
GI: Abdominal pain, dyspepsia, diarrhea
HEMA: Thromboembolism, thrombosis, bleeding, myelofibrosis, erythromelalgia
MS: Myalgia
SYST: Secondary malignancy, antibody formation

PHARMACOKINETICS

Peak 7-50 hr, half-life 1-34 days

INTERACTIONS

- Possible bleeding risk: anticoagulants, NSAIDs, platelet inhibitors, thrombolytics, salicylates

NURSING CONSIDERATIONS

Assess:

- Blood studies: CBC during treatment weekly and for 2 wk after discontinuing
- **Bone marrow suppression:** if cytopenias occur, product should be discontinued; may use a bone marrow biopsy and staining for fibrosis
- **Thromboembolic disease:** do not use to normalize patients; use only in those with thrombocytopenia in idiopathic thrombocytopenic purpura, maintain platelets ≥ 50,000/mm³

Evaluate:

- Therapeutic response: increase in platelet counts, absence of bleeding

Teach patient/family:

- To report bleeding
- About the reason for product and expected results; to avoid hazardous activities that may cause bleeding
- To report a missed dose to prescriber due to increased risk of bleeding
- That lab tests will be done weekly and dose may be changed; if dose is not changed, lab will be checked monthly; after drug is discontinued, labs will be checked weekly × 2 wk
- To advise prescriber if spleen has been removed, bleeding or clotting problems
- To notify prescriber if pregnancy is planned or suspected, pregnancy (C); if pregnancy occurs, call registry 1-877-675-2831

rOPINIRole (Rx)

(roh-pin′ih-role)

Requip, Requip XL

Func. class.: Antiparkinson agent
Chem. class.: DOPamine-receptor agonist, nonergot

Do not confuse:
rOPINIRole/risperiDONE

ACTION:

Selective agonist for D_2 receptors (presynaptic/postsynaptic sites); binding at D_3 receptor contributes to antiparkinson effects

USES:

Parkinson's disease, restless leg syndrome (RLS)

R

CONTRAINDICATIONS:

Hypersensitivity

Precautions: Pregnancy (C), dysrhythmias, affective disorder, psychosis, cardiac/renal/hepatic disease

DOSAGE AND ROUTES

Parkinson's disease

- **Adult: PO (regular release)** Initially, 0.25 mg PO tid × 1 wk; gradually titrate at weekly intervals: **Week 2,** 0.5 mg tid; **Week 3,** 0.75 mg tid; **Week 4,** 1 mg tid; **After week 4,** may increase by 1.5 mg/day each week, max 9 mg/day total dosage, and then by 3 mg/day each week, max 24 mg/day

• **PO (ext rel)** initially, 2 mg/day × 1-2 wk, may increase by mg/day at intervals ≥1 wk based upon response; max 24 mg/day; if significant interruption of therapy occurs, retitration may be necessary

Conversion from immediate-release to extended-release tablets

• **Adult: PO** currently taking 0.75-2.25 mg/day imm rel: give 2 mg/day ext rel

• **PO** currently taking 3-4.5 mg/day imm rel: give 4 mg/day ext rel

• **PO** currently taking 6 mg/day imm rel: give 6 mg/day ext rel

• **PO** currently taking 7.5-9 mg/day imm rel: give 8 mg/day ext rel

• **PO** currently taking 12 mg/day imm rel: give 12 mg/day ext rel

• **PO** currently taking 15-18 mg/day imm rel: give 16 mg/day ext rel

• **PO** currently taking 21 mg/day imm rel: give 20 mg/day ext rel

• **PO** currently taking 24 mg/day imm rel: give 24 mg/day ext rel

Restless legs syndrome

• **Adult: PO (reg rel)** Initially, 0.25 mg every day 1-3 hr before bedtime; days 3-7, may increase to 0.5 mg every day; at the beginning of wk 2 (day 8); the dosage may be increased to 1 mg every day × 1 wk; weeks 3-6, dosage may be titrated up by 0.5 mg each wk (from 1.5-3 mg over the 5-wk period) as needed to achieve desired effect; wk 7, may increase dosage to 4 mg/day; dosage is titrated based on clinical response; give all doses 1-3 hr before bedtime

Available forms: Tabs 0.25, 0.5, 1, 2, 3, 4, 5 mg; ext rel tab 2, 4, 6, 8, 12 mg

Administer:

• Product until NPO before surgery

• Adjust dosage to patient response; taper when discontinuing

• With meals to reduce nausea

• **Extended release:** do not chew, crush, or divide

• Testing for diabetes mellitus, acromegaly if patient receiving long-term therapy

SIDE EFFECTS

CNS: *Agitation, insomnia,* psychosis, hallucination, dystonia, depression, dizziness, somnolence, sleep attacks, impulse control disorders

CV: *Orthostatic hypotension,* tachycardia, hypo/hypertension, syncope, palpitations

EENT: Blurred vision

GI: *Nausea, vomiting, anorexia, dry mouth,* constipation, dyspepsia, flatulence

GU: Impotence, urinary frequency

HEMA: Hemolytic anemia, leukopenia, agranulocytosis

INTEG: Rash, sweating

RESP: Pharyngitis, rhinitis, sinusitis, bronchitis, dyspnea

PHARMACOKINETICS

Peak 1-2 hr, half-life 6 hr, extensively metabolized by liver by P450 CYP1A2 enzyme system, protein binding 40%

INTERACTIONS

Increase: rOPINIRole effect—cimetidine, ciprofloxacin, diltiazem, enoxacin, erythromycin, fluvoxaMINE, mexiletine, norfloxacin, tacrine, digoxin, theophylline, L-dopa

Decrease: rOPINIRole effects—butyrophenones, metoclopramide, phenothiazines, thioxanthenes

NURSING CONSIDERATIONS

Assess:

• **Parkinsonism:** akinesia, tremors, staggering gait, muscle rigidity, drooling

• B/P, respirations during initial treatment; hypo/hypertension should be reported

⚠ **Sleep attacks:** drowsiness, falling asleep without warning even during hazardous activities

• Mental status: affect, mood, behavioral changes, depression; complete suicide assessment; worsening of symptoms in restless leg syndrome

Evaluate:

• Therapeutic response: improvement in movement disorder

⚠ Nurse Alert

Teach patient/family:

• To notify prescriber if pregnancy is planned or suspected, pregnancy (C), breastfeeding

• To take with food to prevent nausea

• To report hallucinations, confusion (usually in geriatric patients)

• That therapeutic effects may take several weeks to a few months

• To change positions slowly to prevent orthostatic hypotension

• To use product exactly as prescribed; if product is discontinued abruptly, parkinsonian crisis may occur

• That drowsiness, sleep attacks may occur; to avoid driving, other hazardous activities until response known

• To avoid alcohol, CNS depressants, cough and cold products

⚠ To notify prescriber if unusual urges occur

⚠ HIGH ALERT

rosiglitazone (Rx)

(ros-ih-glit′ah-zone)

Avandia

Func. class.: Antidiabetic, oral

Chem. class.: Thiazolidinedione

Do not confuse:

rosiglitazone/pioglitazone

Avandia/Prandin

ACTION: Improves insulin resistance by hepatic glucose metabolism, insulin receptor kinase activity, insulin receptor phosphorylation

USES: Type 2 diabetes mellitus, alone or in combination with sulfonylureas, metformin, insulin

CONTRAINDICATIONS: Breastfeeding, children, hypersensitivity to thiazolidinediones, diabetic ketoacidosis, jaundice

Black Box Warning: NYHA III, IV acute heart failure, heart failure

Precautions: Pregnancy (C), geriatric patients, thyroid disease, renal/hepatic disease, heart failure, class I, II NYHA

Black Box Warning: MI

DOSAGE AND ROUTES

• **Adult: PO** 4 mg/day or in 2 divided doses, may increase to 8 mg/day or in 2 divided doses after 12 wk; may be added to metformin, sulfonylurea for adult dose

Available forms: Tabs 2, 4, 8 mg

Administer:

• Conversion from other oral hypoglycemic agents if needed; change may be made without gradual dosage change; monitor blood glucose during conversion

• Store in tight container in cool environment

PO route

• Once or in 2 divided doses, without regard to food

• Tabs crushed and mixed with food or fluids for patients with difficulty swallowing

• Only through the REMS Program 1-800-Avandia

SIDE EFFECTS

CNS: Fatigue, *headache*

CV: **MI, CHF, death (geriatric patients)**

ENDO: Hypo/hyperglycemia

GI: Weight gain, **hepatotoxicity**, increase total, LDL, HDL cholesterol; decrease free fatty acids, diarrhea

MISC: Accidental injury, URI, sinusitis, anemia, back pain, diarrhea, edema, bone fractures (female), pulmonary/macular/peripheral edema

SYST: **Anaphylaxis, Stevens-Johnson syndrome**

PHARMACOKINETICS

Maximal reductions in FBS after 6-12 wk; protein binding 99.8%; excreted in urine, feces; elimination half-life 3-4 hr; may be excreted in breast milk

INTERACTIONS

Increase: hypoglycemia—gemfibrozil, fluvoxaMINE, ketoconazole, trimethoprim; monitor glucose

R

- Avoid concurrent use with insulin, nitrates
- May increase or decrease level: CYP2C5 inducer/inhibitors

Drug/Herb

Increase: antidiabetic effect—garlic, horse chestnut

Drug/Lab Test

Increase: ALT, HDL, LDL, total cholesterol, blood glucose

Decrease: Hgb/Hct

NURSING CONSIDERATIONS

Assess:

Black Box Warning: CHF/MI: dyspnea, crackles, edema, weight gain ≥5 lb, jugular venous distention; may need to change dose or discontinue product, do not use in acute coronary syndrome, NYHA Class 3/IV heart failure

- Hypoglycemic reactions (sweating, weakness, dizziness, anxiety, tremors, hunger), hyperglycemic reactions soon after meals
- ⚠ Systemic reactions: anaphylaxis, Stevens-Johnson syndrome
- ⚠ **Hepatotoxicity:** LFTs periodically AST, ALT (if ALT >2.5 × ULN, do not use product)
- Fasting blood sugar, A1c, plasma lipids/lipoproteins, B/P, body weight during treatment
- To use product provider/patient must be enrolled in the Avandia-Rosiglitazone Medicines Access Program

Evaluate:

- Therapeutic response: decrease in polyuria, polydipsia, polyphagia; clear sensorium; absence of dizziness; stable gait; blood glucose, A1c improvement

Teach patient/family:

- To monitor blood glucose; that periodic liver function tests mandatory; to report edema, weight gain
- About the symptoms of hypo/hyperglycemia, what to do about each
- That product must be continued on daily basis; about the consequences of discontinuing the product abruptly
- To avoid OTC medications, herbal preparations, nitrates, or insulin unless approved by prescriber
- That diabetes is lifelong; that product is not a cure, only controls symptoms
- That all food included in diet plan must be eaten to prevent hypoglycemia
- To carry emergency ID and glucagon emergency kit
- ⚠ To report symptoms of hepatic dysfunction (nausea, vomiting, abdominal pain, fatigue, anorexia, dark urine, jaundice) immediately; to report macular edema (change in vision)
- That 2 wk is needed to see reduction in blood glucose level and 2-3 mo needed to see full effect of product
- To notify prescriber if oral contraceptives are used
- Not to use if breastfeeding, may be secreted in breast milk
- That a medication guide should be dispensed with each prescription/refill

rosuvastatin (Rx)

(roe-soo′va-sta-tin)

Crestor

Func. class.: Antilipemic

Chem. class.: HMG-CoA reductase inhibitor

ACTION: Inhibits HMG-CoA reductase enzyme, which reduces cholesterol synthesis

USES: As an adjunct for primary hypercholesterolemia (types IIa, IIb) and mixed dyslipidemia, elevated serum triglycerides, homozygous/heterozygous familial hypercholesterolemia (FH), slowing of atherosclerosis, CV disease prophylaxis, MI, stroke prophylaxis (normal LDL)

CONTRAINDICATIONS: Pregnancy (X), breastfeeding, hypersensitivity, active hepatic disease

Precautions: Children <10 yr, geriatric patients, past hepatic disease, alcoholism, severe acute infections, trauma, hypotension, uncontrolled seizure disorders, severe metabolic disorders, electrolyte imbalances, severe renal impairment, hypothyroidism, Asian patients

DOSAGE AND ROUTES

Hypercholesterolemia

- **Adult: PO** 5-40 mg/day; initial dose 10 mg/day, reanalyze lipid levels at 2-4 wk, adjust dosage accordingly

Homozygous familial hypercholesterolemia

- **Adult: PO** 20 mg/day, max 40 mg; Asian patients 5 mg/day

Dose in patients taking cycloSPORINE/gemfibrozil/lopinavir/ritonavir/atazanavir

- **Adult: PO** 5 mg/day, max 10 mg/day

Asian patients/patients with predisposition for myopathy

- **Adult: PO** 5 mg/day

Atherosclerosis slowing

- **Adult: PO** 10 mg/day (for those not taking cycloSPORINE or gemfibrozil)

Heterozygous familial hypercholesterolemia

- **Females ≥1 yr postmenarche and ≥10 yr): PO** 5-20 mg/day individualized

MI/stroke prophylaxis (unlabeled)

- **Adult: PO** 20 mg daily

Renal/hepatic dose

- **Adult: PO CCr <30 ml/min, 5 mg/day; max 10 mg/day; avoid use with hepatic disease**

Available forms: Tabs 5, 10, 20, 40 mg

Administer:

- May be taken at any time of day, with/without food
- Store in cool environment in airtight, light-resistant container

SIDE EFFECTS

CNS: *Headache, dizziness,* insomnia, paresthesia, confusion

GI: *Nausea, constipation, abdominal pain, flatus, diarrhea, dyspepsia, heartburn,* **kidney failure, liver dysfunction,** vomiting

HEMA: **Thrombocytopenia, hemolytic anemia, leukopenia**

INTEG: *Rash, pruritus*

MS: *Asthenia, muscle cramps, arthritis, arthralgia, myalgia,* **myositis, rhabdomyolysis;** leg, shoulder, or localized pain

PHARMACOKINETICS

Peak 3-5 hr, minimal live metabolism (about 10%), 88% protein bound, excreted primarily in feces (90%), crosses placenta, half-life 19 hr, not dialyzable

INTERACTIONS

Increase: hepatotoxicity—alcohol

⚠ **Increase: myalgia, myositis, rhabdomyolysis—cycloSPORINE, gemfibrozil, niacin, clofibrate, azole antifungals, antiretroviral protease inhibitors, fibric acid derivatives**

Increase: bleeding risk—warfarin

Drug/Lab Test

Increase: LFTs

NURSING CONSIDERATIONS

Assess:

- Diet; obtain diet history including fat, cholesterol in diet
- Fasting cholesterol, LDL, HDL, triglycerides at baseline and q4-6wk, then periodically
- Liver function: LFTs at baseline, 12 wk, then q6mo; AST, ALT, LFTs may increase
- Renal function in patients with compromised renal system: BUN, creatinine, I&O ratio

⚠ **Rhabdomyolysis: muscle pain, tenderness, obtain CPK; if these occur, product may need to be discontinued; for patients with Asian ancestry: increased blood levels, rhabdomyolysis**

Evaluate:

- Therapeutic response: decreased LDL, cholesterol, triglycerides, increased HDL, slowing CAD

Teach patient/family:

⚠ **To report suspected pregnancy; to use contraception while taking product, pregnancy (X); not to breastfeed**

R

⚠ To report weakness, muscle tenderness, pain, fever, liver injury (jaundice, anorexia, abdominal pain)
- That blood work and follow-up exams will be necessary during treatment
- To report severe GI symptoms, dizziness, headache, muscle pain, weakness
- That previously prescribed regimen will continue: low-cholesterol diet, exercise program, smoking cessation

rufinamide (Rx)

(roo-fin′a-mide)

Banzel

Func. class.: Anticonvulsant

Chem. class.: Triazole derivative

ACTION: May act through action at sodium channels; exact action is unknown

USES: Lennox-Gastaut syndrome

Unlabeled uses: Partial seizures

CONTRAINDICATIONS: Hypersensitivity, familial short QT syndrome

Precautions: Pregnancy (C), breastfeeding, children <16 yr, geriatric patients, renal/hepatic disease, depression, dialysis, hazardous activities, suicidal ideation

DOSAGE AND ROUTES

- **Adult: PO** 400-800 mg/day divided bid; increase by 400-800 mg/day q2days to 3200 mg/day
- **Child ≥4 yr: PO** 10 mg/kg/day divided equally bid; increase by 10 mg/kg/day every other day to 45 mg/kg/day or 3200 mg/day, whichever is less

Available forms: Tabs 200, 400 mg; oral susp 40 mg/ml

Administer:

- **PO tabs:** give with food; may give whole, crushed, or halved
- **Oral susp:** shake well before use; use provided adapter and calibrated oral dosing syringe; insert adapter firmly in neck of bottle before use; keep in place for duration of bottle use; insert dosing syringe into adapter; withdraw dose from inverted bottle; replace cap after each use; use within 90 days of opening; give with food

SIDE EFFECTS

CNS: Dizziness, ataxia, drowsiness, fever, seizures, tremors, fatigue, headache, gait disturbance, suicidal ideation

EENT: Diplopia, blurred vision, nystagmus

GI: Nausea, hepatitis, vomiting, abdominal pain

HEMA: Anemia, leukopenia, neutropenia, thrombocytopenia, lymphadenopathy, DRESS

INTEG: Rash, urticaria, Stevens-Johnson syndrome

MISC: Edema, hematuria, influenzae, nephrolithiasis, back pain, urinary frequency

PHARMACOKINETICS

Peak 4-6 hr, half-life 6-10 hr, metabolized by liver, excreted by kidneys, 34% protein binding

INTERACTIONS

Increase: rufinamide effect—valproate

Decrease: effect of hormonal contraceptives

Decrease: effect of rufinamide—carBAMazepine, phenytoin, primidone, PHENobarbital

Drug/Lab Test

Increase: LFTs

NURSING CONSIDERATIONS

Assess:

- **Seizures:** duration, type, intensity precipitating factors

⚠ Mental status: mood, sensorium, affect, memory (long, short), increased suicidal thoughts/actions

Evaluate:

- Therapeutic response: decrease in severity of seizures

Teach patient/family:

- Not to discontinue product abruptly because seizures may occur

- To avoid hazardous activities until stabilized on product
- To carry emergency ID stating product use
- To notify prescriber if pregnancy is planned or suspected; to use alternative form of contraception because effect of hormonal contraceptives may be decreased
- To consume adequate fluids
- To report suicidal thoughts/behavior immediately
- To report rash/fever to prescriber

R

salicylic acid topical

See Appendix B

salmeterol (Rx)

(sal-met′er-ole)

Serevent ♣, Serevent Diskus

Func. class.: β_2-Adrenergic agonist, bronchodilator

ACTION: Causes bronchodilation by action on β_2 (pulmonary) receptors by increasing levels of cAMP, which relaxes smooth muscle with little effect on heart rate; maintains improvement in FEV from 3 to 12 hr; prevents nocturnal asthma symptoms

USES: Prevention of exercise-induced bronchospasm, COPD, asthma

CONTRAINDICATIONS: Hypersensitivity to sympathomimetics, tachydysrhythmias, severe cardiac disease, monotherapy treatment of asthma

Precautions: Pregnancy (C), breastfeeding, cardiac disorders, hyperthyroidism, diabetes mellitus, hypertension, closed-angle glaucoma, seizures, acute asthma, as a substitute to corticosteroids, QT prolongation

Black Box Warning: Asthma-related death, children <4 yr

DOSAGE AND ROUTES

- **Adult/child ≥4 yr: INH** 50 mcg (1 inhalation as dry powder) q12hr; **exercise-induced bronchospasm** 50 mcg (1 inhalation) ½-1 hr before exercise

Available forms: Inhalation powder 50 mcg/blister

Administer:

- Gum, sips of water for dry mouth
- Use ½ hr before exercise for exercise-induced bronchospasm prevention
- Do not use spacer with this product
- Store in foil pouch; do not expose to temperature >86° F (30° C); discard 6 wk after removal from foil pouch

SIDE EFFECTS

CNS: *Tremors, anxiety,* insomnia, headache, dizziness, fever

CV: Palpitations, tachycardia, hypo/hypertension, angina, dysrhythmias

EENT: Dry nose, irritation of nose and throat

GI: Heartburn, nausea, vomiting, abdominal pain

MS: Muscle cramps

RESP: Bronchospasm, cough

PHARMACOKINETICS

INH: Onset 30-50 min; peak 4 hr; duration 12 hr; metabolized in liver; excreted in urine, breast milk; crosses placenta, blood-brain barrier; protein binding 94%-98%; terminal half-life 3-5 hr

INTERACTIONS

Increase: CV effect—CYP3A4 inhibitors (itraconazole, ketoconazole, nelfinavir, nefazodone, saquinavir)

Increase: action of aerosol bronchodilators

Increase: action of salmeterol—tricyclics, MAOIs

Decrease: salmeterol action—other β-blockers

NURSING CONSIDERATIONS

Assess:

- **Respiratory function:** vital capacity, forced expiratory volume, ABGs, lung sounds, heart rate and rhythm
- ⚠ **Paradoxical bronchospasm:** dyspnea, wheezing, chest tightness

Black Box Warning: Children should not use this product as monotherapy for asthma, use only with persistent asthma in those whose symptoms are not well-controlled with a long-term asthma product

Evaluate:

- Therapeutic response: absence of dyspnea, wheezing

Teach patient/family:

- Not to use for exercise-induced bronchospasm; never to exhale into diskus; to hold level, keep mouthpiece dry
- Not to use OTC medications because extra stimulation may occur
- Review package insert with patient
- To avoid getting powder in eyes
- To avoid smoking, smoke-filled rooms, persons with respiratory infections
- Not for treatment of acute exacerbation, a fast-acting β-blocker should be used instead

⚠ To immediately report dyspnea after use if ≥1 canister is used in 2 mo time

- To notify prescriber if >4 inhalations are needed, or if product is no longer working
- Not to get canister or mouthpiece wet, not to use spacer, not to exhale into mouthpiece
- To take other products as prescribed

TREATMENT OF OVERDOSE:
β_2-Adrenergic blocker

⚠ HIGH ALERT

sargramostim (GM-CSF) (Rx)

(sar-gram′oh-stim)

Leukine, GM-CSF

Func. class.: Biologic modifier

Chem. class.: Granulocyte macrophage colony-stimulating factor (GM-CSF)

Do not confuse:
Leukine/leucovorin/Leukeran

ACTION:
Stimulates proliferation and differentiation of hematopoietic progenitor cells (granulocytes, macrophages)

USES:
Acceleration of myeloid recovery in patients with non–Hodgkin's lymphoma, acute lymphoblastic leukemia, acute myelogenous leukemia, autologous bone marrow transplantation in Hodgkin's disease; bone marrow transplantation failure or engraftment delay, mobilization and transplant of peripheral blood progenitor cells (PBPCs)

Unlabeled uses: Aplastic anemia, Crohn's disease, HIV, ganciclovir- or zidovudine-induced neutropenia, malignant melanoma

CONTRAINDICATIONS:
Neonates; hypersensitivity to GM-CSF, benzyl alcohol, yeast products; excessive leukemic myeloid blast in bone marrow, peripheral blood

Precautions: Pregnancy (C), breastfeeding, children; lung/cardiac/renal/hepatic disease; pleural, pericardial effusions, peripheral edema, leukocytosis, mannitol hypersensitivity, hepatic/renal disease

DOSAGE AND ROUTES

Myeloid recovery in Hodgkin's disease, non-Hodgkin's lymphoma, acute lymphocytic leukemia

Adult: IV 250 mcg/m^2/day over a 2-hr period beginning 2-4 hrs after infusion of bone marrow and not <24 hrs after last dose of chemotherapy or radiotherapy

Child (unlabeled): SUBCUT/IV 250 mcg/m^2/day beginning 2-4 hrs after infusion of bone marrow and not <24 hrs after last dose of chemotherapy

Acceleration of myeloid recovery

- **Adult: IV** 250 mcg/m^2/day × 14 days; give over 2 hr; may repeat in 7 days; may repeat 500 mcg/m^2/day × 14 days after another 7 days if no improvement

Mobilization of PBPCs

- **Adult: IV/SUBCUT** 250 mcg/m^2/day during collection of PBPCs

After PBPC transplantation

- **Adult: IV/SUBCUT** 250 mcg/m^2/day until ANC >1500 cells/mm^3 × 3 days

Aplastic anemia (unlabeled)

- **Adult: SUBCUT** 250-500 mcg/day or 5 mcg/kg/day × 14-90 days, used with erythropoietin or immunosuppressive therapy

HIV (unlabeled)

- **Adult: SUBCUT** 250 mcg/m^2/day 3×/wk for ≤20 mo

S

Available forms: Powder for inj lyophilized 250 mcg; sol for inj 500 mcg/ml

Administer:

- Store in refrigerator; do not freeze

SUBCUT route

- No further dilution of reconstituted sol is needed; take care not to inject intradermally

Intermittent IV INFUSION route

- After reconstituting with 1 ml sterile water for inj without preservative; do not reenter vial; discard unused portion; direct reconstitution sol at side of vial; rotate contents; do not shake
- Dilute in 0.9% NaCl inj to prepare IV infusion; if final concentration is <10 mcg/ml, add human albumin to make final concentration of 0.1% to NaCl before adding sargramostim to prevent adsorption; for a final concentration of 0.1% albumin, add 1 mg human albumin/1 ml 0.9% NaCl inj run over 2 hr **(bone marrow transplant or failure of graft)**; over 4 hr **(chemotherapy for AML)**; over 24 hr as cont infusion **(PBPCs)**; give within 6 hr after reconstitution

Y-site compatibilities: Amikacin, aminophylline, aztreonam, bleomycin, butorphanol, calcium gluconate, CARBOplatin, carmustine, ceFAZolin, cefepime, cefotaxime, cefoTEtan, ceftizoxime, cefTRIAXone, cefuroxime, cimetidine, CISplatin, clindamycin, cyclophosphamide, cycloSPORINE, cytarabine, dacarbazine, DACTINomycin, dexamethasone, diphenhydrAMINE, DOPamine, DOXOrubicin, doxycycline, droperidol, etoposide, famotidine, fentaNYL, floxuridine, fluconazole, fluorouracil, furosemide, gentamicin, granisetron, heparin, IDArubicin, ifosfamide, immune globulin, magnesium sulfate, mannitol, mechlorethamine, meperidine, mesna, methotrexate, metoclopramide, metroNIDAZOLE, minocycline, mitoXANtrone, netilmicin, pentostatin, piperacillin/tazobactam, potassium chloride, prochlorperazine, promethazine, ranitidine, teniposide, ticarcillin, ticarcillin-clavulanate, trimethoprim-sulfamethoxazole, vinBLAStine, vinCRIStine, zidovudine

SIDE EFFECTS

CNS: Fever, malaise, CNS disorder, weakness, chills, dizziness, syncope, headache

CV: Transient supraventricular tachycardia, peripheral edema, pericardial effusion, hypotension, tachycardia

GI: Nausea, vomiting, diarrhea, anorexia, GI hemorrhage, stomatitis, liver damage, hyperbilirubinemia

GU: Urinary tract disorder, abnormal kidney function

HEMA: Blood dyscrasias, hemorrhage

INTEG: Alopecia, rash, peripheral edema

MS: Bone pain, myalgia

RESP: Dyspnea

PHARMACOKINETICS

Half-life elimination: IV 60 min, SUBCUT 2-3 hr; detected within 5 min after administration, peak 2 hr

INTERACTIONS

Increase: myeloproliferation—lithium, corticosteroids

Drug/Lab Test

Increase: bilirubin, BUN, creatinine, eosinophils, LFTs, leukocytes

NURSING CONSIDERATIONS

Assess:

⚠ Blood studies: CBC, differential count before treatment, 2 × weekly; leukocytosis may occur (WBC $>$50,000 cells/mm^3, ANC $>$20,000 cells/mm^3), platelets; if ANC $>$20,000/mm^3 or 10,000/mm^3 after nadir has occurred or platelets $>$500,000/mm^3, reduce dose by ½ or discontinue; if blast cells occur, discontinue

- Renal, hepatic studies before treatment: BUN, creatinine, urinalysis; AST, ALT, alk phos; 2 × weekly monitoring is needed in renal/hepatic disease
- **Hypersensitivity**, rashes, local inj-site reactions; usually transient
- Body weight, hydration status; increased fluid retention in cardiac disease; pulmonary function
- Constitutional symptoms: asthenia, chills, fever, headache, malaise
- Myalgia, arthralgia in legs, feet; use analgesics, antipyretics

• **Gasping syndrome in neonates:** due to benzyl alcohol hypersensitivity, do not use

Evaluate:

• Therapeutic response: WBC and differential recovery

Teach patient/family:

• To report dyspnea to health care provider
• Review all aspects of product use

⚠ HIGH ALERT

saxagliptin (Rx)

(sax-a-glip′tin)

Onglyza

Func. class.: Antidiabetic, oral

Chem. class.: Dipeptidyl-peptidase-4 inhibitor (DPP-4 inhibitor)

Do not confuse:
saxagliptin/sitaGLIPtin

ACTION: Slows the inactivation of incretin hormones; improves glucose homeostasis, improves glucose-dependent insulin synthesis, lowers glucagon secretions, and slows gastric emptying time

USES: In adults, type 2 diabetes mellitus as monotherapy or in combination with other antidiabetic agents

CONTRAINDICATIONS: Hypersensitivity, angioedema

Precautions: Pregnancy (B), geriatric patients, GI obstruction, surgery, thyroid/renal/hepatic disease, trauma, diabetic ketoacidosis (DKA), type 1 diabetes, heart failure

DOSAGE AND ROUTES

• **Adult: PO** 2.5-5 mg; may use with other antidiabetic agents other than insulin; if used with insulin, a lower dose may be needed; max 2.5 mg with strong 3A415 inhibitors

Renal dose

• **Adult: PO** CCr ≤50 ml/min, 2.5 mg daily

Available forms: Tabs 2.5, 5 mg

Administer:

PO route

• May be taken with/without food
• Do not break or cut tabs
• Conversion from other antidiabetic agents; change may be made with gradual dosage change
• Store in tight containers at room temperature

SIDE EFFECTS

CNS: *Headache*
RESP: Upper respiratory infection
ENDO: Hypoglycemia (renal impairment)
GI: *Nausea, vomiting,* abdominal pain, **pancreatitis**
INTEG: Urticaria, **angioedema, anaphylaxis**
MISC: Lymphopenia, peripheral edema
CV: Edema
EENT: Sinusitis
GU: UTI
META: Hypoglycemia

PHARMACOKINETICS

Rapidly absorbed, excreted by the kidneys (unchanged 24%), terminal half-life 2.5 hr, 3.1 hr metabolite, peak 2 hr, duration 24 hr

INTERACTIONS

Increase: hypoglycemia—androgens, insulins, β-blockers, cimetidine, corticosteroids, salicylates, MAOIs, fibric acid derivatives, FLUoxetine, insulin, sulfonylureas, ACE inhibitors; strong CYP3A4/5 inhibitors

Drug/Herb

Increase: antidiabetic effect—garlic, horse chestnut

Drug/Lab Test

Decrease: lymphocytes, glucose

NURSING CONSIDERATIONS

Assess:

• **Hypoglycemic reactions** (sweating, weakness, dizziness, anxiety, tremors, hunger); monitor blood glucose, HbA1c **renal studies:** BUN, creatinine during treatment

S

• **Heart failure:** history of risk factors for heart failure, use cautiously in these patients

• **Pancreatitis:** abdominal pain, nausea, vomiting; discontinue

Evaluate:

• Therapeutic response: decrease in polyuria, polydipsia, polyphagia; clear sensorium; absence of dizziness; stable gait, blood glucose at normal level

Teach patient/family:

• To perform regular self-monitoring of blood glucose using blood-glucose meter

• About the symptoms of hypo/hyperglycemia; what to do about each

• That product must be continued on daily basis; about consequences of discontinuing product abruptly

• To avoid OTC medications, alcohol, digoxin, exenatide, insulins, nateglinide, repaglinide, and other products that lower blood glucose unless approved by prescriber

• That diabetes is lifelong; that this product is not a cure, only controls symptoms

• That all food included in diet plan must be eaten to prevent hypo/hyperglycemia

• To carry emergency ID

• To take product without regard to food

• To notify prescriber when surgery, trauma, stress occurs because dose may need to be adjusted

RARELY USED

scopolamine (Rx)

(skoe-pol′a-meen)

Maldemar, Scopace, Transderm Scop

Func. class.: Cholinergic blocker

Chem. class.: Belladonna alkaloid

USES: Preoperatively to produce amnesia, sedation and to decrease secretions; motion sickness, parkinsonian symptoms

CONTRAINDICATIONS: Hypersensitivity, closed-angle glaucoma, myasthenia gravis, GI/GU obstruction, hypersensitivity to belladonna, barbiturates

DOSAGE AND ROUTES

Motion sickness

• **Adult: TD** 1 patch 4 hr before travel and q3days

Parkinsonian symptoms

• **Adult: PO** 0.4-0.8 mg q8hr

Preoperatively

• **Adult: IM/IV/SUBCUT** 0.32-0.65 mg; **TD** apply 1 patch PM before surgery or 1 hr before c-section

Nausea and vomiting

• **Adult: SUBCUT** 0.6-1 mg

• **Child: SUBCUT** 0.006 mg/kg; max 0.3 mg/dose

selegiline (Rx)

(se-le′ji-leen)

Eldepryl, Emsam, Zelapar

Func. class.: Antiparkinson agent

Chem. class.: MAOI, type B

Do not confuse:

Eldepryl/enalapril

ACTION: Increased dopaminergic activity by inhibition of MAO type B activity; not fully understood

USES: Adjunct management of Parkinson's disease for patients being treated with levodopa/carbidopa who had poor response to therapy; depression (transdermal)

Unlabeled uses: Alzheimer's disease, depression

CONTRAINDICATIONS: Children/adolescents (suicide/hypertensive crisis), hypersensitivity, breastfeeding

Precautions: Pregnancy (C)

DOSAGE AND ROUTES

• **Adult: PO** 10 mg/day given with levodopa/carbidopa in divided doses, 5 mg at breakfast and lunch; after 2-3 days, begin to reduce dose of levodopa/carbidopa 10%-30%; **ORAL DISINTEGRATING** 1.25 mg (1 tab) × 6 wk or more initially, then 2.5 mg (2 tabs) dissolved on tongue daily before breakfast; max 2.5 mg/day; **TRANSDERMAL** 6 mg/24 hr initially, increase by 3 mg/24 hr at ≥2 wk, up to 12 mg/24 hr if needed

Alzheimer's disease (unlabeled)
- **Adult: PO** 5 mg bid AM, PM

Available forms: Tabs 5 mg; caps 5 mg; oral disintegrating tabs 1.25 mg; transdermal 6 mg/24 hr (20 mg/20 cm^2), 9 mg/24 hr (30 mg/30 cm^2), 12 mg/24 hr (40 mg/40 cm^2)

Administer:

PO route

⚠ Do not use in children due to risk for hypertensive crisis
- Product until NPO before surgery
- Adjust dosage to response
- With meals; limit protein taken with product
- Dosing bid in AM and afternoon; avoid PM or bedtime dosing
- At doses of <10 mg/day because of risks associated with nonselective inhibition of MAO
- **Oral disintegrating tab:** peel back foil; remove tab; do not push through foil; place tab on tongue; allow to dissolve; swallow with saliva

Transdermal route
- Apply to dry, intact skin on upper torso, upper thigh, or outer surface of upper arm q12hr

SIDE EFFECTS

CNS: Increased tremors, chorea, restlessness, blepharospasm, increased bradykinesia, grimacing, tardive dyskinesia, dystonic symptoms, involuntary movements, increased apraxia, hallucinations, *dizziness,* mood changes, nightmares, delusions, lethargy, apathy, overstimulation, sleep disturbances, headache, migraine, numbness, muscle cramps, confusion, anxiety, tiredness, vertigo, personality change, back/leg pain, **suicide in child/adolescent, suicidal ideation in adults**

CV: Orthostatic hypotension, hypo/hypertension, dysrhythmia, palpitations, angina pectoris, **tachycardia, edema, sinus bradycardia,** syncope, **hypertensive crisis (children)**

EENT: Diplopia, dry mouth, blurred vision, tinnitus

GI: Nausea, vomiting, constipation, weight loss, anorexia, diarrhea, heartburn, rectal bleeding, poor appetite, dysphagia, xerostomia

GU: Slow urination, nocturia, prostatic hypertrophy, urinary hesitation, retention, frequency, sexual dysfunction

INTEG: Increased sweating, alopecia, hematoma, rash, photosensitivity, facial hair; site reactions (transdermal)

RESP: Asthma, SOB

PHARMACOKINETICS

Absorption (tab) 40-90 min, (oral disintegrating tab) 10-15 min; peak ½-2 hr; rapidly metabolized (active metabolites: *N*-desmethyldeprenyl, amphetamine, methamphetamine); metabolites excreted in urine; half-life 10 hr, orally disintegrating tab 1.3 hr; protein binding up to 85%

INTERACTIONS

⚠ **Fatal interaction: opioids (especially meperidine); do not administer together**

⚠ **Serotonin syndrome (confusion, seizures, fever, hypertension, agitation); death—FLUoxetine, PARoxetine, sertraline, fluvoxaMINE (discontinue 5 wk before selegiline treatment); do not use together**

⚠ **Fatal interaction: do not use with tricyclics**

Increase: side effects of levodopa/carbidopa

Increase: unusual behavior, psychosis—dextromethorphan

Increase: hypotension—antihypertensives

Drug/Lab Test

Decrease: VMA

False positive: urine ketones, urine glucose

False negative: urine glucose (glucose oxidase)

False increase: uric acid, urine protein

NURSING CONSIDERATIONS

Assess:

- **Parkinson's symptoms:** decreased rigidity, unsteady gait, weakness, tremors
- Cardiac status: tachycardia/bradycardia; B/P, respiration throughout treatment
- Mental status: affect, mood, behavioral changes, depression; perform suicide assessment on all patients, suicidal ideation may occur

⚠ Opioids; if patient has received, do not administer selegiline; fatal reactions have occurred

- Assistance with ambulation during beginning therapy

Evaluate:

- Therapeutic response: decrease in akathisia, improved mood

Teach patient/family:

- To change positions slowly to prevent orthostatic hypotension
- **Hypertensive crisis:** nausea, vomiting, sweating, agitation, change in mental status, headache, chest pain; to notify prescriber immediately
- **Serotonin syndrome:** to report twitching, sweating, shivering, diarrhea to prescriber immediately
- To use product exactly as prescribed; if discontinued abruptly, parkinsonian crisis may occur
- **Pregnancy:** to report if pregnancy is planned or suspected, pregnancy (C); to avoid breastfeeding
- To use during the day to prevent insomnia
- To avoid heating pads, hot tubs when using transdermal products
- To avoid hazardous activities until response is known
- To avoid foods high in tyramine: cheese, pickled products, wine, beer, large amounts of caffeine

⚠ Not to exceed recommended dose of 10 mg (PO) because this might precipitate hypertensive crisis; to report severe headache, other unusual symptoms

TREATMENT OF OVERDOSE:

IV fluids for hypertension, IV dilute pressure agent for B/P titration

selenium topical

See Appendix B

sertraline (Rx)

(ser′tra-leen)

Zoloft

Func. class.: Antidepressant

Chem. class.: SSRI

Do not confuse:

Zoloft/Zocor

ACTION:

Inhibits serotonin reuptake in CNS; increases action of serotonin; does not affect dopamine, norepinephrine

USES:

Major depressive disorder, obsessive-compulsive disorder (OCD), posttraumatic stress disorder (PTSD), panic disorder, social anxiety disorder, premenstrual dysphoric disorder (PMDD)

Unlabeled uses: Premature ejaculation, pruritus with cholestatic liver disease, hot flashes during menopause, breast cancer patients taking tamoxifen; men with prostate cancer secondary to androgen-deprivation therapy, separation anxiety disorder

CONTRAINDICATIONS:

Hypersensitivity to this product or SSRIs

Precautions: Pregnancy (C), breastfeeding, geriatric patients, renal/hepatic disease, epilepsy, recent MI, latex sensitivity (dropper of oral concentration)

Black Box Warning: Children, suicidal ideation

DOSAGE AND ROUTES

Major depression/OCD

- **Adult/geriatric patient/adolescent (unlabeled): PO** 25-50 mg/day; may increase to max of 200 mg/day; do not change dose at intervals of <1 wk; administer daily in AM or PM

• **Child 6-12 yr (unlabeled): PO** 25 mg/day, increase by 25-50 mg/wk

Premenstrual dysphoric disorder

• **Adult: PO** 50-150 mg nightly

Premature ejaculation (unlabeled)

• **Adult: PO** 50 mg/day

Pruritus (unlabeled)

• **Adult: PO** 50-100 mg/day

Hepatic dose

• **Adult: PO** use lower dose or less frequent dosing intervals

Available forms: Tabs 25, 50, 100 mg; oral sol 20 mg/ml

Administer:

• Store at room temperature; do not freeze
• Increased fluids, bulk in diet for constipation, urinary retention
• With food, milk for GI symptoms
• Crushed if patient is unable to swallow medication whole
• Sugarless gum, hard candy, frequent sips of water for dry mouth
• **Oral concentration:** dilute before use with 4 oz (½ cup) of water, orange juice, ginger ale, or lemon/lime soda; do not mix with other liquids
• Avoid use with other CNS depressants
• Dropper contains latex

SIDE EFFECTS

CNS: *Insomnia, agitation, somnolence, dizziness, headache, tremors, fatigue,* paresthesia, twitching, confusion, ataxia, gait abnormality (geriatric patients), seizures, neuroleptic malignant-syndrome–like reaction, serotonin syndrome, suicidal ideation, anxiety, drowsiness

CV: Palpitations, chest pain

EENT: Vision abnormalities, yawning, tinnitus, intraocular pressure

ENDO: SIADH (geriatric patients); diabetes mellitus

GI: *Diarrhea, nausea, constipation, anorexia, dry mouth,* dyspepsia, *vomiting, flatulence,* weight gain/loss, hepatitis

GU: *Male sexual dysfunction,* micturition disorder

INTEG: Increased sweating, rash, hot flashes

MISC: Hyponatremia, neonatal abstinence syndrome

PHARMACOKINETICS

PO: Peak 4.5-8.4 hr; steady-state 1 wk; plasma protein binding 98%; elimination half-life 26 hr; extensively metabolized; metabolite excreted in urine, bile; weak inhibitor of CYP3A4, moderate inhibitor of CYP2D6

INTERACTIONS

• Altered lithium levels: lithium
• Disulfiram reaction: disulfiram and oral concentration due to alcohol content

⚠ Fatal reactions: MAOIs, pimozide

Increase: sertraline levels—cimetidine, warfarin, other highly protein-bound products

Increase: effects of antidepressants (tricyclics), diazepam, TOLBUTamide, warfarin, benzodiazepines, SUMAtriptan, phenytoin, cloZAPine

Increase: bleeding risk—anticoagulants, NSAIDs, thrombolytic, platelet inhibitors, salicylates

Increase: serotonin syndrome, neuroleptic malignant syndrome—SSRIs, SNRIs, serotonin-receptor agonists, tricyclics, sibutramine, traZODone, busPIRone, linezolid, traMADol

Drug/Herb

Increase: of SSRI, serotonin syndrome—St. John's wort, SAM-e, tryptophan; do not use together

Increase: CNS effect—kava kava, valerian

Drug/Lab Test

Increase: AST, ALT

False positive: urine screen for benzodiazepines

S

NURSING CONSIDERATIONS

Assess:

Black Box Warning: Mental status: mood, sensorium, affect, suicidal tendencies (child/young adult), increase in psychiatric symptoms, depression, panic attacks, OCD, PTSD, social anxiety disorder

⚠ **Serotonin syndrome** (hyperthermia, hypertension, rigidity, delirium, coma, myoclonus) or neuroleptic malignant-like syndrome (muscle cramps, fever, unstable B/P, agitation, tremors, mental changes)

⚠ **Bleeding** (platelet serotonin depletion): GI bleeding, ecchymoses, epistaxis, hematomas, petechiae, hemorrhage

• LFTs, thyroid function tests, growth rate, weight at baseline and periodically

• B/P (lying/standing), pulse q4hr; if systolic B/P drops 20 mm Hg, hold product, notify prescriber; VS q4hr in patients with CV disease

• Weight weekly; appetite may decrease with product

• Urinary retention, constipation, especially in geriatric patients

• Alcohol consumption; hold dose until morning

Evaluate:

• Therapeutic response: significant improvement in depression, OCD

Teach patient/family:

• That therapeutic effect may take ≥1 wk

• To use caution when driving, performing other activities requiring alertness because drowsiness, dizziness, blurred vision may occur

• Not to discontinue medication quickly after long-term use; may cause nausea, headache, malaise

• To avoid alcohol

• May be taken without regard to food

• **Serotonin syndrome:** agitation, nausea, vomiting, diarrhea, twitching, sweating, shivering; report to prescriber immediately

• To notify prescriber if pregnant or if planning to become pregnant, pregnancy (C) or breastfeeding

Black Box Warning: That suicidal thoughts/behaviors may occur in children/adolescents

sildenafil (Rx)

(sil-den′a-fill)

Revatio, Viagra

Func. class.: Erectile agent, antihypertensive, peripheral vasodilator

Chem. class.: Phosphodiesterase type-5 inhibitor

Do not confuse:

Viagra/Allegra

ACTION: Enhances the effect of nitric oxide (NO) by inhibiting phosphodiesterase type 5 (PDE5), which is necessary for degrading cGMP in the corpus cavernosum

USES: Treatment of erectile dysfunction, improvement in exercise ability, pulmonary hypertension

Unlabeled uses: Sexual dysfunction (women); lower urinary tract symptoms and erectile dysfunction (with alfuzosin); altitude sickness, Raynaud's disease

CONTRAINDICATIONS: Hypersensitivity to this product or nitrates

Precautions: Pregnancy (B), anatomical penile deformities, sickle cell anemia, leukemia, multiple myeloma, retinitis pigmentosa, bleeding disorders, active peptic ulceration, CV/renal/hepatic disease, multiproduct antihypertensive regimens, geriatric patients

DOSAGE AND ROUTES

Erectile dysfunction (Viagra only)

• **Adult male <65 yr: PO** 50 mg 1 hr before sexual activity; may be increased to 100 mg or decreased to 25 mg; max frequency 1×/day

• **Adult ≥65 yr (male): PO** 25 mg as needed about 1 hr before sexual activity

Renal/hepatic dose

• **Adult: PO** (Child-Pugh A, B) 25 mg, take 1 hr before sexual activity; max 1×/day; CCr <30 ml/min, 25 mg starting dose

Pulmonary hypertension (Revatio only)
• **Adult: PO** 20 mg tid; take 4-6 hr apart; **IV BOL** 10 mg tid
Pulmonary hypertension induced by altitude sickness (unlabeled)
• **Adult: PO** 40 mg 6-8 hr after arriving at 14,272 ft, then 40 mg tid × 6 days
Anorgasmy in antidepressant therapy/sexual dysfunction in women (unlabeled)
• **Adult: PO** 50 mg 60-90 min before sexual activity
Available forms: Tabs 20, 25, 50, 100 mg; sol for inj 10 mg/12.5 ml
Administer:
• **Erectile dysfunction:** give approximately 1 hr before sexual activity; do not use more than 1×/day; give on empty stomach for better absorption
• **Pulmonary hypertension:** give 3×/day, 4-6 hr apart

SIDE EFFECTS

CNS: *Headache, flushing, dizziness,* transient global amnesia, seizures
CV: MI, sudden death, CV collapse, TIAs, ventricular dysrhythmias, CV hemorrhage
MISC.: *Dyspepsia, nasal congestion, UTI, abnormal vision, diarrhea, rash,* nonarteritic ischemic optic neuropathy, hearing loss, priapism, sickle cell crisis

PHARMACOKINETICS

Rapidly absorbed; bioavailability 40%; metabolized by P45 CYP3A4, 2C9 in the liver (active metabolites); terminal half-life 4 hr; peak 15-30 min; reduced absorption with high-fat meal; excreted in feces, urine

INTERACTIONS

⚠ Do not use with nitrates; fatal fall in B/P
Increase: sildenafil levels—cimetidine, erythromycin, ketoconazole, itraconazole, antiretroviral protease inhibitors, tacrolimus
Decrease: sildenafil levels—CYP-450 inducers, rifampin, barbiturates, bosentan, carBAMazepine, dexamethasone, phenytoin, nevirapine, rifabutin, troglitazone; antacids
Decrease: B/P—α-blockers, alcohol, amlodipine, angiotensin II receptor blockers
Drug/Food
Increase: product effect—grapefruit
Decrease: absorption—high-fat meal

NURSING CONSIDERATIONS

Assess:
• **Phosphodiesterase type 5 inhibitors with lopinavir/ritonavir (Kaletra):** assess for hypotension, visual changes, prolonged erection, syncope; give only 25 mg q48hr and monitor for adverse reactions
• Erectile dysfunction before use
⚠ Any severe loss of vision while taking this or any similar products; products should not be used
⚠ Use of organic nitrates that should not be used with this product
• **MI, sudden death, CV collapse:** those with an MI within 6 mo, resting hypotension <90/50, resting hypertension >170/100, fluid depletion should use this product cautiously; may occur right after sexual activity to days afterward
• **Sickle cell crisis (vasoocclusive crisis):** when used for pulmonary hypertension, may require hospitalization
• Cardiac status, hemodynamic parameters, exercise tolerance in pulmonary hypertension: B/P, pulse
Evaluate:
• Therapeutic response: decreasing pulmonary hypertension/improved exercise tolerance; ability to perform sexually (male)
Teach patient/family:
• That product does not protect against sexually transmitted diseases, including HIV
• That product absorption is reduced with a high-fat meal
• That product should not be used with nitrates in any form
• That tabs may be split
⚠ To notify prescriber immediately and to stop taking product if vision/hearing loss occurs or erection lasts >4 hr

- That erections lasting >4 hr may occur; report to prescriber immediately
- Do not use more than 100 mg in 24 hr

silodosin (Rx)

(si-lo′do-seen)

Rapaflo

Func. class.: Selective α_1-adrenergic blocker, BPH agent

Chem. class.: Sulfamoylphenethylamine derivative

ACTION: Binds preferentially to α_{1A}-adrenoceptor subtype located mainly in the prostate

USES: Symptoms of benign prostatic hyperplasia (BPH)

CONTRAINDICATIONS: Hypersensitivity, renal failure, hepatic disease

Precautions: Pregnancy (B), breastfeeding, children, females, geriatric patients, renal/hepatic disease, hypotension, ocular surgery, orthostatic hypotension, prostate cancer, syncope

DOSAGE AND ROUTES

- **Adult: PO** 8 mg/day with meal; max 8 mg/day

Renal dose

- **Adult: PO** CCr 30-49 ml/min, 4 mg/day; CCr <30 ml/min, not recommended

Available forms: Cap 4, 8 mg

Administer:

- Give with meal at same time each day
- Cap may be opened and sprinkled in applesauce
- Store at room temperature; protect from light and moisture

SIDE EFFECTS

CNS: *Dizziness, headache,* asthenia, insomnia, syncope

CV: Orthostatic hypotension

EENT: Nasal congestion, rhinorrhea, sinusitis

GI: Diarrhea, abdominal pain, jaundice

GU: Abnormal ejaculation, priapism, urinary incontinence

HEMA: Purpura

PHARMACOKINETICS

Decreased absorption with high-fat/high-calorie meal, half-life of metabolite 24 hr, metabolized in liver, excreted via urine, extensively protein bound (97%)

INTERACTIONS

Increase: silodosin effect—CYP3A4 inhibitors (clarithromycin, itraconazole, ritonavir, antiretroviral protease inhibitors, aprepitant, chloramphenicol, conivaptan, dalfopristin, danazol, delavirdine, efavirenz, fosaprepitant, fluconazole, fluvoxaMINE, imatinib, isoniazid, mifepristone, nefazodone, tamoxifen, telithromycin, troleandomycin, voriconazole, zileuton, zafirlukast)

Drug/Food

Increase: silodosin effect—grapefruit juice

Drug Lab/Test

Increase: LFTs

NURSING CONSIDERATIONS

Assess:

- **Prostatic hyperplasia:** change in urinary patterns at baseline and throughout treatment, testing for prostate cancer, before administration is recommended
- BUN, uric acid, urodynamic studies (urinary flow rates, residual volume)
- I&O ratios, weight daily; edema, report weight gain or edema
- B/P, monitor for orthostatic hypotension

Evaluate:

- Therapeutic response: decreased symptoms of BPH

Teach patient/family

- Not to drive, operate machinery until effect known
- Not to use with grapefruit juice
- To take with same meal each day

silver nitrate 1% ophthalmic

See Appendix B

silver nitrate 1% sulfacetamide sodium ophthalmic

See Appendix B

silver sulfADIAZINE topical

See Appendix B

simeprevir

(sim-e′pre-vir)

Olysio

Func. class.: Antiviral, antihepatitis agent

ACTION: Prevents formation of mature viral proteins by inhibiting hepatitis C viral (HCV) replication by blocking proteolytic activity of the hepatitis C virus NS3/4A protease

USES: Chronic C infection, hepatitis, (HCV, genotype 1) in adults with compensated liver disease

CONTRAINDICATIONS: Hypersensitivity, male-mediated teratogenicity, pregnancy (X) in combination

Precautions: Pregnancy (C), (alone), breastfeeding, Asian patients, liver transplant, UV exposure, hepatic disease, serious rash, children

DOSAGE AND ROUTES

- **Adult: PO** 150 mg daily with food with peginterferon alfa and ribavirin ×12 wk

Available forms: Cap 150 mg

Administer:

- By mouth with food; swallow whole
- Do not use as monotherapy; if peginterferon alfa or ribavirin are discontinued, discontinue simeprevir and do not restart
- Obtain NS3 Q80K polymorphism test before starting treatment
- **Treatment naïve/prior relapse:** after initial 3-drug treatment, give another 12 wk with peginterferon alfa and ribavirin × another 12 wk; if HCV RNA concentrations ≥25 interstitial units/ml, discontinue all 3 drugs
- **Prior nonresponders (partial/null):** after initial 3-drug treatments, give an additional 36 wk of peginterferon alfa and ribavirin; monitor HCV RNA at wk 4, 12, 24; if ≥25 interstitial units/ml, discontinue products
- Keep in original container

SIDE EFFECTS

EENT: Blurred vision, conjunctivitis
GI: Hyperbilirubinemia, nausea
INTEG: Exfoliative dermatitis, pruritus, photosensitivity, vasculitis
MISC: Rash, dyspnea

PHARMACOKINETICS

99.9% protein binding, excreted 91% feces half-life 40 hrs, metabolized primarily by CYP3A4, also a mild inhibitor of intestinal CYP3A4 and CYP1A2

INTERACTIONS

Increase: effects of CYP3A4 inhibitors
Increase: simeprevir effects—bromocriptine, chloramphenicol, cimetidine, dalfopristin/quinupristin, danazol, FLUoxetine, isoniazid, lanreotide, octreotide, zafirlukast, erythromycin, protease inhibitors
Increase: effect of amiodarone, atorvastatin, disopyramide, digoxin, flecainide, mexiletine, propafenone, quinidine, calcium channel blockers, rosuvastatin, PDE_5 inhibitors
Decrease: simeprevir effect—CYP3A4 inducers (carbamazepine, dexamethasone, phenobarbital, rifampin, efavirenz, etravirine)

S

Drug/Herb

Decrease: simeprevir level—St. John's wort

Drug/Food

Food increases bioavailability

NURSING CONSIDERATIONS

Assess:

- Allergic reaction: rash, pruritus, exfoliative dermatitis
- Asian patients: levels may be 3.4-fold higher
- Pregnancy: if planned or suspected; if pregnant call the Pregnancy Registry 800-258-4263, pregnancy (X) in combination
- Liver function tests; serum HCV RNA concentrations at wk 4, 12, and 24 and at end of treatment; pregnancy tests

Evaluate:

- Therapeutic response: decreased symptoms of chronic hepatitis C

Teach patient/family:

- That optimal duration of treatment is unknown; that product is not a cure; that transmission may still occur, to use precautions
- To avoid use with other medications unless approved by prescriber
- To use protective clothing, sunscreen; photosensitivity may occur and can be severe
- Not to stop abruptly unless directed; worsening of hepatitis may occur
- To notify prescriber if pregnancy is planned or suspected; to avoid breastfeeding; use 2 reliable forms of contraception; do not try to conceive for at least 6 mo after discontinuation of this drug combination
- Teach patient to use cautiously in sulfonamide allergy; do not take the drug as single agent; must use as combination therapy
- That periodic laboratory testing, follow-up will be required
- To report nausea, vomiting, rash, trouble breathing to prescriber

simethicone (OTC, Rx)

(si-meth′i-kone)

Barriere ✱, Gas Relief ✱, Gas-Relief, Gas-X, Mylanta Gas Relief, Mylanta Gas, Mylicon, Ovol ✱, Phazyme

Func. class.: Antiflatulent

Do not confuse:

Mylicon/Mylanta Gas

Simethicone/Cimetidine

ACTION: Disperses/prevents mucous gas pockets in GI system, lowers surface tension of gas bubbles

USES: Flatulence

Unlabeled uses: Dyspepsia

CONTRAINDICATIONS: Hypersensitivity, GI obstruction/perforation

Precautions: Pregnancy (C), abdominal pain, fistula, hiatal hernia

DOSAGE AND ROUTES

- **Adult and child >12 yr: PO** 40-125 mg after meals and at bedtime prn, max 500 mg/day
- **Child 2-12 yr: PO** 40-50 mg after meals and at bedtime prn, max 240 mg/day
- **Child <2 yr: PO** 20 mg qid prn

Available forms: Chew tabs 40, 150, 166 mg; tabs 60, 80, 95, 125 mg; drops 20 mg/0.3 ml; caps 95, 180 mg; soft gel caps 125, 180 mg; oral dissolving film 62.5 mg

Administer:

- After meals, at bedtime; shake susp well before giving; chew tabs should be chewed

SIDE EFFECTS

GI: Belching, rectal flatus, diarrhea

NURSING CONSIDERATIONS

Assess:

- Reason for excess gas production, decreased bowel sounds, recent surgery, other GI conditions

Evaluate:

- Therapeutic response: reduction of abdominal gas, discomfort

Teach patient/family:

- That tabs must be chewed
- To shake susp well before pouring

simvastatin (Rx)

(sim-va-sta′tin)

Zocor

Func. class.: Antilipemic

Chem. class.: HMG-CoA reductase inhibitor

Do not confuse:
Zocor/Cozaar/Zoloft

ACTION: Inhibits HMG-CoA reductase enzyme, which reduces cholesterol synthesis

USES: As an adjunct for primary hypercholesterolemia (types IIa, IIb), isolated hypertriglyceridemia (Frederickson type IV), and type III hyperlipoproteinemia, CAD, heterozygous familial hypercholesterolemia; MI/stroke prophylaxis

CONTRAINDICATIONS: Pregnancy (X), breastfeeding, hypersensitivity, active hepatic disease

Precautions: Past hepatic disease, alcoholism, severe acute infections, trauma, severe metabolic disorders, electrolyte imbalances, Chinese patients

DOSAGE AND ROUTES

- **Adult: PO** 20-40 mg/day in PM initially; usual range 5-40 mg/day in PM, max 40 mg/day for most patients, max 80 mg/day for patients taking 80 mg/day chronically without myopathy; dosage adjustments may be made in ≥4-wk intervals; those taking verapamil and amiodarone max 20 mg/day; max <80 mg for Chinese patients taking lipid-modifying niacin doses
- **Child/adolescent ≥10 yr including girls ≥1 yr postmenarche: PO** 10 mg in PM, range 10-40 mg/day

With diltiazem/verapamil/dronedarone

- **Adult: PO** 5-10 mg in PM, max 10 mg/day

With amiodarone, amoLODIPine, ranolazine

- **Adult: PO** 5-20 mg daily in evening, max 20 mg/day

Heterozygous familial hypercholesterolemia

- **Adult: PO** 40 mg daily in evening, make dosage adjustments q4wk

Available forms: Tabs 5, 10, 20, 40, 80 mg

Administer:

- Total daily dose in evening
- Store in cool environment in tight container protected from light

SIDE EFFECTS

CNS: Headache, cognitive impairment

GI: Nausea, constipation, diarrhea, dyspepsia, flatus, abdominal pain, **liver dysfunction, pancreatitis**, hyperglycemia

INTEG: Rash, pruritus

MS: Muscle cramps, myalgia, **myositis, rhabdomyolysis**, myopathy

RESP: Upper respiratory tract infection

PHARMACOKINETICS

Metabolized in liver (active metabolites); >98% protein bound; excreted primarily in bile, feces (60%), kidneys (15%); peak 1-2 hr; half-life 3 hr

INTERACTIONS

⚠ Do not use with cycloSPORINE, gemfibrozil

⚠ **Increase:** effects of warfarin

⚠ **Increase:** rhabdomyolysis, myalgia; do not use concurrently—CYP3A4 inhibitors, niacin, erythromycin, clofibrate, clarithromycin, ketoconazole, itraconazole, protease inhibitors, macrolide antibiotics,

S

danazol, delavirdine, nefazodone, verapamil, diltiazem, amiodarone, azole antifungals, telithromycin, voriconazole
Increase: simvastatin effect—ATP1B1 inhibitors
Increase: serum level of digoxin
Drug/Herb
Increase: effect—red yeast, rice
Decrease: effect—St. John's wort
Drug/Food
Increase: simvastatin level grapefruit juice (large amounts)
Drug/Lab Test
Increase: CK, LFTs, HbA1c

NURSING CONSIDERATIONS

Assess:

- Diet history: fat consumption; baseline and lipid profile: LDL, HDL, TG, cholesterol
- Hepatic studies at baseline, after 4-6 wk, periodically thereafter; AST, ALT, may increase

⚠ **Rhabdomyolysis:** muscle tenderness, increased CPK levels (10× above upper normal limit); therapy should be discontinued, more likely in those receiving >80 mg/day, first year of treatment, those ≥65 yr, females

- Renal studies in patients with compromised renal systems: BUN, I&O ratio, creatinine

Evaluate:

- Therapeutic response: decrease in LDL, total cholesterol, triglycerides; increase in HDL; slowing CAD

Teach patient/family:

- That blood work will be necessary during treatment
- To report severe GI symptoms, headache
- That previously prescribed regimen will continue: low-cholesterol diet, exercise program, smoking cessation
- To notify prescriber if pregnancy is suspected or planned; pregnancy (X); not to breastfeed
- To take in evening
- To report muscle pain, weakness, abdominal pain, dark urine, yellowing of skin, eyes, memory loss

⚠ HIGH ALERT

sirolimus (Rx)

(seer-oh-lie′mus)

Rapamune

Func. class.: Immunosuppressant
Chem. class.: Macrolide

ACTION: Produces immunosuppression by inhibiting T-lymphocyte activation and proliferation

USES: Organ transplants to prevent rejection; recommended use is with cycloSPORINE and corticosteroids

CONTRAINDICATIONS: Breastfeeding, hypersensitivity to this product, components of product
Precautions: Pregnancy (C), children <13 yr, severe cardiac/renal/hepatic disease; diabetes mellitus, hyperkalemia, hyperuricemia, hypertension, interstitial lung disease, hyperlipidemia, soya lecithin hypersensitivity

Black Box Warning: Lymphomas, infection, other malignancies, liver transplant, requires a specialized setting, requires an experienced clinician

DOSAGE AND ROUTES

- **Adult/adolescent ≥40 kg: PO** 2 mg/day with 6 mg loading dose
- **Child >13 yr weighing <40 kg (88 lb): PO** 1 mg/m²/day, 3 mg/m² loading dose

Hepatic dose

- **Adult/child ≥13 yr/<40 kg: PO** reduce by 33% for maintenance dose (mild to moderate hepatic impairment); reduce by 50% for maintenance dose (severe hepatic impairment)

Available forms: Oral sol 1 mg/ml; tabs 0.5 mg, 1 mg, 2 mg
Administer:

- Prophylaxis for *Pneumocystis jiroveci* pneumonia for 1 yr after transplantation;

prophylaxis for CMV is recommended for 90 days after transplantation in those at increased risk for CMV

- All medications PO if possible; avoid IM inj; bleeding may occur
- For 3 days before transplant surgery; patients should be placed in protective isolation; give at same time of day; give 4 hr after cycloSPORINE oral sol or caps; do not give with grapefruit juice
- Use amber oral dose syringe and withdraw amount of oral sol needed from bottle; empty correct dose into plastic/glass container holding 60 ml of water/orange juice; stir vigorously and have patient drink at once; refill container with additional 120 ml water/orange juice; stir vigorously and have patient drink at once; if using a pouch, squeeze entire contents into container; follow above directions
- Store protected from light, refrigerate; stable for 30 days after opening (sol)
- Do not crush, chew; store tabs at room temperature

Black Box Warning: Only those experienced in immunosuppressant therapy and transplant should use this drug, must use in a specialized care setting with adequate medical equipment

SIDE EFFECTS

CNS: *Tremors, headache, insomnia, paresthesia,* chills, fever
CV: Hypertension, *atrial fibrillation, CHF, hypotension, palpitation, tachycardia,* peripheral edema, thrombosis
EENT: Blurred vision, photophobia
GI: Nausea, vomiting, diarrhea, constipation, hepatotoxicity
GU: UTIs, albuminuria, hematuria, proteinuria, renal failure, nephrotic syndrome, increased creatinine
HEMA: Anemia, leukopenia, thrombocytopenia, purpura, pancytopenia
INTEG: *Rash, acne,* photosensitivity
META: Hyperglycemia, increased creatinine, edema, hypercholesterolemia, *hyperlipemia,* hypophosphatemia, weight gain, hypo/hyperkalemia, hyperuricemia, hypomagnesemia, hypertriglyceridemia
MS: Arthralgia
RESP: Pleural effusion, atelectasis, *dyspnea,* pneumonitis, pulmonary embolism/fibrosis
SYST: Lymphoma, exfoliative dermatitis

PHARMACOKINETICS

Rapidly absorbed; peak 1 hr single dose, 2 hr multiple dosing; protein binding 92%; extensively metabolized by CYP3A4 enzyme system, half-life 57-63 hr

INTERACTIONS

⚠ **Increase:** angioedema—ACE inhibitors, angiotensin-II–receptor antagonists, cephalosporins, iodine-containing radiopaque contrast media, neuromuscular blockers, NSAIDs, penicillins, salicylates, thrombolytics
Increase: blood levels—antifungals, calcium channel blockers, cimetidine, danazol, erythromycin, cycloSPORINE, metoclopramide, bromocriptine, HIV-protease inhibitors
Decrease: blood levels—carBAMazepine, PHENobarbital, phenytoin, rifamycin, rifapentine
Decrease: effect of vaccines

Drug/Herb

- St. John's wort: may decrease the effect of sirolimus

Drug/Food

- Alters bioavailability; use consistently with/without food; do not use with grapefruit juice

Drug/Lab Test

Increase: LFTs, alk phos, lipids, triglycerides, total cholesterol, BUN, creatinine, LDH, phosphate
Decrease: platelets, sodium
Increase or decrease: magnesium, glucose, calcium

NURSING CONSIDERATIONS

Assess:

- Blood levels in patients who may have altered metabolism, trough level ≥15 ng/ml are associated with increased adverse reactions; monitor trough concentrations in all patients

S

- Creatinine/BUN, CBC, serum potassium
- **Lipid profile:** cholesterol, triglycerides; lipid-lowering agent may be needed

Black Box Warning: Infection and development of lymphoma; only those experienced in immunosuppressant therapy and organ transplantation should use this product; use only in renal transplant

- **High risk:** those with Baniff grade 3 acute rejection or vascular rejection before cycloSPORINE withdrawal, dialysis dependent, creatinine >4.5 mg/dl, African descent, re-transplants, multiorgan transplant, high panel of reactive antibodies
- **Pulmonary fibrosis, pulmonary effusion, pneumonitis:** dyspnea, cough, hypoxia; some fatal cases have occurred
- **Wound dehiscence and anastomotic disruption:** wound, vascular, airway, ureteral, biliary, inhibition of growth factors; do not combine with corticosteroids, not recommended in lung or liver transplant
- **Anaphylaxis, angioedema, exfoliative dermatitis:** more common when given with ACE inhibitors; do not use if a hypersensitivity reaction occurs

⚠ **Bone marrow suppression:** Hgb, WBC, platelets during treatment each mo; if leukocytes $<3000/mm^3$ or platelets $<100{,}000/mm^3$, product should be discontinued or reduced; decreased hemoglobin level

⚠ **Hepatotoxicity:** alk phos, AST, ALT, amylase, bilirubin, dark urine, jaundice, itching, light-colored stools; product should be discontinued

Evaluate:
- Therapeutic response: absence of graft rejection; immunosuppression with autoimmune disorders

Teach patient/family:

⚠ To report fever, rash, severe diarrhea, chills, sore throat, fatigue; serious infections may occur; clay-colored stools, cramping **(hepatotoxicity)**; fever, chills, sore throat **(infection)**
- To avoid crowds, persons with known infections to reduce risk for infection
- To use contraception before, during, for 12 wk after product discontinued; to avoid breastfeeding
- To use sunscreen, protective clothing to prevent burns, skin cancer
- Not to use with grapefruit juice
- To avoid vaccines
- That lifelong use will be required to prevent rejection
- That continuing follow-up exams and blood work will be required
- Not to get on skin
- How to use product
- To take with or without regard to food, at same time, consistently
- Take 4 hr after cycloSPORINE

⚠ HIGH ALERT

sitaGLIPtin (Rx)

(sit-a-glip′tin)

Januvia

Func. class.: Antidiabetic, oral

Chem. class.: Dipeptidyl-peptidase-4 inhibitor (DPP-4 inhibitor)

ACTION: Slows the inactivation of incretin hormones; improves glucose homeostasis, improves glucose-dependent insulin secretion, lowers glucagon secretions, and slows gastric emptying time

USES: Type 2 diabetes mellitus as monotherapy or in combination with other antidiabetic agents

CONTRAINDICATIONS: Angioedema, diabetic ketoacidosis (DKA)

Precautions: Pregnancy (B), geriatric patients, GI obstruction, surgery, thyroid/renal/hepatic disease, trauma, breastfeeding, pancreatitis, hypercortisolism, hyperglycemia, hyperthyroidism, hypogylcemia, ileus, pituitary insufficiency, surgery, type 1 diabetes mellitus, diabetic ketoacidosis, adrenal insufficiency, burns

DOSAGE AND ROUTES

• **Adult: PO** 100 mg/day; may use with antidiabetic agents other than insulin

Renal dose

• **Adult: PO** CCr 30-50 ml/min, 50 mg daily; CCr <30 ml/min, 25 mg daily

Available forms: Tabs 25, 50, 100 mg

Administer:

• May be taken with/without food
• Do not split, crush, chew; swallow whole
• Conversion from other antidiabetic agents; change may be made with gradual dosage change
• Store in tight container at room temperature

SIDE EFFECTS

CNS: *Headache*

ENDO: Hypoglycemia

GI: *Nausea, vomiting,* abdominal pain, diarrhea, pancreatitis, constipation

GU: Acute renal failure

MISC: *Peripheral edema*

SYST: Anaphylaxis, Stevens-Johnson syndrome, angioedema

PHARMACOKINETICS

Rapidly absorbed, excreted by the kidneys (unchanged 79%), terminal half-life 12.4 hr, peak 1-4 hr

INTERACTIONS

Increase: sitaGLIPtin level—cimetidine, disopyramide

Increase: levels of digoxin

Increase: hypoglycemia—androgens, insulins, β-blockers, cimetidine, corticosteroids, salicylates, MAOIs, fibric acid derivatives, FLUoxetine, sulfonylureas

Decrease: antidiabetic effect—thiazide diuretics, ACE inhibitors, protease inhibitors, sympathomimetics, ARIPiprazole, cloZAPine, OLANZapine, QUEtiapine, risperiDONE, ziprasidone, phenytoin, fosphenytoin, phenothiazines, estrogens, progestins, oral contraceptives

Drug/Herb

Increase: antidiabetic effect—garlic, green tea, horse chestnut

Drug/Lab Test

Increase: creatinine, LFTs

NURSING CONSIDERATIONS

Assess:

• **Hypoglycemic reactions:** sweating, weakness, dizziness, anxiety, tremors, hunger; hyperglycemic reactions soon after meals

⚠ **Serious skin reactions:** swelling of face, mouth, lips, dyspnea, wheezing

⚠ **Pancreatitis:** severe abdominal pain, nausea, vomiting; discontinue product

• **Renal studies:** BUN, creatinine during treatment, especially in geriatric patients or those with renal disease
• Glycosylated hemoglobin A1c; monitor blood glucose (BG) as needed

Evaluate:

• Therapeutic response: decrease in polyuria, polydipsia, polyphagia; clear sensorium; absence of dizziness; stable gait, blood glucose, A1c improvement

Teach patient/family:

• To perform regular self-monitoring of blood glucose using blood-glucose meter
• About the symptoms of hypo/hyperglycemia; what to do about each; to carry emergency ID
• To notify prescriber if pregnancy is planned, suspected
• That product must be continued on daily basis; about consequences of discontinuing product abruptly; to continue health regimen (diet, exercise)
• To avoid OTC medications, alcohol, digoxin, exenatide, insulins, nateglinide, repaglinide, and other products that lower blood glucose unless approved by prescriber
• That diabetes is a lifelong illness; that product is not a cure, only controls symptoms
• That all food included in diet plan must be eaten to prevent hypo/hyperglycemia
• To immediately notify prescriber of hypersensitivity reactions (rash, swelling of face, trouble breathing)

S

sodium bicarbonate (Rx, OTC)

Baking soda, Neut, Sellymin ✦

Func. class.: Alkalinizer

Chem. class.: $NaHCO_3$

ACTION: Orally neutralizes gastric acid, which forms water, NaCl, CO_2; increases plasma bicarbonate, which buffers H^+ ion concentration; reverses acidosis IV

USES: Acidosis (metabolic), cardiac arrest, alkalinization (systemic/urinary) antacid, salicylate poisoning

Unlabeled uses: Contrast media nephrotoxicity prevention

CONTRAINDICATIONS: Metabolic/respiratory alkalosis, hypochloremia, hypocalcemia

Precautions: Pregnancy (C), children, CHF, cirrhosis, toxemia, renal disease, hypertension, hypokalemia, breastfeeding, hypernatremia, Bartter's syndrome, Cushing syndrome, hyperaldosteronism

DOSAGE AND ROUTES

Acidosis, metabolic (not associated with cardiac arrest)

- **Adult and child: IV INFUSION** 2-5 mEq/kg over 4-8 hr depending on CO_2, pH, ABGs

Cardiac arrest

- **Adult and child: IV BOL** 1 mEq/kg of 7.5% or 8.4% sol, then 0.5 mEq/kg q10min, then doses based on ABGs
- **Infant: IV** 1 mEq/kg over several min (use only the 0.5 mEq/ml [4.2%] sol for inj)

Alkalinization of urine

- **Adult: PO** 325 mg to 2 g qid or 48 mEq (4 g), then 12-24 mEq q4hr
- **Child: PO** 84-840 mg/kg/day (1-10 mEq/kg) in divided doses q4-6hr

Antacid

- **Adult: PO** 300 mg to 2 g chewed, taken with water daily-qid

Available forms: Tabs 300, 325, 600, 650 mg; inj 4.2%, 5%, 7.5%, 8.4%

Administer:

PO route

- Chew antacid tablets and drink 8 oz water
- Do not take antacid with milk because milk-alkali syndrome may result

Direct IV route

- Use for cardiac emergencies, not used often in cardiac arrest
- Use ampules or prefilled syringes only; give by rapid bolus dose; flush with NS before, after use

Continuous IV INFUSION route

- Diluted in an equal amount of compatible sol given 2-5 mEq/kg over 4-8 hr, max 50 mEq/hr; slower rate in children
- Extravasation with IV administration (tissue sloughing, ulceration, necrosis)

Y-site compatibilities: Acyclovir, amifostine, asparaginase, aztreonam, bivalirudin, bumetanide, ceFAZolin, cefepime, cefTAZidime, ceftizoxime, cefTRIAXone, chloramphenicol, cimetidine, cladribine, clindamycin, cyclophosphamide, cycloSPORINE, cytarabine, DAPTOmycin, DAUNOrubicin, dexamethasone sodium phosphated exmedetomidine, digoxin, DOCEtaxel, DOXOrubicin, enalaprilat, ertapenem, erythromycin, esmolol, etoposide, etoposide phosphate, famotidine, fentaNYL, filgrastim, fluconazole, fludarabine, furosemide, gallium nitrate, gemcitabine, gentamicin, granisetron, heparin, hydrocortisone sodium succinate, ifosfamide, indomethacin, insulin, ketorolac, labetalol, levofloxacin, lidocaine, linezolid, LORazepam, magnesium sulfate, melphalan, mesna, meperidine, methylPREDNISolone sodium succinate, metoclopramide, metoprolol, metroNIDAZOLE, milrinone, morphine, nafcillin, nitroglycerin, nitroprusside, PACLitaxel, palonosetron, pantoprazole, PEMEtrexed, penicillin G potassium, phenylephrine, phytonadione, piperacillin/tazobactam, potassium chloride, procainamide, propranolol, propofol, protamine, ranitidine, remifentanil, tacrolimus, teniposide, thiotepa, ticarcillin/clavulanate, tirofiban, tobramycin, tolazoline, vasopressin, vit B complex with C, voriconazole

SIDE EFFECTS

CNS: Irritability, headache, confusion, stimulation, tremors, *twitching, hyperreflexia,* tetany, weakness, seizures of alkalosis

CV: Irregular pulse, cardiac arrest, water retention, edema, weight gain

GI: Flatulence, *belching, distention*

META: *Metabolic alkalosis*

MS: Muscular twitching, tetany, irritability

PHARMACOKINETICS

PO: Onset rapid, duration 10 min

IV: Onset 15 min, duration 1-2 hr, excreted in urine

INTERACTIONS

Increase: effects—amphetamines, mecamylamine, quiNINE, quiNIDine, pseudoephedrine, flecainide, anorexiants, sympathomimetics

Increase: sodium and decrease potassium—corticosteroids

Decrease: effects—lithium, chlorproPAMIDE, barbiturates, salicylates, benzodiazepines, ketoconazole, corticosteroids

Drug/Lab Test

Increase: sodium, lactate

Decrease: potassium

NURSING CONSIDERATIONS

Assess:

- Respiratory and pulse rate, rhythm, depth, lung sounds; notify prescriber of abnormalities
- **Fluid balance** (I&O, weight daily, edema); notify prescriber of fluid overload; assess for edema, crackles, shortness of breath
- Electrolytes, blood pH, PO_2, HCO_3^-, during treatment; ABGs frequently during emergencies
- Weight daily with initial therapy
- **Alkalosis:** irritability, confusion, twitching, hyperreflexia stimulation, slow respirations, cyanosis, irregular pulse
- **Milk-alkali syndrome:** confusion, headache, nausea, vomiting, anorexia, urinary stones, hypercalcemia
- For GI perforation secondary to carbon dioxide in GI tract; may lead to perforation if ulcer is severe enough

Evaluate:

- Therapeutic response: ABGs, electrolytes, blood pH, HCO_3^- WNL

Teach patient/family:

- Not to take antacid with milk because milk-alkali syndrome may result; not to use antacid for >2 wk

⚠ To notify prescriber if indigestion accompanied by chest pain; trouble breathing; diarrhea; dark, tarry stools; vomit that looks like coffee grounds; swelling of feet/ankles

- About sodium-restricted diet; to avoid use of baking soda for indigestion

sodium polystyrene sulfonate (Rx)

(po-lee-stye′reen)

Kalexate, Kayexalate, K-Exit ♣, Kionex, SPS

Func. class.: Potassium-removing resin

Chem. class.: Cation exchange resin

ACTION: Removes potassium by exchanging sodium for potassium in body, primarily in large intestine

USES: Hyperkalemia in conjunction with other measures

CONTRAINDICATIONS: Hypersensitivity to saccharin or parabens that may be in some products, GI obstruction, neonate (reduced gut motility)

Precautions: Pregnancy (C), geriatric patients, renal failure, CHF, severe edema, severe hypertension, sodium restriction, constipation, GI bleeding, hypocalcemia

DOSAGE AND ROUTES

- **Adult: PO** 15 g daily-qid; **RECT** enema 30-50 g q1-2hr initially prn, then q6hr prn

S

• **Child (unlabeled): PO** 1 g/kg q6hr prn; **RECT** 1 g/kg q2-6hr prn

Available forms: Powder for susp 453.6 g, 454 g; oral susp 15 g/60 ml

Administer:

PO route

• **Powdered resin:** each dose of the powdered resin is usually given orally as a suspension in water or in a syrup; usually, the amount of fluid ranges from 20 to 100 ml, depending on the dosage, or 3-4 ml/g of resin; suspensions should be freshly prepared and not stored for >24 hr; the suspension may be also be introduced into the stomach via a tube, or the powdered resin may be mixed with the patient's food; the powder should not be mixed with foods or liquids that contain a large amount of potassium (bananas or orange juice)

Rectal route

• Precede retention enema with a cleansing enema

• Instruct patient to lie down on left side with lower leg extended and the upper leg flexed for support, or place the patient in the knee–chest position; gently insert a soft, large (28 Fr) rubber tube into the rectum for a distance of about 20 cm; the tip should be well into the sigmoid colon; tape the tube in place; suspend the sodium polystyrene sulfonate powdered resin in 100 ml of an aqueous vehicle (water or sorbitol) that has been warmed to body temperature and introduce through the tube by gravity; the particles should be kept suspended by stirring the suspension during administration; alternatively, 120-180 ml of a commercially available suspension may be administered as a retention enema after the suspension has been warmed to body temperature; following administration, flush the tube with 50-100 ml of fluid and clamp the tube and leave in place; the suspension should be retained in the colon for at least 30-60 min or for several hours, if possible

• After several hours have passed, administer a cleansing enema using a non–sodium-containing solution at body temperature; up to 2 quarts of fluid may be necessary; drain fluid through a Y-tube connection; observe the drainage if sorbitol was used

SIDE EFFECTS

GI: Constipation, anorexia, nausea, vomiting, diarrhea (sorbitol), fecal impaction, gastric irritation

META: Hypocalcemia, hypokalemia, hypomagnesemia, sodium retention

INTERACTIONS

Increase: hypokalemia—loop diuretics, cardiac glycosides

Increase: metabolic alkalosis—magnesium/calcium antacids

⚠ **Increase:** colonic necrosis—sorbitol; do not use concurrently

Decrease: effect of—lithium, thyroid hormones

NURSING CONSIDERATIONS

Assess:

• **Hyperkalemia:** confusion, dyspnea, weakness, dysrhythmias; ECG for spiked T waves, depressed ST segments, prolonged QT and widening QRS complex

• Bowel function daily; note consistency of stools, times/day

• **Hypotension:** confusion, irritability, muscular pain, weakness

• **Electrolytes:** serum potassium, calcium, magnesium, sodium; acid–base balance

• I&O ratio, weight daily; crackles, dyspnea, jugular venous distension, edema

• **Digoxin toxicity** (nausea, vomiting, blurred vision, anorexia, dysrhythmias) in those receiving digoxin

Evaluate:

• Therapeutic response: potassium level 3.5-5 mg/dl

Teach patient/family:

• About reason for medication and expected results

• To follow a low-potassium diet, provide sample diet

• To avoid laxatives, antacids, electrolyte-based products unless approved by prescriber

sofosbuvir

(soe-fos′bue-vir)

Sovaldi

Func. class.: Antiviral, antihepatitis agent

Chem. class.: Nucleotide analog polymerase inhibitor

ACTION: Inhibits hepatitis C virus RNA polymerase by incorporating the polymerase into the viral RNA; also acts as a chain terminator

USES: Chronic hepatitis C (genotypes 1, 2, 3, 4) with compensated liver disease

CONTRAINDICATIONS: Hypersensitivity, pregnancy (X) in combination; male-mediated teratogenicity

Precautions: Pregnancy (B), breastfeeding, children, hepatic/renal disease

DOSAGE AND ROUTES

Chronic hepatitis C

Genotype 1, 4

- **Adult: PO** 400 mg daily with peginterferon alfa and ribavirin ×12 wk; may consider use for genotype 1 with only ribavirin ×24 wk

Chronic hepatitis C

Genotype 2

- **Adult: PO** 400 mg daily with ribavirin ×12 wk

Chronic hepatitis C

Genotype 3

- **Adult: PO** 400 mg daily with ribavirin or daclatasvir ×24 wk

Chronic hepatitis C with hepatocellular carcinoma in those waiting for liver transplant

Adult: PO 400 mg daily with ribavirin × 48 wks or until transplant

Available forms: Tabs 400 mg

Administer:

- By mouth without regard to food
- Do not use as mono therapy
- Do not crush, break tabs

SIDE EFFECTS

CNS: Headache, chills, weakness, fatigue, fever, insomnia

GI: Diarrhea, hyperbilirubinemia

MISC: Rash, pruritus, neutropenia, anemia, myalgia

PHARMACOKINETICS

PO: Peak ½-2 hr, excreted by kidneys 80%, 61%-65% protein binding; half-life 0.4-27 hr

INTERACTIONS

Decrease: sofosbuvir-P-glycoprotein (P-gp) inducers (carBAMazepine, PHENobarbital, phenytoin, rifampin); OXcarbazepine, rifabutin, rifapentine, tipranavir; avoid concurrent use

Increase: bradycardia—amiodarone, avoid using together

Increase: sofosbuvir level—carvedilol, cobicistat

Drug/Herb

Decrease: sofosbuvir level—St. John's wort, do not use together

NURSING CONSIDERATIONS

Assess:

- Serum HCV-RNA baseline and periodically
- Severe renal disease/GFR <30 ml/min/1.73 m²: monitor BUN, creatinine
- Geriatric patients more carefully; may develop renal, cardiac symptoms more rapidly
- Pregnancy: if planned or suspected; if pregnant call the Pregnancy Registry 800-258-4263; obtain pregnancy test before starting treatment, women who have HIV-1 and HCV who are taking antiretrovirals also should enroll with the registry

Evaluate:

- Therapeutic response: decreased symptoms of chronic hepatitis C

Teach patient/family:

- That optimal duration of treatment is unknown; that product is not a cure; that transmission may still occur
- To avoid use with other medications unless approved by prescriber

S

• Not to stop abruptly unless directed; worsening of hepatitis may occur, not to use alone, keep in original container
• To notify prescriber if pregnancy is planned or suspected; use 2 forms of reliable contraception; avoid breastfeeding

solifenacin (Rx)

(sol-i-fen′a-sin)

VESIcare

Func. class.: Urinary antispasmodic, anticholinergic

Chem. class.: Antimuscarinic

Do not confuse:
Vesicare/Vesanoid

ACTION: Relaxes smooth muscles in urinary tract by inhibiting acetylcholine at postganglionic sites

USES: Overactive bladder (urinary frequency, urgency, incontinence)

CONTRAINDICATIONS: Hypersensitivity, uncontrolled closed-angle glaucoma, urinary retention, gastric retention

Precautions: Pregnancy (C), breastfeeding, children, geriatric patients, renal/hepatic disease, controlled closed-angle glaucoma, bladder outflow obstruction, GI obstruction, decreased GI motility, history of QT prolongation

DOSAGE AND ROUTES

• **Adult: PO** 5 mg/day, max 10 mg/day

Renal/hepatic dose

• **Adult: PO** (Child-Pugh B) max 5 mg/day; CCr ≤30 ml/min, 5 mg/day

Available forms: Tabs 5, 10 mg

Administer:

PO route

• Without regard to meals
• Swallow product whole with water, liquid

SIDE EFFECTS

CNS: Anxiety, paresthesia, fatigue, *dizziness,* headache, confusion, delirium, depression, drowsiness

CV: Chest pain, hypertension, QTc prolongation, peripheral edema, palpitations, sinus tachycardia

EENT: *Vision abnormalities, xerophthalmia,* nasal dryness

GI: *Nausea, vomiting, anorexia,* abdominal pain, *constipation, dry mouth,* dyspepsia

GU: Dysuria, urinary retention, frequency, UTI

INTEG: Rash, pruritus, angioedema, exfoliative dermatitis, erythema multiforme, anaphylaxis

MISC: Hyperthermia

RESP: Bronchitis, cough, pharyngitis, upper respiratory tract infection

PHARMACOKINETICS

90% absorbed; 98% protein bound; extensively metabolized by CYP3A4; excreted in urine 69% (metabolites), feces 22%; terminal half-life 45-68 hr

INTERACTIONS

Increase: QT prolongation—Class IA, III antidysrhythmias

Increase: CNS depression—sedatives, hypnotics, benzodiazepines, opioids

Increase: effects—CYP3A4 inhibitors (ketoconazole, clarithromycin, diclofenac, doxycycline, erythromycin, isoniazid, nefazodone, propofol, protease inhibitors, verapamil), max dose 5 mg

Decrease: effects—CYP3A4 inducers (carBAMazepine, nevirapine, PHENobarbital, phenytoin)

Drug/Herb

Decrease: effects—St. John's wort

Drug/Food

Increase: effect—grapefruit juice

Drug/Lab Test

Increase: LFTs

NURSING CONSIDERATIONS

Assess:

• **Urinary patterns:** distention, nocturia, frequency, urgency, incontinence
• **Allergic reactions:** rash
• **Angioedema:** of the face, lips, tongue, larynx

⚠ Cardiac patients: monitor ECG for QTc prolongation; avoid products that increase QT prolongation

Evaluate:

- Decreasing dysuria, frequency, nocturia, incontinence

Teach patient/family:

- To avoid hazardous activities because dizziness may occur
- That constipation, blurred vision may occur; to notify prescriber if abdominal pain with constipation occurs
- To take without regard to food
- To swallow tab whole; do not split, crush, chew
- To call prescriber if severe abdominal pain or constipation lasts for ≥3 days
- That heat prostration may occur if used in hot environment, sweating is decreased
- About **anticholinergic effects:** blurred vision, constipation, urinary retention, hyperthermia

somatropin (Rx)

(soe-ma-troe′pin)

Genotropin, Humatrope, Norditropin, Norditropin Flexpro, Nutropin, Nutropin AQ, Omnitrope, Saizen, Serostim, Tev-Tropin, Zorbtive

Func. class.: Pituitary hormone

Chem. class.: Growth hormone

Do not confuse:

somatropin/SUMAtriptan/somatrem

ACTION: Stimulates growth; somatropin is similar to natural growth hormone; both preparations were developed with the use of recombinant DNA

USES: Pituitary growth hormone deficiency (hypopituitary dwarfism), children with human growth hormone deficiency/growth failure, AIDS wasting syndrome, cachexia, adults with somatropin deficiency syndrome (SDS), short stature in Noonan syndrome, SHOX deficiency, Turner's syndrome, Prader-Willi syndrome

CONTRAINDICATIONS: Hypersensitivity to benzyl alcohol, creosol; closed epiphyses, intracranial lesions, acute respiratory failure, Prader-Willi syndrome with obesity, trauma

Precautions: Pregnancy (C), breastfeeding, newborn, geriatric patients, diabetes mellitus, hypothyroidism, prolonged treatment in adults, scoliosis, sleep apnea, chemotherapy, respiratory disease, glycerin hypersensitivity (with formulations that contain these products)

DOSAGE AND ROUTES

Genotropin

- **Child: SUBCUT** 0.16-0.24 mg/kg/wk divided into 6 or 7 daily inj; give in abdomen, thigh, buttocks
- **Adult: SUBCUT** 0.04-0.08 mg/kg/wk divided into 6-7 daily doses

Humatrope

- **Adult: IM** 0.006 international units/kg/day, max 0.0125 units/kg/day
- **Child: SUBCUT/IM** 0.18 mg/kg divided into equal doses either on 3 alternate days or 6×/wk, max weekly dose 0.3 mg/kg

Nutropin/Nutropin AQ (growth hormone deficiency)

- **Child: SUBCUT** 0.3 mg/kg/wk

Serostim

- **Adult: SUBCUT** at bedtime >55 kg, 6 mg; 45-55 kg, 5 mg; 35-45 kg, 4 mg

Norditropin

- **Child: SUBCUT** 0.024-0.034 mg/kg 6-7×/wk

Replacement of GH in GH deficiency

- **Adult: SUBCUT** (Saizen) 0.005 mg/kg/day; may increase after 4 wk to max 0.01 mg/kg/day

Available forms: Powder for inj (lyophilized) 1.5 mg (4 international units/ml), 4 mg (12 international units/vial), 5 mg (13 international units/vial), 5 mg

S

(15 international units/vial) rDNA origin, 5.8 mg (15 international units/ml), 6 mg (18 international units/ml), 8 mg (24 international units/vial), 10 mg (26 international units/vial); inj 10 mg (30 international units/vial), 5 mg/1.5 ml, 10 mg/1.5 ml, 15 mg/1.5 ml

Administer:

- Give IM or subcut; do not use IV
- Discontinue therapy if final height is achieved or epiphyseal fusion occurs
- Visually inspect parenteral products for particulate matter and discoloration

Reconstitution and storage

Genotropin:

- Powder, filled in a two-chamber cartridge with the active substance in the front chamber and the diluent in the rear chamber; available in a 5-mg cartridge (green tip) and a 12-mg cartridge (purple tip); the 5- and 12-mg cartridges may be used with the Genotropin Pen or the Genotropin Mixer; also in various doses ranging from 0.2 mg to 2 mg, in single use, auto-mix devices called Genotropin Miniquicks
- **Cartridges:** store cartridges refrigerated before reconstitution, do not freeze; protect from light; a reconstitution device supplied is used to mix the powder and the diluent; after the powder and diluent are mixed, gently tip the cartridge upside down a few times until powder is dissolved; *do not shake;* if solution is cloudy, do not use; following reconstitution, the 5-mg cartridge contains a 5 mg/ml; the 12-mg cartridge contains a 12 mg/ml 5-mg, and 12-mg cartridges contain overfill; the cartridges contain diluent with preservative (m-cresol) and may be stored refrigerated ≤28 days after reconstitution; do not use the 5-mg and 12-mg cartridges in patients with m-cresol hypersensitivity
- **Genotropin Miniquicks:** after dispensing but before reconstitution, store at ≤77° ≤3 mo; a reconstitution device is supplied and is used to mix the powder and diluent; 10 different strengths are available that each deliver a fixed volume of 0.25 ml; this product contains a diluent with no preservative, refrigerate after reconstitution and use within 24 hr; use the reconstituted solution only once and discard any remaining

Humatrope:

- Before reconstitution, store refrigerated
- **Vials:** reconstitute each 5-mg vial with 1.5-5 ml of the diluent (contains m-cresol as a preservative) or bacteriostatic water for injection (contains benzoyl alcohol as a preservative); sterile water for injection may be used for patients with a hypersensitivity to m-cresol and benzoyl alcohol; direct the liquid against the glass vial wall; swirl until contents are dissolved; do not shake; if the solution is cloudy, do not use; small, colorless particles may be present after refrigeration, this is not unusual for solutions containing proteins; vials reconstituted with the diluent or bacteriostatic water are stable for 14 days when refrigerated; for vials reconstituted with sterile water, use the vial only once and discard if not used immediately, refrigerate and use within 24 hr; avoid freezing
- **Cartridges:** reconstitute cartridges using *only* the supplied diluent syringe; the cartridges are designed for use only with the Humatrope injection device; once reconstituted, the cartridges are stable for up to 28 days when stored refrigerated; store the injection device without the needle attached; avoid freezing reconstituted solutions

Norditropin:

- Do not use reconstituted solution if it is cloudy or contains particulate matter
- Before use, store refrigerated
- Reconstitution of the cartridges is not required; the cartridge is intended for use only with the NordiPen injector; a prefilled, disposable pen, NordiFlex Pen injector, is also available; each cartridge size (5 mg, 10 mg, or 15 mg per 1.5-ml

cartridge) has a color-coded corresponding pen, which is graduated to deliver an appropriate dose based on the solution's concentration; NordiPen and NordiFlex Pen allow administration of a minimum 0.25-mg dose to a maximum 4.5-mg dose, depending on cartridge concentrations; follow directions provided in NordiPen injector instruction booklet

- After a cartridge has been inserted into the NordiPen injector or once a NordiFlex pen is in use, the pen should be stored refrigerated and used within 4 wk; alternatively, the 5-mg and 10-mg cartridges may be stored in the pen at room temperature, no higher than 77°, for up to 3 wk; NovoFine needles are recommended for administration; wipe the stopper of the pen cartridge with rubbing alcohol

Nutropin:

- Before reconstitution, store refrigerated
- Reconstitute each 5-mg vial with 1-5 ml bacteriostatic water for injection (benzyl alcohol preserved) and each 10-mg vial with 1-10 ml of bacteriostatic water for injection (benzyl alcohol preserved); if using for newborns, reconstitute with sterile water for injection; direct the liquid against the glass vial wall; swirl vial with a gentle rotary motion until contents are dissolved completely; do not shake; if the solution is cloudy after reconstitution or refrigeration, do not use; small, colorless particles may be present after refrigeration, this is not unusual for solutions containing proteins
- Solutions reconstituted with bacteriostatic water for injection are stable for 14 days refrigerated
- Solutions reconstituted with sterile water for injection should be used immediately and only once; discard any unused portions; avoid freezing reconstituted solutions

Nutropin AQ:

- Does not require reconstitution; solution should be clear; small, colorless particles may be present after refrigeration, this is not unusual for solutions containing proteins; allow vial or pen cartridge to come to room temperature, and gently swirl; if solution is cloudy, do not use
- **Vials:** before inserting needle, wipe the vial septum with rubbing alcohol or antiseptic solution to prevent contamination by microorganisms that may be introduced by repeated needle insertions; administer using sterile disposable syringes and needles; use syringes with small enough volume that the prescribed dose may be drawn from the vial with reasonable accuracy
- **Pen cartridge:** two strengths are available, 10 mg and 20 mg; intended for use only with Nutropin AQ Pen; each pen and cartridge are color coded to ensure accurate placement of the 10-mg or 20-mg cartridge into the appropriate pen; do not use the 20-mg cartridge in the pen intended for the 10-mg cartridge, and vice versa; wipe septum of pen cartridge with rubbing alcohol or antiseptic solution to prevent contamination by microorganisms that may be introduced by repeated needle insertions; administer using sterile, disposable needles; follow the directions provided in the Nutropin AQ Pen Instructions for Use; the Nutropin AQ 10 pen allows administration of a minimum 0.1-mg dose to a maximum 4-mg dose, in 0.1-mg increments; the Nutropin AQ 20 pen allows administration of a minimum 0.2-mg dose to a maximum 8-mg dose, in 0.2-mg increments
- **Prefilled device:** a prefilled multidose, dial-a-dose device is available in 3 strengths; administer using disposable needles; follow the directions provided in the Nutropin AQ NuSpin Instructions for Use; the Nutropin AQ Nuspin 5 allows administration of a minimum dose of 0.05 mg to a maximum dose of 1.75 mg, in increments of 0.05 mg; the Nutropin AQ Nuspin 10 allows administration of a minimum dose of 0.1 mg to a maximum

S

dose of 3.5 mg, in increments of 0.1 mg; the Nutropin AQ Nuspin 20 allows administration of a minimum dose of 0.2 mg to a maximum dose of 7 mg, in increments of 0.2 mg

• After initial use, vials, cartridges, and prefilled devices are stable for 28 days refrigerated; avoid freezing; vials, cartridges, and prefilled devices are light sensitive; protect from light

Omnitrope:

• Before reconstitution, store vials refrigerated; store in the carton; Omnitrope is sensitive to light

• **Vials:** reconstitute the vial with diluent provided using a sterile disposable syringe; swirl the vial gently, but do not shake; if the solution is cloudy after reconstitution, the contents must not be injected; after reconstitution, the 1.5-mg vial may be refrigerated ≤24 hr; the 1.5-mg vial does not contain a preservative and should only be used once; discard any remaining solution; the 5.8-mg vial diluent contains benzoyl alcohol as a preservative; after reconstitution, the contents must be used within 3 wk; after the first injection, store the 5.8-mg vial in the carton, to protect from light, in the refrigerator; avoid freezing

• **Omnitrope Pen 5 cartridge:** each 5-mg cartridge must be inserted into the Omnitrope Pen 5 delivery system; follow the directions provided in the Omnitrope Instructions for Use; the cartridge contains benzoyl alcohol as a preservative; after the first use, store refrigerated ≤28 days; protect from light, avoid freezing

• **Omnitrope Pen 10 cartridge:** each 10-mg cartridge must be inserted into the Omnitrope Pen 10 delivery system; follow the directions provided in the Omnitrope Instructions for Use; after the first use, store refrigerated ≤28 days; protect from light, avoid freezing

Saizen:

• Before reconstitution, store at room temperature

• **Vials:** reconstitute each 5-mg vial with 1-3 ml bacteriostatic water for injection; reconstitute each 8.8-mg vial with 2-3 ml bacteriostatic water for injection (benzoyl alcohol preserved); in patients with hypersensitivity to benzyl alcohol, the vials may be mixed with sterile water for injection; direct the liquid against the glass vial wall; swirl vial with a gentle rotary motion until contents are dissolved completely; do not shake; the solution should be clear; if it is cloudy immediately after reconstitution or refrigeration, do not use; small colorless particles may be present after refrigeration, this is not unusual for solutions containing proteins; after reconstitution, store vials mixed with bacteriostatic water for injection refrigerated and use within 14 days; for vials mixed with sterile water for injection, the solution should be used immediately, and any unused portion should be discarded; avoid freezing

• **Cartridges:** available in 4-mg and 8.8-mg click.easy cartridges for use in a compatible injection device; a reconstitution device supplied by the manufacturer is used to mix the Saizen with accompanying diluent containing metacresol; cartridges reconstituted with the diluent containing metascresol are stable under refrigeration for ≤21 days; avoid freezing

Serostim:

• Before reconstitution, store vials and diluent at room temperature (15-30° C; 59–86° F)

• **Vials:** reconstitute the 5-mg or 6-mg vials with 0.5-1 ml of supplied diluent (sterile water for injection); reconstitute the 4-mg vial with 0.5-1 ml of bacteriostatic water for injection (benzoyl alcohol preserved) and the 8.8-mg vial with 1-2 ml of bacteriostatic water for injection (benzoyl alcohol preserved); direct the liquid against the glass vial wall; swirl vial with a gentle rotary motion until contents are dissolved completely; do not shake; the solution should be clear; if it is cloudy immediately after reconstitution or refrigeration, do not use; small colorless particles may be present after refrigeration, this is not unusual for solutions containing proteins; if reconstituted with sterile water for injection, use within 24 hr; if reconstituted with bacteriostatic water for injection (benzoyl alcohol preserved), the solution is stable for up to 14 days under refrigeration (2-8° C or 36-46° F); avoid freezing

• **Cartridges:** available in 8.8-mg click. easy cartridges for use in a compatible injection device; a reconstitution device is supplied by the manufacturer and is used to mix the Serostim with accompanying diluent containing metacresol; after reconstitution, cartridges are stable under refrigeration for ≤21 days; avoid freezing

Serostim LQ:

• Before use, store refrigerated

• Available in 6-mg single-use cartridges that do not require reconstitution; administer using sterile disposable syringes and needles

• Bring to room temperature before use; discard single-use cartridge after use, even if some drug remains; discard cartridges after the expiration date stated on the product; do not freeze; protect from light

Tev-Tropin:

• Before reconstitution, store refrigerated

• Reconstitute each 5-mg vial with 1-5 ml bacteriostatic 0.9% sodium chloride (benzoyl alcohol preserved) for injection; direct the liquid against the glass vial wall; swirl vial with a gentle rotary motion until contents are dissolved completely; do not shake; the solution should be clear; if it is cloudy immediately after reconstitution, do not inject; small, colorless particles may be present after refrigeration, this is not unusual for solutions containing proteins; when administering to newborns, reconstitute with sterile normal saline for injection that is unpreserved

• Solution reconstituted with bacteriostatic 0.9% sodium chloride is stable for 14 days when stored refrigerated; solution reconstituted with sterile normal saline should be used only once; discard any remaining solution; avoid freezing

Valtropin:

• Before dispensing, store vials and diluent refrigerated; after dispensing to patients, may be stored at or below 77° F for up to 3 mo

• Reconstitute each 5-mg vial with the entire contents of the accompanying diluent, which contains metacresol as a preservative; if patients are allergic to metacresol, sterile water for injection may be used; direct the liquid against the glass vial wall; swirl vial with a gentle rotary motion until contents are dissolved completely; do not shake; the solution should be clear, if it is cloudy or contains particulate matter immediately after reconstitution or after refrigeration, do not inject; the final concentration of the reconstituted solution is 3.33 mg/ml

• After reconstitution with the provided diluent, solutions may be stored refrigerated for up to 14 days; after reconstitution with sterile water for injection, use only one dose of Valtropin per vial and discard the unused portion if not used immediately

Zorbtive:

• Unreconstituted vials of drug and diluent may be stored at room temperature until expiration date

• Reconstitute each vial of 4 mg, 5 mg, or 6 mg with 0.5-1 ml sterile water for injection, USP; reconstitute each 8.8 mg with 1-2 ml bacteriostatic water for injection (0.9% benzyl alcohol preserved); in newborns or patients with a benzoyl alcohol hypersensitivity, sterile water for injection may be used; review manufacturer's labeling for expected concentrations; direct the liquid against the glass vial wall; swirl vial with a gentle rotary motion until contents are dissolved completely; do not shake; the solution should be clear, if it is cloudy after reconstitution or refrigeration, do not use; small colorless particles may be present after refrigeration, this is not unusual for solutions containing proteins

- After reconstitution with sterile water for injection, use the solution immediately and discard any unused portion; when using bacteriostatic water for injection, reconstituted solutions are stable for up to 14 days refrigerated; avoid freezing vials of drug or diluent or reconstituted vials

IM route

- Inject deeply into a large muscle; aspirate before injection; rotate injection sites daily

SUBCUT route

- Volumes >1 ml of reconstituted solution are not recommended; do not inject intradermally
- Allow refrigerated solutions to come to room temperature before injection
- Subcutaneous injections may be given in the thigh, buttocks, or abdomen; rotate injection sites daily

SIDE EFFECTS

CNS: Headache, growth of intracranial tumor, fever, aggressive behavior
ENDO: Hyperglycemia, ketosis, hypothyroidism, thyroid hormone replacement may be needed
GI: Nausea, vomiting, pancreatitis
GU: *Hypercalciuria*
INTEG: Rash, urticaria, pain; inflammation at inj site, hematoma
MS: Tissue swelling, joint and muscle pain
SYST: Antibodies to growth hormone

PHARMACOKINETICS

Half-life 15-60 min, duration 7 days, metabolized in liver

INTERACTIONS

Increase: epiphyseal closure—androgens, thyroid hormones
Decrease: growth—glucocorticosteroids
Decrease: insulin, antidiabetic effect—dosage adjustment may be needed

Drug/Lab Test

Increase: glucose, urine glucose
Decrease: glucose thyroid hormones

NURSING CONSIDERATIONS

Assess:

- Signs/symptoms of diabetes
- Growth hormone antibodies if patient fails to respond to therapy
- Thyroid function tests: T_3, T_4, T_7, TSH to identify hypothyroidism
- **Allergic reaction:** rash, itching, fever, nausea, wheezing
- **Hypercalciuria:** urinary stones; groin, flank pain; nausea, vomiting, urinary frequency, hematuria, chills
- Growth rate, bone age of child at intervals during treatment
- **Respiratory infection:** in those with Prader-Willi syndrome, may have sleep apnea, upper airway obstruction; discontinue if obstruction occurs
- Rapid growth: assess for slipped capital femoral epiphysis may also occur in endocrine disorders
- Monitor ophthalmologic status baseline and periodically; intracranial hypertension may occur

Evaluate:

- Therapeutic response: growth in children

Teach patient/family:

- That treatment may continue for years; that regular assessments are required
- To maintain a growth record; to report knee/hip pain or limping
- That treatment is very expensive
- Identify creosol or benzyl-alcohol hypersensitivity before use

sotalol (Rx)

(sot'ah-lahl)

Betapace, Betapace AF, Rylosol ♣, Sorine

Func. class.: Antidysrhythmic group III
Chem. class.: Nonselective β-blocker

ACTION: Blockade of β_1- and β_2-receptors leads to antidysrhythmic effect, prolongs action potential in myocardial fibers without affecting conduction, prolongs QT interval, no effect on QRS duration

USES:
Life-threatening ventricular dysrhythmias; Betapace AF: to maintain sinus rhythm with symptomatic atrial fibrillation/flutter

Unlabeled uses: Atrial fibrillation prophylaxis, cardiac surgery, PSVT, Wolff-Parkinson-White (WPW) syndrome

CONTRAINDICATIONS:
Hypersensitivity to β-blockers, cardiogenic shock, heart block (2nd/3rd degree), sinus bradycardia, CHF, bronchial asthma, CCr <40 ml/min

Black Box Warning: Congenital or acquired long QT syndrome, hypokalemia

Precautions: Pregnancy (B), breastfeeding, major surgery, diabetes mellitus, renal/thyroid disease, COPD, well-compensated heart failure, CAD, nonallergic bronchospasm, electrolyte disturbances, bradycardia, peripheral vascular disease

Black Box Warning: Cardiac dysrhythmias, torsades de pointes, ventricular dysrhythmias, ventricular fibrillation

DOSAGE AND ROUTES

- **Adult: PO** initial 80 mg bid, may increase to 240-320 mg/day
- **Child >2 yr with normal renal function (unlabeled): PO** 30 mg/m^2 tid, adjust dose gradually after ≥36 hr to max 60 mg/m^2 tid

Renal dose

- **Adult: PO** CCr 30-60 ml/min, give q24hr; CCr 10-29 ml/min, give q36-48hr; CCr <10 ml/min, individualize dose

Life-threatening ventricular dysrhythmias

- **Adult (CCr 40-60 ml/min): IV** 75 mg over 5 hr daily, monitor QTc at end of each infusion during initiation and titration; 80 mg PO = 75 mg IV; 120 mg PO = 112.5 mg IV; 160 mg PO = 150 mg IV

Betapace AF

- **Adult: PO** initial 80 mg bid, titrate upward to 120 mg bid during initial hospitalization, monitor QTc interval for 2-4 hr after each dose

Renal dose (Betapace AF)

- **Adult: PO** CCr >60 ml/min, give q12hr; CCr 40-60 ml/min, give q24hr; CCr <40 ml/min, do not use

Available forms: Tabs 80, 120, 160, 240 mg; (Betapace AF) 80, 120, 160 mg; inj 150 mg/10 ml (15 mg/ml)

Administer:

PO route

- Before, at bedtime; tab may be crushed or swallowed whole; give 1 hr before or 2 hr after meals
- Reduced dosage in renal dysfunction
- Betapace and Betapace AF are not interchangeable
- Do not give within 2 hr of antacids
- Store in dry area at room temperature; do not freeze

IV route

- Dilute to vol of either 120 ml or 300 ml with D_5W, LR
- **75 mg dose:** withdraw 6 ml sotalol inj (90 mg), add 114 ml dilute to make 120 ml (0.75 mg/ml); or withdraw 6 ml sotalol inj (90 mg), add 294 ml dilute to make 300 ml (0.3 mg/ml)
- **112.5 mg dose:** withdraw 9 ml sotalol inj (135 ml), add 111 ml dilute to make 120 ml (1.125 mg/ml); or withdraw 9 ml sotalol (135 mg), add 291 ml dilute to make 300 ml (0.45 mg/ml)
- **150 mg dose:** withdraw 12 ml of sotalol (180 mg), add 108 ml to make 120 ml (1.5 mg/ml); or withdraw 12 ml sotalol (180 mg), add 288 ml to make 300 ml (0.6 mg/ml)
- Use infusion pump and infuse 100 or 250 ml over 5 hr at a constant rate

SIDE EFFECTS

CNS: Dizziness, mental changes, drowsiness, fatigue, headache, catatonia, depression, anxiety, nightmares, paresthesia, lethargy, insomnia, decreased concentration

S

CV: Prodysrhythmia, prolonged QT, orthostatic hypotension, bradycardia, CHF, chest pain, ventricular dysrhythmias, AV block, peripheral vascular insufficiency, palpitations, torsades de pointes; life-threatening ventricular dysrhythmias (Betapace AF)
EENT: Tinnitus, visual changes, sore throat, double vision; dry, burning eyes
GI: Nausea, vomiting, diarrhea, dry mouth, flatulence, constipation, anorexia, indigestion
GU: Impotence, dysuria, ejaculatory failure, urinary retention
HEMA: Agranulocytosis, thrombocytopenic purpura (rare), thrombocytopenia, leukopenia
INTEG: Rash, alopecia, urticaria, pruritus, fever, diaphoresis
MISC: Facial swelling, decreased exercise tolerance, weight change, Raynaud's disease
MS: Joint pain, arthralgia, muscle cramps, pain
RESP: Bronchospasm, dyspnea, wheezing, nasal stuffiness, pharyngitis

PHARMACOKINETICS

PO: Onset 1-2 hr, peak 2-4 hr, duration 8-12 hr, half-life 12 hr, excreted unchanged in urine, crosses placenta, excreted in breast milk, protein binding 0%

INTERACTIONS

Black Box Warning: Increase: QT prolongation—class IA/III antidysrhythmics, some phenothiazines, β agonists, local anesthetics, tricyclics, haloperidol, chloroquine, droperidol, pentamidine; CYP3A4 inhibitors (amiodarone, clarithromycin, erythromycin, telithromycin, troleandomycin), arsenic trioxide, levomethadyl; CYP3A4 substrates (methadone, pimozide, QUEtiapine, quiNIDine, risperiDONE, ziprasidone)

Increase: hypoglycemia effect—insulin
Increase: effects of lidocaine
Increase: hypotension—diuretics, other antihypertensives, nitroglycerin
Decrease: β-blocker effects—sympathomimetics
Decrease: bronchodilating effects of theophylline, β_2-agonists
Decrease: hypoglycemic effects of sulfonylureas

Drug/Lab Test
False increase: urinary catecholamines
Interference: glucose, insulin tolerance tests

Drug/Herb
- Do not use with hawthorn

NURSING CONSIDERATIONS

Assess:
- I&O, weight daily; edema in feet, legs daily
- B/P, pulse q4hr; note rate, rhythm, quality
- Potassium, magnesium levels

Black Box Warning: Requires a specialized care setting: for a minimum of at least 3 days on maintenance dose with continuous ECG monitoring, creatinine clearance; calculate before dosing

Black Box Warning: Cardiogenic shock, acute pulmonary edema: do not use, effect can further depress cardiac output

⚠ **QT syndrome:** apical/radial pulse before administration: notify prescriber of any significant changes; monitor ECG continuously (Betapace AF); use QT interval to determine patient eligibility; baseline QT must be ≤450 msec, if ≥500 msec, frequency or dosage must be decreased or drug discontinued
- Baselines of renal studies before therapy begins
- **Abrupt discontinuation:** do not discontinue abruptly, taper over 1-2 wk
- Dose should be adjusted slowly, with at least 3 days between changes; monitor ECG for QT interval
- Monitor electrolytes (hypokalemia, hypomagnesia) may increase dysrhythmias

Evaluate:
- Therapeutic response: absence of life-threatening dysrhythmias

Teach patient/family:

- Not to discontinue product abruptly; to taper over 2 wk or may precipitate angina; to take exactly as prescribed
- Not to use antacids or OTC products containing α-adrenergic stimulants (nasal decongestants, OTC cold preparations) unless directed by prescriber
- To report bradycardia, dizziness, confusion, depression, fever
- To take pulse at home; advise patient when to notify prescriber
- To avoid alcohol, smoking, sodium intake
- To carry emergency ID to identify product being taken, allergies
- To avoid hazardous activities if dizziness present
- To report symptoms of CHF including difficulty breathing, especially on exertion or when lying down; night cough, swelling of extremities
- To wear support hose to minimize effects of orthostatic hypotension
- To monitor blood glucose if diabetic
- That hospitalization will be required for ≥3 days

TREATMENT OF OVERDOSE:
Lavage, IV atropine for bradycardia, IV theophylline for bronchospasm, digoxin, O_2, diuretic for cardiac failure; hemodialysis is useful for removal; administer vasopressor (norepinephrine) for hypotension, isoproterenol for heart block

spironolactone (Rx)
(speer′on-oh-lak′tone)

Aldactone, Novo-Spiroton ✦

Func. class.: Potassium-sparing diuretic

Chem. class.: Aldosterone antagonist

Do not confuse:
Aldactone/Aldactazide

ACTION:
Competes with aldosterone at receptor sites in distal tubule, thereby resulting in the excretion of sodium chloride and water and the retention of potassium and phosphate

USES:
Edema of CHF, hypertension, diuretic-induced hypokalemia, primary hyperaldosteronism (diagnosis, short-term treatment, long-term treatment), edema of nephrotic syndrome, cirrhosis of liver with ascites

Unlabeled uses: CHF, hirsutism in women, bronchopulmonary dysplasia (BPD), PMS, polycystic ovary syndrome, acne vulgaris, premenstrual syndrome

CONTRAINDICATIONS:
Hypersensitivity, anuria, severe renal disease, hyperkalemia

Precautions: Breastfeeding, dehydration, hepatic disease, renal impairment, electrolyte imbalances, metabolic acidosis, gynecomastia, pregnancy (C)

Black Box Warning: Secondary malignancy

DOSAGE AND ROUTES
Edema/hypertension
- **Adult: PO** 25-200 mg/day in 1-2 divided doses

CHF
- **Adult: PO** 12.5-25 mg/day; max 50 mg/day

Edema
- **Child: PO** 1.5-3.3 mg/kg/day as single dose or in divided doses

Hypertension
- **Child (unlabeled): PO** 1.5-3.3 mg/kg/day in divided doses

Hypokalemia
- **Adult: PO** 25-100 mg/day; if **PO,** potassium supplements must not be used

Primary hyperaldosteronism diagnosis
- **Adult: PO** 400 mg/day × 4 days or 4 wk depending on test, then 100-400 mg/day maintenance

Edema (nephrotic syndrome, CHF, hepatic disease)
- **Adult: PO** 100 mg/day given as single dose or in divided doses, titrate to response

• **Child: PO** 1.5-3.3 mg/kg/day or 60 $mg/m^2/day$ given daily or in 2-4 divided doses

Renal dose

• **Adult: PO** CCr 10-50 ml/min; give dose q12-24hr; CCr <10 ml/min, avoid use

Polycystic ovary syndrome/ hirsutism in women (unlabeled)

• **Adult: PO** 50-200 mg in 1-2 divided doses

Available forms: Tabs 25, 50, 100 mg

Administer:

• In AM to avoid interference with sleep
• With food; if nausea occurs, absorption may be decreased slightly
• Effect may take 2 wk

SIDE EFFECTS

CNS: *Headache,* confusion, drowsiness, lethargy, ataxia

ELECT: Hyperchloremic metabolic acidosis, hyperkalemia, hyponatremia

ENDO: Impotence, gynecomastia, irregular menses, amenorrhea, postmenopausal bleeding, hirsutism, deepening voice, breast pain

GI: *Diarrhea,* cramps, bleeding, gastritis, *vomiting,* anorexia, nausea, hepatocellular toxicity

HEMA: Agranulocytosis

INTEG: *Rash, pruritus,* urticaria

PHARMACOKINETICS

Onset 24-48 hr, peak 48-72 hr, metabolized in liver, excreted in urine, crosses placenta, protein binding >90%, terminal half-life 10-35 hr

INTERACTIONS

Increase: action of antihypertensives, digoxin, lithium

Increase: hyperchloremic acidosis in cirrhosis—cholestyramine

Increase: hyperkalemia—potassium-sparing diuretics, potassium products, ACE inhibitors, salt substitutes

Decrease: effect of anticoagulants, monitor INR/PT

Decrease: effect of spironolactone—ASA, NSAIDs

Drug/Food

Increase: hyperkalemia—potassium-rich foods, potassium salt substitutes

Drug/Herb

Increase: hypotension—hawthorn, horse chestnut

Decrease: antihypertensive effect—ephedra

Increase: severe photosensitivity—St. John's wort

Increase: BUN, potassium

Decrease: sodium, magnesium

Drug/Lab Test

Interference: 17-OHCS, 17-KS, radioimmunoassay, digoxin assay

NURSING CONSIDERATIONS

Assess:

• **Hypokalemia:** polyuria, polydipsia; dysrhythmias, inluding a U wave on ECG
• **Hyperkalemia:** weakness, fatigue, dyspnea, dysrhythmias, confusion, fatigue
• Electrolytes: sodium, chloride, potassium, BUN, serum creatinine, ABGs, CBC
• Weight, I&O daily to determine fluid loss; effect of product may be decreased if used daily; ECG periodically with long-term therapy
• Signs of metabolic acidosis: drowsiness, restlessness
• Confusion, especially in geriatric patients; take safety precautions if needed
• **Hydration:** skin turgor, thirst, dry mucous membranes

Black Box Warning: Secondary malignancy: assess periodically

Evaluate:

• Therapeutic response: improvement in edema of feet, legs, sacral area daily if medication is being used in CHF

Teach patient/family:

• To avoid foods with high potassium content: oranges, bananas, salt substitutes, dried apricots, dates; to avoid potassium salt substitutes
• That drowsiness, ataxia, mental confusion may occur; to observe caution when driving

- To notify prescriber of cramps, diarrhea, lethargy, thirst, headache, skin rash, menstrual abnormalities, deepening voice, breast enlargement
- To take in AM, to prevent sleeplessness
- To avoid hazardous activities until reaction is known
- To notify prescriber if pregnancy is planned or suspected, pregnancy (C); not to breastfeed

TREATMENT OF OVERDOSE:
Lavage if taken orally; monitor electrolytes, administer IV fluids, monitor hydration, renal, CV status

stavudine (d4T) (Rx)
(sta′vyoo-deen)

Zerit

Func. class.: Antiretroviral

Chem. class.: Nucleoside reverse transcriptase inhibitor (NRTI)

ACTION: Prevents replication of HIV by the inhibition of the enzyme reverse transcriptase; causes DNA chain termination

USES: Treatment of HIV-1 in combination with other antiretrovirals

CONTRAINDICATIONS: Hypersensitivity to this product or zidovudine; didanosine, zalcitabine; severe peripheral neuropathy

Black Box Warning: Lactic acidosis

Precautions: Breastfeeding, advanced HIV infection, bone marrow suppression, renal disease, peripheral neuropathy, osteoporosis, obesity

Black Box Warning: Pregnancy (C), hepatic disease, pancreatitis

DOSAGE AND ROUTES
- **Adult >60 kg: PO** 40 mg q12hr
- **Adult <60 kg: PO** 30 mg q12hr
- **Child <30 kg: PO** 1 mg/kg q12hr
- **Child ≥30 kg, ≤60 kg: PO** 30 mg q12hr
- **Child >60 kg: PO** 40 mg q12hr

Renal dose
- **Adult: PO** CCr 26-50 ml/min, reduce by 50%, give q12hr; CCr 10-25 ml/min, reduce by 50%, give q24hr

Available forms: Caps 15, 20, 30, 40 mg; powder for oral sol 1 mg/ml

Administer:
- With/without meals; absorption does not appear to be lowered when taken with food
- Use after hemodialysis
- Every 12 hr around the clock
- Shake suspension well before using

SIDE EFFECTS
CNS: *Peripheral neuropathy,* insomnia, anxiety, depression, dizziness, confusion, *headache,* chills/fever, malaise, neuropathy

CV: Chest pain, vasodilation, hypertension

EENT: Conjunctivitis, abnormal vision

GI: **Hepatotoxicity,** *diarrhea, nausea, vomiting,* anorexia, dyspepsia, constipation, stomatitis, **pancreatitis**

HEMA: **Bone marrow suppression,** leukopenia, macrocytosis

INTEG: *Rash,* sweating, pruritus, benign neoplasms

MISC: **Lactic acidosis,** asthenia, lipodystrophy

MS: Myalgia, arthralgia

RESP: Dyspnea, pneumonia, asthma

S

PHARMACOKINETICS
Excreted in urine, breast milk; peak 1 hr; half-life: elimination 1-1.6 hr

INTERACTIONS
Increase: myelosuppression—other myelosuppressants

Increase: peripheral neuropathy—lithium, dapsone, chloramphenicol didanosine, ethambutol, hydrALAZINE, phenytoin, vinCRIStine, zalcitabine

Increase: stavudine levels—probenecid

Decrease: stavudine effect—methadone, zidovudine

NURSING CONSIDERATIONS

Assess:

Black Box Warning: Lactic acidosis and severe hepatomegaly with steatosis: death may result; monitor LFTs

Black Box Warning: Pancreatitis: severe upper abdominal pain, radiating to back, nausea, vomiting usually when used in combination with didanosine

- Blood studies: WBC, differential, RBC, Hct, Hgb, platelets, serum amylase, lipase, blood glucose, plasma hepatitis C RNA, pregnancy test, serum cholesterol, serum lipids, hepatitis serology, baseline and periodically
- Renal tests: urinalysis, protein, blood, serum creatinine
- Lipoatrophy/lipodystrophy during treatment
- Bowel pattern before, during treatment
- Weakness, tremors, confusion, dizziness; product may have to be decreased, discontinued
- Viral load, CD4 counts, plasma HIV RNA at baseline and throughout treatment
- **Peripheral neuropathy:** tingling, pain in extremities; discontinue product, may not resolve after treatment is discontinued

Evaluate:

- Therapeutic response: decreased symptoms of HIV

Teach patient/family:

- **About the signs of peripheral neuropathy:** burning, weakness, pain, prickling feeling in extremities
- That product should not be given with antineoplastics
- That product is not a cure for AIDS but will control symptoms
- To notify prescriber if sore throat, swollen lymph nodes, malaise, fever occur; that other products may be needed to prevent other infections
- That, even with use of product, patient may pass AIDS virus to others
- That follow-up visits are necessary; that serious toxicity may occur; that blood counts must be done q2wk
- ⚠ That serious product interactions may occur if other medications are ingested; to see prescriber before taking chloramphenicol, dapsone, CISplatin, didanosine, ethambutol, lithium, antifungals, antineoplastics

Black Box Warning: To notify prescriber if pregnancy is planned or suspected, fatal lactic acidosis may occur, pregnancy (C), avoid breastfeeding

- That product may cause fainting or dizziness

⚠ HIGH ALERT

succinylcholine (Rx)

(suk-sin-ill-koe′leen)

Anectine, Quelicin

Func. class.: Neuromuscular blocker (depolarizing, ultra short)

ACTION: Inhibits transmission of nerve impulses by binding with cholinergic receptor sites, thus antagonizing action of acetylcholine; causes release of histamine

USES: Facilitation of endotracheal intubation, skeletal muscle relaxation during orthopedic manipulations

CONTRAINDICATIONS: Hypersensitivity, malignant hyperthermia, trauma

Precautions: Pregnancy (C), breastfeeding, geriatric or debilitated patients, cardiac disease, severe burns, fractures (fasciculations may increase damage) electrolyte imbalances, dehydration, neuromuscular/respiratory/cardiac/renal/hepatic disease, collagen diseases, glaucoma, eye surgery

Black Box Warning: Children <2 yr, hyperkalemia, myopathy, rhabdomyolysis

DOSAGE AND ROUTES

- **Adult: IV** 0.3-1.1 mg/kg, max 150 mg, maintenance 0.04-0.07 mg/kg q5-10min as needed; **CONT IV INFUSION** dilute to concentration of 1-2 mg/ml in D_5W or NS 10-100 mcg/kg/min
- **Child: IV** initially 1-2 mg/kg; **CONT IV INFUSION** not recommended

Available forms: Inj 20, 50, 100 mg/ml; powder for inj 100, 500 mg/vial, 1 g/vial

Administer:

- Give IV or IM; only experienced clinicians familiar with the use of neuromuscular blocking drugs should administer or supervise the use of this product
- Visually inspect parenteral products for particulate matter and discoloration before use
- Monitor heart rate and mechanical ventilator status during use
- Store in refrigerator, powder at room temperature; close tightly

IM route

- Recommended for infants and other patients in whom a suitable vein is not accessible
- Inject into a large muscle, preferably high into the deltoid muscle; aspirate before injection

Rapid IV injection route

- Owing to tachyphylaxis and prolonged apnea, this method is not recommended for prolonged procedures; rapid IV injection of succinylcholine can result in profound bradycardia or asystole in pediatric patients; as with adults, the risk increases with repeated doses; pretreatment with atropine may be needed
- No dilution of injection solution is necessary
- Inject rapidly IV over 10-30 sec

Continuous IV infusion route

- Not recommended for infants and children owing to risk of malignant hyperthermia
- This route is preferred for long surgical procedures owing to possible tachyphylaxis and prolonged apnea associated with administration of repeated fractional doses
- Dilute succinylcholine to a concentration of 1-2 mg/ml with D_5W, D_5NS, NS, or 1/6 M sodium lactate injection; 1 g of the powder for injection or 20 ml of a 50-mg/ml solution may be added to 1 L or 500 ml of diluent to give solutions containing 1 or 2 mg/ml, respectively; alternatively, 500 mg of the powder for injection or 10 ml of a 50 mg/ml solution may be added to 500 ml or 250 ml of diluent to give solutions containing 1 or 2 mg/ml, respectively
- Infuse IV at a rate of 2.5 mg/min (range = 0.5-10 mg/min); adjust rate based on patient's response and requirements

Additive compatibilities: Amikacin, cephapirin, isoproterenol, meperidine, methyldopate, morphine, norepinephrine, scopolamine

Syringe compatibilities: Heparin

Y-site compatibilities: Etomidate, heparin, potassium chloride, propofol, vit B/C

SIDE EFFECTS

CV: Bradycardia, tachycardia; increased, decreased B/P; **sinus arrest, dysrhythmias**, edema

EENT: Increased secretions, intraocular pressure

HEMA: **Myoglobulinemia**

INTEG: Rash, flushing, pruritus, urticaria

MS: Weakness, muscle pain, fasciculations, prolonged relaxation, myalgia, **rhabdomyolysis**

RESP: **Prolonged apnea, bronchospasm, cyanosis, respiratory depression**, wheezing, dyspnea

SYST: **Anaphylaxis, angioedema**

PHARMACOKINETICS

Hydrolyzed in blood, excreted in urine (active/inactive metabolites)

IM: Onset 2-3 min, duration 10-30 min

IV: Onset 1 min, peak 2-3 min, duration 6-10 min

INTERACTIONS

Increase: dysrhythmias: theophylline

Increase: neuromuscular blockade—aminoglycosides, β-blockers, cardiac glycosides, clindamycin, lincomycin, procainamide, quiNIDine, local anesthetics, polymyxin antibiotics, lithium, opioids, thiazides, enflurane, isoflurane, magnesium salts, oxytocin

Drug/Herb

- Blocks succinylcholine: melatonin

NURSING CONSIDERATIONS

Assess:

- Electrolyte imbalances (potassium, magnesium); may lead to increased action of product
- VS (B/P, pulse, respirations, airway) until fully recovered; rate, depth, pattern of respirations, strength of hand grip
- I&O ratio; check for urinary retention, frequency, hesitancy
- **Recovery:** decreased paralysis of face, diaphragm, leg, arm, rest of body
- **Allergic reactions:** rash, fever, respiratory distress, pruritus; product should be discontinued

Black Box Warning: Myopathy, rhabdomyolysis: in pediatric patients (rare)

- Reassurance if communication is difficult during recovery from neuromuscular blockade; postoperative stiffness is normal, soon subsides

Evaluate:

- Therapeutic response: paralysis of jaw, eyelid, head, neck, rest of body

TREATMENT OF OVERDOSE:

Neostigmine, atropine, monitor VS; may require mechanical ventilation

sucralfate (Rx)

(soo-kral′fate)

Carafate, Sulcrate ♣

Func. class.: Protectant, antiulcer

Chem. class.: Aluminum hydroxide, sulfated sucrose

Do not confuse:

Carafate/Cafergot

ACTION: Forms a complex that adheres to ulcer site, adsorbs pepsin

USES: Duodenal ulcer, oral mucositis, stomatitis after radiation of head and neck

Unlabeled uses: Gastric/aphthous ulcers, gastroesophageal reflux, NSAID-induced ulcer prophylaxis, proctitis, stomatitis, stress gastritis prophylaxis, *C. difficile*

CONTRAINDICATIONS: Hypersensitivity

Precautions: Pregnancy (B), breastfeeding, children, renal failure; hypoglycemia (diabetics)

DOSAGE AND ROUTES

Duodenal ulcers

- **Adult: PO** 1 g qid 1 hr before meals, at bedtime
- **Child: PO** 40-80 mg/kg/day divided

Aphthous ulcer/stomatitis (unlabeled)

- **Adult: PO** 5-10 ml (500 mg-1 g) swished in mouth for several min; spit or swallow qid

Gastric ulcer/NSAID-induced ulcer prophylaxis/esophagitis/GERD (unlabeled)

- **Adult: PO** 1 g qid, 1 hr before meals and at bedtime

Available forms: Tabs 1 g; oral susp 1 g/10 ml

Administer:

PO route

- Do not crush or chew tabs; tabs may be broken or dissolved in water
- Do not take antacids 30 min before or after sucralfate
- On an empty stomach 1 hr before meals or other medications and at bedtime
- Store at room temperature

SIDE EFFECTS

CNS: Drowsiness, dizziness

ENDO: Hyperglycemia (diabetes mellitus)

GI: *Dry mouth, constipation,* nausea, gastric pain, vomiting

INTEG: Urticaria, rash, pruritus

PHARMACOKINETICS

PO: Duration up to 6 hr

INTERACTIONS

Decrease: action of tetracyclines, phenytoin, fat-soluble vitamins, digoxin, ketoconazole, theophylline
Decrease: absorption of fluoroquinolones
Decrease: absorption of sucralfate—antacids, cimetidine, ranitidine

NURSING CONSIDERATIONS

Assess:

- **GI symptoms:** abdominal pain, blood in stools
- **Hypoglycemia:** may occur in patients with diabetes mellitus; monitor blood glucose carefully

Evaluate:

- Therapeutic response: absence of pain, GI complaints

Teach patient/family:

- To take on empty stomach
- To take full course of therapy; not to use for >8 wk; to avoid smoking
- To avoid antacids within ½ hr of product
- To increase fluids, bulk, exercise to lessen constipation

sulfamethoxazole-trimethoprim (Rx)

(trye-meth′oh-prim–sul-fa-meth-ox′a-zole)

Bacter-Aid DS, Bactrim DS, Novo-Trimel ✦, Nu-Cotrimox ✦, Septra, Septra DS, Sultrex, SMZ/TMP

Func. class.: Antiinfective
Chem. class.: Sulfonamide—miscellaneous

ACTION: Sulfamethoxazole (SMZ) interferes with the bacterial biosynthesis of proteins by competitive antagonism of PABA when adequate levels are maintained; trimethoprim (TMP) blocks the synthesis of tetrahydrofolic acid; the combination blocks 2 consecutive steps in the bacterial synthesis of essential nucleic acids and protein

USES: UTI, otitis media, acute and chronic prostatitis, shigellosis, chancroid, traveler's diarrhea, *Enterobacter* sp., *Escherichia coli, Haemophilus influenzae (beta-lactamase negative), Haemophilus influenzae (beta-lactamase positive), Klebsiella* sp., *Morganella morganii, Pneumocystis carinii, Pneumocystis jiroveci, Proteus mirabilis, Proteus* sp., *Proteus vulgaris, Shigella flexneri, Shigella sonnei, Streptococcus pneumonia;* **may also be effective for** *Acinetobacter baumannii, Actinomadura madurae, Actinomadura pelletierii, Bordetella pertussis, Burkholderia pseudomallei, Cyclospora cayetanensis, Haemophilus ducreyi, Isospora belli, Klebsiella granulomatis, Legionella micdadei, Legionella pneumophila, Listeria monocytogenes, Moraxella catarrhalis, Neisseria gonorrhoeae, Nocardia asteroides, Nocardia brasiliensis, Nocardia otitidiscaviarum, Pediculus capitis, Plasmodium falciparum, Providencia* sp., *Salmonella* sp., *Serratia* sp., *Shigella* sp., *Staphylococcus aureus (MRSA), Staphylococcus aureus (MSSA), Staphylococcus epidermidis, Stenotrophomonas maltophilia, Streptococcus pyogenes* (group A beta-hemolytic streptococci), *Streptomyces somaliensis, Toxoplasma gondii, Vibrio cholerae, Viridans streptococci, Yersinia enterocolitica*

CONTRAINDICATIONS: Breastfeeding, infants <2 mo; hypersensitivity to trimethoprim or sulfonamides; pregnancy at term, megaloblastic anemia, CCr <15 ml/min
Precautions: Pregnancy (C), geriatric patients, infants, renal disease, G6PD deficiency, impaired hepatic/renal function, possible folate deficiency, severe allergy,

S

bronchial asthma, UV exposure, porphyria, hyperkalemia, hypothyroidism

DOSAGE AND ROUTES

Based on TMP content

UTI

- **Adult: PO** 160 mg TMP q12hr × 10-14 days
- **Child: PO** 8 mg/kg TMP/day in 2 divided doses q12hr (treatment): 2 mg/kg/day (prophylaxis)

Otitis media

- **Child: PO** 8 mg/kg TMP/day in 2 divided doses q12hr × 10 days

Chronic bronchitis

- **Adult: PO** 160 mg TMP q12hr × 10-14 days

***Pneumocystis jiroveci* pneumonitis**

- **Adult and child: PO** 15-20 mg/kg TMP daily in 4 divided doses q6hr × 14-21 days; **IV** 15-20 mg/kg/day (based on TMP) in 3-4 divided doses for ≤14 days
- Dosage reduction necessary in moderate to severe renal impairment (CCr <30 ml/min)

Available forms: Tabs 80 mg trimethoprim/400 mg sulfamethoxazole, 160 mg trimethoprim/800 mg sulfamethoxazole; susp 200 mg-40 mg/5 ml, 800 mg-160 mg/20 ml; IV 16 mg/80 mg/ml

Administer:

PO route

- Medication after C&S; repeat C&S after full course of medication
- With resuscitative equipment, EPINEPHrine available; severe allergic reactions may occur
- Without regard to meals
- With full glass of water to maintain adequate hydration; increase fluids to 2 L/day to decrease crystallization in kidneys
- Store in tight, light-resistant container at room temperature

Intermittent IV INFUSION route

- After diluting 5 ml of product/125 ml D_5W, run over 1-1½ hr, if using Septra ADD-Vantage vials dilute each 10-ml vial in ADD-Vantage diluent containers containing 250 ml of D_5W, infuse over 60-90 min, change site q48-72hr

Y-site compatibilities: Acyclovir, aldesleukin, allopurinol, amifostine, amphotericin B cholesteryl, atracurium, aztreonam, cefepime, cyclophosphamide, diltiazem, DOXOrubicin liposome, enalaprilat, esmolol, filgrastim, fludarabine, gallium, granisetron, HYDROmorphone, labetalol, LORazepam, magnesium sulfate, melphalan, meperidine, morphine, pancuronium, perphenazine, piperacillin/tazobactam, remifentanil, sargramostim, tacrolimus, teniposide, thiotepa, vecuronium, zidovudine

SIDE EFFECTS

CNS: Headache, insomnia, hallucinations, depression, vertigo, fatigue, anxiety, seizures, product fever, chills, aseptic meningitis

CV: Allergic myocarditis

EENT: Tinnitus

GI: *Nausea, vomiting, abdominal pain,* stomatitis, hepatitis, glossitis, pancreatitis, diarrhea, enterocolitis, anorexia, pseudomembranous colitis

GU: Renal failure, toxic nephrosis; increased BUN, creatinine; crystalluria

HEMA: Leukopenia, neutropenia, thrombocytopenia, agranulocytosis, hemolytic anemia, hypoprothrombinemia, Henoch-Schönlein purpura, methemoglobinemia, eosinophilia I

INTEG: Rash, dermatitis, urticaria, Stevens-Johnson syndrome, erythema, photosensitivity, pain, inflammation at inj site, toxic epidermal necrolysis, erythema multiforme

RESP: Cough, SOB

SYST: Anaphylaxis, SLE

PHARMACOKINETICS

PO: Rapidly absorbed; peak 1-4 hr; half-life 8-13 hr; excreted in urine (metabolites and unchanged), breast milk; crosses placenta; 68% bound to plasma proteins; TMP achieves high levels in prostatic tissue and fluid

INTERACTIONS

Increase: thrombocytopenia—thiazide diuretics

Increase: potassium levels—potassium-sparing diuretics, potassium supplements
Increase: hypoglycemic response—sulfonylurea agents
Increase: anticoagulant effects—oral anticoagulants
Increase: levels of dofetilide
Increase: crystalluria—methenamine
Increase: bone marrow depressant effects—methotrexate
Decrease: hepatic clearance of phenytoin, CYP2C9, CYP3A4 inducers
Decrease: response—cycloSPORINE
Drug/Lab Test
Increase: creatinine, bilirubin
Decrease: Hgb, platelets

NURSING CONSIDERATIONS

Assess:

- I&O ratio; note color, character, pH of urine if product administered for UTI; output should be 800 ml less than intake; if urine is highly acidic, alkalization may be needed
- Renal studies: BUN, creatinine, urinalysis with long-term therapy
- Type of infection; obtain C&S before starting therapy
- Blood dyscrasias, skin rash, fever, sore throat, bruising, bleeding, fatigue, joint pain
- **Allergic reaction:** rash, dermatitis, urticaria, pruritus, dyspnea, bronchospasm; product should be discontinued at 1st sign of rash; AIDS patients more susceptible

Evaluate:

- Therapeutic response: absence of pain, fever; C&S negative

Teach patient/family:

- To take each oral dose with full glass of water to prevent crystalluria; to drink 8-10 glasses of water/day; to take product on an empty stomach 1 hr before meals, 2 hr after meals
- To complete full course of treatment to prevent superinfection
- To avoid sunlight; to use sunscreen to prevent burns
- To avoid OTC medications (aspirin, vit C) unless directed by prescriber
- To use alternative contraceptive measures; that decreased effectiveness of oral contraceptives may occur
- To notify prescriber if skin rash, sore throat, fever, mouth sores, unusual bruising, bleeding occur; to notify prescriber of CNS effects: anxiety, depression, hallucinations, seizures

sulfaSALAzine (Rx)

(sul-fa-sal′a-zeen)

Azulfidine, Azulfidine EN-tabs, Salazopyrin ✦

Func. class.: GI antiinflammatory, antirheumatic (DMARD)

Chem. class.: Sulfonamide

Do not confuse:
sulfaSALAzine/sulfiSOXAZOLE

ACTION:
Prodrug to deliver sulfapyridine and 5-aminosalicylic acid to colon; antiinflammatory in connective tissue also

USES:
Ulcerative colitis; RA; juvenile RA (Azulfidine EN-tabs)
Unlabeled uses: Crohn's disease

CONTRAINDICATIONS:
Pregnancy at term, children <2 yr; hypersensitivity to sulfonamides or salicylates; intestinal, urinary obstruction; porphyria
Precautions: Pregnancy (B), breastfeeding, impaired renal/hepatic function, severe allergy, bronchial asthma, megaloblastic anemia

S

DOSAGE AND ROUTES

Bowel disease

- **Adult: PO** 3-4 g/day in divided doses; maintenance 2 g/day in divided doses q6hr
- **Child ≥6 yr: PO** 40-60 mg/kg/day in 4-6 divided doses, then 30 mg/kg/day in 4 doses, max 2 g/day

Rheumatoid arthritis

- **Adult: PO** 0.5-1 g/day, then increase daily dose by 500 mg/wk to 2 g/day in 2-3 divided doses

Juvenile rheumatoid arthritis

- **Child ≥6 yr: PO** 30-50 mg/kg/24 hr in 2 divided doses

Renal dose

- Modify dose based on renal impairment, response

Crohn's disease (unlabeled)

- **Adult: PO** 1 g/15 kg, max 5 g/day

Available forms: Tabs 500 mg; oral susp 250 mg/5 ml; del rel tabs 500 mg

Administer:

- Do not break, crush, chew del rel tabs
- With full glass of water to maintain adequate hydration; increase fluids to 2 L/day to decrease crystallization in kidneys
- Total daily dose in evenly spaced doses and after meals to help minimize GI intolerance
- Store in tight, light-resistant container at room temperature

SIDE EFFECTS

CNS: Headache, confusion, insomnia, hallucinations, depression, vertigo, fatigue, anxiety, seizures, product fever, chills

CV: Allergic myocarditis

GI: *Nausea, vomiting, abdominal pain,* stomatitis, hepatitis, glossitis, pancreatitis, diarrhea

GU: Renal failure, toxic nephrosis, increased BUN, creatinine, crystalluria

HEMA: Leukopenia, neutropenia, thrombocytopenia, agranulocytosis, hemolytic anemia

INTEG: Rash, dermatitis, urticaria, Stevens-Johnson syndrome, erythema, photosensitivity

SYST: Anaphylaxis

PHARMACOKINETICS

PO: Partially absorbed; peak 1½-6 hr; duration 6-12 hr; half-life 6 hr; excreted in urine as sulfaSALAzine (15%), sulfapyridine (60%), 5-aminosalicylic acid, metabolites (20%-33%); excreted in breast milk; crosses placenta

INTERACTIONS

Increase: leukopenia risk—thiopurines (azaTHIOprine, mercaptopurine)

Increase: hypoglycemic response—oral hypoglycemics

Increase: anticoagulant effects—oral anticoagulants

Decrease: effect of cycloSPORINE, digoxin, folic acid

Decrease: renal excretion of methotrexate

Drug/Food

Decrease: iron/folic acid absorption

Drug/Lab Test

False positive: urinary glucose test

NURSING CONSIDERATIONS

Assess:

- Renal studies: BUN, creatinine, urinalysis (long-term therapy)
- ⚠ **Blood dyscrasias:** skin rash, fever, sore throat, bruising, bleeding, fatigue, joint pain; monitor CBC before therapy and q3mo
- ⚠ **Allergic reaction:** rash, dermatitis, urticaria, pruritus, dyspnea, bronchospasm
- **Ulcerative colitis, proctitis, other inflammatory bowel disease:** character, amount consistency of stools; abdominal pain, cramping, blood, mucus
- **Rheumatoid arthritis:** assess mobility, joint swelling, pain, ability to complete activities of daily living

Evaluate:

- Therapeutic response: absence of fever, mucus in stools, pain in joints

Teach patient/family:

- To take each oral dose with full glass of water to prevent crystalluria
- That contact lenses, urine, skin may be yellow-orange
- To avoid sunlight or use sunscreen to prevent burns
- To notify prescriber of skin rash, sore throat, fever, mouth sores, unusual bruising, bleeding

⚠ Nurse Alert

SUMAtriptan (Rx)

(soo-ma-trip′tan)

ALSUMA Auto-injector, Imitrex, Sumavel DosePro, Zecuity

Func. class.: Antimigraine agent

Chem. class.: 5-HT_1B/D receptor agonist, abortive agent, triptan

Do not confuse:
SUMAtriptan/somatropin

ACTION: Binds selectively to the vascular 5-HT_1B/D receptor subtype; exerts antimigraine effect; causes vasoconstriction in cranial arteries

USES: Acute treatment of migraine with/without aura and cluster headache

CONTRAINDICATIONS: Angina pectoris, history of MI, documented silent ischemia, Prinzmetal's angina, ischemic heart disease, IV use, concurrent ergotamine-containing preparations, uncontrolled hypertension, hypersensitivity, basilar or hemiplegic migraine

Precautions: Pregnancy (C), breastfeeding, children <18 yr, geriatric patients, postmenopausal women, men >40 yr, risk factors for CAD, hypercholesterolemia, obesity, diabetes, impaired renal/hepatic function, overuse

DOSAGE AND ROUTES

- **Adult: SUBCUT** ≤6 mg; may repeat in 1 hr; max 12 mg/24 hr; **PO** 25 mg with fluids, if no relief in 2 hr, give another dose, max 200 mg/day; **NASAL** single dose of 5, 10, or 20 mg in 1 nostril, may repeat in 2 hr, max 40 mg/24 hr; 1 puff each nostril q2hr; TD 1 patch (6.5 mg/4 hr) after application push activation button

Hepatic dose

- **Adult: PO** 25 mg; if no response after 2 hr, give ≤50 mg

Available forms: Inj 4, 6 mg/0.5 ml; tabs 25, 50, 100 mg; nasal spray 5 mg/100 mcl-U; dose spray device 20 mg/100 mcl-U; transdermal patch 6.5 mg/4 hr

Administer:

PO route

- Swallow tabs whole; do not break, crush, or chew
- Take tabs with fluids as soon as symptoms appear; may take a 2nd dose >4 hr; max 200 mg/24 hr

SUBCUT route

SUBCUT only just below the skin; avoid IM or IV administration; use only for actual migraine attack

- Give 1st dose supervised by medical staff to patients with coronary artery disease or those at risk for CAD

Nasal route

- May give as 2 sprays of 5 mg in 1 nostril or 1 spray in each nostril (10 mg)

Transdermal route

- Do not cut; apply to upper arm or thigh of dry intact skin; do not use over scars, tattoos, cuts, scratches, burns, abrasions
- Apply another patch if headache is not relieved ≥2 hr after 1st patch; push activation button within 15 min of applying or patch will not work; do not bathe, shower, swim; may be taped with medical tape if needed
- Do not use with MRI
- Remove slowly; cleanse with soap and water; may cause redness
- Dispose of after folding in half

SIDE EFFECTS

CNS: *Tingling, hot sensation, burning, feeling of pressure, tightness, numbness, dizziness, sedation,* headache, anxiety, fatigue, cold sensation
CV: *Flushing,* **MI**, hypo/hypertension
EENT: Throat, mouth, nasal discomfort; vision changes
GI: Abdominal discomfort
INTEG: Inj-site reaction, sweating
MS: *Weakness, neck stiffness,* myalgia
RESP: Chest tightness, pressure

PHARMACOKINETICS

Onset of pain relief 10 min-2 hr, peak 10-20 min; 10%-20% plasma protein binding; metabolized in liver (metabolite); excreted in urine, feces; nasal spray half-life 2 hr

S

INTERACTIONS

Increase: vasospastic effects: ergot, ergot derivatives

Increase: serotonin syndrome—SSRIs, SNRIs, serotonin-receptor agonists, sibutramine

Increase: SUMAtriptan effect—MAOIs

Drug/Herb

- Serotonin syndrome: SAM-e, St. John's wort

NURSING CONSIDERATIONS

Assess:

- **Migraine:** type of pain, aura; alleviating, aggravating factors; sensitivity to light, noise

⚠ **Serotonin syndrome:** delirium, coma, agitation, diaphoresis, hypertension, fever, tremors; may resemble neuroleptic malignant syndrome in patients taking SSRIs, SNRIs

- B/P; signs, symptoms of coronary vasospasms, ECG
- Tingling, hot sensation, burning, feeling of pressure, numbness, flushing, inj-site reaction
- Stress level, activity, recreation, coping mechanisms
- Neurologic status: LOC, blurring vision, nausea, vomiting, tingling in extremities preceding headache
- Ingestion of tyramine foods (pickled products, beer, wine, aged cheese), food additives, preservatives, colorings, artificial sweeteners, chocolate, caffeine, which may precipitate these types of headaches
- Renal function, urinary output
- Quiet, calm environment with decreased stimuli: noise, bright light, excessive talking

Evaluate:

- Therapeutic response: decrease in frequency, severity of migraine

Teach patient/family:

- To report chest pain, tightness; sudden, severe abdominal pain; swelling of eyelids, face, lips; skin rash to prescriber immediately
- Not to use for more than 3-4 headaches per month
- To notify prescriber if pregnancy is planned or suspected; to use contraception while taking product
- **Nasal spray:** to use 1 spray in 1 nostril; may repeat if headache returns; not to repeat if pain continues after 1st dose
- To have a dark, quiet environment
- To avoid hazardous activities if dizziness, drowsiness occur
- To avoid alcohol; may increase headache
- To use SUBCUT inj technique, nasal route if prescribed
- That product does not reduce number of migraines; to be used for acute migraine; to use as symptoms occur

⚠ ***HIGH ALERT***

SUNItinib (Rx)

(soo-nit′-in-ib)

Sutent

Func. class.: Antineoplastic—miscellaneous

Chem. class.: Protein-tyrosine kinase inhibitor

ACTION: Inhibits multiple receptor tyrosine kinases (RTKs); some are responsible for tumor growth

USES: Gastrointestinal stromal tumors (GIST) after disease progression or intolerance to imatinib; advanced renal carcinoma, pancreatic neuroendocrine tumors (pNET) in patients with unresectable locally advanced/metastatic disease

CONTRAINDICATIONS: Pregnancy (D), breastfeeding, hypersensitivity

Precautions: Children, geriatric patients, active infections, QT prolongation, torsades de pointes, stroke, heart failure

Black Box Warning: Hepatic disease

DOSAGE AND ROUTES

Gastrointestinal stromal tumors (GIST)/renal cell cancer

- **Adult: PO** 50 mg/day × 4 wk, then 2 wk off; may increase or decrease dose by 12.5 mg; if administered with CYP3A4 inducers, give 87.5 mg/day; if given with CYP3A4 inhibitors, give 37.5 mg/day

Pancreatic neuroendocrine (pNET)

- **Adult: PO** 37.5 mg daily continuously, increase or decrease by 12.5 mg based on tolerance, avoid potent CYP3A4 inhibitors/inducers; if used with CYP3A4 inhibitors, decrease SUNItinib dose to minimum of 25 mg/day; if used with CYP3A4 inducers, increase SUNItinib to max 62.5 mg/day

Available forms: Caps 12.5, 25, 50 mg

Administer:

- With meal and large glass of water to decrease GI symptoms
- Store at 25° C (77° F)

SIDE EFFECTS

CNS: **CNS hemorrhage,** headache, dizziness, insomnia, **seizures,** fatigue

CV: Hypertension, **left ventricular dysfunction, QT prolongation, cardiotoxicity, torsades de pointes, thrombotic microangiopathy, cardiac arrest, thromboembolism**

ENDO: Hypo/hyperthyroidism

GI: *Nausea,* **hepatotoxicity, vomiting,** dyspepsia, *anorexia, abdominal pain,* altered taste, *constipation,* stomatitis, mucositis, **pancreatitis, diarrhea, GI bleeding/perforation**

GU: **Nephrotic syndrome**

HEMA: **Neutropenia, thrombocytopenia, hemolytic anemia, leukopenia**

INTEG: *Rash, yellow skin discoloration,* depigmentation of hair or skin, alopecia, **necrotizing fasciitis, pyoderma gangrenosum**

MS: Pain, arthralgia, myalgia, **myopathy, rhabdomyolysis**

RESP: Cough, dyspnea, **pulmonary embolism**

SYST: **Bleeding,** electrolyte abnormalities, hand-foot syndrome, **serious infection**

PHARMACOKINETICS

Protein binding 95%; metabolized by CYP3A4; excreted in feces, small amount in urine; peak plasma levels 6-12 hr; terminal half-life 40-60 hr (SUNItinib); active metabolite 80-110 hr

INTERACTIONS

⚠ **Increase:** **microangiopathic hemolytic anemia—bevacizumab; avoid concurrent use**

⚠ **Increase:** **QT prolongation—class IA/III antidysrhythmics, some phenothiazines, β agonists, local anesthetics, tricyclics, haloperidol, chloroquine, droperidol, pentamidine; CYP3A4 inhibitors (amiodarone, clarithromycin, erythromycin, telithromycin, troleandomycin), arsenic trioxide, levomethadyl; CYP3A4 substrates (methadone, pimozide, QUEtiapine, quiNIDine, risperiDONE, ziprasidone)**

Increase: **hepatotoxicity—acetaminophen**

Increase: plasma concentrations of simvastatin, calcium channel blockers; warfarin; avoid use with warfarin, use low-molecular-weight anticoagulants instead

Decrease: SUNItinib concentrations—dexamethasone, phenytoin, carBAMazepine, rifampin, PHENobarbital

Drug/Herb

Decrease: SUNItinib concentration—St. John's wort

Drug/Food

Increase: plasma concentrations—grapefruit juice

NURSING CONSIDERATIONS

S

Assess:

⚠ **ANC and platelets; if ANC <1 × 10^9/L and/or platelets <50 × 10^9/L, stop until ANC >1.5 × 10^9/L and platelets >75 × 10^9/L; if ANC <0.5 × 10^9/L and/or platelets <10 × 10^9/L, reduce dosage by 200 mg; if cytopenia continues, reduce dosage by another 100 mg; if cytopenia continues for 4 wk, stop product until ANC ≥1 × 10^9/L**

⚠ **CV status:** **hypertension, QT prolongation can occur; monitor left ventricular** ejection fraction (LVEF), (MUGA) at baseline, periodically; ECG

⚠ **Renal toxicity:** if bilirubin >3 × IULN, withhold SUNItinib until bilirubin levels return to <1.5 × IULN; electrolytes

Black Box Warning: **Hepatotoxicity:** monitor LFTs before treatment, monthly; if liver transaminases >5 × IULN, withhold SUNItinib until transaminase levels return to <2.5 × IULN

- **CHF:** adrenal insufficiency in those experiencing trauma
- Bleeding: epistaxis; rectal, gingival, upper GI, genital, wound bleeding; tumor-related hemorrhage may occur rapidly
- Nutritious diet with iron, vitamin supplement, low fiber, few dairy products

Evaluate:

- Therapeutic response: decrease in size of tumor

Teach patient/family:

- To report adverse reactions immediately: SOB, bleeding
- About reason for treatment, expected result
- That many adverse reactions may occur: high B/P, bleeding, mouth swelling, taste change, skin discoloration, depigmentation of hair/skin
- To avoid persons with known upper respiratory infections; that immunosuppression is common
- To avoid grapefruit juice

⚠ To report if pregnancy is planned or suspected, pregnancy (D)

⚠ HIGH ALERT

suvorexant

(soo′voe-rex′ant)

Belsomra

Func. class.: Psychotropic—sedative/hypnotic, anxiolytic

Chem. class.: Orexin receptor antagonist

ACTION: Suvorexant alters the signaling of neurotransmitters called orexins, which are responsible for regulating the sleep–wake cycle

USES: The treatment of insomnia characterized by difficulties with sleep onset and/or sleep maintenance

CONTRAINDICATIONS: Narcolepsy, hypersensitivity

Precautions: Preexisting respiratory disease, COPD, breastfeeding, pregnancy (C), labor, geriatrics, hepatic disease, sleep apnea, substance abuse, alcohol use, suicidal ideation, mental changes, depression

DOSAGE AND ROUTES

- **Adults: PO** 10 mg every night within 30 min of going to bed, and with ≥7 hr remaining before the planned time of awakening, may increase to maximum 20 mg every night

Available forms: Tabs 5, 10, 15, 20 mg

Administer:

- Give 30 min before bedtime
- Effect may be delayed if taken with food, take on empty stomach for faster effect

SIDE EFFECTS

CNS: Amnesia, suicidal ideation, anxiety, dizziness, drowsiness, hallucinations, headache, memory impairment

GI: Diarrhea

PHARMACOKINETICS

High-protein binding, peak 2 hr, terminal half-life 12 hr, excreted by feces (66%), urine (23%)

INTERACTIONS

Avoid use with CYP3A inhibitors

Increase: effects of both products—CNS depressants

Decrease: suvorexant effect—CYP3A inducers

Drug/Herb:

Increase: suvorexant effect—kava kava, valerian, melatonin

NURSING CONSIDERATIONS

Assess:

- **Sleeping patterns:** Waking in the night, inability to fall asleep, stay asleep, amnesia

Evaluate:

- Therapeutic response: Normalized sleeping patterns

Teach patient/family:

- To use on an empty stomach for faster effect
- To report immediately suicidal thoughts/behaviors
- To avoid use with other products unless approved by prescriber

tacrolimus (Rx) (PO, IV)

(tak-row'lim-us)

Astagraf XL, Prograf

tacrolimus (topical) (Rx)

Protopic

Func. class.: Immunosuppressant
Chem. class.: Macrolide

ACTION: Produces immunosuppression by inhibiting T-lymphocytes

USES: Organ transplants to prevent rejection; **topical:** atopic dermatitis
Unlabeled uses: Severe recalcitrant psoriasis, contact dermatitis, GVHD prophylaxis/disease, pancreas/heart/kidney/liver/lung/small-bowel transplant rejection, uveitis, ulcerative colitis, nephrotic syndrome, lichen sclerosus

CONTRAINDICATIONS: Children <2 yr (topical); hypersensitivity to this product or to some kinds of castor oil (IV); long-term use (topical)
Precautions: Pregnancy (C), breastfeeding, severe renal/hepatic disease; diabetes mellitus, hyperkalemia, hyperuricemia, hypertension, acute bronchospasm, African American patients, heart failure, seizures, QT prolongation

Black Box Warning: Children <12, lymphomas, infection, neoplastic disease, neonates, infants, requires a specialized setting, requires an experienced clinician; liver transplant (ext rel)

DOSAGE AND ROUTES

Kidney transplant rejection prophylaxis
- **Adult: IV** 0.03-0.05 mg/kg/day as **CONT INFUSION,** give no sooner than 6 hr after transplantation; **Ext Rel Caps** 0.1 mg/kg daily preoperatively on empty stomach, 1st dose 12 hr before reperfusion and 0.2 mg/kg once daily postoperatively, 1st dose within 12 hr of reperfusion but ≥4 hr after preoperative dose in combination with mycophenolate and corticosteroids

Liver transplant rejection prophylaxis
- **Adult: PO** 0.1-0.15 mg/kg/day in 2 divided doses q12hr; give no sooner than 6 hr after transplantation; **IV** 0.03-0.05 mg/kg/day as **CONT INFUSION;** give no sooner than 6 hr after transplantation

Heart transplant rejection prophylaxis
- **Adult: PO** 0.075 mg/kg/day in 2 divided doses q12hr; give no sooner than 6 hr after transplantation; **IV** 0.01 mg/kg/day as **CONT INFUSION;** give no sooner than 6 hr after transplantation

Atopic dermatitis
- **Adult: TOP** use 0.03% or 0.1% ointment; apply bid × 7 days after clearing of signs
- **Child ≥ 2-15 yr: TOP** 0.03% ointment; apply bid × 7 days after clearing of signs

Graft-versus-host disease (Orphan drug)
- **Adult and adolescent: IV** 0.1 mg/kg/day in 2 divided doses given with other immunosuppressants or **PO** 0.3 mg/kg/day in 2 divided doses
- **Child CONT IV INFUSION** 0.1 mg/kg/day

Graft-versus-host prophylaxis (unlabeled)
- **Adult: CONT IV INFUSION** 0.03 mg/kg/day starting 1-2 days before bone marrow transplant; **PO** 0.12 mg/kg/day in 2 divided doses
- **Adolescent and child: PO** 0.12 mg/kg/day in 2 divided doses

Heart transplant rejection (unlabeled)
- **Adult: IV** 0.05 mg/kg/day or **PO** 0.2-0.3 mg/kg/day in 2 divided doses; adjust to maintain whole blood concentration 7-15 ng/ml

Lung transplant rejection (unlabeled)
- **Adult: PO** 0.15 mg/kg/day, maintain 12-hr trough, whole blood concentration 1-1.5 ng/ml

Small-bowel transplant rejection (unlabeled)
- **Adult: IV** 0.1-0.15 mg/kg/day, then **PO** 0.3 mg/kg/day in divided doses

Contact dermatitis (unlabeled)
- **Adult: TOP** 0.1% ointment, apply bid × 8 wk

Available forms: Inj 5 mg/ml; caps 0.5, 1, 5 mg; ext rel cap 0.5, 1, 5 mg; ointment 0.03%, 0.1%

Administer:

PO route
- Give on empty stomach; food decreases absorption
- For several days before transplant surgery, patients should be placed in protective isolation

Extended release
- Take in morning on empty stomach, 1 hr before or 2 hr after a meal
- Swallow whole, do not chew, divide, crush
- Do not use with alcohol
- If dose is missed, up to 14 hr from scheduled dose, take dose, if >14 hr, skip

Topical route
- Apply thin layers to affected skin only; rub in gently
- Do not use occlusive dressings
- Use on small area of skin
- **Topical ointment has risk of developing cancer; use only when other options have failed**

Continuous IV INFUSION route
- After diluting in 0.9% NaCl or D_5W to 0.004 to 0.02 mg/ml as continuous infusion over 24 hr

Y-site compatibilities: Alemtuzumab, alfentanil, amifostine, amikacin, aminophylline, amiodarone, amphotericin B colloidal, amphotericin B liposome, anidulafungin, argatroban, atracurium, aztreonam, benztropine, bivalirudin, bleomycin, bumetanide, buprenorphine, busulfan, butorphanol, calcium acetate/chloride/gluconate, CARBOplatin, carmustine, caspofungin, ceFAZolin, cefoperazone, cefotaxime, cefoTEtan, cefOXitin, cefTAZidime, ceftizoxime, cefTRIAXone, cefuroxime, chloramphenicol, chlorproMAZINE, cimetidine, ciprofloxacin, cisatracurium, CISplatin, clindamycin, cyclophosphamide, cycloSPORINE, cytarabine, DACTINomycin, DAPTOmycin, dexamethasone, dexmedetomidine, dexrazoxane, digoxin, diltiazem, diphenhydrAMINE, DOBUTamine, DOCEtaxel, dolasetron, DOPamine, doripenem, doxacurium, DOXOrubicin hydrochloride, doxycycline, droperidol, enalaprilat, ePHEDrine, EPINEPHrine, epirubicin, ertapenem, erythromycin, esmolol, etoposide, etoposide phosphate, famotidine, fenoldopam, fentaNYL, fluconazole, fludarabine, foscarnet, fosphenytoin, gemcitabine, gentamicin, glycopyrrolate, granisetron, haloperidol, heparin, hydrALAZINE, hydrocortisone, HYDROmorphone, IDArubicin, ifosfamide, imipenem/cilastatin, inamrinone, insulin, isoproterenol, ketorolac, labetalol, leucovorin, levofloxacin, levorphanol, lidocaine, linezolid, LORazepam, magnesium sulfate, mannitol, mechlorethamine, meperidine, meropenem, mesna, metaraminol, methotrexate, methyldopate, methylPREDNISolone, metoclopramide, metoprolol, metroNIDAZOLE, micafungin, midazolam, milrinone, mitoMYcin, mitoXANtrone, mivacurium, morphine, multivitamins, nafcillin, nalbuphine, naloxone, nesiritide, niCARdipine, nitroglycerin, nitroprusside, norepinephrine, octreotide, ondansetron, oxacillin, oxaliplatin, oxytocin, PACLitaxel, palonosetron, pancuronium, PEMEtrexed, penicillin G, pentamidine, pentazocine, perphenazine, phentolamine, phenylephrine, piperacillin/tazobactam, potassium chloride/phosphates, procainamide, prochlorperazine, promethazine, propranolol, quinupristin/dalfopristin, ranitidine, remifentanil, rocuronium, sodium acetate/bicarbonate/phosphates, streptozocin, succinylcholine, SUFentanil, teniposide, theophylline, thiotepa, ticarcillin/clavulanate, tigecycline, tirofiban, tobramycin, tolazoline, trimethobenzamide, vancomycin, vasopressin, vecuronium, verapamil, vinCRIStine, vinorelbine, voriconazole, zidovudine, zoledronic acid

T

SIDE EFFECTS

CNS: *Tremors, headache,* insomnia, paresthesia, chills, fever, seizures, posterior reversible encephalopathy syndrome, BK-virus–associated nephropathy, coma
CV: Hypertension, myocardial hypertrophy, prolonged QTc, cardiomyopathy
EENT: Blurred vision, photophobia
GI: Nausea, vomiting, diarrhea, constipation, GI bleeding
GU: UTIs, albuminuria, hematuria, proteinuria, renal failure, hemolytic uremic syndrome
HEMA: Anemia, leukocytosis, thrombocytopenia, purpura
INTEG: Rash, flushing, itching, alopecia
META: Hyperglycemia, hyperuricemia, hypokalemia, hypomagnesemia, hyperkalemia
MS: Back pain, muscle spasms
RESP: Pleural effusion, atelectasis, dyspnea, interstitial lung disease
SYST: Anaphylaxis, infection, malignancy

PHARMACOKINETICS

PO: Extensively metabolized, half-life 10 hr, 75% protein binding

INTERACTIONS

Increase: QT prolongation—class IA/III antidysrhythmics, some phenothiazines, β agonists, local anesthetics, tricyclics, haloperidol, chloroquine, droperidol, pentamidine; CYP3A4 inhibitors (amiodarone, clarithromycin, erythromycin, telithromycin, troleandomycin), arsenic trioxide, levomethadyl; CYP3A4 substrates (methadone, pimozide, QUEtiapine, quiNIDine, risperiDONE, ziprasidone); do not use together
Increase: toxicity—aminoglycosides, CISplatin, cycloSPORINE
Increase: blood levels—antifungals, calcium channel blockers, cimetidine, danazol, mycophenolate, mofetil
Decrease: blood levels—carBAMazepine, PHENobarbital, phenytoin, rifamycin
Decrease: effect of live-virus vaccines

Drug/Herb
Decrease: immunosuppression—astragalus, echinacea, melatonin, ginseng, St. John's wort

Drug/Food
Increase: effect—grapefruit juice
Decreased absorption: food

Drug/Lab Test
Increase: glucose, BUN, creatinine
Increase or decrease: LFTs, potassium
Decrease: magnesium, Hgb, platelets

NURSING CONSIDERATIONS

Assess:

- Blood studies: Hgb, WBC, platelets during treatment monthly; if leukocytes <3000/mm³ or platelets <100,000/mm³, product should be discontinued or reduced; decreased hemoglobulin level may indicate bone marrow suppression
- Hepatic studies: alk phos, AST, ALT, amylase, bilirubin; for hepatotoxicity: dark urine, jaundice, itching, light-colored stools; product should be discontinued
- Serum creatinine/BUN, serum electrolytes, lipid profile, serum tacrolimus concentration

Anaphylaxis: rash, pruritus, wheezing, laryngeal edema; stop infusion, initiate emergency procedures

- **QT prolongation:** ECG, ejection fraction; assess for chest pain, palpitations, dyspnea

Black Box Warning: Liver transplant: ext rel product should not be used because of increased female mortality rate

Black Box Warning: Specialized care setting, experienced clinician: this product should only be used when equipped and staffed with adequate supportive medical services and by those experienced in immunosuppressive therapy and organ transplantation

Black Box Warning: Children, infants, neonates: not approved use of ointment in those <2 yr, ext rel in those <16 yr; not approved for pediatric kidney/heart transplant

Evaluate:

- Therapeutic response: absence of graft rejection; immunosuppression in patients with autoimmune disorders

Teach patient/family:

PO route

- To report fever, rash, severe diarrhea, chills, sore throat, fatigue; that serious infections may occur; to report clay-colored stools, cramping **(hepatotoxicity), nephrotoxicity,** signs of diabetes mellitus
- To avoid crowds, persons with known infections to reduce risk for infection; to avoid eating raw shellfish
- To avoid exposure to natural or artificial sunlight
- Not to breastfeed while taking product
- That repeated lab tests will be needed during treatment
- To avoid vaccines
- Not to use with alcohol, grapefruit
- To report if pregnancy is planned or suspected

Black Box Warning: To report symptoms of lymphoma

tadalafil (Rx)

(tah-dal′a-fil)

Adcirca, Cialis

Func. class.: Impotence agent

Chem. class.: Phosphodiesterase type 5 inhibitor

ACTION: Inhibits phosphodiesterase type 5 (PDE5); enhances erectile function by increasing the amount of cGMP, which causes smooth muscle relaxation and increased blood flow into the corpus cavernosum; improves erectile function for up to 36 hr

USES: Treatment of erectile dysfunction, benign prostatic hyperplasia (BPH) with or without erectile dysfunction pulmonary arterial hypertension (PAH) (Adcirca only)

Unlabeled uses: Sexual dysfunction in males receiving antidepressants

CONTRAINDICATIONS: Newborns, children, women, hypersensitivity, patients taking organic nitrates either regularly and/or intermittently, patients taking any α-adrenergic antagonist other than 0.4 mg once-daily tamsulosin

Precautions: Pregnancy (B) although not indicated for females, anatomic penile deformities, sickle cell anemia, leukemia, multiple myeloma, CV/renal/hepatic disease, bleeding disorders, active peptic ulcer, prolonged erection

DOSAGE AND ROUTES

Erectile dysfunction

- **Adult: PO** (Cialis) 10 mg taken before sexual activity; dose may be reduced to 5 mg or increased to max 20 mg; usual max dosing frequency is 1×/day; once-daily dosing 2.5 mg/day at same time each day

BPH

- **Adult: PO** 5 mg daily at the same time every day

Renal dose

- **Adult: PO** CCr 51-80 ml/min: no adjustment for erectile dysfunction, 20 mg/day initially for pulmonary hypertension; CCr 31-50 ml/min, 5 mg/day, max 10 mg q48hr; CCr <30 ml/min, max 5 mg q72hr

Hepatic dose

- **Adult: PO** (Child-Pugh A, B) max 10 mg/day or 20 mg/day, (pulmonary hypertension) max 40 mg/day; (Child-Pugh C) not recommended

Concomitant medications

- Ketoconazole, itraconazole, ritonavir, max 10 mg q72hr

Pulmonary hypertension

- **Adult: PO (Adcirca only)** 40 mg daily
- **Adult taking ritonavir: PO** 20 mg daily initially, then increase to 40 mg daily as tolerated

Male sexual dysfunction (from antidepressants) (unlabeled)

- **Adult: PO** (Cialis) 10-20 mg before sexual activity

Available forms: Tabs 2.5, 5, 10, 20 mg; PO tab (Adcirca) 20 mg

Administer:

- Product should not be used with nitrates in any form

T

• **Sexual dysfunction:** give before sexual activity; do not use more than 1×/day
• **Pulmonary hypertension:** give Adcirca with/without meals

SIDE EFFECTS

CNS: *Headache, flushing, dizziness,* seizures, transient global amnesia
CV: Hypotension, QT prolongation
INTEG: Stevens-Johnson syndrome, exfoliative dermatitis, urticaria
MISC: Back pain/myalgia, *dyspepsia, nasal congestion, UTI,* blurred vision, changes in color vision, *diarrhea,* pruritus, priapism, nonarteritic ischemic optic neuropathy (NAION), hearing loss

PHARMACOKINETICS

Rapidly absorbed; metabolized by liver by CYP3A4; terminal half-life 17.5 hr; peak ½-6 hr; excreted primarily as metabolites in feces, urine; excreted 61% in feces, 36% in urine; 94% protein bound; rate and extent of absorption not influenced by food

INTERACTIONS

⚠ Do not use with nitrates because of unsafe drop in B/P, which could result in MI or stroke
Increase: tadalafil levels—itraconazole, ketoconazole, ritonavir (although not studied, may also include other HIV protease inhibitors)
Decrease: B/P—alcohol, α-blockers, amLODIPine, angiotensin II receptor blockers, enalapril
Decrease: effects of tadalafil—bosentan, antacids
Drug/Food
Increase: tadalafil effect—grapefruit

NURSING CONSIDERATIONS

Assess:
• **Cialis:** underlying cause of erectile dysfunction before treatment; use of organic nitrates that should not be used with this product; any severe loss of vision while taking this or any similar products
• **Adcirca:** hemodynamic parameters at baseline and periodically
Evaluate:
• Therapeutic response: ability to engage in sexual intercourse, improvement in exercise ability in pulmonary hypertension
Teach patient/family:
• To take 1 hr before sexual activity
• Not to drink large amounts of alcohol
• That product does not protect against sexually transmitted diseases, including HIV
• That product has no effect in the absence of sexual stimulation; to seek medical help if erection lasts >4 hr
• To notify physician about all medicines, vitamins, herbs being taken, especially ritonavir, indinavir, ketoconozole, itraconazole, erythromycin, nitrates, α-blockers; that tadalafil is contraindicated for use with α-blockers except 0.4 mg/day tamsulosin
⚠ To notify prescriber immediately and to stop taking product if vision, hearing loss occur or if erection lasts >4 hr or if chest pain occurs

⚠ *HIGH ALERT*

tamoxifen (Rx)

(ta-mox′i-fen)
Apo-Tamox ✤, Soltamox, Tamofen ✤, Tamone ✤, Tamoplex ✤
Func. class.: Antineoplastic
Chem. class.: Antiestrogen hormone

ACTION: Inhibits cell division by binding to cytoplasmic estrogen receptors; resembles normal cell complex but inhibits DNA synthesis and estrogen response of target tissue

USES: Advanced breast carcinoma not responsive to other therapy in estrogen-receptor–positive patients (usually postmenopausal), prevention of breast cancer, after breast surgery/radiation for ductal carcinoma in situ

Unlabeled uses: Mastalgia, to reduce pain/size of gynecomastia, ovulation stimulation, malignant carcinoid tumor, carcinoid syndrome, metastatic melanoma, desmoid tumors, McCune-Albright syndrome (female pediatric patients), osteoporosis, bipolar I disorder, infertility, precocious puberty, gynecomastia, mastalgia

CONTRAINDICATIONS:
Pregnancy (D), breastfeeding, hypersensitivity

Black Box Warning: Thromboembolic disease

Precautions: Women of childbearing age, leukopenia, thrombocytopenia, cataracts

Black Box Warning: Endometrial cancer, stroke

DOSAGE AND ROUTES

Breast cancer

- **Adult: PO** 20-40 mg/day for 5 yr; doses >20 mg/day, divide AM/PM

High risk for breast cancer

- **Adult: PO** 20 mg/day × 5 yr

Ductal carcinoma in situ (DCIS)

- **Adult: PO** 20 mg/day × 5 yr

McCune-Albright syndrome/ precocious puberty (unlabeled)

- **Child 2-10 yr (girls): PO** 20 mg/day for ≤1 yr

Bipolar I disorder (unlabeled)

- **Adult: PO** 40 mg bid

Stimulation of ovulation with infertility (unlabeled)

- **Adult: PO** 20-80 mg/day × 5 days

Mastalgia (unlabeled)

- **Adult (female): PO** 10-20 mg/day × 3-6 mo

Mastalgia/gynecomastia in men with prostate cancer (unlabeled)

- **Adult (male): PO** 20 mg/day for ≤1 yr

Available forms: Tabs 10, 20 mg; oral solution 10 mg/5 ml

Administer:

- Do not break, crush, or chew tabs
- Antacid before oral agent; give product after evening meal, before bedtime; give with food or fluids for GI symptoms
- Antiemetic 30-60 min before product to prevent vomiting
- Store in light-resistant container at room temperature

Oral solution: Use calibrated container, dose >20 mg/day should be divided morning and evening, may be used with food for gastric irritation

SIDE EFFECTS

CNS: *Hot flashes, headache, lightheadedness,* depression, mood changes

CV: Chest pain, **stroke**, fluid retention, flushing

EENT: Ocular lesions, retinopathy, cataracts, corneal opacity, blurred vision (high doses)

GI: *Nausea, vomiting,* altered taste (anorexia)

GU: Vaginal bleeding, pruritus vulvae, **uterine malignancies,** *altered menses, amenorrhea*

HEMA: **Thrombocytopenia, leukopenia,** DVT

INTEG: *Rash,* alopecia

META: Hypercalcemia

RESP: **Pulmonary embolism**

PHARMACOKINETICS

PO: Peak 4-7 hr, half-life 7 days (1 wk terminal), metabolized in liver, excreted primarily in feces

INTERACTIONS

⚠ **Increase:** **risk for death from breast cancer—PARoxetine**

Increase: bleeding—anticoagulants

Increase: tamoxifen levels—bromocriptine

Increase: thromboembolic events—cytotoxics

⚠ **Increase:** **toxicity—CYP3A4 inhibitors (aprepitant, antiretroviral protease inhibitors, clarithromycin, danazol, delavirdine, diltiazem, erythromycin, fluconazole, FLUoxetine, fluvoxaMINE, imatinib,**

ketoconazole, mibefradil, nefazodone, telithromycin, voriconazole)
Decrease: tamoxifen levels—aminoglutethimide, rifamycin
Decrease: letrozole levels—letrozole
Decrease: tamoxifen effect—CYP3A4 inducers (barbiturates, bosentan, carBAMazepine, efavirenz, phenytoins, nevirapine, rifabutin, rifampin)
Decrease: tamoxifen effects—CYP2D6 inhibitors (antidepressants)

Drug/Herb
- Avoid use with St. John's wort, dong qui, black cohosh

Drug/Lab Test
Increase: serum calcium, T_4, AST, ALT, cholesterol, triglycerides

NURSING CONSIDERATIONS

Assess:
- CBC, differential, platelet count weekly; withhold product if WBC count is <3500 or platelet count is <100,000; notify prescriber; breast exam, mammogram, pregnancy test, bone mineral density, LFTs, serum calcium, serum lipid profile, periodic eye exams (cataracts, retinopathy)

Black Box Warning: Bleeding q8hr: hematuria, guaiac, bruising, petechiae, mucosa, or orifices

- Effects of alopecia on body image; discuss feelings about body changes

⚠ **Uterine malignancies, symptoms of stroke, pulmonary embolism** that may occur in women with ductal carcinoma in situ (DCIS) and women at high risk for breast cancer

⚠ **Severe allergic reactions:** rash, pruritus, urticaria, purpuric skin lesions, itching, flushing

- Bone pain; may give analgesics; pain usually transient

Evaluate:
- Therapeutic response: decreased tumor size, spread of malignancy

Teach patient/family:
- To use nonhormonal contraception during and for 2 mo after discontinuing treatment, pregnancy (D)
- To notify prescriber of stroke: blurred vision, headache, weakness on one side of the body; PE: chest pain, fainting, sweating, difficulty breathing
- To report any complaints, side effects to prescriber; that use may be 5 yr
- To increase fluids to 2 L/day unless contraindicated
- To wear sunscreen, protective clothing, sunglasses
- That vaginal bleeding, pruritus, hot flashes are reversible after discontinuing treatment
- To immediately report decreased visual acuity, which may be irreversible; about need for routine eye exams; that care providers should be told about tamoxifen therapy
- To report vaginal bleeding immediately
- **Tumor flare**—increase in size of tumor, increased bone pain—may occur and will subside rapidly; may take analgesics for pain
- That premenopausal women must use mechanical birth control because ovulation may be induced
- That hair may be lost during treatment; that a wig or hairpiece may make patient feel better; that new hair may be different in color, texture

tamsulosin (Rx)

(tam-sue-lo′sen)

Flomax

Func. class.: Selective α_1-peripheral adrenergic blocker, BPH agent

Chem. class.: Sulfamoylphenethylamine derivative

Do not confuse:
Flomax/Fosamax/Volmax

ACTION: Binds preferentially to α_{1A}-adrenoceptor subtype, which is located mainly in the prostate

USES: Symptoms of benign prostatic hyperplasia (BPH)

CONTRAINDICATIONS: Hypersensitivity

Precautions: Pregnancy (B), breastfeeding, children, hepatic disease, CAD, severe renal disease, prostate cancer; cataract surgery (floppy iris syndrome)

DOSAGE AND ROUTES

• **Adult: PO** 0.4 mg/day increasing to 0.8 mg/day if required after 2-4 wk

Available forms: Caps 0.4 mg

Administer:

• Without regard to food
• Swallow caps whole; do not break, crush, or chew
• Give ½ hr after same meal each day
• If treatment is interrupted for several days, restart at lowest dose (0.4 mg/day)
• Store in tight container in cool environment

SIDE EFFECTS

CNS: *Dizziness, headache,* asthenia, insomnia
CV: Chest pain, orthostatic hypotension
EENT: Amblyopia, floppy iris syndrome
GI: Nausea, diarrhea, dysgeusia
GU: Decreased libido, abnormal ejaculation, **priapism**
INTEG: Rash, pruritus, urticaria
MS: Back pain
RESP: Rhinitis, pharyngitis, cough
SYST: **Angioedema**

PHARMACOKINETICS

Peak 4-5 hr, duration 9-15 hr, half-life 9-13 hr, metabolized in liver, excreted via urine, extensively protein bound (98%)

INTERACTIONS

Increase: B/P—prazosin, terazosin, doxazosin, α-blockers, vardenafil
Increase: toxicity—cimetidine

NURSING CONSIDERATIONS

Assess:

• **Prostatic hyperplasia:** change in urinary patterns at baseline and throughout treatment; I&O ratios, weight daily; edema; report weight gain or edema
• **Orthostatic hypotension:** monitor B/P, standing, sitting

Evaluate:

• Therapeutic response: decreased symptoms of benign prostatic hyperplasia

Teach patient/family:

• Not to drive or operate machinery for 4 hr after 1st dose or after dosage increase
• To continue to take even if feeling better
• To advise providers of all products, herbs taken
• To make position changes slowly because orthostatic hypotension may occur
• To take ½ hr before same meal each day
• To teach about priapism (rare)
• Not to crush, break, chew

⚠ HIGH ALERT

tapentadol (Rx)

(ta-pen′ta-dol)

Nucynta, Nucynta ER

Func. class.: Analgesic, misc.
Chem. class.: μ-Opioid receptor agonist

Controlled Substance Schedule II

ACTION: Centrally acting synthetic analgesic; μ-opioid agonist activity is thought to result in analgesia; inhibits norepinephrine uptake

USES: Moderate to severe pain, diabetic peripheral neuropathy

CONTRAINDICATIONS: Hypersensitivity, asthma, ileus, respiratory depression

Black Box Warning: Respiratory depression

Precautions: Pregnancy (C), breastfeeding, children <18 yr, increased intracranial pressure, MI (acute), severe heart disease, respiratory depression, renal/hepatic disease, GI obstruction, ulcerative colitis, sleep apnea, seizure disorder

Black Box Warning: Accidental exposure, avoid ethanol, substance abuse, neonatal opioid withdrawal syndrome, potential for overdose, poisoning

DOSAGE AND ROUTES

- **Adult: PO** 50-100 mg q4-6hr, may give 2nd dose ≥1 hr after 1st dose, max 700 mg on day 1, max 600 mg/day thereafter; ext rel 50 mg q12hr (opioid-naive), titrate to 100-250 mg q12hr, max 250 mg q12hr

Hepatic Disease

Adult: PO Immediate rel/oral sol 50 mg q8hr, may titrate to response; ext rel 50 mg daily max 100 mg/day

Available forms: Tabs 50, 75, 100 mg; tabs ext rel 50, 100, 150, 200, 250 mg

Administer:

- With antiemetic if nausea, vomiting occur
- When pain is beginning to return; determine dosage interval by response
- Do not crush, chew, break, or use with alcohol, ext rel product
- Preferred analgesic in those with altered cytochrome P450 or mild hepatic, mild to moderate renal disease
- Store in light-resistant area at room temperature

Black Box Warning: These products have high potential for overdose, poisoning, may be fatal because of respiratory depression

SIDE EFFECTS

CNS: *Drowsiness, dizziness, confusion, headache, euphoria,* hallucinations, restlessness, syncope, anxiety, flushing, psychological dependence, insomnia, lethargy, tremors, seizures

CV: Palpitations, bradycardia, hypo/hypertension, orthostatic hypotension, sinus tachycardia

GI: *Nausea, vomiting, anorexia, constipation, cramps,* gastritis, dyspepsia, biliary spasms

GU: Urinary retention/frequency

INTEG: *Rash,* urticaria, diaphoresis, pruritus

RESP: Respiratory depression, cough

SYST: Anaphylaxis, infection, serotonin syndrome

PHARMACOKINETICS

Bioavailability 32%, extensively metabolized by liver, excreted in urine 99%, terminal half-life 4 hr, protein binding 20%

INTERACTIONS

Increase: effects with other CNS depressants—alcohol, opioids, sedative/hypnotics, antipsychotics, skeletal muscle relaxants

Increase: toxicity—MAOIs

Increase: serotonin syndrome—SSRIs, SNRIs, serotonin-receptor agonists, tricyclics

Black Box Warning: Do not use with alcohol, fatal overdose may occur

Drug/Herb

Increase: sedative effect—kava, St. John's wort, valerian

NURSING CONSIDERATIONS

Assess:

- **Pain:** intensity, location, type, characteristics; need for pain medication by pain/sedation scoring; physical dependence
- I&O ratio; check for decreasing output; may indicate urinary retention
- CNS changes: dizziness, drowsiness, hallucinations, euphoria, LOC, pupil reaction

⚠ **Serotonin syndrome:** increased heart rate, shivering, sweating, dilated pupils, tremors, high B/P, hyperthermia, headache, confusion; if these occur, stop product, administer serotonin antagonist if needed

• Allergic reactions: rash, urticaria, anaphylaxis

Black Box Warning: Addiction risk, previous substance abuse: assess before using ext rel product

Black Box Warning: Identify if alcohol has been used before giving this product, may be fatal if used with tapentadol

Black Box Warning: **Respiratory dysfunction:** respiratory depression, character, rate, rhythm; notify prescriber if respirations are <10/min; B/P, pulse

Evaluate:
• Therapeutic response: decrease in pain

Teach patient/family:
• To report any symptoms of CNS changes, allergic reactions, seizures, serotonin syndrome
• That physical dependency may result from extended use
• That withdrawal symptoms may occur: nausea, vomiting, cramps, fever, faintness, anorexia
• To avoid CNS depressants, alcohol
• To avoid driving, operating machinery if drowsiness, dizziness occur
• To change positions slowly to decrease orthostatic hypotension
• To notify prescriber if pregnancy planned, suspected or if breastfeeding

Black Box Warning: Not to use with alcohol, may be fatal

RARELY USED

tasimelteon
(tas′i-mel′tee-on)

Hetlioz

Func. class.: Anxiolytic/sedative/hypnotics

USES: Sleep-wake disorder in the blind

CONTRAINDICATIONS: Hypersensitivity

DOSAGE AND ROUTES
• **Adults: PO** 20 mg before bedtime at the same time every night; take without food

tavaborole topical
See Appendix B

RARELY USED

tbo-filgrastim
(fil-gras′tim)

Neutrophil

Func. class.: Biologic modifier
Chem. class.: Short-acting granulocyte colony-stimulating factor (G-CSF)

USES: Chemotherapy-induced neutropenia prophylaxis to reduce the duration of severe neutropenia in nonmyeloid malignancies

CONTRAINDICATIONS: Hypersensitivity

DOSAGE AND ROUTES
• **Adult: SUBCUT** 5 mcg/kg/day

teduglutide
(te′due-gloo′tide)

Gattex

Func. class.: Functional GI disorder agent
Chem. class.: Recombinant glucagon-like peptide-2 analog

ACTION: Increases intestinal, portal blood flow, inhibits gastric acid secretion, decreases gastric motility

USES: Short bowel syndrome, dependent on parenteral support

Precautions: Pregnancy (C), breastfeeding, diarrhea, pancreatitis, renal disease, electrolyte imbalances, GI obstruction, heart failure, neoplastic disease, biliary tract disease, cardiac disease, gastric cancer, GI disease

DOSAGE AND ROUTES

- **Adult: SUBCUT** 0.05 mg/kg daily

Available forms: Powder for injection 5 mg

Administer:

Subcut route

- ***Reconstitution:*** Slowly inject the 0.5 ml of preservative-free sterile water for injection provided in the prefilled syringe into the vial; allow to stand for 30 sec and gently roll the vial between your palms for 15 sec; do not shake, allow to stand 2 min; if undissolved powder is present, roll the vial again until all material is dissolved; if the product remains undissolved after the second attempt, do not use; discard unused portion; use within 3 hr after reconstitution
- ***Subcut injection:*** Calculate dose, withdraw into a syringe, and give; do not use IV, IM; if a dose is missed, it should be given as soon as possible on the same day; two doses should not be given on the same day; alternate sites

SIDE EFFECTS

CNS: Headache, fatigue

GI: Nausea, abdominal pain, cholecystitis, cholestasis, GI obstruction, pancreatitis, vomiting

PHARMACOKINETICS

Half-life 2 hr; 1.3 hr (short bowel syndrome)

INTERACTIONS

Increase: absorption of—benzodiazepine, carBAMazepine, cycloSPORINE, digoxin, disopyramide, ethosuximide, flecainide, levothyroxine, lithium, phenytoin, procainamide, quiNIDine, sirolimus, tacrolimus, theophylline, valproic acid, warfarin

NURSING CONSIDERATIONS

Assess:

- GI symptoms: nausea, abdominal pain
- Monitor alk phos, amylase, bilirubin, serum electrolytes, lipase baseline, q6mo

Evaluate:

- Therapeutic response: increased absorption of nutrients

Teach patient/family:

- To notify prescriber of GI symptoms

telaprevir

tel-a'pre-vir

Incivek

Func. class.: Antivirals, antihepatitis agent

Chem. class.: NS3/4A protease inhibitor

ACTION: Prevents hepatitis C viral (HCV) replication by blocking the proteolytic activity of HCV NS3/4A serine protease; hepatitis C virus NS3/4A serine protease is an enzyme responsible for the conversion of HCV-encoded polyproteins to mature/functioning viral proteins; these proteins (NS4A, NS4B, NS5A, NS5B) are needed for viral replication

USES: Chronic hepatitis C

CONTRAINDICATIONS: Pregnancy (X) in combination, male partners of women who are pregnant

Precautions: Breastfeeding, neonates, infants, children, adolescents <18 yr of age, anemia, neutropenia, thrombocytopenia, HIV, hepatitis B, decompensated hepatic disease, liver or other organ transplants

Black Box Warning: Serious rash

DOSAGE AND ROUTES

Chronic hepatitis C infection (genotype 1) in compensated liver disease without cirrhosis who are previously untreated or have relapsed after treatment with interferon and ribavirin therapy

• **Adults: PO** 1125 mg bid with peginterferon alfa and ribavirin; duration is determined by patient's HCV RNA level at treatment wk 4, 12; if the HCV RNA is undetectable at wk 4, 12, give three-drug regimen for 12 wk, then give an additional 12 wk of only peginterferon alfa and ribavirin (24 wk total); if the HCV RNA is detectable but ≤1000 international units/ml at wk 4 or 12, give three-drug regimen × 12 wk, then an additional 36 wk of only peginterferon alfa and ribavirin (48 wk total)

Without cirrhosis who are previously partial or null responders to interferon and ribavirin therapy/ or those with cirrhosis:

• **Adults: PO** 1125 mg bid with peginterferon alfa and ribavirin; give three-drug regimen × 12 wk, then another 36 wk (48 wk total) of only peginterferon alfa and ribavirin

Available forms: Tab 375 mg

Administer:

• Only use in combination with peginterferon alfa and ribavirin; never give as monotherapy

⚠ Discontinue in all patients with hepatitis C virus RNA concentrations ≥1000 IU/ml at wk 4 or 12 or a confirmed detectable HCV RNA concentration at wk 24

⚠ Any contraindication to peginterferon alfa or ribavirin also applies to this product; see ribavirin or peginterferon alfa monographs for additional information regarding contraindications and warning associated with these products

• For relief of mild to moderate rashes, give oral antihistamines and/or topical corticosteroids; treatment with systemic steroids is not recommended

• Give with food, not low-fat

• Store tabs at room temperature

SIDE EFFECTS

CNS: Fatigue

GI: Hemorrhoids, anorectal discomfort, pruritus ani, rectal burning, nausea, diarrhea, vomiting, dysgeusia, hyperbilirubinemia

HEMA: Anemia, decreased Hgb, lymphopenia, leukopenia, neutropenia, thrombocytopenia

INTEG: Drug reaction with eosinophilia and systemic symptoms (DRESS), Stevens-Johnson syndrome (SJS), rash, pruritus, severe rashes (bullous rash, vesicular rash, and skin ulcerations)

META: Increased uric acid

PHARMACOKINETICS

59%-76% plasma protein binding, primarily to α 1-acid glycoprotein and albumin; metabolized extensively in liver by hydrolysis, oxidation, reduction by CYP3A4; excreted in feces (82%), exhaled (9%), excreted in urine (1%); elimination half life 4-4.7 hr; steady-state half life 9-11 hr, peak 4-5 hr; food increases effect; steady-state is reduced by 15% in mild hepatic disease, 46% in moderate hepatic disease (Child-Pugh class B)

INTERACTIONS

⚠ **Increase:** life-threatening reactions of each product—alfuzosin, ergots (dihydroergotamine, ergotamine, ergonovine, methylergonovine), cisapride, pimozide, lovastatin, simvastatin, ezetimibe, niacin with simvastatin and boceprevir; triazolam, oral midazolam; sildenafil, tadalafil (pulmonary arterial hypertension); do not use concurrently

Increase: effect and adverse reactions of each product—phosphodiesterase type 5 (PDE5) inhibitors (for erectile dysfunction), atorvastin, lidocaine, atorvastatin, amiodarone, bepridil, flecainide, propafenone, quiNIDine, digoxin, ketoconazole, itraconazole, posaconazole, voriconazole, desipramine, traZODone, erythromycin, clarithromycin, telithromycin, rifabutin, dexamethasone, felodipine,

T

niCARdipine, NIFEdipine, budesonide, bosentan, warfarin, astemizole, boceprevir, bupivacaine, busPIRone, cevimeline, chloroquine, cilostazol, cinacalcet, clomiPRAMINE, clonazePAM, clopidogrel, cloZAPine, cyclobenzaprine, dapsone, dextromethorphan, diazepam, diclofenac, disopyramide, disulfiram, dolasetron, donepezil, colchicine, cycloSPORINE, tacrolimus, sirolimus, buprenorphine, salmeterol, vardenafil, ALPRAZolam, citalopram, amLODIPine, diltiazem, nisoldipine, verapamil, systemic corticosteroids, acetaminophen, alfentanil, aliskiren, almotriptan, alosetron, ARIPiprazole, dutasteride, ebastine, eplerenone, erlotinib, omeprazole, estazolam, eszopiclone, ethosuximide, exemestane, finasteride, flunitrazepam, flurazepam, galantamine, gefitinib, granisetron, halofantrine, haloperidol, HYDROcodone, ifosfamide, imipramine, indiplon, isradipine, ivermectin, ixabepilone, losartan, meloxicam, mirtazapine, montelukast, nateglinide, oxybutynin, oxyCODONE, palonosetron, paricalcitol, prasugrel, praziquantel, quazepam, QUEtiapine, quinacrine, ramelteon, repaglinide, ropivacaine, selegiline, sibutramine, sitaxsentan, solifenacin, SUFentanil, SUNItinib, theophylline, aminophylline, tiaGABine, tinidazole, tolterodine, traMADol, venlafaxine, amitriptyline, carvedilol, DAUNOrubicin, loratadine, desloratadine, lansoprazole, dexlansoprazole, DOCEtaxel, DOXOrubicin, droperidol, eletriptan, etoposide, fentaNYL, fexofenadine, glyburide, irinotecan, loperamide, maraviroc, mefloquine, mitoMYcin, morphine, nortriptyline, ondansetron, PACLitaxel, plicamycin, risperiDONE, sertraline, silodosin, teniposide, terfenadine, testosterone, tolvaptan, vinBLAStine, vinCRIStine and others; use cautiously, may need to reduce dose

Increase: hyperkalemia—drospirenone

Decrease: estrogen levels—ethinyl estradiol

Decrease: telaprevir effect—CYP3A4 inhibitors (phenytoin, carBAMazepine, PHENobarbital, rifampin)

Decrease: effect of—methadone

Possible treatment failure: efavirenz, ritonavir, atazanavir, lopinavir with ritonavir

Drug/Herb

⚠ Do not use with St. John's wort

NURSING CONSIDERATIONS

Assess:

⚠ **Pregnancy:** pregnancy (X) combination therapy; obtain a pregnancy test before, monthly during, and for 6 mo after treatment is completed; those who are not willing to practice strict contraception should not receive treatment with these products; report any cases of prenatal ribavirin exposure to the Ribavirin Pregnancy registry at (800) 593-2214

⚠ **Anemia:** monitor hemoglobin before, at treatment wk 4, 8, 12, and as needed; if Hgb is <10 g/dL, decrease ribavirin dosage; if Hgb is <8.5 g/dL, discontinuation of therapy is recommended; telaprevir dosage should not be altered based on adverse reactions; anemia may be managed through ribavirin dose modifications; never alter the dose of telaprevir; if anemia persists despite a reduction in ribavirin dose, consider discontinuing telaprevir; if management of anemia requires permanent discontinuation of ribavirin, treatment with telaprevir must also be permanently discontinued; once telaprevir has been discontinued, it must not be restarted; monitor CBC with differential at treatment wk 4, 8, 12, and at other treatment points

Black Box Warning: Serious rash: Toxic epidermal necrolysis, Stevens-Johnson syndrome: eosinophilia, fever, mucosal skin erosion, mucosal ulceration, target lesions; if serious skin reaction occurs, immediately discontinue all components of the three-drug regimen and refer the patient for urgent medical care

• **Hepatitis C:** Hepatitis C RNA baseline, wk 4, and wk 12; thyroid function tests, LFTs, serum bilirubin/creatinine, BUN, bilirubin, serum electrolytes, serum uric acid, baseline and periodically during treatment

Evaluate:

- Decreasing hepatitis C viral infection, HCV-RNA level ≥1000 IU/ml at wk 4 and 12, confirm wk 24

Teach patient/family:

- That 3-drug regimen must be used, not to discontinue unless approved by prescriber
- To take with food with fat for increased absorption
- Transmission of infection may still occur; use precautions
- If dose is missed, take if within 6 hr of when dose should have been used, provide "Medication Guide"
- Drink plenty of fluids to prevent dehydration
- Not to use other products (OTC, Rx, herbs, supplements) unless approved by prescriber

⚠ To use two forms of effective contraception (intrauterine devices and barrier methods) during treatment and for 6 mo after treatment; pregnancy (X), not to breastfeed

Black Box Warning: That if a serious skin reaction occurs, to seek urgent medical care; all components of the triple-drug regimen must be discontinued immediately

telavancin (Rx)

(tel-a-van′sin)

Vibativ

Func. class.: Antiinfective, miscellaneous

Chem. class.: Lipoglycopeptide

ACTION: Inhibits bacterial cell-wall synthesis, disrupts cell membrane integrity, blocks glycopeptides

USES: Skin/skin-structure infections caused by *Enterococcus faecalis, E. faecium, Staphylococcus aureus* (MSRA), *S. aureus* (MSSA), *S. epidermidis, S. haemolyticus, Streptococcus agalactiae* (group B), *S. dysgalactiae, S. pyogenes* (group A β-tremolytic), *S. anginosus, S. intermedius, S. constellates,* nosocomial pneumonia caused by susceptible gram-positive bacteria

Unlabeled uses: Bacteremia

CONTRAINDICATIONS: Hypersensitivity

Precautions: Breastfeeding, children, geriatric patients, renal disease, antimicrobial resistance, diabetes mellitus, diarrhea, GI disease, heart failure, hypertension, pseudomembranous colitis, QT prolongation, vancomycin hypersensitivity

Black Box Warning: Pregnancy (C)

DOSAGE AND ROUTES

Complicated skin/skin-structure infections

- **Adult: IV INFUSION** 10 mg/kg over 60 min q24hr × 7-14 days

Nosocomial pneumonia

- **Adult: IV INFUSION** 10 mg/kg q24hr × 7-21 days

Renal dose

- **Adult: IV** CCr 30-50 ml/min 7.5 mg/kg q24hr; CCr 10-29 ml/min 10 mg/kg q48hr

Available forms: Lyophilized powder for inj 250, 750 mg

Administer:

- Use only for susceptible organisms to prevent drug-resistant bacteria
- Antihistamine if red man syndrome occurs: decreased B/P; flushing of neck, face
- Avoid IM, subcut use

Intermittent IV INFUSION route

- After reconstitution with 15 ml D_5W sterile water for inj; 0.9% NaCl (15 mg/ml) 250-mg vial; add 45 ml to 750-mg vial (15 mg/ml) for dose of 150-800 mg; further dilute with 100-250 ml of compatible sol; for dose <150 mg or >800 mg, further dilute to concentration of 0.6-8 mg/ml with compatible sol; give over 60 min; reconstituted or diluted sol is stable for 4 hr room temperature, 7 hr

T

refrigerated; avoid rapid IV; may cause red man syndrome

Y-site compatibility: Amphotericin B lipid complex (Abelcet), ampicillin-sulbactam, azithromycin, calcium gluconate, caspofungin, cefepime, cefTAZidime, cefTRIAXone, ciprofloxacin, dexamethasone, diltiazem, DOBUTamine, DOPamine, doripenem, doxycycline, ertapenem, famotidine, fluconazole, gentamicin, hydrocortisone, labetalol, magnesium sulfate, mannitol, meropenem, metoclopramide, milrinone, norepinephrine, ondansetron, pantoprazole, phenylephrine, piperacillin-tazobactam, potassium chloride/phosphates, ranitidine, sodium bicarbonate, sodium phosphates, tigecycline, tobramycin, vasopressin

SIDE EFFECTS

CNS: Anxiety, chills, flushing, headache, insomnia, dizziness
CV: QT prolongation, irregular heartbeat
EENT: Hearing loss
GI: Nausea, vomiting, pseudomembranous colitis, abdominal pain, constipation, diarrhea, metallic/soapy taste
GU: Nephrotoxicity, *increased BUN, creatinine,* renal failure, foamy urine
HEMA: Leukopenia, eosinophilia, anemia, thrombocytopenia
INTEG: Chills, fever, rash, thrombophlebitis at inj site; urticaria, pruritus, necrosis (red man syndrome)
SYST: Anaphylaxis, superinfection

PHARMACOKINETICS

Onset rapid, half-life 8-9 hr, excreted in urine (76%), protein binding 90%, hepatic metabolism

INTERACTIONS

⚠ **Increase:** otoxicity or nephrotoxicity—aminoglycosides, cephalosporins, colistin, polymyxin, bacitracin, CISplatin, amphotericin B, nondepolarizing muscle relaxants, cidofovir, tacrolimus, IV pentamine acyclovir, adefovir, cycloSPORINE, foscarnet, ganciclovir, pamidronate, streptozocin, zoledronic acid, NSAIDs, salicylates, ACE inhibitors

⚠ **Increase:** QT prolongation—class IA, III antidysrhythmics; some phenothiazines; chloroquine, clarithromycin, droperidol, dronedarone, erythromycin, haloperidol, levomethadye, methadone, pimozide, ziprasidone

Drug/Lab Test
False increase: INR, PT, PTT

NURSING CONSIDERATIONS

Assess:

- **Infection:** WBC, urine, stools, sputum, characteristics of wound throughout treatment C&S
- I&O ratio; report hematuria, oliguria; nephrotoxicity may occur
- **Pseudomembranous colitis:** Monitor for diarrhea, fever, blood in stools, abdominal pain, may be several wk after therapy ends, report to prescriber immediately
- **Anaphylaxis:** Monitor for rash, itching, wheezing, laryngeal edema, discontinue and notify prescriber immediately, emergency equipment and epinephrine should be nearby

Black Box Warning: Obtain a pregnancy test before use; if a woman has taken this product during pregnancy, the national registry should be notified at 866-658-4228

- Auditory function during, after treatment; hearing loss; ringing, roaring in ears; product should be discontinued
- B/P during administration; sudden drop may indicate red man syndrome; also flushing, pruritus, rash
- Respiratory status: rate, character, wheezing, tightness in chest
- Adequate intake of fluids (2 L/day) to prevent nephrotoxicity

Evaluate:

- Therapeutic response: negative culture

Teach patient/family:

- About all aspects of product therapy; that culture may be taken after completed course of medication
- To notify prescriber if infection continues

• That bitter taste, nausea, vomiting, headache may occur
• To report sore throat, fever, fatigue; could indicate superinfection; diarrhea **(pseudomembranous colitis);** hearing loss; rash, wheezing, tightness of chest, itching, tightening of throat (anaphylaxis)
• To use contraception while taking this product; not to breastfeed; to notify prescriber if pregnancy is planned or suspected

telbivudine (Rx)

(tel-bi′vyoo-deen)

Sebivo ✱, Tyzeka

Func. class.: Antiretroviral

Chem. class.: Nucleoside reverse transcriptase inhibitor (NRTI)

ACTION: Inhibits replication of HBV DNA polymerase, which inhibits HBV replication

USES: Treatment of chronic hepatitis B

CONTRAINDICATIONS: Hypersensitivity, breastfeeding

Precautions: Pregnancy (B), children, severe renal disease, anemia, organ transplant, dialysis, HIV, obesity, alcoholism; Hispanic or African descendents (safety not established)

Black Box Warning: Impaired hepatic function, lactic acidosis

DOSAGE AND ROUTES

• **Adult and adolescent >16 yr: PO** 600 mg/day; max 600 mg/day

Renal dose

• **Adult: PO** CCr 30-49 ml/min, 600 mg tab q48hr or 400 mg oral sol daily; CCr <30 ml/min (not requiring dialysis), 600 mg tab q72hr or 200 mg oral sol daily

Available forms: Tabs 600 mg

Administer:

• With/without food with a full glass of water
• Store at room temperature

SIDE EFFECTS

CNS: *Fever, headache, malaise,* weakness, *dizziness, insomnia*

EENT: Taste change, hearing loss, photophobia

GI: *Nausea, vomiting, diarrhea, anorexia,* abdominal pain, hepatomegaly

INTEG: *Rash*

MISC: Lactic acidosis

MS: Myalgia, arthralgia, muscle cramps

RESP: Cough

PHARMACOKINETICS

Excreted by kidneys (unchanged), steady-state 5-7 days, protein binding 3.3%, terminal half-life 40-49 hr, peak 1-4 hr

INTERACTIONS

• Altered telbivudine levels: any agent altering renal function
• Do not use with pegylated interferon α-2a

Increase: myopathy risk possible—HMG-CoA reductase inhibitors, fibric acid derivatives, penicillamine, zidovudine, ZDV, cycloSPORINE, erythromycin, niacin, azole antifungals, corticosteroids, hydrochloroquine

NURSING CONSIDERATIONS

Assess:

Black Box Warning: LFTs, hepatitis B serology, creatine kinase, periodically, monitor HBV DNA after 24 wk; if viral suppression incomplete (≥300 copies/ml), start alternate therapy; monitor HBV DNA q6mo

Black Box Warning: Lactic acidosis: obtain baseline liver function tests; if elevated, discontinue treatment; discontinue even if liver function tests normal but lactic acidosis, hepatomegaly present; may be fatal

Evaluate:

• Therapeutic response: decreasing hepatitis B serology

Teach patient/family:

• That GI complaints and insomnia may resolve after 3-4 wk of treatment

T

- That product does not cure hepatitis B and does not stop its spread to others
- That follow-up visits must be continued
- That serious product interactions may occur if OTC products are ingested; to check with prescriber before taking
- That product may cause dizziness; to avoid hazardous activities until response is known
- To report symptoms of cough, difficulty sleeping, excessive headache, muscle pain/weakness
- To report progressive liver dysfunction: light-colored stools, dark urine, poor appetite, nausea, yellowing of skin, eyes
- That product will not cure HBV, and precautions should be taken to protect others

telmisartan (Rx)

(tel-mih-sar′tan)

Micardis

Func. class.: Antihypertensive

Chem. class.: Angiotensin II receptor (Type AT_1) antagonist

ACTION: Blocks the vasoconstricting and aldosterone-secreting effects of angiotensin II; selectively blocks the binding of angiotensin II to the AT_1 receptor found in tissues

USES: Hypertension, alone or in combination; stroke, MI prophylaxis (>55 yr) in patients unable to take ACE inhibitors

Unlabeled uses: Heart failure, proteinuria in diabetic nephropathy

CONTRAINDICATIONS: Hypersensitivity

Black Box Warning: Pregnancy (D) 2nd/3rd trimesters

Precautions: Pregnancy (C) 1st trimester, breastfeeding, children, geriatric patients; hypersensitivity to ACE inhibitors; renal/hepatic disease, renal artery stenosis, dialysis, CHF, hyperkalemia, hypotension, hypovolemia, African descent

DOSAGE AND ROUTES

- **Adult: PO** 40 mg/day; range 20-80 mg/day

Stroke, MI prophylaxis

- **Adult >55 yr: PO** 80 mg/day

Available forms: Tabs 20, 40, 80 mg

Administer:

- Without regard to meals
- Increased dose to African American patients or consider alternative agent; B/P response may be reduced
- Do not remove from blister pack until ready to use

SIDE EFFECTS

CNS: Dizziness, insomnia, *anxiety,* headache, fatigue, syncope

GI: Diarrhea, dyspepsia, *anorexia, vomiting*

META: Hyperkalemia

MS: Myalgia, pain

RESP: *Cough, upper respiratory infection,* sinusitis, pharyngitis

SYST: Angioedema

PHARMACOKINETICS

Onset of antihypertensive activity 3 hr, peak 0.5-1 hr, extensively metabolized, terminal half-life 24 hr, protein binding 99.5%, excreted in feces >97%, B/P response is less in African American patients

INTERACTIONS

Increase: digoxin peak/trough concentrations—digoxin

Increase: antihypertensive action—diuretics, other antihypertensives, NSAIDs

Increase: hyperkalemia—potassium-sparing diuretics, potassium salt substitutes, ACE inhibitors

Decrease: antihypertensive effect—NSAIDs, salicylates

Drug/Lab Test

Increase: LFTs

NURSING CONSIDERATIONS

Assess:

Black Box Warning: Pregnancy test, if positive stop treatment

- B/P, pulse standing, lying; note rate, rhythm, quality; if severe hypotension occurs, place in supine position, usually occurs during first few weeks of treatment
- Baselines of renal, hepatic, electrolytes studies before therapy begins
- **CHF:** edema in feet, legs daily; jugular venous distention; dyspnea, crackles

Evaluate:

- Therapeutic response: decreased B/P

Teach patient/family:

- To comply with dosage schedule, even if feeling better; to take at same time of day; that therapeutic effect may take 2-4 wk
- To notify prescriber of mouth sores, fever, swelling of hands or feet, irregular heartbeat, chest pain, decreased urine output
- Not to stop abruptly
- That excessive perspiration, dehydration, vomiting, diarrhea may lead to fall in blood pressure; to consult prescriber if these occur
- That product may cause dizziness, fainting, lightheadedness; to avoid hazardous activities until response is known

Black Box Warning: To notify prescriber if pregnancy is planned or suspected, pregnancy (D) 2nd/3rd trimester

- To notify prescriber of all prescriptions, OTC products, and supplements taken; to rise slowly from sitting to prevent drop in B/P
- **Overdose:** dizziness, bradycardia, or tachycardia

⚠ HIGH ALERT

temazepam (Rx)

(te-maz′e-pam)

Restoril

Func. class.: Sedative/hypnotic

Chem. class.: Benzodiazepine, short to intermediate acting

Controlled Substance Schedule IV (USA), Schedule F (Canada)

Do not confuse:
Restoril/Risperdal

ACTION: Produces CNS depression at limbic, thalamic, hypothalamic levels of the CNS; may be mediated by neurotransmitter γ-aminobutyric acid (GABA); results are sedation, hypnosis, skeletal muscle relaxation, anticonvulsant activity, anxiolytic action

USES: Insomnia, short-term treatment (generally 7-10 days)

CONTRAINDICATIONS: Pregnancy (X), breastfeeding, hypersensitivity to benzodiazepines

Precautions: Children <15 yr, geriatric patients, anemia, renal/hepatic disease, suicidal individuals, drug abuse, psychosis, acute closed-angle glaucoma, seizure disorders, angioedema, sleep-related behaviors (sleepwalking), intermittent porphyria, COPD, dementia, myasthenia gravis

DOSAGE AND ROUTES

- **Adult: PO** 7.5 to 30 mg at bedtime
- **Geriatric: PO** 7.5 mg at bedtime

Available forms: Caps 7.5, 15, 22.5, 30 mg

Administer:

- 15-30 min before bedtime for sleeplessness
- Without regard to food
- Avoid use with CNS depressants; serious CNS depression may result
- Store in tight container in cool environment

SIDE EFFECTS

CNS: *Lethargy, drowsiness, daytime sedation,* dizziness, confusion, light-headedness, headache, anxiety, irritability, complex sleep-related reactions (sleep driving, sleep eating), fatigue
CV: Chest pain, pulse changes, hypotension
EENT: Blurred vision
GI: Nausea, vomiting, diarrhea, heartburn, abdominal pain, constipation, anorexia
SYST: Severe allergic reactions

PHARMACOKINETICS

Onset 30 min, peak 1-2 hr, duration 6-8 hr, half-life 10-20 hr, metabolized by liver, excreted by kidneys, crosses placenta, excreted in breast milk, 98% protein binding

INTERACTIONS

Increase: effects of cimetidine, disulfiram, oral contraceptives
Increase: action of both products—alcohol, CNS depressants
Increase: effect of temazepam—probenecid
Decrease: effect of antacids, theophylline, rifampin
Drug/Herb
Increase: CNS depression—hops, kava, valerian, chamomile, skullcap
Drug/Food
Decrease: temazepam effect—caffeine
Drug/Lab Test
Increase: ALT, AST

NURSING CONSIDERATIONS

Assess:

- Mental status: mood, sensorium, affect, memory (long, short), orientation
- Type of sleep problem: falling asleep, staying asleep, baseline, periodically
- **Dependency:** restrict amount given to patient, assess for physical/psychological dependency; high-level risk for abuse
- Assistance with ambulation after receiving dose

Evaluate:

- Therapeutic response: ability to sleep at night, decreased early morning awakening if taking product for insomnia

Teach patient/family:

- To avoid driving, other activities requiring alertness until stabilized
- To avoid alcohol ingestion, other CNS depressants
- That effects may take 2 nights for benefits to be noticed
- To limit to 7-10 days of continuous use
- About alternative measures to improve sleep: reading, exercise several hours before bedtime, warm bath, warm milk, TV, self-hypnosis, deep breathing
- Not to discontinue abruptly, withdraw gradually
- That complex sleep-related behaviors may occur: sleep driving/eating
- That hangover, memory impairment are common in geriatric patients but less common than with barbiturates

⚠ To notify prescriber if pregnancy is planned or suspected, pregnancy (X); to use contraception while taking this product

TREATMENT OF OVERDOSE:

Lavage, activated charcoal; monitor electrolytes, VS

⚠ HIGH ALERT

temozolomide (Rx)

(tem-oh-zole′oh-mide)

Temodar

Func. class.: Antineoplastic-alkylating agent
Chem. class.: Imidazotetrazine derivative

ACTION:

Prodrug that undergoes conversion to MTIC; MTIC action prevents DNA transcription

USES:

Anaplastic astrocytoma with relapse, glioblastoma multiforme, malignant glioma
Unlabeled uses: Metastatic melanoma

CONTRAINDICATIONS:
Pregnancy (D), breastfeeding; hypersensitivity to this product, carbazine, or gelatin

Precautions: Geriatric patients, radiation therapy, renal/hepatic disease, bone marrow suppression, infection, myelosuppression

DOSAGE AND ROUTES

Anaplastic astrocytoma

- **Adult: PO** adjust dose based on nadir neutrophil and platelet counts 150 mg/m^2/day × 5 days during a 28-day cycle

Glioblastoma multiforme

- **Adult: PO/IV** 75 mg/m^2/day × 42 days with focal radiotherapy, then maintenance of 6 cycles

Refractory anaplastic astrocytoma

- **Adult: IV** 150 mg/m^2/day over 90 min on days 1-5 q28days, may increase to 200 mg/m^2/day on days 1-5 q28days if hematologic parameters permit

Available forms: Caps 5, 20, 100, 140, 180, 250 mg; powder for inj 100 mg

Administer:

PO route

- Do not break, crush, chew, open caps
- Antiemetic 30-60 min before product to prevent vomiting
- Caps 1 at a time with 8 oz of water at same time of day
- Fluids IV or PO before chemotherapy to hydrate patient
- If caps accidentally damaged, do not allow contact with skin or inhale
- Use proper procedures for handling/disposing of chemotherapy products
- Give on empty stomach at bedtime to prevent nausea/vomiting
- Store in light-resistant container in a dry area

IV route

- Bring vial to room temperature; discard if cloudy
- Inject 41 ml sterile water for inj into vial (2.5 mg/ml)
- Gently swirl; do not shake

Intermittent IV INFUSION route

- Withdraw up to 40 ml from each vial to make total dose; transfer to empty 250-ml PVC infusion bag; flush before and after infusion
- Run over 90 min
- Use reconstituted sol within 14 hr, including infusion time
- Do not admix

SIDE EFFECTS

CNS: Seizures, *hemiparesis, dizziness, poor coordination, amnesia, insomnia, paresthesia, somnolence, paresis, ataxia, anxiety, dysphagia, depression, confusion*

GI: *Nausea, anorexia, vomiting,* abdominal pain, constipation

GU: Urinary incontinence, UTI, frequency

HEMA: **Thrombocytopenia, leukopenia,** anemia, **myelosuppression, neutropenia**

INTEG: *Rash, pruritus*

MISC: Headache, fatigue, asthenia, fever, edema, back pain, weight increase, diplopia

RESP: URI, pharyngitis, sinusitis, coughing

SYST: **Anaphylaxis, secondary malignancy**

PHARMACOKINETICS

Absorption complete, rapid; crosses blood-brain barrier; excreted in urine, feces; half-life 1.8 hr; peak 1 hr

INTERACTIONS

Increase: myelosuppression—radiation, other antineoplastics

Increase: bleeding risk—NSAIDs, anticoagulants, platelet inhibitors, thrombolytics

Decrease: antibody reaction—live virus vaccines, toxoids

Decrease: action of digoxin

Drug/Food

Decrease: drug absorption

Drug/Lab Test

Decrease: Hgb, platelets, WBC, neutrophils

NURSING CONSIDERATIONS

Assess:

- Tumor response during treatment
- **CBC on day 22 (21 days after 1st dose), CBC weekly until recovery if ANC is $<1.5 \times 10^9$/L and platelets $<100 \times 10^9$/L; do not administer to patients who**

T

do not tolerate 100 mg/m²; myelosuppression usually occurs late during the treatment cycle

- Seizures throughout treatment; mental status
- Monitor temperature; may indicate beginning infection
- Hepatic studies before, during therapy (bilirubin, AST, ALT, LDH), as needed or monthly
- Bleeding: hematuria, guaiac, bruising, petechiae, mucosa or orifices

Evaluate:

- Therapeutic response: decreased tumor size, spread of malignancy

Teach patient/family:

- To report signs of infection: fever, sore throat, flulike symptoms
- To report signs of anemia: fatigue, headache, faintness, SOB, irritability
- To report bleeding; to avoid use of razors, commercial mouthwash
- To notify prescriber if pregnancy is planned or suspected, pregnancy (D); not to breastfeed

RARELY USED

temsirolimus (Rx)

(tem-sir-oh′li-mus)

Torisel

Func. class.: Biologic response modifier

Chem. class.: Kinase inhibitor, mTOR antagonist

USES: Renal cell carcinoma

CONTRAINDICATIONS: Pregnancy (D), breastfeeding; hypersensitivity to this product or to sirolimus; polysorbate 80

Precautions: Children <13 yr, females, severe pulmonary/renal/hepatic disease (bilirubin >1-1.5×ULN or AST >ULN but bilirubin ≤ULN), diabetes mellitus, hyperkalemia, hyperuricemia, hypertension, bone marrow suppression, hypertriglyceridemia/hyperlipidemia, surgery, brain tumors

DOSAGE AND ROUTES

- **Adult:** **IV** 25 mg over 30-60 min weekly; treat until disease progression or severe toxicity occurs

Hepatic dose

- **Adult:** **IV** (mild impairment) bilirubin >1-1.5×ULN or AST >ULN but bilirubin ≤ULN; reduce to 15 mg/wk; (moderate or severe impairment, do not use)

⚠ HIGH ALERT

tenecteplase (TNK-tPA) (Rx)

(ten-ek′ta-place)

TNKase

Func. class.: Thrombolytic

Chem. class.: Tissue plasminogen activator

ACTION: Activates conversion of plasminogen to plasmin (fibrinolysin): plasmin breaks down clots (fibrin), fibrinogen, factors V, VII; occlusion of venous access lines

USES: Acute myocardial infarction, coronary artery thrombosis

CONTRAINDICATIONS: Hypersensitivity, arteriovenous malformation, aneurysm, active bleeding, intracranial/intraspinal surgery or trauma within 2 mo, CNS neoplasms, severe hypertension, severe renal/hepatic disease, history of CVA, increased ICP/stroke

Precautions: Pregnancy (C), breastfeeding, children, geriatric patients, arterial emboli from left side of heart, hypocoagulation, subacute bacterial endocarditis, rheumatic valvular disease, cerebral embolism/thrombosis/hemorrhage, intraarterial diagnostic procedure or surgery (10 days), recent major surgery, dysrhythmias, hypertension

DOSAGE AND ROUTES

Total dose, max 50 mg based on patient's weight

- **Adult <60 kg IV BOL** 30 mg, give over 5 sec
- **Adult ≥60-<70 kg: IV BOL** 35 mg, give over 5 sec
- **Adult ≥70-<80 kg: IV BOL** 40 mg, give over 5 sec
- **Adult ≥80-<90 kg: IV BOL** 45 mg, give over 5 sec
- **Adult ≥90 kg: IV BOL** 50 mg, give over 5 sec, max 50 mg total dose

Available forms: Powder for inj, lyophilized 50 mg

Administer:

Intermittent IV INFUSION route

- As soon as thrombi identified; not useful for thrombi >1 wk old
- Cryoprecipitate or fresh frozen plasma if bleeding occurs
- Heparin after fibrinogen level >100 mg/dl; heparin infusion to increase PTT to 1.5-2× baseline for 3-7 days; IV heparin with loading dose is recommended
- Aseptically withdraw 10 ml of sterile water for inj from diluent vial; use red cannula syringe-filling device; inject all contents of syringe into product vial; direct into powder, swirl, withdraw correct dose; discard any unused sol; stand shield with dose vertically on flat surface and passively recap red cannula; remove entire shield assembly by twisting counter-clockwise; give by IV BOL
- IV therapy: use upper-extremity vessel that is accessible to manual compression
- If product not used immediately, refrigerate; use within 8 hr; not compatible with dextrose; flush dextrose-containing lines with saline before and after administration

SIDE EFFECTS

CV: Dysrhythmias, hypotension, pulmonary edema, **pulmonary embolism, cardiogenic shock, cardiac arrest, heart failure, myocardial reinfarction, myocardial rupture, tamponade, pericarditis, pericardial effusion, thrombosis, CVA**

HEMA: Decreased Hct, **bleeding**

INTEG: Rash, urticaria, phlebitis at IV infusion site, itching, flushing

SYST: **GI, GU, intracranial, retroperitoneal bleeding, surface bleeding, anaphylaxis**

PHARMACOKINETICS

IV: Onset immediate, half-life 20-24 min, metabolized by liver

INTERACTIONS

Increase: bleeding—aspirin, indomethacin, phenylbutazone, anticoagulants, antithrombolytics, glycoprotein IIb/IIIa inhibitors, dipyridamole, clopidogrel, ticlopidine, NSAIDs, cefamandole, cefoperazone, cefoTEtan, SSRIs, SNRIs

Drug/Herb

Increase: risk of bleeding—feverfew, garlic, ginger, ginkgo, green tea, horse chestnut

Drug/Lab Test

Increase: INR, PT, PTT

NURSING CONSIDERATIONS

Assess:

- **Allergy:** fever, rash, itching, chills; mild reaction may be treated with antihistamines
- **Cholesterol embolism, blue-toe syndrome, renal failure, MI, cerebral/spinal cord/bowel/retinal infarction, hypertension; can be fatal**
- ⚠ **Bleeding during 1st hr of treatment; hematuria, hematemesis, bleeding from mucous membranes, epistaxis, ecchymosis; may require tranfusion (rare), continue to assess for bleeding for 24 hr**
- Blood studies (Hct, platelets, PTT, PT, TT, aPTT) before starting therapy; PT or aPTT must be <2× control before starting therapy; PTT or PT q3-4hr during treatment
- Hypersensitive reactions: fever, rash, dyspnea; product should be discontinued
- VS, B/P, pulse, respirations, neurologic signs, temperature at least q4hr; temperature >104° F (40° C) indicates internal bleeding; systolic pressure increase >25 mm Hg should be reported to prescriber

⚠ Neurologic changes that may indicate intracranial bleeding
⚠ Retroperitoneal bleeding: back pain, leg weakness, diminished pulses
- Bed rest during entire course of treatment
- Avoidance of venous or arterial puncture, inj, rectal temperature, any invasive treatment
- Treatment of fever with acetaminophen or aspirin
- Pressure for 30 sec to minor bleeding sites; inform prescriber if this does not attain hemostasis; apply pressure dressing

Evaluate:
- Therapeutic response: resolution of MI

Teach patient/family:
- About proper dental care to avoid bleeding
- To notify prescriber immediately of sudden, severe headache
- To notify prescriber of bleeding; hypersensitivity; fast, slow, or uneven heart rate; feeling of faintness; blood in urine, stools; nose bleeds

tenofovir (Rx)
(ten-oh-foh′veer)
Viread
Func. class.: Antiretroviral
Chem. class.: Nucleoside reverse transcriptase inhibitor (NRTI)

ACTION: Inhibits replication of HIV virus by competing with the natural substrate and then incorporating into cellular DNA by viral reverse transcriptase, thereby terminating cellular DNA chain

USES: HIV-1 infection with at least 2 other antiretrovirals, hepatitis B

CONTRAINDICATIONS: Hypersensitivity

Black Box Warning: Lactic acidosis

Precautions: Pregnancy (B), breastfeeding, children, geriatric patients, renal disease, CCr <60 ml/min, osteoporosis, immune reconstitution syndrome

Black Box Warning: Hepatic disease, hepatitis

DOSAGE AND ROUTES
- **Adult: PO** 300 mg/day with meal; if used with didanosine, give tenofovir 2 hr before or 1 hr after didanosine
- **Child ≥2 yr: PO** 8 mg/kg daily approximate; ≥35 kg 300 mg daily; 28-34 kg 250 mg daily; 22-27 kg 200 mg daily; 17-21 kg 150 mg daily

Renal dose
- **Adult: PO** CCr 30-49 ml/min, 300 mg q48hr; CCr 10-29 ml/min, 300 mg q72-96hr; CCr <10 ml/min, not recommended

Available forms: Tabs 150, 200, 250, 300 mg; oral powder 40 mg/scoop

Administer:
- Without regard to food
- 2 hr before or 1 hr after didanosine (if used)
- Store at 25° C (77° F)
- **Oral powder:** use scoop provided, mix powder into 2-4 oz (1/4-1/2 cup) of applesauce, yogurt, do not mix with liquid, product will not mix, product is bitter, use immediately after mixing, clean scoop

SIDE EFFECTS
CNS: *Headache, asthenia*
GI: *Nausea, vomiting, diarrhea,* anorexia, *flatulence, abdominal pain,* pancreatitis
GU: Renal failure, renal tubular acidosis/necrosis, Fanconi syndrome
HEMA: Neutropenia, osteopenia
INTEG: *Rash,* angioedema
META: Lactic acidosis, hypokalemia, hypophosphatemia
MS: Myopathy, rhabdomyolysis
SYST: Lipodystrophy

PHARMACOKINETICS

Rapidly absorbed, distributed to extravascular space, excreted unchanged in urine 70%-80%, terminal half-life 17 hr, peak 1-2 hr

INTERACTIONS

Increase: tenofovir level—cidofovir, acyclovir, valacyclovir, ganciclovir, valganciclovir

Increase: level of didanosine when given with tenofovir

Increase: tenofovir level—any product that decreases renal function

NURSING CONSIDERATIONS

Assess:

- Viral load, CD4+ T-cell count, plasma HIV RNA, serum creatinine/BUN/phosphate
- Resistance testing at start of therapy and at treatment failure

Black Box Warning: Hepatitis exacerbations: Monitor hepatic studies: AST, ALT, bilirubin; amylase, lipase, triglycerides periodically during treatment

- Bone, renal toxicity: if bone abnormalities are suspected, obtain tests; serum phosphorus, creatinine

Black Box Warning: Lactic acidosis, severe hepatomegaly with steatosis, Fanconi syndrome: obtain baseline liver function tests; if elevated, discontinue treatment; discontinue even if liver function tests normal but lactic acidosis, hepatomegaly present; may be fatal

Evaluate:

- Therapeutic response: decrease in signs, symptoms of HIV

Teach patient/family:

- To take without regard to food
- That GI complaints resolve after 3-4 wk of treatment
- **Not to breastfeed while taking this product**
- That product must be taken daily even if patient feels better
- That follow-up visits must be continued because serious toxicity may occur; that blood counts must be done q2wk
- That product will control symptoms but is not a cure for HIV; that patient is still infectious, may pass HIV virus on to others
- That other products may be necessary to prevent other infections
- That changes in body fat distribution may occur

Black Box Warning: To notify prescriber of symptoms of lactic acidosis

terazosin (Rx)

(ter-ay′zoe-sin)

Func. class.: Antihypertensive

Chem. class.: α-Adrenergic blocker

ACTION: Decreases total vascular resistance, which is responsible for a decrease in B/P; this occurs by the blockade of α_1-adrenoreceptors

USES: Hypertension, as a single agent or in combination with diuretics or β-blockers; BPH

CONTRAINDICATIONS: Hypersensitivity

Precautions: Pregnancy (C), breastfeeding, children, prostate cancer, syncope

DOSAGE AND ROUTES

Hypertension

- **Adult: PO** 1 mg at bedtime, may increase dose slowly to desired response; max 20 mg/day divided q12hr

Benign prostatic hyperplasia

- **Adult: PO** 1 mg at bedtime, gradually increase up to 5-10 mg; max 20 mg divided q12hr

Available forms: Caps 1, 2, 5, 10 mg

T

Administer:
- Give dose at bedtime; patient should not operate machinery because fainting may occur
- If treatment is interrupted for several days, restart with initial dose
- Without regard to food; feeding tube: place cap in 60 ml of warm tap water; stir until liquid spills from ruptured shell (5 min); stir until cap dissolves; draw solution into oral syringe; give through feeding tube; flush with water
- Store at room temperature

SIDE EFFECTS

CNS: *Dizziness, headache, drowsiness,* anxiety, depression, vertigo, weakness, fatigue, syncope
CV: *Palpitations, orthostatic hypotension,* tachycardia, *edema,* rebound hypertension
EENT: Blurred vision, epistaxis, tinnitus, dry mouth, red sclera, nasal congestion, sinusitis
GI: *Nausea,* vomiting, diarrhea, constipation, abdominal pain
GU: Urinary frequency, incontinence, impotence, priapism
RESP: Dyspnea, cough, pharyngitis, nasal congestion

PHARMACOKINETICS

Half-life 9-12 hr; protein binding 90%-94%; metabolized in liver; excreted in urine, feces, peak 2-3 hr, onset 15 min, duration 24 hr

INTERACTIONS

Increase: hypotensive effects—β-blockers, nitroglycerin, verapamil, other antihypertensives, alcohol, phosphodiesterase (PDE5) inhibitors (vardenafil, tadalafil, sildenafil)
Decrease: hypotensive effects—estrogens, NSAIDs, sympathomimetics, salicylates
Drug/Herb
Increase: antihypertensive effect—hawthorn
Decrease: antihypertensive effect—ephedra
Drug/Lab Test
Decrease: Hgb, WBC, platelets, albumin

NURSING CONSIDERATIONS

Assess:
- **BPH:** urinary patterns (hesitancy, frequency, change in stream, dribbling, dysuria, urgency)
- **Hypertension:** crackles, dyspnea, orthopnea q30min; orthostatic B/P, pulse, jugular venous distention q4hr; weight daily, I&O
- BUN, uric acid if patient receiving long-term therapy

Evaluate:
- Therapeutic response: decreased B/P, edema in feet, legs; decreased symptoms of BPH

Teach patient/family:
- That fainting occasionally occurs after 1st dose; not to drive or operate machinery for 4 hr after 1st dose or after an increase in dose; to take 1st dose at bedtime
- To rise slowly from sitting or lying position
- Not to discontinue abruptly; not to drink alcohol
- **Hypertension:** to continue with regimen including diet, exercise

terbinafine oral (Rx)

(ter-bin′a-feen)
Lamisil
Func. class.: Antifungal
Chem. class.: Synthetic allylamine derivative

Do not confuse:
terbinafine/terbutaline
LamISIL/LaMICtal

ACTION: Interferes with cell-membrane permeability of fungi such as *Trichophyton rubrum, Trichophyton mentagrophytes, Trichophyton tonsurans, Epidermophyton floccosum, Microsporum canis, Microsporum audouinii, Microsporum gypseum, Candida;* broad-spectrum antifungal

USES: (Oral) onychomycosis of toenail or fingernail due to dermatophytes, tinea capititis/corporis/cruris/pedis/versicolor

Unlabeled uses: Cutaneous candidiasis, tinea versicolor

CONTRAINDICATIONS: Hypersensitivity

Precautions: Pregnancy (B), breastfeeding, children, chronic/active hepatic disease, renal disease GFR ≤50 ml/min, immunosuppression

DOSAGE AND ROUTES

- **Adult: PO** 250 mg/day × 6 wk (fingernail); × 12 wk (toenail)

Available forms: Tabs 250 mg; oral granules 125, 187.5 mg

Administer:

- **PO:** without regard to food
- Store at <25° C (77° F); protect from light
- **Granules:** take with food; sprinkle packet contents on pudding or nonacidic soft food; swallow without chewing; do not use fruit-based foods

SIDE EFFECTS

CNS: Depression

EENT: Tinnitus, hearing impairment

GI: Diarrhea, dyspepsia, vertigo, abdominal pain, nausea, hepatitis

HEMA: Neutropenia

INTEG: Rash, pruritus, urticaria, **Stevens-Johnson syndrome**, photosensitivity

MISC: Headache, hepatic enzyme changes, taste, visual/olfactory disturbance

PHARMACOKINETICS

Peak 1-2 hr, >99% protein binding, half-life 36 hr

INTERACTIONS

Increase: levels of dextromethorphan

Increase: terbinafine clearance—rifampin

Increase: clearance of cycloSPORINE

Decrease: terbinafine clearance—cimetidine

Decrease: metabolism of—CYP2D6 (antidysrthymics IC, III, amoxapine, atomoxetine, cloZAPine

Drug/Herb

- Side effects: cola nut, guarana, yerba maté, tea (black, green), coffee

Drug/Lab Test

Increase: LFTs

NURSING CONSIDERATIONS

Assess:

- Hepatic studies (ALT, AST) before beginning treatment; do not use in presence of hepatic disease
- CBC in treatment >6 wk
- Continuing infection: increased size, number of lesions

Evaluate:

- Therapeutic response: decrease in size, number of lesions

Teach patient/family:

- That treatment may take 10 wk (toenail), 4 wk (fingernail)
- **To notify prescriber of nausea, vomiting, fatigue, jaundice, dark urine, clay-colored stool, RUQ pain; may indicate hepatic dysfunction**

terbinafine topical

See Appendix B

terbutaline (Rx)

(ter-byoo′ta-leen)

Bricanyl ♣

Func. class.: Selective β_2-agonist; bronchodilator

Chem. class.: Catecholamine

Do not confuse:

terbutaline/TOLBUTamide/terbinafine

ACTION: Relaxes bronchial smooth muscle by direct action on β_2-adrenergic receptors through the accumulation of cAMP at β-adrenergic receptor sites; bronchodilation, diuresis, CNS, cardiac stimulation occur; relaxes uterine smooth muscle

USES: Bronchospasm

Unlabeled uses: Premature labor, nonresponsive status asthmaticus in children (IV)

CONTRAINDICATIONS: Hypersensitivity to sympathomimetics, closed-angle glaucoma, tachydysrhythmias

Precautions: Pregnancy (B), breastfeeding, geriatric patients, cardiac disorders, hyperthyroidism, diabetes mellitus, prostatic hypertension, hypertension, seizure disorder

Black Box Warning: Labor

DOSAGE AND ROUTES

Bronchospasm

- **Adult and child >12 yr: PO** 2.5-5 mg q8hr; **SUBCUT** 0.25 mg q15-30min, max 0.5 mg in 4 hr
- **Adolescent ≤15 yr and child ≥12 yr: PO** 2.5 mg tid, max 7.5 mg/day
- **Child 6-11 yr (unlabeled): PO** 0.05 mg/kg q8hr, may increase slowly

Renal dose

- **Adult: PO** CCr 10-50 ml/min, 50% of dose; CCr <10 ml/min, avoid use

Tocolytic (preterm labor) (unlabeled)

- **Adult: SUBCUT** 0.25 mg q20min to 6 hr, hold if pulse >120 bpm

Available forms: Tabs 2.5, 5 mg; inj 1 mg/ml

Administer:

- With food; may be crushed
- 2 hr before bedtime to avoid sleeplessness

IV route (unlabeled)

- Only used if subcut is ineffective
- IV after diluting each 5 mg/1 L D_5W for infusion
- IV, run 5 mcg/min; may increase 5 mcg q10min, titrate to response; after ½-1 hr, taper dose by 5 mcg; switch to PO as soon as possible
- Store at room temperature; do not use discolored sol

Y-site compatibilities: Insulin (regular)

SIDE EFFECTS

CNS: Tremors, anxiety, insomnia, headache, dizziness, stimulation

CV: Palpitations, tachycardia, hypertension, dysrhythmias, cardiac arrest, QT prolongation

GI: Nausea, vomiting

META: Hypokalemia, hyperglycemia

RESP: Paradoxical bronchospasm, dyspnea

PHARMACOKINETICS

PO: Onset ½ hr, peak 1-2 hr, duration 4-8 hr, half-life 3.4 hr

SUBCUT: Onset 6-15 min, peak ½-1 hr, duration 1½-4 hr, half-life 5.7 hr

INTERACTIONS

Increase: hypertensive crisis—MAOIs

Increase: effects of both products—other sympathomimetics

Decrease: action—β-blockers; do not use together

Drug/Herb

Increase: effect—green tea (large amounts), guarana

NURSING CONSIDERATIONS

Assess:

- Respiratory function: vital capacity, forced expiratory volume, ABGs, B/P, pulse, respiratory pattern, lung sounds, sputum before and after treatment
- Tolerance in patients receiving long-term therapy; dose may have to be changed; monitor for rebound bronchospasm

⚠ **Paradoxical bronchospasm:** dyspnea, wheezing; keep emergency equipment nearby

Black Box Warning: Labor: maternal heart rate, B/P, contraction, fetal heart rate; can inhibit uterine contractions, labor; monitor for hypoglycemia, do not use injectable product for prevention or treatment over 72 hr in preterm labor, do not use oral product for preterm labor

- Increase in fluids of >2 L/day

Evaluate:

- Therapeutic response: absence of dyspnea, wheezing

Teach patient/family:

- Not to use OTC medications because extra stimulation may occur
- About all aspects of product; to avoid smoking, smoke-filled rooms, persons with respiratory infections
- To increase fluids by >2 L/day; to allow 15 min between inhalation of product and inhaled product containing steroid
- To take on time; if missed, not to make up after 1 hr; to wait until next dose

terconazole vaginal antifungal

See Appendix B

teriflunomide

(ter′i-floo′noe-mide)

Aubagio

Func. class.: Multiple sclerosis agent

Chem. class.: Pyrimidine synthesis inhibitor

ACTION: Antiproliferative effects including peripheral T- and B-lymphocytes, might reduce inflammatory demyelination

USES: Reduction of the frequency of relapses or remitting MS

CONTRAINDICATIONS: Hypersensitivity

Black Box Warning: Pregnancy (X)

Precautions: Breastfeeding, alcoholism, diabetes mellitus, eosinophilic pneumonia, hepatitis, jaundice, male-mediated teratogenicity, pneumonitis, pulmonary disease/fibrosis, sarcoidosis, TB, vaccination

Black Box Warning: Hepatic disease

DOSAGE AND ROUTES

- **Adult: PO** 7 or 14 mg/day

Available forms: Tabs 7, 14 mg

Administer:

PO route

- May be taken without regard to food

SIDE EFFECTS

CNS: Anxiety, headache

CV: Palpitations, hypertension, MI

EENT: Blurred vision, conjunctivitis, sinusitis

GI: Nausea, vomiting, diarrhea, cystitis

HEMA: Leukopenia, lymphopenia, neutropenia

INTEG: Acne vulgaris, alopecia, pruritus

META: Weight loss

MISC: Infection, cystitis

PHARMACOKINETICS

Protein binding >99%, median half-life 18-19 days, peak 1-4 hr

INTERACTIONS

- Do not use with leflunomide, live virus vaccines

Increase: teriflunomide effect—cycloSPORINE, eltrombopag, gefitinib

Increase: hepatotoxicity—methotrexate, HMG-CoA reductase inhibitors

Increase: hematologic toxicity—zidovudine

Increase: effect of—oral contraceptives, repaglinide, pioglitazone, rosiglitazone, PACLitaxel, naproxen, topotecan, bosentan, furosemide

Decrease: effect of—warfarin, alosetron, DULoxetine, theophylline, tiZANidine, quiNINE, tamoxifen, bendamustine, rasagiline, rOPINIRole, selegiline, propafenone, mexiletine, lidocaine, anagrelide, cloZAPine, cinacalcet, caffeine, monitor closely

Decrease: effect of teriflunomide—cholestyramine, activated charcoal

NURSING CONSIDERATIONS

Assess:

- CNS symptoms: anxiety, confusion, vertigo

• GI status: diarrhea, vomiting, abdominal pain
• Cardiac status: tachycardia, palpitations, vasodilation, chest pain

Evaluate:
• Therapeutic response: decreased symptoms of MS

Teach patient/family:
• That blurred vision can occur
• To notify prescriber if pregnancy is planned or suspected, pregnancy (X)
• Not to change dosing or stop taking without advice of prescriber

teriparatide (Rx)
(tah-ree-par′ah-tide)
Forteo
Func. class.: Parathyroid hormone (rDNA)
Chem. class.: Teriparatide

ACTION: Contains human recombinant parathyroid hormone to stimulate new bone growth

USES: Postmenopausal women with osteoporosis, men with primary or hypogonadal osteoporosis who are at high risk for fracture, glucocorticoid-induced osteoporosis
Unlabeled uses: Hypoparathyroidism

CONTRAINDICATIONS: Hypersensitivity, increased baseline risk for osteosarcoma (Paget's disease, open epiphyses; previous bone radiation), bone metastases, history of skeletal malignancies, other metabolic bone diseases, preexisting hypercalcemia
Precautions: Pregnancy (C), breastfeeding, children, urolithiasis, hypotension, use >2 yr, cardiac disease

Black Box Warning: Secondary malignancy

DOSAGE AND ROUTES
• **Adult: SUBCUT** 20 mcg/day up to 2 yr

Available forms: Prefilled pen delivery device (delivers 20 mcg/day)

Administer:
SUBCUT route
• Give by SUBCUT using disposable pen only; inject in thigh or abdomen; lightly pinch fold of skin; insert needle; release skin; inject at 90-degree angle over 5 sec; rotate inj sites
• Have patient sit or lie down; orthostatic hypotension may occur
• Protect from freezing, light; refrigerate pen
• Store refrigerated; do not freeze; may be used for 28 days after first inj

SIDE EFFECTS
CNS: Dizziness, headache, insomnia, depression, vertigo
CV: Hypertension, angina, syncope
GI: Nausea, diarrhea, dyspepsia, vomiting, constipation
INTEG: Rash, sweating
MISC: Pain, asthenia, hyperuricemia
MS: Arthralgia, leg cramps, back/leg pain, weakness, osteosarcoma (rare)
RESP: Rhinitis, cough, pharyngitis, pneumonia, dyspnea

PHARMACOKINETICS
SUBCUT: Extensively and rapidly absorbed, metabolized by liver, excreted by kidneys, terminal half-life 1 hr, onset rapid, peak ½ hr, duration 3 hr

INTERACTIONS
Increase: digoxin toxicity: digoxin
Drug/Lab Test
Increase: calcium, uric acid, urinary calcium
Decrease: phosphorous, magnesium

NURSING CONSIDERATIONS
Assess:

Black Box Warning: Secondary malignancy: osteosarcoma, dependent on length of treatment; those at higher risk for osteosarcoma should not use this product

- Uric acid, magnesium, creatinine, BUN, urine pH, vit D, phosphate for normal serum levels; serum calcium may be transiently increased after dosing (max at 4-6 hr after dose)
- Bone pain, headache, fatigue, changes in LOC, leg cramps
- **Signs of persistent hypercalcemia:** nausea, vomiting, constipation, lethargy, muscle weakness
- Nutritional status: diet for sources of vit D (milk, some seafood), calcium (dairy products, dark green vegetables), phosphates (dairy products)

Evaluate:

- Therapeutic response: increased bone mineral density

Teach patient/family:

- About the symptoms of hypercalcemia
- About foods rich in calcium, vit D
- How to use delivery device, dispose of needles; not to share pen with others; to use at same time of day
- To sit or lie down if dizziness or fast heartbeat occurs after 1st few doses
- To rotate administration sites
- To store pen in refrigerator; pen may be used for 28 days

tesamorelin

Egrifta

Func. class.: Pituitary hormone, growth hormone modifiers

ACTION: Binds to growth hormone (GH) releasing factor receptors on the pituitary somatotroph cells; binding stimulates the production, release of endogenous GH

USES: Treatment of excess abdominal fat in HIV-infected patients with lipodystrophy

CONTRAINDICATIONS: Hypersensitivity to this product or mannitol, neoplastic disease, pregnancy X, *disruption of the hypothalamic-pituitary axis* (hypothalamic-pituitary-adrenal (HPA) suppression) due to hypophysectomy, hypopituitarism, pituitary tumor/surgery, radiation therapy of the head or head trauma, IV/IM administration

Precautions: Breastfeeding, CABG, diabetes, diabetic retinopathy, edema, geriatric patients, children, infants, adolescents

DOSAGE AND ROUTES

- **Adult: SUBCUT** 2 mg/day

Available forms: Powder for injection 1 mg

Administer:

Subcut route:

- Visually inspect parenteral products for particulate matter and discoloration before use
- To reconstitute, use 2, 1 mg vials, inject 2.1 ml sterile water for inj into the first 1 mg vial; use syringe with needle already attached; to avoid foaming, push plunger in slowly with needle on a slight angle so sterile water goes down the inside wall of vial; with needle and syringe attached to vial, keep vial upright and gently roll vial for 30 sec until mixed; do not shake; withdraw 2.1 ml of the reconstituted sol and add to second 1 mg vial; roll, do not shake
- To administer, take syringe out of vial, place needle cap on its side against a clean flat surface, do not touch needle, hold syringe and slide needle into cap, push cap all the way or until it snaps shut; do not touch cap until it covers needle completely; remove needle, insert a 0.5-inch 27-G safety injection needle onto syringe; use immediately; throw away any unused product or used sterile water for inj, sol should be clear, do not use if discolored, cloudy, or has particles; slight foaming is acceptable; inject subcut into abdomen; avoid scar tissues, bruises, or navel; rotate inj sites in abdomen; slowly push plunger down until all sol has been injected
- After removing needle from skin, flip back needle shield until it snaps, covering the injection needle completely; keep pressing until you hear a click, which means the injection needle is protected

• Use a piece of sterile gauze to rub the inj site clean; if bleeding, apply pressure to site with gauze for 30 sec; if bleeding continues, apply a bandage to site
• Properly dispose of used syringe, needles, vial, and sterile water for injection bottle in a sharps container

SIDE EFFECTS

CNS: Depression, peripheral neuropathy paresthesias, hypoesthesia, spasms, flushing, night sweats, insomnia, headache
CV: Chest pain, palpitations, hypertension, edema, peripheral edema
GI: Nausea, vomiting, upper abdominal pain, dyspepsia, diarrhea
INTEG: Pruritus, urticaria, rash, flushing, injection site reactions
MS: Arthralgia, joint swelling, stiffness, myalgias, carpal tunnel syndrome
RESP: Upper respiratory tract infection
SYST: Secondary malignancy

PHARMACOKINETICS

Half-life 26 min in healthy patients, 38 min in those with HIV infection; peak 0.15 hr

INTERACTIONS

Decrease: effect of—simvastatin, ritonavir, cortisone, predniSONE

NURSING CONSIDERATIONS

Assess:
• **Lipodystrophy:** Assess for sunken cheeks, thinning arms and legs, fat accumulation in the abdomen, jaws, and back of neck; after treatment these should lessen
• Monitor glycosylated hemoglobin A1c (HbA1c), serum IGF-1 concentrations, ophthalmologic exam

Evaluate:
• Decreasing lipodystrophy in HIV patients

testosterone cypionate (Rx)

Depo-Testosterone

testosterone enanthate (Rx)

Delatestryl

testosterone gel (Rx)

AndroGel, FORTESTA, Testim

testosterone pellets (Rx)

Testopel

testosterone transdermal (Rx)

Androderm

testosterone buccal (Rx)

Striant

testosterone topical solution, gel

AndroGel, Axiron, Fortesta, Testim, Vogelxo

testosterone nasal gel

Natesto

Func. class.: Androgenic anabolic steroid
Chem. class.: Halogenated testosterone derivative

Controlled Substance Schedule III

ACTION: Increases weight by building body tissue; increases potassium, phosphorus, chloride, nitrogen levels, bone development

USES: Female breast cancer, hypogonadism, eunuchoidism, male climacteric, oligospermia, impotence, vulvar dystrophies, low testosterone levels, delayed male puberty (inj)
Unlabeled uses: Weight loss in AIDS patients, andropause, anemia, cryptorchidism, lichen sclerosis, microphallus, transsexualism

CONTRAINDICATIONS: Pregnancy (X), breastfeeding, severe cardiac/renal/hepatic disease, hypersensitivity, genital bleeding (rare), male breast/prostate cancer

Precautions: Diabetes mellitus, CV disease, MI, urinary tract disorders, prostate cancer, hypercalcemia

Black Box Warning: Children, accidental exposure

DOSAGE AND ROUTES

Replacement

- **Adult: IM (enanthate or cypionate)** 50-400 mg q2-4wk; topical sol (Axiron) 60 mg (2 pump actuations); apply each AM
- **Adult (male) and child: SUBCUT (pellets)** 150-450 mg (2-6 pellets) inserted q3-6mo
- **Adult: TRANSDERMAL (Testoderm, Androderm)** 4-6 mg applied q24hr; **GEL (AndroGel)** 1% 5 mg applied q24hr, once daily; 1.62% 40.5 mg (2 pump actuations) every AM; topical sol **(Axiron)** 30 mg/actuation **BUCCAL** 1 buccal system (30 mg) to the gum region q12hr before meals/PM

Breast cancer

- **Adult: IM** 200-400 mg q2-4wk (cypionate or enanthate)

Delayed male puberty

- **Child >12 yr: IM** ≤100 mg/mo for ≤6 mo

Available forms: Enanthate: inj 200 mg/ml; **cypionate:** inj 100, 200 mg/ml; pellets 75 mg; **transdermal** 2, 4, mg/24 hr; **gel** 1%, 1.62%, 10 mg/actuation; **buccal system** 30 mg; **topical sol** 30 mg/actuation

Administer:

- Titrated dose; use lowest effective dose
- IM inj deep into upper outer quadrant of gluteal muscle
- **Transdermal patches:** Testoderm to skin of scrotum; Androderm to skin of back, upper arms, thighs, abdomen; area must be dry shaved; may be reapplied after bathing, swimming
- **Gel:** products not interchangeable; dosage and administration for AndroGel 1% differs from that of AndroGel 1.62%; apply daily to clean, dry area on shoulders, upper arms, or abdomen; women, children should not touch treated skin

Buccal system route

- Do not chew or swallow buccal system
- Rotate sites; place above incisor tooth on either side of mouth
- Open packet; place rounded side of surface against gum and hold firmly in place with finger over lip for 30 sec; if product falls off, replace with new system; discard in trash can away from children or pets

Topical solution route

- Using the provided applicator, apply the solution to clean, dry, intact skin of the axilla, preferably at the same time each morning; do not apply to any other part of the body; allow the solution to dry completely before dressing; if an antiperspirant or deodorant is used, apply at least 2 min before applying the solution; the pump must be primed before the first use by fully depressing the pump mechanism 3×; discard any solution that is released during the priming; to dispense the solution, position the nozzle over the applicator cup and carefully depress the pump once fully; the cup should be filled with no more than 1 pump actuation (30 mg); with the applicator upright, place it up into the axilla and wipe steadily down and up into the axilla; do not use fingers or hand to rub the solution; if multiple applications are necessary for the required dose, alternate application between the left and right axilla; when repeat application to the same axilla is necessary, allow the solution to dry completely before the next application; after use, rinse the applicator under running water and pat dry with tissue; wash hands with soap and water
- Following application, allow the site to dry before putting on clothing
- Direct contact of the medicated skin with the skin of another person can result in the transfer of residual testosterone

T

and absorption by the other person; to reduce accidental transfer, the patient should cover the application site(s) with clothing (e.g., a T-shirt) after the solution has dried; the application site should be washed with soap and water before any skin-to-skin contact regardless of the length of time since application; in the case of direct contact, the other person should wash the area of contact with soap and water as soon as possible

• Patients should be advised that the topical solution is flammable; therefore, fire, flame, and smoking should be avoided during use

• Advise patients to avoid swimming or washing the application site until 2 hr following application of solution

SIDE EFFECTS

CNS: Dizziness, headache, fatigue, tremors, paresthesias, flushing, sweating, anxiety, lability, insomnia, carpal tunnel syndrome

CV: Increased B/P

EENT: Conjunctival edema, nasal congestion

ENDO: Abnormal glucose tolerance test

GI: Nausea, vomiting, constipation, weight gain, cholestatic jaundice

GU: Hematuria, amenorrhea, vaginitis, decreased libido, decreased breast size, clitoral hypertrophy, testicular atrophy, gynecomastia, large prostate

HEMA: Polycythemia

INTEG: Rash, acneiform lesions, oily hair/skin, flushing, sweating, acne vulgaris, alopecia, hirsutism

MS: Cramps, spasms

PHARMACOKINETICS

PO: Metabolized in liver; excreted in urine, breast milk; crosses placenta

INTERACTIONS

• Edema: ACTH, adrenal steroids, buPROPion

Increase: effects of oxyphenbutazone

Increase: PT—anticoagulants

Decrease: glucose levels may alter need for oral antidiabetics, insulin

Drug/Lab Test

Increase: serum cholesterol, blood glucose, urine glucose

Decrease: serum calcium, serum potassium, T_4, T_3, thyroid ^{131}I uptake test, urine 17-OHCS, 17-KS, PBI

NURSING CONSIDERATIONS

Assess:

• Weight daily; notify prescriber if weekly weight gain >5 lb

• B/P q4hr, Hgb/HCT

• I&O ratio; be alert for decreasing urinary output, increasing edema

• Growth rate, bone age in children; growth rate may be uneven (linear/bone growth) with extended use

• Electrolytes: potassium, sodium, chlorine, calcium; cholesterol

• Hepatic studies: ALT, AST, bilirubin

• Edema, hypertension, cardiac symptoms, jaundice

• Mental status: affect, mood, behavioral changes, aggression

• **Signs of masculinization in female:** increased libido, deepening of voice, decreased breast tissue, enlarged clitoris, menstrual irregularities; male: gynecomastia, impotence, testicular atrophy

• **Hypercalcemia:** lethargy, polyuria, polydipsia, nausea, vomiting, constipation; product may have to be decreased

• **Hypoglycemia** in diabetic patients; oral antidiabetic action is increased

• Diet with increased calories, protein; decrease sodium if edema occurs

Evaluate:

• Therapeutic response: 4-6 wk with osteoporosis

Teach patient/family:

• That product must be combined with complete health plan: diet, rest, exercise

• To notify prescriber if therapeutic response decreases, if edema occurs

• About changes in sex characteristics: priapism, gynecomastia, increased libido

• That women should report menstrual irregularities, voice changes, acne, facial hair growth; if pregnancy is planned or suspected

- That 1-3-mo course is necessary for response with breast cancer
- About the proper application of patches

tetracaine ophthalmic

See Appendix B

tetracaine topical

See Appendix B

tetracycline (Rx)

(tet-ra-sye′kleen)

Func. class.: Broad-spectrum antiinfective

Chem. class.: Tetracycline

ACTION: Inhibits protein synthesis and phosphorylation in microorganisms; bacteriostatic

USES: Syphilis, *Chlamydia trachomatis,* gonorrhea, lymphogranuloma venereum; uncommon gram-positive, gram-negative organisms; rickettsial infections

CONTRAINDICATIONS: Pregnancy (D), breastfeeding, children <8 yr, hypersensitivity to tetracyclines

Precautions: Renal/hepatic disease, UV exposure

DOSAGE AND ROUTES

Susceptible gram-positive/gram-negative infections

- **Adult: PO** 250-500 mg q6hr
- **Child >8 yr: PO** 25-50 mg/kg/day in divided doses q6hr

Chlamydia trachomatis

- **Adult: PO** 500 mg qid × 7 days

Syphilis

- **Adult and adolescent: PO** 500 mg qid × 2 wk; if syphilis duration >1 yr, must treat 28 days

Brucellosis

- **Adult: PO** 500 mg q6hr × 3 wk with **IM** 1 g streptomycin bid × 1st wk, then daily × 2nd wk

Urethral, endocervical, rectal infections *(C. trachomatis)*

- **Adult: PO** 500 mg qid × 7 days

Acne

- **Adult and adolescent: PO** 250 mg q6hr, then 125-500 mg/day or every other day

Renal dose

- **Adult: PO** CCr 51-90 ml/min, give dose q8-12hr; CCr 10-50 ml/min, give dose q12-24hr; CCr <10 ml/min, give dose q24hr

Available forms: Caps 250, 500 mg

Administer:

- After C&S obtained
- 2 hr before or after iron products; 1 hr after antacid products
- Should be given on empty stomach (1 hr before or 2 hr after meals)
- Store in tight, light-resistant container at room temperature

SIDE EFFECTS

CNS: Fever, headache, paresthesia

CV: Pericarditis

EENT: Dysphagia, glossitis, decreased calcification, discoloration of deciduous teeth, oral candidiasis, oral ulcers

GI: *Nausea,* abdominal pain, *vomiting, diarrhea,* anorexia, enterocolitis, **hepatotoxicity,** flatulence, abdominal cramps, epigastric burning, stomatitis, **hepatitis, pseudomembranous colitis**

GU: *Increased BUN,* **azotemia, acute renal failure**

HEMA: Eosinophilia, neutropenia, thrombocytopenia, leukocytosis, hemolytic anemia

INTEG: *Rash, urticaria, photosensitivity, increased pigmentation,* **exfoliative dermatitis,** pruritus, **angioedema, Stevens-Johnson syndrome**

MISC: Increased intracranial pressure, candidiasis

PHARMACOKINETICS

PO: Peak 2-3 hr; duration 6 hr; half-life 6-12 hr; excreted in urine, breast

T

milk; crosses placenta; 65% protein bound

INTERACTIONS

⚠ Fatal nephrotoxicity: methoxyflurane

Increase: effect of warfarin, digoxin

Decrease: effect of tetracycline—antacids, sodium bicarbonate, alkali products, iron, cimetidine

Decrease: effect of penicillins

Drug/Herb

- Photosensitivity: dong quai

Drug/Food

Decrease: tetracycline effect—dairy products

Drug/Lab Test

Increase: BUN, LFTs

NURSING CONSIDERATIONS

Assess:

⚠ **Pseudomembranous colitis:** diarrhea, abdominal pain, fever, fatigue, anorexia; possible anemia, elevated WBC count, low serum albumin; stop product; usually either vancomycin or IV metroNIDAZOLE is given

- Signs of anemia: Hct, Hgb, fatigue
- I&O ratio
- Blood studies: PT, CBC, AST, ALT, BUN, creatinine if on prolonged therapy
- **Allergic reactions:** rash, itching, pruritus
- **Serious skin reactions:** angioedema, Stevens-Johnson syndrome, exfoliative dermatitis; report immediately after stopping product
- Nausea, vomiting, diarrhea; administer antiemetic, antacids as ordered

⚠ **Superinfection:** fever, malaise, redness, pain, swelling, drainage, perineal itching, diarrhea, changes in cough or sputum if on prolonged therapy

Evaluate:

- Therapeutic response: absence of lesions, negative C&S, resolution of infection, prevention of malaria

Teach patient/family:

- To avoid sun exposure; that sunscreen does not seem to decrease photosensitivity
- That all prescribed medication must be taken to prevent superinfection
- To avoid milk products, antacids or to separate by 2 hr; to take with full glass of water; to take 1 hr before bedtime to prevent esophageal ulceration
- That tooth discoloration may occur
- To notify prescriber immediately of diarrhea with pus, mucus, fever, abdominal pain

⚠ To notify prescriber if pregnancy is planned or suspected, pregnancy (D)

- Not to use outdated products, Fanconi syndrome (nephrotoxicity) may occur

tetrahydrozoline nasal agent

See Appendix B

tetrahydrozoline ophthalmic

See Appendix B

theophylline (Rx)

(thee-off′i-lin)

Phyllocontin ✦, Theochron, Theo-24, Uniphyl

Func. class.: Bronchodilator, spasmolytic

Chem. class.: Methylxanthine

ACTION: Exact mechanism unknown, relaxes smooth muscle of respiratory system by blocking phosphodiesterase, which increases cAMP; increased cAMP alters intracellular calcium ion movements; produces bronchodilation, increased pulmonary blood flow, relaxation of respiratory tract

USES: Bronchial asthma, bronchospasm associated with chronic bronchitis, emphysema, apnea during infancy for respiratory/myocardial stimulation

Unlabeled uses: Methotrexate toxicity, sleep apnea, status asthmaticus

CONTRAINDICATIONS:

Hypersensitivity to xanthines, tachydysrhythmias

Precautions: Pregnancy (C), breastfeeding, children, geriatric patients, CHF, cor pulmonale, hepatic disease, diabetes mellitus, hyperthyroidism, hypertension, seizure disorder, irritation of the rectum/lower colon, alcoholism, active peptic ulcer disease

DOSAGE AND ROUTES

Reversible airway obstruction (bronchospasm prophylaxis) associated with asthma or chronic obstructive pulmonary disease (COPD, emphysema, chronic bronchitis)

Calculate initial mg/kg dose based on ideal body weight as theophylline distributes poorly into body fat

Acute exacerbations of the symptoms and reversible airflow obstruction associated with asthma and other chronic lung diseases (COPD) along with inhaled β-2 selective agonists and systemic corticosteroids

- **Adult <60 yr/adolescent ≥16 yr: IV CONT INFUSION** expressed in theophylline; initially, 0.4 mg/kg/hr; max 900 mg/day (otherwise healthy nonsmokers); patients who smoke may require an increased dose; give 0.2 mg/kg/hr (≥400 mg/day) in CHF, cor pulmonale, liver dysfunction, sepsis with multiorgan failure, shock; reduced doses may be needed in patients receiving other drugs that decrease theophylline clearance; adjust dosage based on serum concentrations
- **Adult ≥60 yr: IV CONT INFUSION** initially, 0.3 mg/kg/mg/kg/hr; give 0.2 mg/kg/hr in CHF, cor pulmonale, liver dysfunction, sepsis with multiorgan failure, shock; reduced doses may be needed in patients receiving other drugs that decrease theophylline clearance; adjust dosage based on serum concentrations; max 400 mg/day unless serum concentration and patient condition require a higher dose
- **Child ≥12 yr/adolescent ≤15 yr: IV CONT INFUSION** initially, 0.5 mg/kg/hr (healthy nonsmokers (up to 900 mg/day); 0.7 mg/kg/hr in smokers; 0.2 mg/kg/hr (up to 400 mg/day) in cardiac decompensation, cor pulmonale, liver dysfunction, sepsis with multiorgan failure, or shock); adjust dosage based on serum concentrations
- **Child 9-11 yr: IV CONT INFUSION** initially, 0.7 mg/kg/hr; reduced doses may be needed in patients receiving other drugs that decrease theophylline clearance; give 0.2 mg/kg/hr (up to 400 mg/day) in cardiac decompensation, cor pulmonale, liver dysfunction, sepsis with multiorgan failure, or shock; adjust dosage based on serum concentrations
- **Child 1-8 yr: IV CONT INFUSION** initially, 0.8 mg/kg/hr; reduced doses may be needed in patients receiving other drugs that decrease theophylline clearance; 0.2 mg/kg/hr (up to 400 mg/day) in cardiac decompensation, cor pulmonale, liver dysfunction, sepsis with multiorgan failure, or shock; adjust dosage based on serum concentrations
- **Infant 6-52 wk: IV CONT INFUSION** calculate initial dosage using the following equation: (0.008 × age in wk) + 0.21 = theophylline dosage in mg/kg/hr IV; reduced doses may be needed in patients with risk factors for reduced theophylline clearance (cimetidine therapy, cardiac or liver dysfunction, renal impairment in infant <3 mo); adjust dosage based on serum concentrations

For maintenance therapy of asthma or COPD

- **Adult/adolescent/child >45 kg: PO** (expressed in theophylline and reg release products) PO initially, 300 mg/day in divided doses q6-8hr; after 3 days, if tolerated, increase dose to 400 mg/day in divided doses q6-8hr; after 3 more days, if tolerated, increase dose to 600 mg/day PO in divided doses q6-8hr; adjust dose to maintain therapeutic range; doses of

T

400-1600 mg/day may be needed, max 400 mg/day in patients with risk factors for decreased theophylline clearance (elderly patients >60 yr); NIH recommends initial dose for asthma of 10 mg/kg/day (max: 300 mg/day) titrated to serum concentration of 5-15 mcg/ml (usual max: 800 mg/day in ≥12 yr and 16 mg/kg/day in children 1-11 yr)

- **Child/adolescent ≤15 yr old and ≤45 kg: PO** initially, 12-14 mg/kg (max 300 mg) per day in divided doses q4-6hr; after 3 days, if tolerated, may increase to 16 mg/kg (max 400 mg) per day in divided doses q4-6hr; after 3 more days, if tolerated and if needed, increase dose to 20 mg/kg (max 600 mg) per day in divided doses q4-6hr; adjust dose to maintain therapeutic range (doses of 10-36 mg/kg/day in child 1-9 yr may be needed); max 16 mg/kg (400 mg) per day in patients with risk factors for decreased theophylline clearance or who cannot receive recommended serum concentration monitoring; NIH recommends initial dose for asthma of 10 mg/kg/day (max 300 mg/day) titrated to serum concentration of 5-15 mcg/ml (usual max 800 mg/day in patients ≥12 yr and 16 mg/kg/day in children 1-11 yr)
- **Neonate/infant ≤52 wk: PO** calculate initial dose using the following equation: [(0.2 × age in wk) + 5] × (kg body weight) = theophylline dosage in mg/day; in infants ≤26 wk, divide dose and administer q8hr and in infant >26 wk, divide dose and give q6hr; adjust dose to maintain a steady-state serum concentration of 5-10 mcg/ml in neonates and 10-15 mcg/ml in infants; NIH recommends initial dose for asthma of 10 mg/kg/day titrated to theophylline serum concentration of 5-15 mcg/ml, max in mg/kg/day = [(0.2 × age in weeks) + 5]
- Extended-release products are to be used only for chronic disease management; do not use in treatment of acute symptoms of asthma and reversible bronchospasm
- **Adult/adolescents/child ≥12 yr and >45 kg: (Theo-24 Cap) PO** initially, 300-400 mg/day q24hr; evening dosing is not recommended; after 3 days, if tolerated, increase to 400-600 mg/day q24hr; adjust dose to maintain therapeutic range; doses of 400-1600 mg/day may be needed; max 400 mg/day in patients with decreased theophylline clearance, (elderly >60 yr), and in those who cannot receive recommended serum concentration monitoring
- **Child >12 yr/adolescent <16 yr and <45 kg: (Theo-24 Cap) PO** initially, 12-14 mg/kg (max 300 mg) per day q24hr; evening dosing is not recommended; after 3 days, if tolerated, may increase to 16 mg/kg (max 400 mg) per day; after 3 more days, if tolerated and if needed, increase to 20 mg/kg (max 600 mg) per day; adjust dose to maintain therapeutic range; max 16 mg/kg/day up to 400 mg/day in patients with decreased theophylline clearance

Treatment of methotrexate toxicity (unlabeled)

- **Adult/adolescents/child ≥3 yr: IV** 2.5 mg/kg over 45-60 min

Available forms: Inj 250 mg/10 ml, 500 mg/20 ml, 100 mg/100 ml in 0.45% NaCl, 200 mg/100 ml in 0.45% NaCl; rect supp 250, 500 mg; tabs 100, 200 mg; ext rel tab 100, 200, 300, 400, 450, 600 mg; ext rel cap 100, 200, 300, 400; elixir 80 mg/15 ml

Administer:

- Avoid IM inj; pain and tissue damage may occur

PO route

- Avoid giving with food

Continuous IV INFUSION route

- Only clear sol; flush IV line before dose
- May be **diluted** for IV infusion in 100-200 ml in D_5W, $D_{10}W$, $D_{20}W$, 0.9% NaCl, 0.45% NaCl, LR
- **Give** loading dose over ½ hr; max rate of infusion 25 mg/min, use infusion pump; after loading dose, give by cont infusion
- Store diluted sol for 24 hr if refrigerated

Syringe compatibilities: Heparin, metoclopramide, PENTobarbital, thiopental

Y-site compatibilities: Allopurinol, amifostine, amphotericin B, amrinone, aztreonam, cefTAZidime, cholesteryl sulfate complex, cimetidine, cladribine, DOXOrubicin liposome, enalaprilat, esmolol, famotidine, filgrastim, fluconazole, fludarabine, foscarnet, gallium, granisetron, heparin sodium with hydrocortisone sodium succinate, labetalol, melphalan, meropenem, netilmicin, PACLitaxel, pancuronium, piperacillin/tazobactam, potassium chloride, propofol, ranitidine, remifentanil, sargramostim, tacrolimus, teniposide, thiotepa, tolazoline, vecuronium

SIDE EFFECTS

CNS: Anxiety, restlessness, insomnia, *dizziness,* **seizures**, headache, lightheadedness, muscle twitching, tremors
CV: *Palpitations, sinus tachycardia,* hypotension, flushing, **dysrhythmias**, edema
GI: *Nausea, vomiting,* diarrhea, dyspepsia, anal irritation (suppositories), epigastric pain, reflux, anorexia
GU: Urinary frequency, SIADH
INTEG: Flushing, urticaria
MISC: Hyperglycemia
RESP: Tachypnea, increased respiratory rate

PHARMACOKINETICS

Metabolized by liver (caffeine); excreted in urine; crosses placenta; appears in breast milk; half-life 6.5-10.5 hr; half-life increased in geriatric patients, hepatic disease, CHF, neonates, premature infants; protein binding 40%, crosses into CSF
PO: Onset $^{1}/_{4}$ hr, peak 1-2 hr, duration 6-8 hr, well absorbed
PO-ER: Onset unknown, peak 4-7 hr, duration 8-12 hr, well absorbed slowly
IV: Onset rapid, duration 6-8 hr
RECT: Onset erratic, peak 1-2 hr, duration 6-8 hr, supp absorbed erratically, sol absorbed quickly

INTERACTIONS

- Dose-dependent reversal of neuromuscular blockade
- **Increase:** dysrhythmias: halothane
- May increase or decrease theophylline levels: carBAMazepine, loop diuretics, isoniazid

Increase: action of theophylline, toxicity—cimetidine, nonselective β-blockers, erythromycin, clarithromycin, oral contraceptives, corticosteroids, interferons, fluoroquinolones, disulfiram, mexiletine, fluvoxaMINE, high doses of allopurinol, influenza vaccines, interferon, benzodiazepines
Increase: adverse reactions—tetracyclines
Increase: elimination—smoking
Decrease: effects of lithium
Decrease: effect of theophylline—nicotine products, adrenergics, barbiturates, phenytoin, ketoconazole, rifampin

Drug/Herb
Increase: effects—cola tree, guarana, yerba maté, tea (black, green), horsetail, ginseng, Siberian ginseng
Decrease: effects—St. John's wort

Drug/Food
Increase: effect—xanthines
Increase: elimination by low-carbohydrate, high-protein diet; charcoal-broiled beef
Decrease: elimination by high-carbohydrate, low-protein diet

Drug/Lab Test
Increase: plasma-free fatty acids

NURSING CONSIDERATIONS

Assess:

- Theophylline blood levels (therapeutic level is 10-20 mcg/ml); toxicity may occur with small increase above 20 mcg/ml, especially in geriatric patients; whether theophylline was given recently (24 hr)
- Monitor I&O; diuresis occurs; dehydration may occur in geriatric patients or children
- Liver function tests: periodically, lower doses may be required in those with moderate to severe hepatic disease
- Respiratory rate, rhythm, depth; auscultate lung fields bilaterally; notify prescriber of abnormalities, monitor pulmonary function tests

T

• Allergic reactions: rash, urticaria; if these occur, product should be discontinued

Evaluate:

• Therapeutic response: decreased dyspnea, respiratory stimulation for infants, clear lung fields bilaterally

Teach patient/family:

• To take doses as prescribed; not to skip dose; not to double dose

• To check OTC medications, current prescription medications for ePHEDrine; will increase CNS stimulation; not to drink alcohol or caffeine products (tea, coffee, chocolate, colas); to avoid large amounts of charcoal-grilled beef

• To avoid hazardous activities; dizziness may occur

• If GI upset occurs, to take product with 8 oz water; to avoid food because absorption may be decreased

⚠ To notify prescriber immediately about **toxicity:** insomnia, anxiety, nausea, vomiting, rapid pulse, seizures, flushing, headache, diarrhea

• To notify prescriber about changes in smoking habits because a change in dose may be required; to avoid smoking because it decreases drug blood levels and terminal half-life

• To increase fluids to 2 L/day to decrease secretion viscosity

thiamine (vit B_1) (PO-OTC; IV, IM-Rx)

Vitamin B-1

Func. class.: Vit B_1

Chem. class.: Water soluble

Do not confuse:

thiamine/Tenormin

ACTION: Needed for pyruvate metabolism, carbohydrate metabolism

USES: Vit B_1 deficiency or polyneuritis, cheilosis adjunct with thiamine beriberi, Wernicke-Korsakoff syndrome, pellagra, metabolic disorders, alcoholism

CONTRAINDICATIONS: Hypersensitivity

Precautions: Pregnancy (A)

DOSAGE AND ROUTES

RDA

• **Adult: PO** (males) 1.2-1.5 mg; (females) 1.1 mg; (pregnancy) 1.4 mg; (breastfeeding) 1.4 mg

• **Child 9-13 yr: PO** 0.9 mg

• **Child 4-8 yr: PO** 0.6 mg

• **Child 1-3 yr: PO** 0.5 mg

• **Infant 7 mo-1 yr: PO** 0.3 mg

• **Neonate and infant ≤6 mo: PO** 0.2 mg

Beriberi

• **Adult: PO** 5-30 mg daily or in 3 divided doses × 1 mo; **IM/IV** 5-30 mg daily or in 3 divided doses, then convert to **PO**

• **Infant/child: PO** 10-50 mg daily × 2 wk, then 5-10 mg daily × 1 mo; **IV/IM** 10-25 mg/day × 2 wk, then 5-10 mg daily × 1 mo

Available forms: Tabs 50, 100, 250, 500 mg; inj 100 mg/ml; enteric-coated tabs 20 mg

Administer:

IM route

• By IM inj; rotate sites if pain and inflammation occur; do not mix with alkaline sol; Z-track to minimize pain

Direct IV route

• Undiluted at 100 mg/ml over 5 min

Continuous IV INFUSION route

• Diluted in compatible IV sol

Y-site compatibilities: Famotidine

SIDE EFFECTS

CNS: Weakness, restlessness

CV: Collapse, pulmonary edema, hypotension

EENT: Tightness of throat

GI: Hemorrhage, *nausea, diarrhea*

INTEG: Angioneurotic edema, cyanosis, sweating, warmth

SYST: Anaphylaxis

PHARMACOKINETICS

PO/INJ: Unused amounts excreted in urine (unchanged)

NURSING CONSIDERATIONS

Assess:

- **Anaphylaxis (IV only):** swelling of face, eyes, lips, throat, wheezing
- **Thiamine deficiency:** anorexia, weakness/pain, depression, confusion, blurred vision, tachycardia
- Nutritional status: yeast, beef, liver, whole or enriched grains, legumes
- Application of cold to help decrease pain

Evaluate:

- Therapeutic response: absence of nausea, vomiting, anorexia, insomnia, tachycardia, paresthesias, depression, muscle weakness

Teach patient/family:

- About the necessary foods to be included in diet: yeast, beef, liver, legumes, whole grains

RARELY USED

thioridazine (Rx)

(thye-or-rid′a-zeen)

Func. class.: Antipsychotic (typical)

Chem. class.: Phenothiazine piperidine

Do not confuse:

thioridazine/thiothixene/Thorazine

ACTION: Depresses cerebral cortex, hypothalamus, limbic system, which control activity, aggression; blocks neurotransmission produced by dopamine at synapse; exhibits strong α-adrenergic and anticholinergic blocking action; mechanism for antipsychotic effects is unclear

USES: Psychotic disorders, schizophrenia, behavioral problems in children, anxiety, major depressive disorders, organic brain syndrome

Unlabeled uses: Behavioral symptoms associated with dementia in geriatric patients

CONTRAINDICATIONS: Children <2 yr, hypersensitivity, coma, CNS depression

Black Box Warning: QT prolongation, cardiac dysrhythmias

Precautions: Pregnancy (C), breastfeeding, seizure disorders, hypertension, hepatic/pulmonary disease, renal failure, BPH, glaucoma, phenothiazine hypersensitivity, suicidal ideation, smoking, Reye's syndrome, Parkinson's disease

Black Box Warning: Cardiac disease, dementia, AV block, bundle branch block, torsades de pointes

DOSAGE AND ROUTES

Psychosis

- **Adult: PO** 25-100 mg tid, max 800 mg/day; dose gradually increased to desired response, then reduced to minimum maintenance

Depression/behavioral problems/ organic brain syndrome

- **Adult: PO** 25 mg tid, range from 10 mg bid-qid to 50 mg tid-qid, max 800 mg/day for short period
- **Geriatric: PO** 10-25 mg daily-tid, increase 4-7 days by 10-25 mg to desired dose, max 800 mg/day for short period
- **Child 2-12 yr: PO** 0.5-3 mg/kg/day in divided doses, max 3 mg/kg/day

Available forms: Tabs 10, 25, 50, 100 mg

Administer:

- Antiparkinsonian agent on order from prescriber for EPS
- Avoid use with CNS depressants
- Antacids separated by 2 hr or more
- Store in tight, light-resistant container; avoid contact with skin

SIDE EFFECTS

CNS: *EPS: pseudoparkinsonism, akathisia, dystonia, tardive dyskinesia,* **seizures,** *headache,* confusion, **neuroleptic malignant syndrome,** dizziness, drowsiness

CV: Orthostatic hypotension, **cardiac arrest,** ECG changes, **tachycardia, QT prolongation, torsades de pointes**

EENT: Blurred vision, glaucoma, dry eyes

GI: *Dry mouth, nausea, vomiting, anorexia, constipation,* diarrhea, jaundice, weight gain
GU: Urinary retention, urinary frequency, enuresis, impotence, amenorrhea, gynecomastia, ejaculation dysfunction, priapism
HEMA: Anemia, leukopenia, leukocytosis, agranulocytosis
INTEG: *Rash,* photosensitivity, dermatitis
RESP: Laryngospasm, dyspnea, respiratory depression

PHARMACOKINETICS

PO: Onset erratic; peak 2-4 hr; metabolized by liver; excreted in urine, breast milk; crosses placenta; half-life 26-36 hr; 91%-99% protein binding

INTERACTIONS

⚠ **Increase:** QT prolongation—class IA/III antidysrhythmics, some phenothiazines, β agonists, local anesthetics, tricyclics, haloperidol, chloroquine, droperidol, pentamidine; CYP3A4 inhibitors (amiodarone, clarithromycin, erythromycin, telithromycin, troleandomycin), arsenic trioxide, levomethadyl; CYP3A4 substrates (methadone, pimozide, QUEtiapine, quiNIDine, risperiDONE, ziprasidone), CYP2D6 inhibitors
• Oversedation: other CNS depressants, alcohol, barbiturate anesthetics
Increase: anticholinergic effects—anticholinergics
Decrease: antiparkinson's agent effects
Decrease: thioridazine effect—lithium, barbiturates
Decrease: antihypertensive effect—centrally acting antihypertensives
Decrease: absorption—aluminum hydroxide, magnesium hydroxide antacids

Drug/Lab Test
Increase: LFTs, prolactin, bilirubin, alk phos
Decrease: Hct/Hgb, platelets, granulocytes, leukocytes, neutrocytes, eosinophils

NURSING CONSIDERATIONS

Assess:
• Mental status before 1st dose, affect, orientation, LOC, reflexes, gait, coordination, sleep pattern disturbances
• I&O ratio; palpate bladder if low urinary output occurs, urinary retention may be the cause
• Bilirubin, CBC, LFTs monthly
• Urinalysis recommended before and during prolonged therapy
• B/P standing, lying; include pulse and respirations q4hr during initial treatment; establish baseline before starting treatment; report drops of 30 mm Hg
• Dizziness, faintness, palpitations, tachycardia on rising
• **EPS** including akathisia (inability to sit still, no pattern to movements), tardive dyskinesia (bizarre movements of jaw, mouth, tongue, extremities), pseudoparkinsonism (rigidity, tremors, pill rolling, shuffling gait)
⚠ **Neuroleptic malignancy syndrome:** altered mental status, muscle rigidity, increased CPK, hyperthermia, dyspnea, fatigue
⚠ **QT prolongation:** ECG, ejection fraction; assess for chest pain, palpitations, dyspnea
• Constipation, urinary retention daily; increase bulk, water in diet
• Supervised ambulation if needed until stabilized on medication; do not involve patient in strenuous exercise program because fainting is possible; patient should not stand still for long periods
• Sips of water, candy, gum for dry mouth

Evaluate:
• Therapeutic response: decrease in emotional excitement, hallucinations, delusions, paranoia; reorganization of patterns of thought, speech

Teach patient/family:
• That orthostatic hypotension occurs frequently; to rise from sitting or lying position gradually; to avoid hazardous activities until stabilized on medication
• To avoid hot tubs, hot showers, tub baths because hypotension may occur
• To avoid abrupt withdrawal of thioridazine because EPS may result; that product should be withdrawn slowly
• To avoid OTC preparations (cough, hay fever, cold) unless approved by prescriber; that serious product interactions

may occur; to avoid use with alcohol because increased drowsiness may occur
- To use sunscreen to prevent burns
- About compliance with product regimen
- About the necessity for meticulous oral hygiene because oral candidiasis may occur
- To report sore throat, malaise, fever, bleeding, mouth sores; if these occur, CBC should be drawn and product discontinued; that product may cause vision impairment, should be reported to prescriber
- That in hot weather, heat stroke may occur; to take extra precautions to stay cool
- That product may cause discoloration of urine

TREATMENT OF OVERDOSE:
Lavage if orally ingested, provide an airway; do not induce vomiting; CV monitoring, continuous ECG

RARELY USED

thyroid USP (desiccated) (Rx)

(thye′roid)

Armour Thyroid, Bio-Throid, Nature Thyroid, NP Thyroid

Func. class.: Thyroid hormone

Chem. class.: Active thyroid hormone in natural state and ratio

ACTION: Increases metabolic rates, increases cardiac output, O_2 consumption, body temperature, blood volume; growth, development at cellular level

USES: Hypothyroidism, cretinism (juvenile hypothyroidism), myxedema

CONTRAINDICATIONS: Adrenal insufficiency, MI, thyrotoxicosis, porcine protein hypersensitivity

Black Box Warning: Obesity treatment

Precautions: Pregnancy (A), breastfeeding, geriatric patients, angina pectoris, hypertension, ischemia, cardiac disease

DOSAGE AND ROUTES

Hypothyroidism
- **Adult: PO** 30 mg/day, increased by 15 mg/mo until desired response; maintenance dose 60-120 mg/day
- **Geriatric: PO** 7.5-15 mg/day, increase dose q6-8wk until desired response

Cretinism/juvenile hypothyroidism
- **Child: PO** 15 mg/day, then 30 mg/day after 2 wk, then 60 mg/day after another 2 wk; maintenance dose 60-180 mg/day

Myxedema
- **Adult: PO** 15 mg/day, double dose q2wk, maintenance 60-180 mg/day

Available forms: Tabs 16, 32, 60, 65, 98, 130, 195, 260, 325 mg; enteric-coated tabs 32, 65, 130 mg; sugarcoated tabs 32, 65, 130, 195 mg; caps 65, 130, 195, 325 mg

Administer:
- In AM if possible as single dose to decrease sleeplessness; separate iron, calcium products by 4 hr
- At same time each day to maintain product level
- Only for hormone imbalances; not to be used for obesity, male infertility, menstrual disorders, lethargy
- Lowest dose that relieves symptoms
- Removal of medication 4 wk before RAIU test

SIDE EFFECTS
CNS: *Insomnia, tremors,* headache, thyroid storm

CV: *Tachycardia, palpitations, angina, dysrhythmias,* hypertension, cardiac arrest

GI: Nausea, diarrhea, increased or decreased appetite, cramps

MISC: Menstrual irregularities, weight loss, sweating, heat intolerance, fever

PHARMACOKINETICS
PO: Peak 12-48 hr, half-life 6-7 days

INTERACTIONS

Increase: effects of anticoagulants, sympathomimetics, tricyclics, catecholamines
Decrease: thyroid absorption—bile acid sequestrants, aluminum, magnesium, calcium
Decrease: thyroid effects—estrogens

Drug/Herb

Decrease: thyroid effect—soy

Drug/Lab Test

Increase: CPK, LDH, AST, PBI, blood glucose
Decrease: thyroid function tests

NURSING CONSIDERATIONS

Assess:

> **Black Box Warning: Obesity treatment:** use can lead to serious or life-threatening toxicity

- B/P, pulse before each dose
- I&O ratio
- Weight daily in same clothing, using same scale, at same time of day
- Height, growth rate of child
- T_3, T_4, which are decreased; radioimmunoassay of TSH, which is increased; radio uptake, which is decreased if dosage is too low
- PT may require decreased anticoagulant; check for bleeding, bruising
- **Hyperthyroidism:** increased nervousness, excitability, irritability; may indicate too high of a dose of medication, usually after 1-3 wk of treatment
- **Hypothyroidism:** lethargy, cold intolerance, weight gain, constipation, muscle cramps; may indicate too low of a dose
- Cardiac status: angina, palpitation, chest pain, change in VS

Evaluate:

- Therapeutic response: absence of depression; increased weight loss, diuresis, pulse, appetite; absence of constipation, peripheral edema, cold intolerance; pale, cool, dry skin; brittle nails, alopecia, coarse hair, menorrhagia, night blindness, paresthesias, syncope, stupor, coma, rosy cheeks

Teach patient/family:

- That hair loss will occur in child, is temporary
- To report excitability, irritability, anxiety; indicates overdose
- Not to switch brands unless directed by prescriber
- That strong odor is normal
- That hypothyroid child will show almost immediate behavior/personality change
- That treatment product is not to be taken to reduce weight
- To avoid OTC preparations with iodine; to read labels
- To separate iron, calcium products by 4 hr
- To avoid iodine food, iodized salt, soybeans, tofu, turnips, some seafood, some bread

tiaGABine (Rx)

(tie-ah-ga′been)

Gabitril

Func. class.: Anticonvulsant

Do not confuse:
tiaGABine/tiZANidine

ACTION: Inhibits reuptake and metabolism of GABA, may increase seizure threshold; structurally similar to GABA; tiaGABine binding sites in neocortex, hippocampus

USES: Adjunct treatment of partial seizures in adults and children ≥12 yr

CONTRAINDICATIONS: Hypersensitivity

Precautions: Pregnancy (C), breastfeeding, children <12 yr, geriatric patients, renal/hepatic disease, suicidal thoughts/behaviors, status epilepticus, mania, bipolar disorder, abrupt discontinuation, depression

DOSAGE AND ROUTES

When not given with a CYP3A4 enzyme, effect of tiaGABine is doubled; lower doses are indicated

- **Adult (those receiving an enzyme-inducing antiepileptic product): PO** 4 mg/day in divided doses, may increase by 4-8 mg/wk until desired response, max 56 mg/day
- **Child 12-18 yr: PO** 4 mg/day, may increase by 4 mg at beginning of wk 2; may increase by 4-8 mg/wk until desired response; max 32 mg/day

Hepatic dose

- **Adult: PO** reduce dose or increase dosing interval

Available forms: Tabs 2, 4, 12, 16 mg

Administer:

- Store at room temperature, away from heat and light
- Use with food

SIDE EFFECTS

CNS: *Dizziness, anxiety,* somnolence, ataxia, confusion, *asthenia,* unsteady gait, depression, **suicidal ideation, seizures,** tremors, hostility, EEG changes

CV: Vasodilation, tachycardia, hypertension

ENDO: Goiter, hypothyroidism

GI: Nausea, vomiting, diarrhea, increased appetite

INTEG: Pruritus, rash, **Stevens-Johnson syndrome,** alopecia, hyperhidrosis

MS: Myalgia

RESP: Pharyngitis, coughing

PHARMACOKINETICS

Absorption >95%; peak 45 min; protein binding 96%; metabolized in the liver via CYP3A4; half-life 7-9 hr without enzyme inducers, 2-5 hr with enzyme inducers

INTERACTIONS

- Lower doses may be needed when used with valproate

Increase: CNS depression—CNS depressants, alcohol

Decrease: tiaGABine effect—sevelamer

Decrease: effect—carBAMazepine, PHENobarbital, phenytoin, primidone

Drug/Food

Decrease: rate of absorption—high-fat meal

NURSING CONSIDERATIONS

Assess:

- Renal studies: urinalysis, BUN, urine creatinine q3mo
- Hepatic studies: ALT, AST, bilirubin
- **Seizures:** location, duration, presence of aura; assess for weakness
- Withdraw gradually to prevent seizures
- May cause status epilepticus and unexplained death
- ⚠ Mental status: mood, sensorium, affect, behavioral changes, suicidal thoughts/behaviors; if mental status changes, notify prescriber, hypomania may be present before suicide attempt
- Assistance with ambulation during early part of treatment; dizziness occurs
- Seizure precautions: padded side rails; move objects that may harm patient

Evaluate:

- Therapeutic response: decreased seizure activity; document on patient's chart

Teach patient/family:

- To carry emergency ID stating patient's name, products taken, condition, prescriber's name and phone number
- To avoid driving, other activities that require alertness
- Not to discontinue medication quickly after long-term use
- To take with food
- To notify prescriber if pregnancy is planned or suspected; avoid breastfeeding
- To report suicidal thoughts, behaviors immediately

T

⚠ HIGH ALERT

ticagrelor

Brilinta

Func. class.: Platelet inhibitor

Chem. class.: ADP receptor antagonist

ACTION:

Reversibly bind to the platelet receptor, preventing platelet activation

USES: Arterial thromboembolism prophylaxis in acute coronary syndrome (ACS) (unstable angina, acute MI), including in patients undergoing percutaneous coronary intervention (PCI)

CONTRAINDICATIONS: Hypersensitivity, severe hepatic disease

Black Box Warning: Bleeding, intracranial bleeding

Precautions: Pregnancy (C), breastfeeding, infants, neonates, children, GI bleeding, hepatic disease, abrupt discontinuation

Black Box Warning: Coronary artery bypass graft surgery (CABG), surgery

DOSAGE AND ROUTES

- **Adult: PO** loading dose 180 mg with aspirin (usually 325 mg PO); then give 90 mg bid with aspirin 75-100 mg/day, do not give maintenance doses of aspirin >100 mg/day

Available forms: Tab 90 mg

Administer:

PO route

- May be taken without regard to food
- Discontinue 5-7 days before surgery
- May be crushed (90 mg tab) and mixed with purified water, 100 mg (PO) or 50 ml (NG); ensure entire dose is given by flushing mortar, syringe, NG tube with 2 additional 50 ml of water
- Store at room temperature, in original container in dry place

SIDE EFFECTS

CNS: Headache, dizziness, fatigue

CV: Hypertension, hypotension, chest pain, atrial fibrillation, bradyarrhythmias, syncope, ventricular pauses

GI: Nausea, diarrhea

HEMA: Serious, fatal bleeding

MISC: Back pain, hyperuricemia, gynecomastia

RESP: Dyspnea, cough

PHARMACOKINETICS

Absolute bioavailability 36%, protein binding (>99%), metabolism by CYP3A4, weak P-glycoprotein substrates and inhibitors, elimination for product and metabolite are hepatic and biliary, 84% excreted in feces, 26% in urine, half-life is 7 hr for ticagrelor, 9 hr for metabolite, maximum inhibition of platelet aggregation (IPA) effect 2 hr, maintained ≥8 hr, peak 1.5 hr product, 2.5 hr metabolite

INTERACTIONS

Black Box Warning: Increase: bleeding risk—CYP3A4 inhibitors (ketoconazole, itraconazole, voriconazole, clarithromycin, telithromycin, nefazodone, ritonavir, lopinavir, ritonavir, saquinavir, nelfinavir, indinavir, atazanavir, delavirdine, isoniazid, dalfopristin, quinupristin, tipranavir)

Decrease: ticagrelor action—CYP3A4 inducers (rifampin, dexamethasone, phenytoin, carBAMazepine, PHENobarbital)

Increase: effect of—simvastatin, lovastatin

Increase: bleeding risk—NSAIDs, anticoagulants, platelet inhibitors

Increase or decrease: digoxin

Drug/Lab Test

Increase: serum creatinine

NURSING CONSIDERATIONS

Assess:

- **Thromboembolism:** Monitor CBC with differential with platelet count baseline and periodically during treatment

Black Box Warning: Bleeding: Assess for bleeding that may occur when aspirin is combined with this product; some bleeding can be fatal, usually aspirin doses >100 mg/day; watch for frank bleeding, hypotension

Black Box Warning: CABG: Do not use in those undergoing CABG, discontinue ≥5 days before surgery

• **Abrupt discontinuation:** do not discontinue abruptly, may increase risk for MI, stent thrombosis, death

Evaluate:

• Prevention of thromboembolism

Teach patient/family:

• To take only as prescribed; not to skip or double doses; if a dose is missed, to take next dose at scheduled time

Black Box Warning: To notify prescriber of chills, fever, bruising, bleeding; not to use aspirin ≥100 mg/day

• Not to use any prescription, OTC products, herbs without approval of prescriber; products with aspirin, NSAIDs may cause bleeding
• To notify all health care providers of product use
• That product can be taken without regard to meals
• That it may take longer for bleeding to stop
• Not to breastfeed
• To notify prescriber if pregnancy is planned or suspected

ticarcillin/clavulanate (Rx)

Timentin

Func. class.: Broad-spectrum antiinfective

Chem. class.: Extended-spectrum penicillin, β-lactamase inhibitor

ACTION: Interferes with cell-wall replication of susceptible organisms; osmotically unstable cell-wall swells, bursts from osmotic pressure; clavulanate inhibits β-lactamase and protects against enzymatic degradation of ticarcillin

USES: Respiratory, soft-tissue, and urinary tract infections; bacterial septicemia; effective for gram-positive cocci *(Staphylococcus aureus, Streptococcus faecalis, Streptococcus pneumoniae)*, gram-negative cocci *(Neisseria gonorrhoeae)*, gram-positive bacilli *(Clostridium perfringens, Clostridium tetani)*, gram-negative bacilli *(Bacteroides, Fusobacterium nucleatum, Escherichia coli, Proteus mirabilis, Salmonella, Morganella morganii, Proteus rettgeri, Enterobacter, Pseudomonas aeruginosa, Serratia)*; and *Peptococcus, Peptostreptococcus,* and *Eubacterium*

CONTRAINDICATIONS: Neonates, hypersensitivity to penicillins

Precautions: Pregnancy (B), hypersensitivity to cephalosporins, renal disease

DOSAGE AND ROUTES

Systemic/urinary tract infections, moderate/severe infections

• **Adult ≥60 kg: IV INFUSION** 3.1 g q4-6hr
• **Adult <60 kg: IV INFUSION** 200-300 mg/kg/day q4-6hr
• **Child >60 kg: IV INFUSION** 3.1 g q4-6hr
• **Child <60 kg: IV INFUSION** 200-300 mg/kg/day q4hr
• **Full-term neonates/infants <3 mo (unlabeled): IV** 50 mg/kg q4hr for severe infections; **IV** 50 mg/kg q6hr for mild to moderate infections

Mild to moderate infections

• **Child ≥60 kg: IV INFUSION** 3.1 g q6hr
• **Child <60 kg: IV INFUSION** 200 mg/kg/day q6hr

Renal dose

• **Adult: IV INFUSION** loading dose 3.1 g; CCr 60 ml/min, 3.1 g q4hr; CCr 30-60 ml/min, 2 g q4hr; CCr 10-30 ml/min, 2 g q8hr; CCr <10 ml/min, 2 g q12hr; CCr <10 ml/min with hepatic dysfunction, 2 g q24hr

Available forms: Inj 3 g ticarcillin, 0.1 g clavulanate; IV infusion 3 g ticarcillin, 0.1 g clavulanate; powder for inj 3 g ticarcillin, 0.1 g clavulanate

Administer:

• Product after C&S, give ≥q1hr before bactericidal antiinfectives, change IV site q48hr

T

Intermittent IV INFUSION route
- After diluting ≤3.1 g/13 ml of sterile water or NaCl (200 mg/ml), shake; may further dilute in ≥50-100 ml NS, D_5W, or LR sol and run over ½ hr
- Store reconstituted sol 12-24 hr at room temperature, or 3-7 days refrigerated

Y-site compatibilities: Allopurinol, amifostine, amikacin, anidulafungin, atropine, aztreonam, bivalirudin, bumetanide, ceFAZolin, cefepime, cefotaxime, cefOXitin, cefTAZidime, ceftizoxime, cefTRIAXone, cefuroxime, chloramphenicol, cimetidine, clindamycin, cyclophosphamide, cycloSPORINE, dexamethasone, dexmedetomidine, digoxin, diltiazem, diphenhydrAMINE, DOCEtaxel, DOPamine, DOXOrubicin liposome, doxycycline, enalaprilat, EPINEPHrine, esmolol, etoposide phosphate, famotidine, fenoldopam, filgrastim, fluconazole, furosemide, gemcitabine, gentamicin, granisetron, heparin, hydrocortisone, HYDROmorphone, imipenem/cilastatin, insulin, isoproterenol, labetalol, levofloxacin, lidocaine, linezolid, LORazepam, melphalan, meperidine, methylPREDNISolone, metoclopramide, metoprolol, metroNIDAZOLE, milrinone, morphine, nitroglycerin, nitroprusside, norepinephrine, ondansetron, palonosetron, pantoprazole, PEMEtrexed, penicillin G potassium, perphenazine, phenylephrine, procainamide, propofol, propranolol, ranitidine, remifentanil, sargramostim, sodium bicarbonate, tacrolimus, teniposide, theophylline, thiotepa, tirofiban, tobramycin, vasopressin, verapamil, vinorelbine, voriconazole

SIDE EFFECTS

CNS: Anxiety, seizures, confusion, drowsiness

GI: *Nausea, vomiting, diarrhea;* increased AST, ALT; abdominal pain, glossitis, colitis, pseudomembranous colitis, hepatotoxicity

HEMA: Anemia, increased bleeding time, bone marrow depression, granulocytopenia

INTEG: Rash, urticaria, toxic epidermal necrolysis, pain at injection site

META: Hypokalemia, hypernatremia

SYST: Anaphylaxis, Stevens-Johnson syndrome, overgrowth of organisms

PHARMACOKINETICS

IV: Peak 30-45 min, duration 4 hr, half-life 64-68 min, excreted in urine

INTERACTIONS

▲ **Increase:** bleeding—anticoagulants

Increase: methotrexate level—methotrexate, uric acid, bilirubicin, BUN, creatinining, alk, phos, LDH

Increase: ticarcillin concentrations—probenecid, sulfipyrazone

Decrease: antimicrobial effect of ticarcillin—tetracyclines, aminoglycosides IV, chloramphenicol, macrolides, sulfonamides

Decrease: effect—oral contraceptives, erythromycin

Drug/Lab Test

False positive: urine glucose, urine protein, Coombs' test

Increase: LFTs, sodium, eosinophils, INR bleeding time

Decrease: Hgb, potassium, platelets, WBC, granulocytes

NURSING CONSIDERATIONS

Assess:
- Infection: WBC, wound, temperature, sputum, urine, baseline and periodically

▲ **Pseudomembranous colitis:** diarrhea, abdominal pain, fever, fatigue, anorexia; possible anemia, elevated WBC count, low serum albumin; stop product; usually either vancomycin or IV metroNIDAZOLE is given

▲ **Serious skin reactions:** Stevens-Johnson syndrome, toxic epidermal necrolysis; anaphylaxis: wheezing, rash, laryngeal edema; have emergency equipment nearby

- Hepatic studies: AST, ALT
- Blood studies: WBC, RBC, Hct, Hgb, bleeding time, platelets, baseline and periodically
- Renal studies: BUN, creatinine, sodium, potassium

- Skin eruptions after administration of penicillin to 1 wk after discontinuing product
- EPINEPHrine, suction, tracheostomy set, endotracheal intubation equipment

Evaluate:

- Therapeutic response: resolution of infection

Teach patient/family:

- To report persistent diarrhea with blood, pus, mucus, or fever
- That culture may be taken after completed course of medication
- To report sore throat, fever, fatigue (may indicate superinfection); CNS effects (anxiety, depression, hallucinations, seizures)
- To wear or carry emergency ID if allergic to penicillins
- To use alternative birth control method instead of hormonal

TREATMENT OF OVERDOSE:
Withdraw product, maintain airway, administer EPINEPHrine, O_2, IV corticosteroids for anaphylaxis

ticlopidine (Rx)
(tye-cloe′pi-deen)

Func. class.: Platelet aggregation inhibitor

Chem. class.: Thienopyridine compound

ACTION:
Irreversible inhibition of platelet aggregation through antagonism of ADP

USES:
Reducing the risk for stroke in high-risk patients

Unlabeled uses: Intermittent claudication, chronic arterial occlusion, subarachnoid hemorrhage, uremic patients with AV shunts/fistulas, open heart surgery, coronary artery bypass grafts, primary glomerulonephritis, sickle cell disease, diabetic retinopathy

CONTRAINDICATIONS:
Hypersensitivity, severe hepatic disease, active bleeding, coagulopathy

Black Box Warning: Agranulocytosis, neutropenia, thrombocytopenia, thrombotic thrombocytopenic purpura (TTP)

Precautions: Pregnancy (B), breastfeeding, children, geriatric patients, past hepatic disease, renal disease, increased bleeding risk, peptic ulcer disease, surgery

Black Box Warning: Anemia, hematologic disease

DOSAGE AND ROUTES
- **Adult: PO** 250 mg bid with food

Available forms: Tabs 250 mg

Administer:

- With food to decrease gastric symptoms
- Discontinue when absolute neutrophil count falls during treatment to <1200/mm^3 or platelets <80,000/mm^3; may use methylPREDNISolone IV 20 mg to provide normal bleeding time in 2 hr

SIDE EFFECTS
CNS: Dizziness, headache, weakness

EENT: Tinnitus, epistaxis

GI: Nausea, vomiting, *diarrhea,* GI discomfort, **cholestatic jaundice, hepatitis,** increased cholesterol, LDL, VLDL, triglycerides

GU: Hematuria

HEMA: Bleeding (epistaxis, hematuria, conjunctival hemorrhage, GI bleeding), agranulocytosis, neutropenia, thrombocytopenia, thrombotic thombocytopenic purpura

INTEG: *Rash,* pruritus

META: Hypercholesterolemia, hypertriglyceridemia

PHARMACOKINETICS
Peak 1-3 hr; metabolized by liver; excreted in urine, feces; half-life increases with repeated dosing, initially 12-36 hr; antiplatelet effect 2-5 days; 98% protein binding

INTERACTIONS

Increase: levels of CYP2C19, CYP2DC substrates, phenytoin, fosphenytoin, ambrisentan, theophylline

Increase: bleeding tendencies—anticoagulants, salicylates, thrombolytics, NSAIDs, abciximab, eptifibatide, tirofiban, thrombin inhibitors, SSRIs, aspirin

Increase: effects of ticlopidine—cimetidine

Decrease: plasma levels of ticlopidine—antacids

Decrease: plasma levels of digoxin, cycloSPORINE

Drug/Herb

Increase: bleeding risk—ginger, ginkgo, garlic, feverfew, horse chestnut, green tea

NURSING CONSIDERATIONS

Assess:

- Hepatic studies: AST, ALT, bilirubin, creatinine with long-term therapy

Black Box Warning: Blood dyscrasias, bone marrow depression, do not use in those with a history of these conditions; blood studies: CBC; CBC q2wk × 3 mo, Hct, Hgb, PT with long-term therapy

Black Box Warning: Bleeding time at baseline and throughout treatment; levels may be 2-5× normal limit

Evaluate:

- Therapeutic response: absence of stroke

Teach patient/family:

- That blood work will be necessary during treatment

Black Box Warning: To report any unusual bleeding to prescriber

- To report side effects such as diarrhea, skin rashes, subcut bleeding, signs of cholestasis (jaundiced skin and sclera, dark urine, light-colored stools)
- That product should be discontinued 10-14 days before surgery; not to double a missed dose
- That there are many product and herbal interactions, to avoid all OTC products unless approved by prescriber
- To take with food

tigecycline (Rx)

(tye-ge-sye′kleen)

Tygacil

Func. class.: Broad-spectrum antiinfective

Chem. class.: Glycylcyclines

ACTION: Inhibits protein synthesis and phosphorylation in microorganisms; bacteriostatic structurally similar to the tetracyclines

USES: Complicated skin/skin-structure infections *(Escherichia coli, Enterococcus faecalis* [vancomycin-susceptible only], *Staphylococcus aureus, Streptococcus agalactiae, S. anginosus* group, *S. pyogenes, Bacteroides fragilis;* complicated intraabdominal infections *[Citrobacter freundii] Enterobacter cloacae, E. coli, Klebsiella oxytoca, K. pneumoniae, E. faecalis* [vancomycin-susceptible only], *S. aureus* [methicillin-susceptible only], *S. anginosus* group, *B. fragilis, Bacteroides thetaiotaomicron, B. uniformis, B. vulgatus, Clostridium perfringens, Peptostreptococcus micros);* community-acquired pneumonia

CONTRAINDICATIONS: Pregnancy (D), breastfeeding, children <18 yr, hypersensitivity to tigecycline

Precautions: Renal/hepatic disease, hypersensitivity to tetracyclines, ventilator-associated/hospital-acquired pneumonias

Black Box Warning: Infection

DOSAGE AND ROUTES

- **Adult:** **IV** 100 mg then 50 mg q12hr, **IV INFUSION** given over 30-60 min q12hr; given for 5-14 days, depending on infection

Hepatic dose

- **Adult: IV** (Child-Pugh C) 100 mg, then 25 mg q12hr

Available forms: Powder for inj, lyophilized 50 mg

Administer:

- Tigecycline allergy test before using, obtain C&S, do not begin treatment before results or if susceptible organism is strongly suspected

Intermittent IV INFUSION route

- Reconstitute each vial with 5.3 ml of 0.9% NaCl or D_5 (10 mg/ml); swirl to dissolve; immediately withdraw 5 ml of reconstituted sol and add to 100-ml IV bag for infusion (1 mg/ml); may be yellow or orange; if not, sol should be discarded; do not give if particulate matter is present, use a dedicated IV line or Y-site, flush with NS before and after use, give over ½ hr
- Store in tight, light-resistant container at room temperature, diluted sol at room temperature for up to 24 hr, 6 hr in vial, and remaining time in IV bag, ≤48 hr refrigerated

Y-site compatibilities: Acyclovir, alfentanil, allopurinol, amifostine, amikacin, aminocaproic acid, aminophylline, amphotericin B liposome, ampicillin, ampicillin/sulbactam, argatroban, azithromycin, aztreonam, bivalirudin, bumetanide, buprenorphine, butorphanol, calcium chloride/gluconate, CARBOplatin, carmustine, caspofungin, ceFAZolin, cefepime, cefotaxime, cefoTEtan, cefOXitin, cefTAZidime, ceftizoxime, cefTRIAXone, cefuroxime, cimetidine, ciprofloxacin, cisatracurium, CISplatin, clindamycin, cyclophosphamide, cycloSPORINE, cytarabine, dacarbazine, DACTINomycin, DAPTOmycin, DAUNOrubicin hydrochloride, dexamethasone, dexmedetomidine, dexrazoxane, digoxin, diltiazem, diphenhydrAMINE, DOBUTamine, DOCEtaxel, dolasetron, DOPamine, doripenem, DOXOrubicin hydrochloride, DOXOrubicin liposome, droperidol, enalaprilat, EPINEPHrine, eptifibatide, ertapenem, erythromycin, esmolol, etoposide, etoposide phosphate, famotidine, fenoldopam, fentaNYL, fluconazole, fludarabine, fluorouracil, foscarnet, fosphenytoin, furosemide, ganciclovir, gemcitabine, gentamicin, glycopyrrolate, granisetron, haloperidol, heparin, hydrocortisone, HYDROmorphone, ifosfamide, imipenem/cilastatin, insulin, irinotecan, isoproterenol, ketorolac, labetalol, lansoprazole, lepirudin, leucovorin, levofloxacin, lidocaine, linezolid, LORazepam, magnesium sulfate, mannitol, mechlorethamine, melphalan, meperidine, meropenem, mesna, methohexital, methotrexate, methyldopa, metoclopramide, metoprolol, metroNIDAZOLE, midazolam, milrinone, mitoMYcin, mitoXANtrone, morphine, moxifloxacin, mycophenolate, nafcillin, nalbuphine, naloxone, nesiritide, nitroglycerin, nitroprusside, norepinephrine, octreotide, ondansetron, oxaliplatin, oxytocin, PACLitaxel, palonosetron, pamidronate, pancuronium, pantoprazole, PEMEtrexed, pemtamidine, pentazocin, PENTobarbital, PHENobarbital, phenylephrine, piperacillin/tazobactam, potassium acetate/chloride/phosphate, procainamide, prochlorperazine, promethazine, propofol, propranolol, ranitidine, remifentanil, rocuronium, sodium acetate/bicarbonate/phosphate, streptozocin, succinylcholine, SUFentanil, tacrolimus, teniposide, theophylline, thiopental, thiotepa, ticarcillin/clavulanate, tirofiban, tobramycin, topotecan, trimethoprim/sulfamethoxazole, vancomycin, vasopressin, vecuronium, vinBLAStine, vinCRIStine, vinorelbine, zidovudine, zoledronic acid

SIDE EFFECTS

CNS: Headache, dizziness, insomnia
CV: Hypo/hypertension, phlebitis
EENT: Tooth discoloration
GI: *Nausea, vomiting, diarrhea,* anorexia, constipation, dyspepsia, abdominal pain, **hepatotoxicity, hepatic failure, pseudomembranous colitis**
HEMA: **Anemia, leukocytosis, thrombocytopenia**

T

INTEG: *Rash,* pruritus, sweating, photosensitivity
META: Increased ALT, AST, BUN, lactic acid, alk phos, amylase; hyperglycemia, hypokalemia, hypoproteinemia, bilirubinemia
MISC: Back pain, fever, abnormal healing, abdominal pain, abscess, asthenia, infection, pain, peripheral edema, local reactions
RESP: Cough, dyspnea
SYST: Anaphylaxis

PHARMACOKINETICS

Not extensively metabolized, 22% of unchanged product excreted in urine, terminal half-life 42 hr, primarily biliary excreted, protein binding 71%-89%

INTERACTIONS

Increase: effect of warfarin
Decrease: effect of oral contraceptives
Drug/Lab Test
Increase: amylase, LFTs, alk phos, BUN, creatinine, LDH, WBC, INR, PTT, PT
Decrease: potassium, calcium, sodium, Hgb/Hct, platelets

NURSING CONSIDERATIONS

Assess:

Black Box Warning: Use only with confirmation of strongly suspected bacterial infection, do not use as a prophylactic

⚠ **Pseudomembranous colitis:** diarrhea, abdominal pain, fever, fatigue, anorexia; possible anemia, elevated WBC level, low serum albumin; stop product; usually either vancomycin or IV metroNIDAZOLE is given

- Signs of anemia: Hct, Hgb, fatigue
- Blood studies: PT, CBC, AST, ALT, BUN creatinine

⚠ **Allergic reactions:** rash, itching, pruritus, angioedema

- Serious allergic skin reactions: Stevens-Johnson anaphylaxis
- Nausea, vomiting, diarrhea; administer antiemetic, antacids as ordered
- **Toxicity:** pseudotumor cerebri, photosensitivity, antianabolic actions (azotemia, BUN, hypophosphatemia, metabolic acidosis) tigecycline is structurally similar to tetracycline; pancreatitis, hyperamylasemia; (may be fatal) if these occur, discontinue, improvement usually occurs after product is discontinued
- **Overgrowth of infection:** fever, malaise, redness, pain, swelling, drainage, perineal itching, diarrhea, changes in cough or sputum

Evaluate:

- Therapeutic response: decreased temperature, absence of lesions, negative C&S

Teach patient/family:

- To avoid sun exposure; sunscreen does not seem to decrease photosensitivity

⚠ To avoid pregnancy while taking this product; fetal harm may occur; to avoid breastfeeding

- To report infection, increase in temperature; to report burning, pain at inj site
- To report diarrhea, fatigue, abdominal pain

timolol (Rx)

(tye′moe-lole)

Apo-Timol ♣, Novo-Timol ♣

Func. class.: Antihypertensive
Chem. class.: Nonselective β-blocker

ACTION: Competitively blocks stimulation of β-adrenergic receptor within vascular smooth muscle (decreases rate of SA node discharge, increases recovery time); slows conduction of AV node and decreases heart rate, which decreases O_2 consumption in myocardium; also decreases renin-aldosterone-angiotensin system; at high doses, inhibits β_2-receptors in bronchial system

USES: Mild to moderate hypertension, migraine prophylaxis, to decrease mortality after MI
Unlabeled uses: Tremors, angina pectoris

CONTRAINDICATIONS:
Hypersensitivity to β-blockers, cardiogenic shock, heart block (2nd/3rd degree), sinus bradycardia, CHF, cardiac failure, severe COPD, asthma

Precautions: Pregnancy (C), breastfeeding, major surgery, diabetes mellitus, COPD, well-compensated heart failure, nonallergic bronchospasm, peripheral vascular disease, thyroid/renal/hepatic disease

Black Box Warning: Abrupt discontinuation

DOSAGE AND ROUTES

Hypertension

- **Adult: PO** 10 mg bid or 20 mg/day, may increase by 10 mg q7days, max 60 mg/day
- **Geriatric patients: PO** initiate dose cautiously

Myocardial infarction

- **Adult: PO** 10 mg bid beginning 1-4 wk after MI for ≥2 yr

Migraine headache prevention

- **Adult: PO** 10 mg bid or 20 mg/day; may increase to 30 mg/day, 20 mg in AM, 10 mg in PM; discontinue if not effective after 8 wk

Available forms: Tabs 5, 10, 20 mg

Administer:

- PO before or immediately after meals, at bedtime; tab may be crushed or swallowed whole
- Reduced dosage in renal dysfunction
- Store at room temperature; do not freeze

SIDE EFFECTS

CNS: *Insomnia, dizziness,* hallucinations, anxiety, fatigue, depression, headache

CV: Hypotension, bradycardia, **CHF**, edema, chest pain, claudication, angina, AV block, ventricular dysrhythmias

EENT: *Visual changes;* sore throat; *double vision;* dry, burning eyes

GI: *Nausea,* vomiting, **ischemic colitis,** diarrhea, *abdominal pain,* **mesenteric arterial thrombosis,** flatulence, constipation

GU: Impotence, urinary frequency

HEMA: **Agranulocytosis, thrombocytopenia, purpura**

INTEG: Rash, alopecia, pruritus, fever

META: Hypoglycemia

MUSC: *Joint pain, muscle pain*

RESP: **Bronchospasm,** *dyspnea,* cough, crackles, nasal stuffiness

PHARMACOKINETICS

Peak 1-2 hr; half-life 4 hr; metabolized by liver; excreted in urine, breast milk; protein binding <10%

INTERACTIONS

Increase: hypotension, bradycardia—hydrALAZINE, methyldopa, prazosin, anticholinergics, alcohol, reserpine, nitrates

Increase: effects of β-blockers, calcium channel blockers

Decrease: antihypertensive effects—NSAIDs, sympathomimetics, thyroid, salicylates

Decrease: hypoglycemic effects—insulin, sulfonylureas

Decrease: bronchodilation—theophyllines

Drug/Lab Test

Increase: renal, hepatic studies, uric acid

Interference: glucose, insulin tolerance test

NURSING CONSIDERATIONS

Assess:

Black Box Warning: Abrupt discontinuation: may result in myocardial ischemia, MI, severe hypotension, ventricular dysrhythmias in those with preexisting cardiovascular disease

- **Headaches:** location, severity, duration, frequency at baseline and throughout treatment
- I&O, weight daily
- B/P during initial treatment, periodically thereafter, pulse q4hr; note rate, rhythm, quality
- Apical/radial pulse before administration; notify prescriber of any significant changes

- Baselines of renal, hepatic studies before therapy begins
- Edema in feet, legs daily

Evaluate:

- Therapeutic response: decreased B/P after 1-2 wk

Teach patient/family:

- To take before or immediately after meals

Black Box Warning: Not to discontinue product abruptly; to taper over 2 wk; may cause precipitate angina

- Not to use OTC products containing α-adrenergic stimulants (nasal decongestants, cold preparations) unless directed by prescriber
- To report bradycardia, dizziness, confusion, depression, fever, sore throat, SOB to prescriber
- Product masks hypoglycemia; monitor blood sugar
- To take pulse at home; advise when to notify prescriber
- To avoid alcohol, smoking, sodium intake
- To comply with weight control, dietary adjustments, modified exercise program
- To carry emergency ID to identify product, allergies
- To avoid hazardous activities if dizziness is present
- To report symptoms of **CHF:** difficulty breathing, especially on exertion or when lying down; night cough; swelling of extremities
- To take medication at bedtime; to wear support hose to minimize effect of orthostatic hypotension

TREATMENT OF OVERDOSE:

Lavage, IV atropine for bradycardia, IV theophylline for bronchospasm, digoxin, O_2, diuretic for cardiac failure, hemodialysis; administer vasopressor (norepinephrine)

timolol (ophthalmic)

(tie-moe′lol)

Betimol, Istalol, Timoptic, Timoptic-XE

Func. class.: Antiglaucoma

Chem. class.: β-Blocker

ACTION: Can decrease aqueous humor and increase outflows

USES: Treatment of chronic open-angle glaucoma and ocular hypertension

CONTRAINDICATIONS: Hypersensitivity, AV block, heart failure, bradycardia, sick sinus syndrome, asthma

Precautions: Abrupt discontinuation, pregnancy, breastfeeding, children, COPD, depression, diabetes mellitus, myasthenia gravis, hyperthyroidism, pulmonary disease, angle-closure glaucoma

DOSAGE AND ROUTES

- **Adult:** instill 1 drop in each affected eye bid (0.25% solution) initially; if no response, 1 drop in each affected eye bid (0.5% solution) or 1 drop of gel in each affected eye daily

Available forms: Ophthalmic solution 0.25, 0.5%; ophthalmic gel 0.25%, 0.5%

Administer:

- For ophthalmic use only
- Do not touch the tip of the dropper to the eye, fingertips, or other surface to prevent contamination
- Wash hands before and after use
- Tilt head back slightly and pull the lower eyelid down with the index finger to form a pouch; squeeze the prescribed number of drops into the pouch; close eyes to spread drops; to avoid excessive systemic absorption, apply finger pressure on the lacrimal sac for 1-2 min after use
- If >1 topical ophthalmic drug product is being used, the drugs should be administered at least 5 min apart

- Administer other topically applied ophthalmic medications at least 10 min before timolol gel-forming solution
- To avoid contamination or the spread of infection, do not use dropper for more than one person
- Some products contain the preservative benzalkonium chloride, which can be absorbed by soft contact lenses; remove contact lenses before administration of the solution; lenses may be reinserted 15 min after administration
- Decreased intraocular pressure can take several weeks, monitor IOP after a month

SIDE EFFECTS

CNS: *Insomnia,* headache, *dizziness,* anxiety, depression, headache, nightmares, *fatigue*
CV: Palpitations, heart failure, hypotension
EENT: Eye stinging/burning, tearing, photophobia, visual disturbances
GI: Nausea, dry mouth
PULM: Bronchospasm

PHARMACOKINETICS

Onset 30 min, peak 1-2 hr, duration 12-24 hr

INTERACTIONS

Increase: β-blocking effect—oral β-blockers
Increase: intraocular pressure reduction—topical miotics, dipivefrin, EPINEPHrine, carbonic anhydrase inhibitors; this may be beneficial
Increase: B/P, severe—when abruptly stopping cloNIDine
Increase: depression of AV nodal conduction, bradycardia, or hypotension—adenosine, cardiac glycosides, disopyramide,* other antiarrhythmics, class 1C antiarrhythmic drugs (flecainide, propafenone, moricizine, encainide quiNIDine, calcium-channel blockers, or drugs that significantly depress AV nodal conduction)
Increase: AV block nodal conduction, induce AV block—high doses of procainamide
Increase: antihypertensive effect—other antihypertensives

NURSING CONSIDERATIONS

Assess:

⚠ **Systemic absorption**: When used in the eye, systemic absorption is common with the same adverse reactions and interactions

- Glaucoma: monitor intraocular pressure

Evaluate:

- Decreasing intraocular pressure

Teach patient/family:

- That product is for ophthalmic use only
- Not to touch the tip of the dropper to the eye, fingertips, or other surface to prevent contamination
- To wash hands before and after use
- To tilt the head back slightly and pull the lower eyelid down with the index finger to form a pouch; squeeze the prescribed number of drops into the pouch; close eyes to spread drops
- To apply finger pressure on the lacrimal sac for 1-2 min following use to prevent excessive systemic absorption
- To administer drugs at least 5 min apart if more than one topical ophthalmic drug product is being used
- To administer other topically applied ophthalmic medications at least 10 min before timolol gel-forming solution
- To not use dropper for more than one person to avoid contamination or the spread of infection
- That some products contain the preservative benzalkonium chloride, which may be absorbed by soft contact lenses; to remove contact lenses before administration of the solution; that lenses may be reinserted 15 min after administration

⚠ HIGH ALERT

tinidazole (Rx)

(tye-ni′da-zole)

Tindamax

Func. class.: Antiprotozoal

Chem. class.: Nitroimidazole derivative

ACTION: Interferes with DNA/RNA synthesis in protozoa

USES: Amebiasis, giardiasis, trichomoniasis

Unlabeled uses: *Bacteroides* sp., *Clostridium* sp., *Eubacterium* sp., *Fusobacterium* sp., *Peptococcus* sp., *Peptostreptococcus* sp., gingivitis, urethritis, *Veillonella* sp.

CONTRAINDICATIONS: Pregnancy, breastfeeding; hypersensitivity to this product or nitroimidazole derivative

Precautions: Children, geriatric patients, hepatic disease, CNS depression, blood dyscrasias, candidiasis, seizures, viral infection, alcoholism, pregnancy (C)

Black Box Warning: Secondary malignancy

DOSAGE AND ROUTES

Intestinal amebiasis/amebic involvement of the liver

- **Adult: PO** 2 g daily × 3 days
- **Child ≥3 yr/adolescent: PO** 50 mg/kg/day × 3 days, max 2 g/day

Giardiasis

- **Adult: PO** 2 g as a single dose
- **Child ≥3 yr: PO** 50 mg/kg as a single dose, max 2 g

Trichomoniasis

- **Adult: PO** 2 g as a single dose

Bacterial vaginosis

- **Adult (nonpregnant woman): PO** 2 g/day × 2 days with food or 1 g/day × 5 days with food

Available forms: Tabs 250, 500 mg

Administer:

- Tabs can be crushed and mixed with artificial cherry syrup for children
- With food to increase plasma concentrations, minimize epigastric distress and other GI effects

SIDE EFFECTS

CNS: *Dizziness, headache,* seizures, *peripheral neuropathy,* malaise, fatigue

GI: *Nausea, vomiting,* anorexia, increased AST/ALT, constipation, abdominal pain, indigestion, altered taste

HEMA: Leukopenia, neutropenia

INTEG: Pruritus, urticaria, *rash*, oral candidiasis

SYST: Angioedema, cramping

PHARMACOKINETICS

Peak $1^1/_2$ hr; metabolized extensively in liver; excreted unchanged (20%-25%) in urine, (12%) feces; half-life 12-14 hr; crosses blood-brain barrier

INTERACTIONS

- Do not use within 2 wk of disulfiram

Increase: tinidazole action—CYP3A4 inhibitors (cimetidine, ketoconazole): increased action of tinidazole

Increase: action of anticoagulants, cycloSPORINE, tacrolimus, fluorouracil, hydantoins, lithium

Decrease: tinidazole action—CYP3A4 inducers (PHENobarbital, rifampin, phenytoin); cholestyramine, oxytetracycline: decreased action of tinidazole

Drug/Herb

Increase or decrease: tinidazole level—St. John's wort

Drug/Lab Test

Increase: triglycerides, LDH, AST/ALT, glucose

Decrease: WBCs

NURSING CONSIDERATIONS

Assess:

- **Giardiasis:** obtain 3 stool samples several days apart beginning q3-4wk after treatment
- **Amebic liver abscess:** monitor CBC, ESR, amebic gel diffusion test, ultrasound;

also total and differential leukocyte count

Black Box Warning: Secondary malignancy: avoid unnecessary use

- Signs of infection, anemia
- Bowel pattern before, during treatment

Evaluate:
- Therapeutic response: decrease in infection as evidenced by negative culture

Teach patient/family:
- To take with food to increase plasma concentrations, minimize epigastric distress and other GI effects; not to use alcoholic beverages during or for 3 days after treatment
- **Trichomoniasis:** both partners should be treated at the same time
- To avoid alcohol; may cause disulfiram reaction
- To avoid doing hazardous activities until reaction is known
- That product causes unpleasant taste
- Not to use OTC, Rx, or herbal products unless approved by prescriber

tioconazole vaginal antifungal

See Appendix B

tiotropium (Rx)

(ty-oh′tro-pee-um)

Spiriva HandiHaler, Spiriva Respimat

Func. class.: Anticholinergic, bronchodilator

Chem. class.: Synthetic quaternary ammonium compound

Do not confuse:
Spiriva/Inspra

ACTION: Inhibits interaction of acetylcholine at receptor sites on the bronchial smooth muscle, thereby resulting in decreased cGMP and bronchodilation

USES: COPD; for the long-term treatment and once-daily maintenance of bronchospasm associated with COPD, including chronic bronchitis and emphysema

CONTRAINDICATIONS: Hypersensitivity to this product, atropine, or its derivatives

Precautions: Pregnancy (C), breastfeeding, children, geriatric patients, closed-angle glaucoma, prostatic hypertrophy, bladder neck obstruction, renal disease

DOSAGE AND ROUTES
- **Adult: INH** content of 1 cap/day (18 mcg) using HandiHaler inhalation device or 2 INH (spray) (2.5 mcg each) daily

Available forms: Powder for INH 18 mcg in blister packs containing 6 caps with inhaler; 30 caps with inhaler; spray inhaler (Respimat) 2.5 mcg/spray

Administer:

Inhalation route (caps)
- Caps are for INH only; do not swallow
- Immediately before administration, peel back foil until cap is visible and to "stop" line; remove cap from blister cavity; open dust cap of HandiHaler by pulling upward, then open mouthpiece; place cap in center chamber; firmly close mouthpiece until it clicks, leaving dust cap open
- When finished taking dose, remove used capsule and dispose of it; close mouthpiece and dust cap; store
- Rinse mouth after use

Inhalation route (spray)
- Insert cartridge into inhaler, prime inhaler, must reprime once if not used for >3 days, if not used for >21 days, prime until aerosol is visible, and 3 more times

SIDE EFFECTS
CNS: Depression, paresthesia
CV: Chest pain, increased heart rate

T

EENT: Dry mouth, blurred vision, glaucoma
GI: Vomiting, abdominal pain, constipation, dyspepsia
GU: Urinary difficulty, urinary retention, UTI
INTEG: Rash, angioedema
MISC: Candidiasis, flulike syndrome, herpes zoster, infections, angina pectoris
MS: Arthritis myalgic leg/skeletal pain
RESP: *Cough, sinusitis, upper respiratory tract infection,* epistaxis, pharyngitis

PHARMACOKINETICS

Half-life 5-6 days in animals, does not cross blood-brain barrier, very little metabolized in the liver, excreted in urine, 72% protein binding

INTERACTIONS

- Anticholinergics: avoid use with other anticholinergics

Drug/Lab Test
Increase: cholesterol, glucose

NURSING CONSIDERATIONS

Assess:

- **Respiratory status:** dyspnea, rate, breath sounds before and during treatment; pulmonary function tests at baseline and periodically; upper respiratory infections, cough, sinusitis
- Tolerance over long-term therapy; dose may have to be increased or changed
- Patient's ability to use HandiHaler

Evaluate:

- Therapeutic response: ability to breathe easier

Teach patient/family:

- Signs of closed-angle glaucoma (eye pain, blurred vision, visual halos)
- That product is used for long-term maintenance, not for immediate relief of breathing problems; that effect takes 20 min, lasts 24 hr
- To avoid getting the powder in the eyes; may cause blurred vision and pupil dilation
- To hold HandiHaler with mouthpiece upward; to press button in once, completely, and release; this allows for medication to be released
- To breathe out completely; not to breathe into mouthpiece at any time
- To raise device to mouth and close lips tightly around mouthpiece
- With head upright, to breathe in slowly and deeply, but allow the cap to vibrate; to breathe until the lungs fill; to hold breath and remove mouthpiece; to resume normal breathing
- To rinse mouth after use; to use hard candy or regular oral hygiene to reduce dry mouth
- To report immediately blurred vision, eye pain, halos
- To keep caps in sealed blisters before use; to store at room temperature

tipranavir (Rx)

(ti-pran′a-veer)

Aptivus

Func. class.: Antiretroviral
Chem. class.: Protease inhibitor

ACTION:

Inhibits human immunodeficiency virus (HIV) protease, thereby preventing the maturation of the virus

USES:

HIV in combination with other antiretrovirals

CONTRAINDICATIONS:

Hypersensitivity

Black Box Warning: Hepatic disease (Child-Pugh B, C)

Precautions: Pregnancy (C), breastfeeding, children, renal disease, history of renal stones, sulfa allergy, hemophilia, diabetes mellitus, pancreatitis, alcoholism, immune reconstitution syndrome, surgery, trauma, infection

Black Box Warning: Intracranial bleeding, hepatitis

DOSAGE AND ROUTES

Reduce dose with mild to moderate hepatic impairment and ketoconazole coadministration

- **Adult: PO** 500 mg coadministered with ritonavir 200 mg bid with food
- **Adolescent and child ≥2 yr: PO** 14 mg/kg given with ritonavir 6 mg/kg bid or 375 mg/m² given with ritonavir 150 mg/m² bid, max 500 mg with ritonavir 200 mg bid

Available forms: Caps 250 mg; oral sol 100 mg/ml

Administer:

- Not to be used in those who are treatment-naive
- Swallow cap whole; do not break, crush, chew; store caps in refrigerator before use; after opening, store at room temperature; use within 60 days
- After meals
- In equal intervals around the clock to maintain blood levels
- Give oral sol using calibrated dosing syringe or 5-ml oral syringe provided; store oral sol at room temperature; use within 60 days after opening bottle

SIDE EFFECTS

CNS: *Headache, insomnia,* dizziness, somnolence, fatigue, *fever,* **intracranial bleeding**

GI: *Diarrhea, abdominal pain, nausea, vomiting,* anorexia, dry mouth, **hepatitis B or C, fatalities when given with ritonavir, pancreatitis**

GU: Nephrolithiasis

INTEG: *Rash,* urticaria, lipodystrophy, **serious rash**

MS: Pain

OTHER: Asthenia, **insulin-resistant hyperglycemia,** *hyperlipidemia,* **ketoacidosis**

PHARMACOKINETICS

Terminal half-life 6 hr, peak 3 hr, plasma protein binding 99.9%, steady-state 7-10 days, metabolism CYP3A4, 80% fecal excretion

INTERACTIONS

⚠ **Life-threatening dysrhythmias:** amiodarone, astemizole, cisapride, ergots, flecainide, midazolam, pimozide, propafenone, quiNIDine, rifabutin, rifampin, terfenadine, triazolam

Increase: myopathy, rhabdomyolysis—HMG-CoA reductase inhibitors (lovastatin, simvastatin)

Increase: tipranavir levels—ketoconazole, delavirdine, itraconazole

Increase: levels of both products—clarithromycin, zidovudine

Increase: levels of tipranavir—oral contraception

Decrease: tipranavir levels—rifamycins, fluconazole, nevirapine, efavirenz

Drug/Herb

Decrease: tipranavir levels—St. John's wort; avoid concurrent use

Drug/Food

Decrease: tipranavir absorption—grapefruit juice; high-fat, high-protein foods

Drug/Lab Test

Increase: AST/ALT, cholesterol, blood glucose, amylase, lipase, triglycerides

NURSING CONSIDERATIONS

Assess:

- Signs of infection, anemia; presence of other sexually transmitted diseases

Black Box Warning: Hepatic studies: ALT, AST; total bilirubin, amylase; all may be elevated, discontinue in those with hepatic insufficiency or hepatitis or AST/ALT 10 × upper limit or AST/ALT 5-10 × ULN and total bilirubin 2.5 × ULN; assess for anorexia, nausea, jaundice, hepatomegaly, clay-colored stools

- **HIV:** Viral load, CD4, plasma HIV RNA, serum cholesterol profile, serum triglycerides during treatment
- Bowel pattern before, during treatment; if severe abdominal pain with bleeding occurs, product should be discontinued; monitor hydration

T

• **Serious rash:** if serious rash occurs, product should be discontinued
• **Immune reconstitution syndrome:** has been reported with combination antiretroviral therapy, patients may develop pain (MAC, CMV, PcP, TB) and autoimmune disease months after treatment

Black Box Warning: Intracranial bleeding: more common in those with trauma, surgery, or those taking antiplatelets or anticoagulants; assess for headache, nausea, vomiting, seizures, confusion, inability to speak, can be fatal

• Cushingoid symptoms: buffalo hump, facial/peripheral wasting, breast enlargement, central obesity

Evaluate:
• Therapeutic response: improving CD4 counts, viral load

Teach patient/family:
• To take as prescribed; if dose is missed, to take as soon as remembered up to 1 hr before next dose; not to double dose
• That product must be taken in equal intervals around the clock to maintain blood levels for duration of therapy
⚠ That hyperglycemia may occur; to watch for increased thirst, weight loss, hunger, dry, itchy skin; to notify prescriber
• That product does not cure AIDS, only controls symptoms; not to donate blood
• Not to breastfeed
• That redistribution of body fat may occur
• Not to use with other products unless approved by prescriber, many drug interactions
• That product must be taken in combination with ritonavir
• To stop product and notify prescriber if anorexia, nausea, vomiting, yellowing of skin or eyes, clay-colored stools, fatigue, pain in upper abdomen

⚠ HIGH ALERT

tirofiban (Rx)

(tie-roh-fee′ban)

Aggrastat

Func. class.: Antiplatelet
Chem. class.: Glycoprotein IIb/IIIa inhibitor

ACTION: Antagonist of platelet glycoprotein (GP) IIb/IIIa receptor that prevents binding of fibrinogen and von Willebrand's factor, which inhibits platelet aggregation

USES: Acute coronary syndrome in combination with heparin

CONTRAINDICATIONS: Hypersensitivity, active internal bleeding, stroke, major surgery, severe trauma within 30 days, intracranial neoplasm, aneurysm, hemorrhage, acute pericarditis, platelets $<100,000/mm^3$, history of thrombocytopenia, coagulopathy, systolic B/P >180 mm Hg or diastolic B/P > 110 mm Hg

Precautions: Pregnancy (B), breastfeeding, children, geriatric patients, renal disease, bleeding tendencies, hypertension, platelets $<150,000/mm^3$

DOSAGE AND ROUTES

• **Adult: IV** 0.4 mcg/kg/min × 30 min, then 0.1 mcg/kg/min for 12-24 hr after angioplasty or atherectomy

Renal dose

• **Adult: IV** CCr <30 ml/min, 0.2 mcg/kg/min × 30 min, then 0.05 mcg/kg/min during angiography and for 12-24 hr after angioplasty

Available forms: Inj 50 ml vials; inj premixed bag 50 mcg/ml in 100, 250 ml

Administer:

Intermittent IV INFUSION route
• Do not use if particulates are present
• Dilute inj: withdraw and discard 100 ml from 500-ml bag of sterile 0.9% NaCl

or D_5W and replace this vol with 100 ml of tirofiban inj from 2 vials
- Tirofiban inj for sol is premixed in containers of 500 ml 0.9% NaCl (50 mg/ml), infuse over 30 min
- Minimize other arterial/venous punctures; IM inj, catheter use, intubation, to reduce bleeding risk
- Discard unused solution after 24 hr from start of infusion

Y-site compatibilities: Acyclovir, alfentanil, allopurinol, amifostine, amikacin, aminocaproic acid, aminophylline, amiodarone, ampicillin, ampicillin/sulbactam, anidulafungin, argatroban, arsenic trioxide, atracurium, atropine, azithromycin, aztreonam, bivalirudin, bleomycin, bumetanide, buprenorphine, butorphanol, calcium chloride/gluconate, capreomycin, CARBOplatin, carmustine, caspofungin, ceFAZolin, cefepime, cefotaxime, cefoTEtan, cefOXitin, cefTAZidime, ceftizoxime, cefTRIAXone, cefuroxime, chloramphenicol, chlorproMAZINE, cimetidine, ciprofloxacin, cisatracurium, CISplatin, clindamycin, cyclophosphamide, cycloSPORINE, cytarabine, DACTINomycin, DAPTOmycin, dexamethasone, dexmedetomidine, dexrazoxane, digoxin, diltiazem, diphenhydrAMINE, DOBUTamine, DOCEtaxel, dolasetron, DOPamine, doxacurium, DOXOrubicin, DOXOrubicin liposome, doxycycline, droperidol, enalaprilat, ePHEDrine, EPINEPHrine, epirubicin, eptifibatide, ertapenem, erythromycin, esmolol, etoposide, etoposide phosphate, famotidine, fenoldopam, fentaNYL, fluconazole, fludarabine, fluorouracil, foscarnet, fosphenytoin, furosemide, ganciclovir, gemcitabine, gentamicin, glycopyrrolate, granisetron, haloperidol, heparin, hydrALAZINE, hydrocortisone, HYDROmorphone, IDArubicin, ifosfamide, imipenem/cilastatin, insulin, irinotecan, isoproterenol, ketorolac, labetalol, leucovorin, lidocaine, linezolid, LORazepam, magnesium sulfate, mannitol, mechlorethamine, melphalan, meperidine, meropenem, mesna, methylhexital, methotrexate, methyldopate, methylPREDNISolone, metoclopramide, metoprolol, metroNIDAZOLE, midazolam, milrinone, mitoXANtrone, morphine, mycophenolate, nafcillin, nalbuphine, naloxone, nesiritide, niCARdipine, nitroglycerin, nitroprusside, norepinephrine, octreotide, ondansetron, oxaliplatin, oxytocin, PACLitaxel, palonosetron, pamidronate, pancuronium, pantoprazole, PEMEtrexed, PENTobarbital, PHENobarbital, phentolamine, phenylephrine, piperacillin/tazobactam, potassium acetate, potassium chloride/phosphates, procainamide, prochlorperazine, promethazine, propranolol, quinupristin/dalfopristin, ranitidine, remifentanil, rocuronium, sodium acetate/bicarbonate, streptozocin, succinylcholine, SUFentanil, tacrolimus, teniposide, theophylline, thiopental, thiotepa, ticarcillin/clavulanate, tigecycline, tobramycin, topotecan, vancomycin, vasopressin, vecuronium, verapamil, vinBLAStine, vinCRIStine, vinorelbine, voriconazole, zidovudine, zoledronic acid

SIDE EFFECTS

CNS: Dizziness, headache
CV: Bradycardia, hypotension
GI: Nausea, vomiting
HEMA: **Bleeding, thrombocytopenia**
INTEG: *Rash*
MISC: Dissection, edema, pain in legs/pelvis, sweating
SYST: **Anaphylaxis**

PHARMOCOKINETICS

Half-life 2 hr; excretion via urine, feces; plasma clearance 20%-25% lower in geriatric patients with CAD; renal insufficiency decreases plasma clearance

INTERACTIONS

Increase: bleeding—aspirin, heparin, NSAIDs, abciximab, eptifibatide, clopidogrel, ticlopidine, dipyridamole, cefamandole, cefoTEtan, cefoperazone, valproic acid, heparins, thrombin inhibitors, SSRIs, SNRIs

T

NURSING CONSIDERATIONS

Assess:

⚠ **Bleeding:** platelet counts, Hct, Hgb before treatment, within 6 hr of loading dose, and at least daily thereafter; watch for bleeding from puncture sites, catheters, or in stools, urine; discontinue if platelets <100,000/mm^3

Evaluate:

- Therapeutic response: treatment of acute coronary syndrome

Teach patient/family:

- That it is necessary to quit smoking to prevent excessive vasoconstriction
- About signs, symptoms of bleeding and low platelets
- That there are many product and herbal interactions, do not use unless approved by prescriber

tiZANidine (Rx)

(ti-za′nih-deen)

Zanaflex

Func. class.: Skeletal muscle relaxant, α_2-adrenergic agonist

Chem. class.: Imidazoline

Do not confuse:
tiZANidine/tiaGABine

ACTION: Increases presynaptic inhibition of motor neurons and reduces spasticity by α_2-adrenergic agonism

USES: Acute/intermittent management of increased muscle tone associated with spasticity, symptoms of MS

Unlabeled uses: Tension headache, low back pain, trigeminal neuralgia

CONTRAINDICATIONS: Hypersensitivity

Precautions: Pregnancy (C), breastfeeding, children, geriatric patients, hypotension, renal/hepatic disease

DOSAGE AND ROUTES

- **Adult: PO** 8 mg q6-8hr, max 36 mg/24 hr

Renal dose

- **Adult: PO** CCr <25 ml/min, start with lower dose

Available forms: Tabs 2, 4 mg; caps 2, 4, 6 mg

Administer

- Consistently either with/without food; food may affect absorption
- Titrate doses carefully
- Avoid use with other CNS depressants

SIDE EFFECTS

CNS: Somnolence, dizziness, speech disorder, dyskinesia, nervousness, hallucination, psychosis

CV: Hypotension, bradycardia

GI: Dry mouth, vomiting, increased ALT, abnormal LFTs, constipation

OTHER: Blurred vision, urinary frequency, pharyngitis, rhinitis, tremors, rash, muscle weakness

PHARMACOKINETICS

Completely absorbed, widely distributed, peak 1-2 hr, duration 3-6 hr, half-life 2.5 hr, protein binding 30%, metabolized by liver; excreted in urine, feces

INTERACTIONS

Increase: CNS depression—alcohol, other CNS depressants

Increase: tiZANidine levels—other CYP1A2 inhibitors (acyclovir, amiodarone, famotidine, mexiletine, enoxacin, norfloxacin, propafenone, tacrine, verapamil, zileuton, oral contraceptives ciprofloxacin), fluvoxaMINE; avoid concurrent use

Increase: hypotension—antihypertensives

Increase: effect of rasagiline

Drug/Herb

Increase: CNS depression—kava, St. John's wort

Drug/Lab Test

Increase: alk phos, AST, ALT, serum glucose

NURSING CONSIDERATIONS

Assess:

- **Muscle spasticity** at baseline and throughout treatment

• **Hypotension:** gradual dosage increase should lessen hypotensive effects; have patient rise slowly from supine to upright; watch those patients receiving antihypertensives for increased effects
• Increased sedation, dizziness, hallucinations, psychosis; product may need to be discontinued
• Vision by ophthalmic exam; corneal opacities may occur
• Hepatic studies: 1, 3, 6 mo during treatment and periodically thereafter

Evaluate:
• Therapeutic response: decreased muscle spasticity

Teach patient/family:
• To rise slowly from lying or sitting to upright position to prevent orthostatic hypotension
• To ask for assistance if dizziness, sedation occur; to avoid drinking alcohol; to avoid operating machinery, driving until effects known
• To discontinue gradually
• To avoid hazardous activities until reaction is known
• Not to use other products unless approved by prescriber

tobramycin (Rx)
(toe-bra-mye′sin)
TOBI, TOBI Podhaler
Func. class.: Antiinfective
Chem. class.: Aminoglycoside

ACTION: Interferes with protein synthesis in bacterial cell by binding to ribosomal subunits, thereby causing inaccurate peptide sequences to form in protein chain causing bacterial death

USES: Severe systemic infections of CNS, respiratory, GI, urinary tract, bone, skin, soft tissues; cystic fibrosis (nebulizer) for *Acinetobacter calcoaceticus, Citrobacter* sp., *Enterobacter aerogenes, Enterobacter* sp., *Enterococcus* sp., *Escherichia coli, Haemophilus aegyptius, Haemophilus influenzae (beta-lactamase negative), Haemophilus influenzae (beta-lactamase positive), Klebsiella pneumoniae, Klebsiella* sp., *Moraxella lacunata, Morganella morganii, Neisseria* sp., *Proteus mirabilis, Proteus vulgaris, Providencia* sp., *Pseudomonas aeruginosa, Serratia* sp., *Staphylococcus aureus (MSSA), Staphylococcus epidermidis, Staphylococcus* sp., *Streptococcus pneumoniae, Streptococcus* sp.; may also be used for the following: *Acinetobacter* sp., *Aeromonas* sp., *Bacillus anthracis, Salmonella* sp., *Shigella* sp.

Unlabeled uses: Endocarditis, febrile neutropenia

CONTRAINDICATIONS: Hypersensitivity to aminoglycosides

Black Box Warning: Pregnancy (D), severe renal disease

Precautions: Breastfeeding, geriatric patients, neonates, mild renal disease, myasthenia gravis, Parkinson's disease

Black Box Warning: Hearing deficits, neuromuscular disease

DOSAGE AND ROUTES
• **Adult: IM/IV** 3 mg/kg/day in divided doses q8hr; may give up to 6 mg/kg/day in divided doses q8-12hr; once-daily dosing (pulse dosing) (unlabeled) **IV** 5-7 mg/kg, dosing intervals determined using nomogram, based on random levels drawn 8-12 hr after 1st dose
• **Child: IM/IV** 6-7.5 mg/kg/day in 3-4 equal divided doses
• **Child ≥6 yr: NEB** 300 mg bid in repeating cycles of 28 days on/28 days off of product; give **INH** over 10-15 min using a handheld PARI LC PLUS reusable nebulizer with DeVilbiss Pulmo-Aid compressor
• **Neonate <1 wk: IM/IV** ≤4 mg/kg/day divided q12hr

T

Cystic fibrosis with *Pseudomonas aeruginosa*

• **Adult/adolescent/child ≥6 yr: IV** 2.5-3.3 mg/kg q8hr, **NEB** 300 mg via inhalation bid × 28 days, then 28 days after; **ORAL INH** (TOBI Podhaler) 112 mg bid ×28 day, then 28 days after; may repeat

Renal dose

Conventional dosing:

• Multiply the serum creatinine (mg/100 ml) by 6 to determine the dosing; to decrease the dose, divide the standard dose by the serum creatinine (mg/100 ml) to determine the lower recommended dose

Interval adjustment of extended-interval dosing of 5 or 7 mg/kg (unlabeled):

• Adjust doses based on serum concentrations and organism MIC; CCr 40-59 ml/min: 5 or 7 mg/kg **IV** q36hr; CCr 20-39 ml/min: 5 or 7 mg/kg **IV** q48hr; CCr <20 ml/min: 5 or 7 mg/kg **IV** once, then follow serial levels to determine time of next dose (serum concentration <1 mcg/ml)

Dose adjustment of extended dosing of 5 mg/kg (unlabeled)

• Adjust doses based on serum concentrations and organism MIC: CCr >80 ml/min: no dosage adjustment is needed: CCr 60-79 ml/min: 4 mg/kg **IV** q24hr; CCr 50 ml/min: 3.5 mg/kg **IV** q24hr; CrCl 40 ml/min: 2.5 mg/kg **IV** q24hr; CrCl <30 ml/min: use traditional dosing

Available forms: Inj 10, 40 mg/ml; powder for inj 1.2 g; neb sol 300 mg/5 ml; powder for inh 28 mg

Administer:

• After obtaining specimen for C&S; begin treatment before results

• Product in evenly spaced doses to maintain blood level; separate aminoglycosides and penicillins by ≥1 hr

• Use only on susceptible organisms to prevent development of product-resistant bacteria

IM route

• IM inj in large muscle mass; rotate inj sites, aspirate

• Draw peak 1 hr after dose, trough right before next dose; absorption erratic

Inhalation route: (TOBI Podhaler)

• Use with Podhaler device; do not swallow caps; use device for 7 days, then discard

• Keep caps in blister pack until ready to use; administer other inhaled products or chest physiotherapy before

• While holding base of Podhaler device, unscrew lid, stand upright, unscrew mouthpiece; while holding body, tear blister card in half lengthwise along precut lines, peel back foil, place cap in chamber at top of device, reattach mouthpiece and tighten; with mouthpiece pointed down, press blue button down with thumb, release, exhale completely, place mouth over mouthpiece, close lips, inhale with single breath, hold 5 sec, exhale normally away from device; after a few normal breaths, repeat, unscrew mouthpiece, and remove cap; cap should be empty; repeat process 3 more times (total 4 caps); after use, reattach mouthpiece and wipe with clean, dry cloth

Intermittent IV INFUSION route

• Visually inspect sol; do not use if discolored or particulate is present

• **Vantage vials** are for IV only and only for exactly 60 or 80 mg

• Diluted in 50-100 ml 0.9% NaCl D_5W ($D_{10}W$, Ringer's, LR); infuse over 20-60 min; volume for pediatric patients needs and should be sufficient to allow for 20-60 min infusion

Y-site compatibilities: Acyclovir, aldesleukin, alfentanil, alprostadil, amifostine, aminophylline, amiodarone, amsacrine, anidulafungin, ascorbic acid, atracurium, atropine, aztreonam, bivalirudin, bretylium, bumetanide, buprenorphine, butorphanol, calcium chloride/gluconate, CARBOplatin, caspofungin, chloramphenicol, cimetidine, ciprofloxacin, cisatracurium, CISplatin, clindamycin, cyanocobalamin, cyclophosphamide, cycloSPORINE, cytarabine, DACTINomycin, DAPTOmycin, dexmedetomidine, digoxin, diltiazem, diphenhydrAMINE, DOBUTamine, DOCEtaxel, DOPamine, doripenem, doxacurium, DOXOrubicin hydrochloride, DOXOrubicin liposome, doxycycline, enalaprilat, ePHEDrine, EPINEPHrine, epirubicin, epoetin alfa, ertapenem, esmolol, etoposide, etoposide phosphate, famotidine, fenoldopam, fentaNYL, filgrastim, fluconazole, fludarabine, fluorouracil, foscarnet, furosemide, gemcitabine, gentamicin, glycopyrrolate, granisetron, HYDROmorphone, ifosfamide, imipenem/cilastatin, isoproterenol, ketorolac, labetalol, levofloxacin, lidocaine, linezolid, LORazepam, magnesium sulfate, mannitol, mechlorethamine, melphalan, meperidine, metaraminol, methicillin, methotrexate, methoxamine, methyldopate, methylPREDNISolone, metoclopramide, metoprolol, metroNIDAZOLE, miconazole, midazolam, milrinone, minocycline, mitoXANtrone, morphine, moxalactam, multiple vitamins, nafcillin, nalbuphine, naloxone, niCARdipine, nitroglycerin, nitroprusside, norepinephrine, octreotide, ondansetron, oxaliplatin, oxytocin, PACLitaxel, palonosetron, pantoprazole, papaverine, penicillin G, pentazocine, perphenazine, PHENobarbital, phentolamine, phenylephrine, phytonadione, potassium chloride, procainamide, prochlorperazine, promethazine, propranolol, protamine, pyridoxime, quinupristin/dalfopristin, ranitidine, remifentanil, riTUXimab, rocuronium, sodium acetate/bicarbonate, succinylcholine, SUFentanil, tacrolimus, teniposide, theophylline, thiamine, thiotepa, ticarcillin/clavulanate, tigecycline, tirofiban, tolazoline, trastuzumab, trimethaphan, urokinase, vancomycin, vasopressin, vecuronium, verapamil, vinCRIStine, vinorelbine, voriconazole, zidovudine

SIDE EFFECTS

CNS: Confusion, depression, numbness, tremors, **seizures**, muscle twitching, **neurotoxicity**, dizziness, vertigo

CV: Hypo/hypertension, palpitation

EENT: **Ototoxicity**, deafness, visual disturbances, tinnitus

GI: *Nausea, vomiting, anorexia;* increased ALT, AST, bilirubin, hepatomegaly, **hepatic necrosis**, splenomegaly

GU: **Oliguria, hematuria, renal damage, azotemia, renal failure, nephrotoxicity**

HEMA: **Agranulocytosis, thrombocytopenia, leukopenia, eosinophilia**, anemia

INTEG: *Rash,* burning, urticaria, dermatitis, alopecia

PHARMACOKINETICS

Plasma half-life 2-3 hr, prolonged in neonates; not metabolized; excreted unchanged in urine; crosses placental barrier; poor penetration into CSF

IM: Onset rapid, peak 1 hr, duration 8 hr

IV: Onset immediate, peak 30 min, duration 8 hr

INTERACTIONS

Black Box Warning: Increase: ototoxicity, neurotoxicity, nephrotoxicity—other aminoglycosides, amphotericin B, polymyxin, vancomycin, ethacrynic acid, furosemide, mannitol, methoxyflurane, CISplatin, cephalosporins, bacitracin, acyclovir, penicillins, cidofovir

Drug/Lab Test

Increase: eosinophils, BUN, creatinine, AST, ALT, LDH, alk phos, glucose

Decrease: potassium, calcium, sodium, magnesium, WBC, granulocytes, platelets

NURSING CONSIDERATIONS

Assess:

- Weight before treatment; dosage is usually based on ideal body weight but may be calculated on actual body weight
- I&O ratio, urinalysis daily for proteinuria, cells, casts; report sudden change in urine output
- VS during infusion; watch for hypotension, change in pulse
- IV site for thrombophlebitis, including pain, redness, swelling q30min; change site if needed; apply warm compresses to discontinued site

T

Black Box Warning: Serum aminoglycoside concentration; serum peak drawn at 30-60 min after IV infusion or 60 min after IM inj, trough drawn just before next dose, peak 4-10 mcg/ml, trough 0.5-2 mcg/ml, increased level may lead to serious toxicity

Black Box Warning: Renal impairment: CCr, BUN, serum creatinine; lower dosage should be given in renal impairment (CCr <80 ml/min); monitor electrolytes: potassium, sodium, chloride, magnesium monthly if patient receiving long-term therapy

Black Box Warning: Pregnancy: identify if pregnancy is planned or suspected, pregnancy (D)

Black Box Warning: Deafness by audiometric testing; ringing, roaring in ears; vertigo; assess hearing before, during, after treatment

- **Overgrowth of infection:** fever, malaise, redness, pain, swelling, perineal itching, diarrhea, stomatitis, change in cough, sputum
- **Vestibular dysfunction:** nausea, vomiting, dizziness, headache; product should be discontinued if severe
- Adequate fluids of 2-3 L/day unless contraindicated to prevent irritation of tubules
- Supervised ambulation, other safety measures with vestibular dysfunction

Evaluate:
- Therapeutic response: absence of fever, draining wounds, negative C&S after treatment

Teach patient/family:
- To promptly report headache, dizziness, symptoms of overgrowth of infection, renal impairment

Black Box Warning: To report loss of hearing; ringing, roaring in ears; feeling of fullness in head

Black Box Warning: To notify prescriber if pregnancy is planned or suspected; pregnancy (D)

- To avoid hazardous activities until response is known

Nebulizer
- To use other therapies first, then tobramycin, not to use if cloudy or contains particulates

TREATMENT OF OVERDOSE:
Hemodialysis; monitor serum levels of product

tobramycin ophthalmic
See Appendix B

tocilizumab (Rx)
(toe′si-liz′oo-mab)

Actemra

Func. class.: DMARDs (disease-modifying antirheumatoid drugs)/ tumor necrosis factor (TNF) modifier

ACTION: Interleukin-6 (IL-6) receptor inhibiting monoclonal antibody

USES: Rheumatoid arthritis, active systemic juvenile idiopathic arthritis

CONTRAINDICATIONS: Hypersensitivity

Precautions: Breastfeeding, pregnancy (C); risk for GI perforation, active hepatic disease, severe neutropenia/ thrombocytopenia, demyelinating disorders

Black Box Warning: Invasive fungal infection, active TB

DOSAGE AND ROUTES
Monotherapy with or without methotrexate or other DMARDs, moderate-severe rheumatoid arthritis
- **Adult: IV** 4 mg/kg over 1 hr q4wk, may increase to 8 mg/kg q4wk based on clinical response, max dose 800 mg/infusion; do not initiate if ANC >2000, platelets <100,000
- **Adults <100 kg: SUBCUT** 162 mg every other wk (monotherapy or in

combination); increase to 162 mg weekly based on response

- **Adults ≥100 kg:** **SUBCUT** 162 mg weekly (monotherapy or in combination)

Juvenile idiopathic arthritis

- **Child ≥2 yr/adolescent ≥30 kg:** **IV** 8 mg/kg over 1 hr q2wk
- **Child ≥2 yr/adolescent <30 kg:** **IV** 10 mg/kg over 1 hr

Available forms: Sol for inj 80 mg/4 ml, 200 mg/10 ml, 400 mg/20 ml

Administer:

Intermittent IV INFUSION route

- Visually inspect for particulate matter, discoloration before administration whenever sol and container permit; colorless to pale yellow liquid
- From 100-ml infusion bag or bottle, withdraw vol of 0.9% sodium chloride inj equal to vol of tocilizumab sol required for patient's dose
- Slowly add tocilizumab from each vial into infusion bag or bottle; gently invert bag to avoid foaming; fully diluted sols are compatible with polypropylene, polyethylene, polyvinyl chloride infusion bags and polypropylene, polyethylene, glass infusion bottles
- Fully diluted sol for infusion may be stored refrigerated or at room temperature for ≤24 hr and should be protected from light; do not use unused product remaining in vials; no preservatives
- Allow the fully diluted sol to reach room temperature before infusion
- Give over 60 minutes with infusion set; do not administer as IV push or bolus
- Do not infuse concomitantly in same IV line with other drugs

SIDE EFFECTS

CNS: Headache, dizziness

CV: Hypertension

GI: **Perforation**, abdominal pain, gastritis, mouth ulcerations

HEMA: **Neutropenia, thrombocytopenia**

INTEG: Rash, infusion reactions

RESP: Upper respiratory infections, nasopharyngitis, bronchitis

SYST: **Serious infections, anaphylaxis,** infusion-related reactions, antitocilizumab antibody formation, **secondary malignancy**

INTERACTIONS

Decrease: product level—cycloSPORINE, theophylline warfarin

Decreased: level of CYP3A4 substrates (hormonal contraceptives, omeprazole, atorvastatin, simvastatin)

- **Do not give with live virus vaccines**
- **Avoid use with TNF modifiers, DMARDs, immunosuppressives due to increased risk of infection**

PHARMACOKINETICS

Half-life approx 6 days with single dose, approx 11 days with multiple (steady-state) doses

NURSING CONSIDERATIONS

Assess:

- **Rheumatoid arthritis:** ROM, pain, stiffness at baseline q1-2wk
- Blood studies: CBC with differential, LFTs, platelet count, serum lipid profile at baseline and periodically

Black Box Warning: Infection before treatment and periodically; obtain TB screening before beginning treatment, invasive fungal infections; discontinue if infection occurs during administration; may use antituberculosis therapy before tocilizumab in past history of latent or active TB when adequate course of treatment cannot be confirmed and those with a negative TB with risk factors for infections

- **Secondary malignancy:** assess for malignancy periodically

Evaluate:

- Therapeutic response: ability to move more easily with less pain

Teach patient/family:

- That this treatment must continue unless safety or effectiveness is an issue
- About reason for use and expected results

• To avoid live vaccines, bring immunizations up to date before treatment

Black Box Warning: To report signs, symptoms of infection, including TB and hepatitis B, to avoid others with infections

• To notify prescriber if pregnancy or suspected pregnancy (C); not to use if breastfeeding, consider using a nonhormonal contraceptive because contraception may be decreased

tofacitinib

(toe′fa-sye′ti-nib)

Xeljanz

Func. class.: Antirheumatic agent (disease modifying), immunomodulator/biologic DMARD

Chem. class.: Janus kinase inhibitor

ACTION: Affects the signaling pathway of Janus kinase

USES: Rheumatoid arthritis (moderately to severely active) in those who have taken methotrexate with inadequate response or intolerance

CONTRAINDICATIONS: Hypersensitivity

Precautions: Pregnancy (C), breastfeeding, neonates, infants, children, geriatric patients, neoplastic disease, ulcerative colitis, neutropenia, peptic ulcer disease, active infections, risk of lymphomas/leukemias, TB, posttransplant lymphoproliferative disorder (PTLD), kidney disease, diabetes mellitus, HIV, hypercholesterolemia, herpes virus infection reactivation, Asian patients

Black Box Warning: Infection, secondary malignancy

DOSAGE AND ROUTES

• **Adult: PO** 5 mg bid if receiving potent CYP3A4 inhibitor, then 5 mg/day if receiving moderate CYP3A4 inhibitor and 2C19 inhibitors

Available forms: Tabs 5 mg

Administer:

PO route

• Without regard to food

SIDE EFFECTS

CNS: Headache, paresthesias, insomnia, fatigue

CV: Hypertension

GI: Abdominal pain, nausea, liver damage, dyspepsia, vomiting, diarrhea, gastritis, GI perforation, steatosis

HEMA: Anemia, lymphocytosis, lymphopenia, neutropenia

INTEG: Rash, pruritus

MISC: Increased cancer risk, risk of infection (TB, invasive fungal infections, other opportunistic infections), may be fatal, posttransplant lymphoproliferative disorder (PTLD)

PHARMACOKINETICS

Bioavailability 70%, protein binding 40% (albumin), metabolism mediated by CYP3A4, half-life 3 hr, peak 0.5-1 hr

INTERACTIONS

Black Box Warning: Do not use with TNF modifiers, vaccines, potent immunosuppressants, other biologic DMARDS

Increase: tofacinib effect—CYP3A4 inhibitors (amprenavir, boceprevir, delavirdine, ketoconazole, indinavir, itraconazole, dalfopristin/quinupristin, ritonavir, tipranavir, fluconazole, isoniazid, miconazole)

Decrease: tofacinib effect—CYP3A4 inducers (rifampin, rifapentine, rifabutin, primidone, phenytoin, PHENobarbital, nevirapine, nafcillin, modafinil, griseofulvin, etravirine, efavirenz, barbiturates, bexarotene, bosentan, carBAMazepine, enzalutamide, dexamethasone)

Drug/Lab Test

Increase: LFTs, cholesterol

Decrease: neutrophils, lymphocytes, Hct, Hgb

NURSING CONSIDERATIONS

Assess:

- Monitor lipid profile, Hct/Hgb WBC, LFTs
- **RA:** Pain, stiffness, ROM, swelling of joints before, during treatment

Black Box Warning: Active infection, including localized infection: evaluate and test patients for latent or active TB before use; treat with antimycobacterials before use of product; this product increases the risk of serious including fatal infections (pulmonary or extrapulmonary TB; invasive fungal infections; and bacterial, viral, and opportunistic infections); during and after use, monitor for infection including TB in those who tested negative for latent TB before use; if a serious infection develops, interrupt receipt until the infection is controlled, reactivation of viral infections is higher in Asian patients

Black Box Warning: Secondary malignancy: lymphoma and other malignancies have been noted with product use

⚠ **Epstein–Barr virus–associated post-transplant lymphoproliferative disorder (PTLD):** in kidney transplant patients when used with this product and immunosupressives

- **Liver disease:** not recommended in severe liver disease, impairment; dose modification is needed with moderate liver impairment, monitor LFTs

⚠ **GI perforation:** assess in those with diverticulitis, peptic ulcer disease, or ulcerative colitis

Black Box Warning: Immunosuppression: obtain neutrophil and lymphocyte counts before use; do not start the product in lymphocyte count <500 cells/mm^3 or ANC <1000 cells/mm^3; for ANC >1000 cells/mm^3, monitor neutrophil counts after 4-8 wk and every 3 mo thereafter; lymphocyte count >500 cells/mm^3, monitor lymphocyte counts every 3 mo

⚠ **Anemia:** determine Hgb, do not start in Hgb <9 g/dl; in Hgb ≥ 9 g/dl, monitor Hgb after 4-8 wk and every 3 mo thereafter

⚠ **Pregnancy (C)/breastfeeding:** use during pregnancy only if the potential benefit justifies the potential risk to the fetus; if pregnancy occurs, enrollment in the pregnancy registry is encouraged by calling 1-877-311-8972; discontinue product or breastfeeding; serious adverse reactions can occur in nursing infants

Black Box Warning: Neoplastic disease (lymphomas/leukemias)

Evaluate:

- Therapeutic response: decreased inflammation, pain in joints, decreased joint destruction

Teach patient/family:

- Not to have vaccines while taking this product
- Not to take any live virus vaccines during treatment
- To report signs of infection, allergic reaction

⚠ **Pregnancy (C):** teach patient to report if pregnancy is planned or suspected; do not breastfeed

tolcapone (Rx)

(toll′cah′pone)

Tasmar

Func. class.: Antiparkinson agent

Chem. class.: COMT inhibitor

ACTION: Inhibits COMT; used as adjunct to levodopa/carbidopa therapy

USES: Parkinson's disease

CONTRAINDICATIONS: Hypersensitivity, rhabdomyolysis

Black Box Warning: Hepatic disease

Precautions: Pregnancy (C), breastfeeding, cardiac/renal disease, hypertension, asthma, history of rhabdomyolysis

DOSAGE AND ROUTES

- **Adult: PO** 100-200 mg tid with levodopa/carbidopa therapy; max 600 mg/day, discontinue if no benefit after 3 wk

Available forms: Tabs 100, 200 mg

Administer:

- Only to be used if levodopa/carbidopa does not provide satisfactory results
- Give without regard to food

SIDE EFFECTS

CNS: Dystonia, dyskinesia, dreaming, *fatigue, headache, confusion,* psychosis, hallucination, dizziness, sleep disorders

CV: *Orthostatic hypotension,* chest pain, hypotension

EENT: Cataract, eye inflammation

GI: *Nausea, vomiting, anorexia, abdominal distress,* diarrhea, constipation, fatal hepatic failure, increased LFTs

GU: UTI, urine discoloration, uterine tumor, micturition disorder, hematuria

HEMA: Hemolytic anemia, leukopenia, agranulocytosis

INTEG: Sweating, alopecia

MS: Rhabdomyolysis

PHARMACOKINETICS

Rapidly absorbed, peak 2 hr, protein binding 99%, extensively metabolized, half-life 2-3 hr, excreted in urine (60%)/feces (40%)

INTERACTIONS

Increase: CNS depression—CNS depressants

- May influence pharmacokinetics of α-methyldopa, DOBUTamine, apomorphine, isoproterenol
- Inhibition of normal catecholamine metabolism: MAOIs, MAO-B inhibitor may be used

NURSING CONSIDERATIONS

Assess:

Black Box Warning: **Hepatic disease:** AST, ALT, alk phos, LDH, bilirubin, CBC; monitor ALT, AST q2wk × 1 yr, then q4wk × 6 mo, then q8wk thereafter; if LFTs elevated, product should not be used, if no improvement in 3 wk, discontinue

- Involuntary movements of parkinsonism: akinesia, tremors, staggering gait, muscle rigidity, drooling
- B/P, respiration during initial treatment; hypo/hypertension should be reported
- Mental status: affect, mood, behavioral changes, avoid use in those with dystonia

Evaluate:

- Therapeutic response: decrease in akathisia, increased mood

Teach patient/family:

- To change positions slowly to prevent orthostatic hypotension
- That urine, sweat may change color
- That food taken within 1 hr before meals or 2 hr after meals decreases action of product by 20%; may be taken without regard to food
- To notify prescriber if pregnancy is planned or suspected, pregnancy (C)
- That CNS changes may occur, hallucinations, involuntary movement
- To avoid hazardous activities until reaction is known; dizziness may occur
- That nausea and diarrhea are common

Black Box Warning: **To report signs of hepatic injury:** clay-colored stools, jaundice, fatigue, appetite loss, lethargy, fatigue, itching, right upper abdominal pain

- To report nausea, vomiting, anorexia; that nausea may occur at beginning of treatment

tolnaftate topical

See Appendix B

tolterodine (Rx)

(toll-tehr′oh-deen)

Detrol, Detrol LA

Func. class.: Overactive bladder product

Chem. class.: Muscarinic receptor antagonist

ACTION: Relaxes smooth muscles in urinary tract by inhibiting acetylcholine at postganglionic sites

USES: Overactive bladder (urinary frequency, urgency), urinary incontinence

CONTRAINDICATIONS: Hypersensitivity, uncontrolled closed-angle glaucoma, urinary retention, gastric retention

Precautions: Pregnancy (C), breastfeeding, children, renal/hepatic disease, controlled closed-angle glaucoma, bladder obstruction, QT prolongation, decreased GI motility

DOSAGE AND ROUTES

• **Adult and geriatric: PO** 2 mg bid; may decrease to 1 mg bid; **EXT REL** 4 mg/day, may decrease to 2 mg/day if needed, max 4 mg/day

Hepatic/renal dose

• **Adult: PO** 1 mg bid (50% dose) or **EXT REL** 2 mg/day; CCr ≤30 ml/min, reduce by 50%

Available forms: Tabs 1, 2 mg; ext rel caps 2, 4 mg

Administer:

• Whole; take with liquids; do not crush, chew, or break ext rel product; without regard to meals

SIDE EFFECTS

CNS: Anxiety, paresthesia, fatigue, *dizziness, headache;* increasing dementia, memory impairment

CV: Chest pain, hypertension, QT prolongation

EENT: Vision abnormalities, xerophthalmia

GI: *Nausea, vomiting, anorexia,* abdominal pain, constipation, dry mouth, dyspepsia

GU: Dysuria, urinary retention, frequency, UTI

INTEG: Rash, pruritus

RESP: Bronchitis, cough, pharyngitis, upper respiratory tract infection

SYST: Angioedema, Stevens-Johnson syndrome

PHARMACOKINETICS

Rapidly absorbed; highly protein bound; extensively metabolized by CYP2D6; a portion of the population may be poor metabolizers; excreted in urine, feces

INTERACTIONS

• Do not use in those with known hypersensitivity-festerodine

⚠ **Increase:** QT prolongation—class IA/III antidysrhythmics, some phenothiazines, β-agonists, local anesthetics, tricyclics, haloperidol, methadone, chloroquine, clarithromycin, droperidol, erythromycin, pentamidine

Increase: action of tolterodine—antiretroviral protease inhibitors, macrolide antiinfectives, azole antifungals

Increase: anticholinergic effect—antimuscarinics

Increase: urinary frequency—diuretics

Drug/Food

• Food increases bioavailability of tolterodine

Drug/Lab

Increase: LFTs, bilirubin

NURSING CONSIDERATIONS

Assess:

• **Urinary patterns:** distention, nocturia, frequency, urgency, incontinence

⚠ **Serious skin disorders:** angioedema, Stevens-Johnson syndrome; allergic reactions: rash; if this occurs, product should be discontinued

⚠ **QT prolongation:** ECG, ejection fraction; assess for chest pain, palpitations, dyspnea

Black Box Warning: Fatal hepatic injury: increased LFTs, bilirubin during first 18 mo of therapy in those with autosomal dominant polycystic kidney disease; assess for fatigue, anorexia, right upper abdominal pain, dark urine, jaundice; if these occur, discontinue product and do not restart if cause is liver injury

Evaluate:
- Decreasing dysuria, frequency, nocturia, incontinence

Teach patient/family:
- To avoid hazardous activities; dizziness may occur
- Not to drink liquids before bedtime, to swallow ext rel product whole
- About the importance of bladder maintenance
- Not to breastfeed
- To report signs of infection, skin effects, shortness of breath, urinary retention

tolvaptan (Rx)

(tole-vap′tan)

Samsca

Func. class.: Antihypertensive

Chem. class.: Vasopressin receptor antagonist, V2

ACTION: Arginine vasopressin (AVP) antagonist with affinity for V2 receptors; level of circulating AVP in circulating blood is critical for the regulation of water and the electrolyte balance, and it is usually elevated with euvolemic/hypervolemic hyponatremia

USES: Hypervolemic/euvolemic hyponatremia with heart failure, cirrhosis, SIADH

CONTRAINDICATIONS: Hypersensitivity, hypovolemia, anuria

Precautions: Pregnancy (C), breastfeeding, children, dehydration, geriatric, hyperkalemia, autosomal dominant PKD

Black Box Warning: Alcoholism, malnutrition, hepatic disease

DOSAGE AND ROUTES

- **Adult: PO** 15 mg daily; after 24 hr, may increase to 30 mg daily; max 60 mg/day for ≤30 days

Available forms: Tabs 15, 30 mg

Administer:
- PO with/without food
- Avoid fluid restriction for first 24 hr
- Initiate in hospital setting

SIDE EFFECTS

CNS: Fever, dizziness
CV: Ventricular fibrillation, DIC, stroke, thrombosis
GI: *Nausea,* vomiting, *constipation,* colitis, hepatic injury
GU: Polyuria
HEMA: Bleeding
META: *Dehydration, hyperglycemia,* hyperkalemia, hypernatremia
MS: Rhabdomyolysis
RESP: Respiratory depression, pulmonary embolism

PHARMACOKINETICS

Peak 2-4 hr, protein binding 99%, metabolized by CYP3A4, terminal half-life 12 hr

INTERACTIONS

Increase: concentrations of tolvaptan—CYP3A4 inhibitors (efavirenz, fosamprenavir, quiNINE); P-gp inhibitors (cycloSPORINE, azithromycin, mefloquine, palperidone, propafenone, quiNIDine, testosterone)

Decrease: concentration of tolvaptan—CYP3A4 inducers (carBAMazepine, dexamethasone, etravirine, flutamide, griseofulvin, metyrapsone, modafinil, nafacillin, nevirapine, OXcarbazepine, phenytoin, rifampin, rifabutin, rifapendine, topiramate)

Drug/Herb

Decreased: tolvaptan effect: CYP3A4 inducer (St. John's wort)

Drug/Food

- Grapefruit juice: do not use together

NURSING CONSIDERATIONS

Assess:

- Renal, hepatic function

Black Box Warning: Malnutrition, alcoholism, frequent sodium vol status; overly rapid correction of sodium concentration (12 mEq/L per 24 hr), may result in osmotic demyelination syndrome, may occur in alcoholism, severe malnutrition, advanced liver disease, syndrome of inappropriate antidiuretic hormone, correct sodium levels slowly

- CV status: ventricular fibrillation, hypertension; monitor B/P, pulse
- Monitor electrolytes (sodium, potassium)

Evaluate:

- Therapeutic response: correction of serum sodium levels

Teach patient/family:

- To avoid pregnancy, breastfeeding while taking this product
- About administration procedure and expected results
- To report difficulty swallowing, speaking, seizures, dizziness, drowsiness; embolism may be the cause
- To drink fluid in response to thirst
- Not to use grapefruit juice
- To notify prescriber before using other products

topiramate (Rx)

(toh-pire′ah-mate)

Qudexy XR, Topamax, Topamax Sprinkle, Topiragen, Trokendi XR

Func. class.: Anticonvulsant—miscellaneous

Chem. class.: Monosaccharide derivative

ACTION: May prevent seizure spread as opposed to an elevation of seizure threshold, increases GABA activity

USES: Partial seizures in adults and children 2-16 yr old; tonic-clonic seizures; seizures with Lennox-Gastaut syndrome; migraine prophylaxis

Unlabeled uses: Infantile spasms, bipolar disorder, alcohol dependence, absence seizures, neuropathic pain, cluster headaches, mania, bulimia nervosa

CONTRAINDICATIONS: Hypersensitivity, metabolic acidosis, pregnancy (D)

Precautions: Breastfeeding, children, renal/hepatic disease, acute myopia, secondary closed-angle glaucoma, behavioral disorders, COPD, dialysis, encephalopathy, status asthmaticus, status epilepticus, surgery, paresthesias, maculopathy, nephrolithiasis

DOSAGE AND ROUTES

Adjunctive therapy for seizures

- **Adult/adolescent/child ≥10 yr: PO** 25-50 mg/day initially, titrate by 25-50 mg/wk, up to 200-400 mg/day in 2 divided doses
- **Adult/adolescent/child ≥10 yr: PO** (Qudexy XR, Trokendi XR) 50 mg daily, increase by 50 mg weekly during wk 2, 3, 4, increase by 100 mg weekly, wk 5, 6, final dose 400 mg daily
- **Child 2-9 yr: PO** week 1: 25 mg in PM, then 25 mg bid if tolerated (week 2), then increase by 25-50 mg/day each week as tolerated over 5- to 7-wk titration period, maintenance given in 2 divided doses; <11 kg, minimum 150 mg/day, max 250 mg/day; 12-22 kg, minimum 200 mg/day, max 300 mg/day; 23-31 kg, minimum 200 mg/day, max 350 mg/day; 32-38 kg, minimum 250 mg/day, max 350 mg/day; >38 kg, minimum 250 mg/day, max 400 mg/day; Qudexy XR 25 mg daily at night, may increase to 50 mg wk 2, if tolerated, increase by 25-50 mg each wk over 5- to 7-wk titration period, max dose based on weight
- **Child ≤11 kg: PO** Qudexy XR minimum 150 mg daily, max 250 mg daily
- **Child 12-22 kg:** minimum 200 mg daily, max 300 mg daily

T

- **Child 23-31 kg:** minimum 200 mg daily, max 350 mg daily
- **Child 32-38 kg:** minimum 250 mg daily, max 350 mg daily
- **Child >38 kg:** minimum 250 mg daily, max 400 mg daily

Migraine prophylaxis

- **Adult: PO** 25 mg/day initially, increase by 25 mg/day/wk up to 100 mg/day in 2 divided doses

Renal dose

- **Adult: PO** CCr <70 ml/min, give ½ dose

Atonic/atypical absence/myoclonic seizures (unlabeled)

- **Adult/adolescent >16 yr: PO** 50 mg/day, titrate slowly by 50 mg/wk to 100-300 mg tid
- **Child 2-16 yr: PO** 0.5-1 mg/kg, max 25 mg, initially daily × 7 days, then increase by 0.5-1 mg/kg/day weekly up to 3-6 mg/kg/day in divided doses

Refractory infantile spasms (unlabeled)

- **Child: PO** 25 mg/day, may increase by 25 mg q2-3days until spasms controlled, max 24 mg/kg/day

Alcoholism (unlabeled)

- **Adult: PO** 25 mg/day, titrated to max 300 mg/day in divided doses

Neuropathic pain (unlabeled)

- **Adult: PO** 12.5-25 mg daily or bid × 4 wk, then double dose q4wk to max 100-200 mg/day in divided doses

Bipolar disorder (unlabeled)

- **Adult: PO** 25 mg/day, then increase by 25-mg increments to 200 mg/day

Available forms: Tabs 25, 50, 100, 200 mg; sprinkle caps 15, 25 mg; ext rel caps 25, 50, 100, 200 mg; ext rel cap (sprinkles 24 hr) 25, 50, 100, 150, 200 mg

Administer:

- Swallow tabs whole; do not break, crush, or chew tabs; very bitter
- May take without regard to meals
- Sprinkle cap can be given whole or opened and sprinkled on soft food; do not chew, drink water after sprinkle
- Store at room temperature away from heat, light

SIDE EFFECTS

CNS: *Dizziness, fatigue*, cognitive disorders, insomnia, *anxiety*, depression, paresthesia, *memory loss, tremors,* motor retardation, suicidal ideation, poor balance, ataxia

CV: Flushing, chest pain

EENT: Diplopia, *vision abnormality*

GI: Diarrhea, *anorexia, nausea, dyspepsia*, abdominal pain, constipation, dry mouth, pancreatitis

GU: Breast pain, dysmenorrhea, menstrual disorder

INTEG: Rash, alopecia

MISC: Weight loss, leukopenia, metabolic acidosis, increased body temperature; unexplained death (epilepsy)

RESP: Upper respiratory tract infection, pharyngitis, sinusitis

PHARMACOKINETICS

Well absorbed, peak 2 hr, terminal half-life 19-25 hr, excreted in urine (55%-97% unchanged), crosses placenta, excreted in breast milk, protein binding (9%-17%), steady-state 4 days

INTERACTIONS

Increase: renal stones—carbonic anhydrase inhibitors

Increase: effect of amitriptyline

Increase: CNS depression—alcohol, CNS depressants

Increase: topiramate levels—metformin, hydrochlorothiazide, lamoTRIgine

Decrease: levels of oral contraceptives, estrogen, digoxin, valproic acid, lithium, risperiDONE

Decrease: topiramate levels—phenytoin, carBAMazepine, valproic acid, probenecid

NURSING CONSIDERATIONS

Assess:

- **Seizures:** location, type, duration, aura
- **Bipolar disorder:** mood, behavior
- Renal studies: urinalysis, BUN, urine creatinine, electrolytes q3mo; symptoms of renal colic
- Hepatic studies: ALT, AST, bilirubin if patient receiving long-term treatment

• CBC during long-term therapy (anemia); serum bicarbonate (metabolic acidosis)
• Migraines: pain location, duration; alleviating factors
⚠ Mental status: mood, sensorium, affect, behavioral changes, **suicidal thoughts/behaviors;** if mental status changes, notify prescriber
• Body weight, evidence of cognitive disorder
• Assistance with ambulation during early part of treatment; dizziness occurs
• Seizure precautions: padded side rails, move objects that may harm patient

Evaluate:
• Therapeutic response: decreased seizure activity

Teach patient/family:
• To carry emergency ID stating patient's name, products taken, condition, prescriber's name, and phone number
• To avoid driving, other activities that require alertness, until response is known
• Not to discontinue medication quickly after long-term use
• To notify prescriber immediately of blurred vision, periorbital pain, vision loss may occur
• To maintain adequate fluid intake
• About administration procedure and expected results
• To use nonhormonal contraceptive; that effect of oral contraceptives is decreased, pregnancy (D)
• To drink plenty of fluids to prevent kidney stones
• May need to increase amount of food consumed; weight loss may occur
• To swallow ext rel product whole

⚠ HIGH ALERT

topotecan (Rx)
(toh-poh-tee′kan)
Hycamtin
Func. class.: Antineoplastic, natural; topoisomerase inhibitor
Chem. class.: Camptothecin analog

ACTION: Antitumor product with topoisomerase-I–inhibitory activity; topoisomerase I relieves torsional strain in DNA by causing single-strand breaks; also causes double-strand DNA damage

USES: Metastatic ovarian cancer after failure of traditional chemotherapy; relapsed small-cell lung cancer; cervical cancer
Unlabeled uses: Non–small-cell lung cancer (NSCLC), rhabdomyosarcoma

CONTRAINDICATIONS: Pregnancy (D), breastfeeding, hypersensitivity, severe bone marrow depression

Black Box Warning: Neutropenia

Precautions: Children, renal disease, gelatin hypersensitivity

DOSAGE AND ROUTES
Metastatic carcinoma of the ovary after failure of first or subsequent chemotherapy; SCLC-sensitive disease after failure of first-line therapy
• **Adult: IV INFUSION** 1.5 mg/m^2 over 30 min daily × 5 days starting on day 1 of 21-day course × 4 courses; may be reduced to 0.25 mg/m^2 for subsequent courses if severe neutropenia occurs; relapsed small-cell lung cancer (SCLC) in those with a prior complete or partial response, ≥45 days from end of first-line treatment; **PO** 2.3 mg/m^2/day on days 1-5 of 21-day course

Renal dose

• **Adult: IV** CCr 20-39 ml/min, 0.75 mg/m^2/day × 5 days starting on day 1 of 21-day course

Available forms: Lyophilized powder for inj 4 mg; caps 0.25, 1 mg

Administer:

• Store caps in refrigerator; IV INFUSION unopened at room temperature; protect both from light

PO route

• Do not break, crush, chew, or open caps; protect from light

• Take without regard to food

Intermittent IV INFUSION route

• Visually inspect for particulate matter and discoloration before use

• Reconstitute each 4-mg vial with 4 ml sterile water for injection; use immediately; no preservative

• Withdraw the appropriate volume of the reconstituted solution; dilute further; dilute in 0.9% NaCl or D_5W before administration

• The reconstituted solution is yellow or yellow-green

• Topotecan injection diluted for infusion is stable at room temperature with normal light for 24 hr

• Infuse over 30 min

SIDE EFFECTS

CNS: Arthralgia, *asthenia, headache,* myalgia, *pain,* weakness

GI: *Abdominal pain, constipation,* diarrhea, obstruction, *nausea,* stomatitis, *vomiting;* increased ALT, AST; anorexia

HEMA: Neutropenia, leukopenia, thrombocytopenia, anemia, sepsis

INTEG: *Total alopecia*

RESP: Dyspnea, cough, interstitial lung disease

PHARMACOKINETICS

Rapidly and completely absorbed, excreted in urine and feces as metabolites, half-life 2.8 hr, 7%-35% bound to plasma proteins

INTERACTIONS

• Avoid use with P-glycoprotein, breast cancer resistance protein inhibitors (amiodarone, clarithromycin, diltiazem, erythromycin, indinavir), quiNIDine, testosterone, verapamil, tamoxifen, itraconazole, mefloquine, RU-486, niCARdipine, vaccines, toxoids

Increase: myelosuppression when used with CISplatin

Increase: bleeding risk—NSAIDs, anticoagulants, thrombolytics, platelet inhibitors

Drug/Food

• Avoid use with grapefruit juice

NURSING CONSIDERATIONS

Assess:

• Hepatic studies: AST, ALT, alk phos, which may be elevated; creatinine, BUN

Black Box Warning: CBC, differential, platelet count weekly; withhold product if WBC is $<3500/mm^3$ or platelet count is $<100,000/mm^3$; notify prescriber of results; product should be discontinued

• Buccal cavity for dryness, sores or ulcerations, white patches, oral pain, bleeding, dysphagia

• **Interstitial lung disease (ILD):** fever, cough, dyspnea, hypoxia, may be fatal

• Increased fluid intake to 2-3 L/day to prevent dehydration unless contraindicated

• Rinsing of mouth tid-qid with water, club soda; brushing of teeth bid-tid with soft brush or cotton-tipped applicator for stomatitis; use unwaxed dental floss

Evaluate:

• Therapeutic response: decreased tumor size, spread of malignancy

Teach patient/family:

• That total alopecia may occur; that hair grows back but is different in color and texture

• To avoid foods with citric acid or hot or rough texture if stomatitis is present; to drink adequate fluids

• To report stomatitis and any bleeding, white spots, ulcerations in mouth; to examine mouth daily; to report symptoms

Black Box Warning: To report signs of anemia: fatigue, headache, faintness, SOB, irritability

- To use effective contraception during treatment and for ≤6 mo after, pregnancy (D); to avoid breastfeeding
- To avoid OTC products without approval of prescriber
- To avoid driving or other activities requiring alertness
- To avoid vaccines, toxoids

RARELY USED

toremifene (Rx)

(tor-em′ih-feen)

Fareston

Func. class.: Antineoplastic

Chem. class.: Antiestrogen hormone

USES: Advanced breast carcinoma not responsive to other therapy in estrogen-receptor–positive patients (usually postmenopausal)

CONTRAINDICATIONS: Pregnancy (D), hypersensitivity, history of thromboembolism

Black Box Warning: QT prolongation

DOSAGE AND ROUTES

- **Adult: PO** 60 mg/day

Available forms: Tabs 60 mg

torsemide (Rx)

(tor′suh-mide)

Demadex

Func. class.: Loop diuretic

Chem. class.: Sulfonamide derivative

ACTION: Acts on loop of Henle by inhibiting absorption of chloride, sodium, water

USES: Treatment of hypertension and edema with CHF, ascites

CONTRAINDICATIONS: Infants, hypersensitivity to sulfonamides, anuria

Precautions: Pregnancy (B), breastfeeding, diabetes mellitus, dehydration, severe renal disease, electrolyte depletion, hypovolemia, syncope, ventricular dysrhythmias

DOSAGE AND ROUTES

CHF

- **Adult: PO/IV** 10-20 mg/day, may increase as needed, max 200 mg/day

Edema in chronic renal failure

- **Adult: PO/IV** 20 mg/day, may increase to 200 mg/day

Hepatic cirrhosis in combination with aldosterone antagonist/potassium-sparing diuretic

- **Adult: PO/IV** 5-10 mg/day, may increase as needed, max 40 mg/day

Hypertension

- **Adult: PO** 5 mg/day, may increase to 10 mg/day

Available forms: Tabs 5, 10, 20, 100 mg; inj 10 mg/ml

Administer:

PO route

- In AM to avoid interference with sleep if using product as diuretic
- With food or milk if nausea occurs; absorption may be decreased slightly

IV route

- Visually inspect for particulate matter and discoloration before use
- Give either slowly as an IV bolus or as a continuous IV infusion
- Ampules are single-use containers; discard any unused portion after opening

IV bolus

- No dilution is necessary if given as a slow IV injection; give over 2 min
- If administered through an IV line, flush the line with 0.9% sodium chloride for injection before and after administration

Continuous IV INFUSION

- If administered through an IV line, flush the line with 0.9% sodium chloride for injection before and after use
- Stable for 24 hr at room temperature

T

SIDE EFFECTS

CNS: *Headache, dizziness,* asthenia, insomnia, nervousness

CV: Orthostatic hypotension, chest pain, ECG changes, circulatory collapse, ventricular tachycardia, edema

EENT: *Loss of hearing,* ear pain, tinnitus, blurred vision

ELECT: *Hypokalemia, hypochloremic alkalosis, hyponatremia,* metabolic alkalosis

ENDO: *Hyperglycemia, hyperuricemia*

GI: *Nausea,* diarrhea, dyspepsia, cramps, constipation

GU: *Polyuria,* renal failure, glycosuria

INTEG: *Rash,* photosensitivity, pruritus

MS: Cramps, stiffness

RESP: Rhinitis, cough increase

PHARMACOKINETICS

PO: Rapidly absorbed; duration 6 hr; breast milk; crosses placenta; half-life 3.5 hr; protein binding 97%-99%, cleared through hepatic metabolism

INTERACTIONS

Increase: toxicity—lithium, nondepolarizing skeletal muscle relaxants, digoxin

Increase: action of antihypertensives, oral anticoagulants, nitrates

Increase: ototoxicity—aminoglycosides, CISplatin, vancomycin

Decrease: antihypertensive effect of torsemide—indomethacin, carBAMazepine, PHENobarbital, phenytoin, rifampin, NSAIDs

Drug/Herb

- Severe photosensitivity: St. John's wort

Drug/Lab Test

Increase: BUN, creatinine, uric acid, blood glucose, cholesterol

Decrease: potassium, magnesium, chloride sodium

NURSING CONSIDERATIONS

Assess:

- Hearing when giving high doses
- Weight, I&O daily to determine fluid loss; effect of product may be decreased if used daily
- B/P lying, standing; postural hypotension may occur
- Electrolytes: potassium, sodium, chlorine; include BUN, blood glucose, CBC, serum creatinine, blood pH, ABGs, uric acid, calcium, magnesium
- Glucose in urine of diabetic patients
- **Metabolic alkalosis:** drowsiness, restlessness
- **Hypokalemia:** postural hypotension, malaise, fatigue, tachycardia, leg cramps, weakness
- Rashes, temperature elevation daily
- Confusion, especially in geriatric patients; take safety precautions if needed

Evaluate:

- Therapeutic response: improvement in edema of feet, legs, sacral area daily if medication is being used with CHF

Teach patient/family:

- To rise slowly from lying, sitting position
- To recognize adverse reactions: muscle cramps, weakness, nausea, dizziness, tinnitus
- To take with food or milk for GI symptoms; to limit alcohol use
- To take early during the day to prevent nocturia
- To use sunscreen, protective clothing to prevent sunburn

TREATMENT OF OVERDOSE:

Lavage if taken orally; monitor electrolytes; administer dextrose in saline; monitor hydration, CV, renal status

traMADol (Rx)

(tram′a-dole)

ConZip, Ultram, Ultram ER, Zytram ✤

Func. class.: Analgesic—miscellaneous

Do not confuse:
traMADol/Toradol

ACTION:

Binds to μ-opioid receptors, inhibits reuptake of norepinephrine, serotonin

USES:
Management of moderate to severe pain, chronic pain

Unlabeled uses: Restless leg syndrome (RLS), postoperative shivering, arthralgia/myalgia, bone/dental/neuropathic pain, headache, osteoarthritis

CONTRAINDICATIONS:
Hypersensitivity, acute intoxication with any CNS depressant, alcohol, asthma, respiratory depression

Precautions: Pregnancy (C), breastfeeding, children, geriatric patients, seizure disorder, renal/hepatic disease, respiratory depression, head trauma, increased intracranial pressure, acute abdominal condition, drug abuse, depression, suicidal ideation

DOSAGE AND ROUTES

Mild to moderate pain

- **Adult: PO** 25 mg daily, titrate by 25 mg ≥3 days to 100 mg/day (25 mg qid), then may increase by 50 mg ≥3 days to 200 mg (50 mg qid), then 50-100 mg q4-6hr, max 400 mg/day, use caution in geriatric patients
- **Geriatric >75 years: PO** <300 mg/day in divided doses

Moderate to severe chronic pain

- **Adult: PO-ER** (Ultram ER) 100 mg daily, titrate upward q5days in 100-mg increments, max 300 mg/day; (Ryzolt) 100 mg, titrate upward q2-3days in 100-mg increments, max 300 mg/day; products are not interchangeable

Renal dose

- **Adult: PO** CCr <30 ml/min, give q12hr, max 200 mg/day; do not use ext rel tab

Hepatic dose

- **Adult (Child-Pugh C): PO** 50 mg q12hr; do not use ext rel tab

Restless leg syndrome (RLS) (unlabeled)

- **Adult: PO** 50-150 mg/day × 15-24 mo

Available forms: Tabs 50 mg; ext rel tab 100, 200, 300 mg

Administer:

- Some ext rel products (Ultram ER) are not interchangeable
- Do not break, crush, or chew ext rel product
- With antiemetic for nausea, vomiting
- When pain is beginning to return; determine dosage interval by patient response
- With or without food; ER: always give with food, or always give on empty stomach
- Store in cool environment; protected from sunlight

SIDE EFFECTS

CNS: Dizziness, CNS stimulation, somnolence, headache, anxiety, confusion, euphoria, **seizures**, hallucinations, sedation, **neuroleptic-malignant-syndrome–like reactions**

CV: Vasodilation, orthostatic hypotension, tachycardia, hypertension, abnormal ECG

EENT: Visual disturbances

GI: Nausea, constipation, vomiting, dry mouth, diarrhea, abdominal pain, anorexia, flatulence, **GI bleeding**

GU: Urinary retention/frequency, menopausal symptoms, dysuria, menstrual disorder

INTEG: Pruritus, rash, urticaria, vesicles, flushing

SYST: **Anaphylaxis, Stevens-Johnson syndrome, toxic epidermal necrolysis,** serotonin syndrome

PHARMACOKINETICS

Rapidly and almost completely absorbed, steady-state 2 days, peak 1.5 hr, duration 6 hr, terminal half-life 7.9-8.8 hr, may cross blood-brain barrier, extensively metabolized, 30% excreted in urine as unchanged product, protein binding 20%

INTERACTIONS

- Inhibition of norepinephrine and serotonin reuptake: MAOIs; use together with caution

Increase: CNS depression—alcohol, sedatives, hypnotics, opiates

⚠ **Increase:** serotonin syndrome—**SSRIs, SNRIs, serotonin-receptor agonists**

Increase: traMADol levels—CYP3A4 inhibitors (aprepitant, antiretroviral protease inhibitors, clarithromycin, danazol, delavirdine, diltiazem, erythromycin, fluconazole, FLUoxetine, fluvoxaMINE, imatinib, ketoconazole, mibefradil, nefazodone, telithromycin, voriconazole)
Decrease: traMADol effects—CYP3A4 inducers (barbiturates, bosentan, carBAMazepine, efavirenz, phenytoins, nevirapine, rifabutin, rifampin)
Decrease: levels of traMADol—carBAMazepine

Drug/Herb
- Avoid use with St. John's wort

Increase: CNS depression—chamomile, hops, kava, skullcap, valerian

Drug/Lab Test
Increase: creatinine, hepatic enzymes
Decrease: Hgb

NURSING CONSIDERATIONS

Assess:
- **Pain:** location, type, character, give before pain becomes extreme
- **Respiratory depression:** withhold if respirations <12/min
- I&O ratio: check for decreasing output; may indicate urinary retention
- Need for product; dependency
- Bowel pattern; for constipation, increase fluids, bulk in diet
- CNS changes: dizziness, drowsiness, hallucinations, euphoria, LOC, pupil reaction
- **Hypersensitivity:** usually after beginning treatment
- Increased side effects in renal/hepatic disease

⚠ **Serotonin syndrome, neuroleptic malignant syndrome:** increased heart rate, shivering, sweating, dilated pupils, tremors, high B/P, hyperthermia, headache, confusion; if these occur, stop product, administer serotonin antagonist if needed
- Assistance with ambulation
- Safety measures: side rails, night-light, call bell within easy reach

Evaluate:
- Therapeutic response: decrease in pain

Teach patient/family:
- To report any symptoms of CNS changes, allergic reactions, serotonin syndrome, seizures
- That drowsiness, dizziness, and confusion may occur; to avoid hazardous activities
- To make position changes slowly because orthostatic hypotension may occur
- To avoid OTC medications, herbs, supplements, CNS depressants, and alcohol unless approved by prescriber
- Not to discontinue abruptly, taper

⚠ HIGH ALERT

trametinib

(tra-me′ti-nib)

MeKinist

Func. class.: Antineoplastic biologic response modifiers
Chem. class.: Signal transduction inhibitors (STIs), tyrosine kinase inhibitor

ACTION: Inhibits MEK-1, MEK-2 tyrosine kinase created in patients with malignant melanoma

USES: Unresectable or metastatic BRAD V600E or BRAF V600K mutated malignant melanoma

CONTRAINDICATIONS: Pregnancy (D), hypersensitivity
Precautions: Breastfeeding, children, diarrhea, geriatric patients, hepatic disease, bone marrow suppression, infection, thrombocytopenia, neutropenia, immunosuppression

DOSAGE AND ROUTES

Unresectable or metastatic malignant melanoma (BRAF V600E or V600K mutations) as a single agent
- **Adult: PO** 2 mg daily; may be used in combination with dacarbazine or PACLitaxel in those with BRAF V600E

Unresectable or metastatic malignant melanoma (BRAF V600E or V600K mutations) in combination with dabrafenib

- **Adult: PO** 2 mg daily with dabrafenib 150 mg q12hr until disease progression, take both at same time

Management of treatment-related toxicity

Cutaneous toxicity:

- *Grade 2 rash:* reduce dose by 0.5 mg (e.g., 2 mg/day to 1.5 mg/day) or discontinue in patients who are receiving trametinib 1 mg/day; in patients with an intolerable grade 2 rash that does not improve within 3 wk of a dosage reduction, withhold trametinib for up to 3 wk; if the rash is improved within 3 wk, resume therapy at a lower dose (reduce the previous dose by 0.5 mg); discontinue in patients who are receiving trametinib 1 mg/day; if the rash does not improve within 3 wk, permanently discontinue
- *Grade 3 or 4 rash:* withhold for up to 3 wk; if the rash is improved within 3 wk, resume at a lower dose (reduce the previous dose by 0.5 mg); discontinue in patients who are receiving trametinib 1 mg/day; if the rash does not improve within 3 wk, permanently discontinue therapy

Cardiac toxicity:

- Asymptomatic cardiac toxicity and an absolute decrease in LVEF of ≥10% from baseline and is below institutional lower limits of normal (LLN) from pretreatment value: withhold for up to 4 wk; if the LVEF is improved within 4 wk, resume at a lower dose (reduce the previous dose by 0.5 mg); discontinue in patients who are receiving 1 mg/day; if the LVEF does not improve to normal within 4 wk, permanently discontinue
- Symptomatic CHF or an absolute decrease in LVEF of >20% from baseline and is below institutional LLN: permanently discontinue

Ocular toxicity:

- *Grade 2 or 3 retinal pigment epithelial detachment (RPED):* withhold for up to 3 wk; if the RPED improves to grade 1 or less within 3 wk, resume at a lower dose (reduce the previous dose by 0.5 mg); discontinue therapy in patients who are receiving 1 mg/day; if the RPED does not improve to at least grade 1 within 3 wk, permanently discontinue
- Retinal vein occlusion: permanently discontinue therapy

Pulmonary toxicity

- Interstitial lung disease/pneumonitis: permanently discontinue

Other toxicity:

- *Grade 3 toxicity:* withhold for up to 3 wk: if the toxicity improves to grade 1 or less within 3 wk, resume at a lower dose (reduce the previous dose by 0.5 mg); discontinue in patients who are receiving 1 mg/day; if the toxicity does not improve to at least grade 1 within 3 wk, permanently discontinue
- *Grade 4 toxicity:* permanently discontinue

Available forms: Tabs 0.5, 2 mg

Administer:

- Give 1 hr before or 2 hr after a meal
- If dose is missed, take within 12 hr of missed dose; if >12 hr have passed, skip dose
- Follow cytotoxic handling procedures

SIDE EFFECTS

CNS: Dizziness

CV: Heart failure, hypertension, cardiomyopathy

EENT: Ocular hemorrhage, retinal detachment, blurred vision

GI: Diarrhea, nausea, vomiting, abdominal pain, stomatitis

GU: Hematuria

INTEG: Rash, pruritus, acne, folliculitis, erythema

MS: Rhabdomyolysis

OTHER: Elevated LFTs, hand-foot syndrome

RESP: Cough, dyspnea, pleural effusion, pneumonitis, edema

PHARMACOKINETICS

Protein binding 97.4%, peak 1.5 hr, excreted in feces

T

INTERACTIONS

- None known

NURSING CONSIDERATIONS

Assess:

- LFTs every mo ×3 mo, then as clinically indicated

Evaluate:

- Therapeutic response: decrease in progression of disease

Teach patient/family:

- To report adverse reactions immediately, bleeding
- About reason for treatment, expected results
- To use effective contraception during treatment and up to 30 days after discontinuing treatment

trandolapril (Rx)

(tran-doe′la-prill)

Mavik

Func. class.: Antihypertensive

Chem. class.: Angiotension-converting enzyme inhibitor

ACTION: Selectively suppresses renin-angiotensin-aldosterone system; inhibits ACE; prevents conversion of angiotensin I to angiotensin II, dilates arterial and venous vessels, lowers B/P

USES: Hypertension, heart failure, left ventricular dysfunction post MI

CONTRAINDICATIONS: Breastfeeding, hypersensitivity, history of angioedema

Black Box Warning: Pregnancy (D)

Precautions: Geriatric patients, hyperkalemia, hepatic disease, bilateral renal stenosis, after kidney transplant, aorta/mitral valve stenosis, cirrhosis, severe renal disease, untreated CHF, autoimmune disease, cough, pregnancy (C) 1st trimester, African descent

DOSAGE AND ROUTES

Hypertension

- **Adult: PO** 1 mg/day; 2 mg/day in African Americans; make dosage adjustment ≥1 wk; max 8 mg/day

Heart failure, left ventricular dysfunction post MI

- **Adult: PO** 1 mg/day, titrate upward to 4 mg/day if tolerated, 2-4 yr

Renal/hepatic dose

- **Adult: PO** CCr <30 ml/min or hepatic disease, 0.5 mg/day

Available forms: Tabs 1, 2, 4 mg

Administer:

- Discontinue diuretic 2-3 days before starting this product; if not possible, decrease initial dose to 0.5 mg
- Make dosage changes ≥1 wk
- Give without regard to food
- Space antacids by 2 hr after dose

SIDE EFFECTS

CNS: *Dizziness, syncope,* paresthesias, headache, fatigue, drowsiness, depression, sleep disturbances, anxiety, syncope

CV: *Hypotension,* MI, palpitations, angina, TIAs, stroke, *bradycardia,* dysrhythmias

GI: Nausea, vomiting, cramps, diarrhea, constipation, pancreatitis, *dyspepsia*

GU: Proteinuria, renal failure

HEMA: Agranulocytosis, neutropenia, leukopenia, anemia

INTEG: Rash, purpura, pruritus, angioedema

MISC: Hyperkalemia, hyponatremia, impotence, *myalgia,* angioedema, muscle cramps, *asthenia,* hypocalcemia, gout

RESP: Dyspnea, *cough*

PHARMACOKINETICS

Peak 4-10 hr, duration 24 hr, half-life 6-10 hr, metabolized by liver (active metabolite trandolaprilat), excreted in urine (33%), feces (66%), protein binding 65%-94%

INTERACTIONS

Increase: effects—phenothiazines, diuretics

Increase: severe hypotension—diuretics, other antihypertensives, NSAIDs

Increase: potassium levels—salt substitutes, potassium-sparing diuretics, potassium supplements, ACE inhibitors
Increase: effects of ergots, neuromuscular blocking agents, antihypertensives, hypoglycemics, barbiturates, reserpine, levodopa, lithium
Decrease: effects of trandolapril—antacids, NSAIDs, salicylates
Drug/Lab Test
Increase: potassium, LFTs, BUN, creatinine
Decrease: sodium, WBC

NURSING CONSIDERATIONS
Assess:

Black Box Warning: Pregnancy: Identify if pregnancy is planned or suspected, pregnancy (D)

- **Hepatotoxicity (rare):** increased LFTs, jaundice, fulfillment hepatic necrosis; if jaundice occurs, discontinue product
- **Angioedema** of the face, edema of the extremities, mucous membranes; may need to discontinue
- **Hyperkalemia:** monitor electrolytes, check potassium
- B/P, pulse q4hr; note rate, rhythm, quality
- Baselines of renal, hepatic studies before therapy begins
- Edema in feet, legs daily
- **Symptoms of CHF:** edema, dyspnea, wet crackles

Evaluate:
- Therapeutic response: decreased B/P

Teach patient/family:
- Not to use OTC (cough, cold, or allergy) products unless directed by prescriber, to separate antacids by 2 hr; to avoid salt substitutes
- To comply with dosage schedule even if feeling better
- To notify prescriber of mouth sores, sore throat, fever, swelling of hands/feet, irregular heartbeat, chest pain, signs of angioedema
- That excessive perspiration, dehydration, vomiting, diarrhea may lead to fall in B/P; to consult prescriber if these occur
- That product may cause dizziness, fainting; lightheadedness may occur during 1st few days of therapy
- That product may cause skin rash or impaired perspiration
- Not to discontinue product abruptly, taper
- To rise slowly to sitting or standing position to minimize orthostatic hypotension

Black Box Warning: To notify prescriber if pregnancy is planned or suspected; pregnancy (D)

⚠ HIGH ALERT

trastuzumab (Rx)
(tras-tuz′uh-mab)
Herceptin
Func. class.: Antineoplastic—miscellaneous
Chem. class.: Humanized monoclonal antibody

ACTION: DNA-derived monoclonal antibody selectively binds to extracellular portion of human epidermal growth factor receptor 2; it inhibits the proliferation of cancer cells

USES: Breast cancer; metastatic with overexpression of HER2, early breast cancer (adjuvant, neoadjuvant), gastric cancer; previously untreated HER2 overexpressing metastatic gastric or gastroesophageal junction adenocarcinoma with CISplatin, 5-fluorouracil, or capecitabine

CONTRAINDICATIONS: Pregnancy (D); hypersensitivity to this product, Chinese hamster ovary cell protein
Precautions: Breastfeeding, children, geriatric patients, pulmonary disease, anemia, leukopenia

T

Black Box Warning: Cardiac disease, respiratory distress syndrome, respiratory insufficiency, infusion-related reactions, cardiomyopathy

DOSAGE AND ROUTES

Breast cancer

- Several regimens may be used
- **Adult: IV** 4 mg/kg given over 90 min, then maintenance 2 mg/kg given over 30 min; do not give as IV push or bol; may be given in combination with other antineoplastics

Gastric cancer

- **Adult: IV** 8 mg/kg over 90 min on day 1, then 6 mg/kg over 30-90 min q21days from day 22, give with CISplatin 80 mg/m^2 on day 1 plus 5-fluorouracil 800 mg/m^2 **CONT INFUSION** on days 1-5 or capecitabine 1000 mg/m^2 bid on days 1-14, repeat cycle q3wk

Available forms: Lyophilized powder 440 mg

Administer:

- Acetaminophen as ordered to alleviate fever and headache

Intermittent IV INFUSION route

- After reconstituting vial with 20 ml bacteriostatic water for inj, 1.1% benzyl alcohol preserved (supplied) to yield 21 mg/ml; mark date on vial 28 days from reconstitution date; if patient is allergic to benzyl alcohol, reconstitute with sterile water for inj; use immediately; infuse over 90 min; q3wk give 8 mg/kg loading dose over 90 min; subsequent 6 mg/kg dose may be given over 30-60 min
- Do not mix or dilute with other products or dextrose sol

SIDE EFFECTS

CNS: *Dizziness, numbness, paresthesias,* depression, *insomnia,* neuropathy, peripheral neuritis

CV: Tachycardia, CHF

GI: Nausea, vomiting, *anorexia, diarrhea,* abdominal pain, hepatotoxicity, dysgeusia

HEMA: *Anemia,* leukopenia

INTEG: Rash, acne, herpes simplex

META: Edema, peripheral edema

MISC: *Flulike symptoms; fever, headache, chills*

MS: Arthralgia, *bone pain*

RESP: *Cough, dyspnea, pharyngitis, rhinitis,* sinusitis, pneumonia, pulmonary edema/fibrosis, acute respiratory distress syndrome (ARDS)

SYST: Anaphylaxis, angioedema

PHARMACOKINETICS

Half-life 1-32 days

INTERACTIONS

Increase: bleeding risk—warfarin

Increase: cardiomyopathy—anthracyclines, cyclophosphamide; avoid use

Decrease: immune response—vaccines, toxoids

NURSING CONSIDERATIONS

Assess:

- CBC, HER2 overexpression

Black Box Warning: CHF, other cardiac symptoms: dyspnea, coughing; gallop; obtain full cardiac workup including ECG, echo, multigated acquisition scan

- Symptoms of infection; may be masked by product
- CNS reaction: LOC, mental status, dizziness, confusion
- ⚠ **Hypersensitive reactions, anaphylaxis**

Black Box Warning: **Infusion reactions** that may be fatal: fever, chills, nausea, vomiting, pain, headache, dizziness, hypotension; discontinue product

- **Pulmonary toxicity:** dyspnea, interstitial pneumonitis, pulmonary hypertension, ARDs; can occur after infusion reaction, those with lung disease may have more severe toxicity

Perform/provide:

- Increased fluid intake to 2-3 L/day

Evaluate:

- Therapeutic response: decrease in size of tumors

Teach patient/family:
- To take acetaminophen for fever
- To avoid hazardous tasks because confusion, dizziness may occur
- To report signs of infection: sore throat, fever, diarrhea, vomiting
- That emotional lability is common; to notify prescriber if severe or incapacitating
- To use contraception while taking this product; pregnancy (D); to avoid breastfeeding

Black Box Warning: To report pain at infusion site

travoprost ophthalmic

See Appendix B

traZODone (Rx)

(tray′zoe-done)

Oleptro

Func. class.: Antidepressant—miscellaneous

Chem. class.: Triazolopyridine

Do not confuse:
traZODone/traMADol

ACTION: Selectively inhibits serotonin uptake by brain; potentiates behavorial changes

USES: Depression

Unlabeled uses: Alcoholism, anxiety, panic disorder, insomnia

CONTRAINDICATIONS: Hypersensitivity to tricyclics

Precautions: Pregnancy (C), suicidal patients, severe depression, increased intraocular pressure, closed-angle glaucoma, urinary retention, cardiac/hepatic disease, hyperthyroidism, electroshock therapy, elective surgery, bleeding, abrupt discontinuation, bipolar disorder, breastfeeding, dehydration, hyponatremic, hypovolemia, recovery phase of MI, seizure disorders, prostatic hypertrophy, family history of long QT

Black Box Warning: Suicidal ideation in children/adolescents

DOSAGE AND ROUTES

Depression
- **Adult: PO** 150 mg/day in divided doses, may increase by 50 mg/day q3-4days, max 400 mg/day (outpatient), 600 mg/day (inpatients); **EXT REL** 150 mg in PM, may increase gradually by 75 mg/day q3days, max 375 mg/day
- **Child 6-18 yr (unlabeled): PO** 1.5-2 mg/kg/day in divided doses, may increase q3-4days up to 6 mg/kg/day or 400 mg/day, whichever is less
- **Geriatric: PO** 25-50 mg at bedtime, increase by 25-50 mg q3-7days to desired dose, usually 75-150 mg/day

Alcoholism (unlabeled)
- **Adult: PO** 50-100 mg/day

Panic disorder (unlabeled)
- **Adult: PO** 150 mg in divided doses, may increase by 50 mg/day q3-4days

Insomnia (unlabeled)
- **Adult: PO** 50 mg at bedtime

Available forms: Tabs 50, 100, 150, 300 mg; ext rel tabs 150, 300 mg

Administer:
- Increased fluids, bulk in diet if constipation occurs, especially in geriatric patients
- With food, milk for GI symptoms
- Dosage at bedtime for oversedation during day; may take entire dose at bedtime; geriatric patients may not tolerate daily dosing
- Avoid use of CNS depressants
- Do not crush, break, chew ext rel product
- Store in tight, light-resistant container at room temperature

SIDE EFFECTS

CNS: *Dizziness, drowsiness,* confusion, headache, anxiety, tremors, stimulation,

T

weakness, insomnia, nightmares, EPS (geriatric patients), increase in psychiatric symptoms, suicide in children/adolescents

CV: *Orthostatic hypotension, ECG changes, tachycardia,* hypertension, palpitations

EENT: *Blurred vision,* tinnitus, mydriasis

GI: *Diarrhea, dry mouth,* nausea, vomiting, paralytic ileus, increased appetite, cramps, epigastric distress, jaundice, hepatitis, stomatitis, constipation

GU: *Urinary retention,* acute renal failure, priapism

HEMA: Agranulocytosis, thrombocytopenia, eosinophilia, leukopenia

INTEG: Rash, urticaria, sweating, pruritus, photosensitivity

PHARMACOKINETICS

Peak 1 hr without food, 2 hr with food; metabolized by liver (CYP3A4); excreted by kidneys, in feces; half-life 4.4-7.5 hr

INTERACTIONS

⚠ Hyperpyretic crisis, seizures, hypertensive episode: MAOIs; do not use within 14 days of traZODone

Increase: toxicity, serotonin syndrome—FLUoxetine, nefazodone, other SSRIs, SNRIs, linezolid; methylene blue (IV)

Increase: effects of direct-acting sympathomimetics (EPINEPHrine), alcohol, barbiturates, benzodiazepines, CNS depressants, digoxin, phenytoin, carBAMazepine

Increase: effects of traZODone—CYP3A4, 2D6 inhibitors (phenothiazines, protease inhibitors, azole antifungals)

Increase or decrease: effects of warfarin

Decrease: effects of guanethidine, cloNIDine, indirect-acting sympathomimetics (ePHEDrine)

Drug/Herb

Increase: serotonin syndrome—SAM-e, St. John's wort

Increase: CNS depression—hops, kava, lavender, valerian

Drug/Lab Test

Increase: LFTs

Decrease: Hgb

NURSING CONSIDERATIONS

Assess:

- B/P lying, standing; pulse q4hr; if systolic B/P drops 20 mm Hg, hold product, notify prescriber; take vital signs q4hr in patients with CV disease
- Blood studies: CBC, leukocytes, differential
- Hepatic studies: AST, ALT, bilirubin
- Weight weekly; appetite may increase with product
- ECG for flattening of T wave, bundle branch block, AV block, dysrhythmias in cardiac patients
- EPS, primarily in geriatric patients: rigidity, dystonia, akathisia

Black Box Warning: Mental status changes: mood, sensorium, affect, suicidal tendencies, increase in psychiatric symptoms, depression, panic; observe for suicidal behaviors in children/adolescents, not approved for children

- Urinary retention, constipation; constipation most likely in children
- **Withdrawal symptoms:** headache, nausea, vomiting, muscle pain, weakness; not usual unless product discontinued abruptly
- Alcohol consumption; hold dose until morning

⚠ **Serotonin syndrome, neuroleptic malignant syndrome:** increased heart rate, shivering, sweating, dilated pupils, tremors, high B/P, hyperthermia, headache, confusion; if these occur, stop product, administer serotonin antagonist if needed

- Assistance with ambulation during beginning therapy for drowsiness, dizziness

Evaluate:

- Therapeutic response: decreased depression

Teach patient/family:

- That therapeutic effects may take 2-3 wk; to take product before bedtime; not to crush, chew ext rel product
- To use caution when driving, performing other activities requiring alertness because of drowsiness, dizziness, blurred vision

- To avoid alcohol ingestion
- Not to discontinue medication quickly after long-term use; may cause nausea, headache, malaise
- To report urinary retention, priapism >4 hr immediately
- To wear sunscreen or large hat because photosensitivity occurs

Black Box Warning: That suicidal thoughts/behaviors may occur (adolescents/children)

- To notify prescriber if pregnancy is planned or suspected, pregnancy (C), avoid breastfeeding
- To rise slowly to prevent dizziness

TREATMENT OF OVERDOSE:

ECG monitoring; lavage, activated charcoal; administer anticonvulsant, atropine for bradycardia

treprostinil (Rx)

(treh-prah′stin-ill)

Remodulin, Tyvaso

Func. class.: Antihypertensive, vasodilators

Chem. class.: Tricyclic benzidine prostacyclin analog

ACTION:

Direct vasodilation of pulmonary, systemic arterial vascular beds; inhibition of platelet aggregation

USES:

Pulmonary arterial hypertension (PAH) NYHA class II through IV

Unlabeled uses: Pulmonary arterial hypertension in children/adolescents, pediatric patients transitioning from epoprostenol to treprostinil, claudication

CONTRAINDICATIONS:

Hypersensitivity to this product, other prostacyclin analogs

Precautions: Pregnancy (B), breastfeeding, children, geriatric patients, past renal/hepatic disease, thromboembolic disease, abrupt discontinuation, IV administration

DOSAGE AND ROUTES

Pulmonary arterial hypertension (WHO Group 1)

- **Adult: SUBCUT INFUSION** 1.25 ng/kg/min by **CONT INFUSION,** may reduce to 0.625 ng/kg/min if not tolerated; may increase by 1.25 ng/kg/min weekly for first 4 wk, then 2.5 ng/kg/min/wk for remainder of infusion; **ORAL INH** 3 breaths via Tyvaso inh system qid

Hepatic dose

- **Adult: SUBCUT INFUSION** 0.625 ng/kg ideal body weight/min; increase cautiously

Available forms: Inj 1, 2.5, 5, 10 mg/ml; neb sol 1.74 mg/2.9 ml

Administer:

- Sudden decreased doses, abrupt withdrawal may worsen pulmonary arterial hypertension symptoms

SUBCUT route

- By continuous infusion
- No dilution required
- Subcutaneous infusion rate = [dose (mg/kg/min) × weight (kg) × 0.00006]/treprostinil vial strength (mg/ml)

Oral INH route

- Avoid skin, eyes; do not take orally; use Tyvaso Inhalation System only
- Patient should have backup Optineb-ir device to avoid interruptions
- Follow instructions for use, cleaning
- Do not mix with other medications in Optineb-ir device
- Twist off cap; squeeze total contents into medicine cup; vol is sufficient for 4 treatments

Continuous IV INFUSION route

- By surgically placed CV catheter using ambulatory infusion pump
- IV pump, product, patient education can be obtained from Priority Healthcare in United States
- Must be diluted with sterile water for inj or 0.9% NaCl
- Concentration should be calculated using this formula: diluted concentration = [dose (ng/kg/min) × weight (kg) × 0.00006] / infusion rate (ml/hr)]

SIDE EFFECTS

CNS: Dizziness, headache, syncope
CV: Vasodilation, *hypotension, edema,* right ventricular heart failure
GI: Nausea, *diarrhea*
INTEG: *Rash,* pruritus
OTHER: Jaw pain, cough, throat irritation
SYST: Infusion-site reactions, pain; increased risk for infection

PHARMACOKINETICS

Metabolized by liver; excreted in urine, feces; terminal half-life 2-4 hr; 90% protein binding

INTERACTIONS

- Excessive hypotension: diuretics, antihypertensives, vasodilators, MAOIs, β-blockers, calcium channel blockers

Increase: bleeding tendencies—anticoagulants, aspirin, NSAIDs, thrombin inhibitors, SSRIs

NURSING CONSIDERATIONS

Assess:

- **Hypertension:** monitor B/P, baseline and periodically
- Hepatic studies: AST, ALT, bilirubin, creatinine with long-term therapy
- ⚠ Blood studies: CBC; CBC q2wk × 3 mo, Hct, Hgb, PT with long-term therapy, ABGs
- ⚠ Bleeding time at baseline, throughout treatment; levels may be 2-5× normal limit

Evaluate:

- Avoid abrupt discontinuation
- Therapeutic response: decreased pulmonary arterial hypertension (PAH)

Teach patient/family:

- That blood work will be necessary during treatment; that treatment may last for years
- To report side effects such as diarrhea, skin rashes
- That therapy will be needed for prolonged periods of time, sometimes years
- To prevent infection, aseptic technique must be used for preparation, administration of treprostinil
- That there are many product, herbal interactions
- About signs, symptoms of bleeding; blood in urine, stools
- How to use inhaled solution; how to care for equipment

tretinoin (vit A acid, retinoic acid) (Rx)

(tret′i-noyn)

Avita, Renova, Retin-A, Retin-A Micro, Stieva-A ✱

Func. class.: Vit A acid, acne product; antineoplastic (miscellaneous)
Chem. class.: Tretinoin derivative

ACTION:

(Topical) Decreases cohesiveness of follicular epithelium, decreases microcomedone formation; (PO) induces maturation of acute promyelocytic leukemia, exact action is unknown

USES:

(Topical) Acne vulgaris (grades 1-3); (PO) acute promyelocytic leukemia, facial wrinkles, photoaging

Unlabeled uses: Acne rosacea, actinic keratosis, ichthyosis, Kaposi's sarcoma, keloids, keratosis follicularis, melasma

CONTRAINDICATIONS:

Hypersensitivity to retinoids or sensitivity to parabens

Black Box Warning: Pregnancy (D) (PO)

Precautions: Pregnancy (C) (topical), breastfeeding, eczema, sunburn, sun exposure

Black Box Warning: Rapid-evolving leukocytosis, respiratory compromise, acute promyelocytic leukemia differentiation syndrome, requires a specialized care setting, experienced clinician

DOSAGE AND ROUTES

- **Adult and child: TOP** cleanse area, apply 0.025%-0.1% cream or 0.05% liquid gel at bedtime, cover lightly

Promyelocytic leukemia

• **Adult: PO** 45 mg/m^2/day given as 2 evenly divided doses until remission, discontinue treatment 30 days after remission or 90 days of treatment, whichever is first

Available forms: Cream 0.01%, 0.02%, 0.025%, 0.05%, 0.1%; gel 0.01%, 0.025%, 0.04%, 0.05%, 0.1%; liquid 0.05%; caps 10 mg

Administer:

Topical route

• Once daily before bedtime; cover area lightly using gauze; use gloves to apply
• Store at room temperature
• Handwashing after application

SIDE EFFECTS

PO

CNS: *Headache, fever, sweating,* fatigue

CV: Cardiac dysrhythmias, pericardial effusion

GI: *Nausea, vomiting,* hemorrhage, *abdominal pain, diarrhea, constipation, dyspepsia, distention, hepatitis*

Topical

INTEG: Rash, stinging, warmth, redness, erythema, blistering, crusting, peeling, contact dermatitis, hypo/hyperpigmentation, dry skin, pruritus, scaly skin, retinoic acid syndrome (RAS)

META: Hypercholesterolemia, hypertriglyceridemia

RESP: Pneumonia, upper respiratory tract disease

PHARMACOKINETICS

PO: Terminal half-life 0.5-2 hr

TOPICAL: Poor systemic absorption

INTERACTIONS

• Use with caution: medicated, abrasive soaps; cleansers that have a drying effect; products with high concentration of alcohol astringents (topical)

Increase: peeling—medication containing agents such as sulfur, benzoyl peroxide, resorcinol, salicylic acid (topical)

Increase: plasma concentrations of tretinoin—ketoconazole (PO)

⚠ **Increase:** ICP, risk of pseudotumor cerebri—tetracyclines; do not use together

Increase: photosensitivity—retinoids, quinolones, phenothiazines, sulfonamides, sulfonylureas, thiazide diuretics

Increase: thrombotic complications—aninocaproic acid, aprotinin, tranexamic acid

Drug/Lab Test

Increase: AST, ALT

NURSING CONSIDERATIONS

Assess:

Topical route

• Area of body involved, what helps or aggravates condition; cysts, dryness, itching; lesions may worsen at beginning of treatment

PO route

• Hepatic function, coagulation, hematologic parameters; also cholesterol, triglycerides

Evaluate:

• Therapeutic response: decrease in size, number of lesions

Teach patient/family:

Topical route

• To avoid application on normal skin; to avoid getting cream in eyes, nose, other mucous membranes; not to use product on areas with cuts, scrapes
• To use cream/gel by applying a thin layer to affected skin; to rub gently; to use liquid; to apply with fingertip or cotton swab
• To avoid sunlight, sunlamps; to use protective clothing, sunscreen
• That treatment may cause warmth, stinging; that dryness, peeling will occur
• That cosmetics may be used over product; not to use shaving lotions
• That rash may occur during first 1-3 wk of therapy
• That product does not cure condition, only relieves symptoms
• That therapeutic results may be seen in 2-3 wk but may not be optimal until after 6 wk

T

PO route

Black Box Warning: To notify prescriber if pregnancy is planned or suspected; pregnancy (D) PO

tretinoin topical

See Appendix B

triamcinolone (ophthalmic)

See Appendix B

triamcinolone (Rx)

(trye-am-sin′oh-lone)

Aristospan, Kenalog-10, Kenalog-40, Tac-3, Triesence

Func. class.: Corticosteroid, synthetic

Chem. class.: Glucocorticoid, intermediate acting

ACTION: Decreases inflammation by suppression of migration of polymorphonuclear leukocytes, fibroblasts; reversal of increased capillary permeability and lysosomal stabilization

USES: Severe inflammation, immunosuppression, neoplasms, asthma (steroid dependent); collagen, respiratory, dermatologic/rheumatic disorders

CONTRAINDICATIONS: Hypersensitivity, neonatal prematurity; epidural/intrathecal administration (Triamcinolone acetonide injections [Kenalog]), systemic fungal infections

Precautions: Pregnancy (C), breastfeeding, diabetes mellitus, glaucoma, osteoporosis, seizure disorders, ulcerative colitis, CHF, myasthenia gravis, renal disease, esophagitis, peptic ulcer, acne, cataracts, coagulopathy, head trauma, children <2 yr, psychosis, idiopathic thrombocytopenia, acute glomerulonephritis, amebiasis, fungal infections, nonasthmatic bronchial disease, AIDS, TB, adrenal insufficiency, acute bronchospasm, acne rosacea, Cushing syndrome, acute MI, thromboembolism

DOSAGE AND ROUTES

- **Adult:** IM (acetonide) 40 mg/wk; (acetonide) 5-48 mg into neoplasms; (acetonide) 2-40 mg into joint or soft tissue; (hexacetonide) 0.5 mg/in^2 of affected intralesional skin; (hexacetonide) 2-20 mg into joint or soft tissue

Severe/incapacitating allergic conditions such as asthma

- **Adult:** IM (Trivaris) 60 mg, titrate, usual range 40-80 mg
- **Child:** IM (Trivaris) 0.11-1.6 mg/kg/day (3.2-48 mg/m^2/day) in 3-4 divided doses

Available forms: Inj 3, 10, 40 mg/ml acetonide; inj 20, 5 mg/ml hexacetonide

Administer:

IM route

- After shaking susp (parenteral)
- Titrated dose; use lowest effective dose
- IM inj deep in large muscle mass; rotate sites; avoid deltoid; use 21-G needle
- Avoid SUBCUT administration, may damage tissue

SIDE EFFECTS

CNS: *Depression,* headache, mood changes

CV: *Hypertension,* circulatory collapse, embolism, tachycardia, edema

EENT: Fungal infections, increased intraocular pressure, blurred vision

GI: *Diarrhea, nausea, abdominal distention,* GI hemorrhage, *increased appetite,* pancreatitis

HEMA: Thrombocytopenia

INTEG: Acne, poor wound healing, ecchymosis, petechiae

MS: Fractures, osteoporosis, weakness

PHARMACOKINETICS

PO/IM: Peak 1-2 hr, half-life 2-5 hr

INTERACTIONS

Increase: side effects—alcohol, salicylates, indomethacin, amphotericin B, digoxin, cycloSPORINE, diuretics, quinolones
Increase: action of triamcinolone—salicylates, estrogens, indomethacin, oral contraceptives, ketoconazole, macrolide antiinfectives, carBAMazepine
Decrease: action of triamcinolone—cholestyramine, colestipol, barbiturates, rifampin, ePHEDrine, phenytoin, theophylline
Decrease: effects of anticoagulants, anticonvulsants, antidiabetics, ambenonium, neostigmine, isoniazid, toxoids, vaccines, anticholinesterases, salicylates, somatrem

Drug/Herb

- Hypokalemia: aloe, cascara, senna

Drug/Lab Test

Increase: cholesterol, sodium, blood glucose, uric acid, calcium, urine glucose
Decrease: calcium, potassium, T_4, T_3, thyroid ^{131}I uptake test, urine 17-OHCS, 17-KS, PBI
False negative: skin allergy tests

NURSING CONSIDERATIONS

Assess:

- Potassium, blood glucose, urine glucose while patient receiving long-term therapy; hypokalemia and hyperglycemia
- Weight daily; notify prescriber if weekly gain of >5 lb
- B/P, pulse; notify prescriber if chest pain occurs
- I&O ratio; be alert for decreasing urinary output, increasing edema
- Plasma cortisol levels during long-term therapy (normal level: 138-635 nmol/L SI units when drawn at 8 AM)
- **Infection:** increased temperature, WBC even after withdrawal of medication; product masks infection
- Potassium depletion: paresthesias, fatigue, nausea, vomiting, depression, polyuria, dysrhythmias, weakness
- Edema, hypertension, cardiac symptoms
- Mental status: affect, mood, behavioral changes, aggression
- Assistance with ambulation for patient with bone-tissue disease to prevent fractures

Evaluate:

- Therapeutic response: ease of respirations, decreased inflammation

Teach patient/family:

- That emergency ID as corticosteroid user should be carried; not to discontinue abruptly, taper dose
- To notify prescriber if therapeutic response decreases; that dosage adjustment may be needed
- To avoid OTC products: salicylates, alcohol in cough products, cold preparations unless directed by prescriber; to avoid live vaccines
- About cushingoid symptoms
- About the symptoms of adrenal insufficiency: nausea, anorexia, fatigue, dizziness, dyspnea, weakness, joint pain

triamcinolone nasal agent

See Appendix B

triamcinolone (topical)

(try-am-sin′oh-lone)

Kenalog, Triderm

Func. class.: Corticosteroid, topical

ACTION: Crosses cell membrane to attach to receptors to decrease inflammation, itching; inhibits multiple inflammatory cytokines

USES: Inflammation/itching in corticosteroid-responsive dermatoses on the skin or inflammation in the mouth

CONTRAINDICATIONS: Hypersensitivity, use on face, ear canal, infections
Precautions: Pregnancy (C), breastfeeding, children

T

DOSAGE AND ROUTES

- Apply to the affected areas bid-qid

Available forms: Aerosol 0.2 mg; paste (dental) 0.1%; lotion, cream, ointment 0.025%; ointment 0.05%; lotion, cream, ointment 0.1%; ointment, cream 0.5%

Administer:

Topical route

- May be used with occlusive dressings
- **Cream/Ointment/Lotion:** apply sparingly in a thin film and rub gently into the cleansed, slightly moist affected area; may use gloves to apply cream/ointment/lotion
- **Paste:** apply without rubbing, press into lesion until film develops
- **Spray:** spray a small amount of preparation onto the lesion

SIDE EFFECTS

ENDO: HPA axis suppression, Cushing syndrome

INTEG: Burning, folliculitis, pruritus, dermatitis, hypopigmentation

META: Hyperglycemia; glycosuria

PHARMACOKINETICS

Absorption varies

INTERACTIONS

Increase: blood glucose

NURSING CONSIDERATIONS

Assess:

- Skin reactions: burning, pruritus, folliculitis, mouth lesions

Evaluate:

- Decreasing itching, inflammation on the skin, decreasing mouth lesions

Teach patient/family:

- How to use each product

triamcinolone (topical-oral) (Rx, OTC)

(trye-am-sin′oh-lone)

Kenalog in Orabase, Oralone Dental

Func. class.: Topical anesthetic

Chem. class.: Synthetic fluorinated adrenal corticosteroid

ACTION:
Binds with steroid receptors, decreases inflammation

USES:
Oral pain

CONTRAINDICATIONS:
Hypersensitivity, application to large areas; presence of fungal, viral, or bacterial infections of mouth or throat

Precautions: Pregnancy (C), children <6 yr, sepsis, denuded skin, geriatric patients

DOSAGE AND ROUTES

- **Adult: TOP** Press 1/4 inch into affected area until film appears, repeat bid-tid

Available forms: Paste 0.1%

Administer:

- After cleansing oral cavity after meals

SIDE EFFECTS

INTEG: Rash, irritation, sensitization

NURSING CONSIDERATIONS

Assess:

- Allergy: rash, irritation, reddening, swelling
- Infection: if affected area is infected, do not apply

Evaluate:

- Therapeutic response: absence of pain in affected area

Teach patient/family:

- To report rash, irritation, redness, swelling
- How to apply paste

⚠ HIGH ALERT

triazolam (Rx)

(trye-ay′zoe-lam)

Apo-Triazo ✦, Halcion

Func. class.: Sedative-hypnotic, antianxiety

Chem. class.: Benzodiazepine, short acting

Controlled Substance Schedule IV (USA), Targeted (CDSA IV) (Canada)

Do not confuse:
Halcion/Haldol/halcinonide

ACTION: Produces CNS depression at limbic, thalamic, hypothalamic levels of CNS; may be mediated by neurotransmitter γ-aminobutyric acid (GABA); results are sedation, hypnosis, skeletal muscle relaxation, anticonvulsant activity, anxiolytic action

USES: Insomnia, sedative/hypnotic

CONTRAINDICATIONS: Pregnancy (X), breastfeeding, hypersensitivity to benzodiazepines

Precautions: Children <15 yr, geriatric patients, anemia, renal/hepatic disease, suicidal individuals, drug abuse, psychosis, acute closed-angle glaucoma, seizure disorders, angioedema, respiratory disease, depression, sleep-related behaviors (sleep walking), intermittent porphyria, myasthenia gravis, Parkinson's disease

DOSAGE AND ROUTES

- **Adult: PO** 0.125-0.5 mg at bedtime, max 0.5 mg/day
- **Geriatric: PO** 0.0625-0.125 mg at bedtime, max 0.25 mg/day

Available forms: Tabs 0.125, 0.25 mg

Administer:

- After trying conservative measures for insomnia
- ½ hr before bedtime for sleeplessness
- On empty stomach for fast onset; may be taken with food if GI symptoms occur
- Avoid use with CNS depressants; serious CNS depression may result

SIDE EFFECTS

CNS: *Headache, lethargy, drowsiness, daytime sedation,* dizziness, confusion, lightheadedness, anxiety, irritability, amnesia, poor coordination, **complex sleep-related reactions: sleep driving, sleep eating**

CV: Chest pain, pulse changes, ECG changes

GI: Nausea, vomiting, diarrhea, heartburn, abdominal pain, constipation, **hepatic injury**

SYST: **Severe allergic reactions**

PHARMACOKINETICS

Onset 15-30 min, duration 6-8 hr, metabolized by liver, excreted by kidneys (inactive metabolites), crosses placenta, excreted in breast milk, half-life 1.5-5.5 hr

INTERACTIONS

- Smoking may decrease hypnotic effect

Increase: triazolam levels—CYP3A4 inhibitors, protease inhibitors

⚠ Increase: effects of cimetidine, disulfiram, erythromycin, clarithromycin, probenecid, isoniazid, oral contraceptives; do not use concurrently

Increase: action of both products—alcohol, CNS depressants

Decrease: effect of antacids, theophylline, rifampin, smoking

Drug/Herb

Increase: CNS depression—chamomile, hops, kava, lavender, valerian

Drug/Food

- Grapefruit may increase action, avoid concurrent use

Drug/Lab Test

Increase: ALT, AST, serum bilirubin

Decrease: RAI uptake

False increase: urinary 17-OHCS

NURSING CONSIDERATIONS

Assess:

- Blood studies: Hct, Hgb, RBC if blood dyscrasias suspected (rare)

T

• Hepatic studies: AST, ALT, bilirubin if hepatic damage has occurred
• Mental status: mood, sensorium, affect, memory (long, short term), insomnia, withdrawal symptoms, excessive sedation, impaired coordination
• Blood dyscrasias: fever, sore throat, bruising, rash, jaundice, epistaxis (rare)
• Type of sleep problem: falling asleep, staying asleep
• Assistance with ambulation after receiving dose

Evaluate:
• Therapeutic response: ability to sleep at night, decreased amount of early morning awakening if taking product for insomnia

Teach patient/family:
• To use reliable contraception; pregnancy (X)
• That dependence is possible after long-term use
• To avoid driving, other activities requiring alertness until product is stabilized
• To avoid alcohol ingestion
• That effects may take 2 nights for benefits to be noticed; that product is for short-term use only; to use for 7-10 continuous nights
• About alternative measures to improve sleep: reading, exercise several hours before bedtime, warm bath, warm milk, TV, self-hypnosis, deep breathing
• That complex sleep-related behaviors (sleep eating/driving) may occur
• That hangover common in geriatric patients but less common than with barbiturates; that rebound insomnia may occur for 1-2 nights after discontinuing product; to discontinue by decreasing dose by 50% q2 nights until 0.125 mg for 2 nights, then stop

TREATMENT OF OVERDOSE:
Lavage, activated charcoal; monitor electrolytes, VS

trifluridine ophthalmic
See Appendix B

trimethobenzamide (Rx)
(trye-meth-oh-ben′za-mide)

Tigan

Func. class.: Antiemetic, anticholinergic
Chem. class.: Ethanolamine derivative

ACTION: Acts centrally by blocking chemoreceptor trigger zone, which in turn acts on vomiting center

USES: Nausea, vomiting

CONTRAINDICATIONS: Children (parenterally), hypersensitivity to opioids, shock

Precautions: Pregnancy (C), children, geriatric patients, cardiac dysrhythmias, acute febrile illness, encephalitis, gastroenteritis, dehydration, electrolyte imbalances, Reye's syndrome

DOSAGE AND ROUTES
Nausea/vomiting
• **Adult: IM** 200 mg 3-4×/day; **PO** 300 mg 3-4×/day

Postoperative
• **Adult: IM** 200 mg followed by 2nd dose 1 hr later

Renal dose
• **Adult: IM** CCr 15-30 ml/min, give 50% of dose

Available forms: Caps 300 mg; inj 100 mg/ml

Administer:

PO route
• Capsules may be swallowed whole, chewed, allowed to dissolve

IM route
• Inj in large muscle mass; aspirate to avoid IV administration; inj not to be used in children or infants

Syringe compatibilities: Butorphanol, glycopyrrolate, HYDROmorphone, midazolam, nalbuphine

SIDE EFFECTS
CNS: *Drowsiness,* headache, dizziness, confusion, disorientation, coma, seizures, depression, *vertigo,* EPS

CV: Hypo/hypertension, palpitation, cardiac dysrhythmias
EENT: Dry mouth, blurred vision, photosensitivity
GI: Nausea, diarrhea, vomiting, difficulty swallowing
INTEG: Rash, urticaria, fever, chills, flushing, hyperpyrexia

PHARMACOKINETICS

Metabolized by liver, excreted by kidneys
PO: Onset 20-40 min, duration 3-4 hr
IM: Onset 15-35 min, duration 2-3 hr

INTERACTIONS

Increase: effect—CNS depressants, alcohol

NURSING CONSIDERATIONS

Assess:

- Nausea, vomiting before, after treatment
- VS, B/P; check patients with cardiac disease more often
- Signs of toxicity of other products or masking of symptoms of disease: brain tumor, intestinal obstruction
- Observe for drowsiness, dizziness

Evaluate:

- Therapeutic response: decreased nausea, vomiting

Teach patient/family:

- To avoid hazardous activities, activities requiring alertness because dizziness may occur; to request assistance with ambulation
- To avoid alcohol, other depressants
- To keep out of children's reach

trospium (Rx)

(trose′pee-um)

Sanctura, Sanctura XR

Func. class.: Anticholinergic, urinary antispasmodic

Chem. class.: Muscarinic receptor antagonist

ACTION:
Relaxes smooth muscles in bladder by inhibiting acetylcholine effect on muscarinic receptors

USES:
Overactive bladder (urinary frequency, urgency)

CONTRAINDICATIONS:
Hypersensitivity, uncontrolled closed-angle glaucoma, urinary retention, gastric retention, myasthenia gravis

Precautions: Pregnancy (C), breastfeeding, children, geriatric patients, renal/hepatic disease, controlled closed-angle glaucoma, ulcerative colitis, intestinal atony, bladder outflow obstruction

DOSAGE AND ROUTES

- **Adult <75 yr: PO** 20 mg bid 1 hr before meals or on empty stomach; **ER** 60 mg in AM
- **Geriatric ≥75 yr: PO** titrate down to 20 mg/day based on response and tolerance

Renal dose

- **Adult: PO** CCr <30 ml/min, 20 mg/day at bedtime, ext rel product not recommended

Available forms: Tabs 20 mg; caps ext rel 60 mg

Administer:

- 1 hr before meals or on empty stomach (reg rel); in AM (ext rel) ≥1 hr before meal

SIDE EFFECTS

CNS: Fatigue, dizziness, headache
CV: Tachycardia
EENT: Dry eyes, vision abnormalities

T

GI: Flatulence, abdominal pain, *constipation, dry mouth,* dyspepsia
GU: Urinary retention, UTI
INTEG: Dry skin, angioedema
MISC: Heat stroke, fever

PHARMACOKINETICS

Rapidly absorbed (10%); peak 5-6 hr; protein bound (50%-85%); extensively metabolized; excreted in urine, feces; excreted in urine by active tubular secretion; half-life 20 hr

INTERACTIONS

Increase: drowsiness—CNS depressants, alcohol
Increase or decrease: trospium effect—products excreted by active renal secretion (aMILoride, digoxin, morphine), metformin, quiNIDine, procainamide, ranitidine, tenofovir, triamterene, vancomycin
Drug/Food
Decrease: absorption—high-fat meal

NURSING CONSIDERATIONS

Assess:
- **Urinary patterns:** distention, nocturia, frequency, urgency, incontinence, voiding patterns

Evaluate:
- Therapeutic response: correction of urinary status: absence of dysuria, frequency, nocturia, incontinence

Teach patient/family:
- To avoid hazardous activities because dizziness may occur
- That alcohol may increase drowsiness
- About anticholinergic effects that may occur
- That overheating may occur with strenuous exercise
- To avoid all other products unless approved by prescriber

undecylenic acid topical
See Appendix B

unoprostone ophthalmic
See Appendix B

ustekinumab (Rx)
(us′te-kin′ue-mab)

Stelara

Func. class.: Immune response modifier, antipsoriatic agent

Chem. class.: Monoclonal antibody

ACTION: Interleukin (IL)-12, IL-23 antagonist, binds to an interleukin protein, decreases inflammation

USES: Plaque psoriasis, psoriatic arthritis

CONTRAINDICATIONS: Hypersensitivity, sepsis, active infections

Precautions: Pregnancy (B), breastfeeding, children ≤18 yr, geriatric patients, surgery, TB, diabetes mellitus, immunosuppression

DOSAGE AND ROUTES
Moderate to severe plaque psoriasis
- **Adult ≥100 kg and plaque psoriasis: SUBCUT** 90 mg, repeat in 4 wk, then 90 mg q12wk starting wk 16
- **Adult without plaque psoriasis: SUBCUT** 45 mg, repeat in 4 wk, then 45 mg q12wk starting wk 16

Psoriatic arthritis (monotherapy or methotrexate combination)
- **Adult:** 45 mg repeat subcut in 4 wk, then q12wk maintenance

Psoriatic arthritis with moderate to severe plaque psoriasis (monotherapy or methotrexate combination)
- **Adult ≥100 kg: Subcut** 90 mg, repeat in 4 wk, then q12wk maintenance

Available forms: Solutions for inj 45 mg/0.5 ml, 90 mg/ml single use

Administer:
- Visually inspect for particulate matter or discoloration; solution should be slightly yellow and may contain a few small translucent or white particles; do not use if discolored, cloudy, or if foreign particulate matter is present; do not shake
- Use at 27-G, 0.5-inch needle
- May be administered subcut into upper arm, abdomen, or thigh; rotate inj sites

SIDE EFFECTS
CNS: Headache, leukoencephalopathy, depression, dizziness

HEMA: Bleeding

INTEG: *Inj-site reaction,* pruritus, skin irritation, erythema

SYST: **Serious infections, malignancies**

MS: Myalgia, back pain

RESP: URI

PHARMACOKINETICS
Maximum serum concentration: 13.5 days after a single 45 mg subcut dose, 7 days after a single 90 mg subcut dose; half-life 14.9-45.6 days

INTERACTIONS
- Do not give concurrently with vaccines; immunizations should be brought up to date before treatment
- Avoid use with immunosuppressives

NURSING CONSIDERATIONS
Assess:
- Bring immunizations up to date before starting treatment
- Infection: monitor for fever, sore throat, cough, do not use during active infections
- **Malignancy: skin cancer may occur especially in older patients who have used ultraviolet treatments with immunosuppressants**

• **TB:** TB testing should be done before starting treatment
• For inj-site pain, swelling

Evaluate:

• Therapeutic response: decreased plaque psoriasis

Teach patient/family:

• That product must be continued for prescribed time to be effective, to use as prescribed
• Not to receive live vaccinations during treatment
• To notify prescriber of possible infection (upper respiratory or other) or allergic reactions
• Injection techniques and disposable, not to reuse needles, syringes
• That follow-up will be needed

valACYclovir (Rx)

(val-a-sye′kloh-vir)

Valtrex

Func. class.: Antiviral

Chem. class.: Synthetic purine nucleoside analog

Do not confuse:
valACYclovir/valGANciclovir
Valtrex/Valcyte

ACTION: Interferes with DNA synthesis by conversion to acyclovir, thereby causing decreased viral replication, time of lesional healing

USES: Treatment or suppression of herpes zoster (shingles), genital herpes, herpes labialis (cold sores), varicella, varicella-zoster

Unlabeled uses: CMV with advanced HIV, posttransplant patients, Bell's palsy, herpes simplex virus prophylaxis, acute retinal necrosis (ARN), encephalitis

CONTRAINDICATIONS: Hypersensitivity to this product or acyclovir, valGANciclovir

Precautions: Pregnancy (B), breastfeeding, geriatric patients, hepatic/renal disease, electrolyte imbalance, dehydration, penciclovir, famciclovir, ganciclovir, hypersensitivity, varicella

DOSAGE AND ROUTES

Herpes zoster (shingles)

- **Adult: PO** 1 g tid × 1 wk

Genital herpes (suppressive, initial)

- **Adult: PO** 1 g bid × 10 days initially

Genital herpes (recurrent episodes)

- **Adult: PO** 500 mg bid × 3 days

Genital herpes (suppressive therapy)

- **Adult: PO** 1 g/day with normal immune function; 500 mg/day for those with ≤9 recurrences/yr; 500 mg bid for HIV-infected patients with CD4 count ≥100

Reduction of transmission

- **Adult: PO** 500 mg/day for source partner

Herpes labialis

- **Adult: PO** 2 g bid × 1 day at 1st sign of lesions

Varicella (chickenpox) in immunocompetent patients

- **Adolescent and child ≥2 yr: PO** 20 mg/kg/dose tid × 5 days, max 3 g/day; start at 1st sign, preferably within 24 hr of rash

Renal dose

- **Adult: PO** CCr 30-49 ml/min, 1 g q12hr (for regimens 1 g q8hr); 1 g q12hr × 1 day (herpes labialis); CCr 10-29 ml/min, 1 g q24hr (genital herpes/herpes zoster); 500 mg q24hr (recurrent genital herpes); CCr <10 ml/min, 500 mg q24hr (genital herpes/herpes zoster), 500 mg q24hr (recurrent genital herpes)

Available forms: Tabs 500 mg, 1 g

Administer:

- As soon as possible (herpes labialis, genital herpes); within 24 hr of rash (varicella)
- Within 72 hr of outbreak (herpes zoster)
- Without regard to food
- Caps may be made into susp by pharmacy
- Store at room temperature; protect from light, moisture

SIDE EFFECTS

CNS: Tremors, lethargy, *dizziness, headache,* weakness, depression

ENDO: *Dysmenorrhea*

GI: *Nausea,* vomiting, diarrhea, abdominal pain, constipation, *increased AST*

HEMA: Thrombocytopenic purpura, hemolytic uremic syndrome

INTEG: *Rash*

PHARMACOKINETICS

Onset unknown; terminal half-life 2½-3½ hr; converted to acyclovir that crosses placenta, enters breast milk; excreted in urine primarily as acyclovir; protein binding 13.5%-17.9%

V

INTERACTIONS

Increase: blood levels of valACYclovir—cimetidine, probenecid; only significant with renal disease

Drug/Lab Test

Increase: LFTs, creatinine

Decrease: WBC, platelets

NURSING CONSIDERATIONS

Assess:

- **Infection;** characteristics of lesions; therapy should be started at 1st sign or symptom of herpes; most effective within 72 hr of outbreak

⚠ **Thrombocytopenic purpura, hemolytic uremic syndrome; may be fatal**

- C&S before product therapy; product may be taken as soon as culture is taken; repeat C&S after treatment; determine presence of other sexually transmitted diseases
- Bowel pattern before, during treatment
- Skin eruptions: rash
- Allergies before treatment, reaction of each medication

Evaluate:

- Therapeutic response: absence of itching, painful lesions; crusting and healed lesions

Teach patient/family:

- To take as prescribed; if dose is missed, to take as soon as remembered up to 2 hr before next dose; not to double dose, without regard to meals
- That product may be taken orally before infection occurs; that product should be taken when itching or pain occurs, usually before eruptions
- That partners need to be told that patient has herpes because they can become infected; that condoms must be worn to prevent reinfections
- That product does not cure infection, just controls symptoms; that product does not prevent infection of others
- **To report CNS changes (tremors, weakness, lethargy) immediately**

valGANciclovir (Rx)

(val-gan-sy′kloh-veer)

Valcyte

Func. class.: Antiviral

Chem. class.: Synthetic nucleoside

Do not confuse:

valGANciclovir/valACYclovir

Valcyte/Valtrex

ACTION: Metabolized to ganciclovir; inhibits replication of human cytomegalovirus in vivo and in vitro by selective inhibition of viral DNA synthesis

USES: Cytomegalovirus (CMV) retinitis in immunocompromised persons, including those with AIDS, after indirect ophthalmoscopy confirms diagnosis; prevention of CMV with transplantation; prevention of CMV in at-risk patient going through transplant (kidney, heart, pancreas)

Unlabeled uses: Colitis, Epstein-Barr virus, esophagitis, herpes simplex type 1, 2; human herpesvirus 6, 8; multicentric Castleman's disease, varicella-zoster virus

CONTRAINDICATIONS: Breastfeeding, hypersensitivity to ganciclovir, valACYclovir; absolute neutrophil count $<500/mm^3$; platelet count $<25,000/mm^3$; hemodialysis; liver transplantation

Precautions: Children, geriatric patients, renal function impairment; hypersensitivity to acyclovir, penciclovir, famciclovir

Black Box Warning: Preexisting cytopenias, secondary malignancy, infertility, anemia, pregnancy (C)

DOSAGE AND ROUTES

Treatment of CMV

- **Adult and adolescent (unlabeled): PO** induction 900 mg bid × 21 days with food; maintenance 900 mg/day with food

Transplant (CMV prophylaxis)

• **Adult/adolescent >16 yr: PO** 900 mg/day with food starting 10 days before transplantation until day 100 after transplantation

• **Infant ≥4 mo/child/adolescent ≤16 yr: PO** give within 10 days of heart/kidney transplant; calculate dose as 7 × BSA × CCr, give as single daily dose

Renal dose

• **Adult: PO** CCr ≥60 ml/min, same as above; CCr 40-59 ml/min, 450 mg bid for 21 days, then 450 mg/day; CCr 25-39 ml/min, 450 mg/day, then 450 mg q2days; CCr 10-24 ml/min, 450 mg q2days, then 450 mg 2×/week

Available form: Tabs 450 mg, powder for oral sol 50 mg/ml

Administer:

PO tab

• With food for better absorption; avoid getting product on skin; do not break

Oral sol

• Measure 9 ml purified water in graduated cylinder, shake bottle to loosen powder, add ½ liquid, shake well, add remaining water, shake; remove child-resistant cap and push bottle adapter into neck of bottle, close with cap, give using dispenser provided

• Store liquid in refrigerator; do not freeze; throw away any unused after 49 days

SIDE EFFECTS

CNS: *Fever,* chills, coma, *confusion,* abnormal thoughts, dizziness, bizarre dreams, *headache, insomnia,* psychosis, tremors, somnolence, *paresthesia, weakness,* **seizures**

EENT: Retinal detachment with CMV retinitis

GI: Abnormal LFTs, *nausea, vomiting, anorexia, diarrhea, abdominal pain,* **hemorrhage**

GU: **Hematuria,** increased creatinine, BUN

HEMA: **Granulocytopenia, thrombocytopenia, irreversible neutropenia, anemia, eosinophilia**

INTEG: *Rash,* alopecia, *pruritus,* urticaria, pain at site, phlebitis, **Stevens-Johnson syndrome**

MISC: Local and systemic infections, **sepsis**

PHARMACOKINETICS

Metabolized to ganciclovir, which has a half-life of 3-4½ hr; excreted by kidneys (unchanged); crosses blood-brain barrier, CSF

INTERACTIONS

Increase: Severe granulocytopenia: immunosuppressants, zidovudine, antineoplastics, radiation; do not use together

Increase: toxicity—dapsone, pentamidine, flucytosine, vinCRIStine, vinBLAStine, adriamycin, DOXOrubicin, amphotericin B, trimethoprim-sulfamethoxazole combinations or other nucleoside analogs, cycloSPORINE

Increase: effect of both drugs—mycophenolate

Increase: seizures—imipenem-cilastatin

Increase: effect of didanosine; monitor for adverse effects, toxicity

Decrease: renal clearance of valGANciclovir—probenecid

Drug/Food

Increase: absorption, high-fat meal

Drug/Lab Test

Increase: creatinine

Decrease: RBC/WBC, Hct/Hgb

NURSING CONSIDERATIONS

Assess:

• CMV retinitis by ophthalmoscopy before beginning treatment, q2wk; culture for CMV retinitis

Black Box Warning: Leukopenia/neutropenia/thrombocytopenia: WBCs, platelets q2days during 2×/day dosing, then q1wk; leukopenia with daily WBC count in patients with prior leukopenia with other nucleoside analogs or for whom leukopenia counts are <1000 cells/mm³ at start of treatment

V

Black Box Warning: Malignancy: monitor for malignancy, avoid accidental exposure of broken, crushed tabs, powder, if these were in contact with skin, wash well with soap and water

Black Box Warning: Pregnancy: considered potentially teratogenic; adequate contraception should be used

- Serum creatinine or CCr ≥q2wk

Evaluate:
- Therapeutic response: decreased symptoms of CMV

Teach patient/family:
- That product does not cure condition; that regular ophthalmologic and blood tests necessary
- That major toxicities may necessitate discontinuing product

Black Box Warning: To use contraception during treatment; that infertility may occur; that men should use barrier contraception for 90 days after treatment

- To take with food

⚠ Blood dyscrasias: bruising, bleeding, petechiae; seizures, dizziness; to avoid hazardous activities
- To use sunscreen to prevent burns

valproate (Rx)
(val′proh-ate)

Depacon

valproic acid (Rx)
(val′proh-ik)

Depakene, Stavzor

divalproex sodium (Rx)
(dye-val′proh-ex)

Depakote, Depakote ER, Epival ✦

Func. class.: Anticonvulsant, vascular headache suppressant

Chem. class.: Carboxylic acid derivative

ACTION: Increases levels of γ-aminobutyric acid (GABA) in the brain, which decreases seizure activity

USES: Simple (petit mal), complex (petit mal), absence, mixed, seizures; manic episodes associated with bipolar disorder, prophylaxis of migraine, adjunct for schizophrenia, tardive dyskinesia, aggression in children with ADHD, organic brain syndrome, mania, migraines; tonic-clonic (grand mal), myoclonic seizures

Unlabeled uses: Rectal for seizures (valproic acid)

CONTRAINDICATIONS: Hypersensitivity, urea cycle disorders

Black Box Warning: Pregnancy (D), hepatic disease, pancreatitis

Precautions: Breastfeeding, geriatric patients

Black Box Warning: Children <2 yr

DOSAGE AND ROUTES

Epilepsy
- **Adult and child: PO** 10-15 mg/kg/day in 2-3 divided doses, may increase by

5-10 mg/kg/day weekly, max 60 mg/kg/day in 2-3 divided doses; **IV** ≤20 mg/min over 1 hr

Status epilepticus refractory to diazepam IV (unlabeled)

- **Adult: RECT** 400-600 mg PR as enema or wax-based suppository (not commercially available)
- **Child: RECT** 20 mg/kg/dose

Mania (divalproex sodium)

- **Adult: PO** 750 mg/day in divided doses, max 60 mg/kg/day or 3000 mg/day

Mania (valproic acid: Stavzor)

- **Adult: DEL REL CAP** 750 mg/day in divided doses

Migraine (divalproex sodium)

- **Adult: PO** 250 mg bid, may increase to 1000 mg/day if needed or 500 mg (Depakote ER) daily × 7 days, then 1000 mg/day

Available forms: *Valproate:* inj 100 mg/ml; *valproic acid:* caps 250 mg; oral solution 250 mg/5 ml; del rel cap (Stavzor) 125, 250, 500 mg; *divalproex:* gastro-resistant tabs 125, 250, 500 mg; ext rel tabs 250, 500 mg cap gastro-resistant; sprinkle cap 125 mg

Administer:

PO route

- Swallow tabs or caps whole; do not break, crush, or chew ext rel tabs
- Sprinkle cap contents on food
- Oral solution alone; do not dilute with carbonated beverage; do not give oral solution to patients with sodium restrictions
- Give with food or milk to decrease GI symptoms

IV route

- Dilute dose with ≥50 ml D_5W, NS, LR
- Run over 60 min (20 mg/min)

SIDE EFFECTS

CNS: *Sedation, drowsiness,* dizziness, headache, incoordination, depression, hallucinations, behavioral changes, tremors, aggression, weakness, **coma, suicidal ideation, hypothermia**

CV: Hypo/hypertension, chest pain, palpitations, peripheral edema

EENT: Visual disturbances, taste perversion

GI: *Nausea, vomiting, constipation, diarrhea, dyspepsia,* anorexia, cramps, **hepatic failure, pancreatitis, toxic hepatitis,** stomatitis, weight gain, dry mouth

GU: Enuresis, irregular menses

HEMA: **Thrombocytopenia, leukopenia, lymphocytosis,** increased PT, bruising, epistaxis, **pancytopenia**

INTEG: *Rash,* alopecia, photosensitivity, dry skin

META: Hyperammonemia, SIADH

RESP: Dyspnea

PHARMACOKINETICS

Metabolized by liver; excreted by kidneys, in breast milk; crosses placenta; half-life 6-16 hr; 90% protein binding

PO: Peak 4 hr (regular rel); 4-17 hr (ext rel)

INTERACTIONS

Increase: valproic acid toxicity level—erythromycin, felbamate, salicylates, NSAIDs, rifampin

Increase: CNS depression—alcohol, opioids, barbiturates, antihistamines, MAOIs, sedative/hypnotics, tricyclics

Increase: action of, possible toxicity phenytoin, carBAMazepine, ethosuximide, barbiturates, zidovudine, LORazepam, rufinamide, lamoTRIgine

Increase: bleeding—warfarin

Decrease: seizure threshold—tricyclics

Drug/Lab Test

False positive: ketones, urine

Interference: thyroid function tests

Increase: LFTs, bleeding time, ammonia

Decrease: sodium

NURSING CONSIDERATIONS

Assess:

- **Seizure disorder:** location, aura, activity, duration; seizure precautions should be in place

⚠ **Mental status: bipolar disorder: mood, activity, sleeping/eating, behavior; suicidal thoughts/behaviors**

- **Migraines:** frequency, intensity, alleviating factors

V

• Blood studies: Hct, Hgb, RBC, serum folate, PT/PTT, serum ammonia, platelets, vit D if patient receiving long-term therapy

Black Box Warning: Hepatic studies: AST, ALT, bilirubin; hepatic failure has occurred; monitor for fever, anorexia, vomiting, lethargy, jaundice of skin, eyes that may occur during treatment, those with organic brain disorders, mental retardation, child <2 yr are at greater risk

• **Hyperammonemic encephalopathy:** can be fatal in those with urea cycle disorders (UCD); lethargy, confusion, coma, CV, respiratory changes; discontinue
• Blood levels: therapeutic level 50-125 mcg/ml, during seizures

Black Box Warning: Pancreatitis; may be fatal; report immediately nausea, vomiting, anorexia, abdominal pain; may occur anytime during treatment or for several months/years after discontinuing treatment

Evaluate:
• Therapeutic response: decreased seizures

Teach patient/family:
• That physical dependency may result from extended use
• To avoid driving, other activities that require alertness
• To drink plenty of fluids
• Not to discontinue medication quickly after long-term use because seizures may result

Black Box Warning: To report visual disturbances, rash, diarrhea, abdominal pain, light-colored stools, jaundice, protracted vomiting, weakness to prescriber

• To use contraception while taking this product; pregnancy (D)
• Overdose symptoms: heart block, coma
• To report immediately suicidal thoughts/behaviors

valsartan (Rx)

(val′sahr-tan)

Diovan

Func. class.: Antihypertensive
Chem. class.: Angiotensin II receptor antagonist (Type AT_1)

Do not confuse:
Diovan/Dioval

ACTION: Blocks the vasoconstrictor and aldosterone-secreting effects of angiotensin II; selectively blocks the binding of angiotensin II to the AT_1 receptor found in tissues

USES: Hypertension, alone or in combination in patients >6 yr, CHF, post MI with left ventricular dysfunction/failure in stable patients

CONTRAINDICATIONS: Hypersensitivity, severe hepatic disease, bilateral renal artery stenosis

Black Box Warning: Pregnancy (D)

Precautions: Breastfeeding, children, geriatric patients, hypersensitivity to ACE inhibitors; CHF, hypertrophic cardiomyopathy aortic/mitral valve stenosis, CAD, angioedema, renal/hepatic disease, hyperkalemia, hypovolemia, African descent

DOSAGE AND ROUTES

Hypertension
• **Adult: PO** 80 or 160 mg/day alone or in combination with other antihypertensives, may increase to 320 mg/day
• **Geriatric: PO** adjust on clinical response; may start with lower dose
• **Child and adolescent 6-16 yr: PO** 1.3 mg/kg/day, max 40 mg/day

CHF
• **Adult: PO** 40 mg bid, up to 160 mg bid

Post MI
• **Adult: PO** 20 mg bid as early as 12 hr post MI, may be titrated within 7 days to 40 mg bid, then titrate to maintenance of 160 mg bid

Available forms: Tabs 40, 80, 160, 320 mg

Administer:

- Without regard to meals

SIDE EFFECTS

CNS: *Dizziness, insomnia,* drowsiness, vertigo, headache, fatigue

CV: Angina pectoris, 2nd-degree AV block, **cerebrovascular accident**, hypotension, **MI**, ***dysrhythmias***

EENT: Conjunctivitis

GI: *Diarrhea,* abdominal pain, nausea, **hepatotoxicity**

GU: Impotence, **nephrotoxicity, renal failure**

HEMA: *Anemia,* neutropenia

META: Hyperkalemia

MISC: Vasculitis, **angioedema**

MS: Cramps, myalgia, pain, stiffness

RESP: *Cough*

PHARMACOKINETICS

Onset up to 2 hr; peak 2-4 hr; duration 24 hr; extensively metabolized; protein binding 95%; half-life 6 hr; excreted in feces, urine, breast milk

INTERACTIONS

- **Do not use with aliskiren**

Increase: effects of lithium, antidiabetics

Increase: hyperkalemia—potassium-sparing diuretics, potassium supplements, ACE inhibitors, cycloSPORINE

Increase: Valsartan level—rifampin, ritonavir, gemfibrozil, telithromycin

Decrease: antihypertensive effects—NSAIDs, salicylates

Drug/Herb

Increase: antihypertensive effect—hawthorn

Decrease: antihypertensive effect—ephedra, ma huang

Drug/Food

Increase: hyperkalemia—salt substitutes with potasssium

NURSING CONSIDERATIONS

Assess:

- B/P, pulse q4hr lying, sitting, standing; note rate, rhythm, quality periodically
- Blood studies; BUN, creatinine, LFTs, potassium total/direct bilirubin before treatment
- **Angioedema:** **facial swelling; SOB; edema in feet, legs daily**
- Skin turgor, dryness of mucous membranes for hydration status; correct volume depletion before initiating therapy

Evaluate:

- Therapeutic response: decreased B/P

Teach patient/family:

- To comply with dosage schedule, even if feeling better; that, if dose is missed, to take it as soon as possible unless it is within 1 hr of next dose
- **To notify prescriber of fever, swelling of hands or feet, irregular heartbeat, chest pain, dizziness, persistent cough**
- That excessive perspiration, dehydration, diarrhea may lead to fall in blood pressure; to consult prescriber if these occur; to maintain hydration
- That product may cause dizziness, fainting, lightheadedness; to rise slowly to sitting or standing position to minimize orthostatic hypotension; to take B/P readings
- To avoid potassium supplements and foods, salt substitutes

Black Box Warning: **Not to take product if pregnant (D) or breastfeeding**

- **Overdose symptoms:** **bradycardia or tachycardia, circulatory collapse**

vancomycin (Rx)

(van-koe-mye′sin)

Vancocin

Func. class.: Antiinfective—miscellaneous

Chem. class.: Tricyclic glycopeptide

V

ACTION: Inhibits bacterial cell-wall synthesis, blocks glycopeptides

USES: *Actinomyces* sp., *Bacillus* sp., *Clostridium difficile, Clostridium* sp., *enterococcus faecalis, Enterococcus faecium, Enterococcus* sp., *Lactobacillus* sp., *Listeria monocytogenes, Staphylococcus aureus (MRSA), Staphylococcus aureus (MSSA), Staphylococcus epidermidis, Staphylococcus* sp., *Streptococcus agalactiae (group B streptococci), Streptococcus bovis, Streptococcus pneumoniae, Streptococcus pyogenes (group A beta-hemolytic streptococci), Viridans streptococci;* may be effective against *Corynebacterium jeikeium, Corynebacterium* sp., pseudomembranous colitis, staphylococcal enterocolitis, endocarditis prophylaxis for dental procedures, bacteremia, joint/bone infections, osteomyelitis, pneumonia, septicemia

Unlabeled uses: Bacterial infection prophylaxis, brain abscess, endocarditis prophylaxis, meningitis, orthopedic device related infection, peritonitis, surgical infection prophylaxis, vancomycin desensitization, ventriculitis

CONTRAINDICATIONS:

Hypersensitivity to this product or corn

Precautions: Pregnancy (B) PO, (C) IV; breastfeeding, neonates, geriatric patients, renal disease, hearing loss

DOSAGE AND ROUTES

Serious staphylococcal infections

- **Adult: IV** 500 mg q6-8hr or 1 g q12hr or 15-20 mg/kg q12hr
- **Child: IV** 40-60 mg/kg/day divided q6-8hr
- **Neonate: IV** 15 mg/kg initially, then 10 mg/kg q8-24hr

Pseudomembranous/ staphylococcal enterocolitis

- **Adult: PO** 125 mg qid × 10-14 days
- **Child: PO (unlabeled)** 40 mg/kg/day divided q6hr × 7-10 days, max 2 g/day

Endocarditis prophylaxis

- **Adult: IV** 2 g divided
- **Child: IV** 20 mg/kg over 1 hr given 1 hr before procedure

Renal dose

- **Adult: IV** 15-20 mg/kg loading dose in seriously ill; individualize all other doses

Available forms: Cap 125, 250 mg; powder for inj 500 mg, 1, 5, 10 g; Dextrose sol for inj 500 mg/100 ml, 750 mg/150 ml, 1 g/200 ml

Administer:

- Use only for susceptible organisms to prevent product-resistant bacteria
- Antihistamine if red-man syndrome occurs: decreased B/P, flushing of neck, face; stop or slow infusion
- Dose based on serum concentration
- **PO:** without regard to food, swallow whole
- Store at room temperature for ≤2 wk after reconstitution

Intermittent IV INFUSION route

- After reconstitution with 10 ml sterile water for inj (500 mg/10 ml); further dilution is needed for IV, 500 mg/100 ml 0.9% NaCl, D_5W given as intermittent infusion over 1 hr; decrease rate of infusion if red-man syndrome occurs

Continuous IV INFUSION route (unlabeled)

- May infuse 1-2 g in volume to give over 24 hr if intermittent IV route cannot be used

Y-site compatibilities: Acetylcysteine, acyclovir, alatrofloxacin, aldesleukin, alemtuzumab, alfentanil, allopurinol, alprostadil, amifostine, amikacin, amino acids injection, aminocaproic acid, amiodarone, amoxicillin-clavulanate, amsacrine, anidulafungin, argatroban, ascorbic acid injection, atenolol, atracurium, atropine, azithromycin, benztropine, bleomycin, bretylium, bumetanide, buprenorphine, butorphanol, calcium chloride/ gluconate, CARBOplatin, carmustine, caspofungin, cefpirome, chlorproMAZINE, cimetidine, ciprofloxacin, cisatracurium, CISplatin, clarithromycin, clindamycin, codeine, cyanocobalamin, cyclophosphamide, cycloSPORINE, cytarabine, DACTINomycin, DAUNOrubicin liposome, dexamethasone, dexmedetomidine, dexrazoxane, digoxin, diltiazem, diphenhydrAMINE, DOBUTamine, DOCEtaxel, dolasetron, DOPamine, doripenem, doxacurium, doxapram, DOXOrubicin, DOXOrubicin liposomal, doxycycline, enalaprilat, ePHEDrine, EPINEPHrine, epirubicin, eptifibatide, ertapenem, erythromycin, esmolol, etoposide, etoposide phosphate, famotidine, fenoldopam, fentaNYL, filgrastim, fluconazole, fludarabine, folic acid (as sodium salt), gallium, gemcitabine, gentamicin, glycopyrrolate, granisetron, HYDROmorphone, hydrOXYzine, ifosfamide, insulin, regular, irinotecan, isoproterenol, isosorbide, ketamine, labetalol, lactated Ringer's injection, lepirudin, levofloxacin, lidocaine, linezolid, LORazepam, magnesium sulfate, mannitol, mechlorethamine, melphalan, meperidine, meropenem, metaraminol, methyldopate, metoclopramide, metoprolol, metroNIDAZOLE, midazolam, milrinone, minocycline, mitoXANtrone, morphine, morphine, multiple vitamins injection, mycophenolate, nalbuphine, naloxone, nesiritide, netilmicin, niCARdipine, nitroglycerin, nitroprusside, norepinephrine, octreotide, ofloxacin, ondansetron, oxacillin, oxaliplatin, oxytocin, PACLitaxel (solvent/surfactant), palonosetron, pamidronate, pancuronium, papaverine, PEMEtrexed, penicillin G potassium/sodium, pentamidine, pentazocine, PENTobarbital, perphenazine, PHENobarbital, phentolamine, phenylephrine, phytonadione, piritramide, polymyxin B, potassium acetate/chloride, procainamide, prochlorperazine, promethazine, propranolol, protamine, pyridoxine, quiNIDine, ranitidine, remifentanil, rifampin, Ringer's injection, riTUXimab, sodium acetate/bicarbonate/citrate, succinylcholine, SUFentanil, tacrolimus, teniposide, thiamine, thiotepa, tigecycline, tirofiban, TNA (3-in-1), tobramycin, tolazoline, TPN (2-in-1), trastuzumab, urapidil, vasopressin, vecuronium, verapamil, vinBLAStine, vinCRIStine, vinorelbine, voriconazole, zidovudine, zoledronic acid

SIDE EFFECTS

CNS: Headache
CV: Cardiac arrest, vascular collapse (rare), hypotension, peripheral edema
EENT: *Ototoxicity, permanent deafness,* tinnitus, nystagmus
GI: Nausea, pseudomembranous colitis
GU: Nephrotoxicity, *increased BUN, creatinine, albumin,* fatal uremia
HEMA: Leukopenia, eosinophilia, neutropenia
INTEG: Chills, fever, rash, thrombophlebitis at inj site, urticaria, pruritus, necrosis (red-man syndrome), skin/subcutaneous tissue disorders
MS: Back pain
RESP: Wheezing, dyspnea
SYST: Anaphylaxis, superinfection

PHARMACOKINETICS

PO: Absorption poor
IV: Onset rapid, peak 1 hr, half-life 4-8 hr, excreted in urine (active form)

INTERACTIONS

Increase: ototoxicity or nephrotoxicity—aminoglycosides, cephalosporins, colistin, polymyxin, bacitracin, CISplatin, amphotericin B, methotrexate, NSAIDs, cycloSPORINE, acyclovir, adefovir, capreomycin, foscarnet, ganciclovir, pamidronate, IV pentamidine, streptozocin, tacrolimus, zoledronic acid
• Do not use with cholestyramine, colestipol, cidofovir
Increase: lactic acidosis—metFORMIN
Increase: neuromuscular effects—nondepolarizing muscle relaxants
Drug/Lab Test
Increase: BUN/creatinine, eosinophils
Decrease: WBC

NURSING CONSIDERATIONS

Assess:
• **Infection:** WBC, urine, stools, sputum, characteristics of wound throughout treatment
• I&O ratio; report hematuria, oliguria; nephrotoxicity may occur, BUN, creatinine
• Serum levels: peak 1 hr after 1-hr infusion 25-40 mg/L, trough before next dose 5-10 mg/L, especially in renal disease
• C&S

V

- Auditory function during, after treatment; hearing loss, ringing, roaring in ears; product should be discontinued
- B/P during administration; sudden drop may indicate red-man syndrome
- Skin eruptions
- **Red-man syndrome:** flushing of neck, face, upper body, arms, back, may lead to anaphylaxis; slow IV infusion to >1 hr
- EPINEPHrine, suction, tracheostomy set, endotracheal intubation equipment on unit; anaphylaxis may occur
- Adequate intake of fluids (2 L/day) to prevent nephrotoxicity

Evaluate:

- Therapeutic response: absence of fever, sore throat; negative culture

Teach patient/family:

- About all aspects of product therapy; about the need to complete entire course of medication to ensure organism death (7-10 days); that culture may be taken after completed course of medication
- To report sore throat, fever, fatigue; could indicate superinfection
- That product must be taken in equal intervals around the clock to maintain blood levels

vardenafil (Rx)

(var-den′a-fil)

Levitra, Staxyn

Func. class.: Erectile dysfunction agent

Chem. class.: Phosphodiesterase type 5 inhibitor

ACTION: Inhibits phosphodiesterase type 5 (PDE5), enhances erectile function by increasing the amount of cGMP, which in turn causes smooth muscle relaxation and increased blood flow into the corpus cavernosum

USES: Treatment of erectile dysfunction

CONTRAINDICATIONS: Hypersensitivity, coadministration of α-blockers or nitrates, renal failure, congenital or acquired QT prolongation

Precautions: Pregnancy (B); not indicated for women, children, or newborns; hepatic impairment, retinitis pigmentosa, anatomical penile deformities, sickle cell anemia, leukemia, multiple myeloma, bleeding disorders, active peptic ulceration, CV/renal disease

DOSAGE AND ROUTES

- **Adult: PO** 10 mg taken 1 hr before sexual activity; dose may be reduced to 5 mg or increased to max 20 mg; max dosing frequency once daily; orally disintegrating tab 10 mg 60 min before sexual activity; do not use with potent CYP3A4 inhibitors
- **Geriatric >65 yr: PO** 5 mg initially, titrated as needed/tolerated

Hepatic dose

- **Adult: PO** (Child-Pugh B) 5 mg, max 10 mg/day

Concomitant medications

- Ritonavir, max 2.5 mg q72hr; for indinavir, ketoconazole 400 mg/day and itraconazole 400 mg/day, max 2.5 mg/day; for ketoconazole 200 mg/day, itraconazole 200 mg/day and erythromycin max 5 mg/day

Available forms: Tabs 2.5, 5, 10, 20 mg; orally disintegrating tab 10 mg

Administer:

- Approximately 1 hr before sexual activity; do not use more than once daily; orally disintegrating tabs are not interchangeable with film-coated tabs
- Without regard to food; avoid taking with high-fat meal
- **Oral disintegrating tab:** place on tongue, allow to dissolve, do not use water

SIDE EFFECTS

CNS: *Headache, flushing, dizziness, insomnia,* seizures, transient global amnesia

CV: Hypertension, MI, CV collapse, chest pain

EENT: Conjunctivitis, tinnitus, photophobia, diminished vision, glaucoma, hearing loss

GU: Abnormal ejaculation, priapism
MISC: Rash, GERD, GGTP increased, NAION (nonarteritic ischemic optic neuropathy), dyspepsia
MS: Myalgia, arthralgia, neck pain
RESP: Rhinitis, sinusitis, dyspnea, pharyngitis, epistaxis

PHARMACOKINETICS

Rapidly absorbed, bioavailability 15%, protein binding 95%, metabolized by liver, terminal half-life 4-5 hr, onset 20 min, peak $^1/_2$-$1^1/_2$ hr, duration <5 hr, reduced absorption with high-fat meal, primarily excreted in feces (91%-95%)

INTERACTIONS

⚠ Do not use with nitrates because of unsafe decrease in B/P, which could result in MI or stroke
⚠ Serious dysrhythmias: class IA/III antiarrhythmics, clarithromycin, droperidol, procainamide, quiNIDine, quinolones; do not use concurrently
Increase: hypotension—α-blockers, protease inhibitors, metoprolol, NIFEdipine, alcohol, amLODIPine, angiotensin II receptor blockers; do not use concurrently
Increase: vardenafil levels—erythromycin, azole antifungals (ketoconazole, itraconazole), cimetidine, antiretroviral protease inhibitors
Drug/Food
Decrease: absorption—high-fat meal
Drug/Lab Test
Increase: CK

NURSING CONSIDERATIONS

Assess:
- Erectile dysfunction and cause before treatment

⚠ Any severe loss of vision while taking this or similar products; products should not be used
⚠ Use of organic nitrates that should not be used with this product

Teach patient/family:
- That product does not protect against STDs, including HIV
- That product absorption is reduced with high-fat meal
- That product should not be used with nitrates in any form; to inform physician of all medications being taken
- That product has no effect in the absence of sexual stimulation; that patient should seek immediate medical attention if erections last >4 hr

⚠ To notify prescriber immediately and stop taking product if vision loss occurs

varenicline (Rx)

(var-e-ni′kleen)
Champix ✱, Chantix
Func. class.: Smoking cessation agent
Chem. class.: Nicotine receptor agonist

ACTION: Partial agonist for nicotine receptors; partially activates receptors to help curb cravings; occupies receptors to prevent nicotine binding

USES: Smoking deterrent

CONTRAINDICATIONS: Hypersensitivity, eating disorders

Precautions: Pregnancy (C), breastfeeding, children <18 yr, geriatric patients, renal disease, recent MI, angioedema

Black Box Warning: Bipolar disorder, depression, schizophrenia, suicidal ideation

DOSAGE AND ROUTES

Smoking cessation
- **Adult: PO** therapy should begin 1 wk before smoking stop date (i.e., take product plus tobacco for 7 days); titrate for 1 wk; days 1 through 3, 0.5 mg/day; days 4 through 7, 0.5 mg bid; day 8 through end of treatment, 1 mg bid; treatment is for 12 wk and may be repeated for another 12 wk

Renal dose
- **Adult: PO** CCr ≤50 ml/min, titrate to max 0.5 mg bid

V

Available forms: Tabs 0.5, 1 mg; Chantix continuing month PAK; Chantix starting month PAK

Administer:

- Do not break, crush, or chew tabs
- Increased fluids, bulk in diet if constipation occurs
- After eating with a full glass of water
- Sugarless gum, hard candy, or frequent sips of water for dry mouth

SIDE EFFECTS

CNS: Headache, agitation, dizziness, insomnia, abnormal dreams, fatigue, malaise, behavior changes, depression, suicidal ideation, amnesia, hallucinations, hostility, mania, psychosis, tremors

CV: Dysrhythmias, hypo/hypertension, palpitations, tachycardia, angina, MI

EENT: *Blurred vision,* tinnitus

GI: *Nausea, vomiting,* anorexia, *dry mouth,* increased/decreased appetite, *constipation,* flatulence, GERD

GU: Erectile dysfunction, urinary frequency, menstrual irregularities

INTEG: Rash, pruritus, angioedema, Stevens-Johnson syndrome

MISC: Weight loss or gain

RESP: Dyspnea, rhinorrhea

PHARMACOKINETICS

Elimination half-life 24 hr; metabolism minimal; 93% excreted unchanged in urine; steady state 4 days, onset 4 days, peak 3-4 hr

NURSING CONSIDERATIONS

Assess:

- **Smoking history:** motivation for smoking cessation, years used, amount each day; smoking cessation after 12 wk; if progress not made, product may be used for additional 12 wk
- Renal function in geriatric patients; cardiac status in cardiac disease

Black Box Warning: Neuropsychiatric symptoms: mood, sensorium, affect; behavior changes, agitation, depression, suicidal ideation; suicide has occurred; possible worsening of depression, schizophrenia, bipolar disorder

Evaluate:

- Therapeutic response: smoking cessation

Teach patient/family:

- That treatment for smoking cessation lasts 12 wk and that another 12 wk may be required
- To use caution when driving, performing other activities requiring alertness; blurred vision may occur
- To set a date to quit smoking and to initiate treatment 1 wk before that date
- How to titrate product
- Not to use with nicotine patches unless directed by prescriber; may increase B/P
- To notify prescriber if pregnancy planned or suspected
- About common side effects to be expected

Black Box Warning: To notify prescriber immediately of change in thought/behavior (suicidal ideation, hostility, depression), stop product

vasopressin (Rx)

(vay-soe-press′in)

Pressyn ✦

Func. class.: Pituitary hormone

Chem. class.: Lysine vasopressin

ACTION:
Promotes the reabsorption of water via action on the renal tubular epithelium; causes vasoconstriction

USES:
Diabetes insipidus (nonnephrogenic/nonpsychogenic), abdominal distention postoperatively, bleeding esophageal varices

CONTRAINDICATIONS:
Hypersensitivity, chronic nephritis

Precautions: Pregnancy (C), breastfeeding, CAD, asthma, vascular/renal disease, migraines, seizures

DOSAGE AND ROUTES

Diabetes insipidus

- **Adult: IM/SUBCUT** 5-10 units bid-qid as needed; **CONT IV INFUSION**

0.0005 units/kg/hr (0.05 milliunit/kg/hr), double dose q30min as needed

• **Child: IM/SUBCUT** 2.5-10 units bid-qid as needed; **IM/SUBCUT** 1.25-2.5 units q2-3days (Pitressin Tannate) for chronic therapy

Abdominal distention

• **Adult: IM** 5 units, then q3-4hr, increasing to 10 units if needed (aqueous)

Available forms: sol for inj 20 units/ml

SIDE EFFECTS

CNS: Drowsiness, headache, lethargy, flushing, vertigo

CV: Increased B/P, dysrhythmias, **cardiac arrest, shock, chest pain, MI**

EENT: Nasal irritation, congestion, rhinitis

GI: Nausea, heartburn, cramps, vomiting, flatus

GU: Vulval pain, uterine cramping

MISC: Tremors, sweating, vertigo, urticaria, bronchial constriction

PHARMACOKINETICS

Nasal: Onset 1 hr; duration 3-8 hr; half-life 15 min; metabolized in liver, kidneys; excreted in urine

INTERACTIONS

Increase: antidiuretic effect—tricyclics, carBAMazepine, chloropromide, fludrocortisone, clofibrate, urea

Decrease: antidiuretic effect—lithium, demeclocycline

NURSING CONSIDERATIONS

Assess:

• Pulse, B/P when giving product IV or IM

• I&O ratio, weight daily; fluid/electrolyte balance; check for edema in extremities; if water retention is severe, diuretic may be prescribed

• **Water intoxication: lethargy, behavioral changes, disorientation, neuromuscular excitability**

• Small doses may precipitate coronary adverse effects; keep emergency equipment nearby

Evaluate:

• Therapeutic response: absence of severe thirst, decreased urine output, osmolality

Teach patient/family:

• To measure and record I&O

• To avoid alcohol, all OTC medications unless approved by prescriber

vedolizumab

(ve′-doe-liz′ue-mab)

Entyvio

Func. class.: Immunosuppressive, biologic response modifiers

ACTION:

A specific integrin receptor antagonist that inhibits the migration of specific memory T-lymphocytes across the endothelium into inflamed gastrointestinal parenchymal tissue. The action reduces the chronic inflammatory process present in both ulcerative colitis and Crohn's disease

USES:

For moderately to severely active ulcerative colitis/Crohn's disease to reduce signs and symptoms, and to induce and maintain clinical remission in patients who have an inadequate response to conventional therapy

CONTRAINDICATIONS:

Hypersensitivity

Precautions: Hepatic disease, infections, progressive multifocal leukoencephalopathy (PML), pregnancy (B), breastfeeding

DOSAGE AND ROUTES

• **Adults: IV** INFUSION 300 mg 30 min at weeks 0, 2, and 6 as induction therapy, then 300 mg q8wk

Available forms: Powder for injection 300 mg

Administer:

• Full response is usually observed by 6 wk; those who do not respond by week 14 are unlikely to respond

- Give as IV infusion only, do not use as an IV push or bolus
- Make sure all immunizations are up to date
- Reconstitute with 4.8 ml of sterile water for injection, using a syringe with a 21- to 25-gauge needle
- Insert the syringe needle into the vial and direct the stream of sterile water for injection to the glass wall of the vial, gently swirl the solution for 15 sec, do not shake
- Allow the solution to stand for up to 20 min at room temperature to allow for reconstitution and for any foam to settle
- Once dissolved, product should be clear or opalescent, colorless to light brownish yellow, and free of visible particulates. Discard if discolored or if foreign particles are present
- Before withdrawing solution from vial, gently invert vial 3 times. Withdraw 5 ml (300 mg) of reconstructed product using a 21- to 25-gauge needle. Discard remaining product
- Add the 5 ml (300 mg) of reconstituted product to 250 ml of sterile 0.9% sodium chloride and gently mix infusion bag. Do not mix with other medications. Administer solution as soon as possible; if necessary, may be stored for up to 4 hr refrigerated, do not freeze. Infuse over 30 min; after infusion, flush line with 30 ml of sterile 0.9% sodium chloride injection. Discard any unused infusion solution

SIDE EFFECTS

CNS: Headache, fatigue, dizziness
GI: Nausea, vomiting
MISC: Rash, pruritus, infusion-related reactions
MS: Arthralgia, back pain
SYST: Anaphylaxis, progressive multifocal leukoencephalopathy (PML)

INTERACTIONS

Increase: infection risk—immunosuppressives, natalizumab, antineoplastics
Do not use with tumor necrosis factor (TNF) modifiers
Decrease: immune response—vaccines, toxoids

NURSING CONSIDERATIONS

Assess:

- **Ulcerative colitis/Crohn's disease:** Monitor symptoms before and after treatment
- **Liver dysfunction:** Elevated hepatic enzymes, jaundice, malaise, nausea, vomiting, abdominal pain, and anorexia are predictive of severe liver injury that may be fatal or may require a liver transplant in some patients; if hepatic dysfunction is suspected, discontinue
- **Tuberculosis (TB) latent/active:** Obtain TB skin test both before and during treatment. Do not give in active infection like influenza or sepsis
- **Progressive multifocal leukoencephalopathy (PML):** Increased weakness on one side of the body or clumsiness of limbs, visual disturbance, and changes in thinking, memory, and orientation leading to confusion and personality changes; severe disability or death can come over weeks or months

Evaluate:

- Therapeutic response: lessening of ulcerative colitis and Crohn's disease

Teach patient/family:

- About the symptoms of infection and to report to health care provider immediately
- To report planned or suspected pregnancy, or if breastfeeding

⚠ HIGH ALERT

vemurafenib

Zelboraf

Func. class.: Biologic response modifiers; signal transduction inhibitors (STIs)

ACTION: Inhibitor of some mutated forms of BRAF serine threonine kinase, thereby blocking cellular proliferation in melanoma cells with the mutation; inhibits other kinases including CRAF, ARAF, wild-type BRAF, SRMA, ACK1, MAP4H5, and FGR; potent adenosine triphosphate-competitice inhibitor of RAFs, with a modest preference for mutant BRAF and CRAF compared with wild-type BRAF

USES:
Unresectable or metastatic malignant melanoma with V600E mutation of the BRAF gene

Precautions: Pregnancy (D), breastfeeding, children, infants, neonates, hepatic disease, QT prolongation, secondary malignancy, torsades de pointes, hypokalemia, hypomagnesia, sunlight exposure

DOSAGE AND ROUTES

• **Adult: PO** 960 mg (4 tabs) bid about q12hr

Dose adjustments for toxicity due to symptomatic adverse reactions or QTc prolongation

Grade 1 or tolerable grade 2 adverse events: no dosage change; **intolerable grade 2 or grade 3 adverse events (1st episode):** interrupt treatment until toxicity resolves to grade ≤1, when resuming, reduce dosage to 720 mg (3 tabs) bid; **intolerable grade 2 or grade 3 adverse events (2nd episode):** interrupt treatment until toxicity resolves to grade ≤1, when resuming, reduce dose to 480 mg (2 tabs) bid; **intolerable grade 2 or grade 3 adverse events (3rd episode)** discontinue treatment permanently; **grade 4 adverse events (1st episode):** discontinue permanently or interrupt until toxicity resolves to grade ≤1, when resuming, reduce dose to 480 mg (2 tabs) bid; **grade 4 adverse events (2nd episode):** discontinue permanently

Available forms: Tabs 240 mg

Administer:

• Continue until disease progresses or unacceptable toxicity occurs

• Missed doses can be taken up to 4 hr before the next dose is due; take about 12 hr apart, take without regard to meals

• Swallow whole with a full glass of water; do not crush or chew

• Store at room temperature in original container

SIDE EFFECTS

CNS: *Fatigue, fever, asthenia, headache,* dizziness, peripheral neuropathy, muscle paralysis

CV: **QT prolongation, atrial fibrillation,** peripheral edema, hypotension

EENT: Uveitis, blurred vision, iritis, photophobia

GI: *Nausea, diarrhea, vomiting, constipation, dysgeusia, decreased appetite,* weight loss

INTEG: *Alopecia, pruritus, hyperkeratosis, maculopapular rash, actinic keratosis, xerosis/dry skin, papular rash, palmar-plantar erythrodysesthesia (hand and foot syndrome), photosensitivity*

MS: *Arthralgia, myalgias, extremity pain, musculoskeletal pain, back pain,* arthritis

RESP: Cough

SYST: **Secondary malignancy, anaphylaxis**

PHARMACOKINETICS

>99% protein binding (albumin and alpha-1 acid glycoprotein) an inhibitor of CYP1A2, 2A6, 2C9, 2C19, 2D6, 3A4/5 CYP1A2 inhibitor, a weak CYP2D6 inhibitor, and a CYP3A4 inducer; elimination 94% in feces, 1% in urine, half-life 57 hr

INTERACTIONS

Increase: vemurafenib effect—CYP3A4/CYP1A2 inhibitors (enoxacin, cimetidine, delavirdine, indinavir, isoniazid, itraconazole, dalfopristin, quinupristin, tipranavir)

⚠ **Increase: QT prolongation, torsades de pointes—arsenic trioxide, certain phenothiazines (chlorproMAZINE, mesoridazine, thioridazine), grepafloxacin, levomethadyl, pentamidine, probucol, sparfloxacin, troleandomycin, class IA antiarrhythmics (disopyramide, procainamide, quiNIDine), class III antiarrhythmics (amiodarone, dofetilide, ibutilide, sotalol), clarithromycin, ziprasidone, pimozide, haloperidol, halofantrine, quiNIDine, chloroquine, dronedarone, droperidol, erythromycin, methadone, posaconazole, propafenone, saquinavir, abarelix, amoxapine, apomorphine, asenapine,**

V

β-agonists, ofloxacin, eribulin, ezogabine, flecainide, gatifloxacin, gemifloxacin, halogenated anesthetics, iloperidone, levofloxacin, local anesthetics, magnesium sulfate, potassium sulfate, sodium, maprotiline, moxifloxacin, nilotinib, norfloxacin, ciprofloxacin, OLANZapine, paliperidone, some phenothiazines (fluPHENAZine, perphenazine, prochlorperazine, trifluoperazine), telavancin, tetrabenazine, tricyclic antidepressants, venlafaxine, vorinostat, citalopram, alfuzosin, cloZAPine, cyclobenzaprine, dolasetron, palonosetron, QUEtiapine, rilpivirine, SUNItinib, tacrolimus, vardenafil, indacaterol, dasatinib, fluconazole, lapatinib, lopinavir/ritonavir, mefloquine, octreotide, ondansetron, ranolazine, risperiDONE, telithromycin, vemurafenib

Decrease: vemurafenib effect—CYP3A4 inducers (rifampin, barbiturates, carBAMazepine, phenytoin, erythromycin, ketoconazole, fluvoxaMINE, alcohol, etravirine, ritonavir, bexarotene, rifabutin, OXcarbazepine, nevirapine, modafinil, metyrapone)

Drug/Lab Test:

Increase: serum creatinine, LFTs, alkaline phosphatase, bilirubin

NURSING CONSIDERATIONS

Assess:

- **Hepatic disease:** Liver function test (LFT) abnormalities, altered bilirubin levels, may occur; monitor LFTs and bilirubin levels before treatment, then monthly; more frequent testing is needed in those with grade 2 or greater toxicities; laboratory alterations should be managed with dose reduction, treatment interruption, or discontinuation

⚠ **QT prolongation:** has been reported with the use of this product; therefore, should be avoided in patients with QT prolongation; monitor ECG and electrolytes in those with congestive heart failure, bradycardia, electrolyte imbalance (hypokalemia, hypomagnesemia), or those who are taking concomitant medications known to prolong the QT interval; treatment interruption, dosage adjustment, treatment discontinuation may be needed in those who develop QT prolongation

⚠ **Pregnancy/breastfeeding:** Identify if pregnancy is planned or suspected, pregnancy (D); avoid breastfeeding

- Serum electrolytes

Evaluate:

- Decreased spread of malignancy

Teach patient/family:

- That missed doses can be taken up to 4 hr before the next dose is due to maintain the twice-daily regimen

⚠ Teach patient to use reliable contraception; both women and men of childbearing age should use adequate contraceptive methods during therapy and for at least 90 days after completing treatment, pregnancy (D)

venlafaxine (Rx)

(ven-la-fax′een)

Effexor ✦, Effexor XR

Func. class.: Antidepressant—SNRI

Chem. class.: SNRI

ACTION: Potent inhibitor of neuronal serotonin and norepinephrine uptake, weak inhibitor of dopamine; no muscarinic, histaminergic, or α-adrenergic receptors in vitro

USES: Prevention/treatment of major depression; depression at the end of life; long-term treatment of general anxiety disorder, panic disorder, social anxiety disorder (Effexor XR only)

Unlabeled uses: Hot flashes, premenstrual dysphoric disorder (PMDD), headache, neuropathic pain, fibromyalgia, diabetic neuropathy

CONTRAINDICATIONS: Hypersensitivity

Precautions: Pregnancy (C), breastfeeding, geriatric patients, mania, hypertension, seizure disorder, recent MI, cardiac/renal/hepatic disease, eosinophilic pneumonia, desvenlafaxine hypersensitivity, bipolar disorder, interstitial lung disease

Black Box Warning: Children, suicidal ideation

DOSAGE AND ROUTES

Depression

- **Adult: PO** 75 mg/day in 2-3 divided doses; taken with food, may be increased to 150 mg/day; if needed, may be further increased to 225 mg/day; increments of 75 mg/day at intervals of ≥4 days; some hospitalized patients may require up to 375 mg/day in 3 divided doses; **EXT REL** 37.5-75 mg PO daily, max 225 mg/day; give XR daily

Anxiety disorders

- **Adult: PO** 75 mg/day or 37.5 mg/day × 4-7 days initially, max 225 mg/day

Renal dose

- **Adult: PO** CCr 10-70 ml/min, reduce dose by 25%-50%; CCr <10 ml/min, reduce dose by 50%

Hepatic dose

- **Adult: PO** Moderate impairment, 50% of dose

Hot flashes (unlabeled)

- **Adult (male, prostate cancer): PO** 12.5 mg bid × 4 wk; females 37.5-75 mg/day

Neuropathic pain, diabetic neuropathy, headache, fibromyalgia (unlabeled)

- **Adult: PO** 37.5-75 mg/day, max 75 mg bid (regular rel) or 150 mg/day (ext rel)

Premenstrual dysphoric disorder (PMDD) (unlabeled)

- **Adult female: PO** 50-200 mg/day, start at 50 mg/day for 1st cycle, titrate upward

Available forms: Tabs scored 25, 37.5, 50, 75, 100 mg; ext rel cap (Effexor XR) 37.5, 75, 150 mg

Administer:

- With food, milk for GI symptoms; do not crush, chew caps; caps can be opened and contents sprinkled on applesauce, given with full glass of water
- Sugarless gum, hard candy, frequent sips of water for dry mouth
- Avoid use with CNS depressants
- Give in small amounts because of suicide potential, especially at beginning of therapy
- Store in tight container at room temperature; do not freeze

SIDE EFFECTS

CNS: Emotional lability, *dizziness, weakness,* apathy, ataxia, headache, tremors, hypertonia, euphoria, hallucinations, hostility, insomnia, anxiety, **suicidal ideation in children/adolescents, seizures, neuroleptic-malignant-syndrome–like reaction**

CV: Angina pectoris, hypertension, tachycardia, **change in QTcinterval,** increased cholesterol, extrasystoles, syncope

EENT: *Abnormal vision,* taste, *ear pain*

GI: *Dysphagia, eructation, nausea,* anorexia, dry mouth, colitis, gastritis, gingivitis, *constipation,* stomatitis, stomach and mouth ulceration

GU: *Anorgasmia,* abnormal ejaculation, urinary frequency, decreased libido, impotence, menstrual changes, *impaired urination*

HEMA: **Thrombocytopenia, leukocytosis, leukopenia, abnormal bleeding**

INTEG: Ecchymosis, brittle nails, dry skin, photosensitivity, sweating, **Stevens-Johnson syndrome; angioedema (ext rel)**

META: *Peripheral edema, weight loss,* edema, glycosuria, hyperlipemia, hypokalemia

MS: Arthritis, bone pain, tenosynovitis, arthralgia

RESP: *Bronchitis, dyspnea,* cough

SYST: **Neonatal abstinence syndrome**

PHARMACOKINETICS

Well absorbed; extensively metabolized in liver by CYP2D6 to active metabolite; 87% of product recovered in urine; 27% protein binding; half-life 5, 11 hr (active metabolite), respectively

V

INTERACTIONS

⚠ **Hyperthermia, rigidity, rapid fluctuations of vital signs, mental status changes, neuroleptic malignant syndrome: MAOIs**

Increase: bleeding risk—salicylates, NSAIDs, platelet inhibitors, anticoagulants

Increase: venlafaxine effect—cimetidine
Increase: CNS depression—alcohol, opioids, antihistamines, sedative/hypnotics
Increase: levels of cloZAPine, desipramine, haloperidol, warfarin
Increase: serotonin syndrome—sibutramine, SUMAtriptan, traZODone, traMADol, SSRIs, serotonin receptor agonist, linezolid, methylene blue, tryptophan
Decrease: effect of indinavir
Decrease: venlafaxine effect—cyproheptadine

Drug/Herb

- Serotonin syndrome: St. John's wort, tryptophan

Increase: CNS depression—kava, valerian

Drug/Lab Test

Increase: alk phos, bilirubin, AST, ALT, BUN, creatinine, serum cholesterol, CPK, LDH
False positive: amphetamines, phencyclidine

NURSING CONSIDERATIONS

Assess:

Black Box Warning: Mental status: mood, sensorium, affect, increase in psychiatric symptoms; depression, panic; assess for suicidal ideation in children/adolescents

- B/P lying, standing; pulse q4hr; if systolic B/P drops 20 mm Hg, hold product, notify prescriber; take VS q4hr in patients with CV disease

⚠ **Bleeding:** GI, ecchymosis, epistaxis, hematomas, petechiae, hemorrhage
- Blood studies: CBC, differential, leukocytes, cardiac enzymes if patient is receiving long-term therapy
- Hepatic studies: AST, ALT, bilirubin
- Weight weekly; weight loss or gain; appetite may increase; peripheral edema may occur; monitor cholesterol
- **Withdrawal symptoms:** flulike symptoms, headache, nervousness, agitation, nausea, vomiting, muscle pain, weakness; not usual unless product is discontinued abruptly

⚠ **Serotonin syndrome, neuroleptic malignant syndrome:** increased heart rate, shivering, sweating, dilated pupils, tremors, high B/P, hyperthermia, headache, confusion; if these occur, stop product, administer serotonin antagonist if needed; usually worse if given with linezolid, methylene blue, tryptophan
- Assistance with ambulation during beginning therapy because drowsiness, dizziness occur

Evaluate:

- Therapeutic response: decreased depression, anxiety; increased well-being

Teach patient/family:

- To notify prescriber of rash, hives, allergic reactions, bleeding
- To use with caution when driving, performing other activities requiring alertness because of drowsiness, dizziness, blurred vision

Black Box Warning: That worsening of symptoms, suicidal thoughts/behaviors may occur in children/young adults, discuss with family members

- To avoid alcohol ingestion
- Not to discontinue medication abruptly after long-term use; may cause nausea, headache, malaise, taper over 14 days
- To wear sunscreen or large hat because photosensitivity occurs
- To avoid pregnancy or breastfeeding while taking this product; birth defects have occurred when used in the 3rd trimester
- To monitor B/P with hypertension
- **Serotonin syndrome, neuroleptic malignant syndrome:** Advise patient to report immediately shivering, sweating, tremors, fever, dilated pupils
- To take as prescribed, contents of capsule may be sprinkled on applesauce if unable to swallow whole

TREATMENT OF OVERDOSE:

ECG monitoring; lavage, activated charcoal; administer anticonvulsant; may require whole-bowel irrigation for ext rel product

verapamil (Rx)

(ver-ap′a-mill)

Apo-Verap ♣, Calan, Calan SR, Chronovera ♣, Covera ♣, Isoptin SR, Tarka ♣, Verelan, Verelan PM

Func. class.: Calcium channel blocker; antihypertensive; antianginal, antidysrhythmic (class IV)

Chem. class.: Diphenylalkylamine

ACTION: Inhibits calcium ion influx across cell membrane during cardiac depolarization; produces relaxation of coronary vascular smooth muscle; dilates coronary arteries; decreases SA/AV node conduction; dilates peripheral arteries

USES: Chronic stable, vasospastic, unstable angina; dysrhythmias, hypertension, supraventricular tachycardia, atrial flutter or fibrillation

Unlabeled uses: Prevention of migraine headaches, claudication, mania

CONTRAINDICATIONS: Sick sinus syndrome, 2nd-/3rd-degree heart block, hypotension <90 mm Hg systolic, cardiogenic shock, severe CHF, Lown-Ganong-Levine syndrome, Wolff-Parkinson-White syndrome

Precautions: Pregnancy (C), breastfeeding, children, geriatric patients, CHF, hypotension, hepatic injury, renal disease, concomitant β-blocker therapy

DOSAGE AND ROUTES

Angina

- **Adult: PO** 80-120 mg tid, increase weekly, max 480 mg/day

Dysrhythmias

- **Adult: PO** 240-480 mg/day in 3-4 divided doses in digitalized patients
- **Adult: IV BOL** 5-10 mg (0.075-0.15 mg/kg) over 2 min, may repeat 10 mg (0.15 mg/kg) ½ hr after 1st dose
- **Child 1-15 yr: IV BOL** 0.1-0.3 mg/kg over ≥2 min, repeat in 30 min, max 5 mg in single dose
- **Child 0-1 yr: IV BOL** 0.1-0.2 mg/kg over ≥2 min, may repeat after 30 min

Hypertension

- **Adult: PO** 80 mg tid, may titrate upward; **EXT REL** 120-240 mg/day as single dose, may increase to 240-480 mg/day

Hepatic disease/geriatric patients/compromised ventricular function

- **Adult: PO** 40 mg tid initially, increase as tolerated

Claudication due to PVD (unlabeled)

- **Adult: PO** 120-480 mg/day in divided doses

Mania (unlabeled)

- **Adult: PO** 160-320 mg/day in divided doses, may be given with lithium

Migraine prophylaxis (unlabeled)

- **Adult: PO** 80 mg tid

Available forms: Tabs 40, 80, 120 mg; ext rel tabs 120, 180, 240 mg; inj 2.5 mg/ml in ampules, syringes, vials; ext rel caps 100, 200, 240, 300 mg

Administer:

PO route

- **Reg rel:** Give without regard to food

Ext rel route

- Do not crush or chew ext rel products; caps may be opened and contents sprinkled on food; do not dissolve chew cap contents
- Before meals, at bedtime; give ext rel product with food

Direct IV route

- Undiluted through Y-tube or 3-way stopcock of compatible sol; give over 2 min or 3 min for geriatric patients, with continuous ECG and B/P monitoring, discard unused solution
- Do not use IV with IV β-blockers, may cause AV nodal blockade

Y-site compatibilities: Alfentanil, amikacin, argatroban, ascorbic acid, atracurium, atropine, aztreonam, bivalirudin, bumetanide, buprenorphine, butorphanol, calcium chloride/gluconate, CARBOplatin, caspofungin, ceFAZolin, cefonicid, cefotaxime, cefoTEtan, cefOXitin, ceftizoxime, cefTRIAXone, cefuroxime, chlorproMAZINE, cimetidine, ciprofloxacin,

V

clindamycin, cyanocobalamin, cyclophosphamide, cycloSPORINE, cytarabine, DACTINomycin, DAPTOmycin, dexamethasone, dexmedetomidine, digoxin, diltiazem, diphenhydrAMINE, DOBUTamine, DOCEtaxel, DOPamine, doxacurium, DOXOrubicin hydrochloride, doxycycline, enalaprilat, ePHEDrine, EPINEPHrine, epirubicin, epoetin alfa, eptifibatide, erythromycin, esmolol, etoposide, etoposide phosphate, famotidine, fenoldopam, fentaNYL, fluconazole, fludarabine, gemcitabine, gentamicin, glycopyrrolate, granisetron, heparin, hydrALAZINE, hydrocortisone, HYDROmorphone, ifosfamide, imipenem/cilastatin, inamrinone, insulin, isoproterenol, ketorolac, labetalol, levofloxacin, lidocaine, linezolid, LORazepam, magnesium sulfate, mannitol, mechlorethamine, meperidine, metaraminol, methotrexate, methoxamine, methyldopate, methylPREDNISolone, metoclopramide, metoprolol, metroNIDAZOLE, miconazole, midazolam, milrinone, mitoXANtrone, morphine, multivitamins, nalbuphine, naloxone, nesiritide, nitroglycerin, nitroprusside, norepinephrine, octreotide, ondansetron, oxaliplatin, oxytocin, PACLitaxel, palonosetron, papaverine, PEMEtrexed, penicillin G, pentamidine, pentazocine, phentolamine, phenylephrine, phytonadione, piperacillin/tazobactam, potassium chloride, procainamide, prochlorperazine, promethazine, propranolol, protamine, pyridoxime, quinupristin/dalfopristin, ranitidine, rocuronium, sodium acetate, succinylcholine, SUFentanil, tacrolimus, teniposide, theophylline, thiamine, ticarcillin/clavulanate, tirofiban, tobramycin, tolazoline, trimethaphan, urokinase, vancomycin, vasopressin, vecuronium, vinCRIStine, vinorelbine, voriconazole

SIDE EFFECTS

CNS: *Headache, drowsiness,* dizziness, anxiety, depression, weakness, insomnia, confusion, lightheadedness, asthenia, fatigue

CV: *Edema,* **CHF**, bradycardia, hypotension, palpitations, AV block, **dysrhythmias**

GI: *Nausea,* diarrhea, gastric upset, *constipation,* increased LFTs

GU: Impotence, gynecomastia, nocturia, polyuria

HEMA: Bruising, petechiae, bleeding

INTEG: Rash, bruising

MISC: Gingival hyperplasia

SYST: **Stevens-Johnson syndrome**

PHARMACOKINETICS

Metabolized by liver, excreted in urine (70% as metabolites)

PO: Onset variable; peak 3-4 hr; duration 17-24 hr; half-life (biphasic) 4 min, 3-7 hr (terminal)

IV: Onset 3 min, peak 3-5 min, duration 10-20 min

INTERACTIONS

Increase: hypotension—prazosin, quiNIDine, fentaNYL, other antihypertensives, nitrates

Increase: effects of verapamil—β-blockers, cimetidine, clarithromycin, erythromycin, monitor for CV effects

Increase: levels of digoxin, theophylline, cycloSPORINE, carBAMazepine, nondepolarizing muscle relaxants

Decrease: effects of lithium

Decrease: antihypertensive effects—NSAIDs

Drug/Food

Increase: hypotensive effects—grapefruit juice

Drug/Herb

Increase: verapamil effect—ginseng, ginkgo

Increase: hypertension ephedra (ma huang)

Decrease: verapamil effect—St. John's wort

Drug/Lab Test

Increase: AST, ALT, alk phos, BUN, creatinine, serum cholesterol

NURSING CONSIDERATIONS

Assess:

- **Cardiac status:** B/P, pulse, respiration, ECG intervals (PR, QRS, QT); notify prescriber if pulse <50 bpm, systolic B/P <90 mm Hg

⚠ **CHF:** I&O ratios, weight daily; crackles, weight gain, dyspnea, jugular venous distention

- Renal, hepatic studies during long-term treatment, serum potassium periodically

Evaluate:

- Therapeutic response: decreased anginal pain, decreased B/P, dysrhythmias

Teach patient/family:

- To increase fluids, fiber to counteract constipation
- How to take pulse, B/P before taking product; to keep record or graph
- To avoid hazardous activities until stabilized on product, dizziness no longer a problem
- To limit caffeine consumption; to avoid alcohol products
- To avoid OTC or grapefruit products unless directed by prescriber
- To comply with all areas of medical regimen: diet, exercise, stress reduction, product therapy
- To change positions slowly to prevent syncope
- Not to discontinue abruptly; chest pain may occur

⚠ To report chest pain, palpitations, irregular heart beats, swelling of extremities, skin irritation, rash, tremors, weakness

- To notify prescriber if pregnancy is planned; may breastfeed (American Academy of Pediatrics)

TREATMENT OF OVERDOSE:
Defibrillation, atropine for AV block, vasopressor for hypotension, IV calcium

vigabatrin (Rx)
(vye-ga′ba-trin)

Sabril

Func. class.: Anticonvulsant

Chem. class.: GABA transaminase inhibitor

ACTION:
May inhibit reuptake and metabolism of GABA; may increase seizure threshold; structurally similar to GABA

USES:
Adjunct treatment of partial seizures in adults and children ≥12 yr, infantile spasm

CONTRAINDICATIONS:
Hypersensitivity to this product

Precautions: Pregnancy (C), breastfeeding, children <2 yr, geriatric patients, renal/hepatic disease, suicidal thoughts/behaviors, abrupt discontinuation

Black Box Warning: Visual disturbance

DOSAGE AND ROUTES

Partial seizures

- **Adult: PO** 500 mg bid, titrate in 500-mg increments at weekly intervals up to 1.5 g bid

Infantile spasm

- **Infant >1 mo, child ≤2 yr: PO** 50 mg/kg/day in 2 divided doses, titrate in 25 to 50-mg/kg/day increments q3days, max 150 mg/kg/day

Renal dose

- **Adult: PO** CCr 50-80 ml/min, reduce dose by 25%; CCr 30-50 ml/min, reduce dose by 50%; CCr 10-30 ml/min, reduce dose by 75%

Available forms: Tabs 500 mg; powder for oral solution 500 mg

Administer:

PO route (tab)

- Give without regard to meals

PO route (oral sol)

- Reconstitute immediately before using
- Empty contents of appropriate number of packets into clean cup
- For each packet, dissolve 10 ml water, concentration 50 mg/ml; do not use other liquids
- Stir until dissolved, sol should be clear
- Use calibrated oral syringe to measure correct dosage
- Discard any unused sol
- Store at room temperature

SIDE EFFECTS

CNS: Headache, memory impairment, *dizziness,* irritability, lethargy, malignant hyperthermia, insomnia, suicidal ideation
CV: Edema
EENT: Visual impairment
GI: Nausea, vomiting, diarrhea, increased appetite, abdominal pain, GI bleeding, hemorrhoids, weight gain, constipation
GU: Impotence, dysmenorrhea
HEMA: Anemia
INTEG: Pruritus, rash
RESP: Coughing, respiratory depression, pulmonary embolism

PHARMACOKINETICS

Absorption >95%, no protein binding, widely distributed, not metabolized, excretion in urine 80% parent drug, excretion slowed in renal disease, peak 2 hr, half-life 7.5 hr

INTERACTIONS

Increase: CNS depression—CNS depressants

Increase: Serious ophthalmic effects (glaucoma, retinopathy): azaTHIOprine, chloroquine, corticosteroids, deferoxamine, ethambutol, hydroxychloroquine, interferons, loxapine, mecasermin, rh-IGF-1, pentostatin, phenothiazine, phosphodiesterase inhibitors, tamoxifen, thiothixene; avoid concurrent use

Drug/Lab Test
Decrease: ALT/AST

NURSING CONSIDERATIONS

Assess:

Black Box Warning: Visual impairment: Prescribers must be registered with the SHARE program due to risk of permanent vision loss; if no clinical response in 2-4 wk of pediatric patients or 3 mo in adults discontinue, provide vision assessment before and after ≤ 4 wk at least q3mo, and 3-6 mo after stopping product

- Renal studies: urinalysis, BUN, urine creatinine q3mo in those with renal disease
- Hepatic studies: ALT, AST, bilirubin
- Description of seizures: location, duration, presence of aura
- Mental status: mood, sensorium, affect, behavioral changes; if mental status changes, notify prescriber
- Assistance with ambulation during early part of treatment; dizziness occurs
- Seizure precautions: padded side rails; move objects that may harm patient

Evaluate:

- Therapeutic response: decreased seizure activity; document on patient's chart

Teach patient/family:

- To carry emergency ID stating patient's name, products taken, condition, prescriber's name and phone number
- To avoid driving, other activities that require alertness
- Not to discontinue medication quickly after long-term use
- To notify prescriber if pregnancy is planned or suspected
- To report suicidal thoughts/behaviors immediately
- To avoid alcohol; drowsiness, dizziness may occur

vilazodone (Rx)

(vil-az′oh-done)

Viibryd

Func. class.: Antidepressant, miscellaneous

ACTION: Novel antidepressant unrelated to other antidepressants, enhances serotonergic action by a dual mechanism

USES: Major depression

CONTRAINDICATIONS: Concomitant use of MOA inhibitors or within 14 days after discontinuing MOA inhibitor or within 14 days after discontinuing vilazodone

Precautions: Pregnancy (C), labor, infants, geriatric patients, abrupt discontinuation, bipolar disorder, bleeding, operating machinery, ECT, hepatic disease, hyponatremia, hypovolemia, substance abuse, history of seizures, serotonin syndrome, neuroleptic malignant syndrome; use with serotonin precursors (e.g., tryptophan) or serotonergic drugs; suicidal ideation, worsening depression or behavior

Black Box Warning: Children, suicidal ideation

DOSAGE AND ROUTES

- **Adult: PO** 10 mg × 7 days, then 20 mg × 7 days, then 40 mg/day; if taking potent CYP3A4 inhibitor, max 20 mg/day

Available forms: Tabs 10, 20, 40 mg

Administer:

- With food to increase absorption
- Do not use within 2 wk of MAOIs
- Store at room temperature, away from moisture, heat

SIDE EFFECTS

CNS: Restlessness, dizziness, drowsiness, fatigue, mania, insomnia, migraine, **neuroleptic-malignant–like syndrome,** paresthesias, **seizures, suicidal ideation,** tremors, night sweats, dream disorders

CV: Palpitations, ventricular extrasystole

EENT: Cataracts, blurred vision

GI: *Nausea,* vomiting, flatulence, *diarrhea, xerostomia,* altered taste, gastroenteritis, increased appetite

GU: Decreased libido, ejaculation disorder, increased frequency of urination, sexual dysfunction

HEMA: Bleeding, decreased platelets

INTEG: Sweating

MS: Arthralgia

SYST: **Neonatal abstinence syndrome, withdrawal, serotonin syndrome**

INTERACTIONS

⚠ **Do not use within 2 wk of MAO inhibitors**

⚠ **Increased: serotonin syndrome—SSRIs, SNRIs, serotonin receptor agonists, selegiline, busPIRone, dextromethorphan, ergots, fenfluramine, dexfluramine, lithium, meperidine, fentaNYL, methylphenidate, dexmethylphenidate, metoclopramide, mirtazapine, nefazodone, pentazocine, phenothiazines, haloperidol, loxapine, thiothixene, molindone, amphetamines**

Increased: bleeding—anticoagulants, thrombolytics, platelet inhibitors, salicylates, NSAIDs

Increased: vilazodone levels—CYP3A4 inhibitors (ketoconazole, erythromycin, efavirenz, dronedarone, clarithromycin and others)

Decrease: vilazodone effect—CYP3A4 inducers

Drug/Food

- Avoid use with grapefruit juice

Drug/Herb

Increased: serotonin syndrome—St. John's wort

Drug/Lab Test

Decrease: sodium

PHARMACOKINETICS

Protein binding 96%-99%, metabolized by liver by CYP3A4 (major) and CYP2C19 and CYP2D (minor) and non-CYP pathways, peak 4-5 hr, half-life 25 hr

V

NURSING CONSIDERATIONS

Assess:

Black Box Warning: Mental status: orientation, mood behavior initially and periodically; initiate suicide precautions if indicated; history of seizures, mania

- Renal/hepatic status: hyponatremia
- **Abrupt discontinuation:** do not discontinue abruptly, taper, monitor for symptoms of withdrawal; if intolerable, resume previous dose and decrease more slowly
- **Serotonin syndrome/neuroleptic malignant syndrome:** nausea, vomiting, sedation, sweating, facial flushing, high B/P; discontinue product, notify prescriber

Evaluate:

- Therapeutic response: remission of depressive symptoms

Teach patient/family:

- To take as directed, with food, not to double dose, that follow-up will be needed
- To avoid abrupt discontinuation unless approved by prescriber
- Not to drive or operate machinery until effects are known
- Not to use other products unless approved by prescribed, do not use alcohol

⚠ To contact prescriber regarding the following: allergic reactions; personality changes (aggression, anxiety, anger, hostility); extreme sleepiness or drowsiness; feeling confused, nervous, restless, or clumsy; numbness, tingling, or burning pain in hands, arms, legs, or feet; tremors; unusual behavior or thoughts about hurting oneself

- To notify prescriber if pregnancy is planned or suspected; to avoid breastfeeding

Black Box Warning: Suicidal thoughts/behaviors: discuss with family the possibility of suicidal thoughts/behaviors, to notify prescriber immediately if these occur

⚠ HIGH ALERT

vinBLAStine (VLB) (Rx)

(vin-blast′een)

Func. class.: Antineoplastic

Chem. class.: Vinca alkaloid

Do not confuse:
vinBLAStine/vinCRIStine/vinorelbine

ACTION: Inhibits mitotic activity, arrests cell cycle at metaphase; inhibits RNA synthesis, blocks cellular use of glutamic acid needed for purine synthesis; vesicant

USES: Breast, testicular cancer, lymphomas, neuroblastoma; Hodgkin's/non-Hodgkin's lymphoma; mycosis fungoides, histiocytosis, Kaposi's sarcoma, Langerhans cell histiocytosis

Unlabeled uses: Lung, bladder, prostate cancer; desmoid tumor, malignant melanoma

CONTRAINDICATIONS: Pregnancy (D), breastfeeding, infants, hypersensitivity, leukopenia, granulocytopenia, bone marrow suppression, infection

Black Box Warning: Intrathecal use

Precautions: Renal/hepatic disease, tumor lysis syndrome

Black Box Warning: Extravasation

DOSAGE AND ROUTES

Breast cancer

- **Adult: IV** 4.5 mg/m^2 on day 1 of every 21 days in combination with DOXOrubicin and thiotepa

Hodgkin's disease

- **Adult: IV** 6 mg/m^2 on days 1 and 15 of every 28 days with DOXOrubicin, bleomycin, dacarbazine (ABVD regimen)
- **Child: IV** 2.5-6 mg/m^2/day once q1-2wk × 3-6 wk, max weekly dose 12.5 mg/m^2

Available forms: Inj, powder 10 mg for 10 ml IV; sol for inj 1 mg/ml
Administer:

Black Box Warning: Hyaluronidase 150 units/ml in 1 ml NaCl, warm compress for extravasation for vesicant activity treatment

Black Box Warning: Do not administer intrathecally; fatal

IV inj route
- After diluting 10 mg/10 ml NaCl; give through Y-tube or 3-way stopcock or directly over 1 min

Intermittent IV INFUSION route
- Further dilute in 50-100 ml of NS, infuse over 15-30 min

Additive compatibilities: Bleomycin
Syringe compatibilities: Bleomycin, CISplatin, cyclophosphamide, droperidol, fluorouracil, leucovorin, methotrexate, metoclopramide, mitoMYcin, vinCRIStine
Y-site compatibilities: Allopurinol, amifostine, amphotericin B cholesteryl, aztreonam, bleomycin, CISplatin, cyclophosphamide, DOXOrubicin, DOXOrubicin liposome, droperidol, filgrastim, fludarabine, fluorouracil, granisetron, heparin, leucovorin, melphalan, methotrexate, metoclopramide, mitoMYcin, ondansetron, PACLitaxel, piperacillin/tazobactam, sargramostim, teniposide, thiotepa, vinCRIStine, vinorelbine

SIDE EFFECTS

CNS: Paresthesias, peripheral neuropathy, depression, headache, **seizures**, malaise
CV: Tachycardia, orthostatic hypo/hypertension
GI: *Nausea, vomiting,* ileus, *anorexia, stomatitis, constipation,* abdominal pain, **GI/rectal bleeding, hepatotoxicity,** pharyngitis
GU: Urinary retention, **renal failure,** hyperuricemia
HEMA: **Thrombocytopenia, leukopenia, myelosuppression, agranulocytosis, granulocytosis, aplastic anemia, neutropenia, pancytopenia**
INTEG: *Rash, alopecia,* photosensitivity, **extravasation, tissue necrosis**
META: SIADH
RESP: **Fibrosis, pulmonary infiltrate, bronchospasm**
SYST: **Tumor lysis syndrome (TLS)**

PHARMACOKINETICS

Half-life (triphasic) <5 min, 50-155 min, 23-85 hr; metabolized in liver; excreted in urine, feces; crosses blood-brain barrier

INTERACTIONS

Increase: synergism: bleomycin
Increase: bronchospasm: mitoMYcin
- Do not use with radiation

Increase: bleeding risk—NSAIDs, anticoagulants, thrombolytics, antiplatelets
Increase: toxicity, bone marrow suppression—antineoplastics
Increase: action of methotrexate
Increase: adverse reactions—live virus vaccines
⚠ **Increase:** toxicity—CYP3A4 inhibitors (aprepitant, antiretroviral protease inhibitors, clarithromycin, danazol, delavirdine, diltiazem, erythromycin, fluconazole, FLUoxetine, fluvoxaMINE, imatinib, ketoconazole, mibefradil, nefazodone, telithromycin, voriconazole)
Decrease: vinBLAStine effect—CYP3A4 inducers (barbiturates, bosentan, carBAMazepine, efavirenz, phenytoins, nevirapine, rifabutin, rifampin)

Drug/Herb
- Avoid use with St. John's wort

Drug/Lab Test
Increase: uric acid, bilirubin
Decrease: Hgb, platelets, WBC

NURSING CONSIDERATIONS

V

Assess:
⚠ CBC, differential, platelet count weekly; withhold product if WBC is <2000/mm^3 or platelet count is <75,000/mm^3; notify prescriber; RBC, Hct, Hgb may be decreased, nadir occurs on days 4-10 and continues for another 1-2 wk
- **Tumor lysis syndrome:** monitor for hyperkalemia, hyperphosphatemia,

hyperuricemia; usually occurs with leukemia, lymphoma; alkalinization of the urine, allopurinol should be used to prevent urate nephrophy; monitor electrolytes and renal function (BUN, uric acid, urine CCR)
- Hepatitis: transient hepatitis may occur with continuous IV
- Bleeding: hematuria, guaiac, bruising, petechiae, mucosa or orifices
- **Bronchospasm:** can be life-threatening; usually occurs when giving mitoMYcin
- Effects of alopecia on body image; discuss feelings about body changes
- Sensitivity of feet/hands, which precedes neuropathy
- Jaundiced skin, sclera; dark urine, clay-colored stools, itchy skin, abdominal pain, fever, diarrhea
- Buccal cavity q8hr for dryness, sores, ulcerations, white patches, oral pain, bleeding, dysphagia

Black Box Warning: Local irritation, pain, burning, discoloration at inj site, extravasation

- Symptoms indicating severe allergic reaction: rash, pruritus, urticaria, purpuric skin lesions, itching, flushing
- Increased fluid intake to 2-3 L/day to prevent urate deposits, calculi formation
- Brushing of teeth bid-tid with soft brush or cotton-tipped applicator for stomatitis; use unwaxed dental floss

Evaluate:
- Therapeutic response: decreased tumor size, spread of malignancy

Teach patient/family:
- To report any changes in breathing or coughing; to avoid exposure to persons with infection
- That hair may be lost during treatment; that a wig or hairpiece may make patient feel better; that new hair may be different in color, texture
- To report change in gait or numbness in extremities; may indicate neuropathy
- To avoid foods with citric acid, hot or rough texture
- To report any bleeding, white spots, ulcerations in mouth to prescriber; to examine mouth daily
- To wear sunscreen, protective clothing, sunglasses
- To avoid receiving vaccinations

⚠ **Pregnancy:** pregnancy (D); to avoid breastfeeding; that product may cause male infertility
- To notify prescriber if pregnancy is planned or suspected; to avoid persons with known infections
- **Infection:** to report sore throat, flulike symptoms

⚠ HIGH ALERT

vinCRIStine (VCR) (Rx)

(vin-kris′teen)

Vincasar PFS

VinCRIStine Liposomal (Rx)

Marqibo

Func. class.: Antineoplastic—miscellaneous

Chem. class.: Vinca alkaloid

Do not confuse:
vinCRIStine/vinBLAStine/vinorelbine

ACTION: Inhibits mitotic activity, arrests cell cycle at metaphase; inhibits RNA synthesis, blocks cellular use of glutamic acid needed for purine synthesis; vesicant

USES: Lymphomas, neuroblastoma, Hodgkin's disease, acute lymphoblastic and other leukemias, rhabdomyosarcoma, Wilms' tumor, non-Hodgkin's lymphoma, malignant glioma, soft-tissue sarcoma; liposomal: Philadelphia chromosome-negative ALL in second or greater relapse or that has progressed after ≥2 antileukemia therapies

Unlabeled uses: Lung, breast, colorectal, head/neck, osteogenic sarcomas; small-cell lung cancer, trophoblastic disease

CONTRAINDICATIONS: Pregnancy (D), breastfeeding, infants, hypersensitivity, radiation therapy

Black Box Warning: Intrathecal use

Precautions: Renal/hepatic disease, hypertension, neuromuscular disease

Black Box Warning: Extravasation

DOSAGE AND ROUTES

- **Adult: IV** 0.4-1.4 mg/m²/wk, max 2 mg
- **Child: IV** 1-2 mg/m²/wk, max 2 mg

Liposomal

- **Adult: IV** 2.25 mg/m² over 1 hr q7days

Available forms: Inj 1 mg/ml; liposomal 5 mg/31 ml injection kit

Black Box Warning: Do not give intrathecally; fatal

VinCRIStine

IV route

- After diluting with diluent provided or 1 mg/10 ml sterile water or NaCl; give through Y-tube or 3-way stopcock or directly over 1 min; do not use 5-mg vial for single doses

Black Box Warning: Hyaluronidase 150 units/ml in 1 ml NaCl; apply warm compress for extravasation

IV route

VinCRIStine Liposomal

- Supplied in single-use kit, inspect for particulates after preparation in pharmacy, give using separate line over 1 hr

VinCRIStine Y-site compatibilities Acyclovir, alemtuzumab, alfentanil, allopurinol, amifostine, amikacin, aminocaproic acid, aminophylline, amiodarone, amphotericin B cholesteryl, amphotericin B lipid complex, amphotericin B liposome, ampicillin, ampicillin–sulbactam, anidulafungin, argatroban, arsenic trioxide, asparaginase, atenolol, atracurium, azithromycin, aztreonam, bivalirudin, bleomycin, bumetanide, buprenorphine, butorphanol, calcium chloride/gluconate, capreomycin, CARBOplatin, carmustine, caspofungin, ceFAZolin, cefoperazone, cefoTEtan, cefOXitin, cefTAZidime, ceftizoxime, cefTRIAXone, cefuroxime, chlorproMAZINE, cimetidine, ciprofloxacin, cisatracurium, CISplatin, cladribine, clindamycin, codeine, cyclophosphamide, cycloSPORINE, cytarabine, D5W-dextrose 5%, dacarbazine, DACTINomycin, DAPTOmycin, DAUNOrubicin, DAUNOrubicin citrate liposome, dexamethasone, dexmedetomidine, dexrazoxane, digoxin, diltiazem, diphenhydrAMINE, DOBUTamine, DOCEtaxel, dolasetron, DOPamine, doxacurium, doxapram, DOXOrubicin, DOXOrubicin liposomal, doxycycline, droperidol, enalaprilat, ePHEDrine, EPINEPHrine, epirubicin, ertapenem, erythromycin, esmolol, etoposide, famotidine, fenoldopam, fentaNYL, filgrastim, fluconazole, fludarabine, fluorouracil, foscarnet, fosphenytoin, gallium, ganciclovir, garenoxacin, gatifloxacin, gemcitabine, gentamicin, granisetron, haloperidol, heparin, hydrocortisone sodium phosphate/succinate, HYDROmorphone, hydrOXYzine, ifosfamide, imipenem-cilastatin, inamrinone, insulin, regular, isoproterenol, ketorolac, labetalol, lepirudin, leucovorin, levofloxacin, levorphanol, lidocaine, linezolid, LORazepam, magnesium sulfate, mannitol, mechlorethamine, melphalan, meperidine, meropenem, mesna, methadone, methohexital, methotrexate, methylPREDNISolone, metoclopramide, metoprolol, metroNIDAZOLE, midazolam, milrinone, minocycline, mitoMYcin, mitoXANtrone, mivacurium, morphine, moxifloxacin, nalbuphine, naloxone, nesiritide, niCARdipine, nitroglycerin, nitroprusside, norepinephrine, octreotide, ondansetron, oxaliplatin, PACLitaxel (solvent/surfactant), palonosetron, pamidronate, pancuronium, PEMEtrexed, pentamidine, pentazocine, PENTobarbital, PHENobarbital, phenylephrine, piperacillin, piperacillin–tazobactam, potassium acetate/chloride/phosphates, procainamide, prochlorperazine, promethazine, propranolol, quinupristin-dalfopristin, ranitidine, remifentanil, riTUXimab, rocuronium, sargramostim, sodium acetate/phosphates, succinylcholine, SUFentanil, sulfamethoxazole-trimethoprim, tacrolimus, teniposide, theophylline, thiopental, thiotepa, ticarcillin, ticarcillin–clavulanate, tigecycline, tirofiban, tobramycin, topotecan, trastuzumab, trimethobenzamide, vancomycin, vasopressin, vecuronium, verapamil, vinBLAStine, vinorelbine, voriconazole, zidovudine, zoledronic acid

SIDE EFFECTS

CNS: *Decreased reflexes, numbness, weakness, motor difficulties,* CNS

V

depression, cranial nerve paralysis, seizures, peripheral neuropathy
CV: Orthostatic hypotension
EENT: *Diplopia*
GI: *Nausea, vomiting, anorexia, stomatitis, constipation,* paralytic ileus, *abdominal pain,* hepatotoxicity
GU: Renal tubular obstruction
HEMA: Thrombocytopenia, leukopenia, myelosuppression, anemia
INTEG: *Alopecia,* extravasation
SYST: Tumor lysis syndrome (TLS)

PHARMACOKINETICS

Half-life (triphasic) <5 min, 50-155 min, 23-85 hr; metabolized in liver; excreted in bile, feces; crosses placental, blood-brain barrier

INTERACTIONS

Decrease: immune response—vaccines, toxoids
Decrease: digoxin level—digoxin
Decrease: vinCRIStine effect—CYP3A4 inducers (barbiturates, bosentan, carBAMazepine, efavirenz, phenytoins, nevirapine, rifabutin, rifampin)
Increase: Neurotoxicity: peripheral nervous system products

- Do not use with radiation
- Acute pulmonary reactions: mitoMYcin c

⚠ **Increase:** toxicity—CYP3A4 inhibitors (aprepitant, antiretroviral protease inhibitors, clarithromycin, danazol, delavirdine, diltiazem, erythromycin, fluconazole, FLUoxetine, fluvoxaMINE, imatinib, ketoconazole, mibefradil, nefazodone, telithromycin, voriconazole)

Drug/Herb

- Avoid use with St. John's wort

Drug/Lab Test

Increase: uric acid
Decrease: Hgb, WBC, platelets, sodium

NURSING CONSIDERATIONS

Assess:

- CBC, differential, platelet count before each dose; withhold product if WBC is <4000/mm³ or platelet count is <75,000/mm³; notify prescriber; RBC, Hct, Hgb; may be decreased
- **Bronchospasm:** more common with mitoMYcin
- Hepatic studies before, during therapy (bilirubin, AST, ALT, LDH) as needed or monthly
- Sensitivity of feet/hands, which precedes neuropathy
- **Tumor lysis syndrome:** hyperkalemia, hyperphosphatemia, hyperuricemia, hypocalcemia; more common in leukemia, lymphoma; use alkalinization of urine with allopurinol, monitor electrolytes, renal function (BUN, urine, CCR, uric acid)

Black Box Warning: Extravasation: pain, swelling, poor blood return; if extravasation occurs, local inj of hyaluronidase and moderate heat to area may help disperse product

Intrathecal administration

- **Bleeding:** hematuria, guaiac, bruising, petechiae, mucosa or orifices q8hr
- Effects of alopecia on body image; discuss feelings about body changes
- Buccal cavity q8hr for dryness, sores, ulcerations, white patches, oral pain, bleeding, dysphagia
- Symptoms indicating severe allergic reaction: rash, pruritus, urticaria, purpuric skin lesions, itching, flushing
- Brushing of teeth bid-tid with soft brush or cotton-tipped applicator for stomatitis; use unwaxed dental floss

Evaluate:

- Therapeutic response: decreased tumor size, spread of malignancy

Teach patient/family:

- To report change in gait or numbness in extremities; may indicate neuropathy
- To report any bleeding, white spots, or ulcerations in mouth to prescriber; to examine mouth daily
- To increase bulk, fluids, exercise to prevent constipation
- **Infection:** to report sore throat, fever, flulike symptoms; avoid persons with known infection
- To avoid vaccinations
- That hair may be lost; that hair will grow back but with different texture, color

- **Pregnancy (D):** to notify prescriber if pregnancy is planned or suspected

⚠ To use effective contraception during and for 2 mo after therapy, pregnancy (D), to avoid breastfeeding

⚠ ***HIGH ALERT***

vinorelbine (Rx)

(vi-nor′el-bine)

Navelbine

Func. class.: Antineoplastic—miscellaneous

Chem. class.: Semisynthetic vinca alkaloid

ACTION: Inhibits mitotic spindle activity, arrests cell cycle at metaphase; inhibits RNA synthesis, blocks cellular use of glutamic acid needed for purine synthesis; vesicant

USES: Unresectable advanced non–small-cell lung cancer (NSCLC) stage IV; may be used alone or in combination with CISplatin for stage III or IV NSCLC

Unlabeled uses: Hodgkin's disease, breast/ovarian/head/neck cancer, desmoid tumor

CONTRAINDICATIONS: Pregnancy (D), breastfeeding, infants, hypersensitivity, granulocyte count <1000 cells/mm^3 pretreatment

Black Box Warning: Severe neutropenia, intrathecal administration

Precautions: Children, geriatric patients, renal/hepatic/pulmonary/neurologic disease, anemia, bone marrow suppression

Black Box Warning: Extravasation

DOSAGE AND ROUTES

- **Adult: IV** 30 mg/m^2/wk
- **ANC 1000-1499:** Give 50% of dose; <1000, hold dose; <1000 × 3 wk, discontinue

Hepatic dose

- **Adult: IV** total bilirubin 2.1-3 mg/dl 15 mg/m^2/wk; total bilirubin ≥3 mg/dl 7.5 mg/m^2/day

Available forms: Inj 10 mg/ml

Administer:

Black Box Warning: Do not give intrathecally; fatal

Intermittent IV INFUSION route

- Dilute to 0.5-2 mg/ml with 0.9% NaCl, 0.45% NaCl, D_5W, D_5/0.45% NaCl, LR, Ringer's sol, give over 6-10 min into Y-site or central line, flush line

Black Box Warning: Hyaluronidase 150 units/ml in 1 ml NaCl, warm compress for extravasation for vesicant activity treatment

Continuous IV INFUSION route

- 40 mg/m^2 q3wk after IV bol of 8 mg/m^2; may be given in combination with DOXOrubicin, fluorouracil, CISplatin

Y-site compatibilities: Amikacin, aztreonam, bleomycin, bumetanide, buprenorphine, butorphanol, calcium gluconate, CARBOplatin, carmustine, cefotaxime, cefTAZidime, ceftizoxime, chlorproMAZINE, cimetidine, CISplatin, clindamycin, cyclophosphamide, cytarabine, dacarbazine, DACTINomycin, DAUNOrubicin, dexamethasone, diphenhydrAMINE, DOXOrubicin, DOXOrubicin liposome, doxycycline, droperidol, enalaprilat, etoposide, famotidine, filgrastim, floxuridine, fluconazole, fludarabine, gallium, gentamicin, granisetron, haloperidol, heparin, hydrocortisone, HYDROmorphone, hydrOXYzine, IDArubicin, ifosfamide, imipenem-cilastatin, LORazepam, mannitol, mechlorethamine, melphalan, meperidine, mesna, methotrexate, metoclopramide, metroNIDAZOLE, minocycline, mitoXANtrone, morphine, nalbuphine, netilmicin, ondansetron, plicamycin,

V

streptozocin, teniposide, ticarcillin, ticarcillin-clavulanate, tobramycin, vancomycin, vinBLAStine, vinCRIStine, zidovudine

SIDE EFFECTS

CNS: Paresthesias, peripheral neuropathy, depression, headache, seizures, weakness, jaw pain, asthenia
CV: Chest pain
GI: *Nausea, vomiting,* ileus, *anorexia, stomatitis,* constipation, abdominal pain, *diarrhea,* hepatotoxicity, GI obstruction/perforation
HEMA: Neutropenia, anemia, thrombocytopenia, granulocytopenia
INTEG: *Rash, alopecia,* photosensitivity, inj site reaction, necrosis
META: SIADH
MS: Myalgia
RESP: SOB, dyspnea, pulmonary edema, acute bronchospasm, acute respiratory distress syndrome (ARDS)

PHARMACOKINETICS

Half-life 27-43 hr; peak 1-2 hr; highly bound to platelets, lymphocytes; metabolized in liver; excreted in feces; small amount unchanged in kidneys

INTERACTIONS

Increase: bleeding risk—NSAIDs, anticoagulants
⚠ **Increase:** toxicity—CYP3A4 inhibitors (aprepitant, antiretroviral protease inhibitors, clarithromycin, danazol, delavirdine, diltiazem, erythromycin, fluconazole, FLUoxetine, fluvoxaMINE, imatinib, ketoconazole, mibefradil, nefazodone, telithromycin, voriconazole)
Decrease: vinorelbine effect—CYP3A4 inducers (barbiturates, bosentan, carBAMazepine, efavirenz, phenytoins, nevirapine, rifabutin, rifampin)

Drug/Herb
- Avoid use with St. John's wort

Drug/Lab Test
Increase: LFTs, bilirubin
Decrease: Hgb, WBC, platelets

NURSING CONSIDERATIONS

Assess:
- B/P (baseline, q15min) during administration

Black Box Warning: CBC, differential, platelet count before each dose; withhold product if WBC is <4000/mm³ or platelet count is <75,000/mm³; notify prescriber of results; recovery will take 3 wk

- **Bronchospasm:** more common with mitoMYcin; also dyspnea, wheezing; may be treated with oxygen, bronchodilators, corticosteroids, especially if there is underlying pulmonary disease
- Respiratory status: dyspnea, crackles, unproductive cough, chest pain, tachypnea
- Renal studies: BUN, serum uric acid, urine CCr before, during therapy; I&O ratio; report fall in urine output to <30 ml/hr; decreased hyperuricemia
- **Infection,** cold, fever, sore throat; notify prescriber if these occur; effects of alopecia on body image
- **Bleeding:** hematuria, guaiac, bruising, petechiae, mucosa or orifices, no rectal temperatures; avoid IM inj; apply pressure to venipuncture sites
- Hepatic function tests: AST, ALT, bilirubin, LDH

⚠ **Severe allergic reactions:** rash, pruritus, urticaria, itching, flushing, bronchospasm, hypotension; EPINEPHrine and crash cart should be nearby
- Neurologic status: numbness, pain, tingling, loss of Achilles reflex, weakness, palsies
- Brushing of teeth bid-tid with soft brush or cotton-tipped applicator for stomatitis; unwaxed dental floss

Evaluate:
- Therapeutic response: decreased tumor size, spread of malignancy

Teach patient/family:
- To report change in gait or numbness in extremities, continuing constipation; may indicate neurotoxicity
- To examine mouth daily for bleeding, white spots, ulcerations; to notify prescriber

- **Infection:** report sore throat, fever, flu-like symptoms
- To avoid crowds, people with infections, vaccinations, OTC products

⚠ **Pregnancy:** notify prescriber if pregnancy is planned or suspected; to use effective contraception during treatment and for ≥2 mo after product is discontinued, pregnancy (D); to avoid breastfeeding
- That hair may be lost; that hair will grow back but with different texture, color

⚠ HIGH ALERT

vismodegib

(vis′moe-deg′ib)

Erivedge

Func. class.: Antineoplastic biologic response modifier

Chem. class.: Signal transduction inhibitor (STI)

ACTION: A hedgehog (Hh) signaling pathway inhibitor

USES: Patients who have metastatic basal cell carcinoma, locally advanced, that has recurred after surgery and who are not candidates for surgery/radiation

CONTRAINDICATIONS: Hypersensitivity, breastfeeding

Black Box Warning: Intrauterine fetal death, male-mediated teratogenicity, pregnancy (D)

Precautions: Children, blood donation

DOSAGE AND ROUTES

- **Adult: PO** 150 mg/day

Available forms: Cap 150 mg

Administer:

- Give without regard to food
- Swallow whole, do not open or crush caps
- If a dose is missed, do not take additional dose, take at usual time
- Store at 77°F (25°C)

SIDE EFFECTS

GI: Nausea, vomiting, dysgeusia
GU: Amenorrhea, azotemia
INTEG: Alopecia
META: Hyponatremia
MISC: Fatigue, decreased weight
MS: Arthralgia

PHARMACOKINETICS

Protein binding >99%, elimination half-life 4 days

INTERACTIONS

Increase: effect of each product—Pgp inhibitors (amiodarone, clarithromycin, cycloSPORINE, diltiazem, erythromycin, indinavir, itraconazole, ketoconazole, nelfinavir, niCARdipine, propafenone, quiNIDine, ritonavir, saquinavir, tacrolimus, tamoxifen, verapamil); CYP2C19 substrates (amitriptyline, clomiPRAMINE, imipramine, citalopram, diazepam, phenytoin, PHENobarbital, lansoprazole, omeprazole, pantoprazole, RABEprazole, esomeprazole, clopidogrel, proguanil, propranolol, carisoprodol, chloramphenicol, cyclophosphamide, indomethacin, nelfinavir, nilutamide, progesterone, teniposide, warfarin)

NURSING CONSIDERATIONS

Assess:

Black Box Warning: Pregnancy (D): verify pregnancy status of all women within 7 days before starting therapy; effective contraception is needed during and for 7 mo after treatment; men receiving this product should use condoms with spermicide (even after vasectomy) during sexual intercourse with female partners and for 2 mo after the last dose; report exposure during pregnancy to the Genentech Adverse Event Line

Evaluate:

- Therapeutic response: decreased spread of tumor

V

Teach patient/family:

Black Box Warning: Pregnancy (D): teach patient to notify their provider immediately if pregnancy is suspected (or in a female partner for male patients); effective contraception is needed during and for 7 mo after treatment; men receiving this product should use condoms with spermicide (even after vasectomy) during sexual intercourse with female partners and for 2 mo after the last dose; if product is used during pregnancy or if the patient becomes pregnant during use, the woman (or female partner for male patients) should be apprised of the potential hazard to the fetus; encourage exposed women (either directly or through seminal fluid) to participate in the ERIVEDGE pregnancy pharmacovigilance program

- About reason for treatment, expected results
- If dose is missed, do not take, but resume scheduled doses, swallow whole
- Do not donate blood during therapy or for ≥7 months after conclusion of product

vitamin A (Rx, PO-OTC, Rx-IM)

Aquasol A, Vitamin A

Func. class.: Vitamin, fat soluble

Chem. class.: Retinol

ACTION: Needed for normal bone, tooth development; visual dark adaptation; skin disease; mucosa tissue repair; assists with production of adrenal steroids, cholesterol, RNA

USES: Vit A deficiency

CONTRAINDICATIONS: Pregnancy (X) (IM), hypersensitivity to vit A, malabsorption syndrome, hypervitaminosis A, IV administration

Precautions: Pregnancy (C) (PO), breastfeeding, impaired renal function, children, hepatic disease, infants, alcoholism, hepatitis

DOSAGE AND ROUTES

- **Adult and child >8 yr: PO** 100,000-500,000 international units/day × 3 days then 50,000 international units/day × 2 wk; dose based on severity of deficiency; maintenance 10,000-20,000 international units for 2 mo
- **Child 1-8 yr: IM** 5000-15,000 international units/day × 10 days
- **Infant <1 yr: IM** 5000-15,000 international units × 10 days

Maintenance

- **Child 4-8 yr: IM** 15,000 international units/day × 2 mo
- **Child <4 yr: IM** 10,000 international units/day × 2 mo

Available forms: Caps 10,000, 25,000, 50,000 international units; drops 5000 international units; inj 50,000 international units/ml; tabs 10,000, 25,000, 50,000 international units

Administer:

PO route

- With food (PO) for better absorption
- Do not administer IV because of risk of anaphylactic shock; IM only
- Oral preparations not indicated for vit A deficiency in those with malabsorption syndrome
- Store in tight, light-resistant container

IM route

- Give deep in large muscle mass; do not use deltoid muscle for administration of >1 ml

SIDE EFFECTS

CNS: Headache, increased intracranial pressure, intracranial hypertension, lethargy, malaise

EENT: Gingivitis, papilledema, exophthalmos, inflammation of tongue and lips

GI: Nausea, vomiting, anorexia, abdominal pain, jaundice

INTEG: Drying of skin, pruritus, increased pigmentation, night sweats, alopecia

META: Hypomenorrhea, hypercalcemia

MS: Arthralgia, retarded growth, hard areas on bone

PHARMACOKINETICS

Stored in liver, kidneys, fat; excreted (metabolites) in urine, feces

INTERACTIONS

Increase: levels of vit A—corticosteroids, oral contraceptives
Decrease: absorption of vit A—mineral oil, cholestyramine, colestipol
Drug/Lab Test
False increase: bilirubin, serum cholesterol

NURSING CONSIDERATIONS

Assess:
- Nutritional status: yellow and dark green vegetables, yellow/orange fruits, vit-A–fortified foods, liver, egg yolks
- **Vit A deficiency:** decreased growth; night blindness; dry, brittle nails; hair loss; urinary stones; increased infection; hyperkeratosis of skin; drying of cornea

Evaluate:
- Therapeutic response: increased growth rate, weight; absence of dry skin and mucous membranes, night blindness

Teach patient/family:
- That, if dose is missed, it should be omitted
- That ophthalmic exams may be required periodically throughout therapy
- Not to use mineral oil while taking this product
- To notify prescriber of nausea, vomiting, lip cracking, loss of hair, headache
- Not to take more than prescribed amount

TREATMENT OF OVERDOSE:
Discontinue product

vitamin C (ascorbic acid) (OTC, Rx)
(a-skor′bic)

Acerola C, Apo-C ✦, Ascor L-500, Cenolate, Equaline Vitamin C, Walgreens Gold Seal, and many more

Func. class.: Vit C—water-soluble vitamin

ACTION:
Wound healing, collagen synthesis, antioxidant, carbohydrate metabolism

USES:
Vit C deficiency, scurvy; delayed wound, bone healing; chronic disease; urine acidification; before gastrectomy; dietary supplement
Unlabeled uses: Common cold prevention

CONTRAINDICATIONS:
Tartrazine, sulfite sensitivity; G6PD deficiency
Precautions: Pregnancy (C), gout, diabetes, renal calculi (large doses)

DOSAGE AND ROUTES

Dietary supplementation
- **Adult:** 50-500 mg/day
- **Child 14-18 yr: PO** 65 mg (female), 75 mg (male)
- **Child 9-13 yr: PO** 45 mg/day
- **Child 4-8 yr: PO** 25 mg/day
- **Child 1-3 yr: PO** 15 mg/day
- **Infant: PO** 40-50 mg/day

Scurvy
- **Adult: PO/SUBCUT/IM/IV** 100-250 mg/day × 2 wk, then 50 mg or more daily
- **Child: PO/SUBCUT/IM/IV** 100-300 mg/day × 2 wk, then 35 mg or more daily

Wound healing/chronic disease/fracture (may be given with zinc)
- **Adult: SUBCUT/IM/IV/PO** 200-500 mg/day for 1-2 mo
- **Child: SUBCUT/IM/IV/PO** 100-200 mg added doses for 1-2 mo

Urine acidification
- **Adult:** 4-12 g/day in divided doses
- **Child:** 500 mg q6-8hr

Available forms: Tabs 25, 50, 100, 250, 500, 1000, 1500 mg; effervescent tabs 1000 mg; chewable tabs 100, 250, 500 mg; timed-release tabs 500, 750, 1000, 1500 mg; timed-release caps 500 mg; crys 4 g/tsp; powder 4 g/tsp; liq 35 mg/0.6 ml; sol 100 mg/ml; syr 20 mg/ml, 500 mg/5 ml; inj SUBCUT, IM, IV 100, 250, 500 mg/ml

Administer:

PO route
- Do not crush or chew ext rel tabs or caps
- Caps may be opened and contents mixed with jelly

IV, direct route

- 100 mg undiluted by direct IV over at least 1 min; rapid infusion may cause fainting

Intermittent IV INFUSION route

- Diluted with D_5W, D_5NaCl, NS, LR, Ringer's, sodium lactate and given over 15 min

Syringe compatibilities: Metoclopramide, aminophylline, theophylline

Y-site compatibilities: Warfarin

SIDE EFFECTS

CNS: Headache, insomnia, dizziness, fatigue, flushing

GI: Nausea, vomiting, diarrhea, anorexia, heartburn, cramps

GU: Polyuria, urine acidification, oxalate/urate renal stones, dysuria

HEMA: Hemolytic anemia in patients with G6PD

INTEG: Inflammation at inj site

PHARMACOKINETICS

PO/INJ: Readily absorbed PO, metabolized in liver; unused amounts excreted in urine (unchanged), metabolites; crosses placenta, breast milk

INTERACTIONS

Drug/Lab Test

False negative: occult blood, urine bilirubin, leukocyte determination

NURSING CONSIDERATIONS

Assess:

- I&O ratio; urine pH (acidification)
- Ascorbic acid levels throughout treatment if continued deficiency is suspected
- Nutritional status: citrus fruits, vegetables
- Inj sites for inflammation
- Thrombophlebitis if receiving large dose

Evaluate:

- Therapeutic response: absence of anorexia, irritability, pallor, joint pain, hyperkeratosis, petechiae, poor wound healing

Teach patient/family:

- Necessary foods to include in diet, such as citrus fruits
- That smoking decreases vit C levels; not to exceed prescribed dose; that excesses will be excreted in urine, except when taking timed-release forms

vitamin E (OTC)

Aquasol E

Func. class.: Vit E

Chem. class.: Fat soluble

ACTION: Needed for digestion and metabolism of polyunsaturated fats; decreases platelet aggregation, blood clot formation; promotes normal growth and development of muscle tissue, prostaglandin synthesis

USES: Vit E deficiency, impaired fat absorption, hemolytic anemia in premature neonates, prevention of retrolental fibroplasia, sickle cell anemia, supplement for malabsorption syndrome

CONTRAINDICATIONS: IV use in infants

Precautions: Pregnancy (A), anemia, breastfeeding, hypoprothrombinemia

DOSAGE AND ROUTES

Deficiency

- **Adult: PO** 60-75 international units/day
- **Child: PO** 1 international units/kg (malabsorption)

Prevention of deficiency

- **Adult: PO** 30 international units/day; **TOP** apply to affected areas
- **Infant: PO** 5 international units/day

Available forms: Caps 100, 200, 400, 500, 600, 1000 international units; tabs 100, 200, 400 international units; drops 15 mg/0.3 ml; chew tabs 400 units; ointment; cream; lotion; oil

Administer:

PO route

- Administer with or after meals
- Chew chewable tabs well
- Sol may be dropped in mouth or mixed with food

• Store in tight, light-resistant container

Topical route

• To moisturize dry skin

SIDE EFFECTS

CNS: Headache, fatigue
CV: Increased risk for thrombophlebitis
EENT: Blurred vision
GI: Nausea, cramps, diarrhea
GU: Gonadal dysfunction
INTEG: Sterile abscess, contact dermatitis
META: Altered metabolism of hormones (thyroid, pituitary, adrenal), altered immunity
MS: Weakness

PHARMACOKINETICS

PO: Metabolized in liver, excreted in bile

INTERACTIONS

Increase: action of oral anticoagulants
Decrease: absorption—cholestyramine, colestipol, mineral oil, sucralfate

NURSING CONSIDERATIONS

Assess:

• Nutritional status: wheat germ; dark green, leafy vegetables; nuts; eggs; liver; vegetable oils; dairy products; cereals

Evaluate:

• Therapeutic response: absence of hemolytic anemia, adequate vit E levels, improvement in skin lesions, decreased edema

Teach patient/family:

• About the necessary foods for diet
• To omit dose if missed
• To avoid vitamin supplements unless directed by prescriber

⚠ HIGH ALERT

vorapaxar

(vor′a-pax′ar)

Zontivity

Func. class.: Platelet inhibitor

ACTION:

Antagonizes the protease-activated receptor-1 (PAR-1) expressed on platelets

USES:

Secondary myocardial infarction prophylaxis or stroke prophylaxis or thrombosis prophylaxis for reduction of thrombotic cardiovascular events in patients with a history of myocardial infarction or with peripheral arterial disease

CONTRAINDICATIONS:

Black Box Warning: Bleeding, intracranial bleeding, stroke

Precautions: Breastfeeding, coronary artery bypass graft surgery (CABG), geriatric patients, hepatic disease, labor, obstetric delivery, pregnancy (B), renal impairment, surgery

DOSAGE AND ROUTES

• **Adults: PO** 2.08 mg once daily with aspirin and/or clopidogrel

Available forms: Tab 2.08 mg

Administer:

• May be administered without regard to food

SIDE EFFECTS

CNS: Depression
EENT: Diplopia, retinopathy
HEMA: Anemia, bleeding
MISC: Rash

PHARMACOKINETICS

Within 1 week of treatment reaches ≥80% inhibition of thrombin receptor, half-life 3-4 days, terminal half-life is approximately 8 days, protein binding 99%, primarily eliminated feces; peak 1 hr

INTERACTIONS

Increase: bleeding risk—anticoagulants, aspirin, NSAIDs, other platelet inhibitors, SSRIs, rifampin, SNRIs, thrombolytics, CYP3A inhibitors, ethyl estradiol, calcium channel blockers
Decrease: vorapaxar effect—CYP3A inducers

V

NURSING CONSIDERATIONS

Assess:

Black Box Warning: For bleeding, including intracranial bleeding and stroke during treatment

- Bleeding should be suspected in any patient presenting with hypotension who has recently undergone surgery, coronary angiography, percutaneous coronary intervention (PCI), or CABG

Evaluate:

- Therapeutic response: absence of MI, stroke

Teach patient/family:

- To report any unusual bruising, bleeding to prescriber; that it may take longer to stop bleeding
- To take without regard to food

voriconazole (Rx)

(vohr-i-kahn′a-zol)

Vfend

Func. class.: Antifungal, systemic

Chem. class.: Triazole derivative

Do not confuse:
Vfend/Venofer

ACTION: Inhibits fungal CYP450-mediation demethylation; needed for biosynthesis; causes leakage from cell membrane

USES: Invasive aspergillosis, serious fungal infections (*Candida* sp., *Scedosporium apiospermum, Fusarium* sp., *Monosporium, Apiospermum*)

Unlabeled uses: *Acremonium* sp., *Blastomyces dermatitidis, Coccidioides immitis, Cryptococcus neoformans,* febrile neutropenia, fungal keratitis, *Histoplasma capsulatum,* oropharyngeal candidiasis, *Rhodotorula* sp., *Scedosporium* sp., cutaneous aspergillosis, candidemia (premature neonates), fungal infections in children ≥12 yr

CONTRAINDICATIONS: Pregnancy (D), breastfeeding, children, hypersensitivity, severe bone marrow depression, severe hepatic disease

Precautions: Renal disease (IV); patients of Asian/African descent; cardiomyopathy, cholestasis, chemotherapy, lactase deficiency, visual disturbances, renal failure, pancreatitis, QT prolongation, hypokalemia; ventricular dysrhythmias, torsades de pointes

DOSAGE AND ROUTES

Esophageal candidiasis

- **Adult/geriatric/child ≥12 yr and ≥40 kg: PO** 200 mg q12hr; **<40 kg**, 100 mg q12hr
- **Adult/geriatric/child ≥12 yr: IV INFUSION** Loading dose 6 mg/kg q12hr × 2 dose, then 3-4 mg/kg q12hr; may switch to oral dosing

Candidemia of the skin, kidney, bladder wall, abdomen (nonneutropenic patients)

- **Adult/child ≥12 yr: IV** loading dose 6 mg/kg q12hr × 24 hr, then 3-4 mg/kg q12hr × ≥14 days and ≥7 days after resolution of symptoms; **PO** after loading dose **>40 kg** 200 mg q12hr × ≥14 days and ≥7 days after resolution of symptoms; **<40 kg** 100 mg q12hr × ≥14 days and ≥7 days after resolution of symptoms

Invasive aspergillosis

- **Adults/adolescents: IV** 6 mg/kg q12hr (loading dose), then 4 mg/kg q12hr, may reduce to 3 mg/kg q12hr if intolerable
- **Child ≥12 yr: IV** 6 mg/kg q12hr, then 4 mg/kg q12hr

CNS blastomycosis/blastomycosis meningitis (unlabeled)

- **Adult: PO** 200-400 mg bid × at least 12 mo and until resolution of CSF abnormalities

Renal dose

- **Adult: PO** CCr <50 ml/min, use orally only

Hepatic dose

- **Adult: PO** 6 mg/kg q12hr × 2 doses, then 2 mg/kg q12hr or 100 mg q12hr if >40 kg; 50 mg q12hr if <40 kg

Available forms: Tabs 50, 200 mg; powder for inj, lyophilized 200 mg, powder for oral susp 45 g (40 mg/ml after reconstitution)

Administer:

PO route

- Oral susp: tap bottle; add 46 ml of water to bottle; shake well; remove cap; push bottle adaptor into neck of bottle; replace cap; write expiration date (14 days); shake well before each use; administer using only oral dispenser supplied, 1 hr before or after meals; tabs and susp may be interchanged
- Store at room temperature (powder, tabs)

Intermittent IV INFUSION route

- Product only after C&S confirms organism, product needed to treat condition; make sure product used in life-threatening infections
- Reconstitute powder with 19 ml water for inj to 10 mg/ml; shake until dissolved; infuse over 1-2 hr at concentration of ≤5 mg/ml; do not admix with other products, 4.2% sodium bicarbonate infusion

Y-site compatibilities: Acyclovir, alfentanil, allopurinol, amifostine, amikacin, aminocaproic acid, aminophylline, amiodarone, amphotericin B liposome, ampicillin, ampicillin/sulbactam, anidulafungin, azithromycin, aztreonam, bivalirudin, bleomycin, bumetanide, buprenorphine, butorphanol, calcium acetate/chloride/gluconate, CARBOplatin, carmustine, caspofungin, ceFAZolin, cefotaxime, cefoTEtan, cefOXitin, cefTAZidime, ceftizoxime, cefTRIAXone, chloramphenicol, chlorproMAZINE, cimetidine, ciprofloxacin, cisatracurium, CISplatin, clindamycin, cyclophosphamide, cytarabine, dacarbazine, DACTINomycin, DAPTOmycin, DAUNOrubicin, dexamethasone, dexmedetomidine, dexrazoxane, digoxin, diltiazem, diphenhydrAMINE, DOBUTamine, DOCEtaxel, dolasetron, DOPamine, doripenem, doxacurium, doxycycline, droperidol, enalaprilat, ePHEDrine, EPINEPHrine, epirubicin, ertapenem, erythromycin, esmolol, etoposide, etoposide phosphate, famotidine, fenoldopam, fentaNYL, fluconazole, fludarabine, fluorouracil, foscarnet, fosphenytoin, furosemide, ganciclovir, gemcitabine, gentamicin, glycopyrrolate, granisetron, haloperidol, heparin, hydrALAZINE, hydrocortisone, ifosfamide, imipenem/cilastatin, inamrinone, insulin, irinotecan, isoproterenol, ketorolac, labetalol, leucovorin, levofloxacin, lidocaine, linezolid, LORazepam, magnesium sulfate, mannitol, mechlorethamine, melphalan, meperidine, meropenem, mesna, metaraminol, methohexital, methotrexate, methyldopate, methylPREDNISolone, metoclopramide, metoprolol, metroNIDAZOLE, midazolam, milrinone, mitoMYcin, morphine, nafcillin, nalbuphine, naloxone, niCARdipine, nitroglycerin, norepinephrine, octreotide, ondansetron, oxaliplatin, oxytocin, PACLitaxel, pamidronate, pancuronium, pentamidine, pentazocine, PENTobarbital, PHENobarbital, phentolamine, phenylephrine, piperacillin/tazobactam, potassium chloride/phosphates, procainamide, promethazine, propranolol, quinupristin/dalfopristin, remifentanil, rocuronium, sodium acetate/bicarbonate/phosphates, streptozocin, succinylcholine, SUFentanil, tacrolimus, teniposide, theophylline, thiotepa, ticarcillin/clavulanate, tirofiban, tobramycin, topotecan, trimethobenzamide, trimethoprim/sulfamethoxazole, vancomycin, vasopressin, vecuronium, verapamil, vinBLAStine, vinCRIStine, vinorelbine, zidovudine

SIDE EFFECTS

CNS: *Headache,* paresthesias, peripheral neuropathy, ***hallucinations,*** psychosis, EPS, depression, Guillain-Barré syndrome, insomnia, suicidal ideation, dizziness, fever

CV: **Tachycardia,** hypo/hypertension, vasodilation, **atrial arrhythmias, atrial fibrillation, AV block, bradycardia, CHF, MI, QT prolongation, torsades de pointes,** peripheral edema

EENT: Blurred vision, eye hemorrhage, **visual disturbances**

GI: *Nausea, vomiting, anorexia, diarrhea,* cramps, **hemorrhagic gastroenteritis,**

V

acute hepatic failure, hepatitis, intestinal perforation, pancreatitis
GU: *Hypokalemia,* azotemia, renal tubular necrosis, permanent renal impairment, anuria, oliguria
HEMA: Anemia, eosinophilia, hypomagnesemia, thrombocytopenia, leukopenia, pancytopenia
INTEG: *Burning, irritation,* pain, necrosis at inj site with extravasation, dermatitis, *rash,* photosensitivity
MISC: Respiratory disorder
SYST: Stevens-Johnson syndrome, toxic epidermal necrolysis, sepsis; melanoma, photosensitivity reactions

PHARMACOKINETICS

By CYP3A4, CYP2C9 enzymes; max serum concentration 1-2 hr after dosing; eliminated via hepatic metabolism; protein binding 58%; elimination half-life 6 hr (dose dependent)

INTERACTIONS

Increase: effects of benzodiazepines, calcium channel blockers, cycloSPORINE, ergots, HMG-CoA reductase inhibitors, pimozide, quiNIDine, prednisoLONE, sirolimus, sulfonylureas, tacrolimus, vinca alkaloids, warfarin, rifabutin, proton pump inhibitors, NNRTIs, protease inhibitors, phenytoin
Increase: nephrotoxicity—other nephrotoxic antibiotics (aminoglycosides, CISplatin, vancomycin, cycloSPORINE, polymyxin B)
Increase: hypokalemia—corticosteroids, digoxin, skeletal muscle relaxants, thiazides
⚠ **Increase:** QT prolongation—class IA/III antidysrhythmics, some phenothiazines, β agonists, local anesthetics, tricyclics, haloperidol, chloroquine, droperidol, pentamidine; CYP3A4 inhibitors (amiodarone, clarithromycin, erythromycin, telithromycin, troleandomycin), arsenic trioxide, levomethadyl; CYP3A4 substrates (methadone, pimozide, QUEtiapine, quiNIDine, risperiDONE, ziprasidone)

Drug/Herb
- Do not use with St. John's wort

Drug/Food
- Avoid use with high-fat meals, take 1 hr before or after meal

Drug/Lab Test
Increase: AST/ALT, alk phos, creatinine, bilirubin
Decrease: Hgb/Hct, platelets, WBC

NURSING CONSIDERATIONS

Assess:
- VS q15-30min during first infusion; note changes in pulse, B/P
- I&O ratio; watch for decreasing urinary output, change in specific gravity; discontinue product to prevent permanent damage to renal tubules
- Blood studies: CBC, potassium, sodium, calcium, magnesium, q2wk; BUN, creatinine weekly
- Weight weekly; if weight increases >2 lb/wk, edema is present; renal damage should be considered

⚠ **Renal toxicity:** increasing BUN, serum creatinine; if BUN is >40 mg/dl or if serum creatinine >3 mg/dl, product may be discontinued or dosage reduced
⚠ **Hepatotoxicity:** increasing AST, ALT, alk phos, bilirubin, baseline and periodically
- **Allergic reaction:** dermatitis, rash; product should be discontinued, antihistamines (mild reaction) or epinephrine (severe reaction) administered
- **Hypokalemia:** anorexia, drowsiness, weakness, decreased reflexes, dizziness, increased urinary output, increased thirst, paresthesias
- **Ototoxicity:** tinnitus (ringing, roaring in ears), vertigo, loss of hearing (rare); visual disturbance
- **QT prolongation:** ECG, ejection fraction; assess for chest pain, palpitations, dyspnea

Evaluate:
- Therapeutic response: decreased fever, malaise, rash, negative C&S for infecting organism

Teach patient/family:
- That long-term therapy may be needed to clear infection (2 wk-3 mo, depending on type of infection)
- To notify prescriber of bleeding, bruising, soft-tissue swelling, dark urine, persistent nausea or diarrhea, headache, rash, yellow skin/eyes
- Take 1 hr before or after meal (PO)

- Do not drive at night because of vision changes
- Avoid strong, direct sunlight
- Women of childbearing age should use effective contraceptive, pregnancy (D)

vortioxetine

(vor′tye-ox′e-teen)

Brintellix

Func. class.: Antidepressant

Chem. class.: Serotonin modulator

ACTION: Reuptake inhibition at the serotonin transporter and agonist, or antagonist effects at serotonin receptors

USES: Major depressive disorder in adults

CONTRAINDICATIONS: Hypersensitivity, MAOI therapy

Precautions: Pregnancy (C), breastfeeding, seizure disorder, hypersensitivity, bipolar disorder, hyponatremia, hypovolemia

DOSAGE AND ROUTES

- **Adult: PO** 10 mg/day, may start with 5 mg/day initially, increase to 20 mg/day as tolerated, max 20 mg/day; poor metabolizers of CYP2D6 max 10 mg/day

Available forms: Tabs 5, 10, 20 mg

Administer: Without regard to food

SIDE EFFECTS

CNS: Flushing, mania, serotonin syndrome, vertigo, dizziness, suicidal attempts

GI: Nausea, diarrhea, dyspnea, constipation, vomiting, flatulence

GU: Impotence

INTEG: Pruritus

SYST: Serotonin syndrome, neonatal abstinence syndrome

PHARMACOKINETICS

Protein binding 98%, excreted in urine (59%), feces (26%)

INTERACTIONS

Increase: effect of tricyclics; use cautiously

Increase: serotonin syndrome—serotonin receptor agonists, SSRIs, traMADol, lithium, MAOIs, traZODone, SNRIs (venlafaxine, DULoxetine)

Increase: bleeding risk—NSAIDs, salicylates, thrombolytics, anticoagulants, antiplatelets

Increase: CNS effects—barbiturates, sedative/hypnotics, other CNS depressants

Decrease: vortioxetine levels—carBAMazepine

Drug/Herb:

Increase: serotonin syndrome—St. John's wort

NURSING CONSIDERATIONS

Assess:

Black Box Warning: Mental status: mood, sensorium, affect, suicidal tendencies, increase in psychiatric symptoms, depression, panic

- **Serotonin syndrome:** increased heart rate, sweating, dilated pupils, tremors, twitching, hyperthermia, agitation
- Alcohol consumption; if alcohol is consumed, hold dose until AM
- **Sexual dysfunction:** impotence

Evaluate:

- Therapeutic response: decreased depression
- Children, suicidal ideation

Teach patient/family:

- That therapeutic effect may take several wk
- To use caution when driving, performing other activities that require alertness because of drowsiness, dizziness, blurred vision; to report signs, symptoms or bleeding
- To avoid alcohol, other CNS depressants

Black Box Warning: That suicidal ideas, behaviors may occur in children or young adults

- To notify prescriber if pregnant, planning to become pregnant, or breastfeeding

Black Box Warning: About the effects of serotonin syndrome: nausea/vomiting, tremors; if symptoms occur, to discontinue immediately, notify prescriber

HIGH ALERT

warfarin (Rx)

(war′far-in)

Coumadin, Jantoven

Func. class.: Anticoagulant

Chem. class.: Coumarin derivative

Do not confuse:
Coumadin/Cardura/Compazine

ACTION: Interferes with blood clotting by indirect means; depresses hepatic synthesis of vit-K–dependent coagulation factors (II, VII, IX, X)

USES: Antiphospholipid antibody syndrome, arterial thromboembolism prophylaxis, DVT, MI prophylaxis, after MI, stroke prophylaxis, thrombosis prophylaxis

Unlabeled uses: Angina, unstable angina

CONTRAINDICATIONS: Pregnancy (X), breastfeeding, hypersensitivity, hemophilia, leukemia with bleeding, peptic ulcer disease, thrombocytopenic purpura, hepatic disease (severe), malignant hypertension, subacute bacterial endocarditis, acute nephritis, blood dyscrasias, eclampsia, preeclampsia, hemorrhagic tendencies; surgery of CNS, eye; traumatric surgery with large open surface, bleeding tendencies of GI/GU/respiratory tract, stroke, aneurysms, pericardial effusion, spinal puncture, major regional/lumbar block anesthesia

Black Box Warning: Bleeding

Precautions: Geriatric patients, alcoholism, CHF, debilitated patients, trauma, indwelling catheters, severe hypertension, active infections, protein C deficiency, polycythemia vera, vasculitis, severe diabetes, Asian patients (CYP2C9), protein C, S deficiency

DOSAGE AND ROUTES

- **Adult: PO** 2-10 mg/day × 2-4 days, then titrated to INR/PT
- **Adolescent/child/infant: PO** 0.2 mg/kg/day × 2 days titrated to INR

Available forms: Tabs 1, 2, 2.5, 3, 4, 5, 6, 7.5, 10 mg

Administer:

PO route

- At same time each day to maintain steady blood levels without regard to food; food decreases rate but not extent of absorption; do not change brands
- Tabs whole or crushed
- Avoiding all IM inj that may cause bleeding
- Store in tight container

SIDE EFFECTS

CNS: *Fever,* dizziness, fatigue, headache, lethargy

CV: Angina, chest pain, edema, hypotension, syncope

GI: *Diarrhea,* nausea, vomiting, anorexia, stomatitis, cramps, hepatitis, cholestatic jaundice

GU: Hematuria

HEMA: Hemorrhage, agranulocytosis, leukopenia, eosinophilia, anemia, ecchymosis, petechiae

INTEG: *Rash,* dermatitis, urticaria, alopecia, pruritus

MISC: Epistaxis, hemoptysis, mouth ulcers, taste disturbances, priapism, dyspnea

MS: Bone fractures

SYST: Anaphylaxis, coma, cholesterol, microembolism, exfoliative dermatitis, purple toe syndrome

PHARMACOKINETICS

PO: Onset 12-24 hr, peak 1½-4 days, duration 3-5 days, effective half-life 20-60 hr; metabolized in liver; excreted in urine, feces (active/inactive metabolites); crosses placenta, 99% bound to plasma proteins

INTERACTIONS

Increase: warfarin action—allopurinol, amiodarone, chloral hydrate, chloramphenicol, cimetidine, clofibrate, cotrimoxazole, COX-2 selective inhibitors, dextrothyroxine, diflunisal, disulfiram, erythromycin, ethacrynic acids, furosemide, glucagon, heparin, HMG-CoA reductase inhibitors, indomethacin, isoniazid, mefenamic acid, metroNIDAZOLE, mifepristone, NSAIDs, oxyphenbutazones, penicillins, phenylbutazone, quiNIDine, quinolone antiinfectives, RU-486, salicylates, sulfinpyrazone, sulfonamides, sulindac, SSRIs, steroids, thrombolytics, thyroid, tricyclics

Increase: toxicity—oral sulfonylureas, phenytoin

Decrease: warfarin action—aprepitant, azaTHIOprine, barbiturates, bile acid sequestrants, bosentan, carBAMazepine, dicloxacillin, estrogens, ethchlorvynol, factor IX/VIIa, griseofulvin, nafcillin, oral contraceptives, phenytoin, rifampin, sucralfate, sulfaSALAzine, thyroid, vit K, vit K foods

Drug/Herb

Increase: risk for bleeding—angelica, anise, basil, chamomile, chondroitin, dong quai, evening primrose, feverfew, garlic, ginger, ginkgo, ginseng, horse chestnut, kava, licorice, melatonin, red yeast rice, saw palmetto

Decrease: anticoagulant effect—coenzyme Q10, St. John's wort

Drug/Lab Test

Increase: T_3 uptake, LFTs

Decrease: uric acid

NURSING CONSIDERATIONS

Assess:

Black Box Warning: Blood studies (Hct, PT, platelets, occult blood in stools) q3mo; INR: in hospital daily after 2nd or 3rd dose; when in therapeutic range for 2 consecutive days, monitor 2-3× wk for 1-2 wk, then less frequently, depending on stability of INR results; *Outpatient:* monitor every few days until stable dose then periodically thereafter, depending on stability of INR results, usually at least monthly

Black Box Warning: Bleeding gums, petechiae, ecchymosis, black tarry stools, hematuria; fatal hemorrhage can occur

⚠ Fever, skin rash, urticaria

Evaluate:

- Therapeutic response: decrease in deep venous thrombosis

Teach patient/family:

- To avoid OTC preparations that may cause serious product interactions unless directed by prescriber
- To carry emergency ID identifying product taken
- About the importance of compliance
- To report any signs of bleeding: gums, under skin, urine, stools; to use soft-bristle toothbrush to avoid bleeding gums; to use electric razor
- To avoid hazardous activities (e.g., football, hockey, skiing), dangerous work
- About the importance of avoiding unusual changes in vitamin intake, diet, or lifestyle
- To inform all health care providers of anticoagulant intake

TREATMENT OF OVERDOSE:

Administer vit K

zafirlukast (Rx)

(za-feer′loo-cast)

Accolate

Func. class.: Bronchodilator

Chem. class.: Leukotriene receptor antagonist

Do not confuse:
Accolate/Accupril/Aclovate

ACTION: Antagonizes the contractile action of leukotrienes (LTD_4, LTE_4) in airway smooth muscle; inhibits bronchoconstriction caused by antigens

USES: Prophylaxis and chronic treatment of asthma in adults/children >5 yr
Unlabeled uses: Allergic rhinitis

CONTRAINDICATIONS: Hypersensitivity, hepatic encephalopathy
Precautions: Pregnancy (B), breastfeeding, children, geriatric patients, hepatic disease, Churg-Strauss syndrome, acute bronchospasm

DOSAGE AND ROUTES

- **Adult and child ≥12 yr: PO** 20 mg bid
- **Child 5-11 yr: PO** 10 mg bid

Available forms: Tabs 10, 20 mg
Administer:

- 1 hr before or 2 hr after meals; absorption may be decreased if given with food

SIDE EFFECTS

CNS: Headache, dizziness, suicidal ideation, insomnia, fever
GI: Nausea, diarrhea, abdominal pain, vomiting, dyspepsia, hepatic failure, hepatitis
HEMA: Agranulocytosis
OTHER: Infections, pain, asthenia, myalgia, fever, increased ALT, urticaria, rash, angioedema

PHARMACOKINETICS

Rapidly absorbed, peak 3 hr, 99% protein binding (albumin), extensively metabolized, inhibits CYP2C9 and 3A4 enzyme systems, excreted in feces, clearance reduced in geriatric patients, hepatic impairment, half-life 10 hr

INTERACTIONS

Increase: plasma levels of zafirlukast—aspirin
Increase: PT—warfarin
Decrease: plasma levels of zafirlukast—erythromycin, theophylline
Drug/Food
Decrease: bioavailability

NURSING CONSIDERATIONS

Assess:

⚠ **Adult patients carefully for symptoms of Churg-Strauss syndrome** (rare), including eosinophilia, vasculitic rash, worsening pulmonary symptoms, cardiac complications, neuropathy; may be caused by reducing oral corticosteroids

- Respiratory rate, rhythm, depth; auscultate lung fields bilaterally; notify prescriber of abnormalities; not to be used for acute bronchospasm in acute asthma
- **Hepatic/renal/pancreatic/visual function:** monitor liver function tests

Evaluate:

- Therapeutic response: ability to breathe more easily

Teach patient/family:

- To check OTC medications, current prescription medications that may increase stimulation, do not stop other asthma medications unless instructed to do so
- To avoid hazardous activities because dizziness may occur
- That, if GI upset occurs, to take product with 8 oz water; to avoid taking with food if possible because absorption may be decreased
- To notify prescriber of nausea, vomiting, diarrhea, abdominal pain, fatigue, jaundice, anorexia, flulike symptoms (hepatic dysfunction)
- Not to use for acute asthma episodes
- Not to take if breastfeeding
- To take even if symptom free

⚠ Nurse Alert

⚠ HIGH ALERT

zaleplon (Rx)

(zal′eh-plon)

Sonata

Func. class.: Hypnotic, nonbarbiturate

Chem. class.: Pyrazolopyrimidine

Controlled Substance Schedule IV

ACTION: Binds selectively to omega-1 receptor of the $GABA_A$ receptor complex; results are sedation, hypnosis, skeletal muscle relaxation, anticonvulsant activity, anxiolytic action

USES: Insomnia (short-term treatment)

CONTRAINDICATIONS: Hypersensitivity, severe hepatic disease

Precautions: Pregnancy (C), breastfeeding, children <15 yr, geriatric patients, respiratory/renal/hepatic disease, psychosis, angioedema, depression, sleep-related behaviors (sleep walking), Asian descent, CNS depression

DOSAGE AND ROUTES

- **Adult: PO** 10 mg at bedtime; may increase dose to 20 mg at bedtime if needed; 5 mg may be used in low-weight persons
- **Geriatric: PO** 5 mg at bedtime; may increase if needed

Available forms: Caps 5, 10 mg

Administer:

- Immediately before bedtime for sleeplessness
- On empty stomach for fast onset
- Store in tight container in cool environment

SIDE EFFECTS

CNS: *Lethargy, drowsiness, daytime sedation,* dizziness, confusion, anxiety, amnesia, depersonalization, hallucinations, hyperesthesia, paresthesia, somnolence, tremors, vertigo, **complex sleep-related reactions: sleep driving, sleep eating**

CV: Chest pain, peripheral edema

EENT: Vision change, ear/eye pain, hyperacusis, parosmia

GI: Nausea, abdominal pain, constipation, anorexia, colitis, dyspepsia, dry mouth

MISC: Asthenia, fever, headache, myalgia, dysmenorrhea

MS: Myalgia, back pain, arthritis

RESP: Bronchitis

SYST: **Severe allergic reactions**

PHARMACOKINETICS

Rapid onset, metabolized by liver extensively, excreted by kidneys (inactive metabolites), half-life 1 hr, onset, peak 1 hr, duration 3-4 hr

INTERACTIONS

Increase: effect of zaleplon—cimetidine

Decrease: zaleplon bioavailability—CYP3A4 inducers

Drug/Food

- Prolonged absorption, sleep onset reduced: high-fat/heavy meal

NURSING CONSIDERATIONS

Assess:

- Mental status: mood, sensorium, affect, memory (long, short term), excessive sedation, impaired coordination
- **Sleep disorder:** type of sleep problem: falling asleep, staying asleep; monitor for complex sleep disorders

Evaluate:

- Therapeutic response: ability to sleep at night, decreased amount of early morning awakening

Teach patient/family:

- To avoid driving or other activities requiring alertness until product is stabilized
- To avoid alcohol ingestion
- **That product may cause memory problems, dependence (if used for longer periods of time), changes in behavior/thinking, complex sleep-related behaviors (sleep eating/driving)**
- That product is for short-term use only
- To take immediately before going to bed

Z

• Not to ingest a high-fat/heavy meal before taking

zanamivir (Rx)

(zan′ah-mih-veer)

Relenza

Func. class.: Antiviral

Chem. class.: Neuramidase inhibitor

ACTION: Inhibits neuramidase enzyme needed for influenza virus replication

USES: Treatment of influenza types A and B for patients who have been symptomatic for ≤2 days

CONTRAINDICATIONS: Hypersensitivity

Precautions: Pregnancy (C), breastfeeding, children <7 yr, geriatric patients, respiratory disease, angioedema, milk protein hypersensitivity, Reye's syndrome

DOSAGE AND ROUTES

• **Adult/child >7 yr: INH** 2 inhalations (two 5-mg blisters) q12hr × 5 days; on the 1st day, 2 doses should be taken with at least 2 hr between doses

Available forms: Blisters of powder for inhalation: 5 mg

Administer:

• Within 2 days of symptoms of influenza; continue for 5 days

• Give patient Patient's Instructions for Use, review all points before using delivery system

• Do not use as nebulized sol or in mechanical ventilation

• Store in tight, dry container

SIDE EFFECTS

CNS: *Headache, dizziness,* seizures, fatigue; self-injury, delirium (child)

EENT: Ear, nose, throat infections, throat discomfort

GI: *Nausea, vomiting,* diarrhea

RESP: Nasal symptoms, cough, sinusitis, bronchitis, bronchospasm

SYST: Angioedema

PHARMACOKINETICS

Half-life 2½-5 hr, not metabolized, excreted in urine unchanged

INTERACTIONS

• May decrease intranasal influenzae vaccine; separate by ≥48 hr; do not restart antiviral products for ≥2 wk

NURSING CONSIDERATIONS

Assess:

• Skin eruptions, photosensitivity after administration of product

• Respiratory status: rate, character, wheezing, tightness in chest

• Allergies before initiation of treatment, reaction of each medication

• Signs of infection

Evaluate:

• Therapeutic response: absence of fever, malaise, cough, dyspnea with infection

Teach patient/family:

• That product does not reduce transmission risk of influenza to others

• That patients with asthma or COPD should carry a fast-acting inhaled bronchodilator because bronchospasm may occur; to use scheduled inhaled bronchodilators before using product

• To avoid hazardous activities if dizziness occurs

zidovudine (Rx)

(zye-doe′-vue-deen)

Novo-AZT ♣, Retrovir

Func. class.: Antiretroviral

Chem. class.: Nucleoside reverse transcriptase inhibitor (NRTI)

Do not confuse:

Retrovir/ritonavir

ACTION: Inhibits replication of HIV-1 virus by incorporating into cellular DNA by viral reverse transcriptase, thereby terminating the cellular DNA chain

USES:
Used in combination with at least 2 other antiretrovirals for HIV-1 infection

Unlabeled uses: Epstein-Barr virus, hepatitis B, human T-lymphotropic virus type I (HTLV-I), thrombocytopenia

CONTRAINDICATIONS:
Hypersensitivity

Precautions: Pregnancy (C), breastfeeding, children, granulocyte count $<1000/mm^3$ or Hgb <9.5 g/dl, severe renal disease, obesity

Black Box Warning: Impaired hepatic function, anemia, lactic acidosis, myopathy, neutropenia

DOSAGE AND ROUTES

HIV infections with other antiretrovirals

- **Adult: PO (tabs, caps, syrup)** 600 mg/day in divided doses, either 200 mg tid or 300 mg bid in combination with other antiretrovirals; **IV** 1 mg/kg q4hr, initiate **PO** as soon as possible up to 1000 mg
- **Child 25 kg to <30 kg: PO (tabs/caps)** 500 mg/day divided bid
- **Child 19 kg to <25 kg: PO (tabs/caps)** 400 mg/day divided bid
- **Infant/child ≥4 wk and 13 to <19 kg: PO (tabs/caps)** 300 mg/day divided bid
- **Infant/child ≥4 wk and 7 to <13 kg: PO (tabs/caps)** 200 mg/day divided bid
- **Infant/child ≥4 wk and 5 to <7 kg: PO (tabs/caps)** 150 mg/day divided bid
- **Adolescent/child ≥30 kg: PO (tabs/caps/syrup)** 300 mg bid or 200 mg tid
- **Infant ≥4 wk, child/adolescent ≥9 to <30 kg: PO (syrup)** 18 mg/kg/day divided bid or tid
- **Infant ≥4 wk and 4 to <9 kg: PO (syrup)** 24 mg/kg/day divided bid or tid
- **Neonate (unlabeled): PO (syrup)** 2 mg/kg q6hr
- **Premature neonate (unlabeled): PO (syrup)** 2 mg/kg q12hr, increase to 2 mg/kg q8hr at 2 wk for neonates ≥30 wk gestation or at 4 wk for neonates <30 wk gestation

Prevention of maternal–fetal HIV transmission

- **Neonates ≥34 wk: PO** 2 mg/kg/dose q6hr × 6 wk beginning 8-12 hr after birth; **IV** 1.5 mg/kg/dose over 30 min q6hr until able to take **PO**
- **Maternal (>14 wk gestation): PO** 100 mg 5×/day until start of labor then during labor/delivery **IV** 2 mg/kg over 1 hr followed by **IV INFUSION** 1 mg/kg/hr until umbilical cord clamped

Prevention of HIV after needlestick

- **Adult: PO** 200 mg tid plus lamiVUDine 150 mg bid plus a protease inhibitor for high-risk exposure; begin within 2 hr of exposure

Available forms: Caps 100; tabs 300 mg; inj 10 mg/ml; oral syr 50 mg/5 ml

Administer:

- By mouth; capsules should be swallowed whole
- Trimethoprim-sulfamethoxazole, pyrimethamine, or acyclovir as ordered to prevent opportunistic infections; if these products are given, watch for neurotoxicity
- Store in cool environment; protect from light

Intermittent IV INFUSION route

- After diluting each 1 mg/0.25 ml or more D_5W to ≤4 mg/ml; give over 1 hr
- Protect unopened product from light; use diluted sol within 24 hr room temperature, 48 hr refrigerated

Y-site compatibilities: Acyclovir, alemtuzumab, allopurinol, amifostine, amikacin, amphotericin B, amphotericin B cholesteryl, anidulafungin, argatroban, aztreonam, cefepime, cefTAZidime, cefTRIAXone, cimetidine, cisatracurium, clindamycin, dexamethasone, DOBUTamine, DOPamine, DOXOrubicin liposome, erythromycin, filgrastim, fluconazole, fludarabine, gentamicin, granisetron, heparin, imipenem-cilastatin, LORazepam, melphalan, metoclopramide, morphine, nafcillin, ondansetron, oxacillin, PACLitaxel, pentamidine, phenylephrine, piperacillin,

Z

piperacillin-tazobactam, potassium chloride, ranitidine, remifentanil, sargramostim, tacrolimus, teniposide, thiotepa, tobramycin, trimethoprim-sulfamethoxazole, trimetrexate, vancomycin, vinorelbine, zoledronic acid

SIDE EFFECTS

CNS: *Fever, headache, malaise,* diaphoresis, *dizziness, insomnia,* paresthesia, somnolence, chills, tremors, twitching, anxiety, confusion, depression, lability, vertigo, loss of mental acuity, seizures, malaise

EENT: Taste change, hearing loss, photophobia

GI: *Nausea, vomiting, diarrhea, anorexia,* cramps, *dyspepsia, constipation,* dysphagia, *flatulence,* rectal bleeding, mouth ulcer, abdominal pain, hepatomegaly

GU: Dysuria, polyuria, urinary frequency, hesitancy

HEMA: Granulocytopenia, anemia

INTEG: *Rash,* acne, pruritus, urticaria

MS: Myalgia, arthralgia, muscle spasm

RESP: Dyspnea, cough, wheezing

SYST: Lactic acidosis

PHARMACOKINETICS

PO: Rapidly absorbed from GI tract, peak $\frac{1}{2}$-$1\frac{1}{2}$ hr, metabolized in liver (inactive metabolites), excreted by kidneys, protein binding 38%, terminal half-life $\frac{1}{2}$-3 hr

INTERACTIONS

Increase: bone marrow depression—antineoplastics, radiation, ganciclovir, valganciclovir, trimethoprim-sulfamethoxazole

Increase: zidovudine level—methadone, atovaquone, fluconazole, probenecid, trimethoprim, valproic acid; may need to reduce zidovudine dose

Decrease: zidovudine levels—interferons, NRTIs, DOXOrubicin, ribavirin, stavudine; avoid concurrent use

Drug/Lab Test

Decrease: platelets, granulocytes

Increase: LFTs, amylase, CPK

NURSING CONSIDERATIONS

Assess:

- Blood dyscrasias (anemia, granulocytopenia): bruising, fatigue, bleeding, poor healing

Black Box Warning: Blood counts q2wk; watch for decreasing granulocytes, Hgb; if low, therapy may have to be discontinued and restarted after hematologic recovery; blood transfusions may be required; viral load, CD4 counts, LFTs, plasma HIV RNA, serum creatinine/BUN at baseline and throughout treatment

Black Box Warning: Lactic acidosis, severe hepatomegaly with steatosis: Obtain baseline liver function tests, if elevated, discontinue treatment; discontinue even if liver function tests are normal but lactic acidosis, hepatomegaly are present; may be fatal

Evaluate:

- Therapeutic response: decreased viral load, increased CD4 counts, decreased symptoms of HIV

Teach patient/family:

- That GI complaints and insomnia resolve after 3-4 wk of treatment
- That product not cure for AIDS but will control symptoms, compliance with treatment is required
- To notify prescriber of sore throat, swollen lymph nodes, malaise, fever because other infections may occur
- That patient is still infective, may pass AIDS virus on to others
- That follow-up visits must be continued because serious toxicity may occur; that blood counts must be done q2wk; that blood transfusions may be needed for severe anemia
- That product must be taken bid or tid
- That serious product interactions may occur if OTC products are ingested; to check with prescriber before taking aspirin, acetaminophen, indomethacin
- That other products may be necessary to prevent other infections

- That product may cause fainting or dizziness

zinc (Rx, OTC)

Galzin

Func. class.: Trace element; nutritional supplement

ACTION: Needed for adequate healing, bone and joint development (23% zinc)

USES: Prevention of zinc deficiency, adjunct to vit A therapy

Unlabeled uses: Wound healing

Precautions: Pregnancy (C) parenteral; breastfeeding, neonates, hypocupremia, neonatal prematurity, renal disease

DOSAGE AND ROUTES

Dietary supplement (elemental zinc)

- **Adult/adolescent/pregnant female: PO** 11-13 mg/day
- **Adult/lactating female: PO** 12-14 mg/day × 12 mo
- **Adult/adolescent male ≥14 yr: PO** 11 mg/day
- **Adult female ≥19 yr: PO** 8 mg/day
- **Adolescent female ≥14 yr: PO** 9 mg/day
- **Child 9-13 yr: PO** 8 mg/day
- **Child 4-8 yr: PO** 5 mg/day
- **Child 1-3 yr: PO** 3 mg/day
- **Infant 7-12 mo: PO** 3 mg/day
- **Infant birth to 6 mo: PO** 2 mg/day (adequate intake)

Nutritional supplement (IV)

- **Adult:** 2.5-4 mg/day; may increase by 2 mg/day if needed
- **Child 1-5 yr: IV** 50 mcg/kg/day

Wound healing

- **Adult: PO** 50 mg tid until healed (elemental zinc)

Available forms: Tabs 66, 110 mg; caps 220 mg; inj 1 mg, 5 mg/ml

Administer:

- With meals to decrease gastric upset; avoid dairy products

SIDE EFFECTS

GI: Nausea, vomiting, cramps, heartburn, ulcer formation

OVERDOSE: Diarrhea, rash, dehydration, restlessness

INTERACTIONS

Decrease: absorption of fluoroquinolones—tetracyclines

Drug/Food

Decrease: absorption of PO zinc—dairy products, caffeine

NURSING CONSIDERATIONS

Assess:

- **Zinc deficiency:** poor wound healing, absence of taste, smell, slowing growth
- Alkaline phosphatase, HDL monthly in long term therapy
- Zinc levels during treatment

Evaluate:

- Therapeutic response: absence of zinc deficiency

Teach patient/family:

- That element must be taken for 2-3 mo to be effective
- **To immediately report nausea, diarrhea, rash, severe vomiting, restlessness, abdominal pain, tarry stools**

ziprasidone (Rx)

(zi-praz′ih-dohn)

Geodon, Zeldox ♣

Func. class.: Antipsychotic/neuroleptic

Chem. class.: Benzisoxazole derivative

ACTION: Unknown; may be mediated through both dopamine type 2 (D_2) and serotonin type 2 ($5\text{-}HT_2$) antagonism

USES: Schizophrenia, acute agitation, acute psychosis, bipolar disorder, mania, psychotic depression

CONTRAINDICATIONS: Breastfeeding, hypersensitivity, acute MI, heart failure, QT prolongation

Precautions: Pregnancy (C), children, geriatric patients, cardiac/renal/hepatic

Z

disease, breast cancer, diabetes, seizure disorders, AV block, CNS depression, abrupt discontinuation, agranulocytosis, ambient temperature increase, suicidal ideation, torsades de pointes, strenuous exercise

Black Box Warning: Increased mortality in geriatric patients with dementia-related psychosis

DOSAGE AND ROUTES

Schizophrenia

- **Adult: PO** 20 mg bid with food, adjust dosage every 2 days upward to max of 80 mg bid; **IM** 10-20 mg; may give 10 mg q2hr; doses of 20 mg may be given q4hr; max 40 mg/day (acute episodes); switch to PO as soon as possible

Bipolar disorder

- **Adult: PO** 40 mg bid with food; on day 2 increase to 60 or 80 mg bid, then adjust to response; maintenance as adjunct to lithium/valproate 40-80 mg bid

Available forms: Caps 20, 40, 60, 80 mg; inj 20 mg/ml single-dose vials

Administer:

PO route

- Take cap whole and with food, with plenty of fluid at same time of day
- Reduced dose in geriatric patients
- Anticholinergic agent on order from prescriber to be used for EPS
- Store in tight, light-resistant container

IM route

- Add 1.2 ml sterile water for inj to vial; shake vigorously until dissolved; do not admix; give only IM; give deeply in large muscle; do not mix with other products, do not use if particulates are present, keep patient recumbent for 30 min after injection
- Store injection at room temperature, protect from light, after reconstituting may be stored at room temperature × 24 hr, 7 days refrigerated

SIDE EFFECTS

CNS: *EPS, pseudoparkinsonism, akathisia, dystonia, tardive dyskinesia; drowsiness, insomnia, agitation, anxiety, headache,* seizures, neuroleptic malignant syndrome, dizziness, tremors, facial droop

CV: Orthostatic hypotension, tachycardia, prolonged QT/QTc, hypertension, sudden death, heart failure (geriatric patients), torsades de pointes

EENT: Blurred vision, diplopia

ENDO: Metabolic changes, hyperprolactinemia (rare)

GI: *Nausea,* vomiting, *anorexia, constipation,* jaundice, weight gain, diarrhea, dry mouth, abdominal pain

GU: Enuresis, urinary incontinence, gynecomastia, impotence, priapism

MS: Decreased bone density

RESP: Rhinitis, dyspnea, infection, cough

INTEG: Rash, injection-site pain, sweating

PHARMACOKINETICS

IM: Peak 60 min

PO: Extensively metabolized by liver to major active metabolite, plasma protein binding 99%, peak 6-8 hr, terminal half-life 7 hr

INTERACTIONS

⚠ **Increase:** QT prolongation—class IA/III antidysrhythmics, some phenothiazines, β-agonists, local anesthetics, tricyclics, haloperidol, methadone, chloroquine, clarithromycin, droperidol, erythromycin, pentamidine, moxifloxacin

Increase: sedation—other CNS depressants, alcohol

Increase: EPS, possible neurotoxicity—other antipsychotics, lithium

Increase: ziprasidone excretion—carBAMazepine, barbiturates, phenytoin, rifampin

Increase: ziprasidone level—ketoconazole

Increase: hypotension—antihypertensives

Increase: serotonin syndrome, neuroleptic malignant syndrome—SSRIs, SNRIs

Decrease: ziprasidone effect—carbamazepine

NURSING CONSIDERATIONS

Assess:

- Mental status before initial administration, AIMS assessment

Black Box Warning: Assess geriatric patient with dementia closely; heart failure, sudden death have occurred

- Bilirubin, CBC, LFTs, fasting blood glucose, cholesterol profile; potassium, magnesium when taken with loop/thiazide diuretics monthly
- Urinalysis before, during prolonged therapy
- B/P standing and lying; also pulse, respirations; take these q4hr during initial treatment; establish baseline before starting treatment; report drops of 30 mm Hg; watch for ECG changes; QT prolongation may occur
- Dizziness, faintness, palpitations, tachycardia on rising; metabolic changes, weight gain
- **EPS,** including akathisia (inability to sit still, no pattern to movements), tardive dyskinesia (bizarre movements of the jaw, mouth, tongue, extremities), pseudoparkinsonism (rigidity, tremors, pill rolling, shuffling gait)

⚠ **Neuroleptic malignant syndrome, serotonin syndrome:** hyperthermia, increased CPK, altered mental status, muscle rigidity

- Constipation, urinary retention daily; if these occur, increase bulk and water in diet
- Supervised ambulation until patient is stabilized on medication; do not involve patient in strenuous exercise program because fainting is possible; patient should not stand still for a long time
- Increased fluids to prevent constipation

Evaluate:

- Therapeutic response: decrease in emotional excitement, hallucinations, delusions, paranoia; reorganization of patterns of thought, speech

Teach patient/family:

- That orthostatic hypotension may occur; to rise from sitting or lying position gradually
- To avoid hot tubs, hot showers, tub baths because hypotension may occur
- To avoid abrupt withdrawal of product because EPS may result; that product should be withdrawn slowly
- To avoid OTC preparations (cough, hay fever, cold) unless approved by prescriber because serious product interactions may occur; to avoid use with alcohol because increased drowsiness may occur
- To avoid hazardous activities if drowsy or dizzy
- To report impaired vision, tremors, muscle twitching
- In hot weather, that heat stroke may occur; to take extra precautions to stay cool

TREATMENT OF OVERDOSE:

Lavage if orally ingested; provide airway; *do not induce vomiting*

⚠ HIGH ALERT

ziv-aflibercept

(ziv-a-flih′ber-sept)

Zaltrap

Func. class.: Antineoplastic biologic response modifier

Chem. class.: Signal transduction inhibitor (STI)

ACTION: An angiogenesis inhibitor, a fusion protein that binds to vascular endothelial growth factors (VEGF-A, VEGF-B) and placental growth factor 1 and 2

USES: Metastatic colorectal cancer that is resistant or has progressed after an Oxaliplatin-containing regimen in combination with 5-fluorouracil, leucovorin, irinotecan (FOLFIRI)

CONTRAINDICATIONS: Hypersensitivity

Precautions: Infertility, male-mediated teratogenicity, encephalopathy,

Z

hypertension, dental work, breastfeeding, children, neonates, geriatric patients, infection, neutropenia, pregnancy (C)

Black Box Warning: Bleeding, GI bleeding/perforation, intracranial bleeding, surgery

DOSAGE AND ROUTES

- **Adult: IV** 4 mg/kg over 1 hr on day 1 every 2 wk in combination with the FOLFIRI regimen (irinotecan 180 mg/m^2 over 90 min on day 1 with dl-racemic leucovorin 400 mg/m^2 over 2 hr) (infused at the same time, in same Y-line; then on day 1 by 5-fluorouracil 400 mg/m^2 as a bolus, then 2400 mg/m^2 as a 46-hr cont IV infusion)

Available forms: Solution for injection 100 mg/4 ml; 200 mg/8 ml

Administer:

- Give before FOLFIRI chemotherapy; visually inspect for particulate matter and discoloration before use

Dilution and preparation

- Withdraw the calculated dose; add to 0.9% sodium chloride or dextrose 5% solution to 0.6-8 mg/mL; use polyvinyl chloride (PVC) infusion bags containing bis (2-ethylhexyl) phthalate (DHEP) or polyolefin infusion bags; do not re-enter the vial after first puncture; discard any unused portion; do not mix or combine with other drugs in the same infusion bag; the diluted solution may be stored refrigerated for ≤4 hr; discard any unused portion in the infusion bag

IV infusion

- Give diluted solution over 1 hr using a 0.2-micron polyethersulfone filter; do not use nylon or polyvinylidene fluoride (PVDF) filters; do not give IV push or bolus; do not mix or combine with other drugs in the same IV line; give using an infusion set made of one of the following: PVC containing DEHP, DEHP-free PVC containing trioctyl-trimellitate (TOTM), polypropylene, polyethylene-lined PVC, or polyurethane

Dosage adjustments for recurrent or severe hypertension

⚠ Hold until B/P is controlled and then permanently reduce dose to 2 mg/kg; discontinue in hypertensive crisis or hypertensive encephalopathy

Dosage adjustments for proteinuria (2 g/24 hr)

⚠ Hold until proteinuria is <2 g/24 hr; if proteinuria recurs, hold therapy until proteinuria is <2 g/24 hr, then reduce to 2 mg/kg; discontinue in nephrotic syndrome or thrombotic microangiopathy

SIDE EFFECTS

CNS: Intracranial bleeding, headache, dizziness

CV: Hypertensive crisis, hypertension, stroke

GI: Nausea, hepatotoxicity, dyspepsia, GI hemorrhage, abdominal pain, GI perforation

GU: Proteinuria, hematuria

HEMA: Neutropenia, leukopenia

INTEG: Rash, pruritus, alopecia, hypersensitivity

MISC: Fatigue, epistaxis, night sweats, decreased weight, flulike symptoms, infection

RESP: Dyspnea, pulmonary embolism

PHARMACOKINETICS

Elimination half-life 6 days

NURSING CONSIDERATIONS

Assess:

Black Box Warning: Severe bleeding: GI bleeding, intracranial bleeding, and pulmonary hemorrhage/hemoptysis may be fatal; monitor patients for signs and symptoms of bleeding

Black Box Warning: GI perforation: some cases are fatal; monitor patients for signs and symptoms of GI perforation; discontinue therapy if GI perforation develops

- **Poor wound healing:** hold ≥4 wk before elective surgery; after major surgery, do not restart for ≥4 wk and until the surgical wound is entirely healed

⚠ **Severe hypertension/hypertensive crisis:** usually occurs within the first 2 cycles (grade 3 or 4 hypertension); monitor B/P every 2 wk or more often if needed; treatment with antihypertensives may be needed; product may need to be discontinued

⚠ **Severe proteinuria/nephrotic syndrome/thrombotic microangiopathy (TMA):** monitor urine protein by dipstick analysis and urinary protein–to–creatinine ratio (UPCR); obtain a 24-hr urine collection for a UPCR >1; for proteinuria of 2 g/24 hr, temporarily hold doses until proteinuria is <2 g/24 hr; if proteinuria recurs, hold doses until proteinuria is <2 g/24 hr, then permanently reduce; discontinue in nephrotic syndrome or TMA

⚠ **Febrile neutropenia, neutropenic infection/sepsis:** monitor CBC with differential at baseline and before each cycle; hold FOLFIRI until the neutrophil count is $\geq 1.5 \times 10^9$/L

⚠ **Geriatric toxicity:** assess for diarrhea, dizziness, asthenia, weight loss, and dehydration that can indicate toxicity

⚠ **Pregnancy C/breastfeeding:** highly effective contraception during and up to 3 mo after the last dose is needed for all patients of reproductive potential because infertility and male-mediated teratogenicity can occur; infertility can occur but is reversible within 18 wk after stopping product: do not breastfeed

Evaluate:

- Therapeutic response: decrease in spread of size of tumor

Teach patient/family:

Pregnancy (C)/breastfeeding:

⚠ That highly effective contraception should be used during and up to 3 mo after the last dose in all patients of reproductive potential, infertility and male-mediated teratogenicity can occur; infertility is reversible within 18 wk after stopping product; do not breastfeed

- About reason for treatment, expected results

Black Box Warning: Notify prescriber immediately of bleeding, severe abdominal pain, poor wound healing

zoledronic acid (Rx)

(zoh′leh-drah′nick ass′id)

Reclast, Zometa

Func. class.: Bone-resorption inhibitor

Chem. class.: Bisphosphonate

ACTION: Potent inhibitor of osteoclastic bone resorption; inhibits osteoclastic activity, skeletal calcium release caused by stimulating factors released by tumors; reduction of abnormal bone resorption is responsible for therapeutic effect with hypercalcemia; may directly block dissolution of hydroxyapatite bone crystals

USES: Moderate to severe hypercalcemia associated with malignancy; multiple myeloma; bone metastases from solid tumors (used with antineoplastics); active Paget's disease; osteoporosis, glucocorticoid-induced osteoporosis, osteoporosis prophylaxis in postmenopausal women

CONTRAINDICATIONS: Pregnancy (D), breastfeeding; hypersensitivity to this product or bisphosphonates; hypocalcemia

Precautions: Children, geriatric patients, renal dysfunction, asthmatic patients, acute bronchospasm, anemia, chemotherapy, coagulopathy, dehydration, dental disease, diabetes mellitus, renal disease, electrolyte imbalance, hypertension, hypovolemia, infection, multiple myeloma, phosphate hypersensitivity

DOSAGE AND ROUTES

Hypercalcemia of malignancy

- **Adult: IV INFUSION** 4 mg, given as single infusion over ≥15 min; may retreat with 4 mg if serum calcium does not return to normal within 1 wk

Multiple myeloma/metastatic bone lesions

- **Adult: IV INFUSION** 4 mg, give over 15 min q3-4wk

Z

Osteoporosis

• **Adult: IV INFUSION** 5 mg over ≥15 min q12mo

Active Paget's disease

• **Adult: IV INFUSION** 5 mg over ≥15 min

Osteoporosis prophylaxis (Reclast), postmenopausal women

• **Adult: IV INFUSION** 5 mg every other year

Osteoporosis prophylaxis (Reclast) when taking systemic glucocorticoids

• **Adult: IV** 5 mg every yr

Renal dose

Adult: IV INFUSION CCr 50-60 ml/min, 3.5 mg; CCr 40-49 ml/min, 3.3 mg; CCr 30-39 ml/min, 3 mg; CCr <30 ml/min, do not use

Early breast cancer (unlabeled)

• **Adult: IV** 4 mg q6mo with goserelin 3.6 mg SUBCUT monthly and tamoxifen 20 mg daily or anastrozole 1 mg daily for 3 yr

Available forms: (Zometa) sol for inj 4 mg/5 ml; (Reclast) inj 5 mg/100 ml

Administer:

• Saline hydration must be performed before administration; urine output should be 2 L/day during treatment; do not overhydrate patient

IV route

Zometa

• Administer after reconstituting by adding 5 ml of sterile water for inj to each vial then add to ≥100 ml of sterile 0.9% NaCl, D_5W; run over ≥15 min

• Administer in separate IV line from all other products

Reclast

• No further dilution required

• Infuse over ≥15 min at constant rate; max 5 mg

SIDE EFFECTS

CNS: Dizziness, headache, anxiety, confusion, insomnia, agitation

CV: Hypotension, leg edema, atrial fibrillation, chest pain

GI: Abdominal pain, anorexia, constipation, nausea, diarrhea, vomiting, taste change

GU: UTI, possible reduced renal function, renal damage

META: Anemia, hypokalemia, hypomagnesemia, hypophosphatemia, hypocalcemia, increased serum creatinine

MISC: *Fever, chills, flulike symptoms*

MS: Severe bone pain, *arthralgias, myalgias,* osteonecrosis of jaw

PHARMACOKINETICS

Rapidly cleared from circulation, taken up mainly by bones, not metabolized, eliminated primarily by kidneys, approximately 50% eliminated in urine within 24 hr, max effect 7 days; terminal half-life 167 hr, protein binding 22%

INTERACTIONS

• Hypomagnesemia, hypokalemia: digoxin

Decrease: effect of zoledronic acid—calcium, vit D

Decrease: serum calcium, aminoglycosides, loop diuretics

• Do not mix with calcium-containing infusion sol such as lactated Ringer's sol

Increase: nephrotoxicity—aminoglycosides, NSAIDs, radiopaque contrast agents

Drug/Lab Test

Increase: creatinine

Decrease: calcium, phosphorus, magnesium, potassium, Hct/Hgb, RBC, platelets, WBC

NURSING CONSIDERATIONS

Assess:

• Renal tests, calcium, phosphate, magnesium, potassium; creatinine, BUN; if creatinine elevated, hold treatment

• **Hypocalcemia:** paresthesia, twitching, laryngospasm; Chvostek's/Trousseau's signs

• Dental status; cover with antiinfectives for dental extraction

• Atrial fibrillation

• Sol reconstituted with sterile water may be stored under refrigeration for up to 24 hr

• Acetaminophen before and for 72 hr after to decrease pain

Evaluate:
- Therapeutic response: decreased calcium levels, increased bone density

Teach patient/family:
- To report hypercalcemic relapse: nausea, vomiting, bone pain, thirst
- To continue with dietary recommendations, including calcium and vit D; to take a multiple vitamin daily as well as 500 mg of calcium, 400 international units vit D with multiple myeloma
- If nausea or vomiting occurs, to eat small, frequent meals, to use lozenges or chewing gum
- If bone pain occurs, to notify prescriber to obtain analgesics
- Not to use during pregnancy (D)
- To continue good oral hygiene

ZOLMitriptan (Rx)

(zole-mih-trip′tan)

Zomig, Zomig-ZMT

Func. class.: Migraine agent, abortive

Chem. class.: 5-HT_{1B}/5HT_{1D} receptor agonist (triptan)

ACTION: Binds selectively to the vascular 5-HT_{1B}/5HT_{1D} receptor subtype, exerts antimigraine effect; causes vasoconstriction in cranial arteries

USES: Acute treatment of migraine with/without aura

CONTRAINDICATIONS: Angina pectoris, history of MI, documented silent ischemia, ischemic heart disease, uncontrolled hypertension, hypersensitivity, basilar or hemiplegic migraine, risk of CV events

Precautions: Pregnancy (C), breastfeeding, children, postmenopausal women, men >40 yr, geriatric patients, risk factors for CAD, hypercholesterolemia, obesity, diabetes, impaired renal/hepatic function

DOSAGE AND ROUTES
- **Adult: PO** start at ≤2.5 mg (tab may be broken), may repeat after 2 hr, max 10 mg/24 hr; **NASAL** 1 spray in 1 nostril at onset of migraine, repeat in 2 hr if no relief

Available forms: Tabs 2.5, 5 mg; orally disintegrating tabs 2.5, 5 mg; nasal spray 2.5, 5 mg

Administer:
- Take with fluids as soon as symptoms of migraine occur
- Not approved for more than 3-4 uses in a month
- **Orally disintegrating tab:** do not crush or chew; allow to dissolve on tongue

SIDE EFFECTS
CNS: *Tingling, hot sensation, burning, feeling of pressure, tightness, numbness, dizziness, sedation*

CV: Palpitations, chest pain

GI: Abdominal discomfort, nausea, dry mouth, dyspepsia, dysphagia

MISC: Odd taste (spray)

MS: *Weakness, neck stiffness,* myalgia

RESP: Chest tightness, pressure

PHARMACOKINETICS
Duration 2-3½ hr; 25% plasma protein binding; half-life 3-3½ hr; metabolized in liver (metabolite); excreted in urine (60-80%), feces (20-40%)

INTERACTIONS
⚠ Extended vasospastic effects: ergot, ergot derivatives

⚠ Do not use within 2 wk of MAOIs

⚠ Weakness, hyperreflexia, incoordination: SSRIs (FLUoxetine, fluvoxaMINE, PARoxetine, sertraline), SNRI

Increase: half-life of ZOLMitriptan—cimetidine, oral contraceptives

Increase: ZOLMitriptan levels—sibutramine

Drug/Herb
- Serotonin syndrome: SAM-e, St. John's wort

Drug/Lab Test

Increase: alk phos

Z

NURSING CONSIDERATIONS

Assess:

- Tingling, hot sensation, burning, feeling of pressure, numbness, flushing
- Neurologic status: LOC, blurring vision, nausea, vomiting, tingling in extremities preceding headache
- Ingestion of tyramine foods (pickled products, beer, wine, aged cheese), food additives, preservatives, colorings, artificial sweeteners, chocolate, caffeine, which may precipitate these types of headaches
- **Serotonin syndrome** if also taking SSRI, SNRI

Evaluate:

- Therapeutic response: decrease in frequency, severity of headache

Teach patient/family:

- To report any side effects to prescriber
- To use contraception while taking product
- That product does not prevent or reduce number of migraines
- To report chest pain, rash, swelling of face
- Not to double doses; if second dose is needed, wait at least 2 hr; disintegrating dosage form do not split, break, alter

⚠ HIGH ALERT

zolpidem (Rx)

(zole′pih-dem)

Ambien, Ambien CR, Edluar, Zolpimist

Func. class.: Sedative/hypnotic
Chem. class.: Imidazopyridine

Controlled Substance Schedule IV

ACTION:
Produces CNS depression at limbic, thalamic, hypothalamic levels of CNS; may be mediated by neurotransmitter γ-aminobutyric acid (GABA); results are sedation, hypnosis, skeletal muscle relaxation, anticonvulsant activity, anxiolytic action

USES:
Insomnia, short-term treatment; insomnia with difficulty of sleep onset/maintenance (ext rel)

Unlabeled uses: Head trauma

CONTRAINDICATIONS:
Hypersensitivity to benzodiazepines

Precautions: Pregnancy (C), breastfeeding, children <18 yr, geriatric patients, anemia, hepatic disease, suicidal individuals, drug abuse, seizure disorders, angioedema, depression, respiratory disease, sleep apnea, sleep-related behaviors (sleepwalking), myasthenia gravis, pulmonary disease, next morning impairments; females (lower dose needed)

DOSAGE AND ROUTES

- **Adult: PO** 5 mg (women), 5-10 mg (men) at bedtime × 7-10 days only; total max dose 10 mg; **EXT REL** 6.25 (women), 6.25-12.5 mg (men) immediately before bedtime, may be useful for ≤24 wk in people 18-64 yr with primary insomnia, max 12.5 mg/day; **oral spray** (Zolpimist) 5 mg (women), 5-10 mg (men) immediately before bedtime, max 10 mg/day; **SL** (Edluar) 5 mg (women), 5-10 mg (men) just before bedtime
- **Geriatric: PO** 5 mg at bedtime; **EXT REL** 6.25 mg; SL: 5 mg at bedtime

Available forms: Tabs 5, 10 mg; ext rel tabs 6.25, 12.5 mg; SL: 1.75, 3.5, 5, 10 mg; oral spray 5 mg/spray

Administer:

PO route

- Do not break, crush, or chew ext rel
- Take with full glass of water
- ½-1 hr before bedtime (PO); right before retiring (ext rel)
- On empty stomach for fast onset; may be taken with food if GI symptoms occur
- Store in tight container in cool environment

Spray route

- Prime before first use or if pump is not used for ≥14 days
- Do not use spray with or after a meal

Sublingual route

- Separate blister pack at perforation; peel paper and push product through; place product under tongue; allow to dissolve before swallowing; do not take with water

SIDE EFFECTS

CNS: Headache, lethargy, drowsiness, daytime sedation, dizziness, confusion, lightheadedness, anxiety, irritability, amnesia, poor coordination, complex sleep-related reactions (sleep driving, sleep eating), depression, somnolence, **suicidal ideation**, abnormal thinking/behavioral changes

CV: Chest pain, palpitations

GI: Nausea, vomiting, diarrhea, heartburn, abdominal pain, constipation

HEMA: **Leukopenia, granulocytopenia** (rare)

MISC: Myalgia

SYST: **Severe allergic reactions, angioedema, anaphylaxis**

PHARMACOKINETICS

PO: Onset up to 1.5 hr, metabolized by liver, excreted by kidneys (inactive metabolites), crosses placenta, excreted in breast milk, half-life 2-3 hr

INTERACTIONS

Increase: action of both products—alcohol, CNS depressants

Increase or decrease: zolpidem levels—CYP3A4 inhibitors/inducers

Decrease: zolpidem effect—rifamycins

NURSING CONSIDERATIONS

Assess:

⚠ Mental status: mood, sensorium, affect, memory (long, short term), excessive sedation, impaired coordination, **suicidal thoughts/behaviors**

- Blood dyscrasias: fever, sore throat, bruising, rash, jaundice, epistaxis (rare)
- Type of sleep problem: falling asleep, staying asleep

Evaluate:

- Therapeutic response: ability to sleep at night, decreased amount of early morning awakening if taking product for insomnia

Teach patient/family:

- That dependence is possible after long-term use

⚠ That complex sleep-related behaviors may occur (sleep driving/eating)

- To avoid driving or other activities requiring alertness until dosage is stabilized
- To avoid alcohol ingestion
- That effects may take 2 nights for benefits to be noticed; next morning impairment may occur
- Not to use during pregnancy, breastfeeding
- That hangover is common in geriatric patients but less common than with barbiturates; that rebound insomnia may occur for 1-2 nights after discontinuing product; not to discontinue abruptly; to taper
- Not to crush, chew, break ext rel tabs
- To prime spray pump before using

TREATMENT OF OVERDOSE:

Lavage, activated charcoal; monitor electrolytes, VS

zonisamide (Rx)

(zone-is′a-mide)

Zonegran

Func. class.: Anticonvulsant

Chem. class.: Sulfonamides

ACTION: May act through action at sodium and calcium channels, but exact action is unknown; serotonergic action

USES: Epilepsy, adjunctive therapy for partial seizures

CONTRAINDICATIONS: Hypersensitivity to this product or sulfonamides

Precautions: Pregnancy (C), breastfeeding, children <16 yr, geriatric patients, allergies, renal/hepatic disease; psychiatric condition, hepatic failure, pulmonary disease, suicidal ideation

Z

DOSAGE AND ROUTES

- **Adult and child >16 yr:** 100 mg/day, may increase after 2 wk to 200 mg/day, may increase q2wk, max dose 600 mg/day

Available forms: Caps 25, 50, 100 mg

Administer:

- Without regard to food; swallow whole

SIDE EFFECTS

CNS: Dizziness, insomnia, paresthesias, depression, fatigue, headache, confusion, somnolence, agitation, irritability, speech disturbance, suicidal ideation, seizures, status epilepticus

EENT: Diplopia, verbal difficulty, speech abnormalities, taste perversion, amblyopia, pharyngitis, rhinitis, tinnitus, nystagmus

GI: Nausea, constipation, anorexia, weight loss, diarrhea, dyspepsia, dry mouth, abdominal pain

GU: Kidney stones

HEMA: Aplastic anemia, granulocytopenia (rare); ecchymosis

INTEG: Rash, pruritus

MISC: Flulike symptoms

SYST: Stevens-Johnson syndrome, metabolic acidosis

PHARMACOKINETICS

Peak 2-6 hr, half-life in RBCs 105 hr, metabolized by liver, excreted by kidneys, protein binding 40%

INTERACTIONS

Decrease: half-life of zonisamide—carBAMazepine, phenytoin, PHENobarbital

Altered product levels: CYP3A4 inhibitors/inducers

Increase: CNS depression—alcohol

Drug/Herb

Increase: effect of this product—St. John's wort

Drug/Food

- Do not use with grapefruit

Drug/Lab Test

Increase: BUN, creatinine

NURSING CONSIDERATIONS

Assess:

- **Seizures:** duration, type, intensity, precipitating factors
- Renal function: albumin concentration, BUN, urinalysis, creatinine, serum bicarbonate at baseline and periodically
- ⚠ Mental status: mood, sensorium, affect, memory (long, short term), **suicidal thoughts/behaviors**
- Stevens-Johnson syndrome, aplastic anemia, fulminant hepatic necrosis; may cause death; monitor for rashes and hypersensitive reactions
- Rash, hypersensitivity reactions
- Obtain bicarbonate before treatment/periodically; metabolic acidosis may occur in children

Evaluate:

- Therapeutic response: decrease in severity of seizures

Teach patient/family:

- Not to discontinue product abruptly because seizures may occur
- To avoid hazardous activities until stabilized on product
- To carry emergency ID stating product use
- To notify prescriber of rash immediately; to notify prescriber of back pain, abdominal pain, blood in urine; to increase fluid intake to reduce risk of kidney stones
- To notify prescriber if pregnancy planned, suspected
- To avoid grapefruit
- To notify prescriber of sore throat, fever, easy bruising
- To report suicidal thoughts, behaviors immediately

Appendix A

Selected new drugs

albiglutide (Rx)
(al′-bi-gloo′-tide)
Tanzeum
Func. class.: Antidiabetic
Chem. class.: Incretin mimetic

ACTION: Binds and activates known human GLP-1 receptor, mimics natural physiology for self-regulating glycemic control

USES: Type 2 diabetes mellitus; once-weekly dosing

CONTRAINDICATIONS: Hypersensitivity

Black Box Warning: Medullary thyroid carcinoma, multiple endocrine neoplasia syndrome type 2 (MEN-2), thyroid cancer

Precautions: Pregnancy (C), geriatric patients, severe renal/hepatic/GI disease, pancreatitis, vit D deficiency, breastfeeding, burns, children, colitis, diabetic ketoacidosis, infection, pseudomembranous colitis, surgery, thyroid disease, smoking, trauma, type 1 diabetes mellitus, vomiting

DOSAGE AND ROUTES

• **Adult: SUBCUT 30 mg q7days at any time of day;** may increase to 50 mg q7days if needed

Available forms: Prefilled pen powder for injection 30, 50 mg

Administer:

• Store in refrigerator for unopened pen; may store at room temperature after opening for up to 30 days

SUBCUT route

• Give q7days (weekly); the dose can be given at any time of day without regard to meals

Reconstitution of the Pen:

• The powder contained within the pen must be reconstituted before administration. Twist the clear cartridge on the pen in the direction of the arrow until a *click* is heard. (You will also see a number "2" appear in the number window.) This action mixes the diluent with the powder.

• Slowly and gently rock the pen side to side 5 times to mix. Do NOT shake the pen. Shaking the pen will cause foaming.

• Patients using the product at home must wait 15 min for the 30-mg pen or 30 min for the 50-mg pen to ensure that the medicine is properly mixed and to avoid clogging the pen needle. In health care environments, a health care professional may have to wait up to 10 min after adding the diluent to see complete dissolution

• As long as the needle has not been attached, the pen can be used within 8 hr of reconstitution with the diluent

Preparing the Pen for injection:

• Prime the pen before use

• Slowly rock the pen side to side 5 times. Do NOT shake; inspect for particulate matter, solution will be yellow and free of particles. A small amount of foam is normal

• Holding the pen upright, attach the supplied needle to the pen

• Tap the cartridge to bring bubbles to the top; remove bubbles by twisting until the number "3" appears in window. At the same time, the injection button will be automatically released from the bottom of the pen
• Once the needle is attached, the product must be administered immediately. The product can clog the needle if allowed to dry in the primed pen

Subcutaneous administration using the Pen:
• Inject subcut into the thigh, abdomen, or upper arm. Once the needle is inserted, press the injection button until you hear a *click* and then hold the button for 5 additional seconds to deliver the full dose
• Rotate sites to prevent lipodystrophy

SIDE EFFECTS

GI: Nausea, vomiting, diarrhea, dyspepsia, gastroesophageal reflux, **pancreatitis**
INTEG: Serious injection-site reactions

PHARMACOKINETICS

Peak 3-5 days, increased in renal disease, steady state 4-5 wk, half-life 5 days

INTERACTIONS

Increase: hypoglycemia—ACE inhibitors, disopyramide, sulfonylureas, androgens, fibric acid derivatives, alcohol
Increase: hyperglycemia—phenothiazines, corticosteroids, anabolic steroids, tacrolimus, cyclosporine
Decrease: action of digoxin
Decrease: efficacy—niacin, dextrothyroxine, thiazide diuretics, triamterene, estrogens, progestins, oral contraceptives, MAOIs

NURSING CONSIDERATIONS

Assess:
• Fasting blood glucose, A1c levels during treatment to determine diabetes control

Black Box Warning: Medullary thyroid carcinoma, multiple endocrine neoplasia syndrome 2 (MEN-2), thyroid cancer: monitor patient closely

• **Pancreatitis:** severe abdominal pain, with or without vomiting, product should be discontinued
• Renal studies: urinalysis, creatinine
• Hypo/hyperglycemic reaction that can occur soon after meals; for severe hypoglycemia, give IV $D_{50}W$, then IV dextrose solution
• Nausea, vomiting, diarrhea, ability to tolerate product, may cause dehydration

Evaluate:
• Therapeutic response: decrease in polyuria, polydipsia, polyphagia, clear sensorium, improving A1c, weight

Teach patient/family:
• About the symptoms of hypo/hyperglycemia, what to do about each; to have glucagon emergency kit available; to carry a glucose source (candy, sugar cube) to treat hypoglycemia
• That product must be continued on a weekly basis; about consequences of discontinuing product abruptly
• That diabetes is a lifelong illness; product will not cure disease; to carry emergency ID with prescriber and medication information
• To continue weight control, dietary restrictions, exercise, hygiene
• That regular blood glucose monitoring and A1c testing is needed
• To notify prescriber if pregnant or intending to become pregnant (C)
• About the importance of reading "Information for the Patient" and "Pen User Manual"; about self-injection
• **Pancreatitis: If severe abdominal pain with or without vomiting occurs, seek medical attention immediately**
• To review injection procedure, dispose of pen appropriately

alirocumab (Rx)

(al′-i-rok′-ue-mab)

Praluent

Func. class.: Antilipemic

ACTION: Binds to low-density lipoproteins, a human monoclonal antibody (IgG1)

USES: Heterozygous, familial hypercholesterolemia, atherosclerotic disease

CONTRAINDICATIONS: Hypersensitivity
Precautions: Pregnancy, breastfeeding

DOSAGE AND ROUTES
- **Adult: SUBCUT** 75 mg q2wk, may increase to 150 mg q2wk if needed

Available forms: Prefilled pen 75 mg/1 ml, 150 mg/1 ml
Administer:
- If dose is missed, give within 7 days of next dose; if over 7 days, wait until next scheduled dose
- Visually inspect for particulate matter and discoloration, solution is clear, colorless to pale yellow
- Warm to room temperature for 30-40 min before use. Use as soon as possible after warming
- Do NOT use the prefilled pen or syringe if it has been at room temperature for ≥24 hr
- Give by subcut injection into the thigh, abdomen, or upper arm. Rotate injection site with each injection
- Do NOT inject into areas of active skin disease or injury (sunburn, rash, inflammation, skin infection)
- Do NOT administer with other injectable drugs at the same injection site

SIDE EFFECTS
CNS: Memory impairment, confusion
GI: Diarrhea
MISC: Edema
MS: *Myalgia*
RESP: Pharyngitis, sinusitis, cough
SYST: Infection, antibody formation
INTEG: Pruritus, injection-site reaction, erythema, ecchymosis

PHARMACOKINETICS
Peak 3-7 days; half-life at steady state 17-20 days

INTERACTIONS
None known

Drug/Lab Test
Increase: LFTs

NURSING CONSIDERATIONS
Assess:
- **Hypercholesterolemia:** diet history: fat content, lipid levels (triglycerides, LDL, LDL-C 4-8 wk after start of titration, HDL, cholesterol); LFTs at baseline, periodically during treatment

Evaluate:
- Therapeutic response: decreased cholesterol, LDL; increased HDL

Teach patient/family:
- That compliance is needed
- That risk factors should be decreased: high-fat diet, smoking, alcohol consumption, absence of exercise
- To notify prescriber if pregnancy suspected, planned, or if breastfeeding
- To report confusion, injection-site reactions

⚠ HIGH ALERT

atazanavir/cobicistat (Rx)

(at-a-za-na′veer / koe-bik′-i-stat)

Evotaz

Func. class.: Antiretroviral
Chem. class.: Protease inhibitor

ACTION: Inhibits HIV-1 protease, which prevents maturation of the infectious virus; it combines a protease inhibitor with an enhancer

USES: HIV-1 infection in combination with other antiretroviral agents

CONTRAINDICATIONS: Hypersensitivity, Child-Pugh Class C
Precautions: Pregnancy (B), breastfeeding, children, geriatric patients, hepatic disease, alcoholism, drug resistance, AV block, diabetes, dialysis, female patients, hemophilia, hypercholesterolemia, immune reconstitution syndrome,

lactic acidosis, pancreatitis, cholelithiasis, serious rash

DOSAGE AND ROUTES

- **Adult: PO** 300 mg/150 mg daily in both treatment-naive and treatment-experienced patients
- **Adolescent (unlabeled): PO** 300 mg/150 mg daily in combination with other antiretroviral agents as part of an alternative initial regimen (treatment-naive)

Available forms: Tab 300 mg/150 mg

Administer:

- Antiretroviral drug resistance testing (preferably genotypic testing) is recommended before initiation of therapy in antiretroviral treatment-naive patients and before changing therapy for treatment failure
- With food

SIDE EFFECTS

CNS: Headache, depression, dizziness, insomnia, peripheral neurologic symptoms

CV: Increased PR interval

EENT: Yellowing of sclera

GI: Vomiting, *diarrhea, abdominal pain, nausea,* hepatotoxicity, cholelithiasis

INTEG: Rash, Stevens-Johnson syndrome, photosensitivity, DRESS

MISC: Fatigue, fever, arthralgia, back pain, cough, lipodystrophy, pain, gynecomastia, nephrolithiasis; lactic acidosis, hyperbilirubinemia (pregnancy, female patients, obesity), DRESS

PHARMACOKINETICS

Rapidly absorbed, absorption increased with food, peak 2.5 hr, 86% protein bound, extensively metabolized in liver by CYP3A4, 27% excreted unchanged in urine/feces (minimal), half-life 7 hr

INTERACTIONS

Increase: levels, toxicity of immunosuppressants (cycloSPORINE, sirolimus, tacrolimus, sildenafil), tricyclic antidepressants, warfarin, calcium channel blockers, clarithromycin, chlorazepate, diazepam, irinotecan, HMG-CoA reductase inhibitors, antidysrhythmics, midazolam, triazolam, ergots, pimozide, other protease inhibitors

Increase: effects of estrogens

Increase: atazanavir levels—CYP3A4 substrates, CYP3A4 inhibitors

Increase: hyperbilirubinemia—indinavir

Decrease: telaprevir level when used with atazanavir and ritonavir

Decrease: atazanavir levels—CYP3A4 inducers, rifampin, antacids, didanosine, efavirenz, proton-pump inhibitors, H2-receptor antagonists

Decrease: oral contraceptives

Drug/Herb

Decrease: atazanavir levels—St. John's wort, avoid concurrent use

Increase: myopathy, rhabdomyolysis—red yeast rice

Drug/Lab Test

Increase: AST, ALT, total bilirubin, amylase, lipase, CK

Decrease: Hgb, neutrophils, platelets

Drug/Food

- Increased drug bioavailability (to be taken with food)

NURSING CONSIDERATIONS

Assess:

- For hepatic failure; hepatic studies: ALT, AST, bilirubin
- Immune reconstitution syndrome: when given with combination antiretroviral therapy
- For **lactic acidosis, hyperbilirubinemia** (female patients, pregnancy, obesity); if pregnant, call Antiretroviral Pregnancy Registry 800-258-4263
- PR interval in those taking calcium channel blockers, digoxin
- For signs of infection, anemia, nephrolithiasis
- Bowel pattern before, during treatment; if severe abdominal pain with bleeding occurs, product should be discontinued; monitor hydration
- Viral load, CD4 count throughout treatment
- Serious rash (Stevens-Johnson syndrome, DRESS): most rashes last 1-4 wk; if serious, discontinue product

- Immune reconstitution syndrome: time of onset is variable

Evaluate:

- Therapeutic response: increasing CD4 counts; decreased viral load, resolution of symptoms of HIV-1 infection

Teach patient/family:

- To take as prescribed with other antiretrovirals as prescribed; if dose is missed, to take as soon as remembered up to 1 hr before next dose; not to double dose, share with others
- That product must be taken daily to maintain blood levels for duration of therapy
- To report yellowing of skin, sclera
- To notify prescriber if diarrhea, nausea, vomiting, or rash occurs; dizziness, lightheadedness may occur; ECG may be altered
- That product interacts with many products, including St. John's wort; to advise prescriber of all products, herbal products used
- That redistribution of body fat may occur, the effect is not known
- That product does not cure HIV-1 infection, prevent transmission to others; only controls symptoms
- That, if taking phosphodiesterase type 5 inhibitor with atazanavir, there may be increased risk of phosphodiesterase type 5 inhibitor–associated adverse events (hypotension, prolonged penile erection); to notify physician promptly of these symptoms

cangrelor (Rx)

(kan′grel-or)

Kengreal

Func. class.: Platelet aggregation inhibitor

Chem. class.: ADP receptor antagonist

ACTION: A direct competitive inhibitor of a platelet receptor, prevents further signaling and platelet activation, results in inhibition of platelet activation and aggregation, does not require hepatic conversion to an active metabolite

USES: For use as an adjunct to percutaneous coronary intervention (PCI) for myocardial infarction prophylaxis, repeat coronary revascularization, and stent thrombosis in patients who have not been treated with a P2Y12 platelet inhibitor and are not being given a glycoprotein IIb/IIIa inhibitor

CONTRAINDICATIONS: Hypersensitivity, active bleeding

Precautions: Pregnancy (C), breastfeeding, children, increased bleeding risk, neutropenia, agranulocytosis, renal disease

DOSAGE AND ROUTES

- **Adult: IV BOLUS** 30 mcg/kg as a single, then follow immediately by 4 mcg/kg/min continuous IV infusion; the bolus should be given before PCI and maintenance infusion should be continued for ≥2 hr or for the duration of PCI, whichever is longer; use ticagrelor, prasugrel, or clopidogrel to maintain platelet inhibition

Available forms: Powder for injection 50 mg

Administer:

- Visually inspect parenteral products for particulate matter and discoloration before use, use IV only
- **Reconstitution:** Reconstitute by adding 5 ml sterile water for injection to a 50-mg vial, swirl until dissolved, do not shake, allow foam to settle, solution should be clear and colorless to pale yellow, withdraw contents of one reconstituted 50-mg vial and add to one 250-ml bag of 0.9% sodium chloride injection or dextrose 5% injection resulting in a final infusion concentration of 200 mcg/ml; usually, one bag should be sufficient for most patients for ≥2 hr of dosing, those weighing >100 kg will require a minimum of 2 bags
- Use diluted product immediately. When stored at room temperature, diluted product stable for ≤12 hr in dextrose 5% injection and 24 hr in 0.9% sodium chloride injection, use a dedicated line
- Bolus injection should be administered rapidly (<1 min). The bolus volume may

be withdrawn from the diluted infusion bag and given by IV push or using an infusion pump

• Ensure the bolus dose is completely administered before start of PCI

• Start the continuous IV infusion immediately after administration of the bolus; use infusion pump for the continuous IV infusion

SIDE EFFECTS

CNS: Intracranial bleeding
GI: GI bleeding
GU: Hematuria
HEMA: Bleeding
RESP: Wheezing, dyspnea, bronchospasm
SYST: Anaphylaxis, angioedema

PHARMACOKINETICS

Half-life 3-6 min; plasma protein binding 97%; effect on platelets 2 min, excreted in urine

INTERACTIONS

Do not give clopidogrel or prasugrel until infusion is discontinued

NURSING CONSIDERATIONS

Assess:

• **Bleeding:** intracranial, retroperitoneal, other frank bleeding, after completion of infusion, platelet inhibition decreases rapidly within 1 hr; monitor Hct/Hgb

• **Hypersensitivity:** identify if patient has a known cangrelor hypersensitivity

• **Severe renal impairment:** decreased renal function may occur in those with severe renal impairment creatinine clearance >30 ml/min); however, no dosage change is required

• **Pregnancy (C)/Breastfeeding:** identify whether the patient is pregnant or breastfeeding, it is not known if product is excreted in breast milk

Evaluate:

• Therapeutic response: platelet inhibition during PCI

Teach patient/family:

• Use and expected results

⚠ HIGH ALERT

ceritinib (Rx)

(cerr-ah-tin′ib)

Zykadia

Func. class.: Antineoplastic—miscellaneous

Chem. class.: Protein-tyrosine kinase inhibitor

ACTION:

A tyrosine kinase inhibitor targeting anaplastic lymphoma kinase (ALK); also targets insulin-like growth factor 1 (IFG-1) receptor, insulin receptor (InsR), ROS1

USES:

Anaplastic lymphoma kinase (ALK)–positive metastatic non–small-cell lung cancer (NSCLC) in patients who have progressed on or are intolerant to crizotinib

CONTRAINDICATIONS:

Pregnancy (D), hypersensitivity

Precautions: Breastfeeding, children, geriatric patients, cardiac/hepatic/disease, GI bleeding, bone marrow suppression, infection, diarrhea, hyperglycemia, diabetes mellitus, nausea/vomiting, pancreatitis, pneumonitis, QT prolongation, torsade de pointes, bradycardia, cardiac arrhythmias, electrolyte imbalances, corticosteroid therapy

DOSAGE AND ROUTES

• **Adults: PO** 750 mg daily on an empty stomach until disease progression or unacceptable toxicity. Avoid the concomitant use of strong 3A4 inhibitors or inducers

Hepatic dose

• **Adult: PO** ALT or AST >53 above ULN and total bilirubin ≤2 3 ULN: Hold product. When ALT/AST return to baseline or ≤3 3 ULN, resume with a 150 mg dose reduction. Do not resume in those unable to tolerate 300 mg daily

Available forms: Caps 150 mg

Administer:

Dosage adjustments due to treatment-related toxicity

QTc prolongation

• *QTc >500 msec on at least 2 separate ECGs:* Hold. When QTc returns to <481 msec (or baseline if >481 msec), resume with a 150 mg dose reduction. Do not resume in those unable to tolerate 300 mg daily. Any occurrence of QTc prolongation in combination with torsades de pointes or polymorphic ventricular tachycardia or signs/symptoms of serious arrhythmia: permanently discontinue

• **Bradycardia:** Symptomatic, but not life-threatening: Hold and evaluate other medications that may cause bradycardia. When asymptomatic or heart rate ≥60 bpm, resume with an adjusted dose, do not resume in those unable to tolerate 300 mg daily; life-threatening: discontinue product

• **Lipase or amylase** >2 × **ULN:** Hold product and monitor serum lipase/amylase. When improved to <1.5 × ULN, resume with a 150 mg dose reduction. Do not resume in those unable to tolerate 300 mg daily

• **Any grade interstitial lung disease (ILD) or pneumonitis:** Permanently discontinue

• *Severe or intolerable nausea, vomiting, or diarrhea despite appropriate medical therapy:* Hold dose, when improved, resume with a 150 mg dose reduction. Do not resume in those unable to tolerate 300 mg daily

• **Persistent hyperglycemia >250 mg/dl despite optimal antihyperglycemic therapy:** Hold dose, when hyperglycemia is controlled, resume with a 150 mg dose reduction. Do not resume in those unable to tolerate 300 mg daily. If blood sugars cannot be controlled medically, discontinue

• **Dosage guidance in patients on strong CYP3A4 inducers/inhibitors: Strong CYP3A4 inhibitors:** Avoid concomitant use. If a strong CYP3A4 inhibitor is required, reduce the dose of ceritinib by approximately one-third, rounded to the nearest multiple of 150 mg; close monitoring of the QT interval is recommended. If the strong CYP3A4 inhibitor is discontinued, resume the previous dosage; **strong CYP3A4 inducers:** avoid concomitant use

• Take on an empty stomach. Do not give within 2 hr of a meal; swallow tablets whole; do not crush or dissolve; if a dose is missed, make it up unless the next dose is due within 12 hr. Do not take 2 doses at the same time if missed, if vomiting occurs, do not give an additional dose. Take the next dose at the next scheduled time

SIDE EFFECTS

CNS: Weakness, fatigue, paresthesias

CV: QT prolongation, torsades de pointes, bradycardia

EENT: Blurred vision

GI: *Nausea,* hepatotoxicity, vomiting, *anorexia,* pancreatitis, GERD, *abdominal pain,* diarrhea

INTEG: *Rash*

META: Hyperglycemia, hyperphosphatemia, hyperamylasemia

MISC: Renal failure

RESP: Cough, dyspnea, pneumonitis

PHARMACOKINETICS

Protein binding 97%; metabolized by CYP3A4; peak 4-6 hr; half-life 41 hr

INTERACTIONS

Increase: hepatotoxicity—acetaminophen

Increase: ceritinib concentrations—CYP3A4 inhibitors (ketoconazole, itraconazole, erythromycin, clarithromycin)

Increase: plasma concentrations of simvastatin, calcium channel blockers, ergots

Increase: plasma concentration of warfarin; avoid use with warfarin; use low-molecular-weight anticoagulants instead

Decrease: ceritinib concentrations—CYP3A4 inducers (dexamethasone, phenytoin, carBAMazepine, rifampin, PHENobarbital)

Drug/Herb

Decrease: ceritinib concentration—St. John's wort

Drug/Lab Test
Increase: bilirubin, amylase, LFTs

NURSING CONSIDERATIONS
Assess:
- **Pregnancy:** Assess for pregnancy before starting treatment, pregnancy category (D)
- **QT prolongation:** Assess for a history of cardiac arrhythmias, congestive heart failure, bradycardia, electrolyte imbalance, or congenital long QT syndrome. Correct electrolyte abnormalities before starting product
- **Hyperglycemia:** Monitor for hyperglycemia, may be 6-8–fold in diabetic patients
- **Pancreatitis:** Monitor for nausea, vomiting, severe abdominal pain

Evaluate:
- Therapeutic response: decrease in progression of lung cancer

Teach patient/family:
- To report adverse reactions immediately: abdominal pain, nausea, vomiting, increased blood glucose in diabetic patients
- About reason for treatment, expected results
- To avoid OTC products unless approved by prescriber
- To notify prescriber if pregnancy is planned or suspected, pregnancy (D), do not use

daclatasvir
(dak-lat′-as-vir)
Daklinza
Func. class.: Antiviral, antihepatitis C agent

ACTION: Active against chronic infections caused by genotype 3 hepatitis C virus (HCV); prevents viral RNA replication by impairing protein function

USES: Chronic hepatitis C, genotype 3 with complicated liver disease

CONTRAINDICATIONS: Hypersensitivity
Precautions: Pregnancy (UK), breastfeeding, antimicrobial resistance, hepatic disease, hepatitis C with HIV coinfection, liver transplant

DOSAGE AND ROUTES
Adult: PO 60 mg daily with sofosbuvir 400 mg daily × 12 wk
Adult receiving strong CYP3A inhibitors: PO 30 mg daily with sofosbuvir 400 mg daily × 12 wk
Adult receiving moderate CYP3A inducers: PO 90 mg daily with sofosbuvir 400 mg daily × 12 wk
Available forms: Tabs 30, 60 mg
Administer:
- By mouth without regard to food
- Do not use as monotherapy, must be given with sofosbuvir

SIDE EFFECTS
CNS: Headache, fatigue
GI: Diarrhea, nausea

PHARMACOKINETICS
Peak 2 hr, excreted feces 88%
80%, 99% protein binding; terminal half-life 12-15 hr, metabolized by the liver by CYP3A4, affected by P-glycoprotein (P-gp), organic anion transporting polypeptides (OATP1B1 and OATP1B3), breast cancer resistance protein (BCRP)

INTERACTIONS
- Do not use with potent CYP3A4 inducers

Increase: each product P-glycoprotein (P-gp) substrates
Increase: daclatasvir effect—potent CYP3A4 inhibitors, reduce dose of daclatasvir
Decrease: daclatasvir effect—moderate CYP3A4 inducers, increase dose of daclatasvir

NURSING CONSIDERATIONS
Assess:
- **Liver transplant/cirrhosis:** May have lower sustained virologic response

rates in cirrhosis and use in prior liver transplant is unknown

- **HIV/Hepatitis C coinfection:** All patients with HIV infection should be tested for hepatitis C, with continued annual screening advised for those persons considered at high risk for acquiring hepatitis C. If hepatitis C and HIV coinfection is identified, consider treating both viral infections concurrently
- **Pregnancy/Breastfeeding:** Unknown, give careful consideration for use in pregnancy and breastfeeding
- **Strong CYP3A4 inducers: Do not use concurrently, may lead to treatment failure, review patient's medication profile for potential drug interactions before starting treatment**
- **Hepatitis C:** Monitor plasma hepatitis C RNA and plasma HIV RNA baseline and during treatment

Evaluate:

- Therapeutic response: decreased symptoms of chronic hepatitis C

Teach patient/family:

- That optimal duration of treatment is 12 wk; that product is not a cure; that transmission may still occur and drug must be taken with sofosbuvir
- To avoid use with other medications, herbs, supplements unless approved by prescriber
- Not to stop abruptly unless directed; worsening of hepatitis may occur
- To notify prescriber if pregnancy is planned or suspected or if breastfeeding

darunavir/cobicistat (Rx)

(da-roon′a-veer/koe-bik′i-stat)

Prezcobix

Func. class.: Antiretroviral

Chem. class.: Protease inhibitor

ACTION: Inhibits HIV-1 protease, which prevents maturation of the infectious virus; combines a protease inhibitor with an enhancer

USES: HIV-1 infection in combination with other antiretroviral agents

CONTRAINDICATIONS: Hypersensitivity, Child-Pugh Class C

Precautions: Pregnancy (B), breastfeeding, children, geriatric patients, hepatic disease, alcoholism, drug resistance, AV block, diabetes, dialysis, elderly, females, hemophilia, hypercholesterolemia, immune reconstitution syndrome, lactic acidosis, pancreatitis, cholelithiasis, serious rash

DOSAGE AND ROUTES

- **Adult: PO** 800 mg/150 mg daily in treatment-naive and treatment-experienced adults with no darunavir-resistance–associated substitutions (V11I, V32I, L33F, I47V, I50V, I54L, I54M, T74P, L76V, I84V, L89V)
- **Adolescent (unlabeled): PO** 800 mg/150 mg daily in combination with other antiretroviral agents for treatment-naive adolescents with no darunavir-resistance–associated substitutions (V11I, V32I, L33F, I47V, I50V, I54L, I54M, T74P, L76V, I84V, L89V)

Hepatic dose

- Do not use in severe hepatic disease

Available forms: Tabs 800 mg/150 mg

Administer:

- With food
- Antiretroviral drug resistance testing (preferably genotypic testing) is recommended before initiation of therapy in antiretroviral treatment-naive patients and before changing therapy for treatment failure

SIDE EFFECTS

CNS: Headache, depression, dizziness, insomnia, peripheral neurologic symptoms

CV: Increased PR interval

EENT: Yellowing of sclera

GI: Vomiting, *diarrhea, abdominal pain, nausea,* **hepatotoxicity,** cholelithiasis

INTEG: *Rash,* Stevens-Johnson syndrome, *photosensitivity,* DRESS

MISC: Fatigue, fever, arthralgia, back pain, cough, lipodystrophy, pain, gynecomastia, nephrolithiasis; lactic acidosis, hyperbilirubinemia (pregnancy, female patients, obesity)

PHARMACOKINETICS

Rapidly absorbed, absorption increased with food, peak 2.5 hr, 86% protein bound, extensively metabolized in liver by CYP3A4, 27% excreted unchanged in urine/feces (minimal), half-life 7 hr

INTERACTIONS

Increase: levels, toxicity of immunosuppressants (cycloSPORINE, sirolimus, tacrolimus, sildenafil), tricyclic antidepressants, warfarin, calcium channel blockers, clarithromycin, chlorazepate, diazepam, irinotecan, HMG-CoA reductase inhibitors, antidysrhythmics, midazolam, triazolam, ergots, pimozide, other protease inhibitors
Increase: effects of estrogens with ritonavir
Increase: atazanavir levels—CYP3A4 substrates, CYP3A4 inhibitors
Increase: hyperbilirubinemia—indinavir
Decrease: telaprevir level when used with atazanavir and ritonavir
Decrease: atazanavir levels—CYP3A4 inducers, rifampin, antacids, didanosine, efavirenz, proton-pump inhibitors, H2-receptor antagonists
Decrease: oral contraceptives

Drug/Herb

Decrease: atazanavir levels—St. John's wort, avoid concurrent use
Increase: myopathy, rhabdomyolysis—red yeast rice

Drug/Lab Test

Increase: AST, ALT, total bilirubin, amylase, lipase, CK
Decrease: Hgb, neutrophils, platelets

Drug/Food

- Increased drug bioavailability (to be taken with food)

NURSING CONSIDERATIONS

Assess:

- For hepatic failure; hepatic studies: ALT, AST, bilirubin
- Immune reconstitution syndrome: when given with combination antiretroviral therapy
- For **lactic acidosis, hyperbilirubinemia** (female patients, pregnancy, obesity), if pregnant, call Antiretroviral Pregnancy Registry 800-258-4263
- PR interval in those taking calcium channel blockers, digoxin
- For signs of infection, anemia, nephrolithiasis
- Bowel pattern before, during treatment; if severe abdominal pain with bleeding occurs, product should be discontinued; monitor hydration
- Viral load, CD4 count throughout treatment
- **Serious rash (Stevens-Johnson syndrome, DRESS): most rashes last 1-4 wk; if serious, discontinue product**
- **Immune reconstitution syndrome: time of onset is variable**

Evaluate:

- Therapeutic response: increasing CD4 counts; decreased viral load, resolution of symptoms of HIV-1 infection

Teach patient/family:

- To take as prescribed with other antiretrovirals as prescribed; if dose is missed, to take as soon as remembered up to 1 hr before next dose; not to double dose, share with others
- That product must be taken daily to maintain blood levels for duration of therapy
- To report yellowing of skin, sclera
- To notify prescriber if diarrhea, nausea, vomiting, or rash occurs; dizziness, lightheadedness may occur; ECG may be altered
- That product interacts with many products; St. John's wort; to advise prescriber of all products, herbal products used
- That redistribution of body fat may occur, the effect is not known
- That product does not cure HIV-1 infection, prevent transmission to others; only controls symptoms
- That, if taking phosphodiesterase type 5 inhibitor with atazanavir, there may be increased risk of phosphodiesterase type 5 inhibitor–associated adverse events (hypotension, prolonged penile erection);

to notify physician promptly of these symptoms

RARELY USED

deoxycholic acid
(dee-ox′-i-koe′-lik as′-id)

Kybella ⚠ ✤

Func. class.: Unknown

USES: For the improvement in the appearance of moderate to severe convexity or fullness associated with submental fat

CONTRAINDICATIONS: Infection

DOSAGE AND ROUTES
• **Adult: SUBCUT** 0.2 ml per injection site. A single treatment session consists of up to a maximum of 50 injections (10 ml total dose), with each injection spaced 1 cm apart. Up to 6 single treatments may be given at intervals of no less than 1 mo. Injections are made into the subcutaneous fat of the submental region, between the dermis and the platysma. Do not inject into the platysma.

⚠ HIGH ALERT

dulaglutide (Rx)
(doo-la-gloo′-tide)

Trulicity

Func. class.: Antidiabetic

Chem. class.: Incretin mimetic

ACTION: Binds and activates known human glucagon-like peptide-1 (GLP-1) receptor agonist, mimics natural physiology for self-regulating glycemic control

USES: Type 2 diabetes mellitus, once-weekly dosing

CONTRAINDICATIONS: Hypersensitivity

Black Box Warning: Medullary thyroid carcinoma, multiple endocrine neoplasia syndrome type 2 (men-2), thyroid cancer

Precautions: Pregnancy (C), breastfeeding, children, geriatric patients, severe renal/hepatic/GI disease, pancreatitis, vit D deficiency, burns, colitis, diarrhea, fever, GI bleeding/perforation/obstruction, ileus, infection, pseudomembranous colitis, thyroid disease, trauma, surgery, type 1 diabetes mellitus, tobacco smoking, vomiting

DOSAGE AND ROUTES
• **Adult: SUBCUT** 0.75 mg weekly, may increase to 1.5 mg weekly

Available forms: Injection 0.75 mg/0.5 ml, 1.5 mg/0.5 ml

Administer:

SUBCUT route

• Do not use as first-line therapy for those who have inadequate glycemic control on diet and exercise

• Administer the dose at any time of day, with or without meals

• If a dose is missed, take as soon as remembered, as long as the next dose is due at least 3 days later; if it is more than 3 days after the missed dose, wait until the next regularly scheduled dose

• Give SUBCUT only, do not give IV or IM, inject into the thigh, abdomen, or upper arm, rotate sites with each injection to prevent lipodystrophy

• Properly dispose of the pen or syringe

• Store in refrigerator for unopened pen; may store at room temperature after opening for up to 30 days, do not freeze

• When using concomitantly with insulin, give as separate injections. Never mix them together. The two injections may be injected in the same body region, but not adjacent to each other

Prefilled pen administration: *Part of pen is glass; if dropped on a hard surface, do not use. Uncap the pen after checking* *that it is locked, place base flat, and firmly unlock by turning the lock ring, press and hold green button, click will be heard, continue holding until another click is heard.* Injection is complete when the gray plunger is visible. Remove the pen and dispose of the used pen

SIDE EFFECTS

CNS: Fatigue
ENDO: Hypoglycemia
GI: Nausea, vomiting, diarrhea, anorexia, gastroesophageal reflux, pancreatitis, flatulence, abdominal pain, constipation
SYST: Secondary malignancy
INTEG: Injection-site reactions, rash, urticaria

PHARMACOKINETICS

Peak 24-72 hr, half-life 5 days

INTERACTIONS

Increase: hypoglycemia—ACE inhibitors, disopyramide, sulfonylureas, androgens, fibric acid derivatives, alcohol
Increase: hyperglycemia—phenothiazines, corticosteroids, anabolic steroids
Decrease: effect of dulaglutide—niacin, dextrothyroxine, thiazide diuretics, triamterene, estrogens, progestins, oral contraceptives, MAOIs

NURSING CONSIDERATIONS

Assess:

- Fasting blood glucose, A1c levels, postprandial glucose during treatment to determine diabetes control
- Pancreatitis: severe abdominal pain, with or without vomiting, product should be discontinued
- Hypo/hyperglycemic reaction that can occur soon after meals; for severe hypoglycemia, give IV $D_{50}W$, then IV dextrose solution
- Nausea, vomiting, diarrhea, ability to tolerate product, may cause dehydration

Evaluate:

- Therapeutic response: decrease in polyuria, polydipsia, polyphagia, clear sensorium, improving A1c, weight; absence of dizziness, stable gait

Teach patient/family:

- About the symptoms of hypo/hyperglycemia, what to do about each; to have glucagon emergency kit available; to carry a glucose source (candy, sugar cube) to treat hypoglycemia

RARELY USED

eluxadoline

(el-ux-ad′oh-leen)

Viberzi ⚠ ✤

Func. class.: GI agent

USES: Irritable bowel syndrome with diarrhea

CONTRAINDICATIONS: Hypersensitivity, alcoholism, GI/biliary obstruction, constipation, pancreatitis

DOSAGE AND ROUTES

- **Adult: PO** 100 mg bid with food. Decrease to 75 mg bid with food in those who do not have a gallbladder, are receiving an OATP1B1 inhibitor

⚠ HIGH ALERT

empagliflozin/ metformin (Rx)

(em′pa-gli-floe′ zin / met-for′min)

Synjardy

Func. class.: Antidiabetic

Chem. class.: Biguanide; sodium-glucose cotransporter 2 (SGLT2) inhibitor

ACTION: Combination products containing empagliflozin and metformin improve glycemic control in type 2 diabetes mellitus

Empagliflozin: An inhibitor of sodium-glucose cotransporter 2 (SGLT2), the transporter responsible for reabsorbing the glucose filtered by the tubular lumen in the kidney. By inhibiting SGLT2,

reabsorbs filtered glucose and lowers the renal threshold for glucose (RTG), increases urinary glucose excretion
Metformin: Decreases hepatic gluconeogenesis production, decreases intestinal absorption of glucose, and improves insulin sensitivity by increasing peripheral glucose uptake and utilization

USES: Type 2 diabetes mellitus

CONTRAINDICATIONS: Hypersensitivity, diabetic ketoacidosis, dialysis, metabolic acidosis, radiographic contrast administration, renal failure

Black Box Warning: Lactic acidosis

Precautions: Pregnancy (C), geriatric patients, severe renal/hepatic/GI disease, pancreatitis, vit D deficiency, acidemia, acute heart failure, acute myocardial infarction, alcoholism, balanitis, breastfeeding, burns, cardiac disease, children, dehydration, diarrhea, ethanol intoxication, fever, gastroparesis, hypercholesterolemia, hypercortisolism, hyperglycemia, hyperthyroidism, hypoglycemia, hypotension, hypovolemia, hypoxemia, infection, malnutrition, pernicious anemia, pituitary insufficiency, polycystic ovary syndrome, sepsis, surgery, trauma, type 1 diabetes mellitus, vaginitis, vomiting

DOSAGE AND ROUTES

- **Adult: PO** bid with meals; individualize based on efficacy and tolerability. In geriatric patients, use lowest effective dose. The max dose in normal renal function is empagliflozin 25 mg/day and metformin 2000 mg/day; correct volume depletion before initiation of treatment
- **Patients currently treated with empagliflozin:** Start with metformin 500 mg with a similar total daily dose of empagliflozin; increase gradually to reduce the GI side effects
- **Patients currently treated with metformin:** Start with empagliflozin 5 mg/dose with a similar total daily dose of metformin. Patients taking an evening dose of metformin XR should check with their provider about when to take their last dose before starting empagliflozin; metformin
- **Patients already treated with both empagliflozin and metformin:** May switch to this combination product using the same doses of each component per day, then dividing the daily doses to bid dosing with meals

Renal dose:
Adult: PO eGFR $\geq$ 45 ml/min/1.73 m^2: no change. eGFR $<$ 45 ml/min/1.73 m^2 or CCR $<$ 45 mL/min, including females with a serum creatinine $\geq$ 1.4 mg/dl or males with a serum creatinine $\geq$ 1.5 mg/dl or end-stage renal disease (ESRD): do not use

Available forms: Tabs 5 mg/500 mg, 5 mg/1000 mg, 12.5 mg/500 mg, 12.5 mg/1000 mg

Administer:

- ***Tablets, immediate-release:*** Give bid with meals (usually at morning and evening meals) to reduce GI adverse reactions

SIDE EFFECTS

ENDO: Hypoglycemia, diabetic ketoacidosis
CV: Orthostatic hypotension
GI: Nausea, vomiting, diarrhea, dyspepsia, anorexia, abdominal pain, flatulence, pyrosis (heartburn), polydipsia, metallic taste
GU: Polyuria, vaginitis, phimosis, nocturia, urinary frequency
META: Metabolic acidosis, vitamin B_{12} deficiency, hypercholesterolemia, hyperlipidemia
SYST: Lactic acidosis, infection
MS: Myalgia, arthralgia

PHARMACOKINETICS

Empagliflozin: 86% protein binding, terminal half-life 12.4 hr
Metformin: no protein binding, half-life 6.2 hr

INTERACTIONS

Do not use with gatifloxacin

Increase: hypoglycemia

Increase: hyperglycemia—phenothiazines, corticosteroids, anabolic steroids calcium channel blockers

Decrease: action of digoxin

Decrease: efficacy—niacin, thiazide diuretics, triamterene, estrogens, progestins, oral contraceptives

NURSING CONSIDERATIONS

Assess:

Black Box Warning: Lactic acidosis: Assess for nausea, vomiting, weakness, rapid breathing; notify prescriber immediately

- CBC, serum cholesterol profile, serum electrolytes periodically
- Fasting blood glucose, A1c levels, postprandial glucose during treatment to determine diabetes control
- Renal studies: urinalysis, creatinine
- Hypo/hyperglycemic reaction that can occur soon after meals; for severe hypoglycemia, give IV $D_{50}W$, then IV dextrose solution
- Nausea, vomiting, diarrhea, ability to tolerate product, may cause dehydration

Evaluate:

- Therapeutic response: decrease in polyuria, polydipsia, polyphagia, clear sensorium, improving A1c

Teach patient/family:

- About the symptoms of hypo/hyperglycemia, what to do about each; to have glucagon emergency kit available; to carry a glucose source (candy, sugar cube) to treat hypoglycemia
- That product must be continued daily; about consequences of discontinuing product abruptly
- That diabetes is a lifelong illness; product will not cure disease; to carry emergency ID with prescriber and medication information
- To continue weight control, dietary restrictions, exercise, hygiene
- That regular blood glucose monitoring and A1c testing are needed
- To notify prescriber if pregnant or intending to become pregnant (C)

evolocumab (Rx)

(e′-voe-lok′-ue-mab)

Repatha

Func. class.: Antilipemic

ACTION: Binds to low-density lipoproteins, a human monoclonal antibody (IgG1)

USES: Heterozygous, familial hypercholesterolemia, atherosclerotic disease

CONTRAINDICATIONS: Hypersensitivity

Precautions: Pregnancy, breastfeeding, latex sensitivity

DOSAGE AND ROUTES

Heterozygous familial hypercholesterolemia or primary hyperlipidemia with established clinical atherosclerosis in patients who require additional lowering of LDL-C:

- **Adult: SUBCUT** 140 mg q2wk or 420 mg monthly. If switching dosage regimens, administer the first dose of the new regimen on the next scheduled date of the previous regimen

Homozygous familial hypercholesterolemia in patients who require additional lowering of LDL-C:

- **Adult and adolescent:** 420 mg monthly

Available forms: Auto injector 140 mg/ml, solutions for injection 140 mg/ml

Administer:

- Visually inspect for particulate matter and discoloration, solution is clear, colorless to pale yellow

SUBCUT route

Prefilled Syringe or SureClick Autoinjector

- If stored in the refrigerator, warm to room temperature for ≥30 min before use. Do not shake

• Give into areas of the abdomen (except for a 2-inch area around the umbilicus), thigh, or upper arm that are not tender, bruised, red, or indurated
• To use the 420 mg dose, give 3 injections consecutively within 30 min
• Rotate the site with each injection
• Do not administer with other injectable drugs at the same injection site

Prefilled Syringe Administration

• Do not pick up or pull the prefilled syringe by the plunger rod or gray needle cap. Hold the syringe by the barrel
• Pull the gray needle cap off. It is normal to see a drop of solution at the end of the needle. Do not remove any air bubbles in the syringe
• Pinch the skin injection site to create a firm surface approximately 2 inches wide. Hold the pinch, and insert the needle into the skin using a 45- to 90-degree angle
• Push the plunger rod all the way down until the syringe is empty
• When done, release the plunger and gently lift the syringe off skin

SureClick Autoinjector Administration

• Do not remove the orange cap until you are ready to inject
• Pull the orange cap off
• Stretch (thigh) or pinch (stomach or upper arm) the skin injection site to create a firm surface approximately 2 inch wide. Hold the stretch or pinch, and place the autoinjector on the skin at 90 degrees
• Firmly push down onto the skin when ready to inject, press the gray button. A click should be heard. Keep pushing on the skin and then lift the thumb. The injection could take about 15 sec. The window on the autoinjector will turn from clear to yellow when the injection is complete. A second click may be heard.
• Remove the needle that will be automatically covered

SIDE EFFECTS

CNS: Memory impairment, confusion
GI: Diarrhea
MISC: Edema
MS: *Myalgia*
RESP: Pharyngitis, sinusitis, cough
SYST: Infection, antibody formation
INTEG: Pruritus, injection-site reaction, erythema, ecchymosis

PHARMACOKINETICS

Peak 3-7 days; half-life at steady state 17-20 days

INTERACTIONS

None known

Drug/Lab Test

Increase: LFTs

NURSING CONSIDERATIONS

Assess:

• **Hypercholesterolemia:** diet history: fat content, lipid levels (triglycerides, LDL, HDL, cholesterol); LFTs at baseline, periodically during treatment

Evaluate:

• Therapeutic response: decreased cholesterol, LDL; increased HDL

Teach patient/family:

• That compliance is needed
• That risk factors should be decreased: high-fat diet, smoking, alcohol consumption, absence of exercise
• To notify prescriber if pregnancy suspected, planned, or if breastfeeding
• To report confusion, injection-site reactions

isavuconazonium (Rx)

(eye-sa-vue-koe-na-zoe′nee-un)

Cresemba

Func. class.: Antifungal, systemic
Chem. class.: Triazole derivative

ACTION: Exerts antifungal activity by inhibiting the synthesis of ergosterol, an essential component of the fungal cell membrane. The depletion of ergosterol within the fungal cell membrane results in increased cellular permeability causing leakage of cellular content

USES: Aspergillus flavus, Aspergillus fumigatus, Aspergillus niger, Rhizopus oryzae, Mucormycetes species; do NOT use for infections of Candida, Blastomyces, Histoplasma

CONTRAINDICATIONS:
Hypersensitivity, short QT syndrome

Precautions: Azole hypersensitivity, pregnancy (C), breastfeeding, infusion-related reactions, hepatic disease

DOSAGE AND ROUTES

Invasive aspergillosis and invasive mucormycosis:

- **Adult: PO** loading dose of 2 caps (372 mg) q8hr × 6 doses. Then, 2 caps (372 mg) daily. Start maintenance dosing 12-24 hr after the last loading dose; IV loading dose of 372 mg q8hr × 6 doses, then 372 mg/day; then 12-24 hr after the last loading dose give over 1 hr, use a 0.2- to 1.2-micron in-line filter and administer over a minimum of 1 hr, an additional loading dose is not needed when switching to PO

Administer:

PO route

- Swallow whole, do not chew, crush, dissolve, open the capsules; may be used without regard food

IV route

- Visually inspect for particulate matter and discoloration; diluted solution may contain translucent to white particulates that will be removed by the in-line filter

Reconstitution

- Reconstitute the dry powder with 5 ml sterile water for injection, gently shake until dissolved
- Storage: the reconstituted solution may be stored below 77° F (25° C) for a maximum of 1 hr before further dilution

Dilution

- Remove 5 ml of the reconstituted solution and add it to 250 ml of either 0.9% NaCl or D_5W (1.5 mg/ml)
- Gently mix the solution or roll the bag. DO NOT shake. Do not place in a pneumatic transport system
- Apply an in-line filter (0.2-1.2 microns), adhere an in-line filter reminder sticker to the infusion bag
- Give over ≤6 hr of dilution
- Storage: may be stored immediately after dilution at 36° to 46° F (2° to 8° C); administration MUST be completed within 24 hr of the time of dilution. Do NOT freeze
- Product only after C&S confirms organism, product needed to treat condition; make sure product used in life-threatening infections
- Flush IV lines with 0.9% sodium chloride or 5% dextrose in water before and after administration of the infusion
- Must be administered through a 0.2- to 1.2-micron filter; give over ≥1 hr. Do not give by bolus
- Do not admix

Available forms: Caps 186 mg; powder for injection 382 mg

SIDE EFFECTS

CNS: *Headache,* paresthesias, peripheral neuropathy, *hallucinations,* depression, insomnia, dizziness, fever, vertigo, tremor, confusion

CV: Tachypnea, supraventricular tachycardia, atrial fibrillation/flutter

EENT: Tinnitus

GI: Nausea, vomiting, anorexia, diarrhea, cramps, hepatitis, stomatitis

GU: *Hypokalemia,* renal failure

HEMA: Anemia, eosinophilia, hypomagnesemia, thrombocytopenia, leukopenia

INTEG: *Burning, irritation,* pain, necrosis at inj site with extravasation, *rash*

MISC: Cough

PHARMACOKINETICS

By CYP3A4, CYP3A5, UGT, P-gp, OCT2enzymes; eliminated in urine/feces; peak 2 hr (PO), Chinese patients (levels 40% lower), protein binding >99%

INTERACTIONS

Increase: effects of benzodiazepines, calcium channel blockers, cycloSPORINE, ergots, HMG-CoA reductase inhibitors, pimozide, quiNIDine, prednisoLONE, sirolimus, sulfonylureas, tacrolimus, vinca alkaloids, warfarin, rifabutin, proton pump inhibitors, NNRTIs, protease inhibitors, phenytoin

Increase: effect of CYP3A4 substrates
Decrease: effect of CYP3A4 inhibitors
Drug/Herb
- Do not use with St. John's wort

Drug/Lab Test
Increase: AST/ALT, alk phos, creatinine, bilirubin
Decrease: Hgb/Hct, platelets, WBC

NURSING CONSIDERATIONS
Assess:
- **Pregnancy:** test for pregnancy before starting treatment, pregnancy (C), do not breastfeed
- **Short QT syndrome:** do not use in this condition
- VS q15-30min during first infusion; note changes in pulse, B/P
- Blood studies: CBC, potassium, sodium, calcium, magnesium, q2wk
- **Hepatotoxicity:** increasing AST, ALT, alk phos, bilirubin, baseline and periodically
- **Allergic reaction:** dermatitis, rash; product should be discontinued, antihistamines (mild reaction) or epinephrine (severe reaction) administered
- **Hypokalemia:** anorexia, drowsiness, weakness, decreased reflexes, dizziness, increased urinary output, increased thirst, paresthesias
- **Ototoxicity:** tinnitus (ringing, roaring in ears), vertigo

Evaluate:
- Therapeutic response: resolution of fungal infection, negative C&S

Teach patient/family:
- That long-term therapy may be needed to clear infection (2 wk-3 mo, depending on type of infection)
- To notify prescriber of bleeding, bruising, soft-tissue swelling, dark urine, persistent nausea or diarrhea, headache, rash, yellow skin/eyes
- Women of childbearing age should use effective contraceptive, pregnancy (C), do not breastfeed

RARELY USED
⚠ HIGH ALERT

lenvatinib
(len-va′-ti-nib)
Lenvima ⚠ ✦
Func. class.: Antineoplastic

USES: Locally recurrent or metastatic, progressive, radioactive iodine-refractory differentiated thyroid cancer (DTC)

CONTRAINDICATIONS: Hypersensitivity

DOSAGE AND ROUTES
Adults: PO 24 mg (two 10-mg capsules and one 4-mg capsule) daily
Available forms: Caps 4 mg, 10 mg

RARELY USED

metreleptin
(met′-re-lep′-tin)
Myalept
Func. class.: Hormone replacement-leptin receptor agonist

USES: Complications caused by leptin deficiency in patients with congenital or acquired generalized lipodystrophy

CONTRAINDICATIONS: Hypersensitivity

Black Box Warning: Secondary malignancy, antimetreleptin antibodies

DOSAGE AND ROUTES
- **Adult/adolescent/child >40 kg: SUBCUT: Males:** 2.5 mg/day (0.5 ml) initially, may increase or decrease dose by 1.25-2.5 mg/day (0.25-0.5 ml) as needed, max 10 mg/day (2 ml/day). **Females:** 5 mg/day (1 ml) initially; may

APPENDIX A

increase or decrease dose by 1.25-2.5 mg/day (0.25-0.5 ml) as needed, max 10 mg/day (2 ml/day)

- **Adult/adolescent/child/neonate ≤40 kg: SUBCUT** 0.06 mg/kg/day (0.012 ml/kg) initially. Increase or decrease dose by 0.02 mg/kg/day (0.004 ml/kg) as needed, max 0.13 mg/kg/day (0.026 ml/kg/day). Give daily at the same time every day

RARELY USED

miltefosine

(mil′-te-foe′-seen)

Impavido

Func. class.: Antiprotozoal/Antileishmanial

USES: Treatment of visceral leishmaniasis caused by L. donovani, mucosal leishmaniasis caused by L. braziliensis, and cutaneous leishmaniasis caused by L. braziliensis, L. guyanensis, and L. panamensis

CONTRAINDICATIONS: Hypersensitivity, pregnancy (D)

DOSAGE AND ROUTES

- **Adult/adolescent/child ≥12 yr and ≥45 kg: PO** 50 mg tid × 28 days
- **Adult/adolescent/child ≥12 yr and 30-44 kg: PO** 50 mg bid 3 28 days; HIV guidelines suggest 100 mg daily 3 4 wk in adults and adolescents regardless of weight

RARELY USED
⚠ HIGH ALERT

panobinostat

(pan′-oh-bin′-oh-stat)

Farydak

Func. class.: Antineoplastic: biologic response modifiers

USES: Multiple myeloma in those who have received at least 2 prior therapies (including bortezomib and an immunomodulatory agent), in combination with bortezomib and dexamethasone; an orphan drug

CONTRAINDICATIONS: Hypersensitivity

Precautions:

Black Box Warning: Diarrhea, cardiac dysrhythmias, long QT syndrome, QT prolongation, electrolyte imbalances

DOSAGE AND ROUTES

- **Adult: PO** 20 mg every other day × 3 times per wk (on days 1, 3, 5, 8, 10, and 12) for the first 2 wk of each 21-day cycle. Continue for up to 8 cycles; may give up to another 8 cycles (max of 16 treatment cycles) in those who experience clinical benefit without unresolved severe or medically significant toxicity, give with bortezomib (cycles 1-8: 1.3 mg/m^2 on days 1, 4, 8, and 11; cycles 9-16: 1.3 mg/m^2 on days 1 and 8) and dexamethasone (cycles 1-8: 20 mg PO on days 1, 2, 4, 5, 8, 9, 11, and 12; cycles 9-16: 20 mg PO on days 1, 2, 8, and 9). Avoid concomitant use with strong CYP3A4 inducers

Available forms: Cap 10, 15, 20 mg

secukinumab (Rx)

(sek′-ue-kin′-ue-mab)

Cosentyx

Func. class.: Immune response modifier

Chem. class.: Monoclonal antibody

ACTION: Interleukin (IL)-12, IL-23 antagonist

USES: Plaque psoriasis

CONTRAINDICATIONS: Hypersensitivity, active TB

Precautions: Pregnancy (B), breastfeeding, Crohn's disease, infection, latex hypersensitivity, vaccination

DOSAGE AND ROUTES

Moderate to severe plaque psoriasis
- **Adult: SUBCUT** 300 mg at weeks 0, 1, 2, 3, and 4, then 300 mg q4wk

Available forms: Solution for injection 150 mg/ml (pen, prefilled syringe), 2-pack and single

Administer:
- Visually inspect for particulate matter or discoloration; solution should be slightly yellow and may contain a few small translucent or white particles; do not use if discolored, cloudy, or if foreign particulate matter is present; do not shake
- Use a 27-G, 0.5-inch needle
- May be administered SUBCUT into upper arm, abdomen, or thigh; rotate injection sites
- Use by SUBCUT injection only
- Those with latex hypersensitivity should not handle cap of injection

SUBCUT injection:
- Patients may use the prefilled syringe or Sensoready pen after proper training; the lyophilized powder is for healthcare provider use only
- Each 300 mg dose is used as 2 SUBCUT injections of 150 mg
- Do not administer where skin is tender, bruised, erythematous, indurated, or affected by psoriasis
- *Reconstitution of lyophilized powder:*
- Allow to warm to room temperature for 15-30 min, use 1 ml sterile water for injection to reconstitute, rotate, do not shake or invert vial, allow to stand for 10 min, again rotate vial, allow to stand for another 5 min (150 mg/ml)
- Storage: use immediately or refrigerate for up to 24 hr. Do not freeze. If refrigerated, allow reconstituted solution to reach room temperature (15-30 min) before administration
- *Preparation for use of prefilled syringe or Sensoready pen:*
- Remove prefilled syringe or Sensoready pen from refrigerator and allow 15-30 min to reach room temperature
- Storage: the prefilled syringe or Sensoready should be used within 1 hr

SIDE EFFECTS

EENT: Ocular infections, sinusitis, oral ulceration, rhinitis, sinusitis

GI: Diarrhea

HEMA: Bleeding

INTEG: *Injection-site reaction*, urticaria

SYST: **Serious infections,** anaphylaxis, antibody formation, candidiasis

RESP: URI

PHARMACOKINETICS

Maximum serum concentration: 13.5 days after a single 45 mg SUBCUT dose, 7 days after a single 90 mg SUBCUT dose; half-life 14.9-45.6 days

INTERACTIONS

- Do not give concurrently with vaccines; immunizations should be brought up to date before treatment
- Avoid use with immunosuppressives

Drug/Lab tests

Increase: LFTs

NURSING CONSIDERATIONS

Assess:
- TB: TB testing should be done before starting treatment
- For injection-site pain, swelling
- Bring immunizations up to date before starting treatment
- Infection: monitor for fever, sore throat, cough, do not use during active infections
- **Malignancy:** skin cancer may occur, especially in older patients who have used ultraviolet treatments with immunosuppressants

Evaluate:
- Therapeutic response: decreased plaque psoriasis

Teach patient/family:
- That product must be continued for prescribed time to be effective, to use as prescribed
- Not to receive live vaccinations during treatment
- To notify prescriber of possible infection (upper respiratory or other) or allergic reactions
- Injection techniques and disposal of equipment, not to reuse needles, syringes

RARELY USED
⚠ HIGH ALERT

siltuximab

(sil-tux′-i-mab)

Sylvant ⚠ ✦

Func. class.: Antineoplastic: immune response modifier

USES: Multicentric Castleman disease (MCD) patients who are HIV-negative and human herpesvirus-8 (HHV-8)-negative

CONTRAINDICATIONS: Hypersensitivity

DOSAGE AND ROUTES

• **Adult: IV** 11 mg/kg IV over 1 hr q3wk until treatment failure

RARELY USED
⚠ HIGH ALERT

sonidegib

(soe′-ni-deg′-ib)

Odomzo ⚠ ✦

Func. class.: Antineoplastic

USES: Locally advanced basal cell carcinoma that has recurred after surgery or radiation therapy or in those who are not candidates for surgery or radiation therapy

CONTRAINDICATIONS: Hypersensitivity

Precautions:

Black Box Warning: Pregnancy, intrauterine fetal death, contraceptive requirement

DOSAGE AND ROUTES

• **Adult: PO** 200 mg daily until disease progression or unacceptable toxicity; take on an empty stomach ≥1 hr before or 2 hr after a meal. Avoid use with strong CYP3A inhibitors or strong and moderate CYP3A inducers

Available forms: Cap 200 mg

Appendix B

Ophthalmic, nasal, topical, and otic products

OPHTHALMIC PRODUCTS

ANESTHETICS

lidocaine (Rx)
(lye′doe-kane)
Akten

proparacaine (Rx)
(proe-par′a-kane)
Alcaine, Diocaine ✦, Parcaine

tetracaine (Rx)
(tet′ra-kane)
Minims Tetracaine ✦, Tetracaine, TetraVisc

ANTIHISTAMINES

alcaftadine
(al-caf′tah-deen)
Lastacaft

azelastine (Rx)
(ay-zell′ah-steen)

emedastine (Rx)
(ee-med′a-steen)
Emadine

epinastine (Rx)
(ep-een-as′teen)
Elestat

ketotifen (Rx, OTC)
(kee-toh-tif′en)
Alaway, Claritin Eye, Zaditor, Zyrtec Itchy Eye

levocabastine (Rx)
(lee-voh-cab′ah-steen)
Livostin

olopatadine (Rx)
(oh-loh-pat′ah-deen)
Patanase, Pataday, Pazeo

ANTIINFECTIVES

azithromycin (Rx)
(ay-zi-thro-my′sin)
AzaSite

besifloxacin (Rx)
(be′si-flox′a-sin)
Besivance

ciprofloxacin (Rx)
(sip-ro-floks′a-sin)
Ciloxan

erythromycin (Rx)
(er-ith-roe-mye′sin)
Ilotycin, Romycin

ganciclovir (Rx)
(gan-sye′kloe-vir)
Zirgan

gatifloxacin (Rx)
(gat-ih-floks′ah-sin)
Zymaxid

gentamicin (Rx)
(jen-ta-mye′sin)
Garamycin Ophthalmic, Gentak, Gentasol

levofloxacin (Rx)
(lee-voh-flock′sah-sin)

moxifloxacin (Rx)
(mox-i-flox′a-sin)
Moxeza, Vigamox

natamycin (Rx)
(nat-a-mye′sin)
Natacyn

ofloxacin (Rx)
(oh-floks′a-sin)
Ocuflox

silver nitrate 1% (Rx)

silver nitrate

sulfacetamide sodium (Rx)
(sul-fa-seet′a-mide)
Bleph-10

tobramycin (Rx)
(toe-bra-mye′sin)
Tobrasol, Tobrex

trifluridine (Rx)
(trye-floor′i-deen)
Viroptic

β-ADRENERGIC BLOCKERS

betaxolol (Rx)
(beh-tax′oh-lole)
Betoptic

carteolol (Rx)
(kar-tee′oh-lole)

levobetaxolol (Rx)
(lee-voh-beh-tax′oh-lohl)
Betaxon

levobunolol (Rx)
(lee-voe-byoo′no-lole)
Betagen

metipranolol (Rx)
(met-ee-pran′oh-lole)
OptiPranolol

timolol (Rx)
(tym′moe-lole)
Betimol

CARBONIC ANHYDRASE INHIBITORS

brinzolamide (Rx)
(brin-zoh′la-mide)
Azopt

dorzolamide (Rx)
(dor-zol′a-mide)
Trusopt

CHOLINERGICS (Direct-acting)

acetylcholine (Rx)
(ah-see-til-koe′leen)
Miochol-E

carbachol (Rx)
(kar′ba-kole)
Isopto Carbachol

pilocarpine (Rx)
(pye-loe-kar′peen)
Isopto Carpine

CHOLINESTERASE INHIBITORS

physostigmine (Rx)
(fi-zoe-stig′meen)

CORTICOSTEROIDS

dexamethasone (Rx)
(dex-a-meth′a-sone)
Maxidex

fluorometholone (Rx)
(flure-oh-meth′oh-lone)
Flarex, FML, FML Forte, FML S.O.P.

loteprednol (Rx)
(loe-tee-pred-nole)
Alrex, Lotemax

prednisoLONE (Rx)
(pred-niss′oh-lone)
Econopred Plus, Omnipred, Pred-Forte, Pred Mild

rimexolone (Rx)
(ri-mex′a-lone)
Vexol

MYDRIATICS

atropine (Rx)
(a′troe-peen)

cyclopentolate (Rx)
(sye-kloe-pen′toe-late)
Cyclogyl, Cylate

homatropine (Rx)
(home-a′troe-peen)
Isopto Homatropine

phenylephrine (OTC)
(fen-ill-ef′rin)
Neofrin

NONSTEROIDAL ANTIINFLAMMATORIES

bromfenac (Rx)
(brome′fen-ak)
Prolensa

diclofenac (Rx)
(dye-kloe′fen-ak)

flurbiprofen (Rx)
(flure-bi′pro-fen)
Ocufen

ketorolac (Rx)
(kee-toe′role-ak)
Acular, Acuvail

nepafenac (Rx)
(ne-pa-fen′ak)
Ilevro, Nevanac

SYMPATHOMIMETICS

apraclonidine (Rx)
(a-pra-klon′i-deen)
Iopidine

brimonidine (Rx)
(brem-on′i-dine)
Alphagan P

OPHTHALMIC DECONGESTANTS/ VASOCONSTRICTORS

lodoxamide
(loe-dox′ah-mide)
Alomide

naphazoline (Rx, OTC)
(naf-az′oh-leen)
AK-Con, All Clear Eye Drops, All Clear AR Maximum Strength Opthalmic Solution, CVS Maximum Redness Relief Eye Drops, CVS Redness Relief Lubricant Eye Drops

oxymetazoline (Rx)
(ox-i-met-ah-zoh′leen)
Visine L.R.

tetrahydrozoline (OTC)
(tet-ra-hye-dro′zoe-leen)
Visine Original p0550

MISCELLANEOUS OPHTHALMICS

bimatoprost (Rx)
(bih-mat′o-prost)
Latisse, Lumigan

latanoprost (Rx)
(la-tan′oh-prost)
Xalatan

travoprost (Rx)
(tra′voe-prost)
Travatan

unoprostone (Rx)
(yoo-noe-pros′tone)
Rescula

β-ADRENERGIC BLOCKERS

ACTION: Reduces production of aqueous humor by unknown mechanism

USES: Ocular hypertension, chronic open angle glaucoma

ANESTHETICS

ACTION: Decreases ion permeability by stabilizing neuronal membrane

USES: Cataract extraction, tonometry, gonioscopy, removal of foreign objects, corneal suture removal, glaucoma surgery (ophthalmic); pruritus, sunburn, toothache, sore throat, cold sores, oral pain, rectal pain and irritation, control of gagging (topical)

ANTIINFECTIVES

ACTION: Inhibits folic acid synthesis by preventing PABA use, which is necessary for bacterial growth

USES: Conjunctivitis, superficial eye infections, corneal ulcers, prophylaxis against infection after removal of foreign matter from the eye

ANTIINFLAMMATORIES

ACTION: Decreases inflammation, resulting in decreased pain, photophobia, hyperemia, cellular infiltration

USES: Inflammation of eye, eyelids, conjunctiva, cornea; uveitis, iridocyclitis, allergic conditions, burns, foreign bodies, postoperatively in cataract

CARBONIC ANHYDRASE INHIBITOR

ACTION: Converted to epINEPHrine, which decreases aqueous production and increases outflow

USES: Open angle glaucoma, ocular hypertension

DIRECT-ACTING MIOTIC

ACTION: Acts directly on cholinergic receptor sites; induces miosis, spasm of accommodation, fall in intraocular pressure, caused by stimulation of ciliary, pupillary sphincter muscles, which leads to pulling away of iris from filtration angle, resulting in increased outflow of aqueous humor

USES: Primary glaucoma, early stages of wide angle glaucoma (less useful in advanced stages), chronic open angle glaucoma, acute closed angle glaucoma before emergency surgery; also neutralizes mydriatics used during eye exam; may be used alternately with mydriatics to break adhesions between iris and lens

CONTRAINDICATIONS: Hypersensitivity

Precautions: Pregnancy, breastfeeding, children, aphakia, hypersensitivity to carbonic anhydrase inhibitors, sulfonamides, thiazide diuretics, ocular inhibitors, renal/hepatic insufficiency

Administer

- Storage at room temperature away from light

ADVERSE EFFECTS

CNS: Headache

CV: Hypertension, tachycardia, dysrhythmias

EENT: Burning, stinging

GI: Bitter taste

NURSING CONSIDERATIONS

Assess

- Monitor ophthalmic exams and intraocular pressure readings
- Monitor blood counts; renal/hepatic function tests and serum electrolytes during long-term treatment

Teach patient/family

- Teach how to instill drops
- Advise patient that product may cause burning, itching, blurring, dryness of eye area

Evaluate

Positive therapeutic outcome

- Absence of increased intraocular pressure

NASAL AGENTS

NASAL ANTIHISTAMINES

olopatadine (Rx)
(oh-low-pat′uh-deen)
Patanase

NASAL DECONGESTANTS

azelastine (Rx)
(ay-zell′ah-steen)
Astepro

EPINEPHrine (OTC)
(ep-i-neff′rin)
Adrenalin Nasal Solution

oxymetazoline (OTC)
(ox-i-met-az′oh-leen)
Afrin No Drip, Dristan 12-HR Nasal Spray, Mucinex Moisture, Mucinex Sinus-Max, Vicks QlearQuil, Vicks Sinex

phenylephrine (OTC)
(fen-ill-eff′rin)
4-Way Nasal Spray, Neo-Synephrine

tetrahydrozoline (OTC)
(tet-ra-hye-dro′zoe-leen)
Tyzine, Tyzine Pediatric

NASAL STEROIDS

beclomethasone (Rx)
(be-kloe-meth′a-sone)
Beconase AQ Nasal, Qnasl

budesonide (Rx)
(byoo-des′oh-nide)
Rhinocort Aqua

flunisolide (Rx)
(floo-niss′oh-lide)

fluticasone (Rx)
(floo-tic′a-son)
Veramyst

triamcinolone (Rx)
(trye-am-sin′oh-lone)
Allergy 24 HR Nasal Spray, Nasacort

NONSTEROIDAL ANTIINFLAMMATORY

ketorolac (Rx)
(kee′toe-role-ak)
Sprix

ACTION: Produces vasoconstriction (rapid, long acting) of arterioles, thereby decreasing fluid exudation, mucosal engorgement by stimulation of α-adrenergic receptors in vascular smooth muscle

Therapeutic outcome: Absence of nasal congestion

USES: Nasal congestion

CONTRAINDICATIONS: Hypersensitivity to sympathomimetic amines

Precautions: Pregnancy (C), children <6 yr, geriatric patients, diabetes, CV disease, hypertension, hyperthyroidism, increased ICP, prostatic hypertrophy, glaucoma

Administer

- Have patient tilt head back, squeeze bulb to create a vacuum, and draw correct amount of sol into dropper; insert 2 gtt of sol into nostril; repeat in other nostril
- Store in light-resistant container; do not expose to high temperature or let sol come into contact with aluminum
- Give for <4 consecutive days
- Provide environmental humidification to decrease nasal congestion, dryness

ADVERSE EFFECTS

CNS: Anxiety, restlessness, tremors, weakness, insomnia, dizziness, fever, headache

EENT: Irritation, burning, sneezing, stinging, dryness, rebound congestion

GI: Nausea, vomiting, anorexia
INTEG: Contact dermatitis

NURSING CONSIDERATIONS

Assess

- Assess for redness, swelling, pain in nasal passages before, during treatment
- Assess for systemic absorption; hypertension, tachycardia; notify prescriber; systemic absorption occurs at high doses or after prolonged use

Teach patient/family

- Advise patient that stinging may occur for several applications; drying of mucosa may be decreased by environmental humidification
- Caution patient to notify prescriber if irregular pulse, insomnia, dizziness, or tremors occur
- Teach patient proper administration to avoid systemic absorption
- Advise patient to rinse dropper with very hot water to prevent contamination

Evaluate

Positive therapeutic outcome

- Decreased nasal congestion

TOPICAL GLUCOCORTICOIDS

betamethasone (Rx)
(bay-ta-meth′a-sone)
Beben ✦, Betacort ✦, Betanate, Betnovate ✦, Celestoderm ✦, Del-Beta, Ectosone ✦, Metaderm ✦

betamethasone (augmented) (Rx)
(bay-ta-meth′a-sone)
Diprolene AF

clobetasol (Rx)
(kloe-bay′ta-sol)
Clobex, Cormax, Dermovate ✦, Olux Topical Foam, Temovate

desonide (Rx)
(dess′oh-nide)
Desonate, DesOwen, LoKara, Verdeso Foam

desoximetasone (Rx)
(dess-ox-i-met′a-sone)
Topicort

fluocinolone (Rx)
(floo-oh-sin′oh-lone)
Derma-Smoothe/FS oil, Lidemol ✦, Lyderm ✦, Synalar, Topsyn ✦

flurandrenolide (Rx)
(flure-an-dren′oh-lide)
Cordran, Drenison 1/4 ✦, Drenison Tape ✦

fluticasone (Rx)
(floo-tik′a-sone)
Cutivate

halcinonide (Rx)
(hal-sin′oh-nide)
Halog

hydrocortisone (Rx)
(hye-droe-kor′ti-sone)
Barriere-HC ✦, CaldeCORT, Cortacet ✦, Cortalo, Cortate ✦, Cortef ✦, Corticreme ✦, Cortifoam, Cortoderm ✦, Hyderm ✦, Instacort, Neosporin Eczema Anti-Itch, Novohydrocort ✦, Nutracort , Nuzon, Sarna HC ✦, Unicort ✦

triamcinolone (Rx)
(trye-am-sin′oh-lone)
Dermasorb TA, Kenalog, Pediaderm TA, Trianide ✦, Triderm

ACTION: Antipruritic, antiinflammatory

Therapeutic outcome: Decreased itching, inflammation

USES: Psoriasis, eczema, contact dermatitis, pruritus; usually reserved for severe dermatoses that have not responded to less potent formulation

CONTRAINDICATIONS: Hypersensitivity, viral infections, fungal infections

Precautions: Pregnancy C

DOSAGE AND ROUTES

Adult and child: Apply to affected area

Administer

- Apply only to affected areas; do not get in eyes
- Apply and leave site uncovered or lightly covered; occlusive dressing is not recommended—systemic absorption may occur
- Use only on dermatoses; do not use on weeping, denuded, or infected area
- Cleanse area before application of product
- Continue treatment for a few days after area has cleared
- Store at room temperature

ADVERSE EFFECTS

INTEG: *Acne, atrophy, epidermal thinning, purpura, striae*

NURSING CONSIDERATIONS

Assess

- Monitor temp; if fever develops, product should be discontinued
- Monitor for systemic absorption, increased temp, inflammation, irritation

Teach patient/family

- Teach patient to avoid sunlight on affected area; burns may occur
- Teach patient to limit treatment to 14 days

Evaluate

Positive therapeutic outcome

- Absence of severe itching, patches on skin, flaking

TOPICAL ANTIFUNGALS

clotrimazole (OTC)
(kloe-trye′ma-zole)
Canesten ✱, Clotrimaderm ✱, Cruex, Crux, Desenex, Lotrimin AF, Myclo ✱, Neozol ✱

econazole (OTC)
(ee-kon′a-zole)
Ecoza

efinaconazole
(ef-in-a-kon′a-zole)
Jublia

ketoconazole (OTC)
(kee-toe-kon′a-zole)
Extina, Ketodan, Kuric, Xolegel

luliconazole
(loo-li-kon′a-zole)
Luzu

miconazole (OTC)
(mye-kon′a-zole)
Antifungal, Azolen, Baza, Cruex, Desenex, Micaderm, Novana, Lotrimin AF, Triple Paste AF, Zeasorb-AF

nystatin (OTC)
(nye-stat′in)
Nodostine ✱, Nyamyc, Nyaderm ✱, Nystop, Pediaderm AF

selenium (OTC)
(see-leen′ee-um)

tavaborole
(ta′va-bor′ole)
Kerydin

terbinafine (OTC)
(ter-bin′a-feen)
Lamisil

tolnaftate (OTC)
(tole-naf′tate)
Absorbine Athlete's Foot Cream, Lamasil AF Topical Spray, Ting
undecylenic acid (OTC)
(un-deh-sih-len′ik)

ACTION: Interferes with fungal cell membrane permeability

Therapeutic outcome: Absence of itching and white patches of the skin

USES: Tinea cruris, tinea pedis, diaper rash, minor skin irritations; amphotericin B is used for *Candida* infections

CONTRAINDICATIONS: Hypersensitivity

Precautions: Pregnancy (B), breastfeeding, children

DOSAGE AND ROUTES

Massage into affected area, surrounding area daily or bid, continue for 7-14 days, max 4 wk

Administer

- Apply to affected area, surrounding area; do not cover with occlusive dressings
- Store below 30° C (86° F)

ADVERSE EFFECTS

INTEG: Burning, stinging, dryness, itching, local irritation

NURSING CONSIDERATIONS

Assess

- Assess skin for fungal infections: peeling, dryness, itching before, throughout treatment
- Assess for continuing infection; increased size, number of lesions

Teach patient/family

- Instruct to apply with glove to prevent further infection; not to cover with occlusive dressings
- Teach patient that long-term therapy may be needed to clear infection (2 wk-6 mo depending on organism); compliance is needed even after feeling better
- Teach patient proper hygiene: handwashing technique, nail care, use of concomitant top agents if prescribed
- Caution patient to avoid use of OTC creams, ointments, lotions unless directed by prescriber
- Instruct patient to use medical asepsis (hand washing) before, after each application; to change socks and shoes once a day during treatment of tinea pedis
- Advise patient to report to health care prescriber if infection persists or recurs; if blisters, burning, oozing, swelling occur
- Caution patient to avoid alcohol because nausea, vomiting, hypertension may occur
- Caution patient to use sunscreen or avoid direct sunlight to prevent photosensitivity
- Advise patient to notify prescriber of sore throat, fever, skin rash, which may indicate overgrowth of organisms

Evaluate

Positive therapeutic outcome

- Decrease in size, number of lesions

TOPICAL ANTIINFECTIVES

azelaic acid (Rx)
(a-zuh-lay′ic)
Azelex, Finacea
bacitracin (OTC)
(bass-i-tray′sin)
Bacitin ✦
clindamycin (Rx)
(klin-da-my′sin)
Cleocin T, Clindacin ETZ, Clindaxin PAC, Evocin
erythromycin (Rx, OTC)
(er-ith-roe-mye′sin)
Emgel, Emcin Clear, Ery, Erygel

gentamicin (Rx)
(jen-ta-mye′sin)
mafenide (Rx)
(ma′fe-nide)
Sulfamylon
metronidazole (Rx)
(met-roh-nye′da-zole)
MetroGel, MetroCream, Noritate, Rosaden
mupirocin (Rx)
(myoo-peer′oh-sin)
Bactroban, Centany
retapamulin (Rx)
(re-tap′a-mue′lin)
Altabax
salicylic acid (Rx)
(sal′i-sil′ik)
Bensal HP, Demarest, Keralyt, Salacyn, Salvax, UltraSal-ER
silver sulfADIAZINE (Rx)
(sul-fa-dye′a-zeen)
Flamazine ✦, Silvadene, SSD, Thermazene
tretinoin (Rx)
(treh′tih-noyn)
Atralin, Avita, Refissa, Retin-A, Tretin-X, Renova

ACTION: Interferes with bacterial protein synthesis

Therapeutic outcome: Resolution of infection

USES: Skin infections, minor burns, wounds, skin grafts, primary pyodermas, otitis externa

CONTRAINDICATIONS: Hypersensitivity, large areas, burns, ulcerations

Precautions: Pregnancy (C), breastfeeding, impaired renal function, external ear or perforated eardrum

Administer
- Apply enough medication to cover lesions completely
- Apply after cleansing with soap, water before each application; dry well
- Apply to less than 20% of body surface area when patient has impaired renal function
- Store at room temperature in dry place

ADVERSE EFFECTS
INTEG: Rash, urticaria, scaling, redness

NURSING CONSIDERATIONS
Assess
- Assess for allergic reaction: burning, stinging, swelling, redness
- Assess for signs of nephrotoxicity or ototoxicity

Evaluate

Positive therapeutic outcome
- Decrease in size, number of lesions

TOPICAL ANTIVIRALS

acyclovir (Rx)
(ay-sye′kloe-ver)
Zovirax Topical
penciclovir (Rx)
(pen-sye′kloe-ver)
Denavir

ACTION: Interferes with viral DNA replication

Therapeutic outcome: Resolution of infection

USES: Simple mucocutaneous herpes simplex, in immunocompromised clients with initial herpes genitalis

CONTRAINDICATIONS: Hypersensitivity

APPENDIX B

Precautions: Pregnancy C, breastfeeding

Administer

- Apply with finger cot or rubber glove to prevent further infection
- Apply enough medication to cover lesions completely
- Apply after cleansing with soap, water before each application; dry well
- Store at room temperature in dry place

ADVERSE EFFECTS

INTEG: Rash, urticaria, stinging, burning, pruritus, vulvitis

NURSING CONSIDERATIONS

Assess

- Assess for allergic reaction: burning, stinging, swelling, redness, rash, vulvitis, pruritus
- Assess for signs of nephrotoxicity or ototoxicity

Teach patient/family

- Teach patient not to use in eyes or when there is no evidence of infection
- Advise patient to apply with glove to prevent further infection
- Advise patient to avoid use of OTC creams, ointments, lotions unless directed by prescriber
- Advise patient to use medical asepsis (hand washing) before, after each application and avoid contact with eyes
- Advise patient to adhere strictly to prescribed regimen to maximize successful treatment outcome
- Advise patient to begin taking product when symptoms arise

Evaluate

Positive therapeutic outcome

- Decrease in size, number of lesions

TOPICAL ANESTHETICS

benzocaine (OTC)
(ben′zoe-kane)
Americaine Anesthetic, Anbesol Maximum Strength, Boil-Ease, Ora-Jel

dibucaine (OTC)
(dye′byoo-kane)
Nupercainal

lidocaine (Rx, OTC)
(lye′doe-kane)
EnovaRx, Glydo, LTA, Lidomar, LidoRx, Solarcaine, Zilactin-L

pramoxine (OTC)
(pra-mox′een)
Prax, Proctofoam

tetracaine (OTC, Rx)
(tet′ra-cane)
Pontocaine, Viractin

ACTION: Inhibits conduction of nerve impulses from sensory nerves

Therapeutic outcome: Decreasing inflammation, itching, pain

USES: Oral irritation, sore throat, toothache, cold sore, canker sore, sunburn, minor cuts, insect bites, pain, itching

CONTRAINDICATIONS: Hypersensitivity, infants <1 yr, application to large areas

Precautions: Pregnancy C, children <6 yr, sepsis, denuded skin

DOSAGE AND ROUTES

Adult and child: TOP apply qid as needed; RECT insert tid and after each BM

Administer

- Store in tight, light-resistant container; do not freeze, puncture, or incinerate aerosol container

ADVERSE EFFECTS

INTEG: Rash, irritation, sensitization

NURSING CONSIDERATIONS

Assess

- Assess pain: location, duration, characteristics before, after administration
- Assess for infection: redness, drainage, inflammation; this product should not be used until infection is treated

Teach Patient/Family

- Teach patient to avoid contact with eyes
- Teach patient not to use for prolonged periods: use for <1 wk; if condition remains, prescriber should be contacted

Evaluate

Positive therapeutic outcome

- Decreased redness, swelling, pain

TOPICAL MISCELLANEOUS

docosanol (OTC)
(doh-koh′sah-nohl)
Abreva

pimecrolimus (Rx)
(pim-eh-kroh-ly′mus)
Elidel

ACTION: Docosanol unknown; pimecrolimus may bind with macrophilin and inhibit calcium-dependent phosphatase

Therapeutic outcome: Decreased redness, swelling, pain

USES: Docosanol applied to fever blisters to promote more rapid healing; pimecrolimus used to treat mild to moderate atopic dermatitis in nonimmunocompromised patients ≥2 yr who are unresponsive to other treatment

CONTRAINDICATIONS: Hypersensitivity

Precautions: Pregnancy C, breastfeeding, dermal infections

DOSAGE AND ROUTES

Docosanol

Adult: TOP rub into blisters 5 ×/day until healing occurs

Pimecrolimus

Adult and child ≥2 yr: TOP apply thin layer 2 ×/day and rub in; use as long as needed

Administer

- Apply to skin, rub in gently

ADVERSE EFFECTS

Docosanol

NONE known

Pimecrolimus

INTEG: Burning

NURSING CONSIDERATIONS

Assess

- Assess skin condition (color, pain, inflammation) before, after administration
- Assess for signs and symptoms of skin infections (redness, draining lesions); if present, avoid use of product (pimecrolimus)

Teach patient/family

- Advise patient to avoid contact between medication and eyes
- Instruct patient to discontinue use of product when condition clears

Evaluate

Positive therapeutic outcome

- Decreased inflammation, redness

VAGINAL ANTIFUNGALS

butoconazole (OTC)
(byoo-toh-kone′ah-zole)
Gynazol-1

clotrimazole (OTC)
(kloe-trye′ma-zole)
Canesten ♣, Gyne-Lotrimin 3, Gyne-Lotrimin 7, Myclo ♣

miconazole (OTC)
(mye-kon′a-zole)
Monistat 3, Monistat 7

terconazole (OTC)
(ter-kone′ah-zole)
Terazol 7, Tetrazol 3, Zazole

tioconazole (OTC)
(tye-oh-kone′ah-zole)
Gyno-Trosyd ♣, Monistat 1, Vagistat-1

ACTION: Interferes with fungal DNA replication; binds sterols in fungal cell membranes, which increases permeability, leaking of nutrients

Therapeutic outcome: Fungistatic/fungicidal against susceptible organisms: *Candida* only

USES: Vaginal, vulval, vulvovaginal candidiasis (moniliasis)

CONTRAINDICATIONS: Hypersensitivity

Precautions: Pregnancy, breastfeeding, children <2 yr

Administer
Topical route
- Administer one full applicator every night high into the vagina
- Store at room temperature in dry place

ADVERSE EFFECTS
GU: Vulvovaginal burning, itching, pelvic cramps
INTEG: Rash, urticaria, stinging, burning
MISC: *Headache,* body pain

NURSING CONSIDERATIONS
Assess
- Assess for allergic reaction: burning, stinging, itching, discharge, soreness

Teach patient/family
- Instruct patient in asepsis (hand washing) before, after each application
- Teach patient to apply with applicator only; to avoid use of any other vaginal product unless directed by prescriber; sanitary napkin may prevent soiling of undergarments
- Instruct patient to abstain from sexual intercourse until treatment is completed; reinfection and irritation may occur
- Advise patient to notify prescriber if symptoms persist

Evaluate

Positive therapeutic outcome
- Decrease in itching or white discharge (vaginal)

OTIC ANTIINFECTIVES

ciprofloxacin (Rx)
(sip′roe-flox′a-sin)
Cetraxal, Ofloxacin, Otiprio

ACTION: Inhibits protein synthesis in susceptible microorganisms

USES: Ear infection (external), short-term use

CONTRAINDICATIONS: Hypersensitivity, perforated eardrum

Precautions: Pregnancy (C)

Administer
- After removing impacted cerumen by irrigation
- After cleaning stopper with alcohol
- After restraining child if necessary
- After warming sol to body temp

ADVERSE EFFECTS

EENT: Itching, irritation in ear

INTEG: Rash, urticaria

NURSING CONSIDERATIONS

Assess

• Assess for redness, swelling, fever, pain in ear, which indicates superinfection

Teach patient/family

• Teach patient correct method of instillation using aseptic technique, including not touching dropper to ear

• Inform patient that dizziness may occur after instillation

Evaluate

Positive therapeutic outcome

• Decreased ear pain

Appendix C Vaccines and toxoids

GENERIC NAME	TRADE NAME	USES	DOSAGE AND ROUTES	CONTRAINDICATIONS
anthrax vaccine	BioThrax	Pre-/postexposure prophylaxis	**Preexposure** Adult: SUBCUT 0.5 ml at 0, 2, 4 wk, then 0.5 ml at 6, 12, 18 mo **Postexposure** Adult: SUBCUT 0.5 ml 0, 2, 4 wk, with antibiotics	Hypersensitivity
BCG vaccine	TICE BCG	TB exposure	Adult and child >1 mo: 0.2-0.3 ml Child <1 mo: Reduce dose by 50% using 2 ml of sterile water after reconstituting	Hypersensitivity, hypogammaglobulinemia, positive TB test, burns
diphtheria and tetanus toxoids, adsorbed	Tenivac	Induces antitoxins to provide immunity to diphtheria and tetanus	Adult and child ≥ 7 yr: IM (adult strength) 0.5 ml q4-8wk $\times$ 2 doses, then 3rd dose 6-12 mo after 2nd dose, booster IM 0.5 ml q10yr Child 1-6 yr: IM (pediatric strength) 0.5 ml q4wk $\times$ 2 doses, booster 6-12 mo after 2nd dose Infant 6 wk-1 yr: IM (pediatric strength) 0.5 ml q4wk $\times$ 3 doses, booster 6-12 mo after 3rd dose	Hypersensitivity to mercury, thimerosal; immunocompromised patients; radiation; corticosteroids; acute illness
diphtheria and tetanus toxoids and whole-cell pertussis vaccine (DPT, DTP)	DTwP, Tr-Immunol	Prevention of diphtheria, tetanus, pertussis	Doses vary Check product information	Hypersensitivity, active infection, poliomyelitis outbreak, immunosuppression, febrile illness
diphtheria and tetanus toxoids and acellular pertussis vaccine	Adacel, Boostrix, Daptacel, Infranrix			
diphtheria, tetanus, pertussis, haemophilus, polio IPV	Pentacel	Immunity to diphtheria, tetanus, pertussis, haemophilus, polio IPV	Infant >6 wk and child ≤ 5 yr: IM 0.5 ml at 2, 4, 6, and 15-18 mo	Hypersensitivity, polio outbreak, acute infection, immunosuppression
diphtheria, tetanus, pertussis, polio vaccine IPV	Kinrix, Quadracel	Immunity to diphtheria, tetanus, pertussis, polio vaccine IPV	Child: IM 0.5 ml	Hypersensitivity, polio outbreak, acute infection, immunosuppression

H1N1 influenza A (swine flu) virus vaccine	Influenza A (H1N1)	Immunity to H1N1	Adult <50 yr, adolescent, child ≥2 yr: Intranasal 1 dose (roughly 0.1 ml) into each nostril; child 2-9 repeat dose ≥4 wk later Adult, adolescent, child ≥3 yr: IM 0.5 ml as a single dose; child 3-9 yr repeat dose ≥4 wk later (Sanofi) (CSL); child 4-9 yr repeat dose ≥4 wk later (Novartis); infants ≥6 mo, child <36 mo: IM 0.25 ml, repeat in 4 wk (Sanofi) Adult: IM 0.5 ml as a single dose (GSK)	
haemophilus b conjugate vaccine, diphtheria CRM_{197} protein conjugate (HbOC)	HibTITER	Polysaccharide immunization of children 2-6 yr against *H. influenzae* b, conjugate	**HibTITER (IM only)** Child: IM 0.5 ml Child 2-6 mo: 0.5 ml q2mo × 3 inj	Hypersensitivity, febrile illness, active infection
haemophilus b conjugate vaccine, meningococcal protein conjugate (PRP-OMP)	PedvaxHIB	Immunization of child 2, 4, 6 mo	Child 7-11 mo: Previously unvaccinated 0.5 ml q2mo inj Child 12-14 mo: Previously unvaccinated 0.5 ml × 1 inj **PedvaxHIB (IM only)** Child 2-14 mo: 0.5 ml × 2 inj at 2, 4 mo of age (6 mo dose not needed), then booster at 12-18 mo against invasive disease Child ≥15 mo: Previously unvaccinated 0.5 ml inj	
hepatitis A vaccine, inactivated	Havrix, VAQTA	Active immunization against hepatitis A virus	Adult: IM 1440 EL units (Havrix) or 50 units (VAQTA) as a single dose; booster dose is the same given at 6, 12 mo Child 2-18 yr: IM 720 EL units (Havrix) or 25 units (VAQTA) as a single dose, booster dose is the same given at 6, 12 mo	Hypersensitivity
hepatitis B vaccine, recombinant	Engerix-B, Recombivax HB	Immunization against all subtypes of hepatitis B virus	Varies widely	Hypersensitivity to this vaccine or yeast
human papillomavirus recombinant vaccine, quadrivalent	Gardasil	Prevention of HPV types 6, 11, 16, 18, cervical cancer, genital warts, precancerous dysplasic lesions, anal cancer/anal intraepithelial neoplasia	Adult up to 26 yr and child >9 yr to 26 yr: IM give as 3 separate doses; 1st dose as elected; 2nd dose 2 mo after 1st dose; 3rd dose 6 mo after 1st dose	Child <9 yr, pregnancy, breastfeeding, geriatric patients, active disease, hypersensitivity

Continued

Appendix C Vaccines and toxoids—cont'd

GENERIC NAME	TRADE NAME	USES	DOSAGE AND ROUTES	CONTRAINDICATIONS
influenza virus vaccine	Afluria, FluMist, Fluvirin, Fluzone	Prevention of seasonal influenza	Adult and child >12 yr: IM 0.5 ml in 1 dose Adult 18-64 yr: ID 0.1 ml as a single dose Child 3-12 yr: IM 0.5 ml, repeat in 1 mo (split) unless 1978-1985 vaccine was given; also given nasal Child 6 mo to 3 yr: IM 0.25 ml, repeat in 1 mo (split) unless 1978-1985 vaccine was given; also given nasal child ≤2 yr	Hypersensitivity, active infection, chicken egg allergy, Guillain-Barré syndrome, active neurologic disorders
Japanese encephalitis virus vaccine, inactivated	Ixiaro	Active immunity against Japanese encephalitis (JE)	Adult and child >3 yr: IM 0.5 ml (deltoid), then 0.5 ml 28 days later. Give the second dose ≥1 wk before potential exposure Child ≥2 mo to <3 yr: IM 0.25 ml (anterolateral aspect of the thigh or deltoid for children 1-2 yr with adequate muscle mass), then 0.25 ml 28 days later	Hypersensitivity to murine, thimerosal; allergic reactions to previous dose
measles, mumps, and rubella vaccine, live	M-M-R-II	Prevention of measles, mumps, rubella	Adult: SUBCUT 1 vial; 2 vials separated by 1 mo, in person born after 1957 Child >15 mo and adult: SUBCUT 0.5 ml	Hypersensitivity, blood dyscrasias, anemia, active infection, immunosuppression; egg, chicken allergy; pregnancy, febrile illness, neomycin allergy, neoplasms
measles, mumps, rubella, varicella	ProQuad	Immunity to measles, mumps, rubella, varicella	Child: SUBCUT 0.5 ml	Hypersensitivity to eggs, neomycin, cancer, radiation, corticosteroids, blood dyscrasias, active untreated TB
meningococcal polysaccharide vaccine	Menomune-A/C	Prophylaxis to meningococcal meningitis	Adult and child >2 yr: SUBCUT 0.5 ml	Hypersensitivity to thimerosal, pregnancy, acute illness
pneumococcal 7-valent conjugate vaccine	Prevnar	Immunity against *Streptococcus pneumoniae*	Child: IM 0.5 ml ×3 doses (7-11 mo); × 2 doses (12-23 mo); × 1 dose >2-9 yr	Hypersensitivity to diphtheria toxoid or this product
pneumococcal vaccine, polyvalent	Pneumovax 23	Pneumococcal immunization	Adult and child >2 yr: IM/SUBCUT 0.5 ml	Hypersensitivity, Hodgkin's disease, ARDS
poliovirus vaccine (IPV)	IPOL	Prevention of polio	Adult and child >2 yr: PO 0.5 ml, given q8wk × 2 doses, then 0.5 ml ½-1 yr after dose 2 Infant: PO 0.5 ml at 2, 4, 18 mo; booster at 4-6 yr; may also be given: IPV at 2, 4 mo, then TOPV at 12-18 mo, booster at 4-6 yr	Hypersensitivity, active infection, allergy to neomycin/streptomycin, immunosuppression, vomiting, diarrhea

rabies vaccine, human diploid cell (HDCV)	Imovax, RabAvert	Active immunity to rabies	**Preexposure** Adult and child: IM 1 ml day 0, 7, 21, or 28 (total 4 doses) **Postexposure** Adult and child: IM 1 ml on day 0, 3, 7, 14, 28 (total 5 doses)	No contraindications
rotovirus	RotaTeq, Rotarix	Prevents rotovirus	Infant: PO 3 doses given between 6 and 32 wk of age; 1st dose between 6-12 wk of age; 2nd and 3rd doses q4-10wk	Hypersensitivity to this product or latex, immunocompromised, blood products given within 6 wk, lymphatic disorders
tetanus toxoid, adsorbed	No trade name	Tetanus toxoid: Used for prophylactic treatment of wounds	Adult and child: IM 0.5 ml q4-6wk × 2 doses, then 0.5 ml 1 yr after dose 2 (adsorbed); SUBCUT/IM 0.5 ml q4-8wk × 3 doses, then 0.5 ml $^1/_2$-1 yr after dose 3, booster dose 0.5 ml q10yr	Hypersensitivity, active infection, poliomyelitis outbreak, immunosuppression
typhoid vaccine, parenteral typhoid vaccine, oral	Typhim Vi Vivotif Berna Vaccine	Active immunity to typhoid fever	Adult: PO 1 cap 1 hr before meals × 4 doses, booster q5yr Adult and child >10 yr: SUBCUT 0.5 ml, repeat in 4 wk, booster q3yr Child 6 mo-10 yr: SUBCUT 0.25 ml, repeat in 4 wk, booster q3yr	Parenteral: Systemic or allergic reaction, acute respiratory or other acute infection, intensive physical exercise in high temperatures Oral: Hypersensitivity, acute febrile illness, suppressive or antibiotic products
typhoid Vi polysaccharide vaccine	Typhim Vi	Active immunity to typhoid fever	Adult and child ≥2 yr: IM 0.5 ml as a single dose, reimmunize q2yr 0.5 ml IM, if needed	Hypersensitivity, chronic typhoid carriers
Varicella-Zoster Virus Vaccine	Varivax, Zostavax	Prevention of varicella-zoster (chickenpox)	Adult and child ≥13 yr: SUBCUT 0.5 ml, 2nd dose SUBCUT 0.5 ml 4-8 wk later	Hypersensitivity to neomycin; blood dyscrasias, immunosuppression, active untreated TB, acute illness, pregnancy, diseases of lymphatic system
yellow fever vaccine	YF-Vax	Active immunity to yellow fever	Adult and child ≥9 mo: SUBCUT 0.5 ml deeply, booster q10yr Child 6-9 mo: same as above if exposed	Hypersensitivity to egg or chicken embryo protein, pregnancy, child <6 mo, immunodeficiency

Appendix D

Recent FDA drug approvals

GENERIC	TRADE	USE
Elbasvir/grazoprevir	Zepatier	Hepatitis C infection
Lesinurad	Zurampic	Hyperuricemia
Sebelipase alfa	Kanuma	Lysosomal acid lipase deficiency
Selexipag	Uptravi	Pulmonary arterial hypertension

Index

Drug names and/or monographs denoted with an asterisk are found on your Evolve Resources at: http://evolve.elsevier.com/nursingdrugupdates/Skidmore/NDR

Entries can be identified as follows: DISEASES/DISORDERS, *DRUG CATEGORIES*, generic names, Trade Names.

INDEX

INDEX

Entries can be identified as follows: DISEASES/DISORDERS, *DRUG CATEGORIES*, generic names, Trade Names.

INDEX

INDEX

Entries can be identified as follows: DISEASES/DISORDERS, *DRUG CATEGORIES*, generic names, Trade Names.

Entries can be identified as follows: DISEASES/DISORDERS, *DRUG CATEGORIES*, generic names, Trade Names.

INDEX

Entries can be identified as follows: DISEASES/DISORDERS, *DRUG CATEGORIES*, generic names, Trade Names.

Entries can be identified as follows: DISEASES/DISORDERS, *DRUG CATEGORIES*, generic names, Trade Names.

INDEX

Entries can be identified as follows: DISEASES/DISORDERS, *DRUG CATEGORIES*, generic names, Trade Names.

INDEX

Entries can be identified as follows: DISEASES/DISORDERS, *DRUG CATEGORIES*, generic names, Trade Names.

INDEX

Entries can be identified as follows: DISEASES/DISORDERS, *DRUG CATEGORIES*, generic names, Trade Names.

INDEX

Entries can be identified as follows: DISEASES/DISORDERS, *DRUG CATEGORIES*, generic names, Trade Names.

Entries can be identified as follows: DISEASES/DISORDERS, *DRUG CATEGORIES*, generic names, Trade Names.

INDEX

Entries can be identified as follows: DISEASES/DISORDERS, *DRUG CATEGORIES*, generic names, Trade Names.

INDEX

Entries can be identified as follows: DISEASES/DISORDERS, *DRUG CATEGORIES*, generic names, Trade Names.

INDEX

Entries can be identified as follows: DISEASES/DISORDERS, *DRUG CATEGORIES*, generic names, Trade Names.

Entries can be identified as follows: DISEASES/DISORDERS, *DRUG CATEGORIES*, generic names, Trade Names.

INDEX

Entries can be identified as follows: DISEASES/DISORDERS, *DRUG CATEGORIES*, generic names, Trade Names.

Entries can be identified as follows: DISEASES/DISORDERS, *DRUG CATEGORIES*, generic names, Trade Names.

INDEX

Entries can be identified as follows: DISEASES/DISORDERS, *DRUG CATEGORIES*, generic names, Trade Names.

INDEX

Entries can be identified as follows: DISEASES/DISORDERS, *DRUG CATEGORIES*, generic names, Trade Names.

INDEX

Entries can be identified as follows: DISEASES/DISORDERS, *DRUG CATEGORIES*, generic names, Trade Names.

Entries can be identified as follows: DISEASES/DISORDERS, *DRUG CATEGORIES*, generic names, Trade Names.

INDEX

Entries can be identified as follows: DISEASES/DISORDERS, *DRUG CATEGORIES*, generic names, Trade Names.

Entries can be identified as follows: DISEASES/DISORDERS, *DRUG CATEGORIES*, generic names, Trade Names.

Entries can be identified as follows: DISEASES/DISORDERS, *DRUG CATEGORIES*, generic names, Trade Names.

Entries can be identified as follows: DISEASES/DISORDERS, *DRUG CATEGORIES*, generic names, Trade Names.

INDEX

Entries can be identified as follows: DISEASES/DISORDERS, *DRUG CATEGORIES*, generic names, Trade Names.

Entries can be identified as follows: DISEASES/DISORDERS, *DRUG CATEGORIES*, generic names, Trade Names.

Entries can be identified as follows: DISEASES/DISORDERS, *DRUG CATEGORIES*, generic names, Trade Names.

INDEX

Entries can be identified as follows: DISEASES/DISORDERS, *DRUG CATEGORIES*, generic names, Trade Names.

Entries can be identified as follows: DISEASES/DISORDERS, *DRUG CATEGORIES*, generic names, Trade Names.

INDEX

Entries can be identified as follows: DISEASES/DISORDERS, *DRUG CATEGORIES*, generic names, Trade Names.

INDEX

INDEX

Formulas

Surface area rule:

$$\text{Child dose} = \frac{\text{Surface area (m}^2\text{)}}{1.73\ \text{m}^2} \times \text{Adult dose}$$

Calculating strength of a solution:

Solution Strength: *Desired Solution*:

$$\frac{x}{100} = \frac{\text{Amount of drug desired}}{\text{Amount of finished solution}}$$

Calculating flow rate for IV:

$$\text{Rate of flow} = \frac{\text{Amount of fluid} \times \text{Administration set calibration}}{\text{Running time}}$$

$$\frac{x}{1} = \frac{\text{(ml) (gtt/min)}}{\text{min}}$$

Calculation of medication dosages:

Formula method:

$$\frac{\text{Amount ordered}}{\text{Amount on hand}} \times \text{Vehicle} = \text{Number of tablets, capsules, or amount of liquid}$$

Vehicle is the drug form or amount of liquid containing the dosage. Amounts used in calculation by formula must be in same system.

Ratio–proportion method:

1 tablet:tablet in mg on hand::x tablet order in mg

Know or have::Want to know or order

Multiply means and extremes, divide both sides by known amount to get x. Amounts used in equation must be in same system.

Dimensional analysis method:

$$\text{Order in mg} \times \frac{\text{1 tablet or capsule}}{\text{What 1 tablet or capsule is in mg}} = \text{Tablets or capsules to be given}$$

If amounts are in different systems:

$$\text{Order in mg} \times \frac{\text{1 tablet or capsule}}{\text{What 1 tablet or capsule is in g}} \times \frac{1}{1000\ \text{mg}} = \text{Tablets or capsules to be given}$$

Temperature conversion:

$F = C \times 9/5 + 32$

$C = 5/9\ (F - 32)$

Nomogram for calculation of body surface area

Place a straight edge from the patient's height in the left column to the patient's weight in the right column. The point of intersection on the body surface area column indicates the body surface area (BSA). (Reproduced in Behrman RE, Kliegman RM, Jenson HB: *Nelson textbook of pediatrics,* ed 18, Philadelphia, 2011, WB Saunders; Nomogram modified from data of E. Boyd by CD West.)

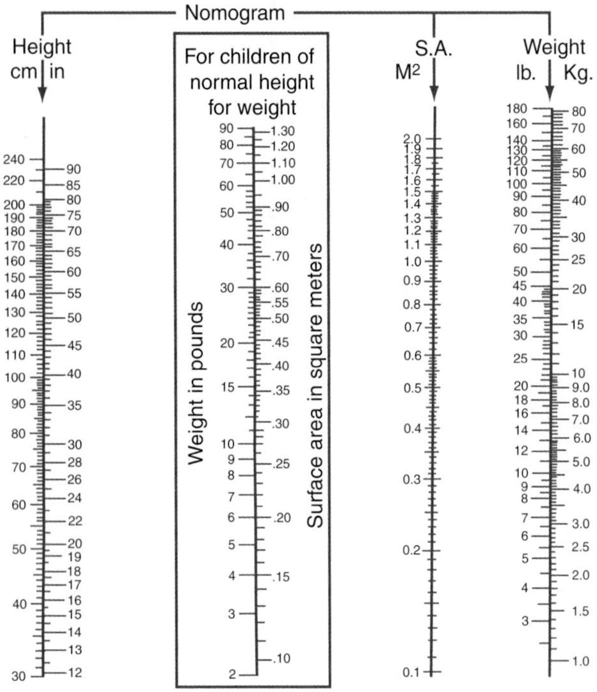

Alternative (Mosteller's formula):

$$\text{Surface area (m}^2\text{)} = \sqrt{\frac{\text{Height (cm)} \times \text{Weight (kg)}}{3600}}$$

Antitoxins and antivenins

GENERIC NAME	TRADE NAME	USES	DOSAGE AND ROUTES	CONTRAINDICATIONS
Black widow spider antivenin *(Lactrodectus mactans)*	No trade name	Black widow spider bite	Adult and child: IM 2.5 ml, 2nd dose may be given if severe; give in anterolateral thigh, obtain test for sensitivity before inj	Hypersensitivity to this product or horse serum
Crotalidae antivenom, polyvalent	No trade name	Rattlesnake bite	Adult and child: IV 20-150 ml depending on seriousness of bite, may give additional doses based on response	Hypersensitivity
Diphtheria antitoxin, equine	No trade name	Diphtheria	Adult and child: IM/slow IV 20,000-120,000 units, may give additional doses after 24 hr	Hypersensitivity
Micrurus fulvius antivenin	No trade name	East/Texas coral snake bite	Adult and child: IV 30-50 ml, give through running IV line of normal saline, give 1st 1-2 ml over 4-5 min, watch for allergic reaction	Hypersensitivity
Scorpion antivenin (centruroides sculpturatus equine)	Anascorp	Scorpion stings	Adult and child: IV 3 vial/50 ml NS given over 10 min, may give other doses 1 vial/50 ml NS over 10 min q30-60min	N/A

Abbreviations

ABG	arterial blood gas
ADA	American Diabetes Association
ADH	antidiuretic hormone
ALT	alanine aminotransferase
ANA	antinuclear antibody
APLA	antiphospholipid antibody syndrome
APTT	activated partial thromboplastin time
ASA	acetylsalicylic acid, aspirin
AST	aspartate aminotransferase (SGOT)
AV	atrioventricular
bid	twice a day
BPH	benign prostatic hypertrophy
BPM	beats per minute
BUN	blood urea nitrogen
CAD	coronary artery disease
CBC	complete blood cell count
CCr	creatinine clearance
CHF	congestive heart failure
CNS	central nervous system
CONT	continuous
COPD	chronic obstructive pulmonary disease
CPAP	continuous positive airway pressure
CPK	creatine phosphokinase
CPS	carbamoyl phosphate synthetase
C&S	culture and sensitivity
CSF	cerebrospinal fluid
CTCL	cutaneous T-cell lymphoma
CV	cardiovascular
CVA	cerebrovascular accident
CVP	central venous pressure
D&C	dilatation and curettage
DIC	diffuse intravascular coagulation
DIR INF	direct infusion
D_5W	5% glucose in distilled water
DVT	deep vein thrombosis
ECG	electrocardiogram (EKG)
EDTA	ethylenediamine tetraacetic acid
EEG	electroencephalogram
EPS	extrapyramidal symptom
ESR	erythrocyte sedimentation rate
EXT REL	extended release
FBS	fasting blood sugar
FHT	fetal heart tones
FSH	follicle-stimulating hormone
GABA	γ-aminobutyric acid
GPC	giant papillary conjunctivitis
gr	grain
GT	glucose tolerance test
GU	genitourinary
GVHD	graft-versus-host disease
H_2	histamine$_2$
hCG	human chorionic gonadotropin
Hct	hematocrit
HDCV	human diploid cell rabies vaccine
Hgb	hemoglobin
H & H	hematocrit and hemoglobin
5-HIAA	5-hydroxyindoleacetic acid
HIV	human immunodeficiency virus (AIDS)
HR	heart rate
IBD	inflammatory bowel disease
IC	intracardiac
ICP	intracranial pressure
ID	intradermal
IgG	immunoglobulin G
IM	intramuscular
INF	infusion
INH	inhalation
inj	injection
I&O	intake and output
INT	intermittent
IPPB	intermittent positive-pressure breathing
IT	intrathecal
ITP	idiopathic thrombocytopenic purpura
IUD	intrauterine device
IV	intravenous
IVP	intravenous pyelogram
K	potassium
LDH	lactic dehydrogenase
LE	lupus erythematosus
LFT	liver function test
LH	luteinizing hormone
LOC	level of consciousness
LR	lactated Ringer's solution
LT	leukotriene
m	minim
m^2	square meter
MAC	monitored anesthesia care
MAOI	monoamine oxidase inhibitor
mcg	microgram
mEq	milliequivalent
mg	milligram
MI	myocardial infarction
ml	milliliter
mm	millimeter
mo	month
Na	sodium
ng	nanogram
NGU	non-gonococcal urethritis